NPF

NURSE
PRESCRIBERS'
FORMULARY

2002-2003

NPF

NURSE PRESCRIBERS' FORMULARY

2002-2003

Incorporating

BNF 43

MARCH 2002

•

British Medical Association

Royal Pharmaceutical Society of Great Britain

In association with

Community Practitioners' and Health Visitors' Association

Royal College of Nursing

Published by the British Medical Association

Tavistock Square, London WC1H 9JP, UK

and the **Royal Pharmaceutical Society of Great Britain**

1 Lambeth High Street, London, SE1 7JN, UK

© 2002 British Medical Association and the Royal Pharmaceutical Society of Great Britain

ISBN: 0 85369 496 6 (Royal Pharmaceutical Society of Great Britain)

ISBN: 0 7279 1735 8 (British Medical Association)

ISSN: 1468-4853

Printed in Great Britain by William Clowes, Beccles, Suffolk

Copies may be obtained through any bookseller or direct from the publishers:

BMJ Books
PO Box 295
London WC1H 9TE
UK
Tel: +44 (0) 20 7383 6244
Fax: +44 (0) 20 7383 6455
E-mail: orders@bmjbookshop.com
www.bmjbookshop.com

Pharmaceutical Press
PO Box 151
Wallingford
Oxon OX10 8QU
UK
Tel: +44 (0) 1491 829272
Fax:+44 (0) 1491 829292
E-mail: rpsgb@cabi.org
www.pharmpress.com

For a list of name changes required by Directive 92/27/EEC, see p. viii

Contents

Preface

The Nurse Prescribers' Formulary for District Nurses and Health Visitors is for use by District Nurses (DN) or Health Visitors (HV) who have received nurse prescriber training. It provides details of preparations that can be prescribed for patients receiving NHS treatment on form FP10P (form FP10(N) in Scotland, form HS21(N) in Northern Ireland). This current edition incorporates BNF No. 43.

From April 2002 nurses who have received specific preparation and training (which is distinct from that provided to District Nurse or Health Visitor nurse prescribers) will be able to prescribe from the *Nurse Prescribers' Extended Formulary,* which includes certain prescription-only medicines. The current edition of the NPF includes a list of the prescription-only medicines and of the conditions that are covered by the Nurse Prescribers' Extended Formulary. Further details may be found on the Department of Health website www.doh.gov.uk/ nurseprescribing.

The NPF forms an appendix to the BNF and as such is termed the Nurse Prescribers' Formulary Appendix (Appendix NPF).

The Nurse Prescribers' Formulary Subcommittee (p. v) oversees the preparation of the NPF and advises the UK health ministers on the list of preparations that may be prescribed by District Nurse or Health Visitor nurse prescribers. The Subcommittee is responsible for the interpretation of the recommendations made by the Advisory Group on Nurse Prescribing (as outlined in the Group's report published in 1989).

The list of preparations from which nurse prescribers (with District Nurse or Health Visitor qualifications) may prescribe is reviewed constantly in the light of comments from nurse prescribers and applications from manufacturers. The Department of Health and MCA are putting in place separate arrangements for the Nurse Prescribers' Extended Formulary.

The Subcommittee records its thanks to C. Dalton, M. Garley, R. Harman, M.G.V. Jenkins, P. Robinson, and M. Williams, for their help with the preparation of this edition. The Subcommittee is grateful to those who have commented on previous editions of the NPF. In order that future editions of the NPF for District Nurses and Health Visitors are able to reflect the requirements of nurse prescribers, users are urged to send comments and constructive criticism to:

Acknowledgements

The Joint Formulary Committee and the Nurse Prescribers' Formulary Subcommittee are grateful to individuals and organisations that have provided advice and information to the NPF/BNF.

The principal contributors for this edition of the BNF were:
P. Abrams, I.H. Ahmed-Jusuf, J.M. Aitken, S.P. Allison, D.G. Arkell, D. Back, T.P. Baglin, A. Bakhai, R.J. Barnes, R.H. Behrens, D. Bowsher, M.J. Brodie, R.J. Buckley, I. Burgess, A.J. Camm, L. Cardozo, D.A. Chamberlain, C. Diamond, R. Dinwiddie, A.J. Duxbury, G.H. Elder, T.S.J. Elliott, B.G. Gazzard, A.M. Geddes, R.H. George, A.H. Ghodse, E.C. Gordon-Smith, I.A. Greer, J. Guillebaud, C.H. Hawkes, C.J. Hawkey, D.F. Hawkins, P.D. Hill, S.H. Jackson, J.R. Kirwan, P.G. Kopelman, M.J.S. Langman, J. Leese, P.N. Leigh, L. Luzzatto, E. Miller, K.E.L. McColl, G.M. Mead, J.M. Neuberger, D. Nutt, D.J. Oliver, L.P. Ormerod, P.A. Poole-Wilson, L.E. Ramsay, P.A. Routledge, D.J. Rowbotham, P.C. Rubin, R. Ryall, R.S. Sawers, M.C. Sheppard, S.D. Shorvon, S.L.R. Stanton, I. Stockley, A.E. Tattersfield, H. Thomas, G.R. Thompson, D.G. Waller, D.A. Warrell.

Members of the British Association of Dermatologists Therapy Guidelines and Audit Subcommittee, C.B. Bunker, N.H. Cox, A.S. Highet, R.H. Meyrick-Thomas, A.D. Ormerod, J.K.L. Schofield, C.H. Smith, and V.A. Preston (Secretariat) have provided valuable advice.

The Joint British Societies' Coronary Risk Prediction Charts have been reproduced with the kind permission of P.N. Durrington who has also provided the BNF with access to the computer program for calculated coronary and stroke risk.

Correspondents in the pharmaceutical industry have provided information on new products and commented on products in the BNF. The Prescription Pricing Authority has supplied the prices of products in the BNF.

Numerous doctors, pharmacists, nurses and others have sent comments and suggestions.

The BNF has valuable access to the *Martindale* data banks by courtesy of S. Sweetman and staff.

S.G. Coleman, A.M. Hargreaves, C.L. Iskander, S.M. Townsend-Smith, E.L. Warrington, L.J. Whitley, and C. Wong provided considerable assistance during the production of this edition of the BNF.

E.I. Connor has assisted with the development of the electronic BNF and publishing software. Quartet Software has provided technical assistance with the editorial database and typesetting software.

Executive Editor, NPF/BNF,
Royal Pharmaceutical Society of Great Britain
1 Lambeth High Street, London SE1 7JN
Email: editor@bnf.org

How to use the NPF/BNF

Nurse Prescribers' Formulary

The NPF part provides information of special relevance to the nurse prescriber. This section includes notes on preparations on the Nurse Prescribers' Formulary for District Nurses and Health Visitors, followed by details of the preparations. An appendix on urinary and stoma appliances and an index for the NPF section are included at the end.

Guidance on prescribing

This part includes information on prescription writing, controlled drugs and dependence, prescribing for children and the elderly, and prescribing in palliative care. Advice is given on the reporting of adverse reactions (see also p. N2).

Emergency treatment of poisoning

This chapter provides information on the management of acute poisoning when first seen in the home, although aspects of hospital-based treatment are mentioned.

Notes on conditions, drugs and preparations

The main text consists of classified notes on clinical conditions, drugs and preparations. These notes are divided into 15 chapters, each of which is related to a particular system of the body or to an aspect of medical care. Each chapter is then divided into sections which begin with appropriate *notes for prescribers*. These notes are intended to provide information to doctors, pharmacists, nurses, and other healthcare professionals to facilitate the selection of suitable treatment. The notes are followed by details of relevant drugs and preparations.

DRUG NAME ◼ ●

Indications: details of uses and indications
Cautions: details of precautions required (with cross-references to appropriate Appendixes) and also any monitoring required
COUNSELLING. Verbal explanation to the patient of specific details of the drug treatment (e.g. posture when taking a medicine)
Contra-indications: details of any contra-indications to use of drug
Side-effects: details of common and more serious side-effects
Dose: dose and frequency of administration (max. dose); CHILD and ELDERLY details of dose for specific age group
By alternative route, dose and frequency

*Approved Name (Non-proprietary) PoM ●
Pharmaceutical form, colour, coating, active ingredient and amount in dosage form, net price, pack size = basic NHS price. Label: (as in Appendix 9)
Proprietary Name® (Manufacturer) PoM
NHS ●
Pharmaceutical form, sugar-free, active ingredient mg/mL, net price, pack size = basic NHS price. Label: (as in Appendix 9)
Excipients: include clinically important excipients or electrolytes
* exceptions to the prescribing status indicated by a footnote.
Note. Specific notes about the product e.g. handling

Preparations
Preparations usually follow immediately after the drug which is their main ingredient.
Preparations are included under a non-proprietary title, if they are marketed under such a title, if they are not otherwise prescribable under the NHS, or if they may be prepared extemporaneously.
If proprietary preparations are of a distinctive colour this is stated.
In the case of compound preparations the indications, cautions, contra-indications, side-effects, and interactions of all constituents should be taken into account for prescribing.

Note. The presentation of preparations in the NPF is slightly different because of the requirements of nurse prescribing.

Drugs
Drugs appear under pharmacopoeial or other non-proprietary titles. When there is an *appropriate current monograph* (Medicines Act 1968, Section 65) preference is given to a name at the head of that monograph; otherwise a British Approved Name (BAN), if available, is used see also p. viii
The symbol ◼ is used to denote those preparations that are considered by the Joint Formulary Committee to be less suitable for prescribing. Although such preparations may not be considered as drugs of first choice, their use may be justifiable in certain circumstances

Prescription-only medicines PoM
This symbol has been placed against those preparations that are available only on medical or dental prescription. For more detailed information see *Medicines, Ethics and Practice*, No. 25, London, Pharmaceutical Press, 2001 (and subsequent editions as available).
The symbol CD indicates that the preparation is subject to the prescription requirements of the Misuse of Drugs Act. For regulations governing prescriptions for such preparations see pages 7–9.

Preparations not available for NHS prescription NHS
This symbol has been placed against those preparations included in the BNF that are not prescribable under the NHS. Those prescribable only for specific disorders have a footnote specifying the condition(s) for which the preparation remains available. Some preparations which are not *prescribable* by brand name under the NHS may nevertheless be *dispensed* using the brand name providing that the prescription shows an appropriate non-proprietary name.

Prices
Prices have been calculated from the basic cost used in pricing NHS prescriptions dispensed in November 2001 or later, see p. vii for further details.

Appendixes and indexes

The appendixes include information on interactions, liver disease, renal impairment, pregnancy, breast-feeding, intravenous additives, borderline substances, wound management products, and cautionary and advisory labels for dispensed medicines. They are designed for use in association with the main body of the text.

The Dental Practitioners' List and the Nurse Prescribers' List are also included in this section. The indexes consist of the Index of Manufacturers and the Main Index.

Prices in the NPF/BNF

Basic **net prices** are given in the NPF/BNF to provide an indication of relative cost. Where there is a choice of suitable preparations for a particular disease or condition the relative cost may be used in making a selection. Cost-effective prescribing must, however, take into account other factors (such as dose frequency and duration of treatment) that affect the total cost. The use of more expensive drugs is justified if it will result in better treatment of the patient or a reduction of the length of an illness or the time spent in hospital.

Prices have generally been calculated from the net cost used in pricing NHS prescriptions dispensed in November 2001, but where available later prices have been included; unless an original pack is available these prices are based on the largest pack size of the preparation in use in community pharmacies. The price for an extemporaneously prepared preparation has been omitted where the net cost of the ingredients used to make it would give a misleadingly low impression of the final price. In Appendix 8 prices stated are for for a single dressing or bandage.

The unit of 20 is still sometimes used as a basis for comparison, but where suitable original packs or patient packs are available these are priced instead.

Gross prices vary as follows:
1. Costs to the NHS are greater than the net prices quoted and include professional fees and overhead allowances;
2. Private prescription charges are calculated on a separate basis;
3. Over-the-counter sales are at retail price, as opposed to basic net price, and include VAT.

> NPF/BNF prices are **not**, therefore, suitable for quoting to patients seeking private prescriptions or contemplating over-the-counter purchases.

A fuller explanation of costs to the NHS may be obtained from the Drug Tariff.

Separate Drug Tariffs apply in England and Wales, Scotland, and Northern Ireland. Prices may vary in the different tariffs.

Patient Packs

On January 1 1994, EC Directive 92/27/EEC came into force, outlining requirements for the labelling of medicines and for the format and content of patient information leaflets to be supplied with each medicine.

All medicines now have approved labelling and patient information leaflets; anyone who supplies a medicine is responsible for providing the relevant information to the patient (see also Appendix 9).

Many medicines are available in manufacturers' original packs complete with patient information leaflets. Where patient packs are available, the NPF/BNF shows the number of dose units in the packs. In certain clinical circumstances, where patient packs need to be split or medicines are provided in bulk dispensing packs, manufacturers will provide additional supplies of patient information leaflets on request.

During the revision of each edition of the BNF careful note is taken of the information that appears on the patient information leaflets. Where it is considered appropriate to alert a prescriber to some specific limitation appearing on the patient information leaflet (for example, in relation to pregnancy) this advice now appears in the BNF.

The patient information leaflet also includes details of all inactive ingredients in the medicine. A list of common E numbers and the inactive ingredients to which they correspond is now therefore included in the BNF (see inside back cover).

Name changes

Directive 92/27/EEC requires use of the Recommended International Non-proprietary Name (rINN) for medicinal substances. In most cases the British Approved Name (BAN) and rINN were identical. Where the two differed, the BAN has been modified to accord with the rINN.

List 1 shows those substances where a change of name was considered to pose the highest potential risk to public health and for which the UK authorities were expected to adopt a system of dual labelling. It was expected that the system would require both the rINN and the former BAN to appear on manufacturers' labels and leaflets (giving precedence to the rINN) for at least 5 years. No such system has been adopted but the BNF shows both names in the main drug entries.

List 2 includes those substances for which the former BAN has been modified to accord with the rINN; the new BAN is required to appear on manufacturers' labels and leaflets. Former BANs have been retained as synonyms.

List 1—Both names to appear

UK name	rINN
[1]adrenaline	epinephrine
amethocaine	tetracaine
bendrofluazide	bendroflumethiazide
benzhexol	trihexyphenidyl
chlorpheniramine	chlorphenamine
dicyclomine	dicycloverine
dothiepin	dosulepin
eformoterol	formoterol
flurandrenolone	fludroxycortide
frusemide	furosemide
hydroxyurea	hydroxycarbamide
lignocaine	lidocaine
methotrimeprazine	levomepromazine
methylene blue	methylthioninium chloride
mitozantrone	mitoxantrone
mustine	chlormethine
nicoumalone	acenocoumarol
[1]noradrenaline	norepinephrine
oxpentifylline	pentoxifylline
procaine penicillin	procaine benzylpenicillin
salcatonin	calcitonin (salmon)
thymoxamine	moxisylyte
thyroxine sodium	levothyroxine sodium
trimeprazine	alimemazine

1. In common with the BP, precedence will continue to be given to the terms adrenaline and noradrenaline

List 2—rINN/new BAN to appear exclusively

former BAN	rINN/new BAN
amfebutamone	bupropion
aminacrine	aminoacridine
amoxycillin	amoxicillin
amphetamine	amfetamine
amylobarbitone	amobarbital
amylobarbitone sodium	amobarbital sodium
beclomethasone	beclometasone
benorylate	benorilate
benzphetamine	benzfetamine
benztropine	benzatropine
busulphan	busulfan
butobarbitone	butobarbital
carticaine	articaine
cephalexin	cefalexin
cephamandole nafate	cefamandole nafate
cephazolin	cefazolin
cephradine	cefradine

List 2 (continued)

former BAN	rINN/new BAN
chloral betaine	cloral betaine
chlorbutol	chlorobutanol
chlormethiazole	clomethiazole
chlorthalidone	chlortalidone
cholecalciferol	colecalciferol
cholestyramine	colestyramine
clomiphene	clomifene
colistin sulphomethate sodium	colistimethate sodium
corticotrophin	corticotropin
cyclosporin	ciclosporin
cysteamine	mercaptamine
danthron	dantron
desoxymethasone	desoximetasone
dexamphetamine	dexamfetamine
dibromopropamidine	dibromopropamidine
dienoestrol	dienestrol
dimethicone(s)	dimeticone
dimethyl sulphoxide	dimethyl sulfoxide
doxycycline hydrochloride (hemihydrate hemiethanolate)	doxycycline hyclate
ethacrynic acid	etacrynic acid
ethamsylate	etamsylate
ethinyloestradiol	ethinylestradiol
ethynodiol	etynodiol
flumethasone	flumetasone
flupenthixol	flupentixol
gestronol	gestonorone
guaiphenesin	guaifenesin
hexachlorophane	hexachlorophene
hexamine hippurate	methenamine hippurate
hydroxyprogesterone hexanoate	hydroxyprogesterone caproate
indomethacin	indometacin
lysuride	lisuride
methyl cysteine	mecysteine
methylphenobarbitone	methylphenobarbital
oestradiol	estradiol
oestriol	estriol
oestrone	estrone
oxethazaine	oxetacaine
pentaerythritol tetranitrate	pentaerithrityl tetranitrate
phenobarbitone	phenobarbital
pipothiazine	pipotiazine
polyhexanide	polihexanide
potassium clorazepate	dipotassium clorazepate
pramoxine	pramocaine
prothionamide	protionamide
quinalbarbitone	secobarbital
riboflavine	riboflavin
sodium calciumedetate	sodium calcium edetate
sodium cromoglycate	sodium cromoglicate
sodium ironedetate	sodium feredetate
sodium picosulphate	sodium picosulfate
sorbitan monostearate	sorbitan stearate
stibocaptate	sodium stibocaptate
stilboestrol	diethylstilbestrol
sulphacetamide	sulfacetamide
sulphadiazine	sulfadiazine
sulphadimidine	sulfadimidine
sulphamethoxazole	sulfamethoxazole
sulphapyridine	sulfapyridine
sulphasalazine	sulfasalazine
sulphathiazole	sulfathiazole
sulphinpyrazone	sulfinpyrazone
tetracosactrin	tetracosactide
thiabendazole	tiabendazole
thioguanine	tioguanine
thiopentone	thiopental
tribavirin	ribavirin
urofollitrophin	urofollitropin

Nurse Prescribers' Formulary

for District Nurses and Health Visitors

Prescription Writing

Further information may be found in BNF pp. 1–5

Prescriptions written by nurse prescribers should:
- be written legibly in ink;
- be dated;
- state patient's full name and address;
- be signed in ink by the prescriber;
- include age and date of birth of patient.

Also recommended:
- Dose and the dose frequency should be stated. For preparations to be taken 'as required' *a minimum dose interval* should be specified, e.g. 'every 4 hours'.
- The unnecessary use of decimal points should be avoided, e.g. 3 mg, not 3.0 mg.
- Strength of the preparation should be stated, e.g. Paracetamol Tablets 500 mg.
- Quantities of 1 gram or more should be written as 1 g etc.
- Quantities of less than 1 gram should be written in milligrams, e.g. 500 mg, not 0.5 g (see inside back cover for conversion guide). It is, however, acceptable to express a range in the decimal form, e.g. 0.5 to 1 g.
- Quantity prescribed should generally be the pack size specified in the NPF under each preparation.
- Names of medicines should be written clearly using approved (generic) titles or proprietary names as specified throughout the NPF and should **not** be abbreviated.
- Directions should be in *English* and should **not** be abbreviated.

Security and validity of prescriptions

In order to ensure the security and validity of prescriptions nurse prescribers should:
- not leave them unattended;
- not leave them in a car where they may be visible;
- keep them locked up when not in use.

When there is any doubt about the authenticity of a prescription, the pharmacist will contact the nurse prescriber; see also Incomplete Prescriptions, below.

Children

Prescriptions should be written according to the guidelines above, stating the child's age.

Children's doses are stated in the NPF where appropriate but nurse prescribers should exercise **special caution** when contemplating prescribing for children and, for laxatives in particular, should consider discussing with the child's medical practitioner before initiating a prescription.

Where a single dose is stated for a given age range, it applies to the middle of the age range and may need to be adjusted to obtain doses for ages at the lower and upper limits of the stated range.

Nurse prescribers are advised to err on the side of caution.

The pharmacist will supply an **oral syringe** with oral liquid preparations if the dose prescribed is less than 5 mL. The oral syringe is marked in 0.5-mL divisions from 1 to 5 mL to measure doses of less than 5 mL. It is provided with an adaptor and an instruction leaflet. A 5-mL spoon will be given for doses of 5 or 10 mL.

Excipients

Where an oral liquid medicine in the NPF is available in a form free of *fructose, glucose,* or *sucrose* a note has been added to say that a sugar-free version may be requested by adding 'sugar free' to the prescription. Preparations containing hydrogenated glucose syrup, mannitol, sorbitol or xylitol are also marked 'sugar-free' since there is evidence that they do not cause dental caries. Whenever possible sugar-free preparations should be requested for children to reduce the risk of dental decay.

Where information on the presence of *aspartame, gluten, tartrazine, arachis (peanut) oil* or *sesame oil* is available, this is indicated against the relevant product entry; if it is essential to check details and the information is not available in the NPF or in the product literature, then the manufacturer should be contacted.

Information is provided on *selected excipients* in skin preparations (see BNF section 13.1).

Prevention of adverse reactions

Adverse reactions may be prevented as follows:
- Never prescribe any medicine unless there is a good indication. If the patient is pregnant do not prescribe any medicine at all (except folic acid) but refer her to the doctor.
- It is very important to recognise allergy as a cause of adverse drug reactions. Ask if the patient has had any previous reactions, particularly when prescribing aspirin or dressings impregnated with iodine.
- Ask if the patient is taking any other medicines **including self medication**; remember that aspirin interacts with warfarin.
- Check whether there are any special instructions in relation to hepatic or renal disease.
- Prescribe as few medicines as possible and give very clear instructions to the elderly or any patient likely to misunderstand complicated instructions. Elderly patients cannot normally cope with more than three different medicines (and ideally they should not need to be taken more than twice daily).

Reporting of adverse reactions. If a patient experiences an adverse reaction to a medicine or dressing, the nurse prescriber should inform the general practitioner. The general practitioner may then decide to notify the Committee on Safety of Medicines using the 'yellow card' scheme for reporting adverse reactions.

Incomplete prescriptions

A pharmacist may need to contact the nurse prescriber if the *quantity, strength* or *dose* are missing from the prescription. The pharmacist will then arrange for the missing details to be added. Under some circumstances the pharmacist will use professional judgement as to what to give and will endorse the prescription.

Labelling of dispensed medicine

The following will appear on the label of a dispensed medicine:
- name of product
- name of patient
- date of dispensing
- name and address of pharmacy
- directions for use
- total quantity of product dispensed
- advice to keep out of reach of children.

Other information (e.g. 'flammable') will be added by the pharmacist as appropriate. Preparation entries in the NPF provide details of any additional cautionary advice that the pharmacist will add.

The *name of the product* will be that which is written on the prescription.

Safety

Patients must be warned to keep all medicines out of reach of children. Medicines will be dispensed in reclosable *child-resistant containers* unless:
- they are in manufacturers' original packs designed for supplying to the patient
- the patient would have difficulty in opening a child-resistant container.

In the latter case the pharmacist will make a particular point of advising that the medicines be kept out of reach of children. The nurse prescriber could usefully *reinforce this advice*.

Patients should be advised to dispose of *unwanted medicines* by returning them to a pharmacist for destruction.

Duplicate medicines

Nurses are well placed to check on whether patients are at risk of taking two medicines with the same action (or which contain the same ingredient) at the same time. This is of special concern in the case of medicines that can also be bought over the counter (e.g. aspirin and paracetamol). Pharmacists reduce this risk to some extent by making sure that the words 'aspirin' *or* 'aspirin and paracetamol' appear on relevant preparations. A check on the patient's medicines (including cough and cold cures) might prevent the patient inadvertently taking duplicate doses of aspirin or paracetamol. A list of preparations on sale to the public that contain aspirin or paracetamol alone or with other ingredients can be found in the BNF (section 4.7.1).

Prices

Net prices have been included in the NPF to provide an indication of relative cost. These prices are **not** suitable for quoting to patients since they do not include the pharmacist's professional fee and other allowances, nor do they include VAT.

PACT and SPA

PACT (Prescribing Analyses and Cost) and SPA (Scottish Prescribing Analysis) provide prescribers with information about their prescribing in comparison with the prescribing figures for the local health authority (or health board in Scotland) and the national average.

This edition of the NPF/BNF is intended as a pocket book for rapid reference and so cannot contain all the information necessary for patient management. For additional information the nurse prescriber should refer to the doctor who will have access to further information including manufacturers' product literature. Supplementary information is also available from pharmacists

Changes to the Nurse Prescribers' List

Additions

Medicinal preparations, appliances, and reagents added to Nurse Prescribers' List since 1999[1]

Applicators, Vaginal
Atomizers, Hand Operated
Auto Inflation Device (for treatment of glue ear)
Breast Reliever
Breast Shields
Chemical Reagents as listed below:
  Reagent solutions (Gerhardt's Reagent and Ammonia Solution, Strong, BP)
Catheter Accessories
Catheter Maintenance Solutions
Chiropody Appliances
Choline Salicylate Dental Gel, BP
Contraceptive Devices
Crotamiton Cream, BP
Crotamiton Lotion, BP
Douches (with vaginal and rectal fittings)
Droppers
Emollients as listed below:
  Arachis Oil, BP
  Cetraben® Emollient Cream
  Doublebase®
  Liquid and White Soft Paraffin Ointment, NPF
  Paraffin, White Soft, BP
  Paraffin, Yellow Soft, BP
Eye Baths
Eye Drops Dispensers
Eye Shades
Finger Cots
Finger Stalls
Hypodermic Equipment (some additions)
Inhaler, Spare Tops
Insufflators
Iodine Brush
Latex Foam, Adhesive
Lubricating Jelly
Methylcellulose Tablets, BP
Nasal Device (nasal dilator)
Nicotine Inhalation Cartridge for Oromucosal Use, NPF
Nicotine Lozenge, NPF
Nicotine Medicated Chewing Gum, NPF
Nicotine Nasal Spray, NPF
Nicotine Sublingual Tablets, NPF
Nicotine Transdermal Patches, NPF
Nipple Shields, Plastic
Peak Flow Meters
Pessaries (some additions)
Protectives (some additions)
Rectal Dilators
Saliva Stimulating Tablets
Sodium Bicarbonate Ear Drops, BP
Sodium Picosulfate Capsules, NPF
Suprapubic Belts (replacements only)
Suprapubic Catheters
Synovial Fluid
Syringes (Bladder/Irrigating, Ear, Enema, Spare Vaginal Pipes)
Tapeless IV Holders
Test Tubes
Tracheostomy and Laryngectomy Appliances
Trusses

1. Some appliances and reagents are not prescribable by nurses in Northern Ireland and Scotland—see full amended list

Wound Management and Related Products as listed below:
  Absorbent Cellulose Dressing with Fluid Repellent Backing
  Absorbent Dressing Pads, Sterile
  Absorbent Perforated Dressing with Adhesive Border
  Belladonna Adhesive Plaster BP 1980
  Boil Dressing Pack
  Boric Acid Lint, BPC 1963
  Chlorhexidine Gauze Dressing, BP
  Conforming Bandage (Synthetic)
  Elastic Diachylon Bandage, Ventilated BPC
  Plaster of Paris Bandage, BP 1988
  Polyester Primary Dressing with Neutral Triglycerides, Knitted
  Skin Adhesive, Sterile
  Standard Dressings
  Surgical Sutures (absorbable and non-absorbable)
  Tapeless Dressing Holders
  Vapour-permeable Adhesive Film Dressing, BP, with absorbent pad
  Wound Drainage Pouch
  Wound Management Dressings (including activated charcoal, capillary-action, and silicone)

Deletions

Preparations deleted from the Nurse Prescribers' List since 1999

Calamine Cream, Aqueous, BP
Calamine Lotion, BP
Calamine Lotion, Oily, BP 1980
Humiderm® Cream
Lactulose Powder, NPF
Piperazine Citrate Elixir, BP

Changes to regulations

The following preparations may only be prescribed in a maximum quantity of 96 tablets with a maximum pack size of 32 tablets:

Aspirin Tablets, Dispersible, 300 mg, BP
Paracetamol Tablets, BP
Paracetamol Tablets, Soluble, BP

Changes of title

Old	New
Emmolate® Bath Oil	*Dermalo*® Bath Emollient
Lignocaine Gel, BP	Lidocaine Gel/ Lignocaine Gel, BP
Lignocaine Ointment, NPF	Lidocaine Ointment/ Lignocaine Ointment, NPF
Lignocaine and Chlorhexidine Gel, BP	Lidocaine and Chlorhexidine Gel/Lignocaine and Chlorhexidine Gel, BP
Miconazole Oral Gel, NPF	Miconazole Oromucosal Gel, BP
Nystatin Pastilles, NPF	Nystatin Pastilles, BP
Titanium Ointment, NPF	Titanium Ointment, BP

Note. The approved names for a number of drugs have changed, see p. viii for further details

Nurse Prescribers' Extended Formulary

Nurses who have received specific training (which is distinct from that provided to District Nurse or Health Visitor Nurse Prescribers) may prescribe from the Nurse Prescribers' Extended Formulary, see p. N8

Nurse Prescribers' Formulary for District Nurses and Health Visitors

List of preparations approved by the Secretary of State which may be prescribed on form FP10P (form GP10 (N) in Scotland, form HS21(N) in Northern Ireland) by Nurses for National Health Service patients.

District Nurse and Health Visitor prescribers who have completed the necessary training may only prescribe items appearing in the nurse prescribers' list set out below.

Medicinal Preparations

Almond Oil Ear Drops, BP
Arachis Oil Enema, NPF
[1]Aspirin Tablets, Dispersible, 300 mg, BP
Bisacodyl Suppositories, BP (includes 5-mg and 10-mg strengths)
Bisacodyl Tablets, BP
Cadexomer–Iodine Ointment, NPF
Cadexomer–Iodine Paste, NPF
Cadexomer–Iodine Powder, NPF
Catheter Maintenance Solution, Chlorhexidine, NPF
Catheter Maintenance Solution, Mandelic Acid, NPF
Catheter Maintenance Solution, Sodium Chloride, NPF
Catheter Maintenance Solution, 'Solution G', NPF
Catheter Maintenance Solution, 'Solution R', NPF
Choline Salicylate Dental Gel, BP
Clotrimazole Cream 1%, BP
Co-danthramer Capsules, NPF
Co-danthramer Capsules, Strong, NPF
Co-danthramer Oral Suspension, NPF
Co-danthramer Oral Suspension, Strong, NPF
Co-danthrusate Capsules, BP
Co-danthrusate Oral Suspension, NPF
Crotamiton Cream, BP
Crotamiton Lotion, BP
Dextranomer Beads, NPF
Dextranomer Paste, NPF
Dimeticone barrier creams containing at least 10%
Docusate Capsules, BP
Docusate Enema, NPF
Docusate Enema, Compound, BP
Docusate Oral Solution, BP
Docusate Oral Solution, Paediatric, BP
Econazole Cream 1%, BP
Emollients as listed below:
    Alcoderm® Cream
    Alcoderm® Lotion
    Aqueous Cream, BP
    Arachis Oil, BP
    Cetraben® Emollient Cream
    Dermamist®
    Diprobase® Cream
    Diprobase® Ointment
    Doublebase®
    E45® Cream
    Emulsifying Ointment, BP
    Epaderm®
    Hydromol® Cream
    Hydrous Ointment, BP
    Keri® Therapeutic Lotion
    LactiCare® Lotion
    Lipobase®
    Liquid and White Soft Paraffin Ointment, NPF
    Neutrogena® Dermatological Cream
    Oilatum® Cream
    Paraffin, White Soft, BP
    Paraffin, Yellow Soft, BP
    Ultrabase®
    Unguentum M®
Emollient Bath Additives as listed below:
    Alpha Keri® Bath Oil
    [2]Balneum®
    [3]Dermalo® Bath Emollient
    Diprobath®
    Hydromol® Emollient
    Oilatum® Emollient
    Oilatum® Fragrance Free
    Oilatum® Gel
Folic Acid 400 micrograms/5 mL Oral Solution, NPF
Folic Acid Tablets 400 micrograms, BP
Glycerol Suppositories, BP
Ispaghula Husk Granules, BP
Ispaghula Husk Granules, Effervescent, BP
Ispaghula Husk Oral Powder, BP
Lactitol Powder, NPF
Lactulose Solution, BP
Lidocaine Gel/Lignocaine Gel, BP
Lidocaine Ointment/Lignocaine Ointment, NPF
Lidocaine and Chlorhexidine Gel/Lignocaine and Chlorhexidine Gel, BP
Macrogol Oral Powder, Compound, NPF
Magnesium Hydroxide Mixture, BP
Magnesium Sulphate Paste, BP
Malathion alcoholic lotions containing at least 0.5%
Malathion aqueous lotions containing at least 0.5%
Mebendazole Oral Suspension, NPF
Mebendazole Tablets, NPF
Methylcellulose Tablets, BP
Miconazole Cream 2%, BP
Miconazole Oromucosal Gel, BP
Mouthwash Solution-tablets, NPF
Nicotine Inhalation Cartridge for Oromucosal Use, NPF
Nicotine Lozenge, NPF
Nicotine Medicated Chewing Gum, NPF
Nicotine Nasal Spray, NPF
Nicotine Sublingual Tablets, NPF
Nicotine Transdermal Patches, NPF
Nystatin Oral Suspension, BP
Nystatin Pastilles, BP
Olive Oil Ear Drops, BP
Paracetamol Oral Suspension, BP (includes 120 mg/5 mL and 250 mg/5 mL strengths—both of which are available as sugar-free formulations)
[1]Paracetamol Tablets, BP
[1]Paracetamol Tablets, Soluble, BP (includes 120-mg and 500-mg tablets)
Permethrin Cream, NPF
Permethrin Cream Rinse, NPF
Phenothrin Alcoholic Lotion, NPF
Phenothrin Aqueous Lotion, NPF
Phenothrin Foam Application, NPF
Phosphates Enema, BP
Piperazine and Senna Powder, NPF
Povidone–Iodine Solution, BP
Senna Granules, Standardised, BP
Senna Oral Solution, NPF
Senna Tablets, BP
Senna and Ispaghula Granules, NPF
Sodium Bicarbonate Ear Drops, BP
Sodium Chloride Solution, Sterile, BP
Sodium Citrate Compound Enema, NPF
Sodium Picosulfate Capsules, NPF
Sodium Picosulfate Elixir, NPF
Sterculia Granules, NPF
Sterculia and Frangula Granules, NPF
Streptokinase and Streptodornase Topical Powder, NPF
Thymol Glycerin, Compound, BP 1988
Titanium Ointment, BP
Zinc and Castor Oil Ointment, BP
Zinc Oxide and Dimeticone Spray, NPF
Zinc Oxide Impregnated Medicated Stocking, NPF

---

1. Max. 96 tablets; max. pack size 32 tablets
2. Except pack sizes that are not to be prescribed under the NHS (see Part XVIIIA of the Drug Tariff, Part XI of the Northern Ireland Drug Tariff)
3. Formerly Emmolate® Bath Oil

Appliances and Reagents (including Wound Management Products)

In the Drug Tariff Appliances and Reagents which may not be prescribed by Nurses are annotated ⊗ (Nx in the Scottish Drug Tariff and ✗ in the Northern Ireland Drug Tariff)

Applicators, Vaginal as listed in Part IXA of the Drug Tariff (Part 3 of the Scottish Drug Tariff, not prescribable by nurses in Northern Ireland)

Atomizers, Hand Operated as listed in Part IXA of the Drug Tariff (Part 3 of the Scottish Drug Tariff, not prescribable by nurses in Northern Ireland)

Auto Inflation Device (for treatment of glue ear) as listed in Part IXA of the Drug Tariff (Part 3 of the Scottish Drug Tariff, Part III of the Northern Ireland Drug Tariff)

Breast Reliever as listed in Part IXA of the Drug Tariff (Part 3 of the Scottish Drug Tariff, not prescribable by nurses in Northern Ireland)

Breast Shields as listed in Part IXA of the Drug Tariff (not prescribable by nurses in Scotland or Northern Ireland)

Chemical Reagents

The following as listed in Part IXR of the Drug Tariff (Part 9 of the Scottish Drug Tariff, Part II of the Northern Ireland Drug Tariff):

Detection Tablets for Glycosuria
Detection Tablets for Ketonuria
Detection Strips for Glycosuria
Detection Strips for Ketonuria
Detection Strips for Proteinuria
Detection Strips for Blood Glucose
Reagent solutions (Gerhardt's Reagent and Ammonia Solution, Strong, BP) (not prescribable by nurses in Northern Ireland)

Also in BNF section 6.1.6. Items not in the Drug Tariff (and thus not prescribable) are described as ⃞ⁿ͟ᴴ͟ˢ *in the BNF. Although glucose for glucose tolerance test is in section 6.1.6 it is not on the Nurse Prescribers' List*

Catheter Accessories as listed in Part IXA of the Drug Tariff (Part 3 of the Scottish Drug Tariff, Part III of the Northern Ireland Drug Tariff)

Catheter Maintenance Solutions as listed in Part IXA of the Drug Tariff (Part 3 of the Scottish Drug Tariff, Part III of the Northern Ireland Drug Tariff)

Note. See also under Medicinal Products

Catheters, Urethral Sterile as listed under Catheters in Part IXA of the Drug Tariff (Part 3 of the Scottish Drug Tariff, Part III of the Northern Ireland Drug Tariff)

Also in Appendix N1: Urethral Catheters

Chiropody Appliances as listed in Part IXA of the Drug Tariff (Part 2 of the Scottish Drug Tariff (except for Corn Plasters), not prescribable by nurses in Northern Ireland)

Contraceptive Devices as listed in Part IXA of the Drug Tariff (Part 3 of the Scottish Drug Tariff, Part III of the Northern Ireland Drug Tariff (fertility (ovulation) thermometers only))

Also in BNF section 7.3.4

Douches (with vaginal and rectal fittings) as listed in Part IXA of the Drug Tariff (Part 3 of the Scottish Drug Tariff, not prescribable by nurses in Northern Ireland)

Droppers as listed in Part IXA of the Drug Tariff (Part 3 of the Scottish Drug Tariff, not prescribable by nurses in Northern Ireland)

Elastic Hosiery including accessories as listed in Part IXA of the Drug Tariff (Part 4 of the Scottish Drug Tariff, Part III of the Northern Ireland Drug Tariff)

Also in BNF Appendix 8 (section A8.3)

Eye Baths as listed in Part IXA of the Drug Tariff (Part 3 of the Scottish Drug Tariff, not prescribable by nurses in Northern Ireland)

Eye-drop Dispensers as listed in Part IXA of the Drug Tariff (Part 3 of the Scottish Drug Tariff, Part III of the Northern Ireland Drug Tariff)

Eye Shades as listed in Part IXA of the Drug Tariff (Part 3 of the Scottish Drug Tariff, not prescribable by nurses in Northern Ireland)

Finger Cots as listed in Part IXA of the Drug Tariff (Part 3 of the Scottish Drug Tariff, not prescribable by nurses in Northern Ireland)

Finger Stalls as listed in Part IXA of the Drug Tariff (Part 3 of the Scottish Drug Tariff, not prescribable by nurses in Northern Ireland)

Hypodermic Equipment as listed in Part IXA of the Drug Tariff (Part 3 of the Scottish Drug Tariff, Part III of the Northern Ireland Drug Tariff (with some exceptions))

Also in BNF section 6.1.1.3. Items not in the Drug Tariff (and thus not prescribable) are described as ⃞ⁿ͟ᴴ͟ˢ *in the BNF*

Incontinence Appliances as listed in Part IXB of the Drug Tariff (Part 5 of the Scottish Drug Tariff, Part III of the Northern Ireland Drug Tariff)

Also in Appendix N1: Incontinence Appliances

Inhaler, Spare Tops as listed in Part IXA of the Drug Tariff (Part 3 of the Scottish Drug Tariff, not prescribable by nurses in Northern Ireland)

Insufflators as listed in Part IXA of the Drug Tariff (Part 3 of the Scottish Drug Tariff, not prescribable by nurses in Northern Ireland)

Iodine Brush as listed under Brushes in Part IXA of the Drug Tariff (Part 3 of the Scottish Drug Tariff, not prescribable by nurses in Northern Ireland)

Irrigation Fluids as listed in Part IXA of the Drug Tariff (Part 2 of the Scottish Drug Tariff, Part III of the Northern Ireland Drug Tariff)

Note. See also under Medicinal Products

Latex Foam, Adhesive as listed in Part IXA of the Drug Tariff (not prescribable by nurses in Scotland or Northern Ireland)

Lubricating Jelly as listed in Part IXA of the Drug Tariff (Part 2 of the Scottish Drug Tariff, not prescribable by nurses in Northern Ireland)

Nasal Device (nasal dilator) as listed in Part IXA of the Druf Tariff (Part 3 of the Scottish Drug Tariff, Part III of the Northern Ireland Drug Tariff)

Nipple Shields, Plastic as listed in Part IXA of the Drug Tariff (Part 3 of the Scottish Drug Tariff, not prescribable by nurses in Northern Ireland)

Peak Flow Meters as listed in Part IXA of the Drug Tariff (Part 3 of the Scottish Drug Tariff, not prescribable by nurses in Northern Ireland)

Also in BNF section 3.1.5

Pessaries as listed in Part IXA of the Drug Tariff (Part 3 of the Scottish Drug Tariff, Part III of the Northern Ireland Drug Tariff (with some exceptions))

Protectives as listed in Part IXA of the Drug Tariff (Part 2 of the Scottish Drug Tariff, Part III of the Northern Ireland Drug Tariff (EMA Disposable Film Gloves only))

Rectal Dilators as listed in Part IXA of the Drug Tariff (Part 3 of the Scottish Drug Tariff, not prescribable by nurses in Northern Ireland)

Saliva Stimulating Tablets as listed in Part IXA of the Drug Tariff (Part 3 of the Scottish Drug Tariff, not prescribable by nurses in Northern Ireland)

Also in BNF section 12.3.5

Stoma Appliances and Associated Products as listed in Part IXC of the Drug Tariff (Part 6 of the Scottish Drug Tariff, Part III of the Northern Ireland Drug Tariff)

Also in Appendix N1: Stoma Appliances

> In the Drug Tariff Appliances and Reagents which may **not** be prescribed by Nurses are annotated Ⓝ
>
> (**Nx** in the Scottish Drug Tariff and **N̶** in the Northern Ireland Drug Tariff)

Suprapubic Belts (replacements only) as listed in Part IXA of the Drug Tariff (Part 3 of the Scottish Drug Tariff, not prescribable by nurses in Northern Ireland)

Suprapubic Catheters as listed in Part IXA of the Drug Tariff (Part 3 of the Scottish Drug Tariff, not prescribable by nurses in Northern Ireland)

Synovial Fluid as listed in Part IXA of the Drug Tariff (Part 3 of the Scottish Drug Tariff, not prescribable by nurses in Northern Ireland)

Note. Mentioned in text of BNF section 10.1

Syringes (Bladder/Irrigating, Ear, Enema, Spare Vaginal Pipes) as listed in Part IXA of the Drug Tariff (Part 3 of the Scottish Drug Tariff, not prescribable by nurses in Northern Ireland)

Tapeless IV Holders as listed in Part IXA of the Drug Tariff (Part 2 of the Scottish Drug Tariff, not prescribable by nurses in Northern Ireland)

Test Tubes as listed in Part IXA of the Drug Tariff (Part 3 of the Scottish Drug Tariff, not prescribable by nurses in Northern Ireland)

Tracheostomy and Laryngectomy Appliances as listed in Part IXA of the Drug Tariff (Part 2 of the Scottish Drug Tariff, not prescribable by nurses in Northern Ireland)

Trusses as listed in Part IXA of the Drug Tariff (Part 3 of the Scottish Drug Tariff, not prescribable by nurses in Northern Ireland)

Urine Sugar Analysis Equipment as listed in Part IXA of the Drug Tariff (Parts 3 and 9 of the Scottish Drug Tariff, Part III of the Northern Ireland Drug Tariff)

Also in BNF section 6.1.6

Wound Management and Related Products (including bandages, dressings, gauzes, lint, stockinette, etc)

The following as listed in Part IXA of the Drug Tariff (Part 2 of the Scottish Drug Tariff, Part III of the Northern Ireland Drug Tariff):

Absorbent Cellulose Dressing with Fluid Repellent Backing

Absorbent Cottons

Absorbent Cotton Gauzes

Absorbent Cotton and Viscose Ribbon Gauze, BP 1988

Absorbent Dressing Pads, Sterile

Absorbent Lint, BPC

Absorbent Perforated Dressing with Adhesive Border

Absorbent Perforated Plastic Film Faced Dressing

Arm Slings

Belladonna Adhesive Plaster, BP 1980

Boil Dressing Pack

Boric Acid Lint, BPC 1963

Cellulose Wadding, BP 1988

Chlorhexidine Gauze Dressing, BP

Cotton Conforming Bandage, BP 1988

Cotton Crêpe Bandage, BP 1988

Cotton Crêpe Bandage, Hospicrepe 239

Cotton, Polyamide and Elastane Bandage

Cotton Stretch Bandage, BP 1988

Crêpe Bandage, BP 1988

Elastic Adhesive Bandage, BP

Elastic Diachylon Bandage, Ventilated BPC

Elastic Web Bandages

Elastomer and Viscose Bandage, Knitted

Gauze and Cotton Tissues

Heavy Cotton and Rubber Elastic Bandage, BP

High Compression Bandages (Extensible)

Knitted Polyamide and Cellulose Contour Bandage, BP 1988

Knitted Viscose Primary Dressing, BP, Type 1

Multi-layer Compression Bandaging

Multiple Pack Dressing No. 1

Open-wove Bandage, BP 1988, Type 1

Paraffin Gauze Dressing, BP

Plaster of Paris Bandage, BP 1988

Polyamide and Cellulose Contour Bandage, BP 1988

Polyester Primary Dressing with Neutral Triglycerides, Knitted

Povidone–Iodine Fabric Dressing, Sterile

Short Stretch Compression Bandage

Skin Adhesive, Sterile

Skin Closure Strips, Sterile

Standard Dressings

Sterile Dressing Packs

Stockinettes

Sub-compression Wadding Bandage

Surgical Adhesive Tapes

Surgical Sutures (absorbable and non-absorbable)

Suspensory Bandages, Cotton

Swabs

Tapeless Dressing Holders

Triangular Calico Bandage, BP 1980

Vapour-permeable Adhesive Film Dressing, BP (including with absorbent pad)

Vapour-permeable Waterproof Plastic Wound Dressing, BP, Sterile

Wound Drainage Pouch

Wound Management Dressings (including activated charcoal, alginate, capillary-action cavity, hydrocolloid, hydrogel, foam and silicone)

Zinc Paste Bandages (including both plain and with additional ingredients)

Also in BNF Appendix 8. Items not in the Drug Tariff (and thus not prescribable) are described as Ⓝ︀Ⓗ︀Ⓢ︀ *in the BNF. Although Framycetin Gauze Dressing, BP is in Appendix 8 it is not on the Nurse Prescribers' List*

Nurse Prescribers' Extended Formulary

List of preparations which may be prescribed by Extended Formulary Nurse Prescribers on Form FP10P, for NHS patients in England (Form GP10(N2) in Scotland).

Independent nurse prescribers who have completed the necessary training and are authorised to prescribe from the Nurse Prescribers' Extended Formulary list may prescribe all General Sales List and Pharmacy medicines currently prescribable by GPs (except Controlled Drugs), together with a list of Prescription Only Medicines. In addition they may prescribe all items in the nurse prescribing list for District Nurses and Health Visitors on pp. N5–7. This will enable them to manage medical conditions, minor ailments, minor injuries, health promotion and palliative care—specified below.

Medical Conditions

Minor Ailments and Injuries	BNF section[1]
General and unspecified	
Infantile colic	1.1.1
Chickenpox	13.3
Circulatory	
Haemorrhoids	1.7.1, 1.7.2
Phlebitis—superficial	–
Digestive	
Aphthous ulcer	12.3.1
Candidiasis—oral	12.3.2
Constipation	1.6
Dental abscess	4.7.1, 10.1.1
Gastroenteritis	1.4
Gingivitis	12.3.4
Heartburn	1.1
Stomatitis	–
Worms—threadworms	5.5.1
Eye	
Blepharitis	11.3.1
Conjunctivitis—allergic	11.4.2
Conjunctivitis—infective	11.3.1
Ear	
Furuncle	–
Otitis externa	12.1.1
Otitis media	12.1.2
Wax in ear	12.1.3
Musculoskeletal	
Back pain—acute, uncomplicated	4.7.1, 10.1.1
Neck pain—acute, uncomplicated	4.7.1, 10.1.1
Soft tissue injury	4.7.1,10.1.1, 10.3.2
Sprains	4.7.1, 10.1.1, 10.3.2
Respiratory	
Acute nasopharyngitis (coryza)	12.2.2
Laryngitis	12.3.1
Pharyngitis	12.3.1
Rhinitis—allergic	12.2.1, 12.2.2, 3.4.1
Sinusitis—acute	12.2.2
Tonsillitis	12.3.1
Skin	
Abrasions	13.10.5
Acne	13.6
Boil/carbuncle	13.10.5
Burn/scald	13.11, App. 8
Candidiasis—skin	13.10.2
Chronic skin ulcer	13.11.7, 13.10.1

Minor Ailments and Injuries	BNF section[1]
Skin	
Dermatitis—atopic	13.5.1
Dermatitis—contact	13.5.1
Dermatitis—seborrhoeic	13.5.1
Dermatophytosis of the skin (ringworm)	13.10.2
Herpes labialis	13.10.3
Impetigo	13.10.1, 5.1 (table 1)
Insect bite/sting	13.3
Lacerations	13.11, App. 8
Nappy rash	13.2.2
Pediculosis (head lice)	13.10.4
Scabies	13.10.4
Urticaria	3.4.1
Warts (including verrucas)	13.7
Urinary system	
Urinary tract infection (women) —lower, uncomplicated	5.1 (table 1), 7.4.3
Female genital system	
Bacterial vaginosis	5.1.11, 7.2.2
Candidiasis—vulvovaginal	7.2.2
Dysmenorrhoea	4.7.1, 10.1.1
Male genital system	
Balanitis	13.10.2

Health Promotion	
Preconceptual counselling	9.1.2
Contraception	7.3
Emergency contraception	7.3
Smoking cessation	4.10
Routine childhood and specific vaccinations	14.1, 14.4

Palliative Care	
Bowel colic	Prescribing in palliative care
Candidiasis—oral	12.3.2
Constipation	Prescribing in palliative care
Cough	Prescribing in palliative care
Dry mouth	Prescribing in palliative care
Excessive respiratory secretions	Prescribing in palliative care
Fungating malodorous tumours	13.10.1.2
Nausea and vomiting	Prescribing in palliative care
Pain control	Prescribing in palliative care

---

1. BNF sections appropriate to the listed conditions are shown. However, not all drugs in the relevant BNF sections are prescribable by nurses. Also, in some cases preparations (including General Sales List and Pharmacy medicines) in other BNF sections may be suitable. Before choosing a Prescription Only Medicine, nurses need to check the Nurse Prescribers' Extended Formulary list and to satisfy themselves that the product is licensed for the condition they wish to prescribe for and that the condition falls within the remit of the Nurse Prescribers' Extended Formulary.

Nurse Prescribers' Extended Formulary

1. All licensed P and GSL Medicines prescribable on the NHS, except controlled drugs
2. Prescription Only Medicines from the list below by the route or form specified

List of prescription only medicines for prescribing by extended formulary nurse prescribers

Oral antibacterials marked * —see separate list below for indications

Drug	Route of administration, use or pharmaceutical form
Aciclovir	External
Acrivastine	Oral
Adapalene	External
Alclometasone dipropionate	External
Alimemazine tartrate (trimeprazine tartrate)	Oral
Amorolfine hydrochloride	External
Amoxicillin trihydrate*	Oral
Aspirin	Oral
Azelaic acid	External
Azelastine hydrochloride	Ophthalmic, nasal
Baclofen	Palliative care—oral
Beclometasone dipropionate	External, nasal
Betamethasone	External
Betamethasone dipropionate	External
Betamethasone sodium phosphate	Aural, nasal
Betamethasone valerate	External, rectal
Budesonide	Nasal
Carbaryl	External
Carbenoxolone sodium	Mouthwash
Cetirizine hydrochloride	Oral
Chloramphenicol	Ophthalmic
Cimetidine	Oral
Cinchocaine hydrochloride	Rectal
Clindamycin phosphate	External, vaginal
Clobetasone butyrate	External
Clotrimazole	External
Cyclizine	Palliative care—parenteral
Dantrolene sodium	Palliative care—oral
Dantron	Oral
Desogestrel	Oral
Desoximetasone	External
Dexamethasone	Aural
Dexamethasone isonicotinate	Nasal
Diclofenac diethylammonium	External
Domperidone	Palliative care—oral and rectal
Domperidone maleate	Palliative care—oral
Doxycycline*	Oral
Econazole nitrate	Vaginal, external
Erythromycin	External
Ethinylestradiol	Oral
Etynodiol diacetate	Oral
Famotidine	Oral
Felbinac	External
Fenticonazole nitrate	Vaginal
Fexofenadine hydrochloride	Oral
Flucloxacillin sodium*	Oral
Fluconazole	Oral
Fludroxycortide (flurandrenolone)	External

Drug	Route of administration, use or pharmaceutical form
Flumetasone pivalate	Aural
Flunisolide	Nasal
Fluocinolone acetonide	External
Fluocinonide	External
Fluocortolone hexanoate	External, rectal
Fluocortolone pivalate	External, rectal
Flurbiprofen	Lozenges
Fluticasone propionate	External, nasal
Fusidic acid	Ophthalmic
Gentamicin sulphate	Aural
Gestodene	Oral
Hydrocortisone	External including rectal
Hydrocortisone acetate	External including rectal
Hydrocortisone butyrate	External
Hydrocortisone sodium succinate	Lozenges
Hyoscine butylbromide	Palliative care—parenteral
Hyoscine hydrobromide	Palliative care—oral, parenteral, transdermal
Ibuprofen	External, oral
Ibuprofen lysine	Oral
Ipratropium bromide	Nasal
Isotretinoin	External
Ketoconazole	External
Ketoprofen	External
Levocabastine hydrochloride	Nasal and ophthalmic
Levomepromazine (methotrimeprazine) maleate	Palliative care—oral
Levomepromazine (methotrimeprazine) hydrochloride	Palliative care—parenteral
Levonorgestrel	Oral
Lithium succinate	External
Lodoxamide trometamol	Ophthalmic
Loperamide hydrochloride	Oral
Loratadine	Oral
Mebendazole	Oral
Medroxyprogesterone acetate	Injection
Mestranol	Oral
Metoclopramide hydrochloride	Palliative care—oral and parenteral
Metronidazole*	Oral, external, vaginal
Miconazole	Dental lacquer
Miconazole nitrate	Vaginal, external
Minocycline*	Oral
Mometasone furoate	External, nasal
Nedocromil sodium	Ophthalmic
Nefopam hydrochloride	Oral
Neomycin sulphate	Aural
Neomycin undecanoate	Aural
Nitrofuratoin*	Oral
Nizatidine	Oral
Norethisterone	Oral
Norethisterone acetate	Oral
Norethisterone enanthate	Parenteral
Norgestimate	Oral
Norgestrel	Oral
Nystatin	External, local mouth treatment, vaginal
Oxytetracycline dihydrate*	Oral
Paracetamol	Oral
Penciclovir	External
Piroxicam	External

Drug	Route of admin-istration, use or pharmaceutical form
Prednisolone hexanoate	Rectal
Prednisolone sodium phosphate	Aural
Ranitidine hydrochloride	Oral
Silver sulfadiazine	External
Sodium cromoglicate	Ophthalmic
Streptodornase	External
Streptokinase	External
Sulconazole nitrate	External
Terbinafine hydrochloride	External
Tetracycline hydrochloride*	Oral, external
Tretinoin	External
Triamcinolone acetonide	Nasal, aural, oral paste, external
Trimethoprim*	Oral
Tuberculin PPD	Injection
Vaccine, Adsorbed Diptheria	Injection
Vaccine, Adsorbed Diptheria and Tetanus	Injection
Vaccine, Adsorbed Diptheria and Tetanus for Adults and Adolescents	Injection
Vaccine, Adsorbed Diptheria for Adults and Adolescents	Injection
Vaccine, Adsorbed Diptheria, Tetanus and Pertussis	Injection
Vaccine, Adsorbed Diptheria, Tetanus and Pertussis (Acellular Component)	Injection
Vaccine, BCG	Injection
Vaccine, BCG Percutaneous	Injection
Vaccine, Haemophilus Influenzae Type B (Hib)	Injection
Vaccine, Haemophilus Influenzae Type B (Hib) with Diptheria, Tetanus and Pertussis	Injection
Vaccine, Haemophilus Influenzae Type B, (Hib) with Diptheria, Tetanus and Acellular Pertussis	Injection
Vaccine, Hepatitis A	Injection
Vaccine, Hepatitis A with Typhoid	Injection
Vaccine, Hepatitis A, Inactivated, with recombinant (DNA) Hepatitis B	Injection
Vaccine, Hepatitis B	Injection
Vaccine, Influenza	Injection
Vaccine, Live Measles, Mumps and Rubella (MMR)	Injection
Vaccine, Meningococcal Group C Conjugate	Injection
Vaccine, Meningococcal Polysaccharide A and C	Injection
Vaccine, Pneumococcal	Injection
Vaccine, Poliomyelitis, Inactivated	Injection
Vaccine, Poliomyelitis, Live (Oral)	Oral
Vaccine, Rubella, Live	Injection
Vaccine, Tetanus, Adsorbed	Injection
Vaccine, Typhoid, Live Attenuated (Oral)	Oral
Vaccine, Typhoid, Polysaccharide	Injection

* Oral antibacterials and indications considered suitable for nurse prescribing

Drug	Indication
Amoxicillin trihydrate	Lower UTI (women)
Nitrofurantoin	Lower UTI (women)
Trimethoprim	Lower UTI (women)
Flucloxacillin sodium	Impetigo
Metronidazole	Fungating malo-dorous tumours; Bacterial vaginosis
Doxycycline	Acne
Minocycline	Acne
Oxytetracycline dihydrate	Acne
Tetracycline hydrochloride	Acne

Laxatives

Corresponds to BNF section 1.6.

Before prescribing laxatives it is important to be sure that the patient *is* constipated and that the constipation is *not* a result of an undiagnosed underlying complaint.

It is also important for those who complain of constipation to understand that bowel habit can vary considerably in frequency without doing harm. Some people may consider themselves constipated if they do not have a bowel movement each day. A useful definition of constipation is the passage of hard stools less frequently than the patient's own normal pattern and this can be explained to the patient.

Misconceptions about bowel habits have led to excessive laxative use. Abuse may lead to hypokalaemia and an atonic non-functioning colon. *Simple constipation* is usually relieved by increasing the intake of dietary fibre.

Laxatives should generally be **avoided** except where straining will exacerbate a condition (such as angina) or increase the risk of rectal bleeding as in haemorrhoids. Laxatives are also of value in *drug-induced constipation*, for the *expulsion of parasites* after anthelmintic treatment, and to clear the alimentary tract *before surgery and radiological procedures*. Prolonged treatment of constipation is seldom necessary except occasionally in the elderly.

CHILDREN. The use of laxatives in children should be discouraged unless prescribed by a doctor. Infrequent defaecation may be normal in breast-fed babies or in response to poor intake of fluid or fibre. Delays of greater than 3 days between stools may increase the likelihood of pain on passing hard stools leading to anal fissure, anal spasm and eventually to a learned response to avoid defaecation. Increased fluid and fibre intake may be sufficient to regulate bowel action.

> Nurse prescribers should discuss with the doctor before prescribing a laxative for a child

Laxatives can be divided into four main groups: *bulk-forming laxatives, stimulant laxatives, faecal softeners,* and *osmotic laxatives.* This simple classification, however, disguises the fact that some laxatives have complex actions.

Bulk-forming laxatives

Bulk-forming laxatives relieve constipation by increasing faecal mass which stimulates peristalsis. Patients should be told that the full effect may take some days to develop. In nursing practice they are particularly useful in the management of patients with *colostomy, ileostomy, haemorrhoids,* and *anal fissure.* Methylcellulose tablets are licensed for other indications including diarrhoea and obesity but nurse prescribers should prescribe them **only** for constipation.

BULK-FORMING LAXATIVES

Indications: constipation, see also notes above

Cautions: adequate fluid intake should be maintained to avoid intestinal obstruction—it may be necessary to supervise elderly or debilitated patients or those with intestinal narrowing or decreased motility

Contra-indications: difficulty in swallowing, intestinal obstruction, colonic atony, faecal impaction; avoid methylcellulose in infective bowel disease

Side-effects: flatulence, abdominal distension; gastro-intestinal obstruction or impaction; hypersensitivity reported

Dose: see preparations, below

> COUNSELLING. Preparations that swell on contact with liquid should always be carefully swallowed with water and should not be taken immediately before going to bed

Prescribe as:

Ispaghula Husk Granules

Granules, brown, sugar- and gluten-free, ispaghula husk 90%, net price 300 g = £3.53. *Proprietary product: Isogel*

Dose: 2 teaspoonfuls in water once or twice daily, preferably at mealtimes; CHILD (but see notes above) 1 teaspoonful

Ispaghula Husk Oral Powder (*Ispagel*)

Powder, beige, sugar-free, ispaghula husk 3.5 g/sachet (orange flavour), net price 30 sachets = £2.10.

Excipients: include aspartame

Dose: 1 sachet in water 1–3 times daily; CHILD (but see notes above) 6–12 years ½ adult dose

Ispaghula Husk Oral Powder (*Konsyl*)

Powder, gluten-free, ispaghula husk (micronised) 3.4 g/sachet, net price 60 sachets (orange flavour) = £3.99.

Note. A sugar-free version containing ispaghula husk 6 g/sachet is also available, net price 30 sachets = £3.99

Dose: 1 sachet in water 1–3 times daily before or after meals; CHILD (but see notes above) over 6 years ½ adult dose or less

Ispaghula Husk Oral Powder (*Regulan*)

Powder, beige, sugar- and gluten-free, ispaghula husk 3.4 g/sachet (orange or lemon/lime flavour), net price 30 sachets = £1.57.

Excipients: include aspartame

Dose: 1 sachet in 150 mL water 1–3 times daily; CHILD (but see notes above) 6–12 years 2.5–5 mL

Effervescent Ispaghula Husk Granules

Granules, buff, effervescent, sugar- and gluten-free, ispaghula husk 3.5 g/sachet, net price 60 sachets (lemon or orange flavour or plain) = £4.24. *Proprietary product: Fybogel*

Excipients: include aspartame 50 mg/sachet

Dose: 1 sachet in water twice daily, preferably after meals; CHILD (but see notes above) 6–12 years 2.5–5 mL

Methylcellulose Tablets

Tablets, pink, scored, methylcellulose '450' 500 mg, net price 112-tab pack = £2.69. *Proprietary products: Celevac* tablets

Dose: 3–6 tablets twice daily with at least 300 mL of water

Sterculia Granules
Granules, coated, gluten-free, sterculia 62%, net price 500 g = £6.05; 60 × 7-g sachets = £5.11.
Proprietary product: Normacol
Dose: 1–2 heaped 5-mL spoonfuls or contents of 1–2 sachets, washed down without chewing with plenty of liquid once or twice daily after meals; CHILD (but see notes above) 6–12 years half adult dose

Sterculia and Frangula Granules
Granules, brown, coated, gluten-free, sterculia 62%, frangula (standardised) 8%, net price 500 g = £6.50; 60 × 7-g sachets = £5.45. *Proprietary product: Normacol Plus*
Dose: 1–2 heaped 5-mL spoonfuls or contents of 1–2 sachets, washed down without chewing with plenty of liquid once or twice daily after meals

Stimulant laxatives

Stimulant laxatives increase intestinal motility and are used in functional constipation that has not responded to dietary measures.

Stimulant laxatives often cause abdominal cramp. They should not be used in intestinal obstruction, and prolonged use can precipitate the onset of an atonic non-functioning colon and hypokalaemia. They should preferably be avoided in children.

BISACODYL
Indications: constipation; tablets act in 10–12 hours; suppositories act in 20–60 minutes
Cautions; Contra-indications; Side-effects: see notes on stimulant laxatives; tablets, griping, suppositories, local irritation
Dose: see under preparations, below

Prescribe as:
Bisacodyl Tablets 5 mg
Tablets, enteric coated, bisacodyl 5 mg. Net price 20 = 59p
Dose: 1–2 tablets at night, occasionally necessary to increase to 3–4; CHILD (but see notes above) under 10 years 1 tablet at night

Bisacodyl Suppositories 10 mg
Suppositories, bisacodyl 10 mg. Net price 12 = 75p
Dose: 1 suppository rectally in the morning

Bisacodyl Paediatric Suppositories 5 mg
Paediatric suppositories, bisacodyl 5 mg. Net price 5 = 89p
Dose: CHILD (but see notes above) under 10 years 1 suppository rectally in the morning

Nurse prescribers should discuss with the doctor before prescribing a laxative for a child

DANTRON
(Danthron)
Indications: in consultation with doctor, only for: constipation in terminally ill patients of all ages; acts within 6–12 hours
Cautions; Contra-indications; Side-effects: see notes on stimulant laxatives; urine may be coloured red; avoid prolonged contact with skin (as in incontinent patients) risk of irritation and excoriation; avoid in pregnancy and breast-feeding; *rodent* studies indicate potential carcinogenic risk
Dose: see under preparations

Prescribe as:
Co-danthramer Capsules PoM
Capsules, co-danthramer 25/200 (dantron 25 mg, poloxamer '188' 200 mg). Net price 60-cap pack = £12.86
Dose: (restricted indications, see above) 1–2 capsules at bedtime; CHILD (terminally ill only) 1 capsule at bedtime

Strong Co-danthramer Capsules PoM
Capsules, co-danthramer 37.5/500 (dantron 37.5 mg, poloxamer '188' 500 mg). Net price 60-cap pack = £15.55
Dose: (restricted indications, see above) 1–2 capsules at bedtime; CHILD under 12 years not recommended

Co-danthramer Oral Suspension PoM
Oral suspension, co-danthramer 25/200 in 5 mL (dantron 25 mg, poloxamer '188' 200 mg/5 mL). Net price 300 mL = £11.27, 1 litre = £37.57
Dose: (restricted indications, see above) 5–10 mL at night; CHILD (terminally ill only) 2.5–5 mL

Strong Co-danthramer Oral Suspension PoM
Strong oral suspension, co-danthramer 75/1000 in 5 mL (dantron 75 mg, poloxamer '188' 1 g/5 mL). Net price 300 mL = £30.13
Dose: (restricted indications, see above) 5 mL at night; CHILD under 12 years not recommended

Co-danthrusate Capsules PoM
Capsules, co-danthrusate 50/60 (dantron 50 mg, docusate sodium 60 mg). Net price 63-cap pack = £13.45
Dose: (restricted indications, see above) 1–3 capsules, usually at night; CHILD 6–12 years (terminally ill only) 1 capsule

Co-danthrusate Oral Suspension PoM
Oral suspension, co-danthrusate 50/60 in 5 mL (dantron 50 mg, docusate sodium 60 mg/5 mL). Net price 200 mL = £8.75. *Proprietary product: Normax*
Dose: (restricted indications, see above) 5–15 mL at night; CHILD 6–12 years (terminally ill only) 5 mL at night

Cross-references to the BNF are provided but nurse prescribers may only prescribe those items that are listed on the Nurse Prescribers' List.

DOCUSATE SODIUM
(Dioctyl Sodium Sulphosuccinate)
Indications: constipation (oral preparations act within 1–2 days)
Cautions; Contra-indications; Side-effects: see notes on stimulant laxatives; do not give with liquid paraffin; rectal preparations not indicated if haemorrhoids or anal fissure
Dose: see under preparations
Note. Docusate preparations probably also have faecal softening effect.

Prescribe as:

Docusate Capsules 100 mg

Capsules, yellow/white, docusate sodium 100 mg, net price 30-cap pack = £1.67, 100-cap pack = £5.00. *Proprietary product: Dioctyl Capsules*
Dose: (acts within 1–2 days) up to 5 capsules daily in divided doses

Docusate Oral Solution 50 mg/5 mL

Oral solution, sugar-free, docusate sodium 50 mg/5 mL. Net price 300-mL = £2.48. *Proprietary product: Docusol Adult Solution*
Dose: (acts within 1–2 days) up to 50 mL daily in divided doses

Paediatric Docusate Oral Solution 12.5 mg/5 mL

Paediatric oral solution, sugar-free, docusate sodium 12.5 mg/5 mL. Net price 300 mL = £1.63. *Propri_ary product: Docusol Paediatric Solution*
Dose: (acts within 1–2 days) CHILD (but see notes above) over 6 months 5 mL 3 times daily, 2–12 years 5–10 mL 3 times daily

Docusate Enema

Enema, docusate sodium 120 mg in 10-g single-dose disposable packs. Net price 10-g unit = 64p. *Proprietary product: Norgalax Micro-enema*
Dose: ADULT and CHILD (but see notes above) over 12 years, 10-g unit

Compound Docusate Enema

Enema, docusate sodium 90 mg, glycerol 3.78 g/5 mL with macrogol and sorbic acid. Net price 5-mL unit = 31p. *Proprietary product: Fletchers' Enemette*
Dose: ADULT and CHILD (but see notes above) over 3 years, 5-mL unit when required

---

GLYCEROL

(Glycerin)
Indications: constipation
Dose: see under preparations

Prescribe as:

Glycerol Suppositories

(Synonym: Glycerin Suppositories)
Suppositories, gelatin 140 mg, glycerol (glycerin) 700 mg/g. Net price 12 × 1-g size (for infants) = 81p; 12 × 2-g size (for children) = 82p; 12 × 4-g size (for adults) = 71p
Dose: 1 suppository moistened with water before use

SENNA

Indications: constipation (acts within 8–12 hours)
Cautions; Contra-indications; Side-effects: see notes on stimulant laxatives
Dose: see under preparations

Prescribe as:

Senna Tablets

Tablets, total sennosides (calculated as sennoside B) 7.5 mg. Net price 20 = 30p
Dose: (acts in 8–12 hours) 2–4 tablets, usually at bedtime; initial dose should be low and then gradually increased; CHILD (but see notes above) over 6 years, half adult dose in the morning (on doctor's advice only)
Note. For senna tablets on general sale to the public lower dose recommended

Senna Granules

Granules, brown, total sennosides (calculated as sennoside B) 15 mg/5 mL or 5.5 mg/g (one 5-mL spoonful = 2.7 g). Net price 100 g = £2.92. *Proprietary product: Senokot Granules*
Dose: (acts in 8–12 hours) 5–10 mL, usually at bedtime; CHILD (but see notes above) over 6 years 2.5–5 mL in the morning
Note. For senna granules on general sale to the public lower dose recommended

Senna Oral Solution

Syrup, brown, total sennosides (calculated as sennoside B) 7.5 mg/5 mL. Net price 100 mL = £2.21. *Proprietary product: Senokot Syrup*
Dose: (acts in 8–12 hours) 10–20 mL, usually at bedtime; CHILD (but see notes above) 2–6 years 2.5–5 mL in the morning (on doctor's advice only), over 6 years, 5–10 mL in the morning
Note. For senna oral solution on general sale to the public lower dose recommended

Senna and Ispaghula Granules

Granules, coated, senna fruit 12.4%, ispaghula 54.2%. Contain ispaghula as a bulk laxative. Net price 400 g = £5.76, 56 × 4-g sachets = £3.80. *Proprietary product: Manevac Granules*
Dose: (acts in 8–12 hours) 1–2 level 5-mL spoonfuls (*or* 1–2 sachets) with water or warm drink after supper and, if necessary, before breakfast *or* every 6 hours in resistant cases for 1–3 days; CHILD (but see notes above) 5–12 years 1 level 5-mL spoonful (*or* 1 sachet) daily
COUNSELLING. Preparations that swell in contact with liquid should always be carefully swallowed with water and should not be taken immediately before going to bed

---

SODIUM PICOSULFATE

(Sodium Picosulphate)
Indications: constipation (acts within 10–14 hours)
Cautions; Contra-indications; Side-effects: see notes on stimulant laxatives
Dose: see under preparations

Prescribe as:

Sodium Picosulfate Capsules

Capsules, sodium picosulfate 2.5 mg, net price 50-cap pack = £2.73. *Proprietary product:* [1]*Dulco-lax Perles*
Dose: 2–4 capsules at night; CHILD (but see notes above) 4–10 years 1–2 capsules at night, over 10 years 2–4 capsules at night

1. The brand name *Dulco-lax*® is also used for bisacodyl tablets and suppositories

Sodium Picosulfate Elixir

Elixir, sodium picosulfate 5 mg/5 mL. Net price 100 mL = £1.85. *Proprietary products:* [2]*Dulco-lax Liquid, Laxoberal* **DHS**
Dose: 5–10 mL at night; CHILD (but see notes above), under 4 years 250 micrograms/kg, 4–10 years 2.5–5 mL at night, over 10 years 5–10 mL at night

2. The brand name *Dulco-lax*® is also used for bisacodyl tablets and suppositories

> Nurse prescribers should discuss with the doctor before prescribing a laxative for a child

Faecal softeners

Faecal softeners, such as enemas containing arachis oil (ground-nut oil, peanut oil), lubricate and soften impacted faeces and promote a bowel movement.

ARACHIS OIL

Indications: constipation, see also notes above
Dose: see under preparation

Prescribe as:
Arachis Oil Enema
Enema, arachis (peanut) oil in 130-mL single-dose disposable packs. Net price 130 mL = £1.02. *Proprietary product: Fletchers' Arachis Oil Retention Enema*
Dose: to soften impacted faeces, 130 mL; the enema should be warmed before use; CHILD on doctor's advice only

Osmotic laxatives

Osmotic laxatives act by retaining fluid in the bowel by osmosis or by changing the pattern of water distribution in the faeces.

Magnesium hydroxide mixture is suitable for occasional use provided an adequate fluid intake is maintained after it has been given. It may be used when a rapid action is required but should be prescribed with caution because it is often abused.

Lactulose is a semi-synthetic disaccharide which is not absorbed from the gastro-intestinal tract. It is contra-indicated in galactosaemia and in intestinal obstruction; side-effects include flatulence, abdominal cramps and discomfort. **Lactitol** is similar to lactulose.

Macrogol (polyethylene glycol) may be used by mouth for constipation and the short-term treatment of faecal impaction. It is important that the initial assessment of faecal impaction is undertaken by a medical practitioner.

Phosphate enemas are useful in bowel clearance before radiology, endoscopy, and surgery.

LACTITOL

Indications; Contra-indications; Side-effects: see under Lactulose
Dose: see under preparation
COUNSELLING. Powder should be mixed with food or liquid and one to two glasses of liquid should be drunk with the meal

Prescribe as:
Lactitol Powder
Powder, lactitol 10 g/sachet. Net price 10-sachet pack = £1.00. Counselling, see above
Dose: initially 2 sachets daily in a single dose with morning or evening meal, then adjusted to produce one stool daily (1 sachet daily may be sufficient); CHILD (but see notes above) 1–6 years ¼–½ sachet, 6–12 years ½–1 sachet, 12–16 years 1–2 sachets daily, subsequently adjusted to produce one stool daily

LACTULOSE

Indications: constipation (may take up to 48 hours to act)
Cautions: lactose intolerance
Contra-indications: galactosaemia, intestinal obstruction
Side-effects: flatulence, cramps, and abdominal discomfort
Dose: see under preparation

Prescribe as:
Lactulose Solution
Solution, lactulose 3.1–3.7 g/5 mL with other ketoses. Net price 500-mL pack = £2.43
Dose: initially 15 mL twice daily, adjusted according to patient's needs; CHILD (but see notes above) under 1 year 2.5 mL twice daily, 1–5 years 5 mL twice daily, 5–10 years 10 mL twice daily

MACROGOLS

(Polyethylene glycols)
Indications: constipation; faecal impaction (**only after** initial assessment by medical practitioner)
Cautions: pregnancy and breast-feeding; discontinue if symptoms of fluid and electrolyte disturbance
Contra-indications: intestinal perforation or obstruction, paralytic ileus, severe inflammatory conditions of the intestinal tract (such as Crohn's disease, ulcerative colitis, and toxic megacolon)
Side-effects: abdominal distension and pain, nausea
Dose: see under preparation below

Prescribe as:
Compound Macrogol Oral Powder (Norgine)
Oral powder, macrogol '3350' (polyethylene glycol '3350') 13.125 g, sodium bicarbonate 178.5 mg, sodium chloride 350.7 mg, potassium chloride 46.6 mg/sachet. Net price 20-sachet pack (lime and lemon flavour) = £4.98, 30-sachet pack = £7.47. *Proprietary product: Movicol*
Note. Not to be confused with a preparation also containing sodium sulphate which is used for bowel cleansing before surgery and bowel procedures
Dose: chronic constipation, 2–3 sachets daily in divided doses; each sachet dissolved in 125 mL water and drunk immediately usually for up to 2 weeks, course repeated if required; ELDERLY initially 1 sachet daily; CHILD not recommended
Faecal impaction (**important**: initial assessment by medical practitioner), 8 sachets daily dissolved in 1 litre water; the solution should be drunk within 6 hours, usually for max. 3 days; CHILD not recommended.
After reconstitution the solution should be kept in a refrigerator and discarded if unused after 6 hours
Caution: patients with impaired cardiovascular function should not take more than 2 sachets in any 1 hour

MAGNESIUM HYDROXIDE

Indications: constipation
Cautions: renal impairment (risk of magnesium accumulation); hepatic impairment; elderly and

debilitated; see also notes above; **interactions:** see BNF Appendix 1 (magnesium salts)

Contra-indications: acute gastro-intestinal conditions

Side-effects: colic

Dose: see under preparation

Prescribe as:

Magnesium Hydroxide Mixture

(Synonym: Cream of Magnesia)

Mixture, containing about 8% of hydrated magnesium oxide

Dose: constipation, 25–50 mL when required

PHOSPHATES (RECTAL)

Indications: rectal use in constipation, see also notes above

Cautions: elderly and debilitated; see also notes above

Contra-indications: acute gastro-intestinal conditions

Side-effects: local irritation

Dose: see under preparations

Prescribe as:

Phosphates Enema (Formula B)

Enema, sodium acid phosphate 12.8 g, sodium phosphate 10.24 g/128 mL. Net price 128 mL with standard tube = 44p, with long rectal tube = 61p.

Dose: 128 mL; CHILD (but see notes above) over 3 years, reduced according to body weight (under 3 years not recommended)

Phosphates Enema (*Fleet*)

Enema, sodium acid phosphate 21.4 g, sodium phosphate 9.4 g/118 mL. Net price single-dose pack (standard tube) = 46p

Dose: ADULT and CHILD over 12 years, 118 mL; CHILD 3–12 years, on doctor's advice only (under 3 years not recommended)

> Nurse prescribers should discuss with the doctor before prescribing a laxative for a child

SODIUM CITRATE (RECTAL)

Indications: rectal use in constipation

Cautions: elderly and debilitated; see also notes above

Contra-indications: acute gastro-intestinal conditions

Dose: see under preparations

Prescribe as:

Sodium Citrate Compound Enema

Enema, sodium citrate 450 mg with other ingredients including glycerol, sorbitol and an anionic surfactant in a 5-mL single-dose disposable pack. *Proprietary products: Micolette Micro-enema* (net price 5-mL pack = 32p), *Micralax Micro-*

enema (5-mL pack = 33p), *Relaxit Micro-enema* (5-mL pack = 32p)

Dose: ADULT and CHILD (but see notes above) over 3 years, 5 mL (under 3 years not recommended)

Gloves

DISPOSABLE FILM GLOVES

EMA Film Gloves, Disposable

Gloves, small, medium, or large. Net price pack of 30 = £2.12. *Proprietary product: Dispos-A-Gloves*

For use as a barrier during manual evacuation of the bowel

Analgesics

Corresponds to BNF section 4.7.1 (non-opioid analgesics)

The **non-opioid** analgesics **aspirin** and **paracetamol** are particularly suitable for pain in musculoskeletal conditions, whereas the opioid analgesics are more suitable for severe visceral pain. Aspirin and paracetamol are effective analgesics for the relief of *mild to moderate pain*. Their familiar role as household remedies should not detract from their considerable value as analgesics; they are also of value in some forms of *severe chronic pain*.

Combinations of aspirin or paracetamol with an opioid analgesic (such as codeine) are commonly used but their advantages have not been substantiated (and they are not on the Nurse Prescribers' List). Any additional pain relief that they might provide can be at the cost of *increased side-effects caused by the opioid component* (constipation, in particular).

> When prescribing aspirin or paracetamol it is important to make sure that the patient is not already taking an aspirin- or a paracetamol-containing preparation (possibly bought over-the-counter). The BNF (section 4.7.1) includes a list of preparations on sale to the public that contain aspirin or paracetamol alone or with other ingredients.

Aspirin

Aspirin is indicated for mild to moderate pain including headache, transient musculoskeletal pain, and dysmenorrhoea; it has anti-inflammatory properties which may be useful, and is an antipyretic. The main side-effect is gastric irritation; rarely, gastric bleeding can be a serious complication. Aspirin increases bleeding time and must **not** be prescribed as an analgesic to patients receiving anticoagulants such as warfarin. Aspirin is also associated with bronchospasm and allergic reactions, particularly in patients with asthma. Aspirin should **not** be prescribed for patients with a history of hypersensitivity to aspirin or any other non-steroidal anti-inflammatory drug (NSAID)—which includes those in whom asthma, angioedema, urticaria or rhinitis have been precipitated by aspirin or another NSAID; it should **not** be prescribed for children **under the age of 12 years** (or for adolescents during fever or viral infection) owing to its association with Reye's syndrome.

> OTHER USES. Since aspirin decreases platelet aggregation, it is prescribed *by doctors* in low doses (e.g. 75–150 mg daily) to prevent cerebrovascular or cardiovascular disease. Aspirin is also occasionally prescribed *by doctors* for rheumatic conditions. Nurse prescribers should **not** prescribe aspirin for these conditions.

ASPIRIN

Indications: mild to moderate pain, pyrexia

Cautions: asthma, allergic disease, impaired renal or hepatic function (avoid if severe), dehydration; preferably avoid during fever or viral infection in adolescents (risk of Reye's syndrome, see below); pregnancy; elderly; G6PD-deficiency (acceptable in a dose of 1 g daily in most G6PD-deficient individuals); **interactions:** see BNF Appendix 1 (aspirin)

Contra-indications: children under 12 years and in breast-feeding (Reye's syndrome—see below); gastro-intestinal ulceration, haemophilia; not for treatment of gout

HYPERSENSITIVITY. Aspirin and other NSAIDs are **contra**-indicated in patients with a history of hypersensitivity to aspirin or any other NSAID—*which includes those* in whom attacks of *asthma, angioedema, urticaria or rhinitis* have been precipitated by aspirin or any other NSAID

REYE'S SYNDROME. Owing to an association with Reye's syndrome aspirin-containing preparations should not be given to children under 12 years, unless specifically indicated, e.g. for juvenile arthritis (Still's disease). Reye's syndrome has also been reported very rarely in children over 12 years and aspirin should preferably be avoided during fever or viral infection in children and adolescents over 12 years.

Side-effects: generally mild and infrequent but high incidence of gastro-intestinal irritation with slight asymptomatic blood loss, increased bleeding time, bronchospasm and skin reactions in hypersensitive patients

Dose: usual, 300–600 mg every 4–6 hours when necessary, not more than 2.4 g daily without doctor's advice; CHILD and ADOLESCENT not recommended (see Reye's syndrome above)

Prescribe as:

¹**Dispersible Aspirin Tablets 300 mg** PoM
Dispersible tablets, aspirin 300 mg. Net price 20 = 19p
Cautionary label added by pharmacist: dissolve or mix with water before taking and take with or after food
1. Nurse prescribers should prescribe packs containing no more than **32 tablets**, a max. of **3** packs of 32 tablets may be prescribed on each occasion; PoM but may be sold to the public under certain circumstances—for details see *Medicines, Ethics and Practice*, No. 25, London, Pharmaceutical Press, 2001 (and subsequent editions as available)

Paracetamol

Paracetamol is similar in efficacy to aspirin, but has no demonstrable anti-inflammatory activity. It is less irritant to the stomach and for that reason paracetamol is now generally preferred to aspirin, particularly in the elderly. It must be remembered, however, that overdosage with paracetamol (alone or as an ingredient of a combination product) is particularly dangerous.

PARACETAMOL

Indications: mild to moderate pain, pyrexia

Cautions: hepatic and renal impairment, alcohol dependence; **interactions**: see BNF Appendix 1 (paracetamol)

Side-effects: side-effects rare, but rashes, blood disorders, and acute pancreatitis reported after prolonged use; **important:** liver damage (and less frequently renal damage) following **overdosage**, immediate transfer to hospital essential

Dose: 0.5–1 g every 4–6 hours; max. 4 g daily CHILD under 3 months on doctor's advice only, 10 mg/kg (5 mg/kg if jaundiced)—post-immunisation pyrexia, see below; 3 months–1 year 60–120 mg; 1–5 years 120–250 mg; 6–12 years 250–500 mg; these doses may be repeated every 4–6 hours when necessary; max. 4 doses in 24 hours

Post-immunisation pyrexia after immunisation with triple vaccine, INFANT 2–3 months, 60 mg followed, if necessary, by second dose after 4–6 hours; if pyrexia persists refer to doctor

Prescribe as:

²Paracetamol Tablets 500 mg PoM

Tablets, paracetamol 500 mg. Net price 20 = 15p
Cautionary label added by pharmacist: Do not take more than 2 tablets at any one time. Do not take more than 8 in 24 hours. Do not take with any other paracetamol products

2. Nurse prescribers should prescribe packs containing no more than **32 tablets**, a max. of **3 packs of 32 tablets** may be prescribed on each occasion; PoM but may be sold to the public under certain circumstances—for details see *Medicines, Ethics and Practice*, No. 25, London, Pharmaceutical Press, 2001 (and subsequent editions as available)

³Soluble Paracetamol Tablets 500 mg PoM

Soluble tablets, paracetamol 500 mg. Net price 20 = 77p
Cautionary label added by pharmacist: Do not take more than 2 tablets at any one time, do not take more than 8 in 24 hours, dissolve in water. Do not take with any other paracetamol products

3. Nurse prescribers should prescribe packs containing no more than **32 tablets**, a max. of **3 packs of 32 tablets** may be prescribed on each occasion; PoM but may be sold to the public under certain circumstances—for details see *Medicines, Ethics and Practice*, No. 25, London, Pharmaceutical Press, 2001 (and subsequent editions as available)

Paracetamol Oral Suspension 120 mg/5 mL

Oral suspension (= paediatric mixture), paracetamol 120 mg/5 mL. Net price 100 mL = 41p
Note. Sugar-free version can be ordered by specifying 'sugar-free' on the prescription
Cautionary label added by pharmacist: Do not take with any other paracetamol products. If a 60-mg dose is required the pharmacist will supply an oral syringe and advise on how to give a 2.5-mL dose

Paracetamol Oral Suspension 250 mg/5 mL

Oral suspension (= mixture), paracetamol 250 mg/5 mL. Net price 100 mL = 73p
Note. Sugar-free version can be ordered by specifying 'sugar-free' on the prescription
Cautionary label added by pharmacist: Do not take with any other paracetamol products.

Local anaesthetics

Corresponds to BNF section 15.2.

Lidocaine

Lidocaine (lignocaine) is effectively absorbed from mucous membranes and is a useful surface anaesthetic in concentrations of 2 to 4%. Except for surface anaesthesia, solutions should not usually exceed 1% in strength.

LIDOCAINE/LIGNOCAINE

Indications: surface anaesthesia (**important:** consult with doctor), see notes above

Cautions: absorbed through mucosa therefore special care if history of epilepsy, cardiac disease, respiratory disease, hepatic impairment or porphyria (BNF section 9.8.2); do **not** use in mouth (risk of choking); also **special care** in infants or young children

Side-effects: include convulsions and cardiac depressant effects; allergic reactions (rarely anaphylaxis)

Administration: see under preparations

Prescribe as:

Lidocaine Gel/Lignocaine Gel

Gel, anhydrous lidocaine hydrochloride in a sterile water-miscible lubricant basis. Net price 1%, 15 mL = 70p; 2%, 15 mL = 70p

Administration: into urethra at least 5 minutes before catheter insertion, men 10 mL followed by further 3–5 mL; women 3–5 mL; CHILD 1–5 mL

Lidocaine Ointment/Lignocaine Ointment

Ointment, lidocaine 5% in a water-miscible basis. Net price 15 g = 75p.

Administration: to be applied very thinly as necessary (max. 3 times daily)

Lidocaine and Chlorhexidine Gel/Lignocaine and Chlorhexidine Gel

Gel, anhydrous lidocaine hydrochloride 1% or 2%, chlorhexidine gluconate solution 0.25% in a sterile lubricant basis. Net price 15 g = 70p.

Administration: into urethra at least 5 minutes before catheter insertion, men 10 mL followed by 3–5 mL; women 3–5 mL; CHILD 1–5 mL

Gel in disposable syringe, lidocaine hydrochloride 2%, chlorhexidine gluconate solution 0.25%, in a sterile lubricant basis in disposable syringe. Net price 6-mL syringe = £1.51, 11-mL syringe = £1.70. *Proprietary product: Instillagel* (6 mL, 11 mL)

Administration: into urethra, 6–11 mL

Prevention of neural tube defects

Corresponds to BNF section 9.1.2.

PREVENTION OF NEURAL TUBE DEFECTS. Recommendations of an expert advisory group of the Department of Health include the advice that:

To prevent *first occurrence of neural tube defect* women who are planning a pregnancy should be advised to take folic acid as a medicinal or food supplement at a dose of 400 micrograms daily before conception and during the first 12 weeks of pregnancy. Women who have not been taking supplements and who suspect they are pregnant should start at once and continue until week 12 of pregnancy.

Women at risk of a recurrence of neural tube defect (in a child of a man or woman with spina bifida or if there is a history of neural tube defect in a previous child) should be referred to a doctor because a higher dose of folic acid is appropriate. Women receiving antiepileptic therapy need individual counselling by their doctor before starting folic acid.

FOLIC ACID

Indications: prevention of neural tube defects, see notes above

Dose: see notes above

Prescribe as:

| **Folic Acid Tablets, 400 micrograms**
Tablets, folic acid 400 micrograms, net price 90-tab pack = £2.13. *Proprietary product: Preconceive and possibly others*

| **Folic Acid Oral Solution 400 micrograms/5 mL**
Oral solution, folic acid 400 micrograms/5 mL, net price 150 mL = £1.56. *Proprietary product: Folicare*
1. Can be sold to the public provided daily doses do not exceed 500 micrograms

Nicotine replacement therapy

Corresponds to BNF section 4.10

Smoking cessation interventions are a cost-effective way of reducing ill health and prolonging life. Smokers should be advised to stop and offered help if interested in doing so, with follow-up where appropriate.

Where possible, smokers should have access to a specialist smokers' clinic for behavioural support. **Nicotine replacement therapy** is an effective aid to smoking cessation for those smoking more than 10 cigarettes a day. The form of nicotine replacement therapy chosen should take into account individual preference and tolerance of side-effects. Combining pharmacotherapy and behavioural support is more successful than either treatment alone.

Nicotine replacement therapy should be prescribed for short durations at a time and the prescriptions repeated only if the attempt at stopping smoking is continuing.

NICOTINE PRODUCTS

Indications: adjunct to smoking cessation

Cautions: cardiovascular disease (avoid if severe); peripheral vascular disease; hyperthyroidism; diabetes mellitus; phaeochromocytoma, renal and hepatic impairment; history of gastritis and peptic ulcers; should not smoke or use nicotine replacement products in combination; *patches*, exercise may increase absorption and side-effects, skin disorders (patches should not be placed on broken skin); **interactions:** BNF Appendix 1 (nicotine and tobacco)

DRIVING. The nasal spray should not be used when driving or operating machinery (sneezing or watering eyes could contribute to accident)

Contra-indications: severe cardiovascular disease (including severe arrhythmias or immediate post-myocardial infarction period); recent cerebrovascular accident (including transient ischaemic attacks); pregnancy and breast-feeding; *patches*, chronic generalised skin disease (patches should not be placed on broken skin); patches not for occasional smokers

Side-effects: nausea, dizziness, headache and cold and influenza-like symptoms, palpitations, dyspepsia and other gastro-intestinal disturbances, hiccups, insomnia, vivid dreams, myalgia; other side-effects reported include chest pain, blood pressure changes, anxiety and irritability, somnolence and impaired concentration, dysmenorrhoea; *with patches*, skin reactions (discontinue if severe)—vasculitis also reported; *with spray*, nasal irritation, nose bleeds, watering eyes, ear sensations; *with gum, sublingual tablets* or *inhalator*, aphthous ulceration (sometimes with swelling of tongue); *with spray, inhalator, sublingual tablets* or *gum*, throat irritation; *with inhalator*, cough, rhinitis, pharyngitis, stomatitis, sinusitis, dry mouth; *with sublingual tablets*, unpleasant taste

Dose: see under preparations, below

Prescribe as:

[1]Nicotine Inhalation Cartridge for Oromucosal Use

Cartridge (for oromucosal use), nicotine 10 mg, net price 6-cartridge (starter) pack = £3.39, 42-cartridge (refill) pack = £11.37. *Proprietary products*: *Nicorette Inhalator*, *Boots Nicotine Inhalator*

1. For use with inhalation mouthpiece; starter pack contains 6 cartridges with inhalator device and holder, refill pack contains 42 cartridges with inhalator device
ADMINISTRATION: Inhale when urge to smoke occurs; initially use 6–12 cartridges daily for up to 8 weeks, then reduce number of cartridges used by half over next 2 weeks and then stop altogether after further 2 weeks; review treatment if abstinence not achieved in 3 months; CHILD and ADOLESCENT under 18 years not recommended

Nicotine Lozenge

Lozenge, nicotine (as bitartrate) 1 mg, net price pack of 12 = £1.71, pack of 36 = £4.27, pack of 96 = £9.12 (*proprietary product*: *Nicotinell Mint Lozenge*) *or* nicotine (as polacrilex) 2 mg, net price pack of 36 = £5.12, pack of 72 = £9.97, 4 mg pack of 36 = £5.12, pack of 72 = £9.97 (*proprietary product*: *NiQuitin CQ Lozenge*)
Excipients: include aspartame (BNF section 9.4.1)
Dose: initially 1 lozenge every 1–2 hours, when urge to smoke occurs; max. 25 lozenges of 1 mg or 15 lozenges of 2 mg or 4 mg daily; withdraw gradually after 3 months; usual max. period of treatment 6 months

Nicotine Sublingual Tablets

Sublingual tablet, nicotine (as a cyclodextrin complex) 2 mg, net price starter pack of 2 × 15-tablet discs with dispenser = £3.57, refill pack of 7 × 15-tablet discs = £9.84. *Proprietary product*: *Nicorette Microtab*
Dose: individuals smoking 20 cigarettes or fewer daily, *sublingually*, 2 mg each hour; patients who fail to stop smoking or have significant withdrawal symptoms, consider increasing to 4 mg each hour
Individuals smoking more than 20 cigarettes daily, 4 mg each hour
Max. 80 mg daily; treatment should be continued for at least 3 months followed by a gradual reduction in dosage; max. period of treatment 6 months
CHILD and ADOLESCENT under 18 years not recommended

Nicotine Medicated Chewing Gum

Chewing gum, nicotine 2 mg, net price pack of 12 = £8.72, pack of 15 = £1.71, pack of 30 = £3.25, pack of 48 = £15.38, pack of 96 = £24.79, pack of 105 = £8.89; 4 mg, net price pack of 12 = £9.41, pack of 15 = £2.11, pack of 30 = £3.99, pack of 48 = £17.09, pack of 96 = £30.77, pack of 105 = £10.83. *Proprietary products*: *Nicorette Gum, Nicorette Plus Gum, Nicotinell Gum, Nicotinell Plus Gum, Boots Nicotine Gum*
Note. Available in various flavours
Dose: individuals smoking 20 cigarettes or fewer daily, initially one 2-mg piece chewed slowly for approx. 30 minutes, when urge to smoke occurs; individuals smoking more than 20 cigarettes daily or needing more than 15 pieces of 2-mg gum

daily may need 4-mg strength; max. 15 pieces of 4-mg strength daily; withdraw gradually after 3 months; CHILD and ADOLESCENT under 18 years not recommended

Nicotine Nasal Spray

Nasal spray, nicotine 500 micrograms/metered spray, net price 200-spray unit = £10.99. *Proprietary product*: *Nicorette Nasal Spray*
ADMINISTRATION: Apply 1 spray into each nostril as required to max. twice an hour for 16 hours daily (max. 64 sprays daily) for 8 weeks, then reduce gradually over next 4 weeks (reduce by half at end of first 2 weeks, stop altogether after further 2 weeks); max. treatment period of 3 months; CHILD and ADOLESCENT under 18 years not recommended

[2]Nicotine Transdermal Patches

Patches, self-adhesive, releasing in each 16 hours, nicotine approx. 5 mg, 10 mg, or 15 mg (*proprietary product*: *Nicorette Patch*) *or* releasing in each 24 hours nicotine approx. 7 mg, 14 mg, or 21 mg (*proprietary products*: *Nicotinell TTS, NiQuitin CQ, Boots NRT Patch*)
Note. for pack sizes and prices, see individual products in BNF section 4.10
2. Prescriber should specify the brand to be dispensed
ADMINISTRATION: see individual products in BNF section 4.10

Cross-references to the BNF are provided but nurse prescribers may only prescribe those items that are listed on the Nurse Prescribers' List.

Drugs for the mouth

Corresponds to BNF sections 12.3.2, 12.3.1, 12.3.4 and 12.3.5

Candida albicans may cause thrush and other forms of stomatitis which sometimes follow the use of broad-spectrum antibacterials or cytotoxics; withdrawal of the causative drug may lead to rapid resolution; alternatively antifungal treatment may be required. Infants may develop thrush which responds to use of an antifungal mouth preparation.

Patients with denture stomatitis may also respond to the use of an antifungal mouth preparation. They should be instructed to cleanse their dentures thoroughly to prevent reinfection; ideally they should leave their dentures out for a few days. Proper dental appraisal may be necessary.

> Patients with an unexplained mouth ulcer of more than 3 weeks' duration require urgent referral to exclude oral cancer.

Oral antifungal drugs

Miconazole and **nystatin** are suitable for the treatment of oral thrush.

MICONAZOLE

Indications: prevention and treatment of oral fungal infections

Cautions: pregnancy and breast feeding; avoid in porphyria (BNF section 9.8.2); **interactions:** see BNF Appendix 1 (antifungals, imidazole and triazole); oral gel may be absorbed enough for interactions to occur after application to the oral mucosa

Contra-indications: hepatic impairment

Side-effects: nausea and vomiting, diarrhoea (with long-term treatment); rarely allergic reactions; isolated reports of hepatitis

Dose: see under preparation

Prescribe as:

³Miconazole Oromucosal Gel PoM

Oral gel, sugar-free, orange-flavoured, miconazole 24 mg/mL (20 mg/g). Net price 15-g tube = £2.27, 80-g tube = £5.00. *Proprietary product: Daktarin Oral Gel*

Dose: place 5–10 mL in the mouth after food and retain near lesions, 4 times daily; CHILD under 2 years 2.5 mL twice daily, 2–6 years 5 mL twice daily, over 6 years 5 mL 4 times daily; treatment continued for 48 hours after lesions have resolved

Localised lesions, smear a small amount of gel on affected area with clean finger (dentures should be removed at night and brushed with gel) (prescribe 15-g tube)

3. 15-g tube can be sold to the public

NYSTATIN

Indications: oral and perioral fungal infections

Side-effects: oral irritation and sensitisation, nausea reported; see also BNF section 5.2

Dose: see under preparations, below

Prescribe as:

Nystatin Pastilles PoM

Pastilles, nystatin 100 000 units. Net price 28-pastille pack = £3.24. *Proprietary product: Nystan Pastilles*

Dose: suck 1 pastille slowly 4 times daily after food usually for 7 days (continued for 48 hours after lesions have resolved)

Note. Only medical practitioners should prescribe for immunosuppressed patients

Nystatin Oral Suspension PoM

Oral suspension, nystatin 100 000 units/mL. Net price 30 mL (with pipette) = £1.96

Note. A sugar-free formulation can be requested

Dose: ADULT and CHILD over 1 month, place 1 mL in the mouth after food and retain near the lesions 4 times daily, usually for 7 days (continued for 48 hours after lesions have resolved); prophylaxis in newborn 1 mL once daily

Note. Only medical practitioners should prescribe for immunosuppressed patients

Thymol

Compound thymol glycerin is a refreshing mouthwash which has a mechanical cleansing action, and helps to alleviate the pain of oral ulceration.

Mouthwash solution-tablets may contain thymol as well as an antimicrobial; they are used to remove unpleasant tastes.

THYMOL

Indications: oral hygiene, see notes above

Dose: see under preparation, below

Prescribe as:

Compound Thymol Glycerin

Mouthwash, glycerol 10%, thymol 0.05% with colouring and flavouring. Net price 100 mL = 40p

Dose: to be used up to 3–4 times daily when necessary; may be used undiluted or diluted with 3 volumes of warm water

Mouthwash Solution-tablets, consist of tablets which may contain antimicrobial, colouring, and flavouring agents in a suitable soluble effervescent basis to make a mouthwash. Net price, 100 = £2.44

Dissolve 1 tablet in a tumblerful of warm water

Drugs for oral ulceration and inflammation

Choline salicylate dental gel has some analgesic action and may provide relief for recurrent mouth ulcers, but excessive application or confinement under a denture irritates the mucosa and can itself cause ulceration. Benefit in teething may merely be due to pressure of application (comparable with biting a teething ring); excessive use can lead to salicylate poisoning.

Removal of earwax

Corresponds to BNF section 12.1.3

> Patients with an unexplained mouth ulcer of more than 3 weeks' duration require urgent referral to exclude oral cancer.

SALICYLATES

Indications: mild oral and perioral lesions

Cautions: frequent application, especially in children, may give rise to salicylate poisoning

Note. CSM warning on aspirin and Reye's syndrome does not apply to non-aspirin salicylates or to topical preparations such as teething gels

Dose: Apply ½-inch of gel with gentle massage not more often than every 3 hours; CHILD over 4 months ¼-inch of gel not more often than every 3 hours; max. 6 applications daily

Prescribe as:

Choline Salicylate Dental Gel

Oral gel, choline salicylate 8.7% in a flavoured gel basis, net price 15 g (sugar-free) = £1.70, 10 g = £1.36. *Proprietary products*: Bonjela, Dinnefords Teejel

Treatment of dry mouth

Dry mouth may be relieved in many patients by simple measures such as frequent sips of cool drinks or sucking pieces of ice or sugar-free fruit pastilles. Sugar-free chewing gum stimulates salivation in patients with residual salivary function.

Saliva stimulating tablets may be prescribed for dry mouth in patients with salivary gland impairment (and patent salivary ducts).

Prescribe as:

Saliva Stimulating Tablets

Tablets, sugar-free, citric acid, malic acid and other ingredients in a sorbitol base, net price 100-tab pack = £4.86. *Proprietary product*: SST tablets

Dose: allow 1 tablet to dissolve slowly in the mouth when required

> Cross-references to the BNF are provided but nurse prescribers may only prescribe those items that are listed on the Nurse Prescribers' List.

Wax is a normal bodily secretion which provides a protective film on the meatal skin and need only be removed if it causes deafness or interferes with a proper view of the eardrum. As a general rule syringing is best avoided in patients with a history of recurring otitis externa, a history of ear drum perforation, or previous ear surgery. A person who has hearing only in one ear should not have that ear syringed because even a very slight risk of damage is unacceptable in this situation.

Wax may be removed by syringing with water (warmed to body temperature). If necessary, wax can be softened before syringing with simple remedies such as **sodium bicarbonate** ear drops, **olive oil** ear drops or **almond oil** ear drops, which are safe, effective and inexpensive. If the wax is hard and impacted the drops may be used twice daily for a few days before syringing; otherwise the wax may be softened on the day of syringing. The patient should lie with the affected ear uppermost for 5 to 10 minutes after a generous amount of the softening remedy has been introduced into the ear.

Prescribe as:

Almond Oil Ear Drops

Ear drops, almond oil in a suitable container. Net price 10 mL = 50p

Application: allow to warm to room temperature and use as indicated above

Note. Do not heat

Olive Oil Ear Drops

Ear drops, olive oil in a suitable container. Net price 10 mL = 50p

Application: allow to warm to room temperature and use as indicated above

Note. Do not heat

Sodium Bicarbonate Ear Drops

Ear drops, sodium bicarbonate 5%. Net price 10 mL = £1.18

Application: allow to warm to room temperature and use as indicated above

Drugs for threadworms

Corresponds to BNF section 5.5.1.

Anthelmintics are effective for threadworm infections (enterobiasis) but their use needs to be combined with hygiene measures to break the cycle of auto-infection. Threadworms are highly infectious therefore all members of the family need to be treated at the same time.

Adult threadworms do not live for longer than 6 weeks; eggs need to be swallowed and subjected to the action of digestive juices for the development of the worms. Adult females lay eggs on the perianal skin, which causes pruritus. Scratching the area leads to eggs being transferred to the fingers and thence to the mouth, starting the cycle afresh. It is therefore important to advise patients to wash their hands and scrub their nails before each meal and after each visit to the toilet. A bath taken immediately after rising will remove eggs laid during the night. Advice for patients is included in the packaging of most preparations, but it is useful to reinforce this advice verbally.

Mebendazole

Mebendazole is the drug of choice for patients over 2 years of age. It is given as a single dose but as reinfection is very common a second dose may be given after 2–3 weeks.

MEBENDAZOLE

Indications: threadworm infection; other infections, on doctor's prescription only

Cautions: pregnancy (toxicity found in *rats*), see package insert information below; breast-feeding see BNF; **interactions:** BNF Appendix 1 (mebendazole)

Side-effects: rarely abdominal pain, diarrhoea; allergic reactions including rash and angioedema reported

Dose: threadworms, ADULT and CHILD over 2 years, 100 mg as a single dose; if reinfection occurs second dose may be needed after 2–3 weeks; CHILD under 2 years not recommended

Prescribe as:

¹Mebendazole Tablets 100 mg [PoM]
Tablets, flavoured, chewable, mebendazole 100 mg. Net price 6-tab pack = £1.53.
Note. The package insert includes the information that the tablets are not suitable for women known to be pregnant or for children under 2 years

¹Mebendazole Oral Suspension 100 mg/5 mL [PoM]
Oral Suspension, mebendazole 100 mg/5 mL. Net price 30 mL = £1.77. *Proprietary product: Vermox*
Note. The package insert includes the information that the suspension is not suitable for women known to be pregnant or for children under 2 years

1. Packs containing no more than 800 mg and labelled to show a max. single dose of 100 mg are on sale to the public for the treatment of threadworm infection

Piperazine

Piperazine is available in combination with sennosides; 2 doses are given for threadworm infection with an interval of 2 weeks between them.

> Mebendazole and piperazine are also prescribed by doctors for other infections (e.g. roundworms). Nurse prescribers should, however, prescribe them for threadworm infection **only**.

PIPERAZINE

Indications: threadworm infection; other infections, on doctor's prescription only

Cautions: renal impairment (avoid if severe), liver disease, neurological disease; epilepsy, pregnancy (see below for warnings in packs and BNF Appendix 4)

Side-effects: nausea, vomiting, colic, diarrhoea; allergic reactions including urticaria, bronchospasm, and rare reports of Stevens-Johnson syndrome and angioedema; rarely dizziness, muscular incoordination ('worm wobble'); drowsiness, confusion and clonic contractions in patients with neurological or renal abnormalities

Dose: threadworms, see under preparation, below

Prescribe as:

Piperazine and Senna Powder
Oral powder, piperazine phosphate 4 g and sennosides 15.3 mg/sachet. Net price two-dose sachet pack = £1.31. *Proprietary product: Pripsen*
Dose: stirred into a small glass of milk or water and drunk immediately, ADULT and CHILD over 6 years 1 sachet, to be repeated after 14 days; INFANT 3 months–1 year (on doctor's advice only), 1 level 2.5-mL spoonful, to be repeated after 14 days; CHILD 1–6 years, 1 level 5-mL spoonful, to be repeated after 14 days
Cautionary label added by pharmacist: dissolve or mix with water before taking
Note. Packs on sale to the public carry a warning to avoid in epilepsy and in pregnancy

Drugs for scabies and head lice

Corresponds to BNF section 13.10.4

Scabies

Malathion, and **permethrin** are used for *scabies* (*Sarcoptes scabiei*).

The following should be noted:
* *alcoholic lotions* are not recommended (owing to irritation of excoriated skin and genitalia);
* it is not necessary to apply preparations *after a hot bath* (a hot bath may even increase absorption into the blood, removing the drug from its site of action on the skin).

All members of the affected household should be treated. Treatment should be applied to the whole body paying particular attention to the webs of the fingers and toes, and brushing lotion under the ends of the nails. In infants and young children (up to the age of about 2 years), the elderly, the immuno-compromised and in those whose treatment has failed, application should be extended to the scalp, neck, face, and ears (if the product packaging does not contra-indicate this). It is now recommended that malathion and permethrin should be applied twice, one week apart. Patients with hyperkeratotic (crusted or 'Norwegian') scabies may require 2 or 3 applications on consecutive days to ensure that enough penetrates the skin crusts to kill all the mites.

It is important to warn users **not** to wash their hands since this would require re-application.

The itch of scabies persists for some weeks after the infestation has been eliminated and antipruritic treatment may be required. Application of **crotamiton** can be used to control itching after treatment with more effective acaricides, but caution is necessary if the skin is excoriated.

Head lice

Malathion, and the **pyrethroids** (permethrin and phenothrin) are effective against *head lice* (*Pediculus humanus capitis*) but lice in some districts have developed resistance; resistance to two or more parasiticidal preparations has also been reported. Lotion, liquid or cream rinse formulations should be used. Shampoos are diluted too much in use to be effective. Aqueous formulations are preferred in severe eczema and for asthmatic patients and small children, to avoid alcoholic fumes. A contact time of 12 hours or overnight treatment is recommended for lotions and liquids. A 2-hour treatment is not sufficient to kill eggs.

In general, a course of treatment for head lice should be 2 applications of product 7 days apart to prevent lice emerging from any eggs that survive the first application.

The policy of rotating insecticides on a district-wide basis is now considered outmoded. To overcome the development of resistance, a mosaic strategy is required whereby, if a course of treatment fails to cure, a different insecticide is used for the next course. If a course of treatment with either permethrin or phenothrin fails, then a non-pyrethroid parasiticidal product should be used for the next course.

A **head lice repellent** containing piperonal 2% (*Rappell®*) is on sale to the public, but its value is uncertain.

Carbaryl is also effective against head lice but in the light of data from animal studies, it would be prudent to consider carbaryl as a human carcinogen. Carbaryl preparations are now restricted to **prescription-only** use although the Department of Health has emphasised that the risk is theoretical (and for intermittent use in head lice, it is likely to be exceedingly small).

WET COMBING METHODS. Several products are available which require the use of a plastic detection comb and hair conditioner. The methods typically involve meticulous combing with the detection comb (probably for at least 30 minutes each time) over the whole scalp at 4-day intervals for a minimum of 2 weeks. However, evidence suggests that treatment with a parasiticidal, such as malathion, is more effective than wet combing.

> Not all preparations included here are licensed for *crab lice* therefore advice on crab lice has not been included

> Individuals can rarely react to certain ingredients in preparations applied to the skin. Special care is required when prescribing skin and scalp products for these individuals—see BNF section 13.1.3. Excipients associated with sensitisation are shown under individual product entries

Malathion

Malathion is recommended for *scabies* and *head lice* (for details see notes above).

The risk of systemic effects associated with 1–2 applications of malathion is considered to be very low; however applications repeated at intervals of less than 1 week *or* application for more than 3 consecutive weeks should be **avoided** since the likelihood of eradication of lice is not increased.

MALATHION

Indications: scabies, head lice

Cautions: avoid contact with eyes; do not use on broken or infected skin; do not use more than once a week for 3 consecutive weeks; use in children under 6 months on doctor's advice only; alcoholic lotions **not** recommended for head lice in severe eczema, asthma or in small children, or for scabies or crab lice (see notes above)

Side-effects: skin irritation

Administration:

Head lice, *lotion,* rub into dry hair and scalp, allow to dry naturally, remove 12 hours later by washing (see also notes above)

Scabies, *lotion,* apply over whole body, wash off after 24 hours; if hands are washed with soap within 24 hours, they should be retreated; see also notes above

Note. For scabies manufacturer recommends application to the body but not necessarily to the head and neck. In young children, however, application may need to be extended to the scalp, neck, face, and ears; this extended application may also be necessary for the elderly, for the immunocompromised and following treatment failure

Prescribe as:

Malathion Alcoholic Lotion 0.5%

Alcoholic lotion, malathion 0.5% in an alcoholic basis. Flammable. *Proprietary products: Prioderm Lotion* (net price 50 mL = £2.22, 200 mL = £5.42), *Suleo-M Lotion* (50 mL = £2.22, 200 mL = £5.42)

Alcohol: alcoholic lotion not recommended for head lice in asthmatics or young children, or for scabies (for details see notes above)

Excipients: include fragrance

Malathion Aqueous Lotion 0.5%

Aqueous lotion, malathion 0.5% in an aqueous basis. *Proprietary products: Derbac-M Liquid* (net price 50 mL = £2.22, 200 mL = £5.42), *Quellada M* (50 mL = £1.85, 200 mL = £4.62)

Excipients: include cetostearyl alcohol, fragrance, hydroxybenzoates (parabens)

Permethrin

Permethrin is effective for *scabies* and *head lice* (for details see notes above).

PERMETHRIN

Indications: scabies, head lice

Cautions: avoid contact with eyes; do not use on broken or infected skin; use for scabies in children under 2 years on doctor's advice only, use for head lice in children under 6 months on doctor's advice only

Side-effects: pruritus, erythema, and stinging; rarely rashes and oedema

Administration: see under preparations

Prescribe as:

Permethrin Cream 5%

Cream, permethrin 5%. Net price 30 g = £5.52. *Proprietary product: Lyclear Dermal Cream*

Excipients: include butylated hydroxytoluene, wool fat derivative

Administration: scabies, apply over whole body and wash off after 8–12 hours; CHILD (see also Cautions above) apply over whole body including face, neck, scalp, and ears; cream should be reapplied to hands if they are washed with soap and water within 8 hours of application

Note. Manufacturer recommends application to the body but to exclude the head and neck. In young children, however, application may need to be extended to the scalp, neck, face, and ears; this extended application may also be necessary for the elderly, for the immunocompromised and for those who have experienced treatment failure.

Larger patients may require up to two 30-g packs for adequate treatment

Permethrin Cream Rinse 1%

Cream rinse, permethrin 1% in basis containing isopropyl alcohol 20%. Net price 59 mL = £2.26, 2 x 59-mL pack = £4.17. Proprietary product: *Lyclear Creme Rinse*

Administration: head lice, apply to clean damp hair and rinse after 10 minutes; not affected by chlorine in swimming pools

Excipients: include cetyl alcohol

> Cross-references to the BNF are provided but nurse prescribers may only prescribe those items that are listed on the Nurse Prescribers' List.

Phenothrin

Phenothrin is recommended for *head lice* (for details see notes above).

PHENOTHRIN

Indications: head lice

Cautions: avoid contact with eyes; do not use on broken or infected skin; do not use more than once a week for 3 weeks at a time; use for children under 6 months on doctor's advice only

Side-effects: skin irritation

Administration: see under preparations

Prescribe as:

Phenothrin Alcoholic Lotion 0.2%

Lotion, phenothrin 0.2% in basis containing isopropyl alcohol 69.3%. Net price 50 mL = £2.22; 200 mL = £5.42. Flammable. *Proprietary product: Full Marks Lotion*

Excipients: include fragrance

Administration: head lice, apply to dry hair and allow to dry naturally; shampoo after 2 hours; comb hair while still wet

Alcohol: alcoholic lotion not recommended for head lice in severe eczema, asthmatics or small children

Phenothrin Aqueous Lotion

Liquid, phenothrin 0.5% in an aqueous basis. Net price 50 mL = £2.22; 200 mL = £5.42. *Proprietary product: Full Marks Liquid*

Excipients: include cetostearyl alcohol, fragrance, hydroxybenzoates (parabens)

Administration: head lice, apply to dry hair, allow to dry naturally; shampoo after 12 hours or next day, comb while still wet

Phenothrin Foam Application

Foam application, phenothrin 0.5% in an alcoholic basis. Net price 50 g = £2.47; 150 g = £5.81. *Proprietary product: Full Marks Mousse*

Excipients: include cetostearyl alcohol

Administration: head lice (alcoholic, see above), apply to dry hair; shampoo after 30 minutes, comb while still wet

Skin preparations

Emollients

Corresponds to BNF section 13.2.1 and 13.2.1.1.

Emollients soothe, smooth and hydrate the skin and are indicated for all dry or scaling disorders. Their effects are short-lived and they should be applied frequently even after improvement occurs. They are useful in dry and eczematous disorders, and to a lesser extent in psoriasis. Light emollients such as **aqueous cream** are suitable for many patients with dry skin but a wide range of more greasy preparations including **white soft paraffin, emulsifying ointment**, and **liquid and white soft paraffin ointment** are available; the severity of the condition, patient preference and site of application will often guide the choice of emollient; emollients should be applied in the direction of hair growth. Some ingredients may occasionally cause sensitisation (BNF section 13.1.3) and this should be suspected if an eczematous reaction occurs.

Preparations such as **aqueous cream** and **emulsifying ointment** can be used as soap substitutes for hand washing and in the bath; the preparation is rubbed on the skin before rinsing off completely. The addition of a bath oil may also be helpful; several proprietary emollient bath additives are available (see below).

Arachis oil (peanut oil) is used for cleansing in dry skin skin conditions (see also BNF section 13.9).

> Individuals can rarely react to certain ingredients in preparations applied to the skin. Special care is required when prescribing skin and scalp products for these individuals—see BNF section 13.1.1. Excipients associated with sensitisation are shown under individual product entries

EMOLLIENTS

Prescribe as:

Aqueous Cream

Cream, emulsifying ointment 30%, [1]phenoxyethanol 1%, in freshly boiled and cooled purified water. Net price 100 g = 21p

1. The BP permits use of alternative antimicrobials provided their identity and concentration are stated on the label

Excipients: include cetostearyl alcohol

Emulsifying Ointment

Ointment, emulsifying wax 30%, white soft paraffin 50%, liquid paraffin 20%. Net price 100 g = 30p

Excipients: include cetostearyl alcohol

Hydrous Ointment

(Also known as Oily Cream)

Ointment, dried magnesium sulphate 0.5%, phenoxyethanol 1%, wool alcohols ointment 50% in freshly boiled and cooled purified water. Net price 100 g = 40p

Liquid and White Soft Paraffin Ointment

Ointment, liquid paraffin 50%, white soft paraffin 50%. Net price 250 g = 88p, 500 g = £1.75

Paraffin, White Soft (white petroleum jelly).

Net price 100 g = 32p

Paraffin, Yellow Soft (yellow petroleum jelly).

Net price 100 g = 32p

Proprietary emollients, prescribe as:

Alcoderm® Cream (Galderma)

Cream, containing liquid paraffin, cetyl alcohol, stearyl alcohol, sodium lauryl sulphate, carbomer, triethanolamine, sorbitan stearate, sorbitol, spermaceti, silicone fluid. Net price 60 g = £2.40

For dry skin conditions

Excipients: include cetyl alcohol, hydroxybenzoates (parabens), isopropyl palmitate, stearyl alcohol

Alcoderm® Lotion (Galderma)

Lotion, water-miscible, ingredients as above. Net price 200 mL = £4.77

For dry skin conditions

Excipients: include cetostearyl alcohol, fragrance, hydroxybenzoates (parabens)

Cetraben® Emollient Cream (Sankyo)

Cream, white soft paraffin 13.2%, light liquid paraffin 10.5%. Net price 50 g = £1.14; 125 g = £2.31; 500-g pump pack = £5.61

For inflamed, damaged, dry or chapped skin including eczema

Excipients: include cetostearyl alcohol, hydroxybenzoates (parabens)

Dermamist® (Yamanouchi)

Spray application, white soft paraffin 10% in a basis containing liquid paraffin, fractionated coconut oil. Net price 250-mL pressurised aerosol unit = £9.17

For dry skin conditions including eczema, ichthyosis, pruritus of the elderly

Caution: flammable

Diprobase® Cream (Schering-Plough)

Cream, cetomacrogol 2.25%, cetostearyl alcohol 7.2%, liquid paraffin 6%, white soft paraffin 15%, water-miscible basis used for *Diprosone®* cream. Net price 50 g = £1.54; 500-g dispenser = £6.61

For dry skin conditions

Excipients: include cetostearyl alcohol, chlorocresol

Diprobase® Ointment (Schering-Plough)

Ointment, liquid paraffin 5%, white soft paraffin 95%, basis used for *Diprosone®* ointment. Net price 50 g = £1.54

For dry skin conditions

Doublebase® (Dermal)

Gel, isopropyl myristate 15%, liquid paraffin 15%, net price 100 g = £2.98; 500 g = £6.55

For dry chapped or itchy skin conditions

E45® Cream (Crookes)

Cream, light liquid paraffin 12.6%, white soft paraffin 14.5%, hypoallergenic hydrous wool fat (hypoallergenic lanolin) 1% in self-emulsifying monostearin. Net price 50 g = £1.18, 125 g = £2.39, 350 g = £4.14, 500 g = £5.61, 500-g pump pack = £6.20

For dry skin conditions

Excipients: include cetyl alcohol, cetostearyl alcohol, hydroxybenzoates (parabens)

Epaderm® (SSL)

Ointment, emulsifying wax 30%, yellow soft paraffin 30%, liquid paraffin 40%, net price 125 g = £3.67; 500 g = £6.21

For use as an emollient or soap substitute

Excipients: include cetostearyl alcohol

Hydromol® Cream (Adams Hlth)

Cream, sodium pidolate 2.5%, net price 50 g = £2.04, 100 g = £3.80, 500 g = £12.60

For dry skin conditions

Excipients: include cetostearyl alcohol, hydroxybenzoates (parabens)

Keri® Therapeutic Lotion (Bristol-Myers Squibb)

Lotion, mineral oil 16%, with lanolin oil. Net price 190-mL pump pack = £3.56; 380-mL pump pack = £5.81

For dry skin conditions and nappy rash

Excipients: include fragrance, hydroxybenzoates (parabens), N-(3-chloroallyl) hexaminium chloride (quaternium 15), propylene glycol

LactiCare® Lotion (Stiefel)

Lotion, lactic acid 5%, sodium pidolate 2.5%. Net price 150 mL = £3.19

For dry skin conditions

Excipients: include cetostearyl alcohol, imidurea, isopropyl palmitate, fragrance

Lipobase® (Yamanouchi)

Cream, fatty cream basis used for *Locoid Lipocream®*. Net price 50 g = £2.05

Excipients: include cetostearyl alcohol, hydroxybenzoates (parabens)

Neutrogena® Dermatological Cream (J&J)

Cream, glycerol 40% in an emollient basis. Net price 100 g = £3.79

For dry skin conditions

Excipients: include cetostearyl alcohol, hydroxybenzoates (parabens)

Oilatum® Cream (Stiefel)

Cream, light liquid paraffin 6%, white soft paraffin 15%. Net price 40 g = £1.79, 150 g = £3.38

For dry skin conditions

Excipients: include benzyl alcohol, cetostearyl alcohol

Ultrabase® (Schering Health)

Cream, water-miscible, containing liquid paraffin and white soft paraffin. Net price 50 g = £1.05; 500-g dispenser = £6.89

For dry skin conditions

Excipients: include fragrance, hydroxybenzoates (parabens), disodium edetate, stearyl alcohol

Unguentum M® (Crookes)

Cream, cetostearyl alcohol, glyceryl monostearate, saturated neutral oil, liquid paraffin, white soft paraffin. Net price 50 g = £1.59;100 g = £3.13; 200 mL dispenser = £6.19; 500 g = £9.55

For dry skin conditions and nappy rash

Excipients: include cetostearyl alcohol, polysorbate 40, propylene glycol, sorbic acid

Proprietary emollient bath additives, prescribe as:

Alpha Keri Bath® Oil (Bristol-Myers Squibb)

Bath oil, liquid paraffin 91.7%, oil-soluble fraction of wool fat 3%. Net price 240 mL = £3.45; 480 mL = £6.43

For dry skin conditions including ichthyosis and pruritus of the elderly, add 10–20 mL /bath (infants 5 mL)

Excipients: include fragrance

¹Balneum® (Crookes)

Balneum® bath oil, soya oil 84.75%. Net price 200 mL = £2.79; 500 mL = £6.06; 1 litre = £11.70

For dry skin conditions including those associated with dermatitis and eczema; add 20 mL/bath (infant 5 mL)

Excipients: include butylated hydroxytoluene, propylene glycol, fragrance

Dermalo® (Dermal)

Bath emollient, acetylated wool alcohols 5%, liquid paraffin 65%. Net price 500 mL = £3.87

For dermatitis, dry skin conditions including ichthyosis and pruritus of the elderly; add 15–20 mL/bath (infant and child 5–10 mL)

Diprobath® (Schering-Plough)

Bath additive, isopropyl myristate 39%, light liquid paraffin 46%. Net price 500 mL = £7.50

For dry skin conditions including dermatitis and eczema; add 25 mL/bath (infant 10 mL)

Hydromol Emollient® (Adams Hlth)

Bath additive, isopropyl myristate 13%, light liquid paraffin 37.8%. Net price 150 mL = £1.87; 350 mL = £3.80; 1 litre = £9.00

For dry skin conditions including eczema, ichthyosis and pruritus of the elderly; add 1–3 capfuls/bath (infant ½–2 capfuls)

Oilatum® Emollient (Stiefel)

Oilatum® Emollient bath additive (emulsion), acetylated wool alcohols 5%, liquid paraffin 63.4%. Net price 250 mL = £2.75; 500 mL = £4.57

For dry skin conditions including dermatitis, pruritus of the elderly and ichthyosis; add 1–3 capfuls/bath (infant 0.5–2 capfuls)

Excipients: include isopropyl palmitate, fragrance

Oilatum® Fragrance Free (Stiefel)

Bath additive, light liquid paraffin 63.4%, net price 500 mL = £5.75

For dry skin conditions including dermatitis, pruritus of the elderly and ichthyosis; add 1–3 capfuls/bath (infant 0.5–2 capfuls)

Excipients: include wool fat, isopropyl palmitate

Oilatum® Gel (Stiefel)

Shower emollient (gel), light liquid paraffin 70%. Net price 125 g = £4.84

For dry skin conditions including dermatitis

Excipients: include fragrance

Barrier preparations

Corresponds to BNF section 13.2.2.

Barrier preparations often contain water-repellent substances such as **dimeticone** (dimethicone) or other silicones. They are used on the skin around stomas, bedsores, and pressure areas in the elderly where the skin is intact. Where the skin has broken down, barrier preparations have a limited role in protecting adjacent skin. They are no substitute for adequate nursing care and it is doubtful if they are any more effective than the traditional **zinc and castor oil ointment**. A spray preparation, **zinc oxide and dimeticone spray**, is also available.

---

1. Some pack sizes may not be prescribed on the NHS and are not listed here

NAPPY RASH. Barrier creams and ointments are used for protection against nappy rash which is usually a local dermatitis. The first line of treatment is to ensure that nappies are changed frequently and that tightly fitting water-proof pants are avoided. The rash may clear when left exposed to the air, and a barrier preparation may be helpful. If the rash is associated with a fungal infection, an antifungal cream such as clotrimazole cream is useful.

DIMETICONE (SILICONE)

Dimeticone barrier creams containing at least 10%

Prescribe as:

Dimeticone Cream (*Conotrane*)

Cream, benzalkonium chloride 0.1%, dimeticone '350' 22%. Net price 100 g = 66p; 500 g = £3.12.

For nappy and urinary rash and pressure sores

Excipients: include cetostearyl alcohol, fragrance

Dimeticone Cream (*Siopel*)

Barrier cream, dimeticone '1000' 10%, cetrimide 0.3%, arachis (peanut) oil. Net price 50 g = 86p.

For protection against water-soluble irritants

Excipients: include butylated hydroxytoluene, cetostearyl alcohol, hydroxybenzoates (parabens)

Dimeticone Cream (*Vasogen*)

Barrier cream, dimeticone 20%, calamine 1.5%, zinc oxide 7.5%. Net price 50 g = 74p; 100 g = £1.30.

For nappy rash, pressure sores, ileostomy and colostomy care

Excipients: include hydroxybenzoates (parabens), wool fat

TITANIUM *or* ZINC

Prescribe as:

Titanium Ointment

Ointment, titanium dioxide 20%, titanium peroxide 5%, titanium salicylate 3% in a basis containing dimeticone, light liquid paraffin, white soft paraffin, and benzoin tincture. Net price 30 g = £1.71.

For nappy rash and related disorders.

Proprietary product: Metanium Ointment

Zinc and Castor Oil Ointment

Ointment, zinc oxide 7.5%, castor oil 50%, arachis (peanut) oil 30.5%, white beeswax 10%, cetostearyl alcohol 2%. Net price 25 g = 14p.

For nappy and urinary rash

Zinc Oxide and Dimeticone Spray

Spray application, dimeticone 1.04%, zinc oxide 12.5%, in a basis containing wool alcohols, cetostearyl alcohol, dextran, white soft paraffin, liquid paraffin, propellants. Net price 115-g pressurised aerosol unit = £3.54.

For urinary rash, pressure sores, leg ulcers, moist eczema, fissures, fistulae and ileostomy care

Caution: flammable

Excipients: include cetostearyl alcohol, hydroxybenzoates (parabens), wool fat

Proprietary product: Sprilon

Pruritus

Corresponds to BNF section 13.3.

Pruritus may be caused by systemic disease (such as drug hypersensitivity, obstructive jaundice, endocrine disease, and certain malignant diseases) as well as by skin disease (e.g. psoriasis, eczema, urticaria, and scabies). Where possible the underlying causes should be treated. An **emollient** may be of value where the pruritus is associated with dry skin (which is common in otherwise healthy elderly people).

Preparations containing **crotamiton** are sometimes used in pruritus. Crotamiton can be used to control itching after treatment with a parasiticidal preparation for scabies (NPF p. N23).

Preparations containing calamine are often ineffective and therefore these preparations are no longer included in the NPF.

CROTAMITON

Indications: pruritus (including pruritus after scabies)

Cautions: avoid use near eyes and broken skin; use on doctor's advice for children under 3 years

Contra-indications: acute exudative dermatoses

Administration: pruritus, apply 2–3 times daily; CHILD below 3 years, apply once daily

Prescribe as:

Crotamiton Cream 10%

Cream, crotamiton 10%. Net price 30 g = £2.27; 100 g = £3.95

Excipients: include beeswax, fragrance, hydroxybenzoates (parabens), stearyl alcohol

Crotamiton Lotion 10%

Lotion, crotamiton 10%. Net price 100 mL = £2.99

Excipients: include cetyl alcohol, fragrance, propylene glycol, sorbic acid, stearyl alcohol

Fungal infections

Corresponds to BNF section 13.10.2.

Fungal skin infections can be prevented by keeping the susceptible area as clean and dry as possible. Established fungal infections such as ringworm infection and candidal skin infection may be treated with **clotrimazole cream, econazole cream** or **miconazole cream**.

CLOTRIMAZOLE

Indications: fungal skin infections

Cautions: avoid contact with eyes and mucous membranes

Side-effects: occasional skin irritation or sensitivity (discontinue if severe)

Administration: apply 2–3 times daily

Prescribe as:

Clotrimazole Cream 1%
Cream, clotrimazole 1%. Net price 20 g = £1.77.

Excipients: not shown because preparation available from several sources; for sensitised individuals, check that version dispensed is free from the sensitising ingredient

ECONAZOLE NITRATE

Indications; Cautions; Side-effects: see under Clotrimazole
Administration: apply twice daily

Prescribe as:

Econazole Cream 1%
Cream, econazole nitrate 1%. *Proprietary products: Ecostatin Cream* (net price 15 g = £1.49, 30 g = £2.75), *Pevaryl Cream* (net price 30 g = £2.65)

Excipients: include butylated hydroxyanisole, fragrance

MICONAZOLE NITRATE

Indications; Cautions; Side-effects: see under Clotrimazole

Administration: apply twice daily continuing for 10 days after lesions have healed

Prescribe as:

Miconazole Cream 2%
Cream, miconazole nitrate 2%. Net price 30 g = £2.07.

Excipients: not shown because preparation available from several sources; for sensitised individuals, check that version dispensed is free from the sensitising ingredient

Boils

Boils are generally treated with an antibacterial, but **magnesium sulphate paste** is a traditional adjunct.

MAGNESIUM SULPHATE

Indications: paste used as an adjunct in the management of boils
Administration: apply under dressing

Prescribe as:

Magnesium Sulphate Paste
Paste, dried magnesium sulphate 45 g, glycerol 55 g, phenol 500 mg. Net price 25 g = 56p, 50 g = 67p
Note. Stir before use

Disinfection and cleansing

Corresponds to BNF section 13.11.

Physiological saline

Sterile **sodium chloride solution 0.9%** is suitable for general cleansing of skin and wounds.

SODIUM CHLORIDE

Indications: skin cleansing
Prescribe as:

Sterile Sodium Chloride Solution 0.9%
Sterile solution, sodium chloride 0.9%. To be used undiluted for topical irrigation of wounds. Net price 10 × 10-mL unit = £3.32; 10 × 20-mL unit = £9.68; 10 × 30-mL unit = £3.00; 25 × 20-mL sachets = £6.83; 25 × 20-mL unit = £6.83, 25 × 25-mL tubes = £6.58 (*Proprietary brands: Saline Steripoules, Steripod and possibly others);* 25 × 25-mL sachets = £5.85, 10 × 100-mL sachets = £7.16, 25 × 25-mL tubes = £6.58 (*Proprietary brands: Normasol and possibly others*); 150 mL container = 83p (*Proprietary brands: Sterac and possibly others*); 1 x 240-mL aerosol can = £2.85 (*Proprietary brand: Irriclens*); other sizes also prescribable if available

Povidone–iodine

Povidone–iodine aqueous solution 10% is useful where skin disinfection is required.

POVIDONE–IODINE

Indications: skin disinfection
Cautions: pregnancy, breast-feeding, broken skin (see below), renal impairment (avoid regular application to inflamed or broken skin)
LARGE OPEN WOUNDS. The application of povidone-iodine to large wounds or severe burns may produce systemic adverse effects such as metabolic acidosis, hypernatraemia and impairment of renal function
Contra-indications: avoid regular use in patients with thyroid disorders or those receiving lithium therapy
Side-effects: rarely sensitivity; may interfere with thyroid function tests

Prescribe as:

Povidone–Iodine Solution 10%
Solution, povidone–iodine 10% in aqueous solution. Net price 500 mL = £1.75. *Proprietary preparation: Betadine Antiseptic Solution. Administration:* apply undiluted in pre- and post-operative skin disinfection; CHILD not recommended for regular use in neonates (and contra-indicated in very low birthweight infants)
Note. Not for body cavity irrigation

Wound management products

See BNF Appendix 8

The following items in BNF Appendix 8 are not on the Nurse Prescribers' List:

- Items not in the Drug Tariff (described as NHS in the BNF)
- Framycetin Gauze Dressing, BP

Desloughing agents

Corresponds to BNF section 13.11.7 and Appendix 8.

> Preparations have been included here because they are licensed as medicinal products. Details of all other wound management products are in BNF Appendix 8.

CADEXOMER–IODINE

Indications; Administration: see under preparations below

Cautions; Contra-indications: avoid in thyroid disorders, in those receiving lithium, and in pregnancy and breast-feeding; caution in patients with severe renal impairment or history of thyroid disorders; iodine may be absorbed particularly if large wounds treated

Prescribe as:

Cadexomer–Iodine Ointment

Ointment, iodine 0.9% as cadexomer–iodine in an ointment basis. Net price 4 × 10-g tubes = £17.24, 2 × 20-g tubes = £17.24. *Proprietary product: Iodosorb Ointment*

Administration: for treatment of chronic exuding wounds, such as leg ulcers, apply to wound surface to depth of approx. 3 mm and cover; renew when saturated (usually 2–3 times weekly, daily for heavily exuding wounds); max. single application 50 g, max. weekly application 150 g; max. duration up to 3 months in any single course of treatment

Cadexomer–Iodine Paste

Paste, iodine 0.9% as cadexomer–iodine in a paste basis with gauze backing. Net price 5 × 5-g units = £19.48, 3 × 10-g units = £23.40, 2 × 17-g units = £24.68. *Proprietary product: Iodoflex*

Administration: for treatment of chronic exuding wounds, such as leg ulcers, apply to wound surface, remove gauze backing and cover; renew when saturated (usually 2–3 times weekly, daily for heavily exuding wounds); max. single application 50 g, max. weekly application 150 g; max. duration up to 3 months in any single course of treatment

Cadexomer–Iodine Powder

Powder, iodine 0.9% as cadexomer–iodine microbeads. Net price 7 x 3-g sachets = £12.89. *Proprietary product: Iodosorb Powder*

Administration: for treatment of chronic exuding wounds, such as leg ulcers, apply to wound surface to depth of approx. 3 mm and cover; renew when saturated (usually 2–3 times weekly, daily for heavily exuding wounds); max. single application 50 g, max. weekly application 150 g; max. duration up to 3 months in any single course of treatment

---

DEXTRANOMER

Indications: see under preparation below

Prescribe as:

Dextranomer Beads

Beads, dextranomer. Net price 60-g castor = £29.01. *Proprietary product: Debrisan*

Administration: for exudative and infected wounds, decubital ulcers, leg ulcers, hand burns, surgical wounds, post-traumatic wounds, sprinkle onto wound to a thickness of at least 3 mm and cover with appropriate dressing, renew before saturation occurs (usually once or twice daily)

Dextranomer Paste

Paste, dextranomer in a soft paste basis. Net price 6 × 10-g pouches = £29.93. *Proprietary product: Debrisan Paste*

Administration: for exudative and infected wounds, decubital ulcers, leg ulcers, surgical wounds, post-traumatic wounds, apply to a thickness of at least 3 mm and cover with appropriate dressing, renew before saturation occurs (usually once or twice daily)

STREPTOKINASE WITH STREPTODORNASE

Indications: removal of clotted blood, fibrinous or purulent accumulation from suppurative surface lesions such as ulcers, pressure sores, amputation sites, diabetic gangrene, radiation necrosis, infected wounds, and surgical incisions

Contra-indications: active haemorrhage

Side-effects: infrequent allergic reactions (reduced by careful and frequent removal of exudate and thorough irrigation with physiological saline); transient burning reported

Administration: reconstitute with 20 mL sterile physiological saline (or water for injections) and apply as wet dressing 1–2 times daily; cover with semi-occlusive dressing; irrigate lesion thoroughly with physiological saline and remove loosened material before next application

Prescribe as:

Streptokinase and Streptodornase Topical Powder PoM

Powder, streptokinase 100 000 units, streptodornase 25 000 units. For preparing solutions for topical use. Net price per vial = £9.44, with sterile physiological saline 20 mL (combi-pack) = £9.92. *Proprietary product: Varidase Topical*

Medicated stocking

Corresponds to BNF Appendix 8.

ZINC OXIDE

Indications; Administration: see under preparation below

Prescribe as:
Zinc Oxide Impregnated Medicated Stocking
Stocking, Sterile rayon, impregnated with ointment containing zinc oxide 20%. Net price 4-pouch carton = £13.33; 10-pouch carton = £33.33. *Proprietary product: Zipzoc*
Administration: chronic leg ulcers; can be used under appropriate compression bandages or hosiery in chronic venous insufficiency

> Cross-references to the BNF are provided but nurse prescribers may only prescribe those items that are listed on the Nurse Prescribers' List.

Elastic hosiery

Corresponds to BNF Appendix 8.

Before elastic hosiery can be dispensed, the quantity (single or pair), article (including accessories), and compression class (I, II, or III) must be specified by the prescriber; for further details see Drug Tariff.

Peak flow meters

Corresponds to BNF section 3.1.5

Measurement of peak flow is particularly helpful for patients who do not readily perceive deterioration in their asthma, and for those with moderate or severe asthma. Patients must be given clear guidance on the action they should take if the peak flow falls below a specified level.

Prescribe as:

Standard-range peak flow meter
Peak flow meter, range 50 to 750 litres/minute, net price = £6.65 (*proprietary product: Asmaplan*), 60 to 800 litres/minute = £6.86 (*proprietary product: Mini-Wright*), 90–710 litres/minute = £6.53 (*proprietary product: Ferraris Pocketpeak*); replacement mouthpieces available (not interchangeable between brands)

Low-range peak flow meter
Peak flow meter, range 25 to 280 litres/minute, net price = £6.65 (*proprietary product: Vitalograph*), 30 to 400 litres/minute = £6.90 (*proprietary product: Mini-Wright*), 40–370 litres/minute = £6.53 (*proprietary product: Ferraris Pocketpeak*); replacement mouthpieces available (not interchangeable between brands)
Note. Low-range peak flow meters are suitable only for adults and children with severely restricted airflow

Urinary catheters and appliances

Urinary appliances

These are listed in Appendix N1. Further details are available in Part IXB of the Drug Tariff (Part 5 of the Scottish Drug Tariff, Part III of the Northern Ireland Drug Tariff).

Urethral catheters

These are listed in Appendix N1. Further details are available in Part IXA of the Drug Tariff (Part 3 of the Scottish Drug Tariff, Part III of the Northern Ireland Drug Tariff).

Catheter patency

Corresponds to BNF section 7.4.4.
The deposition which occurs on catheters is usually chiefly composed of phosphate and to minimise this the catheter (if latex) should be changed at least as often as every 6 weeks. If the catheter is to be left for longer periods a silicone catheter should be used together with the appropriate use of catheter maintenance solutions. Repeated blockage usually indicates that the catheter needs to be changed.

CATHETER PATENCY SOLUTIONS

Indications: catheter care; see also under preparations, below
Administration: to be warmed to body temperature and instilled as required, see also under preparations, below

Prescribe as:

Chlorhexidine 0.02% Catheter Maintenance Solution
Sterile solution, chlorhexidine 0.02%. *Proprietary products: Uro-Tainer Chlorhexidine* (net price 100-mL sachet = £2.60), *Uriflex C* (100-mL sachet = £2.40)
For mechanical cleansing and prevention of bacterial contamination (but not effective against *Pseudomonas* species); discontinue if burning or haematuria occur

Mandelic Acid 1% Catheter Maintenance Solution
Sterile solution, mandelic acid 1%. *Proprietary product: Uro-Tainer Mandelic Acid* (Net price 100-mL sachet = £2.60)
For mechanical cleansing and acidification (and thus prevention of contamination with certain bacteria but chlorhexidine more effective)

Sodium Chloride 0.9% Catheter Maintenance Solution
Sterile solution, sodium chloride 0.9%. *Proprietary products: OptiFlo S* (Net price 50- and 100-mL sachets = £2.94), *Uro-Tainer Sodium Chlor-*

ide (50- and 100-mL sachets = £2.45), *Uriflex S* (100-mL sachet = £2.40)

For removal of clots and other debris, to be instilled as required

'Solution G' Catheter Maintenance Solution

Sterile solution, citric acid 3.23%, magnesium oxide 0.38%, sodium bicarbonate 0.7%, disodium edetate 0.01%. *Proprietary products: OptiFlo G* (Net price 50- and 100-mL sachets = £3.12), *Uro-Tainer Suby G* (50- and 100-mL sachets = £2.60), *Uriflex G* (100-mL sachet = £2.40)

For prevention of catheter encrustation and crystallisation, to be instilled once daily to once weekly according to severity; in very severe cases use 'Solution R'

'Solution R' Catheter Maintenance Solution

Sterile solution, citric acid 6%, gluconolactone 0.6%, magnesium carbonate 2.8%, disodium edetate 0.01%. *Proprietary products: OptiFlo R* (Net price 50- and 100-mL sachets = £3.12), *Uro-Tainer Solution R* (50- and 100-mL sachets = £2.60), *Uriflex R* (100-mL sachet = £2.40)

For prevention of catheter encrustation and dissolution of crystallisation if 'Solution G' unsuccessful, to be instilled once weekly or more frequently up to once daily according to severity

Stoma care products

Corresponds to BNF section 1.8.

Prescribing for patients with stoma calls for special care. The following is a brief account of some of the main points to be borne in mind.

Enemas and washouts should be **not** be prescribed for patients with ileostomies as they may cause rapid and severe dehydration.

Colostomy patients may suffer from constipation and whenever possible should be treated by increasing fluid intake or dietary fibre. **Bulk-forming drugs** (see p. N11) should be tried. If they are insufficient, the smallest possible dose of senna (see under Stimulant Laxatives, p. N12) should be used.

The doctor's advice should be obtained for other complications such as diarrhoea.

See Appendix N1 for brief information on products used in stoma care.

> New patients should be given advice about the use of *cleansing agents, protective creams, lotions, deodorants,* or *sealants.*

Stoma appliances and associated products

These are listed in Appendix N1. Further details are available in Part IXC of the Drug Tariff (Part 6 of the Scottish Drug Tariff, Part III of the Northern Ireland Drug Tariff).

Urostomy pouches

These are listed in Appendix N1. Further details are available in Part IXC of the Drug Tariff (Part 6 of the Scottish Drug Tariff, Part III of the Northern Ireland Drug Tariff).

Appliances and reagents for diabetes

Hypodermic equipment

Corresponds to BNF section 6.1.1.3.

Patients should be advised on the safe disposal of lancets, single-use syringes, and needles. Suitable arrangements for the safe disposal of contaminated waste must be made before these products are prescribed for patients who are carriers of infectious diseases.

> **Lancets** may be used on their own or in an automatic 'finger pricking' device such as *Autolet* NHS or *Glucolet* NHS. Various devices take different lancets; see BNF section 6.1.1.3 for further details

HYPODERMIC EQUIPMENT

See BNF section 6.1.1.3
The following items in BNF section 6.1.1.3 are not on the Nurse Prescribers' List:
- Items not in the Drug Tariff (described as NHS in the BNF)

Monitoring agents

Corresponds to BNF section 6.1.6.

Glucose (for glucose tolerance test) is **not** on the Nurse Prescribers' List.

URINALYSIS

Urine testing for glucose is useful in patients who find blood glucose monitoring difficult. Tests for glucose range from reagent strips specific to glucose to reagent tablets which detect all reducing sugars. Few patients still use *Clinitest; Clinistix* is suitable for screening purposes only.

Reagents are also available to test for ketones and protein in urine but these are usually used in clinics; patients are rarely required to do these tests for themselves unless they become unwell.

■ Reagents
See BNF section 6.1.6
The following items in BNF section 6.1.6 are not on the Nurse Prescribers' List:
- Items not in the Drug Tariff (described as NHS in the BNF)

BLOOD GLUCOSE MONITORING

Blood glucose monitoring gives a direct measure of the glucose concentration at the time of the test and can detect hypoglycaemia as well as hyperglycaemia. Patients should be properly trained in the use of blood glucose monitoring systems and to take appropriate action on the results obtained. Inadequate understanding of the normal fluctuations in blood glucose may lead to confusion and inappropriate action.

Blood glucose monitoring is best carried out by means of a meter. Visual colour comparison is sometimes used but is much less satisfactory. Meters give a more precise reading and are useful for patients with poor eyesight or who are colour blind

Note. In the UK blood glucose concentration is expressed in mmol/litre and the British Diabetic Association advises that these units should be used for self-monitoring of blood glucose. In other European countries units of mg/100 mL (or mg/dL) are commonly used.
It is advisable to check that the meter is pre-set in the correct units.

■ Reagents
See BNF section 6.1.6
The following items in BNF section 6.1.6 are not on the Nurse Prescribers' List:
• Items not in the Drug Tariff (described as NHS in the BNF)

Eye-drop dispensers

Eye-drop dispensers are available to aid the instillation of eye drops especially amongst the elderly, visually impaired, arthritic, or otherwise physically limited patients. Eye-drop dispensers are for use with plastic eye drop bottles, for repeat use by individual patients. Details of products available may be found in the Drug Tariff section IXA (Part 3 of the Scottish Drug Tariff, Part III of the Northern Ireland Drug Tariff).

Fertility and gynaecological products

Fertility (Ovulation) Thermometer
Mercury in glass thermometer, range 35 to 39°C (graduated in 0.1°C). Net price = £1.68
For monitoring ovulation for the fertility awareness method of contraception

Fluid Filled Ring Pessaries
Pessaries, filled with combination fluid, 15 mm thick. Net price 1 pessary, sizes 1–12 = £5.64; other sizes available
Antiseptics: antiseptics containing phenols or cresols should be avoided because absorption may cause severe irritation; pessaries may be washed in soapy water or boiled

Polythene Ring Pessaries
Pessaries, 7.5 mm thick, 50–80 mm (rising in 3 mm), 85–100 mm (rising in 5 mm), and 110 mm. Net price 1 pessary = £1.67
Antiseptics: antiseptics containing phenols or cresols should be avoided because absorption may cause severe irritation; pessaries may be washed in soapy water or boiled

PVC Ring Pessaries
Pessaries, 1.25 cm thick, 50–80 mm (rising in 3 mm), 85–100 mm (rising in 5 mm), and 110 mm. Net price 1 pessary = £1.81
Antiseptics: antiseptics containing phenols or cresols should be avoided as these may be absorbed causing irritation in use

Watch-spring Ring Pessaries
Pessaries, covered with india-rubber, net price 1 pessary, thin, 1.25 cm thick, sizes 1–12 = £4.12; medium 1.4 cm thick, sizes 1–12 = £3.90; other sizes available

Ring Pessaries with Perforated Rubber Diaphragm
Pessaries, 1.3 cm thick, sizes 1–12 (51–86 mm), net price 1 pessary = £3.04; other sizes available

Contraceptive devices

Corresponds to BNF section 7.3.4

Intra-uterine devices

The intra-uterine device (IUD) is suitable for older parous women and as a second-line contraceptive in young nulliparous women who should be carefully screened because they have an increased background risk of pelvic inflammatory disease.
The healthcare professional inserting (or removing) the device should be fully trained in the technique and should provide full counselling backed by the manufacturer's approved leaflet.

INTRA-UTERINE CONTRACEPTIVE DEVICES
Indications: contraception, see BNF section 7.3.4
Cautions: anaemia, heavy menses (progestogen intra-uterine system might be preferable, BNF section 7.3.2.3), endometriosis, severe primary dysmenorrhoea, history of pelvic inflammatory disease, history of ectopic pregnancy or tubal surgery, diabetes, fertility problems, nulliparity and young age, severely scarred uterus (including after endometrial resection) or severe cervical stenosis, valvular heart disease (antibacterial cover needed—BNF section 5.1 table 2)—avoid if prosthetic valve or history of infective endocarditis; drug- or disease-induced immunosuppression (risk of infection—avoid if marked immunosuppression); joint and other prostheses (increased risk of infection); epilepsy; increased risk of expulsion if inserted before uterine involution; gynaecological examination before insertion, 6–8 weeks after then annually but counsel women to see doctor promptly in case of significant symptoms, especially pain; anticoagulant therapy (avoid if possible); remove if pregnancy occurs; if pregnancy occurs, increased likelihood that it may be ectopic
Contra-indications: pregnancy, severe anaemia, recent sexually transmitted infection (if not fully

investigated and treated), unexplained uterine bleeding, distorted or small uterine cavity, genital malignancy, active trophoblastic disease, pelvic inflammatory disease, established or marked immunosuppression; *copper devices:* copper allergy, Wilson's disease, medical diathermy
Side-effects: uterine or cervical perforation, displacement, expulsion; pelvic infection may be exacerbated, heavy menses, dysmenorrhoea, allergy; *on insertion:* pain (alleviated by NSAID such as ibuprofen 30 minutes before insertion) and bleeding, occasionally, epileptic seizure, vasovagal attack

Prescribe as:
Flexi-T® 300
Intra-uterine device, copper wire, surface area approx. 300 mm² wound on vertical stem of T-shaped plastic carrier, impregnated with barium sulphate for radio-opacity, monofilament thread attached to base of vertical stem; preloaded in inserter, net price = £8.65
For uterine length over 5 cm; replacement every 5 years
GyneFix®
Intra-uterine device, 6 copper sleeves with surface area of 330 mm² on polypropylene thread, net price = £24.75
Suitable for all uterine sizes; replacement every 5 years; fitting technique requires additional training
Multiload® Cu250
Intra-uterine device, copper wire, surface area approx. 250 mm² wound on vertical stem of plastic carrier, 3.5 cm length, with 2 down-curving flexible arms, monofilament thread attached to base of vertical stem; preloaded in inserter, net price = £7.13
For uterine length 6–9 cm; replacement every 3 years
Multiload® Cu250 Short
Intra-uterine device, as above, with vertical stem length 2.4 cm, net price = £7.13
For uterine length 5–7 cm; replacement every 3 years
Multiload® Cu375
Intra-uterine device, as above, with copper surface area approx. 375 mm² and vertical stem length 3.5 cm, net price = £9.24
For uterine length 6–9 cm; replacement every 5 years
Nova-T® 380
Intra-uterine device, copper wire with silver core, surface area approx. 380 mm² wound on vertical stem of T-shaped plastic carrier, impregnated with barium sulphate for radio-opacity, threads attached to base of vertical stem, net price = £13.50
For uterine length 6.5–9 cm; replacement every 5 years
T-Safe® CU 380 A
Intra-uterine device, copper wire, wound on vertical stem of T-shaped plastic carrier with copper collar on the distal portion of each arm, total surface area approx. 380 mm², impregnated with barium sulphate for radio-opacity, threads attached to base of vertical stem, net price = £9.40
For uterine length 6.5–9 cm; replacement every 8 years

Other contraceptive devices

■ Contraceptive caps

Prescribe as:
Type A contraceptive pessary
Opaque rubber, sizes 1 to 5 (55–75 mm rising in steps of 5 mm), net price = £6.07. *Proprietary product:* Dumas Vault Cap
Type B contraceptive pessary
Opaque rubber, sizes 22 to 31 mm (rising in steps of 3 mm), net price = £7.18. *Proprietary product:* Prentif Cavity Rim Cervical Cap
Type C contraceptive pessary
Opaque rubber, sizes 1 to 3 (42, 48 and 54 mm), net price = £6.07. *Proprietary product:* Vimule Cap

■ Contraceptive diaphragms

Prescribe as:
Reflexions Flat Spring Diaphragm
Transparent rubber with flat metal spring, sizes 55–95 mm (rising in steps of 5 mm), net price = £5.59. *Proprietary product:* Reflexions
Type B Diaphragm with coiled metal rim
Opaque rubber with coiled metal rim, sizes 60–100 mm (rising in steps of 5 mm), net price = £5.84. *Proprietary product:* Ortho
Type C Arcing Spring Diaphragm
Opaque rubber with arcing spring, sizes 60–95 mm (rising in steps of 5 mm), net price = £6.64. *Proprietary product:* All-Flex

Appendix N1: Urinary and stoma appliances

This Appendix includes incontinence appliances, urethral catheters, and stoma products.

Incontinence appliances and urethral catheters

Incontinence appliances are listed in Part IXB of *Drug Tariff* or Part 5 of *Scottish Drug Tariff*; urethral catheters are included in Part IXA of *Drug Tariff* or Part 3 of *Scottish Drug Tariff*

Drainable dribbling appliances

Re-usable for at least 1 month (with exception of Alexa®)

■ Bullen range
Bags (Bullen)
Net price 10 Dribblet® bags = £22.18; 10 Dribblet® sheath bags = £49.78

■ Coloplast range
Aquadry® (Coloplast)
Drip type urinal. Net price 1 = £51.47

■ Jade-Euro-Med range
Bag (Jade-Euro-Med)
Dribbling bag with loops and tapes. Net price1 = £16.74
Urinal (Jade-Euro-Med)
Drip male urinal with tap. Net price 1 = £44.97; 1 replacement belt = £11.09

■ Rüsch range
Peoplecare® (Rüsch)
Male drip urinal. Net price 1 = £49.39

■ Ward range
Bags (Ward)
Male dribbling bag with diaphragm and belt. Net price 1 = £27.92

Incontinence belts

Average life 6 months

■ Jade-Euro-Med range
Waist belt for kipper bags (Jade-Euro-Med)
Net price 1 = £5.54; 1 (with webbing band) = £5.54

■ Rüsch range
Peoplecare® (Rüsch)
Waist and support strap for kipper bag. Net price 1 = £6.40

■ SIMS Portex range
Belts (SIMS Portex)
Rubber belt. Net price 1 = £5.51
Web belt (small, medium, or large) = £10.82

■ Ward range
Belts (Ward)
Waist belt for black kipper bag. Net price 1 = £5.13
Rubber belt for PP (pubic pressure) urinal. Net price 1 = £4.44

Incontinence sheaths

Unless otherwise indicated the incontinence sheaths (also known as penile sheaths or external catheters) listed below are of the soft, flexible, latex type. Each sheath may be left in place for 1 to 3 days between changes

■ Bard range
Integrity® (Bard)
Incontinence sheath, self-adhesive. Net price 30 sheaths (25, 30, or 35 mm) = £41.03
Reliasheath® (Bard)
Incontinence sheath with adhesive strip. Net price 30 sheaths (20, 25, 30, 35, or 40 mm) = £37.61
Uriplan® (Bard)
Incontinence sheath. Net price 30 sheaths (20, 25, 30, 35, or 40 mm) = £25.20
Uro sheath® (washable; may be used many times). Net price 1 (25, 35, or 40 mm) = £5.26

■ Cliniflex range
Medimates® (CliniFlex)
Incontinence sheath with single-sided adhesive strip. Net price 30 sheaths (straight, 20, 25, 30, 35, or 40 mm; bulb, 25, 30, or 35 mm) = £29.35
Incontinence sheath with double-sided adhesive strip. Net price 30 sheaths (straight, 20, 25, 30, 35, or 40 mm; bulb, 25, 30, or 35 mm) = £31.31

■ Coloplast range
Aquadry® (Coloplast)
Incontinence sheath. Net price 10 sheaths (small, medium, large, or extra-large) = £10.23
Aquadry Freedom® (Coloplast)
Freedom® incontinence sheath, self-adhesive. Net price 30 sheaths (small, medium, standard, large, or extra-large) = £41.90
Freedom Plus® incontinence sheath, self-adhesive. Net price 30 sheaths (small, medium, standard, large, or extra-large) = £41.90
Clear Advantage® (Coloplast)
Incontinence sheath, silicone, self-adhesive . Net price 30 sheaths (small, medium, standard, large, extra-large) = £41.70
Conveen ® (Coloplast)
Incontinence sheath, with anti-kink design and Uriliner® adhesive strip. Net price 30 sheaths (very small, small, medium, large, or extra-large) = £43.95; 30 Security® sheaths (extra small, small, medium, large or extra large) = £44.16
Conveen self-sealing Urisheath® (Coloplast)
Incontinence sheath. Net price 30 sheaths (extra small, small, medium, large or extra large) = £43.50; 30 short sheaths (20, 25, 30, 35 or 40mm) = £43.50; 30 Security® sheaths with anti-kink design (extra small, small, medium, large or extra large) = £43.71
Simpla U-Sheath® (Coloplast)
Incontinence sheath, with Uriseal® liner. Net price 30 sheaths (small, medium, large, or extra-large) = £37.92

■ Hollister range
InCare® (Hollister)
Incontinence sheath, self-adhesive. Net price 30 sheaths (22–25 mm; 26–30 mm; 31–35 mm; 36–39 mm) = £41.39

- Hospital Management and Supplies range

Macrodom® (Hospital Management & Supplies)

Incontinence sheath, including adhesive strip. Net price 30 sheaths (with 2-inch tube) = £22.30; 25 sheaths (with 5-inch tube) = £23.33

- Jade-Euro-Med range

NaturaFlex® (Jade-Euro-Med)

Incontinence sheath, clear, non-adhesive. Net price 30 sheaths (small, medium, intermediate, or large) = £43.17

Ultra Flex® (Jade-Euro-Med)

Incontinence sheath, clear, self-adhesive. Net price 30 sheaths (small, medium, intermediate, large or extra-large) = £43.17

- Kendall range

Texas Catheter® (Kendall)

Incontinence sheath, with adhesive strip. Net price 12 sheaths = £8.64

Uri Drain® (Kendall)

Incontinence sheath, with double-sided adhesive strap (30 mm). Net price 10 = £8.00

- Manfred Sauer range

Comfort sheath® (Manfred Sauer)

Incontinence sheath, non-adhesive without liner. Net price 30 sheaths (18, 20, 22, 24, 26, 28, 30, 32, 35, 37, or 40 mm; extra thin 26, 30, 35, or 40 mm) = £21.74

Comfort Plus® (Manfred Sauer)

Incontinence sheath, latex-free, double sided adhesive liner, net price 30 sheaths (18, 20, 22, 24, 26, 28, 30, 32, 35, 37, or 40mm) = £44.50

- North West Medical range

Uridrop® (North West)

Incontinence sheath. Net price 30 sheaths (paediatric = 42 or 55 mm; sizes 1, 2, 3, or 4 = 70, 80, 100, or 107 mm) = £12.70

Incontinence sheath, with Uristrip® adhesive strip. Net price 30 sheaths (paediatric = 42 or 55 mm; sizes 1, 2, 3, or 4 = 70, 80, 100, or 107 mm) = £25.40

- Payne range

Incontiaid® (Payne)

Incontinence sheath. Net price 10 sheaths, with adhesive strip (sizes 20, 25, 30, 35 or 40 mm) = £13.61; 1 sheath, without adhesive strip (sizes 20, 25, 30, 35 or 40 mm) = 84p; 10 adhesive strips = £5.11

- Rochester Medical range

Silicone Sheath (Jade-Euro-Med)

Natural incontinence sheath, self-adhesive. Net price (25, 29, 32, 36 or 41 mm) = £41.70

Pop-On incontinence sheath, self-adhesive. Net price (25, 29, 32, 36 or 41 mm) = £41.70

Wide Band incontinence sheath, self-adhesive. Net price (25, 29, 32, 36 or 41 mm) = £41.70

- Rüsch range

Dryaid® (Rüsch)

Incontinence sheath. Net price 20 sheaths (with adhesive strip; small, medium, large, or extra-large) = £26.61; 20 sheaths (without adhesive strip; small, medium, large, or extra-large) = £15.42

Portasheath® (Rüsch)

Incontinence sheath. Net price 25 sheaths (25, 30, or 35 mm) = £21.64

Secure external catheter kit, with adhesive strip. Net price 10 sheaths (25, 30, or 35 mm) = £8.86

- Salts range

Heritage Cohesive /Sheath Pack® (Salts)

Incontinence sheath, with adhesive. Net price 30 sheaths (17, 22, 25, 32, or 34 mm) = £34.89

Male continence sheath (Salts)

Incontinence sheath. Net price 10 sheaths (17, 22, 25, 32, or 34 mm) = £7.86

- SIMS Portex range

Continence sheath (SIMS Portex)

Incontinence sheath. Net price 1 sheath (small, medium, large, or extra-large) = £1.45

Male incontinence sheath (SIMS Portex)

Incontinence sheath. Net price 100 sheaths = £65.11

Transfix® (SIMS Portex)

Incontinence sheath, silicone, self-adhesive, 25, 29, 32, 36, or 41 mm. Net price 30 sheaths (style 1 (wide self-adhesive band), style 2 (wide self-adhesive band), style 3 (extra wide self-adhesive band)) = £42.43

Uro Flo® (SIMS Portex)

Incontinence sheath, straight, including adhesive liner. Net price 30 sheaths (small, medium, or large) = £39.30

Uro Flo Mk2® (SIMS Portex)

Incontinence sheath, bulbous, with adhesive liner. Net price 30 sheaths (small, medium or large) = £39.30

Fixing strips and adhesives

Bio Diagnostics®

Urifix® tape. Net price 5 m = £4.90

Camp®

Posey® sheath holder. Net price 12 (adult) = £13.25; 12 (paediatric) = £10.20

CliniFlex®

MediMates® adhesive strips. Net price 30 (double-sided) = £10.00; 30 (single-sided) = £8.00

Coloplast

Aquadry® penile liners. Net price 20 = £8.37

Urifix® tape. Net price 5 m = £6.23

ConvaTec®

Urihesive® strips. Net price 15 = £6.44

North West Medical

Uristrip® adhesive strip. Net price 30 = £12.70

Payne

Incontiaid® sheath holder. Net price 1 = £1.00

Rüsch

Dryaid® strip. Net price 20 strips = £11.19

Salts

Heritage® sheath collar pack. Net price 30 = £4.01

[NHS] Cohesive® strips for use with sheaths. Net price 10 = £4.97

Leg bags

Most plastic bags suitable for use for 5–7 days; rubber bags re-usable for 4–6 months

- Bard range

Uriplan® (Bard)

Leg bag, plastic, shaped, with tap outlet and elastic Velcro straps. Net price 10 bags (350 mL, direct inlet) = £25.18; 10 bags (350 mL, 12 inch inlet tube) = £24.95; 10 bags (500 mL, direct inlet) = £25.37; 10 bags (500 mL, 4 or 12 inch inlet tube) = £25.46; 10 bags (750 mL, direct inlet, or 4, 12, or 15 inch inlet tube) = £25.55

Urisac® (Bard)

Leg bag, plastic. Net price 10 bags (350 mL, short tube) = £12.97; 10 bags (350 mL, long tube) = £13.35; 10 bags (500 mL, short tube) = £14.12; 10 bags (500 mL, long tube) = £14.51; 10 bags (750 mL, short tube) = £14.89; 10 bags (750 mL, long tube) = £15.52

- Beambridge range

Drainage bags (for use with Beambridge urinals), net price 10 = £14.00

- **Coloplast range**
Aquadry® (Coloplast)
Leg bag, plastic. Net price 10 bags (350, 500, or 750 mL, short or long tube) = £22.84
Conveen® (Coloplast)
Security leg bag, plastic. Net price 10 bags (350-, 500-, 750- mL, all 25- or 50-cm tube) = £20.97; 10 sterile bags (500-mL, 25- or 50-cm tube) = £22.29
Contour leg bag, plastic, shaped, sterile with sample port. Net price, with 1 set Velcro bands, 10 bags (600 mL, 5 or 30 cm tube; 800 mL, 45 cm tube) = £25.46; 10 non-sterile bags (600 mL, 45 cm adjustable tube) = £25.46
Leg drainage bags (Coloplast)
Leg bag, plastic. Net price 10 bags (500 mL, short or long tube) = £16.23
Simpla Trident® T1 (Coloplast)
Leg bag, plastic. Net price 10 bags (350 mL, short tube) = £25.30; 10 bags (500 mL, short or long tube) = £25.50; 10 bags (750 mL, short, long, or adjustable long tube) = £25.61
Simpla Trident® T2 (Coloplast)
Leg bag, plastic. Net price 10 bags (350 mL, short tube) = £25.60; 10 bags (500 mL, short tube or long tube) = £25.89; 10 bags (750 mL, short tube, long tube or adjustable long tube) = £26.01

- **ConvaTec range**
Accuseal® (ConvaTec)
Leg bag, plastic. Net price 10 bags (500 mL) = £18.86

- **Flexicare Medical**
Flexicare® (Flexicare)
Leg bag, with tap outlet, overnight connection tube and velcro bands. Net price 10 bags (short or long tube: 350, 500, or 750 mL; 60 cm adjustable tube: 500 mL) = £22.60

- **Incare range**
Urinary leg bag (Incare)
Leg bag, plastic. Net price 10 bags (540 mL, 37 cm tube) = £25.37; 10 bags (540 mL, direct in-let) = £24.76

- **Jade-Euro-Med range**
Leg bags (Jade-Euro-Med)
Kipper bag, black, white, or clear. Net price 1 bag = £25.47
Leg drainage bag, plastic, with tap outlet. Net price 10 bags (350 or 500 mL) = £21.85; 10 bags (750 mL) = £22.80

- **Maersk range**
Careline® (Maersk)
Leg bag, plastic, with tap outlet and overnight connection tube. Net price, with 1 pair Velcro straps, 10 bags (350 mL, short or long tube) = £22.72; 10 bags (500 mL, short or long tube) = £23.32; 10 bags (750 mL, short or long tube) = £23.81

- **Manfred Sauer range**
Discreet® (Manfred Sauer)
Leg bag, female with overnight connection tube and fabric/velcro leg straps. Net price 10 bags (450 mL with inlet tube suitable for suprapubic catheter) = £21.62; 10 bags (400 mL with straight inlet tube) = £21.62
Sauer leg bag (Manfred Sauer)
Leg bag, plastic, with tap outlet and overnight connection tube and fabric/velcro leg straps. Net price 10 bags (700 or 1300 mL, short or long tube) = £20.14; 10 bags, sterile (700 or 1300 mL, short or long tube) = £23.26

- **Payne range**
GU Black Rubber Kipper® Bags (Payne)
Leg bag, single chambered, standard. Net price 1 bag = £40.27; 1 bag with box outlet tap = £49.64; 1 bag (for female use) = £40.27; 1 bag (for night use) = £54.22; 1 bag (Ross type) = £45.97

Incontiaid® (Payne)
Leg bag, plastic. Net price 1 bag (500 or 750 mL) = £2.54
Leg bags (formerly Willis range)
Rubber bag, for catheter drainage, short neck leg strap. Net price 1 bag = £27.60; 1 bag with web belt and support strap) = £32.31
Rubber bag, female, drainage bag, with conical mount. Net price 1 bag = £26.20; 1 bag (with web belt and support strap) = £30.89

- **Rüsch range**
Kipper bags (Rüsch)
Leg bag. Net price 1 bag (clear/white plastic or all black plastic or rubber, with strap and buckle) = £26.73; 1 bag (clear/white plastic, without strap and buckle) = £21.91
Leg bag (Rüsch)
Leg bag, plastic. Net price 10 bags (short tube, 350 or 500 mL) = £13.73; 10 bags (long tube, 350 or 500 mL) = £14.68; 10 bags (750 mL) = £9.82

- **Salts range**
Heritage® (Salts)
Leg bag, plastic. Net price 10 bags (500 mL, short tube) = £14.53; 10 bags (500 mL, long tube) = £14.79; 10 bags (750 mL, short tube) = £16.19; 10 bags (750 mL, long tube) = £16.58; 5 leg bag packs = £10.38

- **SIMS Portex range**
Leg bags (SIMS Portex)
Leg bag, with valve outlet, natural latex straps, and plastic tube. Net price 10 bags (350 mL, short tube) = £24.07; 10 bags (350 mL, long tube) = £24.56; 10 bags (500 mL, short tube) = £24.59; 10 bags (500 mL, long tube) = £25.23; 10 bags (750 mL, short tube) = £24.95; 10 bags (750 mL, long tube) = £25.10
Leg bag, with twist tap, elastic straps, and plastic tube. Net price 10 bags (750 mL, short tube) = £24.99; 10 bags (750 mL, long tube, 30 cm) = £25.14
Tri-form® leg bag, plastic. Net price 10 bags (500 mL, short tube) = £24.32; 10 bags (500 mL, medium tube) = £24.61; 10 bags (500 mL, long tube) = £24.82
PVC drainage bag (SIMS Portex)
Leg bag, plastic. Net price 1 bag (small or large) = £3.81
Rubber bags (SIMS Portex)
Leg bag, rubber, with leg strap. Net price = £36.67

- **Universal range**
Unicorn® (Universal)
Leg bag, plastic. Net price 10 bags (350 mL, short tube) = £17.60; 10 bags (500 mL, short or long tube) = £17.80; 10 bags (750 mL, short or long tube) = £18.00

- **Ward range**
Comfort® (Ward)
Leg bag, plastic. Net price 10 bags (350 mL) = £11.31; 10 bags (500 mL) = £11.63; 10 bags (750 mL) = £12.23
Kipper bag (Ward)
Leg bag, kipper type, rubber. Net price 1 bag (black, clear, or white) = £23.32
Leg drainage bag (Ward)
Leg bag, plastic. Net price 10 bags (350 mL) = £11.26; 10 bags (500 mL) = £11.61; 10 bags (750 mL) = £12.30
St Peters Pattern (Ward)
Leg bag. Net price 5 bags = £31.17

Night drainage bags

Suitable for night-time use for collection of urine from indwelling catheters or from incontinence sheaths; bag hangers normally supplied through community nursing service.

Drainage bags have life of 5–7 nights

Bard
Uriplan® drainage bag. Net price 10 bags = £11.42; Collection bag (non-drainable), 10 bags = £2.27

Coloplast

Aqua® 4, 2 litre urine drainage bag, net price 10 bags = £10.41

Conveen® 1.5 litre drainage bag with 90 cm tube. Net price 10 bags = £12.86

S5 (formerly S4 Plus®) overnight drainage bag. Net price 10 bags = £10.96

Urine drainage bag. Net price 10 bags (S1, non-drainable) = £2.32; 10 bags (S2, non-drainable with non-reflux valve) = £2.44; 10 bags (S4, short tube) = £11.74; 10 bags (S4, long tube) = £12.14

ConvaTec

Surgicare System® 2 litre drainage bag. Net price 5 bags (Accuseal®) = £7.59; 5 bags (night) = £7.59

Dansac

Dansac® 2 litre night drainage bag. Net price 10 bags = £10.78

Flexicare

F4®, 2 litre drainage bag with 100 cm inlet tube, non-reflux valve and tap. Net price 10 bags = £9.50

Jade-Euro-Med

2 litre drainage bag with tap outlet. Net price 1 bag = £1.48

Maersk

Careline® range, 2 litre urine drainage bag with 90 cm inlet tube. Net price 10 bags (Careline® E1, non- drainable) = £2.00; 10 bags (Careline® E2, non-drainable, with non-reflux valve) = £2.14; 10 bags (Careline® E4, with non-reflux valve and tap outlet) = £11.04; 10 bags (Careline® E4, Night Bag with lever tap) = £10.85

Rand Rocket

Urine drainage bag (non-drainable, short or long tube). Net price 25 bags = £3.87

Rüsch

Drainage bags, 2 litre. Net price 10 bags (C) = £10.56; 10 bags with non-reflux valve and plug (CV) = £11.72; 10 bags with non-reflux valve and tap (CVT) = £12.15; 10 bags with non-reflux valve and wide bore tap (DVT) = £11.20

Salts

2 litre H2 urine drainage bag. Net price 10 bags with non-reflux valve and tap = £12.06

SIMS Portex

Inbeds 2 litre drainage bag with twist tap. Net price 10 bags = £13.37

Mirage® night drainage bag. Net price 10 bags = £10.49

Uro-flo® night drainage bag. Net price 10 bags (female or male) = £14.48

Portex TRI-Form, 2 litre drainage bag, 90 cm inlet tube and non-return valve with universal connector, net price 10 = £2.20

Ward

2 litre drainage bag with push/pull outlet. Net price 10 bags = £12.24

Suspensory systems

Drainage bag with support; bags may be used for 5–7 days

Bard

Urisac® Portabag® with belt. Net price 10 bags (plastic) = £12.12; 1 belt = £7.10

Coloplast

Drainage bag for use with Shepheard Sporran belt. Net price 10 bags (plastic) = £17.10; 1 belt = £8.54

Rüsch

Portabag® with *Portabelt®*. Net price 10 bags (plastic) = £15.74; 1 belt = £8.79

SIMS Portex

Holster bag with leg bag holster. Net price 10 bags (400 mL, plastic) = £18.83; 1 holster (24–30, 30–36, or 36–44 inch) = £8.80

Tubing and accessories

Bard

Adaptor for Uro sheath® (penile sheath to leg bag) 8 inch. Net price 1 = £1.14

Foam/Velcro leg bag straps. Net price 10 pairs = £5.16

Latex leg bag straps. Net price 10 pairs = £2.71

Uriplan® leg bag straps (washable). Net price 5 pairs = £13.25

Urisleeve® leg bag holder. Net price 4 (small: 24–39 cm; medium: 36–55 cm; large: 40–70 cm) = £7.40

Beambridge

Beambridge funnel, male urinal director/positioner. Net price 1 funnel = £12.00

Beambridge Lady funnel, female urinal director/positioner. Net price 1 funnel = £12.49

Coloplast

Aquasleeve®. Net price 4 (small: 24–33 cm; standard: 34–39 cm; medium: 40–46 cm; large: 47–64 cm) = £7.03

G-Strap. Net price 'adult' or 'short', 5 = £12.15 'abdomen', 5 = £13.40

Leg bag straps. Net price 5 pairs (elasticated, washable) = £13.27

Velcro bands (washable). Net price 10 pairs = £37.81

ConvaTec

Accuseal® leg bag extension tube. Net price 10 tubes = £6.96

Flexicare

Leg bag straps with velcro fastening, washable. Net price 10 pairs = £11.50

Incare

Leg bag straps. Net price 1 pair (14 inch, calf or 23 inch, thigh) = £2.83

Jade-Euro-Med

Euro J-strap®, net price 5 = £11.96

Eurosleeve®, net price 4 (24–33, 34–39, 40–46, or 47–64 cm) = £7.12

Velcro leg straps. Net price 1 pair = £1.85

Leg bag connecting tube. Net price 1 = £1.44; 1 (with mount) = £2.47

Kendall

Argyle® foam and Velcro strap, washable. Net price 1 (75 cm, leg) = £1.69; 1 (150 cm, abdomen) = £3.17

Argyle Suregrip® general purpose tube, internal diameter 7 mm, length 2.7 m. Net price 50 tubes = £36.00

Argyle Penrose® tubing, internal diameter 6, 8, 10, 13, 16, 19, or 25 mm and length 44 cm. Net price 50 = £30.75

Maersk

Careline® leg bag straps. Net price 10 = £13.16

Payne

Rubber extension tube, 6 inch. Net price = £3.41

Rubber leg strap. Net price 1 = £1.19

Velcro leg strap. Net price 1 = 94p

Rüsch

Connecting tubes, net price 1 tube for kipper bag = £2.66; 14-inch connecting tube for drip urinal = £2.65; 1 connecting tube for all urinals with female connector = £4.04

Salts

Heritage® leg bag extension tube. Net price 2 tubes = £2.08

SIMS Portex

Paul (Penrose) tubing. Net price 10 (6, 13, 19, or 25 mm) = £13.36; 10 (32, 38, 44, or 51 mm) = £13.36

Tapered adaptor (catheter to leg bag). Net price 1 = £6.23; 1(stepped) = £8.80

Stopcock for Chiron plastic urinal bags (in place of screwcap). Net price 1 = £4.52

Rubber extension tube (with mounts). Net price = £4.67

Rubber tubing (length, 1.5 m). Net price 1 = £10.92

Plastic connector with tube. Net price 1 = £3.11

Female connector for Mitcham bag. Net price = £2.09

Night bag connector. Net price 1 = £1.26

Spare 'O' rings for pubic pressure urinal. Net price 5 = £1.19

Uro-Flo® elastic Velcro leg straps. Net price 5 pairs = £4.21

Leg bag extension tube. Net price 10 (30 cm) = £24.37; 10 (60 cm) = £26.81

Silgrip® leg straps. Net price 5 pairs (elasticated or Side-Fix thigh-fitting) = £12.41; 5 pairs (Side-Fix calf-fitting) = £11.79

Urinal systems

Patients generally have two urinal systems (one to wash and one to wear). Each appliance should last for 6 months

Bard

Uriplan Maguire® urinal and adaptor. Net price (waist sizes 66–81 cm, 81–96 cm, or 96–112 cm) = £61.51

Uriplan Maguire® adaptor and tubing. Net price = £8.30

Beambridge

Bridge saddle urinal, net price = £12.99

Bridge urinal, net price = £12.99

Bridge urinal with tap, net price = £12.99

Drainage bags (for use with Beambridge urinals), net price 10 = £14.00

Male draining jug, net price = £12.99

Male draining jug with tap, net price = £12.99

Bell and Croyden

Fridjohn male urinal. Net price 1 = £40.61

Male urinal, day and night use. Net price 1 (with long or short bag) = £37.35

Bullen

Male urinal. Net price 1 (with large-size long bag) = £73.34

Coloplast

Spares

Rubber leg bag connecting tube with female attachment, net price 1 = £2.78

Flange (child: 0.5, 0.675, 0.75, 0.875, 1, 1.125, or 1.25 inch; adult: 1, 1.125, 1.25, 1.375, 1.5, 1.625, or 1.75 inch). Net price 1 = £26.43

Cones. Net price 1 (small, medium, or large; curved or straight) = £11.43

Rubber belt. Net price 1 (24, 28, 36, or 44 inch) = £3.19

Ellis

Hallam modular urinal. Net price 1 = £31.63; 1 spare bag = £1.68; 1 spare belt = £3.75

Hollister

Incare®, retracted penis pouch, net price 10 = £25.88

Jade-Euro-Med

Male day and night urinal with tap, covered bag, with band and suspensory, and leg strap with air vent. Net price 1 = £52.78

Male night urinal with tap, covered bag, with band and suspensory. Net price 1 = £64.23

Male day and night urinal with tap, long tube, covered bag, with band and suspensory with air vent. Net price 1 = £62.41

Male day and night urinal with tap, double bag, air vent, inflating rim, with band understraps. Net price 1 = £66.10

Male day and night urinal with tap, covered bag, diaphragm top, and air vent. Net price 1 = £57.11

Male day and night urinal with tap, improved pattern, inflating rim, short air vent, with band and understrap. Net price 1 = £62.69; 1 (with extension tube) = £66.16

Male day and night urinal with tap, air vent, diaphragm top, with band and understrap. Net price 1 (with long bag) = £60.81; 1 (with short bag) = £56.35

Male day and night urinal with tap, air vent, with band and suspensory. Net price 1 (long bag) = £54.14

Male day urinal with tap, to contain penis and scrotum. Net price 1 (with inner sheath and air vent) = £53.04

Male jockey appliance with tap. Net price 1 = £56.48

Spares

Replacement belt. Net price 1 = £11.09

Outer receiver. Net price 1 = £12.92

Inner sheath. Net price 5 = £12.92

Plastic bags. Net price 5 = £14.23

Rubber bag. Net price 1 = £23.72

Ring. Net price 1 = 94p

Stoke Mandeville male urinal with double bag (specify sheath size). Net price 1 = £71.99; 1 replacement sheath (specify size) = £5.92

Male pubic pressure urinal with tap (specify sheath size). Net price 1 (with rubber bag) = £64.11; 1 (with 5 plastic bags) = £60.34

Spares

Flange with sheaths. Net price 1 = £29.96

Cone. Net price (curved, small, medium, or large; straight, small, medium, large, or extra-large) = £11.88

Plastic bag. Net price 1 (small or large) = £14.23

Rubber bag. Net price 1 = £23.25

Rubber belt. Net price 1 = £4.26

Progress® long life plastic urinal. Net price 1 (inner sheath or scrotal) = £25.33

Fridjohn urinal. Net price 1 = £75.73

YB wet urinal. Net price 1 = £61.46

Essex appliance. Net price 1 = £51.30

One-piece belt. Net price 1 (rubber or plastic bag cover-let) = £51.35

LRC

Dry sheaths. Net price 144 = £14.42

Manfred Sauer

URIbag pocket sized (when not in use) reusable urinal for men and urinary/ostomy appliance users, 1.1 litre capacity, net price 1 = £12.75; URIfem female reusable bottle urinal (for women lying down or in semi-sitting position), 1 litre capacity = 12.75

Payne

Male incontinence appliance with rubber belt. Net price 1 (MK1 with combined rubber flange and understraps) = £63.01; 1 (MK2 with rubber flange and fabric facepiece) = £67.76; 1 (MK3 with combined rubber flange, understraps, and coned top) = £55.92; 1 (MK9, with rubber flange and fabric facepiece) = £70.60

Lightweight male incontinence appliance. Net price 1 (MK4 with fabric facepiece and separate long flanged plastic bag with foam pad) = £39.95; 1 (MK5, with fabric facepiece, with belt combined, separate flange, and long flanged plastic bag) = £56.12; 1 (MK6 with combined flange and understraps and long flanged plastic bag with rubber belt) = £49.21; 1 (MK7) with flange, reinforced coned top and plastic or rubber bag) = £74.38; 1 (MK8, with flange and long plastic bag) = £62.13; 1 (MK10, with fabric facepiece, with belt combined, separate flange, and long flanged plastic bag) = £58.97; 1 (MK11, with flange, soft replaceable diaphragm, facepeice, belt, adjustable rubber understraps, soft coned top, plastic or rubber bag) = £74.38; 1 (MK12 with flange, soft replaceable diaphragm, facepiece, belt, adjustable rubber understraps, long plastic bag) = £62.13

Spares

Rubber flange. Net price 1 (with feathered diaphragm, MK2, MK5, MK9, MK10) = £18.25; 1 (MK1, MK6) = £28.25; 1 (with feathered diaphragm and combined reinforced top, MK3) = £32.04; 1 (MK11 or MK12) 38 mm = £19.23; 45 mm = £18.89; 3 soft replaceable rubber diaphragms = £4.79

Material facepiece. Net price 1 facepiece with belt and loop (MK2, MK4, MK5) = £21.15; 1 facepiece with support belt, loop and scrotal = £24.00

Material facepiece. Net price 1 with belt and adjustable rubber understraps (MK11, MK12) (small, medium, or large) = £25.28

Flange support with wide belt and scrotal support (MK9, MK10). Net price 1 = £24.00

Reinforced cone top (MK1, MK2, MK9). Net price 1 = £12.27

Bag (MK1, MK2, MK3, MK9). Net price 1 plastic bag = £3.08; 1 rubber bag = £18.57

Bag, long flange plastic. Net price 1 MK4 bag = £4.73; 1 MK5, MK6, MK10 bag = £4.17

Belt (MK1, MK3, MK6). Net price 1 (elastic) = £8.42; 1 (web) = £5.89; 1 (rubber) = £3.98

Night connector (MK1, MK2, MK3, MK9). Net price 1 = £3.98

Payne's urine director. Net price 1 = £22.55

Stoke Mandeville condom urinal complete. Net price 1 = £52.00
Spares
Kipper bag. Net price 1 = £29.25
Belt. Net price 1 (38, 46, or 60 inch) = £6.21
Rubber tube and connector. Net price 1 = £2.27; rubber tubing = £4.68 per metre; nylon connector (GU or SM) 1 = £1.32
Dry incontinence sheath, plain or teated end. Net price 100 = £15.13
Pubic pressure urinal complete with bag. Net price 1 (rubber or plastic bag) = £63.01
Spares
Pubic pressure flange with sheath (1-inch flange with 0.5, 0.625, 0.75, or 0.875 inch sheath; 1.25-inch flange with 0.875 or 1 inch sheath; 1.5-inch flange with 1.125 or 1.25 inch sheath; 1.75-inch flange with 1.375, 1.5, or 1.625 inch sheath). Net price 1 = £28.25
Coned top. Net price 1 (straight or curved: small, medium, or large; straight: extra-large) = £12.27
Replacements
Rubber bag with vent tube (MK1, MK2, MK3, MK9). Net price 1 = £22.28
Reinforced cone top with vent tube (MK1, MK2, MK3, MK9). Net price 1 = £16.15
Latex tubing, 8 or 10 mm bore. Net price per metre = £4.68
GU Condom set. Net price 1 = £54.22; 1 (with 40 oz bag) = £67.27
Urinal replacement parts
Nylon stud (GU or SM). Net price 1 = £1.32; 1 (with latex tube) = £2.27
Waist belt for single-chambered bag. Net price 1 (38, 46, or 60 inch) = £6.21
(formerly Willis range)
Male urinal, day and night, air tube to bag, inner sheath and diaphragm to receiver, web belt and cotton suspensory bag. Net price 1 = £51.01; 1 (long narrow Coutil®-covered bag, web belt and cotton suspensory bag) = £53.09
Male urinal, receiver to contain penis and scrotum, web waist band, and tape understraps. Net price 1 (day, night, or small build) = £48.72
Male urinal, long rubber bag with 2 leg straps, loops and straps, flanged receiver, air tube, diaphragm and short conical inner sheath, web band and cotton suspensory bag. Net price 1 (day and night) = £50.40
Male urinal, short rubber bag, detachable bag and night tube, web belt and cotton suspensory bag. Net price 1 (day and night) = £40.61
Spares for above urinals
Suspension bag. Net price 1 (small, medium, or large) = £5.13

Rüsch

Thames urinal with bag and connecting tube. Net price 1 (standard or long bag) = £77.65
Severn urinal with bag and connecting tube. Net price 1 (standard, long, or 5 plastic bags) = £77.65; 5 Severn spare sheaths = £30.44
Mersey urinal with bag and connecting tube. Net price 1 (standard, long, or 5 plastic bags) = £77.65
Wye, male, MkII, light-weight urinal. Net price 1 (with separate connecting tube and on/off valve) = £25.10; 1 (with long night extension tube) = £29.25; 1 (with short or long bag) =£41.79
Arizona male urinal. Net price 1 = £77.65
'55' male urinal for paraplegic patients. Net price 1 = £76.48; 6 spare sheaths = £34.68
Stoke Mandeville pattern male urinal with double chamber rubber collection bag. Net price 1 (20, 24, 25, 28, 32, 35, 38, 42, 45, 48, 51, 54, 57, 60, or 63 mm sheath) =£76.24; 1 spare sheath = £7.03
Sahara one-piece top pubic pressure urinal with bag. Net price 1 paediatric (with small rubber collection bag or 5 small plastic collection bags) = £74.02; 1 standard or large (with standard or long rubber collection bag or 5 medium plastic collection bags, and connecting tube) = £74.02

Peoplecare® pubic pressure male urinal. Net price 1 paediatric (flange 25 mm and sheath 13, 16, 19, or 22 mm; or flange 29 mm and sheath 22 or 25 mm; or flange 32 mm and sheath 19, 22, or 25 mm) = £24.04; 1 adult (flange 38 mm and sheath 19, 22, 25, 29, or 32 mm; or flange 44 mm and sheath 35, 38, or 41 mm) = £24.04
Spares
Pubic pressure bag, standard. Net price 1 (medium) = £12.41; 1 (large) = £15.38; 1 (curved top, small, medium, or large) = £9.36; 1 (straight top, small, medium, large, or extra-large) = £9.36
Transverse rubber bag with tap. Net price 1 = £25.40
Pubic pressure flange for transverse rubber bag with tap. Net price 1 (double-based) = £24.04; 1 (adult, rubber) = £27.71
Kipper inco set with 1 black rubber kipper bag, 10 penile sheaths, waist and support strap, and connecting tube. Net price 1 = £41.60

Salts

Male pubic pressure urinal with rubber bag or 4 plastic bags. Net price 1 = £51.55
Spares
Pubic pressure flange with sheath (25 mm flange with 18 mm sheath; 32 mm flange with 25 mm sheath; 38 mm flange with , 18, 22, 25, 29, or 32 mm sheath; 44 mm flange with 35 or 38 mm sheath), net price 1 = £25.37
Cone. Net price 1 (small, medium, or large: straight or curved; extra-large: straight) = £10.91
Pubic pressure flange belt. Net price 1 = £21.52
Bags. Net price 4 (plastic, child or adult) = £11.99; 1 (rubber, child, adult, or transverse) = £11.99
Belt. Net price = £3.65

SIMS Portex

Male pubic pressure urinal, child, with integral flange. Net price 1 (rubber bag, straight cone, medium) = £61.84; 1 (plastic bag, curved cone, small or medium) = £60.46
Spares
Pubic pressure flange with integral sheath for child. Net price 1 (25-mm flange with 13, 16, 19, or 22 mm sheath; 29-mm flange with 25 mm sheath; 32-mm flange with 25 mm sheath) = £34.04
Cone. Net price 1 (small, medium, or large, straight or curved; extra-large, straight) = £14.39
Pubic pressure flange, double-based. Net price 1 (child, 32 mm; adult, 38 or 44 mm) = £30.42
Chailey male urinal. Net price 1 (child, plastic bag) = £63.64; 1 (adolescent or adult, rubber bag) = £57.06; 1 (adolescent or adult, plastic bag) = £72.27
Spares
Curved top with integral sheath and straps. Net price 1 (child: 22-mm sheath; adult: 22, 25, 29, 32, 35, 38, or 44 mm sheath) = £38.07
Belt, rubber. Net price 1 (61 or 91 cm) = £5.61
Bags, plastic (also suitable for pubic pressure and Chiron® urinals). Net price 1 (wide neck, adult, or child) = £3.74
Bags, rubber (also suitable for pubic pressure and Chiron® urinals). Net price 1 child size = £18.11; 1 adult size = £24.81
Male pubic pressure urinal, adult, with integral flange. Net price 1 (rubber bag, various sizes) = £71.65; 1 (plastic bag, various sizes) = £66.76
Replacement pubic pressure flange. Net price 1 = £34.04
Male pubic pressure urinal, adult, with double-based flange. Net price 1 (rubber bag, various sizes) = £71.65; 1 (plastic bag,various sizes) = £66.76
Replacement sheath. Net price 10 = £1.30
Bag, rubber, for pubic pressure urinals. Net price 1 (adult, with vent tube) = £29.70; 1 (adult, double) = £31.81
Stoke Mandeville urinal. Net price 1 (sheath type) = £65.28; 1 (double rubber bag) = £84.83
Spares
Sheath. Net price 1 = £8.90;10 (for sheath type) = £3.91
Chiron male rubber urinal with webbing belt. Net price 1 = £58.75
Male one-piece urinal. Net price = £55.93
Surrey model lightweight urinal. Net price (MKI or MKII) = £53.14

Spares
Foam pad. Net price 5 (76 mm/32 mm) = £6.59
Chiron urinal. Net price 1 (male, plastic, rubber sheaths) = £30.40; 1 (geriatric, film-type sheaths) = £44.14; 1 (rubber sheaths) = £44.14
Spares
Sheath. Net price 1 (rubber) = £5.61; 10 (non-allergenic film type) = £1.03
Net suspensory. Net price 1 = £13.20
Male urinal for bed use. Net price 1 = £49.59
Pubic flange, large opening. Net price 1 = £22.80
Transverse rubber bag and stopcock. Net price 1 (child) = £33.56

Ward

Jockey male urinal. Net price 1 = £73.14
Varsity male urinal. Net price 1 = £56.46
Male urinal. Net price 1 (day use, covered bag, complete with belt suspensory and thigh strap) = £46.71; 1 (day and night, covered bag, air vent, belt suspensory) = £48.34; 1 (day and night, short bag and belt) = £50.04; 1 (day and night, short covered bag and belt) = £54.24; 1 (day and night, double chamber bag) = £56.38; 1 (day and night, long bag and belt) = £50.04
Paraplegic male urinal. Net price 1 = £68.39
Stoke Mandeville Pattern. Net price 1 = £65.71; 1 (removable rubber sheath, double chamber rubber bag, thigh strap and belt) = £59.02
Spare sheath. Net price 1 = £6.09
Male pubic pressure urinal. Net price 1 (rubber bag) = £61.23; 1 (plastic bag) = £54.25
Spares
Pubic pressure flange. Net price 1 = £28.09
Pubic pressure cone; Net price 1 = £11.10
Bags. Net price 1 (rubber) = £15.21; 1 (plastic) = £3.04
Male urinal. Net price 1 (day, covered bag complete with belt) = £44.46; 1 (day and night or night, covered bag complete with belt, suspensory, and thigh strap) = £58.74; 1 (day and night, long tube, air vent, rubber bag, complete with belt and thigh strap) = £53.33
Male urinal. Net price 1 (night, covered bag complete with belt, suspensory, and thigh strap) = £58.74
Male dribbling bag and tapes. Net price 1 = £21.70
Male urinal. Net price 1 (day and night, short covered bag or short bag and belt) = £50.04
Male urinal. Net price 1 (sheath and disc type with long rubber belt or sheath and suspensory with short or long covered bag) = £54.57
Night urinal. Net price 1 (with long tube) = £26.37
Stoke Mandeville sheath-type urinal, with 30 rubber film sheaths, rubber bag, and thigh strap and belt. Net price 1 = £52.24
Webbing belt. Net price 1 = £9.24
Elastic leg strap. Net price 10 = £5.28
Net suspensory. Net price 1 = £12.15
Spare rubber bag with vent. Net price 1 = £26.39
Spare receiver. Net price 1 = £38.00

Urethral catheters

Urethral catheter sizes are designated by the Charrière (Ch) gauge system; when the size is not stated by the prescriber the Drug Tariff recommends that size 14 or 16 be supplied. For the Foley catheter, if the balloon size is not stated, the 10 mL size should be supplied for adults, 5 mL for paediatric use (balloon sizes are defined as the amount of fluid required to fully inflate the volume of lumen).

■ Foley catheters for short-/medium-term use in adults
Average period of use is 1–3 weeks

Bard

Uriplan®, teflon-coated latex, male or female. Net price, male (12–26 Ch: 10-mL balloon; 16–26 Ch: 30-mL balloon), 1 catheter = £2.31; female (Ch 12–22: 10-mL balloon), 1 catheter = £3.45; pre-filled with sterile water (Ch 12–22: 10-mL balloon), 1 catheter = £2.64

Rüsch

PTFE Aquaflate®, PTFE coated latex with syringe containing sterile water for balloon inflation. Net price, male (12–24 Ch, 10-mL balloon), 1 catheter = £2.06; female (12–24 Ch, 10-mL balloon), 1 catheter = £2.06
Soft Simplastic®, PVC, male or female. Net price, male (12–26 Ch: 10-mL balloon; 16–26 Ch: 30-mL balloon),1 catheter = £4.60; female (12–22 Ch: 10-mL balloon; 16–22 Ch: 30-mL balloon), 1 catheter = £4.60
100 plus®, teflon-coated latex, male or female. Net price male (12–26 Ch: 10-mL balloon; 16–26 Ch: 30-mL balloon), 1 catheter = £1.99; female (12–22 Ch: 10-mL balloon; 16–32 Ch: 30-mL balloon), 1 catheter = £2.53

SIMS Portex

Eschmann Folatex®, latex, male or female. Net price, male (12–28 Ch: 10- or 30-mL balloon), 1 catheter = £2.19; female (12–28 Ch: 10-mL balloon), 1 catheter = £2.19

■ Foley catheters for short-/medium-term use in children
All 8–10 Ch: 5-mL balloon

Bard

Uriplan®, teflon-coated latex. Net price 1 catheter = £6.39

Rüsch

100 plus®, teflon-coated latex. Net price 1 catheter = £4.24

SIMS Portex

Eschmann Folatex ®, latex. Net price 1 catheter = £3.69

■ Foley catheters for long-term use in adults
Average period of use is 3–12 weeks

Bard

Biocath®, hydrogel-coated, male or female. Net price, male (12–26 Ch: 10- or 30-mL balloon), 1 catheter = £7.14; female (12–22 Ch: 10-mL balloon), 1 catheter = £7.23; pre-filled with sterile water, (12–22 Ch: 10-mL balloon), 1 male catheter = £7.34; 1 female catheter = £7.38
Lubri-Sil®, hydrogel-coated silicone, net price (male 12–24 Ch: 10- or 30-mL balloon; female 12–16 Ch: 10-mL balloon) = £8.50
Silastic®, silicone-coated. Net price (12–24 Ch: 10-mL balloon; 16–28 Ch: 30-mL balloon), 1 catheter = £7.40
Bard®, silicone elastomer-coated latex, male or female. Net price, male (12–22 Ch: 10-mL balloon; 16–22 Ch: 30-mL balloon), 1 catheter = £7.85; female (16–22 Ch: 30-mL balloon), 1 catheter = £7.85; pre-filled with sterile water, male or female (12–22 Ch: 10-mL balloon), 1 catheter = £8.48
Bard®, all silicone. Net price male (12–22 Ch: 10-mL balloon; 16–22 Ch: 30-mL balloon), 1 catheter = £8.10; female (12–16 Ch: 10-mL balloon), 1 catheter = £7.77

Coloplast

All silicone, male or female, net price, male (12–14 Ch: 10-mL balloon; 16–20 Ch: 10-mL balloon; 16–18 Ch: 20-mL balloon; 16–26 Ch: 30-mL balloon), 1 catheter = £8.35; female (12–14 Ch: 10-mL balloon; 16–18 Ch: 10-mL balloon; 20 Ch: 30-mL balloon), 1 catheter = £8.27

Kendall

Argyle®, all silicone, male or female. Net price, male (12–22 Ch: 10-mL balloon; 16 Ch: 20-mL balloon; 18–26 Ch: 30-mL balloon), 1 catheter = £5.83; female (12–18 Ch: 10-mL balloon), 1 catheter = £5.83
Ultramer®, polymer-coated, male or female. Net price male (12–26 ch: 5-mL balloon; 16–26 ch: 30-mL balloon), 1 catheter = £6.25; female (12–22 ch: 5-mL balloon; 16–22 ch: 30-mL balloon), 1 catheter = £6.25

Medasil

All silicone, male or female. Net price, male (12–26 Ch: 10-mL balloon; 16–26 Ch: 30-mL balloon), 1 catheter = £4.62; female (12–26 Ch: 10-mL balloon; 16–26 Ch: 30-mL balloon), 1 catheter = £4.62

Rüsch

Brilliant Aquaflate®, all-silicone with syringe containing sterile water for balloon inflation. Net price, male (12–

24 Ch, 10-mL balloon) 1 catheter = £5.85; female (12–24 Ch, 10-mL balloon), 1 catheter = £5.85

Silikon 100®, male or female. Net price, male (12–26 Ch: 10-mL balloon; 18–20 Ch: 20-mL balloon; 22–26 Ch: 30-mL balloon), 1 catheter = £6.62; female (12–22 Ch: 10-mL balloon; 18–20 Ch: 20-mL balloon; 22 Ch: 30-mL balloon), 1 catheter = £6.62

Sympacath®, hydrogel coated. Net price , male (12–30 Ch: 30-mL balloon) 1 catheter = £6.67; female (12–26 Ch: 30-mL balloon), 1 catheter = £6.67; 3-way (16–24 Ch: 30-mL balloon) = £7.12

Sympacath Aquaflate®, hydrogel coated latex with syringe containing sterile water for balloon inflation. Net price, male (12–24 Ch, 10-mL balloon) 1 catheter = £5.85; female (12–24 Ch, 10-mL balloon), 1 catheter = £5.85

Ultrasil®, silicone elastomer-coated latex, male. Net price (12–26 Ch: 10-mL balloon; 16–26 Ch: 30-mL balloon), 1 catheter = £5.52

■ Foley catheters for long-term use in children
All 5-mL balloon

Bard
Biocath®, hydrogel-coated. Net price 1 catheter = £7.23
Lubri-Sil®, hydrogel-coated silicone (8–10 Ch), net price 1 catheter = £8.50

Caremed
All silicone, 2-way, net price 5-catheter pack (6, 8, or 10 Ch) = £7.95

Coloplast
All silicone. Net price 1 catheter = £8.06

Kendall
Argyle®, all silicone. Net price 1 catheter = £6.29

Medasil
All silicone. Net price 1 catheter = £4.62

Rüsch
Silikon 100®. Net price 1 catheter = £6.62
Sympacath®, hydrogel coated, net price (8–10 Ch: 5-mL balloon) 1 catheter = £6.67

■ Intermittent catheter (with introducer tip and urine bag)

Hollister
InstantCath Protect®, net price, Nélaton (6–18 Ch) 25-catheter pack = £62.50; Tiemann tip (12–16 Ch), 25-catheter pack = £62.50

■ Stainless steel catheter for long-term use, reusable for intermittent self catheterisation

Malvern Medical Developments
Biscath® system, stainless steel catheters, brushes, scraper, hard and soft carying case, net price female (8, 10, 12, or 14 Ch), 6-catheter pack = £248.75

■ Nélaton catheters ('ordinary' cylindrical catheter)

Bard
Reliacath®, teflon-coated latex, 14 Ch. Net price 5-catheter pack = £6.91
Reliacath®, plastic, male, female, or paediatric. Net price, male or female (12–18 Ch), 5-catheter pack = £6.37; paediatric (8–10 Ch), 5-catheter pack = £6.37

Coloplast
Aquadry® Self-cath, male, female or paediatric. Net price, male (8–18 Ch), 5-catheter pack = £5.09; female (10–14 Ch), 5-catheter pack = £5.09; paediatric (8–10 Ch), 5-catheter pack = £5.09
PVC, male, female or paediatric. Net price, male (10–18 Ch), 5-catheter pack = £5.00; female (12–18 Ch), 5-catheter pack = £5.33; paediatric (6–10 Ch), 5-catheter pack = £5.33
Simpla PVC, male, female, or paediatric. Net price, male (12–14 Ch), 5-catheter pack = £5.19; female (12–14 Ch), 5-catheter pack = £5.19; paediatric (8–10 Ch), 5-catheter pack = £5.19

Speedicath®, pre-hydrated polyurethane, net price, male (8, 10–14, or 16–18 Ch), female (8, 10–14, or 16 Ch), paediatric (8–10 Ch), *Speedicath* 30 cm (8–12 Ch), Tieman (10–14 Ch) 30-catheter packs all = £39.36

Hunter
SafetyCat®, non-coated ISC, net price male (8–18 Ch), female (8–18 Ch), paediatric (6–10 Ch), 5 catheter packs = £7.10

Maersk
PVC, male, female or paediatric. Net price, male (12–20 Ch), 5-catheter pack = £5.19; female (12–16 Ch), 5-catheter pack = £5.19; male paediatric (6–10 Ch), 5-catheter pack = £5.19; female paediatric (8–10 Ch), 5-catheter pack = £5.19

Pennine
Male, female, or paediatric. Net price, male (12–16 Ch), 10-catheter pack = £3.71; female (10–14 Ch), 10-catheter pack = £3.38; paediatric (6–10 Ch), 10-catheter pack = £3.38

Rüsch
Jacques®, soft red rubber, 8–18 Ch. Net price 1 catheter = £1.18, 5-catheter pack = £5.90
Riplex Jacques®, PVC, male or female, 8–18 Ch. Net price, male, 5-catheter pack = £6.78; female, 5-catheter pack = £6.18
Riplex®, extra-long, PVC, male or female, 8–18 Ch. Net price 5-catheter pack = £6.87

SIMS Portex
PVC, male or female, 8–14 Ch. Net price, male, 5-catheter pack = £7.44; female, 5-catheter pack = £7.18

■ Nélaton catheters (single use)

Astra Tech
Lofric®, PVC, single use, male, female, paediatric, or Tiemann tip. Net price, male (8–24 Ch); female (8–18 Ch); paediatric (6–10 Ch); Tiemann tip (10–20 Ch), 25-catheter pack (all) = £30.00

Coloplast
Aquacath®, single use, male, female, or paediatric. Net price, male (8–18 Ch); female (8–18 Ch); paediatric (6–10 Ch), 25-catheter pack (all) = £25.46
Conveen Easicath®, single use, male, female, paediatric, or Tiemann tip. Net price, male (8–22 Ch); female (8–16 Ch); paediatric (6–10 Ch); EasiCath 30 cm (6–12 Ch); Tiemann tip (10–20 Ch), 25-catheter pack (all) = £25.95
Speedicath®, pre-hydrated polyurethane, net price, male (8, 10–14, or 16–18 Ch); female (8, 10–14, or 16 Ch); paediatric (8–10 Ch); *Speedicath* 30 cm (8–12 Ch); Tiemann tip (10–14 Ch) 30-catheter packs = £39.36

Hollister
Incare® Instant Cath, male (10–16 Ch), female (10–14 Ch), paediatric (6–8 Ch), 25-catheter pack = £28.00

Maersk
Puricat®, male firm or female (8–16 Ch), male soft or Tiemann tip (10–16 Ch). Net price, 25-catheter pack = £27.50

SIMS Portex
Uro-Flo Silky®, single use, male or female, 8–16 Ch. Net price 25-catheter pack = £30.56

■ Nélaton catheters for occasional use

Astra Tech
Lofric® Cath-kit, with urine drainage bag. Net price, male (8–18 Ch), female (8–18 Ch), paediatric (6–10 Ch), Tiemann tip (10–18 Ch), 25-catheter pack (all) = £37.50
Lofric® Hydro-kit, with water container and urine drainage bag. Net price, male (8–18 Ch), female (8–18 Ch), paediatric (6–10 Ch), Tiemann tip (10–18 Ch) 20-catheter pack (all) = £33.60

■ Scott catheters (short curved tubular catheter for women and girls)

SIMS Portex
Polyethylene, female, 8–14 Ch. Net price 5-catheter pack = £11.66

Anal plugs

Coloplast
Conveen® anal plug. Net price 20 (small or large) = £38.66
Note. Should be used only after assessment of suitability by appropriate medical professional

---

Catheter valve

For use with an indwelling catheter after assessment of bladder function by an appropriate medical professional.
It is recommended that the catheter valve is changed every 5–7 days.
Bard
Flip-Flo® catheter valve. Net price 5 = £12.07
Coloplast
Catheter valve. Net price 5 = £11.80
Jade-Euro-Med
Euro catheter valve, net price 5 = £11.19
SIMS Portex
Uro-Flo® catheter valve. Net price 5 = £11.59

Stoma care

The 3 major types of abdominal stoma are:
- colostomy
- ileostomy
- urostomy

Each requires the collection of body waste into an artificial appliance (the 'bag') attached to the body. The bags and accessories are tailored for the different types of stoma.

COLOSTOMY. In a colostomy, a stoma is formed from a cut end of colon. The output depends on the position along the colon from which the stoma is created; the further down the colon's length from which the colostomy is formed, the greater the volume of fluid that can be reabsorbed. The discharge changes from a liquid or paste-like consistency to a nearly fully formed stool mass. The nature of the discharge determines whether the bag can be drainable or non-drainable.

A *permanent colostomy* is formed by surgical removal of the diseased part of the colon. A *temporary colostomy* may be created to allow a distal part of the colon to recover from trauma (e.g. a gunshot wound, stabbing, or road traffic accident). On healing, the colon is surgically rejoined to permit normal faecal output.

ILEOSTOMY. In an ileostomy, a piece of ileum is brought to the abdominal surface following removal of varying lengths of the colon:
- pan-procto colectomy—removal of all parts of the colon
- total colectomy—removal of all of the colon apart from the rectal stump. Later, it may be possible to create an artificial pouch in the abdominal cavity which rejoins the ileum to the rectal stump, permitting normal discharge of faeces.

UROSTOMY. A urostomy (ileal conduit) is created by the diversion of the two ureters into a piece of colon or, more commonly, ileum. The piece of intestine is brought to the abdominal surface to form a stoma.

Normal gastro-intestinal function is resumed after removal of the piece to form the stoma.

Stoma appliances

The only essential prerequisites for stoma management are the collection receptacle (the 'bag') and a means of attaching it to the abdominal wall. However, practical and successful management demands, and the *Drug Tariff* permits, the supply of a range of other components.

STOMA BAGS AND FLANGES. Modern stoma bags are oblong or tapered, rectangular, plastic receptacles. A circular opening is placed over the stoma. Around the opening is a flange that is used to attach the bag to the abdominal wall. A bag may be non-drainable, for use with a descending colostomy with a solid and predictable action; or it may be drainable, having a wide-necked opening with a **bag closure**, for all other types of colostomy and for an ileostomy. A bag for a urostomy has a tap for regular drainage of urine.

A bag may be one- or two-piece, depending on whether the flange is integral with the bag, or separate.

The **flange** may be attached to the abdominal wall by double-sided adhesive rings, or by the separate use of plasters or other adhesives. Skin care is important in stoma management, and a varied range of karaya-based flanges is also available. Non-adhesive flanges are available for stomas that have a solid output only.

As a colostomy stoma is much larger than that formed from ileum, a range of flange sizes is available. However, most flanges have to be cut to size by the patient, for which measuring cards are commonly provided.

A **two-piece bag** is one in which the flange is separate from the bag, and from which the bag can be detached without removing the flange from the skin. The bag is clipped to the flange, and a waist belt can be clipped to the bag. The two-piece bag permits rapid changing should the bag develop a leak.

ACCESSORIES. **Adhesive removers** are available to assist in cleaning the skin after the flange has been removed. Care must be taken to ensure that their use does not cause or aggravate skin soreness.

Bag covers of a wide range of designs and colours are available. They are particularly useful for bags that are made of transparent or semi-transparent material.

Belts are available for use with one- or two-piece bags. Their use may aid the confidence of wearers in the ability of the adhesive to keep the bag attached to the abdomen, and be necessary in wearers with irregularly shaped or distended abdomens.

Deodorants can be placed in the bag to minimise the odour from the discharge.

Filters are integral to many colostomy and ileostomy bags, and are useful for the removal of flatus from the bag. Replacement filters can be incorporated into some designs.

Irrigation/wash-out appliances are available for colostomy patients who evacuate the bowel once every 24 to 48 hours as an alternative to uncontrolled, irregular evacuation through the stoma. A cone-shaped irrigation system is inserted into the stoma, and the distal colon filled with 1–1.5 litres of warm water. Only replacement parts can be prescribed on the NHS; complete systems have to be supplied by a hospital.

Skin fillers and protectives comprise a range of aerosols, barrier creams, gels, lotions, pastes, and wipes. Fillers are used if the abdominal wall is distorted and needs levelling to allow successful attachment of the flange. Protectives are used in cases of skin soreness, but care must be taken to ensure that their use does not compromise the adhesiveness of the flange.

Stoma caps can be clipped to the flange of a two-piece bag for short periods (e.g. during swimming or sports). Their use is practicable only with colostomies that have regular faecal movements.

Tubing that may be prescribed consists of drainage tubing for urostomy bags, for use by immobile patients, or for overnight attachment to night drainage bags.

Stoma appliances

Stoma appliances are listed in Part IXC of *Drug Tariff* or Part 6 of *Scottish Drug Tariff*.

It is not necessary to state an **order number** on a prescription for one of these products provided the **full details** as given in the BNF are included on the **prescription**.

Closed pouches and colostomy sets

Closed pouches are suitable for patients with a **colostomy** and well-formed stools

■ Braun Biotrol range
Biotrol® (Braun Biotrol)

Almarys, one-piece pouch with skin protector adhesive, cover and filter. Net price 30 pouches (clear, starter hole) = £59.32; beige (25, 30, 35, 40, 45, or 50 mm holes) = £59.32

Almarys Optima, one-piece closed pouch with filter and soft cover, Net price 30 pouches, clear (10 mm starter hole) = £57.30; beige (10 mm starter hole, 25, 30, 35, 40, 45, 50 or 60 mm) = £57.30

Almarys Optima Mini, one-piece closed pouch, with filter and soft cover. Net price 30 pouches, beige (20, 25, 30, 35 or 40 mm) = £50.70

Almarys Petite, one-piece pouch with skin protector adhesive, cover and filter, beige. Net price 30 pouches (starter hole, 25, 30, 35, or 40 mm holes) = £51.71

Almarys Preference, one-piece pouch with filter, skin protector, adhesive and soft cover. Net price 30 pouches, clear (10 mm starter hole) = £59.32; beige (10 mm starter hole, 25, 30, 35, 40, 45, or 50 mm holes) = £59.32

Almarys Quiet, one-piece closed pouch with filter and soft cover. Net price 30 pouches, clear (10 mm starter hole) = £57.30; beige (10 mm starter hole, 25, 30, 35, 40, 45, 50 or 60 mm holes) = £57.30

Colo S, one-piece pouch with skin protector adhesive, white. Net price 30 pouches (25, 30, 35, 40, 45, 50, or 60 mm holes) = £64.30

Elite Closed, covered one-piece pouch with skin protector adhesive and filter, white or beige. Net price 30 pouches (starter hole, 25, 30, 35, 40, 45, 50, 60, 70 mm holes) = £67.82; clear (25, 30, 35, 40, 45, 50, 60, 70 mm holes) 30 pouches = £63.00; starter hole, 30 = £63.87

Elite Petite, one-piece pouch with skin protector adhesive and filter, beige. Net price 30 pouches (starter hole, 25, 30, 35, 40 or 45 mm holes) = £57.65

Lockring 2, two-piece pouches with filter and backing, white. Net price 30 pouches (for 35, 50 or 75 mm flanges) = £31.06; paediatric, beige (35 mm hole) 30 pouches = £27.23

Mini S, one-piece pouch with skin protector adhesive and filter, beige. Net price 30 pouches (25, 30, 35, or 40 mm) = £53.05

Integrale, one-piece pouch with skin protector adhesive and filter, white. Net price 30 pouches (starter hole, 25, 30, 35, 40, 45, 50, 60, 70 mm holes) = £67.82

Preference Closed, fabric covered one-piece pouch with skin protector adhesive, porous adhesive collar, and filter, white or beige. Net price 30 pouches (starter hole, 25, 30, 35, 40, 45, 50, 60 mm holes) = £64.50

■ CliniMed range
Welland (CliniMed)

Colostomy, one-piece closed pouch with filter, beige, net price 30 pouches (25, 29, 32, 35, 38, 44, 51, 60 mm holes or 10 mm cut-to-fit holes) = £63.54; with soft backing, beige or clear = £64.62

Impact, one-piece closed pouch with toilet disposable liner, filter and soft backing, beige. Net price 30 pouches (19, 25, 29, 32, 35, 38, 44 or 51 mm holes) standard or maxi = £63.16; mini = £51.90

Ovation, one-piece closed pouch with skin protector, filter and soft backing. Net price 30 pouches, clear or beige (10 mm starter hole), oval flange = £64.53; large vertical flange = £63.42

Silhouette closed, one-piece pouch, beige or clear. Net price 30 pouches (25, 29, 32, 35, 38, 44, 51 mm or 10 mm cut-to-fit holes), short length = £51.90; standard length = £58.50; 30 pouches (60 mm holes), standard length = £58.50

Vogue, one-piece closed pouch with filter and soft backing, beige or clear. Net price 30 pouches (25, 29, 32, 35, 38, 44, 51 mm holes or 10 mm cut-to-fit holes) = £54.39

■ Coloplast range
Assura® (Coloplast)

Conseal, one-piece plug for 20–35 mm or 35–45 mm stoma. Net price 10 plugs (length, 35 or 45 mm) = £21.61

Note. Should be used only after assessment of suitability by appropriate medical professional

Inspire Clear, one-piece closed pouch with filter, adhesive and soft backing. Net price 30 pouches, Midi (20–65 mm starter hole, 25, 30, or 35 mm holes) = £66.03; Maxi (20–75 mm starter hole) = £66.03

Inspire Soft Cover, one-piece closed pouch with filter, adhesive and opaque soft cover front and back. Net price 30 pouches, Midi (20–65 mm starter hole, 25, 30, 35, 40, 45, or 50 mm holes) = £66.03; Maxi (20–75 mm starter hole) = £66.03

Inspire Design, one-piece closed pouch with filter, adhesive and soft cover front and back. Net price 30 pouches, Midi (20–65 mm starter hole, 25, 30, 35, 40, 45, or 50 mm holes) = £66.03; Maxi (20–75 mm starter hole) = £66.03

Maxi, closed pouches, opaque or clear. Net price 30 one-piece pouches (opaque or clear: 10–70 mm starter holes, 20, 25, 30, 35, 40 mm; clear: also 45 or 50 mm holes; 20 mm can be cut to fit up to 55 mm) = £66.03; 30 two-piece pouches, opaque or clear (to fit 40, 50, or 60 mm base plates) = £36.42; 30 one-piece closed pouches with filter and soft cover front and back (opaque: 10–70 mm, 20–55 mm starter holes) = £66.03

Midi, closed pouches with flatus filter, opaque or clear. Net price 30 one-piece pouches (20, 25, 30, 35, 40, 45, or 50 mm holes) = £66.03; 30 two-piece pouches (to fit 40, 50, or 60 mm base plates) = £36.42; base plate (40, 50, or 60 mm), 5 = £14.31; 30 one-piece closed pouches with filter and soft cover front and back (opaque: 20–55 mm starter hole, 25, 30, 35, 40, 45 or 50 mm holes) = £66.03

Mini, closed pouches with filter and soft backing. Net price 30 one-piece pouches (clear: 20 mm cut-to-fit hole; opaque: 20 mm cut-to-fit hole; 25, 30, 35, or 40 mm holes) = £52.86; 30 one-piece closed pouches with filter and soft cover front and back (opaque: 20–55 mm starter hole) = £52.86; 30 two-piece pouches (opaque: to fit 40 or 50 mm base plates) = £29.94

Minicap, closed pouches, opaque. Net price 30 two-piece pouches (to fit 40 or 50 mm base plates) = £34.14

Paediatric, closed pouches with filter and soft backing. Net price 30 one-piece pouches (clear or opaque: 10–35 mm starter hole) = £57.54; 30 two-piece pouches (clear or opaque: to fit 40 mm base plates) = £27.18

Seal Integral Convexity, one-piece closed pouch. Net price 10 maxi or midi pouches (clear: 15, 18, 21, 25, 28, 31, 35, 38 or 41 mm holes) = £21.58; (opaque: 15–33 mm or 15–43 mm starter holes) = £21.58

Note. Should be used only after assessment of suitability by appropriate medical professional

Conseal® System (Coloplast)

Two-piece pouch. Net price 30 bags (to fit 40 or 50 mm base plates) = £38.37; base plate (40 or 50 mm) 5 = £14.19; colostomy plug (40 × 35 or 45 mm, 50 × 35 or 45 mm) 10 = £12.92; discharge bag (40 or 50 mm) 50 = £2.80

K-Flex® (Coloplast)

One-piece closed pouch with karaya skin protector and filter. Net price 30 pouches (opaque: 30 or 40 mm holes) = £68.61

Extra, one-piece closed pouch. Net price, No. 2 (30 or 40 mm holes), 100 = £114.50; No. 3 (30 mm hole), 100 = £137.40

mc2000® (Coloplast)

One-piece pouch with double seal and filter, opaque or clear. Net price 30 pouches (25, 30, 35, 40, 45, 50, 55, or 60 mm holes) = £71.01

mc2002® (Coloplast)

Two-piece pouch with filter, opaque or clear. Net price 30 pouches (to fit 40 or 60 mm base plates) = £40.11; base plate (40 mm × 15 or 25 mm, 60 × 35 or 45 mm) 5 = £14.81; belt plate (40 or 60 mm) 10 = £6.01

pc3000® (Coloplast)

One-piece pouch, opaque or clear. Net price 30 pouches (25, 30, 35, 40, 45, 50, or 55 mm holes; 25 mm can be cut to fit up to 60 mm) = £67.05

Schacht® (Coloplast)

Colostomy bag (= pouch), one-piece closed pouch. Net price 100 pouches = £34.26

Colostomy appliance. Net price 1 appliance = £29.55

■ ConvaTec range

Colodress® (ConvaTec)

Colodress, one-piece closed pouch with textured backing, opaque beige. Net price 30 pouches (19, 32, 38, 45, or 50 mm holes; 19 mm can be cut to fit) = £64.06

Colodress Plus, one-piece closed pouch with single-release paper and filter. Net price 30 pouches (opaque or clear: 19, 25, 32, 38, 45, 50, or 64 mm holes; opaque: 19 mm can be cut to fit) = £64.39; Mini pouches, 30 pouches (19, 25, 32, 38, or 45 mm holes) = £58.08

Colodress Plus Lite, one-piece closed pouch, standard, opaque. Net price 30 pouches (25, 32, 38, 45 or 50 mm holes; 19 mm can be cut to fit) = £59.18

Combihesive Natura® (ConvaTec)

Two-piece closed pouch with filter, opaque. Net price 30 pouches (to fit 32, 38, 45, 57 or 70 mm flanges) = £33.28; Mini pouches, 20 pouches (to fit 32, 38, 45 or 57 mm flanges) = £18.24

Combihesive Natura® Little Ones (ConvaTec)

Stomahesive wafer with flexible collar, net price 5 (32 mm, 75 x 75 mm; 45 mm, 100 x 100 mm) = £14.24 Closed pouch, net price 20 (32 or 45 mm) = £19.10 Drainable pouch, net price 10 (32 or 45 mm) = £11.19

Consecura® (ConvaTec)

Two-piece closed pouch with filter. Net price 50 pouches (clear or opaque to fit 35, 45 or 55 mm flanges) = £54.39

Naturess® (ConvaTec)

Naturess, closed pouches. Net price 50 pouches (standard opaque pouch: 19 mm starter hole, 25, 32, 38, 45 or 50 mm hole; standard clear pouch: 19 mm starter hole) =

£100.53; 50 pouches (small opaque pouch: 19 mm starter hole, 25, 32, 38 or 45 mm holes) = £89.36

Naturess A, closed pouches with absorbent pads. Net price 50 pouches (standard opaque pouch: 19 mm starter hole, 25, 32, 38, 45 or 50 mm hole) = £98.08

Surgicare System ® 2 (ConvaTec)

System 2, two-piece closed pouch, white. Net price 30 pouches (to fit 38, 45, 57, or 70 mm flanges) = £32.39

System 2 Combihesive, two-piece closed pouch with textured backing, beige. Net price 30 pouches (to fit 38, 45, 57, or 70 mm flanges) = £32.39; with filter, 30 pouches (to fit 32, 38, 45, 57, or 70 mm flanges) = £33.28; Mini pouches, 20 pouches (to fit 32, 38, 45 or 57 mm flanges) = £18.61

■ Dansac range

Dansac® (Dansac)

Light Convex, integral convexity, one-piece closed pouch with filter and soft cover. Net price 10 pouches, clear or opaque (15–24 mm, 15–37 mm or 15–46 mm starter holes, 20, 25, 30, 35, 40, or 45 mm pre-cut holes) = £21.40

Note. Should be used only after assessment of suitability by appropriate medical professional

Nova, net price 30 pouches (20–60 mm starter hole, opaque or clear); (25, 30, 35, 40, 45, or 50 mm pre-cut, opaque or clear = £67.16

Nova Mini, opaque, net price (20–50 mm starter hole, 25, 30, 35, or 40 mm pre-cut) = £54.95

Unique, one-piece closed pouch, opaque or clear. Net price 30 pouches (25, 35, 40, 45, 50, 60 mm or cut-to-fit holes) = £60.16; oval flange, opaque or clear, starter hole, net price 30 = £60.16

Unique 2, two-piece closed pouch, opaque or clear. Net price 30 pouches (to fit 36, 43, 55 or 80 mm flange) = £33.34; flange, 36, 43, or 55 mm, net price 5 = £13.64; 80 mm, net price, 5 = £13.91

Unique 2 Mini, two-piece closed pouch with cover, opaque. Net price 30 pouches (to fit 36, 43 or 55 mm flange) = £28.16

Unique 2 MiniCap, two-piece closed pouch, opaque. Net price 30 pouches (to fit 36, 43 or 55 mm flange) = £29.55

Unique 2 Plus, two-piece closed pouch with cover, opaque. Net price 30 pouches (to fit 36, 43, 55 or 80 mm flange) = £33.17

Unique Light, one-piece closed pouch with filter and comfort backing, opaque. Net price 30 pouches (25, 30, 35, 40, 45, 50 or 60 mm holes; 20–60 mm starter hole) = £61.32

Unique Mini, one-piece closed pouch, opaque. Net price 30 pouches (25, 30, 35, or 40 mm holes; 20 mm can be cut to fit up to 50 mm) = £56.45

■ Hollister range

Classic® (Hollister)

All with 25, 32, 38, 44, 51, 64, or 76 mm holes

Karaya seal (series 716), one-piece pouch with karaya skin protector (without filter), must be worn with belt, clear. Net price 30 pouches = £57.54

Karaya 5® Seal (series 331 and 332), one-piece closed pouch with porous adhesive, karaya skin protector seal, and filter, may be worn with belt, opaque or clear. Net price 30 pouches = £68.23

Microporous adhesive (series 314), one-piece compact closed pouch with porous adhesive and filter, may be worn with belt, clear. Net price 50 pouches = £73.21

Compact® (Hollister)

Closed, one-piece pouch with filter and comfort backing. Net price 30 pouches (beige or clear: 13-64 mm cut-to-fit; 25, 32, 38, 44, 51, or 64 mm) = £64.21

Conform 2® (Hollister)

Closed Pouch, two-piece pouch with beige comfort backing. Net price 30 pouches, with or without clear front (45 or 70 mm holes) = £31.50

Guardian® (Hollister)

*Flanges, net price 'S' stationary flange (25, 38, 51, or 64 mm) 5 = £13.22

Impression C® (Hollister)

Closed, one-piece pouch with wafer, filter and bridge, beige (with double side comfort backing) or clear (with single side comfort backing). Net price 10 pouches (19, 22, 25, 29, 32, 35, 38, 41, 44 or 51 mm holes) = £21.94

Impression CPL® (Hollister)

Closed, two-piece pouch with filter and comfort backing, clear or beige. Net price 30 pouches (38, 44, 57 or 70 mm holes) = £32.10

Mini, two-piece closed pouch with filter, opaque. Net price 30 pouches (38, 44, 57 or 70 mm holes) = £27.73

Moderma® (Hollister)

Closed, one-piece pouch with barrier, filter and comfort backing, beige, quiet film. Net price 30 pouches (clear or opaque: 15–50 mm starter hole; opaque: 20, 25, 30, 35, 40, 45 or 50 mm holes) = £59.58

Premium® (Hollister)

Karaya 5® Seal (series 355 and 353), one-piece closed pouch with porous adhesive, karaya skin protector and filter, may be worn with belt, opaque (32, 38, 44, 51, 64, or 76 mm holes) or clear (25, 32, 38, 44, 51, 64, or 76 mm holes), net price 15 pouches = £36.25

■ Jade-Euro-Med range

Rubber bags screwcap (Jade-Euro-Med)

Black butyl, one-piece closed pouch. Net price 1 day pouch = £28.41; 1 night pouch = £33.14

White rubber, one-piece closed pouch. Net price 1 day pouch = £15.79; 1 night pouch = £18.09

Rubber bags spout (Jade-Euro-Med)

Black butyl, one-piece closed pouch. Net price 1 day pouch or night pouch = £30.00

White rubber, one-piece closed pouch. Net price 1 day pouch or night pouch = £14.19

■ Marlen range

Ultra® (Marlen)

All with 12, 16, 19, 22, 25, 29, 32, 34, 38, 41, 44, 48, 50, 54, 57, 60, 63, 70, 73, 76 mm or cut-to-fit holes; opaque or clear; flat or shallow convex.

Closed, one-piece pouch. Net price 15 pouches = £28.80

■ Oakmed range

Option® (Oakmed)

Colostomy Plus, closed, one-piece pouch, clear or opaque. Net price 30 pouches (starter hole, 20, 25, 30, 35, 40, 45, 50, 55 or 60 mm holes) = £57.35

Mini, closed, one-piece pouch, clear or opaque. Net price 30 pouches (10–50 mm cut-to-fit holes) = £50.70

Standard, closed, one-piece pouch, clear or opaque. Net price 30 pouches (starter hole, 20, 25, 30, 35, 40, 45 or 50 mm holes) = £56.00

■ Pelican range

Pelican® (Pelican)

Closed, one-piece pouch (formerly Simplaseel®). Net price 30 pouches (26, 32, 40, 45, 50 mm or cut-to-fit holes) = £73.37; 30 casual pouches (32, 40, or 45 mm holes) = £69.62

Mini, closed, one-piece pouch. Net price 30 pouches (opaque or clear: 20–65mm cut-to-fit holes; opaque: 27, 34, 41, 48 or 55 mm holes) = £53.47

Pelican Select® (Pelican)

Afresh, closed pouch with skin protector, filter, fabric front and back, net price 30 pouches, standard shape, clear or opaque, (cut-to-fit 20–65 mm; pre-cut: 22.5, 25, 27.5, 30, 32.5, 35, 37.5, 40, 45, 50, or 55mm) = £66.14; mini shape, opaque (cut-to-fit 20–65 mm; pre-cut: 22.5, 25, 27.5, 30, 32.5, 35, 37.5, 40, 45, 50, or 55 mm) or clear (cut-to-fit 20–65 mm) = £66.14

Closed, one-piece pouch with skin protector, filter, fabric front and back. Net price 30 pouches, clear or opaque, 20–65 mm (cut-to-fit) = £63.75; clear or opaque (27, 34, 41, 48, or 55 mm holes), 30 = £63.75

Phoenix® (Pelican)

Closed, one-piece closed pouch. Net price (both 32, 40, or 45 mm holes) 100 pouches = £166.70; 100 casual pouches = £155.07

Sassco® (Pelican)

Closed, one-piece closed pouch. Net price 100 pouches (32, 40, or 45 mm holes) = £158.77

■ Rüsch range

Ostopore® (Rüsch)

Colo AV-opaque, one-piece closed pouch with adhesive and vent. Net price 30 pouches (25, 32, 38, or 45 mm holes) with 2 belt flanges = £41.31

Colo KAV-opaque, one-piece closed pouch with karaya seal skin protector, adhesive, and vent. Net price 30 pouches (25, 32, 38, 45, or 51 mm holes) with 5 belt flanges = £56.24

Colo KAV-transparent, one-piece closed pouch with karaya seal skin protector, adhesive, and vent. Net price 30 pouches (32, 38, 45, or 51 mm holes) with 30 belt flanges = £71.81

Rubber bags (Rüsch)

White rubber, one-piece closed pouch with spout outlet. Net price (both 19, 25, or 28 mm holes), 1 day pouch = £11.72; 1 night pouch = £12.65

Translet® (Rüsch)

Premier colostomy set, 1 adhesive ring with 6 bags. Net price 15 (27, 40, or 57 mm hole) = £65.08; spare bags 10 (18 or 28 cm length) = £4.99; adhesive rings or micropo-rous spare adhesive rings (27, 40, or 57 mm) 5 = £6.66

Royal colostomy set, 1 adhesive ring and 6 odourproof bags. Net price 15 (27, 40, or 57 mm) = £90.44; spare bags (18 or 28 cm length) 10 = £7.90

■ Salts range

Cohflex® (Salts)

Closed, one-piece pouch with single-release paper, wafer, and filter, fabric front and back, flesh. Net price 30 pouches (all may be cut to fit; 25, 30, 35, 40, 45, 50, 55, 60 mm or 10–60 mm cut-to-fit holes) = £59.82

Coloset® (Salts)

Closed, one-piece pouch. Net price 30 pouches; (small: 713656) = £10.43; (large: 713658) = £13.14

Confidence® (Salts)

One-piece closed pouch, opaque. Net price 30 pouches (13 mm starter hole, 25, 32, 38, 45, or 52 mm holes) = £60.50

One-piece closed pouch, clear. Net price 30 pouches (13 mm starter hole), with or without overlap film, standard = £57.92, large = £59.67; 30 pouches (25, 32, 38, 45, or 52 mm pre-cut holes) with overlap film, stand-ard = £59.67

Mini, closed pouches. Net price 30 pouches (13 mm starter hole, 25, 32, 38, 45 or 52 mm holes) = £47.67

Eakin® (Salts)

Closed, one-piece pouch, clear. 32, 45, or 64 mm holes, net price 20 pouches = £44.22

Second Nature (Salts)

Second Nature, two-piece closed pouch. Net price 30 pouches (opaque: 32, 38, 45 or 57 mm; clear: 45 or 57mm) = £35.25; clear (with or without overlap) = £34.64

Simplicity® (Salts)

Closed, two-piece closed pouch, clear or pink, medium. Net price, clear (40, 50, 60, or 70 mm) 30 = £16.59; pink (40, 50, or 60 mm holes) 30 = £16.42; flange, standard (30, 40, 50, or 60 mm hole) 5 = £3.01

Simplicity I® (Salts)

Anatomical, closed one-piece pouch. Net price, clear (cut-to-fit), 30 = £66.56; opaque (30, 40, 50, 60 mm, or cut-to-fit holes), 30 = £66.56

Closed, one-piece pouch with porous adhesive, skin pro-tector seal, and filter, fabric front and back. Net price 30 pouches (all may be cut to fit; opaque or pink: 30, 40, 50, or 60 mm holes; opaque, clear or pink: cut-to-fit holes) = £68.15

Simplicity 2® (Salts)

Closed, two-piece closed pouch (may also be applied directly to skin). Net price 30 pouches (40, 50, 60, or 70 mm holes, also 30 mm only for direct application to skin) = £35.23; flange (30, 40, 50, or 60 mm) 5 = £14.85

Supasac® (Salts)

Closed, one-piece pouch. Net price 30 (medium) = £24.72

■ **Shannon range**

Colostomy (Shannon)

Adhesive appliance. Net price, 1 (TJS 948B) = £49.09

Appliance. Net price, 1 appliance (TJS 962) = £17.10

Day bag (= pouch). Net price 1 pouch, TJS 948f = £22.52; TJS 948j = £25.76

Disposable bag (= pouch). Net price TJS 948g, 100 pouches = £11.15

Night bag (= pouch). Net price 1 pouch, TJS 948e = £25.76; TJS 948k = £28.09

Outfit. Net price 1 TJS 948A = £76.03, 1 TJS 948NA = £73.63; 1 TJS 948T = £40.31

Easychange® (Shannon)

Appliance. Net price 1 appliance = £4.51

Spare bag (= pouch). Net price 100 pouches = £44.99

Shannon (Shannon)

Disposable bag (= pouch), closed pouches with plasters. Net price 12 pouches = £6.16

Elastic necks. Net price 50 pouches = £22.50

■ **Shaw range**

Hainsworth® (Shaw)

Hainsworth® bag (= pouch), one-piece closed pouch. Net price (both 25, 32, 38, or 51 mm holes), 20 pouches with body mould adhesive = £42.92; 20 pouches with Healwell® adhesive = £22.53

Shaw (Shaw)

Colostomy outfit, comprising, 4-inch wide elastic belt with groinstrap (26- to 42-inch), 1 flange and 100 colostomy pouches. Net price one NSI 6 outfit with 11 × 6-inch pouches = £39.77; one NSI 7 outfit with 12× 8-inch pouches = £40.57; one NSI 8 outfit with 11× 6-inch pouches = £43.43

Double seal, one-piece closed pouch. Net price 100 11 × 6-inch pouches = £10.27; 100 12 × 8-inch pouches = £11.23

Stick-on bag (= pouch), one-piece closed pouch with plasters. Net price 10 pouches = £8.54

■ **SIMS Portex range**

Adhesive (SIMS Portex)

Stomabag, one-piece closed pouch with adhesive, opaque. Net price (25, 32, 38, 44, 51, or 64 mm holes), 90 pouches = £128.60; with filter, 90 pouches = £144.53

Beta® (SIMS Portex)

Closed, two-piece pouch with filter. Net price, 1 kit comprising 30 pouches and 8 Seel-a-peel sheets (100 × 100 mm) = £53.14; 90 spare pouches = £146.31

Chiron® (SIMS Portex)

Adhesive appliance with spout bag. Net price 1 appliance (Mk I and Mk III) = £69.80

Clearseal bag (= pouch), one-piece closed pouch. Net price 10 pouches (305 × 127 mm: 22 mm hole) = £15.15

Closed bag, one-piece pouch. Net price 10 pouches (305 × 127 mm or 230 × 127 mm: 38 mm hole) = £15.15

Disposable bag (= pouch), one-piece closed pouch. Net price 10 pouches (305 × 102 mm or 305 × 127 mm: 19 mm hole) = £10.09

Reinforced, one-piece disposable pouch. Net price 10 pouches = £15.15

Chironseal® (SIMS Portex)

Closed bag (= pouch), one-piece closed pouch. Net price 10 pouches (305 × 102, 305 × 127, 230 × 127, or 305 × 150 mm: 22 or 38 mm holes) = £11.37; 10 pouches (305 × 205 or 305× 255 mm: 22 or 38 mm hole) = £13.05

Reinforced, one-piece disposable closed pouch. Net price 10 pouches (305 × 102 mm: 25 or 38 mm holes or 305 × 127 mm: 38 mm hole) = £15.15

EC1® (SIMS Portex)

Colo Classic, one-piece closed pouch with wafer, comfort backing, and filter, opaque or clear. Net price 30 pouches (25, 32, 38, 44, 51, 64 mm or 15–64 mm cut-to-fit holes) = £69.06

Mirage® (SIMS Portex)

Closed, one-piece pouch, beige or clear. Net price 30 pouches (25, 32, 38, 44, 51 or 64 mm, or 19–44 mm or 19–64 mm cut-to-fit holes) = £58.36; large (19–90 mm cut-to-fit holes) 10 = £21.08

Closed flushable, one-piece closed pouch with soft backing, beige or clear. Net price 30 pouches (25, 32, 38, 44, 51 mm, or 19–44 mm cut-to-fit holes) = £63.16

Omni® (SIMS Portex)

Closed, one-piece pouch with wafer, porous adhesive, filter. Net price 30 pouches (beige: 25, 32, 38, 44, or 51 mm; beige or clear: 15–44 mm cut-to-fit holes) = £70.06

Redifit® (SIMS Portex)

Continuation bag (= pouch), one-piece closed pouch with karaya skin protector, may be worn with belt, opaque. Net price 20 pouches (32, 38, 44, 51, 64, or 75 mm holes) = £73.22

Non-adhesive bag (= pouch), one-piece closed pouch, opaque, must be worn with belt. Net price 20 pouches with karaya skin protector (44 mm hole) = £73.22; without karaya, 20 pouches (38 mm hole) = £55.57

Rediseal® (SIMS Portex)

Small bag (= pouch), one-piece PVC compact closed pouch, opaque. Net price 10 pouches (38, 44, or 51 mm holes) = £14.30

Serenade® (SIMS Portex)

WC Disposable, two-piece closed pouch. Net price 30 pouches (25, 32, 38, 44, or 51 mm holes) with filter = £34.38; 30 pouches (25, 32, 38, 44, or 51 mm holes) with soft-backing and filter = £35.76; Mini pouches, 30 pouches (15–51 mm) with soft backing and filter = £28.10; base plate (25, 32, 38, 44 or 51 mm), 10 = £28.38

Symphony® (SIMS Portex)

WC Disposable, one-piece closed pouch with wafer and filter. Net price 30 pouches (opaque or clear: 25, 32, 38, 44, or 51 mm holes; opaque: 15–44 mm cut-to-fit holes) = £72.26

Symphony Classic® (SIMS Portex)

WC Disposable, one-piece closed bag with soft backing, beige. Net price 30 pouches (25, 32, 38, 44, 51 mm or 15–51 mm cut-to-fit holes) = £72.26

■ **Ward range**

Ward (Ward)

Disposable bag (= pouch), one-piece closed pouch. Net price 10 pouches (12 × 4-inch) with 4 × 3-inch plasters = £8.87; 10 pouches (12 × 5-inch) with 4 × 4-inch plasters = £8.87

Celluloid colostomy cup, with sponge or solid rim. Net price 1 (small, medium, or large) cup = £36.83; with belt fitting, 1 cup = £42.01; 1 pouch with mount outlet = £15.31

Drainable pouches and ileostomy sets

Drainable pouches are suitable for patients with an **ileostomy** or a **colostomy** with fluid effluent.

■ **Braun Biotrol range**

Biotrol® (Braun Biotrol)

Almarys, one-piece pouch with skin protector adhesive and cover. Net price 30 pouches (beige or clear, starter hole) = £62.73; beige (25, 30, 35, 40, 45, 50 or 60 mm holes) = £62.73

Almarys Optima, one-piece pouch with soft cover. Net price 30 pouches, clear (10 mm starter hole) = £61.50; beige (10 mm starter hole, 25, 30, 35, 40, 45, 50, or 60 mm holes) = £61.50

Almarys Optima Mini, one-piece pouch with soft cover. Net price 30 pouches, beige (20, 25, 30, 35, or 40 mm holes) = £57.20

Almarys Preference, one-piece pouch with skin protector, adhesive and soft cover. Net price 30 pouches, clear or beige (10 mm starter hole) = £63.67

Elite, fabric covered one-piece pouch with skin protector adhesive and clamp closure, white or beige. Net price 30 pouches (starter hole, 20, 25, 30, 35, 40, 45, 50, 60, 70 mm holes) = £69.40; 30 clear pouches (20, 25, 30, 35, 40, 45, 50, 60, 70 mm or cut-to-fit holes) = £64.28; starter hole, 30 = £65.47

Elite Petite, one-piece pouch with skin protector adhesive and fabric backing, beige. Net price 30 pouches (starter hole, 25, 30, 35, 40 or 45 mm holes) = £59.55

Ileo S, one-piece pouch with skin protector adhesive, white. Net price 30 pouches (starter hole, 20, 25, 30, 35, 40, 45, 50, 60, 70 mm holes) = £69.40

Lockring 2, two-piece pouches with backing. Net price 30 pouches (for 35, 50 or 75 mm flanges) = £31.06; paediatric, beige (35 mm hole) 30 pouches = £30.05

Post-op, one-piece pouch with skin protector adhesive, for temporary or permanent colostomies or ileostomies, clear. Net price (cut-to-fit holes) small, 30 pouches = £72.31; large, 30 pouches = £101.57

Preference, fabric covered one-piece pouch with skin protector adhesive, porous adhesive collar, beige. Net price 30 pouches (starter hole, 20, 25, 30, 35, 40, 45, 50, 60 mm or cut-to-fit holes) = £69.40

■ Bullen range
Lenbul® (Bullen)

Day bag (= pouch), one-piece pouch. Net price 1 pouch with screwcap outlet = £12.75

Night bag (= pouch), one-piece pouch. Net price 1 pouch with screwcap outlet = £14.05

■ CliniMed range
Welland® (CliniMed)

Curvex, soft flexible cover, filter, beige or clear, net price 10-pouches (pre-cut 25, 32, or 43 mm) £23.40

Ileostomy pouch, one-piece pouch with wafer and soft backing, beige or clear. Net price 30 pouches (25, 29, 32, 35, 38, 44, 51 mm, or 19 mm cut-to-fit holes) = £63.59

Ovation, one-piece pouch with skin protector and soft backing. Net price 30 pouches, clear or beige (10 mm starter hole) with oval flange = £68.13; 10 pouches beige or clear (10 mm starter hole) with large vertical flange = £22.32

Ovation Mini, one-piece with skin protector and soft backing. Net price 30 pouches, clear or beige. (10 mm starter hole) with oval flange = £58.28; 10 pouches, clear or beige (10 mm starter hole) with large vertical flange = £19.42

Post-op, one-piece pouch with soft backing, clear or beige. Net price (10 mm cut-to-fit hole), 30 pouches = £65.55

Silhouette drainable, one-peice pouch, beige or clear. Net price 30 pouches (25, 29, 32, 35, 38, 44, 51 mm or 19 mm cut-to-fit holes), short length = £54.42; standard length = £63.00

Silhouette Plus, one-piece pouch with filter, beige or clear. Net price 30 pouches (25, 29, 32, 35, 38, 44, 51 mm or 19 mm cut-to-fit holes) = £63.00

Vogue drainable, one-piece pouch, beige, net price 30 pouches (25, 29, 32, 35, 38, 44, 51 mm, or 19 mm cut-to-fit holes) = £54.42

■ Coloplast range
Assura® (Coloplast)

Inspire Clear, one-piece drainable pouch with filter and soft backing. Net price 30 pouches, Mini or Midi (12–55 mm starter hole) = £79.00; Maxi (12–70 mm starter hole) = £79.00

Inspire Soft Cover, one-piece drainable pouch with filter and opaque soft cover front and back. Net price 30 pouches, Mini (12–55 mm starter hole) = £79.00; Midi (12–55 mm starter hole, 25, 30, or 35 mm holes) =

£79.00; Maxi (12–70 mm starter hole, 25, 30, or 35 mm holes) = £79.00

Inspire Design, one-piece drainable pouch with filter and soft cover front and back. Net price 30 pouches, Mini or Midi (10–55 mm starter hole) = £66.78; Maxi (10–70 mm starter hole) = £79.78

Maxi, one-piece pouch, opaque or clear. Net price 30 pouches (10, 25, 30, 35, or 40 mm holes; 10 mm can be cut to fit up to 55 mm) = £66.78; two-piece pouch, opaque or clear. Net price 30 pouches (to fit 40, 50, or 60 mm base plates) = £36.42; 30 one-piece pouches with soft cover front and back (opaque: 10–70 mm starter hole) = £66.78

Midi, one-piece pouch with soft backing. Net price 30 pouches (clear or opaque: 10, 25, 30, 35, or 40 mm holes; 10 mm can be cut to fit up to 55 mm) = £66.78; two-piece pouch, opaque or clear. Net price 30 pouches (to fit 40, 50 or 60 mm base plates) = £36.42; 30 one-piece pouches with soft cover front and back (opaque: 10–55 mm starter hole, 25, 30, 35, 40, 45 or 50 mm holes) = £66.78

Mini, one-piece pouch, opaque. Net price 30 pouches (10 mm hole can be cut to fit up to 55 mm) = £66.78; 30 one-piece pouches with soft cover front and back (opaque: 10–55 mm starter hole) = £66.78

Paediatric, one-piece pouch. Net price 30 pouches (clear or opaque: 10–35 mm starter hole) = £57.75; 30 two-piece pouches, clear or opaque (to fit 40 mm base plates) = £27.18

Post-op, one-piece pouch for high output, clear. Net price 10 large pouches (10–70 mm starter hole) = £25.46

Seal Integral Convexity, one-piece pouch with soft backing. Net price 10 maxi pouches (clear or opaque: 18, 21, 25, 28, 31, 35, 38 or 41 mm holes; clear: 15 mm hole; opaque: 15–33 mm, 15–43 mm starter holes) = £23.06

Note. Should be used only after assessment of suitability by appropriate medical professional

Ileo B® (Coloplast)

One-piece pouch with zinc oxide adhesive, clear or white. Net price 100 pouches (20 mm hole) = £170.60

Mini, one-piece compact pouch with zinc oxide adhesive, white. Net price 100 pouches (20 mm hole) = £169.50

K-Flex® (Coloplast)

One-piece pouch with karaya skin protector, clear. Net price 30 pouches (10 or 40 mm holes) = £76.23

mc2000® (Coloplast)

One-piece pouch with double seal. Net price 30 pouches, clear or opaque (25, 30, 35, 40, or 45 mm holes) = £75.21; clear (20, 50, 55, or 60 mm holes) = £75.21; opaque (10–80 mm holes) = £75.21

Mini, one-piece compact pouch, opaque. Net price 30 pouches (20, 25, 30, 35, or 40 mm holes) = £71.01

mc2002® (Coloplast)

Two-piece pouch, opaque or clear. Net price 30 open pouches (to fit 40 or 60 mm base plates) = £44.25; 30 closed pouches (to fit 40 or 60 mm base plates) = £40.11

pc3000® (Coloplast)

One-piece pouch. Net price 30 pouches, clear or opaque (20, 25, 30, 35, 40, 45, 50, or 60 mm holes) = £68.70; opaque (55 mm hole) = £68.70

Mini starter hole, one-piece pouch. Net price 30 pouches = £62.22

Schacht® (Coloplast)

Ileostomy, one-piece pouches. Net price 50 pouches = £21.00

Ileostomy appliance, odourproof. Net price 1 appliance = £31.03

■ ConvaTec range
Combihesive Natura® (ConvaTec)

Two-piece drainable pouch with or without filter. Net price 10 standard pouches, clear or opaque; small pouches, opaque (to fit 32, 38, 45, 57 or 70 mm flanges) = £11.02; 10 standard size, clear, 100 mm flange = £30.32

Combihesive Natura® High Output (ConvaTec)

Two-piece drainable pouch with filter, opaque, net price 5 pouches (to fit 45, 57 or 70 mm flanges) = £18.24

Consecura® (ConvaTec)

Two-piece drainable pouch. Net price 20 pouches (clear or opaque to fit 35, 45 or 55 mm flanges) = £21.61

Consecura® Low Profile (ConvaTec)

Two-piece drainable pouch, net price 10 pouches (clear or opaque to fit 35, 45, 57, or 70 mm flanges) = £11.00; clear for 100 mm flange) = £18.84

Esteem ® (ConvaTec)

Drainable pouch with integral filter, net price 10 pouches (small, clear or opaque (starter hole 20 mm, pre-cut opaque 25, 30, 40, 50 mm) = £19.57; medium, clear or opaque, (starter hole 20 mm), opaque (pre-cut 25, 30, 40, 50, or 60 mm); large, clear or opaque, (starter hole 20 mm), clear or opaque (pre-cut 25, 30, 40, 50, 60, or 70 mm) = £21.74

Ileodress® (ConvaTec)

Ileodress, one-piece pouch with textured backing. Net price 10 standard pouches (opaque or clear: 19, 38, 45, 50, or 64 mm holes; 19 mm can be cut to fit; opaque only: 25 and 32 mm holes) = £22.41; 10 small pouches with clip, opaque (19, 25, 32, 38, 45, 50, or 64 mm holes; 19 mm can be cut to fit) = £22.15

Ileodress Plus, one-piece pouch single-release paper. Net price 10 standard pouches with clip (opaque or clear: 19, 38, 45, 50, or 64 mm holes; 19 mm can be cut to fit; opaque only: 25 and 32 mm holes) = £22.41; 10 small pouches with clip, opaque (19, 25, 32, 38, 45, or 50 mm holes; 19 mm can be cut-to-fit) = £19.79

Little Ones® (ConvaTec)

Paediatric, one-piece pouch. Net price 15 pouches (8 mm cut-to-fit hole) = £30.83

Naturess® (ConvaTec)

Naturess, one-piece pouch with filter. Net price 20 standard pouches (clear or opaque: 19 mm starter hole; opaque: 25, 32, 38, 45 or 50 mm holes) = £42.74; 20 small pouches (opaque: 19 mm starter hole, 25, 32, 38, 45 or 50 mm holes) = £38.46

Stomadress® (ConvaTec)

One-piece pouch, clear. Net price 10 pouches (8 mm cut-to-fit hole) = £21.79

Surgicare System® 2 (ConvaTec)

System 2, two-piece pouches, white. Net price 10 pouches with clip (to fit 32, 38, 45, 57, or 70 mm flanges) = £11.14

System 2 Combihesive, two-piece pouches with textured backing. Net price 10 standard pouches with clip, beige (to fit 32, 38, 45, 57, or 70 mm flanges) = £11.14; 10 standard pouches with clip, clear, to fit 45, 57, or 70 mm flanges = £11.14, to fit 100 mm flanges = £19.87

■ Dansac range

Dansac® (Dansac)

In Vent, one-piece pouch with filter, anatomically shaped, opaque. Net price 30 pouches (20, 25, 30, 35, 40, 45, 50 mm holes; 15–60 mm cut-to-fit holes) = £64.17

In Vent Convex, integral convexity, one-piece pouch with filter and soft cover, anatomically-shaped. Net price 10 pouches, opaque (15–24 mm, 15–37 mm or 15–46 mm starter holes, 20, 25, 30, 35, 40, or 45 mm pre-cut holes) = £23.00

Note. Should be used only after assessment of suitability by appropriate medical professional

In Vent Symm Convex, integral convexity, one-piece pouch with filter and soft cover, symmetrically-shaped. Net price 10 pouches, clear or opaque (15–24 mm, 15–37 mm or 15–46 mm starter holes, 20, 25, 30, 35, 40, or 45 mm pre-cut holes) = £23.00

InVent Symmetrical, one-piece pouch with filter, symmetrically shaped, clear or opaque. Net price 30 pouches (20, 25, 30, 35, 40, 45 or 50 mm holes; 15–60 mm cut-to-fit holes) = £63.00

Note. Should be used only after assessment of suitability by appropriate medical professional

InVent 2, two-piece drainable pouch with filter, anatomically-shaped, opaque. Net price 10 pouches (36, 43, 55 mm holes) = £11.02

InVent 2 Symmetrical, two-piece pouch with filter, symmetrically-shaped, opaque or clear. Net price 10 pouches (36, 43, 55, 80 mm holes) = £11.02

Nova 2, two-piece drainable pouch, fabric cover, filter, clear or opaque, net price 10 (36, 43, 55 or 70 mm flange) = £11.70

Unique, one-piece pouch, opaque or clear. Net price 30 pouches (20, 25, 30, 35, 40, 45, 50, 60 mm or cut-to-fit holes) = £62.09; oval flange, opaque or clear, starter hole, 30 = £62.09

Unique 2, two-piece pouch, opaque or clear, regular or large. Net price 10 pouches (to fit 36, 43, 55 or 80 mm flange) = £11.02

Unique Infant, one-piece pouch, clear or opaque. Net price 30 pouches (10 mm can be cut to fit 40 mm) = £61.07

Unique Maxi, one-piece pouch. Net price 10 pouches (10 mm can be cut to fit up to 90 mm) = £22.23

Unique Mini, one-piece pouch. Net price 30 pouches (opaque: 20, 25, 30, or 35 mm holes; opaque or clear: 15 mm can be cut to fit up to 50 mm) = £60.11

■ Hollister range

Classic® (Hollister)

Karaya 5® transparent, one-piece pouch with karaya skin protector seal, may be worn with belt. 30- or 40-cm clear pouch with microporous adhesive (series 322 and 327), net price 30 pouches with 1 clamp (25, 32, 38, 44, 51, 64, or 76 mm hole) = £75.37; 30-cm pouches with regular adhesive (series 722) = £75.37

Karaya 5® opaque, one-piece pouch with karaya skin protector seal and porous adhesive, may be worn with belt. Net price 30 pouches with 1 clamp, 23-cm pouches (series 313: 25, 32, 38, 44, or 51 mm holes) = £75.37; 30-cm pouches (series 311: 25, 32, 38, 44, 51, 64, or 76 mm holes) = £73.29

Karaya 5® seal (series 360), one-piece pouch with porous adhesive and karaya skin protector seal, clear. Net price 15 pouches (25, 32, 38, 44, 51, or 64, or 76 mm holes) with 1 clamp = £36.98

Compact® (Hollister)

Drainable, one-piece pouch with comfort backing, net price 10 pouches (beige or clear: 13-64 mm cut-to-fit; 19, 25, 32, 38, 44, 51 or 64 mm) = £22.47

Mini Drainable, one-piece pouch with comfort backing, beige. Net price 10 pouches (13-51 mm cut-to-fit; 19, 25, 32, 38, or 44 mm) = £21.65

Conform 2® (Hollister)

Drainable Pouch, two-piece. Net price 10 pouches, clear (45 or 70 mm holes) = £10.60

Guardian® (Hollister)

Guardian (series 461), two-piece pouch, opaque (64 mm holes with beige non-woven double side backing), net price 10 pouches with 1 clamp = £11.01

Guardian mini-pouch, two-piece compact pouch, opaque. **NHS**: with inner film and replaceable filter (series 463: 25, 38, 51, or 64 mm holes), 10 pouches with pack of filters and 1 clamp

NHS *With replaceable filter* (series 462: 25, 38, 51, or 64 mm holes), two-piece pouch with inner film and replaceable filter, clear. 10 pouches with pack of filters and 1 clamp

Impression® (Hollister)

One-piece pouch with Convex wafer, synthetic seal and Microporous II adhesive, opaque or clear. Net price 10 pouches (19, 22, 25, 29, 32, 35, 38, 41, 44 or 51 mm holes) = £24.28

Impression C® (Hollister)

One-piece pouch with convex wafer, opaque (with double side comfort backing) or clear (with single side comfort backing). Net price 10 pouches (19, 22, 25, 29, 32, 35, 38, 41, 44 or 51 mm holes) = £22.89

Impression CPL® (Hollister)

Two-piece pouch with comfort backing, beige or clear. Net price 10 pouches (38, 44, 57 or 70 mm holes) = £10.81; clear (102 mm hole) = £21.89

Mini Drainable, two-piece pouch with comfort backing, beige. Net price 10 pouches (38, 44, 57 or 70 mm holes) = £10.39

Premium® (Hollister)

Karaya 5® seal with filter (series 366), one-piece pouch with porous adhesive, karaya skin protector seal, and replaceable filter, may be worn with belt, clear. Net price 15 pouches (25, 32, 38, 44, 51, or 64 mm holes) with 1 clamp and filter elements = £40.33

Synthetic seal (series 364), one-piece pouch with porous adhesive and synthetic skin protector seal, clear. Net price 15 pouches (25, 32, 38, 44, 51, or 64 mm holes) with 1 clamp = £36.25

■ **Jade-Euro-Med range**

Rubber bags screwcap (Jade-Euro-Med)

Black butyl, one-piece pouch. Net price 1 day pouch = £28.41; 1 night pouch = £33.14

White rubber, one-piece pouch. Net price 1 day pouch = £15.79; 1 night pouch = £18.09

Rubber bags spout (Jade-Euro-Med)

Black butyl, one-piece pouch. Net price 1 day or night pouch = £30.00

White rubber, one-piece pouch. Net price 1 day pouch = £14.19; 1 night pouch = £14.19

■ **Marlen range**

Ultra® (Marlen)

All with 12, 16, 19, 22, 25, 29, 32, 34, 38, 41, 44, 48, 50, 54, 57, 60, 63, 67, 70, 73, 76 mm or cut-to-fit holes; opaque or clear; small or large

Drainable, one-piece pouch.' Net price 15 pouches = £32.25; with convex flange, 15 pouches = £33.00

■ **Oakmed range**

LOP-F7® (Oakmed)

Ileostomy appliance. Net price 1 appliance = £38.68

Option® (Oakmed)

Mini Ileo, one-piece pouch, opaque or clear, soft cover on both sides. Net price 30 pouches (10–50 mm cut-to-fit holes) = £57.60

Ileostomy, one-piece pouch, opaque or clear. Net price 30 pouches (20, 25, 30, 35, 40, 45 or 50 mm holes) = £57.35

Ileo Oval, one-piece pouch, clear, filter and soft covering on one side, Mackintosh liners, net price 20 (cut-to-fit 20–80 mm) = £65.80

OPR-F® (Oakmed)

Ileostomy appliance. Net price 1 appliance = £80.69

SR-F® (Oakmed)

Ileostomy set. Net price 1 set = £55.60

■ **Pelican range**

Pelican® (Pelican)

Drainable bag (= pouch), formerly Simplaseel®, one-piece pouch, opaque. Net price 30 pouches (26, 32, 40, 45, or 50 mm holes) = £74.15

Paediatric drainable bag (= pouch), one-piece pouch. Net price 30 pouches (7–40 mm cut-to-fit) = £66.43

Pelican Select® (Pelican)

Drainable bag (= pouch), one-piece pouch, with skin protector, clear or opaque. Net price 30 pouches (20–65 mm cut-to-fit; 13, 27, 34, 41, 48 or 55 mm holes) = £64.83

Neonatal pouch, split fabric (plain or printed) front and back, clear or opaque, net price, 30-pouches (10–55 mm cut-to-fit) = £59.02

Paediatric pouch, one-piece pouch with skin protector, fabric both sides, opaque or clear. Net price, 30 pouches (cut-to-fit 10–50 mm) = £58.00

Sassco® (Pelican)

Ileostomy bag (= pouch), one-piece pouch. Net price 100 pouches (26 or 32 mm holes) = £182.28

■ **Rüsch range**

Birkbeck® (Rüsch)

Rubber, one-piece pouch, black or pink. Net price (both 19, 38, or 54 mm holes), 1 day pouch = £27.15; 1 night pouch = £31.05

Disposable, one-piece plastic pouch. Net price 100 pouches = £15.83

Ileostomy appliance. Net price 1 appliance 'A' (19, 38, or 54 mm) = £94.76; 1 appliance 'B' (19, 38, or 54 mm) = £61.17

Ostopore® (Rüsch)

Ileo KAV-opaque, one-piece pouch with karaya seal skin protector, adhesive, and vent, opaque. Net price 30 pouches (25, 32, or 38 mm holes) with 30 belt flanges and 10 clips = £62.92

Rubber bag (Rüsch)

White rubber, one-piece pouch. Net price, 1 day pouch (38, 44, or 51 mm holes) = £12.16; 1 screwcap pouch (38 mm hole) = £13.13; 1 pouch with vent (38 mm hole) = £14.54

White rubber child bag (= pouch), one-piece pouch. Net price (both 19, 25, or 28 mm holes), 1 day pouch = £11.72; 1 night pouch = £14.34

■ **Salts range**

Cohflex® (Salts)

Drainable, one-piece pouch with single-release paper, wafer, and fabric front and back. Net price 30 pouches with integral closure clip (flesh: 25, 30, 35, 40, 45, 50, 55, or 60 mm, flesh or clear, 10–60 mm starter hole) = £64.21

Paediatric drainable, one-piece small pouch with single-release paper, wafer, and fabric backing, opaque/clear/beige. Net price 30 pouches with integral closure clip (10–50 mm cut-to-fit holes) = £56.89

Confidence® (Salts)

Confidence, one-piece pouch, opaque. Net price 30 pouches (13 mm starter hole, 25, 32, 38, 45, or 52 mm holes) = £58.74

Confidence, one-piece pouch, small. Net price 30 pouches (13 mm starter hole, 25, 32, 38, 45 or 52 mm holes) = £46.86

Confidence, one-piece pouch with transparent front. Net price 30 pouches standard (13 mm starter hole) = £56.24; large (13 mm starter hole) = £58.74; with over-lap film (25, 32, 38, 45 or 52 mm holes) = £59.67

Confidence Gold, drainable pouch with hypoallergenic hydrocolloid, and soft beige comfort backing on both sides. Net price 30 pouches, opaque (13 mm starter hole, 25, 32, 35, 38, 45, or 52 mm pre-cut holes) = £60.81, small (13 mm starter hole, 25, 32, 35, 38, 45, or 52 mm pre-cut holes) = £48.51, standard with transparent film (13 mm starter hole) = £58.23, standard with transparent film (25, 32, 38, 45 or 52 mm pre-cut holes) = £61.78, large with transparent film (13 mm starter hole) = £60.81

Confidence Gold with filter, drainable pouch with hypoallergenic hydrocolloid, and soft beige comfort backing on both sides, standard with transparent film, small or opaque. Net price 30 pouches (13 mm starter hole, 25, 32, 35, 38, 45, or 52 mm pre-cut holes) = £63.97

Confidence Gold Easi-Clip, drainable pouch, integral clip and filter, soft beige comfort backing on both sides. Net price 30 pouches small (opaque film) or standard (opaque or transparent film) both (13 mm starter hole, 25, 32, 35, 38, 45, or 52 mm pre-cut holes) = £66.96

Eakin® (Salts)

Drainable, one-piece pouch, clear. Net price 20 small or large pouches (32, 45, or 64 mm holes) = £51.10

Fistula, one-piece pouch with or without remote drainage. Net price 10 infant pouches = £37.45; 10 small pouches = £53.16, 10 medium pouches = £68.76; 10 large pouches = £126.42; 20 wide pouches (90 mm hole) = £105.08

Koenig Rutzen® screwcap (Salts)
All with screwcap outlet
Black butyl all rubber, one-piece pouch. Net price 1 pouch (large: 25, 29, 32, 35, 38, 44, or 51 mm holes; small: 25, 32, 38 or 44 mm holes) = £33.28; with bridge (soft-face Maggie Bag), 1 pouch (large: 25, 32, 38 or 44 mm holes; small: 25, 32, or 38 mm) = £44.65
Black butyl reinforced, one-piece pouch. Net price 1 large or small pouch (25, 32, or 38 mm holes) = £44.65; with bridge (hard-face Maggie Bag), 1 pouch (large: 25, 32, 38, 44, or 51 mm holes; small: 25, 32, or 38 mm) = £52.04

Koenig Rutzen® spout (Salts)
All with spout outlet
Black butyl all rubber, one-piece pouch, net price 1 large pouch (25, 29, 32, 38, 44, or 51 mm holes) or small pouch (25, 32, or 38 mm holes) = £24.89; with bridge, 1 pouch (large: 25, 32, 38, or 51 mm holes) = £32.25
Black butyl reinforced, one-piece pouch. Net price 1 large or small pouch (25, 32, or 38 mm holes) = £33.45; with bridge, 1 pouch (large: 25, 32, 38, 44, or 51 mm holes; small: 25, 32, or 38 mm) = £39.11

Light White® (Salts)
Drainable, one-piece pouch, white. Net price 30 large, small, or medium pouches (all 25, 32, or 38 mm holes) = £50.36
Drainable self-adhesive, one-piece pouch with adhesive, white. Net price 30 pouches (large: 25, 32, 38, or 44 mm holes; small and medium: 25, 32, or 38 mm holes) = £57.01

Rubber bags (Salts)
All must be used with flange
Black butyl screw, one-piece bag with screwcap outlet. Net price 1 large or small pouch = £31.25
Black butyl spout, one-piece bag with spout outlet. Net price 1 large or small pouch = £21.83
White screw, one-piece bag with screwcap outlet. Net price 1 large or small pouch = £10.40
White spout, one-piece bag with spout outlet. Net price 1 large or small pouch = £8.68

Salger® (Salts)
Drainable, one-piece pouch. Net price 10 pouches (40 or 57 mm holes) = £11.73

Second·Nature® (Salts)
Second Nature, two-piece drainable pouch. Net price 30 pouches (opaque: 32, 38, 45 or 57 mm; clear: 45 or 57 mm) = £33.46; secu-ring® to fit 32, 38, 45 or 57 mm flange, 10 = £10.19; wafer (110 × 100 mm to fit 32, 38 or 45 mm flange; 134 × 124 mm to fit 57 mm flange), 5 = £11.47

Simplicity® (Salts)
Drainable, two-piece pouch, clear. Net price 30 230 × 137 mm pouches (40, 50, or 60 mm holes) = £18.91
Post-op, two-piece pouch, clear. Net price 30 300 ×125-mm pouches (40, 50, or 60 mm holes) = £16.42

Simplicity 1® (Salts)
Anatomical, one-piece pouch. Net price clear (cut-to-fit), 30 = £71.37; opaque (30, 40, 50, 60 mm or cut-to-fit holes), 30 = £71.37
Drainable, one-piece pouch with porous adhesive and skin protector seal, fabric front and back. Net price 30 pouches with integral closure clip (opaque or pink: 30, 40, 50, or 60 mm, all may be cut to fit; opaque, clear or pink: 10–60 mm cut-to-fit hole) = £73.22
Paediatric drainable, one-piece pouch with porous adhesive and skin protector seal, clear. Net price 30 pouches (cut-to-fit hole) = £46.16

Simplicity 2® (Salts)
Drainable, two-piece pouch (may also be applied directly to skin). Net price 15 pouches (40, 50, 60, or 70 mm holes, also 30 mm only for direct application to skin) = £19.35
Post-op, two-piece pouch (may also be applied directly to skin). Net price 30 pouches (40, 50, 60, or 70 mm holes, also 30 mm only for direct application to skin) = £39.00
Transverse, two-piece pouch (may also be applied directly to skin). Net price 10 pouches (cut-to-fit hole) = £44.29; 5 flanges = £21.67

■ Shaw range
Rubber bags (Shaw)
Black screwcap, one-piece pouch with screwcap outlet. Net price (both 19, 38 or 54 mm holes), 1 day pouch = £24.13; 1 night pouch = £25.56

■ SIMS Portex range
Adhesive (SIMS Portex)
Stomabag, one-piece pouch with adhesive, opaque. Net price 60 pouches (19, 25, 32, 38, 51 mm or cut-to-fit holes) = £94.01

Cavendish® (SIMS Portex)
Odourproof, one-piece pouch. Net price (all 25, 32, or 38 mm holes), 10 opaque pouches with non-adhesive flange = £31.87; 10 opaque pouches with adhesive flange = £38.15; 10 clear PVC pouches = £31.68

Chiron® screwcap (SIMS Portex)
All with screwcap outlet
Butyl rubber day bag (= pouch), one-piece pouch, black. Net price 1 pouch (38, 44, or 51 mm hole) = £32.95
Butyl rubber night bag (= pouch), one-piece pouch, black. Net price 1 pouch (38 or 44 mm holes) =£39.55
Latex rubber day bag (= pouch), one-piece pouch. Net price 1 pouch (38 mm hole) = £16.74
Latex rubber night bag (= pouch), one-piece pouch. Net price 1 pouch (38 mm hole) = £22.15
White rubber day bag (= pouch), one-piece pouch. Net price 1 pouch (38, 44, or 51 mm) = £18.97, child-size pouch (38 mm hole) = £16.58; body-size outlet, 1 pouch (38 mm hole) = £18.97, child-size pouch (38 mm hole) = £14.97
White rubber night bag (= pouch), one-piece pouch. Net price 1 pouch (38 or 51 mm hole) = £22.15; body-size outlet, 1 pouch (38 mm hole) = £18.13

Chiron® spout (SIMS Portex)
White rubber bag (= pouch), one-piece pouch. Net price 1 day pouch (38 mm hole) = £16.31; 1 night pouch (38 mm hole) = £17.71

EC1® (SIMS Portex)
Ileo classic, one-piece pouch with wafer and comfort backing, opaque. Net price 30 pouches with 1 clamp (19, 25, 32, 38, 44 mm or 10–44 mm cut-to-fit holes) = £72.35
Mini classic, one-piece compact pouch with wafer and comfort backing, opaque or clear. Net price 30 pouches with 1 clamp (10–44 mm cut-to-fit holes) = £72.35
Post-op classic, one-piece pouch with wafer and comfort backing, clear. Net price 30 pouches with 1 clamp, 10–64 mm cut-to-fit holes = £74.63; 10–90 mm cut-to-fit holes = £105.60

Mirage® (SIMS Portex)
Drainable, one-piece pouch, beige or clear. Net price 30 pouches (25, 32, 38, 44, 51 mm or 19–44 mm or 19–64 mm cut-to-fit holes) = £62.64; 10 large outline pouches (beige: 19–90 mm cut-to-fit holes) = £21.82

Omni® (SIMS Portex)
Drainable, one-piece pouch with porous adhesive wafer and replaceable filter. Net price 20 pouches (opaque: 25, 32, 38, 44 mm; opaque or clear: 10–44 mm cut-to-fit hole) = £48.20; ɴʜꜱ opaque (10–90 mm cut-to-fit hole) = £53.39

Redifit® (SIMS Portex)
Opaque, one-piece pouch with karaya skin protector, may be worn with belt. Net price 20 pouches with 2 closure clips (25, 32, 38, 44, 51, or 64 mm holes) = £70.78; small outline pouches, 20 pouches with 2 closure clips (25, 32, or 38 mm holes) = £70.78
Clear fronted, one-piece pouch with karaya skin protector, may be worn with belt. Net price 20 pouches with 2 closure clips (25, 32, 44, 51, or 64 mm holes) = £70.78

■ Ward range
Donald Rose® (Ward)
Bag (= pouch), with celluloid collars, solid, flat or fluid rims. Net price 1 pouch = £19.77
Ileostomy appliance (= pouch). Net price 1 appliance (first stage) = £48.38; 1 appliance (second stage) = £47.86; 1 appliance (new improved) = £50.79

Rubber bags (Ward)

Bag, rubber. Net price 1 pouch, complete with collar = £21.46; 1 pouch, with tap outlet and skirt = £23.98

Night bag (= pouch), shaped rubber with long vertical spring vulcanite screw outlet. Net price 1 pouch = £19.67

Black rubber bag (= pouch), one-piece pouch with screw-cap outlet. Net price (19, 35, or 54 mm hole), 1 day pouch = £18.498 1 night pouch = £19.32

White rubber ileostomy bag (= pouch) with flange, pouch with St. Mark's flange. Net price 1 pouch = £27.95

White rubber ileostomy bag (= pouch), one-piece pouch. Net price 1 day pouch (screwcap or spout outlet) = £12.64; 1 night pouch (screwcap or spout outlet) = £14.21; tap outlet, 1 day pouch = £18.51; 1 night pouch = £20.52

White rubber transverse ileostomy bag (= pouch), one-piece pouch. Net price 1 pouch = £29.54

Urostomy pouches

■ Braun Biotrol range

Biotrol® (Braun Biotrol)

Urostomy bag (= pouch), two-piece pouch, clear. Net price 10 pouches (35, 50 or 75 mm holes) = £23.36

■ Bullen range

Lenbul® (Bullen)

Day bag (= pouch), one-piece pouch. Net price 1 pouch with tap outlet = £14.82; 1 pouch with large opening (for 4-inch flange with tap outlet) = £15.38

Night bag (= pouch). Net price 1 pouch with tap outlet = £16.93; 1 pouch with large opening = £17.57

■ CliniMed range

Welland (CliniMed)

Silhouette 2, urostomy pouch with soft backing and tap, beige or clear, net price (45 mm) 10 pouches = £24.50

Silhouette Uro, urostomy pouch with soft backing. Net price 10 pouches, clear or beige (13, 16, 19, 22, 25, 32, or 38 mm holes) = £40.00

■ Coloplast range

Assura® (Coloplast)

Maxi, urostomy pouch with soft backing, clear or opaque. Net price 30 (one-piece) pouches (10–55 mm hole) = £121.53; two-piece pouch, 30 pouches (to fit 40, 50 or 60 mm base plates) = £72.75

Midi, urostomy pouch with soft backing, clear or opaque. Net price 30 (one-piece) pouches (10–55 mm hole) = £121.53; two-piece pouch, 30 pouches (to fit 40 or 50 mm base plates) = £72.75

Paediatric, urostomy pouches with soft backing, clear or opaque. Net price 30 (one-piece) pouches (10–35 mm hole) = £121.53; two-piece pouch, 30 pouches (to fit 40 mm base plate) = £72.75; 5 paediatric (40 mm) = £14.05

Seal Integral Convexity, urostomy pouch, one-piece, maxi clear or transparent. Net price 10 pouches maxi clear (15, 18, 21, 25, 28 or 31 mm holes) = £39.48; maxi transparent (starter hole (15–33 mm or 15–43 mm) or 35, 38, 41 mm holes) = £39.48

Note. Should be used only after assessment of suitability by appropriate medical professional

Stoma Urine (Coloplast)

Maxi, one-piece pouch with zinc oxide adhesive. Net price 30 pouches (13-mm hole) = £81.54

URO 2002® (Coloplast)

Two-piece pouch. Net price 20 small pouches (100 mL, to fit 40 mm base plate) = £58.80; 20 large pouches (375 mL, to fit 40 or 60 mm base plate) = £58.80

Base plate. Net price 5 plates (40 mm, to fit 10–35 mm stoma) or 5 plates (60 mm, to fit 10–55 mm stoma) = £15.19

■ ConvaTec range

Combihesive Natura® (ConvaTec)

Two-piece drainable pouch with Accuseal® tap. Net price 10 standard pouches (clear or opaque for 32, 38, 45 or 57 mm flange; clear for 70 mm flange); 10 small pouches (opaque for 32, 38, 45 or 57 mm flange) = £24.14

Two-piece drainable pouch with standard tap. Net price 10 small or standard pouches (clear for 32, 38, 45 or 57 mm flange) = £23.56; 10 standard pouches (clear for 70 mm flange) = £25.51; 10 standard pouches (clear for 100 mm flange) = £36.63

Combihesive Natura® Little Ones (ConvaTec)

Urostomy pouch, net price 10 (32 mm) = £24.39

Consecura® Low profile (ConvaTec)

Urostomy pouch with Accuseal® tap, net price 10 pouches (clear or opaque for 35, 45, or 57 mm; opaque for 70 mm flange) = £23.97

Urostomy pouch with fold-up tap, clear, net price 10-pouches (for 35, 45, or 57 mm) = £23.97

Surgicare System® 2 (ConvaTec)

Two-piece pouch, with non-reflux valve, clear. Net price 10 (small or standard) pouches (32, 38, 45, or 57 mm flange) = £23.79; 10 standard pouches (70 mm flange) = £25.76, (100 mm flange) = £38.80

Surgicare System® 2 Combihesive (ConvaTec)

Two-piece pouch with Accuseal® tap, and textured backing, clear. Net price 10 standard pouches (32, 38, 45, or 57 mm flange) = £24.38

Urodress® (ConvaTec)

One-piece pouch with Stomahesive® and tap. Net price 10 pouches (19, 25, 32, 38, or 45 mm holes) = £44.80

Urodress® Deep Convex (ConvaTec)

One-piece pouch, clear, standard. Net price 5 pouches (16, 19, 22, 25, 28, 32, 35 or 38 mm holes) = £19.72

Note. Should be used only after assessment of suitability by appropriate medical professional

■ Dansac range

Unique® 2 (Dansac)

Two-piece pouch, with 1 Dansac® drain tube adaptor, opaque or clear. Net price 10 pouches (to fit 30, 36, 43 or 55 mm flange) = £23.74

■ Hollister range

Classic® (Hollister)

Karaya 5® seal and regular adhesive with attachment for optional belt, one-piece pouch, clear. Net price 20 pouches (series 748, 30-cm pouch: 25, 32, 38, 44, or 51 mm holes) including 1 standard drain tube = £67.91

Regular adhesive with attachment for optional belt, one-piece pouch, clear. Net price 20 pouches (series 747, 30-cm pouch: 25, 32, 38, 44, or 51 mm holes) including 1 standard drain tube = £52.06

Compact® (Hollister)

Urostomy pouch with comfort backing. Net price 10 pouches (13–64 mm cut-to-fit; 13, 16, 19, 25, 32, 38, 44 or 51 mm) = £44.50

First Choice® (Hollister)

Urostomy pouch with synthetic skin barrier and Microporous II® adhesive (series 146). Net price 10 pouches (13–64 mm starter hole, 19, 25, 32, 38, 44, or 51 mm holes) = £46.54

Guardian® (Hollister)

Guardian, two-piece pouch with wide-bore tap and non-reflux valve, clear (with beige, non-woven single side backing) (series 470). Net price 10 pouches (25-cm for max. 25, 38, or 51 mm stomas), including 1 drain tube adaptor = £24.42

Impression® (Hollister)

One-piece pouch with Convex wafer, synthetic seal and Microporous II® adhesive, clear. Net price 10 pouches (13, 16, 19, 22, 25, 29, 32, 35, 38 or 44 mm holes) = £46.54

Impression C® (Hollister)

Closed, one-piece pouch with Convex wafer, comfort backing, clear. Net price 10 pouches (13, 16, 19, 22, 25, 29, 32, 35, 38, 44 or 51 mm holes) = £39.92

Impression CPL® (Hollister)
Two-piece pouch with comfort backing. Net price 10 pouches (38, 44, 57 or 70 mm holes) = £23.79

Lo-profile® (Hollister)
Karaya 5® seal and Microporous II® adhesive with gasket for optional belt, one-piece pouch, with non-reflux valve, clear (series 143). Net price 10 pouches (25-cm pouch: 19, 25, 32, 38, 44, or 51 mm gasket), including 1 Lo-profile® drain tube = £50.28

Moderma Flex® (Hollister)
Urostomy pouch. Net price 10 beige (15–55 mm holes, 20, 25, 30, 35, or 40 mm holes) or clear (15–55 mm holes) = £44.92

■ Jade-Euro-Med range

Rubber bags (Jade-Euro-Med)
Black butyl, one-piece pouch, odourless. Net price 1 day pouch (tap outlet) = £31.59; 1 night pouch (tap outlet) = £33.14
White rubber, one-piece pouch. Net price 1 day pouch (tap outlet) = £15.79; 1 night pouch (tap outlet) = £18.09

■ Marlen range

Ultra® (Marlen)
Urostomy pouch, clear. Net price 10 (small or large; flat or shallow convex) pouches (12 mm starter hole, 12, 16, 19, 22, 25, 29, 32, 34, 38, 41, 44, 48, 50, 54, 57, 60, 63, 67, 70, 73, or 76 mm holes) = £39.24

■ Oakmed range

Urostomy sets (Oakmed)
Urostomy sets. Net price 1 LOP-U appliance (wire ring retainer with 1.5-inch elastic belt for small flange, 10 one-piece flanges and lightweight bags with 1-inch hole, 30 3.5 × 3.5-inch double-sided adhesive plasters) = £38.68; 1 OPR-U appliance (waterproof canvas retaining shield waistband, 2 one-piece flanges and bags with 1- or 2-inch hole and tap outlet, 30 3.5 × 3.5-inch double-sided adhesive plasters) = £80.69; 1 SR-U appliance (plastic retainer ring shield with 1-inch elastic belt for medium flange, Lenbul® 1.5-inch diameter flange, 1 Lenbul® day and 1 night bag with tap outlet, 30 3.5 × 3.5-inch double-sided adhesive plasters) = £60.60

■ Rüsch range

Rubber bags (Rüsch)
Black rubber (Birkbeck®), one-piece pouch with tap outlet. Net price 1 day pouch (19 mm hole) = £31.05; 1 night pouch (19 mm hole) = £33.88
Pink rubber, one-piece pouch with tap outlet. Net price 1 day pouch (19 mm hole) = £31.05; 1 night pouch (19 mm hole) = £33.88
White rubber, one-piece pouch with tap outlet. Net price 1 day pouch (19, 25, or 28 mm holes) = £16.87; 1 night pouch (19, 25, or 28 mm holes) = £17.32
White rubber (Glasgow), one-piece pouch. Net price 1 pouch (small or large tap) = £20.60
White rubber transverse, one-piece pouch. Net price 1 left or right pouch (small, medium, or large) = £20.60

■ Salts range

Confidence® (Salts)
Urostomy pouch, one-piece, with overlap film and 2 drain tube connectors, clear. Net price 10 pouches (13 mm starter hole or 25, 32, 38, 45 mm holes) = £38.00

Koenig Rutzen® (Salts)
All rubber white rubber tap bag (= pouch), one-piece pouch with tap outlet. Net price 1 small or medium pouch (both 25, 32, or 38 mm holes) or 1 large pouch (25, 32, 38, 44, or 51 mm holes) = £16.89
All rubber black butyl bag (= pouch), one-piece pouch with tap outlet and non-reflux valve. Net price 1 medium or large pouch (both 19, 25, 32, or 38 mm holes) = £40.79; special size holes also available to order
All rubber MB black butyl bag (= pouch), one-piece pouch with tap outlet, bridge, and non-reflux valve. Net price 1 small, medium, or large pouch (all 19, 25, 32, or

38 mm holes) = £47.70; special size holes also available to order
Black butyl, reinforced bag (= pouch), one-piece pouch with tap outlet and non-reflux valve. Net price 1 medium or large pouch (both 19, 25, 32, or 38 mm holes) = £50.00; special size holes also available to order
MB black butyl, reinforced bag (= pouch), one-piece pouch with tap outlet and non-reflux valve. Net price 1 medium or large pouch (both 19, 25, 32, or 38 mm holes) = £57.27; special size holes also available to order

Light White® (Salts)
Urostomy pouch with Realistic® washer, one-piece pouch, white. Net price 20 large pouches (all 25, 32, or 38 mm holes) = £110.59
Urostomy pouch with Realistic® washer, one-piece pouch, clear. Net price 20 large or small pouches (all 25, 32, or 38 mm holes) = £110.80
Urostomy pouch, one-piece pouch, white. Net price 20 large pouches (25, 32, or 38 mm holes) = £84.34
Urostomy pouch, one-piece pouch, clear. Net price 20 large or small pouches (25, 32, or 38 mm holes) = £84.34
Urostomy pouch, one-piece pouch with adhesive, white. Net price 20 large pouches (25, 32, or 38 mm holes) = £88.19
Urostomy pouch, one-piece pouch with adhesive, clear. Net price 20 large or small pouches (both 25, 32, or 38 mm holes) = £88.19

Rubber bags (Salts)
Black rubber bag (= pouch) (for use with flange), two-piece pouch with tap outlet. Net price 1 small, medium, or large pouch = £38.51; special size holes also available to order
White rubber bag (= pouch) for use with flange, two-piece pouch with tap outlet. Net price 1 small, medium, or large pouch = £11.25

Second Nature® (Salts)
Urostomy pouch, two-piece, clear. Net price 10 pouches (32, 38, 45 or 57 mm holes), including 1 drain tube connector = £23.30

Simplicity 1® (Salts)
Paediatric Uri-bag, one-piece pouch, 13 mm starter hole. Net price 15 pouches = £42.68

■ SIMS Portex range

Carshalton® (SIMS Portex)
Bag (= pouch), one-piece pouch. Net price 10 oval or triangular pouches (both 25, 32, or 38 mm) with acrylic plaster = £20.10
Set, one-piece pouch. Net price 20 oval or triangular pouches with plasters, bodyplate, clamp, connector, and medium belt (both 25, 32, or 38 mm holes) = £67.39

Chiron® Non-disposable (SIMS Portex)
Butyl rubber bag (= pouch), one-piece pouch with stopcock outlet, odourless, black. Net price 1 day bag (22 mm) = £35.97
Latex rubber bag (= pouch), one-piece pouch with stopcock outlet. Net price (both 38 mm) 1 day bag = £24.92; 1 night bag = £28.26
Rubber child-size bag (= pouch), one-piece pouch with stopcock outlet, white. Net price 1 = £20.91
Rubber day bag (= pouch), one-piece pouch, white with stopcock outlet. Net price 1 (38 mm) = £24.92
Rubber night bag (= pouch), one-piece, white. Net price 1 (38, 44, or 51 mm) = £28.26

Chiron® (SIMS Portex)
Ileal bladder appliance, set comprises 1 web and elastic belt 25 mm wide, 1 wire pressure frame, 1 St Mark's pattern rubber flange (without diaphragm), 2 rubber day pouches with stopcock outlet, 30 double-sided plasters. Net price = £78.04

Mirage® (SIMS Portex)
Urostomy pouch. Net price 10 pouches (beige: up to 44 mm cut-to-fit holes) = £40.77

Mitcham® (SIMS Portex)
Maxi, one-piece pouch. Net price 10 pouches with adhesive flange (25, 32, or 38 mm) = £40.96, 10 pouches with nonadhesive flange (25, 32, or 38 mm) = £33.45
Mini, one-piece pouch. Net price 10 pouches with adhesive flange (19, 25, or 32 mm) = £40.96, 10 pouches with nonadhesive flange (25 mm or 32 mm) = £33.45
Standard, one-piece pouch. Net price 10 pouches with adhesive flange (19, 25, 32 or 38 mm) = £40.96, 10 pouches with nonadhesive flange (19, 25, 32, or 38 mm) = £33.45, 1 pouch with nonadhesive flange and foam pads (25, 32, or 38 mm) = £5.63
Rediflow® (SIMS Portex)
Adhesive set, may be worn with belt. Net price 20 pouches (19, 25, 32, 38, 44, or 51 mm) = £60.18

■ Ward range
Ward® (Ward)
Ureterostomy bag (= pouch) with tap outlet. Net price 1 night pouch = £20.19; 1 day pouch (19, 35, or 54 mm hole) = £18.91

Adhesive preparations, adhesive removers and deodorants

■ Adhesive preparations
Hollister® (Hollister)
Medical adhesive spray (with silicones). Net price 90-g aerosol spray = £14.45
Universal remover wipes, net price (50 wipes) = £12.00
Latex adhesive solution (Salts)
Net price per tube = £1.96. Label: 15
Skin adhesive (Manfred Sauer)
Synthetic. Net price 2 × 28 g tube with long nozzle = £13.95; 45 mL bottle with brush = £13.95
Original Latex. Net price 2 × 28 g tube with long nozzle = £7.95

■ Adhesive removers
Citrus Fresh (Pelican)
Adhesive remover, net price 30-sachets = £8.23
Clear Peel® (CliniMed)
Adhesive remover. Net price 50 mL = £2.10
Hollister® (Hollister)
Adhesive remover spray. Net price 76-g spray = £12.11
Universal remover wipes, net price (50 wipes) = £12.00
Lift® (AlphaMed)
Medical adhesive remover. Net price 30 sachets = £7.95
Salts 'SPR' Plaster Remover (Rezolve)® (Salts)
Adhesive remover spray. Net price 70-g aerosol spray = £2.92. Label: 15

■ Deodorants
Atmocol® is used as a deodorising spray when emptying the appliance. The other deodorants listed are placed in the appliance.
Atmocol® (Adams)
Aerosol deodorant. Net price 1 unit (400 sprays) = £2.01
Chironair Odour Control Liquid® (SIMS Portex)
Deodorant solution. Net price 113 g = £5.85
Citrus Fresh® (Pelican)
Deodorant spray. Net price 50 mL = £3.56
Coloplast OAD® (Coloplast)
Deodorant. Net price 36 mL = £4.16
Colostomy Plus® (Shannon)
Deodorant. Net price 1 unit = £2.73
Day-drop® (Loxley)
Deodorant solution. Net price 7.5 mL = £1.07; 15 mL = £1.78; 30 mL = £3.04 (7.5 and 15 mL also available as Lemon Day-drop®)
Dor® (Pelican)
Deodorant solution. Net price 7 mL = £1.91
Forest Breeze® (Shaw)
Deodorant. Net price 1 unit = £3.40

Friends Ostomy Deodorant Spray (Anglo Venture)
Cinnamon, lemon, or victorian rose, net price 75 mL = £3.55
LiMone® (CliniMed)
Deodorant spray, net price 50 mL = £4.26
NaturCare® (AlphaMed)
Deodorant spray: NaturCare, Fragrant Zest, Grapefruit, or Breeze, net price 50 mL = £3.69
Nodor S® (Dansac)
Deodorant. Net price 50 mL = £3.91; 250 mL = £8.01
Ostobon® (Coloplast)
Deodorant powder. Net price 22 g = £4.17
Saltair No-Roma® (Salts)
Deodorant solution. Net price 28 mL = £2.37; 227 mL = £7.74
Translet Plus One® (Rüsch)
Deodorant solution for men. Net price 7 mL = £2.93
Translet Plus Two® (Rüsch)
Deodorant solution for women. Net price 7 mL = £2.93

Adhesive devices and rings

■ Bullen range
Adhesive plaster, double-sided. Net price 10 zinc oxide plasters 3.5 × 3.5 inch = £4.11, 4 × 4 inch = £5.07, 5 × 5 inch = £8.57; 10 acrylic base plasters 3.5 × 3.5 inch = £3.69, 4 × 4 inch = £4.74, 5 × 5 inch = £7.97
Flange retention strips. Net price 100 strips 4 × 1 inch = £3.68, 4 × 2 inch = £4.98

■ Rüsch range
Ostomy plasters, double-sided. Net price 25 plasters (25 mm hole, or no hole) = £6.61

■ Salts range
Kidney seals. Net price 10 = £4.47
Reliaseal® (Salts)
Adhesive discs, double-sided, round, hypo-allergic. Net price 10 discs (13, 19, 22, 25, 29, 32, or 38 mm) = £17.32
Secuplast® (Salts)
Plasters, circular. Net price 10 plasters (32, 38, 45 or 57 mm) = £9.68
Transacryl® (Salts)
Adhesive plasters, double-sided. Net price 10 plasters (25, 32, or 38 mm) = £5.70
Zopla® (Salts)
Adhesive plasters, double-sided. Net price (both 25, 32, or 38 mm) 10 square plasters = £4.28; 10 round plasters = £4.97

■ Shannon range
Adhesive plasters, double-sided. Net price 25 plasters = £15.17
Rings. Net price 5 rubber retaining rings = £6.06; 1 plastic locking ring = £2.26
Easychange® (Shannon)
Adhesive plasters, with rings (spare). Net price 5 plasters = £6.00

■ Shaw range
Adhesive plasters, double-sided, hole cut-to-size. Net price 10 plasters, 4 × 4 inch = £7.63; 5 × 5 inch = £7.91

■ SIMS Portex range
Adhesive discs, double-sided. Net price 10 discs (76 mm diameter: 19 or 25 mm opening; 90 mm diameter: 32 or 38 mm opening) = £4.88
Rings, elastic, for use with spout bags. Net price 3 rings = £2.26
Carshalton® (SIMS Portex)
Adhesive plasters. Net price both (25, 32, or 38 mm) 10 acrylic plasters = £4.88; 10 zinc oxide plasters = £7.73

Chiron® (SIMS Portex)

Adhesive plasters, double-sided. Net price 10 plasters (90 mm square: 19 or 35 mm hole) = £6.23, (102 mm square: 19 or 35 mm hole) = £7.16, (127 mm square: 19 or 35 mm hole) = £7.89, (150 mm square and 102 × 76 mm: both 19 mm hole) = £8.82, (90 and 102 mm square: both 25 mm hole) = £8.82, (125 mm square: 25 mm hole) = £9.68

Clearseal plasters. Net price 10 plasters (100 mm square: 19 or 35 mm hole) = £7.16

Kidney seals, adhesive flange retaining strips. Net price 10 strips (small or large) = £4.87

■ Ward range

Adhesive plasters, double-sided with opening. Net price 10 plasters = £4.50

Waterproof plasters, single-sided. Net price 10 (100 mm × 25 mm) = £1.23; 10 (100 mm × 50 mm) = £1.85

Bag closures

Clamps

Available from *Braun Biotrol* (Biotrol® for post-op pouches, 1 clamp = £1.01), *CliniMed* (for drainable pouches, 1 clamp = £1.05), *Coloplast* (20 clamps = £18.00), *Hollister* (for drainable pouches, 1 clamp = £1.04, 20 = £17.30; for Premium® pouches, 1 clamp = £1.08, 20 = £18.33), *SIMS Portex* (10 clamps = £8.56; Carshalton®, 5 clamps = £9.95)

Clips

Available from *ConvaTec* (10 beige clips = £2.93; for Surgicare System® 2; drainable, 10 curved clips = £5.19); *Pelican* (drainable, 20 = £6.07); *Salts* (5 clips = £1.89; for drainable pouches, 10 clips = £6.65), *SIMS Portex* (for odourproof pouches, 10 = £6.61)

Closing Tape

Available from *Shannon* (1 reel = £1.47)

Fastening Ring

Rubber pouch fastening ring. Available from *Shaw* (1 ring = £1.10)

Ties

Available from *CliniMed* (30 soft-end ties, white or beige for drainable pouches = £2.56), *ConvaTec* (50 soft wire ties = £5.16), *Dansac* (50 soft wire ties = £5.33); 50 longer soft wire ties = £6.11

Bag covers

Bullen

Bag cover, cloth, for day or night bags. Net price 1 cover = £8.27

CliniMed

Bag cover, cloth for closed or drainable pouches. Net price 5 covers = £8.32

Bag shields, spunbonded polypropylene. Net price 10 shields (small: 25–44 mm; large: 10, 51, or 60 mm) = £3.15

Coloplast

Bag cover, cloth for closed or drainable mc2000® or mc2002® pouches (white or flesh), for mc2000® Mini pouches (decorated: white or flesh), for Ileo B® standard pouches, or for URO2002® pouches (white). Net price 5 covers = £22.65

Cover Care

Bag cover, formerly Surgicare System® 2 pouch covers. Net price 3 covers (for 32/38 mm Mini pouches or 45/57 mm pouches) = £6.81; 3 covers (for standard drainable pouches, urostomy pouches, large urostomy pouches, small closed 38/45 mm pouches: small drainable pouches, combihesive closed pouches, medium closed pouches: 57 and 70 mm) = £7.21

Hollister

Bag cover, non-woven. Net price 5 covers (for closed pouch) = £4.68

Impharm

Ostocover® bag cover, cloth, white or coloured. Net price 3 covers = £6.86

Jade-Euro-Med

Bag cover, cloth. Net price 1 cover = £4.39

Pelican

Bag cover, cotton, for closed pouch. Net price 5 covers, normal = £10.99, casual = £10.93; for drainable pouch, 5 covers = £11.36

Respond Plus

Coversure, bag cover, custom-made (appliance to be stated). Net price 1 cover = £8.27

Rüsch

Bag cover, cloth for Ostopore® pouches. Net price 5 covers (small or large) = £17.38

Salts

Bag covers, cotton, appliance to be stated. Net price 1 cover = £3.71. Cloth, for Eakin® pouches, 1 cover small or large (both 32, 45 or 64 mm) = £4.31

Shaw

Bag covers, cloth. Net price 1 day pouch cover, cotton = £5.01; lycra = £5.29. 1 night cover, cotton = £5.29; lycra = £5.67

SIMS Portex

Bag cover. Net price 1 day or night cotton pouch cover = £10.77; 5 stomabag covers (white or coloured) = £24.16; for Redifit® pouches, 1 cotton cover (25 and 32 mm, 38, 44, and 51 mm, 64, and 75 mm holes) = £7.68; for Symphony® pouches, 5 polyethylene covers = £4.47

Ward

Bag cover, white linen. Net price 1 cover = £6.52

Belts

Braun Biotrol

Almarys, twin belt (support), for two-piece system, net price (120 mm belt) = £4.29

Waist belt for Biotrol® pouches. Net price 1 belt = £4.14

Bullen

Belts. Net price 1.5-inch elastic belt with wire or plastic ring retainer (wire; small, medium, or large) = £9.99; 4-inch belt (wire; small, medium, or large) = £14.21; 1-inch elastic belt with plastic ring shield = £10.57: 1 waterproof canvas retaining shield (small, medium, or large) = £15.33; 1 St Mark's = £41.03

Girdles. Net price 1 Camilla® panty girdle = £18.93; 1 Cloe® roll on girdle = £15.78; 1 Constance® panty girdle = £25.02

J. Chawner

Girdles. Net price 1 ostomy girdle = £31.95; 1 ostomy-panty girdle = £28.90; 1 colostomy belt with understraps = £31.30

Coloplast

Belts. For Ileo B® pouches, net price 1 belt = £7.77; for K-Flex® pouches, 1 belt = £5.93; for Assura® pouches, 1 seal belt = £5.93

ConvaTec

Belt, for Surgicare System® 2. Net price 1 belt = £2.93

Cover Care

Belt. Net price 1 male support belt, small (26–30 inch), medium (31–35 inch), large (36–40 inch), extra large (41–45 inch = £26.10; provision for hole aperture = £5.00

Dansac

Belts. 1 elastic, adjustable (50–90 cm) ostomy belt with soft backing, plus 5 plates. Net price, Ostomy® for one-piece pouches = £36.20; Unique 2 Ostomy® for two-piece pouches = £36.20

Hollister

Belt. Net price 1 adjustable ostomy belt (small, medium, or large) = £6.79; 10 = £56.52

Jade-Euro-Med

Belts. Net price 3-inch belt = £14.80: 3-inch one-piece belt, = £19.31; 4-inch one-piece belt = £19.52; 1-inch web and elastic with button and buckle fastening = £8.21; 2-inch belt = £9.72; 3-inch belt = £11.20: 1 girdle and panti-brief with hole for stoma and suspenders or understrap = £47.92; 1 St Mark's (male or female) = £56.57; 1 St Mark's Coutil ostomy = £38.71

Marlen

Belt. Net price 1 adjustable elastic waist belt = £2.65

Omex

Belt for Schacht® pouches. Net price 36 inch belt = £5.36

Orthotic

Belt. Net price 1 ostomy girdle with hole, zip and suspenders (white) = £31.95

Peacock

Belts. Net price 1 St Mark's belt = £38.15

Respond Plus

Lightweight support belt, 13 cm wide, hook and eye or velcro fastening, with hole. Net price (small, medium, large, or extra large) = £24.14

Ostomy girdle/pantie brief, with hole and suspenders. Net price 1 = £38.31; medium control = £31.67

Otoshield® belt, net price (45/85 cm or 66/124 cm belt) = £3.20

Seamless belt, two-way stretch (unisex), net price (26 cm deep belt available in small, medium, large, X large, or XX large) = £21.00; 33 cm deep belt available in small, medium, large, X large, or XX large) = £23.50

Rüsch

Belts. Net price 5 elastic waistbands (Birkbeck®) = £34.47; 5 elastic waistbands with shields = £45.34; 5 retaining rings (19, 38, or 54 mm) = £8.60. 1 narrow or normal width belts (Ostopore®, waist: 17–34 inch or 28–56 inch) = £5.54. White rubber belting 28 mm = £3.77/ metre, 72 mm = £7.78/metre. White sausage belt per metre = £7.75. 1 waist and support strap = £6.40

Sallis

Belts. Net price 1 night belt, 14b = £10.99; 14c = £5.73; 1 day belt, 15a = £30.27. 1 zipped pocket (to fit 15a and 16) = £5.14; 1 St Mark's = £27.75, 1 shield = £10.05

Salts

Belts. Net price 25 mm elastic belt (single), with 2 loops (standard 35 inch or extra-large 42 inch) = £3.43; with suspender ends = £4.02; double elastic with 4 loops = £5.83; with waterproof panel 102 mm = £14.09, 150 mm = £17.15; with 4 loops and retaining ring = £18.52. 1 rubber belt with straps and buckles = £6.73; with 2 fastening studs = £3.95. 25 mm button belt with or without loop = £3.43. 1 baby lycra belt = £13.84; with Velcro fastening (standard 35 inch or extra-large 42 inch) = £3.49. 1 colostomy belt = £70.54. 1 ileostomy girdle (Saltair®) = £45.06; 1 ileostomy elastic night belt (Salt-air®) = £13.69. For Eakin® pouches, 1 elastic belt (small or large) = £3.39. For Salger® pouches, 1 elastic adjustable belt = £3.52; with Velcro fastening = £3.46

SASH

Belt. Net price 50 mm made to measure stoma hernia support belt, attached to plastic flange with hole over stoma = £30.75

Shannon

Belt. Net price 1 elastic belt with shield and Velcro fastening = £7.45; with button and buckle fastening = £4.53

Shaw

Belts, colostomy, all made to measure. Net price 4 inch elastic web belt = £14.33; with under-strap or suspenders, 6 inch = £19.20, 8 inch = £27.56; with lace fastenings, 6 inch = £25.96; 8 inch = £32.90; 10 inch = £31.29; 12 inch = £34.38; 14 inch = £35.07; with zip panel, 10 inch = £39.49; 12 inch = £41.88; 14 inch = £43.84; elastic with nylon fronts, 10 inch = £36.72; 12 inch = £38.57; 14 inch = £41.04. 1 adjustable colostomy/ ileostomy belt = £8.31; 4 inch (3 sections) = £21.02; 6 inch (3 sections) = £26.50. 1 colostomy night belt (net or rayon, no hole, for use with dressing pad) = £15.30. 4 inch ostomy belt with groin strap = £16.39; with lace fastenings = £17.42; with wire spring = £16.04; double zip panel = £8.31

SIMS Portex

Belts. Net price 25 mm web and elastic belt (WL002 range) = £10.49; 51 mm = £12.23; 75 mm = £13.70; (WL008) 25 mm = £11.46; 1 belt, child (25 mm) = £8.82, 38 mm = £12.28. 1 web and belt with buckle (short) = £7.08. 1 narrow belt (flange diameter: 32, 38, or 51 mm) = £21.81. 1 Redifit adjustable belt (small,

medium, or large) = £8.82. 1 non-slip belt = £17.98; 1 elastic non-slip belt = £12.28. 1 rubber belt ('sausage' or tubular) = £22.91; 1 narrow belt = £6.66. 1 two-way stretch night belt (small, medium, large, or extra-large) = £24.59. 1 stoma belt (small: 17–26 inch or medium: 26–43 inch) = £5.83. 1 Carshalton® belt (small, medium, or large) = £9.30

Ward

Belts. Made to measure, all sizes. Net price 1 day belt = £41.16; 1 night belt = £30.30. 1 nylon elastic colostomy belt, with hook and eye fastening and 2 pairs of suspenders or understraps = £42.52. 1 wide rubberised ileostomy belt with 2 straps and buttonholed ends for use with ileostomy boxes or with celluoid hook ends for use with ileostomy bags = £24.15. 1 belt with understraps or suspenders = £27.15. 1 colostomy belt, with 2 pairs of understraps or suspenders (Gabriel®) = £48.05. 1 web and elastic belt with button and buckle fastening. 1 belt (1 inch) = £7.83; 2 inch = £10.10; 3 inch = £11.47. 1 plastic elastic belt with hook end = £10.93. 1 belt with windows for use with ileostomy bags or colostomy cups or 4 stiched holes for studs of colostomy cups or shields. Net price 35 = £4.38

Filters and bridges

Filters

Available from *Braun Biotrol* (Biotrol®, 50 filters = £11.79), *Coloplast* (Filtrodor®, 50 filters = £19.45; Maclet®, 20 filter washers = £27.48); *Cuxson* (50 patches = £3.12), *Hollister* (replacement filter elements for series 366 drainable bags, 20 = £2.97, 100 = £14.61), *SIMS Portex* (for Beta® and Omni® bags, 20 = £7.44; Doublesure®, 10 filters = £3.52; for Mirage® bags, 20 = £4.07)

Bridges

Available from *Salts* (20 metal bridges ready fixed to lightweight and LWU disposable bags = £9.11; 30 bridges for use with other disposable bags = £13.65), *SIMS Portex* (20 bridges = £3.16)

Flanges

Braun Biotrol

Flanges. Net price 5 flanges for Biotrol® Lockring 2 pouches (35, 50 or 75mm) = £12.47; 5 hydrocolloid flanges (35, 50, 62 or 75 mm) = £12.23

Bullen

Flanges. Net price 1 flange for Lenbul® pouches (1 inch diameter, 2 inch base) = £9.01; 1.5 inch diameter, 3 inch base = £13.71; 2 inch diameter, 4 inch base = £16.00

Coloplast

Flanges for Assura® Seal Integral Convexity pouches. Net price 5 (40 mm flange, 15, 18, 21 mm hole) = £13.94; 5 (50 mm flange, 25, 28, 31 mm hole or 15–33 mm starter hole) = £13.94; 5 (60 mm flange, 35, 38 or 41 mm hole or 15–43 mm starter hole) = £13.94

Note. Should be used only after assessment of suitability by appropriate medical professional

St Mark's flange with inner sheath. Net price 1 flange, all 16 mm deep (76 mm base, 25 or 32 mm diameter; 100 mm base, 35, 38, 45 or 50 mm diameter) = £12.97

ConvaTec

Flanges for Surgicare System® 2. Net price 10 Accordion® flanges, 100 × 100 mm (70 mm hole) = £39.52; 127 ×127 mm (100 mm hole), 10 = £69.77. Combihesive® flexible flanges, 100 × 100 mm (32, 38, or 45 mm hole), 10 = £27.37; 127 × 127 mm (57 or 70 mm hole), 10 = £29.78. Stomahesive® flexible flanges, 100 mm × 100 mm (32, 38, 45 or 57 mm hole), 10 = £24.49. Stomahesive® flanges, 100 × 100 mm (32, 38, 45, 57 or 70 mm holes) 10 = £24.49; 127 ×127 mm (70 mm hole), 10 = £49.14; 152 × 152 mm (100 mm hole), 10 = £58.98. For Combihesive Natura® pouches, 5 flexible flanges (32, 38, 45, 57 or 70 mm holes) = £13.76. For Consecura® pouches, 10 locking flanges (35, 45 or 55 mm holes) = £25.95

Dansac

Convex flanges for Unique® 2 pouches. Net price 5 (36 mm flange: 20, 25 mm or cut-to-fit 15–25 mm hole) = £13.67; 5 (43 mm flange: 25, 30 mm or cut-to-fit 15–32 mm hole) = £13.67; 5 (55 mm flange: 35, 40 mm or cut-to-fit 15–44 mm hole) = £13.67

Flexi flanges for Unique® 2 urostomy pouches. Net price 5 (36 mm flange: 20, 25 mm hole or cut-to-fit 15–28 mm hole); 5 (43 mm flange: 30 mm hole or cut-to-fit 15–35 mm hole); 5 (55 mm flange: 35, 40 mm hole or cut-to-fit 15–47 mm hole) = £13.64; 5 (80 mm flange: 45, 50 mm hole or cut-to-fit 15–70 mm hole) = £13.91.

Nova 2 flange, flange 36 mm, net price 5 (starter hole 15–28 mm, pre-cut 20 or 25 mm); flange 43 mm, 5 (starter hole 15–35 mm, pre-cut 25 or 30 mm); flange 55 mm, 5 (starter hole 15–47 mm, pre-cut 35 or 40 mm); flange 70 mm, 5 (starter hole 15–60 mm, pre-cut 45 or 50 mm) = £13.95

S flanges for Unique® 2 urostomy pouches. Net price 5 (30 mm flange: 15 mm hole or cut-to-fit 10–22 mm hole); 5 (36 mm flange: 20, 25 mm hole or cut-to-fit 15–28 mm hole); 5 (43 mm flange: 30 mm hole or cut-to-fit 15–35 mm hole); 5 (55 mm flange: 35, 40 mm hole or cut-to-fit 15–47 mm hole) = £13.20; 5 (80 mm flange: 45, 50 mm hole or cut-to-fit 15–70 mm hole) = £13.18

Note. Should be used only after assessment of suitability by appropriate medical professional

Hollister

Fixed Flanges for Conform 2® pouches. Net price 5 (45 mm flange: 30, 35, 40 mm or cut-to-fit 13–40 mm hole) = £13.00; (70 mm flange: 45 mm or cut-to-fit 13–55 mm hole) = £13.00

Floating Flanges for Conform 2® pouches. Net price 5 (45 mm flange: cut-to-fit 13–30 mm hole) = £13.00; (70 mm flange: 40, 45 mm or cut-to-fit 13–55 mm hole) = £13.00

Flanges for Impression® pouch. Net price 5 Convex flanges with synthetic seal and Microporous adhesive (13, 16, 19, 22, 25, 29, 32, 35, 38, 41, 44 or 51 mm holes) = £13.90; Impression® CPL convex flange (13, 16, 19, 22, 25, 29, 32, 35, 38, 41, 44 or 51 mm holes), 5 = £14.16; Tandem floating flanges with either barrier and adhesive (19, 25, 32, 38, 44, 51 or 57 mm hole) or barrier only (25, 32, 44, 57 cut-to-fit hole), net price 5 = £13.03 or barrier only (89 mm cut-to-fit hole) 5 = £13.51

Jade-Euro-Med

Flanges. Net price 1 St Mark's soft rubber = £13.41; with diaphragm = £13.41

Omex

Flanges, for Schacht® pouches. Net price 1 Colo flange with locking ring = £5.40; 1 Ileo flange with locking ring = £5.40.

Rüsch

Flange. Net price 2 Birkbeck® white rubber flanges (75 mm base, 16 mm deep, 20 mm diameter); 90 mm base, 16 mm deep, 38 mm diameter; 110 mm base, 16 mm deep, 58 mm diameter = £22.77; St Mark's, in two rubbers with hard centre (76 mm base, 10 or 16 mm deep, 32 or 38 mm diameter), 2 flanges = £34.12; 76 mm base, 13 or 16 mm deep, 25 mm diameter, 2 flanges = £34.12; 102 mm base, 16 mm deep, 44 or 51 mm diameter, 2 flanges = £34.12; in soft honey coloured rubber (51 or 76 mm base, 13 mm deep, 25 mm diameter), 2 flanges = £19.90; (76 mm base, 10 or 16 mm deep, 32 or 38 mm diameter), 2 flanges = £19.90; 102 mm base, 16 mm deep, 44 or 51 mm diameter, 2 flanges = £19.90; with diaphragm, cowl, or dressing retainer at extra cost = £3.24: black, firm rubber (51 mm base, 13 mm deep, 25 mm diameter), 2 flanges = £22.77; 76 mm base, 10 or 16 mm deep, 32 or 38 mm diameter, 2 flanges = £22.77; 102 mm base, 16 mm deep, 44 or 51 mm diameter, 2 flanges = £22.77

Salts

Flange. Net price 1 flange (SF1, soft rubber, 25 mm) = £7.25; SF4, soft rubber, 38 mm = £7.36; SF5, semi-rigid, 38 mm = £12.62; SF6, semi-rigid, hard rubber = £8.41; SF8R, flexible, recessed, 32 mm = £11.65. 1 baby flange

with diaphragm (19 mm) = £9.65. 1 Latex foam diaphragm flange = £41.15; 1 sheath for use with flange = £6.84. For Salger® pouches, 1 polythene flange (40 or 57 mm) = £2.04

Shannon

Flange ring. Net price 1 = £2.27

Shaw

Flange. Net price 1 rubber, adhesive = £6.01; rubber, non-stick = £7.27; with diaphragm = £9.46; non-stick inner diaphragm £2.82; 1 colostomy rubber foam face-piece (face hole diameter: 1.75, 2, 2.5, or 3 inch) = £11.00

SIMS Portex

Flange. Net price 1 rubber flange (16 mm deep, 38 mm diameter) = £16.39; double base hole (38 mm diameter) = £21.72; blue rubber (51 mm base, 13 mm deep, 25 mm diameter or 76 mm base, 10 or 16 mm deep, 38 mm diameter) = £14.83; blue and brown, (76 mm base, 13 mm deep, 25 mm diameter; 10 or 16 mm deep, 38 mm diameter) = £21.52. 1 belt flange (19, 25, 32, 44, 51, or 64 mm) = 27p. For Chiron® pouches, 1 flange (10 or 16 mm deep, 38 mm diameter) = £16.39; 13 mm deep, 25 mm diameter = £16.39; 16 mm deep, 32 mm diameter = £16.39; plastic without diaphragm (13 mm deep, 38 mm diameter) = £8.20. For Redifit® pouches, 1 belt flange = 66p; St Mark's pattern, 1 flange (51 mm base: 13 mm deep, 25 mm diameter; 76 mm base, 13 mm deep, 25 mm diameter; 76 mm base, 10 or 16 mm deep, 32 or 38 mm diameter; 102 mm base, 16 mm deep, 44 or 51 mm diameter) = £13.96: with dressing retainer or with 16 mm canopy, 38 mm = £17.63

Ward

Flange. Net price 1 plastic/rubber air-filled flange = £17.84; 1 St Mark's standard = £11.74; 1 St Mark's with diaphragm = £14.35

Irrigation and wash-out appliances

Available from *Astra Tech* (Medena® 5 ileostomy catheters = £4.60), *Braun Biotrol* (Biotrol®, 50 irrigation sleeves = £40.04 or 1 cone = £2.77), *Coloplast* (30 disposable sleeves (1540 or 1560) = £33.66; 1 colotip = £6.39; 1 irrigator bag = £12.09; 1 supporting plate = £6.08; 1 irrigation belt = £5.93), *Dansac* (1 water container = £17.49; 1 clamp = £7.57; 1 cone = £11.23; 1 brush = £1.90; 1 tube = £1.33; 1 belt = £36.20; Irri-drain® with ring holder for silicone ring, 20 = £22.36; silicone ring, 1 = £4.49; Unique® 2 Irri-drain®, 10 (flange: 36, 43 or 55 mm) = £11.26; 1 stoma cone/irrigator kit = £19.80; 20 irrigator drains = £27.31; 10 replacement cones = £70.23; 1 = £8.59; 1 stoma lubricant = £4.86), *Ward* (1 belt = £8.38)

Pressure plates, shields

Coloplast (1 supporting plate = £5.97; Assura® convex inserts for use with two-piece base plates 40, 50, 60 mm, 5 = £1.30); 5 convex inserts for Combihesive Natura® flanges (38, 45, 57 mm) = £1.34; cotton facepiece with non-slip belt for St. Mark's flange, 45 mm diameter = £18.33, *Salts* (plastic retaining shield, single = £3.21, double = £4.95, large = £3.92; S S Wire retaining ring, large = £3.21, medium = £3.06, small = £2.97; light white anti-sag ring = £1.27, for belt use = £1.45, for vel-cro belt fastening = £1.65; convex plate for light white bag (32, 38, or 44 mm), 5 = £13.84; pressure plate for Kombo®, Simplicity®, or Solo® pouches (30, 40, 50, or 60 mm) = £2.00; Eakin® support frame (32, 45, 64, or 90 mm) = £1.24, convex inserts for use with Second Nature® flanges (38, 45 or 57 mm), 5 = £1.25; *Shannon* (faceplate = £7.66), *SIMS Portex* (plastic pressure plates, Surrey model: 25 or 32 mm or Standard model with attached flange for use with lightweight bags: 25, 32, or 38 mm = £7.38; stainless wire pressure frame, hook, lug, to fit 25, 32, 38, 44, or 51 mm flange) = £8.99; cotton facepiece = £22.38; pressure plates (25, 32, or 38 mm) =

£7.38, *Ward* (celluloid colostomy cup with sponge or solid rim, small, medium, or large = £36.83, with sponge rubber or solid rim, belt fitting = £42.01; St Mark's shield, celluloid with 4 studs = £8.00)

Skin protectives, fillers, and cleansers

Balspray® (Bullen)
Aerosol. Net price 1 unit = £6.87
Bullen Karaya Gum Powder® (Bullen)
Powder. Net price 70 g = £4.56
Cavilon® (3M Healthcare)
Barrier cream, net price 92 g = £7.58
Chiron® (SIMS Portex)
Barrier cream. Net price 52 g = £4.89
CliniShield Wipes® (CliniMed)
Barrier wipes. Net price 50 = £12.28
Coloplast Strip Paste
Paste, net price (10 strips) = £6.91
Comfeel® (Coloplast)
Barrier cream. Net price 60 g = £4.08
Protective film. Net price 30 sachets = £9.33; applicator = £4.43
Dansac® (Dansac)
Soft paste. Net price 50 g = £3.08
Day-Drop® (Loxley)
Barrier Cream. Net price 50 g = £2.15
Derma-gard® (SIMS Portex)
Protective skin wipes. Net price 50 = £14.32
Hollister® (Hollister)
Karaya paste. Net price 128 g = £7.17
   Do not apply to severely excoriated skin
Karaya powder. Net price 71 g = £8.26
Premium paste. Net price 57 g = £3.21
Premium powder. Net price 1 = £2.28
Skin gel. Net price 28 g = £6.22; 50 protective dressing wipes = £12.28. Label: 15
   Do not apply to severely excoriated skin
Orabase® (ConvaTec)
Paste, see section 12.3.1
Orahesive® (ConvaTec)
Powder (with adherent properties), see section 12.3.1
Payne® (Payne)
Barrier cream. Net price 50 g = £3.59
Pelican® (Pelican)
Paste (formerlySimpla® gel). Net price 1 pack = £6.69
Preventox® (Manfred Sauer)
Skin protecting film. Net price 50 wipes = £7.95; with roll-on applicator, 50 mL = £6.52
Saltair® (Salts)
Ostomy cleansing soap (soap spirit). Net price 110-mL = £2.69
Salts® (Salts)
Karaya gum powder. Net price per puffer pack = £4.48
Peri-Prep wipes. Net price 50 = £14.46
Stoma paste. Net price 50 g = £3.18
SIMS Portex® (SIMS Portex)
Karaya gum powder. Net price 100 g = £7.09
Skin shield® Wipes (Coloplast)
Barrier wipes. Net price 50 = £8.36
Stomahesive® (ConvaTec)
Paste. Net price 60 g = £6.72. For filling and sealing skin creases
Superskin® (CliniMed)
Liquid barrier film, net price 10 × 0.7 g = £8.00; 10 × 2 g = £13.00
Translet® (Rüsch)
Wipes. Net price 30 = £5.74

Skin protectors

Braun Biotrol
Biotrol® skin protectors. Net price 10 × 10 cm or 10 cm diameter, 10 = £16.61

Bullen
Karaya gum washers, regular or extra hard. Net price 10 washers (2 inch diameter: 2 × 0.875 inch or 2 × 1.125 inch hole) = £12.41; 2.5 inch diameter: regular 2.5 × 1.25 inch or extra hard 2.5 × 1.5 inch hole = £14.38; 3 inch diameter: 3 × 0.875 inch, 3 × 1.125 inch, 3 × 1.5 inch, or 3 × 2 inch hole = £16.49
CliniMed
Welland Hyperseal® washers, net price 20 small washers = £24.00, 25 = £30.00; 5 large washers = £10.00, 10 = £20.00
Coloplast
Protective sheets. Net price 10 non-sterile sheets (10 × 10 cm) = £20.74; 5 (15 × 15 cm) = £24.56; 5 (20 × 20 cm) = £44.68; 30 rings (10, 15, 20, 25, 30, 40, or 50 mm) = £35.97
ConvaTec
Wafers. Net price 5 Stomahesive® wafers (100 × 100 mm) = £10.12; 3 (200 × 200 mm) = £24.82; 10 Varihesive® wafers (100 × 100 mm) = £8.85
Dansac
GX-tra seals (washers), net price 30 (20, 30, 40, or 50 mm) = £37.96
Hollister
Skin barrier. Net price 5 Hollister® skin barriers (4 × 4 inch) = £10.25; 5 (8 × 8 inch) = £32.23
Omex
Schacht® rings, net price 10 foam, colostomy, or ileostomy rings = £7.52
Pelican
Protectors (formerly Simplaseel® wafers). Net price 10 (100 × 100 mm) = £19.40
Salts
Protectors. Net price 10 karaya gum washers (small) = £7.69; 10 (large) = £12.53; 5 foam cushions (25, 32, 38, or 51 mm) = £2.55; 20 Cohesive® washers (small: 50 mm) = £32.37; 10 (large: 95 mm) = £21.61; 10 protective wafers (10 cm x 10 cm) = £20.10; 10 Realistic® washers (13, 19, 22, 25, 29, 32, or 38 mm) = £15.70; 1 Saltair® twinpack (small) = £9.41; large = £13.17; 10 foam seals (as in twin packs) = £1.91; 5 United® skin barrier wafers (10 × 10 cm) = £10.37; 3 = £24.07; for Salger® pouches, 5 karaya washers with foam (40 or 57 mm) = £13.32
Shannon
Protectors. Net price 1 foam sponge ring = 74p; 10 Kaygee® washers (2.5 inch base: 0.875 or 1.125 inch hole or 2.75 inch base: 0.875 or 1.375 inch hole) = £6.72
Simpla Continence Care
Schacht® rings. Net price 10 foam, colostomy or ileostomy rings = £7.52
Shaw
Protectors. Net price 5 Body Mould® squares (1.0, 1.25, or 1.5 inch hole) = £11.07; 10 washers (1.0 or 1.25 inch hole) = £10.14; 5 rings (1.0, 1.25, or 1.5 inch hole) = £10.14; 12 Healwell® squares (1.0, 1.25 or 1.5 inch hole) = £10.50; 12 rings (1.0, 1.25 or 1.5 inch hole) = £9.07
SIMS Portex
Protectors. Net price 5 foam pads, white (76 mm diameter: 25 mm hole) = £4.82; 76 mm diameter: 29, 32, or 38 mm hole or 90 mm diameter: 32 or 38 mm hole = £6.59; 1 karaya gum sheet (300 × 100 mm) = £7.10: 20 rings (19, 25, 32, 38, or 44 mm) = £23.68; karaya rings (19, 25, 32, 38, or 51 mm) = £25.89: 10 Down's® adhesive karaya gum washers (51 mm base: 22 or 29 mm hole) = £11.53; 70 mm base: 22 or 29 mm hole = £14.22; 10 Redifit® karaya gum washers (25, 32, 38, 44, or 51 mm) = £14.22; 20 Seel-a-peel® squares (100 mm sq) = £39.92; 5 squares (150 mm sq) = £24.58

Stoma caps and dressings

Available from *Braun Biotrol* (30 Biotrol petite®, 15–35 mm starter hole = £33.15, *Coloplast* (100 Colocap® stomacaps = £114.50; Assura Minicap®, 30 opaque stomacaps, 20 mm starter hole, cut to fit up to 55 mm hole = £34.14), *ConvaTec* (Coloplast Plus®, 30 stoma caps

(19 mm hole cut-to-size) = £33.10, *Dansac* (50 Dansac® Combi Mini caps (30 or 40 mm) = £53.25; 50 Dansac® Mini caps (30 or 44 mm) = £55.31; 30 Dansac® Nova Mini caps, opaque stomacaps (25, 30, 40, or 50 mm pre-cut holes; 20–50 mm, cut-to-fit) = £35.00, 30 Dansac® Unique Mini caps, 20 mm starter hole, cut to fit up to 50 mm hole; also 30, 40 or 50 mm = £32.74), *Hollister* (50 stoma caps (51 or 76 mm) = £56.55), *Oakmed* (50 Option® stoma caps = £48.90), *Salts* (30 Confidence® stoma caps with filter, 13 mm starter hole = £30.62; 30 Confidence® Gold stoma caps with filter, 13 mm starter hole = £31.70, 30 stoma caps for Simplicity 1® pouches = £34.46), *SIMS Portex* (20 leisure pouches = £23.30), *Ward* (2 zip fasteners fitted to colostomy belt = £7.95; 1 waterproof front fitted to colostomy belt = £6.56; 1 pair woven understraps with buttonholed ends = £3.04; 1 Donald Rose® ileostomy/colostomy bath belt with internal chamber for dressings and stud fastenings for adjustment = £19.70)

Tubing

Available from *Hollister* (10 urostomy drain tubes = £24.68; 8 tubes for fitting to Lo-Profile® urostomy bags = £22.96; for Premium® urostomy pouches, 10 drain tube adaptors = £19.70), *Salts* (2 night tube adaptors = 97p), *SIMS Portex* (for Carshalton® urostomy pouches, 10 connectors = £4.16), *Ward* (1 metal spring tubing clip = £2.21)

NPF Index

Guidance on prescribing

General guidance

Medicines should be prescribed only when they are necessary, and in all cases the benefit of administering the medicine should be considered in relation to the risk involved. This is particularly important during pregnancy where the risk to both mother and fetus must be considered (for further details see Prescribing in Pregnancy, Appendix 4).

TAKING MEDICINES TO BEST EFFECT. Difficulties in compliance with drug treatment occur regardless of age. Factors contributing to poor compliance with prescribed medicines include:

- Prescription not collected or not dispensed
- Purpose of medicine not clear
- Perceived lack of efficacy
- Real or perceived side-effects
- Instructions for administration not clear
- Physical difficulty in taking medicines (e.g. with swallowing the medicine, with handling small tablets, or with opening medicine containers)
- Unattractive formulation (e.g. unpleasant taste)
- Complicated regimen

The prescriber and the patient should agree on the health outcomes that the patient desires and on the strategy for achieving them ('concordance'). Further information on concordance is available on the Internet (www.concordance.org).

Taking the time to explain to the patient (and relatives) the rationale and the potential adverse effects of treatment may improve compliance. Reinforcement and elaboration of the physician's instructions by the pharmacist also helps. Advising the patient of the possibility of alternative treatments may encourage the patient to seek advice rather than merely abandon unacceptable treatment.

Simplifying the drug regimen may help; the need for frequent administration may reduce compliance although there appears to be little difference in compliance between once-daily and twice-daily administration. Combination products reduce the number of drugs taken but this may be at the expense of the ability to titrate individual doses.

COMPLEMENTARY MEDICINE. An increasing amount of information on complementary ('alternative') medicine is becoming available. However, the scope of the BNF's advice is restricted to the discussion of conventional medicines but where appropriate, reference will be made to complementary treatments if they affect conventional therapy (e.g. interactions with St John's wort—see Appendix 1).

ABBREVIATION OF TITLES. In general, titles of drugs and preparations should be written *in full*. Unofficial abbreviations should not be used as they may be misinterpreted; obsolete titles, such as Mist. Expect. should not be used.

NON-PROPRIETARY TITLES. Where non-proprietary ('generic') titles are given, they should be used in prescribing. This will enable any suitable product to be dispensed, thereby saving delay to the patient and sometimes expense to the health service. The only exception is where bioavailability problems are so important that the patient should always receive the same brand; in such cases, the brand name or the manufacturer should be stated. Non-proprietary titles should **not** be invented for the purposes of prescribing generically since this can lead to confusion, particularly in the case of compound and modified-release preparations.

Titles used as headings for monographs may be used freely in the United Kingdom but in other countries may be subject to restriction.

Many of the non-proprietary titles used in this book are titles of monographs in the European Pharmacopoeia, British Pharmacopoeia or British Pharmaceutical Codex 1973. In such cases the preparations must comply with the standard (if any) in the appropriate publication, as required by the Medicines Act (Section 65).

PROPRIETARY TITLES. Names followed by the symbol ® are or have been used as proprietary names in the United Kingdom. These names may in general be applied only to products supplied by the owners of the trade marks.

DOSES. The doses stated in the BNF are intended for general guidance and represent, unless otherwise stated, the usual range of doses that are generally regarded as being suitable for adults. In general the *doses, indications, cautions, contra-indications and side-effects* in the BNF reflect those in the manufacturers' data sheets or Summaries of Product Characteristics (SPCs) which, in turn, reflect those in the corresponding Marketing Authorisations (formerly known as Product Licences). Where an unlicensed drug is included in the BNF, this is indicated in brackets after the entry. Where a use (or route) is recommended outside the licensed indication ('off-label' use) of an available product this too is indicated.

> It has been noted (*Drug and Therapeutics Bulletin* 1992; **30:** 97–9) that prescribing of licensed medicines outside the recommendations of the Marketing Authorisation alters (and probably increases) the doctor's professional responsibility.

ORAL SYRINGES. An **oral syringe** is supplied when oral liquid medicines are prescribed in doses other than multiples of 5 mL. The oral syringe is marked in 0.5-mL divisions from 1 to 5 mL to measure doses of less than 5 mL. It is provided with an adaptor and an instruction leaflet. The *5-mL spoon* is used for doses of 5 mL (or multiples thereof).

STRENGTHS AND QUANTITIES. The strength or quantity to be contained in capsules, lozenges, tablets, etc. should be stated by the prescriber.

If a pharmacist receives an incomplete prescription for a systemically administered preparation[1] and considers it would not be appropriate for the patient to return to the doctor, the following procedures will apply:

(a) an attempt must always be made to contact the prescriber to ascertain the intention;

(b) if the attempt is successful the pharmacist must, where practicable, subsequently arrange for details of quantity, strength where applicable, and dosage to be inserted by the prescriber on the incomplete form;

(c) where, although the prescriber has been contacted, it has not proved possible to obtain the written intention regarding an incomplete prescription, the pharmacist may endorse the form 'p.c.' (prescriber contacted) and add details of the quantity and strength where applicable of the preparation supplied, and of the dose indicated. The endorsement should be initialled and dated by the pharmacist;

(d) where the prescriber cannot be contacted and the pharmacist has sufficient information to make a professional judgment the preparation may be dispensed. If the quantity is missing the pharmacist may supply sufficient to complete up to 5 days' treatment; except that where a combination pack (i.e. a proprietary pack containing more than one medicinal product) or oral contraceptive is prescribed by name only, the smallest pack shall be dispensed. In all cases the prescription must be endorsed 'p.n.c.' (prescriber not contacted) the quantity, the dose, and the strength (where applicable) of the preparation supplied must be indicated, and the endorsement must be initialled and dated;

(e) if the pharmacist has any doubt about exercising discretion, an incomplete prescription must be referred back to the prescriber.

EXCIPIENTS. Oral liquid preparations that do not contain *fructose, glucose* or *sucrose* are described as 'sugar-free' in the BNF. Preparations containing hydrogenated glucose syrup, mannitol, sorbitol or xylitol are also marked 'sugar-free' since there is evidence that they do not cause dental caries. Patients receiving medicines containing cariogenic sugars should be advised of appropriate dental hygiene measures to prevent caries.

Where information on the presence of *aspartame, gluten, tartrazine, arachis (peanut) oil* or *sesame oil* is available, this is indicated in the BNF against the relevant preparation.

Information is provided on *selected excipients* in skin preparations (see section 13.1.3) and on *selected preservatives* and *excipients* in eye drops and injections. Pressurised metered aerosols containing *chlorofluorocarbons* (CFCs) have also been identified throughout the BNF (see section 3.1.1.1).

The presence of *benzyl alcohol* and *polyoxyl castor oil* (polyethoxylated castor oil) in injections is indicated in the BNF. Benzyl alcohol has been associated with a fatal toxic syndrome in premature infants, and parenteral preparations containing the preservative should not be used in neonates. Polyoxyl castor oils, used as vehicles in intravenous injections, have been associated with severe anaphylactoid reactions.

---

1. With the exception of temazepam, an incomplete prescription is **not** acceptable for controlled drugs in schedules 2 and 3 of the Misuse of Drugs Regulations 2001

In the absence of information on excipients in the BNF and in the product literature, contact the manufacturer (see Index of Manufacturers) if it is essential to check details.

EXTEMPORANEOUS PREPARATION. A product should be dispensed extemporaneously only when no product with a marketing authorisation is available.

The BP direction that a preparation must be *freshly prepared* indicates that it must be made not more than 24 hours before it is issued for use. The direction that a preparation should be *recently prepared* indicates that deterioration is likely if the preparation is stored for longer than about 4 weeks at 15–25° C.

The term **water** used without qualification means either potable water freshly drawn direct from the public supply and suitable for drinking or freshly boiled and cooled purified water. The latter should be used if the public supply is from a local storage tank or if the potable water is unsuitable for a particular preparation (Water for injections, section 9.2.2).

DRUGS AND DRIVING. Prescribers should advise patients if treatment is likely to affect their ability to drive motor vehicles. This applies especially to drugs with sedative effects; patients should be warned that these effects are increased by alcohol. General information about a patient's fitness to drive is available from the Driver and Vehicle Licensing Agency at www.dvla.gov.uk/dvla.htm (see also Appendix 9).

PATENTS. In the BNF certain drugs have been included notwithstanding the existence of actual or potential patent rights. In so far as such substances are protected by Letters Patent, their inclusion in this Formulary neither conveys, nor implies, licence to manufacture.

HEALTH AND SAFETY. When handling chemical or biological materials particular attention should be given to the possibility of allergy, fire, explosion, radiation, or poisoning. Substances, including corticosteroids, some antimicrobials, phenothiazines, and many cytotoxics, are irritant or very potent and should be handled with caution. Contact with the skin and inhalation of dust should be avoided.

SAFETY IN THE HOME. Patients must be warned to keep all medicines out of the reach of children. All solid dose and all oral and external liquid preparations must be dispensed in a reclosable *child-resistant container* unless:

• the medicine is in an original pack or patient pack such as to make this inadvisable;
• the patient will have difficulty in opening a child-resistant container;
• a specific request is made that the product shall not be dispensed in a child-resistant container;
• no suitable child-resistant container exists for a particular liquid preparation.

All patients should be advised to dispose of *unwanted medicines* by returning them to a supplier for destruction.

NAME OF MEDICINE. The name of the medicine should appear on the label unless the prescriber indicates otherwise.

1. Subject to the conditions of paragraphs 4 and 6 below, the name of the prescribed medicine is stated on the label unless the prescriber deletes the letters 'NP' which appear on NHS prescription forms.

2. The strength is also stated on the label in the case of tablets, capsules, and similar preparations that are available in different strengths.

3. If it is the wish of the prescriber that a description such as 'The Sedative Tablets' should appear on the label, the prescriber should write the desired description on the prescription form.

4. The arrangement will extend to approved names, proprietary names or titles given in the BP, BPC, BNF, DPF, or NPF. The arrangement does not apply when a prescription is written so that several ingredients are given.

5. The name written on the label is that used by the prescriber on the prescription.

6. If more than one item is prescribed on one form and the prescriber does not delete the letters 'NP', each dispensed medicine is named on the label, subject to the conditions given above in paragraph 4. If the prescriber wants only selected items on such a prescription to be so labelled this should be indicated by deleting the letters 'NP' on the form and writing 'NP' alongside the medicines to be labelled.

7. When a prescription is written other than on an NHS prescription form the name of the prescribed preparation will be stated on the label of the dispensed medicine unless the prescriber indicates otherwise.

8. The Council of the Royal Pharmaceutical Society advises that the labels of dispensed medicines should indicate the total quantity of the product dispensed in the container to which the label refers. This requirement applies equally to solid, liquid, internal, and external preparations. If a product is dispensed in more than one container, the reference should be to the amount in each container.

SECURITY AND VALIDITY OF PRESCRIPTIONS. The Councils of the British Medical Association and the Royal Pharmaceutical Society have issued a joint statement on the security and validity of prescriptions.

In particular, prescription forms should:
- not be left unattended at reception desks;
- not be left in a car where they may be visible; and
- when not in use, be kept in a locked drawer within the surgery and at home.

Where there is any doubt about the authenticity of a prescription, the pharmacist should contact the prescriber. If this is done by telephone, the number should be obtained from the directory rather than relying on the information on the prescription form, which may be false.

PATIENT GROUP DIRECTION (PGD). In most cases, the most appropriate clinical care will be provided on an individual basis by a prescriber to a specific individual patient. However, a Patient Group Direction for the supply and administration of medicines by other healthcare professionals can be used where it would benefit patient care without compromising safety.

A Patient Group Direction is a written direction relating to supply and administration (or administration only) of a prescription-only medicine by certain classes of healthcare professionals; the Direction is signed by a doctor (or dentist), and by a pharmacist. Further information is available at www.rpsgb.org.uk

---

Non-proprietary names of **compound preparations** which appear in the BNF are those that have been compiled by the British Pharmacopoeia Commission or another recognised body; whenever possible they reflect the names of the active ingredients.

Prescribers should avoid creating their own compound names for the purposes of generic prescribing; such names do not have an approved definition and can be misinterpreted.

Special care should be taken to avoid errors when prescribing compound preparations; in particular the hyphen in the prefix 'co-' should be retained.

Special care should also be taken to avoid creating generic names for **modified-release** preparations where the use of these names could lead to confusion between formulations with different lengths of action.

Prescription writing

Prescriptions[1] should be written legibly in ink or otherwise so as to be indelible[2], should be dated, should state the full name and address of the patient, and should be signed in ink by the prescriber[3]. The age and the date of birth of the patient should preferably be stated, and it is a legal requirement in the case of prescription-only medicines to state the age for children under 12 years.

The following should be noted:

(a) The unnecessary use of decimal points should be avoided, e.g. 3 mg, not 3.0 mg.

Quantities of 1 gram or more should be written as 1 g etc.

Quantities less than 1 gram should be written in milligrams, e.g. 500 mg, not 0.5 g.

Quantities less than 1 mg should be written in micrograms, e.g. 100 micrograms, not 0.1 mg.

When decimals are unavoidable a zero should be written in front of the decimal point where there is no other figure, e.g. 0.5 mL, not .5 mL.

Use of the decimal point is acceptable to express a range, e.g. 0.5 to 1 g.

(b) 'Micrograms' and 'nanograms' should **not** be abbreviated. Similarly 'units' should be **not** be abbreviated.

(c) The term 'millilitre' (ml or mL)[4] is used in medicine and pharmacy, and cubic centimetre, c.c., or cm³ should not be used.

(d) Dose and dose frequency should be stated; in the case of preparations to be taken 'as required' a **minimum dose interval** should be specified.

When doses other than multiples of 5 mL are prescribed for *oral liquid preparations* the dose-volume will be provided by means of an **oral syringe**, see p. 1 (except for preparations intended to be measured with a pipette).

Suitable quantities:

Elixirs, Linctuses, and Paediatric Mixtures (5-mL dose), 50, 100, or 150 mL

Adult Mixtures (10-mL dose), 200 or 300 mL

Ear Drops, Eye drops, and Nasal Drops, 10 mL (or the manufacturer's pack)

Eye Lotions, Gargles, and Mouthwashes, 200 mL

(e) For suitable quantities of dermatological preparations, see section 13.1.2.

(f) The names of drugs and preparations should be written clearly and **not** abbreviated, using approved titles **only** (see also advice in box on p. 3 to **avoid** creating generic titles for modified-release preparations).

(g) The symbol 'NP' on NHS forms should be deleted if it is required that the name of the preparation should not appear on the label. For full details see p. 3.

(h) The quantity to be supplied may be stated by indicating the number of days of treatment required in the box provided on NHS forms. In most cases the exact amount will be supplied. This does not apply to items directed to be used as required—if the dose and frequency are not given the quantity to be supplied needs to be stated.

When several items are ordered on one form the box can be marked with the number of days of treatment provided the quantity is added for any item for which the amount cannot be calculated.

(i) Although directions should preferably be in **English without abbreviation**, it is recognised that some Latin abbreviations are used (for details see Inside Back Cover).

(j) A prescription for a preparation that has been withdrawn or needs to be specially imported for a named patient should be handwritten. The name of the preparation should be endorsed with the prescriber's signature and the letters 'WD' (withdrawn or specially-imported drug); there may be considerable delay in obtaining a withdrawn medicine.

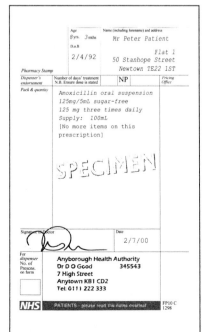

---

1. The above recommendations are acceptable for **prescription-only medicines** (PoM). For items marked CD see also Controlled Drugs and Drug Dependence p. 7.

2. It is permissible to issue carbon copies of NHS prescriptions as long as they are signed in ink.

3. Computer-generated facsimile signatures do not meet the legal requirement.

4. The use of capital 'L' in mL is a printing convention throughout the BNF; both 'mL' and 'ml' are recognised SI abbreviations.

Computer-issued prescriptions

For computer-issued prescriptions the following recommendations of the Joint Computing Group of the General Practitioners Committee and the Royal College of General Practitioners should also be noted:

1. The computer must print out the date,[1] the patient's surname, one forename, other initials, and address, and may also print out the patient's title and date of birth. The age of children under 12 years and of adults over 60 years must be printed in the box available; the age of children under 5 years should be printed in years and months. A facility may also exist to print out the age of patients between 12 and 60 years.

2. The doctor's name must be printed at the bottom of the prescription form; this will be the name of the doctor responsible for the prescription (who will normally sign it). The doctor's surgery address, reference number, and Health Authority (HA)[2] are also necessary. In addition, the surgery telephone number should be printed.

3. When prescriptions are to be signed by general practitioner registrars, assistants, locums, or deputising doctors, the name of the doctor printed at the bottom of the form must still be that of the responsible principal.

4. Names of medicines must come from a dictionary held in the computer memory, to provide a check on the spelling and to ensure that the name is written in full. The computer can be programmed to recognise both the non-proprietary and the proprietary name of a particular drug and to print out the preferred choice, but must not print out both names. For medicines not in the dictionary, separate checks are required—the user must be warned that no check was possible and the entire prescription must be entered in the lexicon.

5. The dictionary may contain information on the usual doses, formulations, and pack sizes to produce standard predetermined prescriptions for common preparations, and to provide a check on the validity of an individual prescription on entry.

6. The prescription must be printed in English without abbreviation; information may be entered or stored in abbreviated form. The dose must be in numbers, the frequency in words, and the quantity in numbers in brackets, thus: 40 mg four times daily (112). It must also be possible to prescribe by indicating the length of treatment required, see (h) above.

7. The BNF recommendations should be followed as in (a), (b), (c), (d), and (e) above.

8. Checks may be incorporated to ensure that all the information required for dispensing a particular drug has been filled in. For instructions such as 'as directed' and 'when required', the maximum daily dose should normally be specified.

9. Numbers and codes used in the system for organising and retrieving data must never appear on the form.

10. Supplementary warnings or advice should be written in full, should not interfere with the clarity of the prescription itself, and should be in line with any warnings or advice in the BNF; numerical codes should not be used.

11. A mechanism (such as printing a series of non-specific characters) should be incorporated to cancel out unused space, or wording such as 'no more items on this prescription' may be added after the last item. Otherwise the doctor should delete the space manually.

12. To avoid forgery the computer may print on the form the number of items to be dispensed (somewhere separate from the box for the pharmacist). The number of items per form need be limited only by the ability of the printer to produce clear and well-demarcated instructions with sufficient space for each item and a spacer line before each fresh item.

13. Handwritten alterations should only be made in exceptional circumstances—it is preferable to print out a new prescription. Any alterations must be made in the doctor's own handwriting and counter-signed; computer records should be updated to fully reflect any alteration. Prescriptions for drugs used for contraceptive purposes (but which are not promoted as contraceptives) may need to be marked in handwriting with the symbol ♀ or endorsed in another way to indicate that the item is prescribed for contraceptive purposes.

14. Prescriptions for controlled drugs must not be printed from the computer. Blank forms may be computer-printed with the doctor's name, surgery address and telephone number, reference number and Health Authority (HA)[2]; the remaining details must be handwritten.[3]

15. The strip of paper on the side of the FP10[4](Comp) may be used for various purposes but care should be taken to avoid including confidential information. It may be advisable for the patient's name to appear at the top, but this should be preceded by 'confidential'.

16. In rural dispensing practices prescription requests (or details of medicines dispensed) will normally be entered in one surgery. The prescriptions (or dispensed medicines) may then need to be delivered to another surgery or location; if possible the computer should hold up to 10 alternatives.

17. Prescription forms that are reprinted or issued as a duplicate should be labelled clearly as such.

---

1. The exemption for own handwriting regulations for phenobarbital does not apply to the date; a computer-generated date need not be deleted but the date must also be added by the prescriber.

2. Health Board in Scotland.

3. Except in the case of phenobarbital (but see also footnote 1) or where the prescriber has been exempted from handwriting requirements, for details see Controlled Drugs and Drug Dependence p. 7.

4. GP10 in Scotland.

Emergency supply of medicines

Pharmacists are sometimes called upon by members of the public to supply medicines in emergencies. For details of emergency supply at the request of a doctor, see *Medicines, Ethics and Practice*, No. 25, London, Pharmaceutical Press, 2001 (and subsequent editions).

The Medicines (Products Other Than Veterinary Drugs) (Prescription Only) Order 1983, as amended, allows exemptions from the Prescription Only requirements for emergency supply to be made by a person lawfully conducting a retail pharmacy business provided:

(a) that the pharmacist has interviewed the person requesting the prescription-only medicine and is satisfied:
   (i) that there is immediate need for the prescription-only medicine and that it is impracticable in the circumstances to obtain a prescription without undue delay;
   (ii) that treatment with the prescription-only medicine has on a previous occasion been prescribed by a doctor[1] for the person requesting it;
   (iii) as to the dose which it would be appropriate for the person to take;
(b) that no greater quantity shall be supplied than will provide 5 days' treatment except when the prescription-only medicine is:
   (i) insulin, an ointment, cream, or preparation for the relief of asthma in an aerosol dispenser when the smallest pack can be supplied;
   (ii) an oral contraceptive when a full cycle may be supplied;
   (iii) an antibiotic in liquid form for oral administration when the smallest quantity that will provide a full course of treatment can be supplied;
(c) that an entry shall be made in the prescription book stating:
   (i) the date of supply;
   (ii) the name, quantity and, where appropriate, the pharmaceutical form and strength;
   (iii) the name and address of the patient;
   (iv) the nature of the emergency;
(d) that the container or package must be labelled to show:
   (i) the date of supply;
   (ii) the name, quantity and, where appropriate, the pharmaceutical form and strength;
   (iii) the name of the patient;
   (iv) the name and address of the pharmacy;
   (v) the words 'Emergency supply'.
(e) that the prescription-only medicine is not a substance specifically excluded from the emergency supply provision, and does not contain a Controlled Drug specified in schedules 1, 2, or 3 to the Misuse of Drugs Regulations 1985 except for phenobarbital or phenobarbital sodium for the treatment of epilepsy: for details see *Medicines, Ethics and Practice*, No. 25, London, Pharmaceutical Press, 2001 (and subsequent editions as available).

Royal Pharmaceutical Society's Guidelines

(1) The pharmacist should consider the medical consequences of *not* supplying.
(2) If the patient is not known to the pharmacist, the patient's identity should be established by way of appropriate documentation.
(3) It may occasionally be desirable to contact the prescriber, e.g. when the medicine requested has a potential for misuse or the prescriber is not known to the pharmacist.
(4) Care should be taken to ask whether the patient's doctor has stopped the treatment, or whether the patient is taking any other medication.
(5) Except for conditions which may occur infrequently (e.g. hay fever, asthma attack or migraine), a supply should not be made if the item requested was last prescribed more than 6 months ago.
(6) Consideration should be given to supplying less than 5 days' quantity if this is justified.
(7) Where a prescription is to be provided later, a record of emergency supply as required by law must still be made. It is good practice to add to the record the date on which the prescription is received. Payment for the medicine supplied is not a legal requirement, but may help to minimise the abuse of the emergency supply exemption. If an NHS prescription is to be provided, a refundable charge may be made.

---

1. The doctor must be a UK-registered doctor.

Controlled drugs and drug dependence

PRESCRIPTIONS. Preparations which are subject to the prescription requirements of the Misuse of Drugs Regulations 1985, i.e. preparations specified in schedules 2 and 3, are distinguished throughout the BNF by the symbol ☐ⒸⒹ (Controlled Drugs). The principal legal requirements relating to medical prescriptions are listed below.

Prescriptions ordering Controlled Drugs subject to prescription requirements must be *signed* and *dated*[1] by the prescriber and specify the prescriber's *address*. The prescription must always state *in the prescriber's own handwriting*[2] in ink or otherwise so as to be indelible:

1. The name and address of the patient;
2. In the case of a preparation, the form[3] and where appropriate the strength[4] of the preparation;
3. The total quantity of the preparation, or the number of dose units, *in both words and figures;*[5]
4. The dose;[6]
5. The words 'for dental treatment only' if issued by a dentist.

A prescription may order a Controlled Drug to be dispensed by instalments; the amount of the instalments and the intervals to be observed must be specified.[7,8] Prescriptions ordering 'repeats' on the same form are **not** permitted. A prescription is valid for 13 weeks from the date stated thereon.

It is an offence for a prescriber to issue an incomplete prescription and a pharmacist is **not** allowed to dispense a Controlled Drug unless all the information required by law is given on the prescription. Failure to comply with the regulations concerning the writing of prescriptions will result in inconvenience to patients and delay in supplying the necessary medicine.

DEPENDENCE AND MISUSE. The most serious drugs of addiction are **cocaine, diamorphine** (heroin), **morphine**, and the **synthetic opioids**. For arrangements for prescribing of diamorphine, dipipanone or cocaine for addicts, see p. 9.

Despite marked reduction in the prescribing of **amphetamines** there is concern that abuse of illicit amfetamine and related compounds is widespread.

Owing to problems of abuse, **flunitrazepam** and **temazepam** are subject to additional controlled drug requirements (but temazepam remains exempt from the additional prescribing requirements).

The principal **barbiturates** are now Controlled Drugs, but phenobarbital (phenobarbitone) and phenobarbital sodium (phenobarbitone sodium) or a preparation containing either of these are exempt from the handwriting requirement but must fulfil all other controlled drug prescription requirements (**important**: the own handwriting exemption does **not** apply to the date; a computer-generated date need not be deleted but the date must also be added by the prescriber). Moreover, for the treatment of epilepsy phenobarbital and phenobarbital sodium are available under the emergency supply regulations (p. 6).

Cannabis (Indian hemp) has no approved medicinal use and cannot be prescribed by doctors. Its use is illegal but has become widespread. Cannabis is a mild hallucinogen seldom accompanied by a desire to increase the dose; withdrawal symptoms are unusual. **Lysergide** (lysergic acid diethylamide, LSD) is a much more potent hallucinogen; its use can lead to severe psychotic states in which life may be at risk.

---

1. A computer-generated date is **not** acceptable; however, the prescriber may use a date stamp.
2. Does not apply to prescriptions for temazepam. Otherwise applies unless the prescriber has been specifically exempted from this requirement or unless the prescription contains no controlled drug other than phenobarbital or phenobarbital sodium or a preparation containing either of these; the exemption does **not** apply to the date—a computer-generated date need not be deleted but the date must also be added by the prescriber.
3. The dosage form (e.g. tablets) must be included on a Controlled Drugs prescription irrespective of whether it is implicit in the proprietary name (e.g. *MST Continus*) or of whether only one form is available.
4. When more than one strength of a preparation exists the strength required must be specified.
5. Does not apply to prescriptions for temazepam.
6. The instruction 'one as directed' constitutes a dose but 'as directed' does not.
7. A total of 14 days' treatment by instalment of any drug listed in Schedule 2 of the Misuse of Drugs Regulations may be prescribed. In *England and Wales*, form FP10HP(AD)1000 (pink—mainly used by hospital-based treatment units) or form FP10MDA1000 (blue—mainly used by general practitioners) should be used; in *Scotland* forms HBP(A) (hospital-based prescribers) or GP10 (general practitioners) should be used.
8. Buprenorphine (Schedule 3) may be prescribed by instalment in England and Wales on form FP10HP(AD)1000 and in England, general practitioners may also prescribe it by instalment on form FP10MDA1000

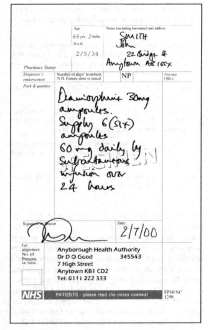

PRESCRIBING DRUGS LIKELY TO CAUSE DEPENDENCE OR MISUSE. The prescriber has three main responsibilities:

1. To avoid creating dependence by introducing drugs to patients without sufficient reason. In this context, the proper use of the morphine-like drugs is well understood. The dangers of other controlled drugs are less clear because recognition of dependence is not easy and its effects, and those of withdrawal, are less obvious. Perhaps the most notable result of uninhibited prescribing is that a very large number of patients in the country take tablets which do them neither much good nor much harm, but are committed to them indefinitely because they cannot readily be stopped.

2. To see that the patient does not gradually increase the dose of a drug, given for good medical reasons, to the point where dependence becomes more likely. This tendency is seen especially with hypnotics and anxiolytics (for CSM advice see section 4.1). The prescriber should keep a close eye on the amount prescribed to prevent patients from accumulating stocks that would enable them to arrange their own dosage or even that of their families and friends. A minimal amount should be prescribed in the first instance, or when seeing a new patient for the first time.

3. To avoid being used as an unwitting source of supply for addicts. Methods include visiting more than one doctor, fabricating stories, and forging prescriptions.

Patients under temporary care should be given only small supplies of drugs unless they present an unequivocal letter from their own doctors. Doctors should also remember that their own patients may be doing a collecting round with other doctors, especially in hospitals. It is sensible to decrease dosages steadily or to issue weekly or even daily prescriptions for small amounts if it is apparent that dependence is occurring.

The stealing and misuse of prescription forms could be minimised by the following precautions:

(a) do not leave unattended if called away from the consulting room or at reception desks; do not leave in a car where they may be visible; when not in use, keep in a locked drawer within the surgery and at home;

(b) draw a diagonal line across the blank part of the form under the prescription;

(c) write the quantity in words and figures when prescribing drugs prone to abuse; this is obligatory for controlled drugs (see Prescriptions, above);

(d) alterations are best avoided but if any are made they should be clear and unambiguous; add initials against altered items;

(e) if prescriptions are left for collection they should be left in a safe place in a sealed envelope.

TRAVELLING ABROAD. Prescribed drugs listed in schedules 4 and 5 to the Misuse of Drugs Regulations 1985 are not subject to import or export licensing but doctors are advised that patients intending to carry Schedule 2 and 3 drugs abroad may require an export licence. This is dependent upon the amount of drug to be exported and further details may be obtained from the Home Office by telephoning (020) 7273 3806. Applications for licences should be sent to the Home Office, Drugs Branch, Queen Anne's Gate, London SW1H 9AT.

There is no standard application form but applications must be supported by a letter from a doctor giving details of:

- the patient's name and current address;
- the quantities of drugs to be carried;
- the strength and form in which the drugs will be dispensed;
- the dates of travel to and from the United Kingdom.

Ten days should be allowed for processing the application.

Individual doctors who wish to take Controlled Drugs abroad while accompanying patients, may similarly be issued with licences. Licences are not normally issued to doctors who wish to take Controlled Drugs abroad solely in case a family emergency should arise.

These import/export licences for named individuals do not have any legal status outside the UK and are only issued to comply with the Misuse of Drugs Act and facilitate passage through UK Customs and Excise control. For clearance in the country to be visited it would be necessary to approach that country's consulate in the UK.

Misuse of Drugs Act

The Misuse of Drugs Act, 1971 prohibits certain activities in relation to 'Controlled Drugs', in particular their manufacture, supply, and possession. The penalties applicable to offences involving the different drugs are graded broadly according to the *harmfulness attributable to a drug when it is misused* and for this purpose the drugs are defined in the following three classes:

Class A includes: alfentanil, cocaine, dextromoramide, diamorphine (heroin), dipipanone, lysergide (LSD), methadone, methylenedioxymethamfetamine (MDMA, 'ecstasy'), morphine, opium, pethidine, phencyclidine, and class B substances when prepared for injection

Class B includes: oral amphetamines, barbiturates, cannabis, cannabis resin, codeine, ethylmorphine, glutethimide, pentazocine, phenmetrazine, and pholcodine

Class C includes: certain drugs related to the amphetamines such as benzfetamine and chlorphentermine, buprenorphine, diethylpropion, mazindol, meprobamate, pemoline, pipradrol, most benzodiazepines, androgenic and anabolic steroids, clenbuterol, chorionic gonadotrophin (HCG), non-human chorionic gonadotrophin, somatotropin, somatrem, and somatropin

The Misuse of Drugs Regulations 2001 define the classes of person who are authorised to supply and possess controlled drugs while acting in their professional capacities and lay down the conditions under which these activities may be carried out. In the regulations drugs are divided into five schedules each specifying the requirements governing such activities as import, export, production, supply, possession, prescribing, and record keeping which apply to them.

Schedule 1 includes drugs such as cannabis and lysergide which are not used medicinally. Possession and supply are prohibited except in accordance with Home Office authority.

Schedule 2 includes drugs such as diamorphine (heroin), morphine, pethidine, secobarbital, glutethimide, amfetamine, and cocaine and are subject to the full controlled drug requirements relating to prescriptions, safe custody (except for secobarbital), the need to keep registers, etc. (unless exempted in schedule 5).

Schedule 3 includes the barbiturates (except secobarbital, now schedule 2), buprenorphine, diethylpropion, flunitrazepam, mazindol, meprobamate, pentazocine, phentermine, and temazepam. They are subject to the special prescription requirements (except for phenobarbital and temazepam, see p. 7) but not to the safe custody requirements (except for buprenorphine, diethylpropion, flunitrazepam, and temazepam) nor to the need to keep registers (although there are requirements for the retention of invoices for 2 years).

Schedule 4 includes in Part I benzodiazepines (except flunitrazepam and temazepam which are in schedule 3) that are subject to minimal control. Part II includes androgenic and anabolic steroids, clenbuterol, chorionic gonadotrophin (HCG), non-human chorionic gonadotrophin, somatotropin, somatrem, and somatropin. Controlled drug prescription requirements do not apply and Schedule 4 Controlled Drugs are not subject to safe custody requirements.

Schedule 5 includes those preparations which, because of their strength, are exempt from virtually all Controlled Drug requirements other than retention of invoices for two years.

Notification of drug misusers

Doctors are expected to report on a standard form cases of drug misuse to their regional or national drug misuse database or centre—see below for contact telephone numbers. The National Drugs Treatment Monitoring System was introduced in England in April 2001; regional centres replace the Regional Drug Misuse Databases. A similar system has been introduced in Wales.

A report (notification) to their regional or national drug misuse database or centre should be made when a patient starts treatment for drug misuse. In England and Wales further information is collected in Spring, including whether or not patients are continuing to receive treatment. All types of problem drug misuse should be reported including opioid, benzodiazepine, and CNS stimulant.

The regional or national drug misuse database or centres are now the only national and local source of epidemiological data on people presenting with problem drug misuse; they provide valuable information to those working with drug misusers and those planning services for them. The databases cannot, however, be used as a check on multiple prescribing for drug addicts because the data are anonymised.

Enquiries about the regional or national drug misuse database or centres (including requests for supplies of notification forms) can be made by contacting one of the centres listed below:

ENGLAND

North West

Merseyside and Cheshire: telephone (0151) 231 4319; fax (0151) 231 4320

North Western: telephone (0161) 772 3782; fax (0161) 772 3445

Northern and Yorkshire
Telephone (0113) 295 1337; fax (0113) 295 1310
South East (West) and Eastern
Telephone (01865) 226734; fax (01865) 226652
South West
Telephone (0117) 918 6880; fax (0117) 918 6883
Thames and South East (East)
Telephone (020) 7594 0811; fax (020) 7594 0866
Trent
Telephone (0116) 225 6360; fax (0116) 225 6370
West Midlands
Telephone (0121) 580 4331; fax (0121) 525 7980

SCOTLAND
Telephone (0131) 551 8715; fax (0131) 551 1392

WALES
Telephone (029) 2082 6260; fax (029) 2082 5473

In **Northern Ireland**, the Misuse of Drugs (Notification of and Supply to Addicts) (Northern Ireland) Regulations 1973 require doctors to send particulars of persons whom they consider to be addicted to certain controlled drugs to Chief Medical Officer of the Department of Health and Social Services. The Northern Ireland contacts are:

Medical contact:
Dr Ian McMaster
C3 Castle Buildings
Belfast BT4 3PP
Telephone (028) 9052 2421
Fax (028) 9052 0781

Administrative contact:
Health Promotion Branch
C4.22 Castle Buildings
Belfast BT4 3PP
Telephone (028) 9052 0532

Prescribing of diamorphine (heroin), dipipanone, and cocaine for addicts

The Misuse of Drugs (Supply to Addicts) Regulations 1997 require that only medical practitioners who hold a special licence issued by the Home Secretary may prescribe, administer or supply diamorphine, dipipanone[1] (*Diconal®*) or cocaine in the treatment of drug addiction; other practitioners must refer any addict who requires these drugs to a treatment centre. Whenever possible the addict will be introduced by a member of staff from the treatment centre to a pharmacist whose agreement has been obtained and whose pharmacy is conveniently sited for the patient. Prescriptions for weekly supplies will be sent to the pharmacy by post and will be dispensed on a daily basis as indicated by the doctor. If any alterations of the arrangements are requested by the addict, the portion of the prescription affected must be represcribed and not merely altered. *General practitioners and other doctors may still prescribe diamorphine, dipipanone, and cocaine for patients (including addicts) for relief of pain due to organic disease or injury without a special licence.*

For guidance on prescription writing, see p. 7.

---

1. Dipipanone in *Diconal®* tablets has been much misused by opioid addicts in recent years. Doctors and others should be suspicious of people who ask for the tablets, especially if temporary residents.

Adverse reactions to drugs

Any drug may produce unwanted or unexpected adverse reactions. Detection and recording of these is of vital importance. Doctors and pharmacists are urged to help by reporting adverse reactions to:

Medicines Control Agency
CSM Freepost
London SW8 5BR
(0800 731 6789)

Prepaid Yellow Cards for reporting are available from the above address and are also bound in this book (inside back cover).

A 24-hour Freefone service is available to all parts of the UK for advice and information on suspected adverse drug reactions; contact the National Yellow Card Information Service at the MCA on 0800 731 6789. Outside office hours a telephone-answering machine will take messages.

The following regional centres also collect data:

CSM Mersey
Freepost
Liverpool L3 3AB
(0151) 794 8206

CSM Wales
Freepost
Cardiff CF4 1ZZ
(029) 2074 4181
(Direct Line)

CSM Northern
Freepost 1085
Newcastle upon Tyne
NE1 1BR
(0191) 232 1525 (Direct Line)

CSM West Midlands
Freepost SW2991
Birmingham B18 7BR
(0121) 507 5672

The MCA's Adverse Drug Reactions On-line Information Tracking (ADROIT) facilitates the monitoring of adverse drug reactions.

Suspected adverse reactions to *any* therapeutic agent should be reported, including drugs (*self-medication* as well as *prescribed* ones), blood products, vaccines, X-ray contrast media, dental or surgical materials, intra-uterine devices, herbal products, and contact lens fluids.

More detailed information on reporting and a list of drugs/products currently under intensive monitoring can be found on the CSM homepage: www.mca.gov.uk/aboutagency/regframework/csm/csmhome.htm.

NEWER DRUGS AND VACCINES. Only limited information is available from clinical trials on the safety of new medicines. Further understanding about the safety of medicines depends on the availability of information from routine clinical practice.

The black triangle symbol (▼) identifies newly licensed medicines that are monitored intensively by the MCA/CSM. Such medicines include those that have been licensed for administration by a new route or drug delivery system, or for significant new indications which may alter the established risks and benefits of that drug. There is no standard time for which products retain a black triangle; safety data are usually reviewed after 2 years.

Spontaneous reporting is particularly valuable for recognising possible new hazards rapidly. For medicines showing the black triangle symbol, the MCA/CSM asks that **all** suspected reactions (including those considered not to be serious) are reported through the Yellow Card scheme. An adverse reaction should be reported even if it is not certain that the drug has caused it, or if the reaction is well recognised, or if other drugs have been given at the same time.

ESTABLISHED DRUGS AND VACCINES. Doctors and pharmacists are asked to report *all* serious suspected reactions, including those that are fatal, life-threatening, disabling, incapacitating, or which result in or prolong hospitalisation; they should be reported even if the effect is well recognised. Examples include anaphylaxis, blood disorders, endocrine disturbances, effects on fertility, haemorrhage from any site, renal impairment, jaundice, ophthalmic disorders, severe CNS effects, severe skin reactions, reactions in pregnant women, and any drug interactions. Reports of serious adverse reactions are required to enable comparison with other drugs of a similar class. Information obtained from overdoses (deliberate or accidental) can complicate the assessment of adverse drug reactions, but provides important information on the potential toxicity of drugs.

For established drugs doctors and pharmacists are asked not to report well-known, relatively minor side-effects, such as dry mouth with tricyclic antidepressants or constipation with opioids.

Special problems

Delayed drug effects. Some reactions (e.g. cancers, chloroquine retinopathy, and retroperitoneal fibrosis) may become manifest months or years after exposure. Any suspicion of such an association should be reported.

The elderly. Particular vigilance is required to identify adverse reactions in the elderly.

Congenital abnormalities. When an infant is born with a congenital abnormality or there is a malformed aborted fetus doctors are asked to consider whether this might be an adverse reaction to a drug and to report all drugs (including self-medication) taken during pregnancy.

Children. Particular vigilance is required to identify and report adverse reactions in children, including those resulting from the unlicensed use of medicines; **all** suspected reactions should be reported (see p. 11).

Prevention of adverse reactions

Adverse reactions may be prevented as follows:

1. Never use any drug unless there is a good indication. If the patient is pregnant do not use a drug unless the need for it is imperative.

2. Allergy and idiosyncrasy are important causes of adverse drug reactions. Ask if the patient had previous reactions.

3. Ask if the patient is already taking other drugs *including self-medication drugs*; interactions may occur.

4. Age and hepatic or renal disease may alter the metabolism or excretion of drugs, so that much smaller doses may be needed. Genetic factors may also be responsible for variations in metabolism, notably of isoniazid and the tricyclic antidepressants.

5. Prescribe as few drugs as possible and give very clear instructions to the elderly or any patient likely to misunderstand complicated instructions.

6. When possible use a familiar drug. With a new drug be particularly alert for adverse reactions or unexpected events.

7. If serious adverse reactions are liable to occur warn the patient.

Defective Medicines

During the manufacture or distribution of a medicine an error or accident may occur whereby the finished product does not conform to its specification. While such a defect may impair the therapeutic effect of the product and could adversely affect the health of a patient, it should **not** be confused with an Adverse Drug Reaction where the product conforms to its specification.

The Defective Medicines Report Centre assists with the investigation of problems arising from licensed medicinal products thought to be defective and co-ordinates any necessary protective action. Reports on suspect defective medicinal products should include the brand or the non-proprietary name, the name of the manufacturer or supplier, the strength and dosage form of the product, the product licence number, the batch number or numbers of the product, the nature of the defect, and an account of any action already taken in consequence. The Centre can be contacted at:

The Defective Medicines Report Centre
Medicines Control Agency
Room 1801, Market Towers
1 Nine Elms Lane
London SW8 5NQ
(020) 7273 0574 (weekdays 9.00 am–5.00 pm)
or (020) 7210 3000 or 5371 (any other time)

Prescribing for children

Children, and particularly neonates, differ from adults in their response to drugs. Special care is needed in the neonatal period (first 30 days of life) and doses should always be calculated with care. At this age, the risk of toxicity is increased by inefficient renal filtration, relative enzyme deficiencies, differing target organ sensitivity, and inadequate detoxifying systems causing delayed excretion.

Whenever possible painful intramuscular injections should be **avoided** in children.

Where possible, medicines for children should be prescribed within the terms of the product licence (marketing authorisation). However, many children may require medicines not specifically licensed for paediatric use.

Although medicines cannot be promoted outside the limits of the licence, the Medicines Act does not prohibit the use of unlicensed medicines. It is recognised that the informed use of unlicensed medicines or of licensed medicines for unlicensed applications ('off-label' use) is often necessary in paediatric practice.

ADVERSE DRUG REACTIONS IN CHILDREN. The reporting of all suspected adverse drug reactions in children is **strongly encouraged** through the Yellow Card scheme (see p. 10) even if the intensive monitoring symbol (▼) has been removed, because experience in children may still be limited.

The identification and reporting of adverse reactions to drugs in children is particularly important because:

- the action of the drug and its pharmacokinetics in children (especially in the very young) may be different from that in adults
- drugs are not extensively tested in children
- many drugs are not specifically licensed for use in children and are used 'off-label'
- suitable formulations may not be available to allow precise dosing in children
- the nature and course of illnesses and adverse drug reactions may differ between adults and children.

PRESCRIPTION WRITING. Prescriptions should be written according to the guidelines in Prescription Writing (p. 4). Inclusion of age is a legal requirement in the case of prescription-only medicines for children under 12 years of age, but it is preferable to state the age for **all** prescriptions for children.

It is particularly important to state the strengths of capsules or tablets. Although liquid preparations are particularly suitable for children, they may contain sugar which encourages dental decay. Sugar-free medicines are preferred for long-term treatment.

Many children are able to swallow tablets or capsules and may prefer a solid dose form; involving the child and parents in choosing the formulation is helpful.

When a prescription for a liquid oral preparation is written and the dose ordered is smaller than 5 mL an **oral syringe** will be supplied (for details, see p. 1). Parents should be advised not to add any medicines to the infant's feed, since the drug may interact with the milk or other liquid in it; moreover the ingested dosage may be reduced if the child does not drink all the contents.

Parents must be warned to keep **all** medicines out of the reach of children, see Safety in the Home, p. 2.

Rare paediatric conditions

Information on substances such as *biotin* and *sodium benzoate* used in rare metabolic conditions can be obtained from:

Drug Information Centre, Alder Hey Children's Hospital, Liverpool L12 2AP. Telephone (0151) 252 5381;

Pharmacy, Great Ormond Street Hospital for Children, Great Ormond St, London, WC1N 3JH. Telephone (020) 7405 9200

Dosage in Children

Children's doses in the BNF are stated in the individual drug entries as far as possible, except where paediatric use is not recommended, information is not available, or there are special hazards.

Doses are generally based on body-weight (in kilograms) or the following age ranges:

first month (neonate)
up to 1 year (infant)
1–5 years
6–12 years

Unless the age is specified, the term 'child' in the BNF includes persons aged 12 years and younger.

DOSE CALCULATION. Children's doses may be calculated from adult doses by using age, body-weight, or body-surface area, or by a combination of these factors. The most reliable methods are those based on body-surface area.

Body-weight may be used to calculate doses expressed in mg/kg. Young children may require a higher dose per kilogram than adults because of their higher metabolic rates. Other problems need to be considered. For example, calculation by body-weight in the obese child may result in much higher doses being administered than necessary; in such cases, dose should be calculated from an ideal weight, related to height and age.

Body-surface area (BSA) estimates are more accurate for calculation of paediatric doses than body-weight since many physiological phenomena correlate better to body-surface area. The average body-surface area of a 70-kilogram human is about $1.8\,m^2$. Thus, to calculate the dose for a child the following formula may be used:

Approximate dose for patient =

$$\frac{\text{surface area of patient } (m^2) \times \text{adult dose}}{1.8}$$

More precise body-surface values may be calculated from height and weight by means of a nomogram (e.g. J. Insley, *A Paediatric Vade-Mecum*, 13th Edition, London, Arnold, 1996); see also BNF Inside back covers.

Where the dose for children is not stated, prescribers should seek advice from a drug information centre or refer to a current edition of a specialist text on the use of medicines in children.

DOSE FREQUENCY. Antibacterials are generally given at regular intervals throughout the day. Some flexibility should be allowed in children to avoid waking them during the night. For example, the night-time dose may be given at the parent's bedtime.

Where new or potentially toxic drugs are used, the manufacturers' recommended doses should be carefully followed.

Prescribing in palliative care

Palliative care is the active total care of patients whose disease is not responsive to curative treatment. Control of pain, of other symptoms, and of psychological, social and spiritual problems, is paramount to provide the best quality of life for patients and their families. Careful assessment of symptoms and needs of the patient should be undertaken by a multidisciplinary team.

Specialist palliative care is available in most areas as day hospice care, home care teams (often known as Macmillan teams), in-patient hospice care, and hospital teams. Many acute hospitals and teaching centres now have consultative, hospital-based teams.

Hospice care of terminally ill patients has shown the importance of symptom control and psychosocial support of the patient and family. Families should be included in the care of the patient if they wish.

Many patients wish to remain at home with their families. Although some families may at first be afraid of caring for the patient at home, support can be provided by community nursing services, social services, voluntary agencies and hospices together with the general practitioner. The family may be reassured by the knowledge that the patient will be admitted to a hospital or hospice if the family cannot cope.

DRUG TREATMENT. The number of drugs should be as few as possible, for even the taking of medicine may be an effort. Oral medication is usually satisfactory unless there is severe nausea and vomiting, dysphagia, weakness, or coma, in which case parenteral medication may be necessary.

Pain

Analgesics are more effective in preventing pain than in the relief of established pain; it is important that they are given regularly.

The non-opioid analgesics **aspirin** or **paracetamol** given regularly will often make the use of opioids unnecessary. Aspirin (or other NSAIDs, if preferred) may also control the pain of *bone secondaries*; naproxen, flurbiprofen, and indometacin (section 10.1.1) are valuable and if necessary can be given rectally. Radiotherapy, bisphosphonates (section 6.6.2) and radioactive isotopes of **strontium** (*Metastron*® available from Amersham) may also be useful for pain due to bone metastases.

An opioid such as **codeine** or **dextropropoxyphene**, alone or in combination with a non-opioid analgesic at adequate dosage, may be helpful in the control of moderate pain if non-opioids alone are not sufficient. If these preparations are not controlling the pain, **morphine** is the most useful opioid analgesic. Alternatives to morphine are **hydromorphone**, **oxycodone** (section 4.7.2) and transdermal **fentanyl** (see below and section 4.7.2). Initiation of an opioid analgesic should not be delayed by concern over a theoretical likelihood of psychological dependence (addiction).

Equivalent single doses of strong analgesics
These equivalences are intended **only** as an approximate guide; patients should be carefully monitored after **any** change in medication and dose titration may be required

Analgesic	Dose
Morphine salts (oral)	10 mg
Diamorphine hydrochloride (intramuscular)	3 mg
Hydromorphone hydrochloride	1.3 mg
Oxycodone	5 mg

ORAL ROUTE. Morphine is given *by mouth* as an oral solution or as standard ('immediate release') tablets regularly every 4 hours, the initial dose depending largely on the patient's previous treatment. A dose of 5–10 mg is enough to replace a weaker analgesic (such as paracetamol or co-proxamol), but 10–20 mg or more is required to replace a strong one (comparable to morphine itself). If the first dose of morphine is no more effective than the previous analgesic, the next dose should be increased by 50%, the aim being to choose the lowest dose which prevents pain. The dose should be adjusted with careful assessment of the pain and the use of adjuvant analgesics (such as NSAIDs) should also be considered. Although morphine in a dose of 5–20 mg is usually adequate there should be no hesitation in increasing it stepwise according to response to 100 mg or occasionally up to 500 mg or higher if necessary. It may be possible to omit the overnight dose if double the usual dose is given at bedtime.

If pain occurs between regular doses ('breakthrough pain'), an additional dose ('rescue dose') should be given. An additional dose should also be given 30 minutes before an activity that causes pain (e.g. wound dressing). Fentanyl lozenges are also licensed for breakthrough pain.

When the pain is controlled and the patient's 24-hour morphine requirement is established, the daily dose can be given as a single dose or in 2 divided doses as a *modified-release preparation*.

Preparations suitable for twice daily administration include *MST Continus*® tablets or suspension, and *Zomorph*® capsules. Preparations that allow administration of the total daily morphine requirement as a single dose include *MXL*® capsules. *Morcap SR*® capsules may be given either twice daily or as a single daily dose.

The starting dose of modified-release preparations designed for twice daily administration is usually 10–20 mg every 12 hours if no other analgesic (or only paracetamol) has been taken previously, but to replace a weaker opioid analgesic (such as co-proxamol) the starting dose is usually 20–30 mg every 12 hours. Increments should be made to the dose, not to the frequency of administration, which should remain at every 12 hours.

The effective dose of modified-release preparations can alternatively be determined by giving the oral solution of morphine every 4 hours in increasing doses until the pain has been controlled, and then transferring the patient to the same total 24-

hour dose of morphine given as the modified-release preparation (divided into two portions for 12-hourly administration). The first dose of the modified-release preparation is given 4 hours after the last dose of the oral solution.[1]

Morphine, as oral solution or standard formulation tablets, should be prescribed for breakthrough pain; the dose should be about one-sixth of the total daily dose of oral morphine.

PARENTERAL ROUTE. If the patient becomes unable to swallow, the equivalent intramuscular dose of morphine is half the oral solution dose; in the case of the modified-release tablets it is half the total 24-hour dose (which is then divided into 6 portions to be given every 4 hours). **Diamorphine** is preferred for injection because, being more soluble, it can be given in a smaller volume. The equivalent intramuscular (or subcutaneous) dose of diamorphine is approximately a third of the oral dose of morphine. *Subcutaneous infusion* of diamorphine via syringe driver can be useful (for details, see p. 15).

If the patient can resume taking medicines by mouth, then oral morphine may be substituted for subcutaneous infusion of diamorphine; see table of equivalent doses of morphine on p. 17 for equivalences between the two opioids.

RECTAL ROUTE. Morphine is also available for *rectal administration* as suppositories; alternatively **oxycodone** suppositories can be obtained on special order. A modified-release preparation of morphine for once-daily administration is available as a rectal tampon (*Moraxen*®). The dose is calculated in the same way as modified-release preparations given by the oral route (see above).

TRANSDERMAL ROUTE. Transdermal preparations of fentanyl are available (section 4.7.2). Careful conversion from oral morphine to transdermal fentanyl is necessary. The following 24-hour doses of morphine are considered to be equivalent to the fentanyl patches shown:

Morphine salt 90 mg daily ≡ fentanyl '25' patch
Morphine salt 180 mg daily ≡ fentanyl '50' patch
Morphine salt 270 mg daily ≡ fentanyl '75' patch
Morphine salt 360 mg daily ≡ fentanyl '100' patch

Morphine (as oral solution or standard formulation tablets) is given for breakthrough pain.

GASTRO-INTESTINAL PAIN. The pain of *bowel colic* may be reduced by loperamide 2–4 mg 4 times daily. Hyoscine hydrobromide may also be helpful, given sublingually at a dose of 300 micrograms 3 times daily as *Kwells*® (Roche Consumer Health) tablets. For the dose by subcutaneous infusion using a syringe driver, see p. 16.

Gastric distension pain due to pressure on the stomach may be helped by a preparation incorporating an antacid with an antiflatulent (section 1.1.1) and by domperidone 10 mg 3 times daily before meals.

MUSCLE SPASM. The pain of muscle spasm can be helped by a muscle relaxant such as diazepam 5–10 mg daily or baclofen 5–10 mg 3 times daily.

NEUROPATHIC PAIN. Patients with neuropathic pain (section 4.7.3) may benefit from a trial of a tricyclic antidepressant for several weeks. An anticonvulsant may be added or substituted if pain persists; gabapentin is licensed for neuropathic pain (section 4.8.1)

Pain due to nerve compression may be reduced by a corticosteroid such as dexamethasone 8 mg daily, which reduces oedema around the tumour, thus reducing compression.

Nerve blocks may be considered when pain is localised to a specific area. **Transcutaneous electrical nerve stimulation** (TENS) may also help.

Miscellaneous conditions

Non-licensed indications or routes

Several recommendations in this section involve non-licensed indications or routes.

RAISED INTRACRANIAL PRESSURE. Headache due to raised intracranial pressure often responds to a high dose of a corticosteroid, such as dexamethasone 16 mg daily for 4 to 5 days, subsequently reduced to 4–6 mg daily if possible; dexamethasone should be given before 6 p.m. to reduce the risk of insomnia.

INTRACTABLE COUGH. Intractable cough may be relieved by moist inhalations or by regular administration of oral morphine in an initial dose of 5 mg every 4 hours. Methadone linctus should be avoided because it has a long duration of action and tends to accumulate.

DYSPNOEA. Dyspnoea may be relieved by regular oral morphine in carefully titrated doses, starting at 5 mg every 4 hours. Diazepam 5–10 mg daily may be helpful; a corticosteroid, such as dexamethasone 4–8 mg daily, may also be helpful if there is bronchospasm or partial obstruction.

EXCESSIVE RESPIRATORY SECRETION. Excessive respiratory secretion (death rattle) may be reduced by subcutaneous injection of hyoscine hydrobromide 400–600 micrograms every 4 to 8 hours; care must however be taken to avoid the discomfort of dry mouth. For the dose by subcutaneous infusion using a syringe driver, see next page.

RESTLESSNESS AND CONFUSION. Restlessness and confusion may require treatment with haloperidol 1–3 mg by mouth every 8 hours. Chlorpromazine 25–50 mg by mouth every 8 hours is an alternative, but causes more sedation. Levomepromazine (methotrimeprazine) is also used occasionally for restlessness. For the dose by subcutaneous infusion using a syringe driver, see next page.

HICCUP. Hiccup due to gastric distension may be helped by a preparation incorporating an antacid with an antiflatulent (section 1.1). If this fails, metoclopramide 10 mg every 6 to 8 hours by mouth or by intramuscular injection can be added; if this also fails, chlorpromazine 10–25 mg every 6 to 8 hours can be tried.

---

1. Studies have indicated that administration of the last dose of the *oral solution* with the first dose of the *modified-release tablets* is not necessary.

ANOREXIA. Anorexia may be helped by prednisolone 15–30 mg daily or dexamethasone 2–4 mg daily.

CONSTIPATION. Constipation is a very common cause of distress and is almost invariable after administration of an opioid. It should be prevented if possible by the regular administration of laxatives; a faecal softener with a peristaltic stimulant (e.g. co-danthramer), or lactulose solution with a senna preparation should be used (section 1.6.2 and section 1.6.3).

FUNGATING GROWTH. Fungating growth may be treated by regular dressing and oral administration of metronidazole; topical application of metronidazole is also used.

CAPILLARY BLEEDING. Capillary bleeding may be reduced by applying gauze soaked in adrenaline (epinephrine) solution 1 mg/mL (1 in 1000).

DRY MOUTH. Dry mouth may be relieved by good mouth care and measures such as the sucking of ice or pineapple chunks or the use of artificial saliva (section 12.3.5); dry mouth associated with candidiasis can be treated by oral preparations of nystatin or miconazole (section 12.3.2); alternatively, fluconazole can be given by mouth (section 5.2). Dry mouth may be caused by certain medication including opioids, antimuscarinic drugs (e.g. hyoscine), antidepressants and some anti-emetics; if possible, an alternative preparation should be considered.

PRURITUS. Pruritus, even when associated with obstructive jaundice, often responds to simple measures such as application of emollients (section 13.2.1). In the case of obstructive jaundice, further measures include administration of colestyramine or an anabolic steroid, such as stanozolol 5–10 mg daily; antihistamines can be helpful (section 3.4.1).

CONVULSIONS. Patients with cerebral tumours or uraemia may be susceptible to convulsions. Prophylactic treatment with phenytoin or carbamazepine (section 4.8.1) should be considered. When oral medication is no longer possible, diazepam as suppositories 10–20 mg every 4 to 8 hours, or phenobarbital by injection 50–200 mg twice daily is continued as prophylaxis. For the use of midazolam by subcutaneous infusion using a syringe driver, see below.

DYSPHAGIA. A corticosteroid such as dexamethasone 8 mg daily may help, temporarily, if there is an obstruction due to tumour. See also under Dry Mouth.

NAUSEA AND VOMITING. Nausea and vomiting are common in patients with advanced cancer. Ideally, the cause should be determined before treatment with anti-emetics (section 4.6) is started.

Nausea and vomiting may occur with opioid therapy particularly in the initial stages but can be prevented by giving an anti-emetic such as haloperidol or metoclopramide. An anti-emetic is usually necessary only for the first 4 or 5 days and therefore combined preparations containing an opioid with an anti-emetic are not recommended because they lead to unnecessary anti-emetic therapy (and associated side-effects when used long-term).

Metoclopramide has a prokinetic action and is used in a dose of 10 mg 3 times daily by mouth for nausea and vomiting associated with gastritis, gastric stasis, and functional bowel obstruction. Drugs with antimuscarinic effects antagonise prokinetic drugs and, where possible, should not therefore be used concurrently.

Haloperidol is used in a dose of 1.5 mg daily (or twice daily if nausea continues) by mouth for most chemical causes of vomiting (e.g. hypercalcaemia, renal failure).

Cyclizine is given in a dose of 50 mg up to 3 times daily by mouth. It is used for nausea and vomiting due to mechanical bowel obstruction, raised intracranial pressure, and motion sickness.

Anti-emetic therapy should be reviewed every 24 hours; it may be necessary to substitute the antiemetic or to add another one.

Levomepromazine (methotrimeprazine) 12.5–25 mg daily by mouth may be used if first-line antiemetics are inadequate. Dexamethasone 8–16 mg daily by mouth may be used as an adjunct.

For the administration of anti-emetics by subcutaneous infusion using a syringe driver, see below.

For the treatment of nausea and vomiting associated with cancer chemotherapy, see section 8.1.

INSOMNIA. Patients with advanced cancer may not sleep because of discomfort, cramps, night sweats, joint stiffness, or fear. There should be appropriate treatment of these problems before hypnotics are used. Benzodiazepines, such as temazepam, may be useful (section 4.1.1).

HYPERCALCAEMIA. See section 9.5.1.2.

Syringe drivers

Although drugs can usually be administered *by mouth* to control the symptoms of advanced cancer, the parenteral route may sometimes be necessary. If the parenteral route is necessary, repeated administration of *intramuscular injections* can be difficult in a cachectic patient. This has led to the use of a portable syringe driver to give a *continuous subcutaneous infusion*, which can provide good control of symptoms with little discomfort or inconvenience to the patient.

> **Syringe driver rate settings.** Staff using syringe drivers should be **adequately trained** and different rate settings should be **clearly identified** and **differentiated**; incorrect use of syringe drivers is a common cause of drug errors.

Indications for the **parenteral route** are:

- the patient is unable to take medicines by mouth owing to *nausea and vomiting, dysphagia, severe weakness,* or *coma;*
- there is *malignant bowel obstruction* in patients for whom further surgery is inappropriate (avoiding the need for an intravenous infusion or for insertion of a nasogastric tube);
- occasionally when the patient *does not wish* to take regular medication by mouth.

NAUSEA AND VOMITING. Haloperidol is given in a *subcutaneous infusion* dose of 2.5–10 mg/24 hours.

Levomepromazine (methotrimeprazine) causes sedation in about 50% of patients; it is given in a *subcutaneous infusion dose* of 25–200 mg/24 hours, although lower doses of 5–25 mg/24 hours may be effective with less sedation.

Cyclizine is particularly liable to precipitate if mixed with diamorphine or other drugs (see under Mixing and Compatibility, below); it is given in a *subcutaneous infusion dose* of 150 mg/24 hours.

Metoclopramide may cause skin reactions; it is given in a *subcutaneous infusion dose* of 30–100 mg/24 hours.

Octreotide (section 8.3.4.3), which stimulates water and electrolyte absorption and inhibits water secretion in the small bowel, can be used by subcutaneous infusion, in a dose of 300–600 micrograms/24 hours to reduce intestinal secretions and vomiting.

BOWEL COLIC AND EXCESSIVE RESPIRATORY SECRETIONS. Hyoscine hydrobromide effectively reduces respiratory secretions and is sedative (but occasionally causes paradoxical agitation); it is given in a *subcutaneous infusion dose* of 0.6–2.4 mg/24 hours.

Hyoscine butylbromide is effective in bowel colic, is less sedative than hyoscine hydrobromide, but is not always adequate for the control of respiratory secretions; it is given in a *subcutaneous infusion dose* of 20–60 mg/24 hours (**important**: this dose of *hyoscine butylbromide* must not be confused with the much lower dose of *hyoscine hydrobromide*, above).

Glycopyrronium 0.6–1.2 mg/24 hours may also be used.

RESTLESSNESS AND CONFUSION. Haloperidol has little sedative effect; it is given in a *subcutaneous infusion dose* of 5–15 mg/24 hours.

Levomepromazine (methotrimeprazine) has a sedative effect; it is given in a *subcutaneous infusion dose* of 50–200 mg/24 hours.

Midazolam is a sedative and an antiepileptic, and is therefore suitable for a very restless patient; it is given in a *subcutaneous infusion dose* of 20–100 mg/24 hours.

CONVULSIONS. If a patient has previously been receiving an antiepileptic *or* has a primary or secondary cerebral tumour *or* is at risk of convulsion (e.g. owing to uraemia) antiepileptic medication should not be stopped. Midazolam is the benzodiazepine antiepileptic of choice for *continuous subcutaneous infusion*, and is given in a dose of 20–40 mg/24 hours.

PAIN CONTROL. Diamorphine is the preferred opioid since its high solubility permits a large dose to be given in a small volume (see under Mixing and Compatibility, below). The table below gives the approximate doses of *morphine by mouth* (as oral solution or standard formulation tablets or as modified-release tablets) equivalent to *diamorphine by injection* (intramuscularly or by subcutaneous infusion).

MIXING AND COMPATIBILITY. The general principle that injections should be given into separate sites (and should not be mixed) does not apply to the use of syringe drivers in palliative care. Provided that there is evidence of compatibility, selected injections can be mixed in syringe drivers. Not all types of medication can be used in a subcutaneous infusion. In particular, chlorpromazine, prochlorperazine and diazepam are **contra-indicated** as they cause skin reactions at the injection site; to a lesser extent cyclizine and levomepromazine (methotrimeprazine) may also sometimes cause local irritation.

In theory injections dissolved in water for injections are more likely to be associated with pain (possibly owing to their hypotonicity). The use of physiological saline (sodium chloride 0.9%) however increases the likelihood of precipitation when more than one drug is used; moreover subcutaneous infusion rates are so slow (0.1–0.3 mL/hour) that pain is not usually a problem when water is used as a diluent.

Diamorphine can be given by subcutaneous infusion in a strength of up to 250 mg/mL; up to a strength of 40 mg/mL either *water for injections* or *physiological saline* (sodium chloride 0.9%) is a suitable diluent—above that strength only *water for injections* is used (to avoid precipitation).

The following can be mixed with *diamorphine:*

Cyclizine[1]	Hyoscine hydrobromide
Dexamethasone[2]	Levomepromazine
Haloperidol[3]	Metoclopramide[4]
Hyoscine butylbromide	Midazolam

Subcutaneous infusion solution should be monitored regularly both to check for precipitation (and discoloration) and to ensure that the infusion is running at the correct rate.

PROBLEMS ENCOUNTERED WITH SYRINGE DRIVERS. The following are problems that may be encountered with syringe drivers and the action that should be taken:

- if the subcutaneous infusion runs *too quickly* check the rate setting and the calculation;
- if the subcutaneous infusion runs *too slowly* check the start button, the battery, the syringe driver, the cannula, and make sure that the injection site is not inflamed;
- if there is an *injection site reaction* make sure that the site does not need to be changed—firmness or swelling at the site of injection is not in itself an indication for change, but pain or obvious inflammation is.

---

1. Cyclizine may precipitate at concentrations above 10 mg/mL *or* in the presence of physiological saline *or* as the concentration of diamorphine relative to cyclizine increases; mixtures of diamorphine and cyclizine are also liable to precipitate after 24 hours.

2. Special care is needed to avoid precipitation of dexamethasone when preparing.

3. Mixtures of haloperidol and diamorphine are liable to precipitate after 24 hours if haloperidol concentration is above 2 mg/mL.

4. Under some conditions metoclopramide may become discoloured; such solutions should be discarded.

Equivalent doses of morphine sulphate by mouth (as oral solution *or* standard tablets *or* as modified-release tablets) *or* of diamorphine hydrochloride by intramuscular injection *or by* subcutaneous infusion

These equivalences are approximate only and may need to be adjusted according to response

ORAL MORPHINE		PARENTERAL DIAMORPHINE	
Morphine sulphate oral solution or standard tablets	Morphine sulphate modified-release tablets	Diamorphine hydrochloride by intramuscular injection	Diamorphine hydrochloride by subcutaneous infusion
every 4 hours	every 12 hours	every 4 hours	every 24 hours
5 mg	20 mg	2.5 mg	15 mg
10 mg	30 mg	5 mg	20 mg
15 mg	50 mg	5 mg	30 mg
20 mg	60 mg	7.5 mg	45 mg
30 mg	90 mg	10 mg	60 mg
40 mg	120 mg	15 mg	90 mg
60 mg	180 mg	20 mg	120 mg
80 mg	240 mg	30 mg	180 mg
100 mg	300 mg	40 mg	240 mg
130 mg	400 mg	50 mg	300 mg
160 mg	500 mg	60 mg	360 mg
200 mg	600 mg	70 mg	400 mg

If breakthrough pain occurs give a subcutaneous (preferable) or intramuscular injection of diamorphine equivalent to one-sixth of the total 24-hour subcutaneous infusion dose. It is kinder to give an intermittent bolus injection *subcutaneously*—absorption is smoother so that the risk of adverse effects at peak absorption is avoided (an even better method is to use a subcutaneous butterfly needle).

To minimise the risk of infection no individual subcutaneous infusion solution should be used for longer than 24 hours.

Prescribing for the elderly

Old people, especially the very old, require special care and consideration from prescribers. *Medicines for Older People*, a component document of the National Service Framework for Older People,[1] describes how to maximise the benefits of medicines and how to avoid excessive, inappropriate, or inadequate consumption of medicines by older people.

POLYPHARMACY. Elderly patients often receive multiple drugs for their multiple diseases. This greatly increases the risk of drug interactions as well as adverse reactions, and may affect compliance (see Taking medicines to best effect under General guidance). Moreover, symptoms such as headache, sleeplessness, and lightheadedness which may be associated with social stress, as in widowhood, loneliness, and family dispersal can lead to further prescribing, especially of psychotropics. The use of drugs in such cases can at best be a poor substitute for effective social measures and at worst pose a serious threat from adverse reactions. Whilst unnecessary medication should be avoided, elderly patients should not be denied effective treatments such as those for stroke prophylaxis in atrial fibrillation or for osteoporosis.

FORM OF MEDICINE. Frail elderly patients may have difficulty swallowing tablets; if left in the mouth, ulceration may develop. They should always be encouraged to take their tablets or capsules with enough fluid, and in some cases it may be helpful to discuss with the patient the possibility of prescribing the drug as a liquid if available.

MANIFESTATIONS OF AGEING. In very old subjects, manifestations of normal ageing may be mistaken for disease and lead to inappropriate prescribing. For example, drugs such as prochlorperazine are commonly misprescribed for giddiness due to age-related loss of postural stability. Not only is such treatment ineffective but the patient may experience serious side-effects such as parkinsonism, postural hypotension, and confusion.

SELF-MEDICATION. Self-medication with over-the-counter products or with drugs prescribed for a previous illness (or even for another person) may be an added complication. Discussion with both the patient and relatives as well as a home visit may be needed to establish exactly what is being taken.

SENSITIVITY. The ageing nervous system shows increased *susceptibility* to many commonly used drugs, such as opioid analgesics, benzodiazepines, antipsychotics, and antiparkinsonian drugs, all of which must be used with caution. Similarly, other organs may also be more susceptible to the effects of drugs such as antihypertensives and NSAIDs.

1. Department of Health. National Service Framework for Older People. London: Department of Health, March 2001

Pharmacokinetics

The most important effect of age is reduction in renal clearance. Many aged patients thus *excrete drugs slowly*, and are *highly susceptible to nephrotoxic drugs*. Acute illness may lead to rapid reduction in renal clearance, especially if accompanied by dehydration. Hence, a patient stabilised on a drug with a narrow margin between the therapeutic and the toxic dose (e.g. digoxin) may rapidly develop adverse effects in the aftermath of a myocardial infarction or a respiratory-tract infection. Metabolism of drugs in the liver may be reduced in the elderly. Furthermore, body composition alters with increasing age and may affect the distribution of drugs.

The net result of pharmacokinetic changes is that the tissue concentration of a drug is commonly increased by over 50%, and debilitated patients may show even larger changes.

Adverse reactions

Adverse reactions often present in the elderly in a vague and non-specific fashion. *Confusion* is often the presenting symptom (caused by almost any of the commonly used drugs). Other common manifestations are *constipation* (with antimuscarinics and many tranquillisers) and postural *hypotension* and *falls* (with diuretics and many psychotropics).

HYPNOTICS. Many hypnotics with long half-lives have serious hangover effects of drowsiness, unsteady gait, and even slurred speech and confusion. Those with short half-lives should be used but they too can present problems (section 4.1.1). Short courses of hypnotics are occasionally useful for helping a patient through an acute illness or some other crisis but every effort must be made to avoid dependence. Benzodiazepines impair balance, which may result in falls.

DIURETICS. Diuretics are overprescribed in old age and should **not** be used on a long-term basis to treat simple gravitational oedema which will usually respond to increased movement, raising the legs, and support stockings. A few days of diuretic treatment may speed the clearing of the oedema but it should rarely need continued drug therapy.

NSAIDs. Bleeding associated with *aspirin* and *other NSAIDs* is more common in the elderly who are more likely to have a fatal or serious outcome. NSAIDs are also a special hazard in patients with cardiac disease or renal impairment which may again place older patients at particular risk.

Owing to the *increased susceptibilty of the elderly* to the *side-effects of NSAIDs* the following recommendations are made:

- for *osteoarthritis, soft-tissue lesions* and *back pain* first try measures such as weight reduction (if obese), warmth, exercise and use of a walking stick;
- for *osteoarthritis, soft-tissue lesions, back pain* and *pain in rheumatoid arthritis*, paracetamol should be used first and can often provide adequate pain relief;
- alternatively, a low-dose NSAID (e.g. ibuprofen up to 1.2 g daily may be given;

- for pain relief when either drug is inadequate, paracetamol in a full dose plus a low-dose NSAID may be given;
- if necessary, the NSAID dose can be increased or an opioid analgesic given with paracetamol;
- do not give two NSAIDs at the same time.

For advice on prophylaxis of NSAID-induced peptic ulcers if continued NSAID treatment is necessary, see section 1.3.

OTHER DRUGS. Other drugs which commonly cause adverse reactions are *antiparkinsonian drugs, antihypertensives, psychotropics,* and *digoxin*. The usual maintenance dose of digoxin in very old patients is 125 micrograms daily (62.5 micrograms in those with renal disease); lower doses are often inadequate but toxicity is common in those given 250 micrograms daily.

Drug-induced blood disorders are much more common in the elderly. Therefore drugs with a tendency to cause bone marrow depression (e.g. *co-trimoxazole, mianserin*) should be avoided unless there is no acceptable alternative.

The elderly generally require a lower maintenance dose of *warfarin* than younger adults; once again, the outcome of bleeding tends to be more serious.

Guidelines

First always question whether a drug is indicated at all.

LIMIT RANGE. It is a sensible policy to prescribe from a limited range of drugs and to be thoroughly familiar with their effects in the elderly.

REDUCE DOSE. Dosage should generally be substantially lower than for younger patients and it is common to start with about 50% of the adult dose. Some drugs (e.g. long-acting antidiabetic drugs such as glibenclamide and chlorpropamide) should be avoided altogether.

REVIEW REGULARLY. Review repeat prescriptions regularly. In many patients it may be possible to stop some drugs, provided that clinical progress is monitored. It may be necessary to reduce the dose of some drugs as renal function declines.

SIMPLIFY REGIMENS. Elderly patients benefit from simple treatment regimens. Only drugs with a clear indication should be prescribed and whenever possible given once or twice daily. In particular, regimens which call for a confusing array of dosage intervals should be avoided.

EXPLAIN CLEARLY. Write full instructions on every prescription (*including* repeat prescriptions) so that containers can be properly labelled with full directions. Avoid imprecisions like 'as directed'. Child-resistant containers may be unsuitable.

REPEATS AND DISPOSAL. Instruct patients what to do when drugs run out, and also how to dispose of any that are no longer necessary. Try to prescribe matching quantities.

If these guidelines are followed most elderly people will cope adequately with their own medicines. If not then it is essential to enrol the help of a third party, usually a relative or a friend.

Drugs and sport

Olympic Movement Anti-Doping Code: Prohibited Classes of Substances and Prohibited Methods 2000

The following are examples of classes and methods prohibited in sport:

Classes	**Stimulants** eg. amphetamine, bromantan, caffeine (above 12mcg/mL), carphedon, cocaine, ephedrine, certain beta$_2$ agonists*. **Narcotics** eg. diamorphine (heroin), morphine, methadone, pethidine. **Anabolic Agents** eg. methandienone, nandrolone, stanozolol, testosterone, clenbuterol, DHEA, androstenedione, 19-norandrostenediol, certain beta$_2$ agonists*. **Diuretics** eg. acetazolamide, frusemide, hydrochlorothiazide, triamterene, mannitol. **Peptide Hormones, Mimetics and Analogues** eg. growth hormone, corticotrophin, chorionic gonadotrophin**, pituitary and synthetic gonadotrophins**, erythropoietin, insulin* and all respective releasing factors and their analogues.
Methods	**Blood Doping** **Administering Artificial Oxygen Carriers or Plasma Expanders** **Pharmacological, Chemical and Physical Manipulation** eg. substances and methods that alter the integrity and validity of the urine, eg. diuretics, probenecid, catheterisation, sample substitution or tampering.
Classes of prohibited substances in certain circumstances	**Alcohol and Cannabinoids** Restricted in certain sports. Refer to regulations of national or international sports federations. **Local Anaesthetics** Route of administration restricted to local or intra-articular injection, when medically justified*. **Glucocorticosteroids** Route of administration restricted to topical (not rectal), inhalation and local or intra-articular injection. All other routes of administration are prohibited. **Beta-blockers** Restricted in certain sports. Refer to regulations of national or international sports federations.

*Written notification of administration to the relevant medical authority may be required, eg. governing body medical officer. Check with your governing body. **Prohibited in males only.

Treatment Guidelines
Examples of permitted & prohibited substances

	ALLOWED	BANNED
Asthma	sodium cromoglycate, theophylline, salbutamol*, terbutaline*, salmeterol*, beclomethasone†, fluticasone†. (*by inhalation only and written notification of administration should be given to relevant medical authority) († by inhalation only).	products containing sympathomimetics eg. ephedrine, isoprenaline, fenoterol, rimiterol, orciprenaline.
Cold/Cough	all antibiotics, steam & menthol inhalations, permitted antihistamines, terfenadine, astemizole, pholcodine, guaiphenesin, dextromethorphan, paracetamol.	products containing sympathomimetics eg. ephedrine, pseudoephedrine, phenylpropanolamine.
Diarrhoea	diphenoxylate, loperamide, products containing electrolytes eg. Dioralyte, Rehidrat.	products containing opioids eg. morphine.
Hayfever	antihistamines, nasal sprays containing a corticosteroid or xylometazoline, eyedrops containing sodium cromoglycate.	products containing ephedrine, pseudoephedrine.
Pain	aspirin, codeine, dihydrocodeine, ibuprofen, paracetamol, all non-steroidal anti-inflammatories, dextropropoxyphene.	products containing opioids, caffeine.
Vomiting	domperidone, metoclopramide.	

WARNING. Prescribed medicines may contain prohibited substances. Some vitamin, herbal and nutritional substances may contain prohibited substances, such as Guarana, Ma Huang, Chinese Ephedra.

The substances listed are only examples of substances permitted or prohibited by the IOC. Not all sports adopt the Olympic Movement Anti-Doping Code. If in doubt check with the relevant governing body or with the UK Sport Drug Information Line (020) 7841 9530. Email: cad@uksport.gov.uk. Website: www.uksport.gov.uk

Supplies of this card are available from: UK Sport, Ethics & Anti-Doping, 40 Bernard Street, London WC1N 1ST.

Similar cards detailing classes of drugs and doping methods prohibited by the Football Association and the Lawn Tennis Association are also available from the respective governing bodies.

General information about drugs and sports together with more comprehensive lists of permitted medications in sport is published in *Competitors and Officials Guide to Drugs and Sport* which may be purchased from UK Sport.

General Medical Council's advice. Doctors who prescribe or collude in the provision of drugs or treatment with the intention of improperly enhancing an individual's performance in sport would be contravening the GMC's guidance, and such actions would usually raise a question of a doctor's continued registration. This does not preclude the provision of any care or treatment where the doctor's intention is to protect or improve the patient's health.

Emergency treatment of poisoning

These notes are only guidelines and it is strongly recommended that **poisons information centres** (see below) be consulted in cases where there is doubt about the degree of risk or about appropriate management.

HOSPITAL ADMISSION. All patients who show features of poisoning should generally be admitted to hospital. Patients who have taken poisons with delayed actions should also be admitted, even if they appear well. Delayed-action poisons include aspirin, iron, paracetamol, tricyclic antidepressants, co-phenotrope (diphenoxylate with atropine, *Lomotil®*), and paraquat; the effects of modified-release preparations are also delayed. A note of what is known and what treatment has been given should accompany the patient to hospital.

TOXBASE

TOXBASE, the primary clinical toxicology database of the National Poisons Information Service, is available on the Internet (http://www.spib.axl.co.uk/). It provides information about routine diagnosis, treatment and management of patients exposed to drugs, household products, and industrial and agricultural chemicals. For further information contact (0131) 536 2298. **Important:** for specialised information telephone the Poisons Information Centres.

TICTAC

TICTAC is a computer-aided tablet and capsule identification system. It is available to authorised users including Regional Medicines Information Centres (see inside front cover) and Poisons Information Centres.

The **poisons information centres** (see below) will provide advice on all aspects of poisoning day and night

Poisons information centres (consult day and night)

The following single number for the UK National Poisons Information Service directs the caller to the relevant local centre:
  (0870) 600 6266

Individual centres can still be contacted directly on the following numbers:

Belfast		(028) 9024 0503
Birmingham		(0121) 507 5588
	or	(0121) 507 5589
Cardiff		(029) 2070 9901
Dublin		Dublin 837 9964
Edinburgh		(0131) 536 2300
London		(020) 7635 9191
Newcastle		(0191) 282 0300

Note. Some of these centres also advise on laboratory analytical services which may be of help in the diagnosis and management of a small number of cases

General care

It is often impossible to establish with certainty the identity of the poison and the size of the dose. Fortunately this is not usually important because only a few poisons (such as opioids, paracetamol, and iron) have specific antidotes; few patients require active removal of the poison. Most patients must be treated symptomatically. Nevertheless, knowledge of the type and timing of poisoning can help in anticipating the course of events. Patients' reports may be of little help, because they may be confused or they may only be able to say that they have taken an undefined amount, possibly of mixed drugs. Parents may think a child has taken something which could be poisonous and may exaggerate or underplay the risks out of anxiety or guilt. Sometimes symptoms are due to an illness such as appendicitis. Accidents can arise from a number of domestic and industrial products (the contents of which are not generally known). A **poisons information centre** should be consulted where there is doubt about any aspect of suspected poisoning.

Respiration

Respiration is often impaired in unconscious patients. An obstructed airway requires immediate attention. Pull the tongue forward, remove dentures and oral secretions, hold the jaw forward, insert an oropharyngeal airway if one is available, and turn the patient semiprone. The risk of inhaling vomit is minimised with the patient positioned semiprone and head down.

Most poisons that impair consciousness also depress respiration. Assisted ventilation by mouth-to-mouth or *Ambu-bag* inflation may be needed. Oxygen is not a substitute for adequate ventilation, though it should be given in the highest concentration possible in poisoning with carbon monoxide and irritant gases.

Respiratory stimulants do not help and are **potentially dangerous**.

Blood pressure

Hypotension is common in severe poisoning with central nervous system depressants. A systolic blood pressure of less than 70 mmHg may lead to irreversible brain damage or renal tubular necrosis. The patient should be carried head downwards on a stretcher and nursed in this position in the ambulance. Oxygen should be given to correct hypoxia and an intravenous infusion set up if practicable. Vasopressor drugs should **not** be used.

Fluid depletion without hypotension is common after prolonged coma and after aspirin poisoning due to vomiting, sweating, and hyperpnoea.

Hypertension, often transient, occurs less frequently than hypotension in poisoning; it may be associated with sympathomimetic drugs such as amphetamines, phencyclidine, and cocaine.

Heart

Cardiac conduction defects and arrhythmias may occur in acute poisoning, notably with tricyclic antidepressants. Arrhythmias often respond to correction of underlying hypoxia, acidosis, or other biochemical abnormalities. Ventricular arrhythmias that have been confirmed by emergency ECG and which are causing serious hypotension may require treatment. If the QT interval is prolonged, specialist advice should be sought because the use of some anti-arrhythmic drugs may be inappropriate. Supraventricular arrhythmias are seldom life-threatening and drug treatment is best withheld until the patient reaches hospital.

Body temperature

Hypothermia may develop in patients of any age who have been deeply unconscious for some hours particularly following overdose with barbiturates or phenothiazines. It may be missed unless core temperature is measured using a low-reading rectal thermometer or by some other means. Hypothermia is best treated by wrapping the patient (e.g. in a 'space blanket') to conserve body heat. A *mild* source of heat (such as water bottles heated to 42°C) may be used but care must be taken to avoid causing burns.

Hyperthermia can develop in patients taking CNS stimulants; children and the elderly are also at risk when taking drugs with antimuscarinic properties at therapeutic doses. It is initially managed by removing all unnecessary clothing. Sponging with tepid water will promote evaporation; iced water should **not** be used.

Both hypothermia and hyperthermia require urgent hospitalisation for assessment and supportive treatment.

Convulsions

Single short-lived convulsions do not require treatment. If convulsions are protracted or recur frequently, lorazepam 4 mg or diazepam (preferably as emulsion) up to 10 mg should be given by slow intravenous injection into a large vein; the benzodiazepines should not be given intramuscularly.

Removal and elimination

Removal from the stomach

The dangers of attempting to empty the stomach have to be balanced against the toxicity of the ingested poison, as assessed by the quantity ingested, the inherent toxicity of the poison, and the time since ingestion. Gastric emptying is clearly unnecessary if the risk of toxicity is small or if the patient presents too late.

Emptying the stomach by **gastric lavage** is of doubtful value if attempted more than 1 hour after ingestion. The chief danger of gastric aspiration and lavage is inhalation of stomach contents, and it should **not** be attempted in drowsy or comatose patients unless there is a good enough cough reflex or the airway can be protected by a cuffed endotracheal tube. Stomach tubes should **not** be passed after corrosive poisoning.

Petroleum products are more dangerous in the lungs than in the stomach and therefore removal from the stomach is **not** advised because of the risk of inhalation.

On balance gastric lavage is seldom practicable or desirable before the patient reaches hospital.

Emesis induced by **ipecacuanha** (Paediatric Ipecacuanha Emetic Mixture BP) has been used in adults and children, but it is of very limited value. There is no evidence that it prevents clinically significant absorption (even if used within 1–2 hours) and its adverse effects may often complicate diagnosis particularly in iron poisoning. Induction of emesis should be considered only if gastric lavage is inadvisable or refused (for advice call a poisons information centre) *and if*:

- the patient is fully conscious;
- the ingested poison is neither corrosive nor a petroleum distillate;
- the poison is not adsorbed by activated charcoal.

Salt solutions, copper sulphate, apomorphine, and mustard are dangerous and should **not** be used to induce emesis.

IPECACUANHA

Indications: induction of emesis in selected patients, see notes above

Cautions: avoid in poisoning with corrosive or petroleum products owing to risk of aspiration (see notes above); also avoid if risk of aspiration, in shock, or if risk of convulsions; cardiovascular disease

Side-effects: excessive vomiting and mucosal damage; cardiac effects if absorbed

Dose: see under preparation below

Ipecacuanha Emetic Mixture, Paediatric, BP
Paediatric Ipecacuanha Emetic
Note. Paediatric Ipecacuanha Emetic Mixture is equivalent in strength to Ipecac Syrup USP
Mixture, ipecacuanha liquid extract 0.7 mL, hydrochloric acid 0.025 mL, glycerol 1 mL, syrup to 10 mL
Dose: ADULT 30 mL; CHILD 6–18 months 10 mL, older children 15 mL; the dose is followed by a tumblerful of water and repeated after 20 minutes if necessary

Prevention of absorption

Given by mouth, **activated charcoal** can bind many poisons in the stomach, thereby *reducing their absorption*. The **sooner** it is given the **more effective** it is, but it may still be effective up to 1 hour after ingestion of the poison—longer in the case of modified-release preparations or of drugs with antimuscarinic (anticholinergic) properties. It is relatively safe and is particularly useful for the prevention of absorption of poisons which are toxic in small amounts, e.g. antidepressants.

For the use of charcoal in active elimination techniques, see below.

CHARCOAL, ACTIVATED

Indications: adsorption of poisons in the gastro-intestinal system; see also active elimination techniques, below

Cautions: drowsy or comatose patient (risk of aspiration); reduced gastro-intestinal motility (risk of obstruction); not for poisoning with petroleum distillates, corrosive substances, alcohols, dicophane (DDT), malathion, and iron and lithium salts

Side-effects: black stools

Dose: see under preparations below

Actidose-Aqua® Advance (Cambridge)
Oral suspension, activated charcoal, net price 50-g pack (240 mL) = £12.50
Note. The brand name *Actidose-Aqua®* was formerly used
Dose: reduction of absorption, 50–100 g; INFANT under 1 year 1 g/kg (approx. 5 mL/kg), CHILD 1–12 years 25–50 g

Active elimination (see below for ADULT dose); INFANT under 1 year, 1 g/kg (approx. 5 mL/kg) every 4–6 hours; CHILD 1–12 years, 25–50 g every 4–6 hours

Carbomix® (Penn)
Powder, activated charcoal, net price 25-g pack = £8.50, 50-g pack = £11.90
Dose: reduction of absorption, 50 g, repeated if necessary; CHILD under 12 years 25 g (50 g in severe poisoning)
Active elimination, see below

Charcodote® (Dominion)
Oral suspension, activated charcoal, net price 50-g pack = £12.50
Dose: reduction of absorption, 50 g, repeated if necessary; CHILD under 12 years 25 g (50 g in severe poisoning)
Active elimination, see below

Liqui-Char® (Oxford Pharmaceuticals)
Oral suspension, activated charcoal, net price 50-g pack = £12.50
Dose: reduction of absorption, 50 g, repeated if necessary; CHILD under 12 years 25 g (50 g in severe poisoning)
Active elimination, see below

Medicoal® (Concord)
Granules, effervescent, activated charcoal 5 g/sachet. Contains Na^+ 17.9 mmol/sachet. Net price 5-sachet pack = £6.52, 30-sachet pack = £30.16
Dose: reduction of absorption, initially 2 sachets repeated every 15–20 minutes until dose of charcoal given is 10 times that of poison ingested (if amount known) or until max. 10 sachets/24 hours have been given; each sachet suspended in approx. 100 mL water (may be administered in divided doses for children)

Active elimination techniques

Repeated doses of **activated charcoal** by mouth *enhance the elimination* of some drugs after they have been absorbed; repeated doses are given after overdosage with:

Carbamazepine	Quinine
Dapsone	Theophylline
Phenobarbital	

The usual adult dose of activated charcoal is 50 g initially then 50 g every 4 hours. Vomiting should be treated (e.g. with an anti-emetic drug) since it may reduce the efficacy of charcoal treatment. In cases of intolerance, the dose may be reduced and the frequency increased (e.g. 25 g every 2 hours *or* 12.5 g every hour) but this may compromise efficacy.

Other techniques intended to enhance the elimination of poisons after absorption are only practicable in hospital and are only suitable for a small number of severely poisoned patients. Moreover, they only apply to a limited number of poisons. Examples include:

Haemodialysis for salicylates, phenobarbital, methyl alcohol (methanol), ethylene glycol, and lithium

Haemoperfusion for medium- and short-acting barbiturates, chloral hydrate, meprobamate, and theophylline.

Alkalinisation of the urine increases elimination of salicylates, but forced alkaline diuresis is no longer recommended.

Specific drugs

Alcohol

Acute intoxication with alcohol (ethanol) is common in adults but also occurs in children. The features include ataxia, dysarthria, nystagmus, and drowsiness, which may progress to coma, with hypotension and acidosis. Aspiration of vomit is a special hazard and hypoglycaemia may occur in children and some adults. Patients are managed supportively with particular attention to maintaining a clear airway and measures to reduce the risk of aspiration of gastric contents. The blood glucose is measured and glucose given if indicated.

Analgesics (non-opioid)

ASPIRIN. The chief features of salicylate poisoning are hyperventilation, tinnitus, deafness, vasodilatation, and sweating. Coma is uncommon but indicates very severe poisoning. The associated acid-base disturbances are complex.

Treatment must be in hospital where plasma salicylate, pH, and electrolytes can be measured. Fluid losses are replaced and sodium bicarbonate (1.26%) given to enhance urinary salicylate excretion when the plasma-salicylate concentration is greater than

500 mg/litre (3.6 mmol/litre) in adults *or*
350 mg/litre (2.5 mmol/litre) in children.

Haemodialysis is the treatment of choice for severe salicylate poisoning and should be given serious consideration when the plasma-salicylate concentration is greater than 700 mg/litre (5.1 mmol/litre) or in the presence of severe metabolic acidosis.

NSAIDs. Mefenamic acid has important consequences in overdosage because it can cause convulsions, which if prolonged or recurrent, require treatment with intravenous lorazepam or diazepam.

Ibuprofen may cause nausea, vomiting, and tinnitus, but more serious toxicity is very uncommon. Gastric emptying is indicated if more than 400 mg/kg has been ingested within the preceding hour, followed by symptomatic measures.

Patients whose plasma-paracetamol concentrations are above the **normal treatment line** should be treated with acetylcysteine by intravenous infusion (or with methionine by mouth, provided the overdose has been taken **within 10–12 hours** and the patient is not vomiting). Patients on enzyme-inducing drugs (e.g. carbamazepine, phenobarbital, phenytoin, rifampicin, and alcohol) or who are malnourished (e.g. in anorexia, in alcoholism, or those who are HIV-positive) should be treated if their plasma-paracetamol concentrations are above the **high-risk treatment line**. The prognostic accuracy after 15 hours is uncertain but a plasma-paracetamol concentration above the relevant treatment line should be regarded as carrying a serious risk of liver damage.
Graph reproduced courtesy of University of Wales College of Medicine Therapeutics and Toxicology Centre

PARACETAMOL. As little as 10–15 g (20–30 tablets) or 150 mg/kg of paracetamol taken within 24 hours may cause severe hepatocellular necrosis and, less frequently, renal tubular necrosis. Nausea and vomiting, the only early features of poisoning, usually settle within 24 hours. Persistence beyond this time, often associated with the onset of right subcostal pain and tenderness, usually indicates development of hepatic necrosis. Liver damage is maximal 3–4 days after ingestion and may lead to encephalopathy, haemorrhage, hypoglycaemia, cerebral oedema, and death.

Therefore, despite a lack of significant early symptoms, patients who have taken an overdose of paracetamol should be transferred to hospital urgently.

Administration of activated charcoal should be considered if paracetamol in excess of 150 mg/kg or 12 g **whichever is the smaller**, is thought to have been ingested within the previous hour.

Antidotes such as **acetylcysteine** and **methionine** protect the liver if given within 10–12 hours of ingestion; acetylcysteine is effective up to and possibly beyond 24 hours.

Patients at risk of liver damage and therefore requiring treatment can be identified from a single measurement of the plasma-paracetamol concentration, related to the time from ingestion, provided this time interval is not less than 4 hours; earlier samples may be misleading. The concentration is plotted on a paracetamol treatment graph of a reference line ('normal treatment line') joining plots of 200 mg/litre (1.32 mmol/litre) at 4 hours and 6.25 mg/litre (0.04 mmol/litre) at 24 hours (see below). Those whose plasma-paracetamol concentrations are above the *normal treatment line* are treated with acetylcysteine by intravenous infusion (or with methionine by mouth, provided the overdose has been taken **within 10–12 hours** *and* the patient is not vomiting). Patients on enzyme-inducing drugs (e.g. carbamazepine, phenobarbital, phenytoin, rifampicin, and alcohol) or who are malnourished (e.g. in anorexia, in alcoholism, or those who are HIV-positive) may develop toxicity at **lower** plasma-paracetamol concentrations and should be treated if concentrations are above the *high-risk treatment line* (which joins plots that are at 50% of the plasma-paracetamol concentrations of the normal treatment line).

The prognostic accuracy after 15 hours is uncertain but a plasma-paracetamol concentration above the relevant treatment line should be regarded as carrying a serious risk of liver damage.

Plasma-paracetamol concentration may be difficult to interpret when paracetamol has been ingested over several hours. If there is doubt about timing or the need for treatment then the patient should be treated with an antidote.

In remote areas methionine (2.5 g) should be given by mouth since it is seldom practicable to give acetylcysteine outside hospital. Once the patient reaches hospital the need to continue treatment with the antidote will be assessed from the plasma-paracetamol concentration (related to the time from ingestion).

See also Co-proxamol, under Analgesics (opioid).

ACETYLCYSTEINE

Indications: paracetamol overdosage, see notes above

Cautions: asthma

Side-effects: rashes, anaphylaxis

Dose: *by intravenous infusion*, in glucose intravenous infusion 5%, initially 150 mg/kg in 200 mL over 15 minutes, followed by 50 mg/kg in 500 mL over 4 hours, then 100 mg/kg in 1000 mL over 16 hours

Parvolex® (Celltech) PoM
Injection, acetylcysteine 200 mg/mL, net price 10-mL amp = £2.65

METHIONINE

Indications: paracetamol overdosage, see notes above

Cautions: hepatic impairment (Appendix 2)

Side-effects: nausea, vomiting, drowsiness, irritability

Dose: ADULT and CHILD over 6 years initially 2.5 g, followed by 3 further doses of 2.5 g every 4 hours, CHILD under 6 years initially 1 g, followed by 3 further doses of 1 g every 4 hours

Methionine (Non-proprietary)
Tablets, DL-methionine 250 mg, net price 200-tab pack = £60.44
Available from Celltech

Analgesics (opioid)

Opioids (narcotic analgesics) cause varying degrees of coma, respiratory depression, and pinpoint pupils. The specific antidote **naloxone** is indicated if there is coma or bradypnoea. Since naloxone has a shorter duration of action than many opioids, close monitoring and repeated injections are necessary according to the respiratory rate and depth of coma. Alternatively, it may be given by continuous intravenous infusion, the rate of administration being adjusted according to response and based on close monitoring of vital signs. The effects of some opioids, such as buprenorphine, are only partially reversed by naloxone. Levacetylmethadol, an opioid used in the treatment of dependence, has a very long duration of action; patients may need to be closely monitored for up to 3 days.

CO-PROXAMOL. A combination of dextropropoxyphene and paracetamol (co-proxamol) is frequently taken in overdose. The initial features are those of acute opioid overdosage with coma, respiratory depression, and pinpoint pupils. Patients may die of acute cardiovascular collapse before reaching hospital (particularly if alcohol has also been consumed) unless adequately resuscitated or given **naloxone** as antidote to the dextropropoxyphene. Paracetamol hepatotoxicity may develop later and should be anticipated and treated as indicated above.

NALOXONE HYDROCHLORIDE

Indications: overdosage with opioids; postoperative respiratory depression (section 15.1.7)

Cautions: physical dependence on opioids; cardiac irritability; naloxone is short-acting, see notes above

Dose: *by intravenous injection*, 0.8–2 mg repeated at intervals of 2–3 minutes to a max. of 10 mg if respiratory function does not improve (then question diagnosis); CHILD 10 micrograms/kg; subsequent dose of 100 micrograms/kg if no response

By subcutaneous or intramuscular injection, as intravenous injection but only if intravenous route not feasible (onset of action slower)

By continuous intravenous infusion, 2 mg diluted in 500 mL intravenous infusion solution at a rate adjusted according to the response
IMPORTANT. Doses used in acute opioid overdosage may not be appropriate for the management of opioid-induced respiratory depression and sedation in those receiving palliative care and in chronic opioid use, see also section 15.1.7 for management of postoperative respiratory depression

Naloxone (Non-proprietary) PoM
Injection, naloxone hydrochloride
400 micrograms/mL, net price 1-mL amp = £6.92
Available from Antigen, Faulding DBL

Min-I-Jet® Naloxone (Celltech) PoM
Injection, naloxone hydrochloride
400 micrograms/mL, net price 1-mL disposable syringe = £5.75; 2-mL disposable syringe = £10.71

Narcan® (Bristol-Myers Squibb) PoM
Injection, naloxone hydrochloride
400 micrograms/mL, net price 1-mL amp = £4.54
Neonatal preparations —section 15.1.7

Antidepressants

Tricyclic and related antidepressants cause dry mouth, coma of varying degree, hypotension, hypothermia, hyperreflexia, extensor plantar responses, convulsions, respiratory failure, cardiac conduction defects, and arrhythmias. Dilated pupils and urinary retention also occur. Metabolic acidosis may complicate severe poisoning; delirium with confusion, agitation, and visual and auditory hallucinations, is common during recovery.

Symptomatic treatment and activated charcoal by mouth may reasonably be given in the home before transfer but hospital admission is strongly advised, and supportive measures to ensure a patent airway and adequate ventilation during transfer are mandatory. Intravenous diazepam may be required for control of convulsions (preferably in emulsion form). Although arrhythmias are worrying, some will respond to correction of hypoxia and acidosis; the use of anti-arrhythmic drugs is best avoided. Diazepam given by mouth is usually adequate to sedate delirious patients but large doses may be required.

Antimalarials

Overdosage with chloroquine and hydroxychloroquine is extremely hazardous and difficult to treat. Urgent advice from a poisons information centre is essential. Life-threatening features include arrhythmias (which can have a very rapid onset) and convulsions (which can be intractable). Quinine overdosage is also a severe hazard and calls for urgent advice from a poisons information centre.

Beta-blockers

Therapeutic overdosages with beta-blockers may cause lightheadedness, dizziness, and possibly syncope as a result of bradycardia and hypotension; heart failure may be precipitated or exacerbated. These complications are most likely in patients with conduction system disorders or impaired myocardial function. Bradycardia is the most common arrhythmia caused by beta-blockers, but sotalol may induce ventricular tachyarrhythmias (sometimes of the torsades de pointes type). The effects of massive overdosage may vary from one beta-blocker to another; propranolol overdosage in particular may cause coma and convulsions.

Acute massive overdosage must be managed in hospital and expert advice should be obtained. Maintenance of a clear airway and adequate ventilation is mandatory. An intravenous injection of atropine is required to treat bradycardia and hypotension (3 mg for an adult, 40 micrograms/kg for a child). Cardiogenic shock unresponsive to atropine is probably best treated with an intravenous injection of glucagon 50–150 micrograms/kg [unlicensed indication and dose] in glucose 5% (with precautions to protect the airway in case of vomi-

ting). A further dose of glucagon (or an intravenous infusion) may be required if the response is not maintained. If glucagon is not available, intravenous isoprenaline or intravenous prenalterol [not on UK market] are alternatives.

Hypnotics and anxiolytics

BARBITURATES. These cause drowsiness, coma, respiratory depression, hypotension, and hypothermia. The duration and depth of cerebral depression vary greatly with the drug, the dose, and the tolerance of the patient. The severity of poisoning is often greater with a large dose of barbiturate hypnotics than with the longer-acting phenobarbital. The majority of patients survive with supportive measures alone. Repeated doses of activated charcoal (see Active Elimination Techniques, above) may be used for phenobarbital poisoning. Charcoal haemoperfusion is the treatment of choice for the small minority of patients with very severe barbiturate poisoning who fail to improve, or who deteriorate despite good supportive care.

BENZODIAZEPINES. Benzodiazepines taken alone cause drowsiness, ataxia, dysarthria, and occasionally minor and short-lived depression of consciousness. They potentiate the effects of other central nervous system depressants taken concomitantly. Flumazenil, a benzodiazepine antagonist, may be used in the *differential diagnosis* of unclear cases of multiple drug overdose but expert advice is **essential** since adverse effects may occur (e.g. convulsions in patients dependent on benzodiazepines).

Iron salts

Iron poisoning is commonest in childhood and is usually accidental. The symptoms are nausea, vomiting, abdominal pain, diarrhoea, haematemesis, and rectal bleeding. Hypotension, coma, and hepatocellular necrosis occur later. Mortality is reduced with intensive and specific therapy with **desferrioxamine**, which chelates iron. The stomach should be emptied at once by gastric lavage. The serum-iron concentration is measured as an emergency and intravenous desferrioxamine given to chelate absorbed iron in excess of the expected iron binding capacity. In **severe toxicity** intravenous desferrioxamine should be given *immediately* without waiting for the result of the serum-iron measurement (contact a poisons information centre for advice).

DESFERRIOXAMINE MESILATE
(Deferoxamine Mesilate)
Indications: iron poisoning; chronic iron overload (section 9.1.3)
Cautions: section 9.1.3
Side-effects: section 9.1.3
Dose: *by continuous intravenous infusion*, up to 15 mg/kg/hour; max. 80 mg/kg in 24 hours

Preparations
Section 9.1.3

Lithium

Most cases of lithium intoxication occur as a complication of long-term therapy and are caused by reduced excretion of the drug due to a variety of factors including dehydration, deterioration of renal function, infections, and co-administration of diuretics or NSAIDs (or other drugs that interact). Acute deliberate overdoses may also occur with delayed onset of symptoms (12 hours or more) due to slow entry of lithium into the tissues and continuing absorption from modified-release formulations.

The early clinical features are non-specific and may include apathy and restlessness which could be confused with mental changes due to the patient's depressive illness. Vomiting, diarrhoea, ataxia, weakness, dysarthria, muscle twitching, and tremor may follow. Severe poisoning is associated with convulsions, coma, renal failure, electrolyte imbalance, dehydration, and hypotension.

Therapeutic lithium concentrations are within the range of 0.4–1.0 mmol/litre; concentrations in excess of 2.0 mmol/litre are usually associated with serious toxicity and such cases may need treatment with haemodialysis (if there is renal failure). In acute overdosage much higher serum concentrations may be present without features of toxicity and all that is usually necessary is to take measures to increase urine production (e.g. by ensuring adequate fluid intake; but avoid diuretics). Otherwise treatment is supportive with special regard to electrolyte balance, renal function, and control of convulsions.

Phenothiazines and related drugs

Phenothiazines cause less depression of consciousness and respiration than other sedatives. Hypotension, hypothermia, sinus tachycardia, and arrhythmias (particularly with thioridazine) may complicate poisoning. Dystonic reactions can occur with therapeutic doses, (particularly with prochlorperazine and trifluoperazine) and convulsions may occur in severe cases. Arrhythmias may respond to correction of hypoxia, acidosis, and other biochemical abnormalities but specialist advice should be sought if arrythmias result from a prolonged QT interval; the use of some anti-arrhythmic drugs may worsen such arrhythmias. Dystonic reactions are rapidly abolished by injection of drugs such as benzatropine or procyclidine (section 4.9.2).

Stimulants

AMPHETAMINES. These cause wakefulness, excessive activity, paranoia, hallucinations, and hypertension followed by exhaustion, convulsions, hyperthermia, and coma. The early stages can be controlled by chlorpromazine and, if necessary, beta-blockers. Later, tepid sponging, anticonvulsants, and artificial respiration may be needed. Amphetamine excretion can be increased by forced acid diuresis but this is seldom necessary.

COCAINE. Cocaine can be smoked, sniffed, or injected. It stimulates the central nervous system causing agitation, dilated pupils, tachycardia, hypertension, hallucinations, hypertonia, and hyperreflexia. Convulsions, coma and metabolic acidosis may develop in the worst cases. Sedation, with intravenous diazepam, may be all that is necessary (and will also control convulsions); intravenous propranolol may be indicated for severe arrhythmias (labetalol may be preferred if there is associated hypertension).

ECSTASY. Ecstasy (methylenedioxymethamfetamine, MDMA) may cause severe reactions, even at doses that were previously tolerated. The most serious effects are delirium, coma, convulsions, ventricular arrhythmias, hyperpyrexia, rhabdomyolysis, acute renal failure, acute hepatitis, disseminated intravascular coagulation, adult respiratory distress syndrome, hyperreflexia, hypotension and intracerebral haemorrhage; hyponatraemia has also been associated with ecstasy use.

Treatment is supportive, with diazepam to control severe agitation or persistent convulsions and close monitoring including ECG. Self-induced water intoxication should be considered in patients with ecstasy poisoning.

Theophylline

Theophylline and related drugs are often prescribed as modified-release formulations and toxicity may therefore be delayed. They cause vomiting (which may be severe and intractable), agitation, restlessness, dilated pupils, sinus tachycardia, and hyperglycaemia. More serious effects are haematemesis, convulsions, and supraventricular and ventricular arrhythmias. Profound **hypokalaemia** may develop rapidly.

The stomach should be emptied if the patient presents within 2 hours. Elimination of theophylline may be enhanced by repeated doses of activated charcoal by mouth (see also under Active Elimination Techniques). Hypokalaemia is corrected by intravenous infusion of potassium chloride and may be so severe as to require 60 mmol/hour (high doses under ECG monitoring). Convulsions should be controlled by intravenous administration of diazepam (emulsion preferred). Sedation with diazepam may be necessary in agitated patients.

Provided the patient does **not** suffer from asthma, **propranolol** (section 2.4) may be administered intravenously to reverse extreme tachycardia, hypokalaemia, and hyperglycaemia.

Other poisons

Consult poisons information services day and night—p. 20.

Cyanides

Cyanide antidotes include dicobalt edetate, given alone, and sodium nitrite followed by sodium thiosulphate. These antidotes are held for emergency use in hospitals as well as in centres where cyanide poisoning is a risk such as factories and laboratories. Hydroxocobalamin is an alternative antidote but its use should ideally be discussed with a poisons information centre; the usual dose is hydroxo-cobalamin 70 mg/kg by intravenous infusion (repeated once or twice according to severity). *Cyanokit®*, which provides hydroxocobalamin 2.5 g/bottle, is available but it is not licensed for use in the UK.

DICOBALT EDETATE

Indications: acute poisoning with cyanides

Cautions: owing to toxicity to be used only when patient tending to lose, or has lost, consciousness; not to be used as a precautionary measure

Side-effects: hypotension, tachycardia, and vomiting

Dose: *by intravenous injection*, 300 mg over 1 minute (5 minutes if condition less serious) followed immediately by 50 mL of glucose intravenous infusion 50%; if response inadequate a second dose of both may be given; if no response after further 5 minutes a third dose of both may be given

Dicobalt Edetate (Cambridge) [PoM]
Injection, dicobalt edetate 15 mg/mL, net price 20-mL (300-mg) amp = £9.08

SODIUM NITRITE

Indications: poisoning with cyanides (used in conjunction with sodium thiosulphate)

Side-effects: flushing and headache due to vasodilatation

Dose: see under preparation below

Sodium Nitrite Injection [PoM]
Injection, sodium nitrite 3% (30 mg/mL) in water for injections
Dose: 10 mL by intravenous injection over 3 minutes, followed by 25 mL of sodium thiosulphate injection 50%, by intravenous injection over 10 minutes
'Special-order' [unlicensed] product: contact Martindale, or regional hospital manufacturing unit

SODIUM THIOSULPHATE

Indications: poisoning with cyanides (used in conjunction with sodium nitrite)

Sodium Thiosulphate Injection [PoM]
Injection, sodium thiosulphate 50% (500 mg/mL) in water for injections
Dose: see above under Sodium Nitrite Injection
'Special-order' [unlicensed] product: contact Martindale, or regional hospital manufacturing unit

Ethylene glycol

Ethanol (by mouth or by intravenous infusion) is used for the treatment of ethylene glycol poisoning. Fomepizole (available on named-patient basis from the UK National Poisons Information Service or from IDIS) has also been used for the treatment of ethylene glycol poisoning. Advice on the treatment of ethylene glycol poisoning should be obtained from Poisons Information Centres.

Heavy metals

Heavy metal antidotes include dimercaprol, penicillamine, and sodium calcium edetate.

DIMERCAPROL
(BAL)

Indications: poisoning by antimony, arsenic, bismuth, gold, mercury, possibly thallium; adjunct (with sodium calcium edetate) in lead poisoning

Cautions: hypertension, renal impairment (discontinue or use with extreme caution if impairment develops during treatment), elderly, pregnancy and breast-feeding

Contra-indications: not indicated for iron, cadmium, or selenium poisoning; severe hepatic impairment (unless due to arsenic poisoning)

Side-effects: hypertension, tachycardia, malaise, nausea, vomiting, salivation, lacrimation, sweating, burning sensation (mouth, throat, and eyes), feeling of constriction of throat and chest, headache, muscle spasm, abdominal pain, tingling of extremities; pyrexia in children; local pain and abscess at injection site

Dose: *by intramuscular injection*, 2.5–3 mg/kg every 4 hours for 2 days, 2–4 times on the third day, then 1–2 times daily for 10 days or until recovery

Dimercaprol (Sovereign) [PoM]
Injection, dimercaprol 50 mg/mL, net price 2-mL amp = £42.73
Note. Contains arachis (peanut) oil as solvent

PENICILLAMINE

Indications: lead poisoning

Cautions: see section 10.1.3

Contra-indications: see section 10.1.3

Side-effects: see section 10.1.3

Dose: 1–2 g daily in divided doses before food until urinary lead is stabilised at less than 500 micrograms/day; CHILD 20 mg/kg daily

Preparations
Section 10.1.3

SODIUM CALCIUM EDETATE
(Sodium Calciumedetate)

Indications: poisoning by heavy metals, especially lead

Cautions: renal impairment

Side-effects: nausea, diarrhoea, abdominal pain, pain at site of injection, thrombophlebitis if given too rapidly, renal damage particularly in overdosage; hypotension, lacrimation, myalgia, nasal congestion, sneezing, malaise, thirst, fever, chills, headache also reported

Dose: *by intravenous infusion*, ADULT and CHILD up to 40 mg/kg twice daily for up to 5 days, repeated if necessary after 48 hours

Ledclair® (Sinclair) [PoM]
Injection, sodium calcium edetate 200 mg/mL, net price 5-mL amp = £6.63

Noxious gases

CARBON MONOXIDE. Carbon monoxide poisoning is usually due to inhalation of smoke, car exhaust, or fumes caused by blocked flues or incomplete combustion of fuel gases in confined spaces. Its toxic effects are entirely due to hypoxia.

Immediate treatment of carbon monoxide poisoning is essential. The person should be removed into the fresh air, the airway cleared, and **oxygen** 100% administered as soon as available. Artificial respiration should be given as necessary and continued until adequate spontaneous breathing starts, or stopped only after persistent and efficient treatment of cardiac arrest has failed. Admission to hospital is desirable because complications may arise after a delay of hours or days. Cerebral oedema should be anticipated in severe poisoning and is treated with an intravenous infusion of mannitol (section 2.2.5). Referral for hyperbaric oxygen treatment should be discussed with the poisons information services if the victim is or has been unconscious, or has a blood carboxyhaemoglobin concentration of more than 20%, or is pregnant.

CS SPRAY. CS spray, which has been used for riot control, irritates the eyes (hence 'tear gas') and the respiratory tract; symptoms normally settle spontaneously within 15 minutes. If symptoms persist, the patient should be removed to a well-ventilated area, and the exposed skin washed with soap and water after removal of contaminated clothing. Contact lenses should be removed and hard ones washed (soft ones should be discarded). Eye symptoms should be treated by irrigating the eyes with physiological saline (or water if saline not available) and advice sought from an ophthalmologist. Patients with features of severe poisoning, particularly respiratory complications, should be admitted to hospital for symptomatic treatment.

SULPHUR DIOXIDE, CHLORINE, PHOSGENE, AMMONIA. All of these gases can cause upper respiratory tract and conjunctival irritation. Pulmonary oedema, with severe breathlessness and cyanosis may develop suddenly up to 36 hours after exposure. Death may occur. Patients are kept under observation and those who develop pulmonary oedema are given corticosteroids and oxygen. Assisted ventilation may be necessary in the most serious cases.

Pesticides

PARAQUAT. Concentrated liquid paraquat preparations (e.g. *Gramoxone®*), available to farmers and horticulturists, contain 10–20% paraquat and are extremely toxic. Granular preparations, for garden use, contain only 2.5% paraquat and have caused few deaths.

Paraquat has local and systemic effects. Splashes in the eyes irritate and ulcerate the cornea and conjunctiva. Copious washing of the eye and instillation of antibacterial eye-drops, should aid healing but it may be a long process. Skin irritation, blistering, and ulceration can occur from prolonged contact both with the concentrated and dilute forms. Inhalation of spray, mist, or dust containing paraquat may cause nose bleeding and sore throat but not systemic toxicity.

Ingestion of concentrated paraquat solutions is followed by nausea, vomiting, and diarrhoea. Painful ulceration of the tongue, lips, and fauces may appear after 36 to 48 hours together with renal failure. Some days later there may be dyspnoea with pulmonary fibrosis due to proliferative alveolitis and bronchiolitis.

Treatment should be started immediately. The single most useful measure is oral administration of repeat-dose **activated charcoal**[1]; the first dose of 100 g is given with a laxative (e.g. magnesium sulphate), followed by activated charcoal 50 g every 4 hours (or more frequently if tolerated) until the charcoal is seen in the stool. Vomiting may preclude the use of activated charcoal and an anti-emetic may be required. Gastric lavage is of doubtful value. Intravenous fluids and analgesics are given as necessary. Oxygen therapy should be avoided in the early stages of management since this may exacerbate damage to the lungs, but oxygen may be required in the late stages to palliate symptoms. Measures to enhance elimination of absorbed paraquat are probably valueless but should be discussed with the poisons information services who will also give guidance on predicting the likely outcome from plasma concentrations. Paraquat absorption can be confirmed by a simple qualitative urine test.

ORGANOPHOSPHORUS INSECTICIDES. Organophosphorus insecticides are usually supplied as powders or dissolved in organic solvents. All are absorbed through the bronchi and intact skin as well as through the gut and inhibit cholinesterase activity thereby prolonging and intensifying the effects of acetylcholine. Toxicity between different compounds varies considerably, and onset may be delayed after skin exposure.

Anxiety, restlessness, dizziness, headache, miosis, nausea, hypersalivation, vomiting, abdominal colic, diarrhoea, bradycardia, and sweating are common. Muscle weakness and fasciculation may develop and progress to generalised flaccid paralysis including the ocular and respiratory muscles. Convulsions, coma, pulmonary oedema with copious bronchial secretions, hypoxia, and arrhythmias occur in severe cases. Hyperglycaemia and glycosuria without ketonuria may also be present.

Further absorption should be prevented by emptying the stomach, removing the patient to fresh air, or removing soiled clothing and washing contaminated skin. In severe poisoning it is vital to ensure a clear airway, frequent removal of bronchial secretions, and adequate ventilation and oxygenation. **Atropine** will reverse the muscarinic effects of acetylcholine and is given in a dose of 2 mg as atropine sulphate (intramuscularly or intravenously according to the severity of poisoning) every 20 to 30 minutes until the skin becomes flushed and dry, the pupils dilate, and tachycardia develops.

---

1. **Fuller's earth** and **bentonite** given by mouth have also been used as adsorbents. A suspension of Fuller's earth 30% was used in 3 doses of 200–500 mL given at 2-hour intervals; magnesium sulphate or mannitol were given with Fuller's earth to promote diarrhoea and empty the gut.

Pralidoxime mesilate (P2S), a cholinesterase reactivator, is indicated, as an adjunct to atropine, in moderate or severe poisoning but is only effective if given within 24 hours. It may be obtained from the National Blood Service, the Welsh Blood Service and designated centres, the names of which are held by the poisons information centres (see p. 20). A dose of 30 mg/kg (diluted with 10–15 mL water for injections) by slow intravenous injection should produce improvement in muscle power within 30 minutes but repeated doses or, in severe cases, an intravenous infusion of up to 500 mg/hour may be required.

PRALIDOXIME MESILATE
(P2S)

Indications: adjunct to atropine in the treatment of organophosphorus poisoning

Cautions: renal impairment, myasthenia gravis

Contra-indications: poisoning due to carbamates and to organophosphorus compounds without anticholinesterase activity

Side-effects: drowsiness, dizziness, disturbances of vision, nausea, tachycardia, headache, hyperventilation, and muscular weakness

Dose: *by slow intravenous injection* (diluted to 10–15 mL with water for injections and given over 5–10 minutes), 30 mg/kg initially followed by 1–2 further doses if necessary; usual max. 12 g in 24 hours

CHILD 20–60 mg/kg as required depending on severity of poisoning and response

Note. Pralidoxime mesilate doses in BNF may differ from those in product literature

Pralidoxime Mesilate PoM

Injection, pralidoxime mesilate 200 mg/mL
Available as 5-mL amps (from designated centres, the National Blood Service and the Welsh Blood Service)

Snake bites and animal stings

SNAKE BITES. Acute envenoming from snake bite is rare in the UK. Many exotic snakes are kept, some illegally, but the only indigenous venomous snake is the adder (*Vipera berus*). The bite may cause local and systemic effects. Local effects include pain, swelling, bruising, and tender enlargement of regional lymph nodes. Systemic effects include early anaphylactoid symptoms (transient hypotension with syncope, angioedema, abdominal colic, diarrhoea, and vomiting), with later persistent or recurrent hypotension, ECG abnormalities, spontaneous systemic bleeding, coagulopathy, adult respiratory distress syndrome, and acute renal failure. There is a small risk of fatal envenoming especially in children and the elderly.

Early anaphylactoid symptoms should be treated with **adrenaline (epinephrine)** (section 3.4.3). Indications for antivenom treatment include systemic envenoming, especially hypotension (see above), ECG abnormalities, vomiting, haemostatic abnormalities, polymorphonuclear leucocytosis, elevated serum creatine kinase and local envenoming if, after bites on the hand or foot, swelling extends beyond the wrist or ankle within 4 hours of the bite. For both **adults** and **children**, the contents of one vial (10 mL) of **European viper venom**

antiserum (available from Farillon) is given *by intravenous injection* over 10–15 minutes or *by intravenous infusion* over 30 minutes after diluting in sodium chloride intravenous infusion 0.9% (use 5 mL diluent/kg body-weight). The **same dose** should be used for **adults** and **children**. The dose can be repeated in 1–2 hours if symptoms of **systemic envenoming** persist. Adrenaline (epinephrine) injection must be immediately to hand for treatment of anaphylactic reactions to the antivenom (for the management of anaphylaxis see section 3.4.3).

Antivenom is available for certain foreign snakes, spiders and scorpions. For information on identification, management, and supply, telephone:

Oxford	(01865) 220 968
or	(01865) 221 332
or	(01865) 741 166
Liverpool	(0151) 708 9393
Liverpool (University Hospital Aintree)	
(emergency supply only)	(0151) 525 5980
London	(020) 7635 9191

INSECT STINGS. Stings from ants, wasps, hornets, and bees cause local pain and swelling but seldom cause direct toxicity unless many stings are inflicted at the same time. If the sting is in the mouth or on the tongue marked swelling may cause respiratory distress. The stings from these insects are usually treated by cleaning the area. Bee stings should be removed as quickly as possible. Anaphylactic reactions require treatment with intramuscular **adrenaline (epinephrine)**; self-administered intramuscular adrenaline (e.g. *EpiPen®*) is the best first-aid treatment for patients with severe hypersensitivity. For the management of anaphylaxis, see section 3.4.3. A short course of an **oral antihistamine** or a **topical corticosteroid** may help to reduce inflammation and relieve itching.

MARINE STINGS. The severe pain of weeverfish stings can be relieved by immersing the stung area in uncomfortably hot, but not scalding, water (not more than 45° C). People stung by jellyfish and Portugese man-of-war around the UK coast should be removed from the sea as soon as possible. Adherent tentacles should be scraped or washed off with seawater. Alcoholic solutions including suntan lotions should not be applied because they may cause further discharge of stinging hairs. Ice packs will reduce pain and sodium bicarbonate, but not vinegar, may be useful for UK species.

1: Gastro-intestinal system

1.1 Dyspepsia and gastro-oesophageal reflux disease

Dyspepsia
Dyspepsia covers pain, fullness, early satiety, bloating, or nausea. It can occur with gastric and duodenal ulceration (section 1.3) and gastric cancer but most commonly it is of uncertain origin.

Helicobacter pylori infection may be present but most individuals with non-ulcer dyspepsia do not generally benefit from *H. pylori* eradication. However, eradication therapy (section 1.3) may be considered for dyspepsia if it is ulcer-like and if it is not accompanied by 'alarm symptoms' (e.g. bleeding or weight loss).

Gastro-oesophageal reflux disease
Gastro-oesophageal reflux disease (including non-erosive gastro-oesophageal reflux and erosive oesophagitis) is characterised by symptoms which include heartburn, acid regurgitation, and sometimes, difficulty in swallowing (dysphagia); oesophageal inflammation (oesophagitis), ulceration, and stricture formation may occur and there is an association with asthma.

The management of gastro-oesophageal reflux disease includes drug treatment, lifestyle changes and, in some cases, surgery. Initial treatment is guided by the severity of symptoms and treatment is then adjusted according to response. The extent of healing depends on the severity of the disease, the treatment chosen, and the duration of therapy.

For *mild symptoms* of gastro-oesophageal reflux disease, initial management may include the use of **antacids** and **alginates**. Alginate-containing antacids form a 'raft' that floats on the surface of the stomach contents to reduce reflux and protect the oesophageal mucosa. **Histamine H$_2$-receptor antagonists** (section 1.3.1) suppress acid secretion and they may relieve symptoms and permit reduction in antacid consumption. For refractory cases, a course of a **proton pump inhibitor** (section 1.3.5) may be considered (as described for severe symptoms, below).

For *severe symptoms* of gastro-oesophageal reflux disease or for patients with a proven or severe pathology (e.g. *oesophagitis, oesophageal ulceration, Barrett's oesophagus*), initial management involves the use of a **proton pump inhibitor** (section 1.3.5); patients need to be reassessed if symptoms persist after 6–8 weeks of treatment with a proton pump inhibitor. When symptoms abate, treatment is titrated down to a level which maintains remission (e.g. by reducing the dose of the proton pump inhibitor or by giving it intermittently, or by substituting treatment with a histamine H$_2$-receptor antagonist). However, for endoscopically confirmed *erosive, ulcerative*, or *stricturing* disease, treatment with a proton pump inhibitor usually needs to be maintained at the minimum effective dose.

A prokinetic drug such as **metoclopramide** (section 4.6) may improve gastro-oesophageal sphincter function and accelerate gastric emptying.

Patients with gastro-oesophageal reflux disease need to be advised about lifestyle changes (avoidance of alcohol and of aggravating foods such as fats); other measures include weight reduction, smoking cessation, and raising the head of the bed.

CHILDREN. Gastro-oesophageal reflux disease is common in infancy but most symptoms resolve between 12 and 18 months of age. Mild or moderate reflux without complications can be managed initially by changes in posture and thickening of liquid feeds (see Appendix 7 for suitable products) followed if necessary by treatment with an alginate-containing product (low sodium and low aluminium content for infants). For older children, life-style changes similar to those for adults (see above) may be helpful followed if necessary by treatment with an alginate-containing product.

Children who do not respond to these measures or who have problems such as respiratory disorders or suspected oesophagitis should be referred to hospital; an H_2-receptor antagonist such as cimetidine (section 1.3.1) may be needed to reduce acid secretion. If the oesophagitis is resistant to H_2-receptor blockade, the proton pump inhibitor omeprazole (section 1.3.5) can be tried.

1.1.1   Antacids and dimeticone

Antacids (usually containing aluminium or magnesium compounds) can often relieve symptoms in *ulcer dyspepsia* and in *non-erosive gastro-oesophageal reflux* (see also section 1.1); they are also sometimes used in non-ulcer dyspepsia but the evidence of benefit is uncertain. Antacids are best given when symptoms occur or are expected, usually between meals and at bedtime, 4 or more times daily; additional doses may be required up to once an hour. Conventional doses e.g. 10 mL 3 or 4 times daily of liquid magnesium–aluminium antacids promote ulcer healing, but less well than antisecretory drugs (section 1.3); proof of a relationship between healing and neutralising capacity is lacking. Liquid preparations are more effective than solids.

Aluminium- and **magnesium-containing** antacids (e.g. aluminium hydroxide, and magnesium carbonate, hydroxide and trisilicate), being relatively insoluble in water, are long-acting if retained in the stomach. They are suitable for most antacid purposes. Magnesium-containing antacids tend to be laxative whereas aluminium-containing antacids may be constipating. Aluminium accumulation does not appear to be a risk if renal function is normal (see also Appendix 3).

Preparations that contain more than one antacid have no clear advantage over simpler preparations: neutralising capacity may be the same. Complexes such as **hydrotalcite** confer no special advantage.

Sodium bicarbonate has been used in the relief of dyspepsia. Some individuals may still use sodium bicarbonate, but it has largely fallen from use as an antacid. However, it retains a place in the

management of urinary-tract disorders (section 7.4.3) and acidosis (section 9.2.1.3 and section 9.2.2). Sodium bicarbonate should be avoided in patients on salt-restricted diets.

Bismuth-containing antacids (unless chelates) are not recommended because absorbed bismuth can be neurotoxic, causing encephalopathy; they tend to be constipating. **Calcium-containing** antacids can induce rebound acid secretion: with modest doses the clinical significance is doubtful, but prolonged high doses also cause hypercalcaemia and alkalosis, and can precipitate the milk alkali syndrome.

Activated **dimeticone** (simethicone) is added to an antacid as an antifoaming agent to relieve flatulence. These preparations may be useful for the relief of hiccup in palliative care. **Alginates** added as protectants against gastro-oesophageal reflux disease (section 1.1) may be useful, but surface anaesthetics (e.g. oxetacaine) added to improve symptom relief are of doubtful efficacy. The amount of additional ingredient or antacid in individual preparations varies widely, as does their sodium content, so that preparations may not be freely interchangeable.

For **preparations** on sale to the public (not prescribable on the NHS), see p. 34.

See also section 1.3 for drugs used in the treatment of peptic ulceration.

INTERACTIONS. Antacids should preferably not be taken at the same time as other drugs since they may impair absorption. Antacids may also damage enteric coatings designed to prevent dissolution in the stomach. See also **Appendix 1** (antacids).

> **Low Na⁺**
> The words low Na⁺ added after some preparations indicate a sodium content of less than 1 mmol per tablet or 10-mL dose.

Aluminium- and magnesium-containing antacids

ALUMINIUM HYDROXIDE

Indications: dyspepsia; hyperphosphataemia (section 9.5.2.2)

Cautions: see notes above; **interactions:** Appendix 1 (antacids)

Contra-indications: hypophosphataemia; porphyria (section 9.8.2)

Side-effects: see notes above

■ Aluminium-only preparations

Aluminium Hydroxide (Non-proprietary)
Tablets, dried aluminium hydroxide 500 mg. Net price 20 = 28p
> *Dose:* 1–2 tablets chewed 4 times daily and at bedtime or as required

Oral suspension, about 4% w/w Al₂O₃ in water, with a peppermint flavour. Net price 200 mL = 41p
> *Dose:* antacid, 5–10 mL 4 times daily between meals and at bedtime or as required; CHILD 6–12 years, up to 5 mL 3 times daily
> *Note.* The brand name *Aludrox®* ▨▨▨ (Pfizer Consumer) is used for aluminium hydroxide mixture; net price 200 mL = £1.42. *Aludrox®* ▨▨▨ tablets also contain magnesium.

Alu-Cap® (3M)

Capsules, green/red, dried aluminium hydroxide 475 mg (low Na⁺). Net price 120-cap pack = £4.03

Dose: antacid, 1 capsule 4 times daily and at bedtime; CHILD not recommended for antacid therapy

■ **Co-magaldrox**

Co-magaldrox is a mixture of aluminium hydroxide and magnesium hydroxide; the proportions are expressed in the form x/y where x and y are the strengths in milligrams per unit dose of magnesium hydroxide and aluminium hydroxide respectively

Maalox TC® (Rhône-Poulenc Rorer)

Tablets, co-magaldrox 300/600 (magnesium hydroxide 300 mg, dried aluminium hydroxide 600 mg (low Na⁺)). Net price 100 = £4.68

Suspension, sugar-free, co-magaldrox 300/600 (magnesium hydroxide 300 mg, dried aluminium hydroxide 600 mg/5 mL (low Na⁺)). Net price 500 mL = £4.68

Dose: antacid, 1–2 tablets chewed or 5–10 mL suspension 4 times daily 20 minutes–1 hour after meals and at bedtime; duodenal ulcer, 3 tablets or 15 mL suspension 4 times daily (treatment) *or* twice daily (prevention of recurrence)

Mucogel® (Forest)

Suspension, sugar-free, co-magaldrox 195/220 (magnesium hydroxide 195 mg, dried aluminium hydroxide 220 mg/5 mL (low Na⁺)). Net price 500 mL = £1.82

Dose: 10–20 mL 3 times daily, 20 minutes–1 hour after meals, and at bedtime or when required; CHILD under 12 years not recommended

For **preparations** containing aluminium and magnesium on sale to the public and not prescribable on the NHS, see p. 34

MAGNESIUM CARBONATE

Indications: dyspepsia

Cautions: renal impairment; see also notes above; **interactions:** Appendix 1 (antacids)

Contra-indications: hypophosphataemia

Side-effects: diarrhoea; belching due to liberated carbon dioxide

Aromatic Magnesium Carbonate Mixture, BP

(Aromatic Magnesium Carbonate Oral Suspension)

Oral suspension, light magnesium carbonate 3%, sodium bicarbonate 5%, in a suitable vehicle containing aromatic cardamom tincture. Contains about 6 mmol Na⁺/10 mL. Net price 200 mL = 61p

Dose: 10 mL 3 times daily in water

For **preparations** also containing aluminium, see above and section 1.1.2.

MAGNESIUM TRISILICATE

Indications: dyspepsia

Cautions: see under Magnesium Carbonate

Contra-indications: see under Magnesium Carbonate

Side-effects: diarrhoea; silica-based renal stones reported on long-term treatment

Magnesium Trisilicate Tablets, Compound, BP

Tablets, magnesium trisilicate 250 mg, dried aluminium hydroxide 120 mg

Dose: 1–2 tablets chewed when required

Magnesium Trisilicate Mixture, BP

(Magnesium Trisilicate Oral Suspension)

Oral suspension, 5% each of magnesium trisilicate, light magnesium carbonate, and sodium bicarbonate in a suitable vehicle with a peppermint flavour. Contains about 6 mmol Na⁺/10 mL

Dose: 10 mL 3 times daily in water

For **preparations** also containing aluminium, see above and section 1.1.2.

Aluminium-magnesium complexes

HYDROTALCITE

Aluminium magnesium carbonate hydroxide hydrate

Indications: dyspepsia

Cautions: see notes above; **interactions:** Appendix 1 (antacids)

Side-effects: see notes above

Hydrotalcite (Peckforton)

Suspension, hydrotalcite 500 mg/5 mL (low Na⁺). Net price 500-mL pack = £1.96

Dose: 10 mL between meals and at bedtime; CHILD under 6 years not recommended, 6–12 years 5 mL

Note. The brand name *Altacite®* NHS is used for hydrotalcite suspension; for *Altacite Plus®* suspension, see below.

Antacid preparations containing dimeticone or local anaesthetics

Altacite Plus® (Peckforton)

Suspension, sugar-free, co-simalcite 125/500 (activated dimeticone 125 mg, hydrotalcite 500 mg)/5 mL (low Na⁺). Net price 500 mL = £1.96

Dose: 10 mL between meals and at bedtime when required; CHILD 8–12 years 5 mL

Tablets NHS, see p. 34

Asilone® (SSL)

Suspension, sugar-free, dried aluminium hydroxide 420 mg, activated dimeticone 135 mg, light magnesium oxide 70 mg/5 mL (low Na⁺). Net price 500 mL = £1.95

Dose: 5–10 mL after meals and at bedtime or when required up to 4 times daily; CHILD under 12 years not recommended

Tablets NHS, see p. 34

Liquid NHS, see p. 34

Maalox Plus® (Rhône-Poulenc Rorer)

Suspension, sugar-free, dried aluminium hydroxide 220 mg, activated dimeticone 25 mg, magnesium hydroxide 195 mg/5 mL (low Na⁺). Net price 500 mL = £2.38

Dose: 5–10 mL 4 times daily (after meals and at bedtime or when required); CHILD under 5 years 5 mL 3 times daily, over 5 years appropriate proportion of adult dose

Tablets NHS, see p. 34

Mucaine® (Wyeth) [PoM] [▨]

Suspension, sugar-free, aluminium hydroxide mixture 4.75 mL, magnesium hydroxide 100 mg, oxetacaine 10 mg/5 mL. Net price 200-mL pack = 76p

Dose: 5–10 mL (without fluid) 3–4 times daily (15 minutes before meals and at bedtime or when required), but evidence of value of local anaesthetic uncertain; CHILD not recommended

> For **preparations** containing aluminium and magnesium on sale to the public and not prescribable on the NHS, see p. 34

Dimeticone alone

Activated **dimeticone** (also known as simethicone) is an antifoaming agent. It is licensed for infantile colic but evidence of benefit is uncertain.

Dentinox® (DDD) [▨]

Colic drops (= emulsion), activated dimeticone 21 mg/2.5-mL dose. Net price 100 mL = £1.40

Dose: gripes, colic or wind pains, INFANT 2.5 mL with or after each feed (max. 6 doses in 24 hours); may be added to bottle feed

Note. The brand name *Dentinox®* is also used for other preparations including teething gel

Infacol® (Forest) [▨]

Liquid, sugar-free, activated dimeticone 40 mg/mL (low Na+). Net price 50 mL = £1.91. Counselling, use of dropper

Dose: gripes, colic or wind pains, INFANT 0.5–1 mL before feeds

Woodward's Colic Drops® (SSL) [▨]

Oral drops, activated dimeticone 20 mg/0.3-mL dose, net price 30 mL = £1.78

Dose: gripes, colic or wind pains, CHILD under 2 years 0.3–0.6 mL 4 times daily before feeds

---

1.1.2   Compound alginates and proprietary indigestion preparations

Alginate-containing antacids form a 'raft' that floats on the surface of the stomach contents to reduce reflux and protect the oesophageal mucosa; they are used in the management of mild symptoms of gastro-oesophageal reflux disease.

Indigestion preparations on sale to the public include antacids with other ingredients such as alginates, dimeticone, and peppermint oil.

Compound alginate preparations

Algicon® (Rhône-Poulenc Rorer)

Tablets, aluminium hydroxide-magnesium carbonate co-gel 360 mg, magnesium alginate 500 mg, heavy magnesium carbonate 320 mg, potassium bicarbonate 100 mg, sucrose 1.5 g (low Na+). Net price 60-tab pack = £2.64

Caution: diabetes mellitus (high sugar content)

Dose: 1–2 tablets 4 times daily (chewed after meals and at bedtime); CHILD under 12 years not recommended

Suspension, yellow, aluminium hydroxide-magnesium carbonate co-gel 140 mg, magnesium alginate 250 mg, magnesium carbonate 175 mg,

potassium bicarbonate 50 mg/5 mL (low Na+). Net price 500 mL (lemon- or mint-flavoured) = £3.07

Dose: 10–20 mL 4 times daily (after meals and at bedtime); CHILD under 12 years not recommended

Gastrocote® (SSL)

Tablets, alginic acid 200 mg, dried aluminium hydroxide 80 mg, magnesium trisilicate 40 mg, sodium bicarbonate 70 mg. Contains about 1 mmol Na+/tablet. Net price 100-tab pack = £3.51

Caution: diabetes mellitus (high sugar content)

Dose: 1–2 tablets chewed 4 times daily (after meals and at bedtime); CHILD under 6 years not recommended

Liquid, sugar-free, peach-coloured, dried aluminium hydroxide 80 mg, magnesium trisilicate 40 mg, sodium alginate 220 mg, sodium bicarbonate 70 mg/5 mL. Contains 1.8 mmol Na+/5 mL. Net price 500 mL = £2.67

Dose: 5–15 mL 4 times daily (after meals and at bedtime)

Gaviscon® (R&C)

Tablets, sugar-free, alginic acid 500 mg, dried aluminium hydroxide 100 mg, magnesium trisilicate 25 mg, sodium bicarbonate 170 mg. Contains 2 mmol Na+/tablet. Net price 60-tab pack (peppermint- or lemon-flavoured) = £2.25

Dose: 1–2 tablets chewed after meals and at bedtime, followed by water; CHILD 2–6 years 1 tablet (on doctor's advice only) and 6–12 years 1 tablet

Liquid, sugar-free, sodium alginate 250 mg, sodium bicarbonate 133.5 mg, calcium carbonate 80 mg/5 mL. Contains about 3 mmol Na+/5 mL. Net price 500 mL (aniseed- or peppermint-flavour) = £2.70

Dose: 10–20 mL after meals and at bedtime; CHILD 2–6 years (on doctor's advice only) and 6–12 years 5–10 mL

Gaviscon 250® [NHS], *Gaviscon 500® Tablets*, and *Gaviscon® Liquid Sachets*, see p. 34

Gaviscon® Advance (R&C)

Suspension, sugar-free, sodium alginate 500 mg, potassium bicarbonate 100 mg/5 mL. Contains 2.3 mmol Na+, 1 mmol K+/5 mL. Net price 500 mL (aniseed- or peppermint-flavour) = £6.44

Dose: ADULT and CHILD over 12 years, 5–10 mL after meals and at bedtime

Gaviscon® Infant (R&C)

Oral powder, sugar-free, sodium alginate 225 mg, magnesium alginate 87.5 mg, with colloidal silica and mannitol/dose (half dual-sachet). Contains 0.92 mmol Na+/dose. Net price 15 dual-sachets (30 doses) = £2.46

Dose: INFANT under 4.5 kg 1 dose (half dual-sachet) mixed with feeds (or water in breast-fed infants) when required; over 4.5 kg 2 doses (1 dual-sachet); CHILD 2 doses (1 dual-sachet) in water after each meal

Note. Not to be used in premature infants, or where excessive water loss likely (e.g. fever, diarrhoea, vomiting, high room temperature), or if intestinal obstruction. Not to be used with other preparations containing thickening agents

IMPORTANT. Each half of the dual-sachet is identified as 'one dose'. To avoid errors prescribe as 'dual-sachet' with directions in terms of 'dose'

Peptac® (IVAX)

Suspension, sugar-free, sodium bicarbonate 133.5 mg, sodium alginate 250 mg, calcium carbonate 80 mg/5 mL. Contains 3.1 mmol Na+/5 mL. Net price 500 mL (aniseed-flavoured) = £2.16

Dose: 10–20 mL after meals and at bedtime; CHILD 6–12 years 5–10 mL

Rennie® Duo (Roche Consumer Health)
Suspension, sugar-free, calcium carbonate
600 mg, magnesium carbonate 70 mg, sodium
alginate 150 mg/5 mL. Contains 2.6 mmol Na$^+$/
5 mL. Net price 500 mL (mint flavour) = £2.67
Dose: ADULT and CHILD over 12 years, 10 mL after
meals and at bedtime; an additional 10 mL may be taken
between doses for heartburn if necessary, max. 80 mL
daily
Excipients: include propylene glycol
Rennie® NHS and *Rennie Deflatine®*, see below

Topal® (Ceuta)
Tablets, alginic acid 200 mg, dried aluminium
hydroxide 30 mg, light magnesium carbonate
40 mg with lactose 220 mg, sucrose 880 mg, sodium bicarbonate 40 mg (low Na$^+$). Net price 42-
tab pack = £1.67
Caution: diabetes mellitus (high sugar content)
Dose: 1–3 tablets chewed 4 times daily (after meals and
at bedtime); CHILD half adult dose

Indigestion preparations

Indigestion **preparations** on sale to the public
(not prescribable on the NHS) include:
Actal® (alexitol = aluminium), **Actonorm Gel**® (aluminium, magnesium, activated dimeticone, peppermint
oil), **Actonorm Powder**® (section 1.2), **Altacite**®
(hydrotalcite = aluminium, magnesium), **Aludrox Liquid**® (aluminium), **Aludrox Tablets**® (aluminium,
magnesium), **Andrews Antacid**® (calcium, magnesium), **APP**® (section 1.2), **Asilone Antacid Liquid**®
(aluminium, activated dimeticone, magnesium; suspension is prescribable), **Asilone Antacid Tablets**® (aluminium, activated dimeticone), **Asilone Heartburn
Liquid**® (sodium alginate, aluminium, magnesium, sodium bicarbonate), **Asilone Heartburn Tablets**®
(alginic acid, aluminium, magnesium, sodium bicarbonate), **Asilone Windcheaters®Capsules** (activated
dimeticone)
Barum Antacid® (calcium), **Birley**® (aluminium,
magnesium), **Bismag**® (magnesium, sodium bicarbonate), **Bisma-Rex**® (bismuth, calcium, magnesium,
peppermint oil), **Bisodol Heartburn Relief Tablets**®
(alginic acid, magaldrate, sodium bicarbonate), **Bisodol
Indigestion Relief Powder**® (magnesium, sodium
bicarbonate), **Bisodol Indigestion Relief Tablets**®
and **Bisodol Extra Strong Mint Tablets**® (calcium,
magnesium, sodium bicarbonate), **Bisodol Wind
Relief Tablets**® (calcium, magnesium, sodium bicarbonate, activated dimeticone), **Boots Heartburn
Relief**® (sodium alginate, calcium, sodium bicarbonate),
Boots Double Action Indigestion Tablets® (alu-
minium, magnesium, activated dimeticone), **Boots
Indigestion Tablets**® (calcium, magnesium, sodium
bicarbonate), **Boots Children's 1 month Plus Gripe
Mixture**® (sodium bicarbonate)
Carbellon® (magnesium, charcoal, peppermint oil),
De Witt's Antacid Powder® (calcium, magnesium,
sodium bicarbonate, light kaolin, peppermint oil), **De
Witt's Antacid Tablets**® (calcium, magnesium,
peppermint oil), **Dijex**® (aluminium, magnesium),
Dynese® (magaldrate = aluminium, magnesium)
Eno®, **Eno Lemon**® (sodium bicarbonate, sodium carb-
onate), **Entrotabs**® (aluminium, attapulgite, pectin)
Gaviscon 250® **Tablets** (alginic acid, aluminium,
magnesium, sodium bicarbonate; **Gaviscon**® and
Gaviscon 500® **Tablets** are prescribable), **Gaviscon®
Liquid Sachets** (sodium alginate, calcium, sodium
bicarbonate), **Gelusil**® (aluminium, magnesium)
Maalox Plus Tablets® (aluminium, magnesium, activated dimeticone; suspension is prescribable), **
Maclean**® (aluminium, calcium, magnesium), **Magna-
tol**® (alexitol, magnesium, potassium bicarbonate, xan-
than gum), **Moorland**® (aluminium, bismuth, calcium,
magnesium, light kaolin)

Nulacin® (calcium, magnesium, peppermint oil; *contains*
gluten)
Opas® (calcium, magnesium, sodium bicarbonate)
Pepto-Bismol® (bismuth), **Phillips' Milk of Magnesia**® (magnesium), **Premiums**® (aluminium, calcium,
magnesium, peppermint oil)
Rap-eze® (calcium), **Remegel**®, **Remegel Alpine
Mint with Lemon**® and **Remegel Freshmint**® (calcium), **Remegel Wind Relief**® (calcium, activated
dimeticone), **Rennie**® (calcium, magnesium), **Rennie
Deflatine**® (calcium, magnesium, activated dimeticone), **Roter**® (bismuth, magnesium, sodium bicarbonate, frangula)
Setlers Antacid® (calcium), **Setlers Heartburn and
Indigestion Liquid**® (calcium, sodium alginate, sodium
bicarbonate), **Setlers Wind-eze**® (activated dimeticone), **Simeco**® (aluminium, magnesium, activated
dimeticone), **Sovol**® (aluminium, magnesium, activated
dimeticone)
Tums® (calcium)

1.2   Antispasmodics and other drugs altering gut motility

The smooth muscle relaxant properties of antimuscarinic and other antispasmodic drugs may be useful in *irritable bowel syndrome* and in *diverticular
disease*. The gastric antisecretory effects of conventional antimuscarinic drugs are of little practical
significance since dosage is limited by atropine-like
side-effects. Moreover, they have been superseded
by more powerful and specific antisecretory drugs,
including the histamine H$_2$-receptor antagonists.

The dopamine-receptor antagonists metoclopramide and domperidone tend to stimulate transit
in the gut.

Antimuscarinics

Antimuscarinics (formerly termed 'anticholinergics') reduce intestinal motility and may be useful
in irritable bowel syndrome and in diverticular disease. Other indications of antimuscarinic drugs
include arrhythmias (section 2.3.1), asthma and airways disease (section 3.1.2), motion sickness (section 4.6), parkinsonism (section 4.9.2), urinary
incontinence (section 7.4.2), mydriasis and
cycloplegia (section 11.5), premedication (section
15.1.3) and as an antidote to organophosphorus
poisoning (p. 28).

Antimuscarinics that are used for gastro-intestinal
smooth muscle spasm include the tertiary amines
atropine sulphate and **dicycloverine hydrochloride (dicyclomine hydrochloride)** and the
quaternary ammonium compounds **propantheline
bromide** and **hyoscine butylbromide**. The quaternary ammonium compounds are less lipid soluble
than atropine and so may be less likely to cross the
blood-brain barrier; they are also less well
absorbed. Although central atropine-like side-
effects, such as confusion, are thereby reduced,
peripheral side-effects are common with quaternary
ammonium compounds.

Propantheline bromide is indicated as an adjunct
in the treatment of gastro-intestinal disorders characterised by smooth muscle spasm (including non-
ulcer dyspepsia and irritable bowel syndrome);
atropine sulphate is also licensed for these indications. Dicycloverine hydrochloride (dicyclomine

hydrochloride) has a much less marked antimuscarinic action than atropine and may also have some direct action on smooth muscle. Hyoscine butylbromide is advocated as a gastro-intestinal antispasmodic, but it is poorly absorbed; the injection is useful in endoscopy and radiology. Non-selective antimuscarinics (e.g. belladonna alkaloids, included in preparations on sale to the public) are outmoded treatments, any clinical virtues being outweighed by atropinic side-effects.

CAUTIONS. Antimuscarinics should be used with caution (due to increased risk of side-effects) in Down's syndrome, in children and in the elderly; they should also be used with caution in gastro-oesophageal reflux disease, diarrhoea, ulcerative colitis, acute myocardial infarction, hypertension, conditions characterised by tachycardia (including hyperthyroidism, cardiac insufficiency, cardiac surgery), pyrexia, pregnancy and breast-feeding. **Interactions:** Appendix 1 (antimuscarinics).

CONTRA-INDICATIONS. Antimuscarinics are contra-indicated in angle-closure glaucoma, myasthenia gravis (but may be used to decrease muscarinic side-effects of anticholinesterases—section 10.2.1), paralytic ileus, pyloric stenosis and prostatic enlargement.

SIDE-EFFECTS. Side-effects of antimuscarinics include constipation, transient bradycardia (followed by tachycardia, palpitations and arrhythmias), reduced bronchial secretions, urinary urgency and retention, dilatation of the pupils with loss of accommodation, photophobia, dry mouth, flushing and dryness of the skin. Side-effects that occur occasionally include confusion (particularly in the elderly), nausea, vomiting and giddiness.

> ◢◣ denotes preparations that are considered to be less suitable for prescribing (see p. vi)

ATROPINE SULPHATE ◢◣

Indications: symptomatic relief of gastro-intestinal disorders characterised by smooth muscle spasm; mydriasis and cycloplegia (section 11.5); pre-medication (section 15.1.3); see also notes above
Cautions: see notes above
Contra-indications: see notes above
Side-effects: see notes above

Atropine (Non-proprietary) PoM
Tablets, atropine sulphate 600 micrograms. Net price 28-tab pack = £6.29
Available from CP
Dose: 0.6–1.2 mg at night

Preparations on sale to the public (not prescribable on the NHS) containing atropine or related alkaloids include:
Actonorm Powder® (atropine, aluminium, calcium, magnesium, sodium bicarbonate, peppermint oil),
APP® (homatropine, aluminium, bismuth, calcium, magnesium)

DICYCLOVERINE HYDROCHLORIDE/ DICYCLOMINE HYDROCHLORIDE

Indications: symptomatic relief of gastro-intestinal disorders characterised by smooth muscle spasm
Cautions: see notes above

Contra-indications: see notes above; infants under 6 months
Side-effects: see notes above
Dose: 10–20 mg 3 times daily; CHILD 6–24 months 5–10 mg up to 3–4 times daily, 15 minutes before feeds, 2–12 years 10 mg 3 times daily

[1] **Merbentyl**® (Florizel) PoM
Tablets, dicycloverine hydrochloride 10 mg, net price 20 = £1.08; 20 mg (*Merbentyl 20*®), 84-tab pack = £9.11
Syrup, dicycloverine hydrochloride 10 mg/5 mL, net price 120 mL = £1.98
1. Dicycloverine hydrochloride can be sold to the public provided that max. single dose is 10 mg and max. daily dose is 60 mg

■ Compound preparations
Kolanticon® (Peckforton)
Gel, sugar-free, dicycloverine hydrochloride 2.5 mg, dried aluminium hydroxide 200 mg, light magnesium oxide 100 mg, activated dimeticone (simethicone USP) 20 mg/5 mL, net price 200 mL = £1.69, 500 mL = £1.85
Dose: 10–20 mL every 4 hours when required

HYOSCINE BUTYLBROMIDE

Indications: symptomatic relief of gastro-intestinal or genito-urinary disorders characterised by smooth muscle spasm; dysmenorrhoea (but see section 4.7.1)
Cautions: see notes above
Contra-indications: see notes above; avoid in porphyria (section 9.8.2)
Side-effects: see notes above
Dose: *by mouth*, 20 mg 4 times daily; CHILD 6–12 years, 10 mg 3 times daily
Irritable bowel syndrome, 10 mg 3 times daily, increased if required up to 20 mg 4 times daily
By intramuscular or intravenous injection, acute spasm and spasm in diagnostic procedures, 20 mg repeated after 30 minutes if necessary (may be repeated more frequently in endoscopy); CHILD not recommended

[1] **Buscopan**® (Boehringer Ingelheim) PoM
Tablets ◢◣, coated, hyoscine butylbromide 10 mg. Net price 56-tab pack = £2.59
1. Hyoscine butylbromide can be sold to the public provided single dose does not exceed 20 mg, daily dose does not exceed 80 mg, and pack does not contain a total of more than 240 mg.
Injection, hyoscine butylbromide 20 mg/mL. Net price 1-mL amp = 20p

PROPANTHELINE BROMIDE

Indications: symptomatic relief of gastro-intestinal disorders characterised by smooth muscle spasm; urinary frequency (section 7.4.2); gustatory sweating (section 6.1.5)
Cautions: see notes above
Contra-indications: see notes above
Side-effects: see notes above
Dose: 15 mg 3 times daily at least 1 hour before meals and 30 mg at night, max. 120 mg daily; CHILD not recommended

Pro-Banthine® (Hansam) PoM
Tablets, pink, s/c, propantheline bromide 15 mg, net price 112-tab pack = £15.32. Label: 23

Other antispasmodics

Alverine, **mebeverine**, and **peppermint oil** are believed to be direct relaxants of intestinal smooth muscle and may relieve pain in *irritable bowel syndrome* and *diverticular disease*. They have no serious adverse effects but, like all antispasmodics, should be avoided in paralytic ileus. Peppermint oil occasionally causes heartburn.

ALVERINE CITRATE

Indications: adjunct in gastro-intestinal disorders characterised by smooth muscle spasm; dysmenorrhoea

Cautions: pregnancy and breast-feeding

Contra-indications: paralytic ileus; when combined with sterculia, intestinal obstruction, faecal impaction, colonic atony

Side-effects: nausea, headache, pruritus, rash and dizziness reported

Dose: 60–120 mg 1–3 times daily; CHILD under 12 years not recommended

Spasmonal® (Norgine)

Capsules, alverine citrate 60 mg (blue/grey), net price 100-cap pack = £11.69; 120 mg (*Spasmonal® Forte*, blue/grey), 60-cap pack = £13.50

Note. A proprietary brand of alverine citrate 60 mg (*Relaxyl®*) is on sale to the public for irritable bowel syndrome

■ Compound preparations

Spasmonal Fibre® (Norgine)

Granules, beige, coated, sterculia 62%, alverine citrate 0.5%. Net price 500 g = £13.70. Label: 25, 27, counselling, see below

Dose: irritable bowel syndrome, 1–2 heaped 5-mL spoonfuls swallowed without chewing with water once or twice daily after meals; CHILD not recommended

COUNSELLING. Preparations that swell in contact with liquid should always be carefully swallowed with water and should not be taken immediately before going to bed

MEBEVERINE HYDROCHLORIDE

Indications: adjunct in gastro-intestinal disorders characterised by smooth muscle spasm

Cautions: pregnancy and breast-feeding; avoid in porphyria (section 9.8.2.)

Contra-indications: paralytic ileus

Side-effects: rarely allergic reactions (including rash, urticaria, angioedema)

Dose: ADULT and CHILD over 10 years 135–150 mg 3 times daily preferably 20 minutes before meals

[1] **Mebeverine Hydrochloride** (Non-proprietary) PoM

Tablets, mebeverine hydrochloride 135 mg, net price 20 = £1.54

Available from Alpharma, APS, Generics, Hillcross, IVAX

1. Mebeverine hydrochloride can be sold to the public for symptomatic relief of irritable bowel syndrome provided that max. single dose is 135 mg and max. daily dose is 405 mg; for uses other than symptomatic relief of irritable bowel syndrome provided that max. single dose is 100 mg and max. daily dose is 300 mg; proprietary brands on sale to the public include *Colofac 100®*, *Colofac IBS®* (135 mg), *Equilon®* (135 mg), *IBS Relief®*

Colofac® (Solvay) PoM

Tablets, s/c, mebeverine hydrochloride 135 mg. Net price 20 = £1.67

Liquid, yellow, sugar-free, mebeverine hydrochloride 50 mg (as embonate)/5 mL. Net price 300 mL = £3.50

■ Modified release

Colofac® MR (Solvay) PoM

Capsules, m/r, mebeverine hydrochloride 200 mg, net price 60-cap pack = £7.41. Label: 25

Dose: irritable bowel syndrome, 1 capsule twice daily preferably 20 minutes before meals; CHILD not recommended

■ Compound preparations

[1] **Fybogel® Mebeverine** (R&C) PoM

Granules, buff, effervescent, ispaghula husk 3.5 g, mebeverine hydrochloride 135 mg/sachet. Contains 7 mmol K+/sachet (caution in renal impairment). Net price 60 sachets = £15.00. Label: 13, 22, counselling, see below

Dose: irritable bowel syndrome, ADULT, 1 sachet in water, morning and evening 30 minutes before food; an additional sachet may also be taken before the midday meal if necessary; CHILD not recommended

COUNSELLING. Preparations that swell in contact with liquid should always be carefully swallowed with water and should not be taken immediately before going to bed

1. 10-sachet pack can be sold to the public

PEPPERMINT OIL

Indications: relief of abdominal colic and distension, particularly in irritable bowel syndrome

Cautions: rarely sensitivity to menthol

Side-effects: heartburn, perianal irritation; rarely, allergic reactions (including rash, headache, bradycardia, muscle tremor, ataxia)

LOCAL IRRITATION. Capsules should not be broken or chewed because peppermint oil may irritate mouth or oesophagus

Colpermin® (Pharmacia)

Capsules, m/r, e/c, light blue/dark blue, blue band, peppermint oil 0.2 mL. Net price 100-cap pack = £10.96. Label: 5, 25

Excipients: include arachis (peanut) oil

Dose: 1–2 capsules, swallowed whole with water, 3 times daily for up to 2–3 months if necessary; CHILD under 15 years not recommended

Mintec® (Shire)

Capsules, e/c, green/ivory, peppermint oil 0.2 mL. Net price 84-cap pack = £7.04. Label: 5, 22, 25

Dose: 1–2 capsules swallowed whole with water, 3 times daily before meals for up to 2–3 months if necessary; CHILD not recommended

Motility stimulants

Metoclopramide and **domperidone** (section 4.6) are dopamine antagonists which stimulate gastric emptying and small intestinal transit, and enhance the strength of oesophageal sphincter contraction. They are used in some patients with *non-ulcer dyspepsia*. Metoclopramide is also used to speed the transit of barium during intestinal follow-through examination, and as accessory treatment for *gastro-oesophageal reflux disease*. Metoclopramide and domperidone are useful in non-specific and in cytotoxic-induced nausea and vomiting. Metoclopramide and occasionally domperidone may induce an acute dystonic reaction, particularly in young women and children—for further details of this and other side-effects, see section 4.6.

1.3 Ulcer-healing drugs

1.3.1 H$_2$-receptor antagonists
1.3.2 Selective antimuscarinics
1.3.3 Chelates and complexes
1.3.4 Prostaglandin analogues
1.3.5 Proton pump inhibitors
1.3.6 Other ulcer-healing drugs

Peptic ulceration commonly involves the stomach, duodenum, and lower oesophagus; after gastric surgery it involves the gastro-enterostomy stoma.

Healing can be promoted by general measures, stopping smoking and taking antacids and by antisecretory drug treatment, but relapse is common when treatment ceases. Nearly all duodenal ulcers and most gastric ulcers not associated with NSAIDs are caused by *Helicobacter pylori*.

The management of *H. pylori* infection and of NSAID-associated ulcers is discussed below.

Helicobacter pylori infection

Long-term healing of duodenal and gastric ulcers can be achieved rapidly by eradicating *Helicobacter pylori*; it is recommended that the presence of *H. pylori* is confirmed before starting eradication treatment. Acid inhibition combined with antibacterial treatment is highly effective in the eradication of *H. pylori*; reinfection is rare. Antibiotic-induced colitis is an uncommon risk.

One-week triple-therapy regimens that comprise a proton pump inhibitor, amoxicillin, and either clarithromycin or metronidazole, eradicate *H. pylori* in over 90% of cases. There is normally **no** need to continue antisecretory treatment (with a proton pump inhibitor or H$_2$-receptor antagonist) unless the ulcer is complicated by haemorrhage or perforation. Resistance to clarithromycin or to metronidazole is much more common than to amoxicillin and can develop during treatment. A regimen containing amoxicillin and clarithromycin is therefore recommended for initial therapy and one containing amoxicillin and metronidazole for eradication failure. Ranitidine bismuth citrate may be substituted for a proton pump inhibitor. Other regimens, including those combining clarithromycin and metronidazole are best used in specialist settings. Treatment failure usually indicates antibacterial resistance or poor compliance.

Two-week triple-therapy regimens offer the possibility of higher eradication rates compared to one-week regimens, but adverse effects are common and poor compliance is likely to offset any possible gain.

Two-week dual-therapy regimens using a proton pump inhibitor and a single antibacterial are licensed, but produce low rates of *H. pylori* eradication and are **not** recommended.

A two-week regimen using tripotassium dicitratobismuthate *plus* a proton pump inhibitor *plus* two antibacterials may have a role in the treatment of resistant cases after confirmation of the presence of *H. pylori*.

Tinidazole or tetracycline are also used occasionally for *H. pylori* eradication; they should be used in combination with antisecretory drugs and other antibacterials.

There is insufficient evidence to support eradication therapy in patients infected with *H. pylori* who continue to take NSAIDs.

Recommended regimens for *Helicobacter pylori* eradication

Acid suppressant	Antibiotic			Price for 7-day course
	Amoxicillin	Clarithromycin	Metronidazole	
Esomeprazole	1 g twice daily	500 mg twice daily	—	£35.43
20 mg twice daily	—	500 mg twice daily	400 mg twice daily	£35.02
Lansoprazole	1 g twice daily	500 mg twice daily	—	£35.06
30 mg twice daily	1 g twice daily	—	400 mg twice daily	£14.35
	—	500 mg twice daily	400 mg twice daily	£37.65
Omeprazole	1 g twice daily	500 mg twice daily	—	£40.46
20 mg twice daily	500 mg 3 times daily	—	400 mg 3 times daily	£17.66
	—	500 mg twice daily	400 mg twice daily	£40.05
Pantoprazole	1 g twice daily	500 mg twice daily	—	£38.01
40 mg twice daily	—	500 mg twice daily	400 mg twice daily	£37.60
Rabeprazole	1 g twice daily	500 mg twice daily	—	£37.56
20 mg twice daily	—	500 mg twice daily	400 mg twice daily	£37.15
Ranitidine bismuth	1 g twice daily	500 mg twice daily	—	£39.18
citrate	1 g twice daily	—	400 mg twice daily	£15.47
400 mg twice daily	—	500 mg twice daily	400 mg twice daily	£38.77

Regimens that include amoxicillin with either clarithromycin or metronidazole are suitable for use in the community. Regimens that combine clarithromycin with metronidazole are best used in specialist settings (see also notes above)

Test for *Helicobacter pylori*

^{13}C-Urea breath test kits are available for the diagnosis of gastro-duodenal infection with *Helicobacter pylori*. The test involves collection of breath samples before and after ingestion of an oral solution of ^{13}C-urea; the samples are sent for analysis by an appropriate laboratory. The test should not be performed within 4 weeks of treatment with an antibacterial or within 2 weeks of treatment with an antisecretory drug.

Helicobacter Test INFAI® (Infai) [PoM]
Oral powder, ^{13}C-urea 75 mg for dissolving in water. Net price 1 kit (including 4 breath sample containers, straws) = £21.01 (analysis included)
Pylobactell® (Torbet) [PoM]
Soluble tablets, ^{13}C-urea 100 mg. Net price 1 kit (including 6 breath sample containers, 30-mL mixing and administration vial, straws) = £20.75 (analysis included)

NSAID-associated ulcers

Gastro-intestinal bleeding and ulceration can occur with NSAID use (section 10.1.1). Wherever possible, NSAIDs should be **withdrawn** if an ulcer occurs.

A proton pump inhibitor or misoprostol may be considered for protection against NSAID-associated gastric and duodenal ulcers; colic and diarrhoea may limit the dose of misoprostol. An H$_2$-receptor antagonist may be effective for protection against NSAID-associated duodenal ulcers only.

NSAID use and *H. pylori* infection are independent risk factors for gastro-intestinal bleeding and ulceration. In patients on an NSAID, eradication of *H. pylori* is not recommended because it is unlikely to reduce the risk of NSAID-induced bleeding or ulceration.

If the *NSAID can be discontinued* in a patient who has developed an ulcer, a proton pump inhibitor usually produces the most rapid healing, but the ulcer can be treated with an H$_2$-receptor antagonist or misoprostol.

If *NSAID treatment needs to continue*, NSAID-associated ulceration is most effectively treated with a proton pump inhibitor (see also guidance issued by NICE, section 1.3.5); on healing, the dose of proton pump inhibitor should be **not** normally be reduced because asymptomatic ulcer deterioration may occur. Misoprostol is an alternative for maintenance treatment.

1.3.1 H$_2$-receptor antagonists

All H$_2$-receptor antagonists heal *gastric and duodenal ulcers* by reducing gastric acid output as a result of histamine H$_2$-receptor blockade; they can also be expected to relieve *gastro-oesophageal reflux disease* (section 1.1). High doses of H$_2$-receptor antagonists have been used in the *Zollinger–Ellison syndrome*, but a proton pump inhibitor may now be preferred.

Maintenance treatment with low doses has largely been replaced in *Helicobacter pylori* positive patients by eradication regimens (section 1.3).

Maintenance treatment may occasionally be used for those with frequent severe recurrences and for the elderly who suffer ulcer complications.

Treatment of *undiagnosed dyspepsia* with H$_2$-receptor antagonists may be acceptable in younger patients but care is required in older people because of the possibility of gastric cancer in these patients.

H$_2$-receptor antagonist therapy can promote healing of *NSAID-associated ulcers* (particularly duodenal) (section 1.3).

Treatment has not been shown to be beneficial in haematemesis and melaena, but prophylactic use reduces the frequency of bleeding from gastroduodenal erosions in hepatic coma, and possibly in other conditions requiring intensive care. Treatment also reduces the frequency of acid aspiration in obstetric patients at delivery (Mendelson's syndrome).

CAUTIONS. H$_2$-receptor antagonists should be used with caution in hepatic impairment (Appendix 2), in renal impairment (Appendix 3), pregnancy (Appendix 4), and in breast-feeding (Appendix 5). H$_2$-receptor antagonists might mask symptoms of gastric cancer; particular care is required in those whose symptoms change and in those who are middle-aged or over.

SIDE-EFFECTS. Side-effects of the H$_2$-receptor antagonists include diarrhoea and other gastro-intestinal disturbances, altered liver function tests (rarely liver damage), headache, dizziness, rash, and tiredness. Rare side-effects include acute pancreatitis, bradycardia, AV block, confusion, depression, and hallucinations particularly in the elderly or the very ill, hypersensitivity reactions (including fever, arthralgia, myalgia, anaphylaxis), and blood disorders (including agranulocytosis, leucopenia, pancytopenia, thrombocytopenia). There have been occasional reports of gynaecomastia and impotence.

INTERACTIONS. Cimetidine retards oxidative hepatic drug metabolism by binding to microsomal cytochrome P450. It should be avoided in patients stabilised on warfarin, phenytoin, and theophylline (or aminophylline), but other interactions (see **Appendix 1**) may be of less clinical relevance. Famotidine, nizatidine, and ranitidine do not share the drug metabolism inhibitory properties of cimetidine.

CIMETIDINE

Indications: benign gastric and duodenal ulceration, stomal ulcer, reflux oesophagitis, Zollinger–Ellison syndrome, other conditions where gastric acid reduction is beneficial (see notes above and section 1.9.4)

Cautions: see notes above; also preferably avoid intravenous injection (use intravenous infusion) particularly in high dosage and in cardiovascular impairment (risk of arrhythmias); **interactions:** Appendix 1 (histamine H$_2$-antagonists) and notes above

Side-effects: see notes above; also alopecia; rarely tachycardia, interstitial nephritis

Dose: *by mouth*, 400 mg twice daily (with breakfast and at night) *or* 800 mg at night (benign gastric and duodenal ulceration) for at least 4 weeks (6 weeks in gastric ulceration, 8 weeks in NSAID-associated ulceration); when necessary the dose may be increased to 400 mg 4 times daily or rarely (as in stress ulceration) to max. 2.4 g daily in divided doses; INFANT under 1 year 20 mg/kg daily in divided doses has been used; CHILD over 1 year 25–30 mg/kg daily in divided doses

Maintenance, 400 mg at night *or* 400 mg morning and night

Reflux oesophagitis, 400 mg 4 times daily for 4–8 weeks

Zollinger–Ellison syndrome (but see notes above), 400 mg 4 times daily or occasionally more

Gastric acid reduction (prophylaxis of acid aspiration; do not use syrup), obstetrics 400 mg at start of labour, then up to 400 mg every 4 hours if required (max. of 2.4 g daily); surgical procedures 400 mg 90–120 minutes before induction of general anaesthesia

Short-bowel syndrome, 400 mg twice daily (with breakfast and at bedtime) adjusted according to response

To reduce degradation of pancreatic enzyme supplements, 0.8–1.6 g daily in 4 divided doses according to response 1–1½ hours before meals

By intramuscular injection, 200 mg every 4–6 hours; max. 2.4 g daily

By slow intravenous injection (but see Cautions above) over at least 5 minutes, 200 mg; may be repeated every 4–6 hours; if larger dose needed or if cardiovascular impairment, dilute and give injection over at least 10 minutes (infusion preferable); max. 2.4 g daily

By intravenous infusion, 400 mg (may be repeated every 4–6 hours) *or by continuous intravenous infusion* usually at a rate of 50–100 mg/hour over 24 hours, max. 2.4 g daily; INFANT under 1 year, *by slow intravenous injection or by intravenous infusion*, 20 mg/kg daily in divided doses has been used; CHILD over 1 year, 25–30 mg/kg daily in divided doses

[1] **Cimetidine** (Non-proprietary) PoM

Tablets, cimetidine 200 mg, net price 120-tab pack = £5.44; 400 mg, 60-tab pack = £5.58; 800 mg, 30-tab pack = £5.71

Available from Alpharma, APS, Ashbourne (*Peptimax*®), Berk (*Ultec*®), BHR (*Phimetin*®), Bioglan, CP, Dexcel Pharma, Eastern (*Zita*®), Galen (*Galenamet*®), Hillcross, IVAX, Opus (*Acitak*®), Sovereign

1. Cimetidine can be sold to the public for adults and children over 16 years (provided packs do not contain more than 2 weeks' supply) for the short-term symptomatic relief of heartburn, dyspepsia, and hyperacidity (max. single dose 200 mg, max. daily dose 800 mg), and for the prophylactic management of nocturnal heartburn (single night-time dose 100 mg); a proprietary brand (*Tagamet 100*® containing cimetidine 100 mg) is on sale to the public

Dyspamet® (Goldshield) PoM

Suspension, sugar-free, cimetidine 200 mg/5 mL. Contains sorbitol 2.79 g/5 mL. Net price 600 mL = £24.08

Tagamet® (SmithKline Beecham) PoM

Tablets, all green, f/c, cimetidine 200 mg, net price 120-tab pack = £19.58; 400 mg, 60-tab pack = £22.62; 800 mg, 30-tab pack = £22.62

Effervescent tablets, sugar-free, cimetidine 400 mg. Contains 17.6 mmol Na$^+$/tablet. Net price 60-tab pack = £20.56. Label: 13

Excipients: include aspartame 70 mg/tablet (section 9.4.1)

Syrup, orange, cimetidine 200 mg/5 mL. Net price 600 mL = £28.49

Injection, cimetidine 100 mg/mL. Net price 2-mL amp = 36p

FAMOTIDINE

Indications: see under Dose

Cautions: see notes above; **interactions:** Appendix 1 (histamine H$_2$-antagonists) and notes above

Side-effects: see notes above; also rarely anxiety, toxic epidermal necrolysis, urticaria, anorexia, dry mouth

Dose: benign gastric and duodenal ulceration, treatment, 40 mg at night for 4–8 weeks; maintenance (duodenal ulceration), 20 mg at night; CHILD not recommended

Reflux oesophagitis, 20–40 mg twice daily for 6–12 weeks; maintenance, 20 mg twice daily

Zollinger–Ellison syndrome (but see notes above), 20 mg every 6 hours (higher dose in those who have previously been receiving another H$_2$-antagonist); up to 800 mg daily in divided doses has been used

[1] **Famotidine** (Non-proprietary) PoM

Tablets, famotidine 20 mg, net price 28-tab pack = £12.02; 40 mg, 28-tab pack = £22.76

Available from APS, Lagap

1. Famotidine can be sold to the public for adults and children over 16 years (provided packs do not contain more than 2 weeks' supply) for the short-term symptomatic relief of heartburn, dyspepsia, and hyperacidity, and for the prevention of these symptoms when associated with consumption of food or drink including when they cause sleep disturbance (max. single dose 10 mg, max. daily dose 20 mg); proprietary brands (*Boots Excess Acid Control*®, *Pepcid*® AC, *Pepcid*® AC Chewable* all containing famotidine 10 mg) are on sale to the public; a combination of famotidine and antacids (*Pepcidtwo*®) is also available for sale to the public

Pepcid® (MSD) PoM

Tablets, f/c, famotidine 20 mg (beige), net price 28-tab pack = £13.37; 40 mg (brown), 28-tab pack = £25.40

NIZATIDINE

Indications: see under Dose

Cautions: see notes above; also avoid rapid intravenous injection (risk of arrhythmias and postural hypotension); **interactions:** Appendix 1 (histamine H$_2$-antagonists) and notes above

Side-effects: see notes above; also sweating; rarely vasculitis, hyperuricaemia, exfoliative dermatitis

Dose: *by mouth*, benign gastric, duodenal or NSAID-associated ulceration, treatment, 300 mg in the evening *or* 150 mg twice daily for 4–8 weeks; maintenance, 150 mg at night; CHILD not recommended

Gastro-oesophageal reflux disease, 150–300 mg twice daily for up to 12 weeks

By intravenous infusion, for short-term use in peptic ulcer hospital inpatients as alternative to oral route, *by intermittent intravenous infusion* over 15 minutes, 100 mg 3 times daily, *or by continuous intravenous infusion*, 10 mg/hour; max. 480 mg daily; CHILD not recommended

¹**Nizatidine** (Non-proprietary) PoM

Capsules, nizatidine 150 mg, net price 60-cap pack = £16.54; 300 mg, 30-cap pack = £16.40

Available from Ashbourne (*Zinga*®)

1. Nizatidine can be sold to the public for the prevention and treatment of symptoms of food-related heartburn and meal-induced indigestion in adults and children over 16 years; max. single dose 75 mg, max. daily dose 150 mg for max. 14 days

Axid® (Lilly) PoM

Capsules, nizatidine 150 mg (pale yellow/dark yellow), net price 28-cap pack = £7.72, 30-cap pack = £8.27; 300 mg (pale yellow/brown), 30-cap pack = £16.40

Injection, nizatidine 25 mg/mL. For dilution and use as an intravenous infusion. Net price 4-mL amp = £1.14

RANITIDINE

Indications: see under Dose, other conditions where reduction of gastric acidity is beneficial (see notes above and section 1.9.4)

Cautions: see notes above; also avoid in porphyria (section 9.8.2); **interactions:** Appendix 1 (histamine H$_2$-antagonists) and notes above

Side-effects: see notes above; also rarely tachycardia, agitation, visual disturbances, erythema multiforme, alopecia

Dose: *by mouth*, 150 mg twice daily *or* 300 mg at night (benign gastric and duodenal ulceration) for 4 to 8 weeks, up to 6 weeks in chronic episodic dyspepsia, and up to 8 weeks in NSAID-associated ulceration (in duodenal ulcer 300 mg can be given twice daily for 4 weeks to achieve a higher healing rate); maintenance, 150 mg at night; CHILD (peptic ulcer) 2–4 mg/kg twice daily, max. 300 mg daily

Duodenal ulceration associated with *H. pylori* (but see p. 37 for recommended regimens), ranitidine 300 mg daily in 1–2 divided doses (plus amoxicillin 750 mg 3 times daily and metronidazole 500 mg 3 times daily) for 2 weeks; ranitidine treatment continued for a further 2 weeks

Prophylaxis of NSAID-induced duodenal ulcer, 150 mg twice daily

Reflux oesophagitis, 150 mg twice daily *or* 300 mg at night for up to 8 weeks, or if necessary 12 weeks (moderate to severe, 150 mg 4 times daily for up to 12 weeks); long-term treatment of healed oesophagitis, 150 mg twice daily

Zollinger–Ellison syndrome (but see notes above), 150 mg 3 times daily; doses up to 6 g daily in divided doses have been used

Gastric acid reduction (prophylaxis of acid aspiration) in obstetrics, *by mouth*, 150 mg at onset of labour, then every 6 hours; surgical procedures, *by intramuscular or slow intravenous injection*, 50 mg 45–60 minutes before induction of anaesthesia (intravenous injection diluted to 20 mL and given over at least 2 minutes), or *by mouth*, 150 mg 2 hours before induction of anaesthesia, and also, when possible on the preceding evening

By intramuscular injection, 50 mg every 6–8 hours

By slow intravenous injection, 50 mg diluted in 20 mL and given over at least 2 minutes; may be repeated every 6–8 hours

By intravenous infusion, 25 mg/hour for 2 hours; may be repeated every 6–8 hours

Prophylaxis of stress ulceration, initial slow intravenous injection of 50 mg (as above) then *continuous infusion*, 125–250 micrograms/kg per hour (may be followed by 150 mg twice daily *by mouth* when oral feeding commences)

¹**Ranitidine** (Non-proprietary) PoM

Tablets, ranitidine (as hydrochloride) 150 mg, net price 60-tab pack = £8.14; 300 mg, 30-tab pack = £8.14

Available from Alpharma, APS, Ashbourne (*Zaedoc*®), Berk (*Rantec*®), CP, Dominion, Galen, Generics, Genus, Goldshield, Hillcross, IVAX, Ranbaxy, Sovereign, Sterwin, Tillomed (*Ranitic*®)

1. Ranitidine can be sold to the public for adults and children over 16 years (provided packs do not contain more than 2 weeks' supply) for the short-term symptomatic relief of heartburn, dyspepsia, and hyperacidity, and for the prevention of these symptoms when associated with consumption of food or drink (max. single dose 75 mg, max. daily dose 300 mg); proprietary brands (*Zantac*® *75, Ranzac*® containing ranitidine (as hydrochloride) 75 mg) are on sale to the public

Zantac® (GlaxoWellcome) PoM

Tablets, f/c, ranitidine (as hydrochloride) 150 mg, net price 60-tab pack = £19.52; 300 mg, 30-tab pack = £19.20

Effervescent tablets, pale yellow, ranitidine (as hydrochloride) 150 mg (contains 14.3 mmol Na⁺/tablet), net price 60-tab pack = £27.88; 300 mg (contains 20.8 mmol Na⁺/tablet), 30-tab pack = £27.42. Label: 13

Note. The effervescent tablets contain aspartame (section 9.4.1)

Syrup, sugar-free, ranitidine (as hydrochloride) 75 mg/5 mL. Net price 300 mL = £22.32

Injection, ranitidine (as hydrochloride) 25 mg/mL. Net price 2-mL amp = 64p

RANITIDINE BISMUTH CITRATE

(Ranitidine Bismutrex)

Indications: see under Dose

Cautions: see notes above; see also under Tripotassium Dicitratobismuthate; **interactions:** Appendix 1 (histamine H$_2$-antagonists) and notes above

Contra-indications: moderate to severe renal impairment; pregnancy (Appendix 4); breastfeeding (Appendix 5); porphyria (section 9.8.2)

Side-effects: see notes above; may darken tongue or blacken faeces; rarely tachycardia, agitation, visual disturbances, erythema multiforme, alopecia

Dose: 400 mg twice daily, preferably with food, for 8 weeks in benign gastric ulceration or 4–8 weeks in duodenal ulceration; CHILD not recommended

Eradication of *Helicobacter pylori*, see eradication regimens on p. 37; ranitidine bismuth citrate treatment may be continued for a total of 4 weeks; long-term (maintenance) treatment not recommended (max. total of 16 weeks treatment in any 1 year); CHILD not recommended

COUNSELLING. May darken tongue and blacken faeces

Pylorid® (GlaxoWellcome) PoM

Tablets, blue, f/c, ranitidine bismuth citrate 400 mg. Net price 14-tab pack = £13.00; Counselling (discoloration of tongue and faeces)

1.3.2   Selective antimuscarinics

Pirenzepine is a selective antimuscarinic drug which was used for the treatment of gastric and duodenal ulcers. It has now been discontinued.

1.3.3   Chelates and complexes

Tripotassium dicitratobismuthate is a bismuth chelate effective in healing gastric and duodenal ulcers, but not on its own in maintaining remission. For the role of tripotassium dicitratobismuthate in a *Helicobacter pylori* eradication regimen for those who have not responded to first-line regimens, see section 1.3.

The bismuth content of tripotassium dicitratobismuthate is low but absorption has been reported; encephalopathy (described with older high-dose bismuth preparations) has not been reported.

Ranitidine bismuth citrate (section 1.3.1) is used in the management of gastric and duodenal ulcers, and in combination with two antibacterials for the eradication of *H. pylori* (section 1.3).

Sucralfate may act by protecting the mucosa from acid-pepsin attack in gastric and duodenal ulcers. It is a complex of aluminium hydroxide and sulphated sucrose but has minimal antacid properties. It should be used with caution in patients under intensive care (**important**: reports of bezoar formation, see CSM advice below)

TRIPOTASSIUM DICITRATOBISMUTHATE
(Bismuth Chelate)

Indications: benign gastric and duodenal ulceration; see also *Helicobacter pylori* infection, section 1.3

Cautions: see notes above; **interactions:** Appendix 1 (tripotassium dicitratobismuthate)

Contra-indications: renal impairment, pregnancy

Side-effects: may darken tongue and blacken faeces; nausea and vomiting reported

De-Noltab® (Yamanouchi)
Tablets, f/c, tripotassium dicitratobismuthate 120 mg. Net price 112-tab pack = £5.88. Counselling, see below
Dose: 2 tablets twice daily *or* 1 tablet 4 times daily; taken for 28 days followed by further 28 days if necessary; maintenance not indicated but course may be repeated after interval of 1 month; CHILD not recommended
COUNSELLING. Each dose to be swallowed with half a tumblerful of water; twice daily dosage to be taken 30 minutes before breakfast and main evening meal; four times daily dosage to be taken as follows: one dose 30 minutes before breakfast, midday meal and main evening meal, and one dose 2 hours after main evening meal; milk should not be drunk by itself during treatment but small quantities may be taken in tea or coffee or on cereal; antacids should not be taken half an hour before or after a dose; may darken tongue and blacken faeces

SUCRALFATE

Indications: see under Dose

Cautions: renal impairment (avoid if severe, see Appendix 3); pregnancy and breast-feeding; administration of sucralfate and enteral feeds should be separated by 1 hour; **interactions:** Appendix 1 (sucralfate)
BEZOAR FORMATION. Following reports of bezoar formation associated with sucralfate, the **CSM** has advised caution in seriously ill patients, especially those receiving concomitant enteral feeds or those with predisposing conditions such as delayed gastric emptying

Side-effects: constipation, diarrhoea, nausea, indigestion, gastric discomfort, dry mouth, rash, hypersensitivity reactions, back pain, dizziness, headache, vertigo and drowsiness, bezoar formation (see above)

Dose: benign gastric and duodenal ulceration and chronic gastritis, 2 g twice daily (on rising and at bedtime) *or* 1 g 4 times daily 1 hour before meals and at bedtime, taken for 4–6 weeks or in resistant cases up to 12 weeks; max. 8 g daily
Prophylaxis of stress ulceration (suspension), 1 g 6 times daily (max. 8 g daily)
CHILD not recommended

Sucralfate (Non-proprietary) [PoM]
Tablets, sucralfate 1 g. Net price 112-tab pack = £9.80. Label: 5
Available from Hillcross

Antepsin® (Chugai) [PoM]
Tablets, scored, sucralfate 1 g. Net price 112-tab pack = £9.80. Label: 5
COUNSELLING. Tablets may be dispersed in water
Suspension, sucralfate, 1 g/5 mL. Net price 560 mL (aniseed- and caramel-flavoured) = £9.80. Label: 5

1.3.4   Prostaglandin analogues

Misoprostol, a synthetic prostaglandin analogue has antisecretory and protective properties, promoting *gastric and duodenal ulcer* healing. It can prevent NSAID-associated ulcers, its use being most appropriate for the frail or very elderly from whom NSAIDs cannot be withdrawn.

For comment on the use of misoprostol to induce abortion or labour [unlicensed indications], see section 7.1.1.

MISOPROSTOL

Indications: see notes above and under Dose

Cautions: conditions where hypotension might precipitate severe complications (e.g. cerebrovascular disease, cardiovascular disease); **interactions:** Appendix 1 (misoprostol)

Contra-indications: pregnancy or planning pregnancy (increases uterine tone)—**important**: women of childbearing age, see also below, and breast-feeding
WOMEN OF CHILDBEARING AGE. Manufacturer advises that misoprostol should not be used in women of childbearing age unless the patient requires non-steroidal anti-inflammatory (NSAID) therapy and is at high risk of complications from NSAID-induced ulceration. In such patients it is advised that misoprostol should only be used if the patient takes *effective contraceptive measures* and has been advised of the *risks of taking misoprostol if pregnant.*

Side-effects: diarrhoea (may occasionally be severe and require withdrawal, reduced by giving single doses not exceeding 200 micrograms and by avoiding magnesium-containing antacids); also reported: abdominal pain, dyspepsia, flatulence, nausea and vomiting, abnormal vaginal bleeding (including intermenstrual bleeding, menorrhagia, and postmenopausal bleeding), rashes, dizziness

Dose: benign gastric and duodenal ulceration and NSAID-associated ulceration, 800 micrograms daily (in 2–4 divided doses) with breakfast (or main meals) and at bedtime; treatment should be continued for at least 4 weeks and may be continued for up to 8 weeks if required

Prophylaxis of NSAID-induced gastric and duodenal ulcer, 200 micrograms 2–4 times daily taken with the NSAID

CHILD not recommended

Cytotec® (Pharmacia) [PoM]
Tablets, scored, misoprostol 200 micrograms, net price 60-tab pack = £11.14. Label: 21

■ With diclofenac or naproxen
Section 10.1.1

| 1.3.5 | **Proton pump inhibitors** |

The proton pump inhibitors **omeprazole**, **esomeprazole**, **lansoprazole**, **pantoprazole** and **rabeprazole** inhibit gastric acid by blocking the hydrogen-potassium adenosine triphosphatase enzyme system (the 'proton pump') of the gastric parietal cell. Proton pump inhibitors are effective short-term treatments for *gastric and duodenal ulcers*; they are also used in combination with antibacterials for the eradication of *Helicobacter pylori* (see p. 37 for specific regimens). An initial short course of a proton pump inhibitor is the treatment of choice in *gastro-oesophageal reflux disease* with severe symptoms; patients with endoscopically confirmed *erosive, ulcerative,* or *stricturing oesophagitis* usually need to be maintained on a proton pump inhibitor (section 1.1).

Proton pump inhibitors are also used in the prevention and treatment of NSAID-associated ulcers (see p. 38 and guidance issued by NICE, below). In patients who need to continue NSAID treatment after an ulcer has healed, the dose of proton pump inhibitor should normally not be reduced because asymptomatic ulcer deterioration may occur.

Omeprazole is effective in the treatment of the *Zollinger–Ellison syndrome* (including cases resistant to other treatment); lansoprazole is also indicated for this condition.

CAUTIONS. Proton pump inhibitors should be used with caution in patients with liver disease (Appendix 2), in pregnancy (Appendix 4) and in breast-feeding. Proton pump inhibitors may mask symptoms of gastric cancer; particular care is required in those whose symptoms change and in those over 45 years of age; the presence of gastric malignancy should be excluded before treatment.

SIDE-EFFECTS. Side-effects of the proton pump inhibitors include gastro-intestinal disturbances (including diarrhoea, nausea and vomiting, constipation, flatulence, abdominal pain), headache, hypersensitivity reactions (including rash, urticaria, angioedema, bronchospasm), pruritus, dizziness, peripheral oedema, muscle and joint pain, malaise, blurred vision, depression and dry mouth. Proton pump inhibitors decrease gastric acidity and may increase the risk of gastro-intestinal infections.

NICE advice (proton pump inhibitors)

The National Institute for Clinical Excellence has provided guidance on the use of proton pump inhibitors for the following indications:

- Gastro-oesophageal reflux disease—use only for severe symptoms (reduce dose when symptoms abate) and in disease complicated by stricture, ulceration, or haemorrhage (full dose should be maintained);

- NSAID-associated ulceration in patients who need to continue NSAID treatment—on healing of the ulcer a lower dose of proton pump inhibitor may be used [but see notes above].

OMEPRAZOLE

Indications: see under Dose

Cautions: see notes above; **interactions:** Appendix 1 (proton pump inhibitors)

Side-effects: see notes above; also reported, bullous eruption, Stevens-Johnson syndrome, toxic epidermal necrolysis, anaphylaxis, fever, photosensitivity, paraesthesia, vertigo, interstitial nephritis, alopecia, somnolence, insomnia, sweating, gynaecomastia, rarely impotence, taste disturbance, stomatitis, liver enzyme changes and liver dysfunction, encephalopathy in severe liver disease; haematological changes (including agranulocytosis, leucopenia, pancytopenia, thrombocytopenia), hyponatraemia; reversible confusion, agitation, and hallucinations in the severely ill; visual impairment reported with high-dose injection

Dose: *by mouth*, benign gastric and duodenal ulcers, 20 mg once daily for 4 weeks in duodenal ulceration or 8 weeks in gastric ulceration; in severe or recurrent cases increase to 40 mg daily; maintenance for recurrent duodenal ulcer, 20 mg once daily; prevention of relapse in duodenal ulcer, 10 mg daily increasing to 20 mg once daily if symptoms return

NSAID-associated duodenal or gastric ulcer and gastroduodenal erosions, 20 mg once daily for 4 weeks, followed by a further 4 weeks if not fully healed; prophylaxis in patients with a history of NSAID-associated duodenal or gastric ulcers, gastroduodenal lesions, or dyspeptic symptoms who require continued NSAID treatment, 20 mg once daily

Duodenal ulcer associated with *Helicobacter pylori*, see eradication regimens on p. 37

Benign gastric ulcer associated with *H. pylori*, omeprazole 40 mg daily in 1–2 divided doses (plus amoxicillin 0.75–1 g twice daily) for 2 weeks

Zollinger–Ellison syndrome, initially 60 mg once daily; usual range 20–120 mg daily (above 80 mg in 2 divided doses)

Gastric acid reduction during general anaesthesia (prophylaxis of acid aspiration), 40 mg on the preceding evening then 40 mg 2–6 hours before surgery

Gastro-oesophageal reflux disease, 20 mg once daily for 4 weeks, followed by a further 4–8 weeks if not fully healed; 40 mg once daily has been given for 8 weeks in gastro-oesophageal reflux disease refractory to other treatment; may be continued at 20 mg once daily

Acid reflux disease (long-term management), 10 mg daily increasing to 20 mg once daily if symptoms return

Acid-related dyspepsia, 10–20 mg once daily for 2–4 weeks according to response

CHILD over 2 years, severe ulcerating reflux oesophagitis, 0.7–1.4 mg/kg daily for 4–12 weeks; max. 40 mg daily (to be initiated by hospital paediatrician)

By intravenous injection over 5 minutes or by intravenous infusion, gastric acid reduction during anaesthesia (prophylaxis of acid aspiration), 40 mg completed 1 hour before surgery

Benign gastric ulcer, duodenal ulcer and gastro-oesophageal reflux, 40 mg once daily until oral administration possible

CHILD not recommended

COUNSELLING. Swallow whole, *or* disperse tablets in water, *or* mix capsule contents or tablets with fruit juice or yoghurt

Losec® (AstraZeneca) [PoM]

MUPS® (= dispersible tablets), f/c, omeprazole 10 mg (light pink), net price 28-tab pack = £18.91 (also 7-tab pack, hosp. only); 20 mg (pink), 28-tab pack = £28.56 (also 7-tab pack, hosp. only); 40 mg (red-brown), 7-tab pack = £14.28. Counselling, administration

Capsules, enclosing e/c granules, omeprazole 10 mg (pink), net price 28-cap pack = £18.91 (also 7-cap pack, hosp. only); 20 mg (pink/brown), 28-cap pack = £28.56 (also 7-cap pack, hosp. only); 40 mg (brown), 7-cap pack = £14.28. Counselling, administration

▼ *Intravenous infusion*, powder for reconstitution, omeprazole (as sodium salt), net price 40-mg vial = £5.21

▼ *Injection*, powder for reconstitution, omeprazole (as sodium salt), net price 40-mg vial (with solvent) = £5.21

ESOMEPRAZOLE

Indications: see under Dose

Cautions: see notes above; renal impairment (Appendix 3); **interactions:** Appendix 1 (proton pump inhibitors)

Side-effects: see notes above; also reported, dermatitis

Dose: duodenal ulcer associated with *Helicobacter pylori*, see eradication regimens on p. 37

Gastro-oesophageal reflux disease, 40 mg once daily for 4 weeks, followed by a further 4 weeks if not fully healed or symptoms persist; maintenance 20 mg daily; symptomatic treatment in the absence of oesophagitis, 20 mg daily for up to 4 weeks, followed by 20 mg daily when required

CHILD not recommended

Nexium® (AstraZeneca) ▼ [PoM]

Tablets, f/c, esomeprazole (as magnesium trihydrate) 20 mg (light pink), net price 28-tab pack =

£18.50; 40 mg (pink), 28-tab pack = £28.56. Label: 25

LANSOPRAZOLE

Indications: see under Dose

Cautions: see notes above; **interactions:** Appendix 1 (proton pump inhibitors)

Side-effects: see notes above; also reported, Stevens-Johnson syndrome, toxic epidermal necrolysis, bullous eruption, erythema multiforme, alopecia, photosensitivity, paraesthesia, interstitial nephritis, anaphylaxis, liver enzyme changes and liver dysfunction, haematological changes (including eosinophilia, leucopenia, pancytopenia, thrombocytopenia), bruising, purpura, petechiae, fatigue, taste disturbance, vertigo, hallucinations, confusion, rarely gynaecomastia, impotence

Dose: benign gastric ulcer, 30 mg daily in the morning for 8 weeks

Duodenal ulcer, 30 mg daily in the morning for 4 weeks; maintenance 15 mg daily

NSAID-associated duodenal or gastric ulcer, 15–30 mg once daily for 4 weeks, followed by a further 4 weeks if not fully healed; prophylaxis, 15–30 mg once daily

Duodenal ulcer associated with *Helicobacter pylori*, see eradication regimens on p. 37

Zollinger-Ellison syndrome (and other hypersecretory conditions), initially 60 mg once daily adjusted according to response; daily doses of 120 mg or more given in two divided doses

Gastro-oesophageal reflux disease, 30 mg daily in the morning for 4 weeks, followed by a further 4 weeks if not fully healed; maintenance 15–30 mg daily

Acid-related dyspepsia, 15–30 mg daily in the morning for 2–4 weeks

CHILD not recommended

Zoton® (Lederle) [PoM]

Capsules, enclosing e/c granules, lansoprazole 15 mg (yellow), net price 28-cap pack = £12.98, 56-cap pack = £25.96; 30 mg (lilac/purple), 14-cap pack = £11.88, 28-cap pack = £23.75, 56-cap pack = £47.50 (also 7-cap pack, hosp. only). Label: 5, 25

Suspension, pink, powder for reconstitution, lansoprazole 30 mg/sachet (strawberry flavour), net price 28-sachet pack = £34.14. Label: 5, 13

■ With antibacterials

For additional cautions, contra-indications and side-effects see Amoxicillin (section 5.1.1), Clarithromycin (section 5.1.5), and Metronidazole (section 5.1.11)

HeliClear® (Wyeth) [PoM]

Triple pack, lansoprazole capsules 30 mg (*Zoton®*), amoxicillin (as trihydrate) capsules 500 mg, clarithromycin tablets 500 mg (*Klaricid®*). Net price 7-day pack (14 × lansoprazole caps, 28 × amoxicillin caps, 14 × clarithromycin tabs) = £36.82. Label: 5, 9, 25

Dose: eradication of *Helicobacter pylori* in patients with duodenal ulcer, lansoprazole 30 mg twice daily, clarithromycin 500 mg twice daily, and amoxicillin 1 g twice daily for 7–14 days; CHILD not recommended

HeliMet® (Wyeth) PoM

Triple pack, lansoprazole capsules 30 mg (*Zoton®*), clarithromycin tablets 500 mg (*Klaricid®*), metronidazole tablets 400 mg, net price 7-day pack (14 × lansoprazole caps, 14 × clarithromycin tabs, 14 × metronidazole tabs) = £35.40. Label: 4, 5, 9, 25, 27

Dose: eradication of *Helicobacter pylori* in patients with duodenal ulcer, lansoprazole 30 mg twice daily, clarithromycin 500 mg twice daily, and metronidazole 400 mg twice daily for 7 days; CHILD not recommended

PANTOPRAZOLE

Indications: see under Dose

Cautions: see notes above; also renal impairment (Appendix 3); **interactions:** Appendix 1 (proton pump inhibitors)

Side-effects: see notes above; also reported fever, liver enzyme changes, raised triglycerides, anaphylaxis

Dose: *By mouth,* benign gastric ulcer, 40 mg daily in the morning for 4 weeks, continued for further 4 weeks if not fully healed

Gastro-oesophageal reflux disease, 40 mg daily in the morning for 4 weeks, continued for further 4 weeks if not fully healed; may be continued at 20 mg daily (long-term management), increased to 40 mg daily if symptoms return

Duodenal ulcer, 40 mg daily in the morning for 2 weeks, continued for further 2 weeks if not fully healed

Duodenal ulcer associated with *Helicobacter pylori*, see eradication regimens on p. 37

CHILD not recommended

By intravenous injection, over 2–15 minutes, duodenal ulcer, gastric ulcer, and gastro-oesophageal reflux, 40 mg daily until oral administration can be resumed

CHILD not recommended

Protium® (Abbott) PoM

Tablets, e/c, pantoprazole (as sodium sesquihydrate) 20 mg, net price 28-tab pack = £12.88; 40 mg 28-tab pack = £23.65. Label: 25

Injection, powder for reconstitution, pantoprazole (as sodium sesquihydrate), net price 40-mg vial = £5.71

RABEPRAZOLE SODIUM

Indications: see under Dose

Cautions: see notes above; **interactions:** Appendix 1 (proton pump inhibitors)

Side-effects: see notes above; also reported, stomatitis, chest pain, cough, rhinitis, sinusitis, leucocytosis, insomnia, nervousness, drowsiness, asthenia, taste disturbance, pharyngitis, anorexia, influenza-like syndrome, sweating, weight gain

Dose: benign gastric ulcer, 20 mg daily in the morning for 6 weeks, followed by a further 6 weeks if not fully healed

Duodenal ulcer, 20 mg daily in the morning for 4 weeks, followed by a further 4 weeks if not fully healed

Gastro-oesophageal reflux disease, 20 mg daily in the morning for 4–8 weeks; may be continued at 10–20 mg daily

Duodenal and benign gastric ulcer associated with *Helicobacter pylori*, see eradication regimens on p. 37

CHILD not recommended

Pariet® (Eisai, Janssen-Cilag) PoM

Tablets, e/c, rabeprazole sodium 10 mg (pink), net price 28-tab pack = £12.43; 20 mg (yellow), 28-tab pack = £22.75. Label: 25

1.3.6   Other ulcer-healing drugs

Carbenoxolone is a synthetic derivative of glycyrrhizinic acid (a constituent of liquorice).

The only oral preparation of carbenoxolone remaining on the UK market is in the form of a combination with antacids for *oesophageal ulceration and inflammation*.

Side-effects of carbenoxolone (commonly sodium and water retention and occasionally hypokalaemia) may cause or exacerbate hypertension, oedema, cardiac failure, and muscle weakness. For these reasons other drugs are preferred; if used, regular monitoring of weight, blood pressure, and electrolytes is advisable during treatment. Carbenoxolone may act by protecting the mucosal barrier from acid–pepsin attack and increasing mucosal mucin production.

CARBENOXOLONE SODIUM ▰

Indications: oesophageal inflammation and ulceration

Cautions: cardiac disease, hypertension, hepatic and renal disease (see contra-indications); elderly (see under preparation); not recommended in children; see also notes above; **interactions:** Appendix 1 (carbenoxolone)

Contra-indications: hypokalaemia, cardiac failure and in those receiving cardiac glycosides (unless electrolyte levels monitored weekly and measures taken to avoid hypokalaemia); hepatic and renal impairment (see Appendixes 2 and 3); pregnancy

Side-effects: sodium and water retention (provoking hypertension and cardiac failure), hypokalaemia (leading to impaired neuromuscular function and muscle damage and to renal damage if prolonged)

Dose: see under preparations

■ Compound preparation

Pyrogastrone® (Sanofi-Synthelabo) PoM ▰

Tablets, chewable, carbenoxolone sodium 20 mg, alginic acid 600 mg, dried aluminium hydroxide 240 mg, magnesium trisilicate 60 mg, sodium bicarbonate 210 mg (Na⁺ 3 mmol/tablet). Net price 100-tab pack = £24.85. Label: 21, 24

Liquid, carbenoxolone sodium 10 mg, dried aluminium hydroxide 150 mg (Na⁺ 0.85 mmol, K⁺ 1.5 mmol)/5 mL when reconstituted with water. Net price 500 mL = £12.39. Label: 21

Dose: for oesophageal inflammation and ulceration, 1 tablet, chewed, 3 times daily after meals, and 2 at night, for 6–12 weeks or 10 mL liquid 3 times daily after meals and 20 mL at night, for 6–12 weeks; not recommended for children or for adults over 75 years

▰ denotes preparations that are considered to be less suitable for prescribing (see p. vi)

1.4 Acute diarrhoea

| 1.4.1 | Adsorbents and bulk-forming drugs |
| 1.4.2 | Antimotility drugs |

The first line of treatment in acute diarrhoea, as in gastro-enteritis, is prevention or treatment of fluid and electrolyte depletion. This is particularly important in infants and in frail and elderly patients. For details of **oral rehydration preparations**, see section 9.2.1.2. Severe dehydration requires immediate admission to hospital and urgent replacement of fluid and electrolytes.

Antimotility drugs (section 1.4.2) relieve symptoms of acute diarrhoea. They are used in the management of uncomplicated acute diarrhoea in adults; fluid and electrolyte replacement may be necessary in case of dehydration. Antimotility drugs are, however, **not** recommended for acute diarrhoea in young children.

Antispasmodics (section 1.2) are occasionally of value in treating abdominal cramp associated with diarrhoea but they should **not** be used for primary treatment. Antispasmodics and antiemetics should be **avoided** in young children with gastro-enteritis since they are rarely effective and have troublesome side-effects.

Antibacterial drugs are generally unnecessary in simple gastro-enteritis, even when a bacterial cause is suspected, because the complaint will usually resolve quickly without such treatment, and infective diarrhoeas in the UK are often caused by viral infections. Systemic bacterial infection does, however, need appropriate systemic treatment; for drugs used in campylobacter enteritis, shigellosis, and salmonellosis, see section 5.1, table 1. **Ciprofloxacin** is occasionally used for prophylaxis against travellers' diarrhoea, but routine use is **not** recommended. Lactobacillus preparations have not been shown to be effective.

Colestyramine (cholestyramine, section 1.9.2) and **aluminium hydroxide mixture** (section 1.1.1), bind unabsorbed bile salts and provide symptomatic relief of diarrhoea following ileal disease or resection.

1.4.1 Adsorbents and bulk-forming drugs

Adsorbents such as kaolin are **not** recommended for *acute diarrhoeas*. Bulk-forming drugs, such as ispaghula, methylcellulose, and sterculia (section 1.6.1) are useful in controlling faecal consistency in ileostomy and colostomy, and in controlling diarrhoea associated with diverticular disease.

KAOLIN, LIGHT ▭

Indications: diarrhoea but see notes above
Cautions: interactions: Appendix 1 (kaolin)

Kaolin Mixture, BP ▭
(Kaolin Oral Suspension)
Oral suspension, light kaolin or light kaolin (natural) 20%, light magnesium carbonate 5%, sodium bicarbonate 5% in a suitable vehicle with a peppermint flavour.
Dose: 10–20 mL every 4 hours
Note. Kaolin-containing preparations on sale to the public include *KLN®*

1.4.2 Antimotility drugs

Antimotility drugs have a role in the management of uncomplicated *acute diarrhoea* in adults but not in young children; see also section 1.4. However, in the case of dehydration, fluid and electrolyte replacement (section 9.2.1.2) are of primary importance.

For comments on their role in *chronic diarrhoeas* see section 1.5.

CODEINE PHOSPHATE

Indications: see notes above; cough suppression (section 3.9.1); pain (section 4.7.2)

Cautions: see section 4.7.2; also not recommended for children; tolerance and dependence may occur with prolonged use; **interactions:** Appendix 1 (opioid analgesics)

Contra-indications: see section 4.7.2; also conditions where inhibition of peristalsis should be avoided, where abdominal distension develops, or in acute diarrhoeal conditions such as acute ulcerative colitis or antibiotic-associated colitis

Side-effects: see section 4.7.2

Dose: see preparations

Codeine Phosphate (Non-proprietary) PoM
Tablets, codeine phosphate 15 mg, net price 28 = £1.02; 30 mg, 28 = £1.45; 60 mg, 28 = £2.59. Label: 2
Dose: acute diarrhoea, 30 mg 3–4 times daily (range 15–60 mg); CHILD not recommended
Note. Travellers needing to take codeine phosphate tablets abroad may require a doctor's letter explaining why they are necessary.

Kaodene® (Sovereign) NHS ▭
Suspension, codeine phosphate 5 mg, light kaolin 1.5 g/5 mL. Net price 250 mL = £2.06
Dose: 20 mL 3–4 times daily; CHILD under 5 years not recommended, over 5 years 10 mL but see cautions and notes above

CO-PHENOTROPE

A mixture of diphenoxylate hydrochloride and atropine sulphate in the mass proportions 100 parts to 1 part respectively

Indications: adjunct to rehydration in acute diarrhoea (but see notes above); chronic mild ulcerative colitis

Cautions: see under Codeine Phosphate; also young children are particularly susceptible to **overdosage** and symptoms may be delayed and observation is needed for at least 48 hours after ingestion; presence of subclinical doses of atropine may give rise to atropine side-effects in susceptible individuals or in overdosage; **interactions:** Appendix 1 (opioid analgesics)

Contra-indications: see under Codeine Phosphate

Side-effects: see under Codeine Phosphate, section 4.7.2

Dose: see preparation

Lomotil® (Goldshield) [PoM]

Tablets, co-phenotrope 2.5/0.025 (diphenoxylate hydrochloride 2.5 mg, atropine sulphate 25 micrograms). Net price 20 = £1.57

Dose: initially 4 tablets, followed by 2 tablets every 6 hours until diarrhoea controlled; CHILD under 4 years not recommended, 4–8 years 1 tablet 3 times daily, 9–12 years 1 tablet 4 times daily, 13–16 years 2 tablets 3 times daily, but see also notes above

Note. Co-phenotrope 2.5/0.025 tablets are also available from Mepra-pharm (*Diarphen®*) and Norgine (*Tropergen®*)

LOPERAMIDE HYDROCHLORIDE

Indications: symptomatic treatment of acute diarrhoea; adjunct to rehydration in acute diarrhoea in adults and children over 4 years (but see notes above); chronic diarrhoea in adults only

Cautions: see notes above; also liver disease; pregnancy (Appendix 4)

Contra-indications: conditions where inhibition of peristalsis should be avoided, where abdominal distension develops, or in conditions such as active ulcerative colitis or antibiotic-associated colitis

Side-effects: abdominal cramps, dizziness, drowsiness, and skin reactions, including urticaria reported; paralytic ileus and abdominal bloating also reported

Dose: acute diarrhoea, 4 mg initially followed by 2 mg after each loose stool for up to 5 days; usual dose 6–8 mg daily; max. 16 mg daily. CHILD under 4 years not recommended, 4–8 years 1 mg 3–4 times daily for up to *3 days only*, 9–12 years 2 mg 4 times daily for up to 5 days

Chronic diarrhoea in adults, initially, 4–8 mg daily in divided doses, subsequently adjusted according to response and given in 2 divided doses for maintenance; max. 16 mg daily

¹ **Loperamide** (Non-proprietary) [PoM]

Capsules, loperamide hydrochloride 2 mg. Net price 30-cap pack = £1.94

Available from Alpharma, APS, Berk (*Diocaps®*), Generics, Hillcross, IVAX, Norgine (*LoperaGen®*), Tillomed (*Norimode®*), Unichem

1. Loperamide can be sold to the public, for adults and children over 12 years, provided it is licensed and labelled for the treatment of acute diarrhoea; proprietary brands including *Arret®* capsules [NHS], *Boots Diareze®* capsules, *Diasorb®* capsules, *Diocalm Ultra®* capsules [NHS] and *Imodium®* [NHS] (8- and 12-cap packs), *Imodium®* liquid and *Normaloe®* tablets are on sale to the public

Imodium® (Janssen-Cilag) [PoM]

Capsules, green/grey, loperamide hydrochloride 2 mg. Net price 30 = £1.22

Syrup, red, sugar-free, loperamide hydrochloride 1 mg/5 mL. Net price 100 mL = £1.05

■ Compound preparations

Imodium®Plus (Janssen-Cilag)

Tablets (chewable), scored, loperamide hydrochloride 2 mg, activated dimeticone 125 mg, net price 6-tab pack = £1.97, 18-tab pack = £4.54. Label: 24.

Dose: acute diarrhoea with abdominal colic, initially 2 tablets (ADOLESCENT 12–18 years 1 tablet) then 1 tablet after each loose stool; max. 4 tablets daily for up to 2 days; CHILD not recommended

MORPHINE

Indications: see notes above

Cautions: see notes above and under Codeine Phosphate (section 4.7.2)

Contra-indications: see notes above and under Codeine Phosphate

Side-effects: see notes above and under Codeine Phosphate (section 4.7.2); sedation and the risk of dependence are greater

Dose: see preparation

Kaolin and Morphine Mixture, BP ◢

(Kaolin and Morphine Oral Suspension)

Oral suspension, light kaolin or light kaolin (natural) 20%, sodium bicarbonate 5% and chloroform and morphine tincture 4% in a suitable vehicle. Contains anhydrous morphine 550–800 micrograms/10 mL.

Dose: 10 mL every 4 hours in water

Preparations on sale to the public containing morphine include:

Diocalm® (attapulgite, morphine)

Enterosan® (belladonna, morphine, kaolin)

Opazimes® (belladonna, morphine, aluminium, kaolin)

◢ denotes preparations that are considered to be less suitable for prescribing (see p. vi)

1.5 Chronic bowel disorders

Once tumours are ruled out individual symptoms of chronic bowel disorders need specific treatment including dietary manipulation as well as drug treatment and the maintenance of a liberal fluid intake.

Irritable bowel syndrome

Irritable bowel syndrome can present with pain, constipation, or diarrhoea, all of which may benefit from a high-fibre diet, with bran or with other agents which increase stool bulk (section 1.6.1). In some patients there may be important psychological aggravating factors which respond to reassurance. Antimotility drugs such as loperamide (section 1.4.2) may relieve diarrhoea and antispasmodic drugs (section 1.2) may relieve pain. Opioids with a central action such as codeine are better avoided because of the risk of dependence.

Malabsorption syndromes

Individual conditions need specific management and also general nutritional consideration. Thus coeliac disease (gluten enteropathy) usually needs a gluten-free diet (Appendix 7) and pancreatic insufficiency needs pancreatin supplements (section 1.9.4).

Inflammatory bowel disease

The chronic inflammatory bowel diseases include *ulcerative colitis* and *Crohn's disease*. Effective management calls for drug therapy, attention to nutrition, and in severe or chronic active disease, surgery.

Aminosalicylates (balsalazide, mesalazine, olsalazine, and sulfasalazine), and **corticosteroids** (hydrocortisone, budesonide, and prednisolone) form the basis of drug treatment.

TREATMENT OF ACUTE ULCERATIVE COLITIS AND CROHN'S DISEASE. Acute mild to moderate disease affecting the rectum (proctitis) or the rectosigmoid (distal colitis) is treated initially with local application of a corticosteroid or an aminosalicylate; foam preparations are especially useful where patients have difficulty retaining liquid enemas.

Diffuse inflammatory bowel disease or disease that does not respond to local therapy requires oral treatment; mild disease affecting the colon may be treated with an aminosalicylate alone but refractory or moderate disease usually requires adjunctive use of an oral corticosteroid such as **prednisolone** for 4–8 weeks. Modified-release **budesonide** is licensed for Crohn's disease affecting the ileum and the ascending colon; it causes fewer systemic side-effects than oral prednisolone.

Severe inflammatory bowel disease calls for hospital admission and treatment with intravenous corticosteroid; other therapy may include intravenous fluid and electrolyte replacement, blood transfusion, and possibly parenteral nutrition and antibiotics. Specialist supervision is required for patients who fail to respond adequately to these measures. Patients with ulcerative colitis may benefit from a short course of ciclosporin [unlicensed indication]. Patients with unresponsive or chronically active Crohn's disease may benefit from azathioprine, mercaptopurine (see below), or once-weekly methotrexate [all unlicensed indications].

Infliximab (*Remicade®*, Schering-Plough) has been introduced for the treatment of severe active Crohn's disease refractory to treatment with a corticosteroid and an immunosuppressant, and for the treatment of refractory fistulas of Crohn's disease. Infliximab is monoclonal antibody which inhibits the pro-inflammatory cytokine, tumour necrosis factor α. Infliximab has been associated with the development of tuberculosis (often in extrapulmonary sites) and with worsening of heart failure. It should be used by specialists where adequate resuscitation facilities are available.

Metronidazole may be beneficial for the treatment of active Crohn's disease particularly with perianal involvement, possibly through its antibacterial activity. Other antibacterials should be given if specifically indicated (e.g. sepsis associated with fistulas and perianal disease) and for managing bacterial overgrowth in the small bowel.

MAINTENANCE OF REMISSION OF ACUTE ULCERATIVE COLITIS AND CROHN'S DISEASE. **Aminosalicylates** are of great value in the maintenance of remission of ulcerative colitis. They are of less value in the maintenance of remission of Crohn's disease; an oral formulation of mesalazine is licensed for the long-term management of ileal disease. Corticosteroids are **not** suitable for maintenance treatment because of side-effects. In resistant or frequently relapsing cases either **azathioprine** (section 8.2.1), 2–2.5 mg/kg daily [unlicensed indication] or **mercaptopurine** (section 8.1.3), 1–1.5 mg/kg daily [unlicensed indication], given under close supervision may be helpful.

ADJUNCTIVE TREATMENT OF INFLAMMATORY BOWEL DISEASE. Due attention should be paid to diet; high-fibre or low-residue diets should be used as appropriate. Irritable bowel syndrome during remission of ulcerative colitis calls for avoidance of a high-fibre diet and possible treatment with an antispasmodic (section 1.2).

Antimotility drugs such as codeine and loperamide, and antispasmodic drugs should **not** be used in active ulcerative colitis because they can precipitate paralytic ileus and megacolon; treatment of the inflammation is more logical. Laxatives may be required in proctitis. Diarrhoea resulting from the loss of bile-salt absorption (e.g. in terminal ileal disease or bowel resection) may improve with **colestyramine** (section 1.9.2), which binds bile salts.

Antibiotic-associated colitis

Antibiotic-associated colitis (pseudomembranous colitis) is caused by colonisation of the colon with *Clostridium difficile* which may follow antibiotic therapy. It is usually of acute onset, but may run a chronic course; it is a particular hazard of clindamycin but few antibiotics are free of this side-effect. Oral **vancomycin** (see section 5.1.7) or **metronidazole** (see section 5.1.11) are used as specific treatment; vancomycin may be preferred for very sick patients.

Diverticular disease

Diverticular disease is treated with a high-fibre diet, **bran supplements**, and **bulk-forming drugs**. **Antispasmodics** may provide symptomatic relief when colic is a problem (section 1.2). **Antibacterials** are used only when the diverticula in the intestinal wall become infected (specialist referral). **Antimotility** drugs which slow intestinal motility, e.g. codeine, diphenoxylate, and loperamide could possibly exacerbate the symptoms of diverticular disease and are **contra-indicated**.

Aminosalicylates

Sulfasalazine is a combination of 5-aminosalicylic acid ('5-ASA') and sulfapyridine; sulfapyridine acts only as a carrier to the colonic site of action but still causes side-effects. In the newer aminosalicylates, **mesalazine** (5-aminosalicylic acid), **balsalazide** (a prodrug of 5-aminosalicylic acid) and **olsalazine** (a dimer of 5-aminosalicylic acid which cleaves in the lower bowel), the sulphonamide-related side-effects of sulfasalazine are avoided, but 5-aminosalicylic acid alone can still cause side-effects including blood disorders (see recommendation below) and lupoid phenomenon also seen with sulfasalazine. Olsalazine may also be particularly prone to cause watery diarrhoea. Some manufacturers of sulfasalazine and mesalazine recommend renal function tests, but evidence of practical value is unsatisfactory.

CAUTIONS. Aminosalicylates should be used with caution during pregnancy (Appendix 4) and breast-feeding (Appendix 5); blood disorders can occur (see recommendation below).

> **Blood disorders**
> It is recommended that patients receiving aminosalicylates should be advised to report any unexplained bleeding, bruising, purpura, sore throat, fever or malaise that occurs during treatment. A blood count should be performed and the drug stopped immediately if there is suspicion of a blood dyscrasia.

CONTRA-INDICATIONS. Aminosalicylates should be avoided in salicylate hypersensitivity and in moderate or severe renal impairment.

SIDE-EFFECTS. Side-effects of the aminosalicylates include diarrhoea, nausea, headache, exacerbation of symptoms of colitis, hypersensitivity reactions (including rash, urticaria, interstitial nephritis and lupus erythematosus-like syndrome); side-effects that occur rarely include acute pancreatitis, hepatitis, nephrotic syndrome, blood disorders (including agranulocytosis, aplastic anaemia, leucopenia, neutropenia, thrombocytopenia—see also recommendation above).

BALSALAZIDE SODIUM

Indications: treatment of mild to moderate ulcerative colitis and maintenance of remission

Cautions: see notes above; also history of asthma; **interactions:** Appendix 1 (aminosalicylates)

Contra-indications: see notes above; also severe hepatic impairment
BLOOD DISORDERS. See recommendation above

Side-effects: see notes above; also abdominal pain, vomiting, cholelithiasis

Dose: acute attack, 2.25 g 3 times daily until remission occurs or for up to max. 12 weeks
Maintenance, 1.5 g twice daily, adjusted according to response (max. 6 g daily)
CHILD not recommended

Colazide® (Shire) PoM
Capsules, beige, balsalazide sodium 750 mg. Net price 130-cap pack = £39.00. Label: 21, 25, counselling, blood disorder symptoms (see recommendation above)

MESALAZINE

Indications: treatment of mild to moderate ulcerative colitis and maintenance of remission; see also under preparations

Cautions: see notes above; elderly; **interactions:** Appendix 1 (aminosalicylates)

Contra-indications: see notes above; also severe hepatic impairment; blood clotting abnormalities
BLOOD DISORDERS. See recommendation above

Side-effects: see notes above; also abdominal pain; rarely allergic lung reactions, allergic myocarditis, methaemoglobinaemia

Dose: see under preparations, below
Note. The delivery characteristics of enteric-coated mesalazine preparations may vary; these preparations should not be considered interchangeable

Asacol® (Procter & Gamble Pharm) PoM
Tablets, red, e/c, mesalazine 400 mg, net price 90-tab pack = £32.69, 120-tab pack = £43.58. Label: 5, 25, counselling, blood disorder symptoms (see recommendation above)
Dose: ulcerative colitis, acute attack, 6 tablets daily in divided doses; maintenance of remission of ulcerative colitis and Crohn's ileo-colitis, 3–6 tablets daily in divided doses; CHILD not recommended
Note. Preparations that lower stool pH (e.g. lactulose) may prevent release of mesalazine

Foam enema, mesalazine 1 g/metered application. Net price 14 g (14 applications) with disposable applicators and plastic bags = £39.60. Counselling, blood disorder symptoms (see recommendation above)
Dose: acute attack affecting the rectosigmoid region, 1 metered application (mesalazine 1 g) into the rectum daily for 4–6 weeks; acute attack affecting the descending colon, 2 metered applications (mesalazine 2 g) once daily for 4–6 weeks; CHILD not recommended

Suppositories, mesalazine 250 mg, net price 20-suppos pack = £7.15; 500 mg, 10 = £7.15. Counselling, blood disorder symptoms (see recommendation above)
Dose: 3–6 suppositories of 250 mg (max. 3 suppositories of 500 mg) daily in divided doses, with last dose at bedtime; CHILD not recommended

Pentasa® (Ferring) PoM
Slow Release tablets, m/r, scored, mesalazine 500 mg (grey), net price 100-tab pack = £25.82. Counselling, administration, see dose, blood disorder symptoms (see recommendation above)
Dose: acute attack, up to 4 g daily in 2–3 divided doses; maintenance, 1.5 g daily in 2–3 divided doses; tablets may be dispersed in water, but should not be chewed; CHILD under 15 years not recommended

Granules, m/r, pale brown, mesalazine 1 g/sachet, net price 50-sachet pack = £31.60. Counselling, administration, see dose, blood disorder symptoms (see recommendation above)
Dose: acute attack, up to 4 g daily in 2–4 divided doses; maintenance, 2 g daily in 2 divided doses; granules should be placed on tongue and washed down with water or orange juice without chewing; CHILD under 12 years not recommended

Retention enema, mesalazine 1 g in 100-mL pack. Net price 7 enemas = £19.45. Counselling, blood disorder symptoms (see recommendation above)
Dose: 1 enema at bedtime; CHILD not recommended

Suppositories, mesalazine 1 g. Net price 28-suppos pack = £44.68. Counselling, blood disorder symptoms (see recommendation above)
Dose: ulcerative proctitis, acute attack, 1 suppository daily for 2–4 weeks; maintenance, 1 suppository daily; CHILD under 15 years not recommended

Salofalk® (Provalis) PoM
Tablets, e/c, yellow, mesalazine 250 mg. Net price 100-tab pack = £18.41. Label: 5, 25, counselling, blood disorder symptoms (see recommendation above)
Dose: acute attack, 6 tablets daily in 3 divided doses; maintenance 3–6 tablets daily in divided doses; CHILD not recommended

Suppositories, mesalazine 500 mg. Net price 30-suppos pack = £16.75. Counselling, blood disorder symptoms (see recommendations above)
Dose: acute attack, 1–2 suppositories 2–3 times daily adjusted according to response; CHILD not recommended

Enema, mesalazine 2 g in 59-mL pack. Net price 7 enemas = £32.95. Counselling, blood disorder symptoms (see recommendations above)
Dose: acute attack *or* maintenance, 1 enema daily at bedtime; CHILD not recommended

OLSALAZINE SODIUM

Indications: treatment of mild ulcerative colitis and maintenance of remission
Cautions: see notes above; **interactions:** Appendix 1 (aminosalicylates)
Contra-indications: see notes above
BLOOD DISORDERS. See recommendation above
Side-effects: see notes above; also watery diarrhoea, arthralgia
Dose: acute attack, 1 g daily in divided doses after meals increased if necessary over 1 week to max. 3 g daily (max. single dose 1 g)
Maintenance, 500 mg twice daily after meals; CHILD not recommended

Dipentum® (Pharmacia) [PoM]
Capsules, brown, olsalazine sodium 250 mg. Net price 112-cap pack = £27.42. Label: 21, counselling, blood disorder symptoms (see recommendation above)
Tablets, yellow, scored, olsalazine sodium 500 mg. Net price 60-tab pack = £29.38. Label: 21, counselling, blood disorder symptoms (see recommendation above)

SULFASALAZINE

(Sulphasalazine)
Indications: treatment of mild to moderate and severe ulcerative colitis and maintenance of remission; active Crohn's disease; rheumatoid arthritis (section 10.1.3)
Cautions: see notes above; also history of allergy; hepatic and renal impairment; G6PD deficiency (section 9.1.5); slow acetylator status; risk of haematological and hepatic toxicity (differential white cell, red cell and platelet counts initially and at monthly intervals for first 3 months, liver function tests at monthly intervals for first 3 months); kidney function tests at regular intervals; upper gastro-intestinal side-effects common over 4 g daily; porphyria (section 9.8.2); **interactions:** Appendix 1 (aminosalicylates)
Contra-indications: see notes above; also sulphonamide hypersensitivity; CHILD under 2 years of age
BLOOD DISORDERS. See recommendation above
Side-effects: see notes above; also loss of appetite; fever; blood disorders (including Heinz body anaemia, megaloblastic anaemia); hypersensitivity reactions (including Stevens-Johnson syndrome, exfoliative dermatitis, epidermal necrolysis, pruritus, photosensitisation, anaphylaxis, serum sickness); lung complications (including eosinophilia, fibrosing alveolitis); ocular complications (including periorbital oedema); stomatitis, parotitis; ataxia, aseptic meningitis; vertigo, tinnitus, alopecia, peripheral neuropathy,

insomnia, depression, hallucinations; kidney reactions (including proteinuria, crystalluria, haematuria); oligospermia; urine may be coloured orange; some soft contact lenses may be stained
Dose: *by mouth*, acute attack 1–2 g 4 times daily (but see **cautions**) until remission occurs (if necessary corticosteroids may also be given), reducing to a maintenance dose of 500 mg 4 times daily; CHILD over 2 years, acute attack 40–60 mg/kg daily, maintenance dose 20–30 mg/kg daily
By rectum, in suppositories, alone or in conjunction with oral treatment 0.5–1 g morning and night after a bowel movement. As an enema, 3 g at night, retained for at least 1 hour

Sulfasalazine (Non-proprietary) [PoM]
Tablets, sulfasalazine 500 mg. Net price 112 = £7.72. Label: 14, counselling, blood disorder symptoms (see recommendation above), contact lenses may be stained
Available from Alpharma, Ashbourne (*Ucine®*), Hillcross
Tablets, e/c, sulfasalazine 500 mg. Net price 112-tab pack = £9.69. Label: 5, 14, 25, counselling, blood disorder symptoms (see recommendation above), contact lenses may be stained
Available from Alpharma (*Sulazine EC®*)
Salazopyrin® (Pharmacia) [PoM]
Tablets, yellow, scored, sulfasalazine 500 mg. Net price 112-tab pack = £7.74. Label: 14, counselling, blood disorder symptoms (see recommendation above), contact lenses may be stained
EN-Tabs® (= tablets e/c), yellow, f/c, sulfasalazine 500 mg. Net price 112-tab pack = £9.69. Label: 5, 14, 25, counselling, blood disorder symptoms (see recommendation above), contact lenses may be stained
Suspension, yellow, sulfasalazine 250 mg/5 mL. Net price 500 mL = £15.70. Label: 14, counselling, blood disorder symptoms (see recommendation above), contact lenses may be stained
Suppositories, yellow, sulfasalazine 500 mg. Net price 10 = £2.75. Label: 14, counselling, blood disorder symptoms (see recommendation above), contact lenses may be stained
Retention enema, sulfasalazine 3 g in 100-mL single-dose disposable packs fitted with a nozzle. Net price 7 × 100 mL = £11.87. Label: 14, counselling, blood disorder symptoms (see recommendation above), contact lenses may be stained

Corticosteroids

BUDESONIDE

Indications: see under preparations
Cautions: see section 6.3.2
Contra-indications: see section 6.3.2
Side-effects: see section 6.3.2
Dose: see under preparations

Budenofalk® (Provalis) [PoM]
Capsules, pink, enclosing e/c pellets, budesonide 3 mg, net price 100-cap pack = £81.20. Label: 5, 10 steroid card, 22, 25
Dose: mild to moderate Crohn's disease affecting the ileum or ascending colon, 3 mg 3 times daily for up to 8 weeks; reduce dose for the last 2 weeks of treatment. See also section 6.3.2
CHILD not recommended

Entocort® (AstraZeneca) PoM
CR Capsules, grey/pink, enclosing e/c, m/r granules budesonide 3 mg, net price 100-cap pack = £90.00. Label: 5, 10 steroid card, 22, 25
Note. Dispense in original container (contains desiccant)
Dose: mild to moderate Crohn's disease affecting the ileum or ascending colon, 9 mg once daily in the morning before breakfast for up to 8 weeks; reduce dose for the last 2–4 weeks of treatment. See also section 6.3.2 CHILD not recommended

Enema, budesonide 2 mg/100 mL when dispersible tablet reconstituted in isotonic saline vehicle, net price pack of 7 dispersible tablets and bottles of vehicle = £30.00
Dose: ulcerative colitis involving rectal and recto-sigmoid disease, 1 enema at bedtime for 4 weeks; CHILD not recommended

HYDROCORTISONE

Indications: ulcerative colitis, proctitis, proctosigmoiditis
Cautions: see section 6.3.2; systemic absorption may occur; prolonged use should be avoided
Contra-indications: use of enemas and rectal foams in obstruction, bowel perforation, and extensive fistulas; untreated infection
Side-effects: see section 6.3.2; local irritation
Dose: rectal, see under Preparations

Colifoam® (Stafford-Miller) PoM
Foam in aerosol pack, hydrocortisone acetate 10%. Net price 20.8 g (14 applications) with applicator = £6.80
Dose: initially 1 metered application (125 mg hydrocortisone acetate) inserted into the rectum once or twice daily for 2–3 weeks, then once on alternate days

PREDNISOLONE

Indications: ulcerative colitis, and Crohn's disease; other indications, see section 6.3.2, see also preparations
Cautions: see under Hydrocortisone and section 6.3.2
Contra-indications: see under Hydrocortisone and section 6.3.2
Side-effects: see under Hydrocortisone and section 6.3.2
Dose: *by mouth*, initially 20–40 mg daily in single or divided doses, until remission occurs, followed by reducing doses
By rectum, see under preparations

■ Oral preparations, section 6.3.2

■ Rectal preparations
Predenema® (Forest) PoM
Retention enema, prednisolone 20 mg (as sodium metasulphobenzoate) in 100-mL single-dose disposable pack. Net price 1 (standard tube) = 76p, 1 (long tube) = £1.29
Dose: ulcerative colitis, initially 1 enema at bedtime for 2–4 weeks, continued if good response; CHILD not recommended

Predfoam® (Forest) PoM
Foam in aerosol pack, prednisolone 20 mg (as metasulphobenzoate sodium)/metered application. Net price 25 g (14 applications) with disposable applicators = £6.74
Dose: proctitis and distal ulcerative colitis, 1 metered application (containing 20 mg prednisolone) inserted

into the rectum once or twice daily for 2 weeks, continued for further 2 weeks if good response; CHILD not recommended

Predsol® (Celltech) PoM
Retention enema, prednisolone 20 mg (as sodium phosphate) in 100-mL single-dose disposable packs fitted with a nozzle. Net price 7 = £5.24
Dose: rectal and rectosigmoidal ulcerative colitis and Crohn's disease, initially 1 enema at bedtime for 2–4 weeks, continued if good response; CHILD not recommended

Suppositories, prednisolone 5 mg (as sodium phosphate). Net price 10 = £1.00
Dose: ADULT and CHILD proctitis and rectal complications of Crohn's disease, 1 suppository inserted night and morning after a bowel movement

Food allergy

Allergy with classical symptoms of vomiting, colic and diarrhoea caused by specific foods such as shellfish should be managed by strict avoidance. The condition should be distinguished from symptoms of occasional food intolerance in those with irritable bowel syndrome. **Sodium cromoglicate** (sodium cromoglycate) may be helpful as an adjunct to dietary avoidance.

SODIUM CROMOGLICATE
(Sodium cromoglycate)

Indications: food allergy (in conjunction with dietary restriction); asthma (section 3.3); allergic conjunctivitis (section 11.4.2); allergic rhinitis (section 12.2.1)
Side-effects: occasional nausea, rashes, and joint pain
Dose: 200 mg 4 times daily before meals; CHILD 2–14 years 100 mg; capsules may be swallowed whole or the contents dissolved in hot water and diluted with cold water before taking. May be increased if necessary after 2–3 weeks to a max. of 40 mg/kg daily and then reduced according to the response

Nalcrom® (Pantheon) PoM
Capsules, sodium cromoglicate 100 mg. Net price 100-cap pack = £66.85. Label: 22, counselling, see dose above

1.6   Laxatives

1.6.1	Bulk-forming laxatives
1.6.2	Stimulant laxatives
1.6.3	Faecal softeners
1.6.4	Osmotic laxatives
1.6.5	Bowel cleansing solutions

Before prescribing laxatives it is important to be sure that the patient *is* constipated and that the constipation is *not* secondary to an underlying undiagnosed complaint.

It is also important for those who complain of constipation to understand that bowel habit can vary considerably in frequency without doing harm. Some people tend to consider themselves constipated if they do not have a bowel movement each day. A useful definition of constipation is the passage of hard stools less frequently than the patient's own normal pattern and this can be explained to the patient.

Misconceptions about bowel habits have led to excessive laxative use. Abuse may lead to hypokalaemia and an atonic non-functioning colon.

Thus, laxatives should generally be **avoided** except where straining will exacerbate a condition (such as angina) or increase the risk of rectal bleeding as in haemorrhoids. Laxatives are also of value in *drug-induced constipation*, for the expulsion of *parasites* after anthelmintic treatment, and to clear the alimentary tract before *surgery and radiological procedures*. Prolonged treatment of constipation is seldom necessary except occasionally in the elderly.

CHILDREN. The use of laxatives in children should be discouraged unless prescribed by a doctor. Infrequent defaecation may be normal in breast-fed babies or in response to poor intake of fluid or fibre. Delays of greater than 3 days between stools may increase the likelihood of pain on passing hard stools leading to anal fissure, anal spasm and eventually to a learned response to avoid defaecation.

If increased fluid and fibre intake is insufficient, an osmotic laxative such as lactulose or a bulk-forming laxative such as methylcellulose may be effective; methylcellulose is given in a dose of 0.5–1 g twice daily for a child over 7 years [unlicensed use]—an appropriate formulation for a younger child is not readily available. If there is evidence of minor faecal retention, the addition of a stimulant laxative such as senna may overcome withholding but may lead to colic or, in the presence of faecal impaction in the rectum, an increase of faecal overflow. Referral to hospital may be needed unless the child evacuates the impacted mass spontaneously. In hospital, enemas or suppositories may clear the mass but their use is frequently distressing for the child and may lead to a persistence of withholding. Enemas may be administered under heavy sedation in hospital or alternatively a bowel cleansing solution (section 1.6.5) may be tried. In severe cases or where the child is afraid, a manual evacuation under anaesthetic may be appropriate.

Long-term use of stimulant laxatives such as senna or sodium picosulfate (sodium picosulphate, section 1.6.2) is essential to prevent recurrence of the faecal impaction. Parents should be encouraged to use them regularly for many months; intermittent use may provoke a series of relapses.

> The laxatives that follow have been divided into 5 main groups (sections 1.6.1–1.6.5). This simple classification disguises the fact that some laxatives have a complex action.

1.6.1 Bulk-forming laxatives

Bulk-forming laxatives relieve constipation by increasing faecal mass which stimulates peristalsis; the full effect may take some days to develop and patients should be told this.

Bulk-forming laxatives are of particular value in those with small hard stools, but should not be required unless fibre cannot be increased in the diet. A balanced diet, including adequate fluid intake and fibre is of value in preventing constipation.

Bulk-forming laxatives are useful in the management of patients with *colostomy*, *ileostomy*, *haemorrhoids*, *anal fissure*, *chronic diarrhoea associated with diverticular disease*, *irritable bowel syndrome*, and as adjuncts in *ulcerative colitis* (section 1.5). Adequate fluid intake must be maintained to avoid intestinal obstruction. Unprocessed wheat **bran**, taken with food or fruit juice, is a most effective bulk-forming preparation. Finely ground bran, though more palatable, has poorer water-retaining properties, but can be taken as bran bread or biscuits in appropriately increased quantities. Oat bran is also used.

Methylcellulose, ispaghula, and **sterculia** are useful in patients who cannot tolerate bran. Methylcellulose also acts as a faecal softener.

BRAN

Indications: see notes above
Cautions: see under Ispaghula Husk
Contra-indications: see under Ispaghula Husk; also gluten enteropathies and coeliac disease
Side-effects: see under Ispaghula Husk
Dose: see preparation below
COUNSELLING. Preparations that swell in contact with liquid should always be carefully swallowed with water and should not be taken immediately before going to bed

Trifyba® (Sanofi-Synthelabo)
Powder, brown, wheat fibre 80%. Net price 56 sachets containing 3.5 g = £3.28. Counselling, see below
Note. Contains gluten
Dose: 1 sachet 2–3 times daily added to food; CHILD (but see section 1.6) half to one sachet 1–2 times daily added to food
COUNSELLING. At least one glass of water or other liquid should be drunk with the meal

---

ISPAGHULA HUSK

Indications: see notes above; hypercholesterolaemia (section 2.12)
Cautions: adequate fluid intake should be maintained to avoid intestinal obstruction—it may be necessary to supervise elderly or debilitated patients or those with intestinal narrowing or decreased motility
Contra-indications: difficulty in swallowing, intestinal obstruction, colonic atony, faecal impaction
Side-effects: flatulence, abdominal distension, gastro-intestinal obstruction or impaction; hypersensitivity reported
Dose: see preparations below
COUNSELLING. Preparations that swell in contact with liquid should always be carefully swallowed with water and should not be taken immediately before going to bed

Fybogel® (R&C)
Granules, buff, effervescent, sugar- and gluten-free, ispaghula husk 3.5 g/sachet (low Na⁺). Net price 60 sachets (plain, lemon, or orange flavoured) = £4.24. Label: 13, counselling, see above
Note. Contains aspartame 50 mg/sachet (see section 9.4.1)
Dose: 1 sachet in water twice daily preferably after meals; CHILD (but see section 1.6) 6–12 years ½–1 level 5-mL spoonful (children under 6 years on doctor's advice only)

Isogel® (Pfizer Consumer)
Granules, brown, sugar- and gluten-free, ispaghula

husk 90%. Net price 300 g = £3.53. Label: 13, counselling, see above

Dose: constipation, 2 teaspoonfuls in water once or twice daily, preferably at mealtimes; CHILD (but see section 1.6) 1 teaspoonful

Diarrhoea (section 1.4.1), 1 teaspoonful 3 times daily

Ispagel® (Richmond)

Powder, beige, sugar-free, ispaghula husk 3.5 g/ sachet, net price 30 sachets (orange flavour) = £2.10. Label: 13, counselling, see above

Excipients: include aspartame (section 9.4.1)

Dose: 1 sachet in water 1–3 times daily; CHILD (but see section 1.6) 6–12 years ½ adult dose (children under 6 years on doctor's advice only)

Konsyl® (Eastern)

Powder, gluten-free, ispaghula husk (micronised), *Konsyl Sugar Free* (6 g/sachet), net price 30-sachet pack = £3.99; *Konsyl Orange* (3.4 g/ sachet), 60-sachet pack = £3.99. Label 13, counselling, see above

Dose: 1 sachet in water 1–3 times daily before or after meals; CHILD (but see section 1.6) over 6 years, ½ adult dose or less (children under 6 years on doctor's advice only)

Diarrhoea (section 1.4.1), 1 sachet in water 3 times daily

Important. Each sachet of *Konsyl Sugar Free* contains almost twice as much ispaghula husk as *Konsyl Orange*

Regulan® (Procter & Gamble)

Powder, beige, sugar- and gluten-free, ispaghula husk 3.4 g/5.85-g sachet (orange or lemon/lime flavour). Net price 30 sachets = £1.05. Label: 13, counselling, see above

Excipients: include aspartame (section 9.4.1)

Dose: 1 sachet in 150 mL water 1–3 times daily; CHILD (but see section 1.6) 6–12 years 2.5–5 mL

METHYLCELLULOSE

Indications: see notes above and section 1.6 [unlicensed dose in children]; adjunct in obesity (but see section 4.5.1)

Cautions: see under Ispaghula Husk

Contra-indications: see under Ispaghula Husk; also infective bowel disease

Side-effects: see under Ispaghula Husk

Dose: see preparations below

COUNSELLING. Preparations that swell in contact with liquid should always be carefully swallowed with water and should not be taken immediately before going to bed

Celevac® (Shire)

Tablets, pink, scored, methylcellulose '450' 500 mg. Net price 112-tab pack = £2.69. Counselling, see above and dose

Dose: constipation and diarrhoea, 3–6 tablets twice daily. In constipation the dose should be taken with at least 300 mL liquid. In diarrhoea, ileostomy, and colostomy control, minimise liquid intake for 30 minutes before and after dose

Adjunct in obesity (but see section 4.5.1), 3 tablets with at least 300 mL warm liquid 30 minutes before food or when hungry

STERCULIA

Indications: see notes above

Cautions: see under Ispaghula Husk

Contra-indications: see under Ispaghula Husk

Side-effects: see under Ispaghula Husk

Dose: see under preparations below

COUNSELLING. Preparations that swell in contact with liquid should always be carefully swallowed with water and should not be taken immediately before going to bed

Normacol® (Norgine)

Granules, coated, gluten-free, sterculia 62%. Net price 500 g = £6.05; 60 × 7-g sachets = £5.11. Label: 25, 27, counselling, see above

Dose: 1–2 heaped 5-mL spoonfuls, or the contents of 1–2 sachets, washed down without chewing with plenty of liquid once or twice daily after meals; CHILD (but see section 1.6) 6–12 years half adult dose

Normacol Plus® (Norgine)

Granules, brown, coated, gluten-free, sterculia 62%, frangula (standardised) 8%. Net price 500 g = £6.50; 60 × 7 g sachets = £5.45. Label: 25, 27, counselling, see above

Dose: constipation and after haemorrhoidectomy, 1–2 heaped 5-mL spoonfuls or the contents of 1–2 sachets washed down without chewing with plenty of liquid once or twice daily after meals

1.6.2 Stimulant laxatives

Stimulant laxatives include **bisacodyl** and members of the **anthraquinone** group, **senna** and **dantron** (danthron). The indications for dantron are limited (see below) by its potential carcinogenicity (based on *rodent* carcinogenicity studies) and evidence of genotoxicity. Powerful stimulants such as **cascara** (an anthraquinone) and **castor oil** are obsolete. **Docusate** sodium probably acts both as a stimulant and as a softening agent.

Stimulant laxatives increase intestinal motility and often cause abdominal cramp; they should be avoided in intestinal obstruction. Prolonged use of stimulant laxatives can precipitate the onset of an atonic non-functioning colon and hypokalaemia; however, prolonged use may be justifiable in some circumstances (see section 1.6 for the use of stimulant laxatives in children).

Glycerol suppositories act as a rectal stimulant by virtue of the mildly irritant action of glycerol.

Soft soap is a more severe irritant; the use of soft soap enema should be **avoided**, especially in pregnancy, as it may inflame the colonic mucosa.

The **parasympathomimetics** bethanechol, distigmine, neostigmine, and pyridostigmine (see section 7.4.1 and section 10.2.1) enhance parasympathetic activity in the gut and increase intestinal motility. They are rarely used for their gastro-intestinal effects. Organic obstruction of the gut must first be excluded and they should not be used shortly after bowel anastomosis.

BISACODYL

Indications: see under Dose; tablets act in 10–12 hours; suppositories act in 20–60 minutes

Cautions: see notes above

Contra-indications: see notes above

Side-effects: see notes above; tablets, griping; suppositories, local irritation

Dose: *by mouth* for constipation, 5–10 mg at night; occasionally necessary to increase to 15–20 mg; CHILD (but see section 1.6) under 10 years 5 mg

By rectum in suppositories for constipation, 10 mg in the morning; CHILD (but see section 1.6) under 10 years 5 mg

Before radiological procedures and surgery, 10 mg by mouth at bedtime for 2 days before examination and, if necessary, a 10-mg suppository 1 hour before examination; CHILD half adult dose

Bisacodyl (Non-proprietary)
Tablets, e/c, bisacodyl 5 mg. Net price 20 = 59p.
Label: 5, 25
Suppositories, bisacodyl 10 mg. Net price 12 = 75p
Paediatric suppositories, bisacodyl 5 mg. Net
price 5 = 89p
Note. The brand name *Dulco-lax®* [NHS] (Boehringer
Ingelheim) is used for bisacodyl tablets, net price 10-tab
pack = 59p; suppositories (10 mg), 10 = £1.48; paed-
iatric suppositories (5 mg), 5 = 89p
The brand names *Dulco-lax® Liquid* and *Dulco-lax Per-
les®* are used for sodium picosulfate preparations

DANTRON
(Danthron)
Indications: only for constipation in terminally ill
patients of all ages
Cautions: see notes above; avoid prolonged contact with skin (as in incontinent patients)—risk of
irritation and excoriation; avoid in pregnancy and
breast-feeding; *rodent* studies indicate potential
carcinogenic risk
Contra-indications: see notes above
Side-effects: see notes above; urine may be coloured red
Dose: see under preparations

■ With poloxamer '188' (as co-danthramer)
Note. Co-danthramer suspension 5 mL = one co-danthramer capsule, **but** strong co-danthramer suspension
5 mL = two strong co-danthramer capsules
Co-danthramer (Non-proprietary) [PoM]
Capsules, co-danthramer 25/200 (dantron 25 mg,
poloxamer '188' 200 mg). Net price 60-cap pack
= £12.86. Label: 14 (urine red)
Dose: 1–2 capsules at bedtime; CHILD 1 capsule at bedtime (restricted indications, see notes above)
Available from Napp
Strong capsules, co-danthramer 37.5/500 (dantron
37.5 mg, poloxamer '188' 500 mg). Net price 60-
cap pack = £15.55. Label: 14 (urine red)
Dose: 1–2 capsules at bedtime (restricted indications,
see notes above); CHILD under 12 years not recommended
Available from Napp
Suspension, co-danthramer 25/200 in 5 mL (dantron 25 mg, poloxamer '188' 200 mg/5 mL). Net
price 300 mL = £11.27, 1 litre = £37.57. Label: 14
(urine red)
Dose: 5–10 mL at night; CHILD 2.5–5 mL (restricted
indications, see notes above)
Available from Galen (*Ailax®*), Hillcross, Napp
(*Codalax®* [NHS]), Sovereign (*Danlax®*)
Strong suspension, co-danthramer 75/1000 in 5 mL
(dantron 75 mg, poloxamer '188' 1 g/5 mL). Net
price 300 mL = £30.13. Label: 14 (urine red)
Dose: 5 mL at night (restricted indications, see notes
above); CHILD under 12 years not recommended
Available from Galen (*Ailax® Forte*), Hillcross, Napp
(*Codalax Forte®* [NHS])

■ With docusate sodium (as co-danthrusate)
Co-danthrusate (Non-proprietary) [PoM]
Capsules, co-danthrusate 50/60 (dantron 50 mg,
docusate sodium 60 mg). Net price 63-cap pack =
£13.45. Label: 14 (urine red)
Dose: 1–3 capsules, usually at night; CHILD 6–12 years 1
capsule (restricted indications, see notes above)
Available from Alpharma, APS, Celltech
(*Normax®* [NHS]), Galen (*Capsuvac®*), Hillcross, IVAX,
Sterwin

Suspension, yellow, co-danthrusate 50/60 (dantron
50 mg, docusate sodium 60 mg/5 mL). Net price
200 mL = £8.75. Label: 14 (urine red)
Dose: 5–15 mL at night; CHILD 6–12 years 5 mL at night
(restricted indications, see notes above)
Available from Celltech (*Normax®*)

DOCUSATE SODIUM
(Dioctyl Sodium Sulphosuccinate)
Indications: constipation (oral preparations act
within 1–2 days); adjunct in abdominal radiological procedures
Cautions: see notes above; do not give with liquid
paraffin; rectal preparations not indicated if
haemorrhoids or anal fissure
Contra-indications: see notes above
Side-effects: see notes above
Dose: *by mouth*, chronic constipation, up to
500 mg daily in divided doses; CHILD (but see
section 1.6) over 6 months 12.5 mg 3 times daily,
2–12 years 12.5–25 mg 3 times daily (use paediatric oral solution only)
With barium meal, 400 mg

Dioctyl® (Schwarz)
Capsules, yellow/white, docusate sodium 100 mg,
net price 30-cap pack = £1.67, 100-cap pack =
£5.00
Docusol® (Typharm)
Adult oral solution, sugar-free, docusate sodium
50 mg/5 mL, net price 300 mL = £2.48
Paediatric oral solution, sugar-free, docusate sodium 12.5 mg/5 mL, net price 300 mL = £1.63

■ Rectal preparations
Fletchers' Enemette® (Forest)
Enema, docusate sodium 90 mg, glycerol 3.78 g/
5 mL with macrogol and sorbic acid. Net price 5-
mL unit = 31p
Dose: ADULT and CHILD (but see section 1.6) over 3
years, 5-mL unit when required
Norgalax Micro-enema® (Norgine)
Enema, docusate sodium 120 mg in 10-g single-
dose disposable packs. Net price 10-g unit = 64p
Dose: ADULT and CHILD (but see section 1.6) over 12
years, 10-g unit

GLYCEROL
(Glycerin)
Indications: constipation
Dose: see below

Glycerol Suppositories, BP
(Glycerin Suppositories)
Suppositories, gelatin 140 mg, glycerol 700 mg,
purified water to 1 g. Net price 12 = 81p (infant),
82p (child), 71p (adult)
Dose: 1 suppository moistened with water before use.
The usual sizes are for *infants* small (1-g mould), *chil-
dren* medium (2-g mould), *adults* large (4-g mould)

SENNA
Indications: constipation; acts in 8–12 hours
Cautions: see notes above
Contra-indications: see notes above
Side-effects: see notes above
Dose: see under preparations

Senna (Non-proprietary)

Tablets, total sennosides (calculated as sennoside B) 7.5 mg. Net price 20 = 30p

Dose: 2–4 tablets, usually at night; initial dose should be low then gradually increased; CHILD (but see section 1.6) over 6 years, half adult dose in the morning (on doctor's advice only)

Note. Lower dose on packs on sale to the public

Available from Alpharma, APS, R&C (*Senokot*® DHS)

Manevac® (Galen)

Granules, coated, senna fruit 12.4%, ispaghula 54.2%. Net price 400 g = £5.76, 56 × 4-g sachets = £3.80. Label: 25, 27, counselling, see Ispaghula Husk

Dose: 1–2 level 5-mL spoonfuls (or sachets) with water or warm drink after supper and, if necessary, before breakfast *or* every 6 hours in resistant cases for 1–3 days; CHILD (but see section 1.6) 5–12 years 1 level 5-mL spoonful (or sachet) daily

Note. One level 5-mL spoonful is equivalent to one 4-g sachet

COUNSELLING. Preparations that swell in contact with liquid should always be carefully swallowed with water and should not be taken immediately before going to bed

Senokot® (R&C)

Tablets DHS, see above

Granules, brown, total sennosides (calculated as sennoside B) 15 mg/5 mL or 5.5 mg/g (one 5-mL spoonful = 2.7 g). Net price 100 g = £2.92

Dose: 5–10 mL, usually at bedtime; CHILD (but see section 1.6) over 6 years 2.5–5 mL in the morning

Note. Lower dose on packs on sale to the public

Syrup, brown, total sennosides (calculated as sennoside B) 7.5 mg/5 mL. Net price 100 mL pack = £2.21

Dose: 10–20 mL, usually at bedtime; CHILD (but see section 1.6) 2–6 years 2.5–5 mL in the morning (doctor's advice only), over 6 years 5–10 mL

Note. Lower dose on packs on sale to the public

SODIUM PICOSULFATE

(Sodium Picosulphate)

Indications: constipation; bowel evacuation before abdominal radiological procedures, endoscopy, and surgery (section 1.6.5); acts within 10–14 hours

Cautions: see notes above

Contra-indications: see notes above

Side-effects: see notes above

Dose: 5–10 mg at night; CHILD (but see section 1.6) under 4 years 250 micrograms/kg, 4–10 years 2.5–5 mg at night, over 10 years 5–10 mg at night

Sodium Picosulfate (Non-proprietary)

Elixir, sodium picosulfate 5 mg/5 mL, net price 100 mL = £1.85

Note. The brand names *Laxoberal*® DHS and *Dulco-lax*® *Liquid* (both Boehringer Ingelheim) are used for sodium picosulfate elixir 5 mg/5 mL

Dulco-lax® (Boehringer Ingelheim)

Perles® (= capsules), sodium picosulfate 2.5 mg, net price 50-cap pack = £2.73

Note. The brand name *Dulco-lax*® is also used for bisacodyl tablets and suppositories

■ Bowel cleansing solutions
Section 1.6.5

Other stimulant laxatives

Unstandardised preparations of cascara, frangula, rhubarb, and senna should be **avoided** as their laxative action is unpredictable. Aloes, colocynth, and jalap should be **avoided** as they have a drastic purgative action.

Stimulant laxative preparations on sale to the public (not prescribable on the NHS) together with their significant ingredients:

Boots Compound Laxative Syrup of Figs® (fig, senna), **Boots Senna Tablets**® (senna)
Califig® (fig, senna), **Calsalettes**® (aloin)
Ex-lax Senna® (senna)
Fam-Lax Senna® (Irish moss, rhubarb, senna)
Juno Junipah Salts® (juniper berry oil, sodium bicarbonate, sodium phosphate, sodium sulphate)
Nylax with Senna® (senna)
Potter's Cleansing Herb® (aloes, cascara, senna)
Rhuaka® (cascara, rhubarb, senna)

1.6.3   Faecal softeners

Liquid paraffin, the classical lubricant, has disadvantages (see below). Bulk laxatives (section 1.6.1) and non-ionic surfactant 'wetting' agents e.g. docusate sodium (section 1.6.2) also have softening properties. Such drugs are useful for oral administration in the management of haemorrhoids and anal fissure; glycerol suppositories (section 1.6.2) are useful for rectal use.

Enemas containing **arachis oil** (ground-nut oil, peanut oil) lubricate and soften impacted faeces and promote a bowel movement.

ARACHIS OIL

Indications: see notes above
Dose: see below

Fletchers' Arachis Oil Retention Enema®
(Forest)

Enema, arachis (peanut) oil in 130-mL single-dose disposable packs. Net price 130 mL = £1.02

Dose: to soften impacted faeces, 130 mL; the enema should be warmed before use; CHILD (but see section 1.6) under 3 years not recommended; over 3 years reduce adult dose in proportion to body-weight (medical supervision only)

LIQUID PARAFFIN

Indications: constipation
Cautions: CSM recommends avoid prolonged use, and has contra-indicated in children less than 3 years of age
Side-effects: anal seepage of paraffin and consequent anal irritation after prolonged use, granulomatous reactions caused by absorption of small quantities of liquid paraffin (especially from the emulsion), lipoid pneumonia, and interference with the absorption of fat-soluble vitamins
Dose: see under preparation

Liquid Paraffin Oral Emulsion, BP

Oral emulsion, liquid paraffin 5 mL, vanillin 5 mg, chloroform 0.025 mL, benzoic acid solution 0.2 mL, methylcellulose-20 200 mg, saccharin sodium 500 micrograms, water to 10 mL

Dose: 10–30 mL at night when required

COUNSELLING. Should not be taken immediately before going to bed

Osmotic laxatives

These act by retaining fluid in the bowel by osmosis or by changing the pattern of water distribution in the faeces.

Saline purgatives such as **magnesium hydroxide** are commonly abused but are satisfactory for occasional use; adequate fluid intake should be maintained. **Magnesium salts** are useful where rapid bowel evacuation is required. **Sodium salts** should be avoided as they may give rise to sodium and water retention in susceptible individuals. **Phosphate enemas** are useful in bowel clearance before radiology, endoscopy, and surgery.

Lactulose is a semi-synthetic disaccharide which is not absorbed from the gastro-intestinal tract. It produces an osmotic diarrhoea of low faecal pH, and discourages the proliferation of ammonia-producing organisms. It is therefore useful in the treatment of *hepatic encephalopathy*. **Lactitol** is a similar disaccharide.

LACTITOL

Indications: see under Lactulose
Contra-indications: see under Lactulose
Side-effects: see under Lactulose
Dose: constipation, initially 20 g daily in a single dose with morning or evening meal, subsequently adjusted to produce one stool daily (dose of 10 g daily may be sufficient); CHILD (but see section 1.6) 1–6 years 2.5–5 g, 6–12 years 5–10 g, 12–16 years 10–20 g daily, subsequently adjusted to produce one stool daily
Hepatic encephalopathy, 500–700 mg/kg daily in 3 divided doses with meals, subsequently adjusted to produce 2 soft stools daily
By nasogastric administration, as a 40% solution (200 g/500 mL), 1–2 mL/kg body-weight daily
COUNSELLING. Powder should be mixed with food or liquid and one to two glasses of liquid should be drunk with the meal

Lactitol (Non-proprietary)
Powder, lactitol 10 g/sachet. Net price 10-sachet pack = £1.00. Counselling, see above
Available from Novartis Consumer Health

LACTULOSE

Indications: constipation (may take up to 48 hours to act), hepatic encephalopathy (portal systemic encephalopathy)
Cautions: lactose intolerance
Contra-indications: galactosaemia, intestinal obstruction
Side-effects: flatulence, cramps, and abdominal discomfort
Dose: see under preparations below

Lactulose (Non-proprietary)
Solution, lactulose 3.1–3.7 g/5 mL with other ketoses. Net price 500-mL pack = £2.43
Dose: constipation, initially 15 mL twice daily, adjusted according to patient's needs; CHILD (but see section 1.6) under 1 year 2.5 mL twice daily, 1–5 years 5 mL twice daily, 5–10 years 10 mL twice daily
Hepatic encephalopathy, 30–50 mL 3 times daily, subsequently adjusted to produce 2–3 soft stools daily
Available from Alpharma, APS, CP, Hillcross, Intrap-

harm (*Lactugal®*), IVAX, Lagap, Novartis Consumer Health (*Regulose®*), Solvay (*Duphalac®* NHS)
Note. A proprietary brand of lactulose 3.3 g/5 mL (*Regulose®*) is on sale to the public

MACROGOLS
(Polyethylene glycols)
Indications: see preparation below
Cautions: pregnancy and breast-feeding; discontinue if symptoms of fluid and electrolyte disturbance
Contra-indications: intestinal perforation or obstruction, paralytic ileus, severe inflammatory conditions of the intestinal tract (such as Crohn's disease, ulcerative colitis, and toxic megacolon)
Side-effects: abdominal distension and pain, nausea
Dose: see preparation below

Movicol® (Norgine)
Oral powder, macrogol '3350' (polyethylene glycol '3350') 13.125 g, sodium bicarbonate 178.5 mg, sodium chloride 350.7 mg, potassium chloride 46.6 mg/sachet. Net price 20-sachet pack (lime and lemon flavour) = £4.98, 30-sachet pack = £7.47. Label: 13
Dose: chronic constipation, 2–3 sachets daily in divided doses; each sachet dissolved in 125 mL water and drunk immediately usually for up to 2 weeks, course repeated if required; ELDERLY initially 1 sachet daily; CHILD not recommended
Faecal impaction, 8 sachets daily dissolved in 1 litre water; the solution should be drunk within 6 hours, usually for max. 3 days; CHILD not recommended.
After reconstitution the solution should be kept in a refrigerator and discarded if unused after 6 hours
Caution: patients with impaired cardiovascular function should not take more than 2 sachets in any 1 hour

MAGNESIUM SALTS
Indications: see under preparations below
Cautions: renal impairment (risk of magnesium accumulation); hepatic impairment (see Appendix 2); elderly and debilitated; see also notes above; **interactions:** Appendix 1 (magnesium salts)
Contra-indications: acute gastro-intestinal conditions
Side-effects: colic
Dose: see under preparations below

■ Magnesium hydroxide
Magnesium Hydroxide Mixture, BP
(Cream of Magnesia)
Aqueous suspension containing about 8% hydrated magnesium oxide. Do not store in cold place
Dose: constipation, 25–50 mL when required

■ Magnesium hydroxide with liquid paraffin
Liquid Paraffin and Magnesium Hydroxide Oral Emulsion, BP ▨
Oral emulsion, 25% liquid paraffin in aqueous suspension containing 6% hydrated magnesium oxide
Dose: constipation, 5–20 mL when required
Note. Liquid paraffin and magnesium hydroxide preparations on sale to the public include: *Milpar®* NHS

▨ denotes preparations that are considered to be less suitable for prescribing (see p. vi)

■ Magnesium sulphate
Magnesium Sulphate. Label: 13, 23
Dose: rapid bowel evacuation (acts in 2–4 hours) 5–10 g in a tumblerful of water preferably before breakfast
Note. Magnesium sulphate is on sale to the public as Epsom Salts; *Andrews Liver Salts*® [NHS] (citric acid, magnesium sulphate, sodium bicarbonate) is also on sale to the public

■ Bowel cleansing solutions
Section 1.6.5

PHOSPHATES (RECTAL)

Indications: rectal use in constipation; bowel evacuation before abdominal radiological procedures, endoscopy, and surgery
Cautions: elderly and debilitated; see also notes above
Contra-indications: acute gastro-intestinal conditions
Side-effects: local irritation
Dose: see below

Carbalax® (Forest)
Suppositories, sodium acid phosphate (anhydrous) 1.3 g, sodium bicarbonate 1.08 g, net price 12 = £2.14
Dose: constipation, 1 suppository, inserted 30 minutes before evacuation required; moisten with water before use; CHILD under 12 years not recommended

Fleet® **Ready-to-use Enema** (De Witt)
Enema, sodium acid phosphate 21.4 g, sodium phosphate 9.4 g/118 mL. Net price single-dose pack (standard tube) = 46p
Dose: ADULT and CHILD (but see section 1.6) over 12 years, 118 mL; CHILD 3–12 years, on doctor's advice only (under 3 years not recommended)

Fletchers' Phosphate Enema® (Forest)
Enema, sodium acid phosphate 12.8 g, sodium phosphate 10.24 g, purified water, freshly boiled and cooled, to 128 mL (corresponds to Phosphates Enema Formula B). Net price 128 mL with standard tube = 44p, with long rectal tube = 61p
Dose: 128 mL; CHILD (but see section 1.6) over 3 years, reduced according to body weight (under 3 years not recommended)

SODIUM CITRATE (RECTAL)

Indications: rectal use in constipation
Cautions: elderly and debilitated; see also notes above
Contra-indications: acute gastro-intestinal conditions
Dose: see below

Micolette Micro-enema® (Dexcel)
Enema, sodium citrate 450 mg, sodium lauryl sulphoacetate 45 mg, glycerol 625 mg, together with citric acid, potassium sorbate, and sorbitol in a viscous solution, in 5-mL single-dose disposable packs with nozzle. Net price 5 mL = 32p
Dose: ADULT and CHILD over 3 years, 5–10 mL (but see section 1.6)

Micralax Micro-enema® (Celltech)
Enema, sodium citrate 450 mg, sodium alkylsulphoacetate 45 mg, sorbic acid 5 mg, together with glycerol and sorbitol in a viscous solution in 5-mL single-dose disposable packs with nozzle. Net price 5 mL = 33p
Dose: ADULT and CHILD over 3 years, 5 mL (but see section 1.6)

Relaxit Micro-enema® (Crawford)
Enema, sodium citrate 450 mg, sodium lauryl sulphate 75 mg, sorbic acid 5 mg, together with glycerol and sorbitol in a viscous solution in 5-mL single-dose disposable packs with nozzle. Net price 5 mL = 32p
Dose: ADULT and CHILD (but see section 1.6) 5 mL (insert only half nozzle length in child under 3 years)

1.6.5   Bowel cleansing solutions

Bowel cleansing solutions are used before colonic surgery, colonoscopy, or radiological examination to ensure the bowel is free of solid contents. They are **not** treatments for constipation.

BOWEL CLEANSING SOLUTIONS

Indications: see above
Cautions: pregnancy; renal impairment; heart disease; ulcerative colitis; diabetes mellitus; reflux oesophagitis; impaired gag reflex; unconscious or semiconscious or possibility of regurgitation or aspiration
Contra-indications: gastro-intestinal obstruction, gastric retention, gastro-intestinal ulceration, perforated bowel, congestive cardiac failure; toxic colitis, toxic megacolon or ileus
Side-effects: nausea and bloating; less frequently abdominal cramps (usually transient—reduced by taking more slowly); vomiting
Dose: see under preparations

Citramag® (Bioglan)
Powder, effervescent, magnesium carbonate 11.57 g, anhydrous citric acid 17.79 g/sachet, net price 10-sachet pack (lemon and lime flavour) = £11.92. Label 10, patient information leaflet, 13, counselling, see below
Dose: bowel evacuation for radiological examination or surgery, on day before procedure, 1 sachet at 8 a.m. and 1 sachet between 2 and 4 p.m.; CHILD 5–9 years one-third adult dose; over 10 years and frail ELDERLY one-half adult dose

COUNSELLING. The patient information leaflet advises that hot water (200 mL) is needed to make the solution and provides guidance on the timing and procedure for reconstitution; it also mentions need for high fluid, low residue diet beforehand (according to hospital advice), and explains that only clear fluids can be taken after *Citramag*® until procedure completed

Fleet Phospho-soda® (De Witt)
Oral solution, sugar-free, sodium dihydrogen phosphate dihydrate 24.4 g, disodium phosphate dodecahydrate 10.8 g/45 mL. Net price 2 × 45-mL bottles = £4.79. Label: 10 patient information leaflet, counselling
Dose: 45 mL diluted with half a glass (120 mL) of cool water, followed by one full glass (240 mL) of cool water
Timing of doses is dependent on the time of the procedure
For morning procedure, first dose should be taken at 7 a.m. and second at 7 p.m. on day before the procedure
For afternoon procedure, first dose should be taken at 7 p.m. on day before and second dose at 7 a.m. on day of the procedure
Solid food must not be taken during dosing period; clear liquids or water should be substituted for meals
CHILD not recommended

Klean-Prep® (Norgine)

Oral powder, macrogol '3350' (polyethylene glycol '3350') 59 g, anhydrous sodium sulphate 5.685 g, sodium bicarbonate 1.685 g, sodium chloride 1.465 g, potassium chloride 743 mg/sachet. Contains aspartame (see section 9.4.1). Net price 4 sachets = £8.39. Label: 10 patient information leaflet, counselling

Four sachets when reconstituted with water to 4 litres provides an iso-osmotic solution for bowel cleansing before surgery, colonoscopy or radiological procedures

Dose: 250 mL (1 tumblerful) of reconstituted solution every 10–15 minutes, or by nasogastric tube 20–30 mL/minute, until 4 litres have been consumed or watery stools are free of solid matter; CHILD not recommended

The solution from all 4 sachets should be drunk within 4–6 hours (250 mL drunk rapidly every 10–15 minutes); flavouring such as clear fruit cordials may be added if required; to facilitate gastric emptying domperidone or metoclopramide may be given 30 minutes before starting.

Alternatively the administration may be divided into two, e.g. taking the solutions from 2 sachets on the evening before examination and the remaining 2 on the morning of the examination

After reconstitution the solution should be kept in a refrigerator and discarded if unused after 24 hours

Note. Allergic reactions reported

Picolax® (Nordic)

Oral powder, sugar-free, sodium picosulfate 10 mg/sachet, with magnesium citrate (for bowel evacuation before radiological procedure, endoscopy, and surgery), net price 2-sachet pack = £3.95, 50-sachet pack (hosp. only) = £14.85. Label: 10, patient information leaflet, 13, counselling, see below

Dose: ADULT and CHILD over 9 years, 1 sachet in water in morning (before 8 a.m.) and a second in afternoon (between 2 and 4 p.m.) of day preceding procedure; CHILD 1–2 years quarter sachet morning and afternoon, 2–4 years half sachet morning and afternoon, 4–9 years 1 sachet morning and half sachet afternoon

Acts within 3 hours of first dose

Note. Low residue diet recommended for 2 days before procedure and copious intake of water or other clear fluids recommended during treatment

COUNSELLING. Patients should be warned that heat is generated on addition to water; for this reason the powder should be added initially to 30 mL (2 tablespoonfuls) of water; after 5 minutes (when reaction complete) the solution should be further diluted to 150 mL (about a tumblerful)

1.7 Local preparations for anal and rectal disorders

1.7.1	Soothing haemorrhoidal preparations
1.7.2	Compound haemorrhoidal preparations with corticosteroids
1.7.3	Rectal sclerosants

Anal and perianal pruritus, soreness, and excoriation are best treated by application of bland ointments and suppositories (section 1.7.1). These conditions occur commonly in patients suffering from haemorrhoids, fistulas, and proctitis. Careful local toilet with attention to any minor faecal soiling, adjustment of the diet to avoid hard stools, the use of bulk-forming materials such as bran (section 1.6.1) and a high residue diet are helpful. In proct-

itis these measures may supplement treatment with corticosteroids or sulfasalazine (see section 1.5).

When necessary topical preparations containing **local anaesthetics** (section 1.7.1) or **corticosteroids** (section 1.7.2) are used provided perianal thrush has been excluded. Perianal thrush is best treated with **nystatin** by mouth and by local application (see section 5.2, section 7.2.2, and section 13.10.2).

The management of *anal fissures* requires stool softening by increasing dietary fibre in the form of bran or by using a bulk-forming laxative. Short-term use of local anaesthetic preparations may help (section 1.7.1). If these measures are inadequate, the patient should be referred for specialist treatment in hospital; surgery or the use of a topical nitrate (e.g. glyceryl trinitrate 0.2–0.3% ointment) may be considered [unlicensed indication].

1.7.1 Soothing haemorrhoidal preparations

Soothing preparations containing mild astringents such as bismuth subgallate, zinc oxide, and hamamelis may give symptomatic relief in haemorrhoids. Many proprietary preparations also contain lubricants, vasoconstrictors, or mild antiseptics.

Local anaesthetics are used to relieve pain associated with *haemorrhoids*, and *pruritus ani* but good evidence is lacking. Lidocaine (lignocaine) ointment (section 15.2) is used before emptying the bowel to relieve pain associated with *anal fissure*. Alternative local anaesthetics include tetracaine (amethocaine), cinchocaine, and pramocaine (pramoxine), but they are more irritant. Local anaesthetic ointments can be absorbed through the rectal mucosa therefore excessive application should be **avoided**, particularly in infants and children. They should be used for short periods only (no longer than a few days) since they may cause sensitisation of the anal skin.

Soothing haemorrhoidal preparations on sale to the public together with their significant ingredients include:

Anacal® (heparinoid, laureth '9'), **Anodesyn®** (allantoin, lidocaine (lignocaine)), **Anusol® cream** (bismuth oxide, Peru balsam, zinc oxide), **Anusol® ointment** and **suppositories** (bismuth oxide, bismuth subgallate, Peru balsam, zinc oxide)

Boots Haemorrhoid Ointment® (lidocaine (lignocaine), zinc oxide), **Boots Suppositories for Haemorrhoids®** (benzyl alcohol, glycol monosalicylate, methyl salicylate, zinc oxide)

Germoloids® (lidocaine (lignocaine), zinc oxide)

Hemocane® (benzoic acid, bismuth oxide, cinnamic acid, lidocaine (lignocaine), zinc oxide)

Lanacane® cream (benzocaine, chlorothymol)

Nupercainal® (cinchocaine)

Preparation H® gel (hamamelis water), **Preparation H® ointment and suppositories** (shark liver oil, yeast cell extract)

1.7.2 Compound haemorrhoidal preparations with corticosteroids

Corticosteroids are often combined with local anaesthetics and soothing agents in preparations for haemorrhoids. They are suitable for occasional short-term use after exclusion of infections, such as herpes simplex; prolonged use can cause atrophy of the anal skin. See section 13.4 for general comments on topical corticosteroids and section 1.7.1 for comment on local anaesthetics.

Haemorrhoids in children are rare. Treatment is usually symptomatic and the use of a locally applied cream is appropriate for short periods; however, local anaesthetics can cause stinging initially and this may aggravate the child's fear of defaecation.

Anugesic-HC® (Parke-Davis) PoM

Cream, benzyl benzoate 1.2%, bismuth oxide 0.875%, hydrocortisone acetate 0.5%, Peru balsam 1.85%, pramocaine hydrochloride 1%, zinc oxide 12.35%. Net price 30 g (with rectal nozzle) = £3.09

Apply night and morning and after a bowel movement; do not use for longer than 7 days; CHILD not recommended

Suppositories, buff, benzyl benzoate 33 mg, bismuth oxide 24 mg, bismuth subgallate 59 mg, hydrocortisone acetate 5 mg, Peru balsam 49 mg, pramocaine hydrochloride 27 mg, zinc oxide 296 mg. Net price 12 = £2.24

Insert 1 suppository night and morning and after a bowel movement; do not use for longer than 7 days; CHILD not recommended

Anusol-HC® (Kestrel) PoM

Ointment, benzyl benzoate 1.25%, bismuth oxide 0.875%, bismuth subgallate 2.25%, hydrocortisone acetate 0.25%, Peru balsam 1.875%, zinc oxide 10.75%. Net price 30 g (with rectal nozzle) = £3.04

Apply night and morning and after a bowel movement; do not use for longer than 7 days; CHILD not recommended

Note. A proprietary brand (*Anusol Plus HC®* ointment) is on sale to the public

Suppositories, benzyl benzoate 33 mg, bismuth oxide 24 mg, bismuth subgallate 59 mg, hydrocortisone acetate 10 mg, Peru balsam 49 mg, zinc oxide 296 mg. Net price 12 = £2.14

Insert 1 suppository night and morning and after a bowel movement; do not use for longer than 7 days; CHILD not recommended

Note. A proprietary brand (*Anusol Plus HC®* suppositories) is on sale to the public

Betnovate® (GlaxoWellcome) PoM

Rectal ointment, betamethasone valerate 0.05%, lidocaine hydrochloride (lignocaine hydrochloride) 2.5%, phenylephrine hydrochloride 0.1%. Net price 30 g (with applicator) = £1.50

Apply 2–3 times daily until inflammation subsides then once daily, externally or by rectum; do not use for longer than 7 days; CHILD under 1 year not recommended

Perinal® (Dermal)

Spray application, hydrocortisone 0.2%, lidocaine hydrochloride (lignocaine hydrochloride) 1%. Net price 30-mL pack = £6.87

Spray twice over the affected area up to 3 times daily; do not use for longer than 1–2 weeks; CHILD under 14 years not recommended

Proctofoam HC® (Stafford-Miller) PoM

Foam in aerosol pack, hydrocortisone acetate 1%, pramocaine hydrochloride 1%. Net price 21.2-g

pack (approx. 40 applications) with applicator = £4.71

Dose: haemorrhoids and proctitis, 1 applicatorful (4–6 mg hydrocortisone acetate, 4–6 mg pramocaine hydrochloride) by rectum 2–3 times daily and after a bowel movement (max. 4 times daily); do not use for longer than 7 days; CHILD not recommended

Proctosedyl® (Hoechst Marion Roussel) PoM

Ointment, cinchocaine (dibucaine) hydrochloride 0.5%, hydrocortisone 0.5%. Net price 30 g = £7.13 (with cannula)

Apply morning and night and after a bowel movement, externally or by rectum; do not use for longer than 7 days

Suppositories, cinchocaine (dibucaine) hydrochloride 5 mg, hydrocortisone 5 mg. Net price 12 = £3.22

Insert 1 suppository night and morning and after a bowel movement; do not use for longer than 7 days

Scheriproct® (Schering Health) PoM

Ointment, cinchocaine (dibucaine) hydrochloride 0.5%, prednisolone hexanoate 0.19%. Net price 30 g = £3.53

Apply twice daily for 5–7 days (3–4 times daily on 1st day if necessary), then once daily for a few days after symptoms have cleared

Suppositories, cinchocaine (dibucaine) hydrochloride 1 mg, prednisolone hexanoate 1.3 mg. Net price 12 = £1.66

Insert 1 suppository daily after a bowel movement, for 5–7 days (in severe cases initially 2–3 times daily)

Ultraproct® (Schering Health) PoM

Ointment, cinchocaine (dibucaine) hydrochloride 0.5%, fluocortolone hexanoate 0.095%, fluocortolone pivalate 0.092%. Net price 30 g (with rectal nozzle) = £4.57

Apply twice daily for 5–7 days (3–4 times daily on 1st day if necessary), then once daily for a few days after symptoms have cleared

Suppositories, cinchocaine (dibucaine) hydrochloride 1 mg, fluocortolone hexanoate 630 micrograms, fluocortolone pivalate 610 micrograms. Net price 12 = £2.15

Insert 1 suppository daily after a bowel movement, for 5–7 days (in severe cases initially 2–3 times daily) then 1 suppository every other day for 1 week

Uniroid-HC® (Chemidex) PoM

Ointment, cinchocaine (dibucaine) hydrochloride 0.5%, hydrocortisone 0.5%. Net price 30 g (with applicator) = £4.23

Apply twice daily and after a bowel movement, externally or by rectum; do not use for longer than 7 days; CHILD under 12 years not recommended

Suppositories, cinchocaine (dibucaine) hydrochloride 5 mg, hydrocortisone 5 mg. Net price 12 = £1.91

Insert 1 suppository twice daily and after a bowel movement; do not use for longer than 7 days; CHILD under 12 years not recommended

Xyloproct® (AstraZeneca) PoM

Ointment (water-miscible), aluminium acetate 3.5%, hydrocortisone acetate 0.275%, lidocaine (lignocaine) 5%, zinc oxide 18%. Net price 30 g (with applicator) = £3.39

Apply several times daily; short-term use only

1.7.3   Rectal sclerosants

Oily phenol injection is used to inject haemorrhoids particularly when unprolapsed.

PHENOL

Indications: see notes above
Side-effects: irritation, tissue necrosis

Oily Phenol Injection, BP, [PoM] phenol 5% in a suitable fixed oil. Net price 5-mL amp = £4.53
Dose: 2–3 mL into the submucosal layer at the base of the pile; several injections may be given at different sites, max. total injected 10 mL at any one time
Available from Celltech

1.8   Stoma care

Prescribing for patients with stoma calls for special care. The following is a brief account of some of the main points to be borne in mind.

Enteric-coated and *modified-release* preparations are **unsuitable**, particularly in patients with ileostomies, as there may not be sufficient release of the active ingredient.

Laxatives. Enemas and washouts should **not** be prescribed for patients with ileostomies as they may cause rapid and severe dehydration.

Colostomy patients may suffer from constipation and whenever possible should be treated by increasing fluid intake or dietary fibre. **Bulk-forming drugs** (section 1.6.1) should be tried. If they are insufficient, as small a dose as possible of senna (section 1.6.2) should be used.

Antidiarrhoeals. Drugs such as **loperamide, codeine phosphate,** or **co-phenotrope** (diphenoxylate with atropine) are effective. Bulk-forming drugs (section 1.6.1) may be tried but it is often difficult to adjust the dose appropriately.

Antibacterials should **not** be given for an episode of acute diarrhoea.

Antacids. The tendency to diarrhoea from magnesium salts or constipation from aluminium salts may be increased in these patients.

Diuretics should be used with caution in patients with ileostomies as they may become excessively dehydrated and potassium depletion may easily occur. It is usually advisable to use a **potassium-sparing** diuretic (see section 2.2.3).

Digoxin. Patients with a stoma are particularly susceptible to hypokalaemia if on digoxin therapy and potassium supplements or a potassium-sparing diuretic may be advisable (for comment see section 9.2.1.1).

Potassium supplements. Liquid formulations are preferred to modified-release formulations (see above).

Analgesics. Opioid analgesics (see section 4.7.2) may cause troublesome constipation in colostomy patients. When a non-opioid analgesic is required **paracetamol** is usually suitable but anti-inflammatory analgesics may cause gastric irritation and bleeding.

Iron preparations may cause loose stools and sore skin in these patients. If this is troublesome and if iron is definitely indicated an intramuscular iron preparation (see section 9.1.1.2) should be used. Modified-release preparations should be **avoided** for the reasons given above.

Patients are usually given advice about the use of *cleansing agents*, *protective creams*, *lotions*, *deodorants*, or *sealants* whilst in hospital, either by the surgeon or by the health authority stoma care nurses. Voluntary organisations offer help and support to patients with stoma.

1.9   Drugs affecting intestinal secretions

1.9.1	Drugs acting on the gall bladder
1.9.2	Bile acid sequestrants
1.9.3	Aprotinin
1.9.4	Pancreatin

1.9.1   Drugs acting on the gall bladder

The use of laparoscopic cholecystectomy and of endoscopic biliary techniques has limited the place of the bile acid **ursodeoxycholic acid** in gallstone disease. Ursodeoxycholic acid is suitable for patients with unimpaired gall bladder function, small or medium-sized radiolucent stones, and whose mild symptoms are not amenable to other treatment; it should be used cautiously in those with liver disease (but see below). Patients should be given dietary advice (including avoidance of excessive cholesterol and calories) and they require radiological monitoring. Long-term prophylaxis may be needed after complete dissolution of the gallstones has been confirmed (preferably with cholecystograms and ultrasound on two separate occasions) because gallstones may recur in up to 25% of patients within one year of stopping treatment.

Ursodeoxycholic acid is also used in primary biliary cirrhosis; liver tests improve in most patients but the effect on overall survival is uncertain. Ursodeoxycholic acid has also been tried in primary sclerosing cholangitis [unlicensed indication].

URSODEOXYCHOLIC ACID

Indications: see under Dose and under preparations
Cautions: see notes above; **interactions:** Appendix 1 (bile acids)
Contra-indications: radio-opaque   stones, pregnancy (Appendix 4), non-functioning gall bladder, inflammatory diseases and other conditions of the small intestine, colon and liver which interfere with entero-hepatic circulation of bile salts
Side-effects: nausea, vomiting, diarrhoea; gallstone calcification; pruritus
Dose: dissolution of gallstones, 8–12 mg/kg daily as a single dose at bedtime *or* in two divided doses, for up to 2 years; treatment is continued for 3–4 months after stones dissolve
Primary biliary cirrhosis, see under *Ursofalk*®

Ursodeoxycholic Acid (Non-proprietary) [PoM]
Tablets, ursodeoxycholic acid 150 mg, net price 60-tab pack = £18.44. Label: 21
Available from Hillcross
Capsules, ursodeoxycholic acid 250 mg, net price 60-cap pack = £34.99. Label: 21
Available from Hillcross

Destolit® (Norgine) PoM
Tablets, scored, ursodeoxycholic acid 150 mg, net price 60-tab pack = £18.07. Label: 21

Urdox® (CP) PoM
Tablets, f/c, ursodeoxycholic acid 300 mg, net price 60-tab pack = £30.24. Label: 21

Ursofalk® (Provalis) PoM
Capsules, ursodeoxycholic acid 250 mg. Net price 60 = £32.95. Label: 21
Suspension, sugar-free, ursodeoxycholic acid 250 mg/5 mL, net price 250 mL = £30.20. Label: 21
Dose: primary biliary cirrhosis, 10–15 mg/kg daily in 2–4 divided doses
Dissolution of gallstones, see Dose, above

Ursogal® (Galen) PoM
Tablets, scored, ursodeoxycholic acid 150 mg, net price 60-tab pack = £17.05. Label: 21
Capsules, ursodeoxycholic acid 250 mg, net price 60-cap pack = £30.50. Label: 21

Other preparations for biliary disorders

A **terpene** mixture (Rowachol®) raises biliary cholesterol solubility. It is not considered to be a useful adjunct.

Rowachol® (Rowa) PoM �
Capsules, green, e/c, borneol 5 mg, camphene 5 mg, cineole 2 mg, menthol 32 mg, menthone 6 mg, pinene 17 mg in olive oil. Net price 50-cap pack = £7.35. Label: 22
Dose: 1–2 capsules 3 times daily before food (but see notes above)
Interactions: Appendix 1 (*Rowachol®*)

1.9.2   Bile acid sequestrants

Colestyramine (cholestyramine) is an anion-exchange resin that is not absorbed from the gastro-intestinal tract. It relieves diarrhoea and pruritus by forming an insoluble complex with bile acids in the intestine. Colestyramine can interfere with the absorption of a number of drugs. Colestyramine is also used in hypercholesterolaemia (section 2.12).

COLESTYRAMINE
(Cholestyramine)
Indications: pruritus associated with partial biliary obstruction and primary biliary cirrhosis; diarrhoea associated with Crohn's disease, ileal resection, vagotomy, diabetic vagal neuropathy, and radiation; hypercholesterolaemia (section 2.12)
Cautions: see section 2.12
Contra-indications: see section 2.12
Side-effects: see section 2.12
Dose: pruritus, 4–8 g daily in water (or other suitable liquid)
Diarrhoea, after initial introduction over 3–4 week period, 12–24 g daily mixed with water (or other suitable liquid) in 1–4 divided doses, then adjusted as required; max. 36 g daily
CHILD 6–12 years, consult product literature
COUNSELLING. Other drugs should be taken at least 1 hour before or 4–6 hours after colestyramine to reduce possible interference with absorption
Preparations
Section 2.12

1.9.3   Aprotinin
Section 2.11.

1.9.4   Pancreatin

Supplements of pancreatin are given by mouth to compensate for reduced or absent exocrine secretion in cystic fibrosis, and following pancreatectomy, total gastrectomy, or chronic pancreatitis. They assist the digestion of starch, fat, and protein.

Pancreatin is inactivated by gastric acid therefore pancreatin preparations are best taken with food (or immediately before or after food). Gastric acid secretion may be reduced by giving cimetidine or ranitidine an hour beforehand (section 1.3). Concurrent use of antacids also reduces gastric acidity. The newer enteric-coated preparations such as *Creon®*, *Nutrizym GR®*, and *Pancrease®* deliver a higher enzyme concentration in the duodenum (provided the granules are swallowed whole without chewing). Higher-strength versions are now also available (**important:** see CSM advice below).

Since pancreatin is also inactivated by heat, excessive heat should be avoided if preparations are mixed with liquids or food; the resulting mixtures should not be kept for more than one hour.

Dosage is adjusted according to size, number, and consistency of stools, so that the patient thrives; extra allowance may be needed if snacks are taken between meals.

Pancreatin can irritate the perioral skin and buccal mucosa if retained in the mouth, and excessive doses can cause perianal irritation. The most frequent side-effects are gastro-intestinal, including nausea, vomiting, and abdominal discomfort; hyperuricaemia and hyperuricosuria have been associated with very high doses. Hypersensitivity reactions occur occasionally and may affect those handling the powder.

PANCREATIN

Note. The pancreatin preparations which follow are all of porcine origin
Indications: see also above
Cautions: see also above and (for higher-strength preparations) see below
Side-effects: see also above and (for higher-strength preparations) see below
Dose: see preparations

Creon® (Solvay)
Granules, brown, e/c, pancreatin, providing: protease 1 125 units, lipase 20 000 units, amylase 22 500 units/sachet. Net price 40-sachet pack = £13.33. Counselling, see dose
Dose: ADULT and CHILD initially 1 sachet with meals either washed down or sprinkled on soft food (then swallowed immediately without chewing); higher doses may be required according to response
Creon® 10 000 (Solvay)
Capsules, brown/clear, enclosing buff-coloured e/c granules of pancreatin, providing: protease 600 units, lipase 10 000 units, amylase 8000 units.

Net price 100-cap pack = £16.66. Counselling, see dose

Dose: ADULT and CHILD initially 1–2 capsules with meals either taken whole or contents mixed with fluid or soft food (then swallowed immediately without chewing)

Nutrizym GR® (Merck)

Capsules, green/orange, enclosing e/c pellets of pancreatin, providing minimum of: protease 650 units, lipase 10 000 units, amylase 10 000 units. Net price 100 = £13.15. Counselling, see dose

Dose: ADULT and CHILD 1–2 capsules with meals swallowed immediately or contents sprinkled on soft food (then swallowed immediately without chewing); higher doses may be required according to response

Nutrizym 10® (Merck)

Capsules, red/yellow, enclosing e/c minitablets of pancreatin providing minimum of: protease 500 units, lipase 10 000 units, amylase 9000 units. Net price 100 = £13.15. Counselling, see dose

Dose: ADULT and CHILD 1–2 capsules with meals and 1 capsule with snacks, swallowed whole or contents taken with water or sprinkled on soft food (then swallowed immediately without chewing); higher doses may be required according to response

Pancrease® (Janssen-Cilag)

Capsules, enclosing e/c beads of pancrelipase USP, providing minimum of: protease 330 units, lipase 5000 units, amylase 2900 units. Net price 100 = £17.07. Counselling, see dose

Dose: ADULT and CHILD 1–2 (occasionally 3) capsules during each meal and 1 capsule with snacks swallowed whole or contents sprinkled on liquid or soft food (then swallowed immediately without chewing); higher doses may be required according to response

Pancrex® (Paines & Byrne)

Granules, pancreatin, providing minimum of: protease 300 units, lipase 5000 units, amylase 4000 units/g. Net price 300 g = £20.39. Label: 25, counselling, see dose

Dose: ADULT and CHILD 5–10 g just before meals washed down or mixed with liquid

Pancrex V® (Paines & Byrne)

Capsules, pancreatin, providing minimum of: protease 430 units, lipase 8000 units, amylase 9000 units. Net price 300-cap pack = £15.80. Counselling, see dose

Dose: ADULT and CHILD over 1 year 2–6 capsules with meals, swallowed whole or sprinkled on food; CHILD up to 1 year 1–2 capsules mixed with feeds

Capsules '125', pancreatin, providing minimum of: protease 160 units, lipase 2950 units, amylase 3300 units. Net price 300-cap pack – £9.72. Counselling, see dose

Dose: NEONATE 1–2 capsules with feeds

Tablets, e/c, s/c, pancreatin, providing minimum of: protease 110 units, lipase 1900 units, amylase 1700 units. Net price 300-tab pack = £4.51. Label: 5, 25, counselling, see dose

Dose: ADULT and CHILD 5–15 tablets before meals

Tablets forte, e/c, s/c, pancreatin, providing minimum of: protease 330 units, lipase 5600 units, amylase 5000 units. Net price 300-tab pack = £13.74. Label: 5, 25, counselling, see dose

Dose: ADULT and CHILD 6–10 tablets before meals

Powder, pancreatin, providing minimum of: protease 1400 units, lipase 25 000 units, amylase

30 000 units/g. Net price 300 g = £24.28. Counselling, see dose

Dose: ADULT and CHILD 0.5–2 g with meals washed down or mixed with liquid; NEONATE 250–500 mg with each feed

■ Higher-strength preparations

The **CSM** has advised of data associating the high-strength pancreatin preparations *Nutrizym 22®* and *Pancreatin HL®* with the development of large bowel strictures (fibrosing colonopathy) in children with cystic fibrosis aged between 2 and 13 years. No association was found with *Creon® 25 000*. The following was recommended:

- *Pancrease HL®*, *Nutrizym 22®*, *Panzytrat® 25 000* [now discontinued] should not be used in children aged 15 years or less with cystic fibrosis;
- the total dose of pancreatic enzyme supplements used in patients with cystic fibrosis should not usually exceed 10 000 units of lipase per kg body-weight daily;
- if a patient on any pancreatin preparation develops new abdominal symptoms (or any change in existing abdominal symptoms) the patient should be reviewed to exclude the possibility of colonic damage.

Possible risk factors are gender (boys at greater risk than girls), more severe cystic fibrosis, and concomitant use of laxatives. The peak age for developing fibrosing colonopathy is between 2 and 8 years.

COUNSELLING. It is important to ensure adequate hydration at all times in patients receiving higher-strength pancreatin preparations.

Creon® 25 000 (Solvay) PoM

Capsules, orange/clear, enclosing brown-coloured e/c pellets of pancreatin, providing: protease (total) 1000 units, lipase 25 000 units, amylase 18 000 units. Net price 100-cap pack = £39.00. Counselling, see above and under dose

Dose: ADULT and CHILD initially 1 capsule with meals either taken whole or contents mixed with fluid or soft food (then swallowed immediately without chewing)

Nutrizym 22® (Merck) PoM

Capsules, red/yellow, enclosing e/c minitablets of pancreatin, providing minimum of: protease 1100 units, lipase 22 000 units, amylase 19 800 units. Net price 100-cap pack = £30.30. Counselling, see above and under dose

Dose: 1–2 capsules with meals and 1 capsule with snacks, swallowed whole or contents taken with water or sprinkled on soft food (then swallowed immediately without chewing)

CHILD under 15 years not recommended

Pancrease HL® (Janssen-Cilag) PoM

Capsules, enclosing light brown e/c minitablets of pancreatin, providing minimum of: protease 1250 units, lipase 25 000 units, amylase 22 500 units. Net price 100 = £36.18. Counselling, see above and under dose

Dose: 1–2 capsules during each meal and 1 capsule with snacks swallowed whole or contents sprinkled on liquid or soft food (then swallowed immediately without chewing)

CHILD under 15 years not recommended

2: Cardiovascular system

2.1 Positive inotropic drugs

2.1.1 Cardiac glycosides
2.1.2 Phosphodiesterase inhibitors

Positive inotropic drugs increase the force of contraction of the myocardium; for sympathomimetics with inotropic activity see section 2.7.1.

2.1.1 Cardiac glycosides

Cardiac glycosides increase the force of myocardial contraction and reduce conductivity within the atrioventricular (AV) node. Digoxin is the most commonly used cardiac glycoside.

Cardiac glycosides are most useful in the treatment of supraventricular tachycardias, especially for controlling ventricular response in persistent atrial fibrillation (section 2.3.1). For reference to the role of digoxin in heart failure, see section 2.5.5.

For management of atrial fibrillation the maintenance dose of the cardiac glycoside can usually be determined by the ventricular rate at rest which should not be allowed to fall below 60 beats per minute except in special circumstances, e.g. with the concomitant administration of a beta-blocker.

When rapid control is desirable, **digoxin** may be given intravenously. However, even with intravenous administration, response may take a number of hours; persistence of tachycardia is therefore not an indication for exceeding the recommended dose. The intramuscular route is **not** recommended.

In patients with mild heart failure a loading dose is not required, and a satisfactory plasma-digoxin concentration can be achieved over a period of about a week, using a dose of digoxin 125 to 250 micrograms twice a day which is then reduced.

Digoxin has a long half-life and maintenance doses need to be given only once daily (although higher doses may be divided to avoid nausea). **Digitoxin** also has a long half-life and maintenance doses need to be given only once daily or on alternate days. Renal function is the most important determinant of digoxin dosage, whereas elimination of digitoxin depends on metabolism by the liver.

Unwanted effects depend both on the concentration of the cardiac glycoside in the plasma and on the sensitivity of the conducting system or of the myocardium, which is often increased in heart disease. Thus plasma concentration alone cannot indicate toxicity reliably but the likelihood of toxicity increases progressively through the range 1.5 to 3 micrograms/litre for digoxin. Cardiac glycosides should be used with special care in the elderly who may be particularly susceptible to digitalis toxicity.

Regular monitoring of plasma-digoxin concentration during maintenance treatment is not necessary unless problems occur. Care should be taken to avoid hypokalaemia if a diuretic is used with a cardiac glycoside because hypokalaemia predisposes the patient to digitalis toxicity. Hypokalaemia is managed by giving a potassium-sparing diuretic or, if necessary, potassium supplements (or foods rich in potassium).

Toxicity can often be managed by discontinuing digoxin and correcting hypokalaemia if appropriate; serious manifestations require urgent specialist management. **Digoxin-specific antibody fragments** are available for reversal of life-threatening overdosage (see below).

CHILDREN. The dose is based on body-weight; they require a relatively larger dose of digoxin than adults.

DIGOXIN

Indications: heart failure, supraventricular arrhythmias (particularly atrial fibrillation)

Cautions: recent infarction; sick sinus syndrome; thyroid disease; reduce dose in the elderly and in renal impairment; avoid hypokalaemia; avoid rapid intravenous administration (nausea and risk of arrhythmias); pregnancy (see also Appendix 4); **interactions:** Appendix 1 (cardiac glycosides)

Contra-indications: intermittent complete heart block, second degree AV block; supraventricular arrhythmias caused by Wolff-Parkinson-White syndrome; hypertrophic obstructive cardiomyopathy (unless concomitant atrial fibrillation and heart failure — but with caution)

Side-effects: usually associated with excessive dosage, include: anorexia, nausea, vomiting, diarrhoea, abdominal pain; visual disturbances, headache, fatigue, drowsiness, confusion, delirium, hallucinations, depression; arrhythmias, heart block; rarely rash, intestinal ischaemia; gynaecomastia on long-term use; thrombocytopenia reported; see also notes above

Dose: *by mouth*, rapid digitalisation, 1–1.5 mg in divided doses over 24 hours; less urgent digitalisation, 250–500 micrograms daily (higher dose may be divided)
Maintenance, 62.5–500 micrograms daily (higher dose may be divided) according to renal function and, in atrial fibrillation, on heart-rate response; usual range, 125–250 micrograms daily (lower dose may be appropriate in elderly)
Emergency loading dose *by intravenous infusion*, 0.75–1 mg over at least 2 hours (see also Cautions)

Note. The above doses may need to be reduced if digoxin (or another cardiac glycoside) has been given in the preceding 2 weeks. Digoxin doses in the BNF may differ from those in product literature. For plasma concentration monitoring, blood should ideally be taken at least 6 hours after a dose

Digoxin (Non-proprietary) PoM
Tablets, digoxin 62.5 micrograms, net price 20 = 54p; 125 micrograms, 20 = 42p; 250 micrograms, 20 = 42p
Injection, digoxin 250 micrograms/mL, net price 2-mL amp = 55p
Available from Antigen
Paediatric injection, digoxin 100 micrograms/mL (hosp. only, available from BCM Specials)

Lanoxin® (GlaxoWellcome) PoM
Tablets, digoxin 125 micrograms, net price 20 = 32p; 250 micrograms (scored), 20 = 32p
Injection, digoxin 250 micrograms/mL. Net price 2-mL amp = 65p

Lanoxin-PG® (GlaxoWellcome) PoM
Tablets, blue, digoxin 62.5 micrograms. Net price 20 = 32p
Elixir, yellow, digoxin 50 micrograms/mL. Do not dilute, measure with pipette. Net price 60 mL = £5.23. Counselling, use of pipette

DIGITOXIN

Indications: heart failure, supraventricular arrhythmias (particularly atrial fibrillation)

Cautions: see under Digoxin but not necessary to reduce dose in mild to moderate renal impairment

Contra-indications: see under Digoxin

Side-effects: see under Digoxin

Dose: maintenance, 100 micrograms daily *or* on alternate days; may be increased to 200 micrograms daily if necessary

Digitoxin (Non-proprietary) PoM
Tablets, digitoxin 100 micrograms, net price 20 = £2.94

Digoxin-specific antibody

Digoxin-specific antibody fragments are indicated for the treatment of known or strongly suspected digoxin or digitoxin overdosage, where measures beyond the withdrawal of the cardiac glycoside and correction of any electrolyte abnormality are felt to be necessary (see also notes above).

Digibind® (GlaxoWellcome) PoM
Injection, powder for preparation of infusion, digoxin-specific antibody fragments (F(ab)) 38 mg. Net price per vial = £83.50 (hosp. and poisons centres only)
Dose: consult product literature

2.1.2 Phosphodiesterase inhibitors

Enoximone and **milrinone** are selective phosphodiesterase inhibitors which exert most of their effect on the myocardium. Sustained haemodynamic benefit has been observed after administration, but there is no evidence of any beneficial effect on survival.

ENOXIMONE

Indications: congestive heart failure where cardiac output reduced and filling pressures increased

Cautions: heart failure associated with hypertrophic cardiomyopathy, stenotic or obstructive valvular disease or other outlet obstruction; monitor blood pressure, heart rate, ECG, central venous pressure, fluid and electrolyte status, renal function, platelet count, hepatic enzymes; renal impairment (Appendix 3); avoid extravasation; pregnancy and breast-feeding

Side-effects: ectopic beats; less frequently ventricular tachycardia or supraventricular arrhythmias (more likely in patients with pre-existing arrhythmias); hypotension; also headache, insomnia, nausea and vomiting, diarrhoea; occasionally, chills, oliguria, fever, urinary retention; upper and lower limb pain

Dose: *by slow intravenous injection* (rate not exceeding 12.5 mg/minute), diluted before use, initially 0.5–1 mg/kg, then 500 micrograms/kg every 30 minutes until satisfactory response or total of 3 mg/kg given; maintenance, initial dose of up to 3 mg/kg may be repeated every 3–6 hours as required

By intravenous infusion, initially 90 micrograms/kg/minute over 10–30 minutes, followed by continuous or intermittent infusion of 5–20 micrograms/kg/minute

Total dose over 24 hours should not usually exceed 24 mg/kg

Perfan® (Aventis Pharma) PoM
Injection, enoximone 5 mg/mL. For dilution before use. Net price 20-mL amp = £15.02
Excipients: include alcohol, propylene glycol
Note. Plastic apparatus should be used; crystal formation if glass used

MILRINONE

Indications: short-term treatment of severe congestive heart failure unresponsive to conventional maintenance therapy (not immediately after myocardial infarction); acute heart failure, including low output states, following heart surgery

Cautions: see under Enoximone; also correct hypokalaemia, monitor renal function

Side-effects: see under Enoximone; also chest pain, tremor, bronchospasm, anaphylaxis and rash reported

Dose: *by intravenous injection* over 10 minutes, diluted before use, 50 micrograms/kg followed by *intravenous infusion* at a rate of 375–750 nanograms/kg/minute, usually for up to 12 hours following surgery or for 48–72 hours in congestive heart failure; max. daily dose 1.13 mg/kg

Primacor® (Sanofi-Synthelabo) PoM
Injection, milrinone (as lactate) 1 mg/mL. For dilution before use. Net price 10-mL amp = £16.61

<table>
<tr><td>**2.2**</td><td>**Diuretics**</td></tr>
<tr><td>2.2.1</td><td>Thiazides and related diuretics</td></tr>
<tr><td>2.2.2</td><td>Loop diuretics</td></tr>
<tr><td>2.2.3</td><td>Potassium-sparing diuretics</td></tr>
<tr><td>2.2.4</td><td>Potassium-sparing diuretics with other diuretics</td></tr>
<tr><td>2.2.5</td><td>Osmotic diuretics</td></tr>
<tr><td>2.2.6</td><td>Mercurial diuretics</td></tr>
<tr><td>2.2.7</td><td>Carbonic anhydrase inhibitors</td></tr>
<tr><td>2.2.8</td><td>Diuretics with potassium</td></tr>
</table>

Thiazides (section 2.2.1) are used to relieve oedema due to chronic heart failure (section 2.5.5) and, in lower doses, to reduce blood pressure.

Loop diuretics (section 2.2.2) are used in pulmonary oedema due to left ventricular failure and in patients with chronic heart failure (section 2.5.5).

Combination diuretic therapy may be effective in patients with oedema resistant to treatment with one diuretic. Vigorous diuresis, particularly with loop diuretics, may induce acute hypotension; rapid reduction of plasma volume should be avoided.

ELDERLY. Lower initial doses of diuretics should be used in the elderly because they are particularly susceptible to the side-effects. The dose should then be adjusted according to renal function. Diuretics should not be used continuously on a long-term basis to treat simple gravitational oedema (which will usually respond to increased movement, raising the legs, and support stockings).

POTASSIUM LOSS. Hypokalaemia may occur with both thiazide and loop diuretics. The risk of hypokalaemia depends on the duration of action as well as the potency and is thus greater with thiazides than with an equipotent dose of a loop diuretic.

Hypokalaemia is dangerous in severe coronary artery disease and in patients also being treated with cardiac glycosides. Often the use of potassium-sparing diuretics (section 2.2.3) avoids the need to take potassium supplements.

In hepatic failure hypokalaemia caused by diuretics can precipitate encephalopathy, particularly in alcoholic cirrhosis; diuretics may also increase the risk of hypomagnesaemia in alcoholic cirrhosis, leading to arrhythmias.

Potassium supplements are seldom necessary when thiazides are used in the routine treatment of hypertension (see also section 9.2.1.1).

2.2.1   Thiazides and related diuretics

Thiazides and related compounds are moderately potent diuretics; they inhibit sodium reabsorption at the beginning of the distal convoluted tubule. They act within 1 to 2 hours of oral administration and most have a duration of action of 12 to 24 hours; they are usually administered early in the day so that the diuresis does not interfere with sleep.

In the management of *hypertension* a low dose of a thiazide, e.g. bendroflumethiazide (bendrofluazide) 2.5 mg daily, produces a maximal or near-maximal blood pressure lowering effect, with very little biochemical disturbance. Higher doses cause more marked changes in plasma potassium, uric acid, glucose, and lipids, with no advantage in blood pressure control, and should not be used. For reference to the use of thiazides in chronic heart failure see section 2.5.5.

Bendroflumethiazide (bendrofluazide) is widely used for mild or moderate heart failure and for hypertension—alone in the treatment of mild hypertension or with other drugs in more severe hypertension.

Chlortalidone (chlorthalidone), a thiazide-related compound, has a longer duration of action than the thiazides and may be given on alternate days to control oedema. It is also useful if acute retention is liable to be precipitated by a more rapid diuresis or if patients dislike the altered pattern of micturition promoted by other diuretics.

Other thiazides and related diuretics (including benzthiazide, clopamide, cyclopenthiazide, hydrochlorothiazide, hydroflumethiazide, and polythiazide) do not offer any significant advantage over those mentioned above, and newer ones are more expensive than the longer-established thiazides.

Metolazone is particularly effective when combined with a loop diuretic (even in renal failure); profound diuresis may occur and the patient should therefore be monitored carefully.

Xipamide and **indapamide** are chemically related to chlortalidone. Indapamide is claimed to lower blood pressure with less metabolic disturbance, particularly less aggravation of diabetes mellitus.

BENDROFLUMETHIAZIDE/ BENDROFLUAZIDE

Indications: oedema, hypertension (see also notes above)

Cautions: may cause hypokalaemia, aggravates diabetes and gout; may exacerbate systemic lupus erythematosus; elderly; pregnancy (Appendix 4) and breast-feeding; hepatic and renal impairment (avoid if severe, see Appendixes 2 and 3); see also notes above; porphyria (section 9.8.2); **interactions:** Appendix 1 (diuretics)

Contra-indications: refractory hypokalaemia, hyponatraemia, hypercalcaemia; severe renal and hepatic impairment; symptomatic hyperuricaemia; Addison's disease

Side-effects: postural hypotension and mild gastro-intestinal effects; impotence (reversible on withdrawal of treatment); hypokalaemia (see also notes above), hypomagnesaemia, hyponatraemia, hypercalcaemia, hypochloraemic alkalosis, hyperuricaemia, gout, hyperglycaemia, and altered plasma lipid concentration; less commonly rashes, photosensitivity; blood disorders (including neutropenia and thrombocytopenia—when given in late pregnancy neonatal thrombocytopenia has been reported); pancreatitis, intrahepatic cholestasis, and hypersensitivity reactions (including pneumonitis, pulmonary oedema, severe skin reactions) also reported

Dose: oedema, initially 5–10 mg in the morning, daily *or* on alternate days; maintenance 5–10 mg 1–3 times weekly

Hypertension, 2.5 mg in the morning; higher doses rarely necessary (see notes above)

Bendroflumethiazide/Bendrofluazide (Non-proprietary) PoM
Tablets, bendroflumethiazide 2.5 mg, net price 20 = 53p; 5 mg, 20 = 52p
Available from Alpharma, APS, Generics, Goldshield (*Neo-NaClex®*, 5 mg only), Hillcross, IVAX, Sovereign (*Aprinox®*)

CHLORTALIDONE
(Chlorthalidone)

Indications: ascites due to cirrhosis in stable patients (under close supervision), oedema due to nephrotic syndrome, hypertension (see also notes above), mild to moderate chronic heart failure; diabetes insipidus (see section 6.5.2)

Cautions: see under Bendroflumethiazide

Contra-indications: see under Bendroflumethiazide

Side-effects: see under Bendroflumethiazide

Dose: oedema, up to 50 mg daily for limited period
Hypertension, 25 mg in the morning, increased to 50 mg if necessary (but see notes above)
Heart failure, 25–50 mg in the morning, increased if necessary to 100–200 mg daily

Hygroton® (Alliance) PoM
Tablets, yellow, scored, chlortalidone 50 mg, net price 28-tab pack = £1.68

CYCLOPENTHIAZIDE

Indications: oedema, hypertension (see also notes above)

Cautions: see under Bendroflumethiazide

Contra-indications: see under Bendroflumethiazide

Side-effects: see under Bendroflumethiazide

Dose: heart failure, 250–500 micrograms daily in the morning increased if necessary to 1 mg daily (reduce to lowest effective dose for maintenance)
Hypertension, initially 250 micrograms daily in the morning, increased if necessary to 500 micrograms daily (but see notes above)
Oedema, up to 500 micrograms daily for a short period

Navidrex® (Goldshield) PoM
Tablets, scored, cyclopenthiazide 500 micrograms. Net price 28-tab pack = £1.27
Excipients: include gluten

INDAPAMIDE

Indications: essential hypertension

Cautions: renal impairment (stop if deterioration); monitor plasma potassium and urate concentrations in elderly, hyperaldosteronism, gout, or with concomitant cardiac glycosides; hyperparathyroidism (discontinue if hypercalcaemia); pregnancy and breast-feeding; **interactions:** Appendix 1 (diuretics)

Contra-indications: recent cerebrovascular accident, severe hepatic impairment

Side-effects: hypokalaemia, headache, dizziness, fatigue, muscular cramps, nausea, anorexia, diarrhoea, constipation, dyspepsia, rashes (erythema multiforme, epidermal necrolysis reported), rarely postural hypotension, palpitations, increase in liver enzymes, blood disorders (including thrombocytopenia), hyponatraemia, metabolic alkalosis, hyperglycaemia, increased plasma urate concentrations, paraesthesia, photosensitivity, impotence, renal impairment, reversible acute myopia; diuresis with doses above 2.5 mg daily

Dose: 2.5 mg in the morning

Indapamide (Non-proprietary) PoM
Tablets, s/c, indapamide 2.5 mg, net price 28-tab pack = £2.81, 56-tab pack = £5.10
Available from Alpharma, APS, Ashbourne (*Nindaxa 2.5®*), Hillcross, IVAX, Sterwin

Natrilix® (Servier) PoM
Tablets, f/c, indapamide 2.5 mg. Net price 30-tab pack = £3.89, 60-tab pack = £7.63

■ Modified release

Natrilix SR® (Servier) [PoM]
Tablets, m/r, indapamide 1.5 mg. Net price 30-tab pack = £4.47. Label: 25
Dose: hypertension, 1 tablet daily, preferably in the morning

METOLAZONE

Indications: oedema, hypertension (see also notes above)
Cautions: see under Bendroflumethiazide; also profound diuresis on concomitant administration with furosemide (monitor patient carefully)
Contra-indications: see under Bendroflumethiazide
Side-effects: see under Bendroflumethiazide
Dose: oedema, 5–10 mg in the morning, increased if necessary to 20 mg daily in resistant oedema, max. 80 mg daily
Hypertension, initially 5 mg in the morning; maintenance 5 mg on alternate days

Metenix 5® (Borg) [PoM]
Tablets, blue, metolazone 5 mg. Net price 100-tab pack = £20.37

POLYTHIAZIDE

Indications: oedema, hypertension (see also notes above)
Cautions: see under Bendroflumethiazide
Contra-indications: see under Bendroflumethiazide
Side-effects: see under Bendroflumethiazide
Dose: usually 1–4 mg daily; in hypertension 500 micrograms daily may be adequate

Nephril® (Pfizer) [PoM]
Tablets, scored, polythiazide 1 mg. Net price 28-tab pack = 79p

XIPAMIDE

Indications: oedema, hypertension (see also notes above)
Cautions: see under Bendroflumethiazide
Contra-indications: see under Bendroflumethiazide
Side-effects: gastro-intestinal disturbances; mild dizziness; hypokalaemia, more rarely other electrolyte disturbances such as hyponatraemia
Dose: oedema, initially 40 mg in the morning, increased to 80 mg in resistant cases; maintenance 20 mg in the morning
Hypertension, 20 mg in the morning

Diurexan® (ASTA Medica) [PoM]
Tablets, scored, xipamide 20 mg. Net price 140-tab pack = £20.92

2.2.2 Loop diuretics

Loop diuretics are used in pulmonary oedema due to left ventricular failure; intravenous administration produces relief of breathlessness and reduces pre-load sooner than would be expected from the time of onset of diuresis. Loop diuretics are also used in patients with chronic heart failure. Diuretic-resistant oedema (except lymphoedema and oedema due to peripheral venous stasis or calcium-channel blockers) can be treated with a loop diuretic combined with a thiazide or related diuretic (e.g. bendroflumethiazide 5–10 mg daily or metolazone 5–20 mg daily).

A loop diuretic is sometimes used to lower blood pressure especially in hypertension resistant to thiazide therapy.

Loop diuretics inhibit reabsorption from the ascending limb of the loop of Henlé in the renal tubule and are powerful diuretics. Hypokalaemia may develop, and care is needed to avoid hypotension. If there is an enlarged prostate, urinary retention may occur; this is less likely if small doses and less potent diuretics are used initially.

Furosemide (frusemide) and **bumetanide** are similar in activity; both act within 1 hour of oral administration and diuresis is complete within 6 hours so that, if necessary, they can be given twice in one day without interfering with sleep. Following intravenous administration they have a peak effect within 30 minutes. The diuresis associated with these drugs is dose related. In patients with impaired renal function very large doses may occasionally be needed; in such doses both drugs can cause deafness and bumetanide can cause myalgia.

Torasemide has properties similar to those of furosemide and bumetanide, and is indicated for oedema and for hypertension.

FUROSEMIDE/FRUSEMIDE

Indications: oedema, oliguria due to renal failure
Cautions: pregnancy and breast-feeding; hypotension; correct hypovolaemia before using in oliguria; liver failure, prostatic enlargement; porphyria (section 9.8.2); although manufacturer advises that rate of intravenous administration should not exceed 4 mg/minute, single doses of up to 50 mg may be administered more rapidly; **interactions:** Appendix 1 (diuretics)
Contra-indications: precomatose states associated with liver cirrhosis; renal failure with anuria
Side-effects: hyponatraemia, hypokalaemia, and hypomagnesaemia (see also section 2.2), hypochloraemic alkalosis, increased calcium excretion, hypotension; less commonly nausea, gastro-intestinal disturbances, hyperuricaemia and gout; hyperglycaemia (less common than with thiazides); temporary increase in plasma cholesterol and triglyceride concentrations; rarely rashes, photosensitivity and bone marrow depression (withdraw treatment), pancreatitis (with large parenteral doses), tinnitus and deafness (usually with large parenteral doses and rapid administration and in renal impairment)
Dose: *by mouth*, oedema, initially 40 mg in the morning; maintenance 20 mg daily *or* 40 mg on alternate days, increased in resistant oedema to 80 mg daily or more; CHILD 1–3 mg/kg daily, max. 40 mg daily
Oliguria, initially 250 mg daily; if necessary larger doses, increasing in steps of 250 mg, may be given every 4–6 hours to a max. of a single dose of 2 g (rarely used)
By intramuscular injection or slow intravenous injection (see Cautions, above), initially 20–50 mg; CHILD 0.5–1.5 mg/kg to a max. daily dose of 20 mg

By intravenous infusion (by syringe pump if necessary), in oliguria, initially 250 mg over 1 hour (rate not exceeding 4 mg/minute), if satisfactory urine output not obtained in the subsequent hour further 500 mg over 2 hours, then if no satisfactory response within subsequent hour, further 1 g over 4 hours, if no response obtained dialysis probably required; effective dose (up to 1 g) can be repeated every 24 hours

Furosemide/Frusemide (Non-proprietary) [PoM]
Tablets, furosemide 20 mg, net price 20 = 35p; 40 mg, 28-tab pack = 78p; 500 mg, 20 = £6.44
Various strengths available from Alpharma, APS, Ashbourne (*Froop®*), CP (including *Rusyde®*), Generics, Hillcross, IVAX, Sovereign
Oral solution, sugar-free, furosemide, net price 4 mg/mL, 150 mL = £12.84; 8 mg/mL, 150 mL = £16.57; 10 mg/mL, 150 mL = £17.91
Available from Rosemont (*Frusol®*)
Injection, furosemide 10 mg/mL, net price 2-mL amp = 52p
Available from Antigen, Celltech, Phoenix (all also 5-mL amp)

Lasix® (Borg) [PoM]
Tablets, all scored, furosemide 20 mg, net price 28-tab pack = £1.57; 40 mg, 28-tab pack = £2.27; 500 mg (yellow), 20 = £21.74
Paediatric liquid, sugar-free, furosemide 1 mg/mL when reconstituted with purified water, freshly boiled and cooled, net price 150 mL = £3.68
Injection, furosemide 10 mg/mL, net price 2-mL amp = 84p
Note. Large volume furosemide injections available from Antigen, Medeva (*Min-I-Jet®*)

BUMETANIDE

Indications: oedema, oliguria due to renal failure
Cautions: see under Furosemide (but has been used in porphyria, see section 9.8.2)
Contra-indications: see under Furosemide
Side-effects: see under Furosemide; also myalgia
Dose: *by mouth*, 1 mg in the morning, repeated after 6–8 hours if necessary; severe cases, increased up to 5 mg or more daily
ELDERLY, 500 micrograms daily may be sufficient
By intravenous injection, 1–2 mg, repeated after 20 minutes; when *intramuscular injection* considered necessary, 1 mg initially then adjusted according to response
By intravenous infusion, 2–5 mg over 30–60 minutes

Bumetanide (Non-proprietary) [PoM]
Tablets, bumetanide 1 mg, net price 28-tab pack = £1.69; 5 mg, 28-tab pack = £11.15
Available from Alpharma, APS, Bioglan, CP, Generics, Hillcross, IVAX
Liquid, bumetanide 1 mg/5 mL, net price 150 mL = £3.17
Available from Leo
Injection, bumetanide 500 micrograms/mL, net price 4-mL amp = 66p
Available from Leo

Burinex® (Leo) [PoM]
Tablets, both scored, bumetanide 1 mg, net price 28-tab pack = £1.64; 5 mg, 28 = £10.45

TORASEMIDE

Indications: oedema, hypertension
Cautions: see under Furosemide
Contra-indications: see under Furosemide; pregnancy and breast-feeding
Side-effects: see under Furosemide; also dry mouth; rarely limb paraesthesia
Dose: oedema, 5 mg once daily, preferably in the morning, increased if required to 20 mg once daily; usual max. 40 mg daily
Hypertension, 2.5 mg daily, increased if necessary to 5 mg once daily

Torem® (Roche) [PoM]
Tablets, torasemide 2.5 mg, net price 28-tab pack = £4.06; 5 mg (scored), 28-tab pack = £5.95; 10 mg (scored), 28-tab pack = £8.75

2.2.3 Potassium-sparing diuretics

Amiloride and **triamterene** on their own are weak diuretics. They cause retention of potassium and are therefore used as a more effective alternative to giving potassium supplements with thiazide or loop diuretics. (See section 2.2.4 for compound preparations with thiazides or loop diuretics.)

Spironolactone is also a potassium-sparing diuretic, and potentiates thiazide or loop diuretics by antagonising aldosterone. It is of value in the treatment of the oedema of cirrhosis of the liver. Low doses of spironolactone are beneficial in severe heart failure, see section 2.5.5.

Spironolactone is also used in primary hyperaldosteronism (Conn's syndrome). It is given before surgery or if surgery is not appropriate, in the lowest effective dose for maintenance.

Potassium supplements must **not** be given with potassium-sparing diuretics. It is also important to bear in mind that administration of a potassium-sparing diuretic to a patient receiving an ACE inhibitor can cause severe hyperkalaemia.

AMILORIDE HYDROCHLORIDE

Indications: oedema, potassium conservation with thiazide and loop diuretics
Cautions: pregnancy and breast-feeding; monitor in renal impairment (avoid if moderate to severe, see also Appendix 3); diabetes mellitus; elderly; **interactions:** Appendix 1 (diuretics)
Contra-indications: hyperkalaemia, renal failure
Side-effects: include gastro-intestinal disturbances, dry mouth, rashes, confusion, postural hypotension, hyperkalaemia, hyponatraemia
Dose: used alone, initially 10 mg daily *or* 5 mg twice daily, adjusted according to response; max. 20 mg daily
With other diuretics, congestive heart failure and hypertension, initially 5–10 mg daily; cirrhosis with ascites, initially 5 mg daily

Amiloride (Non-proprietary) [PoM]
Tablets, amiloride hydrochloride 5 mg, net price 20 = £1.04
Available from Alpharma, APS, CP, Hillcross, IVAX

Oral solution, sugar-free, amiloride hydrochloride 5 mg/5 mL, net price 150 mL = £39.73
Available from Rosemont (*Amilamont®*)

■ Compound preparations with thiazide or loop diuretics, see section 2.2.4

TRIAMTERENE

Indications: oedema, potassium conservation with thiazide and loop diuretics

Cautions: see under Amiloride Hydrochloride; may cause blue fluorescence of urine

Contra-indications: see under Amiloride Hydrochloride

Side-effects: include gastro-intestinal disturbances, dry mouth, rashes; slight decrease in blood pressure, hyperkalaemia, hyponatraemia; photosensitivity and blood disorders also reported; triamterene found in kidney stones

Dose: initially 150–250 mg daily, reducing to alternate days after 1 week; taken in divided doses after breakfast and lunch; lower initial dose when given with other diuretics

COUNSELLING. Urine may look slightly blue in some lights

Dytac® (Goldshield) [PoM]
Capsules, maroon, triamterene 50 mg. Net price 30-cap pack = £16.90. Label: 14 (see above), 21

■ Compound preparations with thiazides or loop diuretics, see section 2.2.4

Aldosterone antagonists

SPIRONOLACTONE

Indications: oedema and ascites in cirrhosis of the liver, malignant ascites, nephrotic syndrome, congestive heart failure (section 2.5.5); primary hyperaldosteronism

Cautions: potential metabolic products carcinogenic in *rodents*; elderly; hepatic impairment; renal impairment (avoid if moderate to severe; Appendix 3); monitor electrolytes (discontinue if hyperkalaemia); porphyria (section 9.8.2); **interactions:** Appendix 1 (diuretics)

Contra-indications: hyperkalaemia, hyponatraemia; pregnancy and breast-feeding; Addison's disease

Side-effects: gastro-intestinal disturbances; impotence, gynaecomastia; menstrual irregularities; lethargy, headache, confusion; rashes; hyperkalaemia (discontinue); hyponatraemia; hepatotoxicity, osteomalacia, and blood disorders reported

Dose: 100–200 mg daily, increased to 400 mg if required; CHILD initially 3 mg/kg daily in divided doses
Heart failure, see section 2.5.5

Spironolactone (Non-proprietary) [PoM]
Tablets, spironolactone 25 mg, net price 20 = £1.50; 50 mg, 20 = £3.21; 100 mg, 20 = £3.31
Available from Alpharma, APS, Ashbourne (*Spirospare®*), Hillcross, IVAX
Oral suspensions, sugar-free, spironolactone 5 mg/5 ml, 10 mg/5 ml, 25 mg/5 ml, 50 mg/5 ml and 100 mg/5 mL available from Rosemont (special order)

Aldactone® (Searle) [PoM]
Tablets, all f/c, spironolactone 25 mg (buff), net price 100-tab pack = £9.88; 50 mg (off-white), 100-tab pack = £19.76; 100 mg (buff), 28-tab pack = £11.07

■ With thiazides or loop diuretics, see section 2.2.4

<table>
<tr><td>**2.2.4**</td><td>**Potassium-sparing diuretics with other diuretics**</td></tr>
</table>

Although it is preferable to prescribe thiazides (section 2.2.1) and potassium-sparing diuretics (section 2.2.3) separately, the use of fixed combinations may be justified if compliance is a problem. Potassium-sparing diuretics are not usually necessary in the routine treatment of hypertension, unless hypokalaemia develops. For **interactions**, see Appendix 1 (diuretics).

■ Amiloride with thiazides

Co-amilozide (Non-proprietary) [PoM]
Tablets, co-amilozide 2.5/25 (amiloride hydrochloride 2.5 mg, hydrochlorothiazide 25 mg), net price 28-tab pack = £1.85
Available from CP, Du Pont (*Moduret 25®*)
Dose: hypertension, initially 1 tablet daily, increased if necessary to max. 2 tablets daily
Congestive heart failure, initially 1 tablet daily, increased if necessary to max. 4 tablets daily
Oedema and ascites in cirrhosis of the liver, initially 2 tablets daily, increased if necessary to max. 4 tablets daily; reduce for maintenance if possible
Tablets, co-amilozide 5/50 (amiloride hydrochloride 5 mg, hydrochlorothiazide 50 mg), net price 28 = £1.99
Available from Alpharma, APS, Ashbourne (*Amilmaxco 5/50®*), CP, Du Pont (*Moduretic®*), Hillcross, IVAX (*Amil-Co®*)
Dose: hypertension, initially ½ tablet daily, increased if necessary to max. 1 tablet daily
Congestive heart failure, initially ½ tablet daily, increased if necessary to max. 2 tablets daily
Oedema and ascites in cirrhosis of the liver, initially 1 tablet daily, increased if necessary to max. 2 tablets daily; reduce for maintenance if possible

Navispare® (Novartis) [PoM]
Tablets, f/c, orange, amiloride hydrochloride 2.5 mg, cyclopenthiazide 250 micrograms. Net price 28-tab pack = £2.25
Excipients: include gluten
Dose: hypertension, 1–2 tablets in the morning

■ Amiloride with loop diuretics

Co-amilofruse (Non-proprietary) [PoM]
Tablets, co-amilofruse 2.5/20 (amiloride hydrochloride 2.5 mg, furosemide 20 mg). Net price 28-tab pack = £4.66, 56-tab pack = £9.49
Available from Alpharma, CP, Helios (*Frumil LS®*), Hillcross, Lagap
Dose: oedema, 1 tablet in the morning

Tablets, co-amilofruse 5/40 (amiloride hydrochloride 5 mg, furosemide 40 mg). Net price 28-
tab pack = £2.58

Available from Alpharma, APS, Ashbourne (*Froop-Co®*),
Borg (*Lasoride®*), CP, Helios (*Frumil®*), Hillcross,
IVAX (*Fru-Co®*), Lagap, Sovereign

Dose: oedema, 1–2 tablets in the morning

Tablets, co-amilofruse 10/80 (amiloride hydrochloride 10 mg, furosemide 80 mg). Net price 28-
tab pack = £7.54, 56-tab pack = £15.08

Available from CP (*Aridil®*), Helios (*Frumil Forte®*)

Dose: oedema, 1 tablet in the morning

Burinex A® (Leo) PoM

Tablets, ivory, scored, amiloride hydrochloride
5 mg, bumetanide 1 mg. Net price 28-tab pack =
£3.06

Dose: oedema, 1–2 tablets daily

■ Triamterene with thiazides

COUNSELLING. Urine may look slightly blue in some lights

Co-triamterzide (Non-proprietary) PoM

Tablets, co-triamterzide 50/25 (triamterene 50 mg,
hydrochlorothiazide 25 mg), net price 30-tab pack
= £1.69. Label: 14 (see above), 21

Dose: hypertension, 1 tablet daily after breakfast,
increased if necessary, max. 4 daily
Oedema, 2 tablets daily (1 after breakfast and 1 after
midday meal) increased to 3 daily if necessary (2 after
breakfast and 1 after midday meal); usual maintenance
in oedema, 1 daily or 2 on alternate days; max. 4 daily

Available from Ashbourne (*TriamaxCo®*), IVAX
(*Triam-Co®*)

Dyazide® (Goldshield) PoM

Tablets, peach, scored, co-triamterzide 50/25
(triamterene 50 mg, hydrochlorothiazide 25 mg).
Net price 30-tab pack = £2.41. Label: 14 (see
above), 21

Dose: hypertension, 1 tablet daily after breakfast,
increased if necessary, max. 4 daily
Oedema, 2 tablets daily (1 after breakfast and 1 after
midday meal) increased to 3 daily if necessary (2 after
breakfast and 1 after midday meal); usual maintenance
in oedema, 1 daily or 2 on alternate days; max. 4 daily

Dytide® (Goldshield) PoM

Capsules, clear/maroon, triamterene 50 mg, benzthiazide 25 mg. Net price 30-cap pack = £16.90.
Label: 14 (see above), 21

Dose: oedema, initially 3 capsules daily (2 after breakfast and 1 after midday meal) for 1 week then 1 or 2 on
alternate days

Kalspare® (Dominion) PoM

Tablets, orange, f/c, scored, triamterene 50 mg,
chlortalidone 50 mg. Net price 28-tab pack =
£3.05. Label: 14 (see above), 21

Dose: hypertension, oedema, 1–2 tablets in the morning

■ Triamterene with loop diuretics

COUNSELLING. Urine may look slightly blue in some lights

Frusene® (Orion) PoM

Tablets, yellow, scored, triamterene 50 mg, furosemide 40 mg. Net price 56-tab pack = £5.67.
Label: 14 (see above), 21

Dose: oedema, ½–2 tablets daily in the morning

■ Spironolactone with thiazides

Co-flumactone (Non-proprietary) PoM ▭

Tablets, co-flumactone 25/25 (hydroflumethiazide
25 mg, spironolactone 25 mg). Net price 100-tab
pack = £16.86

Available from Searle (*Aldactide 25®*)

Dose: congestive heart failure, initially 4 tablets daily;
range 1–8 daily (but not recommended because spironolactone generally given in lower dose)

Tablets, co-flumactone 50/50 (hydroflumethiazide
50 mg, spironolactone 50 mg). Net price 28-tab
pack = £8.92

Available from Searle (*Aldactide 50®*)

Dose: congestive heart failure, initially 2 tablets daily;
range 1–4 daily (but not recommended because spironolactone generally given in lower dose)

■ Spironolactone with loop diuretics

Lasilactone® (Borg) PoM

Capsules, blue/white, spironolactone 50 mg, furosemide 20 mg. Net price 28-cap pack = £8.91

Dose: resistant oedema, 1–4 capsules daily

2.2.5 Osmotic diuretics

Osmotic diuretics are rarely used in heart failure as
they may acutely expand the blood volume. **Mannitol** is used in cerebral oedema—a typical dose is
1 g/kg as a 20% solution given by rapid intravenous
infusion.

MANNITOL

Indications: see notes above; glaucoma (section
11.6)

Cautions: extravasation causes inflammation and
thrombophlebitis

Contra-indications: congestive cardiac failure,
pulmonary oedema

Side-effects: chills, fever

Dose: *by intravenous infusion*, diuresis, 50–200 g
over 24 hours, preceded by a test dose of 200 mg/
kg by slow intravenous injection
Cerebral oedema, see notes above

Mannitol (Non-proprietary) PoM
Intravenous infusion, mannitol 10% and 20%
Available from Baxter

2.2.6 Mercurial diuretics

Mercurial diuretics are effective but are now almost
never used because of their nephrotoxicity.

2.2.7 Carbonic anhydrase inhibitors

The carbonic anhydrase inhibitor **acetazolamide** is
a weak diuretic and is little used for its diuretic
effect. It is used for prophylaxis against mountain
sickness [unlicensed indication] but is not a substitute for acclimatisation.

Acetazolamide and eye drops of dorzolamide and
brinzolamide inhibit the formation of aqueous
humour and are used in glaucoma (section 11.6)

Diuretics with potassium

Many patients on diuretics do not need potassium supplements (section 9.2.1.1). For many of those who do, the amount of potassium in combined preparations may not be enough, and for this reason their use is to be discouraged.

Diuretics with potassium and potassium-sparing diuretics should **not** usually be given together.

COUNSELLING. Modified-release potassium tablets should be swallowed whole with plenty of fluid during meals while sitting or standing

Burinex K® (Leo) [PoM] [image]
Tablets, bumetanide 500 micrograms, potassium 7.7 mmol for modified release. Net price 20 = 81p. Label: 25, 27, counselling, see above

Centyl K® (Leo) [PoM] [image]
Tablets, green, s/c, bendroflumethiazide 2.5 mg, potassium 7.7 mmol for modified release, net price 56-tab pack = £5.44. Label: 25, 27, counselling, see above

Diumide-K Continus® (ASTA Medica) [PoM] [image]
Tablets, f/c, white/orange, furosemide 40 mg, potassium 8 mmol for modified release. Net price 30-tab pack = £2.99. Label: 25, 27, counselling, see above

Lasikal® (Borg) [PoM] [image]
Tablets, white/yellow, f/c, furosemide 20 mg, potassium 10 mmol for modified release. Net price 100-tab pack = £15.21. Label: 25, 27, counselling, see above

Neo-NaClex-K® (Goldshield) [PoM] [image]
Tablets, pink/white, f/c, bendroflumethiazide 2.5 mg, potassium 8.4 mmol for modified release. Net price 20 = £1.59. Label: 25, 27, counselling, see above

[image] denotes preparations that are considered to be less suitable for prescribing (see p. vi)

2.3 Anti-arrhythmic drugs

2.3.1 Management of arrhythmias
2.3.2 Drugs for arrhythmias

2.3.1 Management of arrhythmias

Management of an arrhythmia requires precise diagnosis of the type of arrhythmia, and electrocardiography is essential; underlying causes such as heart failure require appropriate treatment.

ECTOPIC BEATS. If spontaneous with a normal heart, ectopic beats rarely require treatment beyond reassurance. If they are particularly troublesome, beta-blockers are sometimes effective and may be safer than other suppressant drugs.

ATRIAL FIBRILLATION. The ventricular rate at rest can usually be controlled with digoxin. If adequate control at rest or during exercise cannot be achieved readily, a beta-blocker or verapamil may be added; care is needed in the presence of diminished ventricular function. In some cases other classes of drugs may be appropriate. Anticoagulants are indicated especially in valvular or myocardial disease, and in the elderly; in the very elderly the overall benefit and risk needs careful assessment. Younger patients with lone atrial fibrillation in the absence of heart disease probably do not need anticoagulation. Aspirin is less effective than warfarin at preventing emboli but may be appropriate if there are no other risk factors for stroke. Doses of aspirin within the range 75–300 mg daily are used.

ATRIAL FLUTTER. The ventricular rate at rest can sometimes be controlled with digoxin. Reversion to sinus rhythm (if indicated) may be achieved by appropriately synchronised d.c. shock. Alternatively, amiodarone may be used to restore sinus rhythm, and amiodarone or sotalol to maintain it. If the arrhythmia is long-standing a period of treatment with anticoagulants should be considered before cardioversion to avoid the complication of emboli.

PAROXYSMAL SUPRAVENTRICULAR TACHYCARDIA. In most patients this remits spontaneously or can be returned to sinus rhythm by reflex vagal stimulation with respiratory manoeuvres, prompt squatting, or pressure over one carotid sinus (**important:** pressure over carotid sinus should be restricted to monitored patients—it can be dangerous in recent ischaemia, digitalis toxicity, or the elderly).

If vagal stimulation fails, intravenous administration of adenosine is usually the treatment of choice. Intravenous administration of verapamil is useful for patients without myocardial or valvular disease (**important:** never in patients recently treated with beta-blockers, see p. 107). For arrhythmias that are poorly tolerated, synchronised d.c. shock usually provides rapid relief.

In cases of paroxysmal supraventricular tachycardia with block, digitalis toxicity should be suspected. In addition to stopping administration of the cardiac glycoside and giving potassium supplements, intravenous administration of a beta-blocker may be useful. Specific digoxin antibody is available if the toxicity is considered life-threatening (section 2.1.1).

ARRHYTHMIAS AFTER MYOCARDIAL INFARCTION. In patients with a paroxysmal tachycardia or rapid irregularity of the pulse it is best not to administer an antiarrhythmic until an ECG record has been obtained. Bradycardia, particularly if complicated by hypotension, should be treated with atropine sulphate, given intravenously in a dose of 0.3–1 mg. If the initial dose is effective it may be repeated if necessary.

VENTRICULAR TACHYCARDIA. Drug treatment is used both for the treatment of ventricular tachycardia and for prophylaxis of recurrent attacks that merit suppression. Ventricular tachycardia requires treatment most commonly in the acute stage of myocardial infarction, but the likelihood of this and other life-threatening arrhythmias diminishes sharply over the first 24 hours after the attack, especially in patients without heart failure or shock. Lidocaine (lignocaine) is the preferred drug for emergency use. Other drugs are best administered under specialist supervision. Very rapid ventricular tachycardia causes profound circulatory collapse and should be treated urgently with d.c. shock.

Torsades de pointes is a special form of ventricular tachycardia which tends to occur in the presence of a long QT interval (usually drug induced, but other factors including hypokalaemia, severe bradycardia, and genetic predisposition may also be implicated). The episodes are usually self-limiting, but are frequently recurrent and may cause impairment (or loss) of consciousness. If not controlled, the arrhythmia may progress to ventricular fibrillation. Intravenous infusion of magnesium sulphate (section 9.5.1.3) is usually effective. A beta-blocker (but not sotalol) and atrial (or ventricular) pacing may be considered. Anti-arrhythmics (including lidocaine) may further prolong the QT interval, thus worsening the condition.

2.3.2   Drugs for arrhythmias

Anti-arrhythmic drugs can be classified clinically into those that act on supraventricular arrhythmias (e.g. verapamil), those that act on both supraventricular and ventricular arrhythmias (e.g. disopyramide), and those that act on ventricular arrhythmias (e.g. lidocaine (lignocaine)).

They can also be classified according to their effects on the electrical behaviour of myocardial cells during activity:

Class Ia, b, c: membrane stabilising drugs (e.g. quinidine, lidocaine, flecainide respectively)
Class II: beta-blockers
Class III: amiodarone, bretylium, and sotalol (also Class II)
Class IV: calcium-channel blockers (includes verapamil but not dihydropyridines)

This latter classification (the Vaughan Williams classification) is of less clinical significance.

CAUTIONS. The negative inotropic effects of anti-arrhythmic drugs tend to be additive. Therefore special care should be taken if two or more are used, especially if myocardial function is impaired. Most or all drugs that are effective in countering arrhythmias can also provoke them in some circumstances; moreover, hypokalaemia enhances the arrhythmogenic (pro-arrhythmic) effect of many drugs.

Supraventricular arrhythmias

Adenosine is usually the treatment of choice for terminating paroxysmal supraventricular tachycardia. As it has a very short duration of action (half-life only about 8 to 10 seconds, but prolonged in those taking dipyridamole), most side-effects are short lived. Unlike verapamil, adenosine may be used after a beta-blocker. Verapamil may be preferable to adenosine in asthma.

Oral administration of a **cardiac glycoside** (such as digoxin, section 2.1.1) is the treatment of choice in slowing ventricular response in cases of atrial fibrillation and atrial flutter. Intravenous digoxin,

preferably infused slowly, is occasionally required if the ventricular rate needs rapid control. Cardiac glycosides are contra-indicated in supraventricular arrhythmias associated with Wolff-Parkinson-White syndrome.

Verapamil (section 2.6.2) is usually effective for supraventricular tachycardias. An initial intravenous dose (**important**: serious beta-blocker interaction hazard, see p. 107) may be followed by oral treatment; hypotension may occur with larger doses. It should not be used for tachyarrhythmias where the QRS complex is wide (i.e. broad complex) unless a supraventricular origin has been established beyond reasonable doubt. It is also contra-indicated in atrial fibrillation with pre-excitation (e.g. Wolff-Parkinson-White syndrome). It should not be used in children with arrhythmias without specialist advice; some supraventricular arrhythmias in childhood can be accelerated by verapamil with dangerous consequences.

Intravenous administration of a **beta-blocker** (section 2.4) such as esmolol or propranolol, can achieve rapid control of the ventricular rate.

Drugs for both supraventricular and ventricular arrhythmias include **amiodarone**, **beta-blockers**, **disopyramide**, **flecainide**, **procainamide**, **propafenone** and **quinidine**, see below under Supraventricular and Ventricular Arrhythmias.

ADENOSINE

Indications: rapid reversion to sinus rhythm of paroxysmal supraventricular tachycardias, including those associated with accessory pathways (e.g. Wolff-Parkinson-White syndrome); aid to diagnosis of broad or narrow complex supraventricular tachycardias

Cautions: atrial fibrillation or flutter with accessory pathway (conduction down anomalous pathway may increase); heart transplant (see below); **interactions:** Appendix 1 (adenosine)

Contra-indications: second- or third-degree AV block and sick sinus syndrome (unless pacemaker fitted); asthma

Side-effects: include transient facial flush, chest pain, dyspnoea, bronchospasm, choking sensation, nausea, light-headedness; severe bradycardia reported (requiring temporary pacing); ECG may show transient rhythm disturbances

Dose: *by rapid intravenous injection* into central or large peripheral vein, 3 mg over 2 seconds with cardiac monitoring; if necessary followed by 6 mg after 1–2 minutes, and then by 12 mg after a further 1–2 minutes; increments should not be given if high level AV block develops at any particular dose

Note. 3-mg dose ineffective in a number of patients, therefore higher initial dose sometimes used but patients with *heart transplant* are **very** sensitive to effects of adenosine, and should **not** receive higher initial dose. Also if essential to give with dipyridamole reduce initial dose to 0.5–1 mg

Adenocor® (Sanofi-Synthelabo) PoM
Injection, adenosine 3 mg/mL in physiological saline. Net price 2-mL vial = £4.05 (hosp. only)
Note. Intravenous infusion of adenosine (*Adenoscan®*, Sanofi Winthrop) may be used in conjunction with radionuclide myocardial perfusion imaging in patients who cannot exercise adequately or for whom exercise is inappropriate—consult product literature

Supraventricular and ventricular arrhythmias

Amiodarone is used in the treatment of arrhythmias particularly when other drugs are ineffective or contra-indicated. It may be used for paroxysmal supraventricular, nodal and ventricular tachycardias, atrial fibrillation and flutter, and ventricular fibrillation. It should be initiated only under hospital or specialist supervision. Amiodarone may be given by intravenous infusion as well as by mouth, and has the advantage of causing little or no myocardial depression. Unlike oral amiodarone, intravenous amiodarone may act relatively rapidly.

Intravenous injection of amiodarone may be used in cardiopulmonary resuscitation for ventricular fibrillation or pulseless tachycardia unresponsive to other interventions (section 2.7.3).

Amiodarone has a very long half-life (extending to several weeks) and only needs to be given once daily (but high doses may cause nausea unless divided). Many weeks or months may be required to achieve steady-state plasma-amiodarone concentration; this is particularly important when drug interactions are likely (see also Appendix 1).

Most patients taking amiodarone develop corneal microdeposits (reversible on withdrawal of treatment); these rarely interfere with vision, but drivers may be dazzled by headlights at night. Because of the possibility of phototoxic reactions, patients should be advised to shield the skin from light and to use a wide-spectrum sunscreen (section 13.8.1) to protect against both long ultraviolet and visible light.

Amiodarone contains iodine and can cause disorders of thyroid function; both hypothyroidism and hyperthyroidism may occur. Clinical assessment alone is unreliable, and laboratory tests should be performed before treatment and every 6 months. Thyroxine (T4) may be raised in the absence of hyperthyroidism; therefore tri-iodothyronine (T3), T4, and thyroid-stimulating hormone (thyrotrophin, TSH) should all be measured. A raised T3 and T4 with a very low or undetectable TSH concentration suggests the development of thyrotoxicosis. The thyrotoxicosis may be very refractory, and amiodarone should usually be withdrawn at least temporarily to help achieve control; treatment with carbimazole may be required. Hypothyroidism can be treated with replacement therapy without withdrawing amiodarone if it is essential.

Pneumonitis should always be suspected if new or progressive shortness of breath or cough develops in a patient taking amiodarone. Fresh neurological symptoms should raise the possibility of peripheral neuropathy.

Amiodarone is also associated with hepatotoxicity and treatment should be discontinued if severe liver function abnormalities or clinical signs of liver disease develop.

Beta-blockers act as anti-arrhythmic drugs principally by attenuating the effects of the sympathetic system on automaticity and conductivity within the heart, for details see section 2.4. For special reference to the role of **sotalol** in ventricular arrhythmias, see also p. 77.

Disopyramide may be given by intravenous injection to control arrhythmias after myocardial infarction (including those not responding to lidocaine (lignocaine)), but it impairs cardiac contractility. Oral administration of disopyramide is useful but it has an antimuscarinic effect which limits its use in patients with glaucoma or prostatic hypertrophy.

Flecainide belongs to the same general class as lidocaine. It may be of value in serious symptomatic ventricular arrhythmias. It may also be indicated for junctional re-entry tachycardias and for paroxysmal atrial fibrillation. As with quinidine it may precipitate serious arrhythmias in a small minority of patients (including those with otherwise normal hearts).

Procainamide is given by intravenous injection to control ventricular arrhythmias.

Propafenone is used for the prophylaxis and treatment of ventricular arrhythmias and also for some supraventricular arrhythmias. It has complex mechanisms of action, including weak beta-blocking activity (therefore caution is needed in obstructive airways disease—contra-indicated if severe).

Quinidine may be effective in suppressing supraventricular and ventricular arrhythmias. It may itself precipitate rhythm disorders, and is best used on specialist advice; it can cause hypersensitivity reactions and gastro-intestinal upsets.

Drugs for supraventricular arrhythmias include **adenosine**, **cardiac glycosides** and **verapamil**, see above under Supraventricular Arrhythmias. Drugs for ventricular arrhythmias include **bretylium**, **lidocaine**, **mexiletine**, and **phenytoin**, see below under Ventricular Arrhythmias.

AMIODARONE HYDROCHLORIDE

Indications: see notes above (should be initiated in hospital or under specialist supervision)

Cautions: liver-function and thyroid-function tests required before treatment and then every 6 months (see notes above for tests of thyroid function); chest x-ray required before treatment; heart failure; renal impairment; elderly; severe bradycardia and conduction disturbances in excessive dosage; intravenous use may cause moderate and transient fall in blood pressure (circulatory collapse precipitated by rapid administration or overdosage); porphyria (section 9.8.2); **interactions:** Appendix 1 (amiodarone)

Contra-indications: sinus bradycardia, sino-atrial heart block; unless pacemaker fitted avoid in severe conduction disturbances or sinus node disease; history of thyroid dysfunction; pregnancy and breast-feeding (see also Appendixes 4 and 5); iodine sensitivity; avoid *intravenous use* in severe respiratory failure, circulatory collapse, severe arterial hypotension; avoid bolus injection in congestive heart failure or cardiomyopathy

Side-effects: reversible corneal microdeposits (sometimes with night glare), rarely impaired vision due to optic neuritis; peripheral neuropathy and myopathy (usually reversible on withdrawal); bradycardia and conduction disturbances (see Cautions); phototoxicity and rarely persistent slate-grey skin discoloration (see also notes); hypothyroidism, hyperthyroidism, diffuse pulmonary alveolitis, pneumonitis, and fibrosis; raised serum transaminases (may require dose reduction or withdrawal if accompanied by acute liver disorders); jaundice, hepatitis and cirrhosis reported; rarely nausea, vomiting, metallic taste, tremor, hot flushes, sweating, nightmares, vertigo, headache, sleeplessness, fatigue, alopecia, paraesthesia, benign raised intracranial pressure, impotence, epididymo-orchitis; ataxia, rashes (including exfoliative dermatitis), hypersensitivity including vasculitis, renal involvement and thrombocytopenia; haemolytic or aplastic anaemia; anaphylaxis on rapid injection, also bronchospasm or apnoea in respiratory failure

Dose: *by mouth*, 200 mg 3 times daily for 1 week reduced to 200 mg twice daily for a further week; maintenance, usually 200 mg daily or the minimum required to control the arrhythmia

By intravenous infusion via caval catheter, 5 mg/kg over 20–120 minutes with ECG monitoring; max. 1.2 g in 24 hours

Ventricular fibrillation or pulseless ventricular tachycardia, *by intravenous injection* over at least 3 minutes, 300 mg (section 2.7.3)

Amiodarone (Non-proprietary) PoM
Tablets, amiodarone hydrochloride 100 mg, net price 28-tab pack = £4.27; 200 mg, 28-tab pack = £6.45. Label: 11
Available from Alpharma, APS, Generics, Hillcross, IVAX, Sterwin
Injection, amiodarone hydrochloride 30 mg/mL, net price 10-mL prefilled syringe = £10.00
Available from Aurum

Cordarone X® (Sanofi-Synthelabo) PoM
Tablets, both scored, amiodarone hydrochloride 100 mg, net price 28-tab pack = £4.78; 200 mg, 28-tab pack = £7.82. Label: 11
Injection, amiodarone hydrochloride 50 mg/mL. Net price 3-mL amp = £1.43. For dilution and use as an infusion

DISOPYRAMIDE

Indications: ventricular arrhythmias, especially after myocardial infarction; supraventricular arrhythmias

Cautions: discontinue if hypotension, hypoglycaemia, ventricular tachycardia, ventricular fibrillation or torsades de pointes develop; atrial flutter or tachycardia with partial block, bundle branch block, heart failure (avoid if severe); prostatic enlargement; glaucoma; hepatic and renal impairment (see Appendixes 2 and 3); pregnancy and breast-feeding (see Appendixes 4 and 5); **interactions:** Appendix 1 (disopyramide)

Contra-indications: second- and third-degree heart block and sinus node dysfunction (unless pacemaker fitted); cardiogenic shock; severe uncompensated heart failure

Side-effects: ventricular tachycardia, ventricular fibrillation or torsades de pointes (usually associated with prolongation of QRS complex or QT interval—see Cautions above), myocardial depression, hypotension, AV block; antimuscarinic effects include dry mouth, blurred vision, urinary retention; gastro-intestinal irritation; psychosis, cholestatic jaundice, hypoglycaemia also reported (see Cautions above)

Dose: *by mouth*, 300–800 mg daily in divided doses

By slow intravenous injection, 2 mg/kg over at least 5 minutes to a max. of 150 mg, with ECG moni-

toring, followed immediately *either* by 200 mg *by mouth*, then 200 mg every 8 hours for 24 hours *or* 400 micrograms/kg/hour *by intravenous infusion*; max. 300 mg in first hour and 800 mg daily

Disopyramide (Non-proprietary) PoM
Capsules, disopyramide (as phosphate) 100 mg, net price 20 = £3.75; 150 mg, 20 = £4.98
Available from Hillcross, IVAX (100 mg)

Rythmodan® (Borg) PoM
Capsules, disopyramide 100 mg (green/beige), net price 84-cap pack = £15.82; 150 mg, 84-cap pack = £20.99
Injection, disopyramide (as phosphate) 10 mg/mL, net price 5-mL amp = £2.92

■ Modified release

Dirythmin SA® (AstraZeneca) PoM
Durules® (= tablets, m/r), f/c, disopyramide (as phosphate) 150 mg. Net price 20 = £2.47. Label: 25
Dose: 300 mg every 12 hours; max. 750 mg daily

Isomide® **CR** (Tillomed) PoM
Capsules, m/r, disopyramide (as phosphate) 250 mg, net price 56-cap pack = £31.00. Label: 25
Dose: 250 mg every 12 hours

Rythmodan Retard® (Borg) PoM
Tablets, m/r, scored, f/c, disopyramide (as phosphate) 250 mg. Net price 56-tab pack = £31.02. Label: 25
Dose: 250–375 mg every 12 hours

FLECAINIDE ACETATE

Indications: (should be initiated in hospital)
Tablets and injection: AV nodal reciprocating tachycardia, arrhythmias associated with Wolff-Parkinson-White syndrome and similar conditions with accessory pathways, paroxysmal atrial fibrillation in patients with disabling symptoms (arrhythmias of recent onset will respond more readily)
Tablets only: symptomatic sustained ventricular tachycardia, premature ventricular contractions and/or non-sustained ventricular tachycardia causing disabling symptoms in patients resistant to or intolerant of other therapy
Injection only: ventricular tachyarrhythmias resistant to other treatment

Cautions: patients with pacemakers (especially those who may be pacemaker dependent because stimulation threshold may rise appreciably); avoid in sinus node dysfunction, atrial conduction defects, second-degree or greater AV block, bundle branch block or distal block unless pacing rescue available; atrial fibrillation following heart surgery; elderly (accumulation may occur); hepatic impairment (Appendix 2); renal impairment (monitor plasma-flecainide concentration, see also Appendix 3); pregnancy (Appendix 4) and breast-feeding (Appendix 5); **interactions:** Appendix 1 (flecainide)

Contra-indications: heart failure; history of myocardial infarction and either asymptomatic ventricular ectopics or asymptomatic non-sustained ventricular tachycardia; long-standing atrial fibrillation where no attempt has been made to convert to sinus rhythm; haemodynamically significant valvular heart disease

Side-effects: nausea, vomiting; pro-arrhythmic effects; dyspnoea; visual disturbances; less commonly gastro-intestinal disturbances, jaundice, hepatic dysfunction, AV block, heart failure, myocardial infarction, hypotension, pneumonitis, hallucinations, depression, convulsions, peripheral neuropathy, paraesthesia, ataxia, dyskinesia, hypoaesthesia, tinnitus, vertigo, reduction in red blood cells, in white blood cells and in platelets, corneal deposits, rashes, alopecia, sweating, urticaria, photosensitivity, increased antinuclear antibodies

Dose: *by mouth*, ventricular arrhythmias, initially 100 mg twice daily (max. 400 mg daily usually reserved for rapid control or in heavily built patients), reduced after 3–5 days if possible
Supraventricular arrhythmias, 50 mg twice daily, increased if required to max. 300 mg daily

By slow intravenous injection, 2 mg/kg over 10–30 minutes, max. 150 mg, with ECG monitoring; followed if required by *infusion* at a rate of 1.5 mg/kg/hour for 1 hour, subsequently reduced to 100–250 micrograms/kg/hour up to 24 hours; max. cumulative dose in first 24 hours, 600 mg; transfer to *oral* treatment, as above

Note. Plasma-flecainide concentration for optimum response 0.2–1 mg/litre

Flecainide (Non-proprietary) [PoM]
Tablets, flecainide acetate 50 mg, net price 60-tab pack = £15.55; 100 mg, 60-tab pack = £22.21
Available from Alpharma, APS, Generics

Tambocor® (3M) [PoM]
Tablets, flecainide acetate 50 mg, net price 60-tab pack = £15.55; 100 mg (scored), 60-tab pack = £22.21
Injection, flecainide acetate 10 mg/mL. Net price 15-mL amp = £4.73

PROCAINAMIDE HYDROCHLORIDE

Indications: ventricular arrhythmias, especially after myocardial infarction; atrial tachycardia

Cautions: elderly; hepatic and renal impairment, asthma, myasthenia gravis; pregnancy; **interactions:** Appendix 1 (procainamide)

Contra-indications: heart block, heart failure, hypotension; systemic lupus erythematosus; not indicated for torsades de pointes (can exacerbate); breast-feeding

Side-effects: nausea, diarrhoea, rashes, fever, myocardial depression, heart failure, lupus erythematosus-like syndrome, agranulocytosis after prolonged treatment; psychosis and angio-edema also reported

Dose: *by slow intravenous injection*, rate not exceeding 50 mg/minute, 100 mg with ECG monitoring, repeated at 5-minute intervals until arrhythmia controlled; max. 1 g
By intravenous infusion, 500–600 mg over 25–30 minutes with ECG monitoring, followed by maintenance at rate of 2–6 mg/minute, then if necessary oral treatment as above, starting 3–4 hours after infusion

Note. Serum procainamide concentration for optimum response 3–10 mg/litre

Pronestyl® (Squibb) [PoM]
Injection, procainamide hydrochloride 100 mg/mL. Net price 10-mL vial = £1.90

PROPAFENONE HYDROCHLORIDE

Indications: ventricular arrhythmias; paroxysmal supraventricular tachyarrhythmias which include paroxysmal atrial flutter or fibrillation and paroxysmal re-entrant tachycardias involving the AV node or accessory pathway, where standard therapy ineffective or contra-indicated

Cautions: heart failure; hepatic and renal impairment; elderly; pacemaker patients; pregnancy and breast-feeding (see Appendixes 4 and 5); great caution in obstructive airways disease owing to beta-blocking activity (contra-indicated if severe); **interactions:** Appendix 1 (propafenone)

Contra-indications: uncontrolled congestive heart failure, cardiogenic shock (except arrhythmia induced), severe bradycardia, electrolyte disturbances, severe obstructive pulmonary disease, marked hypotension; myasthenia gravis; unless adequately paced avoid in sinus node dysfunction, atrial conduction defects, second degree or greater AV block, bundle branch block or distal block

Side-effects: antimuscarinic effects including constipation, blurred vision, and dry mouth; dizziness, nausea and vomiting, fatigue, bitter taste, diarrhoea, headache, and allergic skin reactions reported; postural hypotension, particularly in elderly; bradycardia, sino-atrial, atrioventricular, or intraventricular blocks; arrhythmogenic (pro-arrhythmic) effect; rarely hypersensitivity reactions (cholestasis, blood disorders, lupus syndrome), seizures; myoclonus also reported

Dose: 70 kg and over, initially 150 mg 3 times daily after food under direct hospital supervision with ECG monitoring and blood pressure control (if QRS interval prolonged by more than 20%, reduce dose or discontinue until ECG returns to normal limits); may be increased at intervals of at least 3 days to 300 mg twice daily and, if necessary, to max. 300 mg 3 times daily; under 70 kg, reduce dose
ELDERLY may respond to lower doses

Arythmol® (Abbott) [PoM]
Tablets, both f/c, propafenone hydrochloride 150 mg, net price 90-tab pack = £21.43; 300 mg (scored), 60-tab pack = £21.43. Label: 21, 25

QUINIDINE

Indications: suppression of supraventricular tachycardias and ventricular arrhythmias (see notes above)

Cautions: 200-mg test dose to detect hypersensitivity reactions; **interactions:** Appendix 1 (quinidine)

Contra-indications: heart block

Side-effects: see under Procainamide Hydrochloride; also ventricular arrhythmias, thrombocytopenia, haemolytic anaemia; rarely granulomatous hepatitis; also cinchonism (see

Quinine, section 5.4.1)

Dose: *by mouth*, quinidine sulphate 200–400 mg 3–4 times daily

Note. Quinidine sulphate 200 mg ≡ quinidine bisulphate 250 mg

Quinidine Sulphate (Non-proprietary) PoM
Tablets, quinidine sulphate 200 mg, net price 100-tab pack = £32.95
Available from Regent

■ Modified release

Kinidin Durules® (AstraZeneca) PoM
Tablets, m/r, f/c, quinidine bisulphate 250 mg. Net price 100-tab pack = £11.05. Label: 25
Dose: 500 mg every 12 hours, adjusted as required

Ventricular arrhythmias

Bretylium is only used as an anti-arrhythmic drug in resuscitation. It is given both intramuscularly and intravenously but can cause severe hypotension, particularly after intravenous administration; nausea and vomiting can occur with either route. The intravenous route should only be used in emergency when there is doubt about absorption because of inadequate circulation.

Lidocaine (lignocaine) is relatively safe when used by slow intravenous injection and should be considered first for emergency use. Though effective in suppressing ventricular tachycardia and reducing the risk of ventricular fibrillation following myocardial infarction, it has not been shown to reduce mortality when used prophylactically in this condition. In patients with cardiac or hepatic failure doses may need to be reduced to avoid convulsions, depression of the central nervous system, or depression of the cardiovascular system.

Mexiletine may be given as a slow intravenous injection if lidocaine is ineffective; it has a similar action. Adverse cardiovascular and central nervous system effects may limit the dose tolerated; nausea and vomiting may prevent an effective dose being given by mouth.

Moracizine (*Ethmozine®*, Shire) is available on a named-patient basis for the prophylaxis and treatment of serious and life-threatening ventricular arrhythmias for patients already stabilised on moracizine.

Phenytoin (section 4.8.2) by slow intravenous injection was formerly used in ventricular arrhythmias particularly those caused by cardiac glycosides, but this use is now obsolete.

Drugs for both supraventricular and ventricular arrhythmias include **amiodarone**, **beta-blockers**, **disopyramide**, **flecainide**, **procainamide**, **propafenone** and **quinidine**, see above under Supraventricular and Ventricular Arrhythmias.

BRETYLIUM TOSILATE

Indications: ventricular arrhythmias resistant to other treatment

Cautions: do not give noradrenaline (norepinephrine) or other sympathomimetic amines; may exacerbate ventricular arrhythmias due to cardiac glycosides; **interactions:** Appendix 1 (adrenergic neurone blockers)

Contra-indications: phaeochromocytoma

Side-effects: hypotension, nausea and vomiting; tissue necrosis reported after intramuscular injection (rotate sites)

Dose: *by slow intravenous injection*, 5–10 mg/kg over 8–10 minutes (preferably 15–30 minutes) with blood pressure and ECG monitoring; may be repeated after 1–2 hours to a total dosage of 30 mg/kg (intravenous dose being diluted to 10 mg/mL in glucose 5% or sodium chloride intravenous infusion)
Maintenance 5–10 mg/kg *by intramuscular injection, by intravenous infusion* (over 15–30 minutes) every 6–8 hours, *or* 1–2 mg/minute *by continuous intravenous infusion*

Min-I-Jet® Bretylium Tosylate (Celltech) PoM
Injection, bretylium tosilate 50 mg/mL, net price 10-mL disposable syringe = £21.73

LIDOCAINE HYDROCHLORIDE/ LIGNOCAINE HYDROCHLORIDE

Indications: ventricular arrhythmias, especially after myocardial infarction

Cautions: lower doses in congestive cardiac failure, in hepatic failure, and following cardiac surgery; elderly; **interactions:** Appendix 1 (lidocaine)

Contra-indications: sino-atrial disorders, all grades of atrioventricular block, severe myocardial depression; porphyria (see section 9.8.2)

Side-effects: dizziness, paraesthesia, or drowsiness (particularly if injection too rapid); other CNS effects include confusion, respiratory depression and convulsions; hypotension and bradycardia (may lead to cardiac arrest); hypersensitivity reported

Dose: *by intravenous injection*, in patients without gross circulatory impairment, 100 mg as a bolus over a few minutes (50 mg in lighter patients or those whose circulation is severely impaired), followed immediately by *infusion* of 4 mg/minute for 30 minutes, 2 mg/minute for 2 hours, then 1 mg/minute; reduce concentration further if infusion continued beyond 24 hours (ECG monitoring and specialist advice for infusion)

IMPORTANT. Following intravenous injection lidocaine has a short duration of action (lasting for 15–20 minutes). If an *intravenous infusion* is not immediately available the initial *intravenous injection* of 50–100 mg can be repeated if necessary once or twice at intervals of not less than 10 minutes

Lidocaine/Lignocaine (Non-proprietary) PoM
Injection 2%, lidocaine hydrochloride 20 mg/mL, net price 2-mL amp = 28p; 5-mL amp = 24p; 10-mL amp = 60p; 20-mL amp = 66p
Available from Braun
Infusion, lidocaine hydrochloride 0.1% (1 mg/mL) and 0.2% (2 mg/mL) in glucose intravenous infusion 5%. 500-mL containers
Available from Baxter

Min-I-Jet® Lignocaine (Celltech) PoM
Injection, lidocaine hydrochloride 1% (10 mg/mL), net price 10-mL disposable syringe = £3.73; 2% (20 mg/mL), 5-mL disposable syringe = £3.37

MEXILETINE HYDROCHLORIDE

Indications: ventricular arrhythmias, especially after myocardial infarction

Cautions: hepatic impairment; close monitoring on initiation of therapy (including ECG, blood pressure, etc.); **interactions:** Appendix 1 (mexiletine)

Contra-indications: bradycardia, cardiogenic shock; high degree AV block (unless pacemaker fitted)

Side-effects: nausea, vomiting, constipation; bradycardia, hypotension, atrial fibrillation, palpitations, conduction defects, exacerbation of arrhythmias, torsades de pointes; drowsiness, confusion, convulsions, psychiatric disorders, dysarthria, ataxia, paraesthesia, nystagmus, tremor; jaundice, hepatitis, and blood disorders reported; see also notes above

Dose: *by mouth*, initial dose 400 mg (may be increased to 600 mg if opioid analgesics also given), followed after 2 hours by 200–250 mg 3–4 times daily

By intravenous injection, 100–250 mg at a rate of 25 mg/minute with ECG monitoring followed by *infusion* of 250 mg as a 0.1% solution over 1 hour, 125 mg/hour for 2 hours, then 500 micrograms/minute

Mexitil® (Boehringer Ingelheim) ▣PoM▣
Capsules, mexiletine hydrochloride 50 mg (purple/red), net price 100-cap pack = £4.95; 200 mg (red), 100-cap pack = £11.87
Injection, mexiletine hydrochloride 25 mg/mL. Net price 10-mL amp = £1.49

■ Modified release

Mexitil PL® (Boehringer Ingelheim) ▣PoM▣
Perlongets® (= capsules, m/r, each enclosing 5 miniature tablets), turquoise/scarlet, mexiletine hydrochloride 360 mg. Net price 60-cap pack = £12.82. Label: 25
Dose: 1 capsule twice daily

2.4 Beta-adrenoceptor blocking drugs

Beta-adrenoceptor blocking drugs (beta-blockers) block the beta-adrenoreceptors in the heart, peripheral vasculature, bronchi, pancreas, and liver.

Many beta-blockers are now available and in general they are all equally effective. There are, however, differences between them which may affect choice in treating particular diseases or individual patients; esmolol and sotalol are used for the management of arrhythmia only (see below).

Intrinsic sympathomimetic activity (ISA, partial agonist activity) represents the capacity of beta-blockers to stimulate as well as to block adrenergic receptors. **Oxprenolol, pindolol, acebutolol** and **celiprolol** have intrinsic sympathomimetic activity; they tend to cause less bradycardia than the other beta-blockers and may also cause less coldness of the extremities.

Some beta-blockers are lipid soluble and some are water soluble. **Atenolol, celiprolol, nadolol,** and **sotalol** are the most water-soluble; they are less likely to enter the brain, and may therefore cause less sleep disturbance and nightmares. Water-soluble beta-blockers are excreted by the kidneys; they accumulate in renal impairment and dosage reduction is therefore often necessary.

Beta-blockers with a relatively short duration of action have to be given two or three times daily. Many of these are, however, available in modified-release formulations so that administration once daily is adequate for hypertension. For angina twice-daily treatment may sometimes be needed even with a modified-release formulation. Some beta-blockers such as atenolol, betaxolol, bisoprolol, carvedilol, celiprolol, and nadolol have an intrinsically longer duration of action and need to be given only once daily.

Beta-blockers slow the heart and can depress the myocardium; they are contra-indicated in patients with second- or third-degree heart block. Beta-blockers should also be avoided in patients with worsening unstable heart failure; care is required when initiating a beta-blocker in those with stable heart failure (see also section 2.5.5). **Sotalol** may prolong the QT interval, and it occasionally causes life-threatening ventricular arrhythmias (**important:** particular care is required to avoid hypokalaemia in patients taking sotalol).

Labetalol, celiprolol, carvedilol and **nebivolol** are beta-blockers which have, in addition, an arteriolar vasodilating action, by diverse mechanisms, and thus lower peripheral resistance. There is no evidence that these drugs have important advantages over other beta-blockers in the treatment of hypertension.

Beta-blockers may precipitate asthma and this effect can be dangerous. Beta-blockers should be **avoided** in patients with a history of asthma or chronic obstructive airways disease; if there is no alternative, a cardioselective beta-blocker may be used with extreme caution under specialist supervision. **Atenolol, betaxolol, bisoprolol, metoprolol, nebivolol** and (to a lesser extent) **acebutolol**, have less effect on the beta$_2$ (bronchial) receptors and are, therefore, relatively *cardioselective*, but they are **not** *cardiospecific*. They have a lesser effect on airways resistance but are **not** free of this side-effect.

Beta-blockers are also associated with fatigue, coldness of the extremities (may be less common with those with ISA, see above), and sleep disturbances with nightmares (may be less common with the water-soluble ones, see above).

Beta-blockers are not contra-indicated in diabetes; however they can lead to a small deterioration of glucose tolerance and interfere with metabolic and autonomic responses to hypoglycaemia. Cardioselective beta-blockers (see above) may be preferable and beta-blockers should be avoided altogether in those with frequent episodes of hypoglycaemia.

HYPERTENSION. Beta-blockers are effective antihypertensives but their mode of action is not understood; they reduce cardiac output, alter baroceptor reflex sensitivity, and block peripheral adrenoceptors. Some beta-blockers depress plasma renin secretion. It is possible that a central effect may also explain their mode of action. Blood pressure can usually be controlled with relatively few side-effects. In general the dose of beta-blocker does not have to be high; for example **atenolol** is given in a dose of 50 mg daily and it is usually not necessary to increase the dose to 100 mg.

Combined thiazide and beta-blocker preparations may help compliance but combined preparations should only be used when blood pressure is not adequately controlled by a thiazide or a beta-blocker alone. Beta-blockers reduce, but do not abolish, the tendency for diuretics to cause hypokalaemia.

Beta-blockers can be used to control the pulse rate in patients with *phaeochromocytoma* (section 2.5.4). However, they should never be used alone as beta-blockade without concurrent alpha-blockade may lead to a hypertensive crisis. For this reason phenoxybenzamine should always be used together with the beta-blocker.

ANGINA. By reducing cardiac work beta-blockers improve exercise tolerance and relieve symptoms in patients with *angina* (for further details on the management of stable and unstable angina see section 2.6). As with hypertension there is no good evidence of the superiority of any one drug, although occasionally a patient will respond better to one beta-blocker than to another. There is some evidence that sudden withdrawal may cause an exacerbation of angina and therefore gradual reduction of dose is preferable when beta-blockers are to be stopped. There is a risk of precipitating heart failure when beta-blockers and verapamil are used together in established ischaemic heart disease (**important**: see p. 107).

MYOCARDIAL INFARCTION. For advice on the management of myocardial infarction see section 2.10.1.

Several studies have shown that some beta-blockers can reduce the recurrence rate of *myocardial infarction*. However, uncontrolled heart failure, hypotension, bradyarrhythmias, and obstructive airways disease render beta-blockers unsuitable in some patients following a myocardial infarction. **Atenolol** and **metoprolol** may reduce early mortality after intravenous and subsequent oral administration in the acute phase, while **acebutolol**, **metoprolol**, **propranolol**, and **timolol** have protective value when started in the early convalescent phase. The evidence relating to other beta-blockers is less convincing; some have not been tested in trials of secondary protection. It is also not known whether the protective effect of beta-blockers continues after 2–3 years; it is possible that sudden cessation may cause a rebound worsening of myocardial ischaemia.

ARRHYTHMIAS. Beta-blockers act as *anti-arrhythmic drugs* principally by attenuating the effects of the sympathetic system on automaticity and conductivity within the heart. They may be used in conjunction with digoxin to control the ventricular response in atrial fibrillation, especially in patients with thyrotoxicosis. Beta-blockers are also useful in the management of supraventricular tachycardias, and are used to control those following myocardial infarction, see above.

Esmolol is a relatively cardioselective beta-blocker with a very short duration of action, used intravenously for the short-term treatment of supraventricular arrhythmias, sinus tachycardia, or hypertension, particularly in the peri-operative period. It may also be used in other situations, such as acute myocardial infarction, where sustained beta blockade might be hazardous.

Sotalol, a non-cardioselective beta-blocker with additional class III anti-arrhythmic activity, is used for prophylaxis in paroxysmal supraventricular arrhythmias. It also suppresses ventricular ectopic beats and non-sustained ventricular tachycardia. It has been shown to be more effective than lidocaine (lignocaine) in the termination of spontaneous sustained ventricular tachycardia due to coronary disease or cardiomyopathy. However, it may induce torsades de pointes in susceptible patients.

HEART FAILURE. Beta-blockers may produce benefit in heart failure by blocking sympathetic activity. **Bisoprolol**, **carvedilol**, and modified-release **metoprolol** [unlicensed indication] reduce mortality in selected patients with stable heart failure. Treatment should be initiated under specialist supervision (see section 2.5.5 for the management of heart failure).

THYROTOXICOSIS. Beta-blockers are used in pre-operative preparation for thyroidectomy. Administration of propranolol can reverse clinical symptoms of *thyrotoxicosis* within 4 days. Routine tests of increased thyroid function remain unaltered. The thyroid gland is rendered less vascular thus making surgery easier (section 6.2.2).

OTHER USES. Beta-blockers have been used to alleviate some symptoms of *anxiety*; probably patients with palpitations, tremor, and tachycardia respond best (see also section 4.1.2 and section 4.9.3). Beta-blockers are also used in the *prophylaxis of migraine* (section 4.7.4.2). Betaxolol, carteolol, levobunolol, metipranolol and timolol are used topically in *glaucoma* (section 11.6).

PROPRANOLOL HYDROCHLORIDE

Indications: see under Dose

Cautions: pregnancy and breast-feeding (see also Appendixes 4 and 5); avoid abrupt withdrawal especially in angina; first-degree AV block; reduce oral dose of propranolol in liver disease; liver function deteriorates in portal hypertension; reduce initial dose in renal impairment; diabetes; myasthenia gravis; history of hypersensitivity—may increase sensitivity to allergens and result in more serious hypersensitivity response, also may reduce response to adrenaline (epinephrine) (see also section 3.4.3); see also notes above; **interactions:** Appendix 1 (beta-blockers), **important:** verapamil interaction, see also p. 107

Contra-indications: asthma or history of obstructive airways disease (**important:** see Bronchospasm below), uncontrolled heart failure, Prinzmetal's angina, marked bradycardia, hypotension, sick sinus syndrome, second- or third-degree AV block, cardiogenic shock, metabolic acidosis, severe peripheral arterial disease; phaeochromocytoma (apart from specific use with alpha-blockers, see also notes above)

BRONCHOSPASM. The CSM has advised that beta-blockers, including those considered to be cardioselective, should not be given to patients with a history of asthma or bronchospasm. However, in these patients there are very rare situations where there is no alternative to the use of a beta-blocker, when a cardioselective one is given with extreme caution and under specialist supervision

Side-effects: bradycardia, heart failure, hypotension, conduction disorders, bronchospasm, peripheral vasoconstriction (including exacerbation of intermittent claudication and Raynaud's phenomenon), gastro-intestinal disturbances, fatigue, sleep disturbances; rare reports of rashes and dry eyes (reversible on withdrawal), exacerbation of psoriasis; see also notes above; **overdosage:** see Emergency Treatment of Poisoning, p. 25

Dose: *by mouth*, hypertension, initially 80 mg twice daily, increased at weekly intervals as required; maintenance 160–320 mg daily

Portal hypertension, initially 40 mg twice daily, increased to 80 mg twice daily according to heartrate; max. 160 mg twice daily

Phaeochromocytoma (only with an alphablocker), 60 mg daily for 3 days before surgery *or* 30 mg daily in patients unsuitable for surgery

Angina, initially 40 mg 2–3 times daily; maintenance 120–240 mg daily

Arrhythmias, hypertrophic obstructive cardiomyopathy, anxiety tachycardia, and thyrotoxicosis (adjunct), 10–40 mg 3–4 times daily

Anxiety with symptoms such as palpitations, sweating, tremor, 40 mg once daily, increased to 40 mg 3 times daily if necessary

Prophylaxis after myocardial infarction, 40 mg 4 times daily for 2–3 days, then 80 mg twice daily, beginning 5 to 21 days after infarction

Migraine prophylaxis and essential tremor, initially 40 mg 2–3 times daily; maintenance 80–160 mg daily

By intravenous injection, arrhythmias and thyrotoxic crisis, 1 mg over 1 minute; if necessary repeat at 2-minute intervals; max. 10 mg (5 mg in anaesthesia)

Note. Excessive bradycardia can be countered with intravenous injection of atropine sulphate 0.6–2.4 mg in divided doses of 600 micrograms; for **overdosage** see Emergency Treatment of Poisoning, p. 25

Propranolol (Non-proprietary) PoM

Tablets, propranolol hydrochloride 10 mg, net price 20 = 42p; 40 mg, 20 = 46p; 80 mg, 20 = 33p 160 mg, 20 = 84p. Label: 8

Available from Alpharma, APS, DDSA (*Angilol®*), Hillcross

Oral solution, propranolol hydrochloride, 5 mg/5 mL, net price 150 mL = £13.30; 10 mg/5 mL, 150 mL = £17.50; 50 mg/5 mL, 150 mL = £21.25

Available from Rosemont (*Syprol®*)

Inderal® (AstraZeneca) PoM

Tablets, all pink, f/c, propranolol hydrochloride 10 mg, net price 100-tab pack = 89p; 40 mg, 100-tab pack = £2.40; 80 mg, 60-tab pack = £2.35. Label: 8

Injection, propranolol hydrochloride 1 mg/mL, net price 1-mL amp = 21p

■ Modified release

Half-Inderal LA® (AstraZeneca) PoM

Capsules, m/r, lavender/pink, propranolol hydrochloride 80 mg. Net price 28-cap pack = £5.40. Label: 8, 25

Note. Modified-release capsules containing propranolol hydrochloride 80 mg also available from APS, Tillomed (*Half Beta Prograne®*)

Inderal-LA® (AstraZeneca) PoM

Capsules, m/r, lavender/pink, propranolol hydrochloride 160 mg. Net price 28-cap pack = £6.67. Label: 8, 25

Note. Modified-release capsules containing propranolol hydrochloride 160 mg also available from APS, Hillcross, Lagap (*Bedranol SR®*), Opus (*Lopranol LA®*), Tillomed (*Beta Prograne®*), Trinity (*Probeta LA®*)

■ With diuretic

Inderetic® (AstraZeneca) PoM

Capsules, propranolol hydrochloride 80 mg, bendroflumethiazide 2.5 mg. Net price 60-cap pack = £5.85. Label: 8

Dose: hypertension, 1 capsule twice daily

Inderex® (AstraZeneca) PoM

Capsules, pink/grey, propranolol hydrochloride 160 mg (m/r), bendroflumethiazide 5 mg. Net price 28-cap pack = £7.45. Label: 8, 25

Dose: hypertension, 1 capsule daily

ACEBUTOLOL

Indications: see under Dose

Cautions: see under Propranolol Hydrochloride

Contra-indications: see under Propranolol Hydrochloride

Side-effects: see under Propranolol Hydrochloride

Dose: hypertension, initially 400 mg once daily *or* 200 mg twice daily, increased after 2 weeks to 400 mg twice daily if necessary

Angina, initially 400 mg once daily *or* 200 mg twice daily; 300 mg 3 times daily in severe angina; up to 1.2 g daily has been used

Arrhythmias, 0.4–1.2 g daily in 2–3 divided doses

Sectral® (Akita) PoM

Capsules, acebutolol (as hydrochloride) 100 mg (buff/white), net price 84-cap pack = £16.10; 200 mg (buff/pink), 56-cap pack = £20.63. Label: 8

Tablets, f/c, acebutolol 400 mg (as hydrochloride). Net price 28-tab pack = £20.02. Label: 8

■ With diuretic

Secadrex® (Akita) PoM

Tablets, f/c, acebutolol 200 mg (as hydrochloride), hydrochlorothiazide 12.5 mg. Net price 28-tab pack = £18.91. Label: 8

Dose: hypertension, 1 tablet daily, increased to 2 daily as a single dose if necessary

ATENOLOL

Indications: see under Dose

Cautions: see under Propranolol Hydrochloride; reduce dose in renal impairment

Contra-indications: see under Propranolol Hydrochloride

Side-effects: see under Propranolol Hydrochloride

Dose: *by mouth*,

Hypertension, 50 mg daily (higher doses rarely necessary)

Angina, 100 mg daily in 1 or 2 doses

Arrhythmias, 50–100 mg daily

By intravenous injection, arrhythmias, 2.5 mg at a rate of 1 mg/minute, repeated at 5-minute intervals to a max. of 10 mg

Note. Excessive bradycardia can be countered with intravenous injection of atropine sulphate 0.6–2.4 mg in divided doses of 600 micrograms; for **overdosage** see Emergency Treatment of Poisoning, p. 25

By intravenous infusion, arrhythmias, 150 micrograms/kg over 20 minutes, repeated every 12 hours if required

Early intervention within 12 hours of myocardial infarction (section 2.10.1), *by intravenous injection* over 5 minutes, 5 mg, then *by mouth*, 50 mg after 15 minutes, 50 mg after 12 hours, then 100 mg daily

Atenolol (Non-proprietary) PoM
Tablets, atenolol 25 mg, net price 28-tab pack = 74p; 50 mg, 28-tab pack = 85p; 100 mg, 28-tab pack = 98p. Label: 8
Various strengths available from Alpharma, APS, Ashbourne (*Atenix*®), CP, Hillcross, IVAX, Sterwin, Tillomed

Tenormin® (AstraZeneca) PoM
'25' tablets, f/c, atenolol 25 mg. Net price 28-tab pack = £4.41. Label: 8
LS tablets, orange, f/c, scored, atenolol 50 mg. Net price 28-tab pack = £5.11. Label: 8
Tablets, orange, f/c, scored, atenolol 100 mg. Net price 28-tab pack = £6.50. Label: 8
Syrup, sugar-free, atenolol 25 mg/5mL. Net price 300 mL = £7.77. Label: 8
Injection, atenolol 500 micrograms/mL. Net price 10-mL amp = 96p (hosp. only)

■ With diuretic

Co-tenidone (Non-proprietary) PoM
Tablets, co-tenidone 50/12.5 (atenolol 50 mg, chlortalidone 12.5 mg), net price 28-tab pack = £2.71; co-tenidone 100/25 (atenolol 100 mg, chlortalidone 25 mg), 28-tab pack = £3.83. Label: 8
Available from Alpharma, APS, Ashbourne (*AtenixCo*®), Berk (*Tenchlor*®), Bioglan, CP (*Totaretic*®), Hillcross, IVAX
Dose: hypertension, 1 tablet daily (but see also under Dose above)

Kalten® (AstraZeneca) PoM
Capsules, red/ivory, atenolol 50 mg, co-amilozide 2.5/25 (anhydrous amilozide hydrochloride 2.5 mg, hydrochlorothiazide 25 mg). Net price 28-cap pack = £8.39. Label: 8
Dose: hypertension, 1 capsule daily

Tenben® (Galen) PoM
Capsules, pink/red, atenolol 25 mg, bendroflumethiazide 1.25 mg, net price 56-cap pack = £4.95. Label: 8
Dose: hypertension, 1–2 capsules daily

Tenoret 50® (AstraZeneca) PoM
Tablets, brown, f/c, co-tenidone 50/12.5 (atenolol 50 mg, chlortalidone 12.5 mg). Net price 28-tab pack = £5.70. Label: 8
Dose: hypertension, 1 tablet daily

Tenoretic® (AstraZeneca) PoM
Tablets, brown, f/c, co-tenidone 100/25 (atenolol 100 mg, chlortalidone 25 mg). Net price 28-tab pack = £8.12. Label: 8
Dose: hypertension, 1 tablet daily (but see also under Dose above)

■ With calcium-channel blocker
Note. Only indicated when calcium-channel blocker or beta-blocker alone proves inadequate

Beta-Adalat® (Bayer) PoM
Capsules, reddish-brown, atenolol 50 mg, nifedipine 20 mg (m/r). Net price 28-cap pack = £10.41. Label: 8, 25
Dose: hypertension, 1 capsule daily, increased if necessary to twice daily; elderly, 1 daily
Angina, 1 capsule twice daily

Tenif® (AstraZeneca) PoM
Capsules, reddish-brown, atenolol 50 mg, nifedipine 20 mg (m/r). Net price 28-cap pack = £10.63. Label: 8, 25
Dose: hypertension, 1 capsule daily, increased if necessary to twice daily; elderly, 1 daily
Angina, 1 capsule twice daily

BETAXOLOL HYDROCHLORIDE

Indications: hypertension; glaucoma (section 11.6)
Cautions: see under Propranolol Hydrochloride
Contra-indications: see under Propranolol Hydrochloride
Side-effects: see under Propranolol Hydrochloride
Dose: 20 mg daily (elderly patients 10 mg), increased to 40 mg if required

Kerlone® (Sanofi-Synthelabo) PoM
Tablets, f/c, scored, betaxolol hydrochloride 20 mg. Net price 28-tab pack = £7.51. Label: 8

BISOPROLOL FUMARATE

Indications: see under Dose
Cautions: see under Propranolol Hydrochloride; reduce dose in hepatic and renal impairment; in heart failure monitor clinical status for 4 hours after initiation (with low dose) and ensure heart failure not worsening before increasing each dose
Contra-indications: see under Propranolol Hydrochloride; also acute or decompensated heart failure requiring intravenous inotropes
Side-effects: see under Propranolol Hydrochloride
Dose: hypertension and angina, usually 10 mg once daily (5 mg may be adequate in some patients); max. 20 mg daily
Stable moderate to severe heart failure, as an adjunct to treatment with an ACE inhibitor, a diuretic and possibly a cardiac glycoside (under specialist supervision), initially 1.25 mg once daily (in the morning) for 1 week then, if well tolerated, increased to 2.5 mg once daily for 1 week, then 3.75 mg once daily for 1 week, then 5 mg once daily for 4 weeks, then 7.5 mg once daily for 4 weeks, then 10 mg once daily; max. 10 mg daily

Bisoprolol Fumarate (Non-proprietary) PoM
Tablets, bisoprolol fumarate 5 mg, net price 28-tab pack = £8.56; 10 mg, 28-tab pack = £9.61. Label: 8
Available from Alpharma, APS, Ashbourne (*Bipranix*®), Dominion, Generics, Genus

Cardicor® (Merck) ▼ PoM
Tablets, f/c, bisoprolol fumarate 1.25 mg, net price 28-tab pack = £8.56; 2.5 mg (scored), 28-tab pack = £8.56; 3.75 mg (scored, white-yellow), 28-tab pack = £8.56; 5 mg (scored, light yellow), 28-tab pack = £8.56; 7.5 mg (scored, yellow), 28-tab pack = £9.09; 10 mg (scored, orange), 28-tab pack = £9.61. Label: 8

Emcor® (Merck) PoM

LS Tablets, yellow, f/c, scored, bisoprolol fumarate 5 mg. Net price 28-tab pack = £8.56. Label: 8

Tablets, orange, f/c, scored, bisoprolol fumarate 10 mg. Net price 28-tab pack = £9.61. Label: 8

Monocor® (Lederle) PoM

Tablets, both f/c, bisoprolol fumarate 5 mg (pink), net price 28-tab pack = £8.56; 10 mg, 28-tab pack £9.61. Label: 8

■ With diuretic

Monozide 10® (Lederle) PoM

Tablets, f/c, bisoprolol fumarate 10 mg, hydrochlorothiazide 6.25 mg. Net price 28-tab pack = £11.20. Label: 8

Dose: hypertension, 1 tablet daily

CARVEDILOL

Indications: hypertension; angina; adjunct to diuretics, digoxin, or ACE inhibitors in symptomatic chronic heart failure

Cautions: see under Propranolol Hydrochloride; before increasing dose ensure renal function and heart failure not deteriorating; severe heart failure, avoid in acute or decompensated heart failure requiring intravenous inotropes

Contra-indications: see under Propranolol Hydrochloride; severe chronic heart failure; hepatic impairment (Appendix 2)

Side-effects: postural hypotension, dizziness, headache, fatigue, gastro-intestinal disturbances, bradycardia; occasionally diminished peripheral circulation, peripheral oedema and painful extremities, dry mouth, dry eyes, eye irritation or disturbed vision, impotence, disturbances of micturition, influenza-like symptoms; rarely angina, AV block, exacerbation of intermittent claudication or Raynaud's phenomenon; allergic skin reactions, exacerbation of psoriasis, nasal stuffiness, wheezing, depressed mood, sleep disturbances, paraesthesia, heart failure, changes in liver enzymes, thrombocytopenia, leucopenia also reported

Dose: hypertension, initially 12.5 mg once daily, increased after 2 days to usual dose of 25 mg once daily; if necessary may be further increased at intervals of at least 2 weeks to max. 50 mg daily in single or divided doses; ELDERLY initial dose of 12.5 mg daily may provide satisfactory control

Angina, initially 12.5 mg twice daily, increased after 2 days to 25 mg twice daily

Heart failure (under specialist supervision), initially 3.125 mg twice daily (with food), dose increased at intervals of at least 2 weeks to 6.25 mg twice daily, then to 12.5 mg twice daily, then to 25 mg twice daily; increase to highest dose tolerated, max. 25 mg twice daily in patients with severe heart failure or body-weight less than 85 kg and 50 mg twice daily in patients over 85 kg

Eucardic® (Roche) ▼ PoM

Tablets, all scored, carvedilol 3.125 mg (pink), net price 28-tab pack = £8.14; 6.25 mg (yellow), 28-tab pack = £9.04; 12.5 mg (peach), 28-tab pack = £10.05; 25 mg, 28-tab pack = £12.56. Label: 8

CELIPROLOL HYDROCHLORIDE

Indications: mild to moderate hypertension

Cautions: see under Propranolol Hydrochloride

Contra-indications: see under Propranolol Hydrochloride; also avoid in severe renal impairment

Side-effects: headache, dizziness, fatigue, nausea and somnolence; also bradycardia, bronchospasm; depression and pneumonitis reported rarely

Dose: 200 mg once daily in the morning, increased to 400 mg once daily if necessary

Celiprolol (Non-proprietary) PoM

Tablets, celiprolol hydrochloride 200 mg, net price 28-tab pack = £17.01; 400 mg, 28-tab pack = £34.38. Label 8, 22

Available from Generics, IVAX, Sovereign

Celectol® (Pantheon) PoM

Tablets, both f/c, scored, celiprolol hydrochloride 200 mg (yellow), net price 28-tab pack = £17.19; 400 mg, 28-tab pack = £34.38. Label: 8, 22

ESMOLOL HYDROCHLORIDE

Indications: short-term treatment of supraventricular arrhythmias (including atrial fibrillation, atrial flutter, sinus tachycardia); tachycardia and hypertension in peri-operative period

Cautions: see under Propranolol Hydrochloride; renal impairment

Contra-indications: see under Propranolol Hydrochloride

Side-effects: see under Propranolol Hydrochloride

Dose: *by intravenous infusion*, usually within range 50–200 micrograms/kg/minute (consult product literature for details of dose titration and doses during peri-operative period)

Brevibloc® (Baxter) PoM

Injection, esmolol hydrochloride 10 mg/mL, net price 10-mL vial = £5.90

Injection concentrate, esmolol hydrochloride 250 mg/mL (for dilution before infusion), 10-mL amp = £65.90

LABETALOL HYDROCHLORIDE

Indications: hypertension (including hypertension in pregnancy, hypertension with angina, and hypertension following acute myocardial infarction); hypertensive crisis (but see section 2.5); controlled hypotension in anaesthesia

Cautions: see under Propranolol Hydrochloride; interferes with laboratory tests for catecholamines; liver damage (see below)

LIVER DAMAGE. Severe hepatocellular damage reported after both short-term and long-term treatment. Appropriate laboratory testing needed at first symptom of liver dysfunction and if laboratory evidence of damage (or if jaundice) labetalol should be stopped and not restarted

Contra-indications: see under Propranolol Hydrochloride

Side-effects: postural hypotension (avoid upright position during and for 3 hours after intravenous administration), tiredness, weakness, headache, rashes, scalp tingling, difficulty in micturition, epigastric pain, nausea, vomiting; liver damage (see above); rarely lichenoid rash

Dose: *by mouth*, initially 100 mg (50 mg in elderly) twice daily with food, increased at intervals of 14

days to usual dose of 200 mg twice daily; up to 800 mg daily in 2 divided doses (3–4 divided doses if higher); max. 2.4 g daily

By intravenous injection, 50 mg over at least 1 minute, repeated after 5 minutes if necessary; max. 200 mg

Note. Excessive bradycardia can be countered with intravenous injection of atropine sulphate 0.6–2.4 mg in divided doses of 600 micrograms; for **overdosage** see Emergency Treatment of Poisoning, p. 25

By intravenous infusion, 2 mg/minute until satisfactory response then discontinue; usual total dose 50–200 mg (**not** recommended for phaeochromocytoma, see notes on phaeochromocytoma, section 2.5.4)

Hypertension of pregnancy, 20 mg/hour, doubled every 30 minutes; usual max. 160 mg/hour

Hypertension following myocardial infarction, 15 mg/hour, gradually increased to max. 120 mg/hour

Labetalol Hydrochloride (Non-proprietary) PoM

Tablets, all f/c, labetalol hydrochloride 100 mg, net price 20 = £1.70; 200 mg, 20 = £2.30; 400 mg, 20 = £3.97. Label: 8, 21

Available from Alpharma, Hillcross, Norton

Trandate® (Celltech) PoM

Tablets, all orange, f/c, labetalol hydrochloride 50 mg, net price 56-tab pack. £5.05; 100 mg, 56-tab pack = £5.56; 200 mg, 56-tab pack = £9.02; 400 mg, 56-tab pack = £12.56. Label: 8, 21

Injection, labetalol hydrochloride 5 mg/mL. Net price 20-mL amp = £2.83

METOPROLOL TARTRATE

Indications: see under Dose

Cautions: see under Propranolol Hydrochloride; reduce dose in hepatic impairment

Contra-indications: see under Propranolol Hydrochloride

Side-effects: see under Propranolol Hydrochloride

Dose: *by mouth*, hypertension, initially 100 mg daily, maintenance 100–200 mg daily in 1–2 doses

Angina, 50–100 mg 2–3 times daily

Arrhythmias, usually 50 mg 2–3 times daily; up to 300 mg daily in divided doses if necessary

Migraine prophylaxis, 100–200 mg daily in divided doses

Hyperthyroidism (adjunct), 50 mg 4 times daily

By intravenous injection, arrhythmias, up to 5 mg at rate 1–2 mg/minute, repeated after 5 minutes if necessary, total dose 10–15 mg

Note. Excessive bradycardia can be countered with intravenous injection of atropine sulphate 0.6–2.4 mg in divided doses of 600 micrograms; for **overdosage** see Emergency Treatment of Poisoning, p. 25

In surgery, 2–4 mg *by slow intravenous injection* at induction or to control arrhythmias developing during anaesthesia; 2-mg doses may be repeated to a max. of 10 mg

Early intervention within 12 hours of infarction, 5 mg *by intravenous injection* every 2 minutes to a max. of 15 mg, followed after 15 minutes by 50 mg *by mouth* every 6 hours for 48 hours; maintenance 200 mg daily in divided doses

Metoprolol Tartrate (Non-proprietary) PoM

Tablets, metoprolol tartrate 50 mg, net price 20 = 63p; 100 mg, 20 = £1.15. Label: 8

Available from Alpharma, APS, Hillcross, IVAX

Betaloc® (AstraZeneca) PoM

Tablets, both scored, metoprolol tartrate 50 mg, net price 100-tab pack = £3.30; 100 mg, 100-tab pack = £6.13. Label: 8

Injection, metoprolol tartrate 1 mg/mL. Net price 5-mL amp = 42p

Lopresor® (Novartis) PoM

Tablets, both f/c, scored, metoprolol tartrate 50 mg (pink), net price 56-tab pack = £2.57; 100 mg (blue), 56-tab pack = £6.68. Label: 8

■ Modified release

Betaloc-SA® (AstraZeneca) PoM

Durules® (= tablets, m/r), metoprolol tartrate 200 mg, net price 28-tab pack = £4.56. Label: 8, 25

Dose: hypertension, angina, 200 mg daily in the morning, increased to 400 mg daily if necessary; migraine prophylaxis, 200 mg daily

Lopresor SR® (Novartis) PoM

Tablets, m/r, yellow, f/c, metoprolol tartrate 200 mg, net price 28-tab pack = £9.80. Label: 8, 25

Dose: hypertension, 200 mg daily; angina, 200-400 mg daily; migraine prophylaxis, 200 mg daily

■ With diuretic

Co-Betaloc® (Searle) PoM

Tablets, scored, metoprolol tartrate 100 mg, hydrochlorothiazide 12.5 mg, net price 28-tab pack = £4.66. Label: 8

Dose: hypertension, 1–3 tablets daily in single or divided doses

Co-Betaloc SA® (Searle) PoM

Tablets, yellow, f/c, metoprolol tartrate (m/r) 200 mg, hydrochlorothiazide 25 mg, net price 28-tab pack = £5.74. Label: 8, 25

Dose: hypertension, 1 tablet daily

NADOLOL

Indications: see under Dose

Cautions: see under Propranolol Hydrochloride; reduce dose in renal impairment

Contra-indications: see under Propranolol Hydrochloride

Side-effects: see under Propranolol Hydrochloride

Dose: hypertension, 80 mg daily, increased at weekly intervals if required; max. 240 mg daily

Angina, 40 mg daily, increased at weekly intervals if required; usual max. 160 mg daily

Arrhythmias, initially 40 mg daily, increased to 160 mg if required; reduce to 40 mg if bradycardia occurs

Migraine prophylaxis, initially 40 mg daily, increased by 40 mg at weekly intervals; usual maintenance dose 80–160 mg daily

Thyrotoxicosis (adjunct), 80–160 mg daily

Corgard® (Sanofi-Synthelabo) PoM

Tablets, both blue, nadolol 40 mg, net price 28-tab pack = £3.76; 80 mg, 28-tab pack = £5.20. Label: 8

■ With diuretic

Corgaretic® (Sanofi-Synthelabo) [PoM]
Tablets, scored, nadolol 40 mg, bendroflumethiazide 5 mg (*Corgaretic 40®*), net price 28-tab pack = £5.92; nadolol 80 mg, bendroflumethiazide 5 mg (*Corgaretic 80®*), 28-tab pack = £8.47. Label: 8
Dose: hypertension, 1–2 tablets daily

NEBIVOLOL
Indications: essential hypertension
Cautions: see under Propranolol Hydrochloride; reduce dose in renal impairment (Appendix 3); elderly
Contra-indications: see under Propranolol Hydrochloride; hepatic impairment
Side-effects: see under Propranolol Hydrochloride; oedema, headache, depression, visual disturbances, paraesthesia, impotence
Dose: 5 mg daily; ELDERLY initially 2.5 mg daily, increased if necessary to 5 mg daily

Nebilet® (Menarini) [PoM]
Tablets, scored, nebivolol (as hydrochloride) 5 mg, net price 28-tab pack = £9.80

OXPRENOLOL HYDROCHLORIDE
Indications: see under Dose
Cautions: see under Propranolol Hydrochloride
Contra-indications: see under Propranolol Hydrochloride
Side-effects: see under Propranolol Hydrochloride
Dose: hypertension, 80–160 mg daily in 2–3 divided doses, increased as required; max. 320 mg daily
Angina, 80–160 mg daily in 2–3 divided doses; max. 320 mg daily
Arrhythmias, 40–240 mg daily in 2–3 divided doses; max. 240 mg daily
Anxiety symptoms (short-term use), 40–80 mg daily in 1–2 divided doses

Oxprenolol (Non-proprietary) [PoM]
Tablets, all coated, oxprenolol hydrochloride 20 mg, net price 20 = 55p; 40 mg, 20 = £1.11; 80 mg, 20 = £2.21; 160 mg, 20 = £2.36. Label: 8
Available from Hillcross, IVAX

Trasicor® (Novartis) [PoM]
Tablets, all f/c, oxprenolol hydrochloride 20 mg (contain gluten), net price 56-tab pack = £1.55; 40 mg (contain gluten), 56-tab pack = £3.11; 80 mg (yellow), 56-tab pack = £6.20. Label: 8

■ Modified release

Slow-Trasicor® (Novartis) [PoM]
Tablets, m/r, f/c, oxprenolol hydrochloride 160 mg. Net price 28-tab pack = £6.63. Label: 8, 25
Dose: hypertension, angina, initially 160 mg once daily; if necessary may be increased to max. 320 mg daily
Note. Modified-release tablets containing oxprenolol hydrochloride 160 mg also available from IVAX

■ With diuretic

Trasidrex® (Novartis) [PoM]
Tablets, red, s/c, co-prenozide 160/0.25 (oxprenolol hydrochloride 160 mg (m/r), cyclopenthiazide 250 micrograms). Net price 28-tab pack = £8.88. Label: 8, 25
Dose: hypertension, 1 tablet daily, increased if necessary to 2 daily as a single dose

PINDOLOL
Indications: see under Dose
Cautions: see under Propranolol Hydrochloride; reduce dose in renal impairment
Contra-indications: see under Propranolol Hydrochloride
Side-effects: see under Propranolol Hydrochloride
Dose: hypertension, initially 5 mg 2–3 times daily *or* 15 mg once daily, increased as required at weekly intervals; usual maintenance 15–30 mg daily; max. 45 mg daily
Angina, 2.5–5 mg up to 3 times daily

Visken® (Novartis) [PoM]
Tablets, both scored, pindolol 5 mg, net price 56-tab pack = £4.88; 15 mg, 28-tab pack = £7.33. Label: 8

■ With diuretic

Viskaldix® (Novartis) [PoM]
Tablets, scored, pindolol 10 mg, clopamide 5 mg. Net price 28-tab pack = £6.70. Label: 8
Dose: hypertension, 1 tablet daily in the morning, increased if necessary to 2 daily; max. 3 daily

SOTALOL HYDROCHLORIDE
Indications: *Tablets and injection:* life-threatening arrhythmias including ventricular tachyarrhythmias, symptomatic non-sustained ventricular tachyarrhythmias
Tablets only: prophylaxis of paroxysmal atrial tachycardia or fibrillation, paroxysmal AV re-entrant tachycardias (both nodal and involving accessory pathways), paroxysmal supraventricular tachycardia after cardiac surgery, maintenance of sinus rhythm following cardioversion of atrial fibrillation or flutter
Injection only: electrophysiological study of inducible ventricular and supraventricular arrhythmias; temporary substitution for tablets
CSM advice. The use of sotalol should be limited to the treatment of ventricular arrhythmias or prophylaxis of supraventricular arrhythmias (see above). It should no longer be used for angina, hypertension, thyrotoxicosis or for secondary prevention after myocardial infarction; when stopping sotalol for these indications, the dose should be reduced gradually
Cautions: see under Propranolol Hydrochloride; reduce dose in renal impairment (avoid if severe); correct hypokalaemia, hypomagnesaemia, or other electrolyte disturbances; severe or prolonged diarrhoea; **interactions:** Appendix 1 (beta-blockers), **important:** verapamil interaction see also p. 107
Contra-indications: see under Propranolol Hydrochloride; congenital or acquired long QT syndrome; torsades de pointes; renal failure
Side-effects: see under Propranolol Hydrochloride; arrhythmogenic (pro-arrhythmic) effect (torsades de pointes—increased risk in women)
Dose: *by mouth* with ECG monitoring and measurement of corrected QT interval, arrhythmias, initially 80 mg daily in 1–2 divided doses increased gradually at intervals of 2–3 days to usual dose of 160–320 mg daily in 2 divided doses; higher doses of 480–640 mg daily for life-threatening ventricular arrhythmias under specialist supervision
By intravenous injection over 10 minutes, acute arrhythmias, 20–120 mg with ECG monitoring,

repeated if necessary with 6-hour intervals between injections

Diagnostic use, see product literature

Note. Excessive bradycardia can be countered with intravenous injection of atropine sulphate 0.6–2.4 mg in divided doses of 600 micrograms; for **overdosage** see Emergency Treatment of Poisoning, p. 25

Sotalol (Non-proprietary) PoM

Tablets, both scored, sotalol hydrochloride 40 mg, net price 20 = 79p; 80 mg, 28-tab pack = £1.64; 160 mg, 28-tab pack = £6.19. Label: 8

Available from Generics, Hillcross, Tillomed

Beta-Cardone® (Celltech) PoM

Tablets, all scored, sotalol hydrochloride 40 mg (green), net price 56-tab pack = £2.22; 80 mg (pink), 56-tab pack = £3.29; 200 mg, 28-tab pack = £4.15. Label: 8

Sotacor® (Bristol-Myers Squibb) PoM

Tablets, sotalol hydrochloride 80 mg, net price 28-tab pack = £3.49; 160 mg, 28-tab pack = £6.89. Label: 8

Injection, sotalol hydrochloride 10 mg/mL. Net price 4-mL amp = £1.76

TIMOLOL MALEATE

Indications: see under Dose; glaucoma (section 11.6)

Cautions: see under Propranolol Hydrochloride

Contra-indications: see under Propranolol Hydrochloride

Side-effects: see under Propranolol Hydrochloride

Dose: hypertension, initially 5 mg twice daily *or* 10 mg once daily; gradually increased if necessary to max. 60 mg daily (given in divided doses above 20 mg daily)

Angina, initially 5 mg 2–3 times daily, usual maintenance 35–45 mg daily (range 15–45 mg daily)

Prophylaxis after myocardial infarction, initially 5 mg twice daily, increased after 2 days to 10 mg twice daily, starting 7 to 28 days after infarction

Migraine prophylaxis, 10–20 mg once daily

Betim® (ICN) PoM

Tablets, scored, timolol maleate 10 mg. Net price 30-tab pack = £2.45. Label: 8

■ With diuretic

Moducren® (MSD) PoM

Tablets, blue, scored, timolol maleate 10 mg, co-amilozide 2.5/25 (amiloride hydrochloride 2.5 mg, hydrochlorothiazide 25 mg). Net price 28-tab pack = £8.00. Label: 8

Dose: hypertension, 1–2 tablets daily as a single dose

Prestim® (ICN) PoM

Tablets, scored, timolol maleate 10 mg, bendroflumethiazide 2.5 mg. Net price 30-tab pack = £4.11. Label: 8

Dose: hypertension, 1–2 tablets daily; max. 4 daily

2.5 Drugs affecting the renin-angiotensin system and some other antihypertensive drugs

2.5.1	Vasodilator antihypertensive drugs
2.5.2	Centrally acting antihypertensive drugs
2.5.3	Adrenergic neurone blocking drugs
2.5.4	Alpha-adrenoceptor blocking drugs
2.5.5	Drugs affecting the renin-angiotensin system
2.5.6	Ganglion-blocking drugs
2.5.7	Tyrosine hydroxylase inhibitors

Lowering raised blood pressure decreases the frequency of stroke, coronary events, heart failure, and renal failure. Advice on antihypertensive therapy in this section reflects the recommendations of the British Hypertension Society (Guidelines for management of hypertension: report of the third working party of the British Hypertension Society. *J Hum Hypertens* 1999; **13**: 569–92).

Possible causes of hypertension (e.g. renal disease, endocrine causes), contributory factors, risk factors, and the presence of any complications of hypertension, such as left ventricular hypertrophy, should be established. Patients should be given advice on lifestyle changes to reduce blood pressure or cardiovascular risk; these include smoking cessation, weight reduction, reduction of alcohol intake, reduction of dietary sodium, reduction of total and saturated fat, increasing exercise, and increasing fruit and vegetable intake.

THRESHOLDS AND TARGETS FOR TREATMENT. The following thresholds for treatment are recommended:

- Accelerated (malignant) hypertension (with papilloedema or fundal haemorrhages and exudates) *or* impending cardiovascular complications, admit for **immediate treatment**;
- Where the initial blood pressure is systolic ≥ 220 mmHg *or* diastolic ≥ 120 mmHg, **treat immediately**;
- Where the initial blood pressure is systolic 200–219 mmHg *or* diastolic 110–119 mmHg, confirm over 1–2 weeks then **treat** if these values are sustained;
- Where the initial blood pressure is systolic 160–199 mmHg *or* diastolic 100–109 mmHg, *and* the patient has cardiovascular complications, end-organ damage (e.g. left ventricular hypertrophy, renal impairment) or diabetes mellitus (type 1 or 2), confirm over 3–4 weeks then **treat** if these values are sustained;
- Where the initial blood pressure is systolic 160–199 mmHg *or* diastolic 100–109 mmHg, but the patient has *no* cardiovascular complications, end-organ damage or diabetes, advise lifestyle changes, reassess weekly initially and **treat** if these values are sustained on repeat measurements over 4–12 weeks;
- Where the initial blood pressure is systolic 140–159 mmHg *or* diastolic 90–99 mmHg *and* the patient has cardiovascular complications, end-organ damage or diabetes, confirm within 4–12 weeks and **treat** if these values are sustained;
- Where the initial blood pressure is systolic 140–159 mmHg *or* diastolic 90–99 mmHg and *no* cardiovascular complications, end-organ damage or dia-

betes, advise lifestyle changes and **reassess** monthly; if mild hypertension persists, **treat** if coronary heart disease risk[1] is ≥ 15% over 10 years.

An optimal target systolic blood pressure < 140 mmHg *and* diastolic blood pressure < 85 mmHg is suggested; the target in diabetes and in renal disease is lower—see below.

DRUG TREATMENT OF HYPERTENSION. Low-dose *thiazides* (section 2.2.1) reduce coronary events, cardiovascular mortality and all-cause mortality. A thiazide is first-line treatment for hypertension unless there is a contra-indication or a specific indication for another drug (see below). A low dose is adequate and higher doses (e.g. more than 2.5 mg bendroflumethiazide (bendrofluazide) or 25 mg hydrochlorthiazide) have no additional antihypertensive effect and increase metabolic side-effects.

A beta-blocker is sometimes preferred as alternative first-line therapy; however, in some individuals there may be contra-indications to these drugs or indications for other antihypertensive drugs. No consistent or important differences have been found between the major classes of antihypertensive drugs in terms of antihypertensive efficacy, side-effects or changes to quality of life (although there have been differences in average response related to age and ethnic group). The choice of antihypertensive drug will depend on the relevant indications or contra-indications for the individual patient; where there are no special considerations, the least expensive drug should be selected. *Some* indications and contra-indications for various antihypertensive drugs are shown below (see also under individual drug entries for details):

- **Thiazides** (section 2.2.1)—particularly indicated for hypertension in the elderly (see below); a contra-indication is gout;
- **Beta-blockers** (section 2.4)—indications include myocardial infarction, angina; compelling contra-indications include asthma, heart block;
- **ACE inhibitors** (section 2.5.5.1)—indications include heart failure, left ventricular dysfunction and diabetic nephropathy; contra-indications include ren-ovascular disease (but see section 2.5.5.1) and pregnancy;
- **Calcium-channel blockers**. There are important differences between calcium-channel blockers (section 2.6.2). **Dihydropyridine calcium-channel blockers** are valuable in isolated systolic hypertension in the elderly when a low-dose thiazide is contra-indicated or not tolerated (see below). 'Rate-limiting' calcium-channel blockers (e.g. diltiazem, verapamil) may be valuable in angina; contra-indications include heart failure and heart block;
- **Alpha-blockers** (section 2.5.4)—a possible indication is prostatism; a contra-indication is urinary incontinence;
- **Angiotensin-II receptor antagonists** (section 2.5.5.2) are alternatives for those who cannot tolerate ACE inhibitors because of persistent dry cough, but they have the same contra-indications as ACE inhibitors.

A single antihypertensive drug is often not adequate and other antihypertensive drugs are usually added in a step-wise manner until control is achieved. Unless it is necessary to lower the blood pressure urgently, an interval of at least 4 weeks should be allowed to determine response. In uncomplicated mild hypertension (systolic blood pressure < 160 mmHg and diastolic < 100 mmHg), drugs may be substituted rather than added.

Response to drug treatment for hypertension may be affected by the patient's ethnic background; in Afro-Caribbean subjects the response to beta-blockers and to ACE inhibitors may be reduced.

OTHER MEASURES TO REDUCE CARDIOVAS-CULAR RISK. **Aspirin** (section 2.9) in a dose of 75 mg daily reduces the risk of cardiovascular events and myocardial infarction; however, concerns about an increased risk of bleeding need to be considered. Unless it is contra-indicated, aspirin is recommended for *secondary prevention* in patients with cardiovascular complications (myocardial infarction, angina, non-haemorrhagic cerebrovascular disease, peripheral vascular disease, or atherosclerotic renovascular disease), and for *primary prevention* in patients aged over 50 years with controlled blood pressure (systolic pressure < 150 mmHg and diastolic pressure < 90 mmHg) who have end-organ damage, type 2 diabetes, or a coronary heart disease risk[1] ≥ 15% over 10 years.

A **statin** (section 2.12) is indicated when serum total cholesterol concentration is ≥ 5 mmol/litre, for *secondary prevention* (in patients with a history of myocardial infarction, coronary artery bypass graft, angioplasty, non-haemorrhagic cerebrovascular disease, peripheral vascular disease or atherosclerotic renovascular disease), for *primary prevention* in patients who have a coronary heart disease risk[1] of ≥ 30% over 10 years, and for *familial hypercholesterolaemia*.

HYPERTENSION IN THE ELDERLY. Benefit from antihypertensive therapy is evident up to at least 85 years of age, but it is probably inappropriate to apply a strict age limit when deciding on drug therapy. Elderly individuals who have a good outlook for longevity should have their blood pressure lowered if they are hypertensive. The thresholds for treatment are diastolic pressure averaging ≥ 90 mmHg *or* systolic pressure averaging ≥ 160 mmHg over 3 to 6 months' observation (despite appropriate non-drug treatment). A low dose of a thiazide is the clear drug of first choice, with addition of a beta-blocker when necessary.

ISOLATED SYSTOLIC HYPERTENSION. Isolated systolic hypertension (systolic pressure ≥ 160 mmHg, diastolic pressure < 90 mmHg) is associated with an increased risk of stroke and coronary events, particularly in those aged over 60 years. Systolic blood pressure averaging 160 mmHg or higher over 3 to 6 months (despite appropriate non-drug treatment) should be lowered in those over 60 years, even if diastolic hypertension is absent. Treatment with a low dose of a thiazide, with addition of a beta-blocker when necessary is effective; a long-acting dihydropyridine calcium-channel blocker is recommended when a thiazide is contra-indicated or not tolerated. Patients with severe postural hypotension should not receive blood pressure lowering drugs.

Isolated systolic hypertension in younger patients is uncommon but treatment may be indicated in those

---

1. Coronary heart disease risk may be formally estimated using the Joint British Societies' 'Cardiac Risk Assessor' computer program or chart (British Cardiac Society, British Hyperlipidaemia Association, British Hypertension Society. *Heart* 1998; **80**(suppl 2): S1–29)

See inside back cover

with a threshold systolic pressure of 160 mmHg (or less if at increased risk of coronary heart disease, see above).

HYPERTENSION IN DIABETES. Hypertension is common in type 2 (non-insulin-dependent) diabetes and treatment prevents both macrovascular and microvascular complications. Systolic blood pressure ≥ 140 mmHg *or* diastolic pressure ≥ 90 mmHg should be lowered to a target systolic blood pressure < 140 mmHg and a diastolic pressure < 80 mmHg. Low-dose thiazides, beta-blockers, ACE inhibitors and dihydropyridine calcium-channel blockers have all shown benefit in type 2 diabetes.

In type 1 (insulin-dependent) diabetes, hypertension usually indicates the presence of diabetic nephropathy and ACE inhibitors have a specific role in this condition (section 6.1.5). The threshold for treatment of hypertension in type 1 diabetes is the same as that for type 2 diabetes, and the target for patients without nephropathy is a systolic blood pressure < 140 mmHg and a diastolic pressure < 80 mmHg; if nephropathy is present the target is a systolic blood pressure < 130 mmHg and a diastolic pressure < 80 mmHg, or even lower if proteinuria exceeds 1 g in 24 hours.

HYPERTENSION IN RENAL DISEASE. The threshold for antihypertensive treatment in patients with renal impairment or persistent proteinuria is a systolic blood pressure ≥ 140 mmHg *or* a diastolic blood pressure ≥ 90 mmHg. Optimal blood pressure is a systolic blood pressure < 130 mmHg and a diastolic pressure < 85 mmHg, or lower if proteinuria exceeds 1 g in 24 hours. Thiazides may be ineffective and high doses of loop diuretics may be required. Specific cautions apply to the use of ACE inhibitors in renal impairment, see section 2.5.5.1.

HYPERTENSION IN PREGNANCY. High blood pressure in pregnancy may usually be due to pre-existing essential hypertension or to pre-eclampsia. Methyldopa (section 2.5.2) is safe in pregnancy. Beta-blockers are effective and safe in the third trimester. Modified-release preparations of nifedipine [unlicensed] are also used for hypertension in pregnancy. Intravenous administration of labetalol (section 2.4) can be used to control hypertensive crises; alternatively hydralazine (section 2.5.1) may be used by the intravenous route. For use of magnesium sulphate in eclampsia, see section 9.5.1.3.

ACCELERATED OR VERY SEVERE HYPERTENSION. Accelerated (or malignant) hypertension or very severe hypertension (e.g. diastolic blood pressure > 140 mmHg) requires urgent treatment in hospital, but it is not an indication for parenteral antihypertensive therapy. Normally treatment should be by mouth with a beta-blocker (atenolol or labetalol) or a long-acting calcium-channel blocker (e.g. amlodipine or modified-release nifedipine). Within the first 24 hours the diastolic blood pressure should be reduced to 100–110 mmHg. Over the next 2 or 3 days blood pressure should be normalised by using beta-blockers, calcium-channel blockers, diuretics, vasodilators, or ACE inhibitors. Very rapid reduction in blood pressure can reduce organ perfusion leading to cerebral infarction and blindness, deterioration in renal function, and myocardial ischaemia. Parenteral antihypertensive drugs are rarely necessary; sodium nitroprusside by infusion is the drug of choice on the rare occasions when parenteral treatment is necessary.

For advice on short-term management of hypertensive episodes in phaeochromocytoma, see notes on phaeochromocytoma (section 2.5.4).

2.5.1 Vasodilator antihypertensive drugs

These are potent drugs, especially when used in combination with a beta-blocker and a thiazide. **Important:** for a warning on the hazards of a very rapid fall in blood pressure, see section 2.5.

Diazoxide has been used by intravenous injection in hypertensive emergencies.

Hydralazine given by mouth is a useful adjunct to other treatment, but when used alone causes tachycardia and fluid retention. Side-effects can be few if the dose is kept below 100 mg daily, but systemic lupus erythematosus should be suspected if there is unexplained weight loss, arthritis, or any other unexplained ill health.

Sodium nitroprusside is given by intravenous infusion to control severe hypertensive crises on the rare occasions when parenteral treatment is necessary.

Minoxidil should be reserved for the treatment of severe hypertension resistant to other drugs. Vasodilatation is accompanied by increased cardiac output and tachycardia and the patients develop fluid retention. For this reason the addition of a beta-blocker and a diuretic (usually furosemide, in high dosage) are mandatory. Hypertrichosis is troublesome and renders this drug unsuitable for women.

Prazosin, doxazosin, and terazosin (section 2.5.4) have alpha-blocking and vasodilator properties.

DIAZOXIDE

Indications: severe hypertension associated with renal disease (but see section 2.5); hypoglycaemia (section 6.1.4)

Cautions: ischaemic heart disease, pregnancy, labour, impaired renal function; **interactions:** Appendix 1 (diazoxide)

Side-effects: tachycardia, hyperglycaemia, sodium and water retention

Dose: *by rapid intravenous injection* (less than 30 seconds), 1–3 mg/kg to max. single dose of 150 mg (see below); may be repeated after 5–15 minutes if required

Note. Single doses of 300 mg have been associated with angina and with myocardial and cerebral infarction

Eudemine® (Goldshield) [PoM] ◢

Injection, diazoxide 15 mg/mL. Net price 20-mL amp = £30.00

◢ denotes preparations that are considered to be less suitable for prescribing (see p. vi)

HYDRALAZINE HYDROCHLORIDE

Indications: moderate to severe hypertension (adjunct); heart failure (with long-acting nitrate, but see section 2.5.5); hypertensive crisis (including during pregnancy) (but see section 2.5)

Cautions: hepatic impairment (Appendix 2), renal impairment (Appendix 3); coronary artery disease (may provoke angina, avoid after myocardial infarction until stabilised), cerebrovascular disease; occasionally blood pressure reduction too rapid even with low parenteral doses; pregnancy (Appendix 4), breast-feeding; manufacturer advises test for antinuclear factor and for proteinuria every 6 months and check acetylator status before increasing dose above 100 mg daily, but evidence of clinical value unsatisfactory; **interactions:** Appendix 1 (hydralazine)

Contra-indications: idiopathic systemic lupus erythematosus, severe tachycardia, high output heart failure, myocardial insufficiency due to mechanical obstruction, cor pulmonale, dissecting aortic aneurysm; porphyria (section 9.8.2)

Side-effects: tachycardia, palpitations, flushing, hypotension, fluid retention, gastro-intestinal disturbances; headache, dizziness; systemic lupus erythematosus-like syndrome after long-term therapy with over 100 mg daily (or less in women and in slow acetylator individuals) (see also notes above); rarely rashes, fever, peripheral neuritis, polyneuritis, paraesthesia, arthralgia, myalgia, increased lacrimation, nasal congestion, dyspnoea, agitation, anxiety, anorexia; blood disorders (including leucopenia, thrombocytopenia, haemolytic anaemia), abnormal liver function, jaundice, raised plasma creatinine, proteinuria and haematuria reported

Dose: *by mouth*, hypertension, 25 mg twice daily, increased to usual max. 50 mg twice daily (see notes above)
Heart failure (initiated in hospital) 25 mg 3–4 times daily, increased every 2 days if necessary; usual maintenance dose 50–75 mg 4 times daily
By slow intravenous injection, hypertension with renal complications and hypertensive crisis, 5–10 mg diluted with 10 mL sodium chloride 0.9%; may be repeated after 20–30 minutes (see Cautions)
By intravenous infusion, hypertension with renal complications and hypertensive crisis, initially 200–300 micrograms/minute; maintenance usually 50–150 micrograms/minute

Hydralazine (Non-proprietary) PoM
Tablets, hydralazine hydrochloride 25 mg, net price 20 = 54p; 50 mg, 20 = £1.05

Apresoline® (Alliance) PoM
Tablets, yellow, s/c, hydralazine hydrochloride 25 mg, net price 84-tab pack = £2.35
Excipients: include gluten
Injection, powder for reconstitution, hydralazine hydrochloride. Net price 20-mg amp = £1.54

MINOXIDIL

Indications: severe hypertension, in addition to a diuretic and a beta-blocker

Cautions: see notes above; angina; after myocardial infarction (until stabilised); lower doses in dialysis patients; pregnancy; porphyria (section 9.8.2); **interactions:** Appendix 1 (minoxidil)

Contra-indications: phaeochromocytoma

Side-effects: sodium and water retention; weight gain, peripheral oedema, tachycardia, hypertrichosis; reversible rise in creatinine and blood urea nitrogen; occasionally, gastro-intestinal disturbances, breast tenderness, rashes

Dose: initially 5 mg (elderly, 2.5 mg) daily, in 1–2 doses, increased by 5–10 mg every 3 or more days; max. usually 50 mg daily

Loniten® (Pharmacia) PoM
Tablets, all scored, minoxidil 2.5 mg, net price 60-tab pack = £7.07; 5 mg, 60-tab pack = £12.59; 10 mg, 60-tab pack = £24.42

SODIUM NITROPRUSSIDE

Indications: hypertensive crisis (but see section 2.5); controlled hypotension in anaesthesia; acute or chronic heart failure

Cautions: hypothyroidism, renal impairment, hyponatraemia, ischaemic heart disease, impaired cerebral circulation, elderly; hypothermia; monitor blood pressure and blood-cyanide concentration and if treatment exceeds 3 days, also blood-thiocyanate concentration; avoid sudden withdrawal—terminate infusion over 15–30 minutes; pregnancy and breast-feeding; **interactions:** Appendix 1 (nitroprusside)

Contra-indications: severe hepatic impairment; severe vitamin B_{12} deficiency; Leber's optic atrophy; compensatory hypertension

Side-effects: associated with over rapid reduction in blood pressure (reduce infusion rate): headache, dizziness, nausea, retching, abdominal pain, perspiration, palpitations, apprehension, retrosternal discomfort; occasionally reduced platelet count, acute transient phlebitis
CYANIDE. Side-effects caused by excessive plasma concentration of the cyanide metabolite include tachycardia, sweating, hyperventilation, arrhythmias, marked metabolic acidosis (discontinue and give antidote, see pp.26–7)

Dose: hypertensive crisis, *by intravenous infusion*, initially 0.5–1.5 micrograms/kg/minute, then increased in steps of 500 nanograms/kg/minute every 5 minutes within range 0.5–8 micrograms/kg/minute (lower doses in patients already receiving other antihypertensives); stop if response unsatisfactory with max. dose in 10 minutes
Note. Lower initial dose of 300 nanograms/kg/minute has been used
Maintenance of blood pressure at 30–40% lower than pretreatment diastolic blood pressure, 20–400 micrograms/minute (lower doses for patients being treated with other antihypertensives)
Controlled hypotension in surgery, *by intravenous infusion*, max. 1.5 micrograms/kg/minute
Heart failure, *by intravenous infusion*, initially 10–15 micrograms/minute, increased every 5–10 minutes as necessary; usual range 10–200 micrograms/minute normally for max. 3 days

Sodium Nitroprusside (Non-proprietary) PoM
Intravenous solution, sodium nitroprusside 10 mg/mL. For dilution and use as an infusion, net price 5-mL vial = £6.64
Available from Faulding DBL

2.5.2 Centrally acting antihypertensive drugs

Methyldopa is a centrally acting antihypertensive; it may be used for the management of hypertension in pregnancy. Side-effects are minimised if the daily dose is kept below 1 g.

Clonidine has the disadvantage that sudden withdrawal may cause a hypertensive crisis. Reserpine and rauwolfia are no longer used in Britain.

Moxonidine, a centrally acting drug, is licensed for mild to moderate essential hypertension. It may have a role when thiazides, beta-blockers, ACE inhibitors and calcium-channel blockers are not appropriate or have failed to control blood pressure.

CLONIDINE HYDROCHLORIDE ◢

Indications: hypertension; migraine (section 4.7.4.2); menopausal flushing (section 6.4.1.1)

Cautions: must be withdrawn gradually to avoid hypertensive crisis; Raynaud's syndrome or other occlusive peripheral vascular disease; history of depression; avoid in porphyria (section 9.8.2); **interactions:** Appendix 1 (clonidine)

DRIVING. Drowsiness may affect performance of skilled tasks (e.g. driving); effects of alcohol may be enhanced

Side-effects: dry mouth, sedation, depression, fluid retention, bradycardia, Raynaud's phenomenon, headache, dizziness, euphoria, nocturnal unrest, rash, nausea, constipation, rarely impotence

Dose: *by mouth,* 50–100 micrograms 3 times daily, increased every second or third day; usual max. dose 1.2 mg daily

By slow intravenous injection, 150–300 micrograms; max. 750 micrograms in 24 hours

Catapres® (Boehringer Ingelheim) PoM ◢
Tablets, both scored, clonidine hydrochloride 100 micrograms, net price 100-tab pack = £5.60; 300 micrograms, 100-tab pack = £13.04. Label: 3, 8

Injection, clonidine hydrochloride 150 micrograms/mL. Net price 1-mL amp = 29p

Dixarit® PoM ◢ (migraine), section 4.7.4.2

◢ denotes preparations that are considered to be less suitable for prescribing (see p. vi)

METHYLDOPA

Indications: hypertension

Cautions: history of liver impairment (Appendix 2); renal impairment (Appendix 3); blood counts and liver-function tests advised; history of depression; positive direct Coombs' test in up to 20% of patients (may affect blood cross-matching); interference with laboratory tests; **interactions:** Appendix 1 (methyldopa)

DRIVING. Drowsiness may affect performance of skilled tasks (e.g. driving); effects of alcohol may be enhanced

Contra-indications: depression, active liver disease, phaeochromocytoma; porphyria (section 9.8.2)

Side-effects: gastro-intestinal disturbances, dry mouth, stomatitis, sialadenitis; bradycardia, exacerbation of angina, postural hypotension, oedema; sedation, headache, dizziness, asthenia, myalgia, arthralgia, paraesthesia, nightmares, mild psychosis, depression, impaired mental acuity, parkinsonism, Bell's palsy; abnormal liver function tests, hepatitis, jaundice; pancreatitis; haemolytic anaemia; bone-marrow depression, leucopenia, thrombocytopenia, eosinophilia; hypersensitivity reactions including lupus erythematosus-like syndrome, drug fever, myocarditis, pericarditis; rashes (including toxic epidermal necrolysis); nasal congestion, failure of ejaculation, impotence, decreased libido, gynaecomastia, hyperprolactinaemia, amenorrhoea

Dose: initially 250 mg 2–3 times daily, increased gradually at intervals of 2 or more days, max. 3 g daily; ELDERLY initially 125 mg twice daily, increased gradually, max. 2 g daily

Methyldopa (Non-proprietary) PoM
Tablets, coated, methyldopa (anhydrous) 125 mg, net price 20 = 54p; 250 mg, 20 = 60p; 500 mg, 20 = £1.23. Label: 3, 8

Available from Alpharma, CP, Hillcross, IVAX, Sovereign

Aldomet® (MSD) PoM
Tablets, all yellow, f/c, methyldopa (anhydrous) 250 mg, net price 20 = 63p; 500 mg, 20 = £1.27. Label: 3, 8

MOXONIDINE

Indications: mild to moderate essential hypertension

Cautions: renal impairment (see Appendix 3); avoid abrupt withdrawal (if concomitant treatment with beta-blocker has to be stopped, discontinue beta-blocker first, then moxonidine after few days); **interactions:** see Appendix 1 (moxonidine)

Contra-indications: history of angioedema; conduction disorders (sick sinus syndrome, sinoatrial block, second- or third-degree AV block); bradycardia; life-threatening arrhythmia; severe heart failure; severe coronary artery disease, unstable angina; severe liver disease or severe renal impairment; also on theoretical grounds: Raynaud's syndrome, intermittent claudication, epilepsy, depression, Parkinson's disease, glaucoma; pregnancy and breast-feeding

Side-effects: dry mouth; headache, fatigue, dizziness, nausea, sleep disturbance (rarely sedation), asthenia, vasodilatation; rarely skin reactions

Dose: 200 micrograms once daily in the morning, increased if necessary after 3 weeks to 400 micrograms daily in 1–2 divided doses; max. 600 micrograms daily in 2 divided doses (max. single dose 400 micrograms)

Physiotens® (Solvay) ▼ PoM
Tablets, f/c, moxonidine 200 micrograms (pink), net price 28-tab pack = £10.45; 300 micrograms (red), 28-tab pack = £12.35; 400 micrograms (red), 28-tab pack = £14.26. Label: 3

2.5.3 Adrenergic neurone blocking drugs

Adrenergic neurone blocking drugs prevent the release of noradrenaline from postganglionic adrenergic neurones. Guanethidine also depletes the nerve endings of noradrenaline. These drugs do not control supine blood pressure and may cause postural hypotension. For this reason they have largely fallen from use, but may be necessary with other therapy in resistant hypertension.

GUANETHIDINE MONOSULPHATE ▰

Indications: hypertensive crisis (but see section 2.5)
Cautions: renal impairment (avoid if creatinine clearance < 40 mL/minute; Appendix 3); coronary or cerebral arteriosclerosis, asthma, history of peptic ulceration; pregnancy; **interactions:** Appendix 1 (adrenergic neurone blockers)
Contra-indications: phaeochromocytoma, heart failure
Side-effects: postural hypotension, failure of ejaculation, fluid retention, nasal congestion, headache, diarrhoea, drowsiness
Dose: *by intramuscular injection,* 10–20 mg, repeated after 3 hours if required

Ismelin® (Alliance) PoM ▰
Injection, guanethidine monosulphate 10 mg/mL. Net price 1-mL amp = £1.56

DEBRISOQUINE ▰

Indications: hypertension
Cautions: see under Guanethidine Monosulphate
Contra-indications: see under Guanethidine Monosulphate
Side-effects: see under Guanethidine Monosulphate (except diarrhoea)
Dose: 10 mg 1–2 times daily, increased by 10 mg every 3 days; usual range 20–60 mg daily (120 mg or higher in severe hypertension)

Debrisoquine (Cambridge) PoM ▰
Tablets, scored, debrisoquine (as sulphate) 10 mg, net price 100-tab pack = £18.55

▰ denotes preparations that are considered to be less suitable for prescribing (see p. vi)

2.5.4 Alpha-adrenoceptor blocking drugs

Prazosin has post-synaptic alpha-blocking and vasodilator properties and rarely causes tachycardia. It may, however, cause a rapid reduction in blood pressure after the first dose and should be introduced with caution. **Doxazosin, indoramin,** and **terazosin** have properties similar to those of prazosin.

Alpha-blockers may be used with other antihypertensive drugs in the treatment of hypertension.

PROSTATIC HYPERPLASIA. Alfuzosin, doxazosin, indoramin, prazosin, tamsulosin and terazosin are indicated for benign prostatic hyperplasia (section 7.4.1).

DOXAZOSIN

Indications: hypertension; benign prostatic hyperplasia (section 7.4.1)
Cautions: care with initial dose (postural hypotension); hepatic impairment (Appendix 2); susceptibility to heart failure; pregnancy (Appendix 4) and breast-feeding (Appendix 5); **interactions:** Appendix 1 (alpha-blockers)
Side-effects: postural hypotension; dizziness, vertigo, headache, fatigue, asthenia, oedema, somnolence, nausea, rhinitis; less frequently abdominal discomfort, diarrhoea, vomiting, agitation, tremor, rash, pruritus; rarely blurred vision, epistaxis, haematuria, thrombocytopenia, purpura, leucopenia, hepatitis, jaundice, cholestasis, and urinary incontinence; isolated cases of priapism and impotence reported
Dose: hypertension, 1 mg daily, increased after 1–2 weeks to 2 mg once daily, and thereafter to 4 mg once daily, if necessary; max. 16 mg daily

Cardura® (Pfizer) PoM
Tablets, doxazosin (as mesilate) 1 mg, net price 28-tab pack = £10.56; 2 mg, 28-tab pack = £14.08

■ Modified-release
Cardura® **XL** (Pfizer) PoM
Tablets, m/r, doxazosin (as mesilate) 4 mg, net price 28-tab pack = £14.08; 8 mg, 28-tab pack = £28.16. Label: 25
Dose: 4 mg once daily, increased to 8 mg once daily after 4 weeks if necessary

INDORAMIN

Indications: hypertension; benign prostatic hyperplasia (section 7.4.1)
Cautions: avoid alcohol (enhances rate and extent of absorption); control incipient heart failure with diuretics and digoxin; hepatic or renal impairment; elderly patients; Parkinson's disease; epilepsy (convulsions in *animal* studies); history of depression; **interactions:** Appendix 1 (alpha-blockers)
DRIVING. Drowsiness may affect performance of skilled tasks (e.g. driving); effects of alcohol may be enhanced
Contra-indications: established heart failure; patients receiving MAOIs
Side-effects: sedation; also dizziness, depression, failure of ejaculation, dry mouth, nasal congestion, extrapyramidal effects, weight gain
Dose: hypertension, initially 25 mg twice daily, increased by 25–50 mg daily at intervals of 2 weeks; max. daily dose 200 mg in 2–3 divided doses

Baratol® (Shire) PoM
Tablets, blue, f/c, indoramin (as hydrochloride) 25 mg, net price 84-tab pack = £9.00. Label: 2

■ Prostatic hyperplasia
Doralese® PoM see section 7.4.1

PRAZOSIN

Indications: see under Dose

Cautions: first dose may cause collapse due to hypotension (therefore should be taken on retiring to bed); elderly; renal impairment (Appendix 3), hepatic impairment (Appendix 2); pregnancy and breast-feeding; **interactions:** Appendix 1 (alpha-blockers)

Contra-indications: not recommended for congestive heart failure due to mechanical obstruction (e.g. aortic stenosis)

Side-effects: postural hypotension, drowsiness, weakness, dizziness, headache, lack of energy, nausea, palpitations; urinary frequency, incontinence and priapism reported

Dose: hypertension, 500 micrograms 2–3 times daily, the initial dose on retiring to bed at night (to avoid collapse, see Cautions); increased to 1 mg 2–3 times daily after 3–7 days; further increased if necessary to max. 20 mg daily

Congestive heart failure (but see section 2.5.5), 500 micrograms 2–4 times daily (initial dose at bedtime, see above), increasing to 4 mg daily in divided doses; maintenance 4–20 mg daily (but rarely used)

Raynaud's syndrome (but efficacy not established, see section 2.6.4.1), initially 500 micrograms twice daily (initial dose at bedtime, see above); maintenance 1–2 mg twice daily

Benign prostatic hyperplasia, section 7.4.1

Prazosin (Non-proprietary) PoM

Tablets, prazosin (as hydrochloride)
500 micrograms, net price 56-tab pack = £2.29; 1 mg, 56-tab pack = £2.82; 2 mg, 56-tab pack = £4.06; 5 mg, 56-tab pack = £8.79. Label: 3, counselling, see dose above

Available from Alpharma, APS, Ashbourne (*Alpha-vase®*), Hillcross, IVAX

Hypovase® (Pfizer) PoM

Tablets, prazosin (as hydrochloride)
500 micrograms, net price 56-tab pack = £2.09; 1 mg (orange, scored), 56-tab pack = 2 mg (scored), 56-tab pack = £3.66; starter pack of 8 × 500-microgram tabs with 32 × 1-mg tabs = £2.52. Label: 3, counselling, see dose above

TERAZOSIN

Indications: mild to moderate hypertension; benign prostatic hyperplasia (section 7.4.1)

Cautions: first dose may cause collapse due to hypotension (within 30–90 minutes, therefore should be taken on retiring to bed) (may also occur with rapid dose increase); **interactions:** Appendix 1 (alpha-blockers)

Side-effects: dizziness, lack of energy, peripheral oedema; urinary frequency and priapism reported

Dose: hypertension, 1 mg at bedtime (compliance with bedtime dose important, see Cautions); dose doubled after 7 days if necessary; usual maintenance dose 2–10 mg once daily; more than 20 mg daily rarely improves efficacy

Hytrin® (Abbott) PoM

Tablets, terazosin (as hydrochloride) 2 mg (yellow), net price 28-tab pack = £8.07; 5 mg (tan), 28-tab pack = £13.07; 10 mg (blue), 28-tab pack =

£26.59: starter pack of 7 × 1-mg tabs with 21 × 2-mg tabs = £13.00. Label: 3, counselling, see dose above

Phaeochromocytoma

Long-term management of phaeochromocytoma involves surgery. Alpha-blockers are used in the short-term management of hypertensive episodes in phaeochromocytoma. Once alpha blockade is established, tachycardia can be controlled by the cautious addition of a beta-blocker (section 2.4); a cardioselective beta-blocker is preferred.

Phenoxybenzamine, a powerful alpha-blocker, is effective in the management of phaeochromocytoma but it has many side-effects. **Phentolamine** is a short-acting alpha-blocker used mainly during surgery of phaeochromocytoma; its use for the diagnosis of phaeochromocytoma has been superseded by measurement of catecholamines in blood and urine.

PHENOXYBENZAMINE HYDROCHLORIDE

Indications: hypertensive episodes in phaeochromocytoma

Cautions: elderly; congestive heart failure; severe heart disease (see also Contra-indications); cerebrovascular disease (avoid if history of cerebrovascular accident); renal impairment; carcinogenic in *animals*; pregnancy; avoid in porphyria (section 9.8.2); avoid infusion in hypovolaemia; avoid extravasation (irritant to tissues)

Contra-indications: history of cerebrovascular accident; during recovery period after myocardial infarction (usually 3–4 weeks)

Side-effects: postural hypotension with dizziness and marked compensatory tachycardia, lassitude, nasal congestion, miosis, inhibition of ejaculation; rarely gastro-intestinal disturbances; decreased sweating and dry mouth after intravenous infusion; idiosyncratic profound hypotension within few minutes of starting infusion

Dose: see under preparations

Phenoxybenzamine (Goldshield) PoM

Injection concentrate, phenoxybenzamine hydrochloride 50 mg/mL. To be diluted before use. Net price 3 × 2-mL amp = £94.88 (hosp. only)

Dose: by intravenous infusion (preferably through large vein), adjunct in severe shock (but rarely used) and phaeochromocytoma, 1 mg/kg daily over at least 2 hours; do not repeat within 24 hours (intensive care facilities needed)

CAUTION. Owing to risk of contact sensitisation healthcare professionals should avoid contamination of hands

Dibenyline® (Goldshield) PoM

Capsules, red/white, phenoxybenzamine hydrochloride 10 mg. Net price 30-cap pack = £10.84

Dose, phaeochromocytoma, 10 mg daily, increased by 10 mg daily; usual dose 1–2 mg/kg daily in 2 divided doses

PHENTOLAMINE MESILATE

Indications: hypertensive episodes due to phaeochromocytoma e.g. during surgery; diagnosis of phaeochromocytoma

Cautions: monitor blood pressure (avoid in hypotension), heart rate; renal impairment; gastritis, peptic ulcer; elderly; pregnancy and breast-feeding; **interactions:** Appendix 1 (alpha-blockers)

ASTHMA. Presence of sulphites in ampoules may (especially in patients with asthma) lead to hypersensitivity (with bronchospasm and shock)

Contra-indications: hypotension; history of myocardial infarction; coronary insufficiency, angina, or other evidence of coronary artery disease

Side-effects: postural hypotension, tachycardia, dizziness, flushing; nausea and vomiting, diarrhoea, nasal congestion; also acute or prolonged hypotension, angina, chest pain, arrhythmias

Dose: hypertensive episodes, *by intravenous injection*, 2–5 mg repeated if necessary

Diagnosis of phaeochromocytoma, consult product literature

Rogitine® (Alliance) PoM

Injection, phentolamine mesilate 10 mg/mL. Net price 1-mL amp = £1.70

2.5.5 Drugs affecting the renin-angiotensin system

2.5.5.1 Angiotensin-converting enzyme inhibitors

2.5.5.2 Angiotensin-II receptor antagonists

Heart failure

The treatment of chronic heart failure aims to relieve symptoms, improve exercise tolerance, reduce the incidence of acute exacerbations and reduce mortality. An **ACE inhibitor** given at an adequate dose[1], together with a diuretic, generally achieves these aims. Digoxin improves symptoms and exercise tolerance and reduces hospitalisation due to acute exacerbations but it does not reduce mortality. Drug treatment of chronic systolic heart failure is covered below; optimal management of diastolic heart failure is less certain but digoxin should probably be avoided.

An ACE inhibitor (section 2.5.5.1) is generally advised for patients with asymptomatic left ventricular dysfunction or symptomatic heart failure.

Patients with fluid overload should also receive either a loop or a thiazide diuretic (with salt or fluid restriction where appropriate). A **thiazide diuretic** (section 2.2.1) may be of benefit in patients with mild heart failure and good renal function; however, thiazide diuretics are ineffective in patients with poor renal function (estimated creatinine clearance less than 30 mL/minute, see Appendix 3) and a **loop diuretic** (section 2.2.2) is preferred. If diuresis with a single diuretic is insufficient, a combination of a loop diuretic and a thiazide diuretic may be tried; addition of metolazone (section 2.2.1) may also be considered but the resulting diuresis may be pro-

---

1. For heart failure the dose of the ACE inhibitor is titrated to a 'target' dose (or to the maximum tolerated dose if lower). Target doses for some ACE inhibitors may exceed licensed ones, e.g. captopril (target dose 50 mg three times daily), enalapril (10–20 mg twice daily), lisinopril (30–35 mg daily), ramipril (5 mg twice daily), trandolapril (4 mg daily [unlicensed indication])

found and care is needed to avoid potentially dangerous electrolyte disturbances.

The aldosterone antagonist **spironolactone** (section 2.2.3) may be considered for patients with severe heart failure who are already receiving an ACE inhibitor and a diuretic; low doses of spironolactone (usually 25 mg daily) have been shown to reduce symptoms and mortality in these patients. Close monitoring of serum creatinine and potassium is necessary with any change in treatment or in the patient's clinical condition.

The **beta-blockers** carvedilol, bisoprolol and modified-release metoprolol [unlicensed indication] (section 2.4) are of value in selected patients with stable heart failure and left-ventricular systolic dysfunction. Beta-blocker treatment should be started under specialist supervision at a very low dose and titrated very slowly over a period of weeks or months. Symptoms may deteriorate initially, calling for adjustment of concomitant therapy.

Digoxin (section 2.1) is given to patients with atrial fibrillation and also to those in sinus rhythm who remain symptomatic despite treatment with an ACE inhibitor, a diuretic, and a beta-blocker.

Patients who cannot tolerate ACE inhibitors or in whom they are contra-indicated may be given **isosorbide dinitrate** (section 2.6.1) with **hydralazine** (section 2.5.1), but this combination may be poorly tolerated. **Angiotensin-II receptor antagonists** (section 2.5.5.2), although not licensed for heart failure, may be useful alternatives for patients who, because of symptoms such as cough, cannot tolerate ACE inhibitors.

2.5.5.1 Angiotensin-converting enzyme inhibitors

Angiotensin-converting enzyme inhibitors (ACE inhibitors) inhibit the conversion of angiotensin I to angiotensin II. They are effective and generally well tolerated.

HEART FAILURE. ACE inhibitors have a valuable role in all grades of heart failure, usually combined with a diuretic (section 2.5). Potassium supplements and potassium-sparing diuretics should be discontinued before introducing an ACE inhibitor because of the risk of hyperkalaemia. However, a low dose of spironolactone may be beneficial in severe heart failure (section 2.5) and can be used with an ACE inhibitor provided serum potassium is monitored carefully. Profound first-dose hypotension may occur when ACE inhibitors are introduced to patients with heart failure who are already taking a high dose of a loop diuretic (e.g. furosemide 80 mg daily or more). Temporary withdrawal of the loop diuretic reduces the risk, but may cause severe rebound pulmonary oedema. Therefore, for patients on high doses of loop diuretics, the ACE inhibitor may need to be initiated under specialist supervision, see below. An ACE inhibitor can be initiated in the community in patients who are receiving a low dose of a diuretic or who are not otherwise at risk of serious hypotension; nevertheless, care is required and a very low dose of the ACE inhibitor is given initially.

HYPERTENSION. ACE inhibitors should be considered for hypertension when thiazides and beta-blockers are contra-indicated, not tolerated, or fail to control blood pressure; they are particularly indicated for hypertension in insulin-dependent diabetics with nephropathy (see also section 6.1.5). ACE inhibitors may cause very rapid falls of blood pressure in some patients particularly in those receiving diuretic therapy (see Cautions, below); the first dose should preferably be given at bedtime.

DIABETIC NEPHROPATHY. For comment on the role of ACE inhibitors in the management of diabetic nephropathy, see section 6.1.5.

MYOCARDIAL INFARCTION. ACE inhibitors are used in the immediate and long-term management of patients who have had a myocardial infarction, see section 2.10.1.

INITIATION UNDER SPECIALIST SUPERVISION. ACE inhibitors should be initiated under specialist supervision and with careful clinical monitoring in those with severe heart failure or in those:

- receiving multiple or high-dose diuretic therapy (e.g. more than 80 mg of furosemide daily or its equivalent);
- with hypovolaemia;
- with hyponatraemia (plasma-sodium concentration below 130 mmol/litre);
- with pre-existing hypotension (systolic blood pressure below 90 mmHg);
- with unstable heart failure;
- with renal impairment (plasma-creatinine concentration above 150 micromol/litre);
- receiving high-dose vasodilator therapy;
- aged 70 years or more.

RENAL EFFECTS. In patients with severe bilateral renal artery stenosis (or severe stenosis of the artery supplying a single functioning kidney), ACE inhibitors reduce or abolish glomerular filtration and are likely to cause severe and progressive renal failure. They are thus contra-indicated in patients known to have these forms of critical renovascular disease.

ACE inhibitor treatment is unlikely to have an adverse effect on overall renal function in patients with severe unilateral renal artery stenosis and a normal contralateral kidney, but glomerular filtration is likely to be reduced (or even abolished) in the affected kidney and the long-term consequences are unknown.

In general, ACE inhibitors are therefore best avoided in patients with known or suspected renovascular disease, unless the blood pressure cannot be controlled by other drugs. If they are used in these circumstances renal function needs to be monitored.

ACE inhibitors should also be used with particular caution in patients who may have undiagnosed and clinically silent renovascular disease. This includes patients with peripheral vascular disease or those with severe generalised atherosclerosis.

Renal function and electrolytes should be checked before starting ACE inhibitors and monitored during treatment (more frequently if features mentioned above present). Although ACE inhibitors now have a specialised role in some forms of renal disease they also occasionally cause impairment of renal function which may progress and become severe in other circumstances (at particular risk are the elderly).

Concomitant treatment with NSAIDs increases the risk of renal damage, and potassium-sparing diuretics (or potassium-containing salt substitutes) increase the risk of hyperkalaemia.

CAUTIONS. ACE inhibitors need to be initiated with care in patients receiving diuretics (**important**: see Concomitant diuretics, below); first doses may cause hypotension especially in patients taking high doses of diuretics, on a low-sodium diet, on dialysis, dehydrated or with heart failure (see above). They should also be used with caution in peripheral vascular disease or generalised atherosclerosis owing to risk of clinically silent renovascular disease (see also above). Renal function should be monitored before and during treatment, and the dose reduced in renal impairment (see also above and Appendix 3). The risk of agranulocytosis is possibly increased in collagen vascular disease (blood counts recommended). ACE inhibitors should be used with care (or avoided) in patients with a history of idiopathic or hereditary angio-edema. Use ACE inhibitors with caution in breast-feeding (see Appendix 5). **Interactions:** Appendix 1 (ACE inhibitors)

ANAPHYLACTOID REACTIONS. To prevent anaphylactoid reactions, ACE inhibitors should be avoided during dialysis with high-flux polyacrylonitrile membranes and during low-density lipoprotein apheresis with dextran sulphate; they should also be withheld before desensitisation with wasp or bee venom

Concomitant diuretics. ACE inhibitors can cause a very rapid fall in blood pressure in volume-depleted patients; treatment should therefore be initiated with very low doses. If the dose of diuretic is greater than 80 mg furosemide or equivalent, the ACE inhibitor should be initiated under close supervision and in some patients the diuretic dose may need to be reduced or the diuretic discontinued at least 24 hours beforehand. If high-dose diuretic therapy cannot be stopped, close observation is recommended after administration of the first dose of ACE inhibitor, for at least 2 hours or until the blood pressure has stabilised.

CONTRA-INDICATIONS. ACE inhibitors are contra-indicated in patients with hypersensitivity to ACE inhibitors (including angioedema) and in known or suspected renovascular disease (see also above), aortic stenosis or outflow tract obstruction. ACE inhibitors should not be used in pregnancy (Appendix 4).

SIDE-EFFECTS. ACE inhibitors can cause profound hypotension (see Cautions) and renal impairment (see Renal effects above), and a persistent dry cough. They may also cause angioedema (onset may be delayed), rash (which may be associated with pruritus and urticaria), pancreatitis and upper respiratory-tract symptoms such as sinusitis, rhinitis and sore throat. Gastro-intestinal effects reported with ACE inhibitors include nausea, vomiting, dyspepsia, diarrhoea and constipation. Altered liver function tests, cholestatic jaundice and hepatitis have been reported. Blood disorders including thrombocytopenia, leucopenia, neutropenia and haemolytic anaemia have also been reported. Other reported side-effects include headache, dizziness, fatigue, malaise, taste disturbance, paraesthesia, bronchospasm, fever, serositis, vasculitis, myalgia, arthralgia, positive antinuclear antibody, raised erythrocyte sedimentation rate, eosinophilia, leuco-cytosis and photosensitivity.

COMBINATION PRODUCTS. A number of products incorporating an ACE inhibitor with a thiazide diuretic are now available for the treatment of hypertension. Use of these combination products should be reserved for patients whose blood pressure has not responded to a thiazide diuretic or an ACE inhibitor alone.

Products combining an ACE inhibitor with a calcium-channel blocker are also available for the management of hypertension. Use of such a combination is rarely justified; the range of adverse effects may be increased considerably. A combination product should be considered only for those patients who have been stabilised on the individual components in the same proportions.

CAPTOPRIL

Indications: mild to moderate essential hypertension alone or with thiazide therapy and severe hypertension resistant to other treatment; congestive heart failure (adjunct—see section 2.5.5); following myocardial infarction, see dose; diabetic nephropathy (microalbuminuria greater than 30 mg/day) in insulin-dependent diabetes

Cautions: see notes above

Contra-indications: see notes above; porphyria (section 9.8.2)

Side-effects: see notes above; tachycardia, serum sickness, weight loss, stomatitis, maculopapular rash, photosensitivity, flushing and acidosis

Dose: hypertension, used alone, initially 12.5 mg twice daily; if used in addition to diuretic (see notes above), or in elderly, initially 6.25 mg twice daily (first dose at bedtime); usual maintenance dose 25 mg twice daily; max. 50 mg twice daily (rarely 3 times daily in severe hypertension)
Heart failure (adjunct), initially 6.25–12.5 mg under close medical supervision (see notes above); usual maintenance dose 25 mg 2–3 times daily (but see section 2.5.5); usual max. 150 mg daily
Prophylaxis after infarction in clinically stable patients with asymptomatic or symptomatic left ventricular dysfunction (radionuclide ventriculography or echocardiography undertaken before initiation), initially 6.25 mg, starting as early as 3 days after infarction, then increased over several weeks to 150 mg daily (if tolerated) in divided doses
Diabetic nephropathy, 75–100 mg daily in divided doses; if further blood pressure reduction required, other antihypertensives may be used in conjunction with captopril; in severe renal impairment, initially 12.5 mg twice daily (if concomitant diuretic therapy required, loop diuretic rather than thiazide should be chosen)

Captopril (Non-proprietary) PoM
Tablets, captopril 12.5 mg, net price 56-tab pack = £2.29; 25 mg, 56-tab pack = £3.21; 50 mg, 56-tab pack = £4.07
Available from Alpharma, Berk (*Kaplon*®), CP, Galen, Generics, Goldshield (*Ecopace*®), Hillcross, IVAX (*Tensopril*®), Lagap, Sovereign, Sterwin, Tillomed

Capoten® (Squibb) PoM
Tablets, captopril 12.5 mg (scored), net price 56-tab pack = £10.56; 25 mg, 56-tab pack = £12.03, 84-tab pack = £18.05; 50 mg (scored), 56-tab pack = £20.50, 84-tab pack = £30.75 (also available as *Acepril*®)

■ With diuretic
Note. For mild to moderate hypertension in patients stabilised on the individual components in the same proportions

Co-zidocapt (Non-proprietary) PoM
Tablets, co-zidocapt 12.5/25 (hydrochlorothiazide 12.5 mg, captopril 25 mg), net price 28-tab pack = £9.00
Available from IVAX (*Capto-co*®)
Tablets, co-zidocapt 25/50 (hydrochlorothiazide 25 mg, captopril 50 mg), net price 28-tab pack = £11.31
Available from Alpharma, IVAX (*Capto-co*®)

Capozide® (Squibb) PoM
LS tablets, scored, co-zidocapt 12.5/25 (hydrochlorothiazide 12.5 mg, captopril 25 mg). Net price 28-tab pack = £11.25
Tablets, scored, co-zidocapt 25/50 (hydrochlorothiazide 25 mg, captopril 50 mg). Net price 28-tab pack = £14.14 (also available as *Acezide*®)

CILAZAPRIL

Indications: essential hypertension; congestive heart failure (adjunct—see section 2.5.5)

Cautions: see notes above; severe hepatic impairment (Appendix 2)

Contra-indications: see notes above; ascites

Side-effects: see notes above; dyspnoea and bronchitis

Dose: hypertension, initially 1 mg once daily (reduced to 500 micrograms daily in those receiving a diuretic, in the elderly, and in renal impairment), then adjusted according to response; usual maintenance dose 2.5–5 mg once daily; max. 5 mg daily
Heart failure (adjunct), initially 500 micrograms once daily under close medical supervision (see notes above), increased to 1 mg once daily; usual maintenance dose 1–2.5 mg daily; max. 5 mg daily

Vascace® (Roche) PoM
Tablets, f/c, cilazapril 500 micrograms (white), net price 28-tab pack = £3.92; 1 mg (yellow), 28-tab pack = £6.46; 2.5 mg (pink), 28-tab pack = £8.21; 5 mg (brown), 28-tab pack = £14.28

ENALAPRIL MALEATE

Indications: essential and renovascular hypertension (but see notes above); congestive heart failure (adjunct—see section 2.5.5); prevention of symptomatic heart failure and prevention of coronary ischaemic events in patients with left ventricular dysfunction

Cautions: see notes above

Contra-indications: see notes above; porphyria (section 9.8.2)

Side-effects: see notes above; also palpitations, arrhythmias, angina, chest pain, syncope, cerebrovascular accident, myocardial infarction; anorexia, ileus, stomatitis, hepatic failure; dermatological side-effects including erythema multiforme, Stevens-Johnson syndrome, toxic epidermal necrolysis, exfoliative dermatitis and pemphigus; confusion, depression, nervousness, asthenia, drowsiness, insomnia, blurred vision, tinnitus, sweating, flushing, impotence, alopecia, dyspnoea, asthma, pulmonary infiltrates and muscle cramps

Dose: hypertension, used alone, initially 5 mg once daily; if used in addition to diuretic (see notes above), in elderly patients, or in renal impairment, initially 2.5 mg daily; usual maintenance dose 10–20 mg once daily; in severe hypertension may be increased to max. 40 mg once daily

Heart failure (adjunct), asymptomatic left ventricular dysfunction, initially 2.5 mg daily under close medical supervision (see notes above); usual maintenance dose 20 mg daily in 1–2 divided doses (but see section 2.5.5)

Enalapril Maleate (Non-proprietary) PoM

Tablets, enalapril maleate 2.5 mg, net price 28-tab pack = £2.61; 5 mg, 28-tab pack = £3.77; 10 mg, 28-tab pack = £5.33; 20 mg, 28-tab pack = £6.15
Available from Alpharma, APS (*Enacard*®), Dexcel, Dominion (*Ednyt*®), IVAX, Opus (*Pralenal*®), Sterwin

Innovace® (MSD) PoM

Tablets, enalapril maleate 2.5 mg, net price 28-tab pack = £5.35; 5 mg (scored), 28-tab pack = £7.51; 10 mg (red), 28-tab pack = £10.53; 20 mg (peach), 28-tab pack = £12.51

■ With diuretic

Note. For mild to moderate hypertension in patients stabilised on the individual components in the same proportions

Innozide® (MSD) PoM

Tablets, yellow, scored, enalapril maleate 20 mg, hydrochlorothiazide 12.5 mg. Net price 28-tab pack = £13.90

FOSINOPRIL

Indications: hypertension; congestive heart failure (adjunct—see section 2.5.5)

Cautions: see notes above

Contra-indications: see notes above

Side-effects: see notes above; chest pain and musculoskeletal pain

Dose: hypertension, initially 10 mg daily, increased if necessary after 4 weeks; usual dose range 10–40 mg (doses over 40 mg not shown to increase efficacy); if used in addition to diuretic see notes above

Heart failure (adjunct), initially 10 mg daily under close medical supervision (see notes above); if initial dose well tolerated, may be increased to up to 40 mg once daily

Staril® (Squibb) PoM

Tablets, fosinopril sodium 10 mg, net price 28-tab pack = £12.04; 20 mg, 28-tab pack = £13.00

IMIDAPRIL HYDROCHLORIDE

Indications: essential hypertension

Cautions: see notes above

Contra-indications: see notes above

Side-effects: see notes above; dry mouth, glossitis, abdominal pain, ileus; bronchitis, dyspnoea; sleep disturbances, depression, confusion, blurred vision, tinnitus, impotence

Dose: initially 5 mg daily before food; if used in addition to diuretic (see notes above), in elderly, in patients with heart failure, angina or cerebrovascular disease, or in renal or hepatic impairment, initially 2.5 mg daily; if necessary increase dose at intervals of at least 3 weeks; usual maintenance dose 10 mg once daily; max. 20 mg daily (elderly, 10 mg daily)

Tanatril (Trinity) ▼ PoM

Tablets, scored, imidapril hydrochloride 5 mg, net price 28-tab pack = £5.65; 10 mg, 28-tab pack = £6.39; 20 mg, 28-tab pack = £7.67

LISINOPRIL

Indications: essential and renovascular hypertension (but see notes above); congestive heart failure (adjunct—see section 2.5.5); following myocardial infarction in haemodynamically stable patients; diabetic nephropathy in normotensive insulin-dependent and hypertensive non-insulin dependent diabetes mellitus

Cautions: see notes above

Contra-indications: see notes above

Side-effects: see notes above; tachycardia, cerebrovascular accident, myocardial infarction; dry mouth, confusion, mood changes, asthenia, sweating, impotence and alopecia

Dose: hypertension, initially 2.5 mg daily; usual maintenance dose 10–20 mg daily; max. 40 mg daily; if used in addition to diuretic see notes above

Heart failure (adjunct), initially 2.5 mg daily under close medical supervision (see notes above); usual maintenance dose 5–20 mg daily (but see section 2.5.5)

Prophylaxis after myocardial infarction, systolic blood pressure over 120 mmHg, 5 mg within 24 hours, followed by further 5 mg 24 hours later, then 10 mg after a further 24 hours, and continuing with 10 mg once daily for 6 weeks (or continued if heart failure); systolic blood pressure 100–120 mmHg, initially 2.5 mg, increasing to maintenance dose of 5 mg once daily

Note. Should not be started after myocardial infarction if systolic blood pressure less than 100 mmHg; temporarily reduce maintenance dose to 5 mg and if necessary 2.5 mg daily if systolic blood pressure 100 mmHg or less during treatment; withdraw if prolonged hypotension occurs (systolic blood pressure less than 90 mmHg for more than 1 hour)

Diabetic nephropathy, initially 2.5 mg daily adjusted to achieve a sitting diastolic blood pressure below 75 mmHg in normotensive insulin-dependent diabetes and below 90 mmHg in hypertensive non-insulin dependent diabetes; usual dose range 10–20 mg daily

Carace® (DuPont) PoM
Tablets, lisinopril 2.5 mg (blue), net price 28-tab pack = £7.30; 5 mg (scored), 28-tab pack = £9.15; 10 mg (yellow, scored), 28-tab pack = £11.30; 20 mg (orange, scored), 28-tab pack = £12.78

Zestril® (AstraZeneca) PoM
Tablets, lisinopril (as dihydrate) 2.5 mg, net price 28-tab pack = £6.26; 5 mg (pink, scored), 28-tab pack = £7.86; 10 mg (pink), 28-tab pack = £9.70; 20 mg (pink), 28-tab pack = £10.97

■ With diuretic

Note. For mild to moderate hypertension in patients stabilised on the individual components in the same proportions

Carace Plus® (DuPont) PoM
Carace 10 Plus tablets, blue, lisinopril 10 mg, hydrochlorothiazide 12.5 mg. Net price 28-tab pack = £11.30
Carace 20 Plus tablets, yellow, scored, lisinopril 20 mg, hydrochlorothiazide 12.5 mg. Net price 28-tab pack = £12.78

Zestoretic® (AstraZeneca) PoM
Zestoretic 10 tablets, peach, lisinopril (as dihydrate) 10 mg, hydrochlorothiazide 12.5 mg. Net price 28-tab pack = £11.83
Zestoretic 20 tablets, lisinopril (as dihydrate) 20 mg, hydrochlorothiazide 12.5 mg. Net price 28-tab pack = £13.38

MOEXIPRIL HYDROCHLORIDE

Indications: essential hypertension
Cautions: see notes above
Contra-indications: see notes above
Side-effects: see notes above; arrhythmias, angina, chest pain, syncope, cerebrovascular accident, myocardial infarction; appetite and weight changes; dry mouth, photosensitivity, flushing, nervousness, mood changes, anxiety, drowsiness, sleep disturbance, tinnitus, influenza-like syndrome, sweating and dyspnoea
Dose: used alone, initially 7.5 mg once daily; if used in addition to diuretic (see notes above), with nifedipine, in elderly, in renal or hepatic impairment, initially 3.75 mg once daily; usual range 15–30 mg once daily; doses above 30 mg daily not shown to increase efficacy

Perdix® (Schwarz) PoM
Tablets, f/c, both pink, scored, moexipril hydrochloride 7.5 mg, net price 28-tab pack = £8.12; 15 mg, 28-tab pack = £9.36

PERINDOPRIL

Indications: essential and renovascular hypertension (but see notes above); congestive heart failure (adjunct—see section 2.5.5)
Cautions: see notes above
Contra-indications: see notes above
Side-effects: see notes above; asthenia, flushing, mood and sleep disturbances
Dose: hypertension, initially 2 mg daily (before food); usual maintenance dose 4 mg once daily; max. 8 mg daily; if used in addition to diuretic see notes above
Heart failure (adjunct), initial dose 2 mg in the morning under close medical supervision (see notes above); usual maintenance 4 mg once daily (before food)

Coversyl® (Servier) PoM
Tablets, perindopril erbumine (= tert-butylamine) 2 mg, net price 30-tab pack = £10.31; 4 mg (scored), 30-tab pack = £10.31

QUINAPRIL

Indications: essential hypertension; congestive heart failure (adjunct—see section 2.5.5)
Cautions: see notes above
Contra-indications: see notes above
Side-effects: see notes above; asthenia, chest pain, oedema, flatulence, nervousness, depression, insomnia, blurred vision, impotence, back pain and myalgia
Dose: hypertension, initially 10 mg once daily; with a diuretic, in elderly, or in renal impairment initially 2.5 mg daily; usual maintenance dose 20–40 mg daily in single or 2 divided doses; up to 80 mg daily has been given
Heart failure (adjunct), initial dose 2.5 mg under close medical supervision (see notes above); usual maintenance 10–20 mg daily in single or 2 divided doses; up to 40 mg daily has been given

Accupro® (Parke-Davis) PoM
Tablets, quinapril (as hydrochloride) 5 mg, net price 28-tab pack = £7.17; 10 mg, 28-tab pack = £7.17; 20 mg, 28-tab pack = £8.99; 40 mg, 28-tab pack = £9.75

■ With diuretic

Note. For hypertension in patients stabilised on the individual components in the same proportions

Accuretic® (Parke-Davis) PoM
Tablets, pink, f/c, scored, quinapril (as hydrochloride) 10 mg, hydrochlorothiazide 12.5 mg. Net price 28-tab pack = £9.79

RAMIPRIL

Indications: mild to moderate hypertension; congestive heart failure (adjunct—see section 2.5.5); following myocardial infarction in patients with clinical evidence of heart failure; in susceptible patients over 55 years, prevention of myocardial infarction, stroke, cardiovascular death or need for revascularisation procedures (consult product literature)
Cautions: see notes above
Contra-indications: see notes above
Side-effects: see notes above; arrhythmias, angina, chest pain, syncope, cerebrovascular accident, myocardial infarction, loss of appetite, stomatitis, dry mouth, skin reactions including erythema multiforme and pemphigoid exanthema; precipitation or exacerbation of Raynaud's syndrome; conjunctivitis, onycholysis, confusion, nervousness, depression, anxiety, impotence, decreased libido, alopecia, bronchitis and muscle cramps
Dose: hypertension, initially 1.25 mg once daily, increased at intervals of 1–2 weeks; usual range 2.5–5 mg once daily; max. 10 mg once daily; if used in addition to diuretic see notes above
Heart failure (adjunct), initially 1.25 mg once daily under close medical supervision (see notes above), increased if necessary at intervals of 1–2 weeks; max. 10 mg daily (daily doses of 2.5 mg or

more may be taken in 1–2 divided doses) (see also section 2.5.5)

Prophylaxis after myocardial infarction (started in hospital 3 to 10 days after infarction), initially 2.5 mg twice daily, increased after 2 days to 5 mg twice daily; maintenance 2.5–5 mg twice daily

Note. If initial 2.5-mg dose not tolerated, give 1.25 mg twice daily for 2 days before increasing to 2.5 mg twice daily, then 5 mg twice daily; withdraw if 2.5 mg twice daily not tolerated

Prophylaxis of cardiovascular events or stroke, initially 2.5 mg once daily, increased after 1 week to 5 mg once daily, then increased after a further 3 weeks to 10 mg once daily

Tritace® (Aventis Pharma) [PoM]
Capsules, ramipril 1.25 mg (yellow/white), net price 28-cap pack = £5.30; 2.5 mg (orange/white), 7-cap pack = £1.88, 28-cap pack = £7.51; 5 mg (red/white), 21-cap pack = £7.17, 28-cap pack = £9.55; 10 mg (blue/white), 28-cap pack = £13.00

■ With calcium-channel blocker
Note. For hypertension in patients stabilised on the individual components in the same proportions, but combination with calcium-channel blocker not first-line treatment. For cautions, contra-indications and side-effects of felodipine, see section 2.6.2

Triapin® (Hoechst Marion Roussel) ▼ [PoM] ▭
Triapin® tablets, f/c, brown, ramipril 5 mg, felodipine 5 mg (m/r), net price 28-tab pack = £24.46. Label: 25
Triapin mite® tablets, f/c, orange, ramipril 2.5 mg, felodipine 2.5 mg (m/r), net price 28-tab pack = £19.37. Label: 25

TRANDOLAPRIL

Indications: mild to moderate hypertension; following myocardial infarction in patients with left ventricular dysfunction; heart failure [unlicensed] see section 2.5.5

Cautions: see notes above

Contra-indications: see notes above

Side-effects: see notes above; tachycardia, arrhythmias, angina, transient ischaemic attacks, cerebral haemorrhage, myocardial infarction; ileus, dry mouth; skin reactions including Stevens-Johnson syndrome, toxic epidermal necrolysis, psoriasis-like efflorescence; asthenia, alopecia, dyspnoea and bronchitis

Dose: hypertension, initially 500 micrograms once daily, increased at intervals of 2–4 weeks; usual range 1–2 mg once daily; max. 4 mg daily; if used in addition to diuretic see notes above

Prophylaxis after myocardial infarction (starting as early as 3 days after infarction), initially 500 micrograms daily, gradually increased to max. 4 mg once daily

Note. If symptomatic hypotension develops during titration, do not increase dose further; if possible, reduce dose of any adjunctive treatment and if this is not effective or feasible, reduce dose of trandolapril

Gopten® (Abbott) [PoM]
Capsules, trandolapril 500 micrograms (red/yellow), net price 14-cap pack = £4.09; 1 mg (red/orange), 28-cap pack = £12.28; 2 mg (red/red), 28-cap pack = £12.28

Odrik® (Hoechst Marion Roussel) [PoM]
Capsules, trandolapril 500 micrograms (red/yellow), net price 28-cap pack = £8.19; 1 mg (red/orange), 28-cap pack = £10.34; 2 mg (red/red), 28-cap pack = £12.29

■ With calcium-channel blocker
Note. For hypertension in patients stabilised on the individual components in the same proportions, but combination with calcium-channel blocker not first-line treatment. For cautions, contra-indications and side-effects of verapamil, see section 2.6.2

Tarka® (Abbott) ▼ [PoM] ▭
Capsules, pink, trandolapril 2 mg, verapamil hydrochloride 180 mg (m/r). Net price 28 cap-pack = £16.23. Label: 25

2.5.5.2 Angiotensin-II receptor antagonists

Losartan and **valsartan** are specific angiotensin-II receptor antagonists with many properties similar to those of the ACE inhibitors; **candesartan**, **eprosartan**, **irbesartan** and **telmisartan** have been introduced more recently. However, unlike ACE inhibitors, they do not inhibit the breakdown of bradykinin and other kinins, and thus do not appear to cause the persistent dry cough which commonly complicates ACE inhibitor therapy. They are therefore a useful alternative for patients who have to discontinue an ACE inhibitor because of persistent cough. Beyond this their role in the management of hypertension remains to be established.

For comment on the role of angiotensin-II receptor antagonists in the management of diabetic nephropathy [unlicensed indication], see section 6.1.5.

CAUTIONS. Angiotensin-II receptor antagonists should be used with caution in renal artery stenosis (see also Renal Effects under ACE Inhibitors, section 2.5.5.1). Monitoring of plasma-potassium concentration is advised, particularly in the elderly and in patients with renal impairment; lower initial doses may be appropriate in these patients. Angiotensin-II receptor antagonists should be used with caution in aortic or mitral valve stenosis and in obstructive hypertrophic cardiomyopathy. **Interactions:** Appendix 1 (as for ACE inhibitors).

CONTRA-INDICATIONS. Angiotensin-II receptor antagonists, like the ACE inhibitors, should be avoided in pregnancy (see also Appendix 4).

SIDE-EFFECTS. Side-effects are usually mild. Symptomatic hypotension may occur, particularly in patients with intravascular volume depletion (e.g. those taking high-dose diuretics). Hyperkalaemia occurs occasionally; angioedema has also been reported with some angiotensin-II receptor antagonists.

CANDESARTAN CILEXETIL

Indications: hypertension (see also notes above)

Cautions: see notes above; hepatic and renal impairment (Appendixes 2 and 3)

Contra-indications: see notes above; breast-feeding (Appendix 5), cholestasis

Side-effects: see notes above; also upper respiratory-tract and influenza-like symptoms including rhinitis and pharyngitis; abdominal pain, back pain, arthralgia, myalgia, nausea, headache, dizziness, peripheral oedema, rash also reported; rarely urticaria, pruritus, blood disorders reported

Dose: initially 4 mg (2 mg in hepatic and renal impairment) once daily adjusted according to response; usual maintenance dose 8 mg once daily; max. 16 mg once daily

Amias® (AstraZeneca, Takeda) [PoM]
Tablets, candesartan cilexetil 2 mg, net price 7-tab pack = £2.99; 4 mg (scored), 7-tab pack = £3.24, 28-tab pack = £12.95; 8 mg (pink, scored), 28-tab pack = £14.95; 16 mg (pink, scored), 28-tab pack = £17.75

EPROSARTAN

Indications: hypertension (see also notes above)
Cautions: see notes above; also renal impairment (Appendix 3); breast-feeding (Appendix 5)
Contra-indications: see notes above; also severe hepatic impairment (Appendix 2)
Side-effects: see notes above; also flatulence, dizziness, arthralgia, rhinitis; hypertriglyceridaemia, rarely anaemia
Dose: 600 mg once daily (elderly over 75 years, mild to moderate hepatic impairment, renal impairment, initially 300 mg once daily); if necessary increased after 2–3 weeks to 800 mg once daily

Teveten® (Solvay) ▼ [PoM]
Tablets, f/c, eprosartan (as mesilate) 300 mg, net price 28-tab pack = £12.50; 400 mg, 56-tab pack = £16.96; 600 mg, 28-tab pack = £14.75. Label: 21

IRBESARTAN

Indications: hypertension (see also notes above)
Cautions: see notes above
Contra-indications: see notes above; breast-feeding (Appendix 5)
Side-effects: see notes above; diarrhoea, dyspepsia, flushing; tachycardia, dizziness, asthenia, myalgia, rash, urticaria, increase in plasma concentration of creatine kinase reported
Dose: 150 mg once daily, increased if necessary to 300 mg once daily (in haemodialysis or in elderly over 75 years, initial dose of 75 mg once daily may be used)

Aprovel® (Bristol-Myers Squibb, Sanofi-Synthelabo) [PoM]
Tablets, irbesartan 75 mg, net price 28-tab pack = £14.80; 150 mg, 28-tab pack = £16.45; 300 mg, 28-tab pack = £22.21

■ With diuretic
Note. For patients with hypertension not adequately controlled on individual components
CoAprovel® (Bristol-Myers Squibb, Sanofi-Synthelabo) [PoM]
Tablets, both peach, irbesartan 150 mg, hydrochlorothiazide 12.5 mg, net price 28-tab pack = £16.45; irbesartan 300 mg, hydrochlorothiazide 12.5 mg, 28-tab pack = £22.21

LOSARTAN POTASSIUM

Indications: hypertension (see also notes above)
Cautions: see notes above; hepatic and renal impairment (Appendixes 2 and 3)
Contra-indications: see notes above; breast-feeding (Appendix 5)
Side-effects: see notes above; diarrhoea, dizziness, taste disturbance, cough, myalgia, migraine, urticaria, pruritus, rash; rarely hepatitis, anaemia (in severe renal disease or following renal transplant), vasculitis (including Henoch-Schoenlein purpura)
Dose: usually 50 mg once daily (elderly over 75 years, moderate to severe renal impairment, intravascular volume depletion, initially 25 mg once daily); if necessary increased after several weeks to 100 mg once daily

Cozaar® (MSD) [PoM]
Tablets, f/c, losartan potassium 25 mg (Half Strength), net price 7-tab pack = £4.31; 50 mg (scored), 28-tab pack = £17.23; 100 mg, 28-tab pack = £22.00

■ With diuretic
Note. For hypertension in patients stabilised on the individual components in the same proportions
Cozaar-Comp® (MSD) [PoM]
Tablets, f/c, yellow, losartan potassium 50 mg, hydrochlorothiazide 12.5 mg. Net price 28-tab pack = £17.23

TELMISARTAN

Indications: hypertension (see also notes above)
Cautions: see notes above; hepatic impairment—avoid if severe (Appendix 2); active gastric or duodenal ulceration or other gastro-intestinal disease (increased risk of gastro-intestinal bleeding)
Contra-indications: see notes above; also severe renal impairment; biliary obstruction; breast-feeding
Side-effects: see notes above; gastro-intestinal disturbances (rarely gastro-intestinal bleeding), pharyngitis, back pain, myalgia; rarely decrease in haemoglobin, increase in uric acid, urticaria
Dose: usually 40 mg once daily, increased if necessary to max. 80 mg once daily

Micardis® (Boehringer Ingelheim) ▼ [PoM]
Tablets, telmisartan 20 mg, net price 28-tab pack = £12.60; 40 mg, 28-tab pack = £12.60; 80 mg, 28-tab pack = £15.75

VALSARTAN

Indications: hypertension (see also notes above)
Cautions: see notes above; mild to moderate hepatic impairment (Appendix 2) and renal impairment (Appendix 3)
Contra-indications: see notes above; severe hepatic impairment (Appendix 2), cirrhosis, biliary obstruction, breast-feeding (Appendix 5)
Side-effects: see notes above; fatigue, rarely epistaxis; neutropenia reported
Dose: usually 80 mg once daily (elderly over 75 years, mild to moderate hepatic impairment, moderate to severe renal impairment, intravascular volume depletion, initially 40 mg once daily); if

necessary increased after at least 4 weeks to 160 mg daily (80 mg daily in hepatic impairment)

Diovan® (Novartis) PoM
Capsules, valsartan 40 mg (grey), net price 7-cap pack = £3.35; 80 mg (grey/pink), 7-cap pack = £3.94 (hosp. only), 28-cap pack = £15.75; 160 mg (dark grey/pink), 7-cap pack = £4.92 (hosp. only), 28-cap pack = £19.69

2.5.6 Ganglion-blocking drugs

TRIMETAPHAN CAMSILATE
Indications: controlled hypotension in surgery
Cautions: hepatic or renal impairment, diabetes mellitus, elderly, cerebral or coronary vascular disease, adrenal insufficiency, Addison's disease, CNS degenerative disease
Contra-indications: severe arteriosclerosis, severe cardiac disease, pyloric stenosis, pregnancy
Side-effects: tachycardia and respiratory depression (particularly with muscle relaxants); constipation, increased intra-ocular pressure, pupillary dilatation
Dose: *by intravenous infusion*, 3–4 mg/minute initially, then adjusted according to response

Trimetaphan Camsilate (Cambridge) PoM
Injection, trimetaphan camsilate 50 mg/mL. Net price 5-mL amp = £17.42. For dilution and use as an infusion

2.5.7 Tyrosine hydroxylase inhibitors

Metirosine (*Demser®*, MSD, available on named-patient basis) inhibits the enzyme tyrosine hydroxylase, and hence the synthesis of catecholamines. It is used in the pre-operative management of phaeochromocytoma, and long term in patients unsuitable for surgery; an alpha-adrenoceptor blocking drug (e.g. phenoxybenzamine, section 2.5.4) may also be required. Metirosine should **not** be used to treat essential hypertension.

2.6 Nitrates, calcium-channel blockers, and potassium-channel activators

2.6.1	Nitrates
2.6.2	Calcium-channel blockers
2.6.3	Potassium-channel activators
2.6.4	Peripheral and cerebral vasodilators

Nitrates, calcium-channel blockers and potassium-channel activators have a vasodilating effect. Vasodilators are known to act in heart failure either by arteriolar dilatation which reduces both peripheral vascular resistance and left ventricular pressure at systole and results in improved cardiac output, *or* venous dilatation which results in dilatation of capacitance vessels, increase of venous pooling, and diminution of venous return to the heart (decreasing left ventricular end-diastolic pressure).

Angina
Stable angina usually results from atherosclerotic plaques in the coronary arteries, whereas *unstable angina* is usually due to plaque rupture and may occur either in patients with a history of stable angina or in those with previously silent coronary artery disease. It is important to distinguish unstable from stable angina; unstable angina is usually characterised by new onset severe angina or sudden worsening of previously stable angina.

STABLE ANGINA. Acute attacks of stable angina should be managed with sublingual **glyceryl trinitrate**. If attacks occur more than twice a week, regular drug therapy is required and should be introduced in a stepwise manner according to response. **Aspirin** (section 2.9) should be given to patients with angina; a dose of 75–150 mg daily is suitable. Revascularisation procedures may also be appropriate.

Patients with mild or moderate stable angina who do not have left ventricular dysfunction, may be managed effectively with sublingual glyceryl trinitrate and regular administration of a **beta-blocker** (section 2.4). If necessary a long-acting **dihydropyridine calcium-channel blocker** (section 2.6.2) and then a **long-acting nitrate** (section 2.6.1) may be added. For those without left ventricular dysfunction and in whom beta-blockers are inappropriate, **diltiazem** or **verapamil** may be given (section 2.6.2) and a long-acting nitrate (section 2.6.1) may be added if symptom control is not adequate. For those intolerant of standard treatment, or where standard treatment has failed, nicorandil may be tried.

For patients with left ventricular dysfunction a long-acting nitrate (section 2.6.1) should be used and a long-acting dihydropyridine calcium-channel blocker (section 2.6.2) may be added if necessary. A **statin** (section 2.12) should be considered for those with an elevated plasma-cholesterol concentration.

UNSTABLE ANGINA. Patients with unstable angina should be admitted to hospital. The aims of management of unstable angina are to provide supportive care and pain relief during the acute attack and to prevent myocardial infarction and death.

Initial management. **Aspirin** (chewed or dispersed in water) is given for its antiplatelet effect at a dose of 300 mg (section 2.9). If aspirin is given before arrival at hospital, a note saying that it has been given should be sent with the patient.

Heparin (section 2.8.1) or the low molecular weight heparins **dalteparin** or **enoxaparin** (section 2.8.1) should also be given.

Nitrates (section 2.6.1) are used to relieve ischaemic pain. If sublingual glyceryl trinitrate is not effective, intravenous or buccal glyceryl trinitrate or intravenous isosorbide dinitrate is given.

Patients without contra-indications should receive intravenous or oral **beta-blockers** (section 2.4). In patients without left ventricular dysfunction and in whom beta-blockers are inappropriate, **diltiazem** or **verapamil** may be given (section 2.6.2).

The glycoprotein IIb/IIIa inhibitors **eptifibatide** and **tirofiban** (section 2.9) are recommended (with aspirin and heparin) for unstable angina in patients with a high risk of developing myocardial infarction.

Abciximab, eptifibatide or tirofiban may also be used with aspirin and heparin in patients undergoing percutaneous coronary intervention, to reduce the immediate risk of vascular occlusion.

Revascularisation procedures are often appropriate for patients with unstable angina.

Long-term management. The importance of lifestyle changes, especially stopping smoking, should be emphasised. Patients should receive low-dose **aspirin** indefinitely—a dose of 75–150 mg daily is suitable. Use of a **statin** (section 2.12) should also be considered. The need for long-term angina treatment or for coronary angiography should be assessed. If there is continuing ischaemia, standard angina treatment should be continued; if not, antianginal treatment may be withdrawn cautiously at least 2 months after the acute attack.

2.6.1   Nitrates

Nitrates have a useful role in *angina* (for details on the management of stable angina, see section 2.6). Although they are potent coronary vasodilators, their principal benefit follows from a reduction in venous return which reduces left ventricular work. Unwanted effects such as flushing, headache, and postural hypotension may limit therapy, especially when angina is severe or when patients are unusually sensitive to the effects of nitrates.

Sublingual **glyceryl trinitrate** is one of the most effective drugs for providing rapid symptomatic relief of angina, but its effect lasts only for 20 to 30 minutes; the 300-microgram tablet is often appropriate when glyceryl trinitrate is first used. The *aerosol spray* provides an alternative method of rapid relief of symptoms for those who find difficulty in dissolving sublingual preparations. Duration of action may be prolonged by *modified-release* and *transdermal* preparations (but tolerance may develop, see below).

Isosorbide dinitrate is active *sublingually* and is a more stable preparation for those who only require nitrates infrequently. It is also effective by mouth for prophylaxis; although the effect is slower in onset, it may persist for several hours. Duration of action of up to 12 hours is claimed for *modified-release* preparations. The activity of isosorbide dinitrate may depend on the production of active metabolites, the most important of which is isosorbide mononitrate. **Isosorbide mononitrate** itself is also licensed for angina prophylaxis; modified-release formulations (for once daily administration) are available.

Glyceryl trinitrate or isosorbide dinitrate may be tried by *intravenous injection* when the sublingual form is ineffective in patients with chest pain due to myocardial infarction or severe ischaemia. Intravenous injections are also useful in the treatment of acute left ventricular failure.

TOLERANCE. Many patients on long-acting or transdermal nitrates rapidly develop tolerance (with reduced therapeutic effects). Reduction of blood-nitrate concentrations to low levels for 4 to 8 hours each day usually maintains effectiveness in such patients. If tolerance is suspected during the use of transdermal patches they should be left off for several consecutive hours in each 24 hours; in the case of modified-release tablets of isosorbide dinitrate (and conventional formulations of isosorbide mononitrate), the second of the two daily doses can be given after about 8 hours rather than after 12 hours. Conventional formulations of isosorbide mononitrate should not usually be given more than twice daily unless small doses are used; modified-release formulations of isosorbide mononitrate should only be given once daily, and used in this way do not produce tolerance.

GLYCERYL TRINITRATE

Indications: prophylaxis and treatment of angina; left ventricular failure

Cautions: severe hepatic or renal impairment; hypothyroidism, malnutrition, or hypothermia; recent history of myocardial infarction; metal-containing transdermal systems should be removed before cardioversion or diathermy; tolerance (see notes above); **interactions:** Appendix 1 (glyceryl trinitrate)

Contra-indications: hypersensitivity to nitrates; hypotensive conditions and hypovolaemia; hypertrophic obstructive cardiomyopathy, aortic stenosis, cardiac tamponade, constrictive pericarditis, mitral stenosis; marked anaemia, head trauma, cerebral haemorrhage, closed-angle glaucoma

Side-effects: throbbing headache, flushing, dizziness, postural hypotension, tachycardia (but paradoxical bradycardia has occurred)

INJECTION. Specific side-effects following injection (particularly if given too rapidly) include severe hypotension, nausea and retching, diaphoresis, apprehension, restlessness, muscle twitching, retrosternal discomfort, palpitations, abdominal pain, syncope; prolonged administration has been associated with methaemoglobinaemia

Dose: *sublingually*, 0.3–1 mg, repeated as required
By mouth, see under preparations
By intravenous infusion, 10–200 micrograms/minute

■ Short-acting tablets and sprays

Glyceryl Trinitrate (Non-proprietary)
Sublingual tablets, glyceryl trinitrate
300 micrograms, net price 100 = £2.91;
500 micrograms, 100 = £1.06; 600 micrograms,
100 = £2.31. Label: 16
Note. Glyceryl trinitrate tablets should be supplied in glass containers of not more than 100 tablets, closed with a foil-lined cap, and containing no cotton wool wadding; they should be discarded after 8 weeks in use
Aerosol spray, glyceryl trinitrate 400 micrograms/ metered dose. Net price 200-dose unit = £3.13
Dose: treatment or prophylaxis of angina, spray 1–2 doses under tongue and then close mouth
Available from Alpharma

Coro-Nitro Pump Spray® (Roche)
Aerosol spray, glyceryl trinitrate 400 micrograms/ metered dose. Net price 200-dose unit = £3.13
Dose: treatment or prophylaxis of angina, spray 1–2 doses under tongue and then close mouth

Glytrin Spray® (Sanofi-Synthelabo)
Aerosol spray, glyceryl trinitrate 400 micrograms/metered dose. Net price 200-dose unit = £3.49
Dose: treatment or prophylaxis of angina, spray 1–2 doses under tongue and then close mouth
Caution: flammable

GTN 300 mcg (Martindale)
Sublingual tablets, glyceryl trinitrate 300 micrograms. Net price 100 = £2.91. Label: 16

Nitrolingual Pumpspray® (Merck)
Aerosol spray, glyceryl trinitrate 400 micrograms/metered dose. Net price 200-dose unit = £3.65; *Duo Pack* (250-dose unit and 75-dose unit) = £4.98
Dose: treatment or prophylaxis of angina, spray 1–2 doses under tongue and then close mouth

Nitromin® (Servier)
Aerosol spray, glyceryl trinitrate 400 micrograms/metered dose, net price 180-dose unit = £2.92, 200-dose unit = £3.13
Dose: treatment or prophylaxis of angina, spray 1–2 doses under tongue and then close mouth

■ Longer-acting tablets

Suscard® (Forest)
Buccal tablets, m/r, glyceryl trinitrate 2 mg, net price 100-tab pack = £13.55; 3 mg, 100-tab pack = £19.56; 5 mg, 100-tab pack = £26.63. Counselling, see administration below
Dose: treatment of angina, 2 mg as required (1 mg in sensitive patients), increased to 3 mg if necessary; prophylaxis 1–3 mg 3 times daily; 5 mg in severe angina
Unstable angina (adjunct), up to 5 mg with ECG monitoring
Congestive heart failure, 5 mg 3 times daily, increased to 10 mg 3 times daily in severe cases
Acute heart failure, 5 mg repeated until symptoms abate
ADMINISTRATION: Tablets have rapid onset of effect; they are placed between upper lip and gum, and left to dissolve; vary site to reduce risk of dental caries

Sustac® (Forest)
Tablets, m/r, all pink, glyceryl trinitrate 2.6 mg, net price 90-tab pack = £5.12; 6.4 mg, 90-tab pack = £7.38; 10 mg, 90-tab pack = £6.85. Label: 25
Dose: prophylaxis of angina, 2.6–12.8 mg 3 times daily or 10 mg 2–3 times daily

■ Parenteral preparations
Note. Glass or polyethylene apparatus is preferable; loss of potency will occur if PVC is used

Glyceryl Trinitrate (Non-proprietary) PoM
Injection, glyceryl trinitrate 5 mg/mL. To be diluted before use. Net price 5-mL amp = £6.49; 10-mL amp = £12.98
Available from Faulding DBL

Nitrocine® (Schwarz) PoM
Injection, glyceryl trinitrate 1 mg/mL. To be diluted before use or given undiluted with syringe pump. Net price 10-mL amp = £7.90; 50-mL bottle = £18.51

Nitronal® (Merck) PoM
Injection, glyceryl trinitrate 1 mg/mL. To be diluted before use or given undiluted with syringe pump. Net price 5-mL vial = £2.06; 50-mL vial = £16.85

■ Transdermal preparations
Deponit® (Schwarz)
Patches, self-adhesive, transparent, glyceryl trinitrate, *'5' patch* (releasing approx. 5 mg/24 hours when in contact with skin), net price 28 = £17.16; *'10' patch* (releasing approx. 10 mg/24 hours), 28 = £18.89
ADMINISTRATION: prophylaxis of angina, apply one '5' or one '10' patch to lateral chest wall, upper arm, or shoulder; replace every 24 hours, siting replacement patch on different area; see also notes above

Minitran® (3M)
Patches, self-adhesive, transparent, glyceryl trinitrate, *'5' patch* (releasing approx. 5 mg/24 hours when in contact with skin), net price 30 = £12.49; *'10' patch* (releasing approx. 10 mg/24 hours), 30 = £13.84; *'15' patch* (releasing approx. 15 mg/24 hours), 30 = £15.26
ADMINISTRATION: prophylaxis of angina, apply one '5' patch to chest or upper arm; replace every 24 hours, siting replacement patch on different area; adjust dose according to response; see also notes above
Maintenance of venous patency ('5' patch only), consult product literature

Nitro-Dur® (Schering-Plough)
Patches, self-adhesive, buff, glyceryl trinitrate, *'0.2 mg/h' patch* (releasing approx. 5 mg/24 hours when in contact with skin), net price 28 = £11.84; *'0.4 mg/h' patch* (releasing approx. 10 mg/24 hours), 28 = £13.10; *'0.6 mg/h' patch* (releasing approx. 15 mg/24 hours), 28 = £14.42
ADMINISTRATION: prophylaxis of angina, apply one '0.2 mg/h' patch to chest or outer upper arm; replace every 24 hours, siting replacement patch on different area: adjust dose according to response; see also notes above

Percutol® (Dominion)
Ointment, glyceryl trinitrate 2%. Net price 60 g = £10.49. Counselling, see administration below
Excipients: include wool fat
ADMINISTRATION: prophylaxis of angina, usual dose 1–2 inches of ointment measured on to *Applirule®*, and applied (usually to chest, arm, or thigh) without rubbing in and secured with surgical tape, every 3–4 hours as required; to determine dose, ½ inch on first day then increased by ½ inch/day until headache occurs, then reduced by ½ inch
Note. Approx. 800 micrograms/hour absorbed from 1 inch of ointment

Transiderm-Nitro® (Novartis)
Patches, self-adhesive, pink, glyceryl trinitrate, *'5' patch* (releasing approx. 5 mg/24 hours when in contact with skin), net price 28 = £19.37; *'10' patch* (releasing approx. 10 mg/24 hours), 28 = £21.30
ADMINISTRATION: prophylaxis of angina, apply one '5' or one '10' patch to lateral chest wall; replace every 24 hours, siting replacement patch on different area; max. two '10' patches daily; see also notes above
Prophylaxis of phlebitis and extravasation ('5' patch only), consult product literature

ISOSORBIDE DINITRATE

Indications: prophylaxis and treatment of angina; left ventricular failure
Cautions: see under Glyceryl Trinitrate
Contra-indications: see under Glyceryl Trinitrate
Side-effects: see under Glyceryl Trinitrate
Dose: *sublingually*, 5–10 mg
By mouth, daily in divided doses, angina 30–120 mg, left ventricular failure 40–160 mg, up to 240 mg if required
By intravenous infusion, 2–10 mg/hour; higher doses up to 20 mg/hour may be required

- Short-acting tablets and sprays

Isosorbide Dinitrate (Non-proprietary)

Tablets, isosorbide dinitrate 10 mg, net price 20 = 28p; 20 mg, 20 = 44p

Available from Alpharma, Hillcross, IVAX

Angitak® (Eastern)

Aerosol spray, isosorbide dinitrate 1.25 mg/metered dose, net price 200-dose unit = £3.95

Dose: treatment or prophylaxis of angina, spray 1–3 doses under tongue whilst holding breath; allow 30 second interval between each dose

Isordil® (Shire)

Tablets (sublingual), pink, isosorbide dinitrate 5 mg. Net price 100-tab pack = £1.43. Label: 26

Tablets, both scored, isosorbide dinitrate 10 mg, net price 112-tab pack = 72p; 30 mg, 112-tab pack = £3.86

- Modified-release preparations

Cedocard Retard® (Pharmacia)

Retard-20 tablets, m/r, yellow, scored, isosorbide dinitrate 20 mg. Net price 60-tab pack = £5.45. Label: 25

Dose: prophylaxis of angina, 1 tablet every 12 hours

Retard-40 tablets, m/r, orange-red, scored, isosorbide dinitrate 40 mg. Net price 60-tab pack = £10.59. Label: 25

Dose: prophylaxis of angina, 1–2 tablets every 12 hours

Isoket Retard® (Schwarz)

Retard-20 tablets, m/r, yellow, scored, isosorbide dinitrate 20 mg. Net price 56-tab pack = £3.47. Label: 25

Retard-40 tablets, m/r, orange, scored, isosorbide dinitrate 40 mg. Net price 56-tab pack = £8.55. Label: 25

Dose: prophylaxis of angina, 20–40 mg every 12 hours

- Parenteral preparations

Isoket® (Schwarz) **PoM**

Injection 0.05%, isosorbide dinitrate 500 micrograms/mL. To be diluted before use or given undiluted with syringe pump. Net price 50-mL bottle = £9.61

Injection 0.1%, isosorbide dinitrate 1 mg/mL. To be diluted before use. Net price 10-mL amp = £3.62; 50-mL bottle = £17.96; 100-mL bottle = £25.98

Note. Glass or polyethylene infusion apparatus is preferable; loss of potency if PVC used

- Transdermal preparations

Isocard® (Eastern)

Transdermal spray, isosorbide dinitrate, 30 mg/metered dose. Net price 65-dose unit = £17.50. Label: 10 patient information leaflet, counselling, administration

Dose: prophylaxis of angina, initially (in those not previously receiving nitrates) 1 spray daily for 3 days, increased if necessary to 2 sprays daily for 3 days and then to 2 sprays twice daily; usual dose, 1–2 sprays in the morning and at night if necessary

COUNSELLING. Apply to clean dry skin on the chest wall holding cane vertically. Spray each dose onto the chest from a distance of about 20 cm and then rub in gently; avoid contact with eyes; do not inhale

Caution: flammable

ISOSORBIDE MONONITRATE

Indications: prophylaxis of angina; adjunct in congestive heart failure

Cautions: see under Glyceryl Trinitrate

Contra-indications: see under Glyceryl Trinitrate

Side-effects: see under Glyceryl Trinitrate

Dose: initially 20 mg 2–3 times daily *or* 40 mg twice daily (10 mg twice daily in those who have not previously received nitrates); up to 120 mg daily in divided doses if required

Isosorbide Mononitrate (Non-proprietary)

Tablets, isosorbide mononitrate 10 mg, net price 56 = £1.13; 20 mg, 56 = £2.09; 40 mg, 56 = £3.69. Label: 25

Various strengths available from Alpharma, APS, Berk (*Dynamin®*), Dominion, Hillcross, IVAX, Opus (*Angeze®*)

Elantan® (Schwarz)

Elantan 10 tablets, scored, isosorbide mononitrate 10 mg. Net price 56 = £3.56; 84 = £5.34. Label: 25

PoM *Elantan 20 tablets*, scored, isosorbide mononitrate 20 mg. Net price 56 = £4.64; 84 = £6.59. Label: 25

PoM *Elantan 40 tablets*, scored, isosorbide mononitrate 40 mg. Net price 56 = £7.56; 84 = £11.35. Label: 25

Ismo® (Roche)

Ismo 10 tablets, isosorbide mononitrate 10 mg. Net price 60-tab pack = £3.24. Label: 25

Ismo 20 tablets, isosorbide mononitrate 20 mg. Net price 60-tab pack = £4.75. Label: 25

Ismo 40 tablets, isosorbide mononitrate 40 mg. Net price 60-tab pack = £7.80. Label: 25

Isotrate® (Bioglan)

Tablets, isosorbide mononitrate 20 mg. Net price 60-tab pack = £7.09. Label: 25

Monit® (Sanofi-Synthelabo)

LS Tablets, isosorbide mononitrate 10 mg. Net price 56-tab pack = £3.22. Label: 25

Tablets, scored, isosorbide mononitrate 20 mg. Net price 56-tab pack = £4.11. Label: 25

- Modified release

Chemydur® 60XL (Sovereign) **PoM**

Tablets, m/r, scored, ivory, isosorbide mononitrate 60 mg, net price 28-tab pack = £15.83. Label: 25

Dose: prophylaxis of angina, 1 tablet in the morning (half a tablet for 2–4 days to minimise possibility of headache), increased if necessary to 2 tablets

Elantan LA® (Schwarz)

Elantan LA 25 capsules, m/r, brown/white, enclosing white micropellets, isosorbide mononitrate 25 mg. Net price 28-cap pack = £6.69. Label: 25

Dose: prophylaxis of angina, 1 capsule in the morning, increased if necessary to 2 capsules

Elantan LA 50 capsules, m/r, brown/pink, enclosing white micropellets, isosorbide mononitrate 50 mg. Net price 28-cap pack = £10.79. Label: 25

Dose: prophylaxis of angina, 1 capsule daily in the morning, increased if necessary to 2 capsules

Imdur® (AstraZeneca)

Durules® (= tablets m/r), yellow, f/c, scored, isosorbide mononitrate 60 mg. Net price 28-tab pack = £11.14. Label: 25

Dose: prophylaxis of angina, 1 tablet in the morning (half a tablet if headache occurs), increased to 2 tablets in the morning if required

Isib 60XL® (Ashbourne)

Tablets, m/r, scored, ivory, isosorbide mononitrate 60 mg. Net price 28-tab pack = £9.47. Label: 25

Dose: prophylaxis of angina, 1 tablet in the morning (half a tablet for 2–4 days if headache occurs), increased if necessary to 2 tablets

Ismo Retard® (Roche)

Tablets, m/r, s/c, isosorbide mononitrate 40 mg. Net price 28-tab pack = £9.78. Label: 25

Dose: prophylaxis of angina, 1 tablet daily in morning

Isodur® (Galen)

Isodur 25XL capsules, m/r, brown/white, isosorbide mononitrate 25 mg, net price 28-cap pack = £6.05. Label: 25

Isodur 50XL capsules, m/r, brown/pink, isosorbide mononitrate 50 mg, net price 28-cap pack = £9.75. Label: 25

Dose: prophylaxis of angina, 25–50 mg daily in the morning, increased if necessary to 50–100 mg once daily

Isotard® (Strakan)

Isotard 25XL tablets, m/r, ivory, isosorbide mononitrate 25 mg, net price 28-tab pack = £6.60. Label: 25

Isotard 40XL tablets, m/r, ivory, isosorbide mononitrate 40 mg, net price 28-tab pack = £7.88. Label: 25

Isotard 50XL tablets, m/r, ivory, isosorbide mononitrate 50 mg, net price 28-tab pack = £7.95. Label: 25

Isotard 60XL tablets, m/r, ivory, isosorbide mononitrate 60 mg, net price 28-tab pack = £8.03. Label: 25

Dose: prophylaxis of angina, 25–60 mg daily in the morning (if headache occurs with 60-mg tablet, half a 60-mg tablet may be given for 2–4 days), increased if necessary to 50–120 mg daily

¹MCR-50® (Pharmacia)

Capsules, m/r, containing white micropellets, isosorbide mononitrate 50 mg. Net price 28-cap pack = £10.52. Label: 25

Dose: prophylaxis of angina, 1 capsule in morning, increased to 2 capsules if required

1. Full product name Mono Cedocard Retard-50®

Modisal XL® (Lagap)

Tablets, m/r, ivory, isosorbide mononitrate 60 mg. Net price 28-tab pack = £15.97. Label: 25

Dose: prophylaxis of angina, 1 tablet daily in the morning (half a tablet for first 2–4 days to minimise possibility of headache), increased if necessary to 2 tablets once daily

Monit SR® (Sanofi-Synthelabo)

Tablets, m/r, s/c, isosorbide mononitrate 40 mg. Net price 28-tab pack = £9.78. Label: 25

Dose: prophylaxis of angina, 1 tablet daily in morning

Monit XL® (Sterwin)

Tablets, m/r, f/c, scored, orange, isosorbide mononitrate 60 mg, net price 28-tab pack = £11.14. Label: 25

Dose: prophylaxis of angina, 1 tablet in the morning (half a tablet if headache occurs), increased to 2 tablets in the morning if required

Monomax SR® (Trinity) [PoM]

Capsules, m/r, isosorbide mononitrate 40 mg, net price 28-cap pack = £8.31; 60 mg, 28-cap pack = £9.03. Label: 25

Dose: prophylaxis of angina, 40 mg once daily, increased if necessary to 60 mg daily

Note. Also available as *Angeze SR®* (Opus)

Monosorb XL 60® (Dexcel) [PoM]

Tablets, m/r, f/c, isosorbide mononitrate 60 mg. Net price 28-tab pack = £16.70. Label: 25

Dose: prophylaxis of angina, 1 tablet daily in the morning (half a tablet for first 2–4 days to minimise possibility of headache), increased if necessary to 2 tablets

Note. Also available from Alpharma and as *Xismox® XL 60* (Genus)

■ **With aspirin**

Note. For prophylaxis of angina and secondary prevention of myocardial infarction; for cautions, contra-indications and side-effects of aspirin see section 2.9

Imazin® XL (Napp)

Tablets, aspirin 75 mg, isosorbide mononitrate 60 mg (m/r), net price 28-tab pack = £10.76. Label: 25, 32

Dose: 1 tablet in the morning, increased to 2 tablets if required

Forte tablets, aspirin 150 mg, isosorbide mononitrate 60 mg (m/r), net price 28-tab pack = £10.76. Label: 25, 32

Dose: 1 tablet in the morning

2.6.2   Calcium-channel blockers

Calcium-channel blockers (less correctly called 'calcium-antagonists') interfere with the inward displacement of calcium ions through the slow channels of active cell membranes. They influence the myocardial cells, the cells within the specialised conducting system of the heart, and the cells of vascular smooth muscle. Thus, myocardial contractility may be reduced, the formation and propagation of electrical impulses within the heart may be depressed, and coronary or systemic vascular tone may be diminished.

Calcium-channel blockers differ in their predilection for the various possible sites of action and, therefore, their therapeutic effects are disparate, with much greater variation than those of beta-blockers. There are important differences between verapamil, diltiazem, and the dihydropyridine calcium-channel blockers (amlodipine, felodipine, isradipine, lacidipine, lercanidipine, nicardipine, nifedipine, nimodipine, and nisoldipine). Verapamil and diltiazem should usually be **avoided** in *heart failure* because they may further depress cardiac function and cause clinically significant deterioration.

Verapamil is used for the treatment of *angina* (section 2.6), *hypertension*, and *arrhythmias* (section 2.3.2). It is a highly negatively inotropic calcium channel-blocker and it reduces cardiac output, slows the heart rate, and may impair atrioventricular conduction. It may precipitate heart failure, exacerbate conduction disorders, and cause hypotension at high doses and should **not** be used with beta-blockers (see p. 107). Constipation is the most common side-effect.

Nifedipine relaxes vascular smooth muscle and dilates coronary and peripheral arteries. It has more influence on vessels and less on the myocardium than does verapamil, and unlike verapamil has no anti-arrhythmic activity. It rarely precipitates heart failure because any negative inotropic effect is off-set by a reduction in left ventricular work. Short-acting formulations of nifedipine are not recommended for angina or long-term management of hypertension; their use may be associated with large variations in blood pressure and reflex tachycardia. **Nicardipine** has similar effects to those of nifedipine and may produce less reduction of myocardial contractility. **Amlodipine** and **felodipine** also resemble nifedipine and nicardipine in their effects and do not reduce myocardial contractility and they do not produce clinical deterioration in heart failure. They have a longer duration of action and can be given once daily. Nifedipine, nicardipine, amlodipine, and felodipine are used for the treatment of angina (section 2.6) or hypertension. All are valuable in forms of *angina associated with coronary vasospasm*. Side-effects associated with vasodilatation such as flushing and headache (which become less obtrusive after a few days), and ankle swelling (which may respond only partially to diuretics) are common.

Isradipine, **lacidipine**, **lercanidipine** and **nisoldipine** have similar effects to those of nifedipine and nicardipine; isradipine, lacidipine, and lercanidipine are only indicated for *hypertension* whereas nisoldipine is indicated for angina and hypertension.

Nimodipine is related to nifedipine but the smooth muscle relaxant effect preferentially acts on cerebral arteries. Its use is confined to prevention of *vascular spasm following subarachnoid haemorrhage.*

Diltiazem is effective in most forms of *angina* (section 2.6); the longer-acting formulation is also used for *hypertension.* It may be used in patients for whom beta-blockers are contra-indicated or ineffective. It has a less negative inotropic effect than verapamil and significant myocardial depression occurs rarely. Nevertheless because of the risk of bradycardia it should be used with caution in association with beta-blockers.

UNSTABLE ANGINA. Calcium-channel blockers do not reduce the risk of myocardial infarction in unstable angina. The use of diltiazem or verapamil should be reserved for patients resistant to treatment with beta-blockers.

WITHDRAWAL. There is some evidence that sudden withdrawal of calcium-channel blockers may be associated with an exacerbation of angina.

AMLODIPINE BESILATE

Indications: hypertension, prophylaxis of angina

Cautions: hepatic impairment; **interactions:** Appendix 1 (calcium-channel blockers)

Contra-indications: cardiogenic shock, unstable angina, significant aortic stenosis; pregnancy and breast-feeding

Side-effects: headache, oedema, fatigue, nausea, flushing, dizziness, gum hyperplasia, rashes (including rarely pruritus and very rarely erythema multiforme); rarely gastro-intestinal disturbances, dry mouth, sweating, palpitations, dyspnoea, drowsiness, mood changes, myalgia, arthralgia, asthenia, peripheral neuropathy, impotence, increased urinary frequency, visual disturbances; also reported, jaundice, pancreatitis, hyperglycaemia, thrombocytopenia, vasculitis, angioedema, alopecia, gynaecomastia

Dose: hypertension or angina, initially 5 mg once daily; max. 10 mg once daily

Istin® (Pfizer) [PoM]

Tablets, amlodipine (as besilate) 5 mg. Net price 28-tab pack = £11.85; 10 mg, 28-tab pack = £17.70

DILTIAZEM HYDROCHLORIDE

Indications: prophylaxis and treatment of angina; hypertension

Cautions: reduce dose in hepatic and renal impairment; heart failure or significantly impaired left ventricular function, bradycardia (avoid if severe), first degree AV block, or prolonged PR interval; **interactions:** Appendix 1 (calcium-channel blockers)

Contra-indications: severe bradycardia, left ventricular failure, second- or third-degree AV block (unless pacemaker fitted), sick sinus syndrome; pregnancy and breast-feeding (see Appendixes 4 and 5)

Side-effects: bradycardia, sino-atrial block, AV block, palpitations, dizziness, hypotension, malaise, asthenia, headache, hot flushes, gastro-intestinal disturbances, oedema (notably of ankles); rarely rashes (including erythema multiforme and exfoliative dermatitis), photosensitivity; hepatitis, gynaecomastia, gum hyperplasia, extrapyramidal symptoms, depression reported

Dose: angina, 60 mg 3 times daily (elderly initially twice daily); increased if necessary to 360 mg daily

Longer-acting formulations, see under preparations below

■ Standard formulations

Note. These formulations are licensed as generics and there is no requirement for brand name dispensing. Although their means of formulation has called for the strict designation 'modified-release' their duration of action corresponds to that of tablets requiring administration 3 times daily

Diltiazem (Non-proprietary) [PoM]

Tablets, m/r (but see note above), diltiazem hydrochloride 60 mg. Net price 100 = £5.24. Label: 25

Available from Alpharma, APS, Ashbourne (*Angiozem®*), Hillcross, IVAX, Opus (*Optil®*), Sterwin

Tildiem® (Sanofi-Synthelabo) [PoM]

Tablets, m/r (but see note above), off-white, diltiazem hydrochloride 60 mg. Net price 90-tab pack = £8.28. Label: 25

■ Longer-acting formulations

Note. Different versions of modified-release preparations may not have the same clinical effect. To avoid confusion between these different formulations of diltiazem, prescribers should specify the brand to be dispensed

Adizem-SR® (Napp) PoM
Capsules, m/r, diltiazem hydrochloride 90 mg (white), net price 56-cap pack = £10.56; 120 mg (brown/white), 56-cap pack = £11.74; 180 mg (brown/white), 56-cap pack = £17.60. Label: 25
Tablets, m/r, f/c, scored, diltiazem hydrochloride 120 mg. Net price 56-tab pack = £17.32. Label: 25
Dose: mild to moderate hypertension, usually 120 mg twice daily (dose form not appropriate for initial dose titration)
Angina, initially 90 mg twice daily (elderly, dose form not appropriate for initial dose titration); increased to 180 mg twice daily if required

Adizem-XL® (Napp) PoM
Capsules, m/r, diltiazem hydrochloride 120 mg (pink/blue), net price 28-cap pack = £10.24; 180 mg (dark pink/blue), 28-cap pack = £11.61; 240 mg (red/blue), 28-cap pack = £12.90; 300 mg (maroon/blue), 28-cap pack = £10.24. Label: 25
Dose: angina and mild to moderate hypertension, initially 240 mg once daily, increased if necessary to 300 mg once daily; in elderly and in hepatic or renal impairment, initially 120 mg daily

Angitil SR® (Trinity) PoM
Capsules, m/r, diltiazem hydrochloride 90 mg (white), net price 56-cap pack = £8.45; 120 mg (brown), 56-cap pack = £9.39; 180 mg (brown), 56-cap pack = £14.08. Label: 25
Dose: angina and mild to moderate hypertension, initially 90 mg twice daily; increased if necessary to 120 mg or 180 mg twice daily
Note. Also available as *Optil® SR* (Opus)

Angitil XL® (Trinity) PoM
Capsules, m/r, diltiazem hydrochloride 240 mg (white), net price 28-cap pack = £10.15; 300 mg (yellow), 28-cap pack = £9.22. Label: 25
Dose: angina and mild to moderate hypertension, initially 240 mg once daily (elderly and in hepatic and renal impairment, dose form not appropriate for initial dose titration); increased if necessary to 300 mg once daily
Note. Also available as *Optil® XL* (Opus)

Calcicard CR® (IVAX) PoM
Tablets, m/r, both f/c, diltiazem hydrochloride 90 mg, net price 56-tab pack = £6.33; 120 mg, 56-tab pack = £7.04. Label: 25
Dose: mild to moderate hypertension, initially 90 mg or 120 mg twice daily; up to 360 mg daily may be required: ELDERLY and in hepatic and renal impairment, initially 120 mg once daily; up to 240 mg daily may be required
Angina, initially 90 mg or 120 mg twice daily; up to 480 mg daily in divided doses may be required; ELDERLY and in hepatic and renal impairment, dose form not appropriate for initial dose titration; up to 240 mg daily may be required
Note. Also available as *Angiozem CR®* (Ashbourne)

Dilcardia SR® (Generics) PoM
Capsules, m/r, diltiazem hydrochloride 60 mg (pink/white), net price 100-cap pack = £14.82; 90 mg (pink/yellow), 56-cap pack = £10.33; 120 mg (pink/orange), 56-cap pack = £11.49. Label: 25
Dose: angina and mild to moderate hypertension, initially 90 mg twice daily; increased if necessary to 180 mg twice daily; ELDERLY and in hepatic or renal impairment, initially 60 mg twice daily, max. 90 mg twice daily

Dilzem SR® (Elan) PoM
Capsules, m/r, all beige, diltiazem hydrochloride 60 mg, net price 56-cap pack = £8.32; 90 mg, 56-

cap pack = £11.23; 120 mg, 56-cap pack = £12.47. Label: 25
Dose: angina and mild to moderate hypertension, initially 90 mg twice daily (elderly 60 mg twice daily); up to 180 mg twice daily may be required

Dilzem XL® (Elan) PoM
Capsules, m/r, diltiazem hydrochloride 120 mg, net price 28-cap pack = £8.32; 180 mg, 28-cap pack = £11.40; 240 mg, 28-cap pack = £11.70. Label: 25
Dose: angina and mild to moderate hypertension, initially 180 mg once daily (elderly and in hepatic and renal impairment, 120 mg once daily); if necessary may be increased to 360 mg once daily

Slozem® (Merck) PoM
Capsules, m/r, diltiazem hydrochloride 120 mg (pink/clear), net price 28-cap pack = £7.00; 180 mg (pink/clear), 28-cap pack = £7.80; 240 mg (red/clear), 28-cap pack = £8.20; 300 mg (red/white), 28-cap pack = £8.50. Label: 25
Dose: angina and mild to moderate hypertension, initially 240 mg once daily (elderly and in hepatic and renal impairment, 120 mg once daily); if necessary may be increased to 360 mg once daily

Tildiem LA® (Sanofi-Synthelabo) PoM
Capsules, m/r, diltiazem hydrochloride 200 mg (pink/grey, containing white pellets), net price 28-cap pack = £11.61; 300 mg (white/yellow, containing white pellets), 28-cap pack = £12.80. Label: 25
Dose: angina and mild to moderate hypertension, initially 200 mg once daily before or with food, increased if necessary to 300–400 mg daily, max. 500 mg daily; ELDERLY and in hepatic or renal impairment, initially 200 mg daily, increased if necessary to 300 mg daily

Tildiem Retard® (Sanofi-Synthelabo) PoM
Tablets, m/r, diltiazem hydrochloride 90 mg, net price 56-tab pack = £9.95; 120 mg, 56-tab pack = £11.06. Label: 25
COUNSELLING. Tablet membrane may pass through gastro-intestinal tract unchanged, but being porous has no effect on efficacy
Dose: mild to moderate hypertension, initially 90 mg or 120 mg twice daily; increased if necessary to 360 mg daily in divided doses; ELDERLY and in hepatic or renal impairment, initially 120 mg once daily; increased if necessary to 120 mg twice daily
Angina, initially 90 mg or 120 mg twice daily; increased if necessary to 480 mg daily in divided doses; ELDERLY and in hepatic or renal impairment, dose form not appropriate for initial titration; up to 120 mg twice daily may be required

Viazem XL® (Genus) PoM
Capsules, m/r, diltiazem hydrochloride 120 mg (lavender), net price 28-cap pack = £6.95; 180 mg (white/blue-green), 28-cap pack = £7.75; 240 mg (blue-green/lavender), 28-cap pack = £8.15; 300 mg (white/lavender), 28-cap pack = £8.45; 360 mg (blue-green), 28-cap pack = £14.95. Label: 25
Dose: mild to moderate hypertension, titrate to usual maintenance dose of 300 mg once daily, adjusted according to response
ELDERLY and in hepatic or renal impairment, initially 120 mg once daily, adjusted according to response

Zemtard® (Galen) PoM
Zemtard 120XL capsules, m/r, brown/orange, diltiazem hydrochloride 120 mg, net price 28-cap pack = £7.65. Label: 25

Zemtard 180XL capsules, m/r, grey/pink, diltiazem hydrochloride 180 mg, net price 28-cap pack = £7.80. Label: 25

Zemtard 240XL capsules, m/r, blue, diltiazem hydrochloride 240 mg, net price 28-cap pack = £8.20. Label: 25

Zemtard 300XL capsules, m/r, white/blue, diltiazem hydrochloride 300 mg, net price 28-cap pack = £8.50. Label: 25

Dose: angina and mild to moderate hypertension, 180–300 mg once daily, increased if necessary to 360 mg once daily in hypertension and to 480 mg once daily in angina; ELDERLY and in hepatic or renal impairment, initially 120 mg once daily

FELODIPINE

Indications: hypertension, prophylaxis of angina

Cautions: withdraw if ischaemic pain occurs or existing pain worsens shortly after initiating treatment or if cardiogenic shock develops; severe left ventricular dysfunction; hepatic impairment; breast-feeding; avoid grapefruit juice (may affect metabolism); **interactions:** Appendix 1 (calcium-channel blockers)

Contra-indications: pregnancy; unstable angina, uncontrolled heart failure; significant aortic stenosis; within 1 month of myocardial infarction

Side-effects: flushing, headache, palpitations, dizziness, fatigue, gravitational oedema; rarely rash, pruritus, cutaneous vasculitis, gum hyperplasia, urinary frequency, impotence, fever

Dose: hypertension, initially 5 mg (elderly 2.5 mg) daily in the morning; usual maintenance 5–10 mg once daily; doses above 20 mg daily rarely needed
Angina, initially 5 mg daily in the morning, increased if necessary to 10 mg once daily

Plendil® (AstraZeneca) [PoM]
Tablets, m/r, f/c, felodipine 2.5 mg (yellow), net price 28-tab pack = £6.09; 5 mg (pink), 28-tab pack = £8.12; 10 mg (brown), 28-tab pack = £10.92. Label: 25

ISRADIPINE

Indications: hypertension

Cautions: tight aortic stenosis; sick sinus syndrome (if pacemaker not fitted); reduce dose in hepatic or renal impairment; pregnancy (may prolong labour); avoid grapefruit juice (may affect metabolism); **interactions:** Appendix 1 (calcium-channel blockers)

Side-effects: headache, flushing, dizziness, tachycardia and palpitations, localised peripheral oedema; hypotension uncommon; rarely weight gain, fatigue, abdominal discomfort, rashes

Dose: 2.5 mg twice daily (1.25 mg twice daily in elderly, hepatic or renal impairment); increased if necessary after 3–4 weeks to 5 mg twice daily (exceptionally up to 10 mg twice daily); maintenance 2.5 or 5 mg once daily may be sufficient

Prescal® (Novartis) [PoM]
Tablets, yellow, scored, isradipine 2.5 mg. Net price 56-tab pack = £15.04

LACIDIPINE

Indications: hypertension

Cautions: cardiac conduction abnormalities; poor cardiac reserve; hepatic impairment; withdraw if ischaemic pain occurs shortly after initiating treatment or if cardiogenic shock develops; avoid grapefruit juice (may affect metabolism); **interactions:** Appendix 1 (calcium-channel blockers)

Contra-indications: aortic stenosis; pregnancy and breast-feeding; avoid within 1 month of myocardial infarction

Side-effects: headache, flushing, oedema, dizziness, palpitations; also asthenia, rash (including pruritus and erythema), gastro-intestinal disturbances, gum hyperplasia, muscle cramps, polyuria, chest pain (see Cautions); mood disturbances

Dose: initially 2 mg as a single daily dose, preferably in the morning; increased after 3–4 weeks to 4 mg daily, then if necessary to 6 mg daily

Motens® (Boehringer Ingelheim) [PoM]
Tablets, both f/c, lacidipine 2 mg, net price 28-tab pack = £10.23; 4 mg (scored), 28-tab pack = £15.30

LERCANIDIPINE HYDROCHLORIDE

Indications: mild to moderate hypertension

Cautions: hepatic and renal impairment (Appendixes 2 and 3); left ventricular dysfunction; sick sinus syndrome (if pacemaker not fitted); avoid grapefruit juice (may affect metabolism); **interactions:** Appendix 1 (calcium-channel blockers)

Contra-indications: aortic stenosis; unstable angina, uncontrolled heart failure; within 1 month of myocardial infarction; pregnancy and breast-feeding

Side-effects: flushing, peripheral oedema, palpitations, tachycardia, headache, dizziness, asthenia; also gastro-intestinal disturbances, hypotension, drowsiness, myalgia, polyuria, rash

Dose: initially 10 mg once daily; increased, if necessary, after at least 2 weeks to 20 mg daily

Zanidip® (Napp) [PoM]
Tablets, yellow, f/c, lercanidipine hydrochloride 10 mg, net price 28-tab pack = £7.80. Label: 22

NICARDIPINE HYDROCHLORIDE

Indications: prophylaxis of angina; mild to moderate hypertension

Cautions: withdraw if ischaemic pain occurs or existing pain worsens within 30 minutes of initiating treatment or increasing dose; congestive heart failure or significantly impaired left ventricular function; elderly; hepatic or renal impairment; avoid grapefruit juice (may affect metabolism); **interactions:** Appendix 1 (calcium-channel blockers)

Contra-indications: cardiogenic shock; advanced aortic stenosis; unstable or acute attacks of angina; pregnancy and breast-feeding; avoid within 1 month of myocardial infarction

Side-effects: dizziness, headache, peripheral oedema, flushing, palpitations, nausea; also gastro-intestinal disturbances, drowsiness, insomnia, tinnitus, hypotension, rashes, dyspnoea, paraesthesia, frequency of micturition; thrombocytopenia, depression and impotence reported

Dose: initially 20 mg 3 times daily, increased, after at least three days, to 30 mg 3 times daily (usual range 60–120 mg daily)

Nicardipine (Non-proprietary) PoM
Capsules, nicardipine hydrochloride 20 mg, net price 56-cap pack = £8.38; 30 mg, 56-cap pack = £9.73
Available from Generics

Cardene® (Yamanouchi) PoM
Capsules, nicardipine hydrochloride 20 mg (blue/white), net price 56-cap pack = £8.38; 30 mg (blue/pale blue), 56-cap pack = £9.73

■ Modified release

Cardene SR® (Yamanouchi) PoM
Capsules, m/r, nicardipine hydrochloride 30 mg, net price 56-cap pack = £9.68; 45 mg (blue), 56-cap pack = £13.44. Label: 25
Dose: mild to moderate hypertension, initially 30 mg twice daily; usual effective dose 45 mg twice daily (range 30–60 mg twice daily)

NIFEDIPINE

Indications: prophylaxis of angina; hypertension; Raynaud's phenomenon

Cautions: withdraw if ischaemic pain occurs or existing pain worsens shortly after initiating treatment; poor cardiac reserve; heart failure or significantly impaired left ventricular function (heart failure deterioration observed); severe hypotension; reduce dose in hepatic impairment; diabetes mellitus; may inhibit labour; pregnancy (Appendix 4); breast-feeding (Appendix 5); avoid grapefruit juice (may affect metabolism); **interactions:** Appendix 1 (calcium-channel blockers)

Contra-indications: cardiogenic shock; advanced aortic stenosis; within 1 month of myocardial infarction; unstable or acute attacks of angina; porphyria (section 9.8.2)

Side-effects: headache, flushing, dizziness, lethargy; tachycardia, palpitations; short-acting preparations may induce an exaggerated fall in blood pressure and reflex tachycardia which may lead to myocardial or cerebrovascular ischaemia; gravitational oedema, rash (erythema multiforme reported), pruritus, urticaria, nausea, constipation or diarrhoea, increased frequency of micturition, eye pain, visual disturbances, gum hyperplasia, paraesthesia, myalgia, tremor, impotence, gynaecomastia; depression, telangiectasia, cholestasis, jaundice reported

Dose: see preparations below

Nifedipine (Non-proprietary) PoM
Capsules, nifedipine 5 mg, net price 84-cap pack = £3.67; 10 mg, 84-cap pack = £4.44
Dose: angina prophylaxis (but not recommended, see notes above) and Raynaud's phenomenon, initially 5 mg 3 times daily, adjusted according to response to 20 mg 3 times daily
Hypertension, not recommended therefore no dose stated
Available from Alpharma, APS, Ashbourne (*Angiopine®*), CP, Hillcross, IVAX

Adalat® (Bayer) PoM
Capsules, both orange, nifedipine 5 mg, net price 90-cap pack = £6.08; 10 mg, 90-cap pack = £7.74
Dose: angina prophylaxis (but not recommended, see notes above) and Raynaud's phenomenon, initially 5 mg 3 times daily, adjusted according to response to 20 mg 3 times daily
Hypertension, not recommended therefore no dose stated

■ Modified release

Note. Different versions of modified-release preparations may not have the same clinical effect. To avoid confusion between these different formulations of nifedipine, prescribers should specify the brand to be dispensed. Modified-release formulations may not be suitable for dose titration in hepatic disease

Adalat® LA (Bayer) PoM
LA 20 tablets, m/r, pink, nifedipine 20 mg, net price 28-tab pack = £8.15. Label: 25
LA 30 tablets, m/r, pink, nifedipine 30 mg, net price 28-tab pack = £9.89. Label: 25
LA 60 tablets, m/r, pink, nifedipine 60 mg, net price 28-tab pack = £15.40. Label: 25
COUNSELLING. Tablet membrane may pass through gastro-intestinal tract unchanged, but being porous has no effect on efficacy
Dose: mild to moderate hypertension, 20 mg once daily, increased if necessary
Angina prophylaxis, 30 mg once daily, increased if necessary; max. 90 mg once daily
Caution: dose form not appropriate for use in hepatic impairment or where there is a history of oesophageal or gastro-intestinal obstruction, decreased lumen diameter of the gastro-intestinal tract, or inflammatory bowel disease (including Crohn's disease)

Adalat® Retard (Bayer) PoM
Retard 10 tablets, m/r, pink, nifedipine 10 mg. Net price 56-tab pack = £8.50. Label: 25
Retard 20 tablets, m/r, pink, nifedipine 20 mg. Net price 56-tab pack = £10.20. Label: 25
Dose: hypertension and angina prophylaxis, 10 mg twice daily, adjusted according to response to 40 mg twice daily

Adipine® MR (Trinity) PoM
Tablets, m/r, nifedipine 10 mg (apricot), net price 56-tab pack = £6.62; 20 mg (pink), 56-tab pack = £8.26. Label: 21, 25
Dose: hypertension and angina prophylaxis, 20 mg twice daily after food (initial titration 10 mg twice daily); max. 40 mg twice daily
Note. Also available as *Nimodrel MR®* (Opus)

Cardilate MR® (IVAX) PoM
Tablets, m/r, nifedipine 10 mg (pink), net price 56-tab pack = £4.97; 20 mg (brown), net price 100-tab pack = £16.62. Label: 25
Dose: hypertension and angina prophylaxis, 20 mg twice daily (initial titration 10 mg twice daily); max. 80 mg daily
Note. Also available as *Angiopine MR®* (Ashbourne)

Coracten SR® (Celltech) PoM
Capsules, m/r, nifedipine 10 mg (grey/pink, enclosing yellow pellets), net price 60-cap pack = £6.25; 20 mg (pink/brown, enclosing yellow pellets), 60-cap pack = £8.67. Label: 25
Dose: hypertension and angina prophylaxis, one 20-mg capsule every 12 hours, adjusted within range 10–40 mg every 12 hours

Coracten XL® (Celltech) [PoM]

Capsules, m/r, nifedipine 30 mg (brown), net price 28-cap pack = £6.73; 60 mg (orange), 28-cap pack = £10.01. Label: 25

Dose: hypertension and angina prophylaxis, 30 mg once daily, increased if necessary; max. 90 mg once daily

Coroday MR® (Generics) [PoM]

Tablets, m/r, red, nifedipine 20 mg, net price 56-tab pack = £9.94. Label: 25

Dose: hypertension and angina prophylaxis, 20 mg every 12 hours, increased if necessary to 40 mg every 12 hours

Fortipine LA 40® (Goldshield) [PoM]

Tablets, m/r, red, nifedipine 40 mg, net price 30-tab pack = £8.00. Label: 21, 25

Dose: hypertension and angina prophylaxis, 40 mg once daily, increased if necessary to 80 mg daily in 1–2 divided doses

Hypolar® Retard 20 (Lagap) [PoM]

Tablets, m/r, red, f/c, nifedipine 20 mg. Net price 56-tab pack = £10.12. Label: 25

Dose: hypertension and angina prophylaxis, 20 mg twice daily, increased if necessary to 40 mg twice daily

Nifedipress® MR (Dexcel) [PoM]

Tablets, m/r, pink, nifedipine 10 mg, net price 56-tab pack = £9.93. Label: 25

Dose: hypertension and angina prophylaxis, initially 10 mg twice daily adjusted according to response to 40 mg twice daily

Nifopress® Retard (Goldshield) [PoM]

Tablets, m/r, pink, nifedipine 20 mg, net price 112-tab pack = £20.00. Label: 21, 25

Dose: mild to moderate hypertension, angina prophylaxis and Raynaud's phenomenon, usually 20 mg twice daily, adjusted according to response to 40 mg twice daily

Slofedipine® (Sterwin) [PoM]

Tablets, m/r, pink, nifedipine 20 mg, net price 56-tab pack = £10.32. Label: 25

Dose: hypertension and angina prophylaxis, initially 20 mg twice daily adjusted according to response to 40 mg twice daily

Slofedipine XL® (Sterwin) [PoM]

Tablets, m/r, brown, nifedipine 30 mg, net price 28-tab pack = £9.89; 60 mg, 28-tab pack = £14.71. Label: 25

Dose: hypertension and angina prophylaxis, 30 mg once daily, increased if necessary to 90 mg once daily

Caution: dose form not appropriate for use in hepatic impairment or where there is a history of oesophageal or gastro-intestinal obstruction, decreased lumen diameter of the gastro-intestinal tract, or inflammatory bowel disease (including Crohn's disease)

Tensipine MR® (Genus) [PoM]

Tablets, m/r, both pink, nifedipine 10 mg, net price 56-tab pack = £4.65; 20 mg, 56-tab pack = £5.99. Label: 21, 25

Dose: hypertension and angina prophylaxis, initially 10 mg twice daily adjusted according to response to 40 mg twice daily

■ With atenolol
Section 2.4

NIMODIPINE

Indications: prevention and treatment of ischaemic neurological deficits following subarachnoid haemorrhage

Cautions: cerebral oedema or severely raised intracranial pressure; hypotension; avoid concomitant administration of nimodipine tablets and infusion, other calcium-channel blockers, or beta-blockers; impaired renal function or nephrotoxic drugs; hepatic impairment (Appendix 2); pregnancy; avoid grapefruit juice (may affect metabolism); **interactions:** Appendix 1 (calcium-channel blockers, alcohol (infusion only))

Contra-indications: within 1 month of myocardial infarction; unstable angina

Side-effects: hypotension, variation in heart-rate, flushing, headache, gastro-intestinal disorders, nausea, sweating and feeling of warmth; thrombocytopenia and ileus reported

Dose: prevention, *by mouth*, 60 mg every 4 hours, starting within 4 days of subarachnoid haemorrhage and continued for 21 days

Treatment, *by intravenous infusion* via central catheter, 1 mg/hour initially, increased after 2 hours to 2 mg/hour, providing no severe decrease in blood pressure; patients with unstable blood pressure or weighing less than 70 kg, 500 micrograms/hour initially or less if necessary; treatment should start as soon as possible; in *aneurysmal* subarachnoid haemorrhage continue intravenous infusion for at least 5 days (max. 14 days); in the event of surgical intervention during treatment continue for at least 5 days after surgery; in *traumatic* subarachnoid haemorrhage continue intravenous infusion for 7–10 days then complete 21-day course by mouth

Max. total duration of treatment 21 days (max. 14 days by intravenous infusion)

Nimotop® (Bayer) [PoM]

Tablets, yellow, f/c, nimodipine 30 mg. Net price 100-tab pack = £38.85

Intravenous infusion, nimodipine 200 micrograms/mL; also contains ethanol 20% and macrogol '400' 17%. Net price 50-mL vial (with polyethylene infusion catheter) = £13.24

Note. Polyethylene, polypropylene or glass apparatus should be used; PVC should be avoided

NISOLDIPINE

Indications: prophylaxis of angina, mild to moderate hypertension

Cautions: elderly; hypotension; avoid grapefruit juice (may affect metabolism); **interactions:** Appendix 1 (calcium-channel blockers)

Contra-indications: cardiogenic shock, aortic stenosis, unstable or acute attacks of angina; within 1 week of myocardial infarction; hepatic impairment (dose form not appropriate); pregnancy and breast-feeding

Side-effects: gravitational oedema, headache, flushing, tachycardia, palpitations; dizziness, asthenia, gastro-intestinal disturbances (including nausea, constipation); less frequently paraesthesia, myalgia, tremor, hypotension, weakness, dyspnoea, allergic skin reactions, increased frequency of micturition; rarely exacerbation of angina, visual disturbances, gynaecomastia, gum hyperplasia

Dose: initially 10 mg daily, preferably before breakfast; if necessary increase at intervals of at least 1 week (usual maintenance in angina 20–40 mg once daily); max. 40 mg daily

Syscor MR® (Forest) PoM

Tablets, m/r, all f/c, yellow, nisoldipine 10 mg, net price 28-tab pack = £9.36; 20 mg, 28-tab pack = £13.10; 30 mg, 28-tab pack = £16.85. Label: 22, 25

VERAPAMIL HYDROCHLORIDE

Indications: see under Dose and preparations

Cautions: first-degree AV block; acute phase of myocardial infarction (avoid if bradycardia, hypotension, left ventricular failure); patients taking beta-blockers **(important:** see below); hepatic impairment (Appendix 2); children, specialist advice only (section 2.3.2); pregnancy (Appendix 4) and breast-feeding (Appendix 5); avoid grapefruit juice (may affect metabolism); **interactions:** Appendix 1 (calcium-channel blockers)

VERAPAMIL AND BETA-BLOCKERS. **Verapamil** injection should not be given to patients recently treated with beta-blockers because of the risk of hypotension and asystole. The suggestion that when verapamil injection has been given first, an interval of 30 minutes before giving a beta-blocker is sufficient has not been confirmed.

It may also be hazardous to give verapamil and a beta-blocker together by mouth (should only be contemplated if myocardial function well preserved).

Contra-indications: hypotension, bradycardia, second- and third-degree AV block, sick sinus syndrome, cardiogenic shock, sino-atrial block; history of heart failure or significantly impaired left ventricular function, even if controlled by therapy; atrial flutter or fibrillation complicating Wolff-Parkinson-White syndrome; porphyria (section 9.8.2)

Side-effects: constipation; less commonly nausea, vomiting, flushing, headache, dizziness, fatigue, ankle oedema; rarely allergic reactions (erythema, pruritus, urticaria, angioedema, Stevens-Johnson syndrome); myalgia, arthralgia, paraesthesia, erythromelalgia; increased prolactin concentration; rarely gynaecomastia and gingival hyperplasia after long-term treatment; after intravenous administration or high doses, hypotension, heart failure, bradycardia, heart block, and asystole

Dose: *by mouth*, supraventricular arrhythmias (but see also Contra-indications), 40–120 mg 3 times daily

Angina, 80–120 mg 3 times daily

Hypertension, 240–480 mg daily in 2–3 divided doses

By slow intravenous injection over 2 minutes (3 minutes in elderly), 5–10 mg (preferably with ECG monitoring); in paroxysmal tachyarrhythmias a further 5 mg after 5–10 minutes if required

Verapamil (Non-proprietary) PoM

Tablets, coated, verapamil hydrochloride 40 mg, net price 20 = 39p; 80 mg, 20 = 50p; 120 mg, 20 = 70p; 160 mg, 20 = £2.02

Various strengths available from Alpharma, APS, Generics, Hillcross, IVAX

Oral solution, verapamil hydrochloride 40 mg/ 5 mL, net price 150 mL = £39.25

Available from Rosemont (*Zolvera®*)

Cordilox® (IVAX) PoM

Tablets, all yellow, f/c, verapamil hydrochloride 40 mg, net price 100-tab pack = £4.57; 80 mg, 84-tab pack = £7.69; 120 mg, 100-tab pack = £13.70; 160 mg, 56-tab pack = £12.77

Injection, verapamil hydrochloride 2.5 mg/mL, net price 2-mL amp = £1.11

Securon® (Abbott) PoM

Tablets, f/c, verapamil hydrochloride 40 mg, net price 100 = £4.57; 120 mg (scored), 60-tab pack = £7.67

Injection, verapamil hydrochloride 2.5 mg/mL. Net price 2-mL amp = £1.08

■ Modified release

Half Securon SR® (Abbott) PoM

Tablets, m/r, f/c, verapamil hydrochloride 120 mg. Net price 28-tab pack = £7.50. Label: 25

Dose: see *Securon SR®*

Securon SR® (Abbott) PoM

Tablets, m/r, pale green, f/c, scored, verapamil hydrochloride 240 mg. Net price 28-tab pack = £10.64. Label: 25

Dose: hypertension, 240 mg daily (new patients initially 120 mg), increased if necessary to max. 480 mg daily (doses above 240 mg daily as 2 divided doses)

Angina, 240 mg twice daily (may sometimes be reduced to once daily)

Prophylaxis after myocardial infarction where beta-blockers not appropriate (started at least 1 week after infarction), 360 mg daily in divided doses, given as 240 mg in the morning and 120 mg in the evening *or* 120 mg 3 times daily

Univer® (Elan) PoM

Capsules, m/r, verapamil hydrochloride 120 mg (yellow/dark blue), net price 28-cap pack = £7.51; 180 mg (yellow), 56-cap pack = £18.15; 240 mg (yellow/dark blue), 28-cap pack = £12.24. Label: 25

Dose: hypertension, 240 mg daily, max. 480 mg daily (new patients, initial dose 120 mg); angina, 360 mg daily, max. 480 mg daily

Verapress MR® (Dexcel) PoM

Tablets, m/r, pale green, f/c, verapamil hydrochloride 240 mg. Net price 28-tab pack = £10.64. Label: 25

Dose: hypertension, 1 tablet daily, increased to twice daily if necessary; angina, 1 tablet twice daily (may sometimes be reduced to once daily)

Note. Also available as *Cordilox® MR* (IVAX), *Ethimil® MR* (Genus)

Vertab® SR 240 (Trinity) PoM

Tablets, m/r, pale green, f/c, scored, verapamil hydrochloride 240 mg, net price 28-tab pack = £8.63. Label: 25

Dose: mild to moderate hypertension, 240 mg daily, increased to twice daily if necessary; angina, 240 mg twice daily (may sometimes be reduced to once daily)

2.6.3   Potassium-channel activators

Nicorandil, a potassium-channel activator with a nitrate component, has both arterial and venous vasodilating properties and is indicated for the prevention and long-term treatment of angina (section 2.6). Nicorandil has similar efficacy to other antianginal drugs in controlling symptoms but there is little evidence about its efficacy in combination with other antianginal drugs. However, when added to maximal therapy with other antianginal drugs in refractory unstable angina [unlicensed indication], it may produce additional benefit.

NICORANDIL

Indications: prophylaxis and treatment of angina

Cautions: hypovolaemia; low systolic blood pressure; acute pulmonary oedema; acute myocardial infarction with acute left ventricular failure and low filling pressures; pregnancy and breast-feeding; **interactions:** Appendix 1 (nicorandil)

DRIVING. Patients should be warned not to drive or operate machinery until it is established that their performance is unimpaired

Contra-indications: cardiogenic shock; left ventricular failure with low filling pressures; hypotension

Side-effects: headache (especially on initiation, usually transitory); cutaneous vasodilatation with flushing; nausea, vomiting, dizziness, weakness also reported; rarely oral ulceration and myalgia; at high dosage, reduction in blood pressure and/or increase in heart rate; angioedema, hepatic dysfunction also reported

Dose: initially 10 mg twice daily (if susceptible to headache 5 mg twice daily); usual dose 10–20 mg twice daily; up to 30 mg twice daily may be used

Ikorel® (Rhône-Poulenc Rorer) PoM
Tablets, both scored, nicorandil 10 mg, net price 60-tab pack = £8.16; 20 mg, 60-tab pack = £15.54

2.6.4 Peripheral and cerebral vasodilators

2.6.4.1 Peripheral vasodilators and related drugs
2.6.4.2 Cerebral vasodilators

2.6.4.1 Peripheral vasodilators and related drugs

Most serious peripheral vascular disorders, such as *intermittent claudication*, are due to occlusion of vessels, either by spasm or sclerotic plaques. Lifestyle changes including smoking cessation and exercise training are the most important measures in the conservative management of intermittent claudication. Low-dose aspirin (75–300 mg daily) should be given as long-term prophylaxis against cardiovascular events and a statin (section 2.12) should be considered if serum total cholesterol is raised. **Naftidrofuryl** 200 mg 3 times daily may alleviate symptoms and improve pain-free walking distance in moderate disease, but it is not known whether naftidrofuryl has any effect on the outcome of the disease. Patients receiving naftidrofuryl should be assessed for improvement after 3–6 months. Inositol nicotinate, pentoxifylline (oxentifylline) and cinnarizine are not established as being effective.

Management of *Raynaud's syndrome* includes avoidance of exposure to cold and stopping smoking. More severe symptoms may require vasodilator treatment, which is most often successful in primary Raynaud's syndrome. **Nifedipine** (section 2.6.2) is useful for reducing the frequency and severity of vasospastic attacks. Alternatively, **naftidrofuryl** may produce symptomatic improvement; **inositol nicotinate** (a nicotinic acid deriva-

tive) may also be considered. Cinnarizine, pentoxifylline, prazosin and moxisylyte (thymoxamine) are not established as being effective.

Vasodilator therapy is not established as being effective for *chilblains* (section 13.14).

CINNARIZINE ⬛

Indications: peripheral vascular disease, Raynaud's syndrome

Cautions: see section 4.6

Contra-indications: see section 4.6

Side-effects: see section 4.6

Dose: initially, 75 mg 3 times daily; maintenance, 75 mg 2–3 times daily

Stugeron Forte® (Janssen-Cilag) ⬛
Capsules, orange/ivory, cinnarizine 75 mg. Net price 100-cap pack = £5.50. Label: 2
Stugeron®: see section 4.6

MOXISYLYTE/THYMOXAMINE ⬛

Indications: primary Raynaud's syndrome (short-term treatment)

Cautions: diabetes mellitus

Contra-indications: active liver disease

Side-effects: nausea, diarrhoea, flushing, headache, dizziness; hepatic reactions including cholestatic jaundice and hepatitis reported to CSM

Dose: initially 40 mg 4 times daily, increased to 80 mg 4 times daily if poor initial response; discontinue after 2 weeks if no response

Opilon® (Hansam) PoM ⬛
Tablets, yellow, f/c, moxisylyte 40 mg (as hydrochloride). Net price 112-tab pack = £79.98. Label: 21

NAFTIDROFURYL OXALATE

Indications: see under Dose

Side-effects: nausea, epigastric pain, rash, hepatitis, hepatic failure

Dose: peripheral vascular disease (see notes above), 100–200 mg 3 times daily; cerebral vascular disease, 100 mg 3 times daily

Naftidrofuryl (Non-proprietary) PoM
Capsules, naftidrofuryl oxalate 100 mg. Net price 84-cap pack = £8.92. Label: 25, 27
Available from Alpharma
Praxilene® (Merck) PoM
Capsules, pink, naftidrofuryl oxalate 100 mg. Net price 84-cap pack = £8.60. Label: 25, 27

NICOTINIC ACID DERIVATIVES ⬛

Indications: peripheral vascular disease; hyperlipidaemia (section 2.12)

Side-effects: flushing, dizziness, nausea, vomiting, hypotension (more frequent with nicotinic acid than derivatives); occasional diabetogenic effect reported with nicotinic acid and nicotinyl alcohol; rarely associated with nodular changes to liver (monitor on prolonged high dosage)

Hexopal® (Sanofi-Synthelabo) ▰

Tablets, scored, inositol nicotinate 500 mg. Net price 20 = £4.10

Dose: 1 g 3 times daily, increased to 4 g daily if required

Tablets forte, scored, inositol nicotinate 750 mg. Net price 112-tab pack = £34.02

Dose: 1.5 g twice daily

Suspension, sugar-free, inositol nicotinate 1 g/5 mL. Net price 300 mL = £20.85

Dose: as for tablets (above)

PENTOXIFYLLINE/OXPENTIFYLLINE ▰

Indications: peripheral vascular disease

Cautions: hypotension, coronary artery disease; renal impairment, severe hepatic impairment; avoid in porphyria (section 9.8.2); **interactions:** Appendix 1 (pentoxifylline)

Contra-indications: cerebral haemorrhage, extensive retinal haemorrhage, acute myocardial infarction; pregnancy and breast-feeding

Side-effects: gastro-intestinal disturbances, dizziness, agitation, sleep disturbances, headache; rarely flushing, tachycardia, angina, hypotension, thrombocytopenia, intrahepatic cholestasis, hypersensitivity reactions including rash, pruritus and bronchospasm

Dose: 400 mg 2–3 times daily

Trental® (Borg) PoM ▰

Tablets, m/r, pink, s/c, pentoxifylline 400 mg. Net price 90-tab pack = £23.81. Label: 21, 25

Other preparations used in peripheral vascular disease

Rutosides (oxerutins, *Paroven®*) are not vasodilators and are not generally regarded as effective preparations as capillary sealants or for the treatment of cramps; side-effects include headache, flushing, rashes, mild gastro-intestinal disturbances.

Paroven® (Novartis Consumer Health) ▰

Capsules, yellow, oxerutins 250 mg. Net price 120-cap pack = £13.05

Dose: relief of symptoms of oedema associated with chronic venous insufficiency, 500 mg twice daily

---

2.6.4.2 Cerebral vasodilators

These drugs are claimed to improve mental function. Some improvements in performance of psychological tests have been reported but the drugs have not been shown clinically to be of much benefit in dementia. For other drugs used in dementia, see section 4.11.

CO-DERGOCRINE MESILATE ▰

A mixture in equal proportions of dihydroergocornine mesilate, dihydroergocristine mesilate, and (in the ratio 2 : 1) α- and β-dihydroergocryptine mesilates

Indications: adjunct in elderly patients with mild to moderate dementia

Cautions: severe bradycardia

Side-effects: gastro-intestinal disturbances, flushing, headache, rash, nasal congestion; dizziness and postural hypotension in hypertensive patients

Dose: 1.5 mg 3 times daily before meals *or* 4.5 mg once daily before a meal

Hydergine® (Novartis) PoM ▰

Tablets, co-dergocrine mesilate 1.5 mg (scored), net price 100-tab pack = £12.94; 4.5 mg, 28-tab pack = £12.94. Label: 22

▰ denotes preparations that are considered to be less suitable for prescribing (see p. vi)

2.7 Sympathomimetics

2.7.1	Inotropic sympathomimetics
2.7.2	Vasoconstrictor sympathomimetics
2.7.3	Cardiopulmonary resuscitation

The properties of sympathomimetics vary according to whether they act on alpha or on beta adrenergic receptors. Adrenaline (epinephrine) (section 2.7.3) acts on both alpha and beta receptors and increases heart rate and contractility (beta$_1$ effects); it can cause peripheral vasodilation (a beta$_2$ effect) or vasoconstriction (an alpha effect).

2.7.1 Inotropic sympathomimetics

The cardiac stimulants **dobutamine** and **dopamine** act on beta$_1$ receptors in cardiac muscle, and increase contractility with little effect on rate. Dosage of dopamine is critical since although low doses induce vasodilatation and increase renal perfusion, higher doses (more than 5 micrograms/kg per minute) lead to vasoconstriction and may exacerbate heart failure.

Dopexamine acts on beta$_2$ receptors in cardiac muscle to produce its positive inotropic effect; and on peripheral dopamine receptors to increase renal perfusion; it is reported not to induce vasoconstriction.

Isoprenaline is less selective and increases both heart rate and contractility; it may prevent Stokes-Adams attacks, but insertion of a pacemaker is preferable. It is now only used as a short-term emergency treatment of heart block or severe bradycardia.

SHOCK. Shock is a medical emergency associated with a high mortality. The underlying causes of shock such as haemorrhage, sepsis or myocardial insufficiency should be corrected. The profound hypotension of shock must be treated promptly to prevent tissue hypoxia and organ failure. Volume replacement is essential to correct the hypovolaemia associated with haemorrhage and sepsis but may be detrimental in cardiogenic shock. Depending on haemodynamic status, cardiac output may be improved by the use of sympathomimetic inotropes such as adrenaline (epinephrine), dobutamine or dopamine (see notes above). In septic shock, when fluid replacement and inotropic support fail to maintain blood pressure, the vasoconstrictor noradrenaline (norepinephrine) (section 2.7.2) may be considered. In cardiogenic shock peripheral resistance is frequently high and to raise it further may worsen myocardial performance and exacerbate tissue ischaemia.

The use of sympathomimetic inotropes and vasoconstrictors should preferably be confined to the intensive care setting and undertaken with invasive haemodynamic monitoring.

For advice on the management of anaphylactic shock, see section 3.4.3.

DOBUTAMINE

Indications: inotropic support in infarction, cardiac surgery, cardiomyopathies, septic shock, and cardiogenic shock

Cautions: severe hypotension complicating cardiogenic shock; **interactions:** Appendix 1 (sympathomimetics)

Side-effects: tachycardia and marked increase in systolic blood pressure indicate overdosage

Dose: *by intravenous infusion*, 2.5–10 micrograms/kg/minute, adjusted according to response

Dobutrex® (Lilly) PoM

Strong sterile solution, dobutamine (as hydrochloride) 12.5 mg/mL. For dilution and use as an intravenous infusion. Net price 20-mL vial = £8.35

Note. Strong sterile solution containing dobutamine (as hydrochloride) 12.5 mg/mL also available in 20-mL amps from Phoenix

Posiject® (Boehringer Ingelheim) PoM

Strong sterile solution, dobutamine (as hydrochloride) 50 mg/mL. For dilution and use as an intravenous infusion. Net price 5-mL amp = £3.85

DOPAMINE HYDROCHLORIDE

Indications: cardiogenic shock in infarction or cardiac surgery

Cautions: correct hypovolaemia; low dose in shock due to acute myocardial infarction—see notes above; **interactions:** Appendix 1 (sympathomimetics)

Contra-indications: tachyarrhythmia, phaeochromocytoma

Side-effects: nausea and vomiting, peripheral vasoconstriction, hypotension, hypertension, tachycardia

Dose: *by intravenous infusion*, 2–5 micrograms/kg/minute initially (see notes above)

Dopamine (Non-proprietary) PoM

Sterile concentrate, dopamine hydrochloride 40 mg/mL, net price 5-mL amp = £3.88; 160 mg/mL, net price 5-mL amp = £14.75. For dilution and use as an intravenous infusion

Available from Antigen, Faulding DBL

Intravenous infusion, dopamine hydrochloride 1.6 mg/mL in glucose 5% intravenous infusion, net price 250-mL container (400 mg) = £11.69; 3.2 mg/mL, 250-mL container (800 mg) = £22.93 (both hosp. only)

Available from Abbott

Select-A-Jet® Dopamine (Celltech) PoM

Strong sterile solution, dopamine hydrochloride 40 mg/mL. Net price 5-mL vial = £4.55; 10-mL vial = £6.65. For dilution and use as an intravenous infusion

DOPEXAMINE HYDROCHLORIDE

Indications: inotropic support and vasodilator in exacerbations of chronic heart failure and in heart failure associated with cardiac surgery

Cautions: myocardial infarction, recent angina, hypokalaemia, hyperglycaemia; correct hypovolaemia before starting, monitor blood pressure, pulse, plasma potassium, blood glucose; avoid abrupt withdrawal; **interactions:** Appendix 1 (sympathomimetics)

Contra-indications: left ventricular outlet obstruction such as hypertrophic cardiomyopathy or aortic stenosis; phaeochromocytoma, thrombocytopenia

Side-effects: tachycardia, other arrhythmias; also reported: nausea, vomiting, anginal pain, tremor, headache

Dose: *by intravenous infusion* into central or large peripheral vein, 500 nanograms/kg/minute, may be increased to 1 microgram/kg/minute and further increased up to 6 micrograms/kg/minute in increments of 0.5–1 microgram/kg/minute at intervals of not less than 15 minutes

Dopacard® (Elan) PoM

Strong sterile solution, dopexamine hydrochloride 10 mg/mL (1%). For dilution and use as an intravenous infusion. Net price 5-mL amp = £21.00

Note. Contact with metal in infusion apparatus should be minimised

ISOPRENALINE HYDROCHLORIDE

Indications: heart block, severe bradycardia

Cautions: ischaemic heart disease, diabetes mellitus, hyperthyroidism; **interactions:** Appendix 1 (sympathomimetics)

Side-effects: tachycardia, arrhythmias, hypotension, sweating, tremor, headache

Dose: *by intravenous infusion*, 0.5–10 micrograms/minute

Min-I-Jet® Isoprenaline (Celltech) PoM

Injection, isoprenaline hydrochloride 20 micrograms/mL. Net price 10-mL disposable syringe = £4.05

Saventrine IV® (Forest) PoM

Strong sterile solution, isoprenaline hydrochloride 1 mg/mL. For dilution and use as an intravenous infusion. Net price 2-mL amp = 42p

2.7.2   Vasoconstrictor sympathomimetics

Vasoconstrictor sympathomimetics raise blood pressure transiently by acting on alpha-adrenergic receptors to constrict peripheral vessels. They are sometimes used as an emergency method of elevating blood pressure where other measures have failed (see also section 2.7.1).

The danger of vasoconstrictors is that although they raise blood pressure they do so at the expense of perfusion of vital organs such as the kidney.

Spinal and epidural anaesthesia may result in sympathetic block with resultant hypotension. Management may include intravenous fluids (which are usually given prophylactically), oxygen, elevation of the legs, and injection of a pressor drug such as ephedrine or methoxamine. As well as constricting peripheral vessels **ephedrine** also accelerates the heart rate (by acting on beta receptors). Use is made of this dual action of ephedrine to manage associated bradycardia (although intravenous injection of atropine sulphate 400 to 600 micrograms may also be required if bradycardia persists). When the hypotension occurs in association with tachycardia the pure alpha-adrenergic stimulant action of **methoxamine** is more appropriate.

EPHEDRINE HYDROCHLORIDE

Indications: see under Dose

Cautions: hyperthyroidism, diabetes mellitus, ischaemic heart disease, hypertension, angle-closure glaucoma, elderly, pregnancy (Appendix 4); may cause acute urine retention in prostatic hypertrophy; **interactions:** Appendix 1 (sympathomimetics)

Contra-indications: breast-feeding (Appendix 5)

Side-effects: nausea, vomiting, anorexia; tachycardia (sometimes bradycardia), arrhythmias, anginal pain, vasoconstriction with hypertension, vasodilation with hypotension, dizziness and flushing; dyspnoea; headache, anxiety, restlessness, confusion, psychoses, insomnia, tremor; difficulty in micturition, urine retention; sweating, hypersalivation; changes in blood-glucose concentration

Dose: reversal of hypotension from spinal or epidural anaesthesia, *by slow intravenous injection* of a solution containing ephedrine hydrochloride 3 mg/mL, 3–6 mg (max. 9 mg) repeated every 3–4 minutes to max. 30 mg

Ephedrine Hydrochloride (Non-proprietary) PoM

Injection, ephedrine hydrochloride 3 mg/mL, net price 10-mL amp = £2.70
Available from Aurum

METARAMINOL

Indications: acute hypotension (see notes above)

Cautions: see under Noradrenaline Acid Tartrate; longer duration of action than noradrenaline (norepinephrine), see below; cirrhosis
HYPERTENSIVE RESPONSE. Metaraminol has a longer duration of action than noradrenaline, and an excessive vasopressor response may cause a prolonged rise in blood pressure

Contra-indications: see under Noradrenaline Acid Tartrate

Side-effects: see under Noradrenaline Acid Tartrate; tachycardia; fatal ventricular arrhythmia reported in Laennec's cirrhosis

Dose: *by intravenous infusion*, 15–100 mg, adjusted according to response
In emergency, *by intravenous injection*, 0.5–5 mg then *by intavenous infusion*, 15–100 mg, adjusted according to response

Aramine® (MSD) PoM

Injection, metaraminol 10 mg (as tartrate)/mL. Net price 1-mL amp = 57p

METHOXAMINE HYDROCHLORIDE

Indications: acute hypotension (see notes above)

Cautions: see under Noradrenaline Acid Tartrate; longer duration of action than noradrenaline (norepinephrine), see below
HYPERTENSIVE RESPONSE. Methoxamine has a longer duration of action than noradrenaline, and an excessive vasopressor response may cause a prolonged rise in blood pressure

Contra-indications: see under Noradrenaline Acid Tartrate

Side-effects: see under Noradrenaline Acid Tartrate

Dose: *by intramuscular injection*, 5–20 mg
By slow intravenous injection, 5–10 mg (rate 1 mg/minute)

Vasoxine® (GlaxoWellcome) PoM

Injection, methoxamine hydrochloride 20 mg/mL. Net price 1-mL amp = 50p

NORADRENALINE ACID TARTRATE/ NOREPINEPHRINE BITARTRATE

Indications: see under dose

Cautions: coronary, mesenteric, or peripheral vascular thrombosis; following myocardial infarction, Prinzmetal's variant angina, hyperthyroidism, diabetes mellitus; hypoxia or hypercapnia; uncorrected hypovolaemia; elderly; extravasation at injection site may cause necrosis; **interactions:** Appendix 1 (sympathomimetics)

Contra-indications: hypertension (monitor blood pressure and rate of flow frequently), pregnancy

Side-effects: hypertension, headache, bradycardia, arrhythmias, peripheral ischaemia

Dose: acute hypotension, *by intravenous infusion*, via central venous catheter, of a solution containing noradrenaline acid tartrate 80 micrograms/mL (equivalent to noradrenaline base 40 micrograms/mL) at an initial rate of 0.16–0.33 mL/minute, adjusted according to response
Cardiac arrest, *by rapid intravenous or intracardiac injection*, 0.5–0.75 mL of a solution containing noradrenaline acid tartrate 200 micrograms/mL (equivalent to noradrenaline base 100 micrograms/mL)

Noradrenaline/Norepinephrine (Non-proprietary) PoM

Injection, noradrenaline acid tartrate 2 mg/mL (equivalent to noradrenaline base 1 mg/mL). For dilution before use. Net price 2-mL amp = 98p, 20-mL amp = £6.35
Available from Abbott

PHENYLEPHRINE HYDROCHLORIDE

Indications: acute hypotension (see notes above)

Cautions: see under Noradrenaline Acid Tartrate; longer duration of action than noradrenaline (norepinephrine), see below; coronary disease
HYPERTENSIVE RESPONSE. Phenylephrine has a longer duration of action than noradrenaline, and an excessive vasopressor response may cause a prolonged rise in blood pressure

Contra-indications: see under Noradrenaline Acid Tartrate; severe hyperthyroidism

Side-effects: see under Noradrenaline Acid Tartrate; tachycardia or reflex bradycardia

Dose: *by subcutaneous or intramuscular injection,* 2–5 mg, followed if necessary by further doses of 1–10 mg

By slow intravenous injection of a 1 mg/mL solution, 100–500 micrograms repeated as necessary after at least 15 minutes

By intravenous infusion, initial rate up to 180 micrograms/minute reduced to 30–60 micrograms/minute according to response

Phenylephrine (Sovereign) PoM
Injection, phenylephrine hydrochloride 10 mg/mL (1%). Net price 1-mL amp = £5.00

2.7.3   Cardiopulmonary resuscitation

The algorithm for cardiopulmonary resuscitation (see inside back cover) reflects the most recent recommendations of the Resuscitation Council (UK). In cardiac arrest **adrenaline (epinephrine)** 1 in 10 000 (100 micrograms/mL) is recommended in a dose of 10 mL by intravenous injection, preferably through a central line. If injected through a peripheral line, the drug must be flushed with at least 20 mL sodium chloride 0.9% injection (to aid entry into the central circulation). Intravenous injection of **amiodarone** 300 mg (from a prefilled syringe *or* diluted in glucose intravenous infusion 5%) should be considered after adrenaline to treat ventricular fibrillation or pulseless ventricular tachycardia in cardiac arrest refractory to defibrillation. **Atropine** 3 mg by intravenous injection (section 15.1.3) as a single dose is also used in cardiopulmonary resuscitation to block vagal activity.

For the management of acute anaphylaxis see section 3.4.3.

ADRENALINE/EPINEPHRINE

Indications: see notes above

Cautions: heart disease, diabetes mellitus, hyperthyroidism, hypertension, arrhythmias, cerebrovascular disease, angle-closure glaucoma, avoid during second stage of labour; **interactions:** Appendix 1 (sympathomimetics)

Side-effects: anxiety, tremor, tachycardia, headache, cold extremities; in overdosage arrhythmias, cerebral haemorrhage, pulmonary oedema; nausea vomiting, sweating, weakness, dizziness and hyperglycaemia also reported

Dose: see notes above

Adrenaline/Epinephrine 1 in 10 000, Dilute
(Non-proprietary) PoM
Injection, adrenaline (as acid tartrate) 100 micrograms/mL. 10-mL amp.

Available from Aurum, Martindale (special order); also from Aurum (1-mL and 10-mL prefilled syringe), Medeva (*Min-I-Jet® Adrenaline* 3- and 10-mL disposable syringes)

2.8   Anticoagulants and protamine

2.8.1   Parenteral anticoagulants
2.8.2   Oral anticoagulants
2.8.3   Protamine sulphate

The main use of anticoagulants is to prevent thrombus formation or extension of an existing thrombus in the slower-moving venous side of the circulation, where the thrombus consists of a fibrin web enmeshed with platelets and red cells. They are therefore widely used in the prevention and treatment of *deep-vein thrombosis in the legs.*

Anticoagulants are of less use in preventing thrombus formation in arteries, for in faster-flowing vessels thrombi are composed mainly of platelets with little fibrin. They are used to prevent thrombi forming on *prosthetic heart valves.*

2.8.1   Parenteral anticoagulants

Heparin

Heparin initiates anticoagulation rapidly but has a short duration of action. It is now often referred to as being **standard** or **unfractionated heparin** to distinguish it from the **low molecular weight heparins** (see p. 113), which have a longer duration of action.

TREATMENT. For the initial treatment of *deep-vein thrombosis and pulmonary embolism* heparin is given as an *intravenous loading dose,* followed by *continuous intravenous infusion* (using an infusion pump) or by *intermittent subcutaneous injection;* the use of *intermittent intravenous injection* is no longer recommended. An oral anticoagulant (usually warfarin, section 2.8.2) is started at the same time as the heparin (the heparin needs to be continued for at least 5 days and until the INR has been in the therapeutic range for 2 consecutive days). Laboratory monitoring is essential—preferably on a daily basis, determination of the activated partial thromboplastin time (APTT) being the most widely used technique. Heparin is also used in regimens for the management of *myocardial infarction* (see also section 2.10.1), the management of *unstable angina* (section 2.6), and the management of *acute peripheral arterial occlusion.*

PROPHYLAXIS. In patients undergoing *general surgery,* low-dose heparin by subcutaneous injection is widely advocated to *prevent postoperative deep-vein thrombosis and pulmonary embolism* in 'high risk' patients (i.e. those with obesity, malignant disease, history of deep-vein thrombosis or pulmonary embolism, patients over 40 years, or those with an established thrombophilic disorder or who are undergoing large or complicated surgical procedures); laboratory monitoring is not required with this *standard prophylactic regimen.*

To combat the increased risk in *major orthopaedic surgery* an *adjusted dose regimen* may be used (with monitoring) or *low molecular weight heparin* (see p. 113) may be selected.

EXTRACORPOREAL CIRCUITS. Heparin is also used in the maintenance of extracorporeal circuits in *cardiopulmonary bypass* and *haemodialysis*.

HAEMORRHAGE. If haemorrhage occurs it is usually sufficient to withdraw heparin, but if rapid reversal of the effects of heparin is required, protamine sulphate (section 2.8.3) is a specific antidote (but only partially reverses the effects of low molecular weight heparins).

HEPARIN

Indications: see under Dose

Cautions: hepatic and renal impairment (Appendix 2 and Appendix 3); pregnancy; hypersensitivity to low molecular weight heparins; spinal or epidural anaesthesia (risk of spinal haematoma); **interactions:** Appendix 1 (heparin)

THROMBOCYTOPENIA. Clinically important thrombocytopenia is immune-mediated, and does not usually develop until after 6 to 10 days; it may be complicated by thrombosis. Platelet counts are recommended for patients receiving heparin (including low molecular weight heparins) for longer than 5 days (heparin should be stopped immediately, and not repeated, in those who develop thrombocytopenia or a 50% reduction of platelet count). Patients requiring continued anticoagulation should preferably be given lepirudin or a heparinoid such as danaparoid

HYPERKALAEMIA. Inhibition of aldosterone secretion by heparin (including low molecular weight heparins) may result in hyperkalaemia; patients with diabetes mellitus, chronic renal failure, acidosis, raised plasma potassium or those taking potassium-sparing drugs seem to be more susceptible. The risk appears to increase with duration of therapy and the CSM has recommended that plasma potassium should be measured in patients at risk before starting heparin and monitored regularly thereafter, particularly if heparin is to be continued for more than 7 days

Contra-indications: haemophilia and other haemorrhagic disorders, thrombocytopenia (including history of heparin-induced thrombocytopenia), peptic ulcer, recent cerebral haemorrhage, severe hypertension, severe liver disease (including oesophageal varices), after major trauma or recent surgery (especially to eye or nervous system), hypersensitivity to heparin

Side-effects: haemorrhage (see notes above), skin necrosis, thrombocytopenia (see Cautions), hyperkalaemia (see Cautions), hypersensitivity reactions (including urticaria, angioedema, and anaphylaxis); osteoporosis after prolonged use (and rarely alopecia)

Dose:

Treatment of deep-vein thrombosis and pulmonary embolism, *by intravenous injection*, loading dose of 5000 units (10 000 units in severe pulmonary embolism) followed by continuous *infusion* of 15–25 units/kg/hour *or* treatment of deep-vein thrombosis, by *subcutaneous injection* of 15 000 units every 12 hours (laboratory monitoring essential—preferably on a daily basis, and dose adjusted accordingly)

SMALL ADULT OR CHILD, lower loading dose *then*, 15–25 units/kg/hour *by intravenous infusion, or* 250 units/kg every 12 hours by *subcutaneous injection*

Unstable angina, acute peripheral arterial occlusion, as intravenous regimen for deep-vein thrombosis and pulmonary embolism, above

Prophylaxis in orthopaedic surgery, see notes above

Prophylaxis in general surgery (see notes above), *by subcutaneous injection*, 5000 units 2 hours before surgery, then every 8–12 hours for 7 days or until patient is ambulant (monitoring not needed); during pregnancy (with monitoring), 5000–10 000 units every 12 hours (**important:** not intended to cover prevention of prosthetic heart valve thrombosis in pregnancy which calls for separate specialist management)

MYOCARDIAL INFARCTION. For the prevention of *coronary re-occlusion after thrombolysis* heparin is used in a variety of regimens according to locally agreed protocols

For the prevention of *mural thrombosis* heparin is considered effective when given by *subcutaneous injection* of 12 500 units every 12 hours for at least 10 days

Prevention of clotting in extracorporeal circuits, consult product literature

---

Note. Doses above reflect the guidelines of the British Society for Haematology; for doses of the low molecular weight heparins, see pp. 114–15

Heparin (Non-proprietary) PoM

Injection, heparin sodium 1000 units/mL, net price 1-mL amp = 19p, 5-mL amp = 57p, 5-mL vial = 46p, 10-mL amp = 61p, 20-mL amp = 91p; 5000 units/mL, 1-mL amp = 37p, 5-mL amp = 99p, 5-mL vial = 92p; 25 000 units/mL, 1-mL amp = £1.02, 5-mL vial = £3.44

Calciparine® (Sanofi-Synthelabo) PoM

Injection (subcutaneous only), heparin calcium 25 000 units/mL. Net price 0.2-mL syringe = 65p; 0.5-mL syringe = £1.46

Minihep® (Leo) PoM

Injection (subcutaneous only), heparin sodium 25 000 units/mL. Net price 0.2-mL amp = 39p

Monoparin® (CP) PoM

Injection, heparin sodium (mucous) 1000 units/mL, net price 1-mL amp = 19p; 5-mL amp = 52p; 10-mL amp = 69p; 20-mL = £1.24; 5000 units/mL, 1-mL amp = 36p; 5-mL amp = £1.00; 25 000 units/mL, 0.2-mL amp = 46p, 1-mL amp = £1.01

Monoparin Calcium® (CP) PoM

Injection, heparin calcium 25 000 units/mL. Net price 0.2-mL amp = 46p

Multiparin® (CP) PoM

Injection, heparin sodium (mucous) 1000 units/mL, net price 5-mL vial = 47p; 5000 units/mL, 5-mL vial = 92p; 25 000 units/mL, 5-mL vial = £3.68

Low molecular weight heparins

Certoparin, **dalteparin**, **enoxaparin**, **reviparin**, and **tinzaparin** are low molecular weight heparins. Low molecular weight heparins are as effective and as safe as unfractionated heparin in the prevention of venous thrombo-embolism; in orthopaedic practice they are probably more effective. They have a longer duration of action than unfractionated heparin; *once-daily subcutaneous* dosage means that they are convenient to use. The standard prophylactic regimen does not require monitoring.

Some low molecular weight heparins are also used in the treatment of deep-vein thrombosis, pulmonary embolism, unstable coronary artery disease (section 2.6) and for the prevention of clotting in extracorporeal circuits.

HAEMORRHAGE. See under Heparin.

CERTOPARIN

Indications: see notes above and under preparations

Cautions: see under Heparin

Contra-indications: see under Heparin

Side-effects: see under Heparin

Dose: see under preparation below

Alphaparin® (Grifols) [PoM]

Injection, certoparin sodium 3000 units/0.3-mL syringe, net price 1 syringe = £2.87

Dose: prophylaxis of deep-vein thrombosis, *by subcutaneous injection,* 3000 units 1–2 hours before surgery, then 3000 units every 24 hours for 7–10 days (or until the patient is mobile)

DALTEPARIN SODIUM

Indications: see notes above and under preparations

Cautions: see under Heparin

Contra-indications: see under Heparin

Side-effects: see under Heparin

Dose: see under preparations below

Fragmin® (Pharmacia) [PoM]

Injection (single-dose syringe), dalteparin sodium 12 500 units/mL, net price 0.2-mL (2500-unit) syringe = £1.86; 25 000 units/mL, 0.2-mL (5000-unit) syringe = £2.82, 0.3-mL (7500-unit) syringe = £4.23, 0.4-mL (10 000-unit) syringe = £5.65, 0.5-mL (12 500-unit) syringe = £7.06, 0.6-mL (15 000-unit) syringe = £8.47, 0.72-mL (18 000-unit) syringe = £10.16

Dose: prophylaxis of deep-vein thrombosis, *by subcutaneous injection,* moderate risk, 2500 units 1–2 hours before surgery then 2500 units every 24 hours for 5–7 days or longer; high risk, 2500 units 1–2 hours before surgery, then 2500 units 8–12 hours later (*or* 5000 units on the evening before surgery, then 5000 units on the following evening), then 5000 units every 24 hours for 5–7 days or longer (5 weeks in hip replacement)

Treatment of deep-vein thrombosis and of pulmonary embolism, *by subcutaneous injection,* as a single daily dose, ADULT body-weight under 46 kg, 7500 units daily; body-weight 46–56 kg, 10 000 units daily; body-weight 57–68 kg, 12 500 units daily; body-weight 69–82 kg, 15 000 units daily; body-weight 83 kg and over, 18 000 units daily, with oral anticoagulant treatment until prothrombin complex concentration in therapeutic range (usually for at least 5 days); monitoring of anti-factor Xa not usually required; for patients at increased risk of haemorrhage, see below

Injection, dalteparin sodium 2500 units/mL (for subcutaneous or intravenous use), net price 4-mL (10 000-unit) amp = £5.12; 10 000 units/mL (for subcutaneous or intravenous use), 1-mL (10 000-unit) amp = £5.12; 25 000 units/mL (for subcutaneous use only), 4-mL (100 000-unit) vial = £48.66

Dose: treatment of deep-vein thrombosis and of pulmonary embolism, *by subcutaneous injection,* 200 units/kg (max. 18 000 units) as a single daily dose (*or* 100 units/kg twice daily if increased risk of haemorrhage) with oral anticoagulant treatment until prothrombin complex concentration in therapeutic range (usually

for at least 5 days)

Note. For monitoring, blood should be taken 3–4 hours after a dose (recommended plasma concentration of anti-Factor Xa 0.5–1 unit/mL); monitoring not required for once-daily treatment regimen and not generally necessary for twice-daily regimen

Unstable coronary artery disease, *by subcutaneous injection,* 120 units/kg every 12 hours (max. 10 000 units twice daily) for 5–8 days

Prevention of clotting in extracorporeal circuits, consult product literature

Injection (graduated syringe), dalteparin sodium 10 000 units/mL, net price 1-mL (10 000-unit) syringe = £5.65

Dose: unstable coronary artery disease, *by subcutaneous injection,* 120 units/kg every 12 hours (max. 10 000 units twice daily) for 5–8 days

ENOXAPARIN

Indications: see notes above and under preparations

Cautions: see under Heparin

Contra-indications: see under Heparin

Side-effects: see under Heparin

Dose: see under preparation below

Clexane® (Rhône-Poulenc Rorer) [PoM]

Injection, enoxaparin 100 mg/mL, net price 0.2-mL syringe (20 mg, 2000 units) = £3.39, 0.4-mL syringe (40 mg, 4000 units) = £4.52, 0.6-mL syringe (60 mg, 6000 units) = £5.11, 0.8-mL syringe (80 mg, 8000 units) = £5.81, 1-mL syringe (100 mg, 10 000 units) = £7.19; 150 mg/mL, 0.8-mL syringe (120 mg, 12 000 units) = £10.51, 1-mL syringe (150 mg, 15 000 units) = £11.94

Dose: prophylaxis of deep-vein thrombosis especially in surgical patients, *by subcutaneous injection, moderate risk,* 20 mg (2000 units) approx. 2 hours before surgery then 20 mg (2000 units) every 24 hours for 7–10 days; *high risk,* 40 mg (4000 units) 12 hours before surgery then 40 mg (4000 units) every 24 hours for 7–10 days

Prophylaxis of deep-vein thrombosis in medical patients, *by subcutaneous injection,* 40 mg (4000 units) every 24 hours for at least 6 days until patient ambulant (max. 14 days)

Treatment of deep-vein thrombosis (with or without pulmonary embolism), *by subcutaneous injection,* 1.5 mg/kg (150 units/kg) every 24 hours, usually for at least 5 days (and until adequate oral anticoagulation established)

Unstable angina and non-Q-wave myocardial infarction, *by subcutaneous injection,* 1 mg/kg (100 units/kg) every 12 hours usually for 2–8 days (minimum 2 days)

Prevention of clotting in extracorporeal circuits, consult product literature

REVIPARIN SODIUM

Indications: see notes above and under preparation

Cautions: see under Heparin; platelet count recommended before treatment, on days 1 and 4 of treatment then twice weekly for first 3 weeks of treatment

Contra-indications: see under Heparin

Side-effects: see under Heparin

Dose: see under preparation below

Clivarine® (ICN) ▼ [PoM]

Injection, reviparin sodium, 1432 units/0.25-mL syringe, net price 1 syringe = £3.63

Dose: prophylaxis of deep-vein thrombosis, *by subcutaneous injection,* 1432 units 2 hours before surgery, then 1432 units every 24 hours for 7 days (or until patient is mobile)

TINZAPARIN SODIUM

Indications: see notes above and under preparations
Cautions: see under Heparin
Contra-indications: see under Heparin
Side-effects: see under Heparin
Dose: see under preparations below

Innohep® (Leo) PoM
 Injection, tinzaparin sodium 10 000 units/mL, net
 price 2500-unit (0.25-mL) syringe = £2.13, 3500-
 unit (0.35-mL) syringe = £2.98, 4500-unit (0.45-
 mL) syringe = £3.83, 20 000-unit (2-mL) vial =
 £11.36
 Dose: prophylaxis of deep-vein thrombosis, *by subcuta-*
 neous injection, general surgery, 3500 units 2 hours
 before surgery, then 3500 units every 24 hours for 7–10
 days; orthopaedic surgery (high risk), 50 units/kg 2
 hours before surgery, then 50 units/kg every 24 hours for
 7–10 days *or* 4500 units 12 hours before surgery, then
 4500 units every 24 hours for 7–10 days
 Prevention of clotting in extracorporeal circuits, consult
 product literature
 Injection, tinzaparin sodium 20 000 units/mL, net
 price 0.5-mL (10 000-unit) syringe = £9.65, 0.7-
 mL (14 000-unit) syringe = £13.52, 0.9-mL
 (18 000-unit) syringe = £17.37, 2-mL (40 000-
 unit) vial = £36.77
 Dose: treatment of deep-vein thrombosis and of pulmonary embolism, *by subcutaneous injection*, 175 units/
 kg once daily for at least 6 days (and until adequate oral
 anticoagulation established)
 Note. This treatment regimen does not require anticoagulation monitoring
 ASTHMA. Presence of sulphites in formulation may
 (especially in patients with asthma) lead to hypersensitivity (with bronchospasm and shock)

Heparinoids

Danaparoid is a heparinoid used for prophylaxis of
deep-vein thrombosis in patients undergoing general or orthopaedic surgery. Providing there is no
evidence of cross-reactivity, it also has a role in
patients who develop thrombocytopenia in association with heparin.

DANAPAROID SODIUM

Indications: prophylaxis of deep-vein thrombosis
 in general and orthopaedic surgery; thromboembolic disease requiring parenteral anticoagulation
 in patients with (or with a history of) heparin-
 induced thrombocytopenia
Cautions: hepatic and renal impairment (avoid for
 prophylaxis if severe); pregnancy and breast-
 feeding
 ASTHMA. Presence of sulphite in ampoules may (especially in patients with asthma) lead to hypersensitivity
 (with bronchospasm and shock)
Contra-indications: see under Heparin; cross-
 reactivity to heparin-induced thrombocytopenia
Side-effects: haemorrhage (see notes above);
 thrombocytopenia (may be cross-reactivity with
 heparin); hypersensitivity reactions (including
 rash); liver enzyme changes; osteoporosis with
 excessive dosage; bruising or pain at injection site
Dose: prophylaxis of deep vein thrombosis, *by
 subcutaneous injection*, 750 units twice daily for
 7–10 days; initiate treatment before operation
 (with last pre-operative dose 1–4 hours before
 surgery)

Heparin-induced thrombocytopenia, *by intravenous
 injection*, 2500 units (1250 units if body-weight
 less than 55 kg, 3750 units if over 90 kg), followed by *intravenous infusion* of 400 units/hour
 for 2 hours, *then* 300 units/hour for 2 hours, *then*
 200 units/hour for 5 days; monitor anti-Xa activity in renal impairment and in patients over 90 kg
 (consult product literature)

Orgaran® (Durbin) PoM
 Injection, danaparoid sodium 1250 units/mL, 0.6-
 mL amp (750 units)
 Note. Currently unlicensed

Hirudins

Lepirudin, a recombinant hirudin, is licensed for
anticoagulation in patients with Type II (immune)
heparin-induced thrombocytopenia who require
parenteral antithrombotic treatment. The dose of
lepirudin is adjusted according to activated partial
thromboplastin time (APTT).

 Desirudin (*Revasc®*, available on a named-
patient basis from Aventis Pharma) is another
recombinant hirudin for the prophylaxis of deep-
vein thrombosis in patients undergoing hip and
knee replacement surgery.

LEPIRUDIN

Indications: thromboembolic disease requiring
 parenteral anticoagulation in patients with heparin-induced thrombocytopenia type II
Cautions: renal impairment (Appendix 3); hepatic
 impairment (Appendix 2); recent bleeding or risk
 of bleeding including recent puncture of large
 vessels, organ biopsy, recent major surgery,
 stroke, haemorrhagic diathesis, severe uncontrolled hypertension, bacterial endocarditis; determine activated partial thromboplastin time 4
 hours after start of treatment (or after infusion
 rate altered) and at least once daily thereafter
Contra-indications: pregnancy and breast-feeding
Side-effects: bleeding manifestations; reduced
 haemoglobin concentration without obvious
 source of bleeding; fever, hypersensitivity reactions (including rash); injection site reactions
Dose: initially *by slow intravenous injection* (of
 5 mg/mL solution), 400 micrograms/kg followed
 by *continuous intravenous infusion* of
 150 micrograms/kg/hour (max. 16.5 mg/hour),
 adjusted according to activated partial thromboplastin time, for 2–10 days (longer if necessary)

Refludan® (Hoechst Marion Roussel) ▼ PoM
 Injection, powder for reconstitution, lepirudin. Net
 price 50-mg vial = £52.30

Heparin flushes

For maintaining patency of peripheral venous catheters, sodium chloride injection 0.9% is as effective
as heparin flushes.

Heparin Sodium (Non-proprietary) PoM
 Solution, heparin sodium 10 units/mL, net price 5-
 mL amp = 28p; 100 units/mL, 2-mL amp = 24p.
 To maintain patency of catheters, cannulas, etc.
 10–200 units flushed through every 4–8 hours.
 Not for therapeutic use
 Available from Leo

Canusal® (CP) [PoM]
Solution, heparin sodium 100 units/mL. Net price
2-mL amp = 28p. To maintain patency of catheters, cannulas, etc., 200 units flushed through every
4 hours or as required. Not for therapeutic use

Hepsal® (CP) [PoM]
Solution, heparin sodium 10 units/mL. Net price 5-
mL amp = 25p. To maintain patency of catheters,
cannulas, etc., 50 units flushed through every 4
hours or as required. Not for therapeutic use

Epoprostenol

Epoprostenol (prostacyclin) can be given to inhibit
platelet aggregation during renal dialysis either
alone or with heparin. It is also licensed for the
treatment of primary pulmonary hypertension
resistant to other treatment, usually with oral anticoagulation. Since its half-life is only about 3 minutes it must be given by continuous intravenous
infusion. It is a potent vasodilator and therefore its
side-effects include flushing, headache, and hypotension.

EPOPROSTENOL
Indications: see notes above
Cautions: anticoagulant monitoring required when
given with heparin; haemorrhagic diathesis; dose
titration for pulmonary hypertension should be in
hospital (risk of pulmonary oedema); pregnancy
(Appendix 4) and breast-feeding (Appendix 5)
Contra-indications: severe left ventricular dysfunction
Side-effects: see notes above; also bradycardia,
tachycardia, pallor, sweating with higher doses;
gastro-intestinal disturbances; lassitude, anxiety,
aggitation; dry-mouth, jaw pain, chest pain; also
reported, hyperglycaemia and injection-site reactions
Dose: see product literature

Flolan® (GlaxoWellcome) [PoM]
Infusion, powder for reconstitution, epoprostenol
(as sodium salt). Net price 500-microgram vial
(with diluent) = £69.43; 1.5-mg vial (with diluent) = £139.86

2.8.2   Oral anticoagulants

Oral anticoagulants antagonise the effects of vitamin K, and take at least 48 to 72 hours for the anticoagulant effect to develop fully; if an immediate
effect is required, heparin must be given concomitantly.

USES. The main indication for an oral anticoagulant
is *deep-vein thrombosis*. Patients with *pulmonary
embolism* should also be treated, as should those
with *atrial fibrillation who are at risk of embolisation* (see also section 2.3.1), and those with
mechanical prosthetic heart valves (to prevent
emboli developing on the valves); an antiplatelet
drug may also be useful in these patients.
Warfarin is the drug of choice; **acenocoumarol
(nicoumalone)** and **phenindione** are seldom
required.
Oral anticoagulants should not be used in cerebral
thrombosis or peripheral arterial occlusion as first-
line therapy; aspirin (section 2.9) is more appropriate for reduction of risk in transient ischaemic
attacks.

DOSE. Whenever possible, the base-line prothrombin time should be determined but the initial dose
should not be delayed whilst awaiting the result.

The usual adult induction dose of warfarin is
10 mg[1] daily for 2 days (higher doses no longer recommended). The subsequent maintenance dose
depends upon the prothrombin time, reported as
INR (international normalised ratio). The daily
maintenance dose of warfarin is usually 3 to 9 mg
(taken at the **same time** each day). The indications
and target INRs[2] currently recommended by the
British Society for Haematology[3] are:

- INR 2–2.5 for prophylaxis of deep-vein thrombosis
  including surgery on high-risk patients;
- INR 2.5 for treatment of deep-vein thrombosis and
  pulmonary embolism (or for recurrence in patients no
  longer receiving warfarin), atrial fibrillation, cardioversion, dilated cardiomyopathy, mural thrombus following myocardial infarction, and rheumatic mitral
  valve disease;
- INR 3.5 for recurrent deep-vein thrombosis and pulmonary embolism (in patients currently receiving warfarin) and mechanical prosthetic heart valves.

MONITORING. It is essential that the INR be determined daily or on alternate days in early days of
treatment, *then* at longer intervals (depending on
response[4]) *then* up to every 12 weeks

HAEMORRHAGE. The main adverse effect of all
oral anticoagulants is haemorrhage. Checking the
INR and omitting doses when appropriate is essential; if the anticoagulant is stopped but not reversed,
the INR should be measured 2–3 days later to
ensure that it is falling. The following recommendations of the British Society for Haematology are
based on the result of the INR and whether there is
major or minor bleeding; the recommendations
apply to patients taking warfarin:

- Major bleeding—stop warfarin; give phytomenadione
  (vitamin K₁) 5 mg by slow intravenous injection; give
  prothrombin complex concentrate (factors II, VII, IX
  and X) 50 units/kg *or* (if no concentrate available) fresh
  frozen plasma 15 mL/kg
- INR > 8.0, no bleeding or minor bleeding—stop warfarin, restart when INR < 5.0; if there are other risk factors for bleeding give phytomenadione (vitamin K₁)
  0.5 mg by slow intravenous injection or 5 mg by mouth
  (for partial reversal of anticoagulation give smaller oral
  doses of phytomenadione e.g. 0.5–2.5 mg using the

---

1. First dose less than 10 mg if base-line prothrombin time
prolonged, if liver-function tests abnormal, or if patient in
cardiac failure, on parenteral feeding, less than average
body weight, elderly, or receiving other drugs known to
potentiate oral anticoagulants.

2. An INR which is within 0.5 units of the target value is
generally satisfactory; larger deviations require dosage
adjustment. Target values (rather than ranges) are now
recommended (except for prophylaxis of deep-vein
thrombosis where a range is still recommended).

3. Guidelines on Oral Anticoagulation: third edition. *Br J
Haematol* 1998; **101**: 374–87

4. Change in patient's clinical condition, particularly associated with liver disease, intercurrent illness, or drug
administration, necessitates more frequent testing. See
also **interactions**, Appendix 1 (warfarin). Major changes
in diet (especially involving salads and vegetables) and in
alcohol consumption may also affect warfarin control.

intravenous preparation orally); repeat dose of phyto-menadione if INR still too high after 24 hours
- INR 6.0–8.0, no bleeding or minor bleeding—stop warfarin, restart when INR < 5.0
- INR < 6.0 but more than 0.5 units above target value—reduce dose or stop warfarin, restart when INR < 5.0
- Unexpected bleeding at therapeutic levels—always investigate possibility of underlying cause e.g. unsuspected renal or gastro-intestinal tract pathology

PREGNANCY. Oral anticoagulants are teratogenic and should not be given in the first trimester of pregnancy. Women at risk of pregnancy should be warned of this danger since stopping warfarin before the sixth week of gestation may largely avoid the risk of fetal abnormality. Oral anticoagulants cross the placenta with risk of placental or fetal haemorrhage, especially during the last few weeks of pregnancy and at delivery. Therefore, if at all possible, oral anticoagulants should be avoided in pregnancy, especially in the first and third trimesters. Difficult decisions may have to be made, particularly in women with prosthetic heart valves or with a history of recurrent venous thrombosis or pulmonary embolism.

TREATMENT BOOKLETS. Anticoagulant treatment booklets should be issued to patients, and are available for distribution to local healthcare professionals from Health Authorities and also from:

England and Wales:
Astron
The Causeway
Oldham Broadway
Business Park
Chadderton
Oldham OL9 9XD
(0161) 683 2376

Scotland:
Banner Business Supplies
20 South Gyle Crescent
Edinburgh EH12 9EB
(0131) 479 3279

Northern Ireland:
Central Services Agency
25 Adelaide St
Belfast BT2 8FH
(028) 9053 5652

These booklets include advice for patients on anticoagulant treatment.

WARFARIN SODIUM

Indications: prophylaxis of embolisation in rheumatic heart disease and atrial fibrillation; prophylaxis after insertion of prosthetic heart valve; prophylaxis and treatment of venous thrombosis and pulmonary embolism; transient ischaemic attacks

Cautions: hepatic or renal disease (Appendixes 2 and 3), recent surgery; breast-feeding (Appendix 5); **interactions:** Appendix 1 (warfarin)

Contra-indications: pregnancy (see notes above), peptic ulcer, severe hypertension, bacterial endocarditis

Side-effects: haemorrhage—see notes above for British Society for Haematology recommendations; other side-effects reported include hypersensitivity, rash, alopecia, diarrhoea, unexplained drop in haematocrit, 'purple toes', skin necrosis, jaundice, hepatic dysfunction; also nausea, vomiting, and pancreatitis

Dose: see notes above

Warfarin (Non-proprietary) PoM
Tablets, warfarin sodium 0.5 mg (white), net price 28-tab pack = £1.00; 1 mg (brown), 20 = £1.01;

3 mg (blue), 20 = £1.14; 5 mg (pink), 20 = £1.22.
Label: 10 anticoagulant card
Available from Alpharma, APS, Generics, Goldshield (*Marevan*®), Hillcross, IVAX

ACENOCOUMAROL/NICOUMALONE

Indications: see under Warfarin Sodium
Cautions: see under Warfarin Sodium
Contra-indications: see under Warfarin Sodium
Side-effects: see under Warfarin Sodium
Dose: 8–12 mg on 1st day; 4–8 mg on 2nd day; maintenance dose usually 1–8 mg daily

Sinthrome® (Alliance) PoM
Tablets, acenocoumarol 1 mg. Net price 20 = 95p.
Label: 10 anticoagulant card

PHENINDIONE

Indications: prophylaxis of embolisation in rheumatic heart disease and atrial fibrillation; prophylaxis after insertion of prosthetic heart valve; prophylaxis and treatment of venous thrombosis and pulmonary embolism

Cautions: see under Warfarin Sodium; **interactions:** Appendix 1 (phenindione)

Contra-indications: see under Warfarin Sodium; avoid breast-feeding

Side-effects: see under Warfarin Sodium; also hypersensitivity reactions including rashes, exfoliative dermatitis, exanthema, fever, leucopenia, agranulocytosis, eosinophilia, diarrhoea, renal and hepatic damage; urine coloured pink or orange

Dose: 200 mg on day 1; 100 mg on day 2; maintenance dose usually 50–150 mg daily

Dindevan® (Goldshield) PoM
Tablets, phenindione 10 mg, net price 20 = 68p; 25 mg (green), 20 = 95p; 50 mg, 20 = £1.21.
Label: 10 anticoagulant card, 14 (urine pink or orange)

2.8.3   Protamine sulphate

Although protamine sulphate is used to counteract overdosage with heparin, if used in excess it has an anticoagulant effect.

PROTAMINE SULPHATE

(Protamine Sulfate)
Indications: see above
Cautions: see above; also if increased risk of allergic reaction to protamine (includes previous treatment with protamine or protamine insulin, allergy to fish, men who are infertile or who have had a vasectomy)

Side-effects: nausea, vomiting, lassitude, flushing, hypotension), bradycardia, dyspnoea; hypersensitivity reactions (including angioedema, anaphylaxis) reported

Dose: *by intravenous injection* over approx. 10 minutes, 1 mg neutralises 80–100 units heparin when given within 15 minutes of heparin; if longer time, less protamine required as heparin rapidly excreted; max. 50 mg

Protamine Sulphate (Non-proprietary) PoM
Injection, protamine sulphate 10 mg /mL, net price 5-mL amp = £1.14, 10-mL amp = £3.30
Available from Celltech, Sovereign

Prosulf® (CP) [PoM]

Injection, protamine sulphate 10 mg/mL. Net price
5-mL amp = 96p (glass), £1.20 (polypropylene)

2.9   Antiplatelet drugs

Antiplatelet drugs decrease platelet aggregation and
may inhibit thrombus formation in the arterial circulation, where anticoagulants have little effect.

A low dose of **aspirin** is used for the *secondary*
prevention of thrombotic cerebrovascular or cardiovascular disease. A single dose of aspirin is given as
soon as possible after an ischaemic event, preferably dispersed in water or chewed; 150–300 mg is
given after myocardial infarction and 300 mg is
given after ischaemic (not haemorrhagic) stroke.
The initial dose is followed by maintenance treatment with aspirin 75–300 mg daily.

A low dose of aspirin is also of benefit in the *primary prevention* of vascular events when the estimated 10-year coronary heart disease risk is 15% or
greater and provided that blood pressure is controlled (see section 2.5).

A low dose of aspirin (75–100 mg daily) is also
given following coronary bypass surgery. For
details on the use of aspirin in atrial fibrillation see
section 2.3.1, for stable angina see section 2.6 and
for intermittent claudication see section 2.6.4.1.

Clopidogrel and **ticlopidine** are licensed for the
prevention of ischaemic events in patients with a
history of symptomatic ischaemic disease.

Dipyridamole is used by mouth as an adjunct to
oral anticoagulation for prophylaxis of thromboembolism associated with prosthetic heart valves.
Modified-release preparations are licensed for secondary prevention of ischaemic stroke and transient
ischaemic attacks.

GLYCOPROTEIN IIb/IIIa INHIBITORS. Glycoprotein IIb/IIIa inhibitors prevent platelet aggregation
by blocking the binding of fibrinogen to receptors
on platelets. **Abciximab** is a monoclonal antibody
which binds to glycoprotein IIb/IIIa receptors and
to other related sites; it is licensed as an adjunct to
heparin and aspirin for the prevention of ischaemic
complications in high-risk patients undergoing percutaneous transluminal coronary intervention.
Abciximab should be used once only. **Eptifibatide**
and **tirofiban** also inhibit glycoprotein IIb/IIIa
receptors; they are licensed for use with heparin and
aspirin to prevent early myocardial infarction in
patients with unstable angina (section 2.6) or non-
Q-wave myocardial infarction (see also NICE guidance, below). Abciximab, eptifibatide and tirofiban
should be used by specialists only.

For use of epoprostenol, see section 2.8.1.

> **NICE guidance (glycoprotein IIb/IIIa inhi-
> bitors).** The National Institute for Clinical Excel-
> lence recommends the use of glycoprotein IIb/IIIa
> inhibitors (in accordance with UK licensing) for high-
> risk patients with unstable angina or non-Q-wave
> myocardial infarction, and for those undergoing
> acute or elective percutaneous coronary interven-
> tion.

ABCIXIMAB

Indications: prevention of ischaemic cardiac complications in patients undergoing percutaneous
coronary intervention; short-term prevention of
myocardial infarction in patients with unstable
angina not responding to conventional treatment
and who are scheduled for percutaneous coronary
intervention (use under specialist supervision)

Cautions: measure baseline prothrombin time,
activated partial thromboplastin time, platelet
count, haemoglobin and haematocrit; monitor
haemoglobin and haematocrit 12 hours and 24
hours after start of treatment and platelet count 2–
4 hours and 24 hours after start of treatment; concomitant use of drugs that increase risk of bleeding; discontinue if uncontrollable serious
bleeding occurs or emergency cardiac surgery
needed; consult product literature for details of
procedures to minimise bleeding; pregnancy
(Appendix 4)

Contra-indications: active internal bleeding,
major surgery, intracranial or intraspinal surgery
or trauma within last 2 months, stroke within last
2 years; intracranial neoplasm, arteriovenous malformation or aneurysm, severe hypertension,
haemorrhagic diathesis, thrombocytopenia, vasculitis, hypertensive or diabetic retinopathy;
severe hepatic or renal impairment (Appendixes 2
and 3); breast-feeding

Side-effects: bleeding manifestations; nausea,
vomiting, hypotension, bradycardia, chest pain,
back pain, headache, fever, puncture site pain,
thrombocytopenia; rarely cardiac tamponade,
adult respiratory distress, hypersensitivity reactions

Dose: ADULT initially *by intravenous injection*
over 1 minute, 250 micrograms/kg, then *by intravenous infusion*, 125 nanograms/kg/minute (max.
10 micrograms/minute); for prevention of
ischaemic complications start 10–60 minutes
before percutaneous coronary intervention and
continue infusion for 12 hours; for unstable
angina start up to 24 hours before possible percutaneous coronary intervention and continue infusion for 12 hours after intervention

ReoPro® (Lilly) [PoM]
Injection, abciximab 2 mg/mL, net price 5-mL vial
= £280.00

ASPIRIN (antiplatelet)

(Acetylsalicylic Acid)

Indications: prophylaxis of cerebrovascular disease or myocardial infarction (see section 2.10.1
and notes above)

Cautions: asthma; uncontrolled hypertension;
pregnancy (but see Appendix 4); **interactions:**
Appendix 1 (aspirin)

Contra-indications: children under 12 years and
in breast-feeding (Reye's syndrome, section
4.7.1); active peptic ulceration; haemophilia and
other bleeding disorders

Side-effects: bronchospasm; gastro-intestinal
haemorrhage (occasionally major), also other
haemorrhage (e.g. subconjunctival)

Dose: see notes above

[1]**Aspirin** (Non-proprietary) PoM
Dispersible tablets, aspirin 75 mg, net price 20 = 11p; 300 mg, see section 4.7.1. Label: 13, 21, 32
Tablets, e/c, aspirin 75 mg, net price 56-tab pack = £3.03; 300 mg, see section 4.7.1. Label: 5, 25, 32
Available from Dexcel (*Micropirin®*), Galen, Genus (*Gencardia®*), Lagap, Lilly (*PostMI 75EC®*)

Angettes 75® (Bristol-Myers Squibb)
Tablets, aspirin 75 mg. Net price 28-tab pack = 94p. Label: 32

Caprin® (Sinclair) PoM
Tablets, e/c, pink, aspirin 75 mg, net price 56-tab pack = £3.08; 300 mg, see section 4.7.1. Label: 5, 25, 32

Nu-Seals® Aspirin (Lilly) PoM
Tablets, e/c, aspirin 75 mg, net price 56-tab pack = £3.09; 300 mg, see section 4.7.1. Label: 5, 25, 32
Note. Tablets may be chewed at diagnosis for rapid absorption

■ With isosorbide mononitrate
Section 2.6.1

CLOPIDOGREL

Indications: prevention of atherosclerotic events in patients with history of symptomatic atherosclerotic disease (ischaemic stroke, myocardial infarction or established peripheral arterial disease)
Cautions: avoid for first few days after myocardial infarction and for 7 days after ischaemic stroke; patients at risk of increased bleeding from trauma, surgery or other pathological conditions; discontinue 7 days before elective surgery if antiplatelet effect not desirable; liver impairment (Appendix 2), renal impairment; pregnancy (Appendix 4); **interactions:** Appendix 1 (clopidogrel)
Contra-indications: active bleeding, breast-feeding
Side-effects: haemorrhage (including gastro-intestinal and intracranial); other side-effects reported include abdominal discomfort, nausea, vomiting, diarrhoea, constipation, gastric and duodenal ulceration; headache, dizziness, vertigo, paraesthesia; rash, pruritus; hepatic and biliary disorders, neutropenia, thrombotic thrombocytopenic purpura, isolated report of aplastic anaemia
Dose: 75 mg once daily

Plavix® (Bristol-Myers Squibb, Sanofi-Synthelabo) ▼ PoM
Tablets, pink, f/c, clopidogrel (as hydrogen sulphate) 75 mg, net price 28-tab pack = £35.31

DIPYRIDAMOLE

Indications: see notes above and under preparations
Cautions: rapidly worsening angina, aortic stenosis, recent myocardial infarction, heart failure; may exacerbate migraine; hypotension; **interactions:** Appendix 1 (dipyridamole)

1. Aspirin tablets 75 mg may be sold to the public in packs of up to 100 tablets; for details relating to other strengths see section 4.7.1 and *Medicines, Ethics and Practice*, No. 25, London, Pharmaceutical Press, 2001 (and subsequent editions as available)

Side-effects: gastro-intestinal effects, dizziness, myalgia, throbbing headache, hypotension, hot flushes and tachycardia; rarely worsening symptoms of coronary heart disease, hypersensitivity reactions such as rash, urticaria, severe bronchospasm and angioedema; increased bleeding during or after surgery; thrombocytopenia reported
Dose: *by mouth*, 300–600 mg daily in 3–4 divided doses before food
Modified-release preparations, see under preparation below
By intravenous injection, diagnostic only, consult product literature

Dipyridamole (Non-proprietary) PoM
Tablets, coated, dipyridamole 25 mg, net price 20 = 40p; 100 mg, 20 = £1.08; 84 = £4.54. Label: 22
Available from Alpharma, Ashbourne (*Cerebrovase®*), Hillcross, IVAX
Oral suspension, dipyridamole 50 mg/5 ml. Available from Rosemont (sugar-free, special order)

Persantin® (Boehringer Ingelheim) PoM
Tablets, both s/c, dipyridamole 25 mg (orange), net price 84-tab pack = £1.70; 100 mg, 84-tab pack = £4.73. Label: 22
Injection, dipyridamole 5 mg/mL. Net price 2-mL amp = 11p

■ Modified release
Persantin® Retard (Boehringer Ingelheim) PoM
Capsules, m/r, red/orange containing yellow pellets, dipyridamole 200 mg. Net price 60-cap pack = £9.75. Label: 21, 25
Dose: secondary prevention of ischaemic stroke and transient ischaemic attacks (used alone or with aspirin), adjunct to oral anticoagulation for prophylaxis of thromboembolism associated with prosthetic heart valves, 200 mg twice daily preferably with food
Note. Dispense in original container (pack contains a desiccant) and discard any capsules remaining 6 weeks after opening

■ With aspirin
For cautions, contra-indications and side-effects of aspirin, see under Aspirin, above
Asasantin® Retard (Boehringer Ingelheim) PoM
Capsules, red/ivory, aspirin 25 mg, dipyridamole 200 mg (m/r), net price 60-cap pack = £9.75. Label: 21, 25
Dose: secondary prevention of ischaemic stroke and transient ischaemic attacks, 1 capsule twice daily
Note. Dispense in original container (pack contains a desiccant) and discard any capsules remaining 6 weeks after opening

EPTIFIBATIDE

Indications: prevention of early myocardial infarction in patients with unstable angina or non-Q-wave myocardial infarction and with last episode of chest pain within 24 hours (use under specialist supervision)
Cautions: renal impairment (Appendix 3); risk of bleeding, concomitant drugs that increase risk of bleeding—discontinue immediately if uncontrolled serious bleeding; measure baseline prothrombin time, activated partial thromboplastin time, platelet count, haemoglobin, haematocrit and serum creatinine; monitor haemoglobin, haematocrit and platelets within 6 hours after start of

treatment then at least once daily; discontinue if thrombolytic therapy, intra-aortic balloon pump or emergency cardiac surgery necessary; pregnancy (Appendix 4)

Contra-indications: abnormal bleeding within 30 days, major surgery or severe trauma within 6 weeks; stroke within last 30 days or any history of haemorrhagic stroke, intracranial disease (aneurysm, neoplasm or arteriovenous malformation), severe hypertension, haemorrhagic diathesis, increased prothrombin time or INR, thrombocytopenia, significant hepatic impairment; breast-feeding

Side-effects: bleeding manifestations

Dose: initially *by intravenous injection*, 180 micrograms/kg, then *by intravenous infusion*, 2 micrograms/kg/minute for up to 72 hours (up to 96 hours if percutaneous coronary intervention during treatment)

Integrilin® (Schering-Plough) ▼ PoM
Injection, eptifibatide 2 mg/mL, net price 10-mL (20-mg) vial = £15.54
Infusion, eptifibatide 750 micrograms/mL, net price 100-mL (75-mg) vial = £48.84

TICLOPIDINE HYDROCHLORIDE

Indications: prophylaxis of major ischaemic events in patients with a history of ischaemic stroke, reversible ischaemic neurological deficit or transient ischaemic attack, and in patients with intermittent claudication (initiate in hospital)

Cautions: hepatic impairment (Appendix 2); renal impairment (Appendix 3); monitor full blood count before treatment and every 2 weeks for first 3 months (and within 2 weeks of discontinuation if before 3 months)—discontinue if neutropenia or thrombocytopenia develop; discontinue at least 10 days before elective surgery; pregnancy (Appendix 4) and breast-feeding (Appendix 5); **interactions:** Appendix 1 (ticlopidine)

BLOOD DISORDERS AND JAUNDICE. Patients and their carers should be told how to recognise signs of blood disorders or jaundice and advised to seek immediate medical attention if symptoms such as fever, sore throat, mouth ulcers, purpura, bruising or bleeding develop

Contra-indications: haemorrhagic diathesis; recent bleeding or risk of bleeding including acute haemorrhagic stroke and active gastroduodenal ulcer; history of leucopenia, thrombocytopenia or agranulocytosis

Side-effects: bleeding manifestations; blood disorders including neutropenia, agranulocytosis, rarely bone marrow aplasia, pancytopenia, thrombotic thrombocytopenic purpura and isolated cases of thrombocytopenia; nausea, diarrhoea (discontinue if severe and persistent); elevated liver enzymes, rarely hepatitis, cholestatic jaundice; increased serum cholesterol and triglyceride concentrations; hypersensitivity reactions including angioedema, vasculitis, lupus syndrome and nephropathy; rashes, pruritus

Dose: 250 mg twice daily

Ticlid (Sanofi-Synthelabo) ▼ PoM
Tablets, f/c, ticlopidine hydrochloride 250 mg, net price 60-tab pack = £100.00. Label: 21

TIROFIBAN

Indications: prevention of early myocardial infarction in patients with unstable angina or non-Q-wave myocardial infarction and with last episode of chest pain within 12 hours (use under specialist supervision)

Cautions: renal impairment (Appendix 3); hepatic impairment (avoid if severe; Appendix 2); major surgery or severe trauma within 3 months (avoid if within 6 weeks); traumatic or protracted cardiopulmonary resuscitation, organ biopsy or lithotripsy within last 2 weeks; risk of bleeding including active peptic ulcer within 3 months; acute pericarditis, aortic dissection, haemorrhagic retinopathy, vasculitis, haematuria, faecal occult blood; severe heart failure, cardiogenic shock, anaemia; puncture of non-compressible vessel within 24 hours; concomitant drugs that increase risk of bleeding (including within 48 hours after thrombolytic); monitor platelet count, haemoglobin and haematocrit before treatment, 2–6 hours after start of treatment and then at least once daily; discontinue if thrombolytic therapy, intra-aortic balloon pump or emergency cardiac surgery necessary; discontinue immediately if serious bleeding uncontrolled by pressure occurs; pregnancy (Appendix 4)

Contra-indications: abnormal bleeding within 30 days, stroke within 30 days or any history of haemorrhagic stroke, intracranial disease (aneurysm, neoplasm or arteriovenous malformation), severe hypertension, haemorrhagic diathesis, increased prothrombin time or INR, thrombocytopenia; breast-feeding

Side-effects: bleeding manifestations; reversible thrombocytopenia

Dose: *by intravenous infusion*, initially 400 nanograms/kg/minute for 30 minutes, then 100 nanograms/kg/minute for at least 48 hours (continue during and for 12–24 hours after percutaneous coronary intervention); max. duration of treatment 108 hours

Aggrastat® (MSD) ▼ PoM
Concentrate for intravenous infusion, tirofiban (as hydrochloride) 250 micrograms/mL. For dilution before use, net price 50-mL (12.5-mg) vial = £146.11

2.10 Myocardial infarction and fibrinolysis

2.10.1   Management of myocardial infarction
2.10.2   Fibrinolytic drugs

2.10.1 Management of myocardial infarction

Local guidelines for the management of myocardial infarction should be followed where they exist

These notes give an overview of the initial and long-term management of myocardial infarction. The aims of management are to provide supportive care and pain relief, to promote revascularisation and to reduce mortality. Oxygen, diamorphine and nitrates provide initial support and pain relief; thrombolytics and aspirin promote revascularisation; long-term use of aspirin, beta-blockers, ACE inhibitors and statins help to reduce mortality further.

INITIAL MANAGEMENT. **Oxygen** (section 3.6) is administered unless the patient has severe chronic obstructive pulmonary disease.

The pain (and anxiety) of myocardial infarction is managed with slow intravenous injection of **diamorphine** (section 4.7.2); an antiemetic such as metoclopramide (or, if left ventricular function is not compromised, cyclizine) by intravenous injection should also be given (section 4.6).

Aspirin (chewed or dispersed in water) is given for its antiplatelet effect (section 2.9); a dose of 150–300 mg is suitable. If aspirin is given prior to arrival at hospital, a note saying that it has been given should be sent with the patient.

Thrombolytic drugs (section 2.10.2) are given to patients unless contra-indicated. Alteplase, reteplase and streptokinase need to be given within 12 hours of a myocardial infarction, ideally within 1 hour; use after 12 hours requires specialist advice. Tenecteplase should be given within 6 hours of a myocardial infarction. Streptokinase remains the drug of choice although antibodies appear after 4 days and streptokinase should not therefore be used again after this time. **Heparin** is used as adjunctive therapy with alteplase, reteplase, and tenecteplase to prevent re-thrombosis; heparin treatment should be continued for at least 24 hours (consult product literature).

Nitrates (section 2.6.1) are used to relieve ischaemic pain. If sublingual glyceryl trinitrate is not effective, intravenous glyceryl trinitrate or isosorbide dinitrate is given.

Early intravenous administration of some **beta-blockers** (section 2.4) has been shown to be of benefit and patients without contra-indications should receive **atenolol** by intravenous injection at a dose of 5 mg over 5 minutes, and the dose repeated once after 10–15 minutes; **metoprolol** by intravenous injection is an alternative.

ACE inhibitors (section 2.5.5.1) are also of benefit to patients who have no contra-indications; in normotensive patients treatment with an ACE inhibitor can be started within 24 hours of the myocardial infarction and continued for at least 5–6 weeks (see below for long-term treatment).

All patients should be closely monitored for hyperglycaemia; those with diabetes or raised blood-glucose concentration should receive **insulin**.

LONG-TERM MANAGEMENT. **Aspirin** (section 2.9) should be given to all patients, unless contra-indicated, at a dose of 75–150 mg daily.

Beta-blockers (section 2.4) should be given to all patients in whom they are not contra-indicated and continued for at least 2–3 years. Acebutolol, metoprolol, propranolol and timolol are suitable; for patients with left ventricular dysfunction, carvedilol, bisoprolol or long-acting metoprolol may be appropriate (section 2.5.5).

Although other calcium-channel blockers (section 2.6.2) have no place in routine management, **verapamil** may be useful in patients in whom beta-blockers are inappropriate.

ACE inhibitors (section 2.5.5.1) are recommended for any patient with evidence of left ventricular dysfunction.

Nitrates (section 2.6.1) are used for patients with angina.

Statins are beneficial in preventing recurrent coronary events, particularly for patients at high risk because of other factors (section 2.12).

2.10.2   Fibrinolytic drugs

Fibrinolytic drugs act as thrombolytics by activating plasminogen to form plasmin, which degrades fibrin and so breaks up thrombi.

Streptokinase is used in the treatment of *life-threatening venous thrombosis*, and in *pulmonary embolism*, but treatment must be started promptly.

The value of thrombolytic drugs for the treatment of *myocardial infarction* has been established (section 2.10.1). **Streptokinase** and **alteplase** have been shown to reduce mortality. **Reteplase**, and more recently, **tenecteplase** are also licensed for acute myocardial infarction; they are given by intravenous injection (tenecteplase is given as a bolus injection). Thrombolytic drugs are indicated for any patient with acute myocardial infarction for whom the benefit is likely to outweigh the risk of treatment. Trials have shown that the benefit is greatest in those with ECG changes that include ST segment elevation (especially in those with anterior infarction) and in patients with bundle branch block. Patients should not be denied thrombolytic treatment on account of age alone because mortality in this group is high and the reduction in mortality is the same as in younger patients.

CAUTIONS. Risk of bleeding including that from venepuncture or invasive procedures, external chest compression, pregnancy (see Appendix 4), abdominal aneurysm or conditions in which thrombolysis might give rise to embolic complications such as enlarged left atrium with atrial fibrillation (risk of dissolution of clot and subsequent embolisation), diabetic retinopathy (very small risk of retinal bleeding), recent or concurrent anticoagulant therapy.

CONTRA-INDICATIONS. Recent haemorrhage, trauma, or surgery (including dental extraction), coagulation defects, bleeding diatheses, aortic dissection, coma, history of cerebrovascular disease especially recent events or with any residual disability, recent symptoms of possible peptic ulceration, heavy vaginal bleeding, severe hypertension, active pulmonary disease with cavitation, acute pancreatitis, severe liver disease, oesophageal varices; also in the case of streptokinase, previous allergic reactions to either streptokinase or anistreplase (no longer available).

Prolonged persistence of antibodies to streptokinase and anistreplase (no longer available) may reduce the effectiveness of subsequent treatment, therefore streptokinase should not be used again beyond 4 days of first administration of either streptokinase or anistreplase.

SIDE-EFFECTS. Side-effects of thrombolytics are mainly nausea and vomiting and bleeding. When thrombolytics are used in myocardial infarction, reperfusion arrhythmias may occur. Hypotension may also occur and can usually be controlled by elevating the patient's legs, or by reducing the rate of infusion or stopping it temporarily. Back pain has been reported. Bleeding is usually limited to the site of injection, but intracerebral haemorrhage or bleeding from other sites may occur. Serious bleeding calls for discontinuation of the thrombolytic and may require administration of coagulation factors and antifibrinolytic drugs (aprotinin or tranexamic acid). Streptokinase may cause allergic reactions (including rash, flushing and uveitis) and anaphylaxis has been reported (for details of management see Allergic Emergencies, section 3.4.3). Guillain-Barré syndrome has been reported rarely after streptokinase treatment.

ALTEPLASE

(rt-PA, tissue-type plasminogen activator)

Indications: acute myocardial infarction (see notes above and section 2.10.1); pulmonary embolism

Cautions: see notes above

Contra-indications: see notes above

Side-effects: see notes above

Dose:

Myocardial infarction, accelerated regimen (initiated within 6 hours), 15 mg by *intravenous injection*, followed by *intravenous infusion* of 50 mg over 30 minutes, then 35 mg over 60 minutes (total dose 100 mg over 90 minutes); lower doses in patients less than 65 kg

Myocardial infarction, initiated within 6–12 hours, 10 mg by *intravenous injection*, followed by *intravenous infusion* of 50 mg over 60 minutes, then 4 *infusions* each of 10 mg over 30 minutes (total dose 100 mg over 3 hours; max. 1.5 mg/kg in patients less than 65 kg)

Pulmonary embolism, 10 mg by *intravenous injection* over 1–2 minutes followed by *intravenous infusion* of 90 mg over 2 hours; max. 1.5 mg/kg in patients less than 65 kg

Actilyse® (Boehringer Ingelheim) [PoM]
Injection, powder for reconstitution, alteplase 10 mg (5.8 million units)/vial, net price per vial (with diluent) = £135.00; 20 mg (11.6 million units)/vial (with diluent and transfer device) = £180.00; 50 mg (29 million units)/vial (with diluent, transfer device, and infusion bag) = £300.00

RETEPLASE

Indications: acute myocardial infarction (see notes above and section 2.10.1)

Cautions: see notes above

Contra-indications: see notes above

Side-effects: see notes above

Dose: *by intravenous injection,* 10 units over not more than 2 minutes, followed after 30 minutes by a further 10 units

Rapilysin® (Roche) [PoM]
Injection, powder for reconstitution, reteplase 10 units (1.16 g)/vial, net price pack of 2 vials (with 2 prefilled syringes of diluent and transfer device) = £716.25

STREPTOKINASE

Indications: deep-vein thrombosis, pulmonary embolism, acute arterial thromboembolism, central retinal venous or arterial thrombosis, thrombosed arteriovenous shunts; acute myocardial infarction (see notes above and section 2.10.1); topical use (section 13.11.7)

Cautions: see notes above

Contra-indications: see notes above

Side-effects: see notes above

Dose: deep-vein thrombosis, pulmonary embolism, acute arterial thromboembolism, central retinal venous or arterial thrombosis, *by intravenous infusion*, 250 000 units over 30 minutes, then 100 000 units every hour for up to 12–72 hours according to condition with monitoring of clotting parameters (consult product literature)

Myocardial infarction, 1 500 000 units over 60 minutes

Thrombosed arteriovenous shunts and intracoronary use in myocardial infarction, consult product literature

Streptokinase (Non-proprietary) [PoM]
Injection, powder for reconstitution, streptokinase, net price 100 000-unit vial = £10.00; 250 000-unit vial = £15.00; 750 000-unit vial = £40.00; 1.5 million-unit vial = £80.00
Available from Braun

Streptase® (Aventis Behring) [PoM]
Injection, powder for reconstitution, streptokinase, net price 250 000-unit vial = £17.11; 750 000-unit vial = £44.86; 1.5 million-unit vial = £89.72 (hosp. only)

TENECTEPLASE

Indications: acute myocardial infarction (see notes above and section 2.10.1)

Cautions: see notes above

Contra-indications: see notes above

Side-effects: see notes above; also fever

Dose: *by intravenous injection* over 10 seconds, 30–50 mg according to body-weight (500–600 micrograms/kg)—consult product literature; max. 50 mg

Metalyse® (Boehringer Ingelheim) ▼ [PoM]
Injection, powder for reconstitution, tenecteplase, net price 40-mg (8000-unit) vial = £700.00; 50-mg (10 000-unit) vial = £770.00 (both with pre-filled syringe of water for injection)

2.11   Antifibrinolytic drugs and haemostatics

Fibrin dissolution can be impaired by the administration of **tranexamic acid**, which inhibits fibrinolysis. It may be useful to prevent bleeding (e.g. in prostatectomy and dental extraction in haemophilia) and can be particularly useful in menorrhagia. Tranexamic acid may also be used in hereditary angioedema, epistaxis and in thrombolytic overdose.

Desmopressin (section 6.5.2) is used in the management of mild to moderate haemophilia.

Aprotinin is a proteolytic enzyme inhibitor acting on plasmin and kallidinogenase (kallikrein). It is indicated for patients at high risk of major blood loss during and after open heart surgery with extracorporeal circulation and for patients in whom optimal blood conservation during open heart surgery is an absolute priority; it is also indicated for the treatment of life-threatening haemorrhage due to hyperplasminaemia (occasionally observed during the mobilisation and dissection of malignant tumours, in acute promyelocytic leukaemia, and following thrombolytic therapy). Aprotinin is also used in liver transplantation [unlicensed].

Etamsylate (ethamsylate) reduces capillary bleeding in the presence of a normal number of platelets. It does not act by fibrin stabilisation, but probably by correcting abnormal platelet adhesion.

APROTININ

Indications: see notes above

Side-effects: occasionally hypersensitivity reactions and localised thrombophlebitis

Dose: *by slow intravenous injection or infusion*
Open heart surgery, loading dose, 2 000 000 units (200 mL) after induction of anaesthesia and before sternotomy—initial 50 000 units (5 mL) *by slow intravenous injection* over several minutes (to detect allergy), remainder *by intravenous infusion* over 20 minutes; maintenance dose, *by intravenous infusion* 500 000 units (50 mL) every hour until end of operation (or early postoperative period in septic endocarditis); pump prime, 2 000 000 units (200 mL) in priming volume of extracorporeal circuit; in septic endocarditis 3 000 000 units (300 mL) added to pump prime
Hyperplasminaemia, *by slow intravenous injection or by intravenous infusion*, initially 500 000–1 000 000 units (50–100 mL) at max. rate 10 mL/minute; followed if necessary by 200 000 units (20 mL) every hour until bleeding stops

Trasylol® (Bayer) PoM
Injection, aprotinin 10 000 kallikrein inactivator units/mL. Net price 50-mL vial = £20.53
Note. Aprotinin injection containing 10 000 kallikrein inactivator units/mL also available from Ferring

ETAMSYLATE
(Ethamsylate)
Indications: see under preparations
Contra-indications: porphyria (see section 9.8.2)
Side-effects: nausea, headache, rashes
Dose: see below

Dicynene® (Delandale) PoM
Tablets, scored, etamsylate 500 mg, net price 100-tab pack = £21.13
Dose: short-term treatment of blood loss in menorrhagia, 500 mg 4 times daily during menstruation
Injection, etamsylate 125 mg/mL. Net price 2-mL amp = 78p
Dose: prophylaxis and treatment of periventricular haemorrhage in low birth-weight infants, by intramuscular or intravenous injection, 12.5 mg/kg every 6 hours
IMPORTANT. The ampoules currently available contain a total of 250 mg in 2 mL volume therefore **small fraction only** required for neonatal use

TRANEXAMIC ACID

Indications: see notes above
Cautions: renal impairment (Appendix 3); massive haematuria (avoid if risk of ureteric obstruction); pregnancy (Appendix 4); regular eye examinations and liver function tests in long-term treatment of hereditary angioedema
Note. Requirement for regular eye examinations during long-term treatment is based on unsatisfactory evidence
Contra-indications: thromboembolic disease
Side-effects: nausea, vomiting, diarrhoea (reduce dose); disturbances in colour vision (discontinue) and thromboembolic events reported rarely; giddiness on rapid intravenous injection
Dose: *by mouth*, local fibrinolysis, 15–25 mg/kg 2–3 times daily
Menorrhagia (initiated when heavy bleeding has started), 1–1.5 g 3–4 times daily for 3–4 days
Hereditary angioedema, 1–1.5 g 2–3 times daily
By slow intravenous injection, local fibrinolysis, 0.5–1 g 3 times daily

Cyklokapron® (Pharmacia) PoM
Tablets, f/c, scored, tranexamic acid 500 mg. Net price 60-tab pack = £14.30
Injection, tranexamic acid 100 mg/mL. Net price 5-mL amp = £1.29

Blood products

ANTITHROMBIN III CONCENTRATE

Dried antithrombin III is prepared from human plasma
Indications: congenital deficiency of antithrombin III
Side-effects: nausea, flushing, headache; rarely, allergic reactions and fever
Available from BPL (Dried Antithrombin III)

FACTOR VIIa (RECOMBINANT)

Recombinant factor VIIa is used in patients with inhibitors to factors VIII and IX
Available from Novo Nordisk (*NovoSeven®*)

FACTOR VIII FRACTION, DRIED
(Human Antihaemophilic Fraction, Dried)
Dried factor VIII fraction is prepared from human plasma by a suitable fractionation technique
Indications: control of haemorrhage in haemophilia A
Cautions: intravascular haemolysis after large or frequently repeated doses in patients with blood groups A, B, or AB—less likely with high potency concentrates
Side-effects: allergic reactions including chills, fever; hyperfibrinogenaemia occurred after massive doses with earlier products but less likely since fibrinogen content has now been substantially reduced
Available from Baxter (*Hemofil M®*), BPL (*Replenate®*, *8Y®*), Aventis Behring (*Monoclate-P®*), Grifols (*Fanhdi®*), SNBTS (*Liberate®*, High Potency Factor VIII Concentrate)
Note. Preparation of recombinant human antihaemophilic factor VIII (octocog alfa) available from Alpha (*Alphanate®*), Baxter Bioscience (*Recombinate®*), Bayer (*Kogenate®*), Wyeth (*ReFacto®* ▼)

FACTOR VIII INHIBITOR BYPASSING FRACTION

Preparations with factor VIII inhibitor bypassing activity are prepared from human plasma

Human Factor VIII Inhibitor Bypassing Fraction (*FEIBA*, Baxter Bioscience) is used in patients with factor VIII inhibitors

> *Note.* A porcine preparation of antihaemophilic factor for patients with inhibitors to human factor VIII is available from Speywood (*Hyate C®*)

FACTOR IX FRACTION, DRIED

Dried factor IX fraction is prepared from human plasma by a suitable fractionation technique; it may also contain clotting factors II, VII, and X.

Indications: congenital factor IX deficiency (haemophilia B)

Cautions: risk of thrombosis—principally with former low purity products

Contra-indications: disseminated intravascular coagulation

Side-effects: allergic reactions, including chills, fever

Available from Alpha (*AlphaNine®*), BPL (Dried Factor IX Fraction, Heat-Treated; *Replenine®-VF*), Aventis Behring (*Mononine®*), SNBTS (Human Factor IX Concentrate, Heat Treated; *HT Defix®*)

> *Note.* Preparation of recombinant coagulation factor IX (nonacog alfa) available from Baxter Bioscience (*Bene-FIX®* ▼)

FRESH FROZEN PLASMA

Fresh frozen plasma is prepared from the supernatant liquid obtained by centrifugation of one donation of whole blood

Indications: to replace coagulation factors or other plasma proteins where their concentration or functional activity is critically reduced, e.g. to reverse warfarin effect

Cautions: avoid in circulatory overload; need for compatibility

Side-effects: allergic reactions including chills, fever, bronchospasm; adult respiratory distress syndrome

Available from Regional Blood Transfusion Services and BPL

> *Note.* A preparation of solvent/detergent treated human plasma (frozen) is available from Octapharma (*Octaplas®* ▼)

PROTEIN C CONCENTRATE

Protein C is prepared from human plasma

Indications: congenital protein C deficiency

Cautions: hypersensitivity to heparin

Side-effects: fever, arrhythmia, bleeding and thrombosis reported; rarely allergic reactions

Available from Baxter (*Ceprotin®*▼)

2.12　Lipid-regulating drugs

Lowering the concentration of low density lipoprotein (LDL) cholesterol and raising high density lipoprotein (HDL) cholesterol reduces the progression of coronary atherosclerosis and may even induce regression.

There is evidence that lowering total cholesterol by 20–25% (or lowering the LDL-cholesterol by about 30%) is effective in both the primary and secondary prevention of clinical manifestations of coronary heart disease. Therefore, treatment with a lipid-regulating drug should be considered in patients with coronary heart disease and in those at high risk of developing it because of multiple risk factors (including smoking, hypertension, diabetes mellitus, and a family history of premature coronary heart disease). Treatment with statins (see Statins, below) has been shown to reduce myocardial infarction, coronary deaths and overall mortality and they are the drugs of choice in patients with a high risk of coronary heart disease. Lipid-regulating drug therapy must be combined with advice on diet and lifestyle measures to reduce coronary risk including, if appropriate, reduction of blood pressure (section 2.5) and use of aspirin (section 2.9).

A number of conditions, some familial, are characterised by very high plasma concentrations of cholesterol, or triglycerides, or both. Statins are drugs of first choice for treating hypercholesterolaemia, fibrates for treating hypertriglyceridaemia, and statins or fibrates can be used, either alone or together, to treat mixed hyperlipidaemia.

Severe hyperlipidaemia often requires a combination of lipid-regulating drugs such as an anion-exchange resin with a fibrate, a statin, or nicotinic acid; such treatment should generally be under specialist supervision. Combinations of a statin with nicotinic acid or a fibrate carry an increased risk of side-effects (including rhabdomyolysis) and should be used with caution. In particular, concomitant administration of gemfibrozil with a statin may increase the risk of rhabdomyolysis considerably (see also below); gemfibrozil and statins should therefore **not** be used concomitantly.

> **CSM advice (muscle effects).** The CSM has advised that rhabdomyolysis associated with lipid-regulating drugs such as the fibrates and statins appears to be rare (approx. 1 case in every 100 000 treatment years) but may be increased in those with renal impairment and possibly in those with hypothyroidism. Concomitant treatment with ciclosporin may increase plasma-statin concentration and the risk of muscle toxicity; concomitant treatment with a fibrate and a statin may also be associated with an increased risk of serious muscle toxicity.

Anion-exchange resins

Colestyramine (cholestyramine) and **colestipol** are anion-exchange resins used in the management of hypercholesterolaemia. They act by binding bile acids, preventing their reabsorption; this promotes hepatic conversion of cholesterol into bile acids; the resultant increased LDL-receptor activity of liver cells increases the breakdown of LDL-cholesterol. Thus both compounds effectively reduce LDL-cholesterol but can aggravate hypertriglyceridaemia.

CAUTIONS. Anion-exchange resins interfere with the absorption of fat-soluble vitamins; supplements of vitamins A, D and K may be required when treatment is prolonged. **Interactions:** Appendix 1 (colestyramine and colestipol).

SIDE-EFFECTS. As colestyramine and colestipol are not absorbed, gastro-intestinal side-effects predominate. Constipation is common, but diarrhoea has occurred, as have nausea, vomiting, and gastro-intestinal discomfort. An increased bleeding tendency has been reported due to hypoprothrombinaemia associated with vitamin K deficiency.

COUNSELLING. Other drugs should be taken at least 1 hour before or 4–6 hours after colestyramine or colestipol to reduce possible interference with absorption.

COLESTYRAMINE

(Cholestyramine)

Indications: hyperlipidaemias, particularly type IIa, in patients who have not responded adequately to diet and other appropriate measures; primary prevention of coronary heart disease in men aged 35–59 years with primary hypercholesterolaemia who have not responded to diet and other appropriate measures; pruritus associated with partial biliary obstruction and primary biliary cirrhosis (section 1.9.2); diarrhoeal disorders (section 1.9.2)

Cautions: see notes above; pregnancy and breast-feeding

Contra-indications: complete biliary obstruction (not likely to be effective)

Side-effects: see notes above; hyperchloraemic acidosis reported on prolonged use

Dose: lipid reduction (after initial introduction over 3–4 weeks) 12–24 g daily in water (or other suitable liquid) in single or up to 4 divided doses; up to 36 g daily if necessary

Pruritus, see section 1.9.2

Diarrhoeal disorders, see section 1.9.2

CHILD 6–12 years, see product literature

Colestyramine (Non-proprietary) PoM
Powder, colestyramine (anhydrous) 4 g/sachet, net price 60-sachet pack = £21.06. Label: 13, counselling, avoid other drugs at same time (see notes above)
Excipients: include aspartame (section 9.4.1)
Available from Dominion

Questran® (Bristol-Myers Squibb) PoM
Powder, orange, colestyramine (anhydrous) 4 g/sachet. Net price 60-sachet pack = £21.06. Label: 13, counselling, avoid other drugs at same time (see notes above)

Questran Light® (Bristol-Myers Squibb) PoM
Powder, orange, colestyramine (anhydrous) 4 g/sachet, net price 60-sachet pack = £22.11. Label: 13, counselling, avoid other drugs at same time (see notes above)
Excipients: include aspartame (section 9.4.1)

COLESTIPOL HYDROCHLORIDE

Indications: hyperlipidaemias, particularly type IIa, in patients who have not responded adequately to diet and other appropriate measures

Cautions: see notes above; pregnancy

Side-effects: see notes above

Dose: 5 g 1–2 times daily in liquid increased if necessary at intervals of 1–2 months to max. of 30 g daily (in single or 2 divided doses)

Colestid® (Pharmacia) PoM
Granules, yellow, colestipol hydrochloride 5 g/sachet. Net price 30 sachets = £11.98. Label: 13, counselling, avoid other drugs at same time (see notes above)
Colestid Orange, granules, yellow/orange, colestipol hydrochloride 5 g/sachet, with aspartame. Net price 30 sachets = £11.98. Label: 13, counselling, avoid other drugs at same time (see notes above)

Fibrates

Bezafibrate, ciprofibrate, fenofibrate, and **gemfibrozil** can be regarded as broad-spectrum lipid-modulating agents in that although their main action is to decrease serum triglycerides they also tend to reduce LDL-cholesterol and to raise HDL-cholesterol. Fibrates may reduce the risk of coronary heart disease events in those with low HDL–cholesterol or with raised triglycerides.

All can cause a myositis-like syndrome, especially in patients with impaired renal function. Also, combination of a fibrate with a statin increases the risk of muscle effects (especially rhabdomyolysis) and should be used with caution (see CSM advice in section 2.12).

BEZAFIBRATE

Indications: hyperlipidaemias of types IIa, IIb, III, IV and V in patients who have not responded adequately to diet and other appropriate measures

Cautions: renal impairment (Appendix 3—see also under Myotoxicity below); **interactions:** Appendix 1 (fibrates)

MYOTOXICITY. Special care needed in patients with renal disease, as progressive increases in serum creatinine concentration or failure to follow dosage guidelines may result in myotoxicity (rhabdomyolysis); discontinue if myotoxicity suspected or creatine kinase concentration increases significantly

Contra-indications: severe hepatic impairment, hypoalbuminaemia, primary biliary cirrhosis, gall bladder disease, nephrotic syndrome, pregnancy and breast-feeding

Side-effects: gastro-intestinal (e.g. nausea, anorexia, gastric pain), pruritus, urticaria, impotence; also headache, dizziness, vertigo, fatigue, hair loss; myotoxicity (with myasthenia or myalgia)—special risk in renal impairment (see Cautions); also reported, anaemia, leucopenia, thrombocytopenia

Dose: see preparations below

Bezafibrate (Non-proprietary) PoM
Tablets, bezafibrate 200 mg, net price 100-tab pack = £9.84. Label: 21
Dose: 200 mg 3 times daily after food
Available from Dominion, Generics

Bezalip® (Roche) PoM
Tablets, f/c, bezafibrate 200 mg. Net price 100-tab pack = £9.84. Label: 21
Dose: 200 mg 3 times daily with or after food

■ Modified release

Bezalip® Mono (Roche) [PoM]
Tablets, m/r, f/c, bezafibrate 400 mg. Net price 30-tab pack = £8.70. Label: 21, 25

Dose: 1 tablet daily after food (dose form not appropriate in renal impairment)

Note. Modified-release tablets containing bezafibrate 400 mg also available from Ashbourne (*Liparol® XL*), Generics (*Bezagen® XL*), Link (*Zimbacol®XL*)

CIPROFIBRATE

Indications: hyperlipidaemias of types IIa, IIb, III, and IV in patients who have not responded adequately to diet

Cautions: see under Bezafibrate

Contra-indications: see under Bezafibrate

Side-effects: see under Bezafibrate

Dose: 100 mg daily

Modalim® (Sanofi-Synthelabo) [PoM]
Tablets, scored, ciprofibrate 100 mg. Net price 28-tab pack = £13.38

FENOFIBRATE

Indications: hyperlipidaemias of types IIa, IIb, III, IV, and V in patients who have not responded adequately to diet and other appropriate measures

Cautions: see under Bezafibrate; renal impairment (Appendix 3); liver function tests recommended every 3 months for first year (discontinue treatment if significantly raised)

Contra-indications: severe renal or hepatic impairment, existing gall bladder disease; pregnancy (Appendix 4) and breast-feeding (Appendix 5); photosensitivity to ketoprofen

Side-effects: see under Bezafibrate; also reported rash, photosensitivity, raised serum transaminases, hepatitis

Dose: see preparations below

Lipantil® (Fournier) [PoM]
Lipantil® Micro 67 capsules, yellow, fenofibrate (micronised) 67 mg, net price 90-cap pack = £23.30. Label: 21

Dose: initially 3 capsules daily in divided doses; usual range 2–4 capsules daily; CHILD 1 capsule/20 kg daily

Lipantil® Micro 200 capsules, orange, fenofibrate (micronised) 200 mg, net price 28-cap pack = £21.75. Label: 21

Dose: initially 1 capsule daily (dose form not appropriate for children or in renal impairment)

Lipantil® Micro 267 capsules, orange/cream, fenofibrate (micronised) 267 mg, net price 28-cap pack = £21.75. Label: 21

Dose: severe hyperlipidaemia, 1 capsule daily (dose form not appropriate for children or in renal impairment)

Note. For an equivalent therapeutic effect, 100 mg previously available non-micronised fenofibrate ≡ 67 mg micronised fenofibrate

■ Modified release

Supralip® 160 (Fournier) [PoM]
Tablets, m/r, f/c, fenofibrate 160 mg, net price 28-tab pack = £14.75. Label: 21, 25

Dose: 160 mg daily (dose form not appropriate for children or in renal impairment)

GEMFIBROZIL

Indications: hyperlipidaemias of types IIa, IIb, III, IV and V in patients who have not responded adequately to diet and other appropriate measures; primary prevention of coronary heart disease in men aged 40–55 years with hyperlipidaemias that have not responded to diet and other appropriate measures

Cautions: lipid profile, blood counts, and liver-function tests before initiating long-term treatment; renal impairment; preferably avoid use with statins (high risk of rhabdomyolysis); **interactions:** Appendix 1 (fibrates)

Contra-indications: alcoholism, hepatic impairment, gallstones; pregnancy and breast-feeding

Side-effects: gastro-intestinal disturbances; also rash, dermatitis, pruritus, urticaria, impotence, headache, dizziness, blurred vision, cholestatic jaundice, angioedema, laryngeal oedema, atrial fibrillation, pancreatitis, myasthenia, myopathy, rhabdomyolysis, painful extremities, myalgia accompanied by increases in creatine kinase

Dose: 1.2 g daily, usually in 2 divided doses; range 0.9–1.5 g daily

Gemfibrozil (Non-proprietary) [PoM]
Tablets, gemfibrozil 600 mg, net price 30-tab pack = £15.20
Available from IVAX

Lopid® (Parke-Davis) [PoM]
'300' capsules, white/maroon, gemfibrozil 300 mg. Net price 112-cap pack = £29.64
'600' tablets, f/c, gemfibrozil 600 mg. Net price 56-tab pack = £29.64

Ispaghula

Ispaghula husk, a form of soluble fibre, can be used as an adjunct to a lipid-lowering diet in patients with mild to moderate hypercholesterolaemia. It probably acts by reducing reabsorption of bile acids; plasma triglycerides remain unchanged.

ISPAGHULA

Indications: primary hypercholesterolaemia in patients with cholesterol concentration of 6.5–7.8 mmol/litre who have not responded adequately to dietary control; constipation, see section 1.6.1

Cautions: maintain adequate fluid intake; diabetes mellitus

Contra-indications: intestinal obstruction, faecal impaction, colonic atony

Side-effects: flatulence, abdominal bloating, particularly on starting treatment (if necessary, reduce dosage to once daily for few days); gastro-intestinal obstruction or impaction

Dose: see under preparation below

Fybozest Orange® (R&C)
Granules, effervescent, sugar-free, ispaghula husk. Net price 265-g tub (with measure) = £6.43. Label: 13, counselling, see below

Note. Contains aspartame 50 mg/3.5-g dose (section 9.4.1) also, sodium 0.4 mmol/3.5-g dose and potassium 0.7 mmol/3.5-g dose

Dose: 3.5 g (1 measure) in at least 150 mL water twice daily; for earlier onset of cholesterol reduction (under medical supervision only), initially 5.25 g (1½ measures) twice daily for 2–3 months

COUNSELLING. Preparations that swell in contact with liquid should always be carefully swallowed with water and should not be taken immediately before going to bed

Statins

The statins (**atorvastatin, fluvastatin, pravastatin** and **simvastatin**) competitively inhibit 3-hydroxy-3-methylglutaryl coenzyme A (HMG CoA) reductase, an enzyme involved in cholesterol synthesis, especially in the liver. They are more effective than other classes of drugs in lowering LDL-cholesterol but less effective than the fibrates in reducing triglycerides and raising HDL-cholesterol.

Statins produce important reductions in coronary events, in all cardiovascular events, and in total mortality in patients aged up to 75 years with coronary heart disease (history of angina or acute myocardial infarction) and with a total serum-cholesterol concentration of 5 mmol/litre or greater. Statins should also be considered for patients who have had coronary artery bypass surgery or angioplasty, or who have other clinically overt atherosclerotic disease such as cerebrovascular disease (non-haemorrhagic stroke or transient ischaemic attacks) or peripheral vascular disease because these patients are at risk of major coronary events. Statins also reduce the incidence of non-haemorrhagic stroke when used for secondary prevention in coronary heart disease.

Statins have a role in primary prevention of coronary events in patients at increased risk. Risk of coronary events is not accurately predicted from cholesterol concentrations alone and methods that take into account factors such as smoking, hypertension and diabetes mellitus should be used to estimate risk. A statin should be considered for patients with a total serum-cholesterol concentration of 5 mmol/litre or greater and a coronary heart disease risk[1] of 30% or greater over 10 years, for primary prevention following a trial of lifestyle measures and other appropriate interventions.

For primary and secondary prevention of coronary heart disease, statin treatment should be adjusted to achieve a target total cholesterol concentration of less than 5 mmol/litre (or a reduction of 20–25% if that produces a lower concentration); in terms of LDL-cholesterol, the target should be below 3 mmol/litre (or a reduction of about 30% if that produces a lower concentration).

Recent evidence suggests that the use of statins may benefit all patients at high risk, including those with a total cholesterol concentration of less than 5 mmol/litre; these findings are awaiting confirmation.

CAUTIONS. Statins should be used with caution in those with a history of liver disease or with a high alcohol intake (use should be avoided in active liver disease). Liver-function tests should be carried out before and within 1–3 months of starting treatment

1. Coronary heart disease risk may be determined using the Joint British Societies' 'Cardiac Risk Assessor' computer program or chart (British Cardiac Society, British Hyperlipidaemia Association, British Hypertension Society. *Heart* 1998; **80**(suppl 2): S1–29) see *inside back cover*

and thereafter at intervals of 6 months for 1 year, unless indicated sooner by signs or symptoms suggestive of hepatotoxicity. Treatment should be discontinued if serum transaminase concentration rises to, and persists at, 3 times the upper limit of the reference range. Patients should be advised to report unexplained muscle pain (see Muscle Effects below). **Interactions:** Appendix 1 (statins).

CONTRA-INDICATIONS. Statins are contra-indicated in active liver disease (or persistently abnormal liver function tests) and in pregnancy (adequate contraception required during treatment and for 1 month afterwards) and breast-feeding (see Appendixes 4 and 5).

SIDE-EFFECTS. Reversible myositis is a rare but significant side-effect of the statins (see also Muscle Effects, p. 124 and below). The statins also cause headache, altered liver-function tests (rarely, hepatitis) and gastro-intestinal effects including abdominal pain, flatulence, diarrhoea, nausea and vomiting. Rash and hypersensitivity reactions (including angioedema and anaphylaxis) have been reported rarely.

MUSCLE EFFECTS. Myalgia, myositis and myopathy have been reported with the statins; if the creatine kinase concentration is markedly elevated (> 10 times upper limit of normal), and myopathy is suspected or diagnosed, treatment should be discontinued. There is an increased incidence of myopathy if the statins are given with a fibrate (see also CSM advice in section 2.12), with lipid-lowering doses of nicotinic acid, or with immunosuppressants such as ciclosporin; close monitoring of liver function and, if symptomatic, of creatine kinase is required in patients receiving these drugs. Rhabdomyolysis with acute renal impairment secondary to myoglobinuria has also been reported.

COUNSELLING. Advise patient to report promptly unexplained muscle pain, tenderness, weakness.

ATORVASTATIN

Indications: primary hypercholesterolaemia, heterozygous familial hypercholesterolaemia, homozygous familial hypercholesterolaemia or combined (mixed) hyperlipidaemia in patients who have not responded adequately to diet and other appropriate measures

Cautions: see notes above

Contra-indications: see notes above

Side-effects: see notes above; also insomnia, angioedema, anorexia, asthenia, paraesthesia, peripheral neuropathy, alopecia, pruritus, rash, impotence, chest pain, hypoglycaemia and hyperglycaemia reported; thrombocytopenia reported rarely

Dose: primary hypercholesterolaemia and combined hyperlipidaemia, usually 10 mg once daily
Familial hypercholesterolaemia, initially 10 mg daily, increased at intervals of 4 weeks to 40 mg once daily; if necessary, further increased to max. 80 mg once daily (or combined with anion-exchange resin in heterozygous familial hypercholesterolaemia)

Lipitor® (Parke-Davis) PoM
Tablets, all f/c, atorvastatin (as calcium trihydrate) 10 mg, net price 28-tab pack = £18.03; 20 mg, 28-tab pack = £29.69; 40 mg 28-tab pack = £29.69; 80 mg, 28-tab pack = £29.69. Counselling, muscle effects, see notes above

FLUVASTATIN

Indications: primary hypercholesterolaemia or combined (mixed) hyperlipidaemia (types IIa and IIb) in patients who have not responded adequately to dietary control; adjunct to diet in retarding progression of coronary atherosclerosis in primary hypercholesterolaemia and concomitant coronary heart disease

Cautions: see notes above

Contra-indications: see notes above; also severe renal impairment

Side-effects: see notes above; also insomnia, paraesthesia

Dose: initially 20–40 mg daily in the evening, adjusted at intervals of 4 weeks; up to 40 mg twice daily may be required

Lescol® (Novartis) PoM

Capsules, fluvastatin (as sodium salt) 20 mg (brown/yellow), net price 28-cap pack = £12.72; 40 mg (brown/orange), 28-cap pack = £12.72, 56-cap pack = £25.44. Counselling, muscle effects, see notes above

■ Modified release

Lescol® XL (Novartis) PoM

Tablets, m/r, yellow, fluvastatin (as sodium salt) 80 mg, net price 28-tab pack = £16.00. Label: 25, counselling, muscle effects, see notes above

Dose: 80 mg once daily (dose form not appropriate for initial dose titration)

PRAVASTATIN SODIUM

Indications: primary hypercholesterolaemia in patients who have not responded adequately to dietary control; adjunct to diet to slow progression of coronary atherosclerosis and reduce incidence of cardiac events in patients with hypercholesterolaemia and atherosclerotic coronary artery disease; adjunct to diet in hypercholesterolaemia without clinically evident coronary heart disease; prevention of stroke, recurrent coronary events (including myocardial infarction), or need for revascularisation procedure in patients with previous myocardial infarction or unstable angina and total serum cholesterol concentration greater than 4.8 mmol/litre (or LDL-cholesterol greater than 3.2 mmol/litre) (see also notes above)

Cautions: see notes above

Contra-indications: see notes above

Side-effects: see notes above; also chest pain, fatigue

Dose: usual range 10–40 mg once daily at night, adjusted at intervals of not less than 4 weeks

Lipostat® (Squibb) PoM

Tablets, all yellow, pravastatin sodium 10 mg, net price 28-tab pack = £16.18; 20 mg, 28-tab pack = £29.69; 40 mg, 28-tab pack = £29.69. Counselling, muscle effects, see notes above

SIMVASTATIN

Indications: primary hypercholesterolaemia, heterozygous familial hypercholesterolaemia, homozygous familial hypercholesterolaemia or combined (mixed) hyperlipidaemia in patients who have not responded adequately to diet and other appropriate measures; prevention of coronary events, need for revascularisation procedures, and to slow progression of coronary atherosclerosis in patients with coronary heart disease and total cholesterol concentration of 5.5 mmol/litre or greater (see also notes above)

Cautions: see notes above; severe renal impairment (Appendix 3)

Contra-indications: see notes above; also porphyria (see section 9.8.2)

Side-effects: see notes above; also alopecia, anaemia, dizziness, paraesthesia, peripheral neuropathy, hepatitis, jaundice, pancreatitis

Dose: primary hypercholesterolaemia, heterozygous familial hypercholesterolaemia, combined hyperlipidaemia, 10 mg daily at night, adjusted at intervals of not less than 4 weeks; usual range 10–80 mg once daily at night

Homozygous familial hypercholesterolaemia, 40 mg daily at night *or* 80 mg daily in 3 divided doses (with largest dose at night)

Coronary heart disease, initially 20 mg once daily at night, adjusted at intervals of not less than 4 weeks; max. 80 mg once daily

Note. Max. 10 mg daily with concomitant ciclosporin, fibrate or lipid-lowering dose of nicotinic acid

Zocor® (MSD) PoM

Tablets, all f/c, simvastatin 10 mg (peach), net price 28-tab pack = £18.03; 20 mg (tan), 28-tab pack = £29.69; 40 mg (red), 28-tab pack = £29.69; 80 mg (red), 28-tab pack = £29.69. Counselling, muscle effects, see notes above

Nicotinic acid group

The value of **nicotinic acid** is limited by its side-effects, especially vasodilatation. In doses of 1.5 to 3 g daily it lowers both cholesterol and triglyceride concentrations by inhibiting synthesis; it also increases HDL-cholesterol. **Acipimox** seems to have fewer side-effects but may be less effective in its lipid-modulating capabilities.

ACIPIMOX

Indications: hyperlipidaemias of types IIa, IIb, and IV in patients who have not responded adequately to diet and other appropriate measures

Cautions: renal impairment (Appendix 3)

Contra-indications: peptic ulcer; pregnancy and breast-feeding

Side-effects: vasodilatation, flushing, itching, rashes, urticaria, erythema; heartburn, epigastric pain, nausea, diarrhoea, headache, malaise, dry eyes; rarely angioedema, bronchospasm, anaphylaxis

Dose: usually 500–750 mg daily in divided doses

Olbetam® (Pharmacia) PoM

Capsules, brown/pink, acipimox 250 mg. Net price 90-cap pack = £36.87. Label: 21

NICOTINIC ACID

Indications: see notes above

Cautions: diabetes mellitus, gout, liver disease, peptic ulcer; **interactions:** Appendix 1 (nicotinic acid)

Contra-indications: pregnancy, breast-feeding

Side-effects: flushing, dizziness, headache, palpitations, pruritus (prostaglandin-mediated symptoms can be reduced by low initial doses taken with meals, or by taking aspirin 75 mg 30 minutes before the dose); nausea, vomiting; rarely impaired liver function and rashes

Dose: initially 100–200 mg 3 times daily (see above), gradually increased over 2–4 weeks to 1–2 g 3 times daily

¹Nicotinic Acid Tablets, [PoM] nicotinic acid 50 mg, net price 100 = £9.25. Label: 21

1. May be sold to the public unless max. daily dose exceeds 600 mg or if intended for treatment of hyperlipidaemia

Fish oils

A fish-oil preparation (*Maxepa®*), rich in omega-3 marine triglycerides, is useful in the treatment of severe hypertriglyceridaemia; however, it can sometimes aggravate hypercholesterolaemia.

OMEGA-3 MARINE TRIGLYCERIDES

Indications: reduction of plasma triglycerides in patients with severe hypertriglyceridaemia judged to be at special risk of ischaemic heart disease or pancreatitis, in conjunction with dietary and other methods (see notes above)

Cautions: haemorrhagic disorders, anticoagulant treatment; aspirin-sensitive asthma; diabetes mellitus

Side-effects: occasional nausea and belching

Dose: see under preparations below

Maxepa® (Seven Seas)
Capsules, 1 g (approx. 1.1 mL) concentrated fish oils containing eicosapentaenoic acid 170 mg, docosahexaenoic acid 115 mg. Vitamin A content less than 100 units/g, vitamin D content less than 10 units/g, net price 200-cap pack = £27.28. Label: 21
Dose: 5 capsules twice daily with food
Liquid, golden-coloured, concentrated fish oils containing eicosapentaenoic acid 170 mg, docosahexaenoic acid 115 mg/g (1.1 mL). Vitamin A content less than 100 units/g, vitamin D content less than 10 units/g, net price 150 mL = £20.46. Label: 21
Dose: 5 mL twice daily with food

2.13 Local sclerosants

Ethanolamine oleate and sodium tetradecyl sulphate are used in sclerotherapy of varicose veins, and phenol is used in haemorrhoids (section 1.7.3).

ETHANOLAMINE OLEATE

(Monoethanolamine Oleate)

Indications: sclerotherapy of varicose veins

Cautions: extravasation may cause necrosis of tissues

Contra-indications: inability to walk, acute phlebitis, oral contraceptive use, obese legs

Side-effects: allergic reactions (including anaphylaxis)

Ethanolamine Oleate Injection, [PoM] ethanolamine oleate 5%. Net price 5-mL amp = £2.12
Available from Medeva
Dose: by slow injection into empty isolated segment of vein, 2–5 mL divided between 3–4 sites; repeated at weekly intervals

SODIUM TETRADECYL SULPHATE

Indications: sclerotherapy of varicose veins

Cautions; Contra-indications; Side-effects: see under Ethanolamine Oleate

Fibro-Vein® (STD Pharmaceutical) [PoM]
Injection, sodium tetradecyl sulphate 0.2%, net price 5-mL amp = £2.34; 0.5%, 2-mL amp = £1.39; 1%, 2-mL amp = £1.50; 3%, 2-mL amp = £1.69, 5-mL vial = £3.25
Dose: by slow injection into empty isolated segment of vein, 0.1–1 mL according to site and condition being treated (consult product literature)

3: Respiratory system

3.1   Bronchodilators

Asthma

Drugs used in the management of asthma include beta$_2$ agonists (section 3.1.1), antimuscarinic bronchodilators (section 3.1.2), theophylline (section 3.1.3), corticosteroids (section 3.2), cromoglicate and nedocromil (section 3.3.1), and leukotriene receptor antagonists (section 3.3.2).

For tables outlining the management of chronic asthma and acute severe asthma see p. 132 and p. 133.

Administration of drugs for asthma

INHALATION. This route delivers the drug directly to the airways; the dose is smaller than that for products given by mouth and side-effects are reduced. *Pressurised metered-dose inhalers* are an effective and convenient method of administering many drugs used for asthma. A spacer device (section 3.1.5) may improve drug delivery, particularly for young children and those who have difficulty using an inhaler; spacers also reduce adverse effects from inhaled corticosteroids. Breath-actuated devices including dry powder inhalers are also available.

Solutions for nebulisation are available for use in acute severe asthma. They are administered over a period of 5–10 minutes from a nebuliser, usually driven by oxygen in hospital. Electric compressors are most suitable for domiciliary use but they are not prescribable on the NHS.

ORAL. The oral route is used when administration by inhalation is not possible. Systemic side-effects occur more frequently when a drug is given orally rather than by inhalation. Drugs given by mouth for the treatment of asthma include beta$_2$ agonists, corticosteroids, theophylline and leukotriene receptor antagonists.

PARENTERAL. Drugs such as beta$_2$ agonists, corticosteroids, and aminophylline may be given by injection in acute severe asthma when administration by nebulisation is inadequate or inappropriate. If the patient is being treated in the community, urgent transfer to hospital should be arranged.

Pregnancy and breast-feeding

It is particularly important that asthma should be well controlled during pregnancy; where this is achieved asthma has no important effects on pregnancy, labour, or on the fetus. Drugs for asthma should preferably be administered by inhalation to minimise exposure of the fetus.

Severe exacerbations of asthma can have an adverse effect on pregnancy and should be treated promptly with conventional therapy, including oral or parenteral administration of a corticosteroid and nebulisation of a beta$_2$ agonist; prednisolone is the preferred corticosteroid for oral administration since very little of the drug reaches the fetus.

Acute severe asthma

Severe asthma can be fatal and **must** be treated promptly and energetically. It is characterised by persistent dyspnoea poorly relieved by broncho-dilators, exhaustion, a high pulse rate (usually over 110/minute), and a very low peak expiratory flow. As asthma becomes more severe, wheezing may be absent. Such patients should be given **oxygen** (if available) and **salbutamol** or **terbutaline** by neb-uliser. This should be followed by a large dose of a **corticosteroid** (section 6.3.2)—for adults, pred-nisolone 30–60 mg by mouth or hydrocortisone 200 mg (preferably as sodium succinate) intrave-nously; for children, prednisolone 1–2 mg/kg by mouth (1–4 years max. 20 mg, 5–15 years max. 40 mg) or hydrocortisone 100 mg (preferably as sodium succinate) intravenously; if vomiting occurs, the parenteral route may be preferred for the first dose. For a table outlining the management of acute severe asthma, see p. 133.

If there is little response the following additional treatment should be considered: **ipratropium** by nebuliser (section 3.1.2), **aminophylline** by slow intravenous injection if the patient has not already been receiving theophylline (section 3.1.3), or the beta₂ agonist by the intravenous route.

Further treatment of these patients is safer in hos-pital where resuscitation facilities are immediately available. Treatment should **never** be delayed for investigations, patients should **never** be sedated, and the possibility of a pneumothorax should be considered.

If the patient deteriorates despite appropriate pharmacological treatment, intermittent positive pressure ventilation may be needed.

Chronic obstructive pulmonary disease

Chronic obstructive pulmonary disease (chronic bronchitis and emphysema) may be helped by an inhaled **short-acting beta₂ agonist** (section 3.1.1.1) used as required *or* when the airways obstruction is more severe, by a regular inhaled **antimuscarinic bronchodilator** (section 3.1.2) *or* an inhaled **long-acting beta₂ agonist** if necessary. Although many patients are treated with an inhaled corticosteroid, long-term studies have shown no reduction in the decline in lung function in patients taking regular inhaled corticosteroids (section 3.2). A limited trial of high-dose inhaled corticosteroid *or* an oral corticosteroid is recommended for patients with moderate airflow obstruction to determine the extent of the airway reversibility and to ensure that asthma has not been overlooked.

Long-term **oxygen** therapy (section 3.6) prolongs survival in some patients with chronic obstructive pulmonary disease. For the management of infec-tions in bronchitis see Table 1, section 5.1.

Croup

Mild croup requires no specific treatment and can be managed in the community. More severe croup calls for hospital admission; a single dose of a corticosteroid (e.g. dexamethasone 150–600 micrograms/kg by mouth) may be administered before transfer to hospital. In hospital, dexamethasone 300–600 micrograms/kg (by mouth or by injection) or budesonide 2 mg (by nebulisa-tion) will often reduce symptoms. For severe croup not effectively controlled with corticosteroid treat-ment, nebulised adrenaline solution 1 in 1000 (1 mg/mL) may be given with close clinical moni-toring in a dose of 400 micrograms/kg (max. 5 mg) repeated after 30 minutes if necessary; the effects of nebulised adrenaline last 2–3 hours.

3.1.1	**Adrenoceptor agonists**
	(Sympathomimetics)
3.1.1.1	Selective beta₂ agonists
3.1.1.2	Other adrenoceptor agonists

The selective beta₂ agonists (selective beta₂-adreno-ceptor agonists, selective beta₂ stimulants) (section 3.1.1.1) such as salbutamol or terbutaline are the safest and most effective beta agonists for asthma. They are recommended over the less selective beta agonists such as orciprenaline (section 3.1.1.2), which should be avoided whenever possible.

Adrenaline (epinephrine) (which has both alpha- and beta-adrenoceptor agonist properties) is used in the emergency management of allergic and anaphy-lactic reactions (section 3.4.3).

3.1.1.1 Selective beta₂ agonists

Mild to moderate symptoms of asthma respond rap-idly to the inhalation of a selective short-acting beta₂ agonist such as **salbutamol** or **terbutaline**. If beta₂ agonist inhalation is needed more often than once daily, prophylactic treatment should be con-sidered, using a stepped approach as outlined on p. 132.

Salmeterol and **formoterol** (eformoterol) are longer-acting beta₂ agonists which are administered by inhalation. They should not be used for the relief of an acute asthma attack. Salmeterol and formot-erol should be added to existing corticosteroid ther-apy and not replace it. They can be useful in nocturnal asthma. Formoterol is also licensed for short-term symptom relief.

REGULAR TREATMENT. Short-acting beta₂ ago-nists should not be prescribed for use on a regular basis in patients with mild or moderate asthma since regular treatment provides no clinical benefit. However, regular use of the longer acting beta₂ ago-nists, salmeterol and formoterol, is of benefit.

Chronic Asthma table, see p. 132
Acute Severe Asthma table, see p. 133

INHALATION. *Pressurised-metered dose inhalers* are an effective and convenient method of drug administration in mild to moderate asthma. At rec-ommended inhaled doses the duration of action of salbutamol, terbutaline and fenoterol is about 3 to 5 hours and for salmeterol and formoterol, 12 hours. The **dose**, the frequency, and the maximum number of inhalations in 24 hours of the beta₂ ago-nist should be **stated explicitly** to the patient. High doses of beta₂ agonists can be dangerous in some patients. Excessive use is usually an indication of **inadequately controlled** asthma and should be

Start at **step most appropriate** to initial severity; **'rescue' course** of prednisolone at **any time** or **any step**

Chronic asthma: adults and schoolchildren

Step 1: occasional relief bronchodilators

Inhaled short-acting beta$_2$ agonist as required (up to once daily)

Note. Move to step 2 if needed more than once daily (or night-time symptoms); check compliance, inhaler technique

Step 2: regular inhaled preventer therapy

Inhaled short-acting beta$_2$ agonist as required
  plus
Either regular standard-dose[1] inhaled corticosteroid
Or regular cromoglicate or nedocromil (but change to inhaled corticosteroid if control not achieved)

Note. Higher dose of inhaled corticosteroid may be required to gain initial control; some individuals benefit from doubling for short period to cover an exacerbation

Step 3: high-dose inhaled corticosteroids or standard-dose inhaled corticosteroids + long-acting inhaled beta$_2$ agonist

Inhaled short-acting beta$_2$ agonist as required
  plus
Either regular high-dose[2] inhaled corticosteroid
Or regular standard-dose[1] inhaled corticosteroid *plus* regular inhaled long-acting beta$_2$ agonist (salmeterol 50 micrograms twice daily *or* in those over 18 years, formoterol 12 micrograms twice daily)

Note. In few who have problems with high-dose inhaled corticosteroid use standard-dose inhaled corticosteroid with *either* inhaled long-acting beta$_2$ agonist option *or* regular modified-release oral theophylline *or* try regular cromoglicate or nedocromil

Step 4: high-dose inhaled corticosteroids + regular bronchodilators

Inhaled short-acting beta$_2$ agonist as required
  with
Regular high-dose[2] inhaled corticosteroid
  plus sequential therapeutic trial of one or more of
  Inhaled long-acting beta$_2$ agonist
  Modified-release oral theophylline
  Inhaled ipratropium or, in adults, oxitropium
  Modified-release oral beta$_2$ agonist
  High-dose inhaled bronchodilators
  Cromoglicate or nedocromil

Step 5: regular corticosteroid tablets

Inhaled short-acting beta$_2$ agonist as required
  with
Regular high-dose[2] inhaled corticosteroid *and* one or more long-acting bronchodilators (see step 4)
  plus
Regular prednisolone tablets (as single daily dose)

Note. In addition to regular prednisolone, continue high-dose inhaled corticosteroid (in exceptional cases may exceed licensed doses); these patients should normally be referred to an asthma clinic

Stepping down

Review treatment every 3–6 months; if control achieved stepwise reduction may be possible; if treatment started recently at step 4 or 5 (or contained corticosteroid tablets) reduction may take place after short interval; in other patients a 1–3 month or longer period of stability needed before slow stepwise reduction is undertaken

1. Standard-dose inhaled corticosteroids are beclometasone dipropionate or budesonide 100–400 micrograms daily *or* fluticasone propionate 50–200 micrograms twice daily
2. High-dose inhaled corticosteroids are beclometasone dipropionate or budesonide 0.8–2 mg daily (in divided doses) *or* fluticasone propionate 0.4–1 mg daily (in divided doses); use a large-volume spacer

Chronic asthma: children under 5 years

Step 1: occasional relief bronchodilators

Short-acting beta$_2$ agonist as required (not more than once daily)

Note. Whenever possible inhaled (less effective and more side-effects when given by mouth); check compliance, technique and that inhaler device is appropriate

Step 2: regular inhaled preventer therapy

Inhaled short-acting beta$_2$ agonist as required
  plus
Either regular inhaled cromoglicate (powder or metered-dose inhaler via large-volume spacer)
Or regular inhaled corticosteroid in standard paediatric dose[3]
    Consider for stabilisation
    5-day course of soluble prednisolone tablets[5] *or* temporary doubling of dose of inhaled corticosteroid

Note. Try cromoglicate for 4–6 weeks. For inhaled corticosteroids assess effect on symptoms after 1 month and adjust doses; if control not adequate consider doubling dose of inhaled corticosteroid for 1 month (alternatively give 5-day course of soluble prednisolone tablets or consider introducing other treatments before increasing dose of inhaled corticosteroid for long periods)

Step 3: increased-dose inhaled corticosteroids

Inhaled short-acting beta$_2$ agonist as required
  plus
Regular inhaled corticosteroid in high paediatric dose[4]
    Consider
    Short course of soluble prednisolone tablets[5]
    Regular inhaled long-acting beta$_2$ agonist *or* regular modified-release oral theophylline

Note. Long-acting beta$_2$ agonist should probably be reserved for supplementing treatment in child already receiving cromoglicate or a corticosteroid; modified-release oral theophylline may be helpful (particularly for nocturnal symptoms), but has appreciable side-effects in up to one-third of children (plasma- or salivary-concentration monitoring recommended)

Step 4: high-dose inhaled corticosteroid + regular bronchodilators

Inhaled short-acting beta$_2$ agonist as required
  with
Regular inhaled corticosteroid in high dose (beclometasone dipropionate or budesonide up to 2 mg daily *via* large-volume spacer)
    Consider (as in step 3)
    Short course of soluble prednisolone[5]
    Regular inhaled long-acting beta$_2$ agonist
    Regular modified-release oral theophylline
    Also nebulised beta$_2$ agonist

Stepping down

Regularly review need for treatment

3. Standard paediatric dose of inhaled corticosteroid is beclometasone dipropionate or budesonide up to 400 micrograms daily (in divided doses) *or* fluticasone propionate up to 200 micrograms daily (in divided doses); initial dose according to age, weight and severity of asthma; use a large-volume spacer
4. High paediatric dose of inhaled corticosteroid is beclomethasone dipropionate or budesonide up to 800 micrograms daily (in divided doses) *or* fluticasone propionate up to 500 micrograms daily (in divided doses); use a large-volume spacer
5. Doses of prednisolone tablets is child under 1 year 1–2 mg/kg daily, 1–5 years 20 mg daily; rescue courses usually for 1–3 days

Based on tables in: British Thoracic Society, the British Paediatric Association and others. Guidelines on the Management of Asthma. *Thorax* 1997; **52** (suppl); S1–S21. Reproduced with permission of BMJ Specialist Journals

MANAGEMENT OF ACUTE SEVERE ASTHMA IN GENERAL PRACTICE

Uncontrolled asthma in adults

— Speech normal
— Pulse <110 beats/minute
— Respiration <25 breaths/minute
— Peak flow >50% of predicted or best

Treat at home but response to treatment **must** be assessed before doctor leaves

Treatment:

Nebulised salbutamol 5 mg or nebulised terbutaline 10 mg

Monitor response 15–30 minutes after nebulisation

If peak flow 50–75% of predicted or best give:

Oral prednisolone 30–60 mg
and step up usual treatment

Alternatively if peak flow >75% of predicted or best:

Step up usual treatment

Follow up

Monitor symptoms and peak flow

Set up self management plan

Review in surgery within 48 hours

Modify treatment at review according to guidelines for chronic asthma (see opposite page)

Important: regard each emergency consultation as being for **acute severe asthma** until shown otherwise.

Important: failure to respond adequately **at any time** requires immediate referral to hospital.

Acute severe asthma in adults

— Cannot complete sentences
— Pulse ≥110 beats/minute
— Respiration ≥25 breaths/minute
— Peak flow ≤50% of predicted or best

Seriously consider hospital admission if more than one of above features present

Treatment:

Oxygen 40–60% if available

Nebulised salbutamol 5 mg or nebulised terbutaline 10 mg

Oral prednisolone 30–60 mg or i/v hydrocortisone 200 mg

Monitor response 15–30 minutes after nebulisation

If any signs of acute asthma persist:

Arrange hospital admission

While awaiting ambulance repeat nebulised beta₂ agonist and give with nebulised ipratropium 500 micrograms

or give subcutaneous terbutaline (or salbutamol)

or give slow intravenous aminophylline 250 mg (**important:** not if taking an oral theophylline)

Alternatively if symptoms have improved, respiration and pulse settling, and peak flow >50% of predicted or best:

Step up usual treatment *and* continue prednisolone

Follow-up

Monitor symptoms and peak flow

Set up self management plan

Review in surgery within 24 hours

Modify treatment at review (see opposite page)

Life-threatening asthma in adults

— Silent chest
— Cyanosis
— Bradycardia or exhaustion
— Peak flow <33% of predicted or best

Arrange IMMEDIATE hospital admission

Treatment:

Oral prednisolone 30–60 mg or i/v hydrocortisone 200 mg (immediately)

Oxygen-driven nebuliser in ambulance

Nebulised¹ beta₂ agonist with nebulised ipratropium or subcutaneous terbutaline (or salbutamol)

or slow intravenous aminophylline 250 mg (**important:** not if taking an oral theophylline)

STAY WITH PATIENT UNTIL AMBULANCE ARRIVES

1. If no nebuliser available give 2 puffs of beta₂ agonist using large-volume spacer and repeat 10–20 times

Important: patients with severe or life-threatening attacks may not be distressed and may not have all these abnormalities; the presence of any should alert doctor.

Important: do not give bolus aminophylline to patient already taking an oral theophylline.

Acute episodes or exacerbations of asthma in young children in primary care

Mild/moderate episode in young children

— short-acting beta₂ agonist from metered dose inhaler *via* large-volume spacer (and face mask in very young), up to 10 puffs (1 puff every 15–30 seconds); alternatively give by nebuliser every 3–4 hours

— if favourable response (respiratory rate reduced, reduced use of accessory muscles, improved 'behaviour' pattern), repeat inhaled beta₂ agonist every 3–4 hours; consider doubling dose of inhaled corticosteroids

— if beta₂ agonist still required every 3–4 hours after 12 hours, start short course of oral prednisolone for 1–3 days (under 1 year 1–2 mg/kg daily; 1–5 years 20 mg daily)

If unresponsive or relapse within 3–4 hours:

— immediately refer to hospital
— increase frequency of beta₂ agonist (give as frequently as needed)
— start oral prednisolone
— give high-flow oxygen *via* face mask

Signs of acute asthma in children

Acute severe asthma:

— too breathless to talk
— too breathless to feed
— respiration >50 breaths/minute (≥40/minute in children over 5 years)
— pulse >140 beats/minute (≥120 beats/minute in children over 5 years)
— in younger children, use of accessory muscles of breathing
— in older children, peak flow ≤50% of predicted or best

Life-threatening features:

— cyanosis, silent chest, or poor respiratory effort
— fatigue or exhaustion
— agitation or reduced level of consciousness
— in older children, peak flow <33% of predicted or best

managed with a prophylactic drug such as an inhaled corticosteroid. The patient should be advised to seek medical advice when the prescribed dose of beta$_2$ agonist fails to provide the usual degree of symptomatic relief because this usually indicates a worsening of the asthma and the patient may require alternative medication (see Chronic Asthma table, p. 132).

CFC-FREE INHALERS. Chlorofluorocarbon (CFC) propellants in pressurised metered-dose inhalers are being replaced by hydrofluoroalkane (HFA) propellants. Patients receiving CFC-free inhalers should be reassured about the efficacy of the new inhalers and counselled that the aerosol may feel and taste different; any difficulty with the new inhaler should be discussed with the doctor or pharmacist.
CSM advice. The CSM has requested reporting of any adverse reaction to the new HFA-containing inhalers and to include the brand name of the inhaler on the yellow card.
Respirator (or nebuliser) solutions of salbutamol and terbutaline are used for the treatment of acute asthma both in hospital and in general practice. Patients with a severe attack of asthma should have oxygen if possible during nebulisation since beta$_2$ agonists can increase arterial hypoxaemia. The dose given by nebuliser is substantially higher than that given by inhaler. Patients should therefore be warned that it is dangerous to exceed the prescribed dose and they should seek medical advice if they fail to respond to the usual dose of the respirator solution. See also guidelines in section 3.1.5.

ORAL. Oral preparations of beta$_2$ agonists may be used by patients who cannot manage the inhaled route. They are sometimes used for children, but inhaled beta$_2$ agonists are generally better and most children can use one of the inhaler systems available. The longer-acting oral preparations including bambuterol may be of value in nocturnal asthma as an alternative to modified-release theophylline preparations (section 3.1.3) but they have a limited role and inhaled long-acting beta $_2$ agonists are usually preferred.

PARENTERAL. Salbutamol or terbutaline are given by intravenous infusion for severe asthma. Although some patients with chronic asthma are treated with a beta$_2$ agonist by subcutaneous injection on a regular basis, this route is not recommended since the evidence of benefit is uncertain and it may be difficult to withdraw such treatment once started. Patients supplied with a selective beta$_2$ agonist injection for severe attacks should be advised to attend hospital immediately after using the injection, for further assessment. Beta$_2$ agonists may also be given by intramuscular injection.

CHILDREN. Selective beta$_2$ agonists are useful even in children under the age of 18 months. They are most effective by the inhaled route; a pressurised metered-dose inhaler should be used with spacer device in children under 5 years (see NICE guidance, section 3.1.5). A beta$_2$ agonist may also be administered by mouth although administration by inhalation is preferred. In severe attacks nebulisation using a selective beta$_2$ agonist or ipratropium is advisable (see also Asthma tables, pp.132-133).

CAUTIONS. Beta$_2$ agonists should be used with caution in hyperthyroidism, cardiovascular disease, arrhythmias, susceptibility to QT-interval prolongation, and hypertension. They should be used with care in pregnancy and breast-feeding (see notes above). Beta$_2$ agonists should be used with caution in diabetes—monitor blood glucose (risk of ketoacidosis, especially when beta$_2$ agonist administered intravenously). **Interactions:** Appendix 1 (sympathomimetics, beta$_2$)
HYPOKALAEMIA. The CSM has advised that potentially serious hypokalaemia may result from beta$_2$ agonist therapy. Particular caution is required in severe asthma, because this effect may be potentiated by concomitant treatment with theophylline and its derivatives, corticosteroids, and diuretics, and by hypoxia. Plasma-potassium concentration should therefore be monitored in severe asthma

SIDE-EFFECTS. Side-effects of the beta$_2$ agonists include fine tremor (particularly in the hands), nervous tension, headache, peripheral dilatation and palpitations. Other side-effects include tachycardia and arrhythmias and disturbances of sleep and behaviour in children. Muscle cramps and hypersensitivity reactions including paradoxical bronchospasm, urticaria, and angioedema have also been reported. Beta$_2$ agonists are associated with hypokalaemia after high doses (for CSM advice see under Cautions). Pain may occur on intramuscular injection.

SALBUTAMOL

Indications: asthma and other conditions associated with reversible airways obstruction; premature labour (section 7.1.3)

Cautions: see notes above

Side-effects: see notes above

Dose: *by mouth*, 4 mg (elderly and sensitive patients initially 2 mg) 3–4 times daily; max. single dose 8 mg (but unlikely to provide much extra benefit or to be tolerated); CHILD under 2 years 100 micrograms/kg 4 times daily [unlicensed]; 2–6 years 1–2 mg 3–4 times daily, 6–12 years 2 mg 3–4 times daily

By subcutaneous or intramuscular injection, 500 micrograms, repeated every 4 hours if necessary

By slow intravenous injection, 250 micrograms, repeated if necessary

By intravenous infusion, initially 5 micrograms/minute, adjusted according to response and heart-rate usually in range 3–20 micrograms/minute, or more if necessary; CHILD 1 month–12 years 0.1–1 microgram/kg/minute [unlicensed]

By aerosol inhalation, 100–200 micrograms (1–2 puffs); for persistent symptoms up to 3–4 times daily (but see also Chronic Asthma table); CHILD 100 micrograms (1 puff), increased to 200 micrograms (2 puffs) if necessary; for persistent symptoms up to 3–4 times daily (but see also Chronic Asthma table)
Prophylaxis in exercise-induced bronchospasm, 200 micrograms (2 puffs); CHILD 100 micrograms (1 puff), increased to 200 micrograms (2 puffs) if necessary

By inhalation of powder (*Ventolin Rotacaps®*, *Ventodisks®*; for *Ventolin Accuhaler®* and *Asmasal®* dose see under preparation), 200–400 micrograms; for persistent symptoms up to 3–4 times daily (but see also Chronic Asthma table); CHILD 200 micrograms

Prophylaxis in exercise-induced bronchospasm (*powder*), 400 micrograms; CHILD 200 micrograms

Note. Bioavailability appears to be lower, so recommended doses for dry powder inhalers are twice those in a metered inhaler

By inhalation of nebulised solution, chronic bronchospasm unresponsive to conventional therapy and severe acute asthma, ADULT and CHILD over 18 months 2.5 mg, repeated up to 4 times daily; may be increased to 5 mg if necessary, but medical assessment should be considered since alternative therapy may be indicated; CHILD under 18 months, [unlicensed] (transient hypoxaemia may occur—consider supplemental oxygen), 1.25–2.5 mg up to 4 times daily but more frequent administration may be needed in severe cases

■ **Oral**

Salbutamol (Non-proprietary) PoM

Tablets, salbutamol (as sulphate) 2 mg, net price 20 = 59p; 4 mg, 20 = £1.08

Available from Alpharma, APS, Hillcross, IVAX

Oral solution, salbutamol (as sulphate) 2 mg/5 mL, net price 150 mL = 64p

Available from Lagap

Ventmax® SR (Trinity) PoM

Capsules, m/r, salbutamol (as sulphate) 4 mg (green/grey), net price 56-cap pack = £8.57; 8 mg (white), 56-cap pack = £10.28. Label: 25

Dose: 8 mg twice daily; CHILD 3–12 years 4 mg twice daily

Ventolin® (A&H) PoM

Syrup, sugar-free, salbutamol (as sulphate) 2 mg/5 mL, net price 150 mL = 64p

Volmax® (A&H) PoM

Tablets, m/r, salbutamol (as sulphate) 4 mg, net price 56-tab pack = £10.55; 8 mg, 56-tab pack = £12.66. Label: 25

Dose: 8 mg twice daily; CHILD 3–12 years 4 mg twice daily

■ **Parenteral**

Salbutamol (Non-proprietary) PoM

Injection, salbutamol (as sulphate) 100 micrograms/mL, net price 50-mL vial = £5.25

Available from Aurum

Ventolin® (A&H) PoM

Injection, salbutamol (as sulphate) 50 micrograms/mL, net price 5-mL amp = 57p; 500 micrograms/mL, 1-mL amp = 43p

Solution for intravenous infusion, salbutamol (as sulphate) 1 mg/mL. Dilute before use. Net price 5-mL amp = £2.78

■ **Inhalation**

COUNSELLING. Advise patients not to exceed prescribed dose and to follow manufacturer's directions; if a previously effective dose of inhaled salbutamol fails to provide at least 3 hours relief, a doctor's advice should be obtained as soon as possible.

Patients receiving CFC-free inhalers should be reassured about their efficacy and counselled that aerosol may feel and taste different

Salbutamol (Non-proprietary) PoM

Aerosol inhalation, salbutamol 100 micrograms/metered inhalation, net price 200-dose unit = £1.91. Counselling, dose

Available from Alpharma, APS, Ashbourne (*Maxivent®*), Hillcross, IVAX

Excipients: include CFC propellants

Aerosol inhalation (CFC-free), salbutamol (as sulphate) 100 micrograms/metered inhalation, net price 200-dose unit = £1.91. Counselling, dose, change to CFC-free inhaler

Available from APS, IVAX (*Salamol®* ▼)

Excipients: include HFA-134a (non-CFC propellant), alcohol

Note. Can be supplied against a generic prescription but if CFC-free not specified will be reimbursed at price for CFC-containing inhaler

Dry powder for inhalation, salbutamol 200 micrograms/metered inhalation, net price 100-dose unit = £5.05

Available from Trinity (*Pulvinal® Salbutamol*)

Nebuliser solution, salbutamol (as sulphate) 1 mg/mL, net price 20 × 2.5 mL (2.5 mg) = £2.49; 2 mg/mL, 20 × 2.5 mL (5 mg) = £4.98. May be diluted with sterile sodium chloride 0.9%

Available from Ashbourne (*Maxivent Steripoules®*), Galen, Generics, IVAX (*Salamol Steri-Neb®*)

Aerolin® Autohaler (3M) PoM

Aerosol inhalation, salbutamol (as sulphate) 100 micrograms/metered inhalation. Net price 200-dose breath-actuated unit = £10.04. Counselling, dose

Excipients: include CFC propellants

Airomir® (3M) PoM

Aerosol inhalation, salbutamol (as sulphate) 100 micrograms/metered inhalation, net price 200-dose unit = £1.97. Counselling, dose, change to CFC-free inhaler

Excipients: include HFA-134a (a non-CFC propellant), alcohol

Also available as *Salbulin®* (3M)

Note. Can be supplied against a generic prescription but if 'CFC-free' not specified will be reimbursed at price for CFC-containing inhaler

Autohaler (breath-actuated aerosol inhalation), salbutamol (as sulphate) 100 micrograms/metered inhalation, net price 200-dose unit = £6.02. Counselling, dose, change to CFC-free inhaler

Excipients: include HFA-134a (a non-CFC propellant), alcohol

Asmasal Clickhaler® (Celltech) PoM

Dry powder for inhalation, salbutamol (as sulphate) 95 micrograms/metered inhalation, net price 200-dose unit = £6.32. Counselling, dose

Dose: acute bronchospasm 1–2 puffs

Persistent symptoms, 2 puffs 3–4 times daily

Prophylaxis in exercise-induced bronchospasm, 2 puffs

Salamol Easi-Breathe® (IVAX) PoM

Aerosol inhalation, salbutamol 100 micrograms/metered inhalation, net price 200-dose breath-actuated unit = £6.30. Counselling, dose

Excipients: include CFC propellants

CFC-Free ▼ *aerosol inhalation*, salbutamol 100 micrograms/metered inhalation, net price 200-dose breath-actuated unit = £6.30. Counselling, dose

Excipients: include alcohol, HFA-134a (a non-CFC propellant)

Ventodisks® (A&H) PoM

Dry powder for inhalation, disks containing 8 blisters of salbutamol (as sulphate) 200 micrograms/blister, net price 14 disks with *Diskhaler®* device = £6.40; 5-disk refill = £2.54 (hosp. only), 14-disk refill = £5.89; 400 micrograms/blister, 14 disks with *Diskhaler®* device = £10.82; 5-disk rcfill – £3.87 (hosp. only), 14-disk refill = £10.30. Counselling, dose

Ventolin® (A&H) PoM

Accuhaler® (dry powder for inhalation), disk containing 60 blisters of salbutamol (as sulphate) 200 micrograms/blister with *Accuhaler®* device, net price = £5.00. Counselling, dose

Dose: by inhalation of powder, 200 micrograms; for persistant symptoms up to 4 times daily (but see also Chronic Asthma table); CHILD 200 micrograms

Prophylaxis in allergen- or exercise-induced bronchospasm, 200 micrograms

Evohaler® ▼ *aerosol inhalation*, salbutamol (as sulphate) 100 micrograms/metered inhalation, net price 200-dose unit = £2.30. Counselling, dose, change to CFC-free inhaler

Excipients: include HFA-134a (a non-CFC propellant)

Note. Can be supplied against a generic prescription but if CFC-free not specified will be reimbursed at price for CFC-containing inhaler

Nebules® (for use with nebuliser), salbutamol (as sulphate) 1 mg/mL, net price 20 × 2.5 mL (2.5 mg) = £3.38; 2 mg/mL, 20 × 2.5 mL (5 mg) = £6.90. May be diluted with sterile sodium chloride 0.9% if administration time in excess of 10 minutes is required

Respirator solution (for use with a nebuliser or ventilator), salbutamol (as sulphate) 5 mg/mL. Net price 20 mL = £2.44 (hosp. only). May be diluted with sterile sodium chloride 0.9%

Rotacaps® (dry powder for inhalation; for use with *Ventolin Rotahaler®*), salbutamol (as sulphate), 200 micrograms (light-blue/clear), net price 112-cap pack = £5.33; 400 micrograms (dark-blue/clear), 112-cap pack = £9.01. Counselling, dose

■ Compound preparations

For some **compound preparations** containing salbutamol, see section 3.1.4

■ Inhaler devices
Section 3.1.5

Chronic Asthma table, see p. 132
Acute Severe Asthma table, see p. 133

TERBUTALINE SULPHATE

Indications: asthma and other conditions associated with reversible airways obstruction; premature labour (section 7.1.3)

Cautions: see notes above

Side-effects: see notes above

Dose: *by mouth*, initially 2.5 mg 3 times daily for 1–2 weeks, then up to 5 mg 3 times daily
CHILD 75 micrograms/kg 3 times daily; 7–15 years 2.5 mg 2–3 times daily

By subcutaneous, intramuscular, or slow intravenous injection, 250–500 micrograms up to 4 times daily; CHILD 2–15 years 10 micrograms/kg to a max. of 300 micrograms

By continuous intravenous infusion as a solution containing 3–5 micrograms/mL, 1.5–5 micrograms/minute for 8–10 hours; reduce dose for children

By aerosol inhalation, ADULT and CHILD 250–500 micrograms (1–2 puffs); for persistent symptoms up to 3–4 times daily (but see also Chronic Asthma table)

By inhalation of powder (*Turbohaler®*), 500 micrograms (1 inhalation); for persistent symptoms up to 4 times daily (but see also Chronic Asthma table)

By inhalation of nebulised solution, 5–10 mg 2–4 times daily; additional doses may be necessary in severe acute asthma; CHILD, up to 3 years 2 mg, 3–6 years 3 mg; 6–8 years 4 mg, over 8 years 5 mg, 2–4 times daily

■ Oral and parenteral

Bricanyl® (AstraZeneca) PoM

Tablets, scored, terbutaline sulphate 5 mg. Net price 20 = 74p

Syrup, sugar-free, terbutaline sulphate 1.5 mg/5 mL. Net price 300 mL = £2.36

Injection, terbutaline sulphate 500 micrograms/mL. Net price 1-mL amp = 27p; 5-mL amp = £1.27

Bricanyl SA® (AstraZeneca) PoM

Tablets, m/r, terbutaline sulphate 7.5 mg. Net price 20 = £1.33. Label: 25

Dose: 7.5 mg twice daily

Monovent® (Lagap) PoM

Syrup, sugar-free, terbutaline sulphate 1.5 mg/5 mL. Net price 300 mL = £2.15

■ Inhalation

COUNSELLING. Advise patients not to exceed prescribed dose and to follow manufacturer's directions; if a previously effective dose of inhaled terbutaline fails to provide at least 3 hours relief, a doctor's advice should be obtained as soon as possible

Terbutaline Sulphate (Non-proprietary) PoM

Nebuliser solution, terbutaline sulphate 2.5 mg/mL, net price 20 × 2 mL (5 mg) = £5.49. May be diluted with sterile sodium chloride 0.9%

Available from Galen

Bricanyl® (AstraZeneca) PoM

Aerosol inhalation, terbutaline sulphate 250 micrograms/metered inhalation. Net price 400-dose unit = £5.31; 400-dose unit with *Spacer* device (collapsible extended mouthpiece) = £7.21. Counselling, dose

Excipients: include CFC propellants

Turbohaler® (= dry powder inhaler), terbutaline sulphate 500 micrograms/inhalation. Net price 100-dose unit = £6.30. Counselling, dose

Respules® (= single-dose units for nebulisation), terbutaline sulphate 2.5 mg/mL. Net price 20 × 2-mL units (5-mg) = £3.67

Respirator solution (for use with a nebuliser or ventilator), terbutaline sulphate 10 mg/mL. Net price 20 mL = £2.64. Before use dilute with sterile sodium chloride 0.9%

■ Inhaler devices
Section 3.1.5

BAMBUTEROL HYDROCHLORIDE

Note. Bambuterol is a pro-drug of terbutaline

Indications: asthma and other conditions associated with reversible airways obstruction

Cautions: see notes above; renal impairment (Appendix 3); avoid in cirrhosis, severe hepatic impairment; manufacturer advises avoid in pregnancy

Side-effects: see notes above
Dose: 20 mg once daily at bedtime if patient has previously tolerated beta₂ agonists; other patients, initially 10 mg once daily at bedtime, increased if necessary after 1–2 weeks to 20 mg once daily; CHILD not recommended

Bambec® (AstraZeneca) PoM
Tablets, both scored, bambuterol hydrochloride 10 mg, net price 28-tab pack = £10.95; 20 mg, 28-tab pack = £13.14

FENOTEROL HYDROBROMIDE

Indications: reversible airways obstruction
Cautions: see notes above
Side-effects: see notes above

■ Compound preparations
For some **compound preparations** containing fenoterol, see section 3.1.4

FORMOTEROL FUMARATE/ EFORMOTEROL FUMARATE

Indications: reversible airways obstruction (including nocturnal asthma and prevention of exercise-induced bronchospasm) in patients requiring long-term regular bronchodilator therapy, see also Chronic Asthma table, p. 132
Note. Formoterol is not for immediate relief of acute attacks and existing corticosteroid therapy should not be reduced or withdrawn
Cautions: see notes above; severe liver cirrhosis; pregnancy (Appendix 4 and notes above); avoid in breast-feeding
Side-effects: see notes above; oropharyngeal irritation, taste disturbances, rash, insomnia, nausea and pruritus also reported; **important:** potential for paradoxical bronchospasm (calling for discontinuation and alternative therapy)
Dose: see under preparations below
COUNSELLING. Advise patients that formoterol should **not** be used for relief of acute attacks, not to exceed prescribed dose, and to follow manufacturer's directions; if a previously effective dose of inhaled formoterol fails to provide adequate relief, a doctor's advice should be obtained as soon as possible

Foradil® (Novartis) PoM
Dry powder for inhalation, formoterol fumarate 12 micrograms/capsule, net price 56-dose unit (with inhaler device) = £24.80. Counselling, dose
Dose: by inhalation of powder, ADULT and CHILD over 5 years, 12 micrograms twice daily, increased to 24 micrograms twice daily in more severe airways obstruction

Oxis® (AstraZeneca) PoM
Turbohaler® (= dry powder inhaler), formoterol fumarate 6 micrograms/inhalation, net price 60-dose unit = £24.80; 12 micrograms/inhalation, 60-dose unit = £24.80. Counselling, dose
Dose: by inhalation of powder, ADULT and CHILD over 12 years, 6–12 micrograms once or twice daily, increased to 24 micrograms twice daily in more severe airways obstruction; for short-term symptom relief (but not acute asthma), additional doses may be taken to a total max. 72 micrograms daily (max. single dose 36 micrograms); reassess treatment if additional doses required on more than 2 days a week

SALMETEROL

Indications: reversible airways obstruction (including nocturnal asthma and prevention of exercise-induced bronchospasm) in patients requiring long-term regular bronchodilator therapy, see also Chronic Asthma table, p. 132
Note. CSM has emphasised that salmeterol is not for immediate relief of acute attacks and that existing corticosteroid therapy should not be reduced or withdrawn
Cautions: see notes above
Side-effects: see notes above; significant incidence of paradoxical bronchospasm—may be clinically important in severe or deteriorating asthma
Dose: *by inhalation*, asthma, 50 micrograms (2 puffs or 1 blister) twice daily; up to 100 micrograms (4 puffs or 2 blisters) twice daily in more severe airways obstruction; CHILD under 4 years not recommended, over 4 years, 50 micrograms (2 puffs or 1 blister) twice daily
Chronic obstructive pulmonary disease 50 micrograms (2 puffs or 1 blister) twice daily
COUNSELLING. Advise patients that salmeterol should **not** be used for relief of acute attacks, not to exceed prescribed dose, and to follow manufacturer's directions; if a previously effective dose of inhaled salmeterol fails to provide adequate relief, a doctor's advice should be obtained as soon as possible

Serevent® (A&H) PoM
Accuhaler® (dry powder for inhalation), disk containing 60 blisters of salmeterol (as xinafoate (= hydroxynaphthoate)) 50 micrograms/blister with *Accuhaler®* device, net price = £28.60. Counselling, dose
Aerosol inhalation, salmeterol (as xinafoate (= hydroxynaphthoate)) 25 micrograms/metered inhalation, net price 60-dose unit = £14.30 (hosp. only), 120-dose unit = £28.60. Counselling, dose
Excipients: include CFC propellants
Diskhaler® (dry powder for inhalation), disks containing 4 blisters of salmeterol (as xinafoate (= hydroxynaphthoate)) 50 micrograms/blister, net price 14 disks with *Diskhaler®* device = £29.97, 5-disk refill = £9.99 (hosp. only), 14-disk refill = £29.40. Counselling, dose

---

3.1.1.2 Other adrenoceptor agonists

Ephedrine and the partially selective beta agonist, orciprenaline, are less suitable and less safe for use as bronchodilators than the selective beta₂ agonists, because they are more likely to cause arrhythmias and other side-effects. They should be avoided whenever possible.

Adrenaline (epinephrine) injection (1 in 1000) is used in the emergency treatment of acute allergic and anaphylactic reactions (section 3.4.3).

EPHEDRINE HYDROCHLORIDE ▱

Indications: reversible airways obstruction, but see notes above
Cautions: hyperthyroidism, diabetes mellitus, ischaemic heart disease, hypertension, renal impairment, elderly; prostatic hypertrophy (risk of acute retention); interaction with MAOIs a dis-

advantage; **interactions:** Appendix 1 (sympatho-mimetics)

Side-effects: tachycardia, anxiety, restlessness, insomnia common; also tremor, arrhythmias, dry mouth, cold extremities

Dose: 15–60 mg 3 times daily; CHILD up to 1 year 7.5 mg 3 times daily, 1–5 years 15 mg 3 times daily, 6–12 years 30 mg 3 times daily

¹ **Ephedrine Hydrochloride** (Non-proprietary)
PoM ▰▰

Tablets, ephedrine hydrochloride 15 mg, net price 28 = £1.59; 30 mg, 28 = £1.66

Elixir, ephedrine hydrochloride 15 mg/5 mL in a suitable flavoured vehicle, containing alcohol 12%. Net price 100 mL = 86p

1. For exemptions see *Medicines, Ethics and Practice*, No. 25, London, Pharmaceutical Press, 2001 (and subsequent editions as available)

For a list of **cough and decongestant preparations on sale to the public**, including those containing ephedrine, see section 3.9.2

ORCIPRENALINE SULPHATE ▰▰

Indications: reversible airways obstruction, but see notes above

Cautions: see section 3.1.1.1 and notes above; **interactions:** Appendix 1 (sympathomimetics)

Side-effects: see section 3.1.1.1 and notes above

Dose: 20 mg 4 times daily; CHILD up to 1 year 5–10 mg 3 times daily, 1–3 years 5–10 mg 4 times daily, 3–12 years 40–60 mg daily in divided doses

Alupent® (Boehringer Ingelheim) PoM ▰▰
Tablets, scored, orciprenaline sulphate 20 mg, net price 100-tab pack = £3.80
Syrup, sugar-free, orciprenaline sulphate 10 mg/5 mL, net price 300 mL = £2.26

▰▰ denotes preparations that are considered to be less suitable for prescribing (see p. vi)

3.1.2 Antimuscarinic bronchodilators

Ipratropium or **oxitropium** may be used by inhalation in the management of chronic asthma in patients who already require high-dose inhaled corticosteroids (see Chronic Asthma table, p. 132). Ipratropium by nebulisation may be added to other standard treatment in life-threatening asthma or where acute asthma fails to improve with standard therapy (see Acute Severe Asthma table, p. 133).

Antimuscarinic bronchodilators are regarded as being more effective in relieving bronchoconstriction associated with chronic obstructive pulmonary disease than in relieving asthma. The aerosol inhalation of ipratropium has a maximum effect 30–60 minutes after use; its duration of action is 3 to 6 hours and bronchodilation can usually be maintained with treatment 3 times a day. **Oxitropium** has a similar action to that of ipratropium.

IPRATROPIUM BROMIDE

Indications: reversible airways obstruction, particularly in chronic obstructive pulmonary disease

Cautions: glaucoma (standard doses unlikely to be harmful but see below); prostatic hypertrophy;

pregnancy (Appendix 4); breast-feeding (Appendix 5)

GLAUCOMA. *Acute angle-closure glaucoma* has been reported in patients given nebulised ipratropium, particularly when used in association with nebulised salbutamol (and possibly other beta₂ agonists). Special caution is needed to protect patient's eyes from nebulised drug

Side-effects: dry mouth occasionally reported; rarely urinary retention, constipation

Dose: *by aerosol inhalation*, 20–40 micrograms, in early treatment up to 80 micrograms at a time, 3–4 times daily; CHILD up to 6 years 20 micrograms 3 times daily, 6–12 years 20–40 micrograms 3 times daily

By inhalation of powder, 40 micrograms 3–4 times daily (may be doubled in less responsive patients); CHILD under 12 years, not recommended

By inhalation of nebulised solution, 100–500 micrograms up to 4 times daily; CHILD 1 month–3 years 62.5–250 micrograms up to 3 times daily [unlicensed]; 3–14 years 100–500 micrograms up to 3 times daily. Dilution of solution is adjusted according to equipment and length of administration. Because paradoxical bronchospasm has occurred, *first dose* should be inhaled under medical supervision

COUNSELLING. Advise patient not to exceed prescribed dose and to follow manufacturer's directions

Ipratropium Bromide (Non-proprietary) PoM
Nebuliser solution, ipratropium bromide 250 micrograms/mL, net price 20 × 1-mL (250-microgram) unit-dose vials = £6.10, 60 × 1-mL = £18.40; 20 × 2-mL (500-microgram) = £6.49, 60 × 2-mL = £21.20. If dilution is necessary use only sterile sodium chloride 0.9%
Available from Ashbourne (*Tropiovent®* Steripoules), Galen, Generics

Atrovent® (Boehringer Ingelheim) PoM
Aerocaps® (dry powder for inhalation; for use with *Atrovent Aerohaler®*), green, ipratropium bromide 40 micrograms, net price pack of 100 caps with *Aerohaler®* = £14.53; 100 caps = £10.53. Counselling, dose
Aerosol inhalation, ipratropium bromide 20 micrograms/metered inhalation, net price 200-dose unit = £4.21. Counselling, dose
Excipients: include CFC propellants
Autohaler® (= breath-actuated aerosol inhalation), ipratropium bromide 20 micrograms/metered inhalation, net price 200-dose unit = £9.39. Counselling, dose
Excipients: include CFC propellants
Forte aerosol inhalation, ipratropium bromide 40 micrograms/metered inhalation, net price 200-dose unit = £6.22. Counselling, dose
Excipients: include CFC propellants
Nebuliser solution, isotonic, ipratropium bromide 250 micrograms/mL, net price 20 × 1-mL unit-dose vials = £6.48, 60 × 1-mL vials = £19.44; 20 × 2-mL vials = £7.60, 60 × 2-mL vials = £22.80. If dilution is necessary use only sterile sodium chloride 0.9%
Note. One *Atrovent Aerocap®* is equivalent to 2 puffs of *Atrovent®* metered aerosol inhalation *or* 1 puff of *Atrovent Forte®* metered aerosol inhalation

Ipratropium Steri-Neb® (IVAX) PoM
Nebuliser solution, isotonic, ipratropium bromide 250 micrograms/mL, net price 20 × 1-mL (250-microgram) unit-dose vials = £4.67; 20 × 2-mL

(500-microgram) = £5.45. If dilution is necessary use only sterile sodium chloride 0.9%

Respontin® (A&H) [PoM]
Nebuliser solution, isotonic, ipratropium bromide 250 micrograms/mL, net price 20 × 1-mL (250-microgram) unit-dose vials = £5.45; 20 × 2-mL (500-microgram) = £6.40. If dilution is necessary use only sterile sodium chloride 0.9%

For some **compound preparations** containing ipratropium, see section 3.1.4

OXITROPIUM BROMIDE

Indications: reversible airways obstruction, particularly in chronic obstructive pulmonary disease
Cautions: see under Ipratropium Bromide
Side-effects: see under Ipratropium Bromide; rarely blurring of vision
Dose: *by aerosol inhalation*, 200 micrograms (2 puffs) 2–3 times daily; CHILD not recommended
COUNSELLING. Advise patient not to exceed prescribed dose and to follow manufacturer's directions

Oxivent® (Boehringer Ingelheim) [PoM]
Aerosol inhalation, oxitropium bromide 100 micrograms/metered inhalation. Net price 200-dose unit = £6.69. Counselling, dose
Excipients: include CFC propellants
Autohaler® (= breath-actuated aerosol inhalation), oxitropium bromide 100 micrograms/metered inhalation. Net price 200-dose unit = £15.72. Counselling, dose
Excipients: include CFC propellants

3.1.3   Theophylline

Theophylline is a bronchodilator used for reversible airways obstruction. It may have an additive effect when used in conjunction with small doses of beta$_2$ agonists; the combination may increase the risk of side-effects, including hypokalaemia (for CSM advice see p. 134).

Theophylline is metabolised in the liver; there is considerable variation in its half-life particularly in smokers, in patients with hepatic impairment or heart failure, or if certain drugs are taken concurrently. The half-life is *increased* in heart failure, cirrhosis, viral infections, in the elderly, and by drugs such as cimetidine, ciprofloxacin, erythromycin, fluvoxamine, and oral contraceptives. The half-life is *decreased* in smokers and in chronic alcoholism, and by drugs such as phenytoin, carbamazepine, rifampicin, and barbiturates. For other interactions of theophylline see Appendix 1.

These differences in half-life are important because theophylline has a narrow margin between the therapeutic and toxic dose. In most subjects a plasma-theophylline concentration of between 10–20 mg/litre is usually required for satisfactory bronchodilation although a plasma-theophylline concentration of 10 mg/litre (or less) may be effective. Adverse effects can occur within the range 10–20 mg/litre and both the frequency and severity increase at concentrations above 20 mg/litre.

Theophylline modified-release preparations are usually able to produce adequate plasma concentrations for up to 12 hours. When given as a single dose at night they have a useful role in controlling nocturnal asthma and early morning wheezing. The use of *rapid-release* oral theophylline preparations has declined because of the high incidence of side-effects associated with rapid absorption.

Theophylline is given by injection as **aminophylline**, a mixture of theophylline with ethylenediamine, which is 20 times more soluble than theophylline alone. Aminophylline must be given by **very slow** intravenous injection (over at least 20 minutes); it is too irritant for intramuscular use.

Intravenous aminophylline has a role in the treatment of severe attacks of asthma that do not respond rapidly to a nebulised beta$_2$ agonist (see also Acute Severe Asthma table, p. 133). Measurement of plasma theophylline concentration may be helpful, and is **essential** if aminophylline is to be given to patients who have been taking oral theophylline preparations, because serious side-effects such as convulsions and arrhythmias can occasionally precede other symptoms of toxicity.

THEOPHYLLINE

Indications: reversible airways obstruction, acute severe asthma; for guidelines see also Asthma tables (pp. 132-133)
Cautions: cardiac disease, hypertension, hyperthyroidism, peptic ulcer, hepatic impairment (Appendix 2), epilepsy, pregnancy and breastfeeding (Appendixes 4 and 5), elderly, fever; **CSM** advice on hypokalaemia risk, p. 134; avoid in porphyria (section 9.8.2); **interactions:** Appendix 1 (theophylline) and notes above
Side-effects: tachycardia, palpitations, nausea and other gastro-intestinal disturbances, headache, CNS stimulation, insomnia, arrhythmias, and convulsions especially if given rapidly by intravenous injection; **overdosage:** see Emergency Treatment of Poisoning, p. 26
Dose: see below
Note. Plasma theophylline concentration for optimum response 10–20 mg/litre (55–110 micromol/litre); narrow margin between therapeutic and toxic dose, see also notes above

Nuelin® (3M)
Tablets, scored, theophylline 125 mg. Net price 90-tab pack = £3.29. Label: 21
Dose: 125 mg 3–4 times daily after food, increased to 250 mg if required; CHILD 7–12 years 62.5–125 mg 3–4 times daily
Liquid, brown, theophylline hydrate (as sodium glycinate) 60 mg/5 mL. Net price 300 mL = £2.93. Label: 21
Dose: 120–240 mg 3–4 times daily after food; CHILD 2–6 years 60–90 mg, 7–12 years 90–120 mg, 3–4 times daily

■ Modified release

Note. The Council of the Royal Pharmaceutical Society of Great Britain advises pharmacists that if a general practitioner prescribes a modified-release, oral theophylline preparation without specifying a brand name, the pharmacist should contact the prescriber and agree the brand to be dispensed. Additionally, it is essential that a patient discharged from hospital should be maintained on the brand on which that patient was stabilised as an in-patient.

Nuelin SA® (3M)
SA tablets, m/r, theophylline 175 mg. Net price 60-tab pack = £3.43. Label: 25
Dose: 175–350 mg every 12 hours; CHILD over 6 years 175 mg every 12 hours

SA 250 tablets, m/r, scored, theophylline 250 mg.
Net price 60-tab pack = £4.80. Label: 25
Dose: 250–500 mg every 12 hours; CHILD over 6 years
125–250 mg every 12 hours

Slo-Phyllin® (Merck)
Capsules, all m/r, theophylline 60 mg (white/clear,
enclosing white pellets), net price 56-cap pack =
£1.92; 125 mg (brown/clear, enclosing white pellets), 56-cap pack = £2.42; 250 mg (blue/clear,
enclosing white pellets), 56-cap pack = £3.02.
Label: 25 *or* counselling, see below
Dose: 250–500 mg every 12 hours; CHILD, every 12
hours, 2–6 years 60–120 mg, 7–12 years 125–250 mg
COUNSELLING. Swallow whole with fluid *or* swallow
enclosed granules with soft food (e.g. yoghurt)

Theo-Dur® (AstraZeneca)
Tablets, m/r, both scored, theophylline 200 mg, net
price 20 = £1.21; 300 mg, 20 = £1.75. Label: 25
Dose: 300 mg every 12 hours, adjust dose by 100–150-
mg steps as required; CHILD up to 35 kg 100 mg, over
35 kg 200 mg, every 12 hours
For nocturnal asthma, total daily requirement may be
given as single evening dose

Uniphyllin Continus® (Napp)
Tablets, m/r, all scored, theophylline 200 mg, net
price 56-tab pack = £4.12; 300 mg, 56-tab pack =
£6.27; 400 mg, 56-tab pack = £7.44. Label: 25
Dose: 200 mg every 12 hours increased after 1 week to
300 mg every 12 hours; over 70 kg 200–300 mg every
12 hours increased after 1 week to 400 mg every 12
hours
May be appropriate to give larger evening or morning
dose to achieve optimum therapeutic effect when symptoms most severe; in patients whose night- or daytime
symptoms persist despite other therapy, who are not currently receiving theophylline, total daily requirement
may be added as single evening or morning dose
CHILD over 7 years, 9 mg/kg twice daily; some children
with chronic asthma may require 10–16 mg/kg every 12
hours

For a list of **cough and decongestant preparations on
sale to the public**, including those containing theophylline, see section 3.9.2

AMINOPHYLLINE

Note. Aminophylline is a stable mixture or combination
of theophylline and ethylenediamine; the ethylenediamine confers greater solubility in water
Indications: reversible airways obstruction, acute
severe asthma
Cautions: see under Theophylline
Side-effects: see under Theophylline; also allergy
to ethylenediamine can cause urticaria, erythema,
and exfoliative dermatitis
Dose: see under preparations, below
Note. Plasma theophylline concentration for optimum
response 10–20 mg/litre (55–110 micromol/litre); narrow margin between therapeutic and toxic dose, see also
notes above

Aminophylline (Non-proprietary)
Tablets, aminophylline 100 mg, net price 20 = 80p.
Label: 21
Dose: by mouth, 100–300 mg, 3–4 times daily, after food
Injection, aminophylline 25 mg/mL, net price 10-
mL amp = 67p [PoM]
Available from Celltech (*Min-I-Jet®*), Phoenix
Dose: deteriorating acute severe asthma **not** previously
treated with theophylline, *by slow intravenous injection*
over at least 20 minutes, 250–500 mg (5 mg/kg), then as

for acute severe asthma; CHILD 5 mg/kg, then as for
acute severe asthma
Acute severe asthma, *by intravenous infusion*,
500 micrograms/kg/hour, adjusted according to plasma-
theophylline concentration; CHILD 6 months–9 years
1 mg/kg/hour, 10–16 years 800 micrograms/kg/hour,
adjusted according to plasma-theophylline concentration
Note. Patients taking oral theophylline or aminophylline
should not normally receive intravenous aminophylline
unless plasma-theophylline concentration is available to
guide dosage

■ **Modified release**
Note. Advice about modified-release theophylline preparations on p. 139 also applies to modified-release aminophylline preparations

Phyllocontin Continus® (Napp)
Tablets, m/r, yellow, f/c, aminophylline hydrate
225 mg. Net price 56-tab pack = £3.34. Label: 25
Dose: 1 tablet twice daily initially, increased after 1
week to 2 tablets twice daily
Forte tablets, m/r, yellow, f/c, aminophylline
hydrate 350 mg. Net price 56-tab pack = £5.55.
Label: 25
Note. Forte tablets are for smokers and other patients
with decreased theophylline half-life (see notes above)
Paediatric tablets, m/r, peach, aminophylline
hydrate 100 mg. Net price 56-tab pack = £2.15.
Label: 25
Dose: CHILD over 3 years, 6 mg/kg twice daily initially,
increased after 1 week to 12 mg/kg twice daily; some
children with chronic asthma may require 13–20 mg/kg
every 12 hours
Note. Modified-release tablets containing aminophylline
225 mg also available from Ashbourne (*Amnivent® 225
SR*), IVAX (*Norphyllin® SR*)

3.1.4

Compound bronchodilator preparations

In general, patients are best treated with single-
ingredient preparations, such as a beta₂ agonist
(section 3.1.1.1) or ipratropium bromide (section
3.1.2), so that the dose of each drug can be adjusted.
This flexibility is lost with combinations, but those
in which both components are effective may have a
role when compliance is a problem.

For **cautions, contra-indications** and **side-
effects** see under individual drugs.

Combivent® (Boehringer Ingelheim) [PoM] [▭]
Aerosol inhalation, ipratropium bromide
20 micrograms, salbutamol (as sulphate)
100 micrograms/metered inhalation. Net price
200-dose unit = £6.45. Counselling, dose
Excipients: include CFC propellants
Dose: bronchospasm associated with chronic obstructive pulmonary disease, 2 puffs 4 times daily; CHILD
under 12 years not recommended
Nebuliser solution, isotonic, ipratropium bromide
500 micrograms, salbutamol (as sulphate) 2.5 mg/
2.5-mL vial, net price 60 unit-dose vials = £33.00
Dose: bronchospasm in chronic obstructive pulmonary
disease, *by inhalation of nebulised solution*, 1 vial 3–4
times daily; CHILD under 12 years not recommended
GLAUCOMA. In addition to other potential side-effects
acute angle-closure glaucoma has been reported with
nebulised ipratropium—for details, see p. 138

Duovent® (Boehringer Ingelheim) [PoM] ▰

Aerosol inhalation, fenoterol hydrobromide 100 micrograms, ipratropium bromide 40 micrograms/metered inhalation. Net price 200-dose unit with mouthpiece = £5.38 (extension tube also available). Counselling, dose

Excipients: include CFC propellants
Dose: reversible airways obstruction in asthma and chronic obstructive pulmonary disease, 1–2 puffs 3–4 times daily; CHILD over 6 years 1 puff 3 times daily

Autohaler® (= breath-actuated aerosol inhalation), fenoterol hydrobromide 100 micrograms, ipratropium bromide 40 micrograms/metered inhalation. Net price 200-dose unit = £10.57. Counselling, dose

Excipients: include CFC propellants
Dose: reversible airways obstruction in asthma and chronic obstructive pulmonary disease, 1–2 puffs 3–4 times daily; CHILD over 6 years 1 puff 3 times daily

Nebuliser solution, isotonic, fenoterol hydrobromide 1.25 mg, ipratropium bromide 500 micrograms/4-mL vial, net price 20 unit-dose vials = £11.00

Dose: acute severe asthma or acute exacerbation of chronic asthma, *by inhalation of nebulised solution*, 1 vial (4 mL); may be repeated up to max. 4 vials in 24 hours; CHILD under 14 years, not recommended

GLAUCOMA. In addition to other potential side-effects acute angle-closure glaucoma has been reported with nebulised ipratropium—for details, see p. 138

▰ denotes preparations that are considered to be less suitable for prescribing (see p. vi)

■ Preparations on sale to the public

For **compound bronchodilator preparations** on sale to the public, see pp. 163–164

For **compound bronchodilator preparations** on sale to the public, see pp. 163–164

3.1.5   Peak flow meters, inhaler devices and nebulisers

Peak flow meters

Measurement of peak flow is particularly helpful for patients who are 'poor perceivers' and hence slow to detect deterioration in their asthma, and for those with moderate or severe asthma. Patients must be given clear guidelines as to the action they should take if their peak flow falls below a certain level. Patients can be encouraged to adjust some of their own treatment (within specified limits) according to changes in peak flow rate.

Ferraris Pocketpeak® (Ferraris)

Peak flow meter, standard (90–710 litres/minute), net price = £6.53, low range (40–370 litres/minute) = £6.53, replacement mouthpiece = 38p (for adult or child)

Mini-Wright® (Clement Clarke)

Peak flow meter, standard (60 to 800 litres/minute), net price = £6.86, low range (30 to 400 litres/minute) = £6.90, replacement mouthpiece = 38p (for adult or child)

Vitalograph® (Vitalograph)

Peak flow meter, standard (50 to 750 litres/minute), now called *Asmaplan®*, net price = £6.65, low range (25 to 280 litres/minute) = £6.65, replacement mouthpiece = 40p (for adult or child)

Drug delivery devices

INHALER DEVICES. These include *pressurised metered-dose inhalers*, *breath-actuated inhalers* and *dry powder inhalers*. Many patients can be taught to use a pressurised metered-dose inhaler effectively but some patients, particularly the elderly and small children find it difficult to use them. *Spacer devices* (see below) can help such patients because they remove the need to co-ordinate actuation with inhalation and are effective even for children under 5 years. Alternatively breath-actuated inhalers or dry powder inhalers (which are activated by patient's inhalation) may be used but they are less suitable for young children. On changing from a pressurised metered-dose inhaler to a dry powder inhaler patients may notice a lack of sensation in the mouth and throat previously associated with each actuation. Coughing may also occur.

The patient should be instructed carefully on the use of the inhaler and it is important to check that the inhaler continues to be used correctly because inadequate inhalation technique may be mistaken for a lack of response to the drug.

NICE Guidance (inhaler devices for children)

The National Institute for Clinical Excellence has advised that in children under the age of 5 years with chronic asthma:

• corticosteroid and bronchodilator therapy should be routinely delivered by pressurised metered-dose inhaler and spacer system, with a facemask if necessary;

• if this is not effective and depending on the child's condition, nebulised therapy may be considered and, in children over 3 years, a dry powder inhaler may also be considered [but see notes above];

• the child's needs and likelihood of good compliance should govern the choice of pressurised metered-dose inhaler and spacer system; only then should cost be considered

SPACER DEVICES. Spacer devices remove the need for co-ordination between actuation of a pressurised metered-dose inhaler and inhalation. The spacer device reduces the velocity of the aerosol and subsequent impaction on the oropharynx. In addition the device allows more time for evaporation of the propellant so that a larger proportion of the particles can be inhaled and deposited in the lungs. The size of the spacer is important, the larger spacers with a one-way valve (*Nebuhaler®*, *Volumatic®*) being most effective. Spacer devices are particularly useful for patients with poor inhalation technique, for children, for patients requiring higher doses, for nocturnal asthma, and for patients prone to develop candidiasis with inhaled corticosteroids.

USE AND CARE OF SPACER DEVICES. Patients should inhale from the spacer device as soon as possible after actuation since the drug aerosol is very short-lived; single-dose actuation is recommended. The device should be cleansed once a week by washing in mild detergent, rinsing and then allowing to dry in air (wiping should be avoided since any electrostatic charge may affect drug delivery). Spacer devices should be replaced every 6–12 months.

Able Spacer® (Clement Clarke)

Spacer device, small-volume device. For use with pressurised (aerosol) inhalers, net price standard device = £4.20; with infant, child or adult mask = £6.86

AeroChamber® (3M)

Spacer device, medium-volume device. For use with *Airomir®*, *Salbulin®*, and *Qvar®* inhalers, net price standard device (blue) = £4.28, with mask (blue) = £7.14; infant device (orange) with mask = £7.14; child device (yellow) with mask = £7.14

Babyhaler® (A&H) [NHS]

Spacer device for paediatric use with *Becotide®-50* and *Ventolin®* inhalers. Net price = £11.34

E-Z Spacer® (Vitalograph) [NHS]

Spacer device, large-volume, collapsible device. For use with pressurised (aerosol) inhalers, price (direct from manufacturer) = £22.50

Haleraid® (GlaxoWellcome) [NHS]

Device to place over standard inhalers as aid to operation by patients with impaired strength in hands (e.g. with arthritis). Available as *Haleraid®-120* for 120-dose inhalers and *Haleraid®-200* for 200-dose inhalers. Net price = 80p

Nebuhaler® (AstraZeneca)

Spacer inhaler, large-volume device. For use with *Bricanyl®* and *Pulmicort®* inhalers, net price = £4.28; with paediatric mask = £4.28

Rotahaler® (A&H)

Breath-actuated device for use with *Rotacaps®*. Available as *Becotide Rotahaler®*, *Ventolin Rotahaler®*, and *Ventide Rotahaler®*. Net price = 78p

Spinhaler® (Rhône-Poulenc Rorer)

Breath-actuated device for use with *Intal Spincaps®*. Net price = £1.92

Volumatic® (A&H)

Spacer inhaler, large-volume device. For use with *Becloforte®*, *Becotide®*, *Flixotide®*, *Serevent®*, *Ventide®*, and *Ventolin®* inhalers, net price = £2.75; with paediatric mask = £2.75

Nebulisers

In England and Wales nebulisers and compressors are not available on the NHS (but they are free of VAT); some nebulisers (but not compressors) are available on form GP10A in Scotland (for details consult Scottish Drug Tariff).

A nebuliser converts a solution of a drug into an aerosol for inhalation. It is used to deliver higher doses of drug to the airways than is usual with standard inhalers. The main indications for use of a nebuliser are:

- to deliver a beta agonist or ipratropium to a patient with an *acute exacerbation* of asthma or of airway obstruction;
- to deliver a beta agonist or ipratropium on a *regular basis* to a patient with severe asthma or reversible airways obstruction who has been shown to benefit from regular treatment with higher doses;
- to deliver *prophylactic medication* such as cromoglicate or a corticosteroid to a patient unable to use other inhalational devices (particularly a young child);
- to deliver an antibiotic (such as colistin) to a patient with chronic purulent infection (as in cystic fibrosis or bronchiectasis);
- to deliver pentamidine for the prophylaxis and treatment of pneumocystis pneumonia to a patient with AIDS.

The proportion of a nebuliser solution that reaches the lungs depends on the type of nebuliser and although it can be as high as 30% it is more frequently close to 10% and sometimes below 10%. The remaining solution is left in the nebuliser as residual volume or it is deposited in the mouthpiece and tubing. The extent to which the nebulised solution is deposited in the airways or alveoli depends on particle size. Particles with a mass median diameter of 1–5 microns are deposited in the airways and are therefore appropriate for asthma whereas a particle size of 1–2 microns is needed for alveolar deposition of pentamidine to combat pneumocystis infection. The type of nebuliser is therefore chosen according to the deposition required and according to the viscosity of the solution (antibiotic solutions usually being more viscous).

Some jet nebulisers are able to increase drug output during inspiration and hence increase efficiency.

The patient should be aware that the dose of a bronchodilator given by nebulisation is usually **much higher** than that from an aerosol inhaler; see below for British Thoracic Society guidelines.

The British Thoracic Society has advised that nebulised bronchodilators may be given to patients with chronic persistent asthma or those with sudden catastrophic severe asthma (brittle asthma). In chronic asthma, nebulised bronchodilators should only be used to relieve persistent daily wheeze (see Chronic Asthma table p. 132). The British Thoracic Society has further recommended that the use of nebulisers in chronic persistent asthma should only be considered:

- after a review of the diagnosis;
- if the airflow obstruction is significantly reversible by bronchodilators without unacceptable side-effects;
- after the patient has been using the usual hand-held inhaler correctly;
- after a larger dose of bronchodilator from a hand-held inhaler (with a spacer if necessary) has been tried for at least 2 weeks;
- if the patient is complying with the prescribed dose and frequency of anti-inflammatory treatment including regular use of high-dose inhaled corticosteroid.

Before prescribing, a home trial should preferably be undertaken to monitor peak flow for up to 2 weeks on standard treatment and up to 2 weeks on nebulised treatment. If prescribed patients must:

- have clear instructions from doctor, specialist nurse or pharmacist on the use of the nebuliser and on peak-flow monitoring;
- be instructed not to treat acute attacks at home without also seeking help;
- receive an education program;
- have regular follow up including peak-flow monitoring and be seen by doctor, specialist nurse or physiotherapist.

■ **Jet nebulisers**

Jet nebulisers are more widely used than ultrasonic nebulisers. Most jet nebulisers require an optimum gas flow rate of 6–8 litres/minute and in hospital can be driven by piped air or oxygen. Domiciliary oxygen cylinders do not provide an adequate flow rate therefore an electrical compressor is required for domiciliary use.

For patients with *chronic obstructive pulmonary disease and hypercapnia*, oxygen can be dangerous and the nebuliser should be driven by air (see also p. 134).

Important: the Department of Health has reminded users of the need to use the correct grade of tubing when connecting a nebuliser to a medical gas supply or compressor.

Medix All Nebuliser® (Medix) ᴅᴴꜱ

Jet nebuliser, disposable; for use with bronchodilators, antimuscarinics, corticosteroids, and antibiotics, replacement recommended every 2–3 months if used 4 times a day. Compatible with **AC 2000 Hi Flo®** ᴅᴴꜱ, **World Traveller Hi Flo®** ᴅᴴꜱ, and **Econoneb®** ᴅᴴꜱ, net price = £1.50

Medix Antibiotic Circuit® (Medix) ᴅᴴꜱ

Jet nebuliser, closed-system; for use with antibiotics and other respiratory drugs. Compatible with **AC 2000 Hi Flo®** ᴅᴴꜱ, **Econoneb®** ᴅᴴꜱ, and **Turboneb®** ᴅᴴꜱ, net price = £7.30

Medix System® (Medix) ᴅᴴꜱ

Jet nebuliser, consisting of mouthpiece, tubing, and nebuliser chamber, net price = £2.80; mask kits with tubing and nebuliser chamber also available, net price (adult) = £2.90; (child) = £2.90

Pari LC Plus Filter® (Pari) ᴅᴴꜱ

Jet nebuliser, closed system, non-disposable, for hospital or home use with low flow compressors; supplied with filter/valve set. Compatible with **Pari TurboBoy®** ᴅᴴꜱ and **Pari JuniorBoy®** ᴅᴴꜱ compressors, net price = £19.90, replacement filters 100 = £33.30

Pari LC Plus® (Pari) ᴅᴴꜱ

Jet nebuliser, non-disposable, for hospital or home use with low flow compressors; for use with bronchodilators, antibiotics, and corticosteroids, replacement recommended yearly if used 4 times a day. Compatible with **Pari TurboBoy®** ᴅᴴꜱ, **Pari JuniorBoy®** ᴅᴴꜱ and **Pari WalkBoy®** ᴅᴴꜱ compressors, net price = £13.90

Pari Baby® (Pari) ᴅᴴꜱ

Jet nebuliser, non-disposable, for hospital or home use with low flow compressors; for use with bronchodilators, antibiotics and corticosteroids; replacement recommended yearly if used 4 times a day. Compatible with **Pari TurboBoy®** ᴅᴴꜱ, **Pari JuniorBoy®** ᴅᴴꜱ, **Pari WalkBoy®** ᴅᴴꜱ compressors. Available separately for children aged less than 1 year, 1–4 years or 4–7 years, net price (with connection hose) = £25.00

Sidestream Durable® (Medic-Aid) ᴅᴴꜱ

Jet nebuliser, non-disposable, for home use; for use with bronchodilators; yearly replacement recommended if 4 six-minute treatments used per day. Compatible with **CR50®** ᴅᴴꜱ, **Freeway Lite®** ᴅᴴꜱ and **Porta-Neb 50®** ᴅᴴꜱ (depending on nebulising solution), net price 10 pack = £94.50; patient pack with **CR50®** ᴅᴴꜱ compressor = £98.50. **Disposable Sidestream®** ᴅᴴꜱ nebuliser also available

Ventstream® (Medic-Aid) ᴅᴴꜱ

Jet nebuliser, closed-system, for use with low flow compressors, compatible with **CR50®** ᴅᴴꜱ, **Porta-Neb 50®** ᴅᴴꜱ, and **Freeway Lite®** ᴅᴴꜱ compressors; for use with antibiotics, bronchodilators, and corticosteroids, replacement recommended yearly if used 4 times a day, net price with filter = £27.00; 10-pack with filter = £250.00; without filter = £23.00; 10-pack with filter = £215.00; patient pack with **CR 50®** ᴅᴴꜱ compressor = £119.95

■ Home compressors with nebulisers
AC 2000 HI FLO® (Medix) ᴅᴴꜱ

Portable, home use, containing 1 **Jet Nebuliser®** ᴅᴴꜱ set with mouthpiece, 1 adult or 1 child mask, 1 spare inlet filter, filter spanner. Mains operated. Nebulises bronchodilators and antibiotics, net price = £117.00; carrying case available

Aquilon® (Henleys) ᴅᴴꜱ

Portable, home use, with 1 adult or 1 child mask and tubing. Mains operated; for use with bronchodilators, corticosteroids and antibiotics, net price = £81.00

Econoneb® (Medix) ᴅᴴꜱ

Home, clinic and hospital use, used with 1 **Jet Nebuliser®** ᴅᴴꜱ set with mouthpiece, 1 adult or 1 child mask, 1 spare inlet filter, filter spanner. Compatible with all types of jet nebuliser sets and also the **Micro Cirrus®** ᴅᴴꜱ nebuliser (recommended for alveolar deposition). Nebulises bronchodilators, corticosteroids, and antibiotics. Mains operated, net price = £99.00

Freeway Lite® (Medic-Aid) ᴅᴴꜱ

Portable, containing 1 **Sidestream Durable®** ᴅᴴꜱ reusable nebuliser, 1 adult or 1 child mask, 1 mouthpiece, 1 Coiled Duratube®, 2 filters, net price = £149.00 with carrying case. **Freeway Lite Luxury®** ᴅᴴꜱ contains additional battery, net price = £198.00

Also compatible with **Ventstream®** ᴅᴴꜱ closed system nebuliser

M-Flo® (Medix) ᴅᴴꜱ

Portable, home use, containing 1 **Jet Nebuliser®** ᴅᴴꜱ set with mouthpiece, spare inlet filter, filter spanner. Mains operated. Nebulises bronchodilators and corticosteroids, net price = £95.00

Medi-Neb® (Timesco) ᴅᴴꜱ

Range of compressors all supplied with adult and child mask, vapourising chamber, and PVC tubing, including: **Medi-Neb Elite®** ᴅᴴꜱ, *home use*. Mains operated, net price = £84.96. **Medi-Neb Companion®** ᴅᴴꜱ, *portable*. Mains/car battery operated, net price = £104.95 (includes car battery adaptor and carrying case). **Medi-Neb Companion Plus®** ᴅᴴꜱ, *portable*. Mains/battery operated, net price = £144.96 (includes rechargeable battery, car battery adaptor, and carrying case). **Medi-Neb Tempest®** ᴅᴴꜱ, *home/hospital use*. Mains operated, net price = £94.96

All used for nebulising antibiotics and bronchodilators

Pari TurboBoy® (Pari) ᴅᴴꜱ

Portable, for hospital or home use, containing **Pari LC Plus** ᴅᴴꜱ with connection tube and mains cable. Filter replacement recommended every 12 months or 550 hours of use. Compatible with **Pari LC Plus®** ᴅᴴꜱ, **Pari LC Plus Filter®** ᴅᴴꜱ, and **Pari Baby®** ᴅᴴꜱ nebulisers, net price = £65.00

Pari JuniorBoy® (Pari) ᴅᴴꜱ

Portable, for hospital or home use, containing **Pari LC Plus** ᴅᴴꜱ with connection tube and mains cable. Filter replacement recommended every 12 months or 550 hours of use. Compatible with **Pari LC Plus®** ᴅᴴꜱ, **Pari LC Plus Filter®** ᴅᴴꜱ, and **Pari Baby®** ᴅᴴꜱ nebulisers, net price = £70.00

Pari WalkBoy® (Pari) ᴅᴴꜱ

Portable, containing 1 **Pari LC Plus®** ᴅᴴꜱ nebuliser with connection tube, mains cable, rechargeable battery and carrying bag. Compatible with **Pari LC Plus®** ᴅᴴꜱ and **Pari Baby®** ᴅᴴꜱ nebulisers, net price = £160.00; car cigarette lighter adapter = £63.00

Porta-Neb® (Medic-Aid) ᴅᴴꜱ

Portable, containing 1 **Sidestream Durable®** ᴅᴴꜱ reusable nebuliser, 1 angled flow-through mouthpiece, 1 adult or 1 child mask, 1 Duratube® supply tubing, 4 spare filters. Mains operated; for use with bronchodilators, net price = £109.50; carrying case available

Also compatible with **Ventstream®** ᴅᴴꜱ closed-system nebuliser; for use with antibiotics, bronchodilators, and corticosteroids

Pulmo-Aide® (De Vilbiss) ᴅᴴꜱ

Home, clinic use, containing disposable nebuliser set, mouthpiece, mask, mains lead, tubing, thumb-valve. For use with bronchodilators, net price = £99.50. **Pulmo-Aide Escort®** ᴅᴴꜱ, *portable*, containing disposable nebuliser set, transformer, rechargeable battery, AC to DC adapter charger, DC lead with car adapter, and carrying case. For use with bronchodilators, net price = £198.50. **Pulmo-Aide AP50®** ᴅᴴꜱ, *home, clinic, hospital use*, net price = £180.00, with anti-pollution kit = £188.50. **Pulmo-Aide Sunmist®** ᴅᴴꜱ, *home use*, containing nebuliser set, mouthpiece, face mask, mains lead, net price = £84.25

SunMist® (De Vilbiss) NHS
Home, clinic and hospital use, with mouthpiece. Mains operated, net price = £89.50. **SunMist Plus®** NHS, *home, clinic and hospital use*, with mouthpiece, higher flow rate. Mains operated, net price = £107.50

Tourer® (Henleys) NHS
Portable, home use. Mains/car battery operated; for use with bronchodilators, corticosteroids and antibiotics, net price = £118.50, rechargeable battery pack = £54.00

Ultima® (Henleys) NHS
Portable, home use. Rechargable or mains/car battery operated. Nebulises bronchodilators and corticosteroids, net price = £184.00 (includes case)

World Traveller HI FLO® (Medix) NHS
Portable, containing 1 **Jet Nebuliser®** NHS set with mouthpiece, 1 adult or 1 child mask, 1 spare inlet filter, filter spanner. Battery/mains operated; rechargeable battery pack available. Nebulises bronchodilators, corticosteroids, and antibiotics, net price excluding battery = £145.00; with battery = £199.00; carrying case available

■ Compressors

System 22 CR50® (Medic-Aid) NHS
Home, clinic and hospital use. Mains operated, net price = £89.50. Also compatible with **Ventstream®** NHS, and **Sidestream Durable®** NHS

System 22 CR60® (Medic-Aid) NHS
Hospital use, high flow compressor. Mains operated, net price = £199.90. Also compatible with **System 22 Antibiotic Tee®** NHS for nebulisation of high viscosity drugs such as antibiotics

Turboneb® (Medix) NHS
Hospital use, high flow compressor. Mains operated, net price = £125.00. Also compatible with **Medix Antibiotic Circuit®** NHS for nebulisation of respiratory drugs in particular viscous antibiotics

■ Ultrasonic nebulisers

Ultrasonic nebulisers produce an aerosol by ultrasonic vibration of the drug solution and therefore do not require a gas flow

AeroSonic® (De Vilbiss) NHS
Portable, containing 1 controlling unit, chamber assembly, carrying case, AC to DC adapter/charger, DC lead, 1 mouthpiece with check valve and adapter, net price = £250.00

F16 Wave® (Parkside) NHS
Portable, adjustable delivery rate. Mains/car battery operated or rechargeable battery pack (supplied), net price = £125.00

Omron U1 MicroAir® (Omron) NHS
Portable. Battery operated/mains adaptor, net price = £325.00

Omron NE U07® (Omron) NHS
Portable. Mains operated or rechargeable battery pack, net price = £166.00 (mains version), £253.00 (rechargeable version)

Sonix 2000® (Medix) NHS
Portable, adjustable delivery rate. Supplied with carrying case and DC lead. Mains/car battery operated; rechargeable battery pack available, net price excluding battery = £150.00, with battery = £215.00

Syst'am® (Vitalograph) NHS
Home and clinic use, adjustable delivery rate, mains operated, carry cases available, net price *Model 230* = £137.00; *Model 260* (fitted with *Flovision®* system indicating inspiratory flow rate) = £174.00; *Model 290* = £154.00

Ultra Neb 2000® (De Vilbiss) NHS
Hospital, clinic and home use, delivery rate adjustable. Supplied with stand, net price = £1125.50

Nebuliser diluent

Nebulisation may be carried out using an undiluted nebuliser solution or it may require dilution beforehand. The usual diluent is sterile sodium chloride 0.9% (physiological saline).

Sodium Chloride (Non-proprietary) PoM
Nebuliser solution, sodium chloride 0.9%, net price 20 × 2.5 mL = £5.49
Available from Galen (*Saline Steripoule®*), IVAX (*Saline Steri-Neb®*)

3.2   Corticosteroids

Corticosteroids are very effective in *asthma*; they reduce airway inflammation (and hence reduce oedema and secretion of mucus into the airway).

Patients with *chronic obstructive pulmonary disease* usually show little or no response to corticosteroids. Long-term studies have shown no reduction in the decline in lung function in chronic obstructive pulmonary disease in patients taking regular inhaled corticosteroids. Higher doses of inhaled corticosteroids may reduce symptoms and exacerbations slightly in patients with more severe chronic obstructive pulmonary disease. A trial of a corticosteroid can distinguish patients who in fact have asthma from those who have chronic obstructive pulmonary disease.

INHALATION. Inhaled corticosteroids are recommended for prophylactic treatment of asthma when patients are using a beta$_2$ agonist more than once daily (see Chronic Asthma table, p. 132).

Corticosteroid inhalers must be used regularly to obtain maximum benefit; alleviation of symptoms usually occurs 3 to 7 days after initiation. **Beclometasone dipropionate** (beclomethasone dipropionate), **budesonide** and **fluticasone propionate** appear to be equally effective. Doses for CFC-free corticosteroid inhalers may be different from those that contain CFCs.

> CFC-FREE INHALERS. Chlorofluorocarbon (CFC) propellants in pressurised aerosol inhalers are being replaced by hydrofluoroalkane (HFA) propellants. Patients receiving CFC-free inhalers should be reassured about the efficacy of the new inhalers and counselled that the aerosol may feel and taste different; any difficulty with the new inhaler should be discussed with the doctor or pharmacist.

> **CSM advice.** The CSM has requested doctors to report any adverse reaction to the new HFA-containing inhalers and to include the brand name of the inhaler on the yellow card.

If the inhaled corticosteroid causes coughing, the use of a beta$_2$ agonist beforehand may help.

Patients who have been taking long-term oral corticosteroids can often be transferred to an inhaled corticosteroid but the transfer must be slow, with gradual reduction in the dose of oral corticosteroid, and at a time when the asthma is well controlled.

High-dose inhalers are available for patients who respond only partially to standard-dose inhalers. High doses should be continued only if there is clear benefit over the lower dose. The recommended maximum doses of inhaled corticosteroids should not generally be exceeded. However, if higher doses are required (e.g. fluticasone in doses above 500 micrograms twice daily), then they should be initiated by specialists.

Systemic therapy may be necessary during episodes of infection or if asthma is worsening, when higher doses are needed and access of inhaled drug to small airways may be reduced; patients may need a reserve supply of tablets.

SIDE-EFFECTS OF INHALED CORTICOSTEROIDS. Inhaled corticosteroids have considerably fewer systemic effects than oral corticosteroids, but adverse effects have been reported including a small increased risk of glaucoma with prolonged high doses of inhaled corticosteroids; cataracts have also been reported with inhaled corticosteroids. Higher doses of inhaled corticosteroids also have the potential to induce adrenal suppression (section 6.3.2) and patients on high doses should be given a 'steroid card'; such patients may need corticosteroid cover during an episode of stress (e.g. an operation). Bone mineral density is reduced following long-term inhalation of higher doses of corticosteroids, and this may predispose patients to osteoporosis (section 6.6). It is therefore sensible to ensure that the dose of inhaled corticosteroid is no higher than necessary to keep a patient's asthma under good control. The dose may therefore be reduced cautiously when the asthma has been well controlled for a few weeks as long as the patient knows that it is necessary to reinstate it should the asthma deteriorate or the peak flow rate fall.

The growth retardation in children associated with oral corticosteroid therapy does not appear to be a significant problem with recommended doses of inhaled therapy; although initial growth velocity may be reduced, there appears to be no effect on normal adult height. However, the CSM recommends that the height of children receiving prolonged treatment is monitored; if growth is slowed, referral to a paediatrician should be considered. Large-volume spacer devices should be used for administering inhaled corticosteroids in children under 5 years (see NICE guidance, section 3.1.5); they are also useful in older children and adults, particularly if high doses are required. Spacer devices increase airway deposition and reduce oropharyngeal deposition, resulting in a marked reduction in the incidence of candidiasis.

Budesonide and fluticasone propionate are both available as suspensions for nebulisation.

ORAL. Acute attacks of asthma should be treated with short courses of oral corticosteroids starting with a high dose, e.g. prednisolone 30 to 60 mg (30 to 40 mg usually adequate) daily for a few days. Patients whose asthma has deteriorated rapidly usually respond quickly to corticosteroids. The dose can usually be stopped abruptly in a mild exacerbation of asthma (see also Withdrawal of Corticosteroids, section 6.3.2) but it should be reduced gradually in those with poorer asthma control, to reduce the possibility of serious relapse. For use of corticosteroids in the emergency treatment of acute severe asthma see table on p. 133.

In chronic continuing asthma, when the response to other anti-asthma drugs has been relatively small, longer term administration of oral corticosteroids

may be necessary; in such cases high doses of an inhaled corticosteroid should be continued to minimise oral corticosteroid requirements. Oral corticosteroids should normally be taken as a single dose in the morning to reduce the disturbance to circadian cortisol secretion. Dosage should always be titrated to the lowest dose that controls symptoms. Regular peak flow measurements often help to optimise the dose.

Alternate-day administration has not been very successful in the management of asthma in adults because control can deteriorate during the second 24 hours. If alternate-day administration is introduced, pulmonary function should be monitored carefully over the 48 hours.

PARENTERAL. For the use of hydrocortisone injection in the emergency treatment of acute severe asthma, see Acute Severe Asthma table, p. 133.

BECLOMETASONE DIPROPIONATE
(Beclomethasone Dipropionate)

Indications: chronic asthma not controlled by short-acting beta$_2$ stimulants (see also Chronic Asthma table p. 132)

Cautions: see notes above; also active or quiescent tuberculosis; systemic therapy may be required during periods of stress or when airways obstruction or mucus prevent drug access to smaller airways

PARADOXICAL BRONCHOSPASM. The potential for paradoxical bronchospasm (calling for discontinuation and alternative therapy) should be borne in mind—if mild it may be prevented by inhalation of a beta$_2$-adrenoceptor stimulant (or by transfer from an aerosol inhalation to a dry powder inhalation)

Side-effects: see notes above; also hoarseness and candidiasis of mouth or throat (usually only with large doses); rarely hypersensitivity reactions including rash and angioedema

CANDIDIASIS. Candidiasis can be reduced by using spacer, see notes above, and responds to antifungal lozenges (section 12.3.2) without discontinuation of therapy—rinsing the mouth with water (or cleaning child's teeth) after inhalation of a dose may also be helpful

Dose: Standard-dose inhalers
By aerosol inhalation (for Qvar® dose see under preparation), 200 micrograms twice daily *or* 100 micrograms 3–4 times daily (in more severe cases initially 600–800 micrograms daily); CHILD 50–100 micrograms 2–4 times daily
By inhalation of powder (Becodisks®, Becotide Rotacaps®; for Asmabec® dose see under preparation), 400 micrograms twice daily *or* 200 micrograms 3–4 times daily; CHILD 100 micrograms 2–4 times daily *or* 200 micrograms twice daily

High-dose inhalers
By aerosol inhalation (for Qvar® dose see under preparation), 500 micrograms twice daily *or* 250 micrograms 4 times daily; if necessary may be increased to 500 micrograms 4 times daily; CHILD not recommended
By inhalation of powder (Becloforte® disks; for Asmabec® dose see under preparation), 400 micrograms twice daily; if necessary may be increased to 800 micrograms twice daily; CHILD not recommended

■ Standard-dose inhalers

Beclometasone (Non-proprietary) PoM
Aerosol inhalation, beclometasone dipropionate
50 micrograms/metered inhalation, net price 200-dose unit = £4.28; 100 micrograms/metered inhalation, 200-dose unit = £8.24; 200 micrograms/metered inhalation, 200-dose unit = £19.61.
Label: 8, counselling, dose
Available from APS, Generics, IVAX (*Beclazone®*), and 3M (*Filair®*)
Excipients: include CFC propellants
Dry powder for inhalation, beclometasone dipropionate 100 micrograms/metered inhalation, net price 100-dose unit = £5.58; 200 micrograms/metered inhalation, 100-dose unit = £10.29.
Label: 8, counselling, dose
Available from Trinity (*Pulvinal® Beclometasone Dipropionate*)

AeroBec® (3M) PoM
AeroBec 50 Autohaler® (breath-actuated aerosol inhalation), beclometasone dipropionate 50 micrograms/metered inhalation, net price 200-dose unit = £10.51. Label: 8, counselling, dose
Excipients: include CFC propellants
AeroBec 100 Autohaler® (breath-actuated aerosol inhalation), beclometasone dipropionate 100 micrograms/metered inhalation, net price 200-dose unit = £12.89. Label: 8, counselling, dose
Excipients: include CFC propellants

Asmabec Clickhaler® (Celltech) PoM
Dry powder for inhalation, beclometasone dipropionate 50 micrograms/metered inhalation, net price 200-dose unit = £7.18; 100 micrograms/metered inhalation, 200-dose unit = £10.55.
Label: 8, counselling, dose
Dose: by inhalation of powder, 200–400 micrograms daily, in 2–4 divided doses (in more severe cases initially 0.8–1.6 mg daily, in 2–4 divided doses—see also High-dose inhalers); CHILD 50–100 micrograms 2–4 times daily

Beclazone Easi-Breathe® (IVAX) PoM
Aerosol inhalation, beclometasone dipropionate 50 micrograms/metered inhalation, net price 200-dose breath-actuated unit = £4.34; 100 micrograms/metered inhalation, 200-dose breath-actuated unit = £8.24. Label: 8, counselling, dose
Excipients: include CFC propellants

Becodisks® (A&H) PoM
Dry powder for inhalation, disks containing 8 blisters of beclometasone dipropionate 100 micrograms/blister, net price 14 disks with *Diskhaler®* device = £10.99, 5-disk refill = £3.93 (hosp. only), 14-disk refill = £10.42; 200 micrograms/blister, 14 disks with *Diskhaler®* device = £20.90, 5-disk refill = £7.46 (hosp. only), 14-disk refill = £20.33; 400 micrograms/blister, 7 disks with *Diskhaler®* device = £20.90, 7-disk refill = £20.33. Label: 8, counselling, dose

Becotide® (A&H) PoM
Becotide®-50 aerosol inhalation, beclometasone dipropionate 50 micrograms/metered inhalation. Net price 200-dose unit = £5.43. Label: 8, counselling, dose
Becotide®-100 aerosol inhalation, beclometasone dipropionate 100 micrograms/metered inhalation. Net price 80-dose unit = £3.82 (hosp. only), 200-dose unit = £10.32. Label: 8, counselling, dose

Becotide®-200 aerosol inhalation, beclometasone dipropionate 200 micrograms/metered inhalation. Net price 200-dose unit = £19.61. Label: 8, counselling, dose, 10 steroid card
Note. Becotide®-200 not indicated for children
Excipients: all include CFC propellants
Rotacaps® (dry powder for inhalation; for use with *Becotide Rotahaler®*), beclometasone dipropionate 100 micrograms (buff/clear), net price 112-cap pack = £8.47; 200 micrograms (brown/clear), 112-cap pack = £16.07; 400 micrograms (dark brown/clear), 112-cap pack = £30.54. Label: 8, counselling, dose

Qvar® (3M) PoM
Qvar® 50 aerosol inhalation, beclometasone dipropionate 50 micrograms/metered inhalation, net price 200-dose unit = £7.87. Label: 8, counselling, dose
Qvar® 100 aerosol inhalation, beclometasone dipropionate 100 micrograms/metered inhalation, net price 200-dose unit = £17.21. Label: 8, counselling, dose, 10 steroid card
Qvar 50 Autohaler® (breath-actuated aerosol inhalation), beclometasone dipropionate 50 micrograms/metered inhalation, net price 200-dose unit = £7.87. Label: 8, counselling, dose
Qvar 100 Autohaler® (breath-actuated aerosol inhalation), beclometasone dipropionate 100 micrograms/metered inhalation, net price 200-dose unit = £17.21. Label: 8, counselling, dose, 10 steroid card
Excipients: include HFA-134a (a non-CFC propellant), ethanol
Dose: by aerosol inhalation, 50–200 micrograms twice daily, if necessary may be increased to max. 400 micrograms twice daily; CHILD not recommended
Note. When transferring a patient from a CFC-containing inhaler (asthma well controlled), initially a 100-microgram metered dose of *Qvar®* should be substituted for:
• 200–250 micrograms of beclometasone dipropionate or budesonide
• 100 micrograms of fluticasone propionate
When transferring a patient from a CFC-containing inhaler (asthma poorly controlled), initially a 100-microgram metered dose of *Qvar®* should be substituted for 100 micrograms of beclometasone dipropionate, budesonide or fluticasone propionate

■ High-dose inhalers
Note. High-dose inhalers not indicated for children

Beclometasone (Non-proprietary) PoM
Aerosol inhalation, beclometasone dipropionate 250 micrograms/metered inhalation, net price 200-dose unit = £17.77. Label: 8, counselling, dose, 10 steroid card
Available from APS, Generics, IVAX (*Beclazone®*), and 3M (*Filair Forte®*)
Excipients: include CFC propellants
Dry powder for inhalation, beclometasone dipropionate 400 micrograms/metered inhalation, net price 100-dose unit = £20.41. Label: 8, counselling, dose, 10 steroid card
Available from Trinity (*Pulvinal® Beclometasone Dipropionate*)

AeroBec Forte® (3M) PoM
Aerosol inhalation, beclometasone dipropionate 250 micrograms/metered inhalation, net price 200-inhalation breath-actuated unit (*Autohaler®*) = £23.97. Label: 8, counselling, dose, 10 steroid card
Excipients: include CFC propellants

Asmabec Clickhaler® (Celltech) [PoM]

Dry powder for inhalation, beclometasone dipropionate 250 micrograms/metered inhalation, net price 100-dose unit = £13.24. Label: 8, counselling, dose, 10 steroid card

Dose: by inhalation of powder, 500 micrograms twice daily *or* 250 micrograms 4 times daily; if necessary may be increased to 500 micrograms 4 times daily; CHILD not recommended

Note. May be difficult to obtain

Beclazone Easi-Breathe® (IVAX) [PoM]

Aerosol inhalation, beclometasone dipropionate 250 micrograms/metered inhalation, net price 200-dose breath-actuated unit = £18.02. Label: 8, counselling, dose, 10 steroid card

Excipients: include CFC propellants

Becloforte® (A&H) [PoM]

Aerosol inhalation, beclometasone dipropionate 250 micrograms/metered inhalation. Net price 80-dose unit = £8.82 (hosp. only), 200-dose unit = £23.10; 200-puff unit with spacer device (*Becloforte Integra®*) = £23.10; 200-dose refill for use with *Becloforte Integra®* = £18.02. Label: 8, counselling, dose, 10 steroid card

Excipients: include CFC propellants

Dry powder for inhalation, disks containing 8 blisters of beclometasone dipropionate 400 micrograms/blister, net price 14 disks with *Diskhaler®* device = £39.70; 14-disk refill = £39.13. Label: 8, counselling, dose, 10 steroid card

Qvar® (3M) [PoM]

See under standard-dose inhalers

■ Compound preparations
(Not recommended)

Ventide® (A&H) [PoM] ▭

Aerosol inhalation, beclometasone dipropionate 50 micrograms, salbutamol 100 micrograms/metered inhalation. Net price 200-dose unit = £5.42. Label: 8, counselling, dose

Excipients: include CFC propellants

Dose: maintenance, 2 puffs 3–4 times daily; CHILD 1–2 puffs 2–4 times daily

Paediatric Rotacaps® (dry powder for inhalation; for use with *Ventide Rotahaler®*), light grey/clear, beclometasone dipropionate 100 micrograms, salbutamol (as sulphate) 200 micrograms. Net price 112-cap pack = £12.68. Label: 8, counselling, dose

Dose: by inhalation of powder, 1 *Paediatric Rotacap®* 2–4 times daily

Rotacaps® (dry powder for inhalation; for use with *Ventide Rotahaler®*), dark grey/clear, beclometasone dipropionate 200 micrograms, salbutamol (as sulphate) 400 micrograms. Net price 112-cap pack = £23.01. Label: 8, counselling, dose

Dose: by inhalation of powder, 1 *Rotacap®* 3–4 times daily

■ Inhaler devices
See section 3.1.5

| Chronic Asthma table, see p. 132 |
| Acute Severe Asthma table, see p. 133 |

BUDESONIDE

Indications: see under Beclometasone Dipropionate

Cautions: see under Beclometasone Dipropionate
Side-effects: see under Beclometasone Dipropionate

Dose: see preparations below

Pulmicort® (AstraZeneca) [PoM]

LS aerosol inhalation, budesonide 50 micrograms/metered inhalation. Net price 200-dose unit with standard or *Spacer* inhaler = £6.66. Label: 8, counselling, dose

Excipients: include CFC propellants

Aerosol inhalation, budesonide 200 micrograms/metered inhalation. Net price 200-dose unit with standard or *Spacer* inhaler = £19.00; 100-dose unit with standard inhaler = £7.60 (hosp. only). Label: 8, counselling, dose, 10 steroid card

Excipients: include CFC propellants

Dose: by aerosol inhalation, 200 micrograms twice daily; may be reduced in well-controlled asthma to not less than 200 micrograms daily; in severe asthma dose may be increased to 1.6 mg daily; CHILD 50–400 micrograms twice daily; in severe asthma may be increased to 800 micrograms daily

Turbohaler® (= dry powder inhaler), budesonide 100 micrograms/inhalation, net price 200-dose unit = £18.50; 200 micrograms/inhalation, 100-dose unit = £18.50; 400 micrograms/inhalation, 50-dose unit = £18.50. Label: 8, counselling, dose, 10 steroid card

Dose: by inhalation of powder, when starting treatment, during periods of severe asthma, and while reducing or discontinuing oral corticosteroid, 0.2–1.6 mg daily in 2 divided doses; in less severe cases 200–400 micrograms once daily (each evening); patients already controlled on inhaled beclometasone dipropionate or budesonide administered twice daily may be transferred to once-daily dosing (each evening) at the same equivalent total daily dose (up to 800 micrograms once daily); CHILD under 12 years 200–800 micrograms daily in 2 divided doses (800 micrograms daily in severe asthma) *or* 200–400 micrograms once daily (each evening)

Respules® (= single-dose units for nebulisation), budesonide 250 micrograms/mL, net price 20 × 2-mL (500-microgram) unit = £32.00; 500 micrograms/mL, 20 × 2-mL (1-mg) unit = £44.64. May be diluted with sterile sodium chloride 0.9%. Label: 8, counselling, dose, 10 steroid card

Dose: by inhalation of nebulised suspension, when starting treatment, during periods of severe asthma, and while reducing or discontinuing oral corticosteroids, 1–2 mg twice daily (may be increased further in very severe asthma); CHILD 3 months–12 years, 0.5–1 mg twice daily

Maintenance, usually half above doses

Croup, 2 mg as a single dose (*or* as two 1-mg doses separated by 30 minutes)

■ Compound preparations

Symbicort® (AstraZeneca) ▼ [PoM]

Symbicort 100/6 Turbohaler® (= dry powder inhaler), budesonide 80 micrograms, formoterol fumarate 4.5 micrograms/metered inhalation, net price 120-dose unit = £33.00. Label: 8, counselling, dose, 10 steroid card

Note. Each metered inhalation of *Symbicort® 100/6* delivers the same quantity of budesonide as a 100-microgram metered inhalation of *Pulmicort Turbohaler®*

and of formoterol as a 6-microgram metered inhalation of *Oxis Turbohaler®*

Symbicort 200/6 Turbohaler® (= dry powder inhaler), budesonide 160 micrograms, formoterol fumarate 4.5 micrograms/metered inhalation, net price 120-dose unit = £38.00. Label: 8, counselling, dose, 10 steroid card

Note. Each metered inhalation of *Symbicort® 200/6* delivers the same quantity of budesonide as a 200-microgram metered inhalation of *Pulmicort Turbohaler®* and of formoterol as a 6-microgram metered inhalation of *Oxis Turbohaler®*

Dose: by inhalation of powder, 1–2 puffs twice daily, may be reduced in well-controlled asthma to 1–2 puffs once daily; CHILD and ADOLESCENT under 17 years not recommended

■ Inhaler devices
Section 3.1.5

FLUTICASONE PROPIONATE

Indications: see under Beclometasone Dipropionate

Cautions: see under Beclometasone Dipropionate

Side-effects: see under Beclometasone Dipropionate

Dose: see preparations below

Flixotide® (A&H) PoM

Accuhaler® (dry powder for inhalation), disk containing 60 blisters of fluticasone propionate 50 micrograms/blister with *Accuhaler®* device, net price = £6.86; 100 micrograms/blister with *Accuhaler®* device = £9.60; 250 micrograms/blister with *Accuhaler®* device = £22.86; 500 micrograms/blister with *Accuhaler®* device = £38.86. Label: 8, counselling, dose; 250- and 500-microgram strengths also label 10 steroid card

Note. Flixotide Accuhaler® 250 micrograms and 500 micrograms are not indicated for children

Dose: by inhalation of powder, ADULT and CHILD over 16 years, 100–250 micrograms twice daily, increased according to severity of asthma to 1 mg twice daily; CHILD 4–16 years, 50–100 micrograms twice daily adjusted as necessary

Aerosol inhalation, fluticasone propionate 25 micrograms/metered inhalation, net price 120-dose unit = £6.86; 50 micrograms/metered inhalation, 120-dose unit = £5.85; 125 micrograms/metered inhalation, 120-dose unit = £11.43 (hosp. only), 120-dose unit = £22.86; 250 micrograms/metered inhalation, 60-dose unit = £19.43 (hosp. only), 120-dose unit = £38.86. Label: 8, counselling, dose; 250-microgram strength also label 10 steroid card

Excipients: include CFC propellants

Note. Flixotide® 125 micrograms and 250 micrograms inhalers not indicated for children

Dose: by aerosol inhalation, ADULT and CHILD over 16 years, 100–250 micrograms twice daily, increased according to severity of asthma to 1 mg twice daily; CHILD 4–16 years, 50–100 micrograms twice daily adjusted as necessary

Diskhaler® (dry powder for inhalation), fluticasone propionate 50 micrograms/blister, net price 14 disks of 4 blisters with *Diskhaler®* device = £8.23, 14-disk refill = £7.66; 100 micrograms/blister, 14 disks of 4 blisters with *Diskhaler®* device = £12.80, 14-disk refill = £12.23;

250 micrograms/blister, 14 disks of 4 blisters with *Diskhaler®* device = £24.23, 5-disk refill = £8.65 (hosp. only), 14-disk refill = £23.66; 500 micrograms/blister, 14 disks of 4 blisters with *Diskhaler®* device = £40.23, 5-disk refill = £14.37 (hosp. only), 14-disk refill = £39.66. Label: 8, counselling, dose; 250- and 500-microgram strengths also label 10 steroid card

Note. Fluticide Diskhaler® 250 micrograms and 500 micrograms are not indicated for children

Dose: by inhalation of powder, ADULT and CHILD over 16 years, 100–250 micrograms twice daily, increased according to severity of asthma to 1 mg twice daily; CHILD 4–16 years, 50–100 micrograms twice daily adjusted as necessary

Evohaler® ▼ *aerosol inhalation,* fluticasone propionate 50 micrograms/metered inhalation, net price 120-dose unit = £5.85; 125 micrograms/metered inhalation, 60-dose unit = £11.43 (hosp. only), 120-dose unit = £22.86; 250 micrograms/metered inhalation, 60-dose unit = £19.43 (hosp. only), 120-dose unit = £38.86. Label: 8, counselling, dose, change to CFC-free inhaler; 250-microgram strength also label 10 steroid card

Excipients: include HFA-134a (a non-CFC propellant)

Note. Fluticide Evohaler® 125 micrograms and 250 micrograms not indicated for children

Dose: by aerosol inhalation, ADULT and CHILD over 16 years, 100–250 micrograms twice daily, increased according to severity of asthma to 1 mg twice daily; CHILD 4–16 years, 50–100 micrograms twice daily adjusted as necessary

Nebules® (= single-dose units for nebulisation) fluticasone propionate 250 micrograms/mL, net price 10×2-mL (500-microgram) unit = £10.04; 1 mg/mL, 10×2-mL (2-mg) unit = £40.16. May be diluted with sterile sodium chloride 0.9%. Label: 8, counselling, dose, 10 steroid card

Dose: by inhalation of nebulised suspension, ADULT and CHILD over 16 years, 0.5–2 mg twice daily

■ Compound preparations

Seretide® (A&H) ▼ PoM

Seretide 100 Accuhaler® (dry powder for inhalation), disk containing 60 blisters of fluticasone propionate 100 micrograms, salmeterol (as xinafoate) 50 micrograms/blister with *Accuhaler®* device, net price = £33.54. Label: 8, counselling, dose

Dose: by inhalation of powder, ADULT and CHILD over 4 years, 1 blister twice daily

Seretide 250 Accuhaler® (dry powder for inhalation), disk containing 60 blisters of fluticasone propionate 250 micrograms, salmeterol (as xinafoate) 50 micrograms/blister with *Accuhaler®* device, net price = £39.41. Label: 8, counselling, dose, 10 steroid card

Dose: by inhalation of powder, ADULT and CHILD over 12 years, 1 blister twice daily

Seretide 500 Accuhaler® (dry powder for inhalation), disk containing 60 blisters of fluticasone propionate 500 micrograms, salmeterol (as xinafoate) 50 micrograms/blister with *Accuhaler®* device, net price = £66.98. Label: 8, counselling, dose, 10 steroid card

Dose: by inhalation of powder, ADULT and CHILD over 12 years, 1 blister twice daily

Seretide 50 Evohaler® (aerosol inhalation), fluticasone propionate 50 micrograms, salmeterol (as xinafoate) 25 micrograms/metered inhalation, net

price 120-dose unit = £19.50. Label: 8, counselling, dose, change to CFC-free inhaler
Excipients: include HFA-134a (a non-CFC propellant)
Dose: by aerosol inhalation, ADULT and CHILD over 12 years, 2 puffs twice daily
Seretide 125 Evohaler® (aerosol inhalation), fluticasone propionate 125 micrograms, salmeterol (as xinafoate) 25 micrograms/metered inhalation, net price 120-dose unit = £39.41. Label: 8, counselling, dose, change to CFC-free inhaler
Excipients: include HFA-134a (a non-CFC propellant)
Dose: by aerosol inhalation, ADULT and CHILD over 12 years, 2 puffs twice daily
Seretide 250 Evohaler® (aerosol inhalation), fluticasone propionate 250 micrograms, salmeterol (as xinafoate) 25 micrograms/metered inhalation, net price 120-dose unit = £66.98. Label: 8, counselling, dose, change to CFC-free inhaler, 10 steroid card
Excipients: include HFA-134a (a non-CFC propellant)
Dose: by aerosol inhalation, ADULT and CHILD over 12 years, 2 puffs twice daily

3.3 Cromoglicate, related therapy and leukotriene receptor antagonists

3.3.1   Cromoglicate and related therapy
3.3.2   Leukotriene receptor antagonists

3.3.1 Cromoglicate and related therapy

Regular inhalation of **sodium cromoglicate** (sodium cromoglycate) can reduce the incidence of asthma attacks and allow dosage reduction of bronchodilators and oral corticosteroids. In general, prophylaxis with sodium cromoglicate is less effective in adults than prophylaxis with corticosteroid inhalations (see Chronic Asthma table, p. 132) but in the long term corticosteroid inhalations may be associated with more side-effects. Children may respond better than adults although there is less evidence of efficacy in those under the age of 4 years. Sodium cromoglicate is of no value in the treatment of acute attacks of asthma.

Sodium cromoglicate is of value in the prevention of exercise-induced asthma, a single dose being inhaled half-an-hour beforehand.

The mode of action of sodium cromoglicate is not completely understood. It may be of value in asthma with an allergic basis, but, in practice, it is difficult to predict who will benefit, therefore it is reasonable to try it for a period of 4 to 6 weeks. Dose frequency is adjusted according to response but is usually 3 to 4 times a day initially; this may subsequently be reduced.

If inhalation of the dry powder form of sodium cromoglicate causes bronchospasm a selective beta$_2$-adrenoceptor stimulant such as salbutamol or terbutaline should be inhaled a few minutes beforehand. The nebuliser solution is an alternative means of delivery for children who cannot manage the dry powder inhaler or the aerosol.

Nedocromil has a pharmacological action similar to that of sodium cromoglicate.

SODIUM CROMOGLICATE
(Sodium Cromoglycate)

Indications: prophylaxis of asthma; food allergy (section 1.5); allergic conjunctivitis (section 11.4.2); allergic rhinitis (section 12.2.1)
Side-effects: coughing, transient bronchospasm, and throat irritation due to inhalation of powder (see also notes above)
Dose: *by aerosol inhalation*, ADULT and CHILD, 10 mg (2 puffs) 4 times daily, increased in severe cases or during periods of risk to 6–8 times daily; additional doses may also be taken before exercise; maintenance 5 mg (1 puff) 4 times daily
By inhalation of powder (Spincaps®), ADULT and CHILD, 20 mg 4 times daily, increased in severe cases to 8 times daily; additional doses may also be taken before exercise
By inhalation of nebulised solution, ADULT and CHILD, 20 mg 4 times daily, increased in severe cases to 6 times daily
COUNSELLING. Regular use is necessary

Sodium Cromoglicate (Non-proprietary) PoM
Aerosol inhalation, sodium cromoglicate 5 mg/metered inhalation. Net price 112-dose unit = £15.30. Label: 8
Available from IVAX (*Cromogen®*)
Excipients: include CFC propellants
Nebuliser solution, sodium cromoglicate 10 mg/mL. Net price 60 × 2-mL unit-dose vials = £11.58
Available from IVAX (*Cromogen Steri-Neb®*)

Cromogen Easi-Breathe® (IVAX) PoM
Aerosol inhalation, sodium cromoglicate 5 mg/metered inhalation. Net price 112-dose breath-actuated unit = £13.91. Label: 8
Excipients: include CFC propellants

Intal® (Rhône-Poulenc Rorer) PoM
Aerosol inhalation, sodium cromoglicate 5 mg/metered inhalation. Net price 112-dose unit = £19.09; 2 × 112-dose unit with spacer device (*Syncroner®*) = £37.98; also available with large volume spacer inhaler (*Fisonair®*), complete unit = £22.06. Label: 8
Excipients: include CFC propellants
Spincaps®, yellow/clear, sodium cromoglicate 20 mg. Net price 112-cap pack = £16.60. Label: 8
Spinhaler insufflator® (for use with Intal Spincaps). Net price = £1.92
Nebuliser solution, sodium cromoglicate 10 mg/mL. Net price 2-mL amp = 34p. For use with power-operated nebuliser

■ Compound preparations
Note. The compound inhalation of sodium cromoglicate with a beta-adrenoceptor stimulant is not recommended as the inhalation is liable to be used inappropriately for relief of bronchospasm rather than for its prophylactic effect

Aerocrom® (Castlemead) PoM ◗
Aerosol inhalation, sodium cromoglicate 1 mg, salbutamol (as sulphate) 100 micrograms/metered inhalation, net price 200-dose unit = £34.42; 200-dose unit with spacer device (*Syncroner®*) = £34.42. Label: 8
Excipients: include CFC propellants
Dose: by aerosol inhalation, 2 inhalations 4 times daily; CHILD, not recommended

◗ denotes preparations that are considered to be less suitable for prescribing (see p. vi)

NEDOCROMIL SODIUM

Indications: prophylaxis of asthma
Side-effects: see under Sodium Cromoglicate; also headache, nausea, vomiting, dyspepsia and abdominal pain; bitter taste (masked by mint flavour)
Dose: *by aerosol inhalation*, ADULT and CHILD over 6 years 4 mg (2 puffs) 4 times daily, when control achieved may be possible to reduce to twice daily
COUNSELLING. Regular use is necessary

Tilade® (Pantheon) [PoM]
Aerosol inhalation, mint-flavoured, nedocromil sodium 2 mg/metered inhalation. Net price 2 × 56-dose units = £42.98; 2 × 112-dose units with spacer device (*Syncroner®*) = £85.96. Label: 8
Excipients: include CFC propellants

Related therapy

Antihistamines are of no value in the treatment of bronchial asthma. **Ketotifen** is an antihistamine with an action said to resemble that of sodium cromoglicate, but it has proved disappointing.

KETOTIFEN

Indications: see notes above
Cautions: previous anti-asthmatic treatment should be continued for a minimum of 2 weeks after initiation of ketotifen treatment; pregnancy and breast-feeding (see Appendixes 4 and 5); **interactions:** Appendix 1 (antihistamines)—also, manufacturer advises avoid with oral antidiabetics (fall in thrombocyte count reported)
DRIVING. Drowsiness may affect performance of skilled tasks (e.g. driving); effects of alcohol enhanced
Side-effects: drowsiness, dry mouth, slight dizziness; CNS stimulation, weight gain also reported
Dose: 1 mg twice daily with food increased if necessary to 2 mg twice daily; initial treatment in readily sedated patients 0.5–1 mg at night; CHILD over 2 years 1 mg twice daily

Zaditen® (Novartis) [PoM]
Capsules, ketotifen (as hydrogen fumarate) 1 mg. Net price 56-cap pack = £9.12. Label: 2, 8, 21
Tablets, scored, ketotifen (as hydrogen fumarate) 1 mg. Net price 60-tab pack = £9.77. Label: 2, 8, 21
Elixir, ketotifen (as hydrogen fumarate) 1 mg/5 mL. Net price 300 mL = £11.57. Label: 2, 8, 21

3.3.2 Leukotriene receptor antagonists

The leukotriene receptor antagonists, **montelukast** and **zafirlukast**, block the effects of cysteinyl leukotrienes in the airways. The role of leukotriene receptor antagonists relative to the long-acting beta$_2$-stimulants is not yet clear but they may be of benefit in exercise-induced asthma and in those with concomitant rhinitis. The benefit of adding a leukotriene antagonist in patients inadequately controlled with an inhaled corticosteroid (with or without a long-acting beta$_2$ agonist) is uncertain; a leukotriene antagonist has not been shown to be beneficial in those with more severe asthma (those requiring high-dose inhaled corticosteroids and regular bronchodilators or those requiring corticosteroid tablets regularly).

The **CSM** has advised that leukotriene receptor antagonists should not be used to relieve an attack of acute severe asthma and that their use does not necessarily allow a reduction in existing corticosteroid treatment.

CHURG-STRAUSS SYNDROME. Churg-Strauss syndrome (characterised by a history of asthma, and often rhinitis and sinusitis, with systemic vasculitis and eosinophilia) has been reported in association with the use of leukotriene receptor antagonists; in many cases the reaction followed the reduction or withdrawal of oral corticosteroid therapy. The CSM has advised that in patients prescribed leukotriene receptor antagonists prescribers should be alert to the development of eosinophilia, vasculitic rash, worsening pulmonary symptoms, cardiac complications or peripheral neuropathy.

MONTELUKAST

Indications: prophylaxis of asthma, see notes above
Cautions: pregnancy (Appendix 4) and breast-feeding (Appendix 5); Churg-Strauss syndrome, see notes above; **interactions:** Appendix 1 (leukotriene antagonists)
Side-effects: gastro-intestinal disturbances, dry mouth, thirst; hypersensitivity reactions including anaphylaxis, angioedema and skin reactions; asthenia, dizziness, irritability, restlessness, headache, sleep disorders (insomnia, drowsiness, abnormal dreams, nightmares); upper respiratory-tract infection, fever; arthralgia, myalgia; increased bleeding tendency, oedema, and seizures also reported
Dose: 10 mg daily at bedtime; CHILD 2–5 years 4 mg daily at bedtime, 6–14 years 5 mg daily at bedtime

Singulair® (MSD) [PoM]
Chewable tablets, both pink, cherry-flavoured, montelukast (as sodium salt) 4 mg, net price 28-tab pack = £25.69; 5 mg, 28-tab pack = £25.69. Label: 23, 24
Excipients: include aspartame equivalent to phenylalanine 674 micrograms/4-mg tablet and 842 micrograms/5-mg tablet (section 9.4.1)
Tablets, beige, f/c, montelukast (as sodium salt) 10 mg, net price 28-tab pack = £25.69

ZAFIRLUKAST

Indications: prophylaxis of asthma, see notes above
Cautions: elderly, pregnancy (Appendix 4), renal impairment (Appendix 3); Churg-Strauss syndrome, see notes above; **interactions:** Appendix 1 (leukotriene antagonists)
HEPATIC DISORDERS. Patients or their carers should be told how to recognise development of liver disorder and advised to seek medical attention if symptoms or signs such as persistent nausea, vomiting, malaise or jaundice develop

Contra-indications: hepatic impairment (Appendix 2); breast-feeding (Appendix 5)

Side-effects: gastro-intestinal disturbances; headache; rarely bleeding disorders, hypersensitivity reactions including angioedema and skin reactions, arthralgia, myalgia, lower limb oedema, raised liver enzymes, hepatitis, thrombocytopenia and very rarely agranulocytosis; also respiratory-tract infection in the elderly

Dose: 20 mg twice daily; CHILD under 12 years, not recommended

Accolate® (AstraZeneca) PoM

Tablets, f/c, zafirlukast 20 mg, net price 56-tab pack = £25.69. Label: 23

3.4 Antihistamines, hyposensitisation, and allergic emergencies

3.4.1	Antihistamines
3.4.2	Hyposensitisation
3.4.3	Allergic emergencies

3.4.1 Antihistamines

All antihistamines are of potential value in the treatment of nasal allergies, particularly seasonal allergic rhinitis (hay fever), and they may be of some value in vasomotor rhinitis. They reduce rhinorrhoea and sneezing but are usually less effective for nasal congestion. Antihistamines are used topically in the eye (section 11.4.2), in the nose (section 12.2.1), and on the skin (section 13.3).

Oral antihistamines are also of some value in preventing urticaria and are used to treat urticarial rashes, pruritus, and insect bites and stings; they are also used in drug allergies. Injections of chlorphenamine (chlorpheniramine) or promethazine are used as an adjunct to adrenaline (epinephrine) in the emergency treatment of anaphylaxis and angioedema (section 3.4.3). For the use of antihistamines (including cinnarizine, cyclizine, and promethazine teoclate) in nausea and vomiting, see section 4.6. Buclizine is included as an anti-emetic in a preparation for migraine (section 4.7.4.1). For reference to the use of antihistamines for occasional insomnia, see section 4.1.1.

Antihistamines differ in their duration of action and incidence of drowsiness and antimuscarinic effects. Many older antihistamines are relatively short acting but some (e.g. promethazine) act for up to 12 hours, while most of the newer non-sedating antihistamines are long acting.

All older antihistamines cause sedation but **alimemazine (trimeprazine)** and **promethazine** may be more sedating whereas **chlorphenamine (chlorpheniramine)** and **cyclizine** (section 4.6) may be less so. This sedating activity is sometimes used to manage the pruritus associated with some allergies. There is little evidence that any one of the older, 'sedating' antihistamines is superior to another and patients vary widely in their response.

Non-sedating antihistamines such as **acrivastine, cetirizine, desloratadine** (an active metabolite of loratadine), **fexofenadine** (an active metabolite of terfenadine), **levocetirizine** (an isomer of cetirizine), **loratadine, mizolastine**, and **terfenadine** cause less sedation and psychomotor impairment than the older antihistamines because they penetrate the blood brain barrier only to a slight extent. Terfenadine is associated with hazardous arrhythmias.

CAUTIONS AND CONTRA-INDICATIONS. Sedating antihistamines have significant antimuscarinic activity and they should therefore be used with caution in prostatic hypertrophy, urinary retention, glaucoma and pyloroduodenal obstruction. Antihistamines should be used with caution in hepatic disease (Appendix 2) and dose reduction may be necessary in renal impairment (Appendix 3). Caution may be required in epilepsy. Children and the elderly are more susceptible to side-effects. Many antihistamines should be avoided in porphyria although some (e.g. chlorphenamine (chlorpheniramine) and cetirizine) are thought to be safe (section 9.8.2). **Interactions:** Appendix 1 (antihistamines); **important:** see also under Terfenadine.

SIDE-EFFECTS. Drowsiness is a significant side-effect with most of the older antihistamines although paradoxical stimulation may occur rarely, especially with high doses or in children and the elderly. Drowsiness may diminish after a few days of treatment and is considerably less of a problem with the newer antihistamines (see also notes above). Side-effects that are more common with the older antihistamines include headache, psychomotor impairment, and antimuscarinic effects such as urinary retention, dry mouth, blurred vision, and gastro-intestinal disturbances.

Other side-effects of antihistamines include palpitations and arrhythmias (**important:** see especially risks associated with *terfenadine,* below), hypotension, hypersensitivity reactions (including bronchospasm, angioedema, and anaphylaxis, rashes and photosensitivity reactions), extrapyramidal effects, dizziness, confusion, depression, sleep disturbances, tremor, convulsions, blood disorders, and liver dysfunction.

Non-sedating antihistamines

DRIVING. Although drowsiness is rare, nevertheless patients should be advised that it can occur and may affect performance of skilled tasks (e.g. driving); excess alcohol should be avoided.

ACRIVASTINE

Indications: symptomatic relief of allergy such as hay fever, urticaria

Cautions: see notes above; pregnancy (Appendix 4) and breast-feeding (Appendix 5)

Contra-indications: see notes above; also avoid in renal impairment; hypersensitivity to triprolidine

Side-effects: see notes above; incidence of sedation and antimuscarinic effects low

Dose: 8 mg 3 times daily; CHILD under 12 years, not recommended; ELDERLY not recommended

¹**Semprex**® (GlaxoWellcome) PoM
Capsules, acrivastine 8 mg. Net price 84-cap pack
= £4.81. Counselling, driving
1. Capsules can be sold to the public for the treatment of
hayfever and allergic skin conditions in adults and children
over 12 years provided packs do not contain over 10 days'
supply (*Benadryl® Allergy Relief*)

CETIRIZINE HYDROCHLORIDE

Indications: symptomatic relief of allergy such as
hay fever, urticaria
Cautions: see notes above
Contra-indications: see notes above; also
pregnancy (Appendix 4) and breast-feeding
(Appendix 5)
Side-effects: see notes above; incidence of sedation and antimuscarinic effects low
Dose: ADULT and CHILD over 6 years, 10 mg daily
or 5 mg twice daily; CHILD 2–6 years, hayfever,
5 mg daily *or* 2.5 mg twice daily

¹**Zirtek**® (UCB Pharma) PoM
Tablets, f/c, scored, cetirizine hydrochloride
10 mg. Net price 30-tab pack = £8.73. Counselling, driving
Oral solution, sugar-free, banana-flavoured, cetirizine hydrochloride 5 mg/5 mL. Net price 200 mL
= £6.10. Counselling, driving
1. Tablets can be sold to the public provided max. daily
dose is 10 mg and packs do not contain more than 10
days' supply (*Zirtek 7*® NHS)

DESLORATADINE

Note. Desloratadine is a metabolite of loratadine
Indications: symptomatic relief of allergy such as
hay fever, urticaria
Cautions: see notes above
Contra-indications: see notes above; also hypersensitivity to loratadine; pregnancy (Appendix 4)
and breast-feeding (Appendix 5)
Side-effects: see notes above; also fatigue; incidence of sedation and antimuscarinic effects low
Dose: ADULT and ADOLESCENT over 12 years,
5 mg daily

Neoclarityn® (Schering-Plough) ▼ PoM
Tablets, blue, f/c, desloratadine 5 mg, net price 30-
tab pack = £7.57. Counselling, driving

FEXOFENADINE HYDROCHLORIDE

Note. Fexofenadine is a metabolite of terfenadine
Indications: see under preparations below
Cautions: see notes above; also pregnancy
(Appendix 4)
Contra-indications: see notes above; also breast-
feeding (Appendix 5)
Side-effects: see notes above; incidence of seda-
tion and antimuscarinic effects low
Dose: see under preparations below

Telfast® 120 (Hoechst Marion Roussel) PoM
Tablets, f/c, peach, fexofenadine hydrochloride
120 mg. Net price 30-tab pack = £7.40. Counselling, driving
Dose: symptomatic relief of seasonal allergic rhinitis,
120 mg once daily; CHILD under 12 years, not recommended

Telfast® 180 (Hoechst Marion Roussel) PoM
Tablets, f/c, peach, fexofenadine hydrochloride
180 mg. Net price 30-tab pack = £9.63. Counselling, driving
Dose: symptomatic relief of chronic idiopathic urticaria,
180 mg once daily; CHILD under 12 years, not recommended

LEVOCETIRIZINE DIHYDROCHLORIDE

Note. Levocetirizine is an isomer of cetirizine
Indications: symptomatic relief of allergy such as
hay fever, urticaria
Cautions: see notes above; also pregnancy
(Appendix 4) and breast-feeding (Appendix 5)
Contra-indications: see notes above; also severe
renal impairment
Side-effects: see notes above; incidence of seda-
tion and antimuscarinic effects low
Dose: ADULT and CHILD over 6 years, 5 mg daily

Xyzal® (UCB Pharma) ▼ PoM
Tablets, f/c, levocetirizine dihydrochloride 5 mg,
net price 30-tab pack =£7.45. Counselling, driving

LORATADINE

Indications: symptomatic relief of allergy such as
hay fever, urticaria
Cautions: see notes above
Contra-indications: see notes above; also
pregnancy (Appendix 4) and breast-feeding
(Appendix 5)
Side-effects: see notes above; incidence of seda-
tion and antimuscarinic effects low
Dose: ADULT and CHILD over 6 years 10 mg daily;
CHILD 2–5 years 5 mg daily

¹**Clarityn**® (Schering-Plough) PoM
Syrup, yellow, loratadine 5 mg/5 mL, net price
100 mL = £7.57. Counselling, driving
1. Tablets and syrup can be sold to the public provided
max. daily dose is 10 mg and packs do not contain more
than 10 days' supply (*Clarityn Allergy*® NHS); another
brand on sale to the public is *Boots Hayfever and Allergy
Relief All Day*®

MIZOLASTINE

Indications: symptomatic relief of allergy such as
hayfever, urticaria
Cautions: see notes above
Contra-indications: see notes above; also susceptibility to QT-interval prolongation (including
cardiac disease and hypokalaemia); significant
hepatic impairment; pregnancy (Appendix 4) and
breast-feeding (Appendix 5)
Side-effects: see notes above; also may cause
weight gain; incidence of sedation and antimuscarinic effects low
Dose: 10 mg daily; CHILD under 12 years, not recommended

Mistamine® (Galderma) ▼ PoM
Tablets, m/r, mizolastine 10 mg, net price 30-
tab pack = £8.55. Label: 25. Counselling, driving
Mizollen® (Schwarz) PoM
Tablets, m/r, f/c, scored, mizolastine 10 mg, net
price 30-tab pack = £8.55. Label: 25. Counselling, driving

TERFENADINE

Indications: symptomatic relief of allergy such as allergic rhinitis, urticaria

Cautions: see notes above: also pregnancy and breast-feeding

Contra-indications: see notes above; avoid grapefruit juice (may inhibit metabolism of terfenadine); **important:** see also Arrhythmias, below

ARRHYTHMIAS. Rare hazardous arrhythmias are associated with terfenadine particularly in association with increased terfenadine blood concentration. Recommendations include:

- not to exceed recommended dose
- avoid in significant hepatic impairment
- avoid in hypokalaemia (or other electrolyte imbalance)
- avoid in known or suspected prolonged QT interval
- avoid concomitant administration of drugs that prolong the QT interval or inhibit the metabolism of terfenadine, or those liable to produce electrolyte imbalance or are potentially arrhythmogenic; for details, see **interactions**: Appendix 1 (antihistamines)
- discontinue if syncope occurs and evaluate for potential arrhythmias

Side-effects: see notes above; incidence of sedation and antimuscarinic effects low; erythema multiforme and galactorrhoea reported; **important:** ventricular arrhythmias (including torsades de pointes) have followed excessive dosage, see also Arrhythmias above

Dose: allergic rhinitis and conjunctivitis, ADULT and CHILD over 50 kg, 60 mg daily increased if necessary to 120 mg daily in single or 2 divided doses

Allergic skin disorders, ADULT and CHILD over 50 kg, 120 mg daily in single or 2 divided doses

Terfenadine (Non-proprietary) PoM
Tablets, terfenadine 60 mg, net price 60-tab pack = £2.17. Counselling, driving
Available from APS

Sedating antihistamines

DRIVING. Drowsiness may affect performance of skilled tasks (e.g. driving); sedating effects enhanced by alcohol.

ALIMEMAZINE TARTRATE/ TRIMEPRAZINE TARTRATE

Indications: urticaria and pruritus, premedication
Cautions: see notes above; also pregnancy (Appendix 4); see also section 4.2.1
Contra-indications: see notes above; also breast-feeding (Appendix 5); see also section 4.2.1
Side-effects: see notes above; see also section 4.2.1
Dose: 10 mg 2–3 times daily, in severe cases up to max. 100 mg daily has been used; ELDERLY 10 mg 1–2 times daily; CHILD under 2 years not recommended, over 2 years 2.5–5 mg 3–4 times daily
Premedication, CHILD 2–7 years up to 2 mg/kg 1–2 hours before operation

Vallergan® (Castlemead) PoM
Tablets, blue, f/c, alimemazine tartrate 10 mg, net price 28-tab pack = £3.24. Label: 2
Syrup, straw-coloured, alimemazine tartrate 7.5 mg/5 mL, net price 100 mL = £3.70. Label: 2
Syrup forte, alimemazine tartrate 30 mg/5 mL, net price 100 mL = £5.72. Label: 2

AZATADINE MALEATE

Indications: symptomatic relief of allergy such as hay fever, urticaria
Cautions: see notes above
Contra-indications: see notes above; also pregnancy (Appendix 4) and breast-feeding (Appendix 5)
Side-effects: see notes above
Dose: 1 mg, increased if necessary to 2 mg, twice daily; CHILD under 1 year not recommended, 1–6 years 250 micrograms twice daily, 6–12 years 0.5–1 mg twice daily

Optimine® (Schering-Plough)
Syrup, blackcurrant-flavoured, azatadine maleate 500 micrograms/5 mL. Net price 120 mL = £1.39. Label: 2

BROMPHENIRAMINE MALEATE

Indications: symptomatic relief of allergy such as hay fever, urticaria
Cautions: see notes above; also pregnancy (Appendix 4)
Contra-indications: see notes above
Side-effects: see notes above
Dose: 4–8 mg 3–4 times daily; CHILD up to 3 years 0.4–1 mg/kg daily in 4 divided doses, 3–6 years 2 mg 3–4 times daily, 6–12 years 2–4 mg 3–4 times daily

Dimotane® (Wyeth)
Elixir, yellow-green, cola-flavoured, brompheniramine maleate 2 mg/5 mL, net price 200 mL = £1.56. Label: 2
For a list of **cough and decongestant preparations on sale to the public**, including those containing brompheniramine, see section 3.9.2.

CHLORPHENAMINE MALEATE/ CHLORPHENIRAMINE MALEATE

Indications: symptomatic relief of allergy such as hay fever, urticaria; emergency treatment of anaphylactic reactions (section 3.4.3)
Cautions: see notes above; also pregnancy (Appendix 4) and breast-feeding (Appendix 5)
Contra-indications: see notes above
Side-effects: see notes above; also exfoliative dermatitis and tinnitus reported; injections may cause transient hypotension or CNS stimulation and may be irritant
Dose: *by mouth*, 4 mg every 4–6 hours, max. 24 mg daily; CHILD under 1 year not recommended, 1–2 years 1 mg twice daily; 2–5 years 1 mg every 4–6 hours, max. 6 mg daily; 6–12 years 2 mg every 4–6 hours, max. 12 mg daily
By subcutaneous or intramuscular injection, 10–20 mg, repeated if required; max. 40 mg in 24 hours
By intravenous injection over 1 minute, 10–20 mg

Chlorphenamine/Chlorpheniramine (Non-proprietary)

Tablets, chlorphenamine maleate 4 mg, net price 20 = 31p. Label: 2

Available from Alpharma, APS, Hillcross

Oral solution, chlorphenamine maleate 2 mg/ 5 mL, net price 150 mL = £2.15. Label: 2

Available from Lagap (sugar-free)

Injection PoM , chlorphenamine maleate 10 mg/ mL, net price 1-mL amp = 1.50

Available from Link

Piriton® (Stafford-Miller)

Tablets, yellow, scored, chlorphenamine maleate 4 mg, net price 20 = 19p. Label: 2

Syrup, chlorphenamine maleate 2 mg/5 mL, net price 150 mL = £2.16. Label: 2

Note. In addition to *Piriton Allergy®* NHS , proprietary brands of chlorphenamine maleate tablets on sale to the public include *Boots Allergy Relief Antihistamine Tablets, Calimal®*

For a list of **cough and decongestant preparations on sale to the public**, including those containing chlorphenamine, see section 3.9.2

CLEMASTINE

Indications: symptomatic relief of allergy such as hay fever, urticaria

Cautions: see notes above; also pregnancy (Appendix 4) and breast-feeding (Appendix 5)

Contra-indications: see notes above

Side-effects: see notes above

Dose: 1 mg twice daily, increased up to 6 mg daily if required; CHILD under 1 year not recommended, 1–3 years 250–500 micrograms twice daily; 3–6 years 500 micrograms twice daily; 6–12 years 0.5–1 mg twice daily

Tavegil® (Novartis)

Tablets, scored, clemastine (as hydrogen fumarate) 1 mg. Net price 60-tab pack = £2.35. Label: 2

Elixir, sugar-free, clemastine (as hydrogen fumarate) 500 micrograms/5 mL. Net price 150 mL = 91p. Label: 2

CYPROHEPTADINE HYDROCHLORIDE

Indications: symptomatic relief of allergy such as hay fever, urticaria; migraine (section 4.7.4.2)

Cautions: see notes above; also pregnancy

Contra-indications: see notes above; also breast-feeding

Side-effects: see notes above

Dose: allergy, usual dose 4 mg 3–4 times daily; usual range 4–20 mg daily, max. 32 mg daily; CHILD under 2 years not recommended, 2–6 years 2 mg 2–3 times daily, max. 12 mg daily; 7–14 years 4 mg 2–3 times daily, max. 16 mg daily

Migraine, 4 mg with a further 4 mg after 30 minutes if necessary; maintenance, 4 mg every 4–6 hours

Periactin® (MSD)

Tablets, scored, cyproheptadine hydrochloride 4 mg. Net price 30 = 86p. Label: 2

DIPHENHYDRAMINE HYDROCHLORIDE

Indications: see under Preparations
Cautions: see notes above
Contra-indications: see notes above
Side-effects: see notes above

Preparations

Proprietary brands of diphenhydramine hydrochloride on sale to the public to aid relief of temporary sleep disturbance in adults include *Dreemon®* (diphenhydramine hydrochloride 10 mg/5 mL), *Medinex®* (diphenhydramine hydrochloride tablets 25 mg), *Medinex®* (diphenhydramine hydrochloride 10 mg/5 mL), *Nightcalm®* (diphenhydramine hydrochloride tablets 25 mg), *Nytol®* NHS (diphenhydramine hydrochloride tablets 25 mg and 50 mg), and *Panadol Night®* (diphenhydramine hydrochloride 25 mg and paracetamol 500 mg, for relief of temporary sleeplessness and night-time pain)

For a list of **cough and decongestant preparations on sale to the public**, including those containing diphenhydramine, see section 3.9.2

DIPHENYLPYRALINE HYDROCHLORIDE

Cautions: see notes above
Contra-indications: see notes above
Side-effects: see notes above

Preparations

For a list of **cough and decongestant preparations on sale to the public**, including those containing diphenylpyraline, see section 3.9.2

DOXYLAMINE

Cautions: see notes above
Contra-indications: see notes above
Side-effects: see notes above

Preparations

Ingredient of **cough and decongestant preparations** (section 3.9.2.) and of **compound analgesics** (section 4.7.1.) on sale to the public

HYDROXYZINE HYDROCHLORIDE

Indications: pruritus, anxiety (short-term) (section 4.1.2)

Cautions: see notes above

Contra-indications: see notes above; also pregnancy (Appendix 4) and breast-feeding (Appendix 5)

Side-effects: see notes above

Dose: pruritus, initially 25 mg at night increased if necessary to 25 mg 3–4 times daily; CHILD 6 months–6 years initially 5–15 mg daily increased if necessary to 50 mg daily in divided doses; over 6 years initially 15–25 mg daily increased if necessary to 50–100 mg daily in divided doses

Anxiety (adults only), 50–100 mg 4 times daily

Atarax® (Pfizer) PoM

Tablets, both s/c, hydroxyzine hydrochloride 10 mg (orange), net price 84-tab pack = £1.52; 25 mg (green), 28-tab pack = £1.02. Label: 2

Ucerax® (UCB Pharma) PoM

Tablets NHS , f/c, scored, hydroxyzine hydrochloride 25 mg, net price 25-tab pack = 91p. Label: 2

Syrup, hydroxyzine hydrochloride 10 mg/5 mL. Net price 200-mL pack = £1.91. Label: 2

PROMETHAZINE HYDROCHLORIDE

Indications: symptomatic relief of allergy such as hay fever, urticaria, premedication; emergency treatment of anaphylactic reactions (section 3.4.3); sedation (section 4.1.1); motion sickness (section 4.6)

Cautions: see notes above; also pregnancy (Appendix 4) and breast-feeding (Appendix 5)

Contra-indications: see notes above

Side-effects: see notes above; intramuscular injection may be painful

Dose: *by mouth*, 25 mg at night increased to 25 mg twice daily if necessary *or* 10–20 mg 2–3 times daily; CHILD under 2 years not recommended, 2–5 years 5–15 mg daily in 1–2 divided doses, 5–10 years 10–25 mg daily in 1–2 divided doses

Premedication, CHILD under 2 years not recommended, 2–5 years 15–20 mg, 5–10 years 20–25 mg

By deep intramuscular injection, 25–50 mg; max. 100 mg; CHILD 5–10 years 6.25–12.5 mg

Premedication, 25–50 mg 1 hour before operation; CHILD 5–10 years, 6.25–12.5 mg

By slow intravenous injection in emergencies, 25–50 mg as a solution containing 2.5 mg/mL in water for injections; max. 100 mg

Phenergan® (Rhône-Poulenc Rorer)
Tablets, both blue, f/c, promethazine hydrochloride 10 mg, net price 56-tab pack = £1.57; 25 mg, 56-tab pack = £2.34. Label: 2

Elixir, sugar-free, golden, promethazine hydrochloride 5 mg/5 mL. Net price 100 mL = £1.49. Label: 2

Injection [PoM], promethazine hydrochloride 25 mg/mL. Net price 1-mL amp = 49p

Promethazine hydrochloride injection 25 mg/mL (1-mL and 2-mL ampoules) also available from Antigen

Note. Proprietary brands of promethazine hydrochloride on sale to the public include *Phenergan Nightime®* (promethazine hydrochloride tablets 25 mg, for occasional insomnia in adults), *Sominex®* [NHS] (promethazine hydrochloride tablets 20 mg, for occasional insomnia in adults)

For a list of **cough and decongestant preparations on sale to the public**, including those containing promethazine, see section 3.9.2

TRIPROLIDINE HYDROCHLORIDE

Cautions: see notes above
Contra-indications: see notes above
Side-effects: see notes above

Preparations
For a list of **cough and decongestant preparations on sale to the public**, including those containing triprolidine, see section 3.9.2

3.4.2   Hyposensitisation

Except for wasp and bee sting allergy, specific hyposensitisation with allergen extract vaccines has usually shown little benefit in asthma. Hyposensitisation may be effective in allergic rhinitis if sensitisation to a particular allergen can be proven. However, the benefit of hyposensitisation needs to be balanced against the significant risk of anaphylaxis, particularly in patients with asthma (see CSM advice below).

Diagnostic skin tests are unreliable and can only be used in conjunction with a detailed history of allergen exposure.

CSM advice. After re-examination of the efficacy and safety of desensitising vaccines, the CSM has concluded that they should only be used for the following indications:

- Seasonal allergic hay fever (which has not responded to anti-allergy drugs) caused by pollens, using licensed products only—patients with *asthma* should not be treated with desensitising vaccines as they are more likely to develop severe adverse reactions.

- Hypersensitivity to wasp and bee venoms—since reactions can be life-threatening, *asthma* is not an absolute contra-indication.

There is an inadequate evidence of benefit from desensitisation to other allergens such as house dust, house dust mite, animal danders and foods and desensitisation is **not** recommended. Desensitising vaccines should be avoided in pregnant women, in children under five years old, and in those taking beta-blockers.

Bronchospasm usually develops within 1 hour and anaphylaxis within 30 minutes of injection. Therefore patients need to be monitored for 1 hour after injection. If symptoms or signs of hypersensitivity develop (e.g. rash, urticaria, bronchospasm, faintness), **even when mild**, the patient should be observed until these have **resolved completely**.

For details of the management of anaphylactic shock, see section 3.4.3.

Each set of allergen extracts usually contains vials for the administration of graded amounts of allergen to patients undergoing hyposensitisation. Maintenance sets containing vials at the highest strength are also available. Product literature must be consulted for details of allergens, vial strengths, and administration.

BEE AND WASP ALLERGEN EXTRACTS

Indications: hypersensitivity to wasp or bee venom (see notes above)

Cautions: see notes above including CSM advice and consult product literature

CSM advice. The CSM has advised that facilities for cardiopulmonary resuscitation must be immediately available and patients monitored closely for one hour after each injection, for full details see above.

Contra-indications: see notes above and consult product literature

Side-effects: consult product literature

Dose: *by subcutaneous injection*, consult product literature

Pharmalgen® (ALK-Abello) [PoM]
Bee venom extract (*Apis mellifera*) or wasp venom extract (*Vespula* spp.). Net price initial treatment set = £59.77 (bee), £73.28 (wasp); maintenance treatment set = £69.54 (bee), £89.45 (wasp)

GRASS AND TREE POLLEN EXTRACTS

Indications: treatment of seasonal allergic hayfever due to grass or tree pollen in patients who have failed to respond to anti-allergy drugs (see notes above)

Cautions: see notes above including CSM advice and consult product literature

CSM advice. The CSM has advised that facilities for cardiopulmonary resuscitation must be immediately available and patients must be monitored closely for one hour after each injection, for full details see above.

Contra-indications: see notes above and consult product literature

Side-effects: consult product literature

Dose: *by subcutaneous injection*, consult product literature

Pollinex® (Allergy) [PoM]
Grass or tree pollen extract, net price initial treatment set (3 vials) = £80.00; extension course treatment (1 vial) = £70.00

3.4.3   Allergic emergencies

Adrenaline (epinephrine) provides physiological reversal of the immediate symptoms (such as laryngeal oedema, bronchospasm, and hypotension) associated with hypersensitivity reactions such as *anaphylaxis* and *angioedema*. See below for full details of adrenaline administration and for adjunctive treatment.

Anaphylaxis

Anaphylactic shock requires prompt energetic treatment of *laryngeal oedema, bronchospasm*, and *hypotension*. Atopic individuals are particularly susceptible. Insect stings are a recognised risk (in particular wasp and bee stings). Certain foods, including eggs, fish, cow's milk protein, peanuts, and nuts may also precipitate anaphylaxis. Medicinal products particularly associated with anaphylaxis include blood products, vaccines, hyposensitising (allergen) preparations, antibiotics, aspirin and other NSAIDs, heparin, and neuromuscular blocking drugs. In the case of drugs, anaphylaxis is more likely after parenteral administration; resuscitation facilities must always be available for injections associated with special risk. Anaphylactic reactions may also be associated with *additives and excipients* in foods and medicines. Refined arachis (peanut) oil, which may be present in some medicinal products, is unlikely to cause an allergic reaction—nevertheless it is wise to check the full formula of preparations which may contain allergenic fats or oils.

First-line treatment includes securing the airway, restoration of blood pressure (laying the patient flat, raising the feet), and administration of **adrenaline (epinephrine)** injection. This is given **intramuscularly** in a dose of 500 micrograms (0.5 mL adrenaline injection 1 in 1000); a dose of 300 micrograms (0.3 mL adrenaline injection 1 in 1000) may be appropriate for *immediate self-administration*. The

dose is repeated if necessary at 5-minute intervals according to blood pressure, pulse and respiratory function [important: possible need for *intravenous route* using *dilute solution*, see below]. **Oxygen** administration is also of primary importance. An antihistamine (e.g. **chlorphenamine (chlorpheniramine)**, given by slow intravenous injection in a dose of 10–20 mg, see p. 153) is a useful adjunctive treatment, given after adrenaline injection and continued for 24 to 48 hours to prevent relapse. Patients receiving beta-blockers or those receiving antidepressants require special consideration (see under Adrenaline, p. 157).

Continuing deterioration requires further treatment including intravenous fluids (section 9.2.2), intravenous aminophylline (see p. 140) or a nebulised beta₂ agonist (such as salbutamol or terbutaline, see p. 134 and p. 136); in addition to oxygen, assisted respiration and possibly emergency tracheotomy may be necessary.

An intravenous corticosteroid e.g. **hydrocortisone** (as sodium succinate) in a dose of 100–300 mg (section 6.3.2) is of secondary value in the initial management of anaphylactic shock because the onset of action is delayed for several hours, but should be given to prevent further deterioration in severely affected patients.

When a patient is so ill that there is doubt as to the adequacy of the circulation, the initial injection of adrenaline may need to be given as a *dilute solution by the intravenous route*, for details of cautions, dose and strength, see under Intravenous Adrenaline (Epinephrine), below.

Some patients with severe allergy to insect stings or foods are encouraged to carry prefilled adrenaline syringes for *self-administration* during periods of risk.

Angioedema

Angioedema is dangerous if *laryngeal oedema* is present. In this circumstance adrenaline (epinephrine) injection and oxygen should be given as described under Anaphylaxis (see above); antihistamines and corticosteroids should also be given (see again above). Tracheal intubation and other measures may be necessary.

The administration of C_1 esterase inhibitor (in fresh frozen plasma or in partially purified form) may terminate acute attacks of *hereditary angioedema*, but is not practical for long-term prophylaxis.

Intramuscular adrenaline (epinephrine)

The *intramuscular route* is the *first choice route* for the administration of adrenaline (epinephrine) in the management of anaphylactic shock. Adrenaline has a rapid onset of action after intramuscular administration and in the shocked patient its absorption from the intramuscular site is faster and more reliable than from the subcutaneous site (the intravenous route should be reserved for extreme emergency when there is doubt as to the adequacy of the circulation, for details of cautions, dose and strength see under Intravenous Adrenaline (Epinephrine), below).

Patients with severe allergy should ideally be instructed in the self-administration of adrenaline by intramuscular injection (for details see under Self-administration of Adrenaline (Epinephrine), below).

Prompt injection of adrenaline is of paramount importance. The following adrenaline doses are based on the revised recommendations of the Project Team of the Resuscitation Council (UK).

Dose of **intramuscular** injection of adrenaline (epinephrine) for anaphylactic shock. Subcutaneous injection **not** generally recommended.

Age	Dose	Volume of adrenaline 1 in 1000 (1 mg/mL)
Under 6 months	50 micrograms	0.05 mL[1]
6 months–6 years	120 micrograms	0.12 mL[1]
6–12 years	250 micrograms	0.25 mL
Adult and adolescent	500 micrograms	0.5 mL

These doses may be repeated several times if necessary at 5-minute intervals according to blood pressure, pulse and respiratory function.

1. Use suitable syringe for measuring small volume

Intravenous adrenaline (epinephrine)

Where the patient is severely ill and there is real doubt about adequacy of the circulation and absorption from the intramuscular injection site, adrenaline (epinephrine) may be given by **slow** *intravenous injection* in a dose of 500 micrograms (5 mL of the dilute 1 in 10 000 adrenaline injection) given at a rate of 100 micrograms (1 mL of the dilute 1 in 10 000 adrenaline injection) per minute, *stopping when a response has been obtained*; children can be given a dose of 10 micrograms/kg (0.1 mL/kg of the dilute 1 in 10 000 adrenaline injection) by **slow** *intravenous injection* over several minutes. Great vigilance is needed to ensure that the *correct strength* is used; anaphylactic shock kits need to make a *very clear distinction* between the 1 in 10 000 strength and the 1 in 1000 strength. It is also important that, where intramuscular injection might still succeed, time should not be wasted seeking intravenous access.

For reference to the use of the intravenous route for *cardiac resuscitation*, see section 2.7.3.

Self-administration of adrenaline (epinephrine)

Individuals at considerable risk of anaphylaxis need to carry adrenaline (epinephrine) at all times and need to be *instructed in advance* how to inject it. In addition, the packs need to be labelled so that in the case of rapid collapse someone else is able to administer the adrenaline. It is important to ensure

that an adequate supply is provided to treat symptoms until medical assistance is available.

Some patients may best cope with a pre-assembled syringe fitted with a needle suitable for very rapid administration (if necessary by a bystander). *Anapen®* and *EpiPen®* consist of a fully assembled syringe and needle delivering a dose of 300 micrograms of adrenaline by *intramuscular injection*; 150-microgram versions (*Anapen®Junior, EpiPen® Jr*) are also available for use in children. Other products for the immediate treatment of anaphylaxis are available but are not licensed for use in the UK. *Ana-Guard®* is a prefilled syringe that delivers two 300-microgram doses of adrenaline by *subcutaneous or intramuscular injection*; it can be adjusted to administer smaller doses for children. *Ana-Kit®* includes a similar prefilled adrenaline syringe, chewable tablets of chlorphenamine maleate (chlorpheniramine maleate) 2 mg, 2 sterile pads impregnated with 70% isopropyl alcohol, and a tourniquet. *Ana-Guard®* and *Ana-Kit®* are available on a named-patient basis from IDIS.

ADRENALINE/EPINEPHRINE

Indications: emergency treatment of acute anaphylaxis; angioedema; cardiopulmonary resuscitation (section 2.7.3)

Cautions: hyperthyroidism, diabetes mellitus, heart disease, hypertension, arrhythmias, cerebrovascular disease, angle-closure glaucoma, second stage of labour, elderly patients

INTERACTIONS. Severe anaphylaxis in patients on non-cardioselective beta-blockers may not respond to adrenaline injection calling for intravenous injection of salbutamol (see p. 134); furthermore, adrenaline may cause severe hypertension in those receiving beta-blockers. Patients on tricyclic antidepressants are considerably more susceptible to arrhythmias calling for a much reduced dose of adrenaline. Other **interactions**, see Appendix 1 (sympathomimetics).

Side-effects: anxiety, tremor, tachycardia, arrhythmias, headache, cold extremities; also hypertension (risk of cerebral haemorrhage) and pulmonary oedema (on excessive dosage or extreme sensitivity); nausea, vomiting, sweating, weakness, dizziness and hyperglycaemia also reported

Dose: acute anaphylaxis, *by intramuscular (or subcutaneous) injection* of 1 in 1000 (1 mg/mL) solution, see notes and table above

Acute anaphylaxis when there is doubt as to the adequacy of the circulation, *by slow intravenous injection* of 1 in 10 000 (100 micrograms/mL) solution (extreme caution), see notes above

IMPORTANT. Intravenous route should be used with **extreme care**, see notes above

■ Intramuscular or subcutaneous

Adrenaline/Epinephrine 1 in 1000 (Non-proprietary) PoM

Injection, adrenaline (as acid tartrate) 1 mg/mL, net price 0.5-mL amp = 49p; 1-mL amp = 34p

Available from Antigen, BCM Specials, Hillcross, Martindale, Phoenix; also available from Aurum (1-mL prefilled syringe)

Excipients:include sulphites

Min-I-Jet® Adrenaline (Celltech) [PoM]

Injection, adrenaline (as hydrochloride) 1 in 1000 (1 mg/mL). Net price 1 mL (with 25 gauge × 0.25 inch needle for subcutaneous injection) = £8.11, 1 mL (with 21 gauge × 1.5 inch needle for intramuscular injection) = £4.40 (both disposable syringes)

Excipients: include sulphites

■ Intravenous

Extreme caution, see notes above

Adrenaline/Epinephrine 1 in 10 000, Dilute (Non-proprietary) [PoM]

Injection, adrenaline (as acid tartrate) 100 micrograms/mL. 10-mL amp.

Available from Aurum, Martindale (special order); also from Aurum (1-mL and 10-mL prefilled syringe) and Medeva (*Min-I-Jet® Adrenaline* 3- and 10-mL disposable syringes)

Excipients:include sulphites

■ Intramuscular injection for self-administration

Anapen® (Lincoln) [PoM]

Anapen® 0.3 mg solution for injection (delivering a single dose of adrenaline 300 micrograms), adrenaline 1 mg/mL (1 in 1000), net price 1.05-mL auto-injector device = £22.44

Excipients: include sulphites

Note. 0.75 mL of the solution remains in the auto-injector device after use

Dose: by intramuscular injection, ADULT and CHILD over 30 kg, 300 micrograms repeated after 10–15 minutes as necessary

Anapen® Junior 0.15 mg solution for injection (delivering a single dose of adrenaline 150 micrograms), adrenaline 500 micrograms/mL (1 in 2000), net price 1.05-mL auto-injector device = £22.44

Excipients: include sulphites

Note. 0.75 mL of the solution remains in the auto-injector device after use

Dose: by intramuscular injection, CHILD 15–30 kg, 150 micrograms repeated after 10–15 minutes as necessary

EpiPen® (ALK-Abello) [PoM]

EpiPen® Auto-injector 0.3 mg (delivering a single dose of adrenaline 300 micrograms), adrenaline 1 mg/mL (1 in 1000), net price 2-mL *Auto-injector* = £28.19

Excipients: include sulphites

Note. 1.7 mL of the solution remains in the *Auto-injector* after use

Dose: by intramuscular injection, ADULT and CHILD over 30 kg, 300 micrograms repeated after 15 minutes as necessary

Epipen® Jr Auto-injector 0.15 mg (delivering a single dose of adrenaline 150 micrograms), adrenaline 500 micrograms/mL (1 in 2000), net price 2-mL *Auto-injector* = £28.19

Excipients: include sulphites

Note. 1.7 mL of the solution remains in the *Auto-injector* after use

Dose: by intramuscular injection, CHILD 15–30 kg, 10 micrograms/kg repeated after 10 minutes as necessary

3.5 Respiratory stimulants and pulmonary surfactants

3.5.1   Respiratory stimulants
3.5.2   Pulmonary surfactants

3.5.1 Respiratory stimulants

Respiratory stimulants (analeptic drugs) have a limited place in the treatment of ventilatory failure in patients with chronic obstructive pulmonary disease. They are effective only when given by intravenous injection or infusion and have a short duration of action. Their use has largely been replaced by ventilatory support including nasal intermittent positive pressure ventilation. However, occasionally when ventilatory support is contraindicated and in patients with hypercapnic respiratory failure who are becoming drowsy or comatose, respiratory stimulants in the short term may arouse patients sufficiently to co-operate and clear their secretions.

Respiratory stimulants can also be harmful in respiratory failure since they stimulate non-respiratory as well as respiratory muscles. They should only be given under **expert supervision** in hospital and must be combined with active physiotherapy. There is at present no oral respiratory stimulant available for long-term use in chronic respiratory failure.

Doxapram is given by continuous intravenous infusion. Frequent arterial blood gas and pH measurements are necessary during treatment to ensure correct dosage.

Nikethamide (now discontinued by most suppliers) is not recommended because the effective doses are close to those causing toxic effects, especially convulsions.

DOXAPRAM HYDROCHLORIDE

Indications: see under Dose

Cautions: give with oxygen in severe irreversible airways obstruction or severely decreased lung compliance (because of increased work load of breathing); give with beta$_2$ agonist in bronchoconstriction; hypertension (avoid if severe), impaired cardiac reserve; hepatic impairment, pregnancy (compelling reasons only); **interactions:** Appendix 1 (doxapram)

Contra-indications: severe hypertension, status asthmaticus, coronary artery disease, thyrotoxicosis, epilepsy, physical obstruction of respiratory tract

Side-effects: perineal warmth, dizziness, sweating, moderate increase in blood pressure and heart rate; side-effects reported in postoperative period (causal effect not established) include muscle fasciculation, hyperactivity, confusion, hallucinations, cough, dyspnoea, laryngospasm, bronchospasm, sinus tachycardia, bradycardia, extrasystoles, nausea, vomiting and salivation

Dose: postoperative respiratory depression, *by intravenous injection* over at least 30 seconds, 1–1.5 mg/kg repeated if necessary after intervals of 1 hour *or* alternatively *by intravenous infusion*, 2–3 mg/minute adjusted according to response; CHILD not recommended

Acute respiratory failure, *by intravenous infusion*, 1.5–4 mg/minute adjusted according to response (given concurrently with oxygen and whenever possible monitor with frequent measurement of blood gas tensions); CHILD not recommended

Dopram® (Anpharm) PoM
Injection, doxapram hydrochloride 20 mg/mL. Net price 5-mL amp = £2.04
Intravenous infusion, doxapram hydrochloride 2 mg/mL in glucose 5%. Net price 500-mL bottle = £21.33

3.5.2 Pulmonary surfactants

Pulmonary surfactants are used in the management of respiratory distress syndrome (hyaline membrane disease) in newborn and preterm infants. They may also be given prophylactically to those considered at risk of developing the syndrome.

CAUTIONS. Continuous monitoring is required to avoid hyperoxaemia (due to rapid improvement in arterial oxygen concentration).

SIDE-EFFECTS. Pulmonary haemorrhage, especially in more premature infants, is a rare complication of therapy; obstruction of the endotracheal tube by mucous secretions has also been reported.

BERACTANT

Indications: treatment of respiratory distress syndrome in neonates over 700 g; prophylaxis of respiratory distress syndrome in preterm infants
Cautions: see notes above
Side-effects: see notes above
Dose: *by endotracheal tube*, phospholipid 100 mg/kg equivalent to a volume of 4 mL/kg, preferably within 8 hours of birth; may be repeated within 48 hours at intervals of at least 6 hours for up to 4 doses

Survanta® (Abbott) PoM
Suspension, beractant (bovine lung extract) providing phospholipid 25 mg/mL, with lipids and proteins, net price 8-mL vial = £306.43

COLFOSCERIL PALMITATE

Indications: treatment and prophylaxis of respiratory distress syndrome
Cautions: see notes above
Side-effects: see notes above
Dose: *by endotracheal tube*, treatment, 67.5 mg/kg; if still intubated, may be repeated after 12 hours; prophylaxis, first dose soon after birth, if still intubated may be repeated 12 and 24 hours later

Exosurf Neonatal® (GlaxoWellcome) PoM
Suspension, colfosceril palmitate 108 mg for reconstitution with 8 mL water for injections (when reconstituted, contains 67.5 mg/5 mL), net price per vial (with endotracheal tube connectors) = £292.64

PORACTANT ALFA

Indications: treatment of respiratory distress syndrome or hyaline membrane disease in neonates over 700 g; prophylaxis of respiratory distress syndrome in preterm infants
Cautions: see notes above
Side-effects: see notes above
Dose: *by endotracheal tube*, treatment, 100–200 mg/kg; further doses of 100 mg/kg may be repeated 12 hours later and after further 12 hours if still intubated; max. total dose 300–400 mg/kg; prophylaxis, 100–200 mg/kg soon after birth (preferably within 15 minutes); further doses of 100 mg/kg may be repeated 6–12 hours later and after further 12 hours if still intubated; max. total dose 300–400 mg/kg

Curosurf® (Trinity) PoM
Suspension, poractant alfa (porcine lung phospholipid fraction) 80 mg/mL, net price 1.5-mL vial = £382.00; 3-mL vial = £764.00

3.6 Oxygen

Oxygen should be regarded as a drug. It is prescribed for hypoxaemic patients to increase alveolar oxygen tension and decrease the work of breathing necessary to maintain a given arterial oxygen tension. The concentration depends on the condition being treated; an inappropriate concentration may have serious or even lethal effects.

High concentration oxygen therapy, with concentrations of up to 60%, is safe in conditions such as pneumonia, pulmonary thromboembolism, and fibrosing alveolitis. In such conditions low arterial oxygen (P_aO_2) is usually associated with low or normal arterial carbon dioxide (P_aCO_2), therefore there is little risk of hypoventilation and carbon dioxide retention.

In acute severe asthma, the arterial carbon dioxide (P_aCO_2) is usually subnormal but as asthma deteriorates it may rise steeply (particularly in children). These patients usually require high concentrations of oxygen and if the arterial carbon dioxide (P_aCO_2) remains high despite other treatment intermittent positive pressure ventilation needs to be considered urgently. Where facilities for blood gas measurements are not immediately available, for example while transferring the patient to hospital, 35% to 50% oxygen delivered through a conventional mask is recommended. Exceptionally, asthma is diagnosed in patients with a long history of chronic bronchitis and probable respiratory failure; in these patients a lower concentration (24% to 28%) may be needed to limit oxygen-induced reduction of respiratory drive.

Low concentration oxygen therapy (controlled oxygen therapy) is reserved for patients with ventilatory failure due to chronic obstructive pulmonary disease or other causes. The concentration should not exceed 28% and in some patients a concentration above 24% may be excessive. The aim is to provide the patient with just enough oxygen to improve hypoxaemia without worsening pre-existing carbon dioxide retention and respiratory acidosis. Treatment should be initiated in hospital as repeated blood gas measurements are required to estimate the correct concentration.

DOMICILIARY OXYGEN. Oxygen should only be prescribed for patients in the home after careful evaluation in hospital by respiratory experts; it should never be prescribed on a placebo basis.

Patients should be **advised of the fire risks** when receiving oxygen therapy.

Intermittent oxygen therapy

Oxygen is occasionally prescribed for intermittent use for episodes of hypoxaemia of short duration, for example asthma. It is important, however, that the patient does not rely on oxygen instead of obtaining medical help or taking more specific treatment.

Alternatively, intermittent oxygen may be prescribed for patients with advanced irreversible respiratory disorders to increase mobility and capacity for exercise and to ease discomfort, for example in chronic obstructive pulmonary disease. Appropriate patients may be prescribed portable equipment through the hospital service, refillable from cylinders in the home.

Under the NHS oxygen may be supplied by pharmacy contractors as **oxygen cylinders**. Oxygen flow can be adjusted as the cylinders are equipped with an oxygen flow meter with 'medium' (2 litres/minute) and 'high' (4 litres/minute) settings. The Health Authorities have lists of pharmacy contractors who provide domiciliary oxygen services.

Patients are supplied with either constant or variable performance masks. The *Intersurgical 010 28%* or *Ventimask Mk IV 28%* are constant performance masks and provide a nearly constant supply of oxygen (28%) despite variations in oxygen flow rate and the patient's breathing pattern. The variable performance masks include the *Intersurgical 005 Mask* and the *Venticaire Mask*; the concentration of oxygen supplied to the patient varies with the rate of flow of oxygen and with the patient's breathing pattern.

PORTABLE OXYGEN CYLINDERS. Portable oxygen sets are not prescribable on the NHS since the fitting is not compatible with the Drug Tariff oxygen equipment. However, Medigas and BOC supply a portable oxygen cylinder called a 'PD oxygen cylinder', which has the same bull-nose fitting as the normal domiciliary headsets (prescriptions must therefore specify 'PD oxygen cylinder'). The PD oxygen cylinder holds about 300 litres of oxygen which will last approximately 2 hours at a standard flow rate of 2 litres/minute.

Long-term oxygen therapy

Long-term administration of oxygen (at least 15 hours daily) prolongs survival in some patients with chronic obstructive pulmonary disease.

The Royal College of Physicians have produced guidelines for oxygen therapy (*Domiciliary oxygen therapy services: Clinical guidelines and advice for prescribers*; June 1999). Assessment for long-term oxygen therapy requires measurement of arterial blood gas tensions. Measurements should be taken on 2 occasions at least 3 weeks apart to demonstrate clinical stability, and not sooner than 4 weeks after an acute exacerbation of the disease. The guidelines recommend that long-term oxygen therapy should be considered for patients with:

- chronic obstructive pulmonary disease with P_aO_2 < 7.3 kPa when breathing air during a period of clinical stability;
- chronic obstructive pulmonary disease with P_aO_2 7.3–8 kPa in the presence of secondary polycythaemia, nocturnal hypoxaemia, peripheral oedema or evidence of pulmonary hypertension;
- interstitial lung disease with P_aO_2 < 8 kPa and in patients with P_aO_2 > 8 kPa with disabling dyspnoea;
- cystic fibrosis when P_aO_2 < 7.3 kPa *or* if P_aO_2 7.3–8 kPa in the presence of secondary polycythaemia, nocturnal hypoxaemia, pulmonary hypertension or peripheral oedema;
- pulmonary hypertension, without parenchymal lung involvement when P_aO_2 < 8 kPa;
- neuromuscular or skeletal disorders, after specialist assessment;
- obstructive sleep apnoea despite continuous positive airways pressure therapy, after specialist assessment;
- pulmonary malignancy or other terminal disease with disabling dyspnoea;
- heart failure with daytime P_aO_2 < 7.3 kPa (on air) or with nocturnal hypoxaemia;
- paediatric respiratory disease, after specialist assessment.

Increased respiratory depression is seldom a problem in patients with stable respiratory failure treated with low concentrations of oxygen although it may occur during exacerbations; patients and relatives should be warned to call for medical help if drowsiness or confusion occur.

Oxygen concentrators are more economical for patients requiring oxygen for long periods, and in England and Wales are now prescribable on the NHS on a regional tendering basis (see below). A concentrator was formerly only provided for a patient who required oxygen for 15 hours a day but it has been found to be cost-effective to provide one for a patient requiring it for 8 hours a day (or 21 cylinders per month).

Prescribing arrangements for oxygen concentrators

Prescribe concentrator and accessories (face mask, nasal cannula, and humidifier) on form FP10. Specify amount of oxygen required (hours per day) and flow rate. If required, prescribe back-up oxygen set and cylinder at same time. Inform patient that the supplier will be in contact to make arrangements and that the prescription form is to be given to the person who installs the concentrator.

Inform supplier by telephone (see table below) that a concentrator has been prescribed. The supplier will send written confirmation of the order to the prescriber, the patient, and the Health Authority.

Follow the same procedure if a back-up oxygen set and cylinder are required later.

Health Authority regional group	Supplier
South Western London South (includes Kent, Surrey, and Sussex)	BOC gases *to order:* Dial 0800 136 603
Eastern London North North Western and North Wales West Midlands	De Vilbiss Medequip Ltd *to order:* Dial 0800 020 202
Central and South Wales Northern Yorkshire (South and West) and Humberside	Oxygen Therapy Co Ltd *to order:* Dial 0800 373 580

In **Scotland** refer the patient for assessment by a respiratory consultant. If the need for a concentrator is confirmed the consultant will arrange for the provision of a concentrator through the Common Services Agency.

3.7   Mucolytics

Mucolytics are sometimes prescribed to facilitate expectoration by reducing sputum viscosity. Regular use of oral mucolytics may be of some benefit in patients with chronic obstructive pulmonary disease who suffer from particularly troublesome exacerbations. Steam inhalation with postural drainage, is good expectorant therapy in bronchiectasis and in some cases of chronic bronchitis.

For reference to dornase alfa, see below.

CARBOCISTEINE

Indications: reduction of sputum viscosity

Contra-indications: active peptic ulceration

Side-effects: occasional gastro-intestinal irritation, rashes

Dose: 750 mg 3 times daily initially, then 1.5 g daily in divided doses; CHILD 2–5 years 62.5–125 mg 4 times daily, 6–12 years 250 mg 3 times daily

* **Carbocisteine Capsules** (Non-proprietary) NHS PoM

Capsules, carbocisteine 375 mg. Net price 30-cap pack = £4.48

* **Carbocisteine Syrup** (Non-proprietary) NHS PoM

Oral liquid, carbocisteine 125 mg/5 mL, net price 300 mL = £4.91; 250 mg/5 mL, 300 mL = £6.28

* NHS except, for patients under the age of 18 years and in whom any condition which, through damage or disease, affects the airways and has required a tracheostomy and endorsed 'SLS'

Note. The brand name *Mucodyne®* NHS (Rhône-Poulenc Rorer) is used for carbocisteine preparations

MECYSTEINE HYDROCHLORIDE
(Methyl Cysteine Hydrochloride)

Indications: reduction of sputum viscosity

Dose: 100–200 mg 3–4 times daily before meals reduced to 200 mg twice daily after 6 weeks; CHILD over 5 years 100 mg 3 times daily Prophylaxis, 100–200 mg 2–3 times every other day during winter months

Visclair® (Sinclair) NHS

Tablets, yellow, s/c, e/c, mecysteine hydrochloride 100 mg. Net price 20 = £3.66. Label: 5, 22, 25

Dornase alfa

Dornase alfa is a genetically engineered version of a naturally occurring human enzyme which cleaves extracellular deoxyribonucleic acid (DNA). It is used in cystic fibrosis and is administered by inhalation using a jet nebuliser (section 3.1.5).

DORNASE ALFA

Phosphorylated glycosylated recombinant human deoxyribonuclease 1 (rhDNase)

Indications: management of cystic fibrosis patients with a forced vital capacity (FVC) of greater than 40% of predicted to improve pulmonary function

Cautions: pregnancy (Appendix 4); breast-feeding (Appendix 5)

Side-effects: pharyngitis, voice changes, chest pain; occasionally laryngitis, rashes, urticaria, conjunctivitis

Dose: *by inhalation of nebulised solution* (by jet nebuliser), 2500 units (2.5 mg) once daily (patients over 21 years may benefit from twice daily dosage); CHILD under 5 years not recommended

Pulmozyme® (Roche) PoM

Nebuliser solution, dornase alfa 1000 units (1 mg)/mL. Net price 2.5-mL (2500 units) vial = £19.47

Note. For use undiluted with jet nebulisers only; ultrasonic nebulisers are unsuitable

3.8   Aromatic inhalations

Inhalations containing volatile substances such as eucalyptus oil are traditionally used and although the vapour may contain little of the additive it encourages deliberate inspiration of warm moist air which is often comforting in bronchitis; boiling water should not be used owing to the risk of scalding. Inhalations are also used for the relief of nasal obstruction in acute rhinitis or sinusitis.

CHILDREN. The use of strong aromatic decongestants (applied as rubs or to pillows) is not advised for infants under the age of 3 months. Mothers with young infants in whom nasal obstruction with mucus is a problem can readily be taught appropriate techniques of suction aspiration.

Benzoin Tincture, Compound, BP
(Friars' Balsam)
Tincture, balsamic acids approx. 4.5%. Label: 15
Directions for use: add one teaspoonful to a pint of hot, **not** boiling, water and inhale the vapour

Menthol and Eucalyptus Inhalation, BP 1980
Inhalation, racementhol or levomenthol 2 g, eucalyptus oil 10 mL, light magnesium carbonate 7 g, water to 100 mL
Directions for use: add one teaspoonful to a pint of hot, **not** boiling, water and inhale the vapour

Karvol® (Crookes) [NHS]
Inhalation capsules, levomenthol 35.55 mg, with chlorobutanol, pine oils, terpineol, and thymol, net price 10-cap pack = £1.34; 20-cap pack = £2.39
Inhalation solution, levomenthol 7.9%, with chlorobutanol, pine oils, terpineol, and thymol, net price 12-mL dropper bottle = £1.75
Administration: express into handkerchief or add to a pint of hot, **not** boiling, water the contents of 1 capsule or 6 drops of solution; avoid in infants under 3 months

3.9   Cough preparations

3.9.1   Cough suppressants
3.9.2   Expectorant and demulcent cough preparations

3.9.1   Cough suppressants

Cough is usually a symptom of an underlying disorder e.g. asthma (section 3.1.1), gastro-oesophageal reflux disease (section 1.1), and 'post-nasal drip'; where there is no identifiable cause, cough suppressants may be useful, for example if sleep is disturbed. They may cause sputum retention and this may be harmful in patients with chronic bronchitis and bronchiectasis.

Codeine may be effective but it is constipating and can cause dependence; **dextromethorphan** and **pholcodine** have fewer side-effects.

Sedating antihistamines, such as diphenhydramine, are used as the cough suppressant component of many compound cough preparations on sale to the public; all tend to cause drowsiness which may reflect their main mode of action.

CHILDREN. The use of cough suppressants containing codeine or similar opioid analgesics is not generally recommended in children and should be avoided altogether in those under 1 year of age.

CODEINE PHOSPHATE

Indications: dry or painful cough; diarrhoea (section 1.4.2); pain (section 4.7.2)
Cautions: asthma; hepatic and renal impairment; history of drug abuse; see also notes above and section 4.7.2; **interactions:** Appendix 1 (opioid analgesics)
Contra-indications: liver disease, ventilatory failure
Side-effects: constipation, respiratory depression in sensitive patients or if given large doses

¹ **Codeine Linctus, BP** [PoM]
Linctus (= oral solution), codeine phosphate 15 mg/5 mL. Net price 100 mL = 40p (diabetic, 73p)
Dose: 5–10 mL 3–4 times daily; CHILD (but not generally recommended) 5–12 years, 2.5–5 mL
Available from Alpharma, APS, Galen (*Galcodine®*, sugar-free), IVAX
Note. BP directs that when Diabetic Codeine Linctus is prescribed, Codeine Linctus formulated with a vehicle appropriate for administration to diabetics, whether or not labelled 'Diabetic Codeine Linctus', shall be dispensed or supplied
1. Can be sold to the public provided the maximum single dose does not exceed 5 mL

Codeine Linctus, Paediatric, BP
Linctus (= oral solution), codeine phosphate 3 mg/5 mL. Net price 100 mL = 21p
Dose: CHILD (but not generally recommended) 1–5 years 5 mL 3–4 times daily
Available from Galen (*Galcodine® Paediatric*, sugar-free), Medeva
Note. BP directs that Paediatric Codeine Linctus may be prepared extemporaneously by diluting Codeine Linctus with a suitable vehicle in accordance with the manufacturer's instructions
For a list of **cough and decongestant preparations on sale to the public**, including those containing codeine, see section 3.9.2

PHOLCODINE

Indications: dry or painful cough
Cautions: see under Codeine Phosphate
Contra-indications: see under Codeine Phosphate
Side-effects: see under Codeine Phosphate

Pholcodine Linctus, BP
Linctus (= oral solution), pholcodine 5 mg/5 mL in a suitable flavoured vehicle, containing citric acid monohydrate 1%. Net price 100 mL = 24p
Dose: 5–10 mL 3–4 times daily; CHILD (but not generally recommended, see notes above) 5–12 years 2.5–5 mL
Available from APS, Boehringer Ingelheim (*Pavacol-D®*, sugar-free), Galen (*Galenphol®*, sugar-free), IVAX

Pholcodine Linctus, Strong, BP
Linctus (= oral solution), pholcodine 10 mg/5 mL in a suitable flavoured vehicle, containing citric acid monohydrate 2%. Net price 100 mL = 33p
Dose: 5 mL 3–4 times daily
Available from APS (sugar-free), IVAX

Galenphol® (Galen)
Paediatric linctus (= oral solution), orange, sugar-free, pholcodine 2 mg/5 mL. Net price 90-mL pack = £1.11
Dose: CHILD (but not generally recommended, see notes above) 1–5 years 5 mL 3 times daily; 6–12 years 5–10 mL

For a list of **cough and decongestant preparations on sale to the public**, including those containing pholcodine, see section 3.9.2

Palliative care

Diamorphine and methadone have been used to control distressing cough in terminal lung cancer although morphine is now preferred (see Prescribing in Palliative Care, p. 14). In other circumstances they are contra-indicated because they induce sputum retention and ventilatory failure as well as causing opioid dependence. Methadone linctus should be avoided because it has a long duration of action and tends to accumulate.

METHADONE HYDROCHLORIDE

Indications: cough in terminal disease
Cautions: see notes in section 4.7.2
Contra-indications: see notes in section 4.7.2
Side-effects: see notes in section 4.7.2; longer-acting than morphine therefore effects may be cumulative
Dose: see below

Methadone Linctus CD ▨

Linctus (= oral solution), methadone hydrochloride 2 mg/5 mL in a suitable vehicle with a tolu flavour. Label: 2
Dose: 2.5–5 mL every 4–6 hours, reduced to twice daily on prolonged use

▰ denotes preparations that are considered to be less suitable for prescribing (see p. vi)

MORPHINE HYDROCHLORIDE

Indications: cough in terminal disease (see also Prescribing in Palliative Care p. 14)
Cautions: see notes in section 4.7.2
Contra-indications: see notes in section 4.7.2
Side-effects: see notes in section 4.7.2
Dose: initially 5 mg every 4 hours

Preparations
Section 4.7.2

3.9.2 Expectorant and demulcent cough preparations

Expectorants are claimed to promote expulsion of bronchial secretions but there is no evidence that any drug can specifically facilitate expectoration. The assumption that sub-emetic doses of expectorants, such as ammonium chloride, ipecacuanha, and squill promote expectoration is a myth. However, a simple expectorant mixture may serve a useful placebo function and has the advantage of being inexpensive.

Demulcent cough preparations contain soothing substances such as syrup or glycerol and certainly some patients believe that such preparations relieve a dry irritating cough. Preparations such as **simple linctus** have the advantage of being harmless and inexpensive; **paediatric simple linctus** is particularly useful in children and sugar-free versions are available.

Compound cough preparations are on sale to the public; the rationale for some is dubious.

Ammonia and Ipecacuanha Mixture, BP

Mixture, ammonium bicarbonate 200 mg, liquorice liquid extract 0.5 mL, ipecacuanha tincture 0.3 mL, concentrated camphor water 0.1 mL, concentrated anise water 0.05 mL, double-strength chloroform water 5 mL, water to 10 mL. It should be recently prepared
Dose: 10–20 mL 3–4 times daily

Simple Linctus, BP

Linctus (= oral solution), citric acid monohydrate 2.5% in a suitable vehicle with an anise flavour. Net price 100 mL = 16p
Dose: 5 mL 3–4 times daily

A sugar-free version is available from Pinewood and various wholesalers.

Simple Linctus, Paediatric, BP

Linctus (= oral solution), citric acid monohydrate 0.625% in a suitable vehicle with an anise flavour. Net price 100 mL = 16p
Dose: CHILD 5–10 mL 3–4 times daily

A sugar-free version is available from Pinewood and various wholesalers.

Systemic cough and decongestant preparations on sale to the public, together with their significant ingredients.

Important: in overdose contact **Poisons Information Services** (p. 20) for full details of the ingredients.

Actifed® (pseudoephedrine, triprolidine), **Actifed Compound Linctus®** (dextromethorphan, pseudoephedrine, triprolidine), **Actifed Expectorant®** (guaifenesin, pseudoephedrine, triprolidine), **Adult Meltus® Expectorant with Decongestant** (guaifenesin, pseudoephedrine, menthol), **Advil Cold and Sinus®** (ibuprofen, pseudoephedrine)

Baby Meltus® (dilute acetic acid), **Beechams All-In-One®** (guaifenesin, paracetamol, phenylephrine), **Beechams Flu-Plus Caplets®** (paracetamol, phenylephrine), **Beechams Hot Lemon®**, **Hot Lemon and Honey®**, **Hot Blackcurrant®**, **Beechams Powders Capsules® with Decongestant** (paracetamol, phenylephrine), **Benylin Chesty Cough®** (diphenhydramine, menthol), **Benylin Children's Chesty Coughs®** (guaifenesin), **Benylin Children's Night Coughs®** (diphenhydramine, menthol), **Benylin Children's Dry Coughs®** (pholcodine), **Benylin Children's Coughs and Colds®** (dextromethorphan, triprolidine), **Benylin with Codeine®** (codeine, diphenhydramine, menthol), **Benylin Cough and Congestion®** (dextromethorphan, diphenhydramine, menthol, pseudoephedrine), **Benylin Dry Cough®** (dextromethorphan, diphenhydramine, menthol), **Benylin Four Flu®** (diphenhydramine, paracetamol, pseudoephedrine), **Benylin Non-drowsy for Chesty Coughs®** (guaifenesin, menthol), **Benylin Non-drowsy for Dry Coughs®** (dextromethorphan), **Benylin Day and Night Cold and Flu Relief®** (*day tablets*, paracetamol, phenylpropanolamine, *night tablets*, paracetamol, diphenhydramine), **Boots Bronchial Cough Mixture®** (ammonium carbonate, ammonium chloride, guaifenesin), **Boots Catarrh Cough Syrup®** (codeine, creosote), **Boots Children's 1 Year Plus Chesty Cough Syrup®** (guaifenesin), **Boots Children's 2 Year Plus Decongestant Syrup®** (pseudoephedrine), **Boots Children's 1 Year Plus Night Time Cough Syrup®** (diphenhydramine, pholcodine), **Boots Children's 2 Years Plus Cough and Cold Syrup with Decongestant®** (guaifenesin, pseudoephedrine), **Boots Children's 3 Months Plus Simple Cough Linctus®** (glycerol), **Boots Children's 6 Months Plus Cough and Congestion Syrup®** (ephedrine, ipecacuanha), **Boots Cold and Flu Relief Tablets®** (paracetamol, phenylephrine), **Boots Decongestant Tablets®** (pseudoephedrine), **Boots Decongestant Tablets with Paracetamol®** (paracetamol, pseudoephedrine), **Bronalin Decongestant Elixir®** (pseudoephedrine), **Bronalin Dry Cough®** (dextromethorphan, pseudoephedrine), **Bronalin Expectorant®** (ammonium chloride, diphenhydramine), **Bronalin Junior Linctus®** (diphenhydramine), **Buttercup Syrup Traditional®** (squill), **Buttercup Honey and Lemon®** (ipecacuanha, menthol)

Cabdrivers® (dextromethorphan, menthol), **CAM®** (ephedrine), **Catarrh-Ex®** (paracetamol, phenylephedrine), **Contac 400®** (phenylpropanolamine, chlorphenamine (chlorpheniramine)), **Covonia Bronchial Balsam®** (dextromethorphan, menthol), **Covonia Mentholated Cough Mixture®** (liquorice, menthol, squill), **Covonia Night Time Formula®** (dextromethorphan, diphenhydramine)

Day Nurse® (dextromethorphan, paracetamol, phenylpropanolamine), **Dimotane Elixir®** (brompheniramine), **Dimotane Expectorant®** (brompheniramine, guaifenesin, pseudoephedrine), **Dimotane Co®** and **Dimotane Co Paediatric®** (brompheniramine, codeine, pseudoephedrine),**Dimotane Plus®** and **Dimotane Plus Paediatric®** (brompheniramine, pseudoephedrine), **Dimotapp®**, **Dimotapp Paediatric®**, and **Dimotapp LA®** (brompheniramine, phenylephrine, phenylpropanolamine), **Do-Do Expectorant®** (guaifenesin), **Do-Do Chesteze®** (ephedrine, theophylline), **Dristan Tablets®** (aspirin, chlorphenamine, phenylephrine)

ES Bronchial® (ammonium bicarbonate, ipecacuanha, senna, squill), **Eskornade®** (diphenylpyraline, phenylpropanolamine), **Expulin®** (chlorphenamine (chlorpheniramine), menthol, pholcodine, pseudoephedrine), **Expulin Chesty Cough®** (guaifenesin, menthol), **Expulin Children's Cough Linctus®** (chlorphenamine (chlorpheniramine), menthol, pholcodine), **Expulin Decongestant for Babies and Children®** (chlorphenamine (chlorpheniramine), ephedrine), **Expulin Dry®** (menthol, pholcodine)

Famel Original® (codeine, creosote), **Fennings Little Healers®** (ipecacuanha), **Franol®** and **Franol Plus®** (both ephedrine, theophylline)

Galcodine® (codeine), **Galcodine Paediatric®** (codeine), **Galenphol®** (pholcodine), **Galenphol Paediatric®** (pholcodine), **Galenphol Strong®** (pholcodine), **Galloway's®** (ipecacuanha, squill), **Galpseud®** (pseudoephedrine), **Galpseud Plus®** (chlorphenamine (chlorpheniramine), pseudoephedrine)

Haymine® (chlorphenamine (chlorpheniramine), ephedrine), **Hill's Balsam Adult Expectorant®** (ipecacuanha, pholcodine), **Hill's Balsam Cough Suppressant®** (pholcodine), **Histalix®** (ammonium chloride, diphenhydramine, menthol)

Jackson's All Fours® (guaifenesin), **Junior Meltus Dry Cough®** (dextromethorphan, pseudoephedrine), **Junior Meltus Expectorant®** (guaifenesin)

Lemsip Lemcaps®, Lemsip Flu Strength®, Lemsip Lemon® or **Blackcurrant®, Lemsip Menthol Extra®** (all paracetamol, phenylephrine), **Lemsip Chesty Cough®** (guaifenesin), **Lemsip Power +®** (ibuprofen, pseudoephedrine), **Liqufruta Garlic®** (guaifenesin)

Medised® (paracetamol, promethazine), **Meltus Baby®** (dilute acetic acid), **Meltus Dry Cough®** (dextromethorphan, pseudoephedrine), **Meltus Expectorant®, Meltus Honey and Lemon®** (guaifenesin), **Mu-Cron Tablets®** (paracetamol, phenylpropanolamine)

Night Nurse® (dextromethorphan, paracetamol, promethazine), **Nirolex for Chesty Coughs with Decongestant®** (guaifenesin, pseudoephedrine), **Nirolex Chesty Cough Linctus®** (guaifenesin), **Nirolex Day Cold Comfort®** (paracetamol, pholcodine, pseudoephedrine), **Nirolex Dry Cough Linctus®** (glycerol), **Nirolex for Dry Coughs with Decongestant®** (dextromethorphan, pseudoephedrine), **Nirolex for Night Time Coughs®** (diphenhydramine, pholcodine), **Non-Drowsy Sudafed Dual Relief Max®** (ibuprofen, pseudoephedrine), **Numark Cold Relief Powders®** (paracetamol), **Nurofen Cold and Flu®** (ibuprofen, pseudoephedrine), **Nurofen Sinus Relief** (ibuprofen, pseudoephedrine), **Nurse Sykes Balsam®** (guaifenesin)

Otrivine® Mu-Cron (paracetamol, pseudoephedrine)

Pavacol D® (pholcodine), **Pulmo Bailly®** (codeine, guaiacol)

Robitussin Chesty Cough® (guaifenesin), **Robitussin Chesty Cough with Congestion®** (guaifenesin, pseudoephedrine), **Robitussin Dry Cough®** (dextromethorphan), **Robitussin Junior Persistant Cough®** (dextromethorphan), **Robitussin Night-Time®** (brompheniramine, codeine, pseudoephedrine)

Sinutab® (paracetamol, phenylpropanolamine), **Strepsils Cough Lozenges®** (dextromethorphan), **Sudafed®** (pseudoephedrine), **Sudafed Co®** (paracetamol, pseudoephedrine), **Sudafed Dual Relief®** (paracetamol, phenylephrine), **Sudafed Expectorant®** (guaifenesin, pseudoephedrine), **Sudafed Linctus®** (dextromethorphan, pseudoephedrine), **Sudafed Plus®** (pseudoephedrine, triprolidine)

Throaties Family Cough Linctus® (ipecacuanha), **Tixycolds®** (diphenhydramine, pseudoephedrine), **Tixylix Catarrh®** (diphenhydramine, menthol), **Tixylix Chesty Cough®** (guaifenesin), **Tixylix Cough and Cold®** (chlorphenamine (chlorpheniramine), pholcodine, pseudoephedrine), **Tixylix Daytime®** (pholcodine), **Tixylix Night-time®** (pholcodine, promethazine), **Tixymol®** (paracetamol)

Uniflu with Gregovite C® (caffeine, codeine, diphenhydramine, paracetamol, phenylephrine)

Venos for Dry Coughs®, Venos Expectorant® (guaifenesin), **Venos Honey and Lemon®, Vicks Medinite®** (dextromethorphan, doxylamine, ephedrine, paracetamol), **Vicks Vaposyrup for Tickly Coughs®** (honey, menthol), **Vicks Vaposyrup Chesty Cough®** (guaifenesin), **Vicks Vaposyrup Dry Cough®** (dextromethorphan)

3.10 Systemic nasal decongestants

Nasal decongestants for administration by mouth may not be as effective as preparations for local application (section 12.2.2) but they do not give rise to rebound nasal congestion on withdrawal. Some systemic nasal decongestants can have unwanted sympathomimetic effects. **Pseudoephedrine** is available over-the-counter; it has few sympathomimetic effects.

Systemic decongestants should be used with caution in diabetes, hypertension, hyperthyroidism, and ischaemic heart disease and **avoided** in patients taking monoamine oxidase inhibitors; **interactions:** Appendix 1 (sympathomimetics). See below for CSM advice on phenylpropanolamine.

CSM advice. The CSM has advised that evidence of a link between phenylpropanolamine and an increased risk of haemorrhagic stroke is weak and is mainly associated with indications that are not licensed in the UK. The CSM has issued a reminder that:

- the maximum daily dose of phenylpropanolamine should not exceed 100 mg;
- patients with high blood pressure, hyperthyroidism, heart disease or who are receiving MAOIs should not take products containing phenylpropanolamine;
- phenylpropanolamine may aggravate conditions such as diabetes, glaucoma or prostatic enlargement.

The main ingredients in systemic nasal decongestant preparations are shown in the list of cough and decongestant preparations on sale to the public (section 3.9.2). Many preparations also contain antihistamines, which may cause drowsiness and affect the ability to drive or operate machinery.

PSEUDOEPHEDRINE HYDROCHLORIDE

Indications: see notes above
Cautions: see under Ephedrine Hydrochloride (section 3.1.1.2)
Side-effects: see under Ephedrine Hydrochloride (section 3.1.1.2)
Dose: see preparations below

Galpseud® (Galen) ◼◼◼◼
Tablets, pseudoephedrine hydrochloride 60 mg.
Net price 20 = 87p
Dose: 1 tablet 4 times daily
Linctus, orange, sugar-free, pseudoephedrine hydrochloride 30 mg/5 mL. Net price 140 mL = £1.70
Dose: 10 mL 3 times daily; CHILD 2–6 years 2.5 mL, 6–12 years 5 mL

Sudafed® (Warner Lambert) ◼◼◼◼
Tablets, red, f/c, pseudoephedrine hydrochloride 60 mg. Net price 20 = 96p
Dose: 1 tablet every 4–6 hours (up to 4 times daily)
Elixir, red, pseudoephedrine hydrochloride 30 mg/5 mL. Net price 100 mL = £1.40
Dose: 10 mL every 4–6 hours (up to 4 times daily); CHILD 2–5 years 2.5 mL, 6–12 years 5 mL

◼◼◼◼ denotes preparations that are considered to be less suitable for prescribing (see p. vi)

■ Preparations on sale to the public
For a list of **cough and decongestant preparations on sale to the public**, including those containing pseudoephedrine, see pp. 163–164

4: Central nervous system

4.1 Hypnotics and anxiolytics

4.1.1   Hypnotics
4.1.2   Anxiolytics
4.1.3   Barbiturates

Most anxiolytics ('sedatives') will induce sleep when given at night and most hypnotics will sedate when given during the day. Prescribing of these drugs is widespread but dependence (both physical and psychological) and tolerance occurs. This may lead to difficulty in withdrawing the drug after the patient has been taking it regularly for more than a few weeks (see Dependence and Withdrawal, below). Hypnotics and anxiolytics should therefore be reserved for short courses to alleviate acute conditions after causal factors have been established.

Benzodiazepines are the most commonly used anxiolytics and hypnotics; they act at benzodiazepine receptors which are associated with gamma-aminobutyric acid (GABA) receptors. Older drugs such as meprobamate and barbiturates (section 4.1.3) are **not** recommended—they have more side-effects and interactions than benzodiazepines and are much more dangerous in overdosage.

PARADOXICAL EFFECTS. A paradoxical increase in hostility and aggression may be reported by patients taking benzodiazepines. The effects range from talkativeness and excitement, to aggressive and antisocial acts. Adjustment of the dose (up or down) usually attenuates the impulses. Increased anxiety and perceptual disorders are other paradoxical effects. Increased hostility and aggression after barbiturates and alcohol usually indicates intoxication.

DRIVING. Hypnotics and anxiolytics may impair judgement and increase reaction time, and so affect ability to drive or operate machinery; they increase the effects of alcohol. Moreover the hangover effects of a night dose may impair driving on the following day. See also Drugs and Driving under General Guidance, p. 2.

DEPENDENCE AND WITHDRAWAL. Withdrawal of a benzodiazepine should be gradual because abrupt withdrawal may produce confusion, toxic psychosis, convulsions, or a condition resembling delirium tremens. Abrupt withdrawal of a barbiturate (section 4.1.3) is even more likely to have serious effects.

The benzodiazepine withdrawal syndrome may develop at any time up to 3 weeks after stopping a long-acting benzodiazepine, but may occur within a few hours in the case of a short-acting one. It is characterised by insomnia, anxiety, loss of appetite and of body-weight, tremor, perspiration, tinnitus, and perceptual disturbances. These symptoms may be similar to the original complaint and encourage further prescribing; some symptoms may continue for weeks or months after stopping benzodiazepines.

A benzodiazepine can be withdrawn in steps of about one-eighth (range one-tenth to one-quarter) of the daily dose every fortnight. A suggested withdrawal protocol for patients who have difficulty is as follows:

1. Transfer patient to equivalent daily dose of diazepam[1] preferably taken at night
2. Reduce diazepam dose in fortnightly steps of 2 or 2.5 mg; if withdrawal symptoms occur, maintain this dose until symptoms improve
3. Reduce dose further, if necessary in smaller fortnightly steps[2]; it is better to reduce too slowly rather than too quickly
4. Stop completely; time needed for withdrawal can vary from about 4 weeks to a year or more

Counselling may help; beta-blockers should **only** be tried if other measures fail; antidepressants should be used **only** for clinical depression or for panic disorder; **avoid** antipsychotics (which may aggravate withdrawal symptoms)

CSM advice

1. Benzodiazepines are indicated for the short-term relief (two to four weeks only) of anxiety that is severe, disabling or subjecting the individual to unacceptable distress, occurring alone or in association with insomnia or short-term psychosomatic, organic or psychotic illness.

2. The use of benzodiazepines to treat short-term 'mild' anxiety is inappropriate and unsuitable.

3. Benzodiazepines should be used to treat insomnia only when it is severe, disabling, or subjecting the individual to extreme distress.

4.1.1 Hypnotics

Before a hypnotic is prescribed the cause of the insomnia should be established and, where possible, underlying factors should be treated. However, it should be noted that some patients have unrealistic sleep expectations, and others understate their alcohol consumption which is often the cause of the insomnia.

Transient insomnia may occur in those who normally sleep well and may be due to extraneous factors such as noise, shift work, and jet lag. If a hypnotic is indicated one that is rapidly eliminated should be chosen, and only one or two doses should be given.

Short-term insomnia is usually related to an emotional problem or serious medical illness. It may last for a few weeks and may recur; a hypnotic can be useful but should not be given for more than three weeks (preferably only one week). Intermittent use is desirable with omission of some doses. A rapidly eliminated drug is generally appropriate.

1. Approximate equivalent doses, diazepam 5 mg
   ≡ chlordiazepoxide 15 mg
   ≡ loprazolam 0.5–1 mg
   ≡ lorazepam 500 micrograms
   ≡ lormetazepam 0.5–1 mg
   ≡ nitrazepam 5 mg
   ≡ oxazepam 15 mg
   ≡ temazepam 10 mg
2. Steps may be adjusted according to initial dose and duration of treatment and can range from diazepam 500 micrograms (one-quarter of a 2-mg tablet) to 2.5 mg

Chronic insomnia is rarely benefited by hypnotics and is more often due to mild dependence caused by injudicious prescribing. Psychiatric disorders such as anxiety, depression, and abuse of drugs and alcohol are common causes. Sleep disturbance is very common in depressive illness and early wakening is often a useful pointer. The underlying psychiatric complaint should be treated, adapting the drug regimen to alleviate insomnia. For example, amitriptyline, mirtazapine, and nefazodone prescribed for depression, will also help to promote sleep if taken at night. Other causes of insomnia include daytime cat-napping and physical causes such as pain, pruritus, and dyspnoea.

Hypnotics should **not** be prescribed indiscriminately and routine prescribing is undesirable. They should be reserved for short courses in the acutely distressed. Tolerance to their effects develops within 3 to 14 days of continuous use and long-term efficacy cannot be assured. A major drawback of long-term use is that withdrawal causes rebound insomnia and precipitates a withdrawal syndrome (section 4.1).

Where prolonged administration is unavoidable hypnotics should be discontinued as soon as feasible and the patient warned that sleep may be disturbed for a few days before normal rhythm is re-established; broken sleep with vivid dreams and increased REM (rapid eye movement) sleep may persist for several weeks.

CHILDREN. The prescribing of hypnotics to children, except for occasional use such as for night terrors and somnambulism (sleep-walking), is not justified.

ELDERLY. Hypnotics should be avoided in the elderly, who are at risk of becoming ataxic and confused and so liable to fall and injure themselves.

Benzodiazepines

Benzodiazepines used as hypnotics include **nitrazepam**, **flunitrazepam**, and **flurazepam** which have a prolonged action and may give rise to residual effects on the following day; repeated doses tend to be cumulative.

Loprazolam, **lormetazepam**, and **temazepam** act for a shorter time and they have little or no hangover effect. Withdrawal phenomena however are more common with the short-acting benzodiazepines.

If insomnia is associated with daytime anxiety then the use of a long-acting benzodiazepine anxiolytic such as **diazepam** given as a single dose at night may effectively treat both symptoms.

For general guidelines on benzodiazepine prescribing see section 4.1.2 and for benzodiazepine withdrawal see section 4.1.

NITRAZEPAM

Indications: insomnia (short-term use)
Cautions: respiratory disease, muscle weakness, history of drug or alcohol abuse, marked personality disorder, pregnancy and breast-feeding (Appendixes 4 and 5); reduce dose in elderly and debilitated, and in hepatic (avoid if severe) and

renal impairment (Appendixes 2 and 3); avoid prolonged use (and abrupt withdrawal thereafter); porphyria (section 9.8.2); **interactions:** Appendix 1 (anxiolytics and hypnotics)

DRIVING. Drowsiness may persist the next day and affect performance of skilled tasks (e.g. driving); effects of alcohol enhanced

Contra-indications: respiratory depression; acute pulmonary insufficiency; severe hepatic impairment, myasthenia gravis, sleep apnoea syndrome; not for use alone to treat depression (or anxiety associated with depression) or chronic psychosis

Side-effects: drowsiness and lightheadedness the next day; confusion and ataxia (especially in the elderly); amnesia may occur; dependence; see also under Diazepam (section 4.1.2); **overdosage:** see Emergency Treatment of Poisoning, p. 25

Dose: 5–10 mg at bedtime; ELDERLY (or debilitated) 2.5–5 mg; CHILD not recommended

Nitrazepam (Non-proprietary) PoM
Tablets, nitrazepam 5 mg, net price 20 = 59p. Label: 19
Available from Alpharma, APS, CP, DDSA (*Remnos*® NHS), ICN (*Mogadon*® NHS)
Oral suspension, nitrazepam 2.5 mg/5 mL. Net price 150 mL = £5.30. Label: 19
Available from Norgine (*Somnite*® NHS)

FLUNITRAZEPAM

Indications: insomnia (short-term use)
Cautions: see under Nitrazepam
Contra-indications: see under Nitrazepam
Side-effects: see under Nitrazepam
Dose: 0.5–1 mg at bedtime; max. 2 mg; ELDERLY (or debilitated) 500 micrograms (max. 1 mg); CHILD not recommended

Rohypnol® (Roche) NHS CD
Tablets, grey-green, f/c, scored, flunitrazepam 1 mg. Net price 30-tab pack = £4.41. Label: 19
WARNING. Flunitrazepam tablets may be particularly subject to abuse

FLURAZEPAM

Indications: insomnia (short-term use)
Cautions: see under Nitrazepam
Contra-indications: see under Nitrazepam
Side-effects: see under Nitrazepam
Dose: 15–30 mg at bedtime; ELDERLY (or debilitated) 15 mg; CHILD not recommended

Dalmane® (ICN) NHS PoM
Capsules, flurazepam (as hydrochloride), 15 mg (grey/yellow), net price 30-cap pack = £5.18; 30 mg (black/grey), 30-cap pack = £6.65. Label: 19

LOPRAZOLAM

Indications: insomnia (short-term use)
Cautions: see under Nitrazepam
Contra-indications: see under Nitrazepam
Side-effects: see under Nitrazepam; shorter acting

Dose: 1 mg at bedtime, increased to 1.5 or 2 mg if required; ELDERLY (or debilitated) 0.5 or 1 mg; CHILD not recommended

Loprazolam (Non-proprietary) PoM
Tablets, loprazolam 1 mg (as mesilate). Net price 28-tab pack = £4.46. Label: 19
Available from Hoechst Marion Roussel (previously *Dormonoct*® NHS)

LORMETAZEPAM

Indications: insomnia (short-term use)
Cautions: see under Nitrazepam
Contra-indications: see under Nitrazepam
Side-effects: see under Nitrazepam; shorter acting
Dose: 0.5–1.5 mg at bedtime; ELDERLY (or debilitated) 500 micrograms; CHILD not recommended

Lormetazepam (Non-proprietary) PoM
Tablets, lormetazepam 500 micrograms, net price 28-tab pack = 76p; 1 mg, 28-tab pack = £1.45. Label: 19
Available from Genus, Wyeth

TEMAZEPAM

Indications: insomnia (short-term use); see also section 15.1.4.1 for peri-operative use
Cautions: see under Nitrazepam
Contra-indications: see under Nitrazepam
Side-effects: see under Nitrazepam; shorter acting
Dose: 10–20 mg at bedtime, exceptional circumstances 30–40 mg; ELDERLY (or debilitated) 10 mg at bedtime, exceptional circumstances 20 mg; CHILD not recommended

¹ **Temazepam** (Non-proprietary) CD
Gel-filled capsules NHS (soft gelatin), temazepam 10 mg, net price 20 = 37p; 15 mg, 20 = 62p; 20 mg, 20 = 60p; 30 mg, 20 = £1.24. Label: 19
WARNING. Gel-filled capsules may be particularly subject to abuse; gangrene has followed abuse by injection
Tablets, temazepam 10 mg, net price 28-tab pack = 89p; 20 mg, 28-tab pack = £1.54. Label: 19
Available from Alpharma, APS, Generics, Genus, IVAX, Hillcross, Lagap, Pharmacia
Oral solution, temazepam 10 mg/5 mL, net price 300 mL = £9.95. Label: 19
Available from Generics (sugar-free), Hillcross (sugar-free), Lagap, Pharmacia (sugar-free), Rosemont (sugar-free)

1. See p. 7 for prescribing requirements for temazepam

Zaleplon, zolpidem, and zopiclone

Zopiclone is a cyclopyrrolone and **zolpidem** is an imidazopyridine. Although neither are benzodiazepines both act on the same receptors (or receptor sub-types) as benzodiazepines. Both have a short duration of action. Zopiclone and zolpidem are not licensed for long-term use and there is evidence of dependence in a small number of patients.

Zaleplon is a pyrazolopyrimidine, which has been introduced recently. It also acts at benzodiazepine receptors and has a very short duration of action.

ZALEPLON

Indications: insomnia (short-term use)

Cautions: respiratory insufficiency (avoid if severe); hepatic impairment (avoid if severe; Appendix 2); history of drug or alcohol abuse; avoid prolonged use (and abrupt withdrawal thereafter); pregnancy (Appendix 4); not for use alone to treat depression

Contra-indications: sleep apnoea syndrome, myasthenia gravis; not for use alone to treat psychosis; breast-feeding

Side-effects: headache, asthenia, drowsiness, dependence, dizziness, amnesia, paradoxical effects (discontinue—see also section 4.1)

Dose: 10 mg at bedtime or after going to bed if difficulty falling asleep; ELDERLY 5 mg; CHILD under 18 years not recommended

Note. Patients should be advised not to take a second dose during a single night

Sonata® (Lundbeck) ▼ PoM

Capsules, zaleplon 5 mg (white/light brown), net price 14-cap pack = £3.08; 10 mg (white), 14-cap pack = £3.70. Label: 2

ZOLPIDEM TARTRATE

Indications: insomnia (short-term use)

Cautions: depression, history of drug or alcohol abuse, hepatic impairment (reduce dose, avoid if severe); renal impairment; elderly; avoid prolonged use (and abrupt withdrawal thereafter); **interactions:** Appendix 1 (anxiolytics and hypnotics)

DRIVING. Drowsiness may persist the next day and affect performance of skilled tasks (e.g. driving); effects of alcohol enhanced

Contra-indications: obstructive sleep apnoea, acute pulmonary insufficiency, respiratory depression, myasthenia gravis, severe hepatic impairment, psychotic illness, pregnancy and breast-feeding

Side-effects: diarrhoea, nausea, vomiting, vertigo, dizziness, headache, drowsiness, asthenia; dependence, memory disturbances, nightmares, nocturnal restlessness, depression, confusion, perceptual disturbances or diplopia, tremor, ataxia, falls reported

Dose: 10 mg at bedtime; ELDERLY (or debilitated) 5 mg; CHILD not recommended

Stilnoct® (Sanofi-Synthelabo) PoM

Tablets, both f/c, zolpidem tartrate 5 mg, net price 28-tab pack = £3.08; 10 mg, 28-tab pack = £4.48. Label: 19

ZOPICLONE

Indications: insomnia (short-term use)

Cautions: hepatic (avoid if severe) and renal impairment (Appendixes 2 and 3); elderly; history of drug abuse, psychiatric illness; avoid prolonged use (and abrupt withdrawal thereafter); **interactions:** Appendix 1 (anxiolytics and hypnotics)

DRIVING. Drowsiness may persist the next day and affect performance of skilled tasks (e.g. driving); effects of alcohol enhanced

Contra-indications: myasthenia gravis, respiratory failure, severe sleep apnoea syndrome, severe hepatic impairment; pregnancy and breast-feeding

Side-effects: bitter or metallic taste; gastro-intestinal disturbances including nausea and vomiting, dry mouth; irritability, confusion, depressed mood; drowsiness, dizziness, lightheadedness, and incoordination, headache; dependence; hypersensitivity reactions reported (including urticaria and rashes); hallucinations, nightmares, amnesia, and behavioural disturbances (including aggression) reported

Dose: 7.5 mg at bedtime; ELDERLY initially 3.75 mg at bedtime increased if necessary; CHILD not recommended

Zopiclone (Non-proprietary) PoM

Tablets, zopiclone 3.75 mg, net price 28-tab pack = £3.06; 7.5 mg, 28-tab pack = £4.48. Label: 19

Available from Alpharma, APS, Dominion, Generics, IVAX, Opus (*Zileze®*)

Zimovane® (Rhône-Poulenc Rorer) PoM

Tablets, f/c, zopiclone 3.75 mg (*Zimovane® LS,* blue), net price 28-tab pack = £3.08; 7.5 mg, 28-tab pack = £4.48. Label: 19

Chloral and derivatives

Chloral hydrate and derivatives were formerly popular hypnotics for children (but the use of hypnotics in children is not usually justified). There is no convincing evidence that they are particularly useful in the elderly and their role as hypnotics is now very limited. **Triclofos** causes fewer gastrointestinal disturbances than chloral hydrate.

CHLORAL HYDRATE ▨

Indications: insomnia (short-term use)

Cautions: respiratory disease, history of drug or alcohol abuse, marked personality disorder; reduce dose in elderly and debilitated; avoid prolonged use (and abrupt withdrawal thereafter); avoid contact with skin and mucous membranes; **interactions:** Appendix 1 (anxiolytics and hypnotics)

DRIVING. Drowsiness may persist the next day and affect performance of skilled tasks (e.g. driving); effects of alcohol enhanced

Contra-indications: cardiac disease, gastritis, hepatic impairment (Appendix 2) or renal impairment; pregnancy and breast-feeding; porphyria

Side-effects: gastric irritation (nausea and vomiting reported), abdominal distention and flatulence; also vertigo, ataxia, staggering gait, rashes, headache, light headedness, malaise, ketonuria, excitement, nightmares, delirium (especially in the elderly), eosinophilia, reduction in white cell count; dependence (may be associated with gastritis and renal damage) on prolonged use

Dose: insomnia, 0.5–1 g (max. 2 g) with plenty of water at bedtime; CHILD 30–50 mg/kg up to a max. single dose of 1 g

Chloral Mixture, BP PoM ▨
(Chloral Oral Solution)

Mixture, chloral hydrate 500 mg/5 mL in a suitable vehicle. Extemporaneous preparations should be recently prepared according to the following formula: chloral hydrate 1 g, syrup 2 mL, water to 10 mL. Net price 100 mL = 44p. Label: 19, 27

Dose: 5–20 mL; CHILD 1–5 years 2.5–5 mL, 6–12 years 5–10 mL, taken well diluted with water at bedtime

Chloral Elixir, Paediatric, BP [PoM] [▰]
(Chloral Oral Solution, Paediatric)

Elixir, chloral hydrate 4% in a suitable vehicle with a blackcurrant flavour. Extemporaneous preparations should be recently prepared according to the following formula: chloral hydrate 200 mg, water 0.1 mL, blackcurrant syrup 1 mL, syrup to 5 mL. Net price 100 mL = 95p. Label: 1, 27

Dose: up to 1 year 5 mL, taken well diluted with water at bedtime

Welldorm® (S&N Hlth.) [PoM] [▰]

Tablets, blue-purple, f/c, cloral betaine 707 mg (≡ chloral hydrate 414 mg). Net price 30-tab pack = £2.43. Label: 19, 27

Dose: 1–2 tablets with water or milk at bedtime, max. 5 tablets (2 g chloral hydrate) daily

Elixir, red, chloral hydrate 143.3 mg/5 mL. Net price 150-mL pack = £2.05. Label: 19, 27

Dose: 15–45 mL (0.4–1.3 g chloral hydrate) with water or milk, at bedtime, max. 70 mL (2 g chloral hydrate) daily; CHILD 1–1.75 mL/kg (30–50 mg/kg chloral hydrate), max. 35 mL (1 g chloral hydrate) daily

TRICLOFOS SODIUM [▰]

Indications: insomnia (short-term use)
Cautions: see Chloral Hydrate
Contra-indications: see Chloral Hydrate
Side-effects: see Chloral Hydrate but less gastric irritation
Dose: see under preparation below

Triclofos Oral Solution, BP [PoM] [▰]
(Triclofos Elixir)

Oral solution, triclofos sodium 500 mg/5 mL. Net price 300 mL = £28.23. Label: 19
Available from Celltech

Dose: 10–20 mL (1–2 g triclofos sodium) at bedtime; CHILD up to 1 year 25–30 mg/kg, 1–5 years 2.5–5 mL (250–500 mg triclofos sodium), 6–12 years 5–10 mL (0.5–1 g triclofos sodium)

> [▰] denotes preparations that are considered to be less suitable for prescribing (see p. vi)

Clomethiazole

Clomethiazole (chlormethiazole) may be a useful hypnotic for elderly patients because of its freedom from hangover but, as with all hypnotics, routine administration is undesirable and dependence occurs. It is indicated for use as a hypnotic only in the elderly (and for *very short-term use* in younger adults to attenuate alcohol withdrawal symptoms, see section 4.10).

CLOMETHIAZOLE
(Chlormethiazole)

Indications: see under Dose; alcohol withdrawal (section 4.10)
Cautions: cardiac and respiratory disease (confusional state may indicate hypoxia); history of drug abuse; marked personality disorder; elderly; excessive sedation may occur (particularly with higher doses); hepatic impairment (especially if severe since sedation can mask hepatic coma); renal impairment; avoid prolonged use (and

abrupt withdrawal thereafter); **interactions:** Appendix 1 (anxiolytics and hypnotics)
DRIVING. Drowsiness may persist the next day and affect performance of skilled tasks (e.g. driving); effects of alcohol enhanced

Contra-indications: acute pulmonary insufficiency; alcohol-dependent patients who continue to drink
Side-effects: nasal congestion and irritation (increased nasopharyngeal and bronchial secretions), conjunctival irritation, headache; rarely, paradoxical excitement, confusion, dependence, gastro-intestinal disturbances, rash, urticaria, bullous eruption, anaphylaxis, alterations in liver enzymes
Dose: severe insomnia in the elderly (short-term use), 1–2 capsules (*or* 5–10 mL syrup) at bedtime; CHILD not recommended
Restlessness and agitation in the elderly, 1 capsule (*or* 5 mL syrup) 3 times daily
Alcohol withdrawal, initially 2–4 capsules, if necessary repeated after some hours;
day 1 (first 24 hours), 9–12 capsules in 3–4 divided doses;
day 2, 6–8 capsules in 3–4 divided doses;
day 3, 4–6 capsules in 3–4 divided doses; then gradually reduced over days 4–6; total treatment for not more than 9 days
Note. For an equivalent therapeutic effect 1 capsule ≡ 5 mL syrup

Heminevrin® (AstraZeneca) [PoM]

Capsules, grey-brown, clomethiazole base 192 mg in an oily basis. Net price 60-cap pack = £4.34. Label: 19

Syrup, sugar-free, clomethiazole edisilate 250 mg/5 mL. Net price 300-mL pack = £3.63. Label: 19

Antihistamines

Some **antihistamines** such as diphenhydramine (section 3.4.1) and promethazine are on sale to the public for occasional insomnia; their prolonged duration of action may often lead to drowsiness the following day. The sedative effect of antihistamines may diminish after a few days of continued treatment; antihistamines are associated with headache, psychomotor impairment and antimuscarinic effects.

Promethazine is also popular for use in children, but the use of hypnotics in children is not usually justified.

PROMETHAZINE HYDROCHLORIDE
[▰]

Indications: night sedation and insomnia (short-term use); other indications (section 3.4.1, section 4.6)
Cautions: section 3.4.1
Contra-indications: section 3.4.1
Side-effects: section 3.4.1
Dose: *by mouth*, 25 mg at bedtime increased to 50 mg if necessary; CHILD under 2 years not recommended, 2–5 years 15–20 mg, 5–10 years 20–25 mg, at bedtime

Preparations
Section 3.4.1

Alcohol

Alcohol is a poor hypnotic because its diuretic action interferes with sleep during the latter part of the night. With chronic use, alcohol disturbs sleep patterns and causes insomnia; **interactions:** Appendix 1 (alcohol).

4.1.2 Anxiolytics

Benzodiazepine anxiolytics can be effective in alleviating anxiety states. Although these drugs are often prescribed to almost anyone with stress-related symptoms, unhappiness, or minor physical disease, their use in many situations is unjustified. In particular, they are not appropriate for treating depression or chronic psychosis. In bereavement, psychological adjustment may be inhibited by benzodiazepines. In children anxiolytic treatment should be used only to relieve acute anxiety (and related insomnia) caused by fear (e.g. before surgery).

Anxiolytic treatment should be limited to the lowest possible dose for the shortest possible time (see CSM advice, section 4.1). Dependence is particularly likely in patients with a history of alcohol or drug abuse and in patients with marked personality disorders.

Anxiolytics, particularly the benzodiazepines, have been termed 'minor tranquillisers'. This term is misleading because not only do they differ markedly from the antipsychotic drugs ('major tranquillisers') but their use is by no means minor. Antipsychotics, in low doses, are also sometimes used in severe anxiety for their sedative action but long-term use should be avoided in view of a possible risk of tardive dyskinesia (section 4.2.1).

Some antidepressants (section 4.3) are licensed for use in anxiety and related disorders; see section 4.3 for a comment on their role in generalised anxiety disorder and panic disorders. The use of antihistamines (e.g. hydroxyzine, section 3.4.1) for their sedative effect in anxiety is not considered to be appropriate.

Benzodiazepines

Benzodiazepines are indicated for the *short-term relief of severe anxiety* but long-term use should be avoided (see p. 166). Diazepam, alprazolam, chlordiazepoxide, clobazam, and clorazepate have a sustained action. Shorter-acting compounds such as **lorazepam** and **oxazepam** may be preferred in patients with hepatic impairment but they carry a greater risk of withdrawal symptoms.

In *panic disorders* (with or without agoraphobia) resistant to antidepressant therapy (section 4.3), a benzodiazepine (lorazepam 3–5 mg daily or clonazepam 1–2 mg daily (section 4.8.1) [both unlicensed]) may be used; alternatively a benzodiazepine may be used as short-term adjunctive therapy at the start of antidepressant treatment to prevent the initial worsening of symptoms.

Diazepam or lorazepam are very occasionally administered intravenously for the *control of panic attacks*. This route is the most rapid but the procedure is not without risk (section 4.8.2) and should be used only when alternative measures have failed. The intramuscular route has no advantage over the oral route.

For guidelines on benzodiazepine withdrawal, see p. 166.

DIAZEPAM

Indications: short-term use in anxiety or insomnia, adjunct in acute alcohol withdrawal; status epilepticus (section 4.8.2); febrile convulsions (section 4.8.3); muscle spasm (section 10.2.2); perioperative use (section 15.1.4.1)

Cautions: respiratory disease, muscle weakness (special care in myasthenia gravis), history of drug or alcohol abuse, marked personality disorder, pregnancy and breast-feeding (Appendixes 4 and 5); reduce dose in elderly and debilitated, and in hepatic impairment (avoid if severe, Appendix 2), renal impairment (Appendix 3); avoid prolonged use (and abrupt withdrawal thereafter); special precautions for intravenous injection (section 4.8.2); porphyria (section 9.8.2); **interactions:** Appendix 1 (anxiolytics and hypnotics)

DRIVING. Drowsiness may affect performance of skilled tasks (e.g. driving); effects of alcohol enhanced

Contra-indications: respiratory depression; acute pulmonary insufficiency; sleep apnoea syndrome; severe hepatic impairment; not for chronic psychosis; should not be used alone in depression or in anxiety with depression; myasthenia gravis; avoid injections containing benzyl alcohol in neonates (see under preparations below)

Side-effects: drowsiness and lightheadedness the next day; confusion and ataxia (especially in the elderly); amnesia; dependence; paradoxical increase in aggression (see also section 4.1); muscle weakness; *occasionally:* headache, vertigo, hypotension, salivation changes, gastrointestinal disturbances, visual disturbances, dysarthria, tremor, changes in libido, incontinence, urinary retention; blood disorders and jaundice reported; skin reactions; on intravenous injection, pain, thrombophlebitis, and rarely apnoea; **overdosage:** see Emergency Treatment of Poisoning, p.25

Dose: *by mouth*, anxiety, 2 mg 3 times daily increased if necessary to 15–30 mg daily in divided doses; ELDERLY (or debilitated) half adult dose

Insomnia associated with anxiety, 5–15 mg at bedtime

CHILD night terrors and somnambulism, 1–5 mg at bedtime

By intramuscular injection or slow intravenous injection (into a large vein, at a rate of not more than 5 mg/minute), for severe acute anxiety, control of acute panic attacks, and acute alcohol withdrawal, 10 mg, repeated if necessary after not less than 4 hours

Note. Only use intramuscular route when oral and intravenous routes not possible; special precautions for intravenous injection see section 4.8.2

By intravenous infusion—section 4.8.2

By rectum as rectal solution, acute anxiety and agitation, 500 micrograms/kg repeated after 12 hours as required; ELDERLY 250 micrograms/kg; CHILD not recommended

CHILD febrile convulsions, see p. 239

By rectum as suppositories, anxiety when oral route not appropriate, 10–30 mg (higher dose divided); dose form not appropriate for less than 10 mg

Diazepam (Non-proprietary) [PoM]

Tablets, diazepam 2 mg, net price 20 = 38p; 5 mg, 20 = 41p; 10 mg, 20 = 60p. Label: 2 *or* 19

Available from Alpharma, APS, DDSA (*Tensium®* [NHS]), IVAX, Ranbaxy (*Rimapam®* [NHS])

Oral solution, diazepam 2 mg/5 mL, net price 100 mL = £2.23. Label: 2 *or* 19

Available from Alpharma, Lagap (*Dialar®* [NHS])

Strong oral solution, diazepam 5 mg/5 mL, net price 100-mL pack = £3.07. Label: 2 *or* 19 [NHS]

Available from Lagap (*Dialar®* [NHS])

Injection (solution), diazepam 5 mg/mL. Do not dilute (except for intravenous infusion). Net price 2-mL amp = 25p

Excipients: may include benzyl alcohol (avoid in neonates, see Excipients, p. 2), ethanol, propylene glycol

Available from CP, Phoenix

Injection (emulsion), diazepam 5 mg/mL. For intravenous injection or infusion. Net price 2-mL amp = 73p

Available from Alpharma (*Diazemuls®*)

Rectal tubes (= rectal solution), diazepam 2 mg/ mL, net price 1.25-mL (2.5-mg) tube = 90p, 2.5-mL (5-mg) tube = £1.34; 4 mg/mL, 2.5-mL (10-mg) tube = £1.73

Available from Alpharma (*Stesolid®* 5 mg, 10 mg), CP (*Diazepam Rectubes®* 2.5 mg, 5 mg, 10 mg), Lagap

Suppositories, diazepam 10 mg, net price 6 = £6.51. Label: 2 *or* 19

Available from Sinclair (*Valclair®*)

ALPRAZOLAM

Indications: anxiety (short-term use)

Cautions: see under Diazepam

Contra-indications: see under Diazepam

Side-effects: see under Diazepam

Dose: 250–500 micrograms 3 times daily (elderly or debilitated 250 micrograms 2–3 times daily), increased if necessary to a total of 3 mg daily; CHILD not recommended

Xanax® (Pharmacia) [NHS] [PoM]

Tablets, both scored, alprazolam 250 micrograms, net price 60-tab pack = £2.75; 500 micrograms (pink), 60-tab pack = £5.27. Label: 2

CHLORDIAZEPOXIDE

Indications: anxiety (short-term use); adjunct in acute alcohol withdrawal (section 4.10)

Cautions: see under Diazepam

Contra-indications: see under Diazepam

Side-effects: see under Diazepam

Dose: anxiety, 10 mg 3 times daily increased if necessary to 60–100 mg daily in divided doses; ELDERLY (or debilitated) half adult dose; CHILD not recommended

Note. The doses stated above refer equally to chlordiazepoxide and to its hydrochloride

Chlordiazepoxide (Non-proprietary) [PoM]

Capsules, chlordiazepoxide hydrochloride 5 mg, net price 20 = 83p; 10 mg, 20 = £1.15. Label: 2

Various strengths available from Alpharma, DDSA (*Tropium®* [NHS]), Hillcross, ICN (*Librium®* [NHS]), Lagap

Chlordiazepoxide Hydrochloride (Non-proprietary) [PoM]

Tablets, chlordiazepoxide hydrochloride 5 mg, net price 20 = 79p; 10 mg, 20 = £1.09; 25 mg, 20 = 70p. Label: 2

CLORAZEPATE DIPOTASSIUM

Indications: anxiety (short-term use)

Cautions: see under Diazepam

Contra-indications: see under Diazepam

Side-effects: see under Diazepam

Dose: 7.5–22.5 mg daily in 2–3 divided doses *or* a single dose of 15 mg at bedtime; ELDERLY (or debilitated) half adult dose; CHILD not recommended

Tranxene® (Boehringer Ingelheim) [NHS] [PoM]

Capsules, clorazepate dipotassium 7.5 mg (maroon/grey), net price 20-cap pack = £2.66; 15 mg (pink/grey), 20-cap pack = £2.78. Label: 2 *or* 19

LORAZEPAM

Indications: short-term use in anxiety or insomnia; status epilepticus (section 4.8.2); peri-operative (section 15.1.4.1)

Cautions: see under Diazepam; short acting; when given parenterally, facilities for managing respiratory depression with mechanical ventilation must be at hand

Contra-indications: see under Diazepam

Side-effects: see under Diazepam

Dose: *by mouth,* anxiety, 1–4 mg daily in divided doses; ELDERLY (or debilitated) half adult dose
Insomnia associated with anxiety, 1–2 mg at bedtime; CHILD not recommended

By intramuscular or slow intravenous injection (into a large vein), acute panic attacks, 25–30 micrograms/kg, repeated every 6 hours if necessary; CHILD not recommended

Note. Only use intramuscular route when oral and intravenous routes not possible

Lorazepam (Non-proprietary) [PoM]

Tablets, lorazepam 1 mg, net price 20 = 88p; 2.5 mg, 20 = 41p. Label: 2 *or* 19

Available from Genus, IVAX, Wyeth (*Ativan®* [NHS])

Injection, lorazepam 4 mg/mL. Net price 1-mL amp = 51p

For intramuscular injection it should be diluted with an equal volume of water for injections or physiological saline (but only use when oral and intravenous routes not possible)

Available from Wyeth (*Ativan®*)

OXAZEPAM

Indications: anxiety (short-term use)

Cautions: see under Diazepam; short acting

Contra-indications: see under Diazepam

Side-effects: see under Diazepam

Dose: anxiety, 15–30 mg (elderly or debilitated 10–20 mg) 3–4 times daily; CHILD not recommended
Insomnia associated with anxiety, 15–25 mg (max. 50 mg) at bedtime; CHILD not recommended

Oxazepam (Non-proprietary) [PoM]

Tablets, oxazepam 10 mg, net price 20 = 23p;
15 mg, 20 = 23p; 30 mg, 20 = 49p. Label: 2

Available from most generic manufacturers

Buspirone

Buspirone is thought to act at specific serotonin
($5HT_{1A}$) receptors. Response to treatment may take
up to 2 weeks. It does not alleviate the symptoms of
benzodiazepine withdrawal. Therefore a patient
taking a benzodiazepine still needs to have the benzodiazepine withdrawn gradually; it is advisable to
do this before starting buspirone. The dependence
and abuse potential of buspirone is low; it is, however, licensed for short-term use only (but specialists occasionally use it for several months).

BUSPIRONE HYDROCHLORIDE

Indications: anxiety (short-term use)

Cautions: does not alleviate benzodiazepine withdrawal (see notes above); history of hepatic or
renal impairment; **interactions:** Appendix 1
(anxiolytics and hypnotics)

DRIVING. May affect performance of skilled tasks (e.g.
driving); effects of alcohol may be enhanced

Contra-indications: epilepsy, severe hepatic or
renal impairment, pregnancy and breast-feeding

Side-effects: nausea, dizziness, headache, nervousness, lightheadedness, excitement; rarely
tachycardia, palpitations, chest pain, drowsiness,
confusion, dry mouth, fatigue, and sweating

Dose: initially 5 mg 2–3 times daily, increased as
necessary every 2–3 days; usual range 15–30 mg
daily in divided doses; max. 45 mg daily; CHILD
not recommended

Buspirone Hydrochloride (Non-proprietary)
[PoM]

Tablets, buspirone hydrochloride 5 mg, net price
100-tab pack = £31.20; 10 mg, 100-tab pack =
£37.47. Counselling, driving

Available from Alpharma, Galen

Buspar® (Bristol-Myers Squibb) [PoM]

Tablets, buspirone hydrochloride 5 mg, net price
90-tab pack = £28.08; 10 mg, 90-tab pack =
£42.12. Counselling, driving

Beta-blockers

Beta-blockers (e.g. propranolol, oxprenolol) (section 2.4) do not affect psychological symptoms,
such as worry, tension, and fear, but they do reduce
autonomic symptoms, such as palpitations and
tremor; they do not reduce non-autonomic symptoms, such as muscle tension. Beta-blockers are
therefore indicated for patients with predominantly
somatic symptoms; this, in turn, may prevent the
onset of worry and fear. Patients with predominantly psychological symptoms may obtain no benefit.

Meprobamate

Meprobamate is **less effective** than the benzodiazepines, more hazardous in overdosage, and can also
induce dependence. It is **not** recommended.

MEPROBAMATE ◣

Indications: short-term use in anxiety, but see
notes above

Cautions: respiratory disease, muscle weakness,
epilepsy (may induce seizures), history of drug
or alcohol abuse, marked personality disorder,
pregnancy; elderly and debilitated; hepatic and
renal impairment; avoid prolonged use, abrupt
withdrawal may precipitate convulsions; **interactions:** Appendix 1 (anxiolytics and hypnotics)

DRIVING. Drowsiness may affect performance of skilled
tasks (e.g. driving); effects of alcohol enhanced

Contra-indications: acute pulmonary insufficiency; respiratory depression; porphyria (section 9.8.2); breast-feeding

Side-effects: see under Diazepam, but incidence
greater and drowsiness most common side-effect;
also gastro-intestinal disturbances, hypotension,
paraesthesia, weakness, CNS effects including
headache, paradoxical excitement, disturbances
of vision; rarely agranulocytosis and rashes

Dose: 400 mg 3–4 times daily; elderly patients half
adult dose or less; CHILD not recommended

Meprobamate (Non-proprietary) [CD] ◣

Tablets, scored, meprobamate 400 mg. Net price
84-tab pack = £9.49. Label: 2

Available from Genus

Equagesic® [CD] ◣

Section 4.7.1

◣ denotes preparations that are considered to
be less suitable for prescribing (see p. vi)

4.1.3   Barbiturates

The intermediate-acting **barbiturates** have a place
only in the treatment of severe intractable insomnia
in patients **already taking** barbiturates; they should
be **avoided** in the elderly. The long-acting barbiturate, phenobarbital is still sometimes of value in
epilepsy (section 4.8.1) but its use as a sedative is
unjustified. The very short-acting barbiturate thiopental is used in anaesthesia (section 15.1.1).

BARBITURATES

Indications: severe intractable insomnia **only** in
patients already taking barbiturates; see also notes
above

Cautions: avoid use where possible; dependence
and tolerance readily occur; abrupt withdrawal
may precipitate serious withdrawal syndrome
(rebound insomnia, anxiety, tremor, dizziness,
nausea, convulsions, delirium, and death);
repeated doses are cumulative and may lead to
excessive sedation; respiratory disease, renal dis-

ease, hepatic impairment; **interactions:** Appendix 1 (barbiturates and primidone)

DRIVING. Drowsiness may persist the next day and affect performance of skilled tasks (e.g. driving); effects of alcohol enhanced

Contra-indications: insomnia caused by pain; porphyria (section 9.8.2), pregnancy, breast-feeding; children, young adults, elderly and debilitated patients, also patients with history of drug or alcohol abuse

Side-effects: include hangover with drowsiness, dizziness, ataxia, respiratory depression, hypersensitivity reactions, headache, particularly in elderly; paradoxical excitement and confusion occasionally precede sleep; **overdosage:** see Emergency Treatment of Poisoning, p. 25

Dose: see under preparations below

Amytal® (Flynn) CD ▰

Tablets, amobarbital (amylobarbitone) 50 mg, net price 20 = £1.84. Label: 19

Dose: 100–200 mg at bedtime (**important:** but see also contra-indications)

Sodium Amytal® (Flynn) CD ▰

Capsules, both blue, amobarbital (amylobarbitone) sodium 60 mg, net price 20 = £3.43; 200 mg, 20 = £6.75. Label: 19

Dose: 60–200 mg at bedtime (**important:** but see also contra-indications)

Soneryl® (Concord) CD ▰

Tablets, pink, scored, butobarbital (butobarbitone) 100 mg. Net price 56-tab pack = £10.65. Label: 19

Dose: 100–200 mg at bedtime (**important:** but see also contra-indications)

■ Preparations containing secobarbital (quinalbarbitone)

Note. Secobarbital (quinalbarbitone) is in schedule 2 of the Misuse of Drugs Regulations 1985; receipt and supply must therefore be recorded in the CD register.

Seconal Sodium® (Flynn) CD ▰

Capsules, both orange, secobarbital (quinalbarbitone) sodium 50 mg, net price 20 = £5.30; 100 mg, 20 = £6.96. Label: 19

Dose: 100 mg at bedtime (**important:** but see also contra-indications)

Tuinal® (Flynn) CD ▰

Capsules, orange/blue, a mixture of amobarbital (amylobarbitone) sodium 50 mg, secobarbital (quinalbarbitone) sodium 50 mg. Net price 20 = £3.88. Label: 19

Dose: 1–2 capsules at bedtime (**important:** but see also contra-indications)

Note. Prescriptions need only specify 'Tuinal capsules'

▰ denotes preparations that are considered to be less suitable for prescribing (see p. vi)

4.2   Drugs used in psychoses and related disorders

4.2.1   Antipsychotic drugs
4.2.2   Antipsychotic depot injections
4.2.3   Antimanic drugs

Advice of Royal College of Psychiatrists on doses above BNF upper limit
Unless otherwise stated, doses in the BNF are licensed doses—any higher dose is therefore **unlicensed** (for an explanation of the significance of this, see p. 1).

1. Consider alternative approaches including adjuvant therapy and newer or atypical neuroleptics such as clozapine.
2. Bear in mind risk factors, including obesity—particular caution is indicated in older patients especially those over 70.
3. Consider potential for drug interactions—see **interactions:** Appendix 1 (antipsychotics).
4. Carry out ECG to exclude untoward abnormalities such as prolonged QT interval; repeat ECG periodically and reduce dose if prolonged QT interval or other adverse abnormality develops.
5. Increase dose slowly and not more often than once weekly.
6. Carry out regular pulse, blood pressure, and temperature checks; ensure that patient maintains adequate fluid intake.
7. Consider high-dose therapy to be for limited period and review regularly; abandon if no improvement after 3 months (return to standard dosage).

Important: When prescribing an antipsychotic for administration on an emergency basis, the intramuscular dose should be **lower** than the corresponding oral dose (owing to absence of first-pass effect), particularly if the patient is very active (increased blood flow to muscle considerably increases the rate of absorption). The prescription should specify the dose for **each route** and should **not** imply that the same dose can be given by mouth or by intramuscular injection. The dose of antipsychotic for emergency use should be reviewed at least **daily**.

4.2.1   Antipsychotic drugs

Antipsychotic drugs are also known as 'neuroleptics' and (misleadingly) as 'major tranquillisers'. Antipsychotic drugs generally tranquillise without impairing consciousness and without causing paradoxical excitement but they should not be regarded merely as tranquillisers. For conditions such as schizophrenia the tranquillising effect is of secondary importance.

In the short term they are used to quieten disturbed patients whatever the underlying psychopathology, which may be schizophrenia, brain damage, mania, toxic delirium, or agitated depression. Antipsychotic drugs are used to alleviate severe anxiety but this too should be a short-term measure.

SCHIZOPHRENIA. Antipsychotic drugs relieve florid psychotic symptoms such as thought disorder, hallucinations, and delusions, and prevent relapse. Although they are usually less effective in apathetic withdrawn patients, they sometimes appear to have an activating influence. For example, haloperidol may restore an acutely ill schizophrenic, who was previously withdrawn or even mute and akinetic, to normal activity and social behaviour. Patients with acute schizophrenia generally respond better than those with chronic symptoms.

Long-term treatment of a patient with a definite diagnosis of schizophrenia may be necessary even after the first episode of illness in order to prevent the manifest illness from becoming chronic. Withdrawal of drug treatment requires careful surveillance because the patient who appears well on medication may suffer a disastrous relapse if treatment is withdrawn inappropriately. In addition the need for continuation of treatment may not become immediately evident because relapse is often delayed for several weeks after cessation of treatment.

Antipsychotic drugs are considered to act by interfering with dopaminergic transmission in the brain by blocking dopamine D_2 receptors, which may give rise to the extrapyramidal effects described below, and also to hyperprolactinaemia. Antipsychotic drugs may also affect cholinergic, alpha-adrenergic, histaminergic, and serotonergic receptors.

CAUTIONS AND CONTRA-INDICATIONS. Antipsychotics should be used with **caution** in patients with hepatic impairment (Appendix 2), renal impairment (Appendix 3), cardiovascular disease, Parkinson's disease (may be exacerbated by antipsychotics), epilepsy (and conditions predisposing to epilepsy), depression, myasthenia gravis, prostatic hypertrophy, or a personal or family history of angle-closure glaucoma (avoid chlorpromazine, pericyazine and prochlorperazine in these conditions). Caution is also required in severe respiratory disease and in patients with a history of jaundice or who have blood dyscrasias (perform blood counts if unexplained infection or fever develops). Antipsychotics should be used with caution in the elderly, who are particularly susceptible to postural hypotension and to hyper- or hypothermia in very hot or cold weather. Serious consideration should be given before prescribing these drugs for elderly patients. As photosensitisation may occur with higher dosages, patients should avoid direct sunlight.

Antipsychotic drugs may be **contra-indicated** in comatose states, CNS depression, and phaeochromocytoma. Most antipsychotics are best avoided during pregnancy, unless essential (Appendix 4) and it is advisable to discontinue breast-feeding during treatment (Appendix 5); **interactions:** Appendix 1 (antipsychotics)

DRIVING. Drowsiness may affect performance of skilled tasks (e.g. driving or operating machinery), especially at start of treatment; effects of alcohol are enhanced

WITHDRAWAL. Withdrawal of antipsychotic drugs after long-term therapy should always be gradual and closely monitored to avoid the risk of acute withdrawal syndromes or rapid relapse.

SIDE-EFFECTS. Extrapyramidal symptoms are the most troublesome. They occur most frequently with the piperazine phenothiazines (fluphenazine, perphenazine, prochlorperazine, and trifluoperazine), the butyrophenones (benperidol, and haloperidol), and the depot preparations. They are easy to recognise but cannot be predicted accurately because they depend on the dose, the type of drug, and on individual susceptibility.

Extrapyramidal symptoms consist of:

- *parkinsonian symptoms* (including tremor), which may occur more commonly in adults or the elderly and may appear gradually;
- *dystonia* (abnormal face and body movements) and *dyskinesia*, which occur more commonly in children or young adults and appear after only a few doses;
- *akathisia* (restlessness), which characteristically occurs after large initial doses and may resemble an exacerbation of the condition being treated; and
- *tardive dyskinesia* (rhythmic, involuntary movements of tongue, face, and jaw), which usually develops on long-term therapy or with high dosage, but it may develop on short-term treatment with low doses—short-lived tardive dyskinesia may occur after withdrawal of the drug.

Parkinsonian symptoms remit if the drug is withdrawn and may be suppressed by the administration of **antimuscarinic** drugs (section 4.9.2). However, routine administration of such drugs is not justified because not all patients are affected and because they may unmask or worsen tardive dyskinesia.

Tardive dyskinesia is of particular concern because it may be irreversible on withdrawing therapy and treatment is usually ineffective. However, some manufacturers suggest that drug withdrawal at the earliest signs of tardive dyskinesia (fine vermicular movements of the tongue) may halt its full development. Tardive dyskinesia occurs fairly frequently, especially in the elderly, and treatment must be carefully and regularly reviewed.

Hypotension and interference with temperature regulation are dose-related side-effects and are liable to cause dangerous falls and hypothermia or hyperthermia in the elderly.

Neuroleptic malignant syndrome (hyperthermia, fluctuating level of consciousness, muscular rigidity, and autonomic dysfunction with pallor, tachycardia, labile blood pressure, sweating, and urinary incontinence) is a rare but potentially fatal side-effect of some drugs. Discontinuation of the antipsychotic is essential because there is no proven effective treatment, but cooling, bromocriptine, and dantrolene have been used. The syndrome, which usually lasts for 5–7 days after drug discontinuation, may be unduly prolonged if depot preparations have been used.

Other side-effects include: drowsiness; apathy; agitation, excitement and insomnia; convulsions; dizziness; headache; confusion; gastro-intestinal disturbances; nasal congestion; antimuscarinic symptoms (such as dry mouth, constipation, difficulty with micturition, and blurred vision); cardiovascular symptoms (such as hypotension, tachycardia, and arrhythmias); ECG changes (cases of sudden death have occurred); endocrine effects such as menstrual disturbances, galactorrhoea, gynaecomastia, impotence, and weight gain; blood dyscrasias (such as agranulocytosis and leucopenia), photosensitisation, contact sensitisation and rashes, and jaundice (including cholestatic); corneal and lens opacities, and purplish pigmentation of the skin, cornea, conjunctiva, and retina

Overdosage: for poisoning with phenothiazines and related compounds, see Emergency Treatment of Poisoning, p. 26.

CLASSIFICATION OF ANTIPSYCHOTICS. The **phenothiazine** derivatives can be divided into 3 main groups.

Group 1: chlorpromazine, levomepromazine (methotrimeprazine), and promazine, generally characterised by pronounced sedative effects and moderate antimuscarinic and extrapyramidal side-effects.

Group 2: pericyazine, pipotiazine, and thioridazine, generally characterised by moderate sedative effects, marked antimuscarinic effects, but fewer extrapyramidal side-effects than groups 1 or 3.

Group 3: fluphenazine, perphenazine, prochlorperazine, and trifluoperazine, generally characterised by fewer sedative effects, fewer antimuscarinic effects, but more pronounced extrapyramidal side-effects than groups 1 and 2.

Drugs of other chemical groups tend to resemble the phenothiazines of *group 3.* They include the **butyrophenones** (benperidol and haloperidol); **diphenylbutylpiperidines** (pimozide); **thioxanthenes** (flupentixol and zuclopenthixol); **substituted benzamides** (sulpiride); **oxypertine**; and **loxapine**.

For details of the newer antipsychotic drugs amisulpride, clozapine, olanzapine, quetiapine, risperidone, sertindole, and zotepine, see under Atypical antipsychotics , p. 181.

CHOICE. As indicated above, the various drugs differ somewhat in predominant actions and side-effects. Selection is influenced by the degree of sedation required and the patient's susceptibility to extrapyramidal side-effects. However, the differences between antipsychotic drugs are less important than the great variability in patient response; moreover, tolerance to secondary effects such as sedation usually develops. The atypical antipsychotics may be appropriate if extrapyramidal side-effects are a particular concern (see under Atypical Antipsychotics, below). Clozapine is used for schizophrenia when other antipsychotics are ineffective or not tolerated.

Prescribing of more than one antipsychotic at the same time is **not** recommended; it may constitute a hazard and there is no significant evidence that side-effects are minimised.

Chlorpromazine is still widely used despite the wide range of adverse effects associated with it. It has a marked sedating effect and is useful for treating violent patients without causing stupor. Agitated states in the elderly can be controlled without confusion, a dose of 10 to 25 mg once or twice daily usually being adequate.

Flupentixol (flupenthixol) and **pimozide** (see CSM advice p. 179) are less sedating than chlorpromazine.

Sulpiride in high doses controls florid positive symptoms, but in lower doses it has an alerting effect on apathetic withdrawn schizophrenics.

Fluphenazine, haloperidol, and **trifluoperazine** are also of value but their use is limited by the high incidence of extrapyramidal symptoms. Haloperidol may be preferred for the rapid control of hyperactive psychotic states. It is less hypotensive than chlorpromazine and is therefore also popular for agitation in the elderly, despite the high incidence of extrapyramidal side-effects.

Thioridazine is associated with rare reports of ventricular arrhythmia and it is now restricted for use as second-line treatment for schizophrenia in adults; it should be prescribed under specialist supervision only.

Promazine is not sufficiently active by mouth to be used as an antipsychotic drug; it has been used to treat agitation and restlessness in the elderly (see Other uses, below).

Loxapine causes relatively little sedation; in overdosage it has a high potential for serious neurological and cardiac toxicity.

OTHER USES. Nausea and vomiting (section 4.6), choreas, motor tics (section 4.9.3), and intractable hiccup (see under Chlorpromazine Hydrochloride and under Haloperidol). **Benperidol** is used in deviant antisocial sexual behaviour but its value is not established.

Psychomotor agitation and, in the elderly, agitation and restlessness, should be investigated for an underlying cause; they can be managed with low doses of chlorpromazine or haloperidol used for short periods. The use of promazine for agitation and restlessness in the elderly has declined. Olanzapine and risperidone may be effective for agitation and restlessness in the elderly [unlicensed].

Equivalent doses of oral antipsychotics

These equivalences are intended **only** as an approximate guide; individual dosage instructions should **also** be checked; patients should be carefully monitored after **any** change in medication

Antipsychotic	Daily dose
Chlorpromazine	100 mg
Clozapine	50 mg
Haloperidol	2–3 mg
Loxapine	10–20 mg
Pimozide	2 mg
Risperidone	0.5–1 mg
Sulpiride	200 mg
Thioridazine	100 mg
Trifluoperazine	5 mg

Important. These equivalences must **not** be extrapolated beyond the max. dose for the drug. Higher doses require careful titration in specialist units and the equivalences shown here may not be appropriate.

DOSAGE. After an initial period of stabilisation, in most patients, the long half-life of antipsychotic drugs allows the total daily oral dose to be given as a single dose. For the advice of The Royal College of Psychiatrists on doses above the BNF upper limit, see p. 174.

BENPERIDOL

Indications: control of deviant antisocial sexual behaviour (but see notes above)

Cautions: see notes above; also manufacturer advises regular blood counts and liver function tests during long-term treatment

Contra-indications: see notes above
Side-effects: see notes above
Dose: 0.25–1.5 mg daily in divided doses, adjusted according to the response; ELDERLY (or debilitated) initially half adult dose; CHILD not recommended

Anquil® (Concord) PoM
Tablets, benperidol 250 micrograms. Net price 100-tab pack = £26.13. Label: 2

CHLORPROMAZINE HYDROCHLORIDE

WARNING. Owing to the risk of contact sensitisation, pharmacists, nurses, and other health workers should avoid direct contact with chlorpromazine; tablets should not be crushed and solutions should be handled with care

Indications: see under Dose; antiemetic in palliative care (section 4.6)
Cautions: see notes above; also patients should remain supine and the blood pressure monitored for 30 minutes after intramuscular injection
Contra-indications: see notes above
Side-effects: see notes above; also intramuscular injection may be painful, cause hypotension and tachycardia, and give rise to nodule formation
Dose: *by mouth*,
  Schizophrenia and other psychoses, mania, short-term adjunctive management of severe anxiety, psychomotor agitation, excitement, and violent or dangerously impulsive behaviour initially 25 mg 3 times daily (*or* 75 mg at night), adjusted according to response, to usual maintenance dose of 75–300 mg daily (but up to 1 g daily may be required in psychoses); ELDERLY (or debilitated) third to half adult dose; CHILD (childhood schizophrenia and autism) 1–5 years 500 micrograms/kg every 4–6 hours (max. 40 mg daily); 6–12 years third to half adult dose (max. 75 mg daily)
  Intractable hiccup, 25–50 mg 3–4 times daily
By deep intramuscular injection, (for relief of acute symptoms but see also Cautions and Side-effects), 25–50 mg every 6–8 hours; CHILD, 1–5 years 500 micrograms/kg every 6–8 hours (max. 40 mg daily); 6–12 years 500 micrograms/kg every 6–8 hours (max. 75 mg daily)
  Induction of hypothermia (to prevent shivering), *by deep intramuscular injection*, 25–50 mg every 6–8 hours; CHILD 1–12 years, initially 0.5–1 mg/kg, followed by maintenance 500 micrograms/kg every 4–6 hours
By rectum in suppositories as chlorpromazine base 100 mg every 6–8 hours [unlicensed]
  Note. For equivalent therapeutic effect 100 mg chlorpromazine base given *rectally* as a suppository ≡ 20–25 mg chlorpromazine hydrochloride *by intramuscular injection* ≡ 40–50 mg of chlorpromazine base or hydrochloride *by mouth*

Chlorpromazine (Non-proprietary) PoM
Tablets, coated, chlorpromazine hydrochloride 10 mg, net price 56-tab pack = 71p; 25 mg, 28-tab pack = 96p; 50 mg, 28-tab pack = 95p; 100 mg, 28-tab pack = £1.15. Label: 2, 11
Available from Antigen, APS, DDSA (*Chloractil®*), Hillcross, IVAX
Oral solution, chlorpromazine hydrochloride 25 mg/5 mL, net price 150 mL = £1.35, 100 mg/5 mL, 150 mL = £3.76. Label: 2, 11
Available from Hillcross, Rosemont

Injection, chlorpromazine hydrochloride 25 mg/mL, net price 1-mL amp = 60p; 2-mL amp = 60p
Available from Antigen
Suppositories, chlorpromazine 100 mg. Label: 2, 11
'Special order' [unlicensed] product; contact Martindale or regional hospital manufacturing unit

Largactil® (Hawgreen) PoM
Tablets, all off-white, f/c, chlorpromazine hydrochloride 10 mg. Net price 56-tab pack = 71p; 25 mg, 56-tab pack = 98p; 50 mg, 56-tab pack = £2.05; 100 mg, 56-tab pack = £3.81. Label: 2, 11
Syrup, brown, chlorpromazine hydrochloride 25 mg/5 mL. Net price 100-mL pack = £1.11. Label: 2, 11
Suspension forte, orange, sugar-free, chlorpromazine hydrochloride 100 mg (as embonate)/5 mL. Net price 100-mL pack = £2.56. Label: 2, 11
Injection, chlorpromazine hydrochloride 25 mg/mL. Net price 2-mL amp = 67p

FLUPENTIXOL

(Flupenthixol)
Indications: schizophrenia and other psychoses, particularly with apathy and withdrawal but not mania or psychomotor hyperactivity; depression (section 4.3.4)
Cautions: see notes above; avoid in porphyria (section 9.8.2)
Contra-indications: see notes above; also excitable and overactive patients
Side-effects: see notes above; less sedating but extrapyramidal symptoms frequent
Dose: psychosis, initially 3–9 mg twice daily adjusted according to the response; max. 18 mg daily; ELDERLY (or debilitated) initially quarter to half adult dose; CHILD not recommended

Depixol® (Lundbeck) PoM
Tablets, yellow, s/c, flupentixol 3 mg (as dihydrochloride). Net price 20 = £2.99. Label: 2
Depot injection (flupentixol decanoate): section 4.2.2

FLUPHENAZINE HYDROCHLORIDE

Indications: see under Dose
Cautions: see notes above
Contra-indications: see notes above
Side-effects: see notes above; less sedating and fewer antimuscarinic or hypotensive symptoms, but extrapyramidal symptoms, particularly dystonic reactions and akathisia, more frequent; systemic lupus erythematosus
Dose: schizophrenia and other psychoses, mania, initially 2.5–10 mg daily in 2–3 divided doses, adjusted according to response to 20 mg daily; doses above 20 mg daily (10 mg in elderly) only with special caution; CHILD not recommended
  Short-term adjunctive management of severe anxiety, psychomotor agitation, excitement, and violent or dangerously impulsive behaviour, initially 1 mg twice daily, increased as necessary to 2 mg twice daily; CHILD not recommended

Moditen® (Sanofi-Synthelabo) PoM
Tablets, all s/c, fluphenazine hydrochloride 1 mg (pink), net price 20 = £1.06; 2.5 mg (yellow), 20 = £1.33; 5 mg, 20 = £1.77. Label: 2
Modecate® PoM
Section 4.2.2

HALOPERIDOL

Indications: see under Dose; motor tics (section 4.9.3)

Cautions: see notes above; also subarachnoid haemorrhage and metabolic disturbances such as hypokalaemia, hypocalcaemia, or hypomagnesaemia

Contra-indications: see notes above

Side-effects: see notes above, but less sedating and fewer antimuscarinic or hypotensive symptoms; pigmentation and photosensitivity reactions rare; extrapyramidal symptoms, particularly dystonic reactions and akathisia especially in thyrotoxic patients; rarely weight loss; hypoglycaemia; inappropriate antidiuretic hormone secretion

Dose: *by mouth,*

Schizophrenia and other psychoses, mania, short-term adjunctive management of psychomotor agitation, excitement, and violent or dangerously impulsive behaviour, initially 1.5–3 mg 2–3 times daily *or* 3–5 mg 2–3 times daily in severely affected or resistant patients; in resistant schizophrenia up to 30 mg daily may be needed; adjusted according to response to lowest effective maintenance dose (as low as 5–10 mg daily); ELDERLY (or debilitated) initially half adult dose; CHILD initially 25–50 micrograms/kg daily (in 2 divided doses) to max. 10 mg

Restlessness and agitation in the elderly, initially 0.5–1.5 mg once or twice daily

Short-term adjunctive management of severe anxiety, 500 micrograms twice daily; CHILD not recommended

Intractable hiccup, 1.5 mg 3 times daily adjusted according to response; CHILD not recommended

By intramuscular or by intravenous injection, initially 2–10 mg, then every 4–8 hours according to response (up to every hour if necessary) to total max. 18 mg; severely disturbed patients may require initial dose of up to 18 mg; ELDERLY (or debilitated) initially half adult dose; CHILD not recommended

Nausea and vomiting, 0.5–2 mg

Haloperidol (Non-proprietary) PoM
Tablets, haloperidol 500 micrograms, net price 28-tab pack = £11.55; 1.5 mg, 20 = £1.03; 5 mg, 20 = £2.55; 10 mg, 20 = £4.79; 20 mg, 20 = £8.47. Label: 2

Dozic® (Rosemont) PoM
Oral liquid, sugar-free, haloperidol 1 mg/mL. Net price 100-mL pack = £7.30. Label: 2

Haldol® (Janssen-Cilag) PoM
Tablets, both scored, haloperidol 5 mg (blue), net price 20 = £1.65; 10 mg (yellow), 20 = £3.21. Label: 2
Oral liquid, sugar-free, haloperidol 2 mg/mL. Net price 100-mL pack (with pipette) = £5.08. Label: 2
Injection, haloperidol 5 mg/mL. Net price 1-mL amp = 33p
Depot injection (haloperidol decanoate): section 4.2.2

Serenace® (IVAX) PoM
Capsules, green, haloperidol 500 micrograms, net price 30-cap pack = 98p. Label: 2

Tablets, haloperidol 1.5 mg, net price 30-tab pack = £1.73; 5 mg (pink), 30-tab pack = £4.90; 10 mg (pale pink), 30-tab pack = £8.81. Label: 2
Oral liquid, sugar-free, haloperidol 2 mg/mL, net price 500-mL pack = £43.83. Label: 2
Injection, haloperidol 5 mg/mL, net price 1-mL amp = 59p; 10 mg/mL, 2-mL amp = £2.03

LEVOMEPROMAZINE/ METHOTRIMEPRAZINE

Indications: see under Dose

Cautions: see notes above; patients receiving large initial doses should remain supine
ELDERLY. Risk of postural hypotension; not recommended for ambulant patients over 50 years unless risk of hypotensive reaction assessed

Contra-indications: see notes above

Side-effects: see notes above; occasionally raised erythrocyte sedimentation rate occurs

Dose: *by mouth,* schizophrenia, initially 25–50 mg daily in divided doses increased as necessary; bedpatients initially 100–200 mg daily usually in 3 divided doses, increased if necessary to 1 g daily; ELDERLY, see Cautions

Adjunctive treatment in palliative care (including management of pain and associated restlessness, distress, or vomiting), 12.5–50 mg every 4–8 hours, but see also Prescribing in Palliative Care, p. 15

By intramuscular injection or by intravenous injection (by intravenous injection after dilution with an equal volume of sodium chloride 0.9% injection), adjunct in palliative care, 12.5–25 mg (severe agitation up to 50 mg) every 6–8 hours if necessary

By continuous subcutaneous infusion, adjunct in palliative care (via syringe driver), diluted in a suitable volume of sodium chloride 0.9% injection, see Prescribing in Palliative Care, p. 16; CHILD (experience limited), 0.35–3 mg/kg daily

Nozinan® (Link) PoM
Tablets, scored, levomepromazine maleate 25 mg. Net price 20 = £4.95. Label: 2
Injection, levomepromazine hydrochloride 25 mg/mL. Net price 1-mL amp = £1.85

LOXAPINE

Indications: acute and chronic psychoses

Cautions: see notes above; avoid in porphyria (section 9.8.2)

Contra-indications: see notes above

Side-effects: see notes above; also weight gain or loss, dyspnoea, ptosis, hyperpyrexia, flushing and headache, paraesthesia, and polydipsia also reported

Dose: initially 20–50 mg daily in 2 divided doses, increased as necessary over 7–10 days to 60–100 mg daily (max. 250 mg) in 2–4 divided doses, then adjusted to usual maintenance dose of 20–100 mg daily; CHILD not recommended

Loxapac® (Lederle) PoM
Capsules, loxapine (as succinate) 10 mg (yellow/green), net price 56-cap pack = £5.86; 25 mg (light green/dark green), 56-cap pack = £11.74; 50 mg (blue/dark green), 28-cap pack = £10.56. Label: 2

OXYPERTINE

Indications: see under Dose
Cautions: see notes above
Contra-indications: see notes above
Side-effects: see notes above; also agitation and hyperactivity with low doses and sedation with high doses; occasionally photophobia
Dose: schizophrenia and other psychoses, mania, short-term adjunctive management of psychomotor agitation, excitement, and violent or dangerously impulsive behaviour, initially 80–120 mg daily in divided doses adjusted according to the response; max. 300 mg daily; CHILD not recommended

Short-term adjunctive management of severe anxiety, initially 10 mg 3–4 times daily preferably after food; max. 60 mg daily; CHILD not recommended

Oxypertine (Sanofi-Synthelabo) PoM
Capsules, oxypertine 10 mg. Net price 20 = £2.12. Label: 2
Tablets, scored, oxypertine 40 mg. Net price 20 = £6.64. Label: 2

PERICYAZINE

(Periciazine)
Indications: see under Dose
Cautions: see notes above
Contra-indications: see notes above
Side-effects: see notes above; more sedating; hypotension common when treatment initiated; respiratory depression
Dose: schizophrenia and other psychoses, initially 75 mg daily in divided doses increased at weekly intervals by steps of 25 mg according to response; usual max. 300 mg daily (elderly initially 15–30 mg daily)

Short-term adjunctive management of severe anxiety, psychomotor agitation, and violent or dangerously impulsive behaviour, initially 15–30 mg (elderly 5–10 mg) daily divided into 2 doses, taking the larger dose at bedtime, adjusted according to response

CHILD (severe mental or behavioural disorders only), initially, 500 micrograms daily for 10-kg child, increased by 1 mg for each additional 5 kg to max. total daily dose of 10 mg; dose may be gradually increased according to response but maintenance should not exceed twice initial dose INFANT under 1 year not recommended

Neulactil® (JHC) PoM
Tablets, all yellow, scored, pericyazine 2.5 mg, net price 84-tab pack = £7.69; 10 mg, 84-tab pack = £20.79. Label: 2
Syrup forte, brown, pericyazine 10 mg/5 mL. Net price 100-mL pack = £10.07. Label: 2

PERPHENAZINE

Indications: see under Dose; anti-emetic (section 4.6)
Cautions: see notes above
Contra-indications: see notes above; also agitation and restlessness in the elderly
Side-effects: see notes above; less sedating; extrapyramidal symptoms, especially dystonia, more frequent, particularly at high dosage; rarely systemic lupus erythematosus
Dose: schizophrenia and other psychoses, mania, short-term adjunctive management of anxiety, severe psychomotor agitation, excitement, and violent or dangerously impulsive behaviour, initially 4 mg 3 times daily adjusted according to the response; max. 24 mg daily; ELDERLY quarter to half adult dose (but see Cautions); CHILD under 14 years not recommended

Fentazin® (Goldshield) PoM
Tablets, both s/c, perphenazine 2 mg, net price 20 = £3.73; 4 mg, 20 = £4.39. Label: 2

PIMOZIDE

Indications: see under Dose
Cautions: see notes above
CSM WARNING. Following reports of sudden unexplained death, the CSM recommends ECG before treatment. The CSM also recommends that patients on pimozide should have an annual ECG (if the QT interval is prolonged, treatment should be reviewed and either withdrawn or dose reduced under close supervision) and that pimozide should **not** be given with other antipsychotic drugs (including depot preparations), tricyclic antidepressants or other drugs which prolong the QT interval, such as certain antimalarials, anti-arrhythmic drugs and certain antihistamines and should **not** be given with drugs which cause electrolyte disturbances (especially diuretics)
Contra-indications: see notes above; history of arrhythmias or congenital QT prolongation
Side-effects: see notes above; less sedating; serious arrhythmias reported; glycosuria and, rarely, hyponatraemia reported
Dose: schizophrenia, initially 2 mg daily, increased according to response in steps of 2–4 mg at intervals of not less than 1 week; usual dose range 2–20 mg daily; ELDERLY half usual starting dose; CHILD not recommended

Monosymptomatic hypochondriacal psychosis, paranoid psychosis, initially 4 mg daily, increased according to response in steps of 2–4 mg at intervals of not less than 1 week; max. 16 mg daily; ELDERLY half usual starting dose; CHILD not recommended

Orap® (Janssen-Cilag) PoM
Tablets, all scored, pimozide 2 mg, net price 20 = £3.17; 4 mg (green), 20 = £6.13; 10 mg, 20 = £11.76. Label: 2

PROCHLORPERAZINE

Indications: see under Dose; anti-emetic (section 4.6)
Cautions: see notes above; also hypotension more likely after intramuscular injection
Contra-indications: see notes above; children, but see section 4.6 for use as anti-emetic
Side-effects: see notes above; less sedating; extrapyramidal symptoms, particularly dystonias, more frequent; respiratory depression may occur in susceptible patients
Dose: *by mouth*, schizophrenia and other psychoses, mania, prochlorperazine maleate or mesilate, 12.5 mg twice daily for 7 days adjusted at

intervals of 4–7 days to usual dose of 75–100 mg daily according to response; CHILD not recommended

Short-term adjunctive management of severe anxiety, 15–20 mg daily in divided doses; max. 40 mg daily; CHILD not recommended

By deep intramuscular injection, psychoses, mania, prochlorperazine mesilate 12.5–25 mg 2–3 times daily; CHILD not recommended

By rectum in suppositories, psychoses, mania, the equivalent of prochlorperazine maleate 25 mg 2–3 times daily; CHILD not recommended

Preparations
Section 4.6

PROMAZINE HYDROCHLORIDE

Indications: see under Dose

Cautions: see notes above; also cerebral arteriosclerosis

Contra-indications: see notes above

Side-effects: see notes above; also haemolytic anaemia

Dose: *by mouth*, short-term adjunctive management of psychomotor agitation, 100–200 mg 4 times daily; CHILD not recommended
Agitation and restlessness in elderly, 25–50 mg 4 times daily

By intramuscular injection, short-term adjunctive management of psychomotor agitation, 50 mg (25 mg in elderly or debilitated), repeated if necessary after 6–8 hours; CHILD not recommended

Promazine (Non-proprietary) PoM
Tablets ▰, coated, promazine hydrochloride 25 mg, net price 20 = 49p; 50 mg, 20 = 87p. Label: 2
Available from Biorex
Oral solution ▰, promazine hydrochloride 25 mg/5 mL, net price 150 mL = £1.60; 50 mg/5 mL, 150 mL = £2.06. Label: 2
Available from Rosemont
Injection, promazine hydrochloride 50 mg/mL. Net price 1-mL amp = 30p
Note. May be difficult to obtain

SULPIRIDE

Indications: schizophrenia

Cautions: see notes above; also excited, agitated, or aggressive patients (even low doses may aggravate symptoms)

Contra-indications: see notes above; also porphyria (section 9.8.2)

Side-effects: see notes above; also hepatitis

Dose: 200–400 mg twice daily; max. 800 mg daily in predominantly negative symptoms, and 2.4 g daily in mainly positive symptoms; ELDERLY, lower initial dose, increased gradually according to response; CHILD under 14 years not recommended

Sulpiride (Non-proprietary) PoM
Tablets, sulpiride 200 mg, net price 100-tab pack = £14.12; 400 mg, 100-tab pack = £36.29. Label: 2
Available from Alpharma, APS, CP, Generics, IVAX

Dolmatil® (Sanofi-Synthelabo) PoM
Tablets, both scored, sulpiride 200 mg, net price 100-tab pack = £13.85; 400 mg (f/c), 100-tab pack = £36.29. Label: 2

Sulpitil® (Pharmacia) PoM
Tablets, scored, sulpiride 200 mg. Net price 28-tab pack = £4.29; 112-tab pack = £12.85. Label: 2

Sulpor® (Rosemont) PoM
Oral solution, sugar-free, lemon- and aniseed-flavoured, sulpiride 200 mg/5 mL, net price 150 mL = £27.00. Label: 2

THIORIDAZINE

Indications: under specialist supervision, second-line treatment of schizophrenia in adults (see Contra-indications, below)

Cautions: see notes above; ECG screening and electrolyte measurement before treatment, after each dose increase and at 6-month intervals; also monitor for visual defects on prolonged use; avoid in porphyria (section 9.8.2)

Contra-indications: see notes above
CARDIOTOXICITY. Thioridazine is associated with QT-interval prolongation and increased risk of ventricular arrhythmias. The CSM has advised that thioridazine should be restricted to second-line treatment of schizophrenia in adults under specialist supervision. Thioridazine is **contra-indicated** in patients with:

* significant cardiac disease, such as angina, bradycardia, second- or third-degree heart block, cardiac failure;
* history of ventricular arrhythmia;
* QT-interval prolongation or a family history of the condition;
* uncorrected hypokalaemia or hypomagnesaemia;
* concomitant use with other drugs known to cause QT-interval prolongation;
* reduced cytochrome P450 2D6 activity;
* concomitant use with drugs that inhibit or are metabolised by cytochrome P450 2D6.

Side-effects: see notes above; less sedating than chlorpromazine, and extrapyramidal symptoms and hypothermia rarely occur; more likely to induce hypotension and increased risk of cardiotoxicity and prolongation of QT interval (see above); pigmentary retinopathy (with reduced visual acuity, brownish colouring of vision, and impaired night vision) occurs rarely with high doses; sexual dysfunction, particularly retrograde ejaculation, may occur

Dose: 50–300 mg daily (initially in divided doses); max. 600 mg daily (in hospital patients only); CHILD not recommended

Thioridazine (Non-proprietary) PoM
Tablets, coated, thioridazine hydrochloride 25 mg, net price 20 = 35p; 50 mg, 20 = £1.02; 100 mg, 20 = £1.57. Label: 2
Available from Alpharma, DDSA (*Rideril®*), Hillcross, IVAX
Oral solution, thioridazine (as hydrochloride) 25 mg/5 mL. Net price 500-mL = £2.67. Label: 2
Available from Hillcross, Rosemont

Melleril® (Novartis) PoM
Tablets, all f/c, thioridazine hydrochloride 10 mg, net price 84-tab pack = £1.01; 25 mg, 84-tab pack = £1.66; 50 mg, 84-tab pack = £3.23; 100 mg, 84-tab pack = £6.24. Label: 2
Suspension 25 mg/5 mL, thioridazine 25 mg/5 mL, net price 300 mL = £1.96. Label: 2

Suspension 100 mg/5 mL, thioridazine 100 mg/ 5 mL, net price 300 mL = £7.14. Label: 2

Note. These suspensions should not be diluted but the two preparations may be mixed with each other to provide intermediate strengths

Syrup, brown, thioridazine (as hydrochloride) 25 mg/5 mL, net price 300 mL = £1.98. Label: 2

TRIFLUOPERAZINE

Indications: see under Dose; anti-emetic (section 4.6)

Cautions: see notes above

Contra-indications: see notes above

Side-effects: see notes above; extrapyramidal symptoms more frequent, especially at doses exceeding 6 mg daily; pancytopenia; thrombocytopenia; hyperpyrexia; anorexia

Dose: *by mouth* (reduce initial doses in elderly by at least half)

Schizophrenia and other psychoses, short-term adjunctive management of psychomotor agitation, excitement, and violent or dangerously impulsive behaviour, initially 5 mg twice daily, *or* 10 mg daily in modified-release form, increased by 5 mg after 1 week, then at intervals of 3 days, according to the response; CHILD up to 12 years, initially up to 5 mg daily in divided doses, adjusted according to response, age, and bodyweight

Short-term adjunctive management of severe anxiety, 2–4 mg daily in divided doses *or* 2–4 mg daily in modified-release form, increased if necessary to 6 mg daily; CHILD 3–5 years up to 1 mg daily, 6–12 years up to 4 mg daily

Trifluoperazine (Non-proprietary) [PoM]

Tablets, coated, trifluoperazine (as hydrochloride) 1 mg, net price 20 = 57p; 5 mg, 20 = 87p. Label: 2

Available from most generic manufacturers

Oral solution, trifluoperazine (as hydrochloride) 5 mg/5 mL. Net price 200-mL = £11.07. Label: 2

Available from Rosemont (sugar-free)

Stelazine® (Goldshield) [PoM]

Tablets, both blue, f/c, trifluoperazine (as hydrochloride) 1 mg, net price 20 = 61p; 5 mg, 20 = 87p. Label: 2

Spansules® (= capsules m/r), all clear/yellow, enclosing dark blue, light blue, and white pellets, trifluoperazine (as hydrochloride) 2 mg, net price 60-cap pack = £4.36; 10 mg, 30-cap pack = £2.83; 15 mg, 30-cap pack = £4.27. Label: 2, 25

Syrup, yellow, sugar-free, trifluoperazine (as hydrochloride) 1 mg/5 mL. Net price 200-mL pack = £2.95. Label: 2

ZUCLOPENTHIXOL ACETATE

Indications: short-term management of acute psychosis, mania, or exacerbations of chronic psychosis

Cautions: see notes above; avoid in porphyria (section 9.8.2)

Contra-indications: see notes above

Side-effects: see notes above

Dose: *by deep intramuscular injection* into the gluteal muscle or lateral thigh, 50–150 mg (elderly 50–100 mg), if necessary repeated after 2–3 days (1 additional dose may be needed 1–2 days after the first injection); max. cumulative dose 400 mg

per course and max. 4 injections; max. duration of treatment 2 weeks—if maintenance treatment necessary change to an oral antipsychotic 2–3 days after last injection, *or* to a longer acting antipsychotic depot injection given concomitantly with last injection of zuclopenthixol acetate; CHILD not recommended

Clopixol Acuphase® (Lundbeck) [PoM]

Injection (oily), zuclopenthixol acetate 50 mg/mL. Net price 1-mL amp = £5.20; 2-mL amp = £10.03

ZUCLOPENTHIXOL DIHYDROCHLORIDE

Indications: schizophrenia and other psychoses, particularly when associated with agitated, aggressive, or hostile behaviour

Cautions: see notes above; avoid in porphyria (section 9.8.2)

Contra-indications: see notes above; apathetic or withdrawn states

Side-effects: see notes above; urinary frequency or incontinence; weight loss (less common than weight gain)

Dose: initially 20–30 mg daily in divided doses, increasing to a max. of 150 mg daily if necessary; usual maintenance dose 20–50 mg daily; ELDERLY (or debilitated) initially quarter to half adult dose; CHILD not recommended

Clopixol® (Lundbeck) [PoM]

Tablets, all f/c, pink, zuclopenthixol (as dihydrochloride) 2 mg, net price 20 = 62p; 10 mg, 20 = £1.73; 25 mg, 20 = £3.47. Label: 2

Depot injection (zuclopenthixol decanoate): section 4.2.2

Atypical antipsychotics

The 'atypical antipsychotics' **amisulpride, clozapine, olanzapine, quetiapine, risperidone,** and **zotepine** may be better tolerated than other antipsychotics; extrapyramidal symptoms and prolactin elevation may be less frequent than with older antipsychotics.

The atypical antipsychotics may be used as first-line treatment for schizophrenia, but clozapine is licensed for the treatment of schizophrenia only in patients unresponsive to, or intolerant of, conventional antipsychotic drugs. It can cause agranulocytosis and its use is restricted to patients registered with the Clozaril Patient Monitoring Service (see under Clozapine, below).

Sertindole has been suspended following reports of arrhythmias and sudden cardiac death; it remains available on a named-patient basis (from Lundbeck—*Serdolect®*) for patients already stabilised on the drug in whom other antipsychotics are inappropriate.

CAUTIONS AND CONTRA-INDICATIONS. While most atypical antipsychotics have not generally been associated with prolongation of the QT interval, caution should be exercised if they are prescribed with other drugs known to increase the QT interval. Atypical antipsychotics should be used with caution in patients with cardiovascular disease, or a history of epilepsy; they should be used with caution in the elderly; **interactions:** Appendix 1 (antipsychotics).

DRIVING. Atypical antipsychotics may affect performance of skilled tasks (e.g. driving); effects of alcohol are enhanced.

SIDE-EFFECTS. Side-effects of the atypical antipsychotics include weight gain, dizziness, postural hypotension (especially during intial dose titration) which may be associated with syncope or reflex tachycardia in some patients, extrapyramidal symptoms (usually mild and transient and which respond to dose reduction or to antimuscarinic drugs), occasionally tardive dyskinesia on long-term administration (discontinue drug on appearance of early signs); neuroleptic malignant syndrome has been reported rarely.

AMISULPRIDE

Indications: schizophrenia

Cautions: see notes above; also renal impairment (Appendix 3); Parkinson's diease; elderly (risk of hypotension or sedation)

Contra-indications: see notes above; also pregnancy (Appendix 4) and breast-feeding (Appendix 5), phaeochromocytoma, prolactin-dependent tumours

Side-effects: see notes above; also insomnia, anxiety, agitation, drowsiness, gastro-intestinal disorders such as constipation, nausea, vomiting, and dry mouth; hyperprolactinaemia (with galactorrhoea, amenorrhoea, gynaecomastia, breast pain, sexual dysfunction), occasionally bradycardia

Dose: acute psychotic episode, 400–800 mg daily in divided doses, adjusted according to response; max. 1.2 g daily
Predominantly negative symptoms, 50–300 mg daily; CHILD under 15 years, not recommended
Note. Doses up to 300 mg may be administered once daily

Solian® (Sanofi-Synthelabo) PoM
Tablets, scored, amisulpride 50 mg, net price 60-tab pack = £18.10, 90-tab pack = £27.16; 200 mg, net price 60-tab pack = £66.00, 90-tab pack = £99.00; 400 mg, 60-tab pack = £132.00. Label: 2

CLOZAPINE

Indications: schizophrenia in patients unresponsive to, or intolerant of, conventional antipsychotic drugs

Cautions: see notes above; initiation must be in hospital in-patients; leucocyte and differential blood counts must be normal before starting treatment and must be monitored weekly for first 18 weeks then at least fortnightly—patients who have received clozapine for 1 year or more and have stable blood counts may have their blood monitoring reduced to every 4 weeks (continue monitoring for 4 weeks after discontinuation); avoid drugs which depress leucopoiesis (Appendix 1) and taper off conventional neuroleptic before starting; withdraw treatment permanently if leucocyte count falls below 3000/mm³ or absolute neutrophil count falls below 1500/mm³; patients should report any symptoms of infection immediately; mild to moderate renal impairment (Appendix 3); prostatic hypertrophy, angle-closure glaucoma

WITHDRAWAL. On planned withdrawal reduce dose gradually over 1–2 weeks to avoid risk of rebound psychosis. If abrupt withdrawal necessary observe patient carefully

GASTRO-INTESTINAL OBSTRUCTION. Following reports of adverse reactions resembling gastro-intestinal obstruction, it is recommended that clozapine should be used with caution in patients receiving concomitant treatment with drugs known to cause constipation (e.g. drugs with antimuscarinic effects) or in patients with a history of colonic disease or previous bowel surgery. Patients receiving clozapine should be monitored for constipation and laxatives prescribed as required.

Contra-indications: severe cardiac disorders (e.g. myocarditis); active liver disease (Appendix 2), severe renal impairment (Appendix 3); history of drug-induced neutropenia or agranulocytosis; bone marrow disorders; alcoholic and toxic psychoses; history of circulatory collapse; drug intoxication; coma or severe CNS depression; uncontrolled epilepsy; pregnancy (Appendix 4) and breast-feeding (Appendix 5)

Side-effects: see notes above; also neutropenia and potentially fatal agranulocytosis (**important:** see Cautions), fever (rule out underlying infection or agranulocytosis), drowsiness, anxiety, agitation, confusion, fatigue, blurred vision, dry mouth, constipation and paralytic ileus (see Gastro-intestinal obstruction, above), nausea and vomiting, dysphagia, headache, dizziness, hypersalivation, urinary incontinence and retention, priapism, impaired temperature regulation, hepatitis, jaundice (discontinue immediately), rarely fulminant hepatic necrosis; arrhythmias, pericarditis, myocarditis (discontinue immediately), cardiomyopathy, delirium; tachycardia, rarely circulatory collapse (but hypertension also reported), respiratory depression, acute pancreatitis; thromboembolism, hyperglycaemia, rash, elevated plasma-creatine kinase concentration, interstitial nephritis, parotid gland enlargement also reported

Dose: (close medical supervision on initiation—risk of collapse due to hypotension) 12.5 mg once or twice on first day then 25–50 mg on second day then increased gradually (if well tolerated) in steps of 25–50 mg over 14–21 days to 300 mg daily in divided doses (larger dose at night, up to 200 mg daily may be taken as a single dose at bedtime); if necessary may be further increased in steps of 50–100 mg once (preferably) or twice weekly; usual antipsychotic dose 200–450 mg daily (max. 900 mg daily); subsequent adjustment to usual maintenance of 150–300 mg; CHILD not recommended

Note. Restarting after *interval of more than 2 days*, 12.5 mg once or twice on first day (but may be feasible to increase more quickly than on initiation)—unless previous respiratory or cardiac arrest with initial dosing in which case extreme caution

ELDERLY AND SPECIAL RISK GROUPS. In *elderly*, 12.5 mg once on first day—subsequent adjustments restricted to 25 mg daily; in *cardiovascular disease, hepatic* or *renal impairment* or if history of *epilepsy*, 12.5 mg on first day—subsequent adjustments slowly and in small steps (if epileptic seizures (see also Cautions), suspend for 24 hours and resume at lower dose)

Clozaril® (Novartis) PoM
Tablets, both yellow, clozapine 25 mg (scored), net price 28-tab pack = £13.70, 84-tab pack (hosp. only) = £41.07; 100 mg, 28-tab pack = £54.75, 84-tab pack (hosp. only) = £164.26. Label: 2, 10 patient information leaflet
Note. Patient, prescriber, and supplying pharmacist must be registered with the Clozaril Patient Monitoring Service—takes several days to do this

OLANZAPINE

Indications: schizophrenia
Cautions: see notes above; also pregnancy, prostatic hypertrophy, paralytic ileus, hepatic impairment (Appendix 2), renal impairment (Appendix 3), diabetes mellitus, low leucocyte or neutrophil count, bone marrow depression, hypereosinophilic disorders, myeloproliferative disease
Contra-indications: angle-closure glaucoma; breast-feeding
Side-effects: see notes above; also mild, transient antimuscarinic effects; drowsiness, increased appetite, oedema, hyperprolactinaemia (but clinical manifestations rare), occasionally blood dyscrasias, rarely bradycardia, rash, photosensitivity, hyperglycaemia, priapism, hepatitis, and elevated creatine kinase concentration
Dose: 10 mg daily adjusted to usual range of 5–20 mg daily; doses of 15 mg daily or greater only after reassessment; CHILD and ADOLESCENT under 18 years not recommended
Note. When one or more factors present that might result in slower metabolism (e.g. female gender, elderly, non-smoker) consider lower initial dose and more gradual dose increase

Zyprexa® (Lilly) PoM
Tablets, f/c, olanzapine 2.5 mg, net price 28-tab pack = £31.70; 5 mg, 28-tab pack = £48.78; 7.5 mg, 56-tab pack = £146.34; 10 mg, 28-tab pack = £97.56, 56-tab pack = £195.11. Label: 2
Orodispersible tablet (*Velotab®*), olanzapine 5 mg, net price 28-tab pack = £56.10; 10 mg, 28-tab pack = £112.19. Label: 2, counselling, administration
Excipients: include aspartame (section 9.4.1)
COUNSELLING. *Velotab®* may be placed on the tongue and allowed to dissolve or dispersed in water, orange juice, apple juice, milk, or coffee

QUETIAPINE

Indications: schizophrenia
Cautions: see notes above; also pregnancy, hepatic impairment (Appendix 2), renal impairment (Appendix 3), cerebrovascular disease
Contra-indications: breast-feeding (Appendix 5)
Side-effects: see notes above; also drowsiness, dyspepsia, constipation, dry mouth, mild asthenia, rhinitis, hypertension, tachycardia; anxiety, fever, myalgia, ear pain, rash; leucopenia, neutropenia and occasionally eosinophilia reported; elevated plasma-triglyceride and cholesterol concentrations, reduced plasma-thyroid hormone concentrations, possible QT interval prolongation; rarely oedema; very rarely priapism
Dose: 25 mg twice daily on day 1, 50 mg twice daily on day 2, 100 mg twice daily on day 3, 150 mg twice daily on day 4, then adjusted according to response, usual range 300–450 mg daily in 2 divided doses; max. 750 mg daily; ELD-

ERLY initially 25 mg daily, increased in steps of 25–50 mg daily; CHILD and ADOLESCENT not recommended

Seroquel® (AstraZeneca) PoM
Tablets, f/c, quetiapine (as fumarate) 25 mg (peach), net price 60-tab pack = £28.20; 100 mg (yellow), 60-tab pack = £113.10; 150 mg (pale yellow), 60-tab pack = £113.10; 200 mg (white), 60-tab pack = £113.10; starter pack of 6 × 25-mg tabs, 2 × 100-mg tabs, and 2 × 150-mg tabs = £10.36. Label: 2

RISPERIDONE

Indications: acute and chronic psychoses
Cautions: see notes above; Parkinson's disease; pregnancy, breast-feeding (Appendix 5); hepatic impairment (Appendix 2), renal impairment (Appendix 3)
Side-effects: see notes above; also insomnia, agitation, anxiety, headache, drowsiness, impaired concentration, fatigue, blurred vision, constipation, nausea and vomiting, dyspepsia, abdominal pain, hyperprolactinaemia (with galactorrhoea, menstrual disturbances, amenorrhoea, gynaecomastia), sexual dysfunction, priapism, urinary incontinence, tachycardia, hypertension, skin rash, rhinitis; neutropenia and thrombocytopenia have been reported; rarely, hyponatraemia, abnormal temperature regulation, oedema
Dose: 2 mg in 1–2 divided doses on first day *then* 4 mg in 1–2 divided doses on second day (slower titration appropriate in some patients); usual dose range 4–6 mg daily; doses above 10 mg daily only if benefit considered to outweigh risk (max. 16 mg daily); ELDERLY (or in hepatic or renal impairment) initially 500 micrograms twice daily increased in steps of 500 micrograms twice daily to 1–2 mg twice daily; CHILD under 15 years not recommended

Risperdal® (Janssen-Cilag, Organon) PoM
Tablets, f/c, scored, risperidone 500 micrograms (brown-red), net price 20-tab pack = £7.67; 1 mg (white), 20-tab pack = £13.45, 60-tab pack = £40.35; 2 mg (orange), 60-tab pack = £79.56; 3 mg (yellow), 60-tab pack = £117.00; 4 mg (green), 60-tab pack = £154.44; 6 mg (yellow), 28-tab pack = £109.20. Label: 2
Liquid, risperidone 1 mg/mL, net price 100 mL = £65.00. Label: 2
Note. Liquid may be diluted with mineral water, orange juice or black coffee (should be taken immediately)

ZOTEPINE

Indications: schizophrenia
Cautions: see notes above; personal or close family history of epilepsy; withdrawal of concomitantly prescribed CNS depressants; QT interval prolongation (ECG required before treatment in patients at risk of arrhythmias); hepatic impairment (Appendix 2); renal impairment (Appendix 3); prostatic hypertrophy, urinary retention, angle-closure glaucoma, paralytic ileus, pregnancy
Contra-indications: acute intoxication with CNS depressants; high doses of concomitantly prescribed antipsychotics; acute gout (avoid for 3 weeks after episode resolves), history of nephrolithiasis; breast-feeding

Side-effects: see notes above; constipation, dyspepsia, dry mouth, tachycardia, QT interval prolongation, rhinitis, agitation, anxiety, depression, asthenia, headache, EEG abnormalities, insomnia, drowsiness, hyperthermia or hypothermia, increased salivation, blood dyscrasias (including leucocytosis, leucopenia), raised erythrocyte sedimentation rate, blurred vision, sweating; less frequently anorexia, diarrhoea, nausea and vomiting, abdominal pain, hypertension, influenza-like syndrome, cough, dyspnoea, confusion, convulsions, decreased libido, speech disorder, vertigo, hyperprolactinaemia, anaemia, thrombocythaemia, increased serum creatinine, hypoglycaemia and hyperglycaemia, hyperlipidaemia, hypouricaemia, oedema, thirst, impotence, urinary incontinence, arthralgia, myalgia, conjunctivitis, acne, dry skin, rash; rarely bradycardia, epistaxis, abdominal enlargement, amnesia, ataxia, coma, delirium, hypaesthesia, myoclonus, thrombocytopenia, abnormal ejaculation, urinary retention, menstrual irregularities, myasthenia, alopecia, photosensitivity

Dose: initially 25 mg 3 times daily increased according to response at intervals of 4 days to max. 100 mg 3 times daily; ELDERLY initially 25 mg twice daily increased according to response to max. 75 mg twice daily; CHILD and ADOLESCENT under 18 years not recommended

Zoleptil® (Orion) ▼ PoM

Tablets, s/c, zotepine 25 mg (white), net price 30-tab pack = £14.33, 90-tab pack = £42.98; 50 mg (yellow), 30-tab pack = £19.10, 90-tab pack = £57.30; 100 mg (pink), 30-tab pack = £31.52, 90-tab pack = £94.55. Label: 2

4.2.2   Antipsychotic depot injections

Long-acting depot injections are used for maintenance therapy especially when compliance with oral treatment is unreliable. However, they may give rise to a higher incidence of extrapyramidal reactions than oral preparations.

ADMINISTRATION. Depot antipsychotics are administered by deep intramuscular injection at intervals of 1 to 4 weeks. Patients should first be given a small test-dose as undesirable side-effects are prolonged. In general not more than 2–3 mL of oily injection should be administered at any one site; correct injection technique (including the use of z-track technique) and rotation of injection sites are essential. If the dose needs to be reduced to alleviate side-effects, it is important to recognise that the plasma-drug concentration may not fall for some time after reducing the dose, therefore it may be a month or longer before side-effects subside.

DOSAGE. Individual responses to neuroleptic drugs are very variable and to achieve optimum effect, dosage and dosage interval must be titrated according to the patient's response. For the advice of The Royal College of Psychiatrists on doses above the BNF upper limit, see p. 174

Equivalent doses of depot antipsychotics

These equivalences are intended **only** as an approximate guide; individual dosage instructions should **also** be checked; patients should be carefully monitored after **any** change in medication

Antipsychotic	Dose (mg)	Interval
Flupentixol decanoate	40	2 weeks
Fluphenazine decanoate	25	2 weeks
Haloperidol (as decanoate)	100	4 weeks
Pipotiazine palmitate	50	4 weeks
Zuclopenthixol decanoate	200	2 weeks

Important. These equivalences must **not** be extrapolated beyond the max. dose for the drug

CHOICE. There is no clear-cut division in the use of these drugs, but **zuclopenthixol** may be suitable for the treatment of agitated or aggressive patients whereas **flupentixol** can cause over-excitement in such patients. The incidence of extrapyramidal reactions is similar for all these drugs.

CAUTIONS. See section 4.2.1. Treatment requires careful monitoring for optimum effect. When transferring from oral to depot therapy, dosage by mouth should be reduced gradually.

CONTRA-INDICATIONS. See section 4.2.1. Do not use in children.

SIDE-EFFECTS. See section 4.2.1. Pain may occur at injection site and occasionally erythema, swelling, and nodules. For side-effects of specific antipsychotics see under the relevant drug.

FLUPENTIXOL DECANOATE

(Flupenthixol Decanoate)

Indications: maintenance in schizophrenia and other psychoses

Cautions: see notes on p. 175 and also under Flupentixol (section 4.2.1) and notes above; an alternative antipsychotic may be necessary if symptoms such as aggression or agitation appear

Contra-indications: see notes on p. 175 and also under Flupentixol (section 4.2.1) and notes above

Side-effects: see notes on p. 175 and also under Flupentixol (section 4.2.1) and notes above, but may have a mood elevating effect

Dose: *by deep intramuscular injection* into the gluteal muscle, test dose 20 mg, then after at least 7 days 20–40 mg repeated at intervals of 2–4 weeks, adjusted according to response; max. 400 mg weekly; usual maintenance dose 50 mg every 4 weeks to 300 mg every 2 weeks; ELDERLY initially quarter to half adult dose; CHILD not recommended

Depixol® (Lundbeck) PoM

Injection (oily), flupentixol decanoate 20 mg/mL. Net price 1-mL amp = £1.63; 2-mL amp = £2.73

Depixol Conc.® (Lundbeck) PoM

Injection (oily), flupentixol decanoate 100 mg/mL. Net price 0.5-mL amp = £3.67; 1-mL amp = £6.72

Depixol Low Volume® (Lundbeck) PoM

Injection (oily), flupentixol decanoate 200 mg/mL. Net price 1-mL amp = £20.99

FLUPHENAZINE DECANOATE

Indications: maintenance in schizophrenia and other psychoses

Cautions: see notes on p. 175 and also notes above

Contra-indications: see notes on p. 175 and also notes above

Side-effects: see notes on p. 175 and also under Fluphenazine Hydrochloride (section 4.2.1) and notes above; also extrapyramidal symptoms usually appear a few hours after injection and continue for about 2 days but may be delayed

Dose: *by deep intramuscular injection* into the gluteal muscle, test dose 12.5 mg (6.25 mg in elderly), then after 4–7 days 12.5–100 mg repeated at intervals of 14–35 days, adjusted according to response; CHILD not recommended

Modecate® (Sanofi-Synthelabo) PoM
Injection (oily), fluphenazine decanoate 25 mg/mL. Net price 0.5-mL amp = £1.35; 1-mL amp = £2.35; 1-mL syringe = £2.72; 2-mL amp = £4.62; 2-mL syringe = £4.93; 10-mL vial = £23.45
Excipients: include sesame oil
Note. Fluphenazine decanoate injection also available from Antigen, Faulding DBL, Hillcross—some versions contain sesame oil

Modecate Concentrate® (Sanofi-Synthelabo) PoM
Injection (oily), fluphenazine decanoate 100 mg/mL. Net price 0.5-mL amp = £4.66; 1-mL amp = £9.10
Excipients: include sesame oil
Note. Fluphenazine decanoate injection also available from Antigen, Faulding DBL, Hillcross—at least some versions contain sesame oil

HALOPERIDOL DECANOATE

Indications: maintenance in schizophrenia and other psychoses

Cautions: see notes on p. 175 and also under Haloperidol (section 4.2.1) and notes above

Contra-indications: see notes on p. 175 and also under Haloperidol (section 4.2.1) and notes above

Side-effects: see notes on p. 175 and also under Haloperidol (section 4.2.1) and notes above

Dose: *by deep intramuscular injection* into the gluteal muscle, haloperidol (as decanoate), initially 50 mg every 4 weeks, if necessary increasing by 50-mg increments to 300 mg every 4 weeks; higher doses may be needed in some patients; ELDERLY, initially 12.5–25 mg every 4 weeks; CHILD not recommended
Note. If 2-weekly administration preferred, doses should be halved

Haldol Decanoate® (Janssen-Cilag) PoM
Injection (oily), haloperidol (as decanoate) 50 mg/mL, net price 1-mL amp = £4.35; 100 mg/mL, 1-mL amp = £5.77
Excipients: include sesame oil

PIPOTIAZINE PALMITATE
(Pipothiazine Palmitate)

Indications: maintenance in schizophrenia and other psychoses

Cautions: see notes on p. 175 and notes above

Contra-indications: see notes on p. 175 and notes above

Side-effects: see notes on p. 175 and notes above

Dose: *by deep intramuscular injection* into the gluteal muscle, test dose 25 mg, then a further 25–50 mg after 4–7 days, then adjusted according to response at intervals of 4 weeks; usual maintenance range 50–100 mg (max. 200 mg) every 4 weeks; ELDERLY initially 5–10 mg; CHILD not recommended

Piportil Depot® (JHC) PoM
Injection (oily), pipotiazine palmitate 50 mg/mL. Net price 1-mL amp = £11.31; 2-mL amp = £18.51
Excipients: include sesame oil

ZUCLOPENTHIXOL DECANOATE

Indications: maintenance in schizophrenia and other psychoses, particularly with aggression and agitation

Cautions: see notes on p. 175 and notes above; avoid in porphyria (section 9.8.2)

Contra-indications: see notes on p. 175 and notes above

Side-effects: see notes on p. 175 and notes above

Dose: *by deep intramuscular injection* into the gluteal muscle, test dose 100 mg, followed after at least 7 days by 200–500 mg or more, repeated at intervals of 1–4 weeks, adjusted according to response; max. 600 mg weekly; ELDERLY quarter to half usual starting dose; CHILD not recommended

Clopixol® (Lundbeck) PoM
Injection (oily), zuclopenthixol decanoate 200 mg/mL. Net price 1-mL amp = £3.39

Clopixol Conc.® (Lundbeck) PoM
Injection (oily), zuclopenthixol decanoate 500 mg/mL. Net price 1-mL amp = £8.00

4.2.3   Antimanic drugs

Drugs are used in mania both to control acute attacks and also to prevent their recurrence.

Benzodiazepines

Use of benzodiazepines (section 4.1) may be helpful in the initial stages of treatment until lithium achieves its full effect; they should not be used for long periods because of the risk of dependence.

Antipsychotic drugs

In an acute attack of mania, treatment with an antipsychotic drug (section 4.2.1) is usually required because it may take a few days for lithium to exert its antimanic effect. Lithium may be given concurrently with the antipsychotic drug, and treatment with the antipsychotic gradually tailed off as lithium becomes effective. Alternatively, lithium therapy may be commenced once the patient's mood has been stabilised with the antipsychotic. However, high doses of haloperidol, fluphenazine, or flupentixol may be hazardous when used with lithium; irreversible toxic encephalopathy has been reported.

Carbamazepine

Carbamazepine (section 4.8.1) may be used for the prophylaxis of bipolar disorder (manic-depressive disorder) in patients unresponsive to lithium; it seems to be particularly effective in patients with rapid cycling manic-depressive illness (4 or more affective episodes per year).

Valproic acid

Valproic acid (as the semisodium salt) has recently been licensed for the treatment of manic episodes associated with bipolar disorder. It may be useful in patients unresponsive to lithium. Sodium valproate (section 4.8.1) has also been used, but it is unlicensed for this indication.

VALPROIC ACID

Indications: treatment of manic episodes associated with bipolar disorder
Cautions: see Sodium Valproate (section 4.8.1); monitor closely if dose greater than 45 mg/kg daily
Contra-indications: see Sodium Valproate (section 4.8.1)
Side-effects: see Sodium Valproate (section 4.8.1)
Dose: initially 750 mg daily in 2–3 divided doses, increased according to response, usual dose 1–2 g daily; CHILD and ADOLESCENT under 18 years not recommended

Depakote® (Sanofi-Synthelabo) ▼ PoM
Tablets, e/c, valproic acid (as semisodium valproate) 250 mg, net price 90-tab pack = £43.19; 500 mg, 90-tab pack = £72.19. Label: 25
Note. Semisodium valproate comprises equimolar amounts of sodium valproate and valproic acid.

Lithium

Lithium salts are used in the prophylaxis and treatment of mania, in the prophylaxis of bipolar disorder (manic-depressive disorder) and in the prophylaxis of recurrent depression (unipolar illness or unipolar depression). Lithium is unsuitable for children.

The decision to give prophylactic lithium usually requires *specialist advice*, and must be based on careful consideration of the likelihood of recurrence in the individual patient, and the benefit weighed against the risks. In long-term use lithium has been associated with thyroid disorders and mild cognitive and memory impairment. Long-term treatment should therefore be undertaken only with careful assessment of risk and benefit, and with regular monitoring of thyroid function. The need for continued therapy should be assessed regularly and patients should be maintained on lithium after 3–5 years only if benefit persists.

SERUM CONCENTRATIONS. Lithium salts have a narrow therapeutic/toxic ratio and should therefore not be prescribed unless facilities for monitoring serum-lithium concentrations are available. There seem few if any reasons for preferring one or other of the salts of lithium available. Doses are adjusted to achieve serum-lithium concentration of 0.4–1 mmol/litre (lower end of the range for maintenance therapy and elderly patients) on samples taken 12 hours after the preceding dose. It is important to determine the optimum range for each individual patient.

Overdosage, usually with serum-lithium concentration of over 1.5 mmol/litre, may be fatal and toxic effects include tremor, ataxia, dysarthria, nystagmus, renal impairment, and convulsions. If these potentially hazardous signs occur, treatment should be stopped, serum-lithium concentrations redetermined, and steps taken to reverse lithium toxicity. In mild cases withdrawal of lithium and administration of generous amounts of sodium and fluid will reverse the toxicity. Serum-lithium concentration in excess of 2 mmol/litre require urgent treatment as indicated under Emergency Treatment of Poisoning, p. 26.

INTERACTIONS. Lithium toxicity is made worse by sodium depletion, therefore concurrent use of diuretics (particularly thiazides) is hazardous and should be avoided. For other **interactions** with lithium, see Appendix 1 (lithium).

WITHDRAWAL. While there is no clear evidence of withdrawal or rebound psychosis, abrupt discontinuation of lithium increases the risk of relapse. If lithium is to be discontinued, the dose should be reduced gradually over a period of a few weeks and patients should be warned of possible relapse if discontinued abruptly.

> LITHIUM CARDS. A lithium treatment card available from pharmacies tells patients how to take lithium preparations, what to do if a dose is missed, and what side-effects to expect. It also explains why regular blood tests are important and warns that some medicines and illnesses can change serum-lithium concentration
>
> Cards may be obtained from NPA Services, 38–42 St. Peter's St, St. Albans, Herts AL1 3NP.

LITHIUM CARBONATE

Indications: treatment and prophylaxis of mania, bipolar disorder, and recurrent depression (see also notes above); aggressive or self-mutilating behaviour
Cautions: measure serum-lithium concentration regularly (every 3 months on stabilised regimens), measure thyroid function every 6–12 months on stabilised regimens and advise patient to seek attention if symptoms of hypothyroidism develop (women are at greater risk) e.g. lethargy, feeling cold; maintain adequate sodium and fluid intake; avoid in renal impairment, cardiac disease, and conditions with sodium imbalance such as Addison's disease; reduce dose or discontinue in diarrhoea, vomiting and intercurrent infection (especially if sweating profusely); caution in pregnancy (Appendix 4), breast-feeding, elderly (reduce dose), diuretic treatment, myasthenia gravis; surgery (section 15.1); if possible avoid abrupt withdrawal (see notes above); **interactions:** Appendix 1 (lithium)
COUNSELLING. Patients should maintain an adequate fluid intake and should avoid dietary changes which

might reduce or increase sodium intake; lithium treatment cards are available from pharmacies (see above)

Side-effects: gastro-intestinal disturbances, fine tremor, polyuria and polydipsia; also weight gain and oedema (may respond to dose reduction); signs of intoxication are blurred vision, increasing gastro-intestinal disturbances (anorexia, vomiting, diarrhoea), muscle weakness, increased CNS disturbances (mild drowsiness and sluggishness increasing to giddiness with ataxia, coarse tremor, lack of co-ordination, dysarthria), and require withdrawal of treatment; with severe **overdosage** (serum-lithium concentration above 2 mmol/litre) hyperreflexia and hyperextension of limbs, convulsions, toxic psychoses, syncope, oliguria, circulatory failure, coma, and occasionally, death; goitre, raised antidiuretic hormone concentration, hypothyroidism, hypokalaemia, ECG changes, exacerbation of psoriasis, and kidney changes may also occur; see also Emergency Treatment of Poisoning, p. 26

Dose: see under preparations below, adjusted to achieve a serum-lithium concentration of 0.4–1 mmol/litre 12 hours after a dose on days 4–7 of treatment, then every week until dosage has remained constant for 4 weeks and every 3 months thereafter; doses are initially divided throughout the day, but once daily administration is preferred when serum-lithium concentration stabilised

Note. **Preparations vary widely in bioavailability**; changing the preparation requires the same precautions as initiation of treatment

Note. Lithium carbonate 200 mg ≡ lithium citrate 509 mg

Camcolit® (Norgine) [PoM]
Camcolit 250® tablets, f/c, scored, lithium carbonate 250 mg (Li⁺ 6.8 mmol), net price 20 = 60p. Label: 10 lithium card, counselling, see above
Camcolit 400® tablets, m/r, f/c, scored, lithium carbonate 400 mg (Li⁺ 10.8 mmol), net price 20 = 79p. Label: 10 lithium card, 25, counselling, see above
Dose (serum monitoring, see above):
Treatment, initially 1–1.5 g daily; prophylaxis, initially 300–400 mg daily; CHILD not recommended
Note. Camcolit 400® also available as *Lithonate®* (Berk)

Liskonum® (SmithKline Beecham) [PoM]
Tablets, m/r, f/c, scored, lithium carbonate 450 mg (Li⁺ 12.2 mmol), net price 60-tab pack = £2.82. Label: 10 lithium card, 25, counselling, see above
Dose (serum monitoring, see above):
Treatment, initially 450–675 mg twice daily (elderly initially 225 mg twice daily); prophylaxis, initially 450 mg twice daily (elderly 225 mg twice daily); CHILD not recommended

Priadel® (Sanofi-Synthelabo) [PoM]
Tablets, both m/r, scored, lithium carbonate 200 mg (Li⁺ 5.4 mmol), net price 20 = 50p; 400 mg (Li⁺ 10.8 mmol), 20 = 82p. Label: 10 lithium card, 25, counselling, see above
Dose (serum monitoring, see above):
Treatment and prophylaxis, initially 0.4–1.2 g daily as a single dose or in 2 divided doses (elderly or patients less than 50 kg, 400 mg daily); CHILD not recommended
Liquid, see under Lithium Citrate, below

LITHIUM CITRATE

Indications: see under Lithium Carbonate and notes above

Cautions: see under Lithium Carbonate and notes above

COUNSELLING. Patients should maintain an adequate fluid intake and should avoid dietary changes which might reduce or increase sodium intake; lithium treatment cards are available from pharmacies (see above)

Side-effects: see under Lithium Carbonate and notes above

Dose: see under preparations below, adjusted to achieve serum-lithium concentration of 0.4–1 mmol/litre as described under Lithium Carbonate

Note. **Preparations vary widely in bioavailability**; changing the preparation requires the same precautions as initiation of treatment

Note. Lithium carbonate 200 mg ≡ lithium citrate 509 mg

Li-Liquid® (Rosemont) [PoM]
Oral solution, lithium citrate 509 mg/5 mL (Li⁺ 5.4 mmol/5 mL), yellow, net price 150-mL pack = £6.16; 1.018 g/5 mL (Li⁺ 10.8 mmol/5 mL), orange, 150-mL pack = £12.32. Label: 10 lithium card, counselling, see above
Dose (plasma monitoring, see above):
Treatment and prophylaxis, initially 1.018–3.054 g daily in 2 divided doses (elderly or patients less than 50 kg, initially 509 mg twice daily); CHILD not recommended

Priadel® (Delandale) [PoM]
Tablets, see under Lithium Carbonate, above
Liquid, sugar-free, lithium citrate 520 mg/5 mL (approx. Li⁺ 5.4 mmol/5 mL), net price 150-mL pack = £6.28. Label: 10 lithium card, counselling, see above
Dose (plasma monitoring, see above):
Treatment and prophylaxis, initially 1.04–3.12 g daily in 2 divided doses (elderly or patients less than 50 kg, 520 mg twice daily); CHILD not recommended

4.3 Antidepressant drugs

4.3.1	Tricyclic and related antidepressant drugs
4.3.2	Monoamine-oxidase inhibitors (MAOIs)
4.3.3	Selective serotonin re-uptake inhibitors
4.3.4	Other antidepressant drugs

Antidepressant drugs are effective in the treatment of major depression of moderate and severe degree including major depression associated with physical illness; they are also effective for dysthymia (lower grade chronic depression). Antidepressant drugs are not generally effective in milder forms of acute depression but a trial may be considered in cases refractory to psychological treatments.

CHOICE. The major classes of antidepressants include the tricyclics and related antidepressants, the selective serotonin re-uptake inhibitors (SSRIs), and the monoamine oxidase inhibitors (MAOIs). A number of more recently introduced antidepressants cannot be accommodated easily into this classification; these are included in section 4.3.4.

Choice of antidepressant should be based on the individual patient's requirements, including the presence of concomitant disease, existing therapy, suicide risk, and previous response to antidepressant therapy.

Either tricyclic and related antidepressants or SSRIs are generally preferred because MAOIs may be less effective and show dangerous interactions with some foods and drugs.

Tricyclic antidepressants may be suitable for many depressed patients. If the potential side-effects of the older tricyclics are of concern, an SSRI or one of the newer classes of antidepressants may be appropriate. Although SSRIs appear to be better tolerated than older drugs, the difference is too small to justify always choosing an SSRI as first-line treatment.

Compared to older **tricyclics** (e.g. amitriptyline), the **tricyclic-related drugs** (e.g. trazodone) have a lower incidence of antimuscarinic side-effects, such as dry mouth and constipation. The related tricyclic drugs may also be associated with a lower risk of cardiotoxicity in overdosage, but some have additional side-effects (for further details see section 4.3.1).

The **selective serotonin re-uptake inhibitors** (SSRIs) have fewer antimuscarinic side-effects than the older tricyclics and they are also less cardiotoxic in overdosage. Therefore, although no more effective, they are preferred where there is a significant risk of deliberate overdosing or where concomitant conditions that preclude the use of other antidepressants. The SSRIs do, however, have characteristic side-effects of their own; gastro-intestinal side-effects such as nausea and vomiting are common.

For severely ill inpatients and those in whom maximising efficacy is of overriding importance, a tricyclic may be more effective than an SSRI or an MAOI. Venlafaxine, at a dose of 150 mg or greater, may also be more effective than SSRIs for major depression of at least moderate severity. Where the depression is very severe electroconvulsive therapy (ECT) may be indicated.

MAOIs may be more effective than tricyclics in non-hospitalised patients with 'atypical depression'.

Although anxiety is often present in depressive illness (and may be the presenting symptom), the use of an antipsychotic or an anxiolytic may mask the true diagnosis. Anxiolytics (section 4.1.2) or antipsychotics (section 4.2.1) should therefore be used with caution in depression but they are useful adjuncts in agitated patients.

See also section 4.2.3 for references to the management of bipolar disorders.

St John's wort (*Hypericum perforatum*) is a popular herbal remedy for treating mild depression. However, preparations of St John's wort can induce drug metabolising enzymes and a number of important interactions with conventional drugs have been identified, see Appendix 1 (St John's wort). The amount of active ingredient can vary between different preparations of St John's wort and switching from one to another can change the degree of enzyme induction. Furthermore, when a patient stops taking St John's wort, concentrations of interacting drugs may increase, leading to toxicity. Antidepressants should **not** be used with St John's wort because of the potential for interaction.

> **CSM advice (hyponatraemia).** Hyponatraemia (usually in the elderly and possibly due to inappropriate secretion of antidiuretic hormone) has been associated with all types of antidepressants and should be considered in all patients who develop drowsiness, confusion or convulsions while taking an antidepressant.

MANAGEMENT. Patients should be reviewed every 1–2 weeks at the start of antidepressant treatment. Treatment should be continued for at least 4 weeks (6 weeks in the elderly) before considering whether to switch antidepressant due to lack of efficacy. In cases of partial response, continue for a further 2 weeks (elderly patients may take longer to respond).

Following remission, antidepressant treatment should be continued at the same dose for at least 4–6 months (about 12 months in the elderly). Patients with a history of recurrent depression should continue to receive maintenance treatment (for at least 5 years and possibly indefinitely). Lithium (section 4.2.3) is an effective second-line alternative for maintenance treatment.

Combination of two antidepressants can be dangerous and is rarely justified (except under specialist supervision).

FAILURE TO RESPOND. Failure to respond to an initial course of antidepressant, may necessitate an increase in the dose, switching to a different antidepressant class, or in patients with 'atypical' major depression, the use of an MAOI. Failure to respond to a second antidepressant may require the addition of an augmenting drug such as lithium or liothyronine (specialist use), psychotherapy, or ECT. Lithium or an MAOI should only be initiated by doctors with special experience of these combinations.

WITHDRAWAL. Gastro-intestinal symptoms of nausea, vomiting, and anorexia, accompanied by headache, giddiness, 'chills', and insomnia, and sometimes by hypomania, panic-anxiety, and extreme motor restlessness may occur if an antidepressant (particularly an MAOI) is stopped suddenly after regular administration for 8 weeks or more. The dose should preferably be reduced gradually over about 4 weeks, or longer if withdrawal symptoms emerge (6 months in patients who have been on long-term maintenance treatment). SSRIs have been associated with a specific withdrawal syndrome (section 4.3.3).

ANXIETY. Management of *acute anxiety* generally involves the use of a benzodiazepine or buspirone (section 4.1.2). For *chronic anxiety* (of longer than 4 weeks' duration), it may be appropriate to use an antidepressant before a benzodiazepine. *Generalised anxiety disorder* which does not respond to buspirone or to a benzodiazepine is treated with an antidepressant. Antidepressants such as SSRIs and venlafaxine may be effective in specific anxiety disorders.

Compound preparations of an antidepressant and an anxiolytic are not recommended because it is not possible to adjust the dosage of the individual components separately. Whereas antidepressants are often given continuously over several months, anxiolytics are generally prescribed on a short-term basis.

PANIC DISORDERS. Antidepressants are generally used for *panic disorders* and *phobias*; clomipramine (section 4.3.1) is licensed for *obsessional and phobic states*; paroxetine (section 4.3.3) and moclobemide (section 4.3.2) are licensed for the management of social phobia. However, in panic disorders (with or without agaraphobia) resistant to antidepressant therapy, a benzodiazepine may be considered (section 4.1.2).

4.3.1 Tricyclic and related antidepressant drugs

This section covers tricyclic antidepressants and also 1-, 2-, and 4-ring structured drugs with broadly similar properties.

These drugs are most effective for treating moderate to severe *endogenous depression* associated with psychomotor and physiological changes such as loss of appetite and sleep disturbances; improvement in sleep is usually the first benefit of therapy. Since there may be an interval of 2 weeks before the antidepressant action takes place electroconvulsive treatment may be required in severe depression when delay is hazardous or intolerable.

Some tricyclic antidepressants are also effective in the management of *panic disorder*.

For reference to the role of some tricyclic antidepressants in some forms of *neuralgia*, see section 4.7.3, and in *nocturnal enuresis* in children, see section 7.4.2.

DOSAGE. About 10 to 20% of patients fail to respond to tricyclic and related antidepressant drugs and inadequate dosage may account for some of these failures. It is important to use doses that are sufficiently high for effective treatment but not so high as to cause toxic effects. Low doses should be used for initial treatment in the **elderly** (see under Side-effects, below).

In most patients the long half-life of tricyclic antidepressant drugs allows **once-daily** administration, usually at night; the use of modified-release preparations is therefore unnecessary.

CHOICE. Tricyclic and related antidepressant drugs can be roughly divided into those with additional sedative properties and those which are less so. Agitated and anxious patients tend to respond best to the sedative compounds whereas withdrawn and apathetic patients will often obtain most benefit from the less sedating ones. Those with **sedative** properties include amitriptyline, clomipramine, dosulepin (dothiepin), doxepin, maprotiline, mianserin, trazodone, and trimipramine. Those with **less sedative** properties include amoxapine, imipramine, lofepramine, and nortriptyline.

Imipramine and **amitriptyline** are well established and relatively safe and effective, but nevertheless have more marked antimuscarinic and cardiac side-effects than compounds such as **doxepin, mianserin, trazodone,** and **viloxazine**; this may be important in individual patients. **Lofepramine** also has a lower incidence of antimuscarinic and sedative side-effects and is less dangerous in overdosage; it is, however, infrequently associated with hepatic toxicity. **Amox-**

apine is related to the antipsychotic loxapine and its side-effects include tardive dyskinesia.

For a comparison of tricyclic and related antidepressants with SSRIs and related antidepressants and MAOIs, see section 4.3.

SIDE-EFFECTS. *Arrhythmias* and *heart block* occasionally follow the use of tricyclic antidepressants, particularly amitriptyline, and may be a factor in the sudden death of patients with cardiac disease. They are also sometimes associated with *convulsions* (and should be prescribed with special caution in epilepsy as they lower the convulsive threshold); maprotiline has particularly been associated with convulsions. *Hepatic* and *haematological* reactions may occur and have been particularly associated with mianserin.

Other side-effects of tricyclic and related antidepressants include *drowsiness, dry mouth, blurred vision, constipation,* and *urinary retention* (all attributed to antimuscarinic activity), and sweating. The patient should be encouraged to persist with treatment as some tolerance to these side-effects seems to develop. They are reduced if low doses are given initially and then gradually increased, but this must be balanced against the need to obtain a full therapeutic effect as soon as possible. Gradual introduction of treatment is particularly important in the elderly, who, because of the hypotensive effects of these drugs, are prone to attacks of *dizziness* or even *syncope*. Another side-effect to which the elderly are particularly susceptible is *hyponatraemia* (see CSM advice on p. 188).

Neuroleptic malignant syndrome (section 4.2.1) may, very rarely, arise in the course of antidepressant treatment.

Limited quantities of tricyclic antidepressants should be prescribed at any one time because they are dangerous in overdosage. For advice on **overdosage** see Emergency Treatment of Poisoning, p. 25.

WITHDRAWAL. If possible tricyclic and related antidepressants should be withdrawn slowly (see also section 4.3).

INTERACTIONS. A tricyclic or related antidepressant (or an SSRI or related antidepressant) should not be started until 2 weeks after stopping an MAOI (3 weeks if starting clomipramine or imipramine). Conversely, an MAOI should not be started until at least 7–14 days after a tricyclic or related antidepressant (3 weeks in the case of clomipramine or imipramine) has been stopped. For guidance relating to the reversible monoamine oxidase inhibitor, moclobemide, see p. 194. For other tricyclic antidepressant **interactions**, see Appendix 1 (antidepressants, tricyclic).

Tricyclic antidepressants

AMITRIPTYLINE HYDROCHLORIDE

Indications: depressive illness, particularly where sedation is required; nocturnal enuresis in children (section 7.4.2)

Cautions: cardiac disease (particularly with arrhythmias, see Contra-indications below), history of epilepsy, pregnancy and breast-feeding (Appendixes 4 and 5), elderly, hepatic impairment (avoid if severe), thyroid disease, phaeochromocytoma, history of mania, psychoses (may aggravate psychotic symptoms), angle-closure glaucoma, history of urinary retention, concurrent electroconvulsive therapy; if possible avoid abrupt withdrawal; anaesthesia (increased risk of arrhythmias and hypotension, see surgery section 15.1); porphyria (section 9.8.2); see section 7.4.2 for additional nocturnal enuresis warnings; **interactions:** Appendix 1 (antidepressants, tricyclic)

DRIVING. Drowsiness may affect performance of skilled tasks (e.g. driving); effects of alcohol enhanced

Contra-indications: recent myocardial infarction, arrhythmias (particularly heart block), not indicated in manic phase, severe liver disease

Side-effects: dry mouth, sedation, blurred vision (disturbance of accommodation, increased intraocular pressure), constipation, nausea, difficulty with micturition; cardiovascular side-effects (such as ECG changes, arrhythmias, postural hypotension, tachycardia, syncope, particularly with high doses); sweating, tremor, rashes and hypersensitivity reactions (including urticaria, photosensitivity), behavioural disturbances (particularly children), hypomania or mania, confusion (particularly elderly), interference with sexual function, blood sugar changes; increased appetite and weight gain (occasionally weight loss); endocrine side-effects such as testicular enlargement, gynaecomastia, galactorrhoea; also convulsions (see Cautions), movement disorders and dyskinesias, fever, agranulocytosis, leucopenia, eosinophilia, purpura, thrombocytopenia, hyponatraemia (may be due to inappropriate antidiuretic hormone secretion) see CSM advice, p. 188, abnormal liver function tests (jaundice); for a general outline of side-effects see also notes above; **overdosage:** see Emergency Treatment of Poisoning, p. 25

Dose: depression, initially 75 mg (elderly and adolescents 30–75 mg) daily in divided doses *or* as a single dose at bedtime increased gradually as necessary to 150–200 mg; CHILD under 16 years not recommended for depression

Nocturnal enuresis, CHILD 7–10 years 10–20 mg, 11–16 years 25–50 mg at night; max. period of treatment (including gradual withdrawal) 3 months—full physical examination before further course

Amitriptyline (Non-proprietary) PoM

Tablets, coated, amitriptyline hydrochloride 10 mg, net price 20 = 56p; 25 mg, 20 = 57p; 50 mg, 20 = 86p. Label: 2

Available from Alpharma, APS, DDSA (*Elavil®*)

Oral solution, amitriptyline (as hydrochloride) 25 mg/5 mL, net price 200 mL = £16.53; 50 mg/ 5 mL, 200 mL = £18.00. Label: 2

Available from Rosemont (sugar-free)

Lentizol® (Parke-Davis) PoM ◪

Capsules, m/r, both enclosing white pellets, amitriptyline hydrochloride 25 mg (pink), net price 56-cap pack = £2.58; 50 mg (pink/red), 56-cap pack = £4.79. Label: 2, 25

■ Compound preparations

Triptafen® (Goldshield) PoM ◪

Tablets, pink, s/c, amitriptyline hydrochloride 25 mg, perphenazine 2 mg. Net price 20 = £4.25. Label: 2

Triptafen-M® (Goldshield) PoM ◪

Tablets, pink, s/c, amitriptyline hydrochloride 10 mg, perphenazine 2 mg. Net price 20 = £3.80. Label: 2

◪ denotes preparations that are considered to be less suitable for prescribing (see p. vi)

AMOXAPINE

Indications: depressive illness

Cautions: see under Amitriptyline Hydrochloride

Contra-indications: see under Amitriptyline Hydrochloride

Side-effects: see under Amitriptyline Hydrochloride; tardive dyskinesia reported; menstrual irregularities, breast enlargement, and galactorrhoea reported in women

Dose: initially 100–150 mg daily in divided doses *or* as a single dose at bedtime increased as necessary to max. 300 mg daily; ELDERLY initially 25 mg twice daily increased as necessary after 5–7 days to max. 50 mg 3 times daily; CHILD under 16 years not recommended

Asendis® (Lederle) PoM

Tablets, amoxapine 50 mg (orange, scored), net price 84-tab pack = £16.78; 100 mg (blue, scored), 56-tab pack = £18.65. Label: 2

CLOMIPRAMINE HYDROCHLORIDE

Indications: depressive illness, phobic and obsessional states; adjunctive treatment of cataplexy associated with narcolepsy

Cautions: see under Amitriptyline Hydrochloride

Contra-indications: see under Amitriptyline Hydrochloride

Side-effects: see under Amitriptyline Hydrochloride

Dose: *by mouth*, initially 10 mg daily, increased gradually as necessary to 30–150 mg daily in divided doses *or* as a single dose at bedtime; max. 250 mg daily; ELDERLY initially 10 mg daily increased carefully over approx. 10 days to 30–75 mg daily; CHILD not recommended

Phobic and obsessional states, initially 25 mg daily (ELDERLY 10 mg daily) increased over 2 weeks to 100–150 mg daily; CHILD not recommended

Adjunctive treatment of cataplexy associated with narcolepsy, initially 10 mg daily gradually increased until satisfactory response (range 10–75 mg daily)

By intramuscular injection, initially 25–50 mg daily, increased by 25 mg daily to 100–150 mg daily; CHILD not recommended

By intravenous infusion (careful monitoring) initially to assess tolerance, 25–50 mg, then increase by 25 mg daily to usual dose of 100 mg daily for 7–10 days—see product literature for details; CHILD not recommended

Clomipramine (Non-proprietary) [PoM]

Capsules, clomipramine hydrochloride 10 mg, net price 28-cap pack = £1.21; 25 mg, 28-cap pack = £1.93; 50 mg, 28-cap pack = £2.42. Label: 2

Available from Alpharma, APS, Generics, Hillcross, IVAX

Anafranil® (Cephalon) [PoM]

Capsules, clomipramine hydrochloride 10 mg (yellow/caramel), net price 84-cap pack = £3.23; 25 mg (orange/caramel), 84-cap pack = £6.35; 50 mg (grey/caramel), 56-cap pack = £8.06. Label: 2

Injection, clomipramine hydrochloride 12.5 mg/mL. Net price 2-mL amp = 56p

Anafranil SR® (Cephalon) [PoM] [image]

Tablets, m/r, grey-red, f/c, clomipramine hydrochloride 75 mg. Net price 28-tab pack = £8.83. Label: 2, 25

DOSULEPIN HYDROCHLORIDE/ DOTHIEPIN HYDROCHLORIDE

Indications: depressive illness, particularly where sedation is required

Cautions: see under Amitriptyline Hydrochloride

Contra-indications: see under Amitriptyline Hydrochloride

Side-effects: see under Amitriptyline Hydrochloride

Dose: initially 75 mg (ELDERLY 50–75 mg) daily in divided doses *or* as a single dose at bedtime, increased gradually as necessary to 150 mg daily (ELDERLY 75 mg may be sufficient); up to 225 mg daily in some circumstances (e.g. hospital use); CHILD not recommended

Dosulepin/Dothiepin (Non-proprietary) [PoM]

Capsules, dosulepin hydrochloride 25 mg, net price 20 = 72p. Label: 2

Available from Alpharma, APS, Ashbourne (*Dothapax®*), Berk (*Prepadine®*), Generics, Hillcross, IVAX, Kent, Lagap, Sanofi-Synthelabo, Sovereign, Sterwin

Tablets, dosulepin hydrochloride 75 mg, net price 28-tab pack = £2.78. Label: 2

Available from Alpharma, APS, Ashbourne (*Dothapax®*), Berk (*Prepadine®*), Generics, Hillcross, IVAX, Kent, Lagap, Sanofi-Synthelabo, Sovereign, Sterwin

Prothiaden® (Abbott) [PoM]

Capsules, red/red-brown, dosulepin hydrochloride 25 mg. Net price 20 = £1.26. Label: 2

Tablets, red, s/c, dosulepin hydrochloride 75 mg. Net price 28-tab pack = £4.20. Label: 2

DOXEPIN

Indications: depressive illness, particularly where sedation is required; skin (section 13.3)

Cautions: see under Amitriptyline Hydrochloride

Contra-indications: see under Amitriptyline Hydrochloride; breast-feeding (Appendix 5)

Side-effects: see under Amitriptyline Hydrochloride

Dose: initially 75 mg daily in divided doses *or* as a single dose at bedtime, increased as necessary to max. 300 mg daily in 3 divided doses (up to 100 mg may be given as a single dose); ELDERLY initially 10–50 mg daily, range of 30–50 mg daily may be adequate; CHILD not recommended

Sinequan® (Pfizer) [PoM]

Capsules, doxepin (as hydrochloride) 10 mg (orange), net price 56-cap pack = £1.21; 25 mg (orange/blue), 28-cap pack = 87p; 50 mg (blue), 28-cap pack = £1.43; 75 mg (yellow/blue), 28-cap pack = £2.26. Label: 2

IMIPRAMINE HYDROCHLORIDE

Indications: depressive illness; nocturnal enuresis in children (see section 7.4.2)

Cautions: see under Amitriptyline Hydrochloride

Contra-indications: see under Amitriptyline Hydrochloride

Side-effects: see under Amitriptyline Hydrochloride, but less sedating

Dose: depression, initially up to 75 mg daily in divided doses increased gradually to 150–200 mg (up to 300 mg in hospital patients); up to 150 mg may be given as a single dose at bedtime; ELDERLY initially 10 mg daily, increased gradually to 30–50 mg daily; CHILD not recommended for depression

Nocturnal enuresis, CHILD 7 years 25 mg, 8–11 years 25–50 mg, over 11 years 50–75 mg at bedtime; max. period of treatment (including gradual withdrawal) 3 months—full physical examination before further course

Imipramine (Non-proprietary) [PoM]

Tablets, coated, imipramine hydrochloride 10 mg, net price 20 = 61p; 25 mg, 20 = 72p. Label: 2

Tofranil® (Novartis) [PoM]

Tablets, red-brown, s/c, imipramine hydrochloride 25 mg, net price 84-tab pack = £3.66. Label: 2

Syrup, imipramine hydrochloride 25 mg/5 mL. Net price 150-mL pack = £3.73. Label: 2

LOFEPRAMINE

Indications: depressive illness

Cautions: see under Amitriptyline Hydrochloride

Contra-indications: see under Amitriptyline Hydrochloride; hepatic and severe renal impairment

Side-effects: see under Amitriptyline Hydrochloride, but less sedating, lower incidence of antimuscarinic effects and less dangerous in overdosage; hepatic disorders reported

Dose: 140–210 mg daily in divided doses; ELDERLY may respond to lower doses; CHILD not recommended

Lofepramine (Non-proprietary) [PoM]

Tablets, lofepramine 70 mg (as hydrochloride). Net price 56-tab pack = £10.19. Label: 2

Available from Alpharma, Ashbourne (*Feprapax®*), Hillcross, Lagap, Sterwin

Oral suspension, lofepramine 70 mg/5 mL (as hydrochloride). Net price 150 mL = £23.64. Label: 2

Available from Rosemont (*Lomont®*, sugar-free)

Gamanil® (Merck) [PoM]

Tablets, f/c, brown-violet, lofepramine 70 mg (as hydrochloride). Net price 56-tab pack = £9.84. Label: 2

NORTRIPTYLINE

Indications: depressive illness; nocturnal enuresis in children (section 7.4.2)

Cautions: see under Amitriptyline Hydrochloride; manufacturer advises plasma-nortriptyline concentration monitoring if dose above 100 mg daily, but evidence of practical value uncertain

Contra-indications: see under Amitriptyline Hydrochloride

Side-effects: see under Amitriptyline Hydrochloride, but less sedating

Dose: depression, low dose initially increased as necessary to 75–100 mg daily in divided doses *or* as a single dose (max. 150 mg daily); ADOLESCENT and ELDERLY 30–50 mg daily in divided doses; CHILD not recommended for depression
Nocturnal enuresis, CHILD 7 years 10 mg, 8–11 years 10–20 mg, over 11 years 25–35 mg, at night; max period of treatment (including gradual withdrawal) 3 months—full physical examination and ECG before further course

Allegron® (Dista) PoM
Tablets, nortriptyline (as hydrochloride) 10 mg, net price 20 = £2.48; 25 mg (orange, scored), 20 = £5.04. Label: 2

■ Compound preparations

Motipress® (Sanofi-Synthelabo) PoM [image]
Tablets, yellow, s/c, fluphenazine hydrochloride 1.5 mg, nortriptyline 30 mg (as hydrochloride). Net price 28-tab pack = £2.83. Label: 2

Motival® (Sanofi-Synthelabo) PoM [image]
Tablets, pink, s/c, fluphenazine hydrochloride 500 micrograms, nortriptyline 10 mg (as hydrochloride). Net price 20 = 67p. Label: 2

> [image] denotes preparations that are considered to be less suitable for prescribing (see p. vi)

TRIMIPRAMINE

Indications: depressive illness, particularly where sedation required

Cautions: see under Amitriptyline Hydrochloride

Contra-indications: see under Amitriptyline Hydrochloride

Side-effects: see under Amitriptyline Hydrochloride

Dose: initially 50–75 mg daily in divided doses *or* as a single dose at bedtime, increased as necessary to 150–300 mg daily; ELDERLY initially 10–25 mg 3 times daily, maintenance half adult dose may be sufficient; CHILD not recommended

Surmontil® (Aventis Pharma) PoM
Capsules, green/white, trimipramine 50 mg (as maleate). Net price 28-cap pack = £8.51. Label: 2
Tablets, trimipramine (as maleate) 10 mg, net price 28-tab pack = £3.84, 84-tab pack = £11.49; 25 mg, 28-tab pack = £5.06, 84-tab pack = £15.16. Label: 2

Related antidepressants

MAPROTILINE HYDROCHLORIDE

Indications: depressive illness, particularly where sedation is required

Cautions: see under Amitriptyline Hydrochloride

Contra-indications: see under Amitriptyline Hydrochloride; history of epilepsy

Side-effects: see under Amitriptyline Hydrochloride, antimuscarinic effects may occur less frequently but rashes common and increased risk of convulsions at higher dosage

Dose: initially 25–75 mg (elderly 30 mg) daily in 3 divided doses *or* as a single dose at bedtime, increased gradually as necessary to max. 150 mg daily; CHILD not recommended

Ludiomil® (Novartis) PoM
Tablets, all f/c, maprotiline hydrochloride 10 mg (pale yellow), net price 30-tab pack = £1.26; 25 mg (greyish-red), 28-tab pack = £2.53; 50 mg (light orange), 28-tab pack = £5.02; 75 mg (brownish-orange), 28-tab pack = £7.46. Label: 2
Excipients: include gluten

MIANSERIN HYDROCHLORIDE

Indications: depressive illness, particularly where sedation is required

Cautions: see under Amitriptyline Hydrochloride; **interactions:** Appendix 1 (mianserin)
BLOOD COUNTS. A full **blood count** is recommended every 4 weeks during the first 3 months of treatment; clinical monitoring should continue subsequently and treatment should be stopped and a full blood count obtained if *fever, sore throat, stomatitis,* or other signs of infection develop.

Contra-indications: see under Amitriptyline Hydrochloride

Side-effects: see under Amitriptyline Hydrochloride, fewer and milder antimuscarinic and cardiovascular effects; leucopenia, agranulocytosis and aplastic anaemia (particularly in the elderly); jaundice; arthritis, arthralgia

Dose: initially 30–40 mg (elderly 30 mg) daily in divided doses *or* as a single dose at bedtime, increased gradually as necessary; usual dose range 30–90 mg; CHILD not recommended

Mianserin (Non-proprietary) PoM
Tablets, mianserin hydrochloride 10 mg, net price 20 = £1.94; 20 mg, 20 = £2.97; 30 mg, 20 = £3.44. Label: 2, 25
Available from Alpharma, IVAX

TRAZODONE HYDROCHLORIDE

Indications: depressive illness, particularly where sedation is required; anxiety

Cautions: see under Amitriptyline Hydrochloride; **interactions:** Appendix 1 (trazodone)

Contra-indications: see under Amitriptyline Hydrochloride

Side-effects: see under Amitriptyline Hydrochloride but fewer antimuscarinic and cardiovascular effects; rarely priapism (discontinue immediately)

Dose: depression, initially 150 mg (elderly 100 mg) daily in divided doses after food *or* as a single dose at bedtime; may be increased to

300 mg daily; hospital patients up to max. 600 mg daily in divided doses

Anxiety, 75 mg daily, increasing if necessary to 300 mg daily

CHILD not recommended

Trazodone (Non-proprietary) PoM
Capsules, trazodone hydrochloride 50 mg, net price 84-cap pack = £17.12; 100 mg, 56-cap pack = £20.07. Label: 2, 21
Available from APS, Generics
Tablets, trazodone hydrochloride 150 mg, net price 28-tab pack = £11.44. Label: 2, 21
Available from APS, Generics

Molipaxin® (Hoechst Marion Roussel) PoM
Capsules, trazodone hydrochloride 50 mg (violet/green), net price 84-cap pack = £19.04; 100 mg (violet/fawn), 56-cap pack = £22.42. Label: 2, 21
Tablets, pink, f/c, trazodone hydrochloride 150 mg. Net price 28-tab pack = £12.78. Label: 2, 21
Liquid, sugar-free, trazodone hydrochloride 50 mg/5 mL, net price 120 mL = £8.51. Label: 2, 21

4.3.2 Monoamine-oxidase inhibitors
(MAOIs)

Monoamine-oxidase inhibitors are used much less frequently than tricyclic and related antidepressants, or SSRIs and related antidepressants because of the dangers of dietary and drug interactions and the fact that it is easier to prescribe MAOIs when tricyclic antidepressants have been unsuccessful than vice versa. **Tranylcypromine** is the most **hazardous** of the MAOIs because of its stimulant action. The drugs of choice are **phenelzine** or **isocarboxazid** which are less stimulant and therefore safer.

Phobic patients and depressed patients with atypical, hypochondriacal, or hysterical features are said to respond best to MAOIs. However, MAOIs should be tried in any patients who are refractory to treatment with other antidepressants as there is occasionally a dramatic response. Response to treatment may be delayed for 3 weeks or more and may take an additional 1 or 2 weeks to become maximal.

WITHDRAWAL. If possible MAOIs should be withdrawn slowly (see also section 4.3).

INTERACTIONS. MAOIs inhibit monoamine oxidase, thereby causing an accumulation of amine neurotransmitters. The metabolism of some amine drugs such as *indirect-acting sympathomimetics* (present in many cough and decongestant preparations, see section 3.10) is also inhibited and their pressor action may be potentiated; the pressor effect of tyramine (in some foods, such as cheese, pickled herring, broad bean pods, and *Bovril®*, *Oxo®*, *Marmite®* or any similar meat or yeast extract or fermented soya bean extract) may also be dangerously potentiated. These interactions may cause a dangerous rise in blood pressure. An early warning symptom may be a throbbing headache. Patients should be advised to eat only fresh foods and avoid food that is suspected of being stale or 'going off'. This

is especially important with meat, fish, poultry or offal; game should be avoided. The danger of interaction persists for up to 2 weeks after treatment with MAOIs is discontinued. Patients should also avoid alcoholic drinks or de-alcoholised (low alcohol) drinks.

Other antidepressants should **not** be started for 2 weeks after treatment with MAOIs has been stopped (3 weeks if starting clomipramine or imipramine). Some psychiatrists use selected tricyclics in conjunction with MAOIs but this is hazardous, indeed potentially lethal, except in experienced hands and there is no evidence that the combination is more effective than when either constituent is used alone. The combination of tranylcypromine with clomipramine is particularly **dangerous**.

Conversely, an MAOI should not be started until at least 7–14 days after a tricyclic or related antidepressant (3 weeks in the case of clomipramine or imipramine) has been stopped.

In addition, an MAOI should not be started for at least 2 weeks after a previous MAOI has been stopped (then started at a reduced dose).

For other interactions with MAOIs including those with opioid analgesics (notably pethidine), see Appendix 1 (MAOIs). For guidance on interactions relating to the reversible monoamine oxidase inhibitor, moclobemide, see p. 194; for guidance on interactions relating to SSRIs, see p. 195.

PHENELZINE

Indications: depressive illness

Cautions: diabetes mellitus, cardiovascular disease, epilepsy, blood disorders, concurrent electroconvulsive therapy; elderly (great caution); monitor blood pressure (risk of postural hypotension and hypertensive responses—discontinue if palpitations or frequent headaches); if possible avoid abrupt withdrawal; severe hypertensive reactions to certain drugs and foods; avoid in agitated patients; porphyria (section 9.8.2); pregnancy and breast-feeding; surgery (section 15.1); **interactions:** Appendix 1 (MAOIs)
DRIVING. Drowsiness may affect performance of skilled tasks (e.g. driving)

Contra-indications: hepatic impairment or abnormal liver function tests (Appendix 2), cerebrovascular disease, phaeochromocytoma; not indicated in manic phase

Side-effects: commonly postural hypotension (especially in elderly) and dizziness; less common side-effects include drowsiness, insomnia, headache, weakness and fatigue, dry mouth, constipation and other gastro-intestinal disturbances, oedema, myoclonic movement, hyperreflexia, elevated liver enzymes; agitation and tremors, nervousness, euphoria, arrhythmias, blurred vision, nystagmus, difficulty in micturition, sweating, convulsions, rashes, purpura, leucopenia, sexual disturbances, and weight gain with inappropriate appetite may also occur; psychotic episodes with hypomanic behaviour, confusion, and hallucinations, may be induced in susceptible persons; jaundice has been reported and, on rare occasions, fatal progressive hepatocellular necrosis; paraesthesia, peripheral neuritis, peripheral neuropathy may be due to pyridoxine deficiency;

for CSM advice on possible hyponatraemia, see p. 188 (hypernatraemia also reported)

Dose: 15 mg 3 times daily, increased if necessary to 4 times daily after 2 weeks (hospital patients, max. 30 mg 3 times daily), then reduced gradually to lowest possible maintenance dose (15 mg on alternate days may be adequate); CHILD not recommended

Nardil® (Hansam) PoM [symbol]
Tablets, orange, f/c, phenelzine 15 mg (as sulphate). Net price 20 = £3.99. Label: 3, 10 patient information leaflet

ISOCARBOXAZID [symbol]

Indications: depressive illness
Cautions: see under Phenelzine
Contra-indications: see under Phenelzine
Side-effects: see under Phenelzine
Dose: initially 30 mg daily in single or divided doses until improvement occurs (increased after 4 weeks if necessary to max. 60 mg daily for 4–6 weeks under close supervision), then reduced to usual maintenance dose 10–20 mg daily (but up to 40 mg daily may be required); ELDERLY 5–10 mg daily; CHILD not recommended

Isocarboxazid (Cambridge) PoM [symbol]
Tablets, pink, scored, isocarboxazid 10 mg. Net price 50 = £24.29. Label: 3, 10 patient information leaflet

TRANYLCYPROMINE [symbol]

Indications: depressive illness
Cautions: see under Phenelzine
Contra-indications: see under Phenelzine; hyperthyroidism
Side-effects: see under Phenelzine; insomnia if given in evening; hypertensive crises with throbbing headache requiring discontinuation of treatment more frequent than with other MAOIs; liver damage less frequent than with phenelzine
Dose: initially 10 mg twice daily not later than 3 p.m., increasing the second daily dose to 20 mg after 1 week if necessary; doses above 30 mg daily under close supervision only; usual maintenance dose 10 mg daily; CHILD not recommended

Parnate® (Goldshield) PoM [symbol]
Tablets, red, s/c, tranylcypromine 10 mg (as sulphate). Net price 28-tab pack = £1.27. Label: 3, 10 patient information leaflet

> [symbol] denotes preparations that are considered to be less suitable for prescribing (see p. vi)

Reversible MAOIs

Moclobemide is indicated for major depression and social phobia; it is reported to act by reversible inhibition of monoamine oxidase type A (it is therefore termed a RIMA). It should be reserved as a second-line treatment.

INTERACTIONS. Moclobemide is claimed to cause less potentiation of the pressor effect of tyramine than the traditional (irreversible) MAOIs, but patients should avoid consuming large amounts of tyramine-rich food (such as mature cheese, yeast extracts and fermented soya bean products).

The risk of drug interactions is also claimed to be less but patients still need to avoid sympathomimetics such as ephedrine, pseudoephedrine, and phenylpropanolamine. In addition, moclobemide should not be given with another antidepressant. Owing to its short duration of action no treatment-free period is required after it has been stopped but it should not be started until at least a week after a tricyclic or related antidepressant or an SSRI or related antidepressant has been stopped (2 weeks in the case of paroxetine and sertraline, and at least 5 weeks in the case of fluoxetine), or for at least a week after an MAOI has been stopped. For other interactions, see Appendix 1 (moclobemide).

MOCLOBEMIDE

Indications: depressive illness; social phobia
Cautions: avoid in agitated or excited patients (or give with sedative for up to 2–3 weeks), thyrotoxicosis, hepatic impairment (Appendix 2), may provoke manic episodes in bipolar disorders, pregnancy and breast-feeding (patient information leaflet advises avoid); **interactions:** see notes above and Appendix 1 (moclobemide)
Contra-indications: acute confusional states, phaeochromocytoma
Side-effects: sleep disturbances, dizziness, gastrointestinal disorders, headache, restlessness, agitation; paraesthesia, dry mouth, visual disturbances, oedema, skin reactions, confusional states reported; rarely raised liver enzymes, galactorrhoea; for CSM advice on possible hyponatraemia, see p. 188
Dose: depression, initially 300 mg daily usually in divided doses after food, adjusted according to response; usual range 150–600 mg daily; CHILD not recommended
Social phobia, initially 300 mg daily increased on fourth day to 600 mg daily in 2 divided doses, continued for 8–12 weeks to assess efficacy; CHILD not recommended

Manerix® (Roche) PoM
Tablets, yellow, f/c, scored, moclobemide 150 mg, net price 30-tab pack = £10.03; 300 mg, 30-tab pack = £15.04. Label: 10 patient information leaflet, 21

4.3.3 Selective serotonin re-uptake inhibitors

Citalopram, fluoxetine, fluvoxamine, paroxetine, and **sertraline** selectively inhibit the re-uptake of serotonin (5-hydroxytryptamine, 5-HT); they are termed selective serotonin re-uptake inhibitors (SSRIs). For a general comment on the management of depression and on the comparison between *tricyclic and related antidepressants* and the *SSRIs and related antidepressants*, see section 4.3.

CAUTIONS. SSRIs should be used with caution in patients with epilepsy (avoid if poorly controlled, discontinue if convulsions develop), concurrent electroconvulsive therapy (prolonged seizures reported with fluoxetine), history of mania, cardiac disease, diabetes mellitus, angle-closure glaucoma, history of bleeding disorders (especially gastro-intestinal bleeding), hepatic and renal impairment (Appendixes 2 and 3), pregnancy and breast-feeding (Appendixes 4 and 5). SSRIs may also impair performance of skilled tasks (e.g. driving). Abrupt withdrawal of SSRIs should be avoided (associated with headache, nausea, paraesthesia, dizziness and anxiety); **interactions:** see below and Appendix 1 (antidepressants, SSRI).

INTERACTIONS. An SSRI or related antidepressant should not be started until 2 weeks after stopping an MAOI. Conversely, an MAOI should not be started until at least a week after an SSRI or related antidepressant has been stopped (2 weeks in the case of paroxetine and sertraline, at least 5 weeks in the case of fluoxetine). For guidance relating to the reversible monoamine oxidase inhibitor, moclobemide, see above. For other SSRI antidepressant interactions, see Appendix 1 (antidepressants, SSRI).

CONTRA-INDICATIONS. SSRIs should not be used if the patient enters a manic phase.

SIDE-EFFECTS. SSRIs are less sedating and have fewer antimuscarinic and cardiotoxic effects than tricyclic antidepressants (section 4.3). Side-effects of the SSRIs include gastro-intestinal effects (dose-related and fairly common—include nausea, vomiting, dyspepsia, abdominal pain, diarrhoea, constipation), anorexia with weight loss (increased appetite and weight gain also reported) and hypersensitivity reactions including rash (consider discontinuation—may be sign of impending serious systemic reaction, possibly associated with vasculitis), urticaria, angioedema, anaphylaxis, arthralgia, myalgia and photosensitivity; other side-effects include dry mouth, nervousness, anxiety, headache, insomnia, tremor, dizziness, asthenia, hallucinations, drowsiness, convulsions (see Cautions above), galactorrhoea, sexual dysfunction, urinary retention, sweating, hypomania or mania (see Cautions above), movement disorders and dyskinesias, visual disturbances, hyponatraemia (may be due to inappropriate antidiuretic hormone secretion—see CSM warning, section 4.3), and cutaneous bleeding disorders including ecchymoses and purpura. Suicidal ideation has been linked with SSRIs but causality has not been established.

CITALOPRAM

Indications: depressive illness, panic disorder
Cautions: see notes above
Contra-indications: see notes above
Side-effects: see notes above; palpitations, tachycardia, postural hypotension, coughing, yawning, confusion, impaired concentration, amnesia, migraine, paraesthesia, taste disturbance, increased salivation, rhinitis, tinnitus, micturition disorders also reported
Dose: see preparations below

Cipramil® (Lundbeck) PoM
Tablets, f/c, citalopram (as hydrobromide) 10 mg, net price 28-tab pack = £9.64; 20 mg (scored), 28-tab pack = £16.03; 40 mg, 28-tab pack = £27.10. Counselling, driving
Dose: depressive illness, 20 mg daily as a single dose in the morning or evening increased if necessary to max.

60 mg daily (ELDERLY max. 40 mg daily); CHILD not recommended
Panic disorder, initially 10 mg daily increased to 20 mg after 7 days, usual dose 20–30 mg daily; max. 60 mg daily (ELDERLY max. 40 mg daily); CHILD not recommended
Oral drops, sugar-free, citalopram (as hydrochloride) 40 mg/mL, net price 15 mL = £21.68. Counselling, driving, administration
Dose: depressive illness, 16 mg daily as a single dose in the morning or evening increased if necessary to max. 48 mg daily (ELDERLY max. 32 mg daily); CHILD not recommended
Panic disorder, initially 8 mg daily as a single dose increased to 16 mg daily after 7 days, usual dose 16–24 mg daily; max. 48 mg daily; (ELDERLY max. 32 mg daily); CHILD not recommended
Excipients: include alcohol
Note. 8 mg (4 drops) *Cipramil®* oral drops may be considered to be equivalent in therapeutic effect to 10-mg *Cipramil®* tablet
Mix with water, orange juice, or apple juice before taking

FLUOXETINE

Indications: see under Dose
Cautions: see notes above
Contra-indications: see notes above
Side-effects: see notes above; possible changes in blood sugar, fever, neuroleptic malignant syndrome-like event; also reported (no causal relationship established): abnormal bleeding, aplastic anaemia, cerebrovascular accident, ecchymoses, eosinophilic pneumonia, gastro-intestinal haemorrhage, haemolytic anaemia, pancreatitis, pancytopenia, thrombocytopenia, thrombocytopenic purpura, vaginal bleeding on withdrawal, violent behaviour; hair loss also reported
Dose: depressive illness, 20 mg daily; CHILD not recommended
Bulimia nervosa, 60 mg daily; CHILD not recommended
Obsessive-compulsive disorder, initially 20 mg daily, dose increase may be considered if no response after several weeks; max. 60 mg daily; CHILD not recommended
Premenstrual dysphoric disorder, 20 mg daily for 6 months then reassess for benefit before continuing
LONG DURATION OF ACTION. Consider the long half-life of fluoxetine when adjusting dosage (or in overdosage)

Fluoxetine (Non-proprietary) PoM
Capsules, fluoxetine (as hydrochloride) 20 mg, net price 30-cap pack = £8.06. Counselling, driving
Available from Alpharma, APS, Bioglan, CP, Generics, Genus (*Oxactin®*), IVAX, Lagap, Opus (*Felicium®*), Sterwin

Prozac® (Dista) PoM
Capsules, fluoxetine (as hydrochloride) 20 mg (green/yellow), net price 30-cap pack = £17.76; 60 mg (yellow), 30-cap pack = £59.51. Counselling, driving
Liquid, fluoxetine (as hydrochloride) 20 mg/5 mL. Net price 70-mL pack = £16.58. Counselling, driving

FLUVOXAMINE MALEATE

Indications: depressive illness, obsessive-compulsive disorder

Cautions: see notes above

CSM ADVICE. The CSM has advised that concomitant use of fluvoxamine and theophylline or aminophylline should usually be avoided; see also **interactions:** Appendix 1 (antidepressants, SSRIs)

Contra-indications: see notes above

Side-effects: see notes above; palpitations, tachycardia (may also cause bradycardia), rarely postural hypotension, confusion, ataxia, rarely abnormal liver function tests, usually symptomatic (discontinue treatment)

Dose: initially 100 mg daily increased if necessary to max. 300 mg daily (over 100 mg in divided doses); CHILD not recommended

Note. If no improvement in obsessive-compulsive disorder within 10 weeks, treatment should be reconsidered

Fluvoxamine Maleate (Non-proprietary) PoM
Tablets, fluvoxamine maleate 50 mg, net price 60-tab pack = £17.92; 100 mg, 30-tab pack = £17.96. Counselling, driving
Available from Alpharma, IVAX

Faverin® (Solvay) PoM
Tablets, f/c, scored, fluvoxamine maleate 50 mg, net price 60-tab pack = £19.00; 100 mg, 30-tab pack = £19.00. Counselling, driving

PAROXETINE

Indications: depressive illness, obsessive-compulsive disorder, panic disorder; social phobia; post-traumatic stress disorder; generalised anxiety disorder

Cautions: see notes above

IMPORTANT. During initial treatment of panic disorder, there is potential for worsening of panic symptoms

CSM ADVICE. Extrapyramidal reactions (including orofacial dystonias) and withdrawal syndrome are reported to the CSM more commonly with paroxetine than with other SSRIs

Contra-indications: see notes above

Side-effects: see notes above; postural hypotension, arthralgia, myalgia; very rarely hepatic disorders (e.g. hepatitis)

Dose: depressive illness, post-traumatic stress disorder, usually 20 mg each morning, if necessary increased gradually in steps of 10 mg; max. 50 mg daily (elderly 40 mg daily); CHILD not recommended

Obsessive-compulsive disorder, initially 20 mg each morning, if necessary increased gradually in weekly steps of 10 mg to usual dose of 40 mg daily; max. 60 mg daily (elderly 40 mg daily); CHILD not recommended

Panic disorder, initially 10 mg each morning, if necessary increased gradually in weekly steps of 10 mg to usual dose of 40 mg daily; max. 50 mg daily (elderly 40 mg daily); CHILD not recommended

Social phobia, initially 20 mg each morning; if no improvement after at least 2 weeks, increase in steps of 10 mg at intervals of at least 1 week; max. 50 mg daily (elderly 40 mg daily); CHILD not recommended

Generalised anxiety disorder, 20 mg each morning; CHILD not recommended

Seroxat® (SmithKline Beecham) PoM
Tablets, both f/c, scored, paroxetine (as hydrochloride) 20 mg, net price 30-tab pack = £17.76; 30 mg (blue), 30-tab pack = £31.16. Label: 21, counselling, driving
Liquid, orange, sugar-free, paroxetine (as hydrochloride) 10 mg/5 mL. Net price 150-mL pack = £20.77. Label: 21, counselling, driving

SERTRALINE

Indications: depressive illness, obsessive-compulsive disorder (under specialist supervision in children)

Cautions: see notes above

Contra-indications: see notes above

Side-effects: see notes above; tachycardia, confusion, amnesia, aggressive behaviour, psychosis, pancreatitis, hepatitis, jaundice, liver failure, menstrual irregularities, paraesthesia; thrombocytopenia also reported (causal relationship not established)

Dose: depressive illness, initially 50 mg daily, increased if necessary by increments of 50 mg over several weeks to max. 200 mg daily; usual maintenance dose 50 mg daily; CHILD not recommended

Obsessive-compulsive disorder, ADULT and ADOLESCENT over 13 years initially 50 mg daily, increased if necessary in steps of 50 mg over several weeks; usual dose range 50–200 mg daily; CHILD 6–12 years initially 25 mg daily, increased to 50 mg daily after 1 week, further increased if necessary in steps of 50 mg at intervals of at least 1 week (max. 200 mg daily); CHILD under 6 years not recommended

Lustral® (Pfizer) PoM
Tablets, both f/c, sertraline (as hydrochloride) 50 mg (scored), net price 28-tab pack = £16.20; 100 mg, 28-tab pack = £26.51. Counselling, driving

4.3.4 Other antidepressant drugs

The thioxanthene **flupentixol** (Fluanxol®) has antidepressant properties, and low doses (1 to 3 mg daily) are given by mouth for this purpose. Flupentixol is also used for the treatment of psychoses (section 4.2.1 and section 4.2.2)

Mirtazapine, a presynaptic α_2-antagonist, increases central noradrenergic and serotonergic neurotransmission. It has few antimuscarinic effects, but causes sedation during initial treatment.

Nefazodone inhibits re-uptake of serotonin and also selectively blocks serotonin receptors.

Reboxetine, a selective inhibitor of noradrenaline re-uptake, has been introduced for the treatment of depressive illness.

Tryptophan appears to benefit some patients with resistant depression when given as adjunctive therapy but tryptophan products have been associated with the eosinophilia-myalgia syndrome; Optimax® (Merck) is available for patients for whom no alternative treatment is suitable.

Venlafaxine is a serotonin and noradrenaline re-uptake inhibitor (SNRI); it lacks the sedative and antimuscarinic effects of the tricyclic antidepressants.

FLUPENTIXOL
(Flupenthixol)

Indications: depressive illness; psychoses (section 4.2.1)

Cautions: cardiovascular disease (including cardiac disorders and cerebral arteriosclerosis), senile confusional states, parkinsonism, renal and hepatic disease; avoid in excitable and overactive patients; porphyria (section 9.8.2); **interactions:** Appendix 1 (antipsychotics)

Side-effects: restlessness, insomnia; hypomania reported; rarely dizziness, tremor, visual disturbances, headache, hyperprolactinaemia, extrapyramidal symptoms

Dose: initially 1 mg (elderly 500 micrograms) in the morning, increased after 1 week to 2 mg (elderly 1 mg) if necessary; max. 3 mg (elderly 2 mg) daily, doses above 2 mg (elderly 1 mg) being divided in 2 portions, second dose not after 4 p.m. Discontinue if no response after 1 week at max. dosage; CHILD not recommended

COUNSELLING. Although drowsiness may occur, can also have an alerting effect so should not be taken in the evening

Fluanxol® (Lundbeck) PoM
Tablets, both red, s/c, flupentixol (as dihydrochloride) 500 micrograms, net price 60-tab pack = £3.10; 1 mg, 60-tab pack = £5.23. Label: 2, counselling, administration

MIRTAZAPINE

Indications: depressive illness

Cautions: epilepsy, hepatic or renal impairment, cardiac disorders, hypotension, history of urinary retention, angle-closure glaucoma, diabetes mellitus, psychoses (may aggravate psychotic symptoms), history of bipolar depression, avoid abrupt withdrawal; manufacturer advises avoid in pregnancy and in breast-feeding (Appendix 5); **interactions:** Appendix 1 (mirtazapine)

BLOOD DISORDERS. Patients should be advised to report any fever, sore throat, stomatitis or other signs of infection during treatment. Blood count should be performed and the drug stopped immediately if blood dyscrasia suspected

Side-effects: increased appetite and weight gain, sedation; less commonly oedema, dizziness, headache, rarely postural hypotension, abnormal dreams, mania, convulsions, tremor, myoclonus, paraesthesia, arthralgia, myalgia, restless legs, exanthema, reversible agranulocytosis (see Cautions above)

Dose: initially 15 mg daily at bedtime increased according to response up to 45 mg daily as a single dose at bedtime or in 2 divided doses; CHILD not recommended

Zispin® (Organon) PoM
Tablets, scored, red/brown, mirtazapine 30 mg. Net price 28-tab pack = £22.92. Label: 2, 25

NEFAZODONE HYDROCHLORIDE

Indications: depressive illness

Cautions: epilepsy, concurrent electroconvulsive therapy (no studies), history of mania or hypomania, elderly (especially female), hepatic and renal impairment (give lower end of dose range), pregnancy; **interactions:** Appendix 1 (nefazodone)

DRIVING. May impair performance of skilled tasks (e.g. driving)

Contra-indications: breast-feeding

Side-effects: asthenia, dry mouth, nausea, somnolence, dizziness; less frequently, chills, fever, postural hypotension, constipation, lightheadedness, paraesthesia, confusion, ataxia, amblyopia and other minor visual disturbances; rarely syncope, liver damage

Dose: initially 50–100 mg twice daily increased after 5–7 days to 200 mg twice daily, may be increased gradually if necessary to max. 300 mg twice daily (ELDERLY usual max. 100–200 mg twice daily); ADOLESCENT and CHILD under 18 years not recommended

Dutonin® (Bristol-Myers Squibb) PoM
Tablets, both scored, nefazodone hydrochloride 100 mg (white), net price 56-tab pack = £16.80; 200 mg (yellow), 56-tab pack = £16.80; treatment initiation pack consisting of 14 × 50 mg (pink) tablets, 14 × 100 mg tablets and 28 × 200 mg tablets = £16.80. Label: 3

REBOXETINE

Indications: depressive illness

Cautions: severe renal impairment (Appendix 3), hepatic impairment (Appendix 2), history of cardiovascular disease and epilepsy, bipolar disorders, urinary retention, prostatic hypertrophy, glaucoma; **interactions:** Appendix 1 (reboxetine)

Contra-indications: pregnancy (Appendix 4) and breast-feeding (Appendix 5)

Side-effects: insomnia, sweating, dizziness, postural hypotension, vertigo, paraesthesia, impotence, dysuria, urinary retention (mainly in men), dry mouth, constipation, tachycardia; lowering of plasma-potassium concentration on prolonged administration in the elderly

Dose: 4 mg twice daily increased if necessary after 3–4 weeks to 10 mg daily in divided doses, max. 12 mg daily; CHILD and ELDERLY not recommended

Edronax® (Pharmacia) PoM
Tablets, scored, reboxetine (as mesilate) 4 mg. Net price 60-tab pack = £18.91. Counselling, driving

TRYPTOPHAN
(L-Tryptophan)

Indications: restricted to use by hospital specialists *only* for patients with severe and disabling depressive illness of more than 2 years continuous duration, *only* after an adequate trial of standard antidepressant drug treatment, and *only* as an adjunct to other antidepressant medication

Cautions: eosinophilia-myalgia syndrome has been reported with tryptophan-containing products therefore close and regular surveillance required; monitor eosinophil count, haematological changes and muscle symptomatology; pregnancy and breast-feeding; **interactions:** Appendix 1 (tryptophan)

Contra-indications: history of eosinophilia-myalgia syndrome following use of tryptophan

Side-effects: drowsiness, nausea, headache, light-headedness; eosinophilia-myalgia syndrome, see Cautions

Dose: 1 g 3 times daily; max. 6 g daily; ELDERLY lower dose may be appropriate especially where renal or hepatic impairment; CHILD not recommended

Optimax® (Merck) PoM

Tablets, scored, tryptophan 500 mg. Net price 84-tab pack = £16.30. Label: 3

Important. Patient and prescriber must be registered with the *Optimax®* Information and Clinical Support (OPTICS) Unit (Tel 0845 7626902). A **safety questionnaire** is sent to the prescriber after **3** and **6 months** of treatment and **every 6 months** thereafter. The information is reviewed by the CSM—it is **important** that the questionnaires should be completed

VENLAFAXINE

Indications: depressive illness; generalised anxiety disorder

Cautions: history of myocardial infarction or unstable heart disease, blood pressure monitoring advisable if dose exceeds 200 mg daily, history of epilepsy, mania, hepatic or renal impairment (Appendixes 2 and 3), avoid abrupt withdrawal (if taken for more than 1 week; withdraw over at least 1 week); glaucoma; **interactions:** Appendix 1 (venlafaxine)

DRIVING. May affect performance of skilled tasks (e.g. driving)

SKIN REACTIONS. Advise patients to contact doctor if rash, urticaria or related allergic reaction develops

Contra-indications: severe hepatic or renal impairment; pregnancy and breast-feeding

Side-effects: nausea, headache, insomnia, drowsiness, dry mouth, dizziness (and occasionally hypotension), dyspnoea, constipation, asthenia, sweating, nervousness, convulsions (discontinue), diarrhoea, ecchymosis, arthralgia, myalgia, increased urinary frequency, visual disturbances, tinnitus; other side-effects reported include anorexia, dyspepsia, abdominal pain, anxiety, sexual dysfunction, vasodilatation, vomiting, tremor, abnormal dreams, paraesthesia, chills, hypertension (see Cautions, above), menstrual irregularities, palpitations, weight changes, agitation, hypertonia, rash (see Skin reactions, above); hepatitis, taste disturbances, arrhythmias, haemorrhage, thrombocytopenia, movement disorders, psychiatric disturbances, urinary retention, galactorrhoea, angioedema, Stevens-Johnson syndrome, photosensitivity, neuroleptic malignant syndrome, hyponatraemia, and alterations in serum cholesterol also reported

Dose: depression, initially 75 mg daily in 2 divided doses increased if necessary after several weeks to 150 mg daily in 2 divided doses

Severely depressed or hospitalised patients, initially 150 mg daily in 2 divided doses increased if necessary in steps of up to 75 mg every 2–3 days to max. 375 mg daily then gradually reduced; ADOLESCENT and CHILD under 18 years not recommended

Generalised anxiety disorder, see under preparations below

Efexor® (Wyeth) PoM

Tablets, all peach, venlafaxine (as hydrochloride) 37.5 mg, net price 56-tab pack = £23.97; 50 mg, 42-tab pack = £23.97; 75 mg, 56-tab pack = £39.97. Label: 21, counselling, driving, skin reactions

■ Modified release

Efexor® XL (Wyeth) PoM

Capsules, m/r, venlafaxine (as hydrochloride) 75 mg (peach), net price 28-cap pack = £23.97; 150 mg (orange), 28-cap pack = £39.97. Label: 21, 25, counselling, driving, skin reactions

Dose: depression, 75 mg daily as a single dose, increased if necessary after at least 2 weeks to 150 mg once daily; max. 225 mg once daily; ADOLESCENT and CHILD under 18 years not recommended

Generalised anxiety disorder, 75 mg daily as a single dose; discontinue if no response after 8 weeks; ADOLESCENT and CHILD under 18 years not recommended

4.4 Central nervous system stimulants

Central nervous system stimulants include the **amphetamines** (notably dexamfetamine) **and related drugs** (e.g. methylphenidate). They have very few indications and in particular, should **not** be used to treat depression, obesity, senility, debility, or for relief of fatigue.

Caffeine is a weak stimulant present in tea and coffee. It is included in many analgesic preparations (section 4.7.1) but does not contribute to their analgesic or anti-inflammatory effect. Over-indulgence may lead to a state of anxiety.

The **amphetamines** have a limited field of usefulness and their use should be **discouraged** as they may cause dependence and psychotic states. They have **no place** in the management of **depression** or **obesity**.

Patients with *narcolepsy* may derive benefit from treatment with dexamfetamine.

Methylphenidate is used for the management of *attention deficit/hyperactivity disorder* (ADHD) (see NICE guidance below); growth may be retarded and it is advisable to monitor growth during treatment. **Dexamfetamine** (dexamphetamine) is an alternative in children who do not respond to methylphenidate. Drug treatment of attention deficit/hyperactivity disorder should be supervised by specialists.

Modafinil is used for the treatment of narcolepsy; dependence with long-term use cannot be excluded and it should therefore be used with caution

NICE guidance (methylphenidate). The National Institute for Clinical Excellence has recommended that methylphenidate should be used as part of a comprehensive treatment programme for children and adolescents with a diagnosis of severe attention deficit/hyperactivity disorder (ADHD). Treatment should be initiated by a specialist in ADHD but may be continued by general practitioners, under a shared-care arrangement. When a child receiving methylphenidate shows improvement and the condition appears stable, treatment can be suspended periodically in order to assess the need for continuation of therapy.

DEXAMFETAMINE SULPHATE

(Dexamphetamine Sulphate)

Indications: narcolepsy, adjunct in the management of refractory hyperkinetic states in children (under specialist supervision)

Cautions: mild hypertension (contra-indicated if moderate or severe)—monitor blood pressure; history of epilepsy (discontinue if convulsions occur); tics and Tourette syndrome (use with caution)—discontinue if tics occur; monitor growth in children (see also below); avoid abrupt withdrawal; data on safety and efficacy of long-term use not complete; porphyria (see section 9.8.2); **interactions:** Appendix 1 (sympathomimetics)

SPECIAL CAUTIONS IN CHILDREN. Monitor height and weight as growth retardation may occur during prolonged therapy (drug free periods may allow catch-up in growth but withdraw slowly to avoid inducing depression or renewed hyperactivity). In psychotic children may exacerbate behavioural disturbances and thought disorder

Contra-indications: cardiovascular disease including moderate to severe hypertension, hyperexcitability or agitated states, hyperthyroidism, history of drug or alcohol abuse, glaucoma, pregnancy and breast-feeding

DRIVING. May affect performance of skilled tasks (e.g. driving); effects of alcohol unpredictable

Side-effects: insomnia, restlessness, irritability and excitability, nervousness, night terrors, euphoria, tremor, dizziness, headache; convulsions (see also Cautions); dependence and tolerance, sometimes psychosis; anorexia, gastrointestinal symptoms, growth retardation in children (see also under Cautions); dry mouth, sweating, tachycardia (and anginal pain), palpitations, increased blood pressure; visual disturbances; cardiomyopathy reported with chronic use; central stimulants have provoked choreoathetoid movements, tics and Tourette syndrome in predisposed individuals (see also Cautions above); **overdosage:** see Emergency Treatment of Poisoning, p. 26

Dose: narcolepsy, 10 mg (elderly, 5 mg) daily in divided doses increased by 10 mg (elderly, 5 mg) daily at intervals of 1 week to a max. of 60 mg daily

Hyperkinesia, CHILD under 6 years not recommended, over 6 years 5–10 mg daily, increased if necessary by 5 mg at intervals of 1 week to usual max. 20 mg daily (older children have received max. 40 mg daily)

Dexedrine® (Celltech) CD

Tablets, scored, dexamfetamine sulphate 5 mg. Net price 28-tab pack = 96p. Counselling, driving

METHYLPHENIDATE HYDROCHLORIDE

Indications: part of a comprehensive treatment programme for attention-deficit hyperactivity disorder when remedial measures alone prove insufficient (under specialist supervision)

Cautions: see under Dexamfetamine Sulphate; also manufacturer recommends periodic complete and differential blood and platelet counts; **interactions:** Appendix 1 (sympathomimetics)

Contra-indications: see under Dexamfetamine Sulphate

Side-effects: see under Dexamfetamine Sulphate; also rash, urticaria, fever, arthralgia, alopecia, exfoliative dermatitis, erythema multiforme, thrombocytopenic purpura, thrombocytopenia, leucopenia, and abnormal liver function reported

Dose: CHILD under 6 years not recommended, over 6 years, initially 5 mg 1–2 times daily, increased if necessary at weekly intervals by 5–10 mg daily to max. 60 mg daily in divided doses; discontinue if no response after 1 month, also suspend periodically to assess child's condition (usually finally discontinued during or after puberty)

EVENING DOSE. If effect wears off in evening (with rebound hyperactivity) a dose at bedtime may be appropriate (establish need with trial bedtime dose)

Equasym® (Celltech) CD

Tablets, scored, methylphenidate hydrochloride 5 mg, net price 30-tab pack = £2.78; 10 mg, net price 30-tab pack = £4.99; 20 mg, net price 30-tab pack = £9.98

Ritalin® (Cephalon) CD

Tablets, scored, methylphenidate hydrochloride 10 mg, net price 30-tab pack = £5.57

MODAFINIL

Indications: narcolepsy

Cautions: hepatic impairment (Appendix 2); renal impairment (Appendix 3); monitor blood pressure and heart rate in hypertensive patients (but see below); possibility of dependence; **interactions:** Appendix 1 (modafinil)

Contra-indications: pregnancy and breast-feeding; moderate to severe hypertension; history of left ventricular hypertrophy or of clinically significant signs of CNS stimulant-induced mitral valve prolapse (including ischaemic ECG changes, chest pain and arrhythmias)

Side-effects: anorexia, abdominal pain, headache, personality disorder, CNS stimulation including insomnia, excitation, euphoria, nervousness, dry mouth, palpitation, tachycardia, hypertension, tremor; gastro-intestinal disturbances (including nausea, gastric discomfort); rashes, pruritus, rarely buccofacial dyskinesia, dose-related increase in alkaline phosphatase

Dose: 200–400 mg daily, *either* in 2 divided doses morning and at noon *or* as a single dose in the morning; ELDERLY initiate at 100 mg daily; CHILD not recommended

Provigil® (Cephalon) PoM

Tablets, modafinil 100 mg. Net price 30-tab pack = £60.00

Cocaine

Cocaine is a drug of addiction which causes central nervous stimulation. Its clinical use is mainly as a topical local anaesthetic (section 15.2). It has been included in analgesic elixirs for the relief of pain in palliative care but this use is obsolete. For management of cocaine poisoning, see p. 26.

4.5   Drugs used in the treatment of obesity

4.5.1   Anti-obesity drugs acting on the gastro-intestinal tract

4.5.2   Centrally acting appetite suppressants

Obesity is associated with many health problems including cardiovascular disease, diabetes mellitus, gallstones and osteoarthritis. Factors that aggravate obesity may include depression, other psychosocial problems, and some drugs.

The main treatment of the obese individual is a suitable diet, carefully explained to the individual, with appropriate support and encouragement; the individual should also be advised to increase physical activity. Smoking cessation (while maintaining body weight) may be worthwhile before attempting supervised weight loss since cigarette smoking may be more harmful than obesity. Attendance at groups (e.g. 'weight-watchers') helps some individuals.

Severe obesity should be managed in an appropriate setting by staff who have been trained in the management of obesity; the individual should receive advice on diet and lifestyle modification and be monitored for changes in weight as well as in blood pressure, blood lipids and other associated conditions.

An anti-obesity drug should be considered only for those with a body mass index (BMI, individual's body-weight divided by the square of the individual's height) of $30 \, kg/m^2$ or greater in whom at least 3 months of managed care involving supervised diet, exercise and behaviour modification fails to achieve a realistic reduction in weight. In the presence of risk factors (such as diabetes, coronary heart disease, hypertension, and obstructive sleep apnoea), it may be appropriate to prescribe a drug to individuals with a BMI of $27 \, kg/m^2$ or greater, provided that such use is permitted by the drug's marketing authorisation. Drugs should **never** be used as the sole element of treatment. The individual should be monitored on a regular basis; drug treatment should be discontinued if weight loss is less than 5% after the first 12 weeks or if the individual regains weight at any time whilst receiving drug treatment.

Drugs specifically licensed for the treatment of obesity are **orlistat** (section 4.5.1) and **sibutramine** (section 4.5.2). There is little evidence to guide selection between the two drugs, but it may be appropriate to choose orlistat for those who have a high intake of fats whereas sibutramine may be chosen for those who cannot control their eating; the cautions, contra-indications and side-effects of the two drugs should also be considered.

Combination therapy involving more than one anti-obesity drug is **contra-indicated** until further information about efficacy and long-term safety is available.

Thyroid hormones have **no** place in the treatment of obesity except in biochemically proven hypothyroid patients. The use of diuretics, chorionic gonadotrophin, or amphetamines is **not** appropriate for weight reduction.

4.5.1   Anti-obesity drugs acting on the gastro-intestinal tract

Orlistat, a pancreatic lipase inhibitor, reduces the absorption of dietary fat. It is used in conjunction with a mildly hypocaloric diet. Some of the weight loss in those taking orlistat probably results from individuals reducing their fat intake to avoid severe gastro-intestinal effects including steatorrhoea. Vitamin supplementation (especially of vitamin D) may be considered if there is concern about deficiency of fat-soluble vitamins. Orlistat is not licensed for use longer than 2 years because there is insufficient experience beyond this period. However, on stopping orlistat, there may be a gradual reversal of weight loss.

> **NICE guidance (orlistat).** The National Institute for Clinical Excellence has recommended that orlistat should be prescribed under the following conditions:
>
> - only for individuals with a body mass index (BMI) of $30 \, kg/m^2$ or more (and no associated co-morbidity) *or* for individuals with a BMI of $28 \, kg/m^2$ or more in the presence of other risk factors (e.g. type 2 diabetes, hypertension, hypercholesterolaemia)
>
> - only for individuals who have lost at least 2.5 kg body-weight by dietary control and increased physical activity in the preceding month
>
> - only for individuals aged between 18 and 75 years
>
> - arrangements should exist for primary care staff (mostly practice nurses) supported by community dieticians to offer specific advice, support and counselling on diet, physical activity, and behavioural strategies to those receiving orlistat
>
> - treatment should continue beyond 3 months only if weight loss is greater than 5% from start of treatment
>
> - treatment should continue beyond 6 months only if weight loss is greater than 10% from start of treatment
>
> - treatment should not usually continue beyond 1 year and never beyond 2 years [see also notes above]

The most commonly used bulk-forming drug is **methylcellulose** (section 1.6.1). It is claimed to reduce intake by producing a feeling of satiety but there is little evidence to support its use in the management of obesity.

ORLISTAT

Indications: adjunct in obesity (see notes above)

Cautions: diabetes mellitus; may impair absorption of fat-soluble vitamins; **interactions:** Appendix 1 (orlistat)

MULTIVITAMINS. If a multivitamin supplement is required, it should be taken at least 2 hours after orlistat dose or at bedtime

Contra-indications: chronic malabsorption syndrome; cholestasis; pregnancy and breast-feeding

Side-effects: liquid oily stools, faecal urgency, flatulence, less frequently abdominal and rectal pain (gastro-intestinal effects minimised by reduced fat diet); headache; menstrual irregularities; anxiety, fatigue; rarely hepatitis

Dose: 120 mg taken immediately before, during, or up to 1 hour after each main meal (up to max. 360 mg daily); max. period of treatment 2 years; CHILD not recommended

Note. If a meal is missed or contains no fat, the dose of orlistat should be omitted

Xenical® (Roche) ▼ PoM
Capsules, turquoise, orlistat 120 mg, net price 84-cap pack = £41.16

4.5.2 Centrally acting appetite suppressants

Sibutramine inhibits the re-uptake of noradrenaline and serotonin. It is used in the adjunctive management of obesity in individuals with a body mass index (BMI) of 30 kg/m² or more (and no associated co-morbidity) *or* in individuals with a BMI of 27 kg/m² or more in the presence of other risk factors such as type 2 diabetes or hypercholesterolaemia.

Dexfenfluramine, **fenfluramine** and, most recently, **phentermine** have been withdrawn following reports of valvular heart disease associated with their use; these drugs were also associated with the rare but serious risk of pulmonary hypertension.

NICE guidance (sibutramine). The National Institute for Clinical Excellence has recommended that sibutramine should be prescribed in accordance with the summary of product characteristics and under the following conditions:

• only for individuals who have attempted seriously to lose weight by diet, exercise, and other behavioural modifications;

• arrangements should exist for appropriate healthcare professionals to offer specific advice, support, and counselling on diet, physical activities, and behavioural strategies to those receiving sibutramine.

SIBUTRAMINE HYDROCHLORIDE

Indications: adjunct in obesity (see notes above)
Cautions: monitor blood pressure and pulse rate (every 2 weeks for the first 3 months *then* monthly for 3 months *then* at least every 3 months)—discontinue if blood pressure or pulse rate raised at 2 consecutive visits; sleep apnoea syndrome (increased risk of hypertension); epilepsy; hepatic impairment (avoid if severe; Appendix 2); renal impairment (avoid if severe); monitor for pulmonary hypertension (but effect not reported with sibutramine); family history of motor or vocal tics; **interactions:** Appendix 1 (sibutramine)

DURATION OF TREATMENT. Treatment should be discontinued if:

• weight loss after 3 months less than 5% of initial body-weight;
• weight loss stabilises at less than 5% of initial body-weight;
• individuals regain 3 kg or more after previous weight loss

In individuals with co-morbid conditions, treatment should be continued only if weight loss is associated with other clinical benefits

Contra-indications: history of major eating disorders; psychiatric illness, Gilles de la Tourette syndrome; history of coronary artery disease, congestive heart failure, tachycardia, peripheral arterial occlusive disease, arrhythmias, and of cerebrovascular disease; uncontrolled hypertension; hyperthyroidism; prostatic hypertrophy; phaeochromocytoma; angle closure glaucoma; history of drug or alcohol abuse; pregnancy (Appendix 4); breast-feeding (Appendix 5)

Side-effects: most commonly constipation, anorexia, dry mouth, insomnia; also nausea, tachycardia, palpitations, hypertension, vasodilation, light-headedness, paraesthesia, headache, anxiety, sweating, taste disturbance; rarely blurred vision

Dose: initially 10 mg daily in the morning, increased if weight loss less than 2 kg after 4 weeks to 15 mg daily; discontinue if weight loss less than 2 kg after 4 weeks at higher dose (see also Duration of Treatment above); max. period of treatment 1 year; CHILD, ADOLESCENT under 18 years, and ELDERLY over 65 years not recommended

Reductil® (Abbott) ▼ PoM
Capsules, sibutramine hydrochloride 10 mg (blue/yellow), net price 28-cap pack = £35.00; 15 mg (blue/white), 28-cap pack = £39.09

4.6 Drugs used in nausea and vertigo

Anti-emetics should be prescribed only when the cause of vomiting is known because otherwise they may delay diagnosis, particularly in children. Anti-emetics are unnecessary and sometimes harmful when the cause can be treated, such as in diabetic ketoacidosis, or in digoxin or antiepileptic overdose.

If anti-emetic drug treatment is indicated, the drug is chosen according to the aetiology of vomiting.

Antihistamines are effective against nausea and vomiting resulting from many underlying conditions. There is no evidence that any one antihistamine is superior to another but their duration of action and incidence of adverse effects (drowsiness and antimuscarinic effects) differ.

The **phenothiazines** are dopamine antagonists and act centrally by blocking the chemoreceptor trigger zone. They are of considerable value for the prophylaxis and treatment of nausea and vomiting associated with diffuse neoplastic disease, radiation sickness, and the emesis caused by drugs such as opioids, general anaesthetics, and cytotoxics. **Prochlorperazine**, **perphenazine**, and **trifluoperazine** are less sedating than **chlorpromazine**; severe dystonic reactions sometimes occur with phenothiazines, especially in children. Other antipsychotic drugs including **haloperidol** and **levomepromazine (methotrimeprazine)** (section 4.2.1) are also used for the relief of nausea. Some phenothiazines are available as rectal suppositories, which can be useful in patients with persistent vomiting or with severe nausea; **prochlorperazine** can also be administered as a buccal tablet which is placed between the upper lip and the gum.

Metoclopramide is an effective anti-emetic and its activity closely resembles that of the phenothiazines. Metoclopramide also acts directly on the gastro-intestinal tract and it may be superior to the phenothiazines for emesis associated with gastro-duodenal, hepatic, and biliary disease. In postoperative nausea and vomiting, metoclopramide in a dose of 10 mg has limited efficacy. High-dose metoclopramide injection is now less commonly used for cytotoxic-induced nausea and vomiting. As with the phenothiazines, metoclopramide can induce acute dystonic reactions involving facial and skeletal muscle spasms and oculogyric crises. These dystonic effects are more common in the young (especially girls and young women) and the very old; they usually occur shortly after starting treatment with metoclopramide and subside within 24 hours of stopping it. Injection of an antiparkinsonian drug such as procyclidine (section 4.9.2) will abort dystonic attacks.

Domperidone acts at the chemoreceptor trigger zone; it is used for the relief of nausea and vomiting, especially when associated with cytotoxic therapy. It has the advantage over metoclopramide and the phenothiazines of being less likely to cause central effects such as sedation and dystonic reactions because it does not readily cross the blood-brain barrier. In Parkinson's disease, it is used during the initiation of apomorphine treatment and it may also be given for the treatment of levodopa- and bromocriptine-induced vomiting (section 4.9.1). Domperidone is also used to treat vomiting due to emergency hormonal contraception (section 7.3.1).

Granisetron, **ondansetron**, and **tropisetron** are specific $5HT_3$ antagonists which block $5HT_3$ receptors in the gastro-intestinal tract and in the CNS. They are of value in the management of nausea and vomiting in patients receiving cytotoxics and in postoperative nausea and vomiting.

Nabilone is a synthetic cannabinoid with anti-emetic properties. It may be used for nausea and vomiting caused by cytotoxic chemotherapy that is unresponsive to conventional anti-emetics. Side-effects such as drowsiness and dizziness occur frequently with standard doses.

Dexamethasone (section 6.3.2) has anti-emetic effects and it is used in vomiting associated with cancer chemotherapy. It can be used alone or with metoclopramide, prochlorperazine, lorazepam, or a $5HT_3$ antagonist (see also section 8.1).

Vomiting of pregnancy

Nausea in the first trimester of pregnancy is generally mild and does not require drug therapy. On rare occasions if vomiting is severe, short-term treatment with an antihistamine, such as **promethazine**, may be required. **Prochlorperazine** or **metoclopramide** may be considered as second-line treatments. If symptoms do not settle in 24 to 48 hours then specialist opinion should be sought. Hyperemesis gravidarum is a more serious condition, which requires intravenous fluid and electrolyte replacement and sometimes nutritional support. Supplementation with thiamine must be considered to reduce the risk of Wernicke's encephalopathy.

Postoperative nausea and vomiting

The incidence of postoperative nausea and vomiting depends on many factors including the anaesthetic used, the type and duration of surgery, and the patient's sex. The aim is to prevent postoperative nausea and vomiting from occurring. Drugs used include some **phenothiazines** (e.g. prochlorperazine), **metoclopramide** (but 10-mg dose has limited efficacy and higher parenteral doses associated with greater side-effects), **$5HT_3$ antagonists**, **antihistamines** (such as cyclizine), and **dexamethasone**. A combination of two anti-emetic drugs acting at different sites may be considered in resistant postoperative nausea and vomiting.

Motion sickness

Anti-emetics should be given prophylactically for the prevention of motion sickness rather than after nausea or vomiting develop. The most effective drug for the prevention of motion sickness is **hyoscine**. A transdermal hyoscine patch provides prolonged activity but it needs to be applied several hours before travelling. The sedating antihistamines are slightly less effective against motion sickness, but are generally better tolerated than hyoscine. If a sedative effect is desired **promethazine** is useful, but generally a slightly less sedating antihistamine such as **cyclizine** or **cinnarizine** is preferred. The $5HT_3$ antagonists, domperidone, metoclopramide, and the phenothiazines (except the antihistamine phenothiazine promethazine) are **ineffective** in motion sickness.

Other vestibular disorders

Management of vestibular diseases is aimed at treating the underlying cause as well as treating symptoms of the balance disturbance and associated nausea and vomiting. Vertigo and nausea associated with Ménière's disease and middle-ear surgery may be difficult to treat.

Betahistine is an analogue of histamine and is claimed to reduce endolymphatic pressure by improving the microcirculation. Betahistine is licensed for vertigo, tinnitus, and hearing loss associated with Ménière's disease.

A **diuretic** alone or combined with salt restriction may provide some benefit in vertigo associated with Ménière's disease. **Antihistamines** (such as cinnarizine), and **phenothiazines** (such as prochlorperazine) are effective for prophylaxis and treatment.

For advice to avoid the inappropriate prescribing of drugs (notably phenothiazines) for dizziness in the elderly, see Prescribing for the Elderly, p. 17.

Cytotoxic chemotherapy

For the management of nausea and vomiting induced by cytotoxic chemotherapy, see section 8.1.

Palliative care

For the management of nausea and vomiting in palliative care, see p. 15 and p 16.

Migraine

For the management of nausea and vomiting associated with migraine, see section 4.7.4.1.

Antihistamines

CINNARIZINE

Indications: vestibular disorders, such as vertigo, tinnitus, nausea, and vomiting in Ménière's disease; motion sickness; vascular disease (section 2.6.4)

Cautions: see under Cyclizine; risk of hypotension with high doses; avoid in porphyria (section 9.8.2)

Contra-indications: see under Cyclizine

Side-effects: see under Cyclizine; allergic skin reactions, fatigue; rarely, extrapyramidal symptoms in elderly on prolonged therapy

Dose: vestibular disorders, 30 mg 3 times daily; CHILD 5–12 years half adult dose
Motion sickness, 30 mg 2 hours before travel then 15 mg every 8 hours during journey if necessary; CHILD 5–12 years half adult dose

Cinnarizine (Non-proprietary)
Tablets, cinnarizine 15 mg. Net price 20 = £1.09. Label: 2
Available from Alpharma, Ashbourne (*Cinazière®*), Hillcross, IVAX

Stugeron® (Janssen-Cilag)
Tablets, scored, cinnarizine 15 mg. Net price 20 = 75p. Label: 2

Stugeron Forte®: see section 2.6.4

CYCLIZINE

Indications: nausea, vomiting, vertigo, motion sickness, labyrinthine disorders

Cautions: see section 3.4.1; severe heart failure; may counteract haemodynamic benefits of opioids; **interactions:** Appendix 1 (antihistamines)
DRIVING. Drowsiness may affect performance of skilled tasks (e.g. driving); effects of alcohol enhanced

Contra-indications: see section 3.4.1

Side-effects: drowsiness, occasional dry mouth and blurred vision; see also section 3.4.1

Dose: *by mouth*, cyclizine hydrochloride 50 mg up to 3 times daily; CHILD 6–12 years 25 mg up to 3 times daily
By intramuscular or intravenous injection, cyclizine lactate 50 mg 3 times daily

Valoid® (CeNeS)
Tablets, scored, cyclizine hydrochloride 50 mg. Net price 20 = 95p. Label: 2
Injection PoM, cyclizine lactate 50 mg/mL. Net price 1-mL amp = 54p

MECLOZINE HYDROCHLORIDE

Indications: see under preparations
Cautions: see under Cyclizine
Contra-indications: see under Cyclizine
Side-effects: see under Cyclizine

Preparations
A proprietary brand of meclozine hydrochloride tablets 12.5 mg (*Sea-legs®*) is on sale to the public for motion sickness

PROMETHAZINE HYDROCHLORIDE

Indications: nausea, vomiting, vertigo, labyrinthine disorders, motion sickness; other indications (section 3.4.1, section 4.1.1, section 15.1.4.1)

Cautions: see under Cyclizine; avoid in porphyria (section 9.8.2)

Contra-indications: see under Cyclizine

Side-effects: see under Cyclizine but more sedating; intramuscular injection may be painful

Dose: motion sickness prevention, 20–25 mg at bedtime on night before travel, repeat following morning if necessary; CHILD under 2 years not recommended, 2–5 years 5 mg at night and following morning if necessary, 5–10 years 10 mg at night and following morning if necessary

Preparations
Section 3.4.1

PROMETHAZINE TEOCLATE

Indications: nausea, vertigo, labyrinthine disorders, motion sickness (acts longer than the hydrochloride)

Cautions: see under Promethazine Hydrochloride

Contra-indications: see under Promethazine Hydrochloride

Side-effects: see under Promethazine Hydrochloride

Dose: 25–75 mg, max. 100 mg, daily; CHILD 5–10 years, 12.5–37.5 mg daily
Motion sickness prevention, 25 mg at bedtime on night before travel *or* 25 mg 1–2 hours before travel; CHILD 5–10 years half adult dose
Severe vomiting in pregnancy, 25 mg at bedtime, increased if necessary to max. 100 mg daily (but see also Vomiting of Pregnancy in notes above)

Avomine® (Manx)
Tablets, scored, promethazine teoclate 25 mg. Net price 10-tab pack = £1.11; 28-tab pack = £3.05. Label: 2

Phenothiazines and related drugs

CHLORPROMAZINE HYDROCHLORIDE

Indications: nausea and vomiting of terminal illness (where other drugs have failed or are not available); other indications (section 4.2.1 and section 15.1.4.1)

Cautions: see Chlorpromazine Hydrochloride, section 4.2.1

Contra-indications: see Chlorpromazine Hydrochloride, section 4.2.1

Side-effects: see Chlorpromazine Hydrochloride, section 4.2.1

Dose: *by mouth*, 10–25 mg every 4–6 hours; CHILD 500 micrograms/kg every 4–6 hours (1–5 years max. 40 mg daily, 6–12 years max. 75 mg daily)

By deep intramuscular injection initially 25 mg then 25–50 mg every 3–4 hours until vomiting stops; CHILD 500 micrograms/kg every 6–8 hours (1–5 years max. 40 mg daily, 6–12 years max. 75 mg daily)

By rectum in suppositories, chlorpromazine 100 mg every 6–8 hours [unlicensed]

Preparations
Section 4.2.1

PERPHENAZINE

Indications: severe nausea, vomiting (see notes above); other indications (section 4.2.1)

Cautions: see Perphenazine (section 4.2.1)

Contra-indications: see Perphenazine (section 4.2.1)

Side-effects: see Perphenazine (section 4.2.1); extrapyramidal symptoms particularly in young adults, elderly, and debilitated

Dose: 4 mg 3 times daily, adjusted according to response; max. 24 mg daily (chemotherapy-induced); ELDERLY quarter to half adult dose; CHILD under 14 years not recommended

Preparations
Section 4.2.1

PROCHLORPERAZINE

Indications: severe nausea, vomiting, vertigo, labyrinthine disorders (see notes above); other indications, section 4.2.1

Cautions: see under Prochlorperazine (section 4.2.1); oral route only for children (avoid if under 10 kg); elderly (see notes above)

Contra-indications: see under Prochlorperazine (section 4.2.1)

Side-effects: see under Prochlorperazine (section 4.2.1); extrapyramidal symptoms, particularly in children, elderly, and debilitated

Dose: *by mouth*, nausea and vomiting, prochlorperazine maleate or mesilate, acute attack, 20 mg initially then 10 mg after 2 hours; prevention 5–10 mg 2–3 times daily; CHILD (over 10 kg only) 250 micrograms/kg 2–3 times daily

Labyrinthine disorders, 5 mg 3 times daily, gradually increased if necessary to 30 mg daily in divided doses, then reduced after several weeks to 5–10 mg daily; CHILD not recommended

By deep intramuscular injection, nausea and vomiting, 12.5 mg when required followed if necessary after 6 hours by an oral dose, as above; CHILD not recommended

By rectum in suppositories, nausea and vomiting, 25 mg followed if necessary after 6 hours by oral dose, as above; *or* due to migraine, 5 mg 3 times daily; CHILD not recommended

Prochlorperazine (Non-proprietary) PoM
Tablets, prochlorperazine maleate 5 mg, net price 20 = £1.05. Label: 2
Available from Alpharma, APS, Ashbourne (*Prozière®*), Generics, Hillcross, IVAX

Stemetil® (Castlemead) PoM
Tablets, prochlorperazine maleate 5 mg (off-white), net price 84-tab pack = £6.65; 25 mg (scored), 56-tab pack = £11.73. Label: 2
Syrup, straw-coloured, prochlorperazine mesilate 5 mg/5 mL. Net price 100-mL pack = £3.74. Label: 2
Eff sachets, granules, effervescent, sugar-free, prochlorperazine mesilate 5 mg/sachet. Net price 21-sachet pack = £6.95. Label: 2, 13
Injection, prochlorperazine mesilate 12.5 mg/mL. Net price 1-mL amp = 59p
Suppositories, prochlorperazine maleate (as prochlorperazine), 5 mg, net price 10 = £9.40; 25 mg, 10 = £12.32. Label: 2

■ Buccal preparation
¹ **Buccastem®** (R&C) PoM
Tablets (buccal), pale yellow, prochlorperazine maleate 3 mg. Net price 5 × 10-tab pack = £5.75. Label: 2, counselling, administration, see under Dose below
Dose: 1–2 tablets twice daily; tablets are placed high between upper lip and gum and left to dissolve; CHILD not recommended
1. Prochlorperazine maleate can be sold to the public for adults over 18 years (provided packs do not contain more than 24 mg) for the treatment of nausea and vomiting in previously diagnosed migraine only (max. daily dose 12 mg); a proprietary brand (*Buccastem® M*) is on sale to the public

TRIFLUOPERAZINE

Indications: severe nausea and vomiting (see notes above); other indications (section 4.2.1)

Cautions: see under Trifluoperazine (section 4.2.1)

Contra-indications: see under Trifluoperazine (section 4.2.1)

Side-effects: see under Trifluoperazine (section 4.2.1); extrapyramidal symptoms, particularly in children, elderly, and debilitated

Dose: 2–4 mg daily in divided doses *or* as a single dose of a modified-release preparation; max. 6 mg daily; CHILD 3–5 years up to 1 mg daily, 6–12 years up to 4 mg daily

Preparations
Section 4.2.1

Domperidone and metoclopramide

DOMPERIDONE

Indications: see under Dose
CHILDREN. Use in children is restricted to nausea and vomiting following cytotoxics or radiotherapy

Cautions: pregnancy and breast-feeding; not recommended for routine prophylaxis of post-operative vomiting or for chronic administration; **interactions:** Appendix 1 (domperidone)

Side-effects: raised prolactin concentrations (possible galactorrhoea and gynaecomastia), reduced libido reported; rashes and other allergic reactions; acute dystonic reactions reported

Dose: *by mouth*, acute nausea and vomiting, (including nausea and vomiting induced by levodopa and bromocriptine), 10–20 mg every 4–8 hours, max. period of treatment 12 weeks; CHILD, nausea and vomiting following cytotoxic therapy or radiotherapy only, 200–400 micrograms/kg every 4–8 hours

Functional dyspepsia, 10–20 mg 3 times daily before food and 10–20 mg at night; max. period of treatment 12 weeks; CHILD not recommended

By rectum in suppositories, nausea and vomiting, 30–60 mg every 4–8 hours; CHILD over 2 years (following cytotoxic therapy or radiotherapy only), body-weight 10–15 kg max. 15 mg twice daily, body-weight 15.5–25 kg max. 30 mg twice daily, body-weight 25.5–35 kg max. 30 mg 3 times daily, body-weight 35.5–45 kg max. 30 mg 4 times daily; since dose needs to be divided throughout day, suppositories may be cut in half for younger children

¹ **Domperidone** (Non-proprietary) [PoM]
Tablets, 10 mg (as maleate), net price 30-tab pack = £2.50; 100-tab pack = £8.31

Available from CP, Generics, Hillcross, Sterwin

1. Domperidone can be sold to the public (provided packs do not contain more than 200 mg) for the relief of postprandial symptoms of excessive fullness, nausea, epigastric bloating and belching occasionally accompanied by epigastric discomfort and heartburn (max. single dose 10 mg, max. daily dose 40 mg); a proprietary brand (*Motilium® 10*) is on sale to the public

Motilium® (Sanofi-Synthelabo) [PoM]
Tablets, f/c, domperidone 10 mg (as maleate). Net price 30-tab pack = £2.35; 100-tab pack = £7.84
Suspension, sugar-free, domperidone 5 mg/5 mL. Net price 200-mL pack = £1.80
Suppositories, domperidone 30 mg. Net price 10 = £2.65

■ Compound preparations (for migraine), section 4.7.4.1

METOCLOPRAMIDE HYDROCHLORIDE

Indications: adults, nausea and vomiting, particularly in gastro-intestinal disorders (section 1.2) and treatment with cytotoxics or radiotherapy; migraine (section 4.7.4.1)

PATIENTS UNDER 20 YEARS. Use restricted to severe intractable vomiting of known cause, vomiting of radiotherapy and cytotoxics, aid to gastro-intestinal intubation, pre-medication; also, dose should be determined on the basis of body-weight

Cautions: hepatic and renal impairment; elderly, young adults, and children (measure dose accurately, preferably with a pipette); may mask underlying disorders such as cerebral irritation; epilepsy; pregnancy; porphyria (see section 9.8.2); **interactions:** Appendix 1 (metoclopramide)

Contra-indications: gastro-intestinal obstruction, perforation or haemorrhage; 3–4 days after gastro-intestinal surgery; phaeochromocytoma; breast-feeding (Appendix 5)

Side-effects: extrapyramidal effects (especially in children/young adults), hyperprolactinaemia, occasionally tardive dyskinesia on prolonged administration; also reported, drowsiness, restlessness, diarrhoea, depression, neuroleptic malignant syndrome, rashes, pruritus, oedema; cardiac conduction abnormalities reported following intravenous administration; rarely methaemoglobinaemia (more severe in G6PD deficiency)

Dose: *by mouth, or by intramuscular injection or by intravenous injection* over 1–2 minutes, 10 mg (5 mg in young adults 15–19 years under 60 kg) 3 times daily; CHILD up to 1 year (up to 10 kg) 1 mg twice daily, 1–3 years (10–14 kg) 1 mg 2–3 times daily, 3–5 years (15–19 kg) 2 mg 2–3 times daily, 5–9 years (20–29 kg) 2.5 mg 3 times daily, 9–14 years (30 kg and over) 5 mg 3 times daily

Note. Daily dose of metoclopramide should not normally exceed 500 micrograms/kg, particularly for children and young adults (restricted use, see above)

For diagnostic procedures, as a single dose 5–10 minutes before examination, 10–20 mg (10 mg in young adults 15–19 years); CHILD under 3 years 1 mg, 3–5 years 2 mg, 5–9 years 2.5 mg, 9–14 years 5 mg

Metoclopramide (Non-proprietary) [PoM]
Tablets, metoclopramide hydrochloride 10 mg, net price 28-tab pack = 86p

Available from Alpharma, Antigen, Ashbourne (*Gastroflux®*), Berk (*Primperan®*), CP, IVAX

Oral solution, metoclopramide hydrochloride 5 mg/5 mL, net price 100-mL pack = £1.10

Available from Berk (*Primperan®*, sugar-free), Lagap, Rosemont (sugar-free)

Injection, metoclopramide hydrochloride 5 mg/mL, net price 2-mL amp = 34p

Available from Antigen, Phoenix

Maxolon® (Shire) [PoM]
Tablets, scored, metoclopramide hydrochloride 5 mg, net price 84-tab pack = £4.69; 10 mg, 84-tab pack = £9.38

Syrup, sugar-free, metoclopramide hydrochloride 5 mg/5 mL. Net price 200-mL pack = £3.83

Paediatric liquid, sugar-free, metoclopramide hydrochloride 1 mg/mL. Net price 15-mL pack with pipette = £1.51. Counselling, use of pipette

Injection, metoclopramide hydrochloride 5 mg/mL. Net price 2-mL amp = 27p

■ High-dose (with cytotoxic chemotherapy only)

Maxolon High Dose® (Shire) [PoM]
Injection, metoclopramide hydrochloride 5 mg/mL. Net price 20-mL amp = £2.67.

For dilution and use as an intravenous infusion in nausea and vomiting associated with cytotoxic chemotherapy only

Dose: by continuous intravenous infusion (preferred method), initially (before starting chemotherapy), 2–4 mg/kg over 15–20 minutes, then 3–5 mg/kg over 8–12 hours; max. in 24 hours, 10 mg/kg

By intermittent intravenous infusion, initially (before starting chemotherapy), up to 2 mg/kg over at least 15 minutes then up to 2 mg/kg over at least 15 minutes every 2 hours; max. in 24 hours, 10 mg/kg

Note. Injection of metoclopramide hydrochloride 5 mg/mL also available in 20-mL ampoules from Phoenix

■ Modified-release preparations

Note. All unsuitable for patients under 20 years

Gastrobid Continus® (Napp) PoM ▗▅▆◣

Tablets, m/r, metoclopramide hydrochloride
15 mg. Net price 56-tab pack = £10.33. Label: 25

Dose: patients over 20 years, 1 tablet twice daily

Maxolon SR® (Shire) PoM ▗▅▆◣

Capsules, m/r, clear, enclosing white granules,
metoclopramide hydrochloride 15 mg. Net price
56-cap pack = £7.01. Label: 25

Dose: patients over 20 years, 1 capsule twice daily

> ▗▅▆◣ denotes preparations that are considered to
> be less suitable for prescribing (see p. vi)

■ Compound preparations (for migraine), section 4.7.4.1

5HT₃ antagonists

GRANISETRON

Indications: see under Dose

Cautions: pregnancy and breast-feeding

Side-effects: constipation, headache, rash; transient increases in liver enzymes; hypersensitivity
reactions reported

Dose: nausea and vomiting induced by cytotoxic
chemotherapy or radiotherapy, *by mouth*, 1–2 mg
within 1 hour before start of treatment, then 2 mg
daily in 1–2 divided doses during treatment; when
intravenous infusion also used, max. combined
total 9 mg in 24 hours; CHILD 20 micrograms/kg
(max. 1 mg) within 1 hour before start of treatment, then 20 micrograms/kg (max. 1 mg) twice
daily for up to 5 days during treatment

By intravenous injection (diluted in 15 mL sodium chloride 0.9% and given over not less than 30
seconds) *or by intravenous infusion* (over 5 minutes, see Appendix 6), prevention, 3 mg before
start of cytotoxic therapy (up to 2 additional 3-mg
doses may be given within 24 hours); treatment,
as for prevention (the two additional doses must
not be given less than 10 minutes apart); max.
9 mg in 24 hours; CHILD, *by intravenous infusion*,
(over 5 minutes), prevention, 40 micrograms/kg
(max. 3 mg) before start of cytotoxic therapy;
treatment, as for prevention—one additional dose
of 40 micrograms/kg (max. 3 mg) may be given
within 24 hours (not less than 10 minutes after
initial dose)

Postoperative nausea and vomiting, *by intravenous
injection* (diluted to 5 mL and given over 30 seconds), prevention, 1 mg before induction of
anaesthesia; treatment, 1 mg, given as for prevention; max. 2 mg in one day; CHILD not recommended

Kytril® (Roche) PoM

Tablets, f/c, granisetron (as hydrochloride) 1 mg,
net price 10-tab pack = £87.32; 2 mg, 5-tab pack
= £87.32

Paediatric liquid, sugar-free, granisetron (as
hydrochloride) 1 mg/5 mL, net price 30 mL =
£52.39

Sterile solution, granisetron (as hydrochloride)
1 mg/mL, for dilution and use as injection or infusion, net price 1-mL amp = £11.46, 3-mL amp =
£34.38

ONDANSETRON

Indications: see under Dose

Cautions: pregnancy and breast-feeding; moderate
or severe hepatic impairment (max. 8 mg daily)

Side-effects: constipation; headache, sensation of
warmth or flushing, hiccups; occasional alterations in liver enzymes; hypersensitivity reactions
reported; occasional transient visual disturbances
and dizziness following intravenous administration; involuntary movements, hiccups, chest pain,
arrhythmias, hypotension and bradycardia also
reported; suppositories may cause rectal irritation

Dose: moderately emetogenic chemotherapy or
radiotherapy, *by mouth*, 8 mg 1–2 hours before
treatment *or by rectum*, 16 mg 1–2 hours before
treatment *or by intramuscular injection or slow
intravenous injection*, 8 mg immediately before
treatment

then by mouth, 8 mg every 12 hours for up to 5
days *or by rectum*, 16 mg daily for up to 5 days

Severely emetogenic chemotherapy, *by intramuscular injection or slow intravenous injection*, 8 mg
immediately before treatment, where necessary
followed by 8 mg at intervals of 2–4 hours for 2
further doses (*or followed by* 1 mg/hour *by continuous intravenous infusion* for up to 24 hours)

then by mouth, 8 mg every 12 hours for up to 5
days *or by rectum*, 16 mg daily for up to 5 days

alternatively, by intravenous infusion over at least
15 minutes, 32 mg immediately before treatment
or by rectum, 16 mg 1–2 hours before treatment

then by mouth, 8 mg every 12 hours for up to 5
days *or by rectum*, 16 mg daily for up to 5 days

Note. Efficacy may be enhanced by addition of a single
dose of dexamethasone sodium phosphate 20 mg by
intravenous injection

CHILD, *by slow intravenous injection or by intravenous infusion* over 15 minutes, 5 mg/m² immediately before chemotherapy then, 4 mg *by mouth*
every 12 hours for up to 5 days

Prevention of postoperative nausea and vomiting,
by mouth, 16 mg 1 hour before anaesthesia *or*
8 mg 1 hour before anaesthesia followed by 8 mg
at intervals of 8 hours for 2 further doses

*alternatively, by intramuscular or slow intra-
venous injection*, 4 mg at induction of anaesthesia; CHILD over 2 years, *by slow intravenous
injection*, 100 micrograms/kg (max. 4 mg) before,
during, or after induction of anaesthesia

Treatment of postoperative nausea and vomiting, *by
intramuscular or slow intravenous injection*,
4 mg; CHILD over 2 years, *by slow intravenous
injection*, 100 micrograms/kg (max. 4 mg)

Zofran® (GlaxoWellcome) PoM

Tablets, both yellow, f/c, ondansetron (as hydrochloride) 4 mg, net price 30-tab pack = £116.03;
8 mg, 10-tab pack = £77.36

Oral lyophilisates (*Zofran Melt®*), ondansetron
4 mg, net price 10-tab pack = £38.68; 8 mg, 10-
tab pack = £77.36. Counselling, administration

COUNSELLING. Tablets should be placed on the tongue,
allowed to disperse and swallowed

Excipients: include aspartame (section 9.4.1)

Syrup, sugar-free, ondansetron (as hydrochloride)
4 mg/5 mL. Net price 50-mL pack = £38.68

Injection, ondansetron (as hydrochloride) 2 mg/mL, net price 2-mL amp = £6.45; 4-mL amp = £12.89

Suppositories, ondansetron 16 mg. Net price 5 = £77.35

TROPISETRON

Indications: see under Dose

Cautions: uncontrolled hypertension (has been aggravated by doses higher than recommended); cardiac conduction disorders; arrhythmias, concomitant administration of drugs that prolong QT interval; pregnancy and breast-feeding; **interactions:** Appendix 1 (tropisetron)

DRIVING. Dizziness or drowsiness may affect performance of skilled tasks (e.g. driving)

Side-effects: constipation, diarrhoea, abdominal pain; headache, dizziness, fatigue; hypersensitivity reactions reported (including facial flushing, urticaria, chest tightness, dyspnoea, bronchospasm and hypotension); collapse, syncope, bradycardia, cardiovascular collapse also reported (causal relationship not established)

Dose: prevention of nausea and vomiting induced by cytotoxic chemotherapy, *by slow intravenous injection or by intravenous infusion*, 5 mg shortly before chemotherapy, then 5 mg *by mouth* every morning at least 1 hour before food for 5 days; CHILD over 2 years, *by intravenous injection* over at least 1 minute or *by intravenous infusion*, 200 micrograms/kg (max. 5 mg) shortly before chemotherapy, then 200 micrograms/kg daily for 4 days; CHILD 25 kg and over, *by intravenous injection* over at least 1 minute or *by intravenous infusion*, 5 mg shortly before chemotherapy, then *by mouth* (preferably) or *by intravenous injection* over at least 1 minute or *by intravenous infusion*, 5 mg daily for 5 days

Postoperative nausea and vomiting, *by slow intravenous injection or by intravenous infusion*, prevention, 2 mg shortly before induction of anaesthesia; treatment, 2 mg within 2 hours of the end of anaesthesia

Navoban® (Novartis) [PoM]

Capsules, white/yellow, tropisetron (as hydrochloride) 5 mg, net price 5-cap pack = £53.86; 50-cap pack = £538.60. Label: 23

Injection, tropisetron (as hydrochloride), 1 mg/mL, net price 2-mL amp = £4.86, 5-mL amp = £12.16

Cannabinoid

NABILONE

Indications: nausea and vomiting caused by cytotoxic chemotherapy, unresponsive to conventional anti-emetics (under close observation, preferably in in-patient setting)

Cautions: history of psychiatric disorder; elderly; hypertension; heart disease; adverse effects on mental state can persist for 48–72 hours after stopping; **interactions:** Appendix 1 (nabilone)

DRIVING. Drowsiness may affect performance of skilled tasks (e.g. driving); effects of alcohol enhanced

Contra-indications: severe hepatic impairment; pregnancy and breast-feeding

Side-effects: drowsiness, vertigo, euphoria, dry mouth, ataxia, visual disturbance, concentration difficulties, sleep disturbance, dysphoria, hypotension, headache and nausea; also confusion, disorientation, hallucinations, psychosis, depression, decreased coordination, tremors, tachycardia, decreased appetite, and abdominal pain

BEHAVIOURAL EFFECTS. Patients should be made aware of possible changes of mood and other adverse behavioural effects

Dose: initially 1 mg twice daily, increased if necessary to 2 mg twice daily, throughout each cycle of cytotoxic therapy and, if necessary, for 48 hours after the last dose of each cycle; max. 6 mg daily given in 3 divided doses. The first dose should be taken the night before initiation of cytotoxic treatment and the second dose 1–3 hours before the first dose of cytotoxic drug; ADOLESCENT and CHILD under 18 years not recommended

Nabilone (Cambridge) [PoM]

Capsules, blue/white, nabilone 1 mg. Net price 20-cap pack = £114.40 (hosp. only). Label: 2, counselling, behavioural effects

Hyoscine

HYOSCINE HYDROBROMIDE

(Scopolamine Hydrobromide)

Indications: motion sickness; premedication (section 15.1.3)

Cautions: elderly, urinary retention, cardiovascular disease, gastro-intestinal obstruction, hepatic or renal impairment; porphyria (see section 9.8.2); pregnancy and breast-feeding; **interactions:** Appendix 1 (antimuscarinics)

DRIVING. Drowsiness may affect performance of skilled tasks (e.g. driving) and may persist for up to 24 hours or longer after removal of patch: effects of alcohol enhanced

Contra-indications: closed-angle glaucoma

Side-effects: drowsiness, dry mouth, dizziness, blurred vision, difficulty with micturition

Dose: motion sickness, *by mouth*, 300 micrograms 30 minutes before start of journey followed by 300 micrograms every 6 hours if required; max. 3 doses in 24 hours; CHILD 4–10 years 75–150 micrograms, over 10 years 150–300 micrograms

Note. Proprietary brands of hyoscine hydrobromide tablets (*Joy-rides®, Kwells®*) are on sale to the public for motion sickness

Injection, see section 15.1.3

Scopoderm TTS® (Novartis Consumer Health) [PoM]

Patch, self-adhesive, pink, releasing hyoscine approx. 1 mg/72 hours when in contact with skin. Net price 2 = £4.30. Label: 19, counselling, see below

Administration: motion sickness prevention, apply 1 patch to hairless area of skin behind ear 5–6 hours before journey; replace if necessary after 72 hours, siting replacement patch behind other ear; CHILD under 10 years not recommended

COUNSELLING. Explain accompanying instructions to patient and in particular emphasise advice to wash hands after handling and to wash application site after removing, and to use one at a time

Other drugs for Ménière's disease

Betahistine has been promoted as a specific treatment for Ménière's disease.

BETAHISTINE DIHYDROCHLORIDE

Indications: vertigo, tinnitus and hearing loss associated with Ménière's disease

Cautions: asthma, history of peptic ulcer; pregnancy and breast-feeding; **interactions:** Appendix 1 (betahistine)

Contra-indications: phaeochromocytoma

Side-effects: gastro-intestinal disturbances; headache, rashes and pruritus reported

Dose: initially 16 mg 3 times daily, preferably with food; maintenance 24–48 mg daily; CHILD not recommended

Betahistine Dihydrochloride (Non-proprietary) PoM

Tablets, betahistine dihydrochloride 8 mg, net price 120-tab pack = £6.51; 16 mg, 84-tab pack = £14.60. Label: 21

Serc® (Solvay) PoM

Tablets, betahistine dihydrochloride 8 mg (Serc®-8), net price 120-tab pack = £10.04; 16 mg (Serc®-16), 84-tab pack = £14.06. Label: 21

4.7   Analgesics

4.7.1	Non-opioid analgesics
4.7.2	Opioid analgesics
4.7.3	Neuropathic pain
4.7.4	Antimigraine drugs

The non-opioid drugs (section 4.7.1), paracetamol and aspirin (and other NSAIDs), are particularly suitable for pain in musculoskeletal conditions, whereas the opioid analgesics (section 4.7.2) are more suitable for moderate to severe pain, particularly of visceral origin.

PAIN IN PALLIATIVE CARE. For advice on pain relief in palliative care see Prescribing in Palliative Care, pp. 13–17.

PAIN IN SICKLE-CELL DISEASE. The pain of mild sickle-cell crises is managed with paracetamol, an NSAID, codeine, or dihydrocodeine. Severe crises may require the use of morphine or diamorphine; concomitant use of an NSAID may potentiate analgesia and allow lower doses of the opioid to be used. Pethidine should be avoided if possible because accumulation of a neurotoxic metabolite can precipitate seizures; the relatively short half-life of pethidine necessitates frequent injections.

DYSMENORRHOEA. Use of an oral contraceptive prevents the pain of dysmenorrhoea which is generally associated with ovulatory cycles. If treatment is necessary paracetamol or an NSAID (section 10.1.1) will generally provide adequate relief of pain. The vomiting and severe pain associated with dysmenorrhoea in women with endometriosis may call for an antiemetic (in addition to an analgesic). Antispasmodics (such as alverine citrate, section 1.2) have been advocated for dysmenorrhoea but the antispasmodic action does not generally provide significant relief. Hyoscine butylbromide (section 1.2) has also been advocated for its antispasmodic action despite poor absorption following oral administration.

4.7.1   Non-opioid analgesics

Aspirin is indicated for headache, transient musculoskeletal pain, dysmenorrhoea and pyrexia. In inflammatory conditions, most physicians prefer anti-inflammatory treatment with another NSAID which may be better tolerated and more convenient for the patient. Aspirin is used increasingly for its antiplatelet properties (section 2.9). Aspirin tablets or dispersible aspirin tablets are adequate for most purposes as they act rapidly.

Gastric irritation may be a problem; it is minimised by taking the dose after food. Enteric coated preparations are available, but have a slow onset of action and are therefore unsuitable for single-dose analgesic use (though their prolonged action may be useful for night pain).

Aspirin interacts significantly with a number of other drugs and its interaction with warfarin is a **special hazard**, see **interactions:** Appendix 1 (aspirin).

Paracetamol is similar in efficacy to aspirin, but has no demonstrable anti-inflammatory activity; it is less irritant to the stomach and for that reason is now generally preferred to aspirin, particularly in the elderly. **Overdosage** with paracetamol is particularly dangerous as it may cause hepatic damage which is sometimes not apparent for 4 to 6 days (see Emergency Treatment of Poisoning, p. 23–24). **Benorilate** (section 10.1.1) is an aspirin–paracetamol ester.

Nefopam may have a place in the relief of persistent pain unresponsive to other non-opioid analgesics. It causes little or no respiratory depression, but sympathomimetic and antimuscarinic side-effects may be troublesome.

Non-steroidal anti-inflammatory analgesics (NSAIDs, section 10.1.1) are particularly useful for the treatment of patients with chronic disease accompanied by pain and inflammation. Some of them are also used in the short-term treatment of mild to moderate pain including transient musculoskeletal pain but paracetamol is now often preferred, particularly in the elderly (see also p. 18). They are also suitable for the relief of pain in dysmenorrhoea and to treat pain caused by secondary bone tumours, many of which produce lysis of bone and release prostaglandins (see Prescribing in Palliative Care, p. 13). NSAIDs including ketorolac are also used for peri-operative analgesia (section 15.1.4.2).

Compound analgesic preparations

Compound analgesic preparations that contain a simple analgesic (such as aspirin or paracetamol) with an opioid component reduce the scope for effective titration of the individual components in the management of pain of varying intensity.

Compound analgesic preparations containing paracetamol or aspirin with a low dose of an opioid analgesic (e.g. 8 mg of codeine phosphate per compound tablet) are commonly used, but the advantages have not been substantiated. The low dose of the opioid may be enough to cause opioid side-effects (in particular, constipation) and can complicate the treatment of **overdosage** (see p. 24) yet may not provide significant additional relief of pain.

A *full dose* of the opioid component (e.g. 60 mg codeine phosphate) in compound analgesic preparations effectively augments the analgesic activity but is associated with the full range of opioid side-effects (including nausea, vomiting, severe constipation, drowsiness, respiratory depression, and risk of dependence on long-term administration). For details of the **side-effects**, **cautions** and **contra-indications** of opioid analgesics, see p. 214 (**important**: the elderly are particularly susceptible to opioid side-effects and should receive lower doses).

In general, when assessing pain, it is necessary to weigh up carefully whether there is a need for a non-opioid and an opioid analgesic to be taken simultaneously.

Caffeine is a weak stimulant that is often included, in small doses, in analgesic preparations. It is claimed that the addition of caffeine may enhance the analgesic effect, but the alerting effect, mild habit-forming effect and possible provocation of headache may not always be desirable. Moreover, in excessive dosage or on withdrawal caffeine may itself induce headache.

ASPIRIN

(Acetylsalicylic Acid)

Indications: mild to moderate pain, pyrexia; see also section 10.1.1; antiplatelet (section 2.9)

Cautions: asthma, allergic disease, impaired renal or hepatic function (avoid if severe), dehydration; preferably avoid during fever or viral infection in adolescents (risk of Reye's syndrome, see below); pregnancy; elderly; G6PD-deficiency (section 9.1.5); **interactions:** Appendix 1 (aspirin)

Contra-indications: children under 12 years and in breast-feeding (Reye's syndrome, see below); gastro-intestinal ulceration, haemophilia; not for treatment of gout

HYPERSENSITIVITY. Aspirin and other NSAIDs are **contra-indicated** in patients with a history of hypersensitivity to aspirin or any other NSAID—*which includes those* in whom attacks of *asthma, angioedema, urticaria or rhinitis* have been precipitated by aspirin or any other NSAID

REYE'S SYNDROME. Owing to an association with Reye's syndrome aspirin-containing preparations should not be given to children under 12 years, unless specifically indicated, e.g. for juvenile arthritis (Still's disease). Reye's syndrome has also been reported very rarely in children over 12 years and aspirin should preferably be avoided during fever or viral infection in children and adolescents over 12 years

Side-effects: generally mild and infrequent but high incidence of gastro-intestinal irritation with slight asymptomatic blood loss, increased bleeding time, bronchospasm and skin reactions in hypersensitive patients. Prolonged administration, see section 10.1.1. **Overdosage:** see Emergency Treatment of Poisoning, p. 22

Dose: 300–900 mg every 4–6 hours when necessary; max. 4 g daily; CHILD and ADOLESCENT not

recommended (see Reye's syndrome above)
Rectal route, see below

Aspirin (Non-proprietary)
Tablets PoM [1], aspirin 300 mg. Net price 20 = 19p. Label: 21, 32
Available from most generic manufacturers
Tablets PoM [1], e/c, aspirin 300 mg, net price 100-tab pack = £5.44; 75 mg, see section 2.9. Label: 5, 25, 32
Available from Ashbourne, Galen
Dispersible tablets PoM [1], aspirin 300 mg, net price 20 = 22p; 75 mg, see section 2.9. Label: 13, 21, 32
Available from most generic manufacturers
Note. BP directs that no strength is stated the 300-mg strength should be dispensed, and that when soluble aspirin tablets are prescribed, dispersible aspirin tablets shall be dispensed.
Suppositories, aspirin 300 mg, net price 10 = £9.13. Label: 32
Dose: 2–3 suppositories inserted every 4 hours when necessary (max. 12 suppositories in 24 hours); CHILD not recommended (see above)
Available from Aurum (who also supply a 150-mg strength)

Caprin® (Sinclair)
Tablets PoM [1], e/c, f/c, pink, aspirin 300 mg, net price 30-tab pack = £1.66, 100-tab pack = £4.89; 75 mg, see section 2.9. Label: 5, 25, 32

Nu-Seals® Aspirin (Lilly)
Tablets PoM [1], e/c, aspirin 300 mg, net price 100-tab pack = £5.80; 75 mg, see section 2.9. Label: 5, 25, 32

■ With codeine phosphate 8 mg

[1]**Co-codaprin** (Non-proprietary) PoM ▱
Tablets, co-codaprin 8/400 (codeine phosphate 8 mg, aspirin 400 mg). Net price 20 = 33p. Label: 21, 32
Dose: 1–2 tablets every 4–6 hours when necessary; max. 8 tablets daily
Dispersible tablets, co-codaprin 8/400 (codeine phosphate 8 mg, aspirin 400 mg). Net price 20 = 73p. Label: 13, 21, 32
Dose: 1–2 tablets in water every 4–6 hours; max. 8 tablets daily
Available from Alpharma
When co-codaprin tablets or dispersible tablets are prescribed and no strength is stated, tablets or dispersible tablets, respectively, containing codeine phosphate 8 mg and aspirin 400 mg should be dispensed

> ▰ denotes preparations that are considered to be less suitable for prescribing (see p. vi)

■ Other compound preparations

Aspav® (Alpharma) PoM ▱
Dispersible tablets, aspirin 500 mg, papaveretum 7.71 mg (providing the equivalent of 5 mg of anhydrous morphine). Net price 30-tab pack = £4.60. Label: 2, 13, 21, 32
Dose: 1–2 tablets in water every 4–6 hours if necessary; max. 8 tablets daily

---

1. May be sold to the public provided packs contain no more than 32 capsules or tablets; pharmacists can sell multiple packs up to a total quantity of 100 capsules or tablets in justifiable circumstances; for details see *Medicines, Ethics and Practice*, No. 25, London, Pharmaceutical Press, 2001 (and subsequent editions as available)

Equagesic® (Wyeth) NHS CD ▰

Tablets, pink/white/yellow, ethoheptazine citrate 75 mg, meprobamate 150 mg, aspirin 250 mg. Net price 100-tab pack = £5.40. Label: 2, 21, 32

Dose: muscle pain, 1–2 tablets 3–4 times daily

■ Preparations on sale to the public

For a list of **preparations** containing aspirin and paracetamol **on sale to the public**, see p. 212.

PARACETAMOL
(Acetaminophen)

Indications: mild to moderate pain, pyrexia

Cautions: hepatic and renal impairment, alcohol dependence; **interactions:** Appendix 1 (paracetamol)

Side-effects: side-effects rare, but rashes, blood disorders; acute pancreatitis reported after prolonged use; **important:** liver damage (and less frequently renal damage) following **overdosage**, see Emergency Treatment of Poisoning, p. 23

Dose: *by mouth*, 0.5–1 g every 4–6 hours to a max. of 4 g daily; CHILD 2 months 60 mg for post-immunisation pyrexia; otherwise under 3 months (on doctor's advice only), 10 mg/kg (5 mg/kg if jaundiced); 3 months–1 year 60–120 mg, 1–5 years 120–250 mg, 6–12 years 250–500 mg; these doses may be repeated every 4–6 hours when necessary (max. of 4 doses in 24 hours)

For full Joint Committee on Vaccination and Immunisation recommendation on post-immunisation pyrexia, see section 14.1

Rectal route, see below

Paracetamol (Non-proprietary)

Tablets PoM [1], paracetamol 500 mg. Net price 20 = 15p. Label: 29, 30

Available from Alpharma, APS, IVAX, Sterling Health (Panadol® NHS)

Soluble Tablets (= Dispersible tablets) PoM [2], paracetamol 500 mg. Net price 60-tab pack = £2.82. Label: 13, 29, 30

Available from Sterling Health (Panadol Soluble® NHS)

Paediatric Soluble Tablets (= Paediatric dispersible tablets), paracetamol 120 mg. Net price 24-tab pack = 82p. Label: 13, 30

Available from R&C (Disprol® Soluble Paracetamol NHS)

Paediatric Oral Solution (= Paediatric Elixir), paracetamol 120 mg/5 mL. Net price 100 mL = 29p. Label: 30

Note. Sugar-free versions are available and can be ordered by specifying 'sugar-free' on the prescription.

Available from IVAX, Rosemont (Paldesic® NHS)

Oral Suspension 120 mg/5 mL (= Paediatric Mixture), paracetamol 120 mg/5 mL. Net price 100 mL = 41p. Label: 30

Note. BP directs that when Paediatric Paracetamol Oral Suspension or Paediatric Paracetamol Mixture is prescribed Paracetamol Oral Suspension 120 mg/5 mL should be dispensed; sugar-free versions can be ordered by specifying 'sugar-free' on the prescription

Available from Cupal (Medinol® Paediatric, sugar-free), IVAX, R&C (Disprol® Paediatric, sugar-free), Rosemont (Paldesic®), Sterling Health (Panadol®, sugar-free), Warner Lambert (Calpol® Paediatric, Calpol® Paediatric sugar-free)

Oral Suspension 250 mg/5 mL (= Mixture), paracetamol 250 mg/5 mL. Net price 100 mL = 73p. Label: 30

Available from Cupal (Medinol® Over 6 NHS), Hillcross, Rosemont (Paldesic®), Warner Wellcome (Calpol® 6 Plus NHS)

Suppositories, paracetamol 60 mg, net price 10 = £9.96; 125 mg, 10 = £11.50; 250 mg, 10 = £23.00; 500 mg, 10 = £9.53. Label: 30

Dose: by rectum, ADULT and CHILD over 12 years 0.5–1 g up to 4 times daily, CHILD 1–5 years 125–250 mg, 6–12 years 250–500 mg

Available from AstraZeneca (Alvedon®, 60 mg, 125 mg, 250 mg), Aurum (120 mg, 240 mg, 500 mg)

■ Co-codamol 8/500

When co-codamol tablets, dispersible (or effervescent) tablets, or capsules are prescribed and **no strength is stated** tablets, dispersible (or effervescent) tablets, or capsules, respectively, containing codeine phosphate **8 mg** and paracetamol **500 mg** should be dispensed.

Co-codamol 8/500 PoM [2](Non-proprietary) ▰

Tablets, co-codamol 8/500 (codeine phosphate 8 mg, paracetamol 500 mg) Net price 20 = 23p. Label: 29, 30

Dose: 1–2 tablets every 4–6 hours; max. 8 tablets daily; CHILD 6–12 years ½–1 tablet

Available from Alpharma, APS, CP, Galen, (Parake® NHS), Generics, IVAX, Sterling Health (Panadeine® NHS), Sterwin

Effervescent or *dispersible tablets*, co-codamol 8/500 (codeine phosphate 8 mg, paracetamol 500 mg). Net price 20 = £1.03. Label: 13, 29, 30

Dose: 1–2 tablets in water every 4–6 hours, max. 8 tablets daily; CHILD 6–12 years ½–1 tablet, max 4 daily

Available from Generics, Lagap, Roche Consumer Health (Paracodol®), Sterwin

Note. The Drug Tariff allows tablets of co-codamol labelled 'dispersible' to be dispensed against an order for 'effervescent' and *vice versa*

Capsules, co-codamol 8/500 (codeine phosphate 8 mg, paracetamol 500 mg). Net price 30 = £2.46. Label: 29, 30

Dose: 1–2 capsules every 4 hours; max. 8 capsules daily

Available from Roche Consumer Health (Paracodol® NHS)

■ Co-codamol 30/500

When co-codamol tablets, dispersible (or effervescent) tablets, or capsules are prescribed and **no strength is stated** tablets, dispersible (or effervescent) tablets, or capsules, respectively, containing codeine phosphate **8 mg** and paracetamol **500 mg** should be dispensed (see preparations above).

See warnings and notes on p. 208 (**important:** special care in elderly—reduce dose)

1. May be sold to the public provided packs contain no more than 32 capsules or tablets; pharmacists can sell multiple packs up to a total quantity of 100 capsules or tablets in justifiable circumstances; for details see *Medicines, Ethics and Practice*, No. 25, London, Pharmaceutical Press, 2001 (and subsequent editions as available)

2. May be sold to the public under certain circumstances; for exemptions see *Medicines, Ethics and Practice*, No. 25, London, Pharmaceutical Press, 2001 (and subsequent editions as available)

Co-codamol 30/500 (Non-proprietary) PoM ◢

Tablets, co-codamol 30/500 (codeine phosphate 30 mg, paracetamol 500 mg), net price 100-tab pack = £7.52. Label: 2, 29, 30

Dose: 1–2 tablets every 4 hours; max. 8 tablets daily; CHILD not recommended

Available from CP

Capsules, co-codamol 30/500 (codeine phosphate 30 mg, paracetamol 500 mg), net price 100-cap pack = £8.21. Label: 2, 29, 30

Dose: 1–2 capsules every 4 hours; max. 8 capsules daily; CHILD not recommended

Available from Goldshield (*Zapain®*), Schwarz (*Medocodene®*)

Kapake® (Galen) PoM ◢

Tablets, scored, co-codamol 30/500 (codeine phosphate 30 mg, paracetamol 500 mg). Net price 30-tab pack = £2.26 (hosp. only), 100-tab pack = £7.53. Label: 2, 29, 30

Dose: 1–2 tablets every 4 hours; max. 8 tablets daily; CHILD not recommended

Capsules, co-codamol 30/500 (codeine phosphate 30 mg, paracetamol 500 mg), net price 100-cap pack = £7.53. Label: 2, 29, 30

Dose: 1–2 capsules every 4 hours; max. 8 capsules daily; CHILD not recommended

Sachets (*Kapake Insts®*), co-codamol 30/500 (codeine phosphate 30 mg, paracetamol 500 mg), net price 30-sachet pack (hosp. only) = £2.56, 100-sachet pack = £8.53. Label: 2, 13, 29, 30

Dose: 1–2 sachets every 4 hours; max. 8 sachets daily; CHILD not recommended

Note. Higher strength also available, see under Co-codamol 60/1000

Solpadol® (Sanofi-Synthelabo) PoM ◢

Caplets (= tablets), co-codamol 30/500 (codeine phosphate 30 mg, paracetamol 500 mg). Net price 100-tab pack = £7.54. Label: 2, 29, 30

Dose: 2 tablets every 4 hours; max. 8 daily; CHILD not recommended

Capsules, grey/purple, co-codamol 30/500 (codeine phosphate 30 mg, paracetamol 500 mg). Net price 100-cap pack = £7.54. Label: 2, 29, 30

Dose: 1–2 capsules every 4 hours; max. 8 capsules daily; CHILD not recommended

Effervescent tablets, co-codamol 30/500 (codeine phosphate 30 mg, paracetamol 500 mg). Contains Na⁺ 18.6 mmol/tablet; avoid in *renal impairment*. Net price 100-tab pack = £9.05. Label: 2, 13, 29, 30

Dose: 2 tablets in water every 4 hours; max. 8 daily; CHILD not recommended

Tylex® (Schwarz) PoM ◢

Capsules, co-codamol 30/500 (codeine phosphate 30 mg, paracetamol 500 mg). Net price 100-cap pack = £8.21. Label: 2, 29, 30

Dose: 1–2 capsules every 4 hours; max. 8 capsules daily; CHILD not recommended

Effervescent tablets, co-codamol 30/500 (codeine phosphate 30 mg, paracetamol 500 mg). Contains Na⁺ 13.6 mmol/tablet; avoid in *renal impairment*. Net price 90-tab pack = £8.15. Label: 2, 13, 29, 30

Excipients: include aspartame 25 mg/tablet (see section 9.4.1)

Dose: 1–2 tablets in water every 4 hours; max. 8 tablets daily; CHILD not recommended

---

■ Co-codamol 60/1000

See warnings and notes on p. 208 (**important**: special care in elderly—reduce dose)

Kapake® (Galen) PoM ◢

Sachets (*Kapake Insts®*), co-codamol 60/1000 (codeine phosphate 60 mg, paracetamol 1 g), net price 50-sachet pack = £8.53. Label: 2, 13, 30

Dose: 1 sachet every 4 hours; max. 4 sachets daily; CHILD not recommended

Note. Lower strength also available, see under Co-codamol 30/500

■ With methionine (co-methiamol)

A mixture of methionine and paracetamol; methionine has no analgesic activity but may prevent paracetamol-induced liver toxicity if overdose taken

Paradote® (Penn)

Tablets, f/c, co-methiamol 100/500 (DL-methionine 100 mg, paracetamol 500 mg). Net price 24-tab pack = £1.05, 96-tab pack = £2.77. Label: 29, 30

Dose: 2 tablets every 4 hours; max. 8 tablets daily; CHILD 12 years and under, not recommended

■ With dihydrocodeine tartrate 10 mg

See notes on p. 208

Co-dydramol (Non-proprietary) PoM ◢

Tablets, scored, co-dydramol 10/500 (dihydrocodeine tartrate 10 mg, paracetamol 500 mg). Net price 20 = 27p. Label: 21, 29, 30

Dose: 1–2 tablets every 4–6 hours; max. 8 tablets daily; CHILD not recommended

Available from Alpharma, APS, CP, Galen (*Galake®* NHS), Generics, IVAX, Sterwin

When co-dydramol tablets are prescribed and no strength is stated tablets containing dihydrocodeine tartrate 10 mg and paracetamol 500 mg should be dispensed.

Note. Tablets containing paracetamol 500 mg and dihydrocodeine 7.46 mg (*Paramol®* NHS) are on sale to the public. The name *Paramol®* was formerly applied to a brand of co-dydramol tablets

■ With dihydrocodeine tartrate 20 or 30 mg

See warnings and notes on p. 208 (**important**: special care in elderly—reduce dose)

Remedeine® (Napp) PoM ◢

Tablets, paracetamol 500 mg, dihydrocodeine tartrate 20 mg. Net price 112-tab pack = £12.42. Label: 2, 21, 29, 30

Dose: 1–2 tablets every 4–6 hours; max. 8 tablets daily; CHILD not recommended

Forte tablets, paracetamol 500 mg, dihydrocodeine tartrate 30 mg. Net price 56-tab pack = £7.67. Label: 2, 21, 29, 30

Dose: 1–2 tablets every 4–6 hours; max. 8 tablets daily; CHILD not recommended

■ Other compound preparations

See warnings and notes on p. 208 (**important**: special care in elderly—reduce dose)

Co-proxamol (Non-proprietary) PoM ◢

Tablets, co-proxamol 32.5/325 (dextropropoxyphene hydrochloride 32.5 mg, paracetamol 325 mg). Net price 20 = 24p. Label: 2, 10 patient information leaflet (if available), 29, 30

Dose: 2 tablets 3–4 times daily; max. 8 tablets daily; CHILD not recommended

Available from Alpharma (*Cosalgesic®* NHS), APS, Dista (*Distalgesic®* NHS), IVAX, Sovereign, Sterwin

When co-proxamol tablets are prescribed and no strength is stated tablets containing dextropropoxyphene hydrochloride 32.5 mg and paracetamol 325 mg should be dispensed.

◢ denotes preparations that are considered to be less suitable for prescribing (see p. vi)

■ Preparations on Sale to the Public

The following is a list of preparations on sale to the public that contain **aspirin** or **paracetamol, alone** or with **other ingredients**. Other significant ingredients (such as codeine and caffeine) are listed. See p. 164 for CSM advice on phenylpropanolamine. For details of preparations containing ibuprofen on sale to the public, see section 10.1.1.

Important: in overdose contact **Poisons Information Services** (p. 20) for full details of the ingredients

Alka-Seltzer® (aspirin), **Alka-Seltzer® XS** (aspirin, caffeine, paracetamol), **Alka XS Go®** (aspirin, caffeine, paracetamol), **Anadin®** (aspirin, caffeine), **Anadin Cold Control®** (paracetamol, caffeine, phenylephrine), **Anadin Extra®**, **Anadin Extra Soluble®** (both aspirin, caffeine, paracetamol), **Anadin Maximum Strength®** (aspirin, caffeine), **Anadin Paracetamol®** (paracetamol), **Angettes 75®** (aspirin), **Askit®** (aspirin, aloxiprin = polymeric product of aspirin, caffeine), **Aspro Clear®** (aspirin)

Beechams-All-In-One® (paracetamol, guaifenesin, phenylephrine), **Beechams Cold & Flu®**, **Beechams Flu-Plus Hot Berry Fruits®**, **Beechams Flu-Plus Powder®**, **Beechams Hot Lemon®**, **Hot Lemon and Honey®**, **Hot Blackcurrant®** (all paracetamol, phenylephrine), **Beechams Flu-Plus Caplets®** (paracetamol, caffeine, phenylephrine), **Beechams Lemon Tablets®** (aspirin), **Beechams Powders®** (aspirin, caffeine), **Beechams Powders Capsules®** (paracetamol, caffeine, phenylephrine), **Benylin 4 Flu®** (paracetamol, diphenhydramine, pseudoephedrine), **Benylin Day and Night®** (*day tablets*, paracetamol, phenylpropanolamine, *night tablets*, paracetamol, diphenhydramine), **Boots Cold & Flu Relief Tablets®** (paracetamol, caffeine, phenylephrine), **Boots Children's 3 Months Plus Pain Relief®** (paracetamol), **Boots Cold Relief Hot Blackcurrant®**, **Hot Lemon®** (paracetamol), **Boots Migraine Relief®** (paracetamol, codeine), **Boots Seltzer®** (aspirin), **Boots Tension Headache Relief®** (paracetamol, caffeine, codeine, doxylamine)

Calpol Fast Melts®, **Calpol Infant®**, **Calpol 6 Plus®** (all paracetamol), **Caprin®** (aspirin), **Catarrh-Ex®** (paracetamol, caffeine, phenylephrine), **Codis 500®** (aspirin, codeine), **Mrs. Cullen's®** (aspirin)

Day Nurse® (paracetamol, dextromethorphan, phenylpropanolamine, caffeine), **De Witt's Analgesic Pills®** (paracetamol, caffeine), **Disprin®**, **Disprin CV®**, **Disprin Direct®** (all aspirin), **Disprin Extra®** (aspirin, paracetamol), **Disprol®** (paracetamol), **Doans Backache Pills®** (paracetamol, sodium salicylate), **Dolvan®** (paracetamol, diphenhydramine, ephedrine, caffeine), **Dozol®** (paracetamol, diphenhydramine), **Dristan Tablets®** (aspirin, caffeine, chlorphenamine, phenylephrine)

Feminax® (paracetamol, caffeine, codeine, hyoscine), **Fennings Children's Cooling Powders®** (paracetamol)

Galpamol® (paracetamol)

Hedex® (paracetamol), **Hedex Extra®** (paracetamol, caffeine)

Infadrops® (paracetamol)

Lemsip Cold + Flu Breathe Easy® (paracetamol, phenylephrine), **Lemsip Cold + Flu Combined Relief Capsules®** (paracetamol, caffeine, phenylephrine), **Lemsip Cold + Flu Max Strength®** (paracetamol, phenylephrine), **Lemsip Lemon®** or **Blackcurrant®**, **Lemsip Max Strength®** (all paracetamol, phenylephrine), **Lemsip Power & Paracetamol®** (paracetamol, pseudoephedrine)

Mandanol® (paracetamol), **Maximum Strength Aspro Clear®** (aspirin), **Medinol®** (paracetamol), **Medised®** (paracetamol, promethazine), **Medised® Infant** (paracetamol, diphenhydramine), **Midrid®** (paracetamol, isometheptene mucate), **Migraleve®** (*pink tablets*, paracetamol, codeine, buclizine, *yellow tablets*, paracetamol, codeine)

Night Nurse® (paracetamol, dextromethorphan, promethazine), **Nirolex Day Cold Comfort®** (paracetamol, pholcodine, pseudoephedrine), **Nirolex Night Cold Comfort®** (paracetamol, pseudoephedrine, diphenhydramine, pholcodine), **Nurse Sykes' Powders®** (aspirin, caffeine, paracetamol)

Panadol® (paracetamol), **Panadol Extra®** (paracetamol, caffeine), **Panadol Night®** (paracetamol, diphenhydramine), **Panadol Soluble®** (paracetamol), **Panadol Ultra®** (paracetamol, codeine), **Panaleve Junior®**, **Panaleve 6+®** (both paracetamol), **Paracets®** (paracetamol), **Paracets Plus®** (paracetamol, caffeine, phenylephrine), **Paraclear®** (paracetamol), **Paracodol®** (paracetamol, codeine), **Paradote®** (co-methiamol (paracetamol, DL-methionine), **Paramol®** (paracetamol, dihydrocodeine), **Phensic®** (aspirin, caffeine), **Placidex®** (paracetamol), **Propain®** (paracetamol, caffeine, codeine, diphenhydramine)

Resolve® (paracetamol)

Sinutab® (paracetamol, phenylpropanolamine), **Sinutab Nightime®** (paracetamol, phenylpropanolamine, phenyltoloxamine), **Solpadeine®** (paracetamol, caffeine, codeine), **Solpadeine Max®** (paracetamol, codeine), **Solpadeine Soluble®** (paracetamol, caffeine, codeine), **Sudafed-Co®** (paracetamol, pseudoephedrine), **Syndol®** (paracetamol, caffeine, codeine, doxylamine)

Tixymol® (paracetamol)

Ultramol Soluble® (paracetamol, codeine, caffeine), **Uniflu®** (paracetamol, caffeine, codeine, diphenhydramine, phenylephrine) **with Gregovite C®**

Veganin® (aspirin, paracetamol, codeine), **Vicks Medinite®** (paracetamol, dextromethorphan, doxylamine, ephedrine)

NEFOPAM HYDROCHLORIDE

Indications: moderate pain

Cautions: hepatic or renal disease, elderly, urinary retention; pregnancy and breast-feeding; **interactions:** Appendix 1 (nefopam)

Contra-indications: convulsive disorders; not indicated for myocardial infarction

Side-effects: nausea, nervousness, urinary retention, dry mouth, lightheadedness; less frequently vomiting, blurred vision, drowsiness, sweating, insomnia, tachycardia, headache; confusion and hallucinations also reported; may colour urine (pink)

Dose: *by mouth*, initially 60 mg (elderly, 30 mg) 3 times daily, adjusted according to response; usual range 30–90 mg 3 times daily; CHILD not recommended

By intramuscular injection, 20 mg every 6 hours; CHILD not recommended

Note. Nefopam hydrochloride 20 mg by injection ≡ 60 mg by mouth

Acupan® (3M) [PoM]
Tablets, f/c, nefopam hydrochloride 30 mg. Net price 90-tab pack = £10.93. Label: 2, 14
Injection, nefopam hydrochloride 20 mg/mL. Net price 1-mL amp = 69p

4.7.2   Opioid analgesics

Opioid analgesics are usually used to relieve moderate to severe pain particularly of visceral origin. Repeated administration may cause dependence and tolerance, but this is no deterrent in the control of pain in terminal illness, for guidelines see Prescribing in Palliative Care, p. 13. Regular use of a potent opioid may be appropriate for certain cases of chronic non-malignant pain; treatment should be supervised by a specialist and the patient should be assessed at regular intervals.

SIDE-EFFECTS. Opioid analgesics share many side-effects though qualitative and quantitative differences exist. The most common include nausea, vomiting, constipation, and drowsiness. Larger doses produce respiratory depression and hypotension. **Overdosage**, see Emergency Treatment of Poisoning, p. 24.

INTERACTIONS. See Appendix 1 (opioid analgesics) (**important**: special hazard with *pethidine and possibly other opioids* and MAOIs).

DRIVING. Drowsiness may affect performance of skilled tasks (e.g. driving); effects of alcohol enhanced.

CHOICE. **Morphine** remains the most valuable opioid analgesic for severe pain although it frequently causes nausea and vomiting. It is the standard against which other opioid analgesics are compared. In addition to relief of pain, morphine also confers a state of euphoria and mental detachment.

Morphine is the opioid of choice for the oral treatment of *severe pain in palliative care*. It is given regularly every 4 hours (or every 12 or 24 hours as modified-release preparations). For guidelines on dosage adjustment in palliative care, see p. 13.

Buprenorphine has both opioid agonist and antagonist properties and may precipitate withdrawal symptoms, including pain, in patients dependent on other opioids. It has abuse potential and may itself cause dependence. It has a much longer duration of action than morphine and sublingually is an effective analgesic for 6 to 8 hours. Vomiting may be a problem. Unlike most opioid analgesics its effects are only partially reversed by naloxone.

Codeine is effective for the relief of mild to moderate pain but is too constipating for long-term use.

Dextromoramide is less sedating than morphine and has a short duration of action.

Diphenoxylate (in combination with atropine, as co-phenotrope) is used in acute diarrhoea (see section 1.4.2).

Dipipanone used alone is less sedating than morphine but the only preparation available contains an anti-emetic and is therefore not suitable for regular regimens in palliative care (see p.15).

Dextropropoxyphene given alone is a very mild analgesic somewhat less potent than codeine. Combinations of dextropropoxyphene with paracetamol (co-proxamol) or aspirin have little more analgesic effect than paracetamol or aspirin alone. An important disadvantage of co-proxamol is that **overdosage** (which may be combined with alcohol) is complicated by respiratory depression and acute heart failure due to the dextropropoxyphene and by hepatotoxicity due to the paracetamol. Rapid treatment is essential (see Emergency Treatment of Poisoning, p. 24).

Diamorphine (heroin) is a powerful opioid analgesic. It may cause less nausea and hypotension than morphine. In *palliative care* the greater solubility of diamorphine allows effective doses to be injected in smaller volumes and this is important in the emaciated patient.

Dihydrocodeine has an analgesic efficacy similar to that of codeine. The dose of dihydrocodeine by mouth is usually 30 mg every 4 hours; doubling the dose to 60 mg may provide some additional pain relief but this may be at the cost of more nausea and vomiting. A 40-mg tablet is now also available.

Alfentanil, fentanyl and **remifentanil** are used by injection for intra-operative analgesia (section 15.1.4.3); fentanyl is available in a transdermal drug delivery system as a self-adhesive patch which is changed every 72 hours.

Meptazinol is claimed to have a low incidence of respiratory depression. It has a reported length of action of 2 to 7 hours with onset within 15 minutes.

Methadone is less sedating than morphine and acts for longer periods. In prolonged use, methadone should not be administered more often than twice daily to avoid the risk of accumulation and opioid overdosage. Methadone may be used instead of morphine in the occasional patient who experiences excitation (or exacerbation of pain) with morphine.

Nalbuphine has a similar efficacy to that of morphine for pain relief, but may have fewer side-effects and less abuse potential. Nausea and vomiting occur less than with other opioids but respiratory depression is similar to that with morphine.

Oxycodone has an efficacy and side-effect profile similar to that of morphine. It is used primarily for control of *pain in palliative care*. It is used as the pectinate in suppositories (special order from BCM Specials).

Pentazocine has both agonist and antagonist properties and precipitates withdrawal symptoms, including pain in patients dependent on other opioids. By injection it is more potent than dihydrocodeine or codeine, but hallucinations and thought disturbances may occur. It is not recommended and, in particular, should be avoided after myocardial infarction as it may increase pulmonary and aortic blood pressure as well as cardiac work.

Pethidine produces prompt but short-lasting analgesia; it is less constipating than morphine, but even in high doses is a less potent analgesic. It is not suitable for severe continuing pain. It is used for analgesia in labour; however, other opioids, such as morphine or diamorphine, are often preferred for obstetric pain.

Phenazocine is effective in severe pain and has less tendency to increase biliary pressure than other opioid analgesics. It can be administered sublingually if nausea and vomiting are a problem.

Tramadol produces analgesia by two mechanisms: an opioid effect and an enhancement of serotoninergic and adrenergic pathways. It has fewer of the typical opioid side-effects (notably, less respiratory depression, less constipation and less addiction potential); psychiatric reactions have been reported.

DOSE. The dose of opioids in the BNF may need to be **adjusted individually** according to the degree of analgesia and side-effects; patients' response to opioids varies widely.

POSTOPERATIVE ANALGESIA. The use of intra-operative opioids affects the prescribing of post-operative analgesics and in many cases delays the need for a postoperative analgesic. A postoperative opioid analgesic should be given with care since it may potentiate any residual respiratory depression (for the treatment of opioid-induced respiratory depression, see section 15.1.7). Non-opioid analgesics are also used for postoperative pain (section 15.1.4.2).

Morphine and **papaveretum** are used most widely. **Tramadol** is not as effective in severe pain as other opioid analgesics. **Buprenorphine** may antagonise the analgesic effect of previously admin-istered opioids and is generally not recommended. **Pethidine** is metabolised to norpethidine which may accumulate, particularly in renal impairment; norpethidine stimulates the central nervous system and may cause convulsions. **Meptazinol** and **nal-buphine** are rarely used.

Opioids are also given epidurally [unlicensed route] in the postoperative period but are associated with side-effects such as pruritus, urinary retention, nausea and vomiting; respiratory depression can be delayed, particularly with morphine.

For details of patient-controlled analgesia (PCA) to relieve postoperative pain, consult hospital proto-cols. Formulations specifically designed for PCA are available (*Pharma-Ject® Morphine Sulphate*).

ADDICTS. Although caution is necessary addicts (and ex-addicts) may be treated with analgesics in the same way as other people when there is a real clinical need. Doctors are reminded that they do not require a special licence to prescribe opioid anal-gesics for addicts for relief of pain due to organic disease or injury.

MORPHINE SALTS

Indications: see notes above and under Dose; acute diarrhoea (section 1.4.2); cough in terminal care (section 3.9.1)

Cautions: hypotension, hypothyroidism, asthma (avoid during attack) and decreased respiratory reserve, prostatic hypertrophy; pregnancy and breast-feeding; may precipitate coma in hepatic impairment (reduce dose or avoid but many such patients tolerate morphine well); reduce dose or avoid in renal impairment (see also Appendix 3), elderly and debilitated (reduce dose); convulsive disorders, dependence (severe withdrawal symp-toms if withdrawn abruptly); use of cough sup-pressants containing opioid analgesics not generally recommended in children and should be avoided altogether in those under at least 1 year; **interactions:** Appendix 1 (opioid analgesics)

PALLIATIVE CARE. In the control of pain in terminal ill-ness these cautions should not necessarily be a deterrent to the use of opioid analgesics

Contra-indications: avoid in acute respiratory depression, acute alcoholism and where risk of paralytic ileus; also avoid in raised intracranial pressure or head injury (in addition to interfering with respiration, affect pupillary responses vital for neurological assessment); avoid injection in phaeochromocytoma (risk of pressor response to histamine release)

Side-effects: nausea and vomiting (particularly in initial stages), constipation, and drowsiness;

larger doses produce respiratory depression and hypotension; other side-effects include difficulty with micturition, ureteric or biliary spasm, dry mouth, sweating, headache, facial flushing, vertigo, bradycardia, tachycardia, palpitations, postural hypotension, hypothermia, hallucina-tions, dysphoria, mood changes, dependence, miosis, decreased libido or potency, rashes, urti-caria and pruritus; **overdosage:** see Emergency Treatment of Poisoning, p. 24; for reversal of opioid-induced respiratory depression, see section 15.1.7.

Dose: acute pain, *by subcutaneous injection* (not suitable for oedematous patients) *or by intramus-cular injection*, 10 mg every 4 hours if necessary (15 mg for heavier well-muscled patients); CHILD up to 1 month 150 micrograms/kg, 1–12 months 200 micrograms/kg, 1–5 years 2.5–5 mg, 6–12 years 5–10 mg
By slow intravenous injection, quarter to half cor-responding intramuscular dose

Premedication, *by subcutaneous or intramuscular injection*, up to 10 mg 60–90 minutes before oper-ation; CHILD, *by intramuscular injection*, 150 micrograms/kg

Postoperative pain, *by subcutaneous or intramuscu-lar injection*, 10 mg every 2–4 hours if necessary (15 mg for heavier well-muscled patients); CHILD up to 1 month 150 micrograms/kg, 1–12 months 200 micrograms/kg, 1–5 years 2.5–5 mg, 6–12 years 5–10 mg
Note. In the postoperative period, the patient should be closely monitored for pain relief as well as for side-effects especially respiratory depression

Patient controlled analgesia (PCA), consult hospital protocols

Myocardial infarction, *by slow intravenous injec-tion* (2 mg/minute), 10 mg followed by a further 5–10 mg if necessary; elderly or frail patients, reduce dose by half

Acute pulmonary oedema, *by slow intravenous injection* (2 mg/minute) 5–10 mg

Chronic pain, *by mouth or by subcutaneous injec-tion* (not suitable for oedematous patients) *or by intramuscular injection*, 5–20 mg regularly every 4 hours; dose may be increased according to needs; oral dose should be approx. double corre-sponding intramuscular dose and approximately triple corresponding intramuscular *diamorphine* dose (see also Prescribing in Palliative Care, p. 13); *by rectum*, as suppositories, 15–30 mg reg-ularly every 4 hours
Note. The doses stated above refer equally to morphine hydrochloride, sulphate, and tartrate; see below for doses of **modified-release** preparations.

■ Oral solutions
Note. For advice on transfer from oral solutions of mor-phine to modified-release preparations of morphine, see Prescribing in Palliative Care, p. 13

Morphine Oral Solutions ⃞PoM⃞ or ⃞CD⃞
Oral solutions of morphine can be prescribed by writing the formula:
Morphine hydrochloride 5 mg
Chloroform water to 5 mL
Note. The proportion of morphine hydrochloride may be altered when specified by the prescriber; if above 13 mg per 5 mL the solution becomes CD. For sample prescrip-tion see Controlled Drugs and Drug Dependence, p. 7. It is usual to adjust the strength so that the dose volume is 5 or 10 mL.

Oramorph® (Boehringer Ingelheim)

Oramorph® oral solution [PoM], morphine sulphate 10 mg/5 mL. Net price 100-mL pack = £2.08; 300-mL pack = £5.79; 500-mL pack = £8.73. Label: 2

Oramorph® Unit Dose Vials 10 mg [PoM] (oral vials), sugar-free, morphine sulphate 10 mg/5-mL vial, net price 25 vials = £3.31. Label: 2

Oramorph® Unit Dose Vials 30 mg [CD] (oral vials), sugar-free, morphine sulphate 30 mg/5-mL vial, net price 25 vials = £9.30. Label: 2

Oramorph® concentrated oral solution [CD], sugar-free, morphine sulphate 100 mg/5 mL. Net price 30-mL pack = £5.82; 120-mL pack = £21.74 (both with calibrated dropper). Label: 2

Oramorph® Unit Dose Vials 100 mg [CD] (oral vials), sugar-free, morphine sulphate 100 mg/5-mL vial, net price 25 vials = £31.00. Label: 2

Sevredol® (Napp)

Oral solution [PoM], morphine sulphate 10 mg/5 mL, net price 100 mL = £1.99, 300 mL = £5.53, 500 mL = £8.34. Label: 2

Concentrated oral solution [CD], morphine sulphate 20 mg/mL, net price 30 mL = £5.56, 120 mL = £20.76 (both with dropper or oral syringe). Label: 2

Dose: severe pain uncontrolled by weaker opioid, 10-20 mg every 4 hours (dose adjusted according to response); CHILD 1–5 years, 5 mg every 4 hours; 6–12 years, 5–10 mg

■ Tablets

Sevredol® (Napp) [CD]

Tablets, f/c, scored, morphine sulphate 10 mg (blue), net price 56-tab pack = £6.03; 20 mg (pink), 56-tab pack = £12.05; 50 mg (pale green), 56-tab pack = £30.13. Label: 2

Dose: severe pain uncontrolled by weaker opioid, 10–50 mg every 4 hours (dose adjusted according to response); CHILD 3–5 years, 5 mg every 4 hours; 6–12 years, 5–10 mg

■ Modified-release oral preparations

Morcap® SR (Sanofi-Synthelabo) [CD]

Capsules, m/r, clear enclosing ivory and brown pellets, morphine sulphate 20 mg, net price 30-cap pack = £5.45, 60-cap pack = £10.91; 50 mg, 30-cap pack = £13.22, 60-cap pack = £26.43; 100 mg, 30-cap pack = £26.43, 60-cap pack = £52.88. Label: 2, counselling, see below

Dose: adjusted according to daily morphine requirements, for further advice on determining dose, see Prescribing in Palliative Care, p. 13; dosage requirements may need to be reviewed if the brand is altered

COUNSELLING. Swallow whole or open capsule and sprinkle contents on soft food

Note. Prescription must also specify 'capsules' (i.e. 'Morcap SR capsules')

MST Continus® (Napp) [CD]

Tablets, m/r, f/c, morphine sulphate 5 mg (white), net price 60-tab pack = £4.30; 10 mg (brown), 60-tab pack = £7.17; 15 mg (green), 60-tab pack = £12.57; 30 mg (purple), 60-tab pack = £17.22; 60 mg (orange), 60-tab pack = £33.58; 100 mg (grey), 60-tab pack = £53.16; 200 mg (green), 60-tab pack = £106.34. Label: 2, 25

Suspension (= sachet of granules to mix with water), m/r, pink, morphine sulphate 20 mg/sachet, net price 30-sachet pack = £27.31; 30 mg/sachet, 30-sachet pack = £28.38; 60 mg/sachet, 30-sachet pack = £56.77; 100 mg/sachet, 30-sachet pack = £94.61; 200 mg/sachet pack, 30-sachet pack = £189.22. Label: 2, 13

Dose: adjusted according to daily morphine requirements, for further advice on determining dose, see Prescribing in Palliative Care, p. 13; dosage requirements may need to be reviewed if the brand is altered

Note. Prescriptions must also specify 'tablets' or 'suspension' (i.e. 'MST Continus tablets' or 'MST Continus suspension').

MXL® (Napp) [CD]

Capsules, m/r, morphine sulphate 30 mg (light blue), net price 28-cap pack = £11.73; 60 mg (brown), 28-cap pack = £16.07; 90 mg (pink), 28-cap pack = £23.70; 120 mg (green), 28-cap pack = £31.34; 150 mg (blue), 28-cap pack = £39.17; 200 mg (red-brown), 28-cap pack = £49.62. Label: 2, counselling, see below

Dose: adjusted according to daily morphine requirements, for further advice on determining dose, see Prescribing in Palliative Care, p. 13; dosage requirements may need to be reviewed if the brand is altered

COUNSELLING. Swallow whole or open capsule and sprinkle contents on soft food

Note. Prescriptions must also specify 'capsules' (i.e. 'MXL capsules')

Zomorph® (Link) [CD]

Capsules, m/r, morphine sulphate 10 mg (yellow/clear enclosing pale yellow pellets), net price 60-cap pack = £4.31; 30 mg (pink/clear enclosing pale yellow pellets), 60-cap pack = £10.33; 60 mg (orange/clear enclosing pale yellow pellets), 60-cap pack = £20.15; 100 mg (white/clear enclosing pale yellow pellets), 60-cap pack = £31.90; 200 mg (clear enclosing pale yellow pellets), 60-cap pack = £63.79. Label: 2, counselling, see below

Dose: adjusted according to daily morphine requirements, for further advice on determining doses, see Prescribing in Palliative Care, p. 13; dosage requirements may need to be reviewed if the brand is altered

COUNSELLING. Swallow whole or open capsule and sprinkle contents on soft food

Note. Prescriptions must also specify 'capsules' (i.e. 'Zomorph capsules')

■ Modified-release rectal preparations

Moraxen® (Schwarz) [CD]

Rectal tampons (= non-dissolving suppositories), m/r, morphine sulphate 35 mg, net price 7 = £10.00; 50 mg, 7 = £10.50; 75 mg, 7 = £15.75; 100 mg, 7 = £21.00. Label: 2, counselling, administration

Dose: adjusted according to daily morphine requirements; for further advice on determining dose, see prescribing in Palliative Care, p. 13; more than one tampon may be used simultaneously

COUNSELLING. Tampon (or tampons) to be expelled after 24 hours before replacing with another dose; if not expelled after 30 hours, use glycerol suppositories or remove manually

Note. Prescriptions must also specify 'rectal tampons' (i.e. 'Moraxen rectal tampons').

■ Suppositories

Morphine (Non-proprietary) CD

Suppositories, morphine hydrochloride or sulphate 10 mg, net price 12 = £6.12; 15 mg, 12 = £6.80; 20 mg, 12 = £7.45; 30 mg, 12 = £9.73. Label: 2

Available from Aurum, Celltech, Martindale

Note. Both the strength of the suppositories and the morphine salt contained in them must be specified by the prescriber

■ Injections

Morphine Sulphate (Non-proprietary) CD

Injection, morphine sulphate 10, 15, 20, and 30 mg/mL, net price 1- and 2-mL amp (all) = 72–£1.59

Intravenous infusion, morphine sulphate 1 mg/mL, net price 50-mL vial = £4.75; 2 mg/mL, 50-mL vial = £4.85

Available from Aurum, Faulding DBL

Morphine and Atropine Injection (Non-proprietary) CD

Injection, morphine sulphate 10 mg, atropine sulphate 600 micrograms/mL. Net price 1-mL amp = £4.65

Dose: premedication, by subcutaneous injection, 0.5–1 mL

■ Injection with anti-emetic

CAUTION. In myocardial infarction cyclizine may aggravate severe heart failure and counteract the haemodynamic benefits of opioids, see section 4.6. **Not recommended** in palliative care, see p. 13

Cyclimorph® (CeNeS) CD

Cyclimorph-10® Injection, morphine tartrate 10 mg, cyclizine tartrate 50 mg/mL. Net price 1-mL amp = £1.22

Dose: moderate to severe pain (short-term use only) by subcutaneous, intramuscular, or intravenous injection, 1 mL, repeated not more often than every 4 hours, with not more than 3 doses in any 24-hour period

Cyclimorph-15® Injection, morphine tartrate 15 mg, cyclizine tartrate 50 mg/mL. Net price 1-mL amp = £1.26

Dose: moderate to severe pain (short-term use only) by subcutaneous, intramuscular, or intravenous injection, 1 mL, repeated not more often than every 4 hours, with not more than 3 doses in any 24-hour period

BUPRENORPHINE

Indications: moderate to severe pain; peri-operative analgesia; opioid dependence (section 4.10)

Cautions: see under Morphine Salts and notes above; effects only partially reversed by naloxone; **interactions:** Appendix 1 (opioid analgesics)

Contra-indications: see under Morphine Salts and notes above

Side-effects: see under Morphine Salts and notes above; can give rise to mild withdrawal symptoms in patients dependent on opioids

Dose: moderate to severe pain, *by sublingual administration*, initially 200–400 micrograms every 8 hours, increasing if necessary to 200–400 micrograms every 6–8 hours; CHILD over 6 months, 16–25 kg, 100 micrograms; 25–37.5 kg, 100–200 micrograms; 37.5–50 kg, 200–300 micrograms

By intramuscular or slow intravenous injection, 300–600 micrograms every 6–8 hours; CHILD over 6 months 3–6 micrograms/kg every 6–8 hours (max. 9 micrograms/kg)

Premedication, by sublingual administration, 400 micrograms

By intramuscular injection, 300 micrograms

Intra-operative analgesia, by slow intravenous injection, 300–450 micrograms

Temgesic® (Schering-Plough) CD

Tablets (sublingual), buprenorphine (as hydrochloride), 200 micrograms, net price 50-tab pack = £5.73; 400 micrograms, 50-tab pack = £11.46. Label: 2, 26

Injection, buprenorphine (as hydrochloride) 300 micrograms/mL, net price 1-mL amp = 53p

CODEINE PHOSPHATE

Indications: mild to moderate pain; diarrhoea (section 1.4.2); cough suppression (section 3.9.1)

Cautions: see under Morphine Salts and notes above; use of cough suppressants containing codeine or similar opioid analgesics not generally recommended in children and should be avoided altogether in those under 1 year; **interactions:** Appendix 1 (opioid analgesics)

Contra-indications: see under Morphine Salts and notes above

Side-effects: see under Morphine Salts and notes above

Dose: *by mouth*, 30–60 mg every 4 hours when necessary, to a max. of 240 mg daily; CHILD 1–12 years, 3 mg/kg daily in divided doses

By intramuscular injection, 30–60 mg every 4 hours when necessary

Codeine Phosphate (Non-proprietary)

Tablets PoM, codeine phosphate 15 mg, net price 20 =73p; 30 mg, 20 = £1.04; 60 mg, 20 = £1.85. Label: 2

Note. As for schedule 2 controlled drugs, travellers needing to take codeine phosphate preparations abroad may require a doctor's letter explaining why they are necessary

Syrup PoM, codeine phosphate 25 mg/5 mL. Net price 100 mL = 89p. Label: 2

Injection CD, codeine phosphate 60 mg/mL. Net price 1-mL amp = £2.15

Codeine Linctuses

Section 3.9.1

Note. Codeine is an ingredient of some compound analgesic preparations, section 4.7.1 and section 10.1.1 (*Codafen Continus®*)

DEXTROMORAMIDE

Indications: severe pain

Cautions: see under Morphine Salts and notes above; short duration of action (2–3 hours); **interactions:** Appendix 1 (opioid analgesics)

Contra-indications: see under Morphine Salts and notes above; obstetric analgesia (increased risk of neonatal depression)

Side-effects: see under Morphine Salts and notes above

Dose: *by mouth*, 5 mg increasing to 20 mg, when required

Palfium® (Roche) CD

Tablets, both scored, dextromoramide (as tartrate) 5 mg (white), net price 60-tab pack = £4.45; 10 mg (peach), 60-tab pack = £8.80. Label: 2

DEXTROPROPOXYPHENE HYDROCHLORIDE

Indications: mild to moderate pain

Cautions: see under Morphine Salts and notes above; compound preparations special hazard in overdose, see notes above; **interactions:** Appendix 1 (opioid analgesics)

Contra-indications: see under Morphine Salts and notes above; those who are suicidal or addiction prone; porphyria (section 9.8.2)

Side-effects: see under Morphine Salts and notes above; also occasional hepatotoxicity; convulsions reported in overdose

Dose: 65 mg every 6–8 hours when necessary; CHILD not recommended

Note. 65 mg dextropropoxyphene hydrochloride ≡ 100 mg dextropropoxyphene napsilate

Dextropropoxyphene (Non-proprietary) PoM

Capsules, pink, the equivalent of dextropropoxyphene hydrochloride 65 mg (as napsilate). Net price 100-tab pack = £8.20. Label: 2

Available from Lilly (Doloxene® NHS)

Note. Dextropropoxyphene is an ingredient of some compound analgesic preparations, section 4.7.1

DIAMORPHINE HYDROCHLORIDE

(Heroin Hydrochloride)

Indications: see notes above; acute pulmonary oedema

Cautions: see under Morphine Salts and notes above; **interactions:** Appendix 1 (opioid analgesics)

Contra-indications: see under Morphine Salts and notes above

Side-effects: see under Morphine Salts and notes above

Dose: acute pain, *by subcutaneous or intramuscular injection*, 5 mg repeated every 4 hours if necessary (up to 10 mg for heavier well-muscled patients)

By slow intravenous injection, quarter to half corresponding intramuscular dose

Myocardial infarction, *by slow intravenous injection* (1 mg/minute), 5 mg followed by a further 2.5–5 mg if necessary; elderly or frail patients, reduce dose by half

Acute pulmonary oedema, *by slow intravenous injection* (1 mg/minute) 2.5–5 mg

Chronic pain, *by mouth or by subcutaneous or intramuscular injection*, 5–10 mg regularly every 4 hours; dose may be increased according to needs; intramuscular dose should be approx. half corresponding oral dose, and approx. one third corresponding oral *morphine* dose—see also Prescribing in Palliative Care, p. 13; *by subcutaneous infusion* (using syringe driver), see Prescribing in Palliative Care, p. 15

Diamorphine (Non-proprietary) CD

Tablets, diamorphine hydrochloride 10 mg. Net price 100-tab pack = £12.30. Label: 2

Available from Aurum

Injection, powder for reconstitution, diamorphine hydrochloride. Net price 5-mg amp = £1.18, 10-mg amp = £1.36, 30-mg amp = £1.62, 100-mg amp = £4.50, 500-mg amp = £20.68

Available from Celltech, CP, Hillcross

DIHYDROCODEINE TARTRATE

Indications: moderate to severe pain

Cautions: see under Morphine Salts and notes above; **interactions:** Appendix 1 (opioid analgesics)

Contra-indications: see under Morphine Salts and notes above

Side-effects: see under Morphine Salts and notes above

Dose: *by mouth*, 30 mg every 4–6 hours when necessary (see also notes above); CHILD over 4 years 0.5–1 mg/kg every 4–6 hours

By deep subcutaneous or intramuscular injection, up to 50 mg repeated every 4–6 hours if necessary; CHILD over 4 years 0.5–1 mg/kg every 4–6 hours

Dihydrocodeine (Non-proprietary)

Tablets PoM, dihydrocodeine tartrate 30 mg. Net price 20 = 71p. Label: 2, 21

Available from most generic manufacturers

Oral solution PoM, dihydrocodeine tartrate 10 mg/5 mL. Net price 150 mL = £3.20. Label: 2, 21

Available from Martindale

Injection CD, dihydrocodeine tartrate 50 mg/mL. Net price 1-mL amp = £1.98

Available from Aurum

DF 118 Forte® (Martindale) PoM

Tablets, dihydrocodeine tartrate 40 mg. Net price 100-tab pack = £11.51. Label: 2, 21

Dose: severe pain, 40–80 mg 3 times daily; max. 240 mg daily; CHILD not recommended

■ Modified release

DHC Continus® (Napp) PoM

Tablets, m/r, dihydrocodeine tartrate 60 mg, net price 56-tab pack = £6.69; 90 mg, 56-tab pack = £10.53; 120 mg, 56-tab pack = £14.07. Label: 2, 25

Dose: chronic severe pain, 60–120 mg every 12 hours; CHILD not recommended

Note. Dihydrocodeine is an ingredient of some compound analgesic preparations, see section 4.7.1

DIPIPANONE HYDROCHLORIDE

Indications: moderate to severe pain

Cautions: see under Morphine Salts and notes above; **interactions:** Appendix 1 (opioid analgesics)

Contra-indications: see under Morphine Salts and notes above

Side-effects: see under Morphine Salts and notes above

Dose: see preparation below

Diconal® (CeNeS) [CD]

Tablets, pink, scored, dipipanone hydrochloride 10 mg, cyclizine hydrochloride 30 mg. Net price 50-tab pack = £7.25. Label: 2

Dose: acute pain, 1 tablet gradually increased to 3 tablets every 6 hours; CHILD not recommended

CAUTION. **Not recommended** in palliative care, see p. 15

FENTANYL

Indications: breakthrough pain in patients already receiving opioid therapy for chronic pain (lozenges); chronic intractable cancer pain (patches); other indications (section 15.1.4.3)

Cautions: see under Morphine Salts and notes above; **interactions:** Appendix 1 (opioid analgesics)

FEVER OR EXTERNAL HEAT. Monitor patients using patches for increased side-effects if fever present (increased absorption possible); avoid exposing application site to external heat (may also increase absorption)

Contra-indications: see under Morphine Salts and notes above

Side-effects: see under Morphine Salts and notes above; with patches, local reactions such as rash, erythema and itching reported

Dose: see under preparation, below

CONVERSION (from oral morphine to transdermal fentanyl). See Prescribing in palliative care, p. 14

Actiq® (Elan) ▼ [CD]

Lozenge, (with integral oromucosal applicator), fentanyl (as citrate) 200 micrograms, net price 3 = £19.44, 30 = £194.40; 400 micrograms, 3 = £19.44, 30 = £194.40; 600 micrograms, 3 = £19.44, 30 = £194.40; 800 micrograms, 3 = £19.44, 30 = £194.40; 1.2 mg, 3 = £19.44, 30 = £194.40; 1.6 mg, 3 = £19.44, 30 = £194.40. Label: 2

Dose: initially 200 micrograms (over 15 minutes) repeated if necessary 15 minutes after first dose (no more than 2 dose units for each pain episode); adjust dose according to response; max. 4 dose units daily

Note. If more than 4 episodes of breakthrough pain each day, adjust dose of background analgesic

Durogesic® (Janssen-Cilag) [CD]

Patches, self-adhesive, transparent, fentanyl, '25' patch (releasing approx. 25 micrograms/hour for 72 hours), net price 5 = £28.97; '50' patch (releasing approx. 50 micrograms/hour for 72 hours), 5 = £54.11; '75' patch (releasing approx. 75 micrograms/hour for 72 hours), 5 = £75.43; '100' patch (releasing approx. 100 micrograms/hour for 72 hours), 5 = £92.97. Label: 2

ADMINISTRATION. apply to dry, non-irritated, non-irradiated, non-hairy skin on torso or upper arm, removing after 72 hours and siting replacement patch on a different area (avoid using the same area for several days). Patients who have not previously received a strong opioid analgesic, initial dose, one '25 micrograms/hour' patch replaced after 72 hours; patients who have received a strong opioid analgesic, initial dose based on previous 24-hour opioid requirement (oral morphine sulphate 90 mg over 24 hours ≈ one '25 micrograms/hour' patch, consult product literature for details); CHILD not recommended

Note. When starting, evaluation of the analgesic effect should **not** be made before the system has been worn for **24 hours** (to allow for the gradual increase in plasma-fentanyl concentration)—previous analgesic therapy should be phased out gradually from time of first patch

application; dose adjustment should normally be carried out in 72-hour steps of '25 micrograms/hour'. More than one patch may be used at a time for doses greater than '100 micrograms/hour' (but applied at *same time* to avoid confusion)—consider additional or alternative analgesic therapy if dose required exceeds 300 micrograms/hour (**important:** it may take 17 hours or longer for the plasma-fentanyl concentration to decrease by 50%, therefore replacement opioid therapy should be initiated at a low dose, increasing gradually).

LONG DURATION OF ACTION. In view of the long duration of action, patients who have experienced severe side-effects should be monitored for up to 24 hours after patch removal

---

HYDROMORPHONE HYDROCHLORIDE

Indications: severe pain in cancer

Cautions: see under Morphine Salts and notes above; **interactions:** Appendix 1 (opioid analgesics)

Contra-indications: see Morphine Salts and notes above

Side-effects: see Morphine Salts and notes above

Dose: see under preparations below

Palladone® (Napp) [CD]

Capsules, hydromorphone hydrochloride 1.3 mg (orange/clear), net price 56-cap pack = £8.82; 2.6 mg (red/clear), 56-cap pack = £17.64. Label: 2, counselling, see below

Dose: 1.3 mg every 4 hours, increased if necessary according to severity of pain; CHILD under 12 years not recommended

COUNSELLING. Swallow whole or open capsule and sprinkle contents on soft food

■ Modified release

Palladone® SR (Napp) [CD]

Capsules, m/r, hydromorphone hydrochloride 2 mg (yellow/clear), net price 56-cap pack = £18.73; 4 mg (pale blue/clear), 56-cap pack = £25.67; 8 mg (pink/clear), 56-cap pack = £50.07; 16 mg (brown/clear), 56-cap pack = £95.12; 24 mg (dark blue/clear), 56-cap pack = £142.70. Label: 2, counselling, see below

Dose: 4 mg every 12 hours, increased if necessary according to severity of pain; CHILD under 12 years not recommended

COUNSELLING. Swallow whole or open capsule and sprinkle contents on soft food

---

MEPTAZINOL

Indications: moderate to severe pain, including postoperative and obstetric pain and renal colic; peri-operative analgesia, see section 15.1.4.3

Cautions: see under Morphine Salts and notes above; effects only partially reversed by naloxone; **interactions:** Appendix 1 (opioid analgesics)

Contra-indications: see under Morphine Salts and notes above

Side-effects: see under Morphine Salts and notes above

Dose: *by mouth,* 200 mg every 3–6 hours as required; CHILD not recommended

By intramuscular injection, 75–100 mg every 2–4 hours if necessary; obstetric analgesia, 100–150 mg according to patient's weight (2 mg/kg); CHILD not recommended

By slow intravenous injection, 50–100 mg every 2–4 hours if necessary; CHILD not recommended

Meptid® (Shire) PoM
Tablets, orange, f/c, meptazinol 200 mg, net price
112-tab pack = £22.11. Label: 2
Injection, meptazinol 100 mg (as hydrochloride)/
mL, net price 1-mL amp = £1.92

METHADONE HYDROCHLORIDE

Indications: severe pain, see notes above; cough
in terminal disease (section 3.9.1); adjunct in
treatment of opioid dependence (section 4.10)
Cautions: see under Morphine Salts and notes
above; **interactions:** Appendix 1 (opioid analgesics)
Contra-indications: see under Morphine Salts
and notes above
Side-effects: see under Morphine Salts and notes
above
Dose: *by mouth or by subcutaneous or intramuscular injection*, 5–10 mg every 6–8 hours, adjusted
according to response; CHILD not recommended

Methadone (Non-proprietary) CD
Tablets, scored, methadone hydrochloride 5 mg.
Net price 50 = £2.97. Label: 2
Available from Martindale (*Physeptone®*)
Injection, methadone hydrochloride 10 mg/mL,
net price 1-mL amp = 86p, 2-mL amp = £1.45,
3.5-mL amp = £1.78, 5-mL amp = £1.92
Available from CP, Martindale (*Physeptone®*)

NALBUPHINE HYDROCHLORIDE

Indications: moderate to severe pain; premedication; peri-operative analgesia; myocardial infarction
Cautions: see under Morphine Salts and notes
above; **interactions:** Appendix 1 (opioid analgesics)
Contra-indications: see under Morphine Salts
and notes above
Side-effects: see under Morphine Salts and notes
above
Dose: moderate to severe pain, *by subcutaneous,
intramuscular, or intravenous injection*, 10–
20 mg for 70 kg patient, adjusted as required;
CHILD up to 300 micrograms/kg repeated once or
twice as necessary
Premedication, *by subcutaneous, intramuscular, or
intravenous injection*, 100–200 micrograms/kg
Induction, *by intravenous injection*, 0.3–1 mg/kg
over 10–15 minutes
Intra-operative analgesia, *by intravenous injection*,
250–500 micrograms /kg at 30-minute intervals
Myocardial infarction, *by slow intravenous injection*, 10–20 mg repeated after 30 minutes if necessary

Nubain® (Bristol-Myers Squibb) PoM
Injection, nalbuphine hydrochloride 10 mg/mL.
Net price 1-mL amp = 70p; 2-mL amp = £1.08

OXYCODONE HYDROCHLORIDE

Indications: moderate to severe pain in patients
with cancer; postoperative pain
Cautions: see under Morphine Salts and notes
above; avoid in porphyria (section 9.8.2); **interactions:** Appendix 1 (opioid analgesics)

Contra-indications: see under Morphine Salts
and notes above
Side-effects: see under Morphine Salts and notes
above
Dose: see under Preparations below

OxyNorm® (Napp) ▼ CD
Capsules, oxycodone hydrochloride 5 mg (orange/
beige), net price 56-cap pack = £10.56; 10 mg
(white/beige), 56-cap pack = £21.12; 20 mg
(pink/beige), 56-cap pack = £42.24. Label: 2
Liquid (= oral solution), sugar-free, oxycodone
hydrochloride 5 mg/5 mL, net price 250 mL =
£9.43. Label: 2
Concentrate (= concentrated oral solution), sugar-
free, oxycodone hydrochloride 10 mg/mL, net
price 120 mL = £45.25. Label: 2
Dose: 5 mg every 4–6 hours, increased if necessary
according to severity of pain, usual max. 400 mg daily,
but some patients may require higher doses; CHILD
under 18 years not recommended

■ Modified release
OxyContin® (Napp) ▼ CD
Tablets, f/c, m/r, oxycodone hydrochloride 10 mg
(white), net price 56-tab pack = £21.43; 20 mg
(pink), 56-tab pack = £42.86; 40 mg (yellow), 56-
tab pack = £85.73; 80 mg (green), 56-tab pack =
£171.46. Label: 2, 25
Dose: 10 mg every 12 hours, increased if necessary
according to severity of pain, usual max. 200 mg every
12 hours, but some patients may require higher doses;
CHILD under 18 years not recommended

PAPAVERETUM

IMPORTANT. Do **not** confuse with papaverine (section
7.4.5)
A mixture of 253 parts of morphine hydrochloride,
23 parts of papaverine hydrochloride and 20 parts
of codeine hydrochloride
The CSM has advised that to avoid confusion the figures
of 7.7 mg/mL or 15.4 mg/mL should be used for prescribing purposes.
Indications: premedication; enhancement of
anaesthesia (but see section 15.1.4.3); postoperative analgesia; severe chronic pain
Cautions: see Morphine Salts and notes above
Contra-indications: see Morphine Salts and
notes above
Side-effects: see Morphine Salts and notes above
Dose: *by subcutaneous, intramuscular, or intravenous injection*, 7.7–15.4 mg repeated every 4
hours if necessary (ELDERLY initially 7.7 mg);
CHILD up to 1 month 115 micrograms/kg, 1–12
months 154 micrograms/kg, 1–5 years 1.93–
3.85 mg, 6–12 years, 3.85–7.7 mg
INTRAVENOUS DOSE. In general the intravenous dose
should be 25–50% of the corresponding subcutaneous or
intramuscular dose

Papaveretum (Non-proprietary) CD
Injection, papaveretum 15.4 mg/mL (providing the
equivalent of 10 mg of anhydrous morphine/mL),
net price 1-mL amp = £1.24
Available from Martindale
Note. The name *Omnopon®* was formerly used for papaveretum preparations.

■ With hyoscine
Papaveretum and Hyoscine Injection CD
papaveretum 15.4 mg (providing the equivalent of 10 mg of anhydrous morphine), hyoscine hydrobromide 400 micrograms/mL. Net price 1-mL amp = £1.98

Dose: premedication, by subcutaneous or intramuscular injection, 0.5–1 mL

Available from Martindale

■ With aspirin
Section 4.7.1

PENTAZOCINE

Indications: moderate to severe pain, but see notes above

Cautions: see under Morphine Salts and notes above; avoid in porphyria (section 9.8.2); **interactions:** Appendix 1 (opioid analgesics)

Contra-indications: see under Morphine Salts and notes above; patients dependent on opioids; arterial or pulmonary hypertension, heart failure

Side-effects: see under Morphine Salts and notes above; occasional hallucinations

Dose: *by mouth,* pentazocine hydrochloride 50 mg every 3–4 hours preferably after food (range 25–100 mg); max. 600 mg daily; CHILD 6–12 years 25 mg

By subcutaneous, intramuscular, or intravenous injection, moderate pain, pentazocine 30 mg, severe pain 45–60 mg every 3–4 hours when necessary; CHILD over 1 year, *by subcutaneous or intramuscular injection,* up to 1 mg/kg, *by intravenous injection* up to 500 micrograms/kg

By rectum in suppositories, pentazocine 50 mg up to 4 times daily; CHILD not recommended

Pentazocine (Non-proprietary) CD
Capsules, pentazocine hydrochloride 50 mg. Net price 20 = £3.90. Label: 2, 21
Tablets, pentazocine hydrochloride 25 mg. Net price 20 = £1.58. Label: 2, 21
Injection, pentazocine 30 mg (as lactate)/mL. Net price 1-mL amp = £1.67; 2-mL amp = £3.21
Suppositories, pentazocine 50 mg (as lactate). Net price 20 = £19.93. Label: 2
Note. The brand name *Fortral®* NHS (Sanofi-Synthelabo) is used for all the above preparations of pentazocine

> denotes preparations that are considered to be less suitable for prescribing (see p. vi)

PETHIDINE HYDROCHLORIDE

Indications: moderate to severe pain, obstetric analgesia; peri-operative analgesia

Cautions: see under Morphine Salts and notes above; not suitable for severe continuing pain; **interactions:** Appendix 1 (opioid analgesics)

Contra-indications: see under Morphine Salts and notes above; severe renal impairment

Side-effects: see under Morphine Salts and notes above; convulsions reported in **overdosage**

Dose: acute pain, *by mouth,* 50–150 mg every 4 hours; CHILD 0.5–2 mg/kg

By subcutaneous or intramuscular injection, 25–100 mg, repeated after 4 hours; CHILD, *by intramuscular injection,* 0.5–2 mg/kg

By slow intravenous injection, 25–50 mg, repeated after 4 hours

Obstetric analgesia, *by subcutaneous or intramuscular injection,* 50–100 mg, repeated 1–3 hours later if necessary; max. 400 mg in 24 hours

Premedication, *by intramuscular injection,* 25–100 mg 1 hour before operation; CHILD 0.5–2 mg/kg

Postoperative pain, *by subcutaneous or intramuscular injection,* 25–100 mg, every 2–3 hours if necessary; CHILD, *by intramuscular injection,* 0.5–2 mg/kg

Note. In the postoperative period, the patient should be closely monitored for pain relief as well as for side-effects especially respiratory depression

Pethidine (Non-proprietary) CD
Tablets, pethidine hydrochloride 50 mg, net price 20 = £1.97. Label: 2
Available from Martindale
Injection, pethidine hydrochloride 50 mg/mL, net price 1-mL amp = 53p, 2-mL amp = 56p; 10 mg/mL, 5-mL amp = £1.50, 10-mL amp =£1.58
Various strengths available from Martindale

Pamergan P100® (Martindale) CD
Injection, pethidine hydrochloride 50 mg, promethazine hydrochloride 25 mg/mL. Net price 2-mL amp = 70p
Dose: by intramuscular injection, premedication, 2 mL 60–90 minutes before operation; CHILD 8–12 years 0.75 mL, 13–16 years 1 mL
Obstetric analgesia, 1–2 mL every 4 hours if necessary
Severe pain, 1–2 mL every 4–6 hours if necessary
Note. Although usually given intramuscularly, may be given intravenously after dilution to at least 10 mL with water for injections

PHENAZOCINE HYDROBROMIDE

Indications: severe pain

Cautions: see under Morphine Salts and notes above; **interactions:** Appendix 1 (opioid analgesics)

Contra-indications: see under Morphine Salts and notes above

Side-effects: see under Morphine Salts and notes above

Dose: *by mouth or sublingually,* 5 mg every 4–6 hours when necessary; single doses may be increased to 20 mg; CHILD not recommended

Narphen® (Napp) CD
Tablets, phenazocine hydrobromide 5 mg. Net price 100-tab pack = £27.23. Label: 2

TRAMADOL HYDROCHLORIDE

Indications: moderate to severe pain

Cautions: see under Morphine Salts and notes above; history of epilepsy (convulsions reported, usually after rapid intravenous injection); manufacturer advises avoid in pregnancy and breastfeeding; not suitable as substitute in opioid-dependent patients; **interactions:** Appendix 1 (opioid analgesics)

GENERAL ANAESTHESIA. Not recommended for analgesia during potentially very light planes of general anaesthesia (possibly increased operative recall reported)

Contra-indications: see under Morphine Salts and notes above

Side-effects: see under Morphine Salts and notes above; also hypotension and occasionally hypertension; anaphylaxis, hallucinations, and confusion reported

Dose: *by mouth*, 50–100 mg not more often than every 4 hours; total of more than 400 mg daily by mouth not usually required; CHILD not recommended

By intramuscular injection or by intravenous injection (over 2–3 minutes) *or by intravenous infusion*, 50–100 mg every 4–6 hours
Postoperative pain, 100 mg initially then 50 mg every 10–20 minutes if necessary during first hour to total max. 250 mg (including initial dose) in first hour, *then* 50–100 mg every 4–6 hours; max. 600 mg daily; CHILD not recommended

Tramadol Hydrochloride (Non-proprietary) PoM

Capsules, tramadol hydrochloride 50 mg. Net price 30-cap pack = £2.63, 100-cap pack = £9.89. Label: 2

Available from Alpharma, APS, Dominion, Galen (*Tramake®*), Generics, Genus, IVAX, Sovereign, Sterwin, Tillomed

Tramake Insts® (Galen) PoM

Sachets, effervescent powder, sugar-free, lemon-flavoured, tramadol hydrochloride 50 mg (contains Na$^+$ 9.7 mmol/sachet), net price 60-sachet pack = £8.95; 100 mg (contains Na$^+$ 14.6 mmol/sachet), 60-sachet pack = £17.90. Label: 2, 13
Excipients: include aspartame (section 9.4.1)

Zamadol® (ASTA Medica) PoM

Capsules, tramadol hydrochloride 50 mg, net price 100-cap pack = £14.52. Label: 2

Injection, tramadol hydrochloride 50 mg/mL, net price 2-mL amp = £1.18

Zydol® (Searle) PoM

Capsules, green/yellow, tramadol hydrochloride 50 mg. Net price 100-cap pack = £16.91. Label: 2
Soluble tablets, tramadol hydrochloride 50 mg, net price 20-tab pack = £3.05, 100-tab pack = £15.23. Label: 2, 13
Injection, tramadol hydrochloride 50 mg/mL. Net price 2-mL amp = £1.24

■ Modified release

Dromadol® SR (IVAX) PoM

Tablets, m/r, tramadol hydrochloride 75 mg (grey), net price 60-tab pack = £12.33; 100 mg (white), 60-tab pack = £16.00; 150 mg (beige), 60-tab pack = £24.00; 200 mg (orange), 60-tab pack = £32.00. Label: 2, 25
Dose: initially 75 mg twice daily increased if necessary; usual max. 400 mg daily in 2 divided doses; CHILD under 12 years not recommended

Dromadol® XL (IVAX) PoM

Tablets, m/r, tramadol hydrochloride 150 mg, 30-tab pack = £13.70; 200 mg, 30-tab pack = £18.26; 300 mg, 30-tab pack = £27.36; 400 mg, 30-tab pack = £36.53. Label: 2, 25
Dose: 150 mg daily increased if necessary; more than 400 mg once daily not usually required; CHILD under 12 years not recommended

Zamadol® SR (ASTA Medica) PoM

Capsules, m/r, tramadol hydrochloride 50 mg (green), net price 60-cap pack = £8.21; 100 mg, net price 60-cap pack = £16.43; 150 mg (dark

green), 60-cap pack = £24.64; 200 mg (yellow), 60-cap pack = £32.85. Label: 2
Dose: 50–100 mg twice daily increased if necessary to 150–200 mg twice daily; total of more than 400 mg daily not usually required; CHILD under 12 years not recommended
COUNSELLING. Swallow whole or open capsule and swallow contents immediately without chewing

Zydol SR® (Searle) PoM

Tablets, m/r, f/c, tramadol hydrochloride 100 mg, net price 60-tab pack = £18.26; 150 mg (beige), 60-tab pack = £27.39; 200 mg (orange), 60-tab pack = £36.52. Label: 2, 25
Dose: 100 mg twice daily increased if necessary to 150–200 mg twice daily; total of more than 400 mg daily not usually required; CHILD not recommended

Zydol XL® (Searle) PoM

Tablets, m/r, f/c, tramadol hydrochloride 150 mg, net price 30-tab pack = £15.22; 200 mg, 30-tab pack = £20.29; 300 mg, 30-tab pack = £30.44; 400 mg, 30-tab pack = £40.59. Label: 2, 25
Dose: 150 mg daily increased if necessary; more than 400 mg once daily not usually required; CHILD not recommended

4.7.3   Neuropathic pain

Neuropathic pain, which occurs as a result of damage to neural tissue, includes *postherpetic neuralgia, phantom limb pain, complex regional pain syndrome* (reflex sympathetic dystrophy, causalgia), *compression neuropathies, peripheral neuropathies* (e.g. due to diabetes, haematological malignancies, rheumatoid arthritis, alcoholism, drug misuse), *trauma, central pain* (e.g. pain following stroke, spinal cord injury and syringomyelia) and *idiopathic neuropathy*. The pain occurs in an area of sensory deficit and may be described as burning, shooting or scalding and is often accompanied by pain that is evoked by a non-noxious stimulus (allodynia).

Trigeminal neuralgia is also caused by dysfunction of neural tissue, but its management is distinct from other forms of neuropathic pain.

Neuropathic pain is generally managed with a tricyclic antidepressant and certain antiepileptic drugs. Neuropathic pain may respond only partially to opioid analgesics. Of the opioids, dextropropoxyphene, methadone, tramadol, and oxycodone are probably the most effective for neuropathic pain and they may be considered when other measures fail. Nerve blocks, transcutaneous electrical nerve stimulation (TENS) and, in selected cases, central electrical stimulation may help. Many patients with chronic neuropathic pain require multidisciplinary management, including physiotherapy and psychological support.

Amitriptyline is prescribed most frequently [unlicensed indication], initially at 10–25 mg each night. The dose may be increased gradually to about 75 mg daily if required (higher doses under specialist supervision); **nortriptyline**, a metabolite of amitriptyline, also given at an initial dose of 10–25 mg at night may produce fewer side-effects. **Gabapentin** (section 4.8.1) is licensed for the treatment of neuropathic pain.

Capsaicin (section 10.3.2) is licensed for neuropathic pain (but the intense burning sensation during initial treatment may limit use). Drugs that are now generally reserved for use under specialist supervision include **sodium valproate** and occasionally **phenytoin**. **Ketamine** (section 15.1.1), an NMDA antagonist, or **lidocaine (lignocaine)** by intravenous infusion may also be useful in some forms of neuropathic pain [both unlicensed indication; specialist use only].

A **corticosteroid** may help to relieve pressure in compression neuropathy and thereby reduce pain. The management of trigeminal neuralgia and postherpetic neuralgia are outlined below; for the management of neuropathic pain in *palliative care*, see p. 14; for the management of diabetic neuropathy, see section 6.1.5.

Trigeminal neuralgia

Surgery may be the treatment of choice in many patients; a neurological assessment will identify those who stand to benefit. **Carbamazepine** (section 4.8.1) taken during the acute stages of trigeminal neuralgia, reduces the frequency and severity of attacks. Plasma-carbamazepine concentration should be monitored when high doses are given. Small doses should be used initially to reduce the incidence of side-effects e.g. dizziness. **Oxcarbazepine** [unlicensed indication] is an alternative to carbamazepine. **Gabapentin** and **lamotrigine** [unlicensed indication] are also used in trigeminal neuralgia. Some cases respond to **phenytoin** (section 4.8.1); the drug may be given by intravenous infusion (possibly as fosphenytoin) in a crisis (specialist use only).

Postherpetic neuralgia

Postherpetic neuralgia follows acute herpes zoster infection (shingles), particularly in the elderly. If **amitriptyline** fails to manage the pain adequately, **gabapentin** may improve control. A topical analgesic preparation containing **capsaicin** 0.075% (section 10.3.2) is licensed for use in postherpetic neuralgia. Application of topical local anaesthetic preparations may be helpful in some patients.

4.7.4	**Antimigraine drugs**
4.7.4.1	Treatment of the acute migraine attack
4.7.4.2	Prophylaxis of migraine

4.7.4.1   Treatment of the acute migraine attack

Treatment of a migraine attack should be guided by response to previous treatment and the severity of the attacks. A **simple analgesic** such as aspirin, paracetamol (preferably in a soluble or dispersible form) or an NSAID is often effective; concomitant **anti-emetic** treatment may be required. If treatment with an analgesic is inadequate, an attack may be treated with a specific antimigraine compound such as a **5HT₁ agonist** ('triptan'). **Ergot alkaloids** are rarely required now; oral and rectal preparations are associated with many side-effects (including 'ergot headache') and they should be avoided in cerebrovascular or cardiovascular disease.

Analgesics

Most migraine headaches respond to analgesics such as **aspirin** or **paracetamol** (section 4.7.1) but because peristalsis is often reduced during migraine attacks the medication may not be sufficiently well absorbed to be effective; dispersible or effervescent preparations are therefore preferred.

The NSAID **tolfenamic acid** is licensed specifically for the treatment of an acute attack of migraine; **diclofenac potassium**, **flurbiprofen**, **ibuprofen**, and **naproxen sodium** (section 10.1.1) are also licensed for use in migraine.

ANALGESICS

■ Aspirin
Section 4.7.1

■ Paracetamol
Section 4.7.1

■ Non-steroidal   anti-inflammatory   drugs (NSAIDs)
Section 10.1.1

■ With anti-emetics

Domperamol® (Servier) PoM
Tablets, f/c, paracetamol 500 mg, domperidone (as maleate) 10 mg, net price 16-tab pack = £7.00. Label: 17, 30
Dose: 2 tablets at onset of attack then up to every 4 hours; max. 8 tablets daily; CHILD not recommended

Migraleve® (Pfizer Consumer)
Tablets, all f/c, *pink tablets*, buclizine hydrochloride 6.25 mg, paracetamol 500 mg, codeine phosphate 8 mg; *yellow tablets*, paracetamol 500 mg, codeine phosphate 8 mg. Net price 48-tab *Migraleve* PoM (32 pink + 16 yellow) = £5.10; 48 pink (*Migraleve Pink*) = £5.56; 48 yellow (*Migraleve Yellow*) = £4.70. Label: 2 (*Migraleve Pink*), 17, 30
Dose: 2 pink tablets at onset of attack, or if it is imminent, then 2 yellow tablets every 4 hours if necessary; max. in 24 hours 2 pink and 6 yellow; CHILD under 10 years, only under close medical supervision; 10–14 years, half adult dose

MigraMax® (Elan) PoM
Oral powder, aspirin (as lysine acetylsalicylate) 900 mg, metoclopramide hydrochloride 10 mg/ sachet, net price 6-sachet pack = £7.00, 20-sachet pack = £23.33. Label: 13, 21, 32
Dose: ADULT over 20 years 1 sachet in water at onset of attack, repeated after 2 hours if necessary (max. 3 sachets in 24 hours); YOUNG ADULT (under 20 years) and CHILD not recommended
IMPORTANT. Metoclopramide can cause **severe extrapyramidal effects**, particularly in children and young adults (for further details, see p. 205)
Excipients: include aspartame (section 9.4.1)

Paramax® (Sanofi-Synthelabo) PoM
Tablets, scored, paracetamol 500 mg, metoclopramide hydrochloride 5 mg. Net price 42-tab pack = £6.69. Label: 17, 30
Sachets, effervescent powder, sugar-free, the contents of 1 sachet = 1 tablet; to be dissolved in ¼ tumblerful of liquid before administration. Net

price 42-sachet pack = £8.69. Label: 13, 17, 30
Dose: (tablets or sachets): 2 at onset of attack then every 4 hours when necessary to max. of 6 in 24 hours;
YOUNG ADULT 12–19 years, 1 at onset of attack then 1 every 4 hours when necessary to max. of 3 in 24 hours (max. dose of metoclopramide 500 micrograms/kg daily)
IMPORTANT. Metoclopramide can cause **severe extra-pyramidal effects**, particularly in children and young adults (for further details, see p. 205)

TOLFENAMIC ACID

Indications: treatment of acute migraine attacks
Cautions: see NSAIDs, section 10.1.1
Contra-indications: see NSAIDs, section 10.1.1
Side-effects: see NSAIDs, section 10.1.1; also dysuria (most commonly in men), tremor, euphoria, and fatigue reported
Dose: 200 mg at onset repeated once after 1–2 hours if necessary

Clotam® (Provalis) PoM
  Rapid Tablets, tolfenamic acid 200 mg. Net price 10-tab pack = £15.00

5HT₁ agonists

Sumatriptan is a 5HT₁ agonist of considerable value in the treatment of an acute attack. It may be used during the established headache phase of an attack and should be regarded as preferred treatment in those who fail to respond to conventional analgesics. Sumatriptan is also of value in cluster headache.

Almotriptan, **naratriptan**, **rizatriptan** and **zolmitriptan** have been introduced more recently. Given orally, rizatriptan appears to have a faster onset of action than sumatriptan.

CAUTIONS. 5HT₁ agonists should be used with caution in conditions which predispose to coronary artery disease (pre-existing cardiac disease, see Contra-indications below); hepatic impairment (see Appendix 2); pregnancy and breast-feeding. 5HT₁ agonists are recommended as monotherapy and should not be taken concurrently with other acute migraine therapies.

CONTRA-INDICATIONS. 5HT₁ agonists should not be used for prophylaxis and are contra-indicated in ischaemic heart disease; previous myocardial infarction; coronary vasospasm (including Prinzmetal's angina); uncontrolled hypertension.

SIDE-EFFECTS. Side-effects of the 5HT₁ agonists include sensations of tingling, heat, heaviness, pressure, or tightness—of any part of the body (including throat and chest—discontinue if intense, may be due to coronary vasoconstriction or to anaphylaxis; see also CSM advice under Sumatriptan); flushing, dizziness, feeling of weakness; fatigue; nausea and vomiting also reported.

ALMOTRIPTAN

Indications: treatment of acute migraine attacks
Cautions: see under 5HT₁ agonists above; hepatic impairment (avoid if severe); severe renal impairment (Appendix 3); sensitivity to sulphonamides;

not to be taken until 24 hours after stopping an ergotamine-type preparation (ergotamine-type preparations not to be taken until 6 hours after almotriptan); other **interactions:** Appendix 1 (5HT₁ agonists)
Contra-indications: see under 5HT₁ agonists above; previous cerebrovascular accident or transient ischaemic attack; peripheral vascular disease
Side-effects: see under 5HT₁ agonists above; transient increase in blood pressure, drowsiness; also paraesthesia, diarrhoea, dyspepsia, dry mouth, myalgia, headache, tinnitus
Dose: 12.5 mg as soon as possible after onset repeated after 2 hours if migraine recurs (patient not responding should not take second dose for same attack); max. 25 mg in 24 hours; CHILD and ADOLESCENT under 18 years not recommended

Almogran® (Lundbeck) ▼ PoM
  Tablets, f/c, almotriptan (as hydrogen malate) 12.5 mg, net price 3-tab pack = £9.75; 6-tab pack = £19.50; 9-tab pack = £29.25. Label: 3

NARATRIPTAN

Indications: treatment of acute migraine attacks
Cautions: see under 5HT₁ agonists above; renal impairment; sensitivity to sulphonamides; **interactions:** Appendix 1 (5HT₁ agonists)
DRIVING. Drowsiness may affect performance of skilled tasks (e.g. driving)
Contra-indications: see under 5HT₁ agonists above; peripheral vascular disease
Side-effects: see under 5HT₁ agonists above, bradycardia or tachycardia; visual disturbances
Dose: 2.5 mg as soon as possible after onset; if migraine recurs after initial response, dose may be repeated after 4 hours (patient not responding should not take second dose for same attack); max. 5 mg in 24 hours; CHILD under 18 years not recommended

Naramig® (GlaxoWellcome) PoM
  Tablets, f/c, green, naratriptan (as hydrochloride) 2.5 mg, net price 6-tab pack = £24.00, 12-tab pack = £48.00. Label: 3

RIZATRIPTAN

Indications: treatment of acute migraine attacks
Cautions: see under 5HT₁ agonists above; renal impairment (Appendix 3); not to be taken until 24 hours after stopping an ergotamine-type preparation (ergotamine-type preparations not to be taken until 6 hours after rizatriptan); other **interactions:** Appendix 1 (5HT₁ agonists)
DRIVING. Drowsiness may affect performance of skilled tasks (e.g. driving)
Contra-indications: see under 5HT₁ agonists above; previous cerebrovascular accident or transient ischaemic attack; peripheral vascular disease
Side-effects: see under 5HT₁ agonists above; drowsiness, palpitations, tachycardia, dry mouth, diarrhoea, dyspepsia, thirst, pharyngeal discomfort, dyspnoea, headache, paraesthesia, decreased alertness, insomnia, tremor, ataxia, nervousness, vertigo, confusion, myalgia and muscle weak-

ness, sweating, urticaria, pruritus, blurred vision; rarely syncope, hypertension; hypersensitivity reactions (including rash, angioedema, and toxic epidermal necrolysis) and taste disturbance reported

Dose: 10 mg as soon as possible after onset repeated after 2 hours if migraine recurs (patient not responding should not take second dose for same attack); max. 20 mg in 24 hours

CHILD under 18 years not recommended

Note. Halve dose in patients taking propranolol; not to be taken within 2 hours of taking propranolol

Maxalt® (MSD) PoM

Tablets, pink, rizatriptan (as benzoate) 5 mg, net price 6-tab pack = £26.74; 10 mg, 3-tab pack = £13.37, 6-tab pack = £26.74. Label: 3

Wafers (*Maxalt® Melt*), rizatriptan (as benzoate) 10 mg, net price 3-wafer pack = £13.37, 6-wafer pack = £26.74. Label: 3, counselling administration

COUNSELLING. *Maxalt® Melt* wafers should be placed on the tongue and allowed to dissolve

Excipients: include aspartame equivalent to phenylalanine 2.1 mg (section 9.4.1)

SUMATRIPTAN

Indications: treatment of acute migraine attacks; cluster headache (subcutaneous injection only)

Cautions: see under 5HT$_1$ agonists above; renal impairment; sensitivity to sulphonamides; should not be taken until 24 hours after stopping an ergotamine-containing preparation (ergotamine-containing preparations should not be taken until 6 hours after sumatriptan); other **interactions:** Appendix 1 (5HT$_1$ agonists)

DRIVING. Drowsiness may affect performance of skilled tasks (e.g. driving)

Contra-indications: see under 5HT$_1$ agonists above; previous cerebrovascular accident or transient ischaemic attack; peripheral vascular disease

Side-effects: see under 5HT$_1$ agonists above; drowsiness, transient increase in blood pressure, hypotension, bradycardia or tachycardia, altered liver function tests, seizures reported

CSM advice. Following reports of chest pain and tightness (coronary vasoconstriction) CSM has emphasised that sumatriptan should **not** be used in ischaemic heart disease or Prinzmetal's angina, and that use with ergotamine should be **avoided** (see also Cautions).

Dose: *by mouth*, 50 mg (some patients may require 100 mg) as soon as possible after onset (patient not responding should not take second dose for same attack); dose may be repeated if migraine recurs; max. 300 mg in 24 hours; CHILD not recommended

By subcutaneous injection using auto-injector, 6 mg as soon as possible after onset (patients not responding should not take second dose for same attack); dose may be repeated once after not less than 1 hour if migraine recurs; max. 12 mg in 24 hours; CHILD not recommended

IMPORTANT. **Not** for intravenous injection which may cause coronary vasospasm and angina

Intranasally, 20 mg (1 spray) into one nostril as soon as possible after onset (patient not responding should not take a second dose for same attack); dose may be repeated once after not less than two hours if migraine recurs; max. 40 mg in 24 hours; CHILD not recommended

Imigran® (GlaxoWellcome) PoM

Tablets, f/c, sumatriptan (as succinate) 50 mg, net price 6-tab pack = £29.70, 12-tab pack = £56.43; 100 mg, 6-tab pack = £48.00, 12-tab pack = £96.00. Label: 3, 10 patient information leaflet

Injection, sumatriptan (as succinate) 12 mg/mL (= 6 mg/0.5-mL syringe), net price, treatment pack (2 × 0.5-mL pre-filled syringes and auto-injector) = £41.14; refill pack (2 × 0.5-mL pre-filled syringes) = £39.14. Label: 3, 10 patient information leaflet

Nasal spray, sumatriptan 20 mg/0.1-mL unit-dose spray device, net price 2 unit-dose vials with applicator = £12.00, 6 unit-dose vials = £36.00. Label: 3, 10 patient information leaflet

ZOLMITRIPTAN

Indications: treatment of acute migraine attacks

Cautions: see under 5HT$_1$ agonists above; should not be taken within 12 hours of any other 5HT$_1$ agonist; **interactions:** Appendix 1 (5HT$_1$ agonists)

Contra-indications: see under 5HT$_1$ agonists above; Wolff-Parkinson-White syndrome or arrhythmias associated with accessory cardiac conduction pathways

Side-effects: see under 5HT$_1$ agonists above; drowsiness, transient increase in blood pressure; dry mouth, myalgia and muscle weakness, dysaesthesia reported

Dose: 2.5 mg as soon as possible after onset repeated after 2 hours if migraine persists or recurs (increase to 5 mg for subsequent attacks in patients not achieving satisfactory relief with 2.5-mg dose); max. 15 mg in 24 hours; CHILD not recommended

Zomig® (AstraZeneca) ▼ PoM

Tablets, f/c, yellow, zolmitriptan 2.5 mg, net price 6-tab pack = £24.00, 12-tab pack = £48.00

Orodispersible tablets (*Zomig Rapimelt®*), zolmitriptan 2.5 mg, net-price 6-tab pack = £24.00. Counselling, administration

COUNSELLING. *Zomig Rapimelt®* should be placed on the tongue, to disperse and swallowed

Excipients: include aspartame equivalent to phenylalanine 2.81 mg/tablet (section 9.4.1)

Ergot alkaloids

The value of **ergotamine** for migraine is limited by difficulties in absorption and by its side-effects, particularly nausea, vomiting, abdominal pain, and *muscular cramps*; it is best avoided. The recommended doses of ergotamine preparations should **not** be exceeded and treatment should **not** be repeated at intervals of less than 4 days.

To avoid habituation the frequency of administration of ergotamine should be limited to **no more than** twice a month. It should **never** be prescribed prophylactically but in the management of cluster headache a low dose (e.g. ergotamine 1 mg at night for 6 nights in 7) is occasionally given for 1 to 2 weeks [unlicensed indication].

ERGOTAMINE TARTRATE ◢

Indications: treatment of acute migraine attacks and migraine variants unresponsive to analgesics

Cautions: risk of peripheral vasospasm (see advice below); elderly; dependence (see Ergot alkaloids above), should not be used for migraine prophylaxis; **interactions:** Appendix 1 (ergotamine) and under Sumatriptan (Cautions), below

PERIPHERAL VASOSPASM. Warn patient to stop treatment immediately if numbness or tingling of extremities develops and to contact doctor.

Contra-indications: peripheral vascular disease, coronary heart disease, obliterative vascular disease and Raynaud's syndrome, hepatic and renal impairment, sepsis, severe or inadequately controlled hypertension, hyperthyroidism, pregnancy and breast-feeding, porphyria (section 9.8.2)

Side-effects: nausea, vomiting, vertigo, abdominal pain, diarrhoea, muscle cramps, and occasionally increased headache; precordial pain, myocardial ischaemia, rarely myocardial infarction; repeated high dosage may cause ergotism with gangrene and confusion; pleural and peritoneal fibrosis may occur with excessive use

Dose: see under preparations below

Cafergot® (Alliance) [PoM] ◢
Tablets, ergotamine tartrate 1 mg, caffeine 100 mg. Net price 30-tab pack = £5.90. Label: 18, counselling, dosage

Dose: 1–2 tablets at onset; max. 4 tablets in 24 hours; not to be repeated at intervals of less than 4 days; max. 8 tablets in one week (but see also notes above); CHILD not recommended

Suppositories, ergotamine tartrate 2 mg, caffeine 100 mg. Net price 30 = £13.50. Label: 18, counselling, dosage

Dose: 1 suppository at onset; max. 2 in 24 hours; not to be repeated at intervals of less than 4 days; max. 4 suppositories in one week (but see also notes above); CHILD not recommended

Migril® (CP) [PoM] ◢
Tablets, scored, ergotamine tartrate 2 mg, cyclizine hydrochloride 50 mg, caffeine hydrate 100 mg. Net price 20 = £11.67. Label: 2, 18, counselling, dosage

Dose: 1 tablet at onset, followed after 30 minutes by ½–1 tablet, repeated every 30 minutes if necessary; max. 4 tablets per attack and 6 tablets in one week (but see also notes above); CHILD not recommended

> ◢ denotes preparations that are considered to be less suitable for prescribing (see p. vi)

Anti-emetics

Anti-emetics (section 4.6), such as **metoclopramide** or **domperidone**, or phenothiazine and antihistamine anti-emetics, relieve the nausea associated with migraine attacks. Anti-emetics may be given by intramuscular injection or rectally if vomiting is a problem. Metoclopramide and domperidone have the added advantage of promoting gastric emptying and normal peristalsis; a single dose should be given at the onset of symptoms. Oral analgesic preparations containing metoclopramide or domperidone are a convenient alternative (**important:** for warnings relating to extrapyramidal effects of metoclopramide particularly in children and young adults, see p. 205).

Other drugs for migraine

Isometheptene mucate (in combination with paracetamol) is licensed for the treatment of acute attacks of migraine; other effective treatments are however available now.

ISOMETHEPTENE MUCATE ◢

Indications: treatment of acute migraine attacks

Cautions: cardiovascular disease, hepatic and renal impairment, diabetes mellitus, hyperthyroidism; **interactions:** Appendix 1 (sympathomimetics)

Contra-indications: glaucoma, severe cardiac, hepatic and renal impairment, severe hypertension, pregnancy and breast-feeding; porphyria (section 9.8.2)

Side-effects: dizziness, circulatory disturbances, rashes, blood disorders also reported

¹**Midrid®** (Shire) [PoM] ◢
Capsules, red, isometheptene mucate 65 mg, paracetamol 325 mg. Net price 100-cap pack = £13.11. Label: 30, counselling, dosage

Dose: migraine, 2 capsules at onset of attack, followed by 1 capsule every hour if necessary; max. 5 capsules in 12 hours; CHILD not recommended

1. A pack containing 15 capsules may be sold to the public

4.7.4.2   Prophylaxis of migraine

Where migraine attacks are frequent, search should be made for provocative factors such as stress or diet (e.g. chocolate, cheese, alcohol); combined oral contraceptives may also provoke migraine; see section 7.3.1 for advice. Benzodiazepines should be avoided because of the risk of dependence. In patients with more than one attack a month, one of four prophylactic agents may be tried: pizotifen, beta-blockers, tricyclic antidepressants (even when the patient is not obviously depressed), or sodium valproate. Long-term treatment with any of these prophylactic drugs is undesirable; the need for continuing therapy should be reviewed at intervals of about 6 months.

Pizotifen is an antihistamine and serotonin antagonist structurally related to the tricyclic antidepressants. It affords good prophylaxis but may cause weight gain. To avoid undue drowsiness treatment may be started at 500 micrograms at night and gradually increased to 3 mg; it is rarely necessary to exceed this dose.

The **beta-blockers** propranolol, metoprolol, nadolol, and timolol (section 2.4) are all effective. Propranolol is the most commonly used in an initial dose of 40 mg 2 to 3 times daily by mouth. Beta-blockers may also be given as a single daily dose of a long-acting preparation. The value of beta-blockers is limited by their contra-indications (section 2.4) and also by their interactions (see Appendix 1, beta-blockers).

Tricyclic antidepressants (section 4.3.1) [unlicensed] may usefully be prescribed in a dose, for example, of amitriptyline 10 mg at night, increasing to a maintenance dose of 50 to 75 mg at night.

Sodium valproate (section 4.8.1) [unlicensed] may be effective in a dose of 300 mg twice daily.

There is some evidence that the **calcium-channel blockers** (section 2.6.2), e.g. verapamil and nifedipine may be useful in migraine prophylaxis.

Cyproheptadine (section 3.4.1), an antihistamine with serotonin-antagonist and calcium channel-blocking properties, may also be tried in refractory cases.

Clonidine (*Dixarit®*) is **not** recommended and may aggravate depression or produce insomnia. **Methysergide**, a semi-synthetic ergot alkaloid, has dangerous side-effects (retroperitoneal fibrosis and fibrosis of the heart valves and pleura); **important:** it should only be administered under hospital supervision.

PIZOTIFEN

Indications: prevention of vascular headache including classical migraine, common migraine, and cluster headache

Cautions: urinary retention; angle-closure glaucoma, renal impairment; pregnancy and breast-feeding; **interactions:** Appendix 1 (pizotifen)

DRIVING. Drowsiness may affect performance of skilled tasks (e.g. driving); effects of alcohol enhanced

Side-effects: antimuscarinic effects, drowsiness, increased appetite and weight gain; occasionally nausea, dizziness; rarely depression; CNS stimulation may occur in children

Dose: 1.5 mg at night *or* 500 micrograms 3 times daily (but see also notes above), adjusted according to response; max. single dose 3 mg, max. daily dose 4.5 mg; CHILD up to 1.5 mg daily in divided doses; max. single dose at night 1 mg

Pizotifen (Non-proprietary) PoM
Tablets, pizotifen (as hydrogen malate), 500 micrograms, net price 28-tab pack = £1.20; 1.5 mg, 28-tab pack = £4.18. Label: 2
Available from Alpharma, APS, IVAX

Sanomigran® (Novartis) PoM
Tablets, both ivory-yellow, s/c, pizotifen (as hydrogen malate), 500 micrograms, net price 60-tab pack = £2.57; 1.5 mg, 28-tab pack = £4.28. Label: 2
Elixir, pizotifen (as hydrogen malate) 250 micrograms/5 mL, net price 300 mL = £4.51. Label: 2

CLONIDINE HYDROCHLORIDE ▭

Indications: prevention of recurrent migraine (but see notes above), vascular headache, menopausal flushing; hypertension (section 2.5.2)

Cautions: depressive illness, concurrent antihypertensive therapy; porphyria (section 9.8.2); **interactions:** Appendix 1 (clonidine)

Side-effects: dry mouth, sedation, dizziness, nausea, nocturnal restlessness; occasionally rashes

Dose: 50 micrograms twice daily, increased after 2 weeks to 75 micrograms twice daily if necessary; CHILD not recommended

Dixarit® (Boehringer Ingelheim) PoM ▭
Tablets, blue, s/c, clonidine hydrochloride 25 micrograms. Net price 112-tab pack = £7.11

Catapres® PoM ▭ (hypertension), section 2.5.2

METHYSERGIDE ▭

Indications: prevention of severe recurrent migraine, cluster headache and other vascular headaches in patients who are refractory to other treatment and whose lives are seriously disrupted (**important:** hospital supervision only, see notes above); diarrhoea associated with carcinoid syndrome

Cautions: history of peptic ulceration; avoid abrupt withdrawal of treatment; after 6 months withdraw (gradually over 2 to 3 weeks) for reassessment for at least 1 month (see also notes above); **interactions:** Appendix 1 (ergotamine)

Contra-indications: renal, hepatic, pulmonary, and cardiovascular disease, severe hypertension, collagen disease, cellulitis, urinary-tract disorders, cachectic or septic conditions, pregnancy, breast-feeding

Side-effects: nausea, vomiting, heartburn, abdominal discomfort, drowsiness, and dizziness occur frequently in initial treatment; mental and behavioural disturbances, insomnia, oedema, weight gain, rashes, loss of scalp hair, cramps, arterial spasm (including coronary artery spasm with angina and possible myocardial infarction), paraesthesias of extremities, postural hypotension, and tachycardia also occur; retroperitoneal and other abnormal fibrotic reactions may occur on prolonged administration, requiring immediate withdrawal of treatment

Dose: initially 1 mg at bedtime, increased gradually over about 2 weeks to 1–2 mg 3 times daily with food (see notes above); CHILD not recommended
Diarrhoea associated with carcinoid syndrome, usual range, 12–20 mg daily (hospital supervision); CHILD not recommended

Deseril® (Alliance) PoM ▭
Tablets, s/c, methysergide (as maleate) 1 mg, net price 60-tab pack = £13.80. Label: 2, 21

> ▭ denotes preparations that are considered to be less suitable for prescribing (see p. vi)

4.8   Antiepileptics

4.8.1   Control of epilepsy
4.8.2   Drugs used in status epilepticus
4.8.3   Febrile convulsions

4.8.1   Control of epilepsy

The object of treatment is to prevent the occurrence of seizures by maintaining an effective dose of one or more antiepileptic drugs. Careful adjustment of doses is necessary, starting with low doses and increasing gradually until seizures are controlled or there are overdose effects.

The frequency of administration is often determined by the plasma half-life, and should be kept as low as possible to encourage better patient compliance. Most antiepileptics, when used in average dosage, may be given twice daily. Phenobarbital and sometimes phenytoin, which have long half-lives, may often be given as a daily dose at bedtime.

However, with large doses, some antiepileptics may need to be administered 3 times daily to avoid adverse effects associated with high peak plasma concentrations. Young children metabolise antiepileptics more rapidly than adults and therefore require more frequent doses and a higher amount per kilogram body-weight.

COMBINATION THERAPY. Therapy with two or more antiepileptic drugs concurrently may be necessary; it should preferably only be used when monotherapy with several alternative drugs has proved ineffective. Combination therapy enhances toxicity and drug interactions may occur between antiepileptics (see below).

INTERACTIONS. Interactions between antiepileptics are complex and may enhance toxicity without a corresponding increase in antiepileptic effect. Interactions are usually caused by *hepatic enzyme induction* or *hepatic enzyme inhibition*; *displacement from protein binding sites* is not usually a problem. These interactions are highly variable and unpredictable. Plasma monitoring is therefore often advisable with combination therapy.

Significant interactions that occur **between antiepileptics** themselves are as follows:

> *Note.* Check under each drug for possible interactions when two or more antiepileptic drugs are used

Carbamazepine
often lowers plasma concentration of *clobazam, clonazepam, lamotrigine, an active metabolite of oxcarbazepine*, and of *phenytoin* (but may also raise phenytoin concentration), *tiagabine, topiramate, and valproate*
sometimes lowers plasma concentration of *ethosuximide, and primidone* (but tendency for corresponding increase in phenobarbital level)

Ethosuximide
sometimes raises plasma concentration of *phenytoin*

Gabapentin
no interactions with gabapentin reported

Lamotrigine
sometimes raises plasma concentration of *an active metabolite of carbamazepine* (but evidence is conflicting)

Levetiracetam
no interactions with levetiracetam reported

Oxcarbazepine
sometimes lowers plasma concentration of *carbamazepine* (but may raise concentration of *an active metabolite of carbamazepine*)
sometimes raises plasma concentration of *phenytoin*
often raises plasma concentration of *phenobarbital*

Phenobarbital *or* Primidone
often lowers plasma concentration of *carbamazepine, clonazepam, lamotrigine, an active metabolite of oxcarbazepine*, and of *phenytoin* (but may also raise phenytoin concentration), *tiagabine, and valproate*
sometimes lowers plasma concentration of *ethosuximide*

Phenytoin
often lowers plasma concentration of *clonazepam, carbamazepine, lamotrigine, an active metabolite of oxcarbazepine*, and of *tiagabine, topiramate, and valproate*
often raises plasma concentration of *phenobarbital*
sometimes lowers plasma concentration of *ethosuximide, and primidone* (by increasing conversion to phenobarbital)

Topiramate
sometimes raises plasma concentration of *phenytoin*

Valproate
sometimes lowers plasma concentration of *an active metabolite of oxcarbazepine*
often raises plasma concentration of *an active metabolite of carbamazepine*, and of *lamotrigine, primidone, phenobarbital, and phenytoin* (but may also lower)
sometimes raises plasma concentration of *ethosuximide, and primidone* (and tendency for significant increase in phenobarbital level)

Vigabatrin
often lowers plasma concentration of *phenytoin*
sometimes lowers plasma concentration of *phenobarbital, and primidone*

For other important interactions see **Appendix 1**, and for FPA guidelines on enzyme-inducing antiepileptics and **oral contraceptives**, see section 7.3.1.

WITHDRAWAL. Abrupt withdrawal of antiepileptics, particularly the barbiturates and benzodiazepines, should be avoided, as this may precipitate severe rebound seizures. Reduction in dosage should be carried out in stages and, in the case of the barbiturates, the withdrawal process may take months. The changeover from one antiepileptic drug regimen to another should be made cautiously, withdrawing the first drug only when the new regimen has been largely established.

The decision to withdraw all antiepileptics from a seizure-free patient, and its timing, is often difficult and may depend on individual patient factors. Even in patients who have been seizure-free for several years, there is a significant risk of seizure recurrence on drug withdrawal.

In patients receiving several antiepileptic drugs, only one drug should be withdrawn at a time.

DRIVING. Patients suffering from epilepsy may drive a motor vehicle (but not a heavy goods or public service vehicle) provided that they have had a seizure-free period of one year or, if subject to attacks only while asleep, have established a 3-year period of asleep attacks without awake attacks. Patients affected by drowsiness should not drive or operate machinery.

Guidance issued by the Drivers Medical Unit of the Driver and Vehicle Licensing Agency (DVLA) recommends that patients should be advised not to drive during withdrawal of antiepileptic drugs, or for 6 months afterwards (see also Drugs and Driving under General Guidance, p. 2).

PREGNANCY AND BREAST-FEEDING. During pregnancy, total plasma concentrations of antiepileptics (particularly of phenytoin) may fall, particularly in the later stages but free plasma concentrations may remain the same (or even rise). There is an increased risk of teratogenicity associated with the use of antiepileptic drugs (reduced if treatment is limited to a single drug). In view of the increased risk of neural tube and other defects associated, in particular, with **carbamazepine, oxcarbazepine, phenytoin** and **valproate** women taking antiepileptic drugs who *may become pregnant* should be **informed of the possible consequences**. Those who *wish to become pregnant* should be referred to an appropriate specialist for advice. Women who become pregnant should be **counselled** and offered **antenatal screening** (alpha-fetoprotein measurement and a second trimester ultrasound scan).

To counteract the risk of neural tube defects adequate folate supplements are advised for women before and during pregnancy; to prevent recurrence of neural tube defects, women should receive folic acid 5 mg daily (section 9.1.2)—this dose may also be appropriate for women receiving antiepileptic drugs.

In view of the risk of neonatal bleeding associated with carbamazepine, phenobarbital and phenytoin, prophylactic vitamin K_1 (section 9.6.6) is recommended for the mother before delivery (as well as for the neonate).

Breast-feeding is acceptable with all antiepileptic drugs, taken in normal doses, with the possible exception of the barbiturates and ethosuximide, and also some of the more recently introduced ones, see Appendix 5.

Partial seizures with or without secondary generalisation

Carbamazepine, lamotrigine, sodium valproate and **phenytoin** can be used in monotherapy for secondarily generalised tonic-clonic seizures and for partial (focal) seizures. **Phenobarbital** and **primidone** are also effective but they are more sedating and are not used as first-line drugs.

Where a single drug has failed to control the seizures, combination therapy can be tried with the above drugs or with additional drugs, such as gabapentin, oxcarbazepine, tiagabine, topiramate, or vigabatrin; alternatives include acetazolamide, clobazam, and clonazepam.

Generalised seizures

TONIC-CLONIC SEIZURES (GRAND MAL). The drugs of choice for tonic-clonic seizures are **carbamazepine, lamotrigine, phenytoin**, and **sodium valproate**. For those patients who have tonic-clonic seizures as part of the syndrome of primary generalised epilepsy, **sodium valproate** is the drug of choice. **Phenobarbital** (phenobarbitone) and **primidone** are also effective but may be more sedating.

ABSENCE SEIZURES (PETIT MAL). **Ethosuximide** and **sodium valproate** are the drugs of choice in simple absence seizures. Sodium valproate is also highly effective in treating the tonic-clonic seizures which may co-exist with absence seizures in primary generalised epilepsy.

MYOCLONIC SEIZURES. Myoclonic seizures (myoclonic jerks) occur in a variety of syndromes, and response to treatment varies considerably. **Sodium valproate** is the drug of choice and **clonazepam, ethosuximide**, or **lamotrigine** may be used. For reference to the adjunctive use of piracetam, see section 4.9.3.

ATYPICAL ABSENCE, ATONIC, AND TONIC SEIZURES. These seizure types are usually seen in childhood, in specific epileptic syndromes, or associated with cerebral damage or mental retardation. They may respond poorly to the traditional drugs. **Phenytoin, sodium valproate, lamotrigine, clonazepam, ethosuximide**, and **phenobarbital** may be tried. Second-line antiepileptic drugs that are occasionally helpful, include **acetazolamide** and **corticosteroids**.

Carbamazepine and oxcarbazepine

Carbamazepine is a drug of choice for simple and complex partial seizures and for tonic-clonic seizures secondary to a focal discharge. It has a wider therapeutic index than phenytoin and the relationship between dose and plasma-carbamazepine concentration is linear, but monitoring of plasma-carbamazepine concentrations may be helpful in determining optimum dosage. It has generally fewer side-effects than phenytoin or the barbiturates, but reversible blurring of vision, dizziness, and unsteadiness are dose-related, and may be dose-limiting. These side-effects may be reduced by altering the timing of medication; use of modified release tablets also significantly lessens the incidence of dose-related side-effects. It is essential to initiate carbamazepine therapy at a low dose and build this up slowly with increments of 100–200 mg every two weeks.

Oxcarbazepine is licensed for the treatment of partial seizures with or without secondarily generalised tonic-clonic seizures. Oxcarbazepine induces hepatic enzymes to a lesser extent than carbamazepine.

CARBAMAZEPINE

Indications: partial and secondary generalised tonic-clonic seizures, some primary generalised seizures; trigeminal neuralgia; prophylaxis of bipolar disorder unresponsive to lithium

Cautions: hepatic or renal impairment; cardiac disease (see also Contra-indications), skin reactions (see also Blood, hepatic or skin disorders below and under Side-effects), history of haematological reactions to other drugs; manufacturer recommends blood counts and hepatic and renal function tests (but evidence of practical value unsatisfactory); glaucoma; pregnancy (**important:** see p. 227 and Appendix 4 (neural tube screening)), breast-feeding (see p. 227); avoid abrupt withdrawal; **interactions:** see p. 227 and Appendix 1 (carbamazepine)

BLOOD, HEPATIC or SKIN DISORDERS. Patients or their carers should be told how to recognise signs of blood, liver, or skin disorders, and advised to seek immediate medical attention if symptoms such as fever, sore throat, rash, mouth ulcers, bruising, or bleeding develop. Leucopenia which is severe, progressive or associated with clinical symptoms requires withdrawal (if necessary under cover of suitable alternative).

Contra-indications: AV conduction abnormalities (unless paced); history of bone marrow depression, porphyria (section 9.8.2)

Side-effects: nausea and vomiting, dizziness, drowsiness, headache, ataxia, confusion and agitation (elderly), visual disturbances (especially double vision and often associated with peak plasma concentrations); constipation or diarrhoea, anorexia; mild transient generalised erythematous rash may occur in a large number of patients (withdraw if worsens or is accompanied by other symptoms); leucopenia and other blood disorders (including thrombocytopenia, agranulocytosis and aplastic anaemia); other side-effects include cholestatic jaundice, hepatitis and acute renal failure, Stevens-Johnson syndrome, toxic epidermal necrolysis, alopecia, thromboembolism, arthralgia, fever, proteinuria, lymph node enlargement, cardiac conduction disturbances (sometimes arrhythmias), dyskinesias, paraesthesia, depression, impotence (and impaired fertility), gynaecomastia, galactorrhoea, aggression, activation of psychosis; photosensitivity, pulmonary hypersensitivity (with dyspnoea and pneumonitis), hyponatraemia, oedema, and disturbances of bone metabolism (with osteomalacia) also reported; suppositories may cause occasional rectal irritation

Dose: *by mouth*, epilepsy, initially, 100–200 mg 1–2 times daily, increased slowly (see notes above) to usual dose of 0.8–1.2 g daily in divided doses; in some cases 1.6–2 g daily may be needed; ELDERLY reduce initial dose; CHILD daily in divided doses, up to 1 year 100–200 mg, 1–5 years 200–400 mg, 5–10 years 400–600 mg, 10–15 years 0.6–1 g

Trigeminal neuralgia, initially 100 mg 1–2 times daily (but some patients may require higher initial dose), increased gradually according to response; usual dose 200 mg 3–4 times daily, up to 1.6 g daily in some patients

Prophylaxis of bipolar disorder unresponsive to lithium (see also section 4.2.3), initially 400 mg daily in divided doses increased until symptoms controlled; usual range 400–600 mg daily; max. 1.6 g daily

By rectum, as suppositories, see below

Note. Plasma concentration for optimum response 4–12 mg/litre (20–50 micromol/litre)

Carbamazepine (Non-proprietary) PoM
Tablets, carbamazepine 100 mg, net price 20 = 58p; 200 mg, 20 = £1.07; 400 mg, 20 = £2.11. Label: 3, 8, counselling, blood, hepatic or skin disorder symptoms (see above), driving (see notes above)

Available from Alpharma, APS, Generics (*Carbagen®*), Hillcross, IVAX (*Epimaz®*)

Note. Different preparations may vary in bioavailability; to avoid reduced effect or excessive side-effects, it may be prudent to avoid changing the formulation (see also notes above on how side-effects may be reduced)

Tegretol® (Cephalon) PoM
Tablets, all scored, carbamazepine 100 mg, net price 84-tab pack = £2.43; 200 mg, 84-tab pack = £4.50; 400 mg, 56-tab pack = £5.90. Label: 3, 8, counselling, blood, hepatic or skin disorder symptoms (see above), driving (see notes above)

Chewtabs, orange, carbamazepine 100 mg, net price 56-tab pack = £3.54; 200 mg, 56-tab pack = £6.59. Label: 3, 8, 21, 24, counselling, blood, hepatic or skin disorder symptoms (see above), driving (see notes above)

Liquid, sugar-free, carbamazepine 100 mg/5 mL. Net price 300-mL pack = £6.86. Label: 3, 8, counselling, blood, hepatic or skin disorder symptoms (see above), driving (see notes above)

Suppositories, carbamazepine 125 mg, net price 5 = £9.00; 250 mg, 5 = £12.00. Label: 3, 8, counselling, blood, hepatic or skin disorder symptoms (see above), driving (see notes above)

Dose: epilepsy, for short-term use (max. 7 days) when oral therapy temporarily not possible; suppositories of 125 mg may be considered to be approximately equivalent in therapeutic effect to tablets of 100 mg but final adjustment should always depend on clinical response (plasma concentration monitoring recommended); max. by rectum 1 g daily in 4 divided doses

■ Modified release

Tegretol® Retard (Novartis) PoM
Tablets, m/r, both scored, carbamazepine 200 mg (beige-orange), net price 56-tab pack = £5.26; 400 mg (brown-orange), 56-tab pack = £10.34. Label: 3, 8, 25, counselling, blood, hepatic or skin disorder symptoms (see above), driving (see notes above)

Dose: epilepsy (ADULT and CHILD over 5 years), as above; trigeminal neuralgia, as above; total daily dose given in 2 divided doses

Teril® CR (Taro) PoM
Tablets, m/r, scored, carbamazepine 200 mg, net price 56-tab pack = £3.85; 400 mg, 56-tab pack = £7.58. Label: 3, 8, 25, counselling, blood, hepatic or skin disorder symptoms (see above), driving (see notes above)

Dose: epilepsy (ADULT and CHILD over 5 years), as above; trigeminal neuralgia, as above; total daily dose given in 1–2 divided doses; bipolar disorder, as above

Timonil® retard (CP) PoM
Tablets, m/r, scored, carbamazepine 200 mg, net price 100-tab pack = £8.50; 400 mg, 100-tab pack = £16.83. Label: 3, 8, 25, counselling, blood, hepatic or skin disorder symptoms (see above), driving (see notes above)

Dose: epilepsy (ADULT and CHILD over 1 year), as above; bipolar disorder, as above; trigeminal neuralgia, as above; total daily dose given in 1–2 divided doses

OXCARBAZEPINE

Indications: monotherapy and adjunctive treatment of partial seizures with or without secondarily generalised tonic-clonic seizures

Cautions: hypersensitivity to carbamazepine; avoid abrupt withdrawal; hepatic impairment (Appendix 2), renal impairment (Appendix 3); pregnancy (see p. 227 and Appendix 4), breast-feeding (Appendix 5); elderly, hyponatraemia (monitor plasma-sodium concentration in patients at risk), heart failure (monitor body-weight), cardiac conduction disorders; **interactions:** Appendix 1 (oxcarbazepine)

BLOOD, HEPATIC OR SKIN DISORDERS. Patients or their carers should be told how to recognise signs of blood, liver, or skin disorders, and advised to seek immediate medical attention if symptoms such as lethargy, confusion, muscular twitching, fever, sore throat, rash, blistering, mouth ulcers, bruising, or bleeding develop

Side-effects: nausea, vomiting, constipation, diarrhoea, abdominal pain, dizziness, headache, drowsiness, agitation, amnesia, asthenia, ataxia, confusion, impaired concentration, depression, tremor, hyponatraemia, acne, alopecia, rash, vertigo, nystagmus, visual disorders including diplopia; less commonly urticaria, leucopenia; rarely arrhythmias, Stevens-Johnson syndrome, systemic lupus erythematosus, hepatitis, thrombocytopenia, angioedema, hypersensitivity reactions

Dose: initially 300 mg twice daily increased according to response in steps of up to 600 mg daily at weekly intervals; usual dose range 0.6–2.4 g daily in divided doses; CHILD 6 years and over, 8–10 mg/kg daily in 2 divided doses increased according to response in steps of up to 10 mg/kg daily at weekly intervals (in adjunctive therapy, maintenance dose approx. 30 mg/kg daily); max. 46 mg/kg daily in divided doses

Note. In adjunctive therapy, patients may require dose reduction of concomitant antiepileptics when using high doses of oxcarbazepine

Trileptal® (Novartis) ▼ PoM

Tablets, f/c, scored, all yellow, oxcarbazepine 150 mg, net price 50-tab pack = £10.00; 300 mg, 50-tab pack = £20.00; 600 mg, 50-tab pack = £40.00. Label: 3, 8, counselling, blood, hepatic or skin disorder symptoms (see above), driving (see notes above)

Ethosuximide

Ethosuximide is sometimes used in simple absence seizures; it may also be used in myoclonic seizures and in atypical absence, atonic, and tonic seizures.

ETHOSUXIMIDE

Indications: absence seizures

Cautions: see notes above; hepatic and renal impairment; manufacturer recommends blood counts and hepatic and renal function tests (but evidence of practical value unsatisfactory); pregnancy and breast-feeding (see notes above); avoid sudden withdrawal; porphyria (see section 9.8.2); **interactions:** Appendix 1 (ethosuximide)

BLOOD DISORDERS. Patients or their carers should be told how to recognise signs of blood disorders, and advised to seek immediate medical attention if symptoms such as fever, sore throat, mouth ulcers, bruising or bleeding develop

Side-effects: gastro-intestinal disturbances, weight loss, drowsiness, dizziness, ataxia, dyskinesia, hiccup, photophobia, headache, depression, and mild euphoria. Psychotic states, rashes, hepatic and renal changes (see Cautions), and haematological disorders such as agranulocytosis and aplastic anaemia occur rarely (blood counts required if signs or symptoms of infection); systemic lupus erythematosus and erythema multiforme (Stevens-Johnson syndrome) reported; other side-effects reported include gum hypertrophy, swelling of tongue, irritability, hyperactivity, sleep disturbances, night terrors, inability to concentrate, aggressiveness, increased libido, myopia, vaginal bleeding

Dose: ADULT and CHILD over 6 years initially, 500 mg daily, increased by 250 mg at intervals of 4–7 days to usual dose of 1–1.5 g daily; occasionally up to 2 g daily may be needed; CHILD up to 6 years initially 250 mg daily, increased gradually to usual dose of 20 mg/kg daily

Note. Plasma concentration for optimum response 40–100 mg/litre (300–700 micromol/litre)

Emeside® (LAB) PoM

Capsules, orange, ethosuximide 250 mg. Net price 112-cap pack = £11.15. Label: 8, counselling, blood disorders (see above), driving (see notes above)

Syrup, blackcurrant, ethosuximide 250 mg/5 mL. Net price 200-mL pack = £6.00. Label: 8, counselling, blood disorders (see above), driving (see notes above)

Zarontin® (Parke-Davis) PoM

Capsules, yellow, ethosuximide 250 mg. Net price 56-cap pack = £4.51. Label: 8, counselling, blood disorders (see above), driving (see notes above)

Syrup, yellow, ethosuximide 250 mg/5 mL. Net price 200-mL pack = £3.73. Label: 8, counselling, blood disorders (see above), driving (see notes above)

Gabapentin

Gabapentin can be given as adjunctive therapy in partial epilepsy with or without secondary generalisation. It is also licensed for the treatment of neuropathic pain (section 4.7.3).

GABAPENTIN

Indications: adjunctive treatment of partial seizures with or without secondary generalisation not satisfactorily controlled with other antiepileptics; neuropathic pain (section 4.7.3)

Cautions: avoid sudden withdrawal (taper off over at least 1 week); history of psychotic illness, elderly (may need to reduce dose), renal impairment (Appendix 3), diabetes mellitus, false positive readings with some urinary protein tests; pregnancy (see p. 227 and Appendix 4) and breast-feeding (see p. 227 and Appendix 5); **interactions:** Appendix 1 (gabapentin)

Side-effects: somnolence, dizziness, ataxia, fatigue; also nystagmus, tremor, diplopia, amblyopia; pharyngitis, dysarthria, weight gain, dyspepsia, amnesia, nervousness, coughing, asthenia, paraesthesia, arthralgia, purpura, leucopenia; rhinitis, myalgia, headache, rarely pancreatitis, altered liver function tests, and Stevens-Johnson syndrome; nausea and vomiting reported

Dose: epilepsy, 300 mg on day 1, then 300 mg twice daily on day 2, then 300 mg 3 times daily (approx. every 8 hours) on day 3, then increased according to response in steps of 300 mg daily (in 3 divided doses) to max. 2.4 g daily, usual range 0.9–1.2 g daily; CHILD 6–12 years (specialist use only) 10 mg/kg on day 1, then 20 mg/kg on day 2, then 25–35 mg/kg daily (in 3 divided doses approx. every 8 hours), maintenance 900 mg daily (body-weight 26–36 kg) or 1.2 g daily (body-weight 37–50 kg)

Neuropathic pain, 300 mg on day 1, then 300 mg twice daily on day 2, then 300 mg 3 times daily on day 3, then increased according to response in steps of 300 mg daily (in 3 divided doses) to max. 1.8 g daily

Neurontin® (Parke-Davis) PoM
Capsules, gabapentin 100 mg (white), net price 100-cap pack = £22.86; 300 mg (yellow), 100-cap pack = £53.00; 400 mg (orange), 100-cap pack = £61.33. Label: 3, 5, 8, counselling, driving (see notes above)
Tablets, gabapentin 600 mg, net price 100-tab pack = £106.00; 800 mg, 100-tab pack = £122.66. Label: 3, 5, 8, counselling, driving (see notes above)

Lamotrigine

Lamotrigine is an antiepileptic for partial seizures and primary and secondarily generalised tonic-clonic seizures. It is also used for myoclonic seizures and may be tried for atypical absence, atonic, and tonic seizures in the Lennox-Gastaut syndrome. Lamotrigine may cause serious skin rash especially in children; dose recommendations should be adhered to closely.

Lamotrigine is used either as sole treatment or as an adjunct to treatment with other antiepileptic drugs. Valproate increases plasma-lamotrigine concentration whereas the enzyme inducing antiepileptics reduce it; care is therefore required in choosing the appropriate initial dose and subsequent titration. Where the potential for interaction is not known, treatment should be initiated with lower doses such as those used with valproate.

LAMOTRIGINE

Indications: monotherapy and adjunctive treatment of partial seizures and primary and secondarily generalised tonic-clonic seizures; seizures associated with Lennox-Gastaut syndrome

Cautions: closely monitor (including hepatic, renal and clotting parameters) and consider withdrawal if rash, fever, influenza-like symptoms, drowsiness, or worsening of seizure control develops (although causal relationship not established, lamotrigine given with other antiepileptics has been associated with rapidly progressive illness with status epilepticus, multi-organ dysfunction, disseminated intravascular coagulation and death); avoid abrupt withdrawal (taper off over 2 weeks or longer) unless serious skin reaction occurs; hepatic impairment (Appendix 2); renal impairment (Appendix 3); elderly; pregnancy and breast-feeding; monitor body-weight in children and review dose if necessary; **interactions**: see p. 227 and Appendix 1 (lamotrigine)

BLOOD DISORDERS. The CSM has advised prescribers to be alert for symptoms and signs suggestive of bone-marrow failure such as anaemia, bruising, or infection. Aplastic anaemia, bone-marrow depression and pancytopenia have been associated rarely with lamotrigine.—

Side-effects: commonly rashes (see also below)– fever, malaise, influenza-like symptoms, drowsiness and rarely hepatic dysfunction, lymphadenopathy, leucopenia, and thrombocytopenia reported in conjunction with rash; angioedema,

and photosensitivity also reported; diplopia, blurred vision, conjunctivitis, dizziness, drowsiness, insomnia, headache, ataxia, tiredness, gastro-intestinal disturbances (including vomiting), irritability, aggression, tremor, agitation, confusion; headache, nausea, dizziness, diplopia and ataxia in patients also taking carbamazepine usually resolve when dose of either drug reduced

SKIN REACTIONS. Serious skin reactions including Stevens-Johnson syndrome and toxic epidermal necrolysis (rarely with fatalities) have developed especially in children; most rashes occur in the first 8 weeks. The CSM has advised that factors associated with increased risk of serious skin reactions include concomitant use of valproate, initial lamotrigine dosing higher than recommended, and more rapid dose escalation than recommended.

COUNSELLING. Warn patients to see their doctor immediately if rash or influenza-like symptoms associated with hypersensitivity develop

Dose: IMPORTANT. Do not confuse the different combinations; see also notes above

Monotherapy, initially 25 mg daily for 14 days, increased to 50 mg daily for further 14 days, then increased by max. of 50–100 mg every 7–14 days; usual maintenance as monotherapy, 100–200 mg daily in 1–2 divided doses (up to 500 mg daily has been required)

Adjunctive therapy *with valproate*, initially 25 mg every other day for 14 days then 25 mg daily for further 14 days, thereafter increased by max. of 25–50 mg every 7–14 days; usual maintenance, 100–200 mg daily in 1–2 divided doses

Adjunctive therapy (with enzyme inducing drugs) *without valproate*, initially 50 mg daily for 14 days then 50 mg twice daily for further 14 days, thereafter increased by max. of 100 mg every 7–14 days; usual maintenance 200–400 mg daily in 2 divided doses (up to 700 mg daily has been required)

CHILD under 12 years, *monotherapy*, not recommended

CHILD 2–12 years, adjunctive therapy *with valproate*, initially 150 micrograms/kg daily for 14 days (those weighing 17–33 kg may receive 5 mg on alternate days for first 14 days) then 300 micrograms/kg daily for further 14 days, thereafter increased by 300 micrograms/kg every 7–14 days; usual maintenance 1–5 mg/kg daily in 1–2 divided doses

CHILD 2–12 years adjunctive therapy (with enzyme inducing drugs) *without valproate*, initially 600 micrograms/kg daily in 2 divided doses for 14 days then 1.2 mg/kg daily in 2 divided doses for further 14 days, thereafter increased by 1.2 mg/kg every 7–14 days; usual maintenance 5–15 mg/kg daily in 2 divided doses

Lamictal® (GlaxoWellcome) PoM
Tablets, all yellow, lamotrigine 25 mg, net price 21-tab pack (*'Valproate Add-on therapy' Starter Pack*) = £8.23, 42-tab pack (*'Monotherapy' Starter Pack*) = £16.45, 56-tab pack = £21.95; 50 mg, 42-tab pack (*'Non-valproate Add-on therapy' Starter Pack*) = £27.98, 56-tab pack = £37.31; 100 mg, 56-tab pack = £64.37; 200 mg, 56-tab pack = £109.42. Label: 8, counselling, driving (see notes above)
Dispersible tablets, chewable, lamotrigine 5 mg (scored), net price 28-tab pack = £8.75; 25 mg,

56-tab pack = £21.95; 100 mg, 56-tab pack = £64.37. Label: 8, 13, counselling, driving (see notes above)

Levetiracetam

Levetiracetam is licensed for the adjunctive treatment of partial seizures.

LEVETIRACETAM

Indications: adjunctive treatment of partial seizures with or without secondary generalisation

Cautions: hepatic impairment (Appendix 2); renal impairment (Appendix 3); pregnancy (see p. 227 and Appendix 4); breast-feeding (Appendix 5); avoid sudden withdrawal

Side-effects: drowsiness, asthenia, dizziness; less commonly, anorexia, diarrhoea, dyspepsia, nausea, amnesia, ataxia, depression, emotional lability, aggression, insomnia, nervousness, tremor, vertigo, headache, diplopia, rash

Dose: initially 1 g daily in 2 divided doses, adjusted in increments of 1 g every 2 to 4 weeks; max. 3 g daily in 2 divided doses; CHILD under 16 years not recommended

Keppra® (UCB Pharma) ▼ PoM
Tablets, f/c, levetiracetam 250 mg (blue), net price 60-tab pack = £27.00; 500 mg (yellow), 60-tab pack = £49.50; 1 g (white), 60-tab pack = £94.50. Label: 8

Phenobarbital and other barbiturates

Phenobarbital (phenobarbitone) is effective for tonic-clonic and partial seizures but may be sedative in adults and cause behavioural disturbances and hyperkinesia in children. It may be tried for atypical absence, atonic, and tonic seizures. Rebound seizures may be a problem on withdrawal. Monitoring plasma concentrations is less useful than with other drugs because tolerance occurs. **Primidone** is largely converted to phenobarbital and this is probably responsible for its antiepileptic action. A small starting dose of primidone (125 mg) is essential, and the drug should be introduced over several weeks.

PHENOBARBITAL

(Phenobarbitone)
Indications: all forms of epilepsy except absence seizures; status epilepticus (section 4.8.2)

Cautions: elderly, debilitated, children, impaired renal or hepatic function, respiratory depression (avoid if severe), pregnancy and breast-feeding (see notes above); avoid sudden withdrawal; see also notes above; avoid in porphyria (see section 9.8.2); **interactions:** see p. 227 and Appendix 1 (barbiturates and primidone)

Side-effects: drowsiness, lethargy, mental depression, ataxia and allergic skin reactions; paradoxical excitement, restlessness and confusion in the elderly and hyperkinesia in children; megaloblastic anaemia (may be treated with folic acid); **overdosage:** see Emergency Treatment of Poisoning, p. 25

Dose: *by mouth*, 60–180 mg at night; CHILD 5–8 mg/kg daily

By intramuscular injection, 200 mg, repeated after 6 hours if necessary; CHILD 15 mg/kg

Status epilepticus, *by intravenous injection* (dilute injection 1 in 10 with water for injections), 10 mg/kg at a rate of not more than 100 mg/minute; max. 1 g

Note. For therapeutic purposes phenobarbital and phenobarbital sodium may be considered equivalent in effect. Plasma concentration for optimum response 15–40 mg/litre (60–180 micromol/litre)

¹**Phenobarbital** (Non-proprietary) CD
Tablets, phenobarbital 15 mg, net price 20 = 45p; 30 mg, 20 = 48p; 60 mg, 20 = 52p. Label: 2, 8, counselling, driving (see notes above)

Elixir, phenobarbital 15 mg/5 mL in a suitable flavoured vehicle, containing alcohol 38%, net price 100 mL = 77p. Label: 2, 8, counselling, driving (see notes above)

Note. Some hospitals supply **alcohol-free** formulations of varying phenobarbital strengths

Injection, phenobarbital sodium 200 mg/mL in propylene glycol 90% and water for injections 10%, net price 1-mL amp = £1.57

Note. Must be diluted before intravenous administration (see under Dose)

Available from Concord (¹*Gardenal Sodium*® CD), Martindale; other strengths also available from Martindale.

1. See p. 7 for prescribing requirements for phenobarbital

PRIMIDONE

Indications: all forms of epilepsy except absence seizures; essential tremor (also section 4.9.3)

Cautions: see under Phenobarbital; **interactions:** see p. 227 and Appendix 1 (barbiturates and primidone)

Side-effects: see under Phenobarbital; drowsiness, ataxia, nausea, visual disturbances, and rashes, particularly at first, usually reversible on continued administration

Dose: epilepsy, ADULT and CHILD over 9 years, initially, 125 mg daily at bedtime, increased by 125 mg every 3 days to 500 mg daily in 2 divided doses then increased by 250 mg every 3 days to max. 1.5 g daily in divided doses; CHILD under 2 years, 250–500 mg daily in 2 divided doses; 2–5 years, 500–750 mg daily in 2 divided doses; 6–9 years 0.75–1 g daily in 2 divided doses

Essential tremor, initially 50 mg daily increased gradually over 2–3 weeks according to response; max. 750 mg daily

Note. Monitor plasma concentrations of derived phenobarbital. Optimum range as for phenobarbital

Mysoline® (AstraZeneca) PoM
Tablets, scored, primidone 250 mg. Net price 100-tab pack = £1.77. Label: 2, 8, counselling, driving (see notes above)

Phenytoin

Phenytoin is effective in tonic-clonic and partial seizures. It has a narrow therapeutic index and the relationship between dose and plasma concentration is non-linear; small dosage increases in some patients may produce large rises in plasma concentrations with acute toxic side-effects. Monitoring of plasma concentration greatly assists dosage adjustment. A few missed doses or a small change in drug absorption may result in a marked change in plasma concentration.

Phenytoin may cause coarse facies, acne, hirsutism, and gingival hyperplasia and so may be particularly undesirable in adolescent patients.

When only parenteral administration is possible, **fosphenytoin** (section 4.8.2), a pro-drug of phenytoin, may be convenient to give. Whereas phenytoin can be given intravenously only, fosphenytoin may also be given by intramuscular injection.

PHENYTOIN

Indications: all forms of epilepsy except absence seizures; trigeminal neuralgia if carbamazepine inappropriate (see also section 4.7.3)

Cautions: hepatic impairment (reduce dose), pregnancy (**important:** see notes above and Appendix 4), breast-feeding (see notes above); avoid sudden withdrawal; manufacturer recommends blood counts (but evidence of practical value unsatisfactory); avoid in porphyria (section 9.8.2); see also notes above; **interactions:** see p. 227 and Appendix 1 (phenytoin)

BLOOD OR SKIN DISORDERS. Patients or their carers should be told how to recognise signs of blood or skin disorders, and advised to seek immediate medical attention if symptoms such as fever, sore throat, rash, mouth ulcers, bruising, or bleeding develop. Leucopenia which is severe, progressive or associated with clinical symptoms requires withdrawal (if necessary under cover of suitable alternative)

Side-effects: nausea, vomiting, mental confusion, dizziness, headache, tremor, transient nervousness, insomnia occur commonly; rarely dyskinesias, peripheral neuropathy; ataxia, slurred speech, nystagmus and blurred vision are signs of overdosage; rashes (discontinue; if mild re-introduce cautiously but discontinue immediately if recurrence), gingival hypertrophy and tenderness, coarse facies, acne and hirsutism, fever and hepatitis; lupus erythematosus, Stevens-Johnson syndrome, toxic epidermal necrolysis, polyarteritis nodosa; lymphadenopathy; rarely haematological effects, including megaloblastic anaemia (may be treated with folic acid), leucopenia, thrombocytopenia, agranulocytosis, and aplastic anaemia; plasma-calcium concentration may be lowered (rickets and osteomalacia)

Dose: *by mouth,* initially 3–4 mg/kg daily *or* 150–300 mg daily (as a single dose *or* in 2 divided doses) increased gradually as necessary (with plasma-phenytoin concentration monitoring); usual dose 200–500 mg daily (exceptionally, higher doses may be used); CHILD initially 5 mg/kg daily in 2 divided doses, usual dose range 4–8 mg/kg daily (max. 300 mg)

By intravenous injection—section 4.8.2
Note. Plasma concentration for optimum response 10–20 mg/litre (40–80 micromol/litre)
COUNSELLING. Take preferably with or after food

Phenytoin (Non-proprietary) PoM
Capsules, phenytoin sodium 50 mg, net price 20 = 40p; 100 mg, 20 = 56p. Label: 8, counselling, administration, blood or skin disorder symptoms (see above), driving (see notes above)
Tablets, coated, phenytoin sodium 50 mg, net price 20 = 89p; 100 mg, 20 = £1.21. Label: 8, counselling, administration, blood or skin disorder symptoms (see above), driving (see notes above)
Available from APS— 50-mg tablets may be difficult to obtain
Note. On the basis of single dose tests there are no clinically relevant differences in bioavailability between available phenytoin sodium tablets and capsules but there may be a pharmacokinetic basis for maintaining the same brand of phenytoin in some patients

Epanutin® (Parke-Davis) PoM
Capsules, phenytoin sodium 25 mg (white/purple), net price 20 = 39p; 50 mg (white/pink), 20 = 40p; 100 mg (white/orange), 20 = 56p; 300 mg (white/green), 20 = £1.69. Label: 8, counselling, administration, blood or skin disorder symptoms (see above), driving (see notes above)
Infatabs® (= chewable tablets), yellow, scored, phenytoin 50 mg. Net price 20 = £1.10. Label: 8, 24, counselling, blood or skin disorder symptoms (see above), driving (see notes above)
Note. Contain phenytoin 50 mg (as against phenytoin sodium) therefore care is needed on changing to capsules or tablets containing phenytoin sodium
Suspension, red, phenytoin 30 mg/5 mL. Net price 100 mL = 71p. Label: 8, counselling, administration, blood or skin disorder symptoms (see above), driving (see notes above)
Note. Suspension of phenytoin 90 mg in 15 mL may be considered to be approximately equivalent in therapeutic effect to capsules or tablets containing phenytoin sodium 100 mg, but nevertheless care is needed in making changes

Tiagabine

Tiagabine is used as adjunctive treatment for partial seizures, with or without secondary generalisation.

TIAGABINE

Indications: adjunctive treatment for partial seizures with or without secondary generalisation not satisfactorily controlled with other antiepileptics

Cautions: hepatic impairment (Appendix 2); avoid abrupt withdrawal
DRIVING. May impair performance of skilled tasks (e.g. driving)

Side-effects: diarrhoea, dizziness, tiredness, nervousness, tremor, concentration difficulties, emotional lability, speech impairment; rarely, confusion, depression, drowsiness, psychosis; leucopenia reported

Dose: adjunctive therapy, with *enzyme-inducing* drugs, 5 mg twice daily for 1 week, then increased at weekly intervals in steps of 5–10 mg daily; usual maintenance dose 30–45 mg daily (doses above 30 mg given in 3 divided doses); in patients receiving *non-enzyme-inducing* drugs, initial maintenance dose should be 15–30 mg daily; CHILD under 12 years not recommended

Gabitril® (Sanofi-Synthelabo) [PoM]
Tablets, f/c, scored, tiagabine (as hydrochloride) 5 mg, net price 100-tab pack = £45.37; 10 mg, 100-tab pack = £90.74; 15 mg, 100-tab pack = £136.11. Label: 21

Topiramate

Topiramate can be given as adjunctive treatment for partial seizures with or without secondary generalisation not satisfactorily controlled with other antiepileptics, for seizures associated with Lennox-Gastaut syndrome, and for primary generalised tonic-clonic seizures

TOPIRAMATE

Indications: adjunctive treatment of partial seizures with or without secondary generalisation not satisfactorily controlled with other antiepileptics; seizures associated with Lennox-Gastaut syndrome; primary generalised tonic-clonic seizures

Cautions: avoid abrupt withdrawal; ensure adequate hydration (especially if predisposition to nephrolithiasis); pregnancy (see notes above); hepatic impairment (Appendix 2); renal impairment (Appendix 3); **interactions:** see p. 227 and Appendix 1 (topiramate)

Contra-indications: breast-feeding

Side-effects: abdominal pain, nausea, anorexia, weight loss; impaired concentration and memory, confusion, impaired speech, emotional lability with mood disorders and depression, altered behaviour, ataxia, abnormal gait, paraesthesia, dizziness, drowsiness, fatigue, asthenia, visual disturbances, diplopia, nystagmus, acute myopia with angle-closure glaucoma (withdraw treatment—see also Cautions above), taste disorder, hypersalivation, also psychotic symptoms, aggression, cognitive problems, leucopenia

Dose: initially 25 mg daily for 1 week *then* increased in steps of 25–50 mg daily at intervals of 1–2 weeks and taken in 2 divided doses; usual dose 200–400 mg daily in 2 divided doses; max. 800 mg daily; CHILD 2–16 years, initially 25 mg at night for one week then increased in steps of 1–3 mg/kg daily according to response at intervals of 1–2 weeks and taken in 2 divided doses; recommended dose range 5–9 mg/kg daily in 2 divided doses

Note. If patient cannot tolerate titration regimen recommended above then smaller steps or longer interval between steps may be used

Topamax® (Janssen-Cilag) [PoM]
Tablets, f/c, topiramate 25 mg, net price 60-tab pack = £22.02; 50 mg (light yellow), 60-tab pack = £36.17; 100 mg (yellow), 60-tab pack = £64.80; 200 mg (salmon), 60-tab pack £125.83. Label: 3, 8, counselling, driving (see notes above)

Sprinkle capsules, topiramate 15 mg, net price 60-cap pack = £16.88; 25 mg, 60-cap pack = £25.32; 50 mg, 60-cap pack = £41.60. Label: 3, 8, counselling, administration, driving (see notes above)
COUNSELLING. Swallow whole or open capsule and sprinkle contents on soft food

Valproate

Sodium valproate is effective in controlling tonic-clonic seizures, particularly in primary generalised epilepsy. It is a drug of choice in primary generalised epilepsy, generalised absences and myoclonic seizures, and may be tried in atypical absence, atonic, and tonic seizures. Controlled trials in partial epilepsy suggest that it has similar efficacy to that of carbamazepine and phenytoin. Plasma-valproate concentrations are not a useful index of efficacy, therefore routine monitoring is unhelpful. The drug has widespread metabolic effects, and may have dose-related side-effects.

Valproic acid (as semisodium valproate) (section 4.2.3) has been licensed recently for acute mania associated with bipolar disorder.

SODIUM VALPROATE

Indications: all forms of epilepsy

Cautions: monitor liver function before therapy and during first 6 months especially in patients most at risk (see also below), ensure no undue potential for bleeding before starting and before surgery; renal impairment (Appendix 3); pregnancy (**important** see notes above and Appendix 4 (neural tube screening)); breast-feeding; systemic lupus erythematosus; false-positive urine tests for ketones; avoid sudden withdrawal; see also notes above; **interactions:** see p. 227 and Appendix 1 (valproate)

LIVER TOXICITY. Liver dysfunction (including fatal hepatic failure) has occurred in association with valproate (especially in children under 3 years of age and those with metabolic or degenerative disorders, organic brain disease or severe seizure disorders associated with mental retardation) usually in the first 6 months of therapy and usually involving multiple antiepileptic therapy (monotherapy preferred). Raised liver enzymes are not uncommon during valproate treatment and are usually transient but patients should be reassessed clinically and liver function (including prothrombin time) monitored until return to normal—an abnormally prolonged prothrombin time (particularly in association with other relevant abnormalities) requires discontinuation of treatment. Any concomitant use of salicylates should be stopped.

BLOOD OR HEPATIC DISORDERS. Patients or their carers should be told how to recognise signs of blood or liver disorders, and advised to seek immediate medical attention if symptoms develop (advice is given on patient information leaflet).

PANCREATITIS. Patients or their carers should be told how to recognise signs of pancreatitis, and advised to seek immediate medical attention if symptoms such as abdominal pain, nausea and vomiting develop; discontinue sodium valproate if pancreatitis is diagnosed

Contra-indications: active liver disease, family history of severe hepatic dysfunction, porphyria (section 9.8.2)

Side-effects: gastric irritation, nausea, ataxia and tremor; hyperammonaemia, increased appetite and weight gain; transient hair loss (regrowth may be curly), oedema, thrombocytopenia, and inhibition of platelet aggregation; impaired hepatic function leading rarely to fatal hepatic failure (see also under Cautions—withdraw treatment immediately if vomiting, anorexia, jaundice, drowsiness, or loss of seizure control occurs); rashes; sedation reported (rarely lethargy and confusion associated with too high an initial dose) and also increased alertness (occasionally aggression, hyperactivity and behavioural disturbances); rarely pancreatitis (measure plasma amylase in acute abdominal pain; see also Pancreatitis under Cautions above), extrapyramidal symptoms, dementia, leucopenia, pancytopenia, red cell hypoplasia, fibrinogen reduction; irregular periods, amenorrhoea, gynaecomastia, hearing loss, Fanconi's syndrome, toxic epidermal necrolysis, Stevens-Johnson syndrome, vasculitis, hirsutism and acne also reported

Dose: *by mouth*, initially, 600 mg daily given in 2 divided doses, preferably after food, increasing by 200 mg/day at 3-day intervals to a max. of 2.5 g daily in divided doses, usual maintenance 1–2 g daily (20–30 mg/kg daily); CHILD up to 20 kg, initially 20 mg/kg in divided doses, may be increased provided plasma concentrations monitored (above 40 mg/kg daily also monitor clinical chemistry and haematological parameters); over 20 kg, initially 400 mg daily in divided doses increased until control (usually in range of 20–30 mg/kg daily); max. 35 mg/kg daily

By intravenous injection (over 3–5 minutes) or *by intravenous infusion*, continuation of valproate treatment when oral therapy not possible, same as current dose by oral route

Initiation of valproate therapy (when oral valproate not possible), *by intravenous injection* (over 3–5 minutes), 400–800 mg (up to 10 mg/kg) followed by *intravenous infusion* up to max. 2.5 g daily; CHILD, usually 20–30 mg/kg daily, may be increased provided plasma concentrations monitored (above 40 mg/kg daily also monitor clinical chemistry and haematological parameters)

Sodium Valproate (Non-proprietary) PoM
Tablets, e/c, sodium valproate 200 mg, net price 20 = £1.12; 500 mg, 20 = £2.96. Label: 5, 8, 25, counselling, blood or hepatic disorder symptoms (see above), driving (see notes above)
Available from Alpharma, APS, CP (*Orlept*®), Hillcross, IVAX, Sterwin
Oral solution, sodium valproate 200 mg/5 mL. Net price 100 mL = £1.82. Label: 8, counselling, blood or hepatic disorder symptoms (see above), driving (see notes above)
Available from CP, (*Orlept*®, sugar-free), Hillcross, IVAX (sugar-free), Sterwin

Epilim® (Sanofi-Synthelabo) PoM
Tablets (crushable), scored, sodium valproate 100 mg. Net price 20 = 78p. Label: 8, counselling, blood or hepatic disorder symptoms (see above), driving (see notes above)
Note. Sodium valproate crushable tablets also available from Hillcross
Tablets, both e/c, lilac, sodium valproate 200 mg, net price 20 = £1.28; 500 mg, 20 = £3.21. Label: 5, 8, 25, counselling, blood or hepatic disorder symptoms (see above), driving (see notes above)
Liquid, red, sugar-free, sodium valproate 200 mg/5 mL. Net price 300-mL pack = £5.89. Label: 8,

counselling, blood or hepatic disorder symptoms (see above), driving (see notes above)
Syrup, red, sodium valproate 200 mg/5 mL. Net price 300-mL pack = £5.89. Label: 8, counselling, blood or hepatic disorder symptoms (see above), driving (see notes above)

Epilim Chrono® (Sanofi-Synthelabo) PoM
Tablets, m/r, all lilac, sodium valproate 200 mg (as sodium valproate and valproic acid), net price 100-tab pack = £8.09; 300 mg, 100-tab pack = £12.13; 500 mg, 100-tab pack = £20.21. Label: 8, 25, counselling, blood or hepatic disorder symptoms (see above), driving (see notes above)
Dose: ADULT and CHILD over 20 kg, as above, total daily dose given in 1–2 divided doses

Epilim® **Intravenous** (Sanofi-Synthelabo) PoM
Injection, powder for reconstitution, sodium valproate. Net price 400-mg vial (with 4-mL amp water for injections) = £8.77

■ Valproic acid

Convulex® (Pharmacia) PoM
Capsules, e/c, valproic acid 150 mg, net price 100-cap pack = £3.68; 300 mg, 100-cap pack = £7.35; 500 mg, 100-cap pack = £12.25. Label: 8, 25, counselling, blood or hepatic disorder symptoms (see above), driving (see notes above)
Dose: ADULT and CHILD initially 15 mg/kg daily in 2–4 divided doses, gradually increasing in steps of 5–10 mg/kg up to 30 mg/kg daily

EQUIVALENCE TO SODIUM VALPROATE. Manufacturer advises that *Convulex*® has a 1:1 dose relationship with products containing sodium valproate, but nevertheless care is needed in making changes.

Vigabatrin

For partial epilepsy with or without secondary generalisation, **vigabatrin** is given in combination with other antiepileptic treatment; its use is restricted to patients in whom all other combinations are inadequate or are not tolerated. It can be used as sole therapy in the management of infantile spasms in West's syndrome.

About one-third of patients treated with vigabatrin have suffered visual field defects; counselling and **careful monitoring** for this side-effect are required (see also Visual Field Defects under Cautions below). Vigabatrin has prominent behavioural side-effects in some patients.

VIGABATRIN

Indications: initiated and supervised by appropriate specialist, adjunctive treatment of partial seizures with or without secondary generalisation not satisfactorily controlled with other antiepileptics; monotherapy for management of infantile spasms (West's syndrome)

Cautions: renal impairment; elderly; closely monitor neurological function; avoid sudden withdrawal (taper off over 2–4 weeks); history of psychosis, depression or behavioural problems; pregnancy (see p. 227 and Appendix 4) and breast-feeding; absence seizures (may be exacerbated); **interactions:** see p. 227 and Appendix 1 (vigabatrin)

VISUAL FIELD DEFECTS. Vigabatrin is associated with visual field defects. The CSM has advised that onset of symptoms varies from 1 month to several years after starting. In most cases, visual field defects have persisted despite discontinuation. Product literature advises visual field testing before treatment and at 6-month intervals; a procedure for testing visual fields in those with a developmental age of less than 9 years is available from the manufacturers. Patients should be warned to report any new visual symptoms that develop and those with symptoms should be referred for an urgent ophthalmological opinion. Gradual withdrawal of vigabatrin should be considered.

Contra-indications: visual field defects

Side-effects: drowsiness (rarely marked sedation, stupor, and confusion with non-specific slow wave EEG), fatigue, visual field defects (see also under Cautions), dizziness, nervousness, irritability, behavioural effects such as excitation and agitation especially in children; depression, abnormal thinking, headache, nystagmus, ataxia, tremor, paraesthesia, impaired concentration; less commonly confusion, aggression, psychosis, mania, memory disturbance, visual disturbance (e.g. diplopia); also weight gain, oedema, gastrointestinal disturbances, alopecia, rash; less commonly, urticaria, occasional increase in seizure frequency (especially if myoclonic), decrease in liver enzymes, slight decrease in haemoglobin; photophobia and retinal disorders (e.g. peripheral retinal atrophy); optic neuritis, optic atrophy also reported

Dose: with current antiepileptic therapy, initially 1 g daily in single or 2 divided doses then increased according to response in steps of 500 mg at weekly intervals; usual range 2–3 g daily (max. 3 g daily); CHILD initially 40 mg/kg daily in single or 2 divided doses then adjusted according to body-weight 10–15 kg, 0.5–1 g daily; body-weight 15–30 kg, 1–1.5 g daily; body-weight 30–50 kg, 1.5–3 g daily; body-weight over 50 kg, 2–3 g daily

Infantile spasms (West's syndrome), *monotherapy*, 50 mg/kg daily, adjusted according to response over 7 days; up to 150 mg/kg daily used with good tolerability

Sabril® (Hoechst Marion Roussel) [PoM]
Tablets, f/c, scored, vigabatrin 500 mg, net price 100-tab pack = £44.85. Label: 3, 8, counselling, driving (see notes above)
Powder, sugar-free, vigabatrin 500 mg/sachet. Net price 50-sachet pack = £24.33. Label: 3, 8, 13, counselling, driving (see notes above)
Note. The contents of a sachet should be dissolved in water or a soft drink immediately before taking

Benzodiazepines

Clonazepam is occasionally used in tonic-clonic or partial seizures, but its sedative side-effects may be prominent. **Clobazam** may be used as adjunctive therapy in the treatment of epilepsy (section 4.1.2), but the effectiveness of these and other **benzodiazepines** may wane considerably after weeks or months of continuous therapy.

CLOBAZAM

Indications: adjunct in epilepsy; anxiety (short-term use)

Cautions: see under Diazepam (section 4.1.2)

Contra-indications: see under Diazepam (section 4.1.2)

Side-effects: see under Diazepam (section 4.1.2)

Dose: epilepsy, 20–30 mg daily; max. 60 mg daily; CHILD over 3 years, not more than half adult dose
Anxiety, 20–30 mg daily in divided doses or as a single dose at bedtime, increased in severe anxiety (in hospital patients) to a max. of 60 mg daily in divided doses; ELDERLY (or debilitated) 10–20 mg daily

¹ **Clobazam** (Non-proprietary) [NHS] [PoM]
Tablets, clobazam 10 mg. Net price 30-tab pack = £10.98. Label: 2 *or* 19, 8, counselling, driving (see notes above)

1. [NHS] except, for epilepsy and endorsed 'SLS'

Note. The brand name *Frisium®* [NHS] (Hoechst Marion Roussel) is used for clobazam tablets

CLONAZEPAM

Indications: all forms of epilepsy; myoclonus; status epilepticus (section 4.8.2)

Cautions: see notes above; respiratory disease; hepatic and renal impairment; elderly and debilitated; pregnancy and breast-feeding (see notes above); avoid sudden withdrawal; porphyria (section 9.8.2); **interactions:** see p. 227 and Appendix 1 (clonazepam)

DRIVING. Drowsiness may affect performance of skilled tasks (e.g. driving); effects of alcohol enhanced

Contra-indications: respiratory depression; acute pulmonary insufficiency

Side-effects: drowsiness, fatigue, dizziness, muscle hypotonia, coordination disturbances; hypersalivation in infants, paradoxical aggression, irritability and mental changes; rarely, blood disorders, abnormal liver-function tests; **overdosage:** see Emergency Treatment of Poisoning, p. 25

Dose: 1 mg (elderly, 500 micrograms), initially at night for 4 nights, increased over 2–4 weeks to a usual maintenance dose of 4–8 mg daily in divided doses; CHILD up to 1 year 250 micrograms increased as above to 0.5–1 mg, 1–5 years 250 micrograms increased to 1–3 mg, 5–12 years 500 micrograms increased to 3–6 mg

Rivotril® (Roche) [PoM]
Tablets, both scored, clonazepam 500 micrograms (beige), net price 20 = 84p; 2 mg (white), 20 = £1.12. Label: 2, 8, counselling, driving (see notes above)

Injection, section 4.8.2

Other drugs

Acetazolamide (section 11.6), a carbonic anhydrase inhibitor, is a second-line drug for both tonic-clonic and partial seizures. It is occasionally helpful in atypical absence, atonic, and tonic seizures.

Piracetam (section 4.9.3) is used as adjunctive treatment for cortical myoclonus.

4.8.2 Drugs used in status epilepticus

Initial management of status epilepticus includes positioning the patient to avoid injury, supporting respiration including the provision of oxygen, maintaining blood pressure, and the correction of any hypoglycaemia. The use of parenteral **thiamine** should be considered if alcohol abuse is suspected; **pyridoxine** should be administered if the status epilepticus is caused by pyridoxine deficiency.

Major status epilepticus should be treated initially with intravenous **lorazepam**. Intravenous **diazepam** may also be used, but lorazepam has a longer duration of antiepileptic action. Diazepam is associated with a high risk of venous thrombophlebitis which is reduced by using an emulsion (*Diazemuls®*).

Where facilities for resuscitation are not immediately available, small doses of lorazepam or diazepam can be given intravenously, or diazepam can be administered as a rectal solution. Absorption from intramuscular injection or from suppositories is too slow for treatment of status epilepticus.

Clonazepam can also be used as an alternative.

If seizures recur or fail to respond after 30 minutes, phenytoin sodium, fosphenytoin, or phenobarbital sodium should be used.

Phenytoin sodium may be given by slow intravenous injection, with ECG monitoring, followed by the maintenance dosage. Intramuscular use of phenytoin is not recommended (absorption is slow and erratic).

Alternatively, **fosphenytoin**, a pro-drug of phenytoin, can be given more rapidly and when given intravenously causes fewer injection site reactions compared to phenytoin. Intravenous administration requires ECG monitoring. Although it can also be given intramuscularly, absorption is too slow by this route for treatment of status epilepticus. Doses of fosphenytoin should be expressed in terms of phenytoin sodium.

Alternatively, **phenobarbital sodium** can be given by intravenous injection (section 4.8.1).

Paraldehyde also remains a valuable drug. Given rectally it causes little respiratory depression and is therefore useful where facilities for resuscitation are poor.

If the above measures fail to control seizures, anaesthesia with thiopental [unlicensed indication] (section 15.1.1) or in adults, a non-barbiturate anaesthetic such as propofol [unlicensed indication] (section 15.1.1), should be instituted with full intensive care support.

DIAZEPAM

Indications: status epilepticus; convulsions due to poisoning (see Emergency Treatment of Poisoning); other indications (section 4.1.2, section 10.2.2, and section 15.1.4.1)

Cautions: see section 4.1.2; when given intravenously facilities for reversing respiratory depression with mechanical ventilation must be at hand (but see also notes above)

SPECIAL CAUTIONS FOR INTRAVENOUS INFUSION. Intravenous infusion of diazepam is potentially hazardous (especially if prolonged), calling for close and constant observation and best carried out in specialist centres with intensive care facilities. Prolonged infusion may lead to accumulation and delay recovery

Contra-indications: see section 4.1.2

Side-effects: see section 4.1.2; hypotension and apnoea

Dose: *by intravenous injection*, 10–20 mg at a rate of 0.5 mL (2.5 mg) per 30 seconds, repeated if necessary after 30–60 minutes; may be followed by *intravenous infusion* to max. 3 mg/kg over 24 hours; CHILD 200–300 micrograms/kg *or* 1 mg per year of age

By rectum as rectal solution, ADULT and CHILD over 10 kg 500 micrograms/kg; ELDERLY 250 micrograms/kg

Diazepam (Non-proprietary) PoM

Injection (solution), diazepam 5 mg/mL. See Appendix 6. Net price 2-mL amp = 25p

Available from CP, Roche (*Valium®*)

Injection (emulsion), diazepam 5 mg/mL (0.5%). See Appendix 6. Net price 2-mL amp = 73p

Available from Alpharma (*Diazemuls®*)

Rectal tubes (= rectal solution), diazepam 2 mg/mL, net price 1.25-mL (2.5-mg) tube = 90p, 2.5-mL (5-mg) tube = £1.34; 4 mg/mL, 2.5-mL (10-mg) tube = £1.73, 5-mL (20-mg) tube = £2.92

Available from Alpharma (*Stesolid®* 5 mg, 10 mg), CP (*Diazepam Rectubes®* 2.5 mg, 5 mg, 10 mg), Lagap

■ Oral preparations, section 4.1.2

CLONAZEPAM

Indications: status epilepticus; other forms of epilepsy, and myoclonus (section 4.8.1)

Cautions: see section 4.8.1; facilities for reversing respiratory depression with mechanical ventilation must be at hand (but see also notes above)

INTRAVENOUS INFUSION. Intravenous infusion of clonazepam is potentially hazardous (especially if prolonged), calling for close and constant observation and best carried out in specialist centres with intensive care facilities. Prolonged infusion may lead to accumulation and delay recovery

Contra-indications: see section 4.8.1; avoid injections containing benzyl alcohol in neonates (see under preparations below)

Side-effects: see section 4.8.1; hypotension and apnoea

Dose: *by intravenous injection* into a large vein (over 30 seconds) *or by intravenous infusion*, 1 mg, repeated if necessary; CHILD all ages, 500 micrograms

Rivotril® (Roche) PoM

Injection, clonazepam 1 mg/mL in solvent, for dilution with 1 mL water for injections immediately before injection or as described in Appendix 6. Net price 1-mL amp (with 1 mL water for injections) = 68p

Excipients: include benzyl alcohol (avoid in neonates, see Excipients, p. 2), ethanol, propylene glycol

■ Oral preparations, section 4.8.1

FOSPHENYTOIN SODIUM

Note. Fosphenytoin is a pro-drug of phenytoin

Indications: status epilepticus; seizures associated with neurosurgery or head injury; when phenytoin by mouth not possible

Cautions: see Phenytoin Sodium; liver impairment (Appendix 2); renal impairment (Appendix 3); resuscitation facilities must be available; **interactions:** see p. 227 and Appendix 1 (phenytoin)

Contra-indications: see Phenytoin Sodium

Side-effects: see Phenytoin Sodium

CSM ADVICE. Intravenous infusion of fosphenytoin has been associated with severe cardiovascular reactions including asystole, ventricular fibrillation, and cardiac arrest. Hypotension, bradycardia, and heart block have also been reported. The CSM advises:

- monitor heart rate, blood pressure, and respiratory function for duration of infusion
- observe patient for at least 30 minutes after infusion
- if hypotension occurs, reduce infusion rate or discontinue
- reduce dose or infusion rate in elderly, and in renal or hepatic impairment

Dose: expressed as **phenytoin sodium equivalent** (PE); fosphenytoin sodium 1.5 mg ≡ phenytoin sodium 1 mg

Status epilepticus, *by intravenous infusion* (at a rate of 100–150 mg(PE)/minute), initially 15 mg(PE)/kg then *by intramuscular injection* or *by intravenous infusion* (at a rate of 50–100 mg(PE)/minute), 4–5 mg(PE)/kg daily in 1–2 divided doses, dose adjusted according to response and trough plasma-phenytoin concentration

CHILD 5 years and over, *by intravenous infusion* (at a rate of 2–3 mg(PE)/kg/minute), initially 15 mg(PE)/kg then *by intravenous infusion* (at a rate of 1–2 mg(PE)/kg/minute), 4–5 mg(PE)/kg daily in 1–4 divided doses, dose adjusted according to response and trough plasma-phenytoin concentration

Prophylaxis or treatment of seizures associated with neurosurgery or head injury, *by intramuscular injection* or *by intravenous infusion* (at a rate of 50–100 mg(PE)/minute), initially 10–15 mg(PE)/kg then *by intramuscular injection* or *by intravenous infusion* (at a rate of 50–100 mg(PE)/minute), 4–5 mg(PE)/kg daily (in 1–2 divided doses), dose adjusted according to response and trough plasma-phenytoin concentration

CHILD 5 years and over, *by intravenous infusion* (at a rate of 1–2 mg(PE)/kg/minute), initially 10–15 mg(PE)/kg then 4–5 mg(PE)/kg daily in 1–4 divided doses, dose adjusted according to response and trough plasma-phenytoin concentration

Temporary substitution for oral phenytoin, *by intramuscular injection* or *by intravenous infusion* (at a rate of 50–100 mg(PE)/minute), same dose and dosing frequency as oral phenytoin therapy; CHILD 5 years and over, *by intravenous infusion* (at a rate of 1–2 mg(PE)/kg/minute), same dose and dosing frequency as oral phenytoin therapy

ELDERLY consider 10–25% reduction in dose or infusion rate

> *Note.* Prescriptions for fosphenytoin sodium should state the dose in terms of phenytoin sodium equivalent (PE)

Pro-Epanutin® (Parke-Davis) ▼ PoM

Injection concentrate, fosphenytoin sodium 75 mg/mL (equivalent to phenytoin sodium 50 mg/mL), net price 10-mL vial = £40.00

Electrolytes: phosphate 3.7 micromol/mg fosphenytoin sodium (phosphate 5.6 micromol/mg phenytoin sodium)

LORAZEPAM

Indications: status epilepticus; other indications (section 4.1.2)

Cautions: see section 4.1.2; facilities for reversing respiratory depression with mechanical ventilation must be at hand

Contra-indications: see section 4.1.2

Side-effects: see section 4.1.2; hypotension and apnoea

Dose: *by intravenous injection* (into large vein), 4 mg; CHILD 2 mg

Preparations

Section 4.1.2

PARALDEHYDE

Indications: status epilepticus

Cautions: bronchopulmonary disease, hepatic impairment; pregnancy (Appendix 4) and breast-feeding (Appendix 5)

Contra-indications: gastric disorders; rectal administration in colitis

Side-effects: rashes; rectal irritation after enema

Dose: *by rectum*, usually 10–20 mL; CHILD up to 3 months 0.5 mL, 3–6 months 1 mL, 6–12 months 1.5 mL, 1–2 years 2 mL, 3–5 years 3–4 mL, 6–12 years 5–6 mL

ADMINISTRATION. Administer as an enema containing 1 part paraldehyde diluted with 9 parts physiological saline (some centres mix paraldehyde with an equal volume of arachis (peanut) oil instead)

Note. Do not use paraldehyde if it has a brownish colour or an odour of acetic acid. Avoid contact with rubber and plastics.

Paraldehyde (Non-proprietary) PoM

Injection, sterile paraldehyde, net price 5-mL amp = £9.49

Available from Faulding DBL

PHENYTOIN SODIUM

Indications: status epilepticus; seizures in neurosurgery; arrhythmias, but now obsolete (section 2.3.2)

Cautions: hypotension and heart failure; resuscitation facilities must be available; injection solutions alkaline (irritant to tissues); see also section 4.8.1; **interactions:** see p. 227 and Appendix 1 (phenytoin)

Contra-indications: sinus bradycardia, sino-atrial block, and second- and third-degree heart block; Stokes-Adams syndrome; porphyria (section 9.8.2)

Side-effects: intravenous injection may cause cardiovascular and CNS depression (particularly if injection too rapid) with arrhythmias, hypotension, and cardiovascular collapse; alterations in respiratory function (including respiratory arrest)

Dose: *by slow intravenous injection or infusion* (with blood pressure and ECG monitoring), status epilepticus, 15 mg/kg at a rate not exceeding 50 mg per minute, as a loading dose (see also notes above); maintenance doses of about 100 mg should be given thereafter at intervals of every 6–8 hours, monitored by measurement of plasma concentrations; rate and dose reduced according to weight; CHILD 15 mg/kg as a loading dose (neonate 15–20 mg/kg at rate of 1–3 mg/kg/minute)

Ventricular arrhythmias (but use now obsolete), *by intravenous injection* via caval catheter, 3.5–5 mg/kg at a rate not exceeding 50 mg/minute, with blood pressure and ECG monitoring; repeat once if necessary

Note. Phenytoin is licensed for administration by intravenous infusion (at the same rate of administration as the injection—not exceeding 50 mg/minute, for further details of the infusion, see Appendix 6). To avoid local venous irritation each injection or infusion should be preceded and followed by an injection of sterile physiological saline through the same needle or catheter

By intramuscular injection, not recommended (see notes above)

Phenytoin (Non-proprietary) PoM
Injection, phenytoin sodium 50 mg/mL with propylene glycol 40% and alcohol 10% in water for injections, net price 5-mL amp = £3.63
Available from Antigen, Faulding DBL

Epanutin® Ready-Mixed Parenteral (Parke-Davis) PoM
Injection, phenytoin sodium 50 mg/mL with propylene glycol 40% and alcohol 10% in water for injections. Net price 5-mL amp = £4.07
Note. Phenytoin injection also available from Antigen, Faulding DBL

■ Oral preparations, section 4.8.1

4.8.3 Febrile convulsions

Brief febrile convulsions need only simple treatment such as tepid sponging or bathing, or antipyretic medication, e.g. **paracetamol** (section 4.7.1). *Prolonged febrile convulsions* (those lasting 15 minutes or longer), *recurrent convulsions*, or those occurring in a child at known risk must be treated more actively, as there is the possibility of resulting brain damage. **Diazepam** is the drug of choice given either by slow intravenous injection in a dose of 250 micrograms/kg (section 4.8.2) or preferably rectally in solution (section 4.8.2) in a dose of 500 micrograms/kg (max. 10 mg), repeated if necessary. The rectal route is preferred as satisfactory absorption is achieved within minutes and administration is much easier. Suppositories are not suitable because absorption is too slow.

Intermittent prophylaxis (i.e. the anticonvulsant administered at the onset of fever) is possible in only a small proportion of children. Again **diazepam** is the treatment of choice, orally or rectally.

The exact role of continuous prophylaxis in children at risk from prolonged or complex febrile convulsions is controversial. It is probably indicated in only a small proportion of children, including those whose first seizure occurred at under 14 months or who have pre-existing neurological abnormalities or who have had previous prolonged or focal convulsions. Thus long-term anticonvulsant prophylaxis is rarely indicated.

4.9 Drugs used in parkinsonism and related disorders

4.9.1 Dopaminergic drugs used in parkinsonism
4.9.2 Antimuscarinic drugs used in parkinsonism
4.9.3 Drugs used in essential tremor, chorea, tics, and related disorders

In idiopathic Parkinson's disease, progressive degeneration of pigment-containing cells of the substantia nigra leads to deficiency of the neurotransmitter dopamine. This, in turn, results in a neurohumoral imbalance in the basal ganglia, causing the characteristic signs and symptoms of the illness to appear. The pathogenesis of this process is still obscure and current drug therapy aims simply to correct the imbalance. Although this approach fails to prevent the progression of the disease, it greatly improves the quality and expectancy of life of most patients.

The patient should be advised at the outset of the limitations of treatment and possible side-effects. About 10 to 20% of patients are unresponsive to treatment.

ELDERLY. Antiparkinsonian drugs carry a special risk of inducing confusion in the elderly. It is particularly important to initiate treatment with low doses and to use small increments.

4.9.1 Dopaminergic drugs used in parkinsonism

Levodopa in combination with a **dopa-decarboxylase inhibitor** is the treatment of choice for patients disabled by idiopathic Parkinson's disease. It is least valuable in elderly patients and in those with long-standing disease who may not tolerate a dose large enough to overcome their deficit. It is also less valuable in patients with post-encephalitic disease who are particularly susceptible to the side-effects. Parkinsonism caused by generalised degenerative brain disease does not normally respond to levodopa. It should not be used for neuroleptic-induced parkinsonism.

Levodopa, the amino-acid precursor of dopamine, acts mainly by replenishing depleted striatal dopamine. It improves bradykinesia and rigidity more than tremor. It is administered in conjunction with an extracerebral dopa-decarboxylase inhibitor that prevents the peripheral degradation of levodopa to dopamine but, unlike levodopa, does not cross the blood-brain barrier. Effective brain concentrations of dopamine can thereby be achieved with lower doses of levodopa. At the same time the reduced peripheral formation of dopamine decreases peripheral side-effects such as nausea and vomiting and cardiovascular effects. There is also less delay in onset of therapeutic effect and a smoother clinical response. A disadvantage is an increased incidence of abnormal involuntary movements.

The extracerebral dopa-decarboxylase inhibitors used with levodopa are benserazide (in **co-benel-dopa**) and carbidopa (in **co-careldopa**).

When co-careldopa 10/100 (10 mg of carbidopa for each 100 mg of levodopa) is used the dose of carbidopa may be insufficient to achieve full inhibition of extracerebral dopa-decarboxylase; co-careldopa 25/100 (25 mg of carbidopa for each 100 mg of levodopa) should then be used so that the daily dose of carbidopa is at least 75 mg.

Levodopa therapy should be initiated with low doses and gradually increased, by small increments, at intervals of 2 to 3 days. The final dose is usually a compromise between increased mobility and dose-limiting side-effects. Intervals between doses may be critical and should be chosen to suit the needs of the individual patient. Nausea and vomiting are rarely dose-limiting but doses should be taken after meals. Domperidone (section 4.6) may be useful in controlling vomiting. The most frequent dose-limiting side-effects of levodopa are involuntary movements and psychiatric complications. As the patient ages, the maintenance dose may need to be reduced.

During the first 6 to 18 months of levodopa therapy there may be a slow improvement in the response of the patient which is maintained for 1½ to 2 years; thereafter a slow decline may occur. Particularly troublesome is the 'on-off' effect, the incidence of which increases as the treatment progresses. This is characterised by fluctuations in performance with normal performance during the 'on' period and weakness and akinesia lasting for 2 to 4 hours during the 'off' period.

'End-of-dose' deterioration may also occur where the duration of benefit after each dose becomes progressively shorter. Modified-release preparations may help with 'end-of-dose' deterioration or nocturnal immobility and rigidity.

Selegiline is a monoamine-oxidase-B inhibitor used in severe parkinsonism in conjunction with levodopa to reduce 'end-of-dose' deterioration. Early treatment with selegiline may delay the need for levodopa therapy but there is no convincing evidence that it delays disease progression. Selegiline given with levodopa may be associated with increased mortality in the longer term, but this remains to be confirmed. Selegiline need not necessarily be withdrawn from patients stabilised on treatment; sudden withdrawal of selegiline may exacerbate symptoms.

Entacapone is licensed for use as an adjunct to co-beneldopa or co-careldopa for patients with Parkinson's disease who experience 'end-of-dose' deterioration and cannot be stabilised on these combinations.

The ergot derivatives, **bromocriptine, cabergoline, lisuride** (lysuride), and **pergolide** act by direct stimulation of surviving dopamine receptors; they are termed dopamine receptor agonists. Although effective, they have no advantages over levodopa. They should be reserved for patients in whom levodopa alone is no longer adequate or who despite careful titration cannot tolerate levodopa. Ergot derivatives are sometimes useful in reducing 'off'

periods and in ameliorating fluctuations in the later stage of Parkinson's disease. Their use is often limited by their side-effects and when used with levodopa, abnormal involuntary movements and confusional states are common; occasionally, ergot derivatives may cause neuropsychiatric effects and retroperitoneal fibrosis.

Ropinirole is a dopamine D_2 receptor agonist which improves the symptoms and signs in Parkinson's disease. It is likely to be most useful as an adjunct to levodopa. Dopamine agonists such as ropinirole are often used as monotherapy, particularly in younger patients who are at risk of developing disabling dyskinesia with long-term levodopa therapy.

Pramipexole is a non-ergot dopamine D_2 and D_3 receptor agonist with antiparkinsonian activity. Side-effects are similar to those of other dopamine agonists. It can be used alone or as adjunctive therapy with levodopa.

Amantadine has modest antiparkinsonian effects. It improves mild bradykinetic disabilities as well as tremor and rigidity. Unfortunately only a small proportion of patients derive much benefit from this drug and tolerance to its effects occurs. However it has the advantage of being relatively free from side-effects.

Apomorphine is a potent stimulator of D_1 and D_2 receptors, which is sometimes helpful in stabilising patients experiencing unpredictable 'off' periods with levodopa treatment. It is essential to establish patients on domperidone for at least 2 days before starting apomorphine. Long-term specialist supervision is advisable throughout apomorphine treatment.

SUDDEN ONSET OF SLEEP. Excessive daytime sleepiness can occur with co-careldopa, co-beneldopa, and the dopamine receptor agonists.
Sudden onset of sleep has been observed with dopamine agonists such as pramipexole and ropinirole. Patients starting treatment with any dopamine agonist should be warned of the possibility of excessive daytime sleepiness

---

LEVODOPA

Indications: parkinsonism (but not drug-induced extrapyramidal symptoms), see notes above

Cautions: pulmonary disease, peptic ulceration, cardiovascular disease, diabetes mellitus, osteomalacia, open-angle glaucoma, skin melanoma, psychiatric illness (avoid if severe); warn patients about excessive drowsiness (see notes above); in prolonged therapy, psychiatric, hepatic, haematological, renal, and cardiovascular surveillance is advisable; warn patients to resume normal activities gradually; avoid abrupt withdrawal; pregnancy (toxicity in *animals*) and breast-feeding; **interactions:** Appendix 1 (levodopa)

Contra-indications: closed-angle glaucoma

Side-effects: anorexia, nausea and vomiting, insomnia, agitation, postural hypotension (rarely labile hypertension), dizziness, tachycardia, arrhythmias, reddish discoloration of urine and other body fluids, rarely hypersensitivity; abnormal involuntary movements and psychiatric symptoms which include hypomania and psychosis may be dose-limiting; depression, drowsiness, headache, flushing, sweating, gastro-intestinal

bleeding, peripheral neuropathy, taste disturbance, pruritus, rash, and liver enzyme changes
also reported; syndrome resembling neuroleptic
malignant syndrome reported on withdrawal

Dose: initially 125–500 mg daily in divided doses
after meals, increased according to response (but
rarely used alone, see notes above)

Levodopa (Non-proprietary) PoM ◾◾
Tablets, levodopa 500 mg. Net price 20 = £7.44.
Label: 14, 21
Available from Cambridge

◾◾ denotes preparations that are considered to
be less suitable for prescribing (see p. vi)

CO-BENELDOPA

A mixture of benserazide hydrochloride and levodopa in
mass proportions corresponding to 1 part of benserazide
and 4 parts of levodopa

Indications: see under Levodopa and notes above

Cautions: see under Levodopa and notes above

Contra-indications: see under Levodopa

Side-effects: see under Levodopa and notes above

Dose: expressed as levodopa, initally 50 mg 3–4
times daily (100 mg 3 times daily in advanced
disease), increased by 100 mg once or twice
weekly according to response; usual maintenance
dose 400–800 mg daily in divided doses after
meals; ELDERLY initially 50 mg once or twice
daily, increased by 50 mg every 3–4 days according to response

Note. When transferring patients from other levodopa
preparations, it is recommended that the previous preparation should be discontinued 12 hours beforehand
(although interval can be shorter); 3 capsules co-beneldopa 25/100 (*Madopar 125®*) should be substituted for
2 g levodopa; if transferring from another levodopa/
dopa-decarboxylase inhibitor preparation, initial dose,
expressed as levodopa, should be 50 mg 3–4 times daily

Madopar® (Roche) PoM
Capsules 62.5, blue/grey, co-beneldopa 12.5/50
(benserazide 12.5 mg (as hydrochloride), levodopa 50 mg). Net price 100-cap pack = £6.67.
Label: 14, 21
Capsules 125, blue/pink, co-beneldopa 25/100
(benserazide 25 mg (as hydrochloride), levodopa
100 mg). Net price 100-cap pack = £9.29. Label:
14, 21
Capsules 250, blue/caramel, co-beneldopa 50/200
(benserazide 50 mg (as hydrochloride), levodopa
200 mg). Net price 100-cap pack = £15.84. Label:
14, 21
Dispersible tablets 62.5, scored, co-beneldopa
12.5/50 (benserazide 12.5 mg (as hydrochloride),
levodopa 50 mg). Net price 100-tab pack = £7.92.
Label: 14, 21, counselling, administration, see
below
Dispersible tablets 125, scored, co-beneldopa 25/
100 (benserazide 25 mg (as hydrochloride) levodopa 100 mg). Net price 100-tab pack = £14.04.
Label: 14, 21, counselling, administration, see
below
Note. The tablets may be dispersed in water or orange
squash (not orange juice) or swallowed whole

Madopar® CR (Roche) PoM
Capsules 125, m/r, dark green/light blue, co-beneldopa 25/100 (benserazide 25 mg (as hydro-

chloride), levodopa 100 mg). Net price 100-cap
pack = £17.16. Label: 5, 14, 25
Dose: Patients not receiving levodopa therapy, initially 1
capsule 3 times daily (max. initial dose 6 capsules daily)
Fluctuations in response related to plasma-levodopa
concentration or to timing of dose, initially 1 capsule
substituted for every 100 mg of levodopa and given at
same dosage frequency, subsequently increased every 2–
3 days according to response; average increase of 50%
needed over previous levodopa dose and titration may
take up to 4 weeks
Supplementary dose of conventional *Madopar®* may be
needed with first morning dose; if response still poor to
total daily dose of *Madopar® CR* plus *Madopar®* corresponding to 1.2 g levodopa, consider alternative therapy

CO-CARELDOPA

A mixture of carbidopa and levodopa; the proportions are
expressed in the form x/y where x and y are the strengths
in milligrams of carbidopa and levodopa respectively

Indications: see under Levodopa and notes above

Cautions: see under Levodopa and notes above

Contra-indications: see under Levodopa

Side-effects: see under Levodopa and notes above

Dose: expressed as levodopa, initially 100 mg
(with carbidopa 25 mg, as *Sinemet-Plus®*) 3 times
daily, increased by 50–100 mg (with carbidopa
12.5–25 mg, as *Sinemet-62.5®* or *Sinemet-Plus®*)
daily or on alternate days according to response,
up to 800 mg (with carbidopa 200 mg) daily in
divided doses
Note. Carbidopa 70–100 mg daily is necessary to
achieve full inhibition of peripheral dopa-decarboxylase
Alternatively, initially 50–100 mg (with carbidopa
10–12.5 mg, as *Sinemet-62.5®* or *Sinemet-110®*)
3–4 times daily, increased by 50–100 mg daily or
on alternate days according to response, up to
800 mg (with carbidopa 80–100 mg) daily in
divided doses
Alternatively, initially 125 mg (with carbidopa
12.5 mg, as ½ tablet of *Sinemet-275®*) 1–2 times
daily, increased by 125 mg (with carbidopa
12.5 mg) daily or on alternate days according to
response
Note. When transferring patients from levodopa, 1 tablet
co-careldopa 25/250 (*Sinemet-275®*) 3–4 times daily
should be substituted for patients receiving more than
1.5 g levodopa daily; 1 tablet co-careldopa 25/100
(*Sinemet-Plus®*) 3–4 times daily should be substituted
for patients receiving less than 1.5 g levodopa daily;
levodopa should be discontinued 12 hours beforehand

Sinemet® (Bristol-Myers Squibb) PoM
Sinemet-62.5® tablets, yellow, scored, co-careldopa 12.5/50 (carbidopa 12.5 mg (as monohydrate), levodopa 50 mg), net price 90-tab pack
= £7.03. Label: 14, 21
Note. 2 tablets *Sinemet-62.5®* ≡ 1 tablet *Sinemet Plus®*;
Sinemet-62.5® previously known as *Sinemet LS®*
Sinemet-110® tablets, blue, scored, co-careldopa
10/100 (carbidopa 10 mg (as monohydrate), levodopa 100 mg), net price 90-tab pack = £7.35.
Label: 14, 21
Sinemet-Plus® tablets, yellow, scored, co-careldopa 25/100 (carbidopa 25 mg (as monohydrate),
levodopa 100 mg), net price 90-tab pack =
£10.81. Label: 14, 21
Note. The daily dose of carbidopa required to achieve
full inhibition of extracerebral dopa-decarboxylase is
75 mg; co-careldopa 25/100 provides an adequate dose
of carbidopa when low doses of levodopa are needed

Sinemet-2/5® tablets, blue, scored, co-careldopa 25/250 (carbidopa 25 mg (as monohydrate), levodopa 250 mg), net price 90-tab pack = £15.36. Label: 14, 21

■ Modified release

Half Sinemet® CR (Bristol-Myers Squibb) [PoM]
Tablets, m/r, pink, co-careldopa 25/100 (carbidopa 25 mg (as monohydrate), levodopa 100 mg), net price 60-tab pack = £18.99. Label: 14, 25
Dose: for fine adjustment of *Sinemet®* CR dose (see below)

Sinemet® CR (Bristol-Myers Squibb) [PoM]
Tablets, m/r, peach, co-careldopa 50/200 (carbidopa 50 mg (as monohydrate), levodopa 200 mg), net price 60-tab pack = £22.35. Label: 14, 25
Dose: initial treatment or fluctuations in response to conventional levodopa therapy, 1 *Sinemet®* CR tablet twice daily; both dose and interval then adjusted according to response at intervals of not less than 3 days; if transferring from existing levodopa therapy withdraw 8 hours beforehand; 1 tablet *Sinemet®* CR twice daily can be substituted for a daily dose of levodopa 300–400 mg in conventional *Sinemet®* tablets

AMANTADINE HYDROCHLORIDE

Indications: Parkinson's disease (but not drug-induced extrapyramidal symptoms); antiviral (section 5.3)

Cautions: hepatic, or renal impairment (Appendix 3), congestive heart disease (may exacerbate oedema), confused or hallucinatory states, elderly; avoid abrupt discontinuation in Parkinson's disease; **interactions:** Appendix 1 (amantadine)
DRIVING. May affect performance of skilled tasks (e.g. driving)

Contra-indications: epilepsy, history of gastric ulceration, severe renal impairment; pregnancy (toxicity in *animals*), breast-feeding

Side-effects: anorexia, nausea, nervousness, inability to concentrate, insomnia, dizziness, convulsions, hallucinations or feelings of detachment, blurred vision, gastro-intestinal disturbances, livedo reticularis and peripheral oedema; rarely leucopenia, rashes

Dose: 100 mg daily increased after one week to 100 mg twice daily, usually in conjunction with other treatment; some patients may require higher doses, max. 400 mg daily
ELDERLY 65 years and over, 100 mg daily adjusted according to response

Symmetrel® (Alliance) [PoM]
Capsules, red-brown, amantadine hydrochloride 100 mg. Net price 56-cap pack = £15.35. Counselling, driving
Note. Also available as *Lysovir®* for the prophylaxis and treatment of influenza A
Syrup, amantadine hydrochloride 50 mg/5 mL. Net price 150-mL pack = £5.05. Counselling, driving

APOMORPHINE HYDROCHLORIDE

Indications: refractory motor fluctuations in Parkinson's disease ('off' episodes) inadequately controlled by levodopa or other dopaminergics (for capable and motivated patients under specialist supervision); erectile dysfunction (section 7.4.5)

Cautions: tendency to nausea and vomiting; pulmonary, cardiovascular or endocrine disease, renal impairment; elderly and debilitated, history of postural hypotension (special care on initiation); hepatic, haemopoietic, renal, and cardiovascular monitoring; *on administration with levodopa* test initially and every 6 months for haemolytic anaemia (development calls for specialist haematological care with dose reduction and possible discontinuation); **interactions:** Appendix 1 (apomorphine)

Contra-indications: respiratory or CNS depression, hepatic impairment, hypersensitiviy to opioids; neuropsychiatric problems or dementia; not suitable if 'on' response to levodopa marred by severe dyskinesia, hypotonia or psychiatric effects; pregnancy and breast-feeding; not for intravenous administration

Side-effects: nausea and vomiting (see below under Dose), dyskinesias during 'on' periods (may require discontinuation); postural instability and falls (impaired speech and balance may not improve), increasing cognitive impairment, and personality change during 'on' phase; confusion and hallucinations (if continued, specialist observation required with possible gradual dose reduction), sedation, postural hypotension; also euphoria, light-headedness, restlessness, tremors; haemolytic anaemia with levodopa (see Cautions) and rarely eosinophilia; local reactions common (include nodule formation and possible ulceration)—rotate injection sites, dilute with sodium chloride 0.9%, consider ultrasound, ensure no infection

Dose: *by subcutaneous injection*, usual range (after initiation as below) 3–30 mg daily in divided doses; subcutaneous infusion may be preferable in those requiring division of injections into more than 10 doses daily; max. single dose 10 mg; ADOLESCENT (under 18 years) and CHILD not recommended
By continuous subcutaneous infusion (those requiring division into more than 10 injections daily) initially 1 mg/hour daily increased according to response (not more often than every 4 hours) in max. steps of 500 micrograms/hour to max. 4 mg/hour (15–60 micrograms/kg/hour); change infusion site every 12 hours and give during waking hours only (24-hour infusions not advised unless severe night-time symptoms)—intermittent bolus boosts also usually needed (in those with severe dyskinesias only when absolutely necessary)
Total daily dose by either route (or combined routes) max. 100 mg

REQUIREMENTS FOR INITIATION. *Hospital admission* and at least 2 days of pretreatment with domperidone for nausea and vomiting, *after at least 3 days* withhold existing antiparkinsonian medication overnight to provoke 'off' episode, *determine* threshold dose, *re-establish* other antiparkinsonian drugs, *determine* effective apomorphine regimen, *teach* to administer by subcutaneous injection into lower abdomen or outer thigh at first sign of 'off' episode, *discharge* from hospital, *monitor* frequently and *adjust* dosage regimen as appropriate (domperidone may normally be withdrawn over several weeks or longer)—for full details of initiation requirements, consult product literature

APO-go® (Britannia) [PoM]
Injection, apomorphine hydrochloride 10 mg/mL,
net price 2-mL amp = £7.59, 5-mL amp = £15.23

Britaject® (Britannia) [PoM]
Injection, apomorphine hydrochloride 10 mg/mL,
net price 3-mL pen injector = £24.78

BROMOCRIPTINE

Indications: parkinsonism (but not drug-induced
extrapyramidal symptoms); endocrine disorders,
section 6.7.1

Cautions: section 6.7.1
HYPOTENSIVE REACTIONS. Hypotensive reactions may
be disturbing in some patients during the first few days
of treatment and particular care should be exercised
when driving or operating machinery; tolerance may be
reduced by alcohol

Contra-indications: section 6.7.1

Side-effects: section 6.7.1

Dose: first week 1–1.25 mg at night, second week
2–2.5 mg at night, third week 2.5 mg twice daily,
fourth week 2.5 mg 3 times daily then increasing
by 2.5 mg every 3–14 days according to response
to a usual range of 10–40 mg daily; taken with
food

Preparations
Section 6.7.1

CABERGOLINE

Indications: adjunct to levodopa (with dopa-
decarboxylase inhibitor) in Parkinson's disease;
endocrine disorders (section 6.7.1)

Cautions: section 6.7.1
HYPOTENSIVE REACTIONS. Hypotensive reactions may
be disturbing in some patients during the first few days
of treatment and particular care should be exercised
when driving or operating machinery; tolerance may be
reduced by alcohol

Contra-indications: section 6.7.1

Side-effects: section 6.7.1

Dose: initially 1 mg daily, increased by increments
of 0.5–1 mg at 7 or 14 day intervals; usual range
2–6 mg daily
Note. Concurrent dose of levodopa may be decreased
gradually while dose of cabergoline is increased

Cabaser® (Pharmacia) [PoM]
Tablets, all scored, cabergoline 1 mg, net price 20-
tab pack = £75.45; 2 mg, 20-tab pack = £75.45;
4 mg, 16-tab pack = £60.36. Label: 21, counselling, hypotensive reactions
Note. Dispense in original container (contains desiccant)

ENTACAPONE

Indications: adjunct to levodopa with dopa-decarboxylase inhibitor in Parkinson's disease and
'end-of-dose' motor fluctuations

Cautions: concurrent levodopa dose may need to
be reduced by about 10–30%; **interactions:**
Appendix 1 (entacapone)

Contra-indications: pregnancy and breast-feeding; hepatic impairment; phaeochromocytoma;
history of neuroleptic malignant syndrome or
non-traumatic rhabdomyolysis

Side-effects: nausea, vomiting, abdominal pain,
constipation, diarrhoea, urine may be coloured
reddish-brown, dry mouth, dyskinesias; dizzi-

ness; anaemia reported; rarely elevated liver
enzymes

Dose: 200 mg with each dose of levodopa with
dopa-decarboxylase inhibitor; max. 2 g daily

Comtess® (Orion) [PoM]
Tablets, f/c, brown/orange, entacapone 200 mg, net
price 30-tab pack = £19.62, 100-tab pack =
£65.41. Label: 14 (urine reddish-brown)

LISURIDE MALEATE
(Lysuride Maleate)

Indications: Parkinson's disease, used alone or as
an adjunct to levodopa

Cautions: history of pituitary tumour; history of
psychotic disturbance; pregnancy; porphyria (section 9.8.2); **interactions:** Appendix 1 (lysuride)
HYPOTENSIVE REACTIONS. Hypotensive reactions may
be disturbing in some patients during the first few days
of treatment and particular care should be exercised
when driving or operating machinery

Contra-indications: severe disturbances of
peripheral circulation; coronary insufficiency

Side-effects: see notes above; nausea and vomiting; dizziness; headache, lethargy, malaise,
drowsiness, psychotic reactions (including hallucinations); occasionally severe hypotension,
rashes; rarely abdominal pain and constipation;
Raynaud's phenomenon reported

Dose: initially 200 micrograms at bedtime with
food increased as necessary at weekly intervals to
200 micrograms twice daily (midday and bedtime) then to 200 micrograms 3 times daily
(morning, midday, and bedtime); further increases
made by adding 200 micrograms each week first
to the bedtime dose, then to the midday dose and
finally to the morning dose; max. 5 mg daily in 3
divided doses after food

Lisuride Maleate (Non-proprietary) [PoM]
Tablets, scored, lisuride maleate 200 micrograms.
Net price 100-tab pack = £41.92. Label: 21, coun-
selling, hypotensive reactions
Available from Cambridge
Note. The brand name *Revanil®* was formerly used for
lisuride maleate tablets

PERGOLIDE

Indications: Parkinson's disease, used alone or as
adjunct to levodopa

Cautions: arrhythmias or underlying cardiac disease, history of confusion or hallucinations, dyskinesia (may exacerbate), pregnancy (Appendix
4), breast-feeding (Appendix 5); increase dose
gradually and avoid abrupt withdrawal; porphyria
(section 9.8.2); **interactions:** Appendix 1 (pergolide)
HYPOTENSIVE REACTIONS. Hypotensive reactions may
be disturbing in some patients during the first few days
of treatment and particular care should be exercised
when driving or operating machinery

Side-effects: see notes above; hallucinations, confusion, dizziness, dyskinesia, drowsiness, abdominal pain, nausea, vomiting, dyspepsia, diplopia,
rhinitis, dyspnoea, pleuritis, pleural effusion,
pleural fibrosis, pericarditis, pericardial effusion
and retroperitoneal fibrosis, insomnia, constipation or diarrhoea, hypotension, syncope, tachycardia and atrial premature contractions, rash,

fever reported; neuroleptic malignant syndrome also reported

Dose: monotherapy, 50 micrograms at night on day 1, then 50 micrograms twice daily on days 2–4, then increased by 100–250 micrograms daily every 3–4 days (given in 3 divided doses) up to a daily dose of 1.5 mg at day 28; after day 30, further increases of up to 250 micrograms twice a week; usual maintenance dose approx. 2–2.5 mg daily (above 5 mg daily not evaluated)

Adjunctive therapy with levodopa, 50 micrograms daily for 2 days, increased gradually by 100–150 micrograms every 3 days over next 12 days, usually given in 3 divided doses; further increases of 250 micrograms every 3 days; usual maintenance dose 3 mg daily (above 5 mg daily not evaluated); during pergolide titration levodopa dose may be reduced cautiously

Celance® (Lilly) PoM

Tablets, all scored, pergolide (as mesilate) 50 micrograms (ivory), net price 100-tab pack = £27.03; 250 micrograms (green), 100-tab pack = £40.77; 1 mg (pink), 100-tab pack = £147.15; 14-day starter pack of 75 × 50-microgram tablets with 6 × 250-microgram tablets = £22.49. Counselling, hypotensive reactions

PRAMIPEXOLE

Indications: Parkinsons disease, used alone or as adjunct to levodopa

Cautions: renal impairment (Appendix 3); psychotic disorders; ophthalmological testing recommended (risk of visual disorders); severe cardiovascular disease; pregnancy (Appendix 4); avoid abrupt withdrawal (risk of neuroleptic malignant syndrome); **interactions:** Appendix 1 (pramipexole)

HYPOTENSIVE REACTIONS. Hypotensive reactions may be disturbing in some patients during the first few days of treatment

DRIVING. Drowsiness (including sudden onset of sleep) may affect performance of skilled tasks; patients should **not** drive or undertake potentially dangerous activities

Contra-indications: breast-feeding (Appendix 5)

Side-effects: nausea, constipation, drowsiness (including sudden onset of sleep) and insomnia, dizziness, hallucinations (mostly visual), dyskinesia during initial dose titration (more frequent in women—reduce levodopa dose), peripheral oedema

Dose: initially, 264 micrograms daily in 3 divided doses, doubling the dose every 5–7 days to 1.08 mg daily in 3 divided doses; further increased if necessary by 540 micrograms daily at weekly intervals; max. 3.3 mg daily in 3 divided doses

Note. During pramipexole dose titration and maintenance, levodopa dose may be reduced

Important. Doses and strengths are stated in terms of pramipexole (base); equivalent strengths in terms of pramipexole dihydrochloride monohydrate (salt) are as follows: 88 micrograms base ≡ 125 micrograms salt; 180 micrograms base ≡ 250 micrograms salt; 700 micrograms base ≡ 1 mg salt

Mirapexin® (Pharmacia) ▼ PoM

Tablets, pramipexole (as hydrochloride) 88 micrograms, net price 30-tab pack = £7.96; 180 micrograms (scored), 30-tab pack = £15.92, 100-tab pack = £53.06; 700 micrograms (scored), 30-tab pack = £63.67, 100-tab pack = £212.24. Counselling, hypotensive reactions, driving

ROPINIROLE

Indications: Parkinson's disease, either used alone or as an adjunct to levodopa; see also notes above

Cautions: hepatic impairment (Appendix 2); renal impairment (Appendix 3); severe cardiovascular disease, major psychotic disorders, avoid abrupt withdrawal; **interactions:** Appendix 1 (ropinirole)

DRIVING. Drowsiness (including sudden onset of sleep) may affect performance of skilled tasks; patients should **not** drive or undertake potentially dangerous activities

Contra-indications: pregnancy and breast-feeding

Side-effects: nausea, drowsiness (including sudden onset of sleep), leg oedema, abdominal pain, vomiting and syncope; dyskinesia, hallucinations and confusion reported in adjunctive therapy; occasionally severe hypotension and bradycardia

Dose: initially 750 micrograms daily in 3 divided doses, increased by increments of 750 micrograms at weekly intervals to 3 mg daily; further increased by increments of up to 3 mg at weekly intervals according to response; usual range 3–9 mg daily (but higher doses may be required if used with levodopa); max. 24 mg daily

Note. When administered as adjunct to levodopa, concurrent dose of levodopa may be reduced by approx. 20%

Requip® (SmithKline Beecham) PoM

Tablets, f/c, ropinirole (as hydrochloride) 250 micrograms (white), net price 210-tab starter pack = £43.12; 1 mg (green), 84-tab pack = £46.20; 2 mg (pink), 84-tab pack = £92.40; 5 mg (blue), 84-tab pack = £184.80. Label: 21, counselling, driving

SELEGILINE HYDROCHLORIDE

Indications: Parkinson's disease or symptomatic parkinsonism (but not drug-induced extrapyramidal symptoms), used alone (in early disease) or as adjunct to levodopa (but see notes above)

Cautions: gastric and duodenal ulceration (avoid in active ulceration), uncontrolled hypertension, arrhythmias, angina, psychosis, pregnancy and breast-feeding, side-effects of levodopa may be increased, concurrent levodopa dosage may need to be reduced by 10–50%; **interactions:** Appendix 1 (selegiline)

Side-effects: constipation, diarrhoea, nausea and vomiting, dry mouth, stomatitis, sore throat, hypotension, depression, confusion, psychosis, agitation, headache, tremor, dizziness, vertigo, sleep disturbances; back pain, muscle cramps, joint pain, difficulty in micturition, skin reactions transient increase in liver enzymes reported; mouth ulceration reported with oral lyophilisate

Dose: 10 mg in the morning, or 5 mg at breakfast and midday; ELDERLY see below

ELDERLY. To avoid initial confusion and agitation, it may be appropriate to start treatment with a dose of 2.5 mg daily, particularly in the elderly

Selegiline Hydrochloride (Non-proprietary) PoM

Tablets, selegiline hydrochloride 5 mg, net price 56-tab pack = £10.75; 10 mg, 30-tab pack = £11.52

Available from Alpharma, APS, Bioglan, Generics, Hillcross, IVAX, Lagap, Sanofi-Synthelabo, Sterwin

Eldepryl® (Orion) PoM

Tablets, both scored, selegiline hydrochloride 5 mg, net price 60-tab pack = £20.70; 10 mg, 30-tab pack = £20.19

Oral liquid, selegiline hydrochloride 10 mg/5 mL, net price 200-mL = £37.44

■ Oral lyophilisate

Zelapar® (Athena) PoM

Oral lyophilisates (= freeze-dried tablets), yellow, selegiline hydrochloride 1.25 mg, net price 30-tab pack = £55.50. Counselling, administration

Dose: initially 1.25 mg daily before breakfast

COUNSELLING. Tablets should be placed on the tongue and allowed to dissolve. Advise patient not to drink, rinse, or wash mouth out for 5 minutes after taking the tablet

Excipients: include aspartame (section 9.4.1)

Note. Patients receiving 10 mg conventional selegiline hydrochloride tablets can be switched to *Zelapar®* 1.25 mg

4.9.2 Antimuscarinic drugs used in parkinsonism

Antimuscarinic drugs (less correctly termed 'anticholinergics') are less effective than levodopa in idiopathic Parkinson's disease although they may supplement its action. Patients with mild symptoms, particularly where tremor predominates, may be treated initially with antimuscarinic drugs (alone or with selegiline, section 4.9.1), levodopa being added or substituted as symptoms progress. They have value in post-encephalitic parkinsonism.

Antimuscarinic drugs exert their antiparkinsonian effect by correcting the relative central cholinergic excess thought to occur in parkinsonism as a result of dopamine deficiency. They reduce tremor and rigidity but have little effect on bradykinesia. They are useful in reducing sialorrhoea.

The antimuscarinic drugs also reduce the symptoms of drug-induced parkinsonism as seen, for example, with antipsychotic drugs (section 4.2.1) but there is no justification for giving them with antipsychotics unless parkinsonian side-effects occur. Tardive dyskinesia is not improved by the antimuscarinic drugs and may be made worse.

No important differences exist between the many synthetic antimuscarinic drugs available but some patients appear to tolerate one better than another. They may be taken before food if dry mouth is troublesome, or after food if gastro-intestinal symptoms predominate. Those most commonly used are **orphenadrine** and **trihexyphenidyl (benzhexol)**; **benzatropine** and **procyclidine** are also used. Benzatropine is similar to trihexyphenidyl but is

excreted more slowly; changes in dose therefore need to be carried out very gradually.

Procyclidine and benzatropine may be given parenterally and are effective emergency treatment for acute drug-induced dystonic reactions which may be severe.

BENZATROPINE MESILATE
(Benztropine mesylate)

Indications: see Trihexyphenidyl Hydrochloride
Cautions: see Trihexyphenidyl Hydrochloride
Contra-indications: see Trihexyphenidyl Hydrochloride; avoid in children under 3 years
Side-effects: see Trihexyphenidyl Hydrochloride, but causes sedation rather than stimulation
Dose: *by mouth*, 0.5–1 mg daily usually at bedtime, gradually increased; max. 6 mg daily; usual maintenance dose 1–4 mg daily in single or divided doses; ELDERLY preferably lower end of range

By intramuscular or intravenous injection, 1–2 mg, repeated if symptoms reappear; ELDERLY preferably lower end of range

Cogentin® (MSD) PoM

Tablets, scored, benzatropine mesilate 2 mg. Net price 20 = 29p. Label: 2

Injection, benzatropine mesilate 1 mg/mL. Net price 2-mL amp = 92p

BIPERIDEN HYDROCHLORIDE

Indications: see Trihexyphenidyl Hydrochloride
Cautions: see Trihexyphenidyl Hydrochloride
Contra-indications: see Trihexyphenidyl Hydrochloride
Side-effects: see Trihexyphenidyl Hydrochloride, but may cause drowsiness
Dose: 1 mg twice daily, increased gradually to 2 mg 3 times daily; usual maintenance dose 3–12 mg daily in divided doses; ELDERLY preferably lower end of range

Akineton® (Abbott) PoM

Tablets, scored, biperiden hydrochloride 2 mg. Net price 100-tab pack = £4.60. Label: 2

ORPHENADRINE HYDROCHLORIDE

Indications: see Trihexyphenidyl Hydrochloride
Cautions: see Trihexyphenidyl Hydrochloride
Contra-indications: see Trihexyphenidyl Hydrochloride; porphyria (section 9.8.2)
Side-effects: see Trihexyphenidyl Hydrochloride, but more euphoric; may cause insomnia
Dose: 150 mg daily in divided doses, increased gradually; max. 400 mg daily; ELDERLY preferably lower end of range

Orphenadrine Hydrochloride (Non-proprietary) PoM

Oral solution, orphenadrine hydrochloride 50 mg/5 mL. Net price 200 mL = £9.47. Counselling, driving

Available from Rosemont (sugar-free)

Biorphen® (Alliance) PoM

Elixir, sugar-free, orphenadrine hydrochloride 25 mg/5 mL. Net price 200 mL = £7.25. Counselling, driving

Disipal® (Yamanouchi) PoM

Tablets, yellow, s/c, orphenadrine hydrochloride 50 mg. Net price 20 = 69p. Counselling, driving

Excipients: include tartrazine

PROCYCLIDINE HYDROCHLORIDE

Indications: see Trihexyphenidyl Hydrochloride

Cautions: see Trihexyphenidyl Hydrochloride

Contra-indications: see Trihexyphenidyl Hydrochloride

Side-effects: see Trihexyphenidyl Hydrochloride

Dose: *by mouth*, 2.5 mg 3 times daily, increased gradually if necessary; usual max. 30 mg daily (60 mg daily in exceptional circumstances); ELD-ERLY preferably lower end of range

Acute dystonia, *by intramuscular injection*, 5–10 mg repeated if necessary after 20 minutes; max. 20 mg daily; *by intravenous injection*, 5 mg (usually effective in 5 minutes); an occasional patient may need 10 mg or more and may require up to half an hour to obtain relief; ELD-ERLY preferably lower end of dose range

Procyclidine (Non-proprietary) PoM

Tablets, procyclidine hydrochloride 5 mg. Net price 20 = £1.08. Counselling, driving
Available from Alpharma, APS, Opus (*Mucinil®*)

Arpicolin® (Rosemont) PoM

Syrup, sugar-free, procyclidine hydrochloride 2.5 mg/5 mL, net price 150 mL = £4.49; 5 mg/5 mL, 150 mL pack = £8.02. Counselling, driving

Kemadrin® (GlaxoWellcome) PoM

Tablets, scored, procyclidine hydrochloride 5 mg. Net price 20 = £1.17. Counselling, driving

Injection, procyclidine hydrochloride 5 mg/mL. Net price 2-mL amp = £1.49

TRIHEXYPHENIDYL HYDROCHLORIDE/BENZHEXOL HYDROCHLORIDE

Indications: parkinsonism; drug-induced extra-pyramidal symptoms (but not tardive dyskinesia, see notes above)

Cautions: cardiovascular disease, hepatic or renal impairment; elderly; avoid abrupt discontinuation of treatment; liable to abuse (may produce euphoric effect); **interactions:** Appendix 1 (antimuscarinics)

DRIVING. May affect performance of skilled tasks (e.g. driving)

Contra-indications: untreated urinary retention, angle-closure glaucoma, gastro-intestinal obstruction

Side-effects: dry mouth, gastro-intestinal disturbances, dizziness, blurred vision; less commonly urinary retention, tachycardia, hypersensitivity, nervousness, and with high doses in susceptible patients, mental confusion, excitement, and psychiatric disturbances which may necessitate discontinuation of treatment

Dose: 1 mg daily, increased gradually; usual maintenance dose 5–15 mg daily in 3–4 divided doses; ELDERLY preferably lower end of range

Trihexyphenidyl/Benzhexol (Non-proprietary) PoM

Tablets, trihexyphenidyl hydrochloride 2 mg, net price 20 = 59p; 5 mg, 20 = 78p. Counselling, before or after food (see notes above), driving
Available from Genus

Broflex® (Alliance) PoM

Syrup, pink, trihexyphenidyl hydrochloride 5 mg/5 mL. Net price 200 mL = £6.36. Counselling, before or after food (see notes above), driving
Note. May temporarily be unavailable

4.9.3 Drugs used in essential tremor, chorea, tics, and related disorders

Tetrabenazine is mainly used to control movement disorders in Huntington's chorea and related disorders. It may act by depleting nerve endings of dopamine. It has useful action in only a proportion of patients and its use may be limited by the development of depression.

Haloperidol may be useful in improving motor tics and symptoms of Gilles de la Tourette syndrome and related choreas. **Pimozide** (see section 4.2.1 for CSM warning), **clonidine** (section 4.7.4.2) and **sulpiride** (section 4.2.1) are also used in Gilles de la Tourette syndrome. **Trihexyphenidyl (benzhexol)** (section 4.9.2) at high dosage may also improve some movement disorders; it is sometimes necessary to build the dose up over many weeks, to 20 to 30 mg daily or higher. **Chlorpromazine** and **haloperidol** are used to relieve intractable hiccup (section 4.2.1).

Propranolol or another beta-adrenoceptor blocking drug (section 2.4) may be useful in treating essential tremor or tremors associated with anxiety or thyrotoxicosis. Propranolol is given in a dosage of 40 mg 2 or 3 times daily, increased if necessary; 80 to 160 mg daily is usually required for maintenance.

Primidone (section 4.8.3) in some cases provides relief from benign essential tremor; the dose is increased slowly to reduce side-effects.

Piracetam is used as an adjunctive treatment for myoclonus of cortical origin.

Riluzole is used to extend life or the time to mechanical ventilation in patients with motor neurone disease who have amyotrophic lateral sclerosis.

> **NICE guidance (riluzole).** The National Institute for Clinical Excellence has recommended riluzole to treat individuals with the amyotrophic lateral sclerosis (ALS) form of motor neurone disease (MND). Treatment should be initiated by a specialist in MND but it can then be supervised under a shared-care arrangement involving the general practitioner.

HALOPERIDOL

Indications: motor tics, adjunctive treatment in choreas and Gilles de la Tourette syndrome; other indications, section 4.2.1

Cautions: section 4.2.1

Contra-indications: section 4.2.1

Side-effects: section 4.2.1

Dose: *by mouth*, 0.5–1.5 mg 3 times daily adjusted according to the response; 10 mg daily or more may occasionally be necessary in Gilles de la Tourette syndrome; CHILD, Gilles de la Tourette syndrome up to 10 mg daily

Preparations
Section 4.2.1

PIRACETAM

Indications: adjunctive treatment of cortical myoclonus

Cautions: avoid abrupt withdrawal; elderly; renal impairment (avoid if severe)

Contra-indications: hepatic and severe renal impairment; pregnancy and breast-feeding

Side-effects: diarrhoea, weight gain; somnolence, insomnia, nervousness, depression; hyperkinesia; rash

Dose: initially 7.2 g daily in 2–3 divided doses, increased according to response by 4.8 g daily every 3–4 days to max. 20 g daily (subsequently, attempts should be made to reduce dose of concurrent therapy); CHILD under 16 years not recommended

ORAL SOLUTION. Follow the oral solution with a glass of water (or soft drink) to reduce bitter taste.

Nootropil® (UCB Pharma) ▼ PoM
Tablets, f/c, scored, piracetam 800 mg, net price 90-tab pack = £15.80; 1.2 g, 56-tab pack = £14.74. Label: 3
Oral solution, piracetam, 333.3 mg/mL, net price 300-mL pack = £21.93. Label: 3

RILUZOLE

Indications: to extend life or the time to mechanical ventilation for patients with amyotrophic lateral sclerosis, initiated by specialists experienced in the management of motor neurone disease

Cautions: history of abnormal hepatic function (consult product literature for details); **interactions:** Appendix 1 (riluzole)

BLOOD DISORDERS. Patients or their carers should be told how to recognise signs of neutropenia and advised to seek immediate medical attention if symptoms such as fever occur; white blood cell counts should be determined in febrile illness; neutropenia requires discontinuation of riluzole

DRIVING. Dizziness or vertigo may affect performance of skilled tasks (e.g. driving)

Contra-indications: hepatic and renal impairment; pregnancy and breast-feeding

Side-effects: nausea, vomiting, asthenia, tachycardia, somnolence, headache, dizziness, vertigo, abdominal pain, circumoral paraesthesia, alterations in liver function tests

Dose: 50 mg twice daily; CHILD not recommended

Rilutek® (Rhône-Poulenc Rorer) PoM
Tablets, f/c, riluzole 50 mg. Net price 56-tab pack = £286.00. Counselling, blood disorders, driving

TETRABENAZINE

Indications: movement disorders due to Huntington's chorea, hemiballismus, senile chorea, and related neurological conditions

Cautions: pregnancy; avoid in breast-feeding; **interactions:** Appendix 1 (tetrabenazine)

DRIVING. May affect performance of skilled tasks (e.g. driving)

Side-effects: drowsiness, gastro-intestinal disturbances, depression, extrapyramidal dysfunction, hypotension; rarely parkinsonism; neuroleptic malignant syndrome reported

Dose: initially 12.5 mg twice daily (elderly 12.5 mg daily) gradually increased to 12.5–25 mg 3 times daily; max. 200 mg daily

Xenazine® 25 (Cambridge) PoM
Tablets, pale yellow-buff, scored, tetrabenazine 25 mg. Net price 112-tab pack = £100.00. Label: 2

Torsion dystonias and other involuntary movements

BOTULINUM A TOXIN-HAEMAGGLUTININ COMPLEX

Indications: dynamic equinus foot deformity due to spasticity in ambulant paediatric cerebral palsy patients over 2 years; blepharospasm; hemifacial spasm; spasmodic torticollis (all specialist use only)

Cautions: potential for anaphylaxis; **interactions:** Appendix 1 (botulinum toxin)

SPECIFIC CAUTIONS FOR BLEPHAROSPASM OR HEMIFACIAL SPASM. Avoid deep or misplaced injections—relevant anatomy (and any alterations due to previous surgery) must be understood before injecting; reduced blinking can lead to corneal exposure, persistent epithelial defect and corneal ulceration (especially in those with VIIth nerve disorders)—careful testing of corneal sensation in previously operated eyes, avoidance of injection in lower lid area to avoid ectropion and vigorous treatment of epithelial defect needed

SPECIFIC CAUTIONS FOR TORTICOLLIS. Patients with defective neuromuscular transmission (risk of excessive muscle weakness)

COUNSELLING. All patients should be alerted to possible side-effects

Contra-indications: generalised disorders of muscle activity (e.g. myasthenia gravis); bleeding disorders; pregnancy and breast-feeding

Side-effects: increased electrophysiologic jitter in some distant muscles; misplaced injections may paralyse nearby muscle groups and excessive doses may paralyse distant muscles; influenza-like syndrome, rash; antibody formation (substantial deterioration in response); transient burning sensation after injection

SPECIFIC SIDE-EFFECTS IN PAEDIATRIC CEREBRAL PALSY. Leg pain, weakness, urinary incontinence; rarely leg cramps, fever, knee and ankle pain, lethargy

SPECIFIC SIDE-EFFECTS IN BLEPHAROSPASM OR HEMIFACIAL SPASM. Ptosis, lacrimation and irritation (including dry eye, lagophthalmos and photophobia); also ectropion, keratitis, diplopia and entropion; angle-closure glaucoma reported; bruising and ecchymosis in soft eyelid tissues minimised by applying gentle pressure at injection site immediately after injection

SPECIFIC SIDE-EFFECTS IN TORTICOLLIS. Dysphagia and pooling of saliva (occurs most frequently after injection into sternomastoid muscle); dry mouth, voice changes, weakness of neck muscles; generalised muscle weakness, malaise, nausea, diplopia and blurred vision; rarely respiratory difficulties (associated with high doses), drowsiness, numbness, stiffness, ptosis, headache, fever; CSM has warned of persistent dysphagia and sequelae (including death)—**important**, see also under Cautions

Dose: consult product literature (**important:** specific to **each individual preparation** and **not interchangeable**)

Botox® (Allergan) [PoM]

Injection, powder for reconstitution, botulinum A toxin-haemagglutinin complex, net price 100-unit vial = £128.93

Dysport® (Ipsen) [PoM]

Injection, powder for reconstitution, botulinum A toxin-haemagglutinin complex, net price 500-unit vial = £164.74

BOTULINUM B TOXIN

Indications: spasmodic torticollis (cervical dystonia)—specialist use only

Cautions: inadvertent injection into a blood vessel; tolerance may occur; **interactions:** Appendix 1 (botulinum toxin)

Contra-indications: neuromuscular or neuromuscular junctional disorders; pregnancy and breast-feeding

Side-effects: increased electrophysiologic jitter in some distant muscles; dry mouth, dysphagia; also dyspepsia, worsening torticollis, neck pain, myasthenia, voice changes, taste disturbances

Dose: *by intramuscular injection*, initially 5000–10 000 units divided between 2–4 most affected muscles; adjust dose and frequency according to response; **important**: **not** interchangeable with other botulinum toxin preparations

NeuroBloc® (Elan) ▼ [PoM]

Injection, botulinum B toxin 5000 units/mL, net price 0.5-mL vial = £111.20; 1-mL vial = £148.27; 2-mL vial = £197.69

Note. May be diluted with sodium chloride 0.9%

4.10   Drugs used in substance dependence

This section includes drugs used in alcohol dependence, cigarette smoking, and opioid dependence.

The health departments of the UK have produced a report, *Drug Misuse and Dependence* which contains guidelines on clinical management.

Drug Misuse and Dependence, London, The Stationery Office, 1999 can be obtained from:

> The Publications Centre
> PO Box 276, London SW8 5DT
> Telephone orders (087) 0600 5522
> Fax (087) 0600 5533

or from The Stationery Office bookshops and through all good booksellers.

It is **important** to be aware that *people who misuse drugs* may be at risk not only from the intrinsic toxicity of the drug itself but also from the practice of injecting preparations intended for administration by mouth. Excipients used in the production of oral dose forms are usually insoluble and may lead to *abscess formation at the site of injection*, or even to *necrosis and gangrene*; moreover, deposits in the heart or lungs may lead to *severe cardiac or pulmonary toxicity*. Additional hazards include *infection* following the use of a dirty needle or an unsterilised diluent.

Alcohol dependence

Disulfiram is used as an adjunct to the treatment of alcohol dependence. It gives rise to extremely unpleasant systemic reactions after the ingestion of even a small amount of alcohol because it leads to accumulation of acetaldehyde in the body. Reactions include flushing of the face, throbbing headache, palpitations, tachycardia, nausea, vomiting, and, with large doses of alcohol, arrhythmias, hypotension, and collapse. Small amounts of alcohol included in many oral medicines may be sufficient to precipitate a reaction (even toiletries and mouthwashes that contain alcohol should be avoided). It may be advisable for patients to carry a card warning of the danger of administration of alcohol.

Long-acting **benzodiazepines** (section 4.1) are used to attenuate withdrawal symptoms but they also have a dependence potential. To minimise the risk of dependence, administration should be for a limited period only (e.g. **chlordiazepoxide** 10–50 mg 4 times daily, gradually reducing over 7–14 days). Benzodiazepines should not be prescribed if the patient is likely to continue drinking alcohol.

Clomethiazole (chlormethiazole) (section 4.1.1) should be used for the management of withdrawal in an **in-patient setting only**. It is associated with a risk of dependence and should not be prescribed if the patient is likely to continue drinking alcohol.

Acamprosate, in combination with counselling, may be helpful in maintaining abstinence in alcohol-dependent patients. It should be initiated as soon as possible *after* abstinence has been achieved and should be maintained if the patient relapses. Continued alcohol abuse, however, negates the therapeutic benefit of acamprosate.

ACAMPROSATE CALCIUM

Indications: maintenance of abstinence in alcohol dependence

Cautions: continued alcohol abuse (risk of treatment failure)

Contra-indications: renal and severe hepatic impairment; pregnancy and breast-feeding

Side-effects: diarrhoea, nausea, vomiting, abdominal pain, pruritus, occasionally maculopapular rash, rarely bullous skin reactions; fluctuation in libido

Dose: ADULT 18–65 years, 60 kg and over, 666 mg 3 times daily; less than 60 kg, 666 mg at breakfast, 333 mg at midday and 333 mg at night

TREATMENT COURSE. Treatment should be initiated as soon as possible after alcohol withdrawal period and maintained if patient relapses; recommended treatment period 1 year

Campral EC® (Merck) [PoM]

Tablet, e/c, acamprosate calcium 333 mg. Net price 168-tab pack = £28.92. Label: 21, 25

Electrolytes: Ca^{2+} 0.8 mmol/tablet

DISULFIRAM

Indications: adjunct in the treatment of chronic alcohol dependence (under specialist supervision)

Cautions: ensure that alcohol not consumed for at least 24 hours before initiating treatment; see also notes above; alcohol challenge **not** recommended on routine basis (if considered essential—specialist units only with resuscitation facilities); hepatic or renal impairment, respiratory disease, diabetes mellitus, epilepsy; **interactions:** Appendix 1 (disulfiram)

ALCOHOL REACTION. Patients should be warned of unpredictable and occasionally severe nature of disulfiram-alcohol interactions. Reactions can occur within 10 minutes and last several hours (may require intensive supportive therapy—oxygen should be available). Patients should not ingest alcohol at all and should be warned of possible presence of alcohol in liquid medicines, remedies, tonics, foods and even in toiletries (alcohol should also be avoided for at least 1 week after stopping)

Contra-indications: cardiac failure, coronary artery disease, history of cerebrovascular accident, hypertension, psychosis, severe personality disorder, suicide risk, pregnancy, breast-feeding

Side-effects: initially drowsiness and fatigue; nausea, vomiting, halitosis, reduced libido; rarely psychotic reactions (depression, paranoia, schizophrenia, mania), allergic dermatitis, peripheral neuritis, hepatic cell damage

Dose: 800 mg as a single dose on first day, reducing over 5 days to 100–200 mg daily; should not be continued for longer than 6 months without review; CHILD not recommended

Antabuse® (Alpharma) PoM
Tablets, scored, disulfiram 200 mg. Net price 50-tab pack = £18.38. Label: 2, counselling, alcohol reaction

Cigarette smoking

Smoking cessation interventions are a cost-effective way of reducing ill health and prolonging life. Smokers should be advised to stop and offered help if interested in doing so, with follow-up where appropriate.

Where possible, smokers should have access to a specialist smokers' clinic for behavioural support. **Nicotine replacement therapy** or **bupropion** (amfebutamone) are effective aids to smoking cessation for those smoking more than 10 cigarettes a day. The form of nicotine replacement therapy chosen should take into account individual preference and tolerance of side-effects. Combining pharmacotherapy and behavioural support is more successful than either method alone.

Bupropion and nicotine replacement therapy should be prescribed for short durations at a time and the prescriptions repeated only if the attempt at stopping smoking is continuing.

CSM advice (bupropion). The CSM has issued a reminder that bupropion is contra-indicated in patients with a history of seizures or of eating disorders, a CNS tumour, or who are experiencing acute symptoms of alcohol or benzodiazepine withdrawal. Bupropion should not be prescribed to patients with other risk factors for seizures unless the potential benefit of smoking cessation clearly outweighs the risk. Factors that increase the risk of seizures include concomitant administration of drugs that can lower the seizure threshold (e.g. antidepressants, antimalarials, antipsychotics, quinolones, sedating antihistamines, systemic corticosteroids, theophylline, tramadol), alcohol abuse, history of head trauma, diabetes, and use of anorectics.

BUPROPION
(Amfebutamone)

Indications: adjunct to smoking cessation in combination with motivational support

Cautions: elderly; hepatic impairment (Appendix 2, avoid in severe hepatic cirrhosis), renal impairment (Appendix 3); predisposition to seizures (see CSM advice above); **interactions:** Appendix 1 (bupropion)

DRIVING. May impair performance of skilled tasks (e.g. driving)

Contra-indications: history of epilepsy, of eating disorders (see CSM advice above) and of bipolar disorder; pregnancy (Appendix 4); breast-feeding (Appendix 5)

Side-effects: dry mouth, gastro-intestinal disturbances, insomnia, tremor, impaired concentration, headache, dizziness, depression, agitation, anxiety, rash, pruritus, sweating, hypersensitivity reactions (may resemble serum sickness), fever, taste disturbances; less commonly chest pain, asthenia, tachycardia, hypertension, flushing, anorexia, tinnitus, visual disturbances; rarely postural hypotension, seizures, Stevens-Johnson syndrome

Dose: initially 150 mg daily for 6 days then 150 mg twice daily (max. single dose 150 mg, max. daily dose 300 mg); max. period of treatment 7–9 weeks; discontinue if abstinence not achieved at 7 weeks; consider 150 mg daily throughout treatment in patients with risk factors for seizures (see CSM advice above); ELDERLY max. 150 mg daily; CHILD and ADOLESCENT under 18 years not recommended

Zyban® (GlaxoWellcome) ▼ PoM
Tablets, m/r, f/c, bupropion (as hydrochloride) 150 mg, net price 60-tab pack = £42.85. Label: 25

NICOTINE PRODUCTS
Indications: adjunct to smoking cessation

Cautions: cardiovascular disease (avoid if severe); peripheral vascular disease; hyperthyroidism; diabetes mellitus; phaeochromocytoma, renal and hepatic impairment; history of gastritis and peptic ulcers; should not smoke or use nicotine replacement products in combination; *patches*, exercise may increase absorption and side-effects, skin disorders (patches should not be placed on broken skin); **interactions:** Appendix 1 (nicotine and tobacco)

DRIVING. The nasal spray should not be used when driving or operating machinery (sneezing or watering eyes could contribute to accident)

Contra-indications: severe cardiovascular disease (including severe arrhythmias or immediate post-myocardial infarction period); recent cerebrovascular accident (including transient ischaemic attacks); pregnancy and breast-feeding; *patches*, chronic generalised skin disease (patches should not be placed on broken skin); patches not for occasional smokers

Side-effects: nausea, dizziness, headache and cold and influenza-like symptoms, palpitations, dyspepsia and other gastro-intestinal disturbances, hiccups, insomnia, vivid dreams, myalgia; other side-effects reported include chest pain, blood pressure changes, anxiety and irritability, somnolence and impaired concentration, dysmenorhoca; *with patches*, skin reactions (discontinue if severe)—vasculitis also reported; *with spray*, nasal irritation, nose bleeds, watering eyes, ear sensations; *with gum, sublingual tablets* or *inhalator*, aphthous ulceration (sometimes with swelling of tongue); *with spray, inhalator, sublingual tablets* or *gum*, throat irritation; *with inhalator*, cough, rhinitis, pharyngitis, stomatitis, sinusitis, dry mouth; *with sublingual tablets*, unpleasant taste

Dose: see under preparations, below

Note. Proprietary brands of nicotine products on sale to the public include *Boots Nicotine Gum* 2 mg, 4 mg, *Boots Nicotine Inhalator* 10 mg, and *Boots NRT Patch* 7 mg/24 hours, 14 mg/24 hours, 21 mg/24 hours

Nicorette® (Pharmacia)

Nicorette Microtab (sublingual), nicotine (as a cyclodextrin complex) 2 mg, net price starter pack of 2 × 15-tablet discs with dispenser = £3.57; refill pack of 7 × 15-tablet discs = £9.84. Label: 26

Dose: individuals smoking 20 cigarettes or less daily, *sublingually*, 2 mg each hour; for patients who fail to stop smoking or have significant withdrawal symptoms, consider increasing to 4 mg each hour

Individuals smoking more than 20 cigarettes daily, 4 mg each hour

Max. 80 mg daily; treatment should be continued for at least 3 months followed by a gradual reduction in dosage; max. period of treatment should not exceed 6 months

CHILD under 18 years not recommended

Nicorette chewing gum, sugar-free, nicotine (as resin) 2 mg, net price pack of 15 = £1.71, pack of 30 = £3.25, pack of 105 = £8.89; 4 mg, net price pack of 15 = £2.11, pack of 30 = £3.99, pack of 105 = £10.83

Note. Also available in citrus and mint flavour

Dose: individuals smoking 20 cigarettes or fewer daily, initially one 2-mg piece chewed slowly for approx. 30 minutes, when urge to smoke occurs; individuals smoking more than 20 cigarettes daily or needing more than 15 pieces of 2-mg gum daily may need the 4-mg strength; max. 15 pieces of 4-mg strength daily; withdraw gradually after 3 months; CHILD under 18 years not recommended

Nicorette patches, self-adhesive, all beige, nicotine, '*5 mg' patch* (releasing approx. 5 mg/16 hours), net price 7 = £9.07; '*10 mg' patch* (releasing approx. 10 mg/16 hours), 7 = £9.07; '*15 mg' patch* (releasing approx. 15 mg/16 hours), 7 = £9.07,

ADMINISTRATION: apply on waking to dry, non-hairy skin on hip, chest or upper arm, removing after approx. 16 hours, usually when retiring to bed; site next patch on different area (avoid using same area on consecutive days); initially '15-mg' patch for 16 hours daily for 8 weeks then if abstinence achieved '10-mg' patch for 16 hours daily for 2 weeks then '5-mg' patch for 16 hours daily for 2 weeks; review treatment if abstinence not achieved in 3 months—further courses may be given if considered beneficial; CHILD under 18 years not recommended

Nicorette nasal spray, nicotine 500 micrograms/metered spray. Net price 200-spray unit = £10.99

ADMINISTRATION: Apply 1 spray into each nostril as required to max. twice an hour for 16 hours daily (max. 64 sprays daily) for 8 weeks, then reduce gradually over next 4 weeks (reduce by half at end of first 2 weeks, stop altogether at end of next 2 weeks); max. treatment length 3 months; CHILD under 18 years not recommended

Nicorette inhalator (nicotine-impregnated plug for use in inhalator mouthpiece), nicotine 10 mg/cartridge. Net price 6-cartridge (starter) pack = £3.39, 42-cartridge (refill) pack = £11.37

ADMINISTRATION: Inhale when urge to smoke occurs; initially use between 6 and 12 cartridges daily for up to 8 weeks, then reduce number of cartridges used by half over next 2 weeks and then stop altogether at end of further 2 weeks; review treatment if abstinence not achieved in 3 months; CHILD under 18 years not recommended

Nicotinell® (Novartis Consumer Health)

Chewing gum, sugar-free, nicotine 2 mg, net price pack of 12 = £8.72, pack of 48 = £15.38, pack of 96 = £24.79; 4 mg, pack of 12 = £9.41, pack of 48 = £17.09, pack of 96 = £30.77

Note. Also available in fruit and mint flavours

Dose: initially one 2-mg piece chewed slowly for approx. 30 minutes, when urge to smoke occurs; max. 15 pieces daily; withdraw gradually after 3 months; CHILD under 18 years not recommended

Nicotinell mint lozenge, sugar-free, nicotine (as bitartrate) 1 mg, net price pack of 12 = £1.71, pack of 36 = £4.27, pack of 96 = £9.12. Label: 24

Excipients: include aspartame (section 9.4.1)

Dose: initially 1 lozenge every 1–2 hours, when urge to smoke occurs; max. 25 lozenges daily; withdraw gradually after 3 months; max. period of treatment should not usually exceed 6 months

TTS Patches, self-adhesive, all yellowish-ochre, nicotine, '*10' patch* (releasing approx. 7 mg/24 hours), net price 7 = £9.12; '*20' patch* (releasing approx. 14 mg/24 hours), net price 2 = £2.57, 7 = £9.40; '*30' patch* (releasing approx. 21 mg/24 hours), net price 2 = £2.85, 7 = £9.97, 21 = £24.51

ADMINISTRATION: apply to dry, non-hairy skin on trunk or upper arm, removing after 24 hours and siting replacement patch on a different area (avoid using the same area for several days); individuals smoking 20 cigarettes daily or fewer, initially '20' patch daily; individuals smoking more than 20 cigarettes daily, initially '30' patch daily; withdraw gradually, reducing dose every 3–4 weeks; review treatment if abstinence not achieved in 3 months; CHILD under 18 years not recommended

NiQuitin CQ® (GSK Consumer Healthcare)

Patches, self-adhesive, pink/beige, nicotine '*7 mg' patch* (releasing approx. 7 mg/24 hours), net price 7 = £9.97; '*14 mg' patch* (releasing approx. 14 mg/24 hours), 7 = £9.97; '*21 mg' patch* (releasing approx. 21 mg/24 hours), 7 = £9.97, 14 = £18.79

ADMINISTRATION: apply on waking to dry, non-hairy skin site, removing after 24 hours and siting replacement patch on different area (avoid using same area for 7 days); individuals smoking 10 or more cigarettes daily, initially '21-mg' patch daily for 6 weeks then '14-mg' patch daily for 2 weeks then '7-mg' patch daily for 2 weeks; review treatment if abstinence not achieved in 10 weeks

Individuals smoking less than 10 cigarettes daily, initially '14-mg' patch daily for 6 weeks then '7-mg' patch daily for 2 weeks

CHILD not recommended

Note. Patients using the '21-mg' patch who experience excessive side-effects, which do not resolve within a few days, should change to '14-mg' patch for the remainder of the initial 6 weeks before switching to the '7-mg' patch for the final 2 weeks

Opioid dependence

Methadone, an opioid *agonist*, can be substituted for opioids such as diamorphine, preventing the onset of withdrawal symptoms; it is itself addictive and should only be prescribed for those who are physically dependent on opioids. It is administered in a single daily dose usually as methadone oral solution 1 mg/mL. The dose is adjusted according to the degree of dependence with the aim of gradual reduction.

Buprenorphine is an opioid partial agonist. Because of its abuse and dependence potential it should be prescribed only for those who are already physically dependent on opioids. It can be used as substitution therapy for patients with moderate opioid dependence. In patients dependent on high doses of opioids, buprenorphine may precipitate withdrawal due to its partial antagonist properties; in these patients, the daily opioid dose should be reduced gradually before initiating therapy with buprenorphine.

Naltrexone, an opioid *antagonist*, blocks the action of opioids and precipitates withdrawal symptoms in opioid-dependent subjects. Because the euphoric action of opioid agonists is blocked by naltrexone it is given to former addicts as an aid to prevent relapse.

Lofexidine is used for the alleviation of symptoms in patients undergoing opioid withdrawal. Like clonidine it appears to act centrally to produce a reduction in sympathetic tone but reduction in blood pressure is less marked.

BUPRENORPHINE

Indications: adjunct in the treatment of opioid dependence; premedication, peri-operative analgesia, analgesia in other situations (section 4.7.2)

Cautions: see section 4.7.2 and notes above; effects only partially reversed by naloxone

Contra-indications: see section 4.7.2; breast-feeding (Appendix 5)

Side-effects: see section 4.7.2

Dose: *by sublingual administration*, initially, 0.8–4 mg as a single daily dose, adjusted according to response; max. 32 mg daily; withdraw gradually; CHILD under 16 years not recommended

Note. In those who have not undergone opioid withdrawal, buprenorphine should be administered at least 4 hours after last use of opioid or when signs of craving appear

For those receiving methadone, dose of methadone should be reduced to max. 30 mg daily before starting buprenorphine

Subutex® (Schering-Plough) ▼ CD
Tablets (sublingual), buprenorphine (as hydrochloride) 400 micrograms, net price 7-tab pack = £1.60; 2 mg, 7-tab pack = £6.72; 8 mg, 7-tab pack = £20.16. Label: 2, 26

LOFEXIDINE HYDROCHLORIDE

Indications: management of symptoms of opioid withdrawal

Cautions: severe coronary insufficiency, recent myocardial infarction, cerebrovascular disease, marked bradycardia (monitor pulse rate fre-

quently); renal impairment; history of depression (on longer treatment); pregnancy and breast-feeding; withdraw gradually over 2–4 days (or longer) to minimise risk of rebound hypertension and associated symptoms; **interactions:** Appendix 1 (lofexidine)

Side-effects: drowsiness, dry mucous membranes (particularly dry mouth, throat and nose), hypotension, bradycardia, rebound hypertension on withdrawal (see Cautions); sedation and coma in overdosage

Dose: initially, 200 micrograms twice daily, increased as necessary in steps of 200–400 micrograms daily to max. 2.4 mg daily; recommended duration of treatment 7–10 days if no opioid use (but longer may be required); withdraw gradually over 2–4 days or longer; CHILD not recommended

BritLofex® (Britannia) PoM
Tablets, peach, f/c, lofexidine hydrochloride 200 micrograms. Net price 60-tab pack = £74.44. Label: 2

METHADONE HYDROCHLORIDE

Indications: adjunct in treatment of opioid dependence, see notes above; analgesia (section 4.7.2); cough in terminal disease (section 3.9.1)

Cautions: section 4.7.2

Contra-indications: section 4.7.2

Side-effects: section 4.7.2; **overdosage:** see Emergency Treatment of Poisoning, p. 24

IMPORTANT. Methadone, even in low doses is a **special hazard** for children; non-dependent adults are also at risk of toxicity; dependent adults are at risk if tolerance is incorrectly assessed during induction

INCOMPATIBILITY. Syrup preserved with hydroxybenzoate (parabens) esters may be incompatible with methadone hydrochloride.

Dose: initially 10–20 mg daily, increased by 10–20 mg daily until no signs of withdrawal or intoxication; usual dose 40–60 mg daily; CHILD not recommended (see also important note above)

Methadone (Non-proprietary) CD
Oral solution 1 mg/mL, methadone hydrochloride 1 mg/mL, net price 30 mL = 44p, 50 mL = 73p, 100 mL = £1.45, 500 mL = £7.59. Label: 2
Available from Generics (*Methex®*), Hillcross, Martindale (*Physeptone*, also as sugar-free), Rosemont (*Metharose®*, sugar-free), Thornton & Ross—taste and colour of different formulations may vary slightly
IMPORTANT. This preparation is 2½ times the strength of Methadone Linctus; many preparations of this strength are licensed for opioid drug addiction only but some are also licensed for analgesia in severe pain
Injection, section 4.7.2

Methadose® (Rosemont) CD
Oral concentrate, methadone hydrochloride 10 mg/mL (blue), net price 150 mL = £12.78; 20 mg/mL (brown), 150 mL = £25.56. Label: 2
Note. The final strength of the methadone mixture to be dispensed to the patient must be specified on the prescription
IMPORTANT. Care is required in prescribing and dispensing the **correct strength** since any confusion could lead to an overdose; this preparation should be dispensed only **after dilution** as appropriate with *Methadose® Diluent* (life of diluted solution 3 months) and is for drug dependent persons (see also p. 7)

NALTREXONE HYDROCHLORIDE

Indications: adjunct to prevent relapse in detoxified formerly opioid-dependent patients (who have remained opioid-free for at least 7–10 days)

Cautions: hepatic and renal impairment; liver function tests needed before and during treatment; test for opioid dependence with naloxone; avoid concomitant use of opioids but increased dose of opioid analgesic may be required for pain (monitor for opioid intoxication); pregnancy, breast-feeding

WARNING FOR PATIENTS. Patients need to be warned that an attempt to overcome the block could result in acute opioid intoxication

Contra-indications: patients currently dependent on opioids; acute hepatitis or liver failure

Side-effects: nausea, vomiting, abdominal pain; anxiety, nervousness, sleeping difficulty, headache, reduced energy; joint and muscle pain; less frequently, loss of appetite, diarrhoea, constipation, increased thirst; chest pain; increased sweating and lacrimation; increased energy, 'feeling down', irritability, dizziness, chills; delayed ejaculation, decreased potency; rash; occasionally, liver function abnormalities; reversible idiopathic thrombocytopenia reported

Dose: (initiate in specialist clinics only) 25 mg initially then 50 mg daily; the total weekly dose may be divided and given on 3 days of the week for improved compliance (e.g. 100 mg on Monday and Wednesday, and 150 mg on Friday); CHILD not recommended

Nalorex® (Bristol-Myers Squibb) [PoM]

Tablets, yellow, f/c, scored, naltrexone hydrochloride 50 mg. Net price 28-tab pack = £42.51

4.11   Drugs for dementia

Acetylcholinesterase inhibiting drugs are used in the treatment of Alzheimer's disease, specifically for mild to moderate disease. The evidence to support the use of these drugs relates to their cognitive enhancement.

Treatment with acetylcholinesterase inhibitors should be initiated and supervised only by a specialist experienced in the management of dementia.

Benefit is assessed by repeating the cognitive assessment at around 3 months. Such assessment cannot demonstrate how the disease may have progressed in the absence of treatment but it can give a good guide to response. Up to half the patients given these drugs will show a slower rate of cognitive decline. The drug should be discontinued in those thought not to be responding. Many specialists repeat the cognitive assessment 4 to 6 weeks after discontinuation to assess deterioration; if significant deterioration occurs during this short period, consideration should be given to restarting therapy.

Donepezil is a reversible inhibitor of acetylcholinesterase that can be given once daily.

Rivastigmine is a reversible non-competitive inhibitor of acetylcholinesterase, which is given twice daily.

Galantamine is a reversible inhibitor of acetylcholinesterase and it also has nicotinic receptor agonist properties. It is given twice daily.

All three drugs can cause unwanted dose-related cholinergic effects and should be started at a low dose and the dose increased according to response and tolerability.

> **NICE guidance (Alzheimer's disease).** The National Institute for Clinical Excellence has recommended that, for the adjunctive treatment of mild and moderate Alzheimer's disease in those whose mini mental-state examination (MMSE) score is above 12 points, donepezil, galantamine, and rivastigmine should be available under the following conditions:
>
> - Alzheimer's disease must be diagnosed in a specialist clinic; the clinic should also assess cognitive, global and behavioural functioning, activities of daily living, and the likelihood of compliance with treatment;
>
> - treatment should be initiated by specialists but may be continued by general practitioners under a shared-care protocol;
>
> - the carers' views of the condition should be sought before and during drug treatment;
>
> - the patient should be assessed 2–4 months after maintenance dose is established; drug treatment should continue only if MMSE score has improved or has not deteriorated *and* if behavioural or functional assessment shows improvement;
>
> - the patient should be assessed every 6 months and drug treatment should normally continue only if MMSE score remains above 12 points and if treatment is considered to have a worthwhile effect on the global, functional and behavioural condition.

DONEPEZIL HYDROCHLORIDE

Indications: mild to moderate dementia in Alzheimer's disease

Cautions: sick sinus syndrome or other supraventricular conduction abnormalities; susceptibility to peptic ulcers; asthma, chronic obstructive pulmonary disease; may exacerbate extrapyramidal symptoms; **interactions:** Appendix 1 (parasympathomimetics)

Contra-indications: pregnancy and breast-feeding

Side-effects: nausea, vomiting, diarrhoea, fatigue, insomnia, muscle cramps, less frequently headache, dizziness, syncope, bradycardia, rarely sino-atrial block, AV block, and convulsions; anorexia, gastric and duodenal ulcers, gastro-intestinal haemorrhage, psychiatric disturbances, hepatitis, urinary incontinence reported, potential for bladder outflow obstruction

Dose: 5 mg once daily at bedtime, increased if necessary after one month to 10 mg daily; max. 10 mg daily

Aricept® (Eisai, Pfizer) [PoM]

Tablets, f/c, donepezil hydrochloride 5 mg, net price 28-tab pack = £68.32; 10 mg (yellow), 28-tab pack = £95.76.

GALANTAMINE

Indications: mild to moderate dementia in Alzheimer's disease

Cautions: hepatic impairment (Appendix 2—avoid if severe); sick sinus syndrome or other supraventricular conduction abnormalities; susceptibility to peptic ulcers; asthma, chronic obstructive pulmonary disease; pregnancy (Appendix 4); avoid in urinary retention and gastro-intestinal obstruction; **interactions:** Appendix 1 (parasympathomimetics)

Contra-indications: severe renal impairment; breast-feeding (Appendix 5); metabolic disorders of galactose metabolism

Side-effects: nausea, vomiting (transient), diarrhoea, abdominal pain, dyspepsia, anorexia, fatigue, dizziness, headache, drowsiness, weight loss; less commonly confusion, insomnia, rhinitis, urinary tract infection; tremor; syncope and severe bradycardia reported; potential for bladder outflow obstruction, convulsions

Dose: initially 4 mg twice daily for 4 weeks increased to 8 mg twice daily for 4 weeks; maintenance 8–12 mg twice daily

Reminyl® (Shire) ▼ PoM

Tablets, all f/c, galantamine (as hydrobromide) 4 mg (white), net price 56-tab pack = £54.60; 8 mg (pink), 56-tab pack = £68.32; 12 mg (orange-brown), 56-tab pack = £84.00, 168-tab pack = £252.00. Label: 21

RIVASTIGMINE

Indications: mild to moderate dementia in Alzheimer's disease

Cautions: renal impairment, mild to moderate hepatic impairment (Appendix 2); sick sinus syndrome, conduction abnormalities; gastric or duodenal ulcers (and those at risk of developing ulcers); history of asthma or chronic obstructive pulmonary disease; pregnancy (Appendix 4); monitor body-weight; **interactions:** Appendix 1 (parasympathomimetics)

Note. If treatment interrupted for more than several days, re-introduce with initial dose and increase gradually (see Dose)

Contra-indications: breast-feeding

Side-effects: asthenia, anorexia, weight loss, dizziness, nausea, vomiting, drowsiness, abdominal pain, agitation and confusion, depression, diarrhoea, dyspepsia, headache, insomnia, sweating, malaise, tremor; rarely angina pectoris, bradycardia, gastro-intestinal haemorrhage, syncope; potential for bladder outflow obstruction, convulsions, rash; rarely AV block reported

Note. Gastro-intestinal side-effects may occur more commonly in women

Dose: initially 1.5 mg twice daily, increased in steps of 1.5 mg twice daily at intervals of at least 2 weeks according to response and tolerance; usual range 3–6 mg twice daily; max. 6 mg twice daily

Exelon® (Novartis) PoM

Capsules, rivastigmine (as hydrogen tartrate) 1.5 mg (yellow), net price 28-cap pack = £31.50, 56-cap pack = £63.00; 3 mg (orange), 28-cap pack = £31.50, 56-cap pack = £63.00; 4.5 mg (red), 28-cap pack = £31.50, 56-cap pack = £63.00; 6 mg (red/orange), 28-cap pack = £31.50, 56-cap pack = £63.00. Label: 21, 25

Oral solution, rivastigmine (as hydrogen tartrate) 2 mg/mL, net price 120 mL (with oral syringe) = £108.00. Label: 21

5: Infections

Notifiable diseases

Doctors must notify the Proper Officer of the local authority (usually the consultant in communicable disease control) when attending a patient suspected of suffering from any of the diseases listed below; a form is available from the Proper Officer.

Anthrax	Mumps
Cholera	Ophthalmia neonatorum
Diphtheria	Paratyphoid fever
Dysentery (amoebic or bacillary)	Plague
	Poliomyelitis, acute
Encephalitis, acute	Rabies
Food poisoning	Relapsing fever
Haemorrhagic fever (viral)	Rubella
Hepatitis, viral	Scarlet fever
Leprosy	Smallpox
Leptospirosis	Tetanus
Malaria	Tuberculosis
Measles	Typhoid fever
Meningitis	Typhus
Meningococcal septicaemia (without meningitis)	Whooping cough
	Yellow fever

Note. It is good practice for doctors to also inform the consultant in communicable disease control of instances of other infections (e.g. psittacosis) where there could be a public health risk.

5.1   Antibacterial drugs

CHOICE OF A SUITABLE DRUG. Before selecting an antibacterial the clinician must first consider two factors—the patient and the known or likely causative organism. Factors related to the patient which must be considered include history of allergy, renal and hepatic function, resistance to infection (i.e. whether immunocompromised), ability to tolerate drugs by mouth, severity of illness, ethnic origin, age and, if female, whether pregnant, breast-feeding or taking an oral contraceptive.

The known or likely organism and its antibacterial sensitivity, in association with the above factors, will suggest one or more antibacterials, the final choice depending on the microbiological, pharmacological, and toxicological properties.

An example of a rational approach to the selection of an antibacterial is treatment of a urinary-tract infection in a patient complaining of nausea in early pregnancy. The organism is reported as being resistant to ampicillin but sensitive to nitrofurantoin (can cause nausea), gentamicin (can only be given by injection and best avoided in pregnancy), tetracycline (causes dental discoloration) and co-trimoxazole (folate antagonist therefore theoretical teratogenic risk), and cefalexin. The safest antibiotics in pregnancy are the penicillins and cephalosporins; therefore, cefalexin would be indicated for this patient.

The principles involved in selection of an antibacterial must allow for a number of variables including changing renal and hepatic function, increasing bacterial resistance, and new information on side-effects. Duration of therapy, dosage, and route of administration depend on site, type and severity of infection and response.

ANTIBACTERIAL POLICIES. Local policies often limit the antibacterials that may be used to achieve reasonable economy consistent with adequate cover, and to reduce the development of resistant organisms. A policy may indicate a range of drugs for general use, and permit other drugs only on the advice of the microbiologist or physician responsible for the control of infectious diseases.

BEFORE STARTING THERAPY. The following precepts should be considered before starting:

• Viral infections should not be treated with antibacterials;

• Samples should be taken for culture and sensitivity testing; 'blind' antibacterial prescribing for unexplained pyrexia usually leads to further difficulty in establishing the diagnosis;

• Knowledge of **prevalent organisms** and their current sensitivity is of great help in choosing an antibacterial before bacteriological confirmation is available;

• The **dose** of an antibacterial varies according to a number of factors including age, weight, renal function, and severity of infection. The prescribing of the so-called 'standard' dose in serious infections may result in failure of treatment or even death of the patient; therefore it is important to prescribe a dose appropriate to the condition. An inadequate dose may also increase the likelihood of antibacterial resistance. On the other hand, for an antibacterial with a narrow margin between the toxic and therapeutic dose (e.g. an aminoglycoside) it is also important to avoid an excessive dose and

the concentration of the drug in plasma may need to be monitored;

• The **route** of administration of an antibacterial often depends on the severity of the infection. Life-threatening infections require intravenous therapy. Whenever possible painful intramuscular injections should be avoided in children;

• **Duration** of therapy depends on the nature of the infection and the response to treatment. Courses should not be unduly prolonged because they encourage resistance, they may lead to side-effects and they are costly; in many cases a 5-day course is sufficient. However, in certain infections such as tuberculosis or chronic osteomyelitis it is necessary to treat for prolonged periods. Conversely a single dose of an antibacterial may cure uncomplicated urinary-tract infections.

SUPERINFECTION. In general, broad-spectrum antibacterial drugs such as the cephalosporins are more likely to be associated with adverse reactions related to the selection of resistant organisms e.g. *fungal infections* or *antibiotic-associated colitis* (pseudomembranous colitis); other problems associated with superinfection include vaginitis and pruritus ani.

THERAPY. Suggested treatment is shown in table 1. When the pathogen has been isolated treatment may be changed to a more appropriate antibacterial if necessary. If no bacterium is cultured the antibacterial can be continued or stopped on clinical grounds. Infections for which prophylaxis is useful are listed in table 2.

Table 1. Summary of antibacterial therapy

If treating a patient suspected of suffering from a notifiable disease, the consultant in communicable disease control should be informed (see p. 254)

Gastro-intestinal system

Gastro-enteritis
Antibacterial not usually indicated
Frequently self-limiting and may not be bacterial
Campylobacter enteritis
Ciprofloxacin *or* erythromycin
Invasive salmonellosis
Ciprofloxacin *or* trimethoprim
Includes severe infections which may be invasive
Shigellosis
Ciprofloxacin *or* trimethoprim
Antibacterial not indicated for mild cases. Ciprofloxacin should be used for trimethoprim-resistant strains
Typhoid fever
Ciprofloxacin *or* cefotaxime *or* chloramphenicol
Infections from Indian subcontinent, Middle-East, and South-East Asia may be multiple-antibacterial-resistant and sensitivity should be tested
Antibiotic-associated colitis (pseudomembranous colitis)
Oral metronidazole *or* oral vancomycin
Give metronidazole by intravenous infusion if oral treatment inappropriate
Biliary-tract infection
A cephalosporin *or* gentamicin
Peritonitis
A cephalosporin (*or* gentamicin) + metronidazole (*or* clindamycin)

Peritoneal dialysis-associated peritonitis
Vancomycin[1] + gentamicin (*or* ceftazidime) added to dialysis fluid (*or* vancomycin added to dialysis fluid + oral ciprofloxacin)
Discontinue any antibacterial not required when sensitivity known; treat usually for 14 days or longer

Cardiovascular system

Endocarditis caused by streptococci (e.g. viridans streptococci)
Benzylpenicillin (*or* vancomycin[1] if penicillin-allergic) + low-dose gentamicin (i.e. 80 mg twice daily)
Treat for up to 4 weeks; stop after 2 weeks if organism fully sensitive to penicillin; treat penicillin-allergic patients with vancomycin for 4 weeks + low-dose gentamicin for first 2 weeks
Endocarditis caused by enterococci (e.g. *Enterococcus faecalis*)
Amoxicillin[2] (*or* vancomycin[1] if penicillin-allergic) + low-dose gentamicin (i.e. 80 mg twice daily)
Treat for 4 weeks; if gentamicin-resistant, substitute streptomycin for gentamicin and treat for at least 6 weeks
Endocarditis caused by staphylococci (including *Staph. aureus*, *Staph. epidermidis*)
Flucloxacillin (*or* benzylpenicillin if penicillin-sensitive *or* vancomycin if penicillin-allergic or if methicillin-resistant staphylococci) + gentamicin (*or* fusidic acid)
Treat for 4 weeks; stop gentamicin (or fusidic acid) after 1 week

Footnote—*see next page*

Respiratory system

Haemophilus influenzae epiglottitis
Cefotaxime *or* chloramphenicol
Give intravenously

Exacerbations of chronic bronchitis
Amoxicillin[2] *or* tetracycline (*or* erythromycin[3])
Some pneumococci and *Haemophilus influenzae* strains tetracycline-resistant; 15% *H. influenzae* strains amoxicillin-resistant

Uncomplicated community-acquired pneumonia
Amoxicillin[2] (*or* benzylpenicillin if previously healthy chest *or* erythromycin[3] if penicillin-allergic)
Add flucloxacillin if staphylococcus suspected, e.g. in influenza or measles; add erythromycin[3] if atypical pneumonia suspected; pneumococci with decreased penicillin sensitivity being isolated but not yet common in UK

Severe community-acquired pneumonia of unknown aetiology
Erythromycin[3] + cefuroxime *or* cefotaxime
Add flucloxacillin if staphylococcus suspected

Suspected atypical pneumonia
Erythromycin[3]
Severe Legionella infections may require addition of rifampicin; tetracycline is an alternative for chlamydia and mycoplasma infections; treat for at least 10–14 days

Hospital-acquired pneumonia
A broad-spectrum cephalosporin (e.g. cefotaxime or ceftazidime) *or* an antipseudomonal penicillin
An aminoglycoside may be added in severe illness

Central nervous system

Meningitis: Initial 'blind' therapy
- Transfer patient urgently to hospital.
- If bacterial meningitis and especially if *meningococcal disease* suspected, general practitioners should give benzylpenicillin (see p. 260 for dose) before urgent transfer to hospital; cefotaxime (section 5.1.2) may be an alternative in penicillin allergy; chloramphenicol (section 5.1.7) may be used if history of anaphylaxis to penicillin or to cephalosporins

Meningitis caused by meningococci
Benzylpenicillin *or* cefotaxime
Treat for at least 5 days; substitute chloramphenicol if history of anaphylaxis to penicillin or to cephalosporins; give rifampicin for 2 days before hospital discharge

Meningitis caused by pneumococci
Cefotaxime
Treat for 10–14 days; substitute benzylpenicillin if organism penicillin-sensitive; if organism highly penicillin- and cephalosporin-resistant, add vancomycin or rifampicin

Meningitis caused by *Haemophilus influenzae*
Cefotaxime
Treat for at least 10 days; substitute chloramphenicol if history of anaphylaxis to penicillin or to cephalosporins or if organism resistant to cefotaxime; for *H. influenzae* type b give rifampicin for 4 days before hospital discharge

Meningitis caused by Listeria
Amoxicillin[2] + gentamicin
Treat for 10–14 days

Urinary tract

Acute pyelonephritis
A broad-spectrum cephalosporin *or* a quinolone
Treat for 14 days; longer treatment may be necessary in complicated pyelonephritis

Acute prostatitis
A quinolone *or* trimethoprim
Treat for 28 days; in severe infection, start treatment with a high-dose broad-spectrum cephalosporin (e.g. cefuroxime or cefotaxime) + gentamicin

'Lower' urinary-tract infection
Trimethoprim *or* amoxicillin[2] *or* nitrofurantoin *or* oral cephalosporin
A short course (e.g. 3 days) is usually adequate for uncomplicated urinary-tract infections in women

Genital system

Syphilis
Procaine benzylpenicillin [unlicensed] *or* doxycycline *or* erythromycin
Treat early syphilis for 14 days (10 days with procaine benzylpenicillin); treat late latent syphilis with procaine benzylpenicillin for 17 days (or with doxycycline for 28 days); contact tracing recommended

Uncomplicated gonorrhoea
Ciprofloxacin *or* ofloxacin *or* cefotaxime
Single-dose treatment in uncomplicated infection; choice depends on locality where infection acquired; contact-tracing recommended; remember chlamydia; pharyngeal infection requires treatment with ciprofloxacin *or* ofloxacin

Uncomplicated genital chlamydial infection, non-gonococcal urethritis and non-specific genital infection
Doxycycline *or* azithromycin
Treat with doxycycline for 7 days or with azithromycin as a single dose; alternatively treat with erythromycin for 14 days; contact tracing recommended

Pelvic inflammatory disease
Ofloxacin + metronidazole
Treat for at least 14 days; in severely ill patients substitute initial treatment with doxycycline + cefoxitin, then switch to oral treatment with doxycycline + metronidazole to complete 14 days' treatment; contact tracing recommended; remember gonorrhoea

Blood

Septicaemia: Initial 'blind' therapy
Community-acquired septicaemia, aminoglycoside + a broad-spectrum penicillin *or* a broad-spectrum cephalosporin alone (e.g. cefotaxime)
Hospital-acquired septicaemia, aminoglycoside + a broad-spectrum antipseudomonal penicillin (*or* ceftazidime), *or* meropenem alone, *or* imipenem (with cilastatin as *Primaxin®*) alone
Choice depends on local resistance patterns and clinical presentation; use aminoglycoside + broad-spectrum antipseudomonal penicillin if pseudomonas suspected; add metronidazole if anaerobic infection suspected; add flucloxacillin or vancomycin[1] if Gram-positive infection suspected

Meningococcal septicaemia
Benzylpenicillin *or* cefotaxime
If meningococcal disease suspected, general practitioners advised to give a single dose of benzylpenicillin before urgent transportation to hospital (see under Benzylpenicillin, section 5.1.1.1); give rifampicin for 2 days before hospital discharge

Musculoskeletal system

Osteomyelitis and septic arthritis
Clindamycin alone *or* flucloxacillin + fusidic acid.
If *Haemophilus influenzae* give amoxicillin[2] *or* cefuroxime
Under 5 years of age may be *H. influenzae*. Treat acute disease for at least 6 weeks and chronic infection for at least 12 weeks

---

1. Where vancomycin is suggested teicoplanin may be used.
2. Where amoxicillin is suggested ampicillin may be used.
3. Where erythromycin is suggested another macrolide (e.g. azithromycin or clarithromycin) may be used.

Eye

Purulent conjunctivitis
Chloramphenicol *or* gentamicin eye-drops

Ear, nose, and oropharynx

Dental infections
Phenoxymethylpenicillin (*or* amoxicillin[2]) *or* erythromycin *or* metronidazole
Tetracycline for chronic destructive forms of periodontal disease

Sinusitis
Amoxicillin[2] *or* doxycycline *or* erythromycin[3]
Treat for 3–10 days

Otitis externa
Flucloxacillin
Use ciprofloxacin (or an aminoglycoside) if pseudomonas suspected, see section 12.1.1

Otitis media
Amoxicillin[2] (*or* erythromycin[3] if penicillin-allergic)
Initial parenteral therapy (in severe infections) with benzylpenicillin, then oral therapy with phenoxymethylpenicillin; treat for 3–7 days; under 5 years of age may be *Haemophilus influenzae*; many infections are caused by viruses and most uncomplicated cases resolve without antibacterial treatment

Throat infections
Phenoxymethylpenicillin (*or* erythromycin[3] if penicillin-allergic) *or* oral cephalosporin
Most throat infections are caused by viruses and many do not require antibiotic therapy; restrict antibiotic prescribing for specific infections e.g. beta-haemolytic streptococcal pharyngitis (treat for at least 10 days); **avoid** amoxicillin if possibility of glandular fever, see section 5.1.1.3; initial parenteral therapy (in severe infection) with benzylpenicillin, then oral therapy with phenoxymethylpenicillin *or* amoxicillin[2]

Skin

Impetigo
Topical fusidic acid or mupirocin; oral flucloxacillin *or* erythromycin if widespread
Topical treatment for 7 days usually adequate; max. duration of topical treatment 10 days; add phenoxymethylpenicillin to flucloxacillin if streptococcal infection suspected

Erysipelas
Phenoxymethylpenicillin
Add flucloxacillin if staphylococcus suspected

Cellulitis
Phenoxymethylpenicillin + flucloxacillin (*or* erythromycin alone if penicillin-allergic) *or* co-amoxiclav alone
Severe cellulitis may require parenteral benzylpenicillin + flucloxacillin or co-amoxiclav alone

Animal bites
Co-amoxiclav
Cleanse wound thoroughly; for tetanus prone wound, give human tetanus immunoglobulin (with adsorbed tetanus vaccine if necessary, according to immunisation history), see under Tetanus Vaccines, section 14.4

Acne—see section 13.6

---

1. Where vancomycin is suggested teicoplanin may be used.
2. Where amoxicillin is suggested ampicillin may be used.
3. Where erythromycin is suggested another macrolide (e.g. azithromycin or clarithromycin) may be used.

Table 2. Summary of antibacterial prophylaxis

Prevention of recurrence of rheumatic fever
Phenoxymethylpenicillin 250 mg twice daily *or* sulfadiazine 1 g daily (500 mg daily for patients under 30 kg)

Prevention of secondary case of meningococcal meningitis[1]
Rifampicin 600 mg every 12 hours for 2 days; CHILD 10 mg/kg (under 1 year, 5 mg/kg) every 12 hours for 2 days
or ciprofloxacin 500 mg as a single dose [not licensed for this indication]; CHILD obtain further advice[1]
or i/m ceftriaxone 250 mg as a single dose [not licensed for this indication]; CHILD under 12 years 125 mg

Prevention of secondary case of *Haemophilus influenzae* type b disease[1]
Rifampicin 600 mg once daily for 4 days (regimen of choice for adults); CHILD 1–3 months 10 mg/kg once daily for 4 days, over 3 months 20 mg/kg once daily for 4 days (max. 600 mg daily)

Prevention of secondary case of diphtheria in non-immune patient
Erythromycin 500 mg every 6 hours for 7 days; CHILD up to 2 years 125 mg every 6 hours, 2–8 years 250 mg every 6 hours
Treat for further 10 days if nasopharyngeal swabs positive after first 7 days' treatment

Prevention of pertussis
ADULT and CHILD erythromycin 50 mg/kg (max. 2 g) daily in 4 divided doses for 7–14 days
Note. Pertussis vaccine inappropriate for outbreak since 3 injections are required for protection

Prevention of pneumococcal infection in asplenia or in patients with sickle cell disease
Phenoxymethylpenicillin 500 mg every 12 hours; CHILD under 5 years 125 mg every 12 hours, 6–12 years 250 mg every 12 hours—if cover also needed for *H. influenzae* in CHILD give amoxicillin instead (under 5 years 125 mg every 12 hours, over 5 years 250 mg every 12 hours)
Note. Antibiotic prophylaxis is not fully reliable

Prevention of endocarditis[2] in patients with heart-valve lesion, septal defect, patent ductus, or prosthetic valve

Dental procedures[3] *under local or no anaesthesia,*

patients who have not received more than a single dose of a penicillin[4] in the previous month, including those with a prosthetic valve (but not those who have had endocarditis), oral amoxicillin 3 g 1 hour before procedure; CHILD under 5 years quarter adult dose; 5–10 years half adult dose

patients who are penicillin-allergic or have received more than a single dose of a penicillin[4] in the previous month, oral clindamycin[5] 600 mg 1 hour before procedure; CHILD under 5 years clindamycin[5] 150 mg *or* azithromycin[6] 200 mg; 5–10 years clindamycin[5] 300 mg *or* azithromycin[6] 300 mg

patients who have had endocarditis, amoxicillin + gentamicin, as under general anaesthesia

---

Footnote—*see next page*

Dental procedures[3] *under general anaesthesia,*

no special risk (including patients who have not received more than a single dose of a penicillin in the previous month),

either i/v amoxicillin 1 g at induction, then oral amoxicillin 500 mg 6 hours later; CHILD under 5 years quarter adult dose; 5–10 years half adult dose *or* oral amoxicillin 3 g 4 hours before induction then oral amoxicillin 3 g as soon as possible after procedure; CHILD under 5 years quarter adult dose; 5–10 years half adult dose

special risk (patients with a prosthetic valve or who have had endocarditis), i/v amoxicillin 1 g + i/v gentamicin 120 mg at induction, then oral amoxicillin 500 mg 6 hours later; CHILD under 5 years amoxicillin quarter adult dose, gentamicin 2 mg/kg; 5–10 years amoxicillin half adult dose, gentamicin 2 mg/kg

patients who are penicillin-allergic or who have received more than a single dose of a penicillin in the previous month,

either i/v vancomycin 1 g over at least 100 minutes then i/v gentamicin 120 mg at induction or 15 minutes before procedure; CHILD under 10 years vancomycin 20 mg/kg, gentamicin 2 mg/kg *or* i/v teicoplanin 400 mg + gentamicin 120 mg at induction or 15 minutes before procedure; CHILD under 14 years teicoplanin 6 mg/kg, gentamicin 2 mg/kg *or* i/v clindamycin[5] 300 mg over at least 10 minutes at induction or 15 minutes before procedure then oral or i/v clindamycin 150 mg 6 hours later; CHILD under 5 years quarter adult dose; 5–10 years half adult dose

Upper respiratory-tract procedures, as for dental procedures; post-operative dose may be given parenterally if swallowing is painful

Genito-urinary procedures, as for *special risk* patients undergoing dental procedures under general anaesthesia except that clindamycin is not given, see above; if urine infected, prophylaxis should also cover infective organism

Obstetric, gynaecological and gastro-intestinal procedures (prophylaxis required for patients with prosthetic valves or those who have had endocarditis only), as for genito-urinary procedures

---

Joint prostheses and dental treatment

Advice of a Working Party of the British Society for Antimicrobial Chemotherapy is that patients with prosthetic joint implants (including total hip replacements) do not require antibiotic prophylaxis for dental treatment. The Working Party considers that it is unacceptable to expose patients to the adverse effects of antibiotics when there is no evidence that such prophylaxis is of any benefit, but that those who develop any intercurrent infection require prompt treatment with antibiotics to which the infecting organisms are sensitive.

The Working Party has commented that joint infections have rarely been shown to follow dental procedures and are even more rarely caused by oral streptococci.

Dermatological procedures

Advice of a Working Party of the British Society for Antimicrobial Chemotherapy is that patients who undergo dermatological procedures[*] do not require antibacterial prophylaxis against endocarditis.

[*] The British Association of Dermatologists Therapy Guidelines and Audit Subcommittee advise that such dermatological procedures include skin biopsies and excision of moles or of malignant lesions

---

Immunosuppression and indwelling intraperitoneal catheters

Advice of a Working Party of the British Society for Antimicrobial Chemotherapy is that patients who are immunosuppressed (including transplant patients) and patients with indwelling intraperitoneal catheters do not require antibiotic prophylaxis for dental treatment provided there is no other indication for prophylaxis.

The Working Party has commented that there is little evidence that dental treatment is followed by infection in immunosuppressed and immunodeficient patients nor is there evidence that dental treatment is followed by infection in patients with indwelling intraperitoneal catheters.

Prevention of **gas-gangrene** in high lower-limb amputations or following major trauma

Benzylpenicillin 300–600 mg every 6 hours for 5 days *or* if penicillin-allergic metronidazole 500 mg every 8 hours

---

1. For details of those who should receive chemoprophylaxis contact a consultant in communicable disease control (or a consultant in infectious diseases or the local public health laboratory). Unless there has been mouth-to-mouth contact (or direct exposure to infectious droplets from a patient with meningococcal disease), healthcare workers do not generally require chemoprophylaxis.

2. Advice on the prevention of endocarditis reflects the recommendations of a Working Party of the British Society for Antimicrobial Chemotherapy, *Lancet*, 1982, **2**, 1323–26; *idem*, 1986, **1**, 1267; *idem*, 1990, **335**, 88–9; *idem*, 1992, **339**, 1292–93; *idem*, 1997, **350**, 1100; also *J Antimicrob Chemother*, 1993; **31**, 437–8

3. Dental procedures that require antibiotic prophylaxis are, *extractions, scaling,* and *surgery involving gingival tissues.* Antibiotic prophylaxis for dental procedures may be supplemented with *chlorhexidine gluconate gel 1%* or *chlorhexidine gluconate mouthwash 0.2%,* used 5 minutes before procedure

4. For multistage procedures a max. of 2 single doses of a penicillin may be given in a month; alternative drugs should be used for further treatment and the penicillin should not be used again for 3–4 months

5. If **clindamycin** is used, periodontal or other multistage procedures should not be repeated at intervals of less than 2 weeks; clindamycin is not licensed for use in endocarditis prophylaxis

6. Azithromycin is not licensed for use in endocarditis prophylaxis

Prevention of **tuberculosis** in susceptible close contacts or those who have become tuberculin positive[1]

Isoniazid 300 mg daily for 6 months; CHILD 5–10 mg/kg daily (max. 300 mg daily)

or isoniazid 300 mg daily + rifampicin 600 mg daily (450 mg if less than 50 kg) for 3 months; CHILD isoniazid 5–10 mg/kg daily (max. 300 mg daily) + rifampicin 10 mg/kg daily (max. 600 mg daily)

Prevention of infection in **abdominal** surgery

Operations on stomach or oesophagus for carcinoma, or cholecystectomy in patients with possibly infected bile

Single dose[2] of i/v gentamicin *or* i/v cefuroxime

Resections of colon and rectum for carcinoma, and resections in inflammatory bowel disease

Single dose[2] of i/v gentamicin + i/v metronidazole[3]

or i/v cefuroxime + i/v metronidazole[3]

or i/v co-amoxiclav alone

Hysterectomy

Single dose[2] of i/v cefuroxime + i/v metronidazole[3] *or* i/v gentamicin + i/v metronidazole[3] *or* i/v co-amoxiclav alone

---

Prevention of infection in **orthopaedic** surgery

Joint replacement including hip and knee

Single dose[2] of i/v cefuroxime *or* i/v flucloxacillin

Substitute vancomycin if history of allergy to penicillins or to cephalosporins

---

5.1.1   Penicillins

5.1.1.1   Benzylpenicillin and phenoxymethylpenicillin
5.1.1.2   Penicillinase-resistant penicillins
5.1.1.3   Broad-spectrum penicillins
5.1.1.4   Antipseudomonal penicillins
5.1.1.5   Mecillinams

The penicillins are bactericidal and act by interfering with bacterial cell wall synthesis. They diffuse well into body tissues and fluids, but penetration into the cerebrospinal fluid is poor except when the meninges are inflamed. They are excreted in the urine in therapeutic concentrations.

The most important side-effect of the penicillins is hypersensitivity which causes rashes and anaphylaxis and can be fatal. Individuals with a history of anaphylaxis, urticaria, or rash immediately after penicillin administration are at risk of immediate hypersensitivity to a penicillin; these individuals should not receive a penicillin, a cephalosporin or another beta-lactam antibiotic. Patients who are allergic to one penicillin will be allergic to all because the hypersensitivity is related to the basic penicillin structure. Individuals with a history of a minor rash (i.e. non-confluent rash restricted to a small area of the body) or a rash that occurs more than 72 hours after penicillin administration are

probably not allergic to penicillin and in these individuals a penicillin should not be withheld unnecessarily for serious infections; the possibility of an allergic reaction should, however, be borne in mind.

A rare but serious toxic effect of the penicillins is encephalopathy due to cerebral irritation. This may result from excessively high doses or in patients with severe renal failure. The penicillins should **not** be given by intrathecal injection because they can cause encephalopathy which may be fatal.

Another problem relating to high doses of penicillin, or normal doses given to patients with renal failure, is the accumulation of electrolyte since most injectable penicillins contain either sodium or potassium.

Diarrhoea frequently occurs during oral penicillin therapy. It is most common with broad-spectrum penicillins, which can also cause antibiotic-associated colitis.

5.1.1.1   Benzylpenicillin and phenoxymethylpenicillin

Benzylpenicillin (Penicillin G) remains an important and useful antibiotic but is inactivated by bacterial beta-lactamases. It is effective for many streptococcal (including pneumococcal), gonococcal, and meningococcal infections and also for anthrax (section 5.1.12), diphtheria, gas-gangrene, leptospirosis, and treatment of Lyme disease (section 5.1.1.3) in children. Pneumococci, meningococci, and gonococci which have decreased sensitivity to penicillin have been isolated; benzylpenicillin is no longer the drug of first choice for pneumococcal meningitis. Although benzylpenicillin is effective in the treatment of tetanus, metronidazole (section 5.1.11) is preferred. Benzylpenicillin is inactivated by gastric acid and absorption from the gut is low; therefore it is best given by injection.

Procaine benzylpenicillin (procaine penicillin) (available on a named-patient basis from IDIS) is used for the treatment of early syphilis and late latent syphilis; it is given in a dose of 600 mg daily by intramuscular injection.

Phenoxymethylpenicillin (Penicillin V) has a similar antibacterial spectrum to benzylpenicillin, but is less active. It is gastric acid-stable, so is suitable for oral administration. It should not be used for serious infections because absorption can be unpredictable and plasma concentrations variable. It is indicated principally for respiratory-tract infections in children, for streptococcal tonsillitis, and for continuing treatment after one or more injections of benzylpenicillin when clinical response has begun. It should not be used for meningococcal or gonococcal infections. Phenoxymethylpenicillin is used for prophylaxis against streptococcal infections following rheumatic fever and against pneumococcal infections following splenectomy or in sickle cell disease.

---

1. The Joint Tuberculosis Committee recommends chemoprophylaxis for patients with documented recent tuberculin conversion, for some tuberculin-positive children identified in BCG schools programme, for children under 2 years in close contact with smear-positive tuberculosis (including those previously vaccinated with BCG but now showing strongly positive Heaf test), for children under 16 years showing a positive Heaf test at new immigrant or contact screening; chemoprophylaxis should be considered in immigrant adults 16–34 years without a BCG scar but with strongly positive Heaf test. See also section 5.1.9, for advice on immunocompromised patients and prevention of tuberculosis.

2. An additional intra-operative dose of antibacterial may be given for prolonged procedures or if there is major blood loss

3. Metronidazole may alternatively be given by suppository but to allow adequate absorption, it should be given 2 hours before surgery

BENZYLPENICILLIN

(Penicillin G)

Indications: throat infections, otitis media, streptococcal endocarditis, meningococcal disease, pneumonia (Table 1, section 5.1); anthrax; prophylaxis in limb amputation (Table 2, section 5.1)

Cautions: history of allergy; renal impairment (Appendix 3); **interactions:** Appendix 1 (penicillins)

Contra-indications: penicillin hypersensitivity

Side-effects: hypersensitivity reactions including urticaria, fever, joint pains, rashes, angioedema, anaphylaxis, serum sickness-like reactions, haemolytic anaemia and interstitial nephritis; neutropenia, thrombocytopenia, coagulation disorders and central nervous system toxicity including convulsions reported (especially with high doses or in severe renal impairment); diarrhoea and antibiotic-associated colitis

Dose: *by intramuscular or by slow intravenous injection or by infusion,* 2.4–4.8 g daily in 4 divided doses, increased if necessary in more serious infections (see also below); PREMATURE INFANT and NEONATE, 50 mg/kg daily in 2 divided doses; INFANT 1–4 weeks, 75 mg/kg daily in 3 divided doses; CHILD 1 month–12 years, 100 mg/kg daily in 4 divided doses (higher doses may be required, see also below)

Bacterial endocarditis, *by slow intravenous injection or by infusion,* 7.2 g daily in 6 divided doses

Anthrax (see also section 5.1.12), *by slow intravenous injection or by infusion,* 2.4 g every 4 hours; CHILD 150 mg/kg daily in 4 divided doses

Meningococcal disease, *by slow intravenous injection or by infusion,* 2.4 g every 4 hours; PREMATURE INFANT and NEONATE, 100 mg/kg daily in 2 divided doses; INFANT 1–4 weeks, 150 mg/kg daily in 3 divided doses; CHILD 1 month–12 years, 180–300 mg/kg daily in 4–6 divided doses

Important. If bacterial meningitis and especially if meningococcal disease is suspected general practitioners are advised to give a single injection of benzylpenicillin by intravenous injection (or by intramuscular injection) before transferring the patient urgently to hospital. Suitable doses are: ADULT 1.2 g; INFANT 300 mg; CHILD 1–9 years 600 mg, 10 years and over as for adult. In **penicillin allergy**, cefotaxime (section 5.1.2) may be an alternative; chloramphenicol may be used if there is a history of anaphylaxis to penicillins

By intrathecal injection, **not** recommended

Note. Benzylpenicillin doses in BNF may differ from those in product literature

Crystapen® (Britannia) PoM

Injection, powder for reconstitution, benzylpenicillin sodium (unbuffered), net price 600-mg vial = 42p, 2-vial 'GP pack' = £1.90; 1.2-g vial = 84p

Electrolytes: Na⁺ 1.68 mmol/600-mg vial; 3.36 mmol/1.2-g vial

PHENOXYMETHYLPENICILLIN

(Penicillin V)

Indications: tonsillitis, otitis media, erysipelas; rheumatic fever and pneumococcal infection prophylaxis (Table 2, section 5.1)

Cautions: see under Benzylpenicillin; **interactions:** Appendix 1 (penicillins)

Contra-indications: see under Benzylpenicillin

Side-effects: see under Benzylpenicillin

Dose: 500 mg every 6 hours increased up to 1 g every 6 hours in severe infections; CHILD, every 6 hours, up to 1 year 62.5 mg, 1–5 years 125 mg, 6–12 years 250 mg

Note. Phenoxymethylpenicillin doses in the BNF may differ from those in product literature

Phenoxymethylpenicillin (Non-proprietary) PoM

Tablets, phenoxymethylpenicillin (as potassium salt) 250 mg, net price 28-tab pack = £1.78. Label: 9, 23

Available from Alpharma, APS (*Apsin®*), Berk, Generics, Kent (*Tenkicin®*), Sovereign

Oral solution, phenoxymethylpenicillin (as potassium salt) for reconstitution with water, net price 125 mg/5 mL, 100 mL = £1.66; 250 mg/5 mL, 100 mL = £2.28. Label: 9, 23

Available from Alpharma, APS (*Apsin®*), Generics, Kent (*Tenkicin®*), Lagap, Sovereign

5.1.1.2   Penicillinase-resistant penicillins

Most staphylococci are now resistant to benzylpenicillin because they produce penicillinases. **Flucloxacillin,** however, is not inactivated by these enzymes and is thus effective in infections caused by penicillin-resistant staphylococci, which is the sole indication for its use. Flucloxacillin is acid-stable and can, therefore, be given by mouth as well as by injection.

Flucloxacillin is well absorbed from the gut. For CSM warning on cholestatic jaundice see under Flucloxacillin.

MRSA. *Staphylococcus aureus* strains resistant to methicillin [now discontinued] (methicillin-resistant *Staph. aureus*, MRSA) and to flucloxacillin have emerged in many hospitals; some of these organisms are sensitive only to vancomycin or teicoplanin (section 5.1.7). Strains may be susceptible to rifampicin, sodium fusidate, tetracyclines, aminoglycosides, and macrolides. Rifampicin or sodium fusidate should not be used alone because resistance may develop rapidly. Trimethoprim alone may be used for urinary-tract infections caused by some MRSA strains. Linezolid (section 5.1.7) and the combination of the streptogramin antibiotics quinupristin and dalfopristin (section 5.1.7) are active against MRSA but these antibacterial drugs should be reserved for organisms resistant to other antibacterials or for patients who cannot tolerate other antibacterial drugs. Treatment is guided by the sensitivity of the infecting strain. For eradication of nasal carriage of MRSA see section 12.2.3.

FLUCLOXACILLIN

Indications: infections due to beta-lactamase-producing staphylococci including otitis externa; adjunct in pneumonia, impetigo, cellulitis, osteomyelitis and in staphylococcal endocarditis (Table 1, section 5.1)

Cautions: see under Benzylpenicillin (section 5.1.1.1); porphyria (section 9.8.2)

CHOLESTATIC JAUNDICE. CSM has advised that cholestatic jaundice may occur up to several weeks after treatment with flucloxacillin has been stopped. Administration for more than 2 weeks and increasing age are risk factors

Contra-indications: see under Benzylpenicillin (section 5.1.1.1)

Side-effects: see under Benzylpenicillin (section 5.1.1.1); also hepatitis and cholestatic jaundice reported (see also CSM advice above)

Dose: *by mouth*, 250–500 mg every 6 hours, at least 30 minutes before food; CHILD under 2 years quarter adult dose; 2–10 years half adult dose

By intramuscular injection, 250–500 mg every 6 hours; CHILD under 2 years quarter adult dose; 2–10 years half adult dose

By slow intravenous injection or by intravenous infusion, 0.25–2 g every 6 hours; CHILD under 2 years quarter adult dose; 2–10 years half adult dose

Endocarditis (see Table 1, section 5.1), 12 g daily in 6 divided doses for 4 weeks

Osteomyelitis (see Table 1, section 5.1), up to 8 g daily in 3–4 divided doses

Note. Flucloxacillin doses in BNF may differ from those in product literature

Flucloxacillin (Non-proprietary) PoM
Capsules, flucloxacillin (as sodium salt) 250 mg, net price 20 = £2.09; 500 mg, 20 = £3.38. Label: 9, 23

Available from Alpharma, APS, Ashbourne (*Fluclomix®*), Berk (*Ladropen®*), Galen (*Galfloxin®*), IVAX, Kent

Oral solution (= elixir or syrup), flucloxacillin (as sodium salt) for reconstitution with water, 125 mg/5 mL, net price 100 mL = £3.23. Label: 9, 23

Available from Alpharma, APS, Berk (*Ladropen®*), IVAX, Kent, Lagap

Injection, powder for reconstitution, flucloxacillin (as sodium salt). Net price 250-mg vial = £1.02; 500-mg vial = £2.04; 1-g vial = £4.08

Available from Berk (*Ladropen®*), CP

Floxapen® (SmithKline Beecham) PoM
Capsules, both black/caramel, flucloxacillin (as sodium salt) 250 mg, net price 28-cap pack = £6.79; 500 mg, 28-cap pack = £13.61. Label: 9, 23

Syrup, flucloxacillin (as magnesium salt) for reconstitution with water, 125 mg/5 mL, net price 100 mL = £3.49; 250 mg/5 mL, 100 mL = £6.97. Label: 9, 23

Excipients: include sucrose

Injection, powder for reconstitution, flucloxacillin (as sodium salt). Net price 250-mg vial = 98p; 500-mg vial = £1.95; 1-g vial = £3.90

Electrolytes: Na+ 0.57 mmol/250-mg vial, 1.13 mmol/500-mg vial, 2.26 mmol/1-g vial

5.1.1.3　Broad-spectrum penicillins

Ampicillin is active against certain Gram-positive and Gram-negative organisms but is inactivated by penicillinases including those produced by *Staphylococcus aureus* and by common Gram-negative bacilli such as *Escherichia coli*. Almost all staphylococci, 50% of *E. coli* strains and 15% of *Haemophilus influenzae* strains are now resistant. The likelihood of resistance should therefore be considered before using ampicillin for the 'blind' treatment of infections; in particular, it should not be used for hospital patients without checking sensitivity.

Ampicillin is well excreted in the bile and urine. It is principally indicated for the treatment of exacerbations of chronic bronchitis and middle ear infections, both of which are usually due to *Streptococcus pneumoniae* and *H. influenzae*, and for urinary-tract infections (section 5.1.13).

Ampicillin can be given by mouth but less than half the dose is absorbed, and absorption is further decreased by the presence of food in the gut.

Maculopapular rashes commonly occur with ampicillin (and amoxicillin) but are not usually related to true penicillin allergy. They almost always occur in patients with glandular fever; broad-spectrum penicillins should not therefore be used for 'blind' treatment of a sore throat. Rashes are also common in patients with chronic lymphocytic leukaemia or in cytomegalovirus infection.

Amoxicillin (amoxycillin) is a derivative of ampicillin and has a similar antibacterial spectrum. It is better absorbed than ampicillin when given by mouth, producing higher plasma and tissue concentrations; unlike ampicillin, absorption is not affected by the presence of food in the stomach. Amoxicillin is used for endocarditis prophylaxis (section 5.1, table 2); it may also be used for the treatment of Lyme disease [not licensed], see below.

Co-amoxiclav consists of amoxicillin with the beta-lactamase inhibitor clavulanic acid. Clavulanic acid itself has no significant antibacterial activity but, by inactivating beta-lactamases, it makes the combination active against beta-lactamase-producing bacteria that are resistant to amoxicillin. These include resistant strains of *Staph. aureus*, *E. coli*, and *H. influenzae*, as well as many *Bacteroides* and *Klebsiella* spp. Co-amoxiclav should be reserved for infections likely, or known, to be caused by amoxicillin-resistant beta-lactamase-producing strains; for CSM warning on cholestatic jaundice see under Co-amoxiclav.

A combination of ampicillin with flucloxacillin (as co-fluampicil) is available to treat infections involving either streptococci or staphylococci (e.g. cellulitis).

LYME DISEASE. Lyme disease should generally be treated by those experienced in its management. **Doxycycline** is the antibacterial of choice for *early* Lyme disease. **Amoxicillin** [unlicensed indication], **cefuroxime axetil**, or **azithromycin** [unlicensed indication] are alternatives if doxycycline is contra-indicated. Intravenous administration of **benzylpenicillin**, **cefotaxime**, or of **ceftriaxone** [unlicensed indication] is recommended for Lyme disease associated with moderate to severe *cardiac* or *neurological abnormalities*, *late Lyme disease*, and *Lyme arthritis*. The duration of treatment is generally 2–4 weeks; Lyme arthritis requires longer treatment with oral antibacterial drugs.

AMOXICILLIN
(Amoxycillin)

Indications: see under Ampicillin; also endocarditis prophylaxis (Table 2, section 5.1) and treatment (Table 1, section 5.1); treatment and prophylaxis of anthrax; adjunct in listerial meningitis (Table 1, section 5.1); *Helicobacter pylori* eradication (section 1.3)

Cautions: see under Ampicillin

Contra-indications: see under Ampicillin

Side-effects: see under Ampicillin

Dose: *by mouth*, 250 mg every 8 hours, doubled in severe infections; CHILD up to 10 years, 125 mg every 8 hours, doubled in severe infections

Severe or recurrent purulent respiratory infection, 3 g every 12 hours

Anthrax (treatment and post-exposure prophylaxis; see also section 5.1.12) 500 mg every 8 hours; CHILD body-weight under 20 kg, 40 mg/kg daily in 3 divided doses; body-weight over 20 kg, adult dose

Short-course oral therapy

Dental abscess, 3 g repeated after 8 hours

Urinary-tract infections, 3 g repeated after 10–12 hours

Otitis media, CHILD 3–10 years, 750 mg twice daily for 2 days

By intramuscular injection, 500 mg every 8 hours; CHILD, 50–100 mg/kg daily in divided doses

By intravenous injection or infusion, 500 mg every 8 hours increased to 1 g every 6 hours; CHILD, 50–100 mg/kg daily in divided doses

Listerial meningitis (in combination with another antibiotic, see Table 1, section 5.1), *by intravenous infusion*, 2 g every 4 hours for 10–14 days

Enterococcal endocarditis (in combination with another antibiotic if necessary, see Table 1, section 5.1), *by intravenous infusion*, 2 g every 4 hours

Note. Amoxicillin doses in BNF may differ from those in product literature

Amoxicillin (Non-proprietary) PoM

Capsules, amoxicillin (as trihydrate) 250 mg, net price 21 = £1.25; 500 mg, 21 = £1.84. Label: 9

Available from Alpharma, APS, Ashbourne (*Amix®*), Berk (*Almodan®*), DDSA, Eastern (*Amoram®*), Galen (*Galenamox®*), Hillcross, IVAX, Kent, Ranbaxy (*Rimoxallin®*)

Oral suspension, amoxicillin (as trihydrate) for reconstitution with water, 125 mg/5 mL, net price 100 mL = £1.14; 250 mg/5 mL, 100 mL = £1.79. Label: 9

Note. Sugar-free versions are available and can be ordered by specifying 'sugar-free' on the prescription

Available from Alpharma, APS, Ashbourne (*Amix®*), Berk (*Almodan®*), Eastern (*Amoram®*), Galen (*Galenamox®*), Hillcross, IVAX, Kent, Ranbaxy (*Rimoxallin®*)

Sachets, sugar-free, amoxicillin (as trihydrate) 3 g/sachet, net price 2-sachet pack = £4.68, 14-sachet pack = £31.94. Label: 9, 13

Available from Hillcross, IVAX, Kent

Injection, powder for reconstitution, amoxicillin (as sodium salt), net price 250-mg vial = 34p; 500-mg vial = 63p; 1-g vial = £1.25

Available from CP

Amoxil® (Bencard) PoM

Capsules, both maroon/gold, amoxicillin (as trihydrate), 250 mg, net price 21-cap pack = £3.86; 500 mg, 21-cap pack = £7.73. Label: 9

Syrup SF, both sugar-free, amoxicillin (as trihydrate) for reconstitution with water, 125 mg/5 mL, net price 100 mL = £2.31; 250 mg/5 mL, 100 mL = £4.62. Label: 9

Paediatric suspension, amoxicillin 125 mg (as trihydrate)/1.25 mL when reconstituted with water, net price 20 mL = £3.63. Label: 9, counselling, use of pipette

Excipients: include sucrose 600 mg/1.25 mL

Sachets SF, powder, sugar-free, amoxicillin (as trihydrate) 3 g/sachet, 2-sachet pack = £4.97. Label: 9, 13

Injection, powder for reconstitution, amoxicillin (as sodium salt), net price 250-mg vial = 34p; 500-mg vial = 63p; 1-g vial = £1.25

Electrolytes: Na⁺ 3.3 mmol/g

AMPICILLIN

Indications: urinary-tract infections, otitis media, sinusitis, bronchitis, uncomplicated community-acquired pneumonia (Table 1, section 5.1), *Haemophilus influenzae* infections, invasive salmonellosis; listerial meningitis (Table 1, section 5.1)

Cautions: history of allergy; renal impairment (Appendix 3); erythematous rashes common in glandular fever, cytomegalovirus infection, and chronic lymphocytic leukaemia (see notes above); **interactions:** Appendix 1 (penicillins)

Contra-indications: penicillin hypersensitivity

Side-effects: nausea, vomiting, diarrhoea; rashes (discontinue treatment); rarely, antibiotic-associated colitis; see also under Benzylpenicillin (section 5.1.1.1)

Dose: *by mouth*, 0.25–1 g every 6 hours, at least 30 minutes before food; CHILD under 10 years, half adult dose

Urinary-tract infections, 500 mg every 8 hours; CHILD under 10 years, half adult dose

By intramuscular injection or intravenous injection or infusion, 500 mg every 4–6 hours; CHILD under 10 years, half adult dose

Listerial meningitis (in combination with another antibiotic), *by intravenous infusion*, 2 g every 4 hours for 10–14 days; INFANT under 1 month, 50 mg/kg every 6 hours; 1–3 months, 50–100 mg/kg every 6 hours; CHILD 3 months–12 years, 100 mg/kg every 6 hours (max. 12 g daily)

Note. Ampicillin doses in BNF may differ from those in product literature

Ampicillin (Non-proprietary) PoM

Capsules, ampicillin 250 mg, net price 20 = 62p; 500 mg, 20 = £1.20. Label: 9, 23

Available from Alpharma, IVAX, Kent, Ranbaxy (*Rimacillin®*)

Oral suspension, ampicillin 125 mg/5 mL when reconstituted with water, net price 100 mL = £1.75; 250 mg/5 mL, 100 mL = £3.24. Label: 9, 23

Available from Alpharma, IVAX, Kent, Ranbaxy (*Rimacillin®*)

Penbritin® (SmithKline Beecham) PoM

Capsules, both black/red, ampicillin (as trihydrate) 250 mg, net price 28-cap pack = £2.26. Label: 9, 23

Injection, powder for reconstitution, ampicillin (as sodium salt). Net price 500-mg vial = 74p

Electrolytes: Na⁺ 1.47 mmol/500-mg vial

■ With flucloxacillin

See Co-fluampicil

CO-AMOXICLAV

A mixture of amoxicillin (as the trihydrate or as the sodium salt) and clavulanic acid (as potassium clavulanate); the proportions are expressed in the form *x/y* where *x* and *y* are the strengths in milligrams of amoxicillin and clavulanic acid respectively

Indications: infections due to beta-lactamase-producing strains (where amoxicillin alone not appropriate) including respiratory-tract infections, genito-urinary and abdominal infections, cellulitis, animal bites, severe dental infection with spreading cellulitis

Cautions: see under Ampicillin and notes above; also caution in hepatic impairment (monitor hepatic function), pregnancy

CHOLESTATIC JAUNDICE. CSM has advised that cholestatic jaundice has been identified as an adverse reaction occuring either during, or shortly after, the use of co-amoxiclav. An epidemiological study has shown that the risk of acute liver toxicity was about 6 times greater with co-amoxiclav than with amoxicillin. Cholestatic jaundice is more common in patients above the age of 65 years and in males; these reactions have only rarely been reported in children. Jaundice is usually self-limiting and very rarely fatal. The duration of treatment should be appropriate to the indication and should not usually exceed 14 days

Contra-indications: penicillin hypersensitivity, history of co-amoxiclav-associated or penicillin-associated jaundice or hepatic dysfunction

Side-effects: see under Ampicillin; hepatitis, cholestatic jaundice (see above); erythema multiforme (including Stevens-Johnson syndrome), toxic epidermal necrolysis, exfoliative dermatitis, vasculitis reported; rarely prolongation of bleeding time, dizziness, headache, convulsions (particularly with high doses or in renal impairment); superficial staining of teeth with suspension, phlebitis at injection site

Dose: *by mouth*, expressed as amoxicillin, 250 mg every 8 hours, dose doubled in severe infections; CHILD see under preparations below (under 6 years *Augmentin®* '125/31 SF' suspension; 6–12 years *Augmentin®* '250/62 SF' suspension *or* for short-term treatment with twice daily dosage in CHILD 2 months–12 years *Augmentin-Duo®* 400/57 suspension)

Severe dental infections (but not generally first-line, see notes above), expressed as amoxicillin, 250 mg every 8 hours for 5 days

By intravenous injection over 3–4 minutes *or by intravenous infusion*, expressed as amoxicillin, 1 g every 8 hours increased to 1 g every 6 hours in more serious infections; INFANTS up to 3 months 25 mg/kg every 8 hours (every 12 hours in the perinatal period and in premature infants); CHILD 3 months–12 years, 25 mg/kg every 8 hours increased to 25 mg/kg every 6 hours in more serious infections

Surgical prophylaxis, expressed as amoxicillin, 1 g at induction; for high risk procedures (e.g. colorectal surgery) a further 2–3 doses may be given every 8 hours in first 24 hours

Co-amoxiclav (Non-proprietary) PoM
Tablets, co-amoxiclav 250/125 (amoxicillin 250 mg as trihydrate, clavulanic acid 125 mg as potassium salt), net price 21-tab pack = £9.73. Label: 9
Available from Alpharma, Ashbourne (*Amiclav®*), Generics, IVAX

Tablets, co-amoxiclav 500/125 (amoxicillin 500 mg as trihydrate, clavulanic acid 125 mg as potassium salt), net price 21-tab pack = £15.72. Label: 9
Available from IVAX

Oral suspension, co-amoxiclav 125/31 (amoxicillin 125 mg as trihydrate, clavulanic acid 31.25 mg as potassium salt)/5 mL when reconstituted with water, net price 100 mL = £4.57. Label: 9
Excipients: include aspartame 12.5 mg/5 mL (section 9.4.1)
Available from IVAX

Oral suspension, co-amoxiclav 250/62 (amoxicillin 250 mg as trihydrate, clavulanic acid 62.5 mg as potassium salt)/5 mL when reconstituted with water, net price 100 mL = £6.42. Label: 9
Excipients: include aspartame 12.5 mg/5 mL (section 9.4.1)
Available from IVAX

Augmentin® (SmithKline Beecham) PoM
Tablets 375 mg, f/c, co-amoxiclav 250/125 (amoxicillin 250 mg as trihydrate, clavulanic acid 125 mg as potassium salt), net price 21-tab pack = £9.79. Label: 9
Tablets 625 mg, f/c, co-amoxiclav 500/125 (amoxicillin 500 mg as trihydrate, clavulanic acid 125 mg as potassium salt). Net price 21-tab pack = £15.73. Label: 9
Dispersible tablets, sugar-free, co-amoxiclav 250/125 (amoxicillin 250 mg as trihydrate, clavulanic acid 125 mg as potassium salt). Net price 21-tab pack = £10.99. Label: 9, 13
Suspension '125/31 SF', sugar-free, co-amoxiclav 125/31 (amoxicillin 125 mg as trihydrate, clavulanic acid 31 mg as potassium salt)/5 mL when reconstituted with water. Net price 100 mL = £4.57. Label: 9
Excipients: include aspartame 12.5 mg/5 mL (section 9.4.1)
Dose: CHILD 1–6 years (10–18 kg) 5 mL every 8 hours *or* INFANT and CHILD up to 6 years 0.8 mL/kg daily in 3 divided doses; in severe infections dose increased to 1.6 mL/kg daily in 3 divided doses
Suspension '250/62 SF', sugar-free, co-amoxiclav 250/62 (amoxicillin 250 mg as trihydrate, clavulanic acid 62 mg as potassium salt)/5 mL when reconstituted with water. Net price 100 mL = £6.42. Label: 9
Excipients: include aspartame 12.5 mg/5 mL (section 9.4.1)
Dose: CHILD 6–12 years (18–40 kg) 5 mL every 8 hours *or* 0.4 mL/kg daily in 3 divided doses; in severe infections dose increased to 0.8 mL/kg daily in 3 divided doses
Injection 600 mg, powder for reconstitution, co-amoxiclav 500/100 (amoxicillin 500 mg as sodium salt, clavulanic acid 100 mg as potassium salt). Net price per vial = £1.49
Electrolytes: Na⁺ 1.6 mmol, K⁺ 0.5 mmol/600-mg vial
Injection 1.2 g, powder for reconstitution, co-amoxiclav 1000/200 (amoxicillin 1 g as sodium salt, clavulanic acid 200 mg as potassium salt). Net price per vial = £2.97
Electrolytes: Na⁺ 3.1 mmol, K⁺ 1 mmol/1.2-g vial

Augmentin-Duo® (SmithKline Beecham) PoM
Suspension '400/57', sugar-free, co-amoxiclav 400/57 (amoxicillin 400 mg as trihydrate, clavulanic acid 57 mg as potassium salt)/5 mL when reconstituted with water. Net price 35 mL = £4.71, 70 mL = £6.61. Label: 9
Excipients: include aspartame 12.5 mg/5 mL (section 9.4.1)
Dose: CHILD 2 months–2 years 0.15 mL/kg twice daily, 2–6 years (13–21 kg) 2.5 mL twice daily, 7–12 years (22–40 kg) 5 mL twice daily, doubled in severe infections

CO-FLUAMPICIL

A mixture of equal parts by mass of flucloxacillin and ampicillin

Indications: mixed infections involving beta-lactamase-producing staphylococci

Cautions: see under Ampicillin and Flucloxacillin

Contra-indications: see under Ampicillin and Flucloxacillin

Side-effects: see under Ampicillin and Flucloxacillin

Dose: *by mouth*, co-fluampicil, 250/250 every 6 hours, dose doubled in severe infections; CHILD under 10 years half adult dose, dose doubled in severe infections

By intramuscular or slow intravenous injection or by intravenous infusion, co-fluampicil 250/250 every 6 hours, dose doubled in severe infections; CHILD under 2 years quarter adult dose, 2–10 years half adult dose, dose doubled in severe infections

Co-fluampicil (Non-proprietary) [PoM]
Capsules, co-fluampicil 250/250 (flucloxacillin 250 mg as sodium salt, ampicillin 250 mg as trihydrate), net price 28-cap pack = £8.73. Label: 9, 22
Available from Alpharma, Generics (*Flu-Amp*®), IVAX, Kent

Magnapen® (CP) [PoM]
Capsules, black/turquoise, co-fluampicil 250/250 (flucloxacillin 250 mg as sodium salt, ampicillin 250 mg as trihydrate), net price 20-cap pack = £6.15. Label: 9, 22

Syrup, co-fluampicil 125/125 (flucloxacillin 125 mg as magnesium salt, ampicillin 125 mg as trihydrate) /5 mL when reconstituted with water, net price 100 mL = £4.99. Label: 9, 22
Excipients: include sucrose 3.14 g/5 mL

Injection 500 mg, powder for reconstitution, co-fluampicil 250/250 (flucloxacillin 250 mg as sodium salt, ampicillin 250 mg as sodium salt), net price per vial = £1.33
Electrolytes: Na⁺ 1.3 mmol/vial

5.1.1.4 Antipseudomonal penicillins

The carboxypenicillin, **ticarcillin**, is principally indicated for serious infections caused by *Pseudomonas aeruginosa* although it also has activity against certain other Gram-negative bacilli including *Proteus* spp. and *Bacteroides fragilis*.

Ticarcillin is now available only in combination with clavulanic acid (section 5.1.1.3); the combination (*Timentin*®) is active against beta-lactamase-producing bacteria resistant to ticarcillin.

The ureidopenicillin, **piperacillin**, has a broad spectrum and it is more active than ticarcillin against *Ps. aeruginosa*.

Tazocin® (piperacillin with the beta-lactamase inhibitor tazobactam) is active against beta-lactamase-producing bacteria resistant to the ureidopenicillins; it has a spectrum of activity comparable to the carbapenems, imipenem and meropenem (section 5.1.2).

For pseudomonas septicaemias (especially in neutropenia or endocarditis) these antipseudomonal penicillins should be given with an aminoglycoside (e.g. gentamicin or netilmicin, section 5.1.4) since they have a synergistic effect. Penicillins and aminoglycosides must not, however, be mixed in the same syringe or infusion.

Owing to the sodium content of many of these antibiotics, high doses may lead to hypernatraemia.

PIPERACILLIN

Indications: infections due to *Pseudomonas aeruginosa*, see notes above; surgical prophylaxis

Cautions: see under Benzylpenicillin (section 5.1.1.1); renal impairment (Appendix 3)

Contra-indications: see under Benzylpenicillin (section 5.1.1.1)

Side-effects: see under Benzylpenicillin (section 5.1.1.1); rarely Stevens-Johnson syndrome, hepatitis, cholestatic jaundice

Dose: *by deep intramuscular injection or by intravenous injection* over 3–5 minutes *or by intravenous infusion*, 100–150 mg/kg daily (in divided doses), increased to 200–300 mg/kg daily in severe infections, and to at least 16 g daily in life-threatening infections; single doses over 2 g intravenous route only; NEONATE *by intravenous injection* over 3–5 minutes *or by intravenous infusion*, aged up to 7 days *or* over 7 days but under 2 kg, 150 mg/kg daily in 3 divided doses; aged over 7 days and over 2 kg, 300 mg/kg daily in 3–4 divided doses; CHILD 1 month–12 years, 100–200 mg/kg daily in 3–4 divided doses, increased in severe infections to 200–300 mg/kg daily in 3–4 divided doses

Surgical prophylaxis, *by deep intramuscular injection or by intravenous injection* over 3–5 minutes *or by intravenous infusion*, 2 g at induction (or in caesarean section, when umbilical cord clamped); further doses may be given at intervals of 4–6 hours for high-risk procedures

Pipril® (Lederle) [PoM]
Injection, powder for reconstitution, piperacillin (as sodium salt). Net price 1-g vial = £3.07; 2-g vial = £6.08; 4-g vial = £12.02
Electrolytes: Na⁺ 1.85 mmol/g
Note. May be difficult to obtain

■ With tazobactam
Tazocin® (Lederle) [PoM]
Injection 2.25 g, powder for reconstitution, piperacillin 2 g (as sodium salt), tazobactam 250 mg (as sodium salt). Net price per vial = £7.96
Electrolytes: Na⁺ 4.69 mmol/2.25-g vial

Injection 4.5 g, powder for reconstitution, piperacillin 4 g (as sodium salt), tazobactam 500 mg (as sodium salt). Net price per vial = £14.48; infusion pack (4.5-g infusion bottle, 50-mL bottle water for injections and transfer needle) = £15.93
Electrolytes: Na⁺ 9.37 mmol/4.5-g vial
Dose: lower respiratory-tract, urinary-tract, intra-abdominal and skin infections, and septicaemia, ADULT and CHILD over 12 years, *by intravenous injection* over 3–5 minutes *or by intravenous infusion*, 2.25–4.5 g every 6–8 hours, usually 4.5 g every 8 hours

Complicated appendicitis, *by intravenous injection* over 3–5 minutes *or by intravenous infusion*, CHILD 2–12 years, 112.5 mg/kg every 8 hours (max. 4.5 g every 8 hours) for 5–14 days; CHILD under 2 years, not recommended

Infections in neutropenic patients (in combination with an aminoglycoside), *by intravenous injection* over 3–5 minutes *or by intravenous infusion*, ADULT and CHILD over 50 kg, 4.5 g every 6 hours; CHILD less than 50 kg, 90 mg/kg every 6 hours

TICARCILLIN

Indications: infections due to *Pseudomonas* and *Proteus* spp, see notes above

Cautions: see under Benzylpenicillin (section 5.1.1.1)

Contra-indications: see under Benzylpenicillin (section 5.1.1.1)

Side-effects: see under Benzylpenicillin (section 5.1.1.1)

Dose: see under preparation

■ With clavulanic acid

Note. For a CSM warning on cholestatic jaundice possibly associated with clavulanic acid, see under Co-amoxiclav p. 263.

Timentin® (SmithKline Beecham) [PoM]

Injection 3.2 g, powder for reconstitution, ticarcillin 3 g (as sodium salt), clavulanic acid 200 mg (as potassium salt). Net price per vial = £6.08

Electrolytes: Na⁺ 16 mmol, K⁺ 1 mmol /3.2-g vial

Dose: by intravenous infusion, 3.2 g every 6–8 hours increased to every 4 hours in more severe infections; CHILD 80 mg/kg every 6–8 hours (every 12 hours in neonates)

5.1.1.5 Mecillinams

Pivmecillinam has significant activity against many Gram-negative bacteria including *Escherichia coli*, klebsiella, enterobacter, and salmonellae. It is not active against *Pseudomonas aeruginosa* or enterococci. Pivmecillinam is hydrolysed to mecillinam, which is the active drug.

PIVMECILLINAM HYDROCHLORIDE

Indications: see under Dose below

Cautions: see under Benzylpenicillin (section 5.1.1.1); also liver and renal function tests required in long-term use; pregnancy; **interactions:** Appendix 1 (penicillins)

Contra-indications: see under Benzylpenicillin (section 5.1.1.1); also carnitine deficiency, oesophageal strictures, gastro-intestinal obstruction, infants under 3 months

Side-effects: see under Benzylpenicillin (section 5.1.1.1); nausea, vomiting, dyspepsia; also reduced serum and total body carnitine (especially with long-term or repeated use)

Dose: acute uncomplicated cystitis, ADULT and CHILD over 40 kg, initially 400 mg then 200 mg every 8 hours for 3 days

Chronic or recurrent bacteriuria, ADULT and CHILD over 40 kg, 400 mg every 6–8 hours

Urinary-tract infections, CHILD under 40 kg, 20–40 mg/kg daily in 3–4 divided doses

Salmonellosis, not recommended therefore no dose stated

COUNSELLING. Tablets should be swallowed whole with plenty of fluid during meals while sitting or standing

Selexid® (Leo) [PoM]

Tablets, f/c, pivmecillinam hydrochloride 200 mg, net price 10-tab pack = £4.50. Label 9, 21, 27, counselling, posture (see Dose above)

5.1.2 Cephalosporins, cephamycins, and other beta-lactams

Antibiotics in this section include the **cephalosporins**, such as cefotaxime, ceftazidime, cefuroxime, cefalexin and cefradine, the **cephamycin**, cefoxitin, the **monobactam**, aztreonam, and the **carbapenems**, imipenem (a thienamycin derivative) and meropenem.

Cephalosporins and cephamycins

The cephalosporins are broad-spectrum antibiotics which are used for the treatment of septicaemia, pneumonia, meningitis, biliary-tract infections, peritonitis, and urinary-tract infections. All have a similar antibacterial spectrum although individual agents have differing activity against certain organisms. The pharmacology of the cephalosporins is similar to that of the penicillins, excretion being principally renal. Cephalosporins penetrate the cerebrospinal fluid poorly unless the meninges are inflamed; cefotaxime is a suitable cephalosporin for infections of the CNS (e.g meningitis).

The principal side-effect of the cephalosporins is hypersensitivity and about 10% of penicillin-sensitive patients will also be allergic to the cephalosporins. Haemorrhage due to interference with blood clotting factors has been associated with several cephalosporins.

Cefradine (cephradine) and **cefazolin** (cephazolin) have generally been replaced by the newer cephalosporins mentioned below.

Cefuroxime and **cefamandole** (cephamandole) are 'second generation' cephalosporins and are less susceptible than the earlier cephalosporins to inactivation by beta-lactamases. They are, therefore, active against certain bacteria which are resistant to the other drugs and have greater activity against *Haemophilus influenzae* and *Neisseria gonorrhoeae*.

Cefotaxime, **ceftazidime** and **ceftriaxone** are 'third generation' cephalosporins with greater activity than the 'second generation' cephalosporins against certain Gram-negative bacteria. However, they are less active than cefuroxime and cefamandole against Gram-positive bacteria, most notably *Staphylococcus aureus*. Their broad antibacterial spectrum may encourage superinfection with resistant bacteria or fungi.

Ceftazidime has good activity against pseudomonas. It is also active against other Gram-negative bacteria.

Ceftriaxone has a longer half-life and therefore only needs once daily administration. Indications include serious infections such as septicaemia, pneumonia, and meningitis. The calcium salt of ceftriaxone forms a precipitate in the gall bladder which may rarely cause symptoms but these usually resolve when the antibiotic is stopped.

Cefpirome is indicated for urinary-tract, lower respiratory-tract and skin infections, bacteraemia, and infections associated with neutropenia.

Cefoxitin, a cephamycin antibiotic, is active against bowel flora including *Bacteroides fragilis* and because of this it has been recommended for abdominal sepsis such as peritonitis.

ORALLY ACTIVE CEPHALOSPORINS. The orally active 'first generation' cephalosporins, **cefalexin** (cephalexin), **cefradine**, and **cefadroxil** and the 'second generation' cephalosporins, **cefaclor** and **cefprozil**, have a similar antimicrobial spectrum. They are useful for urinary-tract infections which do not respond to other drugs or which occur in pregnancy, respiratory-tract infections, otitis media, sinusitis, and skin and soft-tissue infections. Cefaclor has good activity against *H. influenzae*, but it is associated with protracted skin reactions especially in children. Cefadroxil has a long duration of action and can be given twice daily; it has poor activity against *H. influenzae*. **Cefuroxime axetil**, an ester of the 'second generation' cephalosporin cefuroxime, has the same antibacterial spectrum as the parent compound; it is poorly absorbed.

Cefixime has a longer duration of action than the other cephalosporins that are active by mouth. It is presently only licensed for acute infections.

Cefpodoxime proxetil, is more active than the other oral cephalosporins against respiratory bacterial pathogens and it is licensed for upper and lower respiratory-tract infections.

For treatment of Lyme disease, see section 5.1.1.3.

CEFACLOR

Indications: infections due to sensitive Gram-positive and Gram-negative bacteria, but see notes above

Cautions: penicillin sensitivity; renal impairment (Appendix 3); pregnancy and breast-feeding (but appropriate to use); false positive urinary glucose (if tested for reducing substances) and false positive Coombs' test; **interactions:** Appendix 1 (cephalosporins)

Contra-indications: cephalosporin hypersensitivity; porphyria (section 9.8.2)

Side-effects: diarrhoea and rarely antibiotic-associated colitis (CSM has warned both more likely with higher doses), nausea and vomiting, abdominal discomfort, headache; allergic reactions including rashes, pruritus, urticaria, serum sickness-like reactions with rashes, fever and arthralgia, and anaphylaxis; erythema multiforme, toxic epidermal necrolysis reported; disturbances in liver enzymes, transient hepatitis and cholestatic jaundice; other side-effects reported include eosinophilia and blood disorders (including thrombocytopenia, leucopenia, agranulocytosis, aplastic anaemia and haemolytic anaemia); reversible interstitial nephritis, hyperactivity, nervousness, sleep disturbances, confusion, hypertonia, and dizziness

Dose: 250 mg every 8 hours, doubled for severe infections; max. 4 g daily; CHILD over 1 month, 20 mg/kg daily in 3 divided doses, doubled for severe infections, max. 1 g daily; *or* 1 month–1 year, 62.5 mg every 8 hours; 1–5 years, 125 mg; over 5 years, 250 mg; doses doubled for severe infections

Cefaclor (Non-proprietary) PoM
Capsules, cefaclor (as monohydrate) 250 mg, net price 21-cap pack = £6.80; 500 mg 50-cap pack = £44.25. Label: 9
Available from Alpharma, APS, Galen (*Keftid*®), Hillcross, Kent

Suspension, cefaclor (as monohydrate) for reconstitution with water, 125 mg/5 mL, net price 100 mL = £4.19; 250 mg/5 mL, 100 mL = £7.46. Label: 9
Note. Sugar-free versions are available and can be ordered by specifying 'sugar-free' on the prescription
Available from Alpharma, APS, Galen (*Keftid*®), Generics, Genus, Hillcross

Distaclor® (Dista) PoM
Capsules, cefaclor (as monohydrate) 500 mg (violet/grey), net price 20 = £21.66. Label: 9
Suspension, both pink, cefaclor (as monohydrate) for reconstitution with water, 125 mg/5 mL, net price 100 mL = £5.16; 250 mg/5 mL, 100 mL = £10.32. Label: 9

Distaclor MR® (Dista) PoM
Tablets, m/r, both blue, cefaclor (as monohydrate) 375 mg. Net price 14-tab pack = £6.93. Label: 9, 21, 25
Dose: 375 mg every 12 hours with food, dose doubled for pneumonia
Lower urinary-tract infections, 375 mg every 12 hours with food
Note. Modified-release tablets containing cefaclor (as monohydrate) 375 mg available from Ranbaxy

CEFADROXIL

Indications: see under Cefaclor; see also notes above

Cautions: see under Cefaclor

Contra-indications: see under Cefaclor

Side-effects: see under Cefaclor

Dose: patients over 40 kg, 0.5–1 g twice daily; skin, soft tissue, and simple urinary-tract infections, 1 g daily; CHILD under 1 year, 25 mg/kg daily in divided doses; 1–6 years, 250 mg twice daily; over 6 years, 500 mg twice daily

Baxan® (Bristol-Myers Squibb) PoM
Capsules, cefadroxil (as monohydrate) 500 mg, net price 20 = £5.64. Label: 9
Suspension, cefadroxil (as monohydrate) for reconstitution with water, 125 mg/5 mL, net price 60 mL = £1.75; 250 mg/5 mL, 60 mL = £3.48; 500 mg/5 mL, 60 mL = £5.21. Label: 9

CEFALEXIN
(Cephalexin)

Indications: see under Cefaclor

Cautions: see under Cefaclor

Contra-indications: see under Cefaclor

Side-effects: see under Cefaclor

Dose: 250 mg every 6 hours *or* 500 mg every 8–12 hours increased to 1–1.5 g every 6–8 hours for severe infections; CHILD 25 mg/kg daily in divided doses, doubled for severe infections, max. 100 mg/kg daily; *or* under 1 year 125 mg every 12 hours, 1–5 years 125 mg every 8 hours, 6–12 years 250 mg every 8 hours
Prophylaxis of recurrent urinary-tract infection, ADULT 125 mg at night

Cefalexin (Non-proprietary) PoM
Capsules, cefalexin 250 mg, net price 28-cap pack = £2.61; 500 mg, 21-cap pack = £3.90. Label: 9
Available from Alpharma, APS, Generics, Hillcross, IVAX, Kent (*Tenkorex*®), Ranbaxy

Tablets, cefalexin 250 mg, net price 20 = £1.90; 500 mg, 20 = £3.48. Label: 9

Available from Alpharma, APS, Berk (*Kiflone®*), Hillcross, IVAX, Kent (*Tenkorex®*)

Oral suspension, cefalexin for reconstitution with water, 125 mg/5 mL, net price 100 mL = £1.33; 250 mg/5 mL, 100 mL = £2.32. Label: 9

Available from Alpharma, APS, Hillcross, IVAX, Kent (*Tenkorex®*)

Ceporex® (Galen) [PoM]

Capsules, both caramel/grey, cefalexin 250 mg, net price 28-cap pack = £4.47; 500 mg, 28-cap pack = £8.72. Label: 9

Tablets, all pink, f/c, cefalexin 250 mg, net price 28-tab pack = £4.47; 500 mg, 28-tab pack = £8.72; 1 g (scored), 14-tab pack = £8.72. Label: 9

Syrup, all orange, cefalexin for reconstitution with water, 125 mg/5 mL, net price 100 mL = £1.59; 250 mg/5 mL, 100 mL = £3.19; 500 mg/5 mL, 100 mL = £6.19. Label: 9

Keflex® (Lilly) [PoM]

Capsules, cefalexin 250 mg (green/white), net price 28-cap pack = £3.57; 500 mg (pale green/dark green), 21-cap pack = £5.23. Label: 9

Tablets, both peach, cefalexin 250 mg, net price 28-tab pack = £3.57; 500 mg (scored), 21-tab pack = £5.23. Label: 9

Suspension, cefalexin for reconstitution with water, 125 mg/5 mL (pink), net price 100 mL = £1.27; 250 mg/5 mL (orange), 100 mL = £2.55. Label: 9

CEFAMANDOLE

(Cephamandole)

Indications: see under Cefaclor; surgical prophylaxis

Cautions: see under Cefaclor

Contra-indications: see under Cefaclor

Side-effects: see under Cefaclor

Dose: *by deep intramuscular injection or by intravenous injection* over 3–5 minutes *or by intravenous infusion*, 0.5–2 g every 4–8 hours; CHILD over 1 month, 50–100 mg/kg daily in 3–6 divided doses increased to 150 mg/kg daily for severe infections

Surgical prophylaxis, *by intramuscular or intravenous injection*, 1–2 g at induction; further doses may be given every 6 hours for high-risk procedures

Kefadol® (Dista) [PoM]

Injection, powder for reconstitution, cefamandole (as nafate) with sodium carbonate. Net price 1-g vial = £3.91

Electrolytes: Na⁺ 3.35 mmol/1-g vial

CEFAZOLIN

(Cephazolin)

Indications: see under Cefaclor; surgical prophylaxis

Cautions: see under Cefaclor

Contra-indications: see under Cefaclor

Side-effects: see under Cefaclor

Dose: *by intramuscular injection or intravenous injection or infusion*, 0.5–1 g every 6–12 hours; CHILD, 25–50 mg/kg daily (in divided doses), increased to 100 mg/kg daily in severe infections

Kefzol® (Lilly) [PoM]

Injection, powder for reconstitution, cefazolin (as sodium salt). Net price 500-mg vial = £2.45; 1-g vial = £4.63

Electrolytes: Na⁺ 2.1 mmol/g

CEFIXIME

Indications: see under Cefaclor (acute infections only)

Cautions: see under Cefaclor

Contra-indications: see under Cefaclor

Side-effects: see under Cefaclor

Dose: ADULT and CHILD over 10 years, 200–400 mg daily in 1–2 divided doses; CHILD over 6 months 8 mg/kg daily in 1–2 divided doses *or* 6 months–1 year 75 mg daily; 1–4 years 100 mg daily; 5–10 years 200 mg daily

Suprax® (Rhône-Poulenc Rorer) [PoM]

Tablets, f/c, scored, cefixime 200 mg. Net price 7-tab pack = £12.03. Label: 9

Paediatric oral suspension, cefixime 100 mg/5 mL when reconstituted with water. Net price 37.5 mL (with double-ended spoon for measuring 3.75 mL or 5 mL since dilution not recommended) = £7.90; 75 mL = £14.18. Label: 9

CEFOTAXIME

Indications: see under Cefaclor; gonorrhoea (section 5.1, table 1); surgical prophylaxis; Haemophilus epiglottitis and meningitis (section 5.1, table 1); see also notes above

Cautions: see under Cefaclor

Contra-indications: see under Cefaclor

Side-effects: see under Cefaclor; rarely arrhythmias following rapid injection reported

Dose: *by intramuscular or intravenous injection or by intravenous infusion*, 1 g every 12 hours increased in severe infections (e.g. meningitis) to 8 g daily in 4 divided doses; higher doses (up to 12 g daily in 3–4 divided doses) may be required; NEONATE 50 mg/kg daily in 2–4 divided doses increased to 150–200 mg/kg daily in severe infections; CHILD 100–150 mg/kg daily in 2–4 divided doses increased up to 200 mg/kg daily in very severe infections

Gonorrhoea, 500 mg as a single dose

Important. If bacterial meningitis and especially if meningococcal disease is suspected the patient should be transferred urgently to hospital. If benzylpenicillin cannot be given (e.g. because of an allergy), a single dose of cefotaxime may be given (if available) before urgent transfer to hospital. Suitable doses of cefotaxime by intravenous injection (or by intramuscular injection) are ADULT and CHILD over 12 years 1 g; CHILD under 12 years 50 mg/kg; chloramphenicol (section 5.1.7) may be used if there is a history of anaphylaxis to penicillins or cephalosporins

Cefotaxime (Non-proprietary) [PoM]

Injection, powder for reconstitution, cefotaxime (as sodium salt), net price 500-mg vial = £2.41; 1-g vial = £4.85; 2-g vial = £9.65

Available from Genus

Claforan® (Hoechst Marion Roussel) [PoM]

Injection, powder for reconstitution, cefotaxime (as sodium salt), net price 500-mg vial = £2.41; 1-g vial (with or without infusion connector) =

£4.85; 2-g vial (with or without infusion connector) = £9.65
Electrolytes: Na⁺ 2.09 mmol/g

CEFOXITIN

Indications: see under Cefaclor; surgical prophylaxis; more active against Gram-negative bacteria
Cautions: see under Cefaclor
Contra-indications: see under Cefaclor
Side-effects: see under Cefaclor
Dose: *by deep intramuscular or by slow intravenous injection or by infusion*, 1–2 g every 6–8 hours, increased up to 12 g daily in divided doses for infections requiring higher doses; CHILD up to 1 week 20–40 mg/kg every 12 hours, 1–4 weeks 20–40 mg/kg every 8 hours, over 1 month 20–40 mg/kg every 6–8 hours, increased up to 200 mg/kg daily in divided doses (max. 12 g daily) in severe infections; intravenous route recommended for children
Uncomplicated urinary-tract infection, *by deep intramuscular injection*, 1 g every 12 hours for 10 days
Surgical prophylaxis, *by deep intramuscular injection or by intravenous injection or infusion*, 2 g at induction; further doses may be given every 6 hours for high-risk procedures; CHILD 30–40 mg/kg at induction; further doses may be given every 6 hours (every 8–12 hours in NEONATES) for high-risk procedures; intravenous route recommended for children

Mefoxin® (MSD) PoM
Injection, powder for reconstitution, cefoxitin (as sodium salt). Net price 1-g vial = £4.92; 2-g vial = £9.84
Electrolytes: Na⁺ 2.3 mmol/g

CEFPIROME

Indications: see under Cefaclor and notes above
Cautions: see under Cefaclor; interference with creatinine assays using picrate method
Contra-indications: see under Cefaclor
Side-effects: see under Cefaclor; taste disturbance shortly after injection reported
Dose: *by intravenous injection or infusion*, complicated upper and lower urinary-tract, skin and soft-tissue infections, 1 g every 12 hours increased to 2 g every 12 hours in very severe infections
Lower respiratory-tract infections, 1–2 g every 12 hours
Severe infections including bacteraemia and septicaemia and infections in neutropenic patients, 2 g every 12 hours
CHILD under 12 years not recommended

Cefrom® (Hoechst Marion Roussel) PoM
Injection, powder for reconstitution, cefpirome (as sulphate), net price 1-g vial = £10.75; 2-g vial = £21.50

CEFPODOXIME

Indications: see under Dose
Cautions: see under Cefaclor
Contra-indications: see under Cefaclor
Side-effects: see under Cefaclor

Dose: upper respiratory-tract infections (but in pharyngitis and tonsillitis reserved for infections which are recurrent, chronic, or resistant to other antibacterials), 100 mg twice daily (200 mg twice daily in sinusitis)
Lower respiratory-tract infections (including bronchitis and pneumonia), 100–200 mg twice daily
Skin and soft tissue infections, 200 mg twice daily
Uncomplicated urinary-tract infections, 100 mg twice daily (200 mg twice daily in uncomplicated upper urinary-tract infections)
Uncomplicated gonorrhoea, 200 mg as a single dose
CHILD 15 days–6 months 4 mg/kg every 12 hours, 6 months–2 years 40 mg every 12 hours, 3–8 years 80 mg every 12 hours, over 9 years 100 mg every 12 hours

Orelox® (Hoechst Marion Roussel) PoM
Tablets, f/c, cefpodoxime 100 mg (as proxetil), net price 10-tab pack = £9.26. Label: 5, 9, 21
Oral suspension, cefpodoxime (as proxetil) for reconstitution with water, 40 mg/5 mL, net price 50 mL = £6.50, 100 mL = £10.89. Label: 5, 9, 21
Excipients: include aspartame (section 9.4.1)

CEFPROZIL

Indications: see under Dose
Cautions: see under Cefaclor
Contra-indications: see under Cefaclor
Side-effects: see under Cefaclor
Dose: upper respiratory-tract infections and skin and soft tissue infections, 500 mg once daily usually for 10 days; CHILD 6 months–12 years, 20 mg/kg (max. 500 mg) once daily
Acute exacerbation of chronic bronchitis, 500 mg every 12 hours usually for 10 days
Otitis media, CHILD 6 months–12 years, 20 mg/kg (max. 500 mg) every 12 hours

Cefzil® (Bristol-Myers Squibb) ▼ PoM
Tablets, cefprozil, 250 mg (orange), net price 20-tab pack = £14.95; 500 mg, 10-tab pack = £14.95. Label: 9
Suspension, cefprozil, 250 mg/5 mL when reconstituted with water, net price 100 mL = £15.22. Label: 9
Excipients: include aspartame equivalent to phenylalanine 28 mg/5 mL (section 9.4.1)

CEFRADINE
(Cephradine)

Indications: see under Cefaclor; surgical prophylaxis
Cautions: see under Cefaclor
Contra-indications: see under Cefaclor
Side-effects: see under Cefaclor
Dose: *by mouth*, 250–500 mg every 6 hours *or* 0.5–1 g every 12 hours; up to 1 g every 6 hours in severe infections; CHILD, 25–50 mg/kg daily in 2–4 divided doses
By deep intramuscular injection or by intravenous injection over 3–5 minutes *or by intravenous infusion*, 0.5–1 g every 6 hours, increased to 8 g daily in severe infections; CHILD 50–100 mg/kg daily in 4 divided doses
Surgical prophylaxis, *by deep intramuscular injection or by intravenous injection* over 3–5 minutes, 1–2 g at induction

Cefradine (Non-proprietary) PoM
Capsules, cefradine 250 mg, net price 20-cap pack
= £3.51; 500 mg, 20-cap pack = £6.74. Label: 9
Available from APS, Galen (*Nicef®*), Generics, IVAX

Velosef® (Squibb) PoM
Capsules, cefradine 250 mg (orange/blue), net
price 20-cap pack = £3.55; 500 mg (blue), 20-cap
pack = £7.00. Label: 9
Syrup, cefradine 250 mg/5 mL when reconstituted
with water. Net price 100 mL = £4.22. Label: 9
Injection, powder for reconstitution, cefradine. Net
price 500-mg vial = 99p; 1-g vial = £1.95

CEFTAZIDIME

Indications: see under Cefaclor; see also notes
above

Cautions: see under Cefaclor

Contra-indications: see under Cefaclor

Side-effects: see under Cefaclor

Dose: *by deep intramuscular injection or intravenous injection or infusion*, 1 g every 8 hours *or*
2 g every 12 hours; 2 g every 8–12 hours in severe
infections; single doses over 1 g intravenous route
only; elderly usual max. 3 g daily; CHILD, up to 2
months 25–60 mg/kg daily in 2 divided doses,
over 2 months 30–100 mg/kg daily in 2–3 divided
doses; up to 150 mg/kg daily (max. 6 g daily) in 3
divided doses if immunocompromised or meningitis; intravenous route recommended for children
Urinary-tract and less serious infections, 0.5–1 g
every 12 hours
Pseudomonal lung infection in cystic fibrosis,
ADULT with normal renal function 100–150 mg/
kg daily in 3 divided doses; CHILD up to 150 mg/
kg daily (max. 6 g daily) in 3 divided doses; intravenous route recommended for children
Surgical prophylaxis, prostatic surgery, 1 g at
induction of anaesthesia repeated if necessary
when catheter removed

Fortum® (GlaxoWellcome) PoM
Injection, powder for reconstitution, ceftazidime
(as pentahydrate), with sodium carbonate, net
price 250-mg vial = £2.37, 500-mg vial = £4.73,
1-g vial = £9.45, 2-g vial (for injection and for
infusion, both) = £18.91, 3-g vial (for injection or
infusion) = £27.70; *Monovial*, 2 g vial (with transfer needle) = £18.91
Electrolytes: Na⁺ 2.3 mmol/g

Kefadim® (Lilly) PoM
Injection, powder for reconstitution, ceftazidime
(as pentahydrate), with sodium carbonate, net
price 500-mg vial = £4.95, 1-g vial = £9.90, 2-g
vial (for injection and for infusion, both) = £19.80
Electrolytes: Na⁺ 2.3 mmol/g

CEFTRIAXONE

Indications: see under Cefaclor and notes above;
surgical prophylaxis; prophylaxis of meningococcal meningitis [unlicensed indication] (Table
2, section 5.1)

Cautions: see under Cefaclor; severe renal impairment (Appendix 3); hepatic impairment if accompanied by renal impairment (Appendix 2);
premature neonates; may displace bilirubin from
serum albumin, administer over 60 minutes in
neonates (see also Contra-indications)

Contra-indications: see under Cefaclor; neonates
with jaundice, hypoalbuminaemia, acidosis or
impaired bilirubin binding

Side-effects: see under Cefaclor; calcium ceftriaxone precipitates in urine (particularly in very
young, dehydrated or those who are immobilised)
or in gall bladder—consider discontinuation if
symptomatic; rarely prolongation of prothrombin
time, pancreatitis

Dose: *by deep intramuscular injection, or by intravenous injection* over at least 2–4 minutes, *or by
intravenous infusion*, 1 g daily; 2–4 g daily in
severe infections; intramuscular doses over 1 g
divided between more than one site
INFANT and CHILD 20–50 mg/kg daily; up to
80 mg/kg daily in severe infections; doses of
50 mg/kg and over by intravenous infusion only;
NEONATES *by intravenous infusion* over 60 minutes, 20–50 mg/kg daily (max. 50 mg/kg daily)
Uncomplicated gonorrhoea, *by deep intramuscular
injection*, 250 mg as a single dose
Surgical prophylaxis, *by deep intramuscular injection or by intravenous injection* over at least 2–4
minutes, 1 g at induction; colorectal surgery, *by
deep intramuscular injection or by intravenous
injection* over at least 2–4 minutes *or by intravenous infusion*, 2 g at induction; intramuscular
doses over 1 g divided between more than one site

Ceftriaxone (Non-proprietary) PoM
Injection, powder for reconstitution, ceftriaxone
(as sodium salt), net price 1-g vial = £9.95; 2-g
vial = £19.95
Available from Genus

Rocephin® (Roche) PoM
Injection, powder for reconstitution, ceftriaxone
(as sodium salt), net price 250-mg vial = £2.74; 1-
g vial = £10.94; 2-g vial = £21.89
Electrolytes: Na⁺ 3.6 mmol/g

CEFUROXIME

Indications: see under Cefaclor; surgical prophylaxis; more active against *Haemophilus influenzae* and *Neisseria gonorrhoeae*; Lyme disease

Cautions: see under Cefaclor

Contra-indications: see under Cefaclor

Side-effects: see under Cefaclor

Dose: *by mouth* (as cefuroxime axetil), 250 mg
twice daily in most infections including mild to
moderate lower respiratory-tract infections (e.g.
bronchitis); doubled for more severe lower respiratory-tract infections or if pneumonia suspected
Urinary-tract infection, 125 mg twice daily, doubled in pyelonephritis
Gonorrhoea, 1 g as a single dose
CHILD over 3 months, 125 mg twice daily, if necessary doubled in child over 2 years with otitis
media
Lyme disease, ADULT and CHILD over 12 years,
500 mg twice daily for 20 days
*By intramuscular injection or intravenous injection
or infusion*, 750 mg every 6–8 hours; 1.5 g every
6–8 hours in severe infections; single doses over
750 mg intravenous route only
CHILD usual dose 60 mg/kg daily (range 30–
100 mg/kg daily) in 3–4 divided doses (2–3
divided doses in neonates)
Gonorrhoea, 1.5 g as a single dose by intramuscu-

lar injection (divided between 2 sites)
Surgical prophylaxis, 1.5 g by intravenous injection at induction; further doses of 750 mg may be given by intramuscular injection every 8 hours for high-risk procedures
Meningitis, 3 g intravenously every 8 hours; CHILD, 200–240 mg/kg daily (in 3–4 divided doses) reduced to 100 mg/kg daily after 3 days or on clinical improvement; NEONATE, 100 mg/kg daily reduced to 50 mg/kg daily

Zinacef® (GlaxoWellcome) PoM
Injection, powder for reconstitution, cefuroxime (as sodium salt). Net price 250-mg vial = 84p; 750-mg vial = £2.52; 1.5-g vial = £5.05
Electrolytes: Na⁺ 1.8 mmol/750-mg vial

Zinnat® (GlaxoWellcome) PoM
Tablets, both f/c, cefuroxime (as axetil) 125 mg, net price 14-tab pack = £4.73; 250 mg, 14-tab pack = £9.45. Label: 9, 21, 25
Suspension, cefuroxime (as axetil) 125 mg/5 mL when reconstituted with water, net price 70 mL = £5.40. Label: 9, 21
Sachets, cefuroxime (as axetil) 125 mg/sachet, net price 14-sachet pack = £5.40. Label: 9, 13, 21

Other beta-lactam antibiotics

Aztreonam is a monocyclic beta-lactam ('monobactam') antibiotic with an antibacterial spectrum limited to Gram-negative aerobic bacteria including *Pseudomonas aeruginosa*, *Neisseria meningitidis*, and *Haemophilus influenzae*; it should not be used alone for 'blind' treatment since it is not active against Gram-positive organisms. Aztreonam is also effective against *Neisseria gonorrhoeae* (but not against concurrent chlamydial infection). Side-effects are similar to those of the other beta-lactams although aztreonam may be less likely to cause hypersensitivity in penicillin-sensitive patients.

Imipenem, a carbapenem, has a broad spectrum of activity which includes many aerobic and anaerobic Gram-positive and Gram-negative bacteria. Imipenem is partially inactivated in the kidney by enzymatic activity and is therefore administered in combination with **cilastatin**, a specific enzyme inhibitor, which blocks its renal metabolism. Side-effects are similar to those of other beta-lactam antibiotics; neurotoxicity has been observed at very high dosage or in renal failure. **Meropenem** is similar to imipenem but is stable to the renal enzyme which inactivates imipenem and therefore can be given without cilastatin. Meropenem has less seizure-inducing potential and can be used to treat central nervous system infection.

AZTREONAM

Indications: Gram-negative infections including *Pseudomonas aeruginosa*, *Haemophilus influenzae*, and *Neisseria meningitidis*
Cautions: hypersensitivity to beta-lactam antibiotics; hepatic impairment; reduce dose in renal impairment; breast-feeding (Appendix 5); **interactions:** Appendix 1 (aztreonam)
Contra-indications: aztreonam hypersensitivity; pregnancy

Side-effects: nausea, vomiting, diarrhoea, abdominal cramps; mouth ulcers, altered taste; jaundice and hepatitis; blood disorders (including thrombocytopenia and neutropenia); urticaria and rashes
Dose: *by deep intramuscular injection or by intravenous injection* over 3–5 minutes *or by intravenous infusion*, 1 g every 8 hours *or* 2 g every 12 hours; 2 g every 6–8 hours for severe infections (including systemic *Pseudomonas aeruginosa* and lung infections in cystic fibrosis); single doses over 1 g intravenous route only
CHILD over 1 week, *by intravenous injection or infusion*, 30 mg/kg every 6–8 hours increased in severe infections for child of 2 years or older to 50 mg/kg every 6–8 hours; max. 8 g daily
Urinary-tract infections, 0.5–1 g every 8–12 hours
Gonorrhoea/cystitis, *by intramuscular injection*, 1 g as a single dose

Azactam® (Squibb) PoM
Injection, powder for reconstitution, aztreonam. Net price 500-mg vial = £4.48; 1-g vial = £8.95; 2-g vial = £17.90

IMIPENEM WITH CILASTATIN

Indications: aerobic and anaerobic Gram-positive and Gram-negative infections; surgical prophylaxis; hospital-acquired septicaemia (Table 1, section 5.1); not indicated for CNS infections
Cautions: renal impairment (Appendix 3); CNS disorders (e.g. epilepsy); pregnancy (Appendix 4); **interactions:** Appendix 1 (*Primaxin®*)
Contra-indications: hypersensitivity to beta-lactam antibiotics; breast-feeding (Appendix 5)
Side-effects: nausea, vomiting, diarrhoea (antibiotic-associated colitis reported), taste disturbances, tooth or tongue discoloration, hearing loss; blood disorders, positive Coombs' test; allergic reactions (with rash, pruritus, urticaria, Stevens-Johnson syndrome, fever, anaphylactic reactions, rarely toxic epidermal necrolysis, exfoliative dermatitis); myoclonic activity, convulsions, confusion and mental disturbances reported; slight increases in liver enzymes and bilirubin reported, rarely hepatitis; increases in serum creatinine and blood urea; red coloration of urine in children reported; local reactions: erythema, pain and induration, and thrombophlebitis
Dose: *by deep intramuscular injection*, mild to moderate infections, in terms of imipenem, 500–750 mg every 12 hours
By intravenous infusion, in terms of imipenem, 1–2 g daily (in 3–4 divided doses); less sensitive organisms, up to 50 mg/kg daily (max. 4 g daily) in 3–4 divided doses; CHILD 3 months and older, 60 mg/kg (up to max. of 2 g) daily in 4 divided doses; over 40 kg, adult dose
Surgical prophylaxis, *by intravenous infusion*, 1 g at induction of anaesthesia repeated after 3 hours, supplemented in high risk (e.g. colorectal) surgery by doses of 500 mg 8 and 16 hours after induction

Primaxin® (MSD) PoM
Intramuscular injection, powder for reconstitution, imipenem (as monohydrate) 500 mg with cila-

statin (as sodium salt) 500 mg, net price per vial = £12.00

Electrolytes: Na⁺ 1.47 mmol/vial

Intravenous infusion, powder for reconstitution, imipenem (as monohydrate) 500 mg with cilastatin (as sodium salt) 500 mg, net price per vial = £12.00; *Monovial* (vial with transfer needle) = £12.00

Electrolytes: Na⁺ 1.72 mmol/vial

MEROPENEM

Indications: aerobic and anaerobic Gram-positive and Gram-negative infections

Cautions: hypersensitivity to penicillins, cephalosporins and other beta-lactam antibiotics; hepatic impairment (monitor liver function); renal impairment (Appendix 3); pregnancy and breast-feeding; **interactions:** Appendix 1 (meropenem)

Contra-indications: hypersensitivity to meropenem

Side-effects: nausea, vomiting, diarrhoea (antibiotic-associated colitis reported), abdominal pain; disturbances in liver function tests; thrombocytopenia (reduction in partial thromboplastin time reported), positive Coombs' test, eosinophilia, leucopenia, neutropenia; headache, paraesthesia; hypersensitivity reactions including rash, pruritus, urticaria, angioedema, and anaphylaxis; also reported, convulsions, Stevens-Johnson syndrome and toxic epidermal necrolysis; local reactions including pain and thrombophlebitis at injection site

Dose: *by intravenous injection* over 5 minutes *or by intravenous infusion,* 500 mg every 8 hours, dose doubled in hospital-acquired pneumonia, peritonitis, septicaemia and infections in neutropenic patients; CHILD 3 months–12 years [not licensed for infection in neutropenia] 10–20 mg/kg every 8 hours, over 50 kg body weight adult dose

Meningitis, 2 g every 8 hours; CHILD 3 months–12 years 40 mg/kg every 8 hours, over 50 kg body weight adult dose

Exacerbations of chronic lower respiratory-tract infection in cystic fibrosis, up to 2 g every 8 hours; CHILD 4–18 years 25–40 mg/kg every 8 hours

Meronem® (AstraZeneca) [PoM]

Injection, powder for reconstitution, meropenem (as trihydrate) net price 500-mg vial = £14.33; 1-g vial = £28.65

Electrolytes: Na⁺ 3.9 mmol/g

5.1.3 Tetracyclines

The tetracyclines are broad-spectrum antibiotics whose value has decreased owing to increasing bacterial resistance. They remain, however, the treatment of choice for infections caused by chlamydia (trachoma, psittacosis, salpingitis, urethritis, and lymphogranuloma venereum), rickettsia (including Q-fever), brucella (doxycycline with either streptomycin or rifampicin), and the spirochaete, *Borrelia burgdorferi* (Lyme disease—see also section 5.1.1.3). They are also used in respiratory and genital mycoplasma infections, in acne, in destructive (refractory) periodontal disease, in exacerbations of

chronic bronchitis (because of their activity against *Haemophilus influenzae*), and for leptospirosis in penicillin hypersensitivity (as an alternative to erythromycin).

Microbiologically, there is little to choose between the various tetracyclines, the only exception being **minocycline** which has a broader spectrum; it is active against *Neisseria meningitidis* and has been used for meningococcal prophylaxis but is no longer recommended because of side-effects including dizziness and vertigo (see section 5.1, table 2 for current recommendations).

The tetracyclines are deposited in growing bone and teeth (being bound to calcium) causing staining and occasionally dental hypoplasia, and should **not** be given to children under 12 years or to pregnant or breast-feeding women. With the exception of **doxycycline** and **minocycline** the tetracyclines may exacerbate renal failure and should **not** be given to patients with kidney disease. Absorption of tetracyclines is decreased by milk (except doxycycline, lymecycline and minocycline), antacids, and calcium, iron, magnesium and zinc salts.

TETRACYCLINE

Indications: exacerbations of chronic bronchitis; brucellosis (see also notes above), chlamydia, mycoplasma, and rickettsia; acne vulgaris, rosacea (section 13.6)

Cautions: hepatic impairment; **interactions:** Appendix 1 (tetracyclines)

Contra-indications: renal impairment (Appendix 3), pregnancy and breast-feeding (see also Appendixes 4 and 5), children under 12 years

Side-effects: nausea, vomiting, diarrhoea, dysphagia, oesophageal irritation; hypersensitivity reactions (including rash, exfoliative dermatitis, urticaria, angioedema, anaphylaxis, pericarditis); exacerbation of systemic lupus erythematosus and of myasthenia gravis; headache and visual disturbances may indicate benign intracranial hypertension; hepatotoxicity, pancreatitis and antibiotic-associated colitis reported; rarely photosensitivity, skin discoloration, blood dyscrasias; see also notes above

Dose: *by mouth,* 250 mg every 6 hours, increased in severe infections to 500 mg every 6–8 hours

Acne, see section 13.6.2

Non-gonococcal urethritis, 500 mg every 6 hours for 7–14 days (21 days if failure or relapse after first course)

COUNSELLING. Tablets or capsules should be swallowed whole with plenty of fluid while sitting or standing

Tetracycline (Non-proprietary) [PoM]

Capsules, tetracycline hydrochloride 250 mg, net price 20 = 96p. Label: 7, 9, 23, counselling, posture

Available from DDSA (*Economycin®*)

Tablets, coated, tetracycline hydrochloride 250 mg, net price 28-tab pack = £1.04. Label: 7, 9, 23, counselling, posture

Available from Alpharma, Hillcross, IVAX, Kent

Achromycin® (Lederle) [PoM]

Capsules, orange, tetracycline hydrochloride 250 mg, net price 28-cap pack = £1.34. Label: 7, 9, 23, counselling, posture

■ Compound preparations

Deteclo® (Lederle) PoM
Tablets, blue, f/c, tetracycline hydrochloride
115.4 mg, chlortetracycline hydrochloride
115.4 mg, demeclocycline hydrochloride 69.2 mg,
net price 14-tab pack = £1.83. Label: 7, 9, 11, 23,
counselling, posture
Dose: 1 tablet every 12 hours; 3–4 tablets daily in more
severe infections

DEMECLOCYCLINE HYDROCHLORIDE

Indications: see under Tetracycline; also inappropriate secretion of antidiuretic hormone, section 6.5.2
Cautions: see under Tetracycline, but photosensitivity more common (avoid exposure to sunlight or sun lamps)
Contra-indications: see under Tetracycline
Side-effects: see under Tetracycline; reversible nephrogenic diabetes insipidus reported
Dose: 150 mg every 6 hours *or* 300 mg every 12 hours

Ledermycin® (Lederle) PoM
Capsules, red, demeclocycline hydrochloride
150 mg, net price 28-cap pack = £5.78. Label: 7, 9, 11, 23

DOXYCYCLINE

Indications: see under Tetracycline; brucellosis (with rifampicin); also chronic prostatitis and sinusitis; syphilis; pelvic inflammatory disease (Table 1, section 5.1); treatment and prophylaxis of anthrax; malaria treatment and prophylaxis (section 5.4.1)
Cautions: see under Tetracycline, but may be used in renal impairment; alcohol dependence; photosensitivity reported (avoid exposure to sunlight or sun lamps); avoid in porphyria (section 9.8.2)
Contra-indications: see under Tetracycline
Side-effects: see under Tetracycline; anorexia
Dose: 200 mg on first day, then 100 mg daily; severe infections (including refractory urinary-tract infections), 200 mg daily
Early syphilis, 200 mg twice daily for 14 days; late latent syphilis 200 mg twice daily for 28 days
Uncomplicated genital chlamydia, non-gonococcal urethritis, 100 mg twice daily for 7 days (14 days in pelvic inflammatory disease, see also Table 1, section 5.1)
Anthrax (treatment or post-exposure prophylaxis; see also section 5.1.12), 100 mg twice daily; CHILD (only if alternative antibacterial cannot be given) [unlicensed dose] 5 mg/kg daily in 2 divided doses
COUNSELLING. Capsules should be swallowed whole with plenty of fluid during meals while sitting or standing
Note. Doxycycline doses in BNF may differ from those in product literature

Doxycycline (Non-proprietary) PoM
Capsules, doxycycline (as hyclate) 50 mg, net price 28-cap pack = £6.77; 100 mg, 8-cap pack = £2.49. Label: 6, 9, 11, 27, counselling, posture
Available from Alpharma, APS, Ashbourne (*Demix®*), Berk (*Cyclodox®*), Dominion, Hillcross, IVAX, Kent, Lagap (*Doxylar®*)

Vibramycin® (Pfizer) PoM
Capsules, doxycycline (as hyclate) 50 mg (green/ivory), net price 28-cap pack = £7.74, 56-cap pack (*Acne Pack*) = £17.80; 100 mg (green), 8-cap pack = £4.18. Label: 6, 9, 11, 27, counselling, posture

Vibramycin-D® (Pfizer) PoM
Dispersible tablets, off-white, doxycycline (as monohydrate) 100 mg. Net price 8-tab pack = £4.91. Label: 6, 9, 11, 13

LYMECYCLINE

Indications: see under Tetracycline
Cautions: see under Tetracycline
Contra-indications: see under Tetracycline
Side-effects: see under Tetracycline
Dose: 408 mg every 12 hours, increased to 1.224–1.632 g daily in severe infections
Acne, 408 mg daily for at least 8 weeks

Tetralysal 300® (Galderma) PoM
Capsules, lymecycline 408 mg (≡ tetracycline 300 mg). Net price 28-cap pack = £4.97. Label: 6, 9

MINOCYCLINE

Indications: see under Tetracycline; also meningococcal carrier state
Cautions: see under Tetracycline, but may be used in renal impairment; if treatment continued for longer than 6 months, monitor for hepatotoxicity, pigmentation and for systemic lupus erythematosus—discontinue if these develop or if pre-existing systemic lupus erythematosus worsens
Contra-indications: see under Tetracycline
Side-effects: see under Tetracycline; also anorexia, dizziness, tinnitus and vertigo (more common in women); pigmentation (sometimes irreversible), discoloration of conjunctiva, tears and sweat, systemic lupus erythematosus
Dose: 100 mg twice daily
Acne, see section 13.6.2
Prophylaxis of asymptomatic meningococcal carrier state (but no longer recommended, see notes above), 100 mg twice daily for 5 days usually followed by rifampicin
COUNSELLING. Tablets or capsules should be swallowed whole with plenty of fluid while sitting or standing

Minocycline (Non-proprietary) PoM
Capsules, minocycline (as hydrochloride) 50 mg, net price 56-cap pack = £17.20; 100 mg, 28-cap pack = £14.74. Label: 6, 9, counselling, posture
Available from Crookes (*Aknemin®*)
Tablets, minocycline (as hydrochloride) 50 mg, net price 28-tab pack = £7.65, 84-tab pack = £26.99; 100 mg, 28-tab pack = £11.45. Label: 6, 9, counselling, posture
Available from Alpharma, Ashbourne (*Blemix®*), CP, Generics, Hillcross, IVAX, Kent, Lederle (*Minocin®*)

Minocin MR® (Lederle) PoM
Capsules, m/r, orange/brown (enclosing yellow and orange pellets), minocycline (as hydrochloride) 100 mg. Net price 56-cap pack = £35.23. Label: 6, 25
Dose: acne, 1 capsule daily

OXYTETRACYCLINE

Indications: see under Tetracycline
Cautions: see under Tetracycline; porphyria (section 9.8.2)
Contra-indications: see under Tetracycline
Side-effects: see under Tetracycline
Dose: 250–500 mg every 6 hours
Acne, see section 13.6.2

Oxytetracycline (Non-proprietary) PoM
Tablets, coated, oxytetracycline dihydrate 250 mg, net price 28-tab pack = 81p. Label: 7, 9, 23
Available from Alpharma, APS, Ashbourne (*Oxytetramix*®), DDSA (*Oxymycin*®), IVAX, Kent

Terramycin® (Pfizer) PoM
Tablets, yellow, s/c, oxytetracycline (as dihydrate) 250 mg, net price 28-tab pack = 96p. Label: 7, 9, 23

5.1.4   Aminoglycosides

These include amikacin, gentamicin, neomycin, netilmicin, streptomycin, and tobramycin. All are bactericidal and active against some Gram-positive and many Gram-negative organisms. Amikacin, gentamicin, and tobramycin are also active against *Pseudomonas aeruginosa*; streptomycin is active against *Mycobacterium tuberculosis* and is now almost entirely reserved for tuberculosis (section 5.1.9).

The aminoglycosides are not absorbed from the gut (although there is a risk of absorption in inflammatory bowel disease and liver failure) and must therefore be given by injection for systemic infections.

Excretion is principally via the kidney and accumulation occurs in renal impairment.

Most side-effects of this group of antibiotics are dose-related therefore care must be taken with dosage and whenever possible treatment should not exceed 7 days. The important side-effects are ototoxicity, and nephrotoxicity; they occur most commonly in the elderly and in patients with renal failure.

If there is impairment of renal function (or high pre-dose serum concentrations) the interval between doses must be increased; if the renal impairment is severe the dose itself should be reduced as well.

Aminoglycosides may impair neuromuscular transmission and should not be given to patients with myasthenia gravis; large doses given during surgery have been responsible for a transient myasthenic syndrome in patients with normal neuromuscular function.

Aminoglycosides should preferably not be given with potentially ototoxic diuretics (e.g. furosemide (frusemide)); if concurrent use is unavoidable administration of the aminoglycoside and of the diuretic should be separated by as long a period as practicable.

SERUM CONCENTRATIONS. Serum concentration monitoring avoids both excessive and subtherapeutic concentrations thus preventing toxicity and ensuring efficacy. In patients with normal renal function, aminoglycoside concentrations should be measured after 3 or 4 doses; patients with renal impairment may require earlier and more frequent measurement of aminoglycoside concentration.

Blood samples should be taken approximately 1 hour after intramuscular or intravenous administration ('peak' concentration) and also just before the next dose ('trough' concentration).

Serum aminoglycoside concentrations should be measured in all patients and **must** be determined in infants, in the elderly, in obesity, and in cystic fibrosis, *or* if high doses are being given, *or* if there is renal impairment.

ONCE DAILY DOSAGE. Although aminoglycosides are generally given in 2–3 divided doses during the 24 hours, *once daily administration* is more convenient (while ensuring adequate serum concentration) but **expert advice** about dosage and serum concentrations should be obtained.

ENDOCARDITIS. **Gentamicin** is used in combination with other antibiotics for the treatment of bacterial endocarditis (Table 1, section 5.1). Serum-gentamicin concentration should be determined twice each week (more often in renal impairment).

For *streptococcal* and *enterococcal endocarditis* see under Gentamicin. **Streptomycin** may be used as an alternative in gentamicin-resistant enterococcal endocarditis.

In *staphylococcal endocarditis*, gentamicin is given in conventional doses to achieve a one-hour ('peak') serum-gentamicin concentration of 5–10 mg/litre and a pre-dose ('trough') concentration of less than 2 mg/litre.

Gentamicin is the aminoglycoside of choice in the UK and is used widely for the treatment of serious infections. It has a broad spectrum but is inactive against anaerobes and has poor activity against haemolytic streptococci and pneumococci. When used for the 'blind' therapy of undiagnosed serious infections it is usually given in conjunction with a penicillin or metronidazole (or both). Gentamicin is used together with another antibiotic for the treatment of endocarditis (see above and Table 1, section 5.1).

The dose of gentamicin for most infections is up to 5 mg/kg daily given in divided doses every 8 hours (if renal function is normal); whenever possible treatment should not exceed 7 days. Higher doses are occasionally indicated for serious infections, especially in the neonate or the immunocompromised patient. Loading and maintenance doses may be calculated on the basis of the patient's weight and renal function (e.g. using a nomogram); adjustments are then made according to serum-gentamicin concentrations.

Amikacin is a derivative of kanamycin and has one important advantage over gentamicin in that it is more stable than gentamicin to enzyme inactivation. Amikacin is used in the treatment of serious infections caused by gentamicin-resistant Gram-negative bacilli.

Netilmicin has similar activity to gentamicin, but may cause less ototoxicity in those needing treatment for longer than 10 days. Netilmicin is active against a number of gentamicin-resistant Gram-negative bacilli but is less active against *Ps. aeruginosa* than gentamicin or tobramycin.

Tobramycin has similar activity to gentamicin. It is slightly more active against *Ps. aeruginosa* but shows less activity against certain other Gram-negative bacteria. Tobramycin may be administered by nebuliser on a cyclical basis (28 days of tobramycin followed by a 28-day tobramycin-free interval) for the treatment of chronic pulmonary *Ps. aeruginosa* infection in cystic fibrosis; however, resistance may develop and some patients do not respond to treatment.

Neomycin is too toxic for parenteral administration and can only be used for infections of the skin or mucous membranes or to reduce the bacterial population of the colon prior to bowel surgery or in hepatic failure. Oral administration may lead to malabsorption. Small amounts of neomycin may be absorbed from the gut in patients with hepatic failure and, as these patients may also be uraemic, cumulation may occur with resultant ototoxicity.

GENTAMICIN

Indications: septicaemia and neonatal sepsis; meningitis and other CNS infections; biliary-tract infection, acute pyelonephritis or prostatitis, endocarditis (see notes above); pneumonia in hospital patients, adjunct in listerial meningitis (Table 1, section 5.1)

Cautions: pregnancy (Appendix 4), renal impairment, infants and elderly (adjust dose and monitor renal, auditory and vestibular function together with serum gentamicin concentrations); avoid prolonged use; conditions characterised by muscular weakness; see also notes above; **interactions:** Appendix 1 (aminoglycosides)

Contra-indications: myasthenia gravis

Side-effects: vestibular and auditory damage, nephrotoxicity; rarely, hypomagnesaemia on prolonged therapy, antibiotic-associated colitis; also reported, nausea, vomiting, rash; see also notes above

Dose: *by intramuscular or by slow intravenous injection* over at least 3 minutes *or by intravenous infusion*, 3–5 mg/kg daily (in divided doses every 8 hours), see also notes above

CHILD up to 2 weeks, 3 mg/kg every 12 hours; 2 weeks–12 years, 2 mg/kg every 8 hours

Streptococcal or enterococcal endocarditis in combination with other drugs, 80 mg twice daily

Endocarditis prophylaxis, Table 2, section 5.1

By intrathecal injection, seek specialist advice, 1 mg daily (increased if necessary to 5 mg daily)

Note. One-hour ('peak') serum concentration should be 5–10 mg/litre (3–5 mg/litre for streptococcal or enterococcal endocarditis); pre-dose ('trough') concentration should be less than 2 mg/litre (less than 1 mg/litre for streptococcal or enterococcal endocarditis)

Gentamicin (Non-proprietary) PoM
Injection, gentamicin (as sulphate), net price 40 mg/mL, 1-mL amp = £1.40, 2-mL amp = £1.54, 2-mL vial = £1.54, 6-mL vial = £4.62
Available from Faulding DBL

Cidomycin® (Hoechst Marion Roussel) PoM
Injection, gentamicin 40 mg (as sulphate)/mL. Net price 2-mL amp or vial = £1.55
Paediatric injection, gentamicin 10 mg (as sulphate)/mL. Net price 2-mL vial = 65p
Intrathecal injection, gentamicin 5 mg (as sulphate)/mL. Net price 1-mL amp = 77p

Genticin® (Roche) PoM
Injection, gentamicin 40 mg (as sulphate)/mL. Net price 2-mL amp = £1.51

Isotonic Gentamicin Injection (Baxter) PoM
Intravenous infusion, gentamicin 800 micrograms (as sulphate)/mL in sodium chloride intravenous infusion 0.9%. Net price 100-mL (80-mg) Viaflex® bag = £1.61
Electrolytes: Na+ 15.4 mmol/100-mL bag

AMIKACIN

Indications: serious Gram-negative infections resistant to gentamicin

Cautions: see under Gentamicin

Contra-indications: see under Gentamicin

Side-effects: see under Gentamicin

Dose: *by intramuscular or by slow intravenous injection or by infusion*, 15 mg/kg daily in 2 divided doses, increased to 22.5 mg/kg daily in 3 divided doses in severe infections; max. 1.5 g daily for up to 10 days (max. cumulative dose 15 g); CHILD 15 mg/kg daily in 2 divided doses; NEONATE 10 mg/kg initially then 15 mg/kg daily in 2 divided doses

Note. One-hour ('peak') serum concentration should not exceed 30 mg/litre; pre-dose ('trough') concentration should be less than 10 mg/litre

Amikacin (Non-proprietary) PoM
Injection, amikacin (as sulphate) 250 mg/mL. Net price 2-mL vial = £9.64
Electrolytes: Na+ 0.56 mmol/500-mg vial
Available from Faulding DBL

Amikin® (Bristol-Myers Squibb) PoM
Injection, amikacin (as sulphate) 250 mg/mL. Net price 2-mL vial = £10.14
Electrolytes: Na+ <0.5 mmol/vial
Paediatric injection, amikacin (as sulphate) 50 mg/mL. Net price 2-mL vial = £2.36
Electrolytes: Na+ <0.5 mmol/vial

NEOMYCIN SULPHATE

Indications: bowel sterilisation before surgery, see also notes above

Cautions: see under Gentamicin but too toxic for systemic use, see notes above

Contra-indications: see under Gentamicin; intestinal obstruction

Side-effects: see under Gentamicin but poorly absorbed on oral administration; increased salivation, stomatitis

Dose: *by mouth*, pre-operative bowel sterilisation, 1 g every hour for 4 hours, then 1 g every 4 hours for 2–3 days
Hepatic coma, up to 4 g daily in divided doses usually for max. 14 days

Nivemycin® (Sovereign) PoM
Tablets, neomycin sulphate 500 mg. Net price 20 = £3.44

NETILMICIN

Indications: serious Gram-negative infections resistant to gentamicin

Cautions: see under Gentamicin

Contra-indications: see under Gentamicin

Side-effects: see under Gentamicin

Dose: *by intramuscular injection or by intravenous injection over 3–5 minutes or by intravenous infusion*, 4–6 mg/kg daily, as a single daily dose or in divided doses every 8 or 12 hours; in severe infections, up to 7.5 mg/kg daily in divided doses every 8 hours (reduced as soon as clinically indicated, usually within 48 hours) NEONATE up to 1 week, 3 mg/kg every 12 hours; INFANT over 1 week, 2.5–3 mg/kg every 8 hours; CHILD 2–2.5 mg/kg every 8 hours

Urinary-tract infection, 150 mg as a single daily dose for 5 days

Gonorrhoea, 300 mg as a single dose

Note. For divided daily dose regimens, one-hour ('peak') serum concentration should not exceed 12 mg/litre; pre-dose ('trough') concentration should be less than 2 mg/litre

Netillin® (Schering-Plough) PoM
Injection, netilmicin (as sulphate) 10 mg/mL, net price 1.5-mL (15-mg) amp = £1.42; 50 mg/mL, 1-mL (50-mg) amp = £2.11; 100 mg/mL, 1-mL (100-mg) amp = £2.75; 1.5-mL (150-mg) amp = £3.92, 2-mL (200-mg) amp = £5.09

TOBRAMYCIN

Indications: see under Gentamicin and notes above

Cautions: see under Gentamicin
SPECIFIC CAUTIONS FOR INHALED TREATMENT. Other inhaled drugs should be administered before tobramycin; monitor for bronchospasm with initial dose, measure peak flow before and after nebulisation—if bronchospasm occurs, repeat test using bronchodilator; monitor renal function before treatment and then every 6 months; severe haemoptysis

Contra-indications: see under Gentamicin

Side-effects: see under Gentamicin; *on inhalation*, voice alteration, cough

Dose: *by intramuscular injection or by slow intravenous injection or by intravenous infusion*, 3 mg/kg daily in divided doses every 8 hours, see also notes above; in severe infections up to 5 mg/kg daily in divided doses every 6–8 hours (reduced to 3 mg/kg as soon as clinically indicated); NEONATE 2 mg/kg every 12 hours; CHILD over 1 week 2–2.5 mg/kg every 8 hours

Urinary-tract infection, *by intramuscular injection*, 2–3 mg/kg daily as a single dose

Note. One-hour ('peak') serum concentration should not exceed 10 mg/litre; pre-dose ('trough') concentration should be less than 2 mg/litre

Chronic pulmonary *Pseudomonas aeruginosa* infection in cystic fibrosis patients, *by inhalation of nebulised solution*, ADULT and CHILD over 6 years, 300 mg every 12 hours for 28 days, courses repeated after 28-day interval

Tobramycin (Non-proprietary) PoM
Injection, tobramycin (as sulphate) 40 mg/mL, net price 1-mL (40-mg) vial = £2.46, 2-mL (80-mg) vial = £3.77, 6-mL (240-mg) vial = £12.47
Available from Alpharma, Faulding DBL

Nebcin® (King) PoM
Injection, tobramycin (as sulphate) 10 mg/mL, net price 2-mL (20-mg) vial = £2.27; 40 mg/mL, 2-mL (80-mg) vial = £5.52

Tobi® (PathoGenesis) ▼ PoM
Nebuliser solution, tobramycin 60 mg/mL, net price 56 × 5-mL (300-mg) unit = £1540.00

Erythromycin has an antibacterial spectrum that is similar but not identical to that of penicillin; it is thus an alternative in penicillin-allergic patients.

Indications for erythromycin include respiratory infections, whooping cough, legionnaires' disease, and campylobacter enteritis. It is active against many penicillin-resistant staphylococci but some are now also resistant to erythromycin; it has poor activity against *Haemophilus influenzae*. Erythromycin is also active against chlamydia and mycoplasmas.

Erythromycin causes nausea, vomiting, and diarrhoea in some patients; in mild to moderate infections this can be avoided by giving a lower dose (250 mg 4 times daily) but if a more serious infection, such as Legionella pneumonia, is suspected higher doses are needed.

Azithromycin is a macrolide with slightly less activity than erythromycin against Gram-positive bacteria but enhanced activity against some Gram-negative organisms including *H. influenzae*. Plasma concentrations are very low but tissue concentrations are much higher. It has a long tissue half-life and once daily dosage is recommended. For treatment of Lyme disease, see section 5.1.1.3.

Clarithromycin is an erythromycin derivative with slightly greater activity than the parent compound. Tissue concentrations are higher than with erythromycin. It is given twice daily.

Azithromycin and clarithromycin cause fewer gastro-intestinal side-effects than erythromycin.

Spiramycin is also a macrolide (section 5.4.7).

ERYTHROMYCIN

Indications: alternative to penicillin in hypersensitive patients; campylobacter enteritis, pneumonia, legionnaires' disease, syphilis, non-gonococcal urethritis, chronic prostatitis, diphtheria and whooping cough prophylaxis; acne vulgaris and rosacea (section 13.6)

Cautions: hepatic and renal impairment; prolongation of QT interval (ventricular tachycardia reported); porphyria (section 9.8.2); pregnancy (not known to be harmful) and breast-feeding (only small amounts in milk); **interactions:** Appendix 1 (erythromycin and other macrolides)
ARRHYTHMIAS. Avoid concomitant administration with pimozide or terfenadine [other interactions, Appendix 1]

Side-effects: nausea, vomiting, abdominal discomfort, diarrhoea (antibiotic-associated colitis reported); urticaria, rashes and other allergic reactions; reversible hearing loss reported after large doses; cholestatic jaundice, cardiac effects (including chest pain and arrhythmias), myasthenia-like syndrome, Stevens-Johnson syndrome, and toxic epidermal necrolysis also reported

Dose: *by mouth*, ADULT and CHILD over 8 years, 250–500 mg every 6 hours *or* 0.5–1 g every 12 hours (see notes above); up to 4 g daily in severe infections; CHILD up to 2 years 125 mg every 6 hours, 2–8 years 250 mg every 6 hours, doses doubled for severe infections

Early syphilis, 500 mg 4 times daily for 14 days

Uncomplicated genital chlamydia, non-gonococcal urethritis, 500 mg twice daily for 14 days

By intravenous infusion, ADULT and CHILD severe infections, 50 mg/kg daily by continuous infusion *or* in divided doses every 6 hours; mild infections (oral treatment not possible), 25 mg/kg daily

Erythromycin (Non-proprietary) PoM
Tablets, e/c, erythromycin 250 mg, net price 20 = £2.20. Label: 5, 9, 25
Available from Alpharma, APS, Ashbourne (*Rommix®*), Generics, IVAX, Kent

Erythromycin Ethyl Succinate (Non-proprietary) PoM
Oral suspension, erythromycin (as ethyl succinate) for reconstitution with water 125 mg/5 mL, net price 100 mL = £1.16; 250 mg/5 mL, 100 mL = £1.88; 500 mg/5 mL, 100 mL = £2.99. Label: 9
Note. Sugar-free versions are available and can be ordered by specifying 'sugar-free' on the prescription
Available from Alpharma, APS, Generics, Hillcross, IVAX, Kent

Erythromycin Lactobionate (Non-proprietary) PoM
Intravenous infusion, powder for reconstitution, erythromycin (as lactobionate), net price 1-g vial = £9.90
Available from Abbott, Faulding DBL

Erymax® (Elan) PoM
Capsules, opaque orange/clear orange, enclosing orange and white e/c pellets, erythromycin 250 mg, net price 28-cap pack = £5.41, 112-cap pack = £21.65. Label: 5, 9, 25
Dose: 1 capsule every 6 hours *or* 2 capsules every 12 hours; acne, 1 capsule twice daily for 1 month then 1 capsule daily

Erythrocin® (Abbott) PoM
Tablets, both f/c, erythromycin (as stearate), 250 mg, net price 20 = £2.72; 500 mg, 20 = £5.46. Label: 9

Erythroped® (Abbott) PoM
Suspension SF, sugar-free, banana-flavoured, erythromycin (as ethyl succinate) for reconstitution with water, 125 mg/5 mL (*Suspension PI SF*), net price 140 mL = £2.89; 250 mg/5 mL, 140 mL (*Suspension SF Forte*), 140 mL = £9.99. Label: 9

Erythroped A® (Abbott) PoM
Tablets, yellow, f/c, erythromycin 500 mg (as ethyl succinate). Net price 28-tab pack = £10.19. Label: 9

Tiloryth® (Tillomed) PoM
Capsules, enclosing e/c microgranules, erythromycin 250 mg. Net price 30-cap pack = £6.08. Label 5, 9, 25

AZITHROMYCIN

Indications: respiratory-tract infections; otitis media; skin and soft-tissue infections; uncomplicated genital chlamydial infections and non-gonococcal urethritis (Table 1, section 5.1)
Cautions: see under Erythromycin; pregnancy and breast-feeding; **interactions:** Appendix 1 (erythromycin and other macrolides)
Contra-indications: hepatic impairment
Side-effects: see under Erythromycin; anorexia, dyspepsia, constipation; dizziness, headache, drowsiness; photosensitivity; hepatitis, interstitial nephritis, acute renal failure, asthenia, paraesthesia, convulsions and mild neutropenia

reported; rarely tinnitus, hepatic necrosis, hepatic failure, Stevens-Johnson syndrome, toxic epidermal necrolysis and taste disturbances
Dose: 500 mg once daily for 3 days; CHILD over 6 months 10 mg/kg once daily for 3 days; *or* body-weight 15–25 kg, 200 mg once daily for 3 days; body-weight 26–35 kg, 300 mg once daily for 3 days; body-weight 36–45 kg, 400 mg once daily for 3 days
Uncomplicated genital chlamydial infections and non-gonococcal urethritis, 1 g as a single dose

Zithromax® (Pfizer) PoM
Capsules, azithromycin (as dihydrate) 250 mg, net price 4-cap pack = £8.95, 6-cap pack = £13.43. Label: 5, 9, 23
Tablets, f/c, azithromycin (as dihydrate) 500 mg, net price 3-tab pack = £10.99. Label: 5, 9
Oral suspension, cherry/banana-flavoured, azithromycin (as dihydrate) 200 mg/5 mL when reconstituted with water. Net price 15-mL pack = £5.08, 22.5-mL pack = £7.62, 30-mL pack = £13.80. Label: 5, 9

CLARITHROMYCIN

Indications: respiratory-tract infections, mild to moderate skin and soft tissue infections, otitis media; *Helicobacter pylori* eradication (section 1.3)
Cautions: see under Erythromycin; reduce dose in renal impairment; pregnancy and breast-feeding; **interactions:** Appendix 1 (erythromycin and other macrolides)
ARRHYTHMIAS. Avoid concomitant administration with pimozide or terfenadine [other interactions, Appendix 1]
Side-effects: see under Erythromycin; also reported, dyspepsia, headache, smell and taste disturbances, tooth and tongue discoloration, stomatitis, glossitis, arthralgia, myalgia, dizziness, vertigo, tinnitus, anxiety, insomnia, nightmares, confusion, psychosis, hypoglycaemia, cholestasis, jaundice, hepatitis, and Stevens-Johnson syndrome; on intravenous infusion, local tenderness; phlebitis
Dose: *by mouth,* 250 mg every 12 hours for 7 days, increased in severe infections to 500 mg every 12 hours for up to 14 days; CHILD body-weight under 8 kg, 7.5 mg/kg twice daily; 8–11 kg (1–2 years), 62.5 mg twice daily; 12–19 kg (3–6 years), 125 mg twice daily; 20–29 kg (7–9 years), 187.5 mg twice daily; 30–40 kg (10–12 years), 250 mg twice daily
By intravenous infusion into larger proximal vein, 500 mg twice daily; CHILD not recommended

Klaricid® (Abbott) PoM
Tablets, both yellow, f/c, clarithromycin 250 mg, net price 14-tab pack = £11.24; 500 mg, 14-tab pack = £22.49, 20-tab pack = £32.13. Label: 9
Paediatric suspension, clarithromycin for reconstitution with water 125 mg/5 mL, net price 70 mL = £6.00, 100 mL = £10.32; 250 mg/5 ml, 70ml = £12.00. Label: 9
Granules, clarithromycin 250 mg/sachet, net price 14-sachet pack = £12.00. Label: 9, 13
Intravenous infusion, powder for reconstitution, clarithromycin. Net price 500-mg vial = £10.93
Electrolytes: Na⁺ < 0.5 mmol/500-mg vial

Klaricid XL® (Abbott) PoM
Tablets, m/r, yellow, clarithromycin 500 mg, net price 7-tab pack = £10.68, 14-tab pack = £21.36. Label: 9, 21, 25
  Dose: 500 mg once daily (doubled in severe infections) for 7–14 days

5.1.6 Clindamycin

Clindamycin has only a limited use because of serious side-effects. Its most serious toxic effect is antibiotic-associated colitis (section 1.5) which may be fatal and is most common in middle-aged and elderly women, especially following operation. Although it can occur with most antibacterials it is more frequently seen with clindamycin. Patients should therefore discontinue treatment immediately if diarrhoea develops.

Clindamycin is active against Gram-positive cocci, including penicillin-resistant staphylococci and also against many anaerobes, especially *Bacteroides fragilis*. It is well concentrated in bone and excreted in bile and urine.

Clindamycin is recommended for staphylococcal joint and bone infections such as osteomyelitis, and intra-abdominal sepsis. Clindamycin is also used for endocarditis prophylaxis (section 5.1, table 2).

CLINDAMYCIN

Indications: staphylococcal bone and joint infections, peritonitis; endocarditis prophylaxis [unlicensed indication], Table 2, section 5.1

Cautions: discontinue immediately if diarrhoea or colitis develops; hepatic or renal impairment; monitor liver and renal function on prolonged therapy and in neonates and infants; pregnancy; breast-feeding (Appendix 5); avoid rapid intravenous administration; **interactions:** Appendix 1 (clindamycin)

Contra-indications: diarrhoeal states; avoid injections containing benzyl alcohol in neonates (see under preparations below)

Side-effects: diarrhoea (discontinue treatment), abdominal discomfort, nausea, vomiting, antibiotic-associated colitis; jaundice and altered liver function tests; neutropenia, eosinophilia, agranulocytosis and thrombocytopenia reported; rash, urticaria, erythema multiforme, exfoliative and vesiculobullous dermatitis reported; pain, induration, and abscess after intramuscular injection; thrombophlebitis after intravenous injection

Dose: *by mouth,* 150–300 mg every 6 hours; up to 450 mg every 6 hours in severe infections; CHILD, 3–6 mg/kg every 6 hours
  COUNSELLING. Patients should discontinue immediately and contact doctor if diarrhoea develops; capsules should be swallowed with a glass of water.
By deep intramuscular injection or by intravenous infusion, 0.6–2.7 g daily (in 2–4 divided doses); life-threatening infection, up to 4.8 g daily; single doses above 600 mg by intravenous infusion only; single doses by intravenous infusion not to exceed 1.2 g
  CHILD over 1 month, 15–40 mg/kg daily in 3–4 divided doses; severe infections, at least 300 mg daily regardless of weight

Dalacin C® (Pharmacia) PoM
Capsules, clindamycin (as hydrochloride) 75 mg (lavender), net price 24-cap pack = £5.93;

150 mg, (lavender/maroon), 24-cap pack = £10.92. Label: 9, 27, counselling, see above (diarrhoea)
Injection, clindamycin (as phosphate) 150 mg/mL, net price 2-mL amp = £4.94; 4-mL amp = £9.83
  Excipients: include benzyl alcohol (avoid in neonates, see Excipients, p. 2)

5.1.7 Some other antibacterials

Antibacterials discussed in this section include chloramphenicol, fusidic acid, glycopeptide antibiotics (vancomycin and teicoplanin), the streptogramins (quinupristin and dalfopristin) and the polymyxin, colistin.

Chloramphenicol

Chloramphenicol is a potent broad-spectrum antibiotic; however, it is associated with serious haematological side-effects when given systemically and should therefore be reserved for the treatment of life-threatening infections, particularly those caused by *Haemophilus influenzae*, and also for typhoid fever.

Chloramphenicol eye drops (section 11.3.1) and chloramphenicol ear drops (section 12.1.1) are also available.

CHLORAMPHENICOL

Indications: see notes above

Cautions: avoid repeated courses and prolonged treatment; reduce doses in hepatic impairment (Appendix 2); renal impairment (Appendix 3); blood counts required before and periodically during treatment; monitor plasma-chloramphenicol concentration in neonates (see below); **interactions:** Appendix 1 (chloramphenicol)

Contra-indications: pregnancy (see also Appendix 4), breast-feeding, porphyria (section 9.8.2)

Side-effects: blood disorders including reversible and irreversible aplastic anaemia (with reports of resulting leukaemia), peripheral neuritis, optic neuritis, erythema multiforme, nausea, vomiting, diarrhoea, stomatitis, glossitis; nocturnal haemoglobinuria reported; grey syndrome (abdominal distension, pallid cyanosis, circulatory collapse) may follow excessive doses in neonates with immature hepatic metabolism

Dose: *by mouth or by intravenous injection or infusion,* 50 mg/kg daily in 4 divided doses (exceptionally, can be doubled for severe infections such as septicaemia and meningitis, providing high doses reduced as soon as clinically indicated); CHILD, haemophilus epiglottitis and pyogenic meningitis, 50–100 mg/kg daily in divided doses (high dosages decreased as soon as clinically indicated); INFANTS under 2 weeks 25 mg/kg daily (in 4 divided doses), 2 weeks–1 year 50 mg/kg daily (in 4 divided doses)
  Note. Plasma concentration monitoring required in neonates and preferred in those under 4 years of age and in hepatic impairment; recommended peak plasma concentration (approx. 1 hour after intravenous injection or infusion) 15–25 mg/litre; pre-dose ('trough') concentration should not exceed 15 mg/litre

Chloramphenicol (Non-proprietary) [PoM]

Capsules, chloramphenicol 250 mg. Net price 60 = £20.73

Available from Sussex

Kemicetine® (Pharmacia) [PoM]

Injection, powder for reconstitution, chloramphenicol (as sodium succinate). Net price 1-g vial = £1.16

Electrolytes: Na⁺ 3.14 mmol/g

Fusidic acid

Fusidic acid and its salts are narrow-spectrum antibiotics. The only indication for their use is in infections caused by penicillin-resistant staphylococci, especially osteomyelitis, as they are well concentrated in bone; they are also used for staphylococcal endocarditis (section 5.1, table 1). A second antistaphylococcal antibiotic is usually required to prevent emergence of resistance.

SODIUM FUSIDATE

Indications: penicillin-resistant staphylococcal infection including osteomyelitis; staphylococcal endocarditis (in combination with other antibacterials (Table 1, section 5.1)

Cautions: hepatic impairment (Appendix 2)— monitor liver-function with high doses, on prolonged therapy or in hepatic impairment; elimination may be reduced in hepatic impairment or biliary disease or biliary obstruction; pregnancy (Appendix 4); breast-feeding (Appendix 5)

Side-effects: nausea, vomiting, reversible jaundice, especially after high dosage or rapid infusion (withdraw therapy if persistent); rarely rashes, acute renal failure (usually with jaundice), blood disorders

Dose: see under Preparations, below

Fucidin® (Leo) [PoM]

Tablets, f/c, sodium fusidate 250 mg, net price 10-tab pack = £6.47. Label: 9

Dose: as sodium fusidate, 500 mg every 8 hours, doubled for severe infections
Skin infection, as sodium fusidate, 250 mg every 12 hours for 5–10 days

Suspension, off-white, banana- and orange-flavoured, fusidic acid 250 mg/5 mL, net price 50 mL = £7.24. Label: 9, 21

Dose: as fusidic acid, ADULT 750 mg every 8 hours; CHILD up to 1 year 50 mg/kg daily (in 3 divided doses), 1–5 years 250 mg every 8 hours, 5–12 years 500 mg every 8 hours

Note. Fusidic acid is incompletely absorbed and doses recommended for suspension are proportionately higher than those for sodium fusidate tablets

Intravenous infusion, powder for reconstitution, sodium fusidate 500 mg (≡ fusidic acid 480 mg), with buffer, net price per vial (with diluent) = £7.78

Electrolytes: Na⁺ 3.1 mmol/vial when reconstituted with buffer

Dose: as sodium fusidate, by intravenous infusion, ADULT over 50 kg, 500 mg 3 times daily; ADULT under 50 kg and CHILD, 6–7 mg/kg 3 times daily

---

Vancomycin and teicoplanin

The glycopeptide antibiotics vancomycin and teicoplanin have bactericidal activity against aerobic and anaerobic Gram-positive bacteria.

Vancomycin is used *by the intravenous route* in the prophylaxis and treatment of endocarditis and other serious infections caused by Gram-positive cocci including multi-resistant staphylococci; however, there are increasing reports of vancomycin-resistant enterococci. It has a relatively long duration of action and can therefore be given every 12 hours. Vancomycin (added to dialysis fluid) is also used in the treatment of peritonitis associated with peritoneal dialysis [unlicensed route] (Table 1 section 5.1).

Vancomycin given *by mouth* is effective in the treatment of antibiotic-associated colitis (pseudomembranous colitis, see also section 1.5); a dose of 125 mg every 6 hours for 7 to 10 days is considered adequate (higher dose may be considered if the infection fails to respond or if it is severe). Vancomycin should **not** be given by mouth for systemic infections since it is not significantly absorbed.

Teicoplanin is very similar to vancomycin but has a significantly longer duration of action allowing once-daily administration. Unlike vancomycin, teicoplanin can be given by intramuscular as well as by intravenous injection; it is not given by mouth.

VANCOMYCIN

Indications: see notes above

Cautions: avoid rapid infusion (risk of anaphylactoid reactions, see Side-effects); rotate infusion sites; renal impairment (Appendix 3); elderly; avoid if history of deafness; all patients require plasma-vancomycin measurement (after 3 or 4 doses if renal function normal, earlier if renal impairment), blood counts, urinalysis, and renal function tests; monitor auditory function in elderly or if renal impairment; pregnancy and breast-feeding (Appendixes 4 and 5); systemic absorption may follow oral administration especially in inflammatory bowel disorders or following multiple doses; **interactions:** Appendix 1 (vancomycin)

Side-effects: after parenteral administration: nephrotoxicity including renal failure and interstitial nephritis; ototoxicity (discontinue if tinnitus occurs); blood disorders including neutropenia (usually after 1 week or cumulative dose of 25 g), rarely agranulocytosis and thrombocytopenia; nausea; chills, fever; eosinophilia, anaphylaxis, rashes (including exfoliative dermatitis, Stevens-Johnson syndrome, toxic epidermal necrolysis, and vasculitis); phlebitis (irritant to tissue); on rapid infusion, severe hypotension (including shock and cardiac arrest), wheezing, dyspnoea, urticaria, pruritus, flushing of the upper body ('red man' syndrome), pain and muscle spasm of back and chest

Dose: *by mouth*, antibiotic-associated colitis, 125 mg every 6 hours for 7–10 days, see notes above; CHILD 5 mg/kg every 6 hours, over 5 years, half adult dose

Note. Oral paediatric dose is lower than that on product literature but is adequate

By intravenous infusion, 500 mg over at least 60 minutes every 6 hours *or* 1 g over at least 100 minutes every 12 hours; NEONATE up to 1 week, 15 mg/kg initially then 10 mg/kg every 12 hours; INFANT 1–4 weeks, 15 mg/kg initially then 10 mg/kg every 8 hours; CHILD over 1 month, 10 mg/kg every 6 hours

Endocarditis prophylaxis, section 5.1, table 2

Note. Plasma concentration monitoring required; pre-dose ('trough') concentration should be 5–10 mg/litre

Vancomycin (Non-proprietary) PoM
Capsules, vancomycin (as hydrochloride) 125 mg, net price 28-cap pack = £66.23; 250 mg, 28-cap pack = £132.47. Label: 9
Available from Alpharma
Injection, powder for reconstitution, vancomycin (as hydrochloride), for use as an infusion, net price 500-mg vial = £6.67; 1-g vial = £13.41
Note. Can be used to prepare solution for oral administration
Available from Alpharma, Faulding DBL

Vancocin® (Lilly) PoM
Matrigel capsules, vancomycin (as hydrochloride) 125 mg (blue/peach), net price 20-cap pack = £63.08; 250 mg (blue/grey), 20-cap pack = £126.16. Label: 9
Injection, powder for reconstitution, vancomycin (as hydrochloride), for use as an infusion, net price 500-mg vial = £8.66; 1-g vial = £17.32
Note. Can be used to prepare solution for oral administration

TEICOPLANIN

Indications: potentially serious Gram-positive infections including endocarditis, dialysis-associated peritonitis, and serious infections due to *Staphylococcus aureus*; prophylaxis in endocarditis [unlicensed indication] and in orthopaedic surgery at risk of infection with Gram-positive organisms

Cautions: vancomycin sensitivity; blood counts and liver and kidney function tests required; renal impairment (Appendix 3)—monitor renal and auditory function on prolonged administration or if other nephrotoxic or neurotoxic drugs given; pregnancy (Appendix 4) and breast-feeding

Side-effects: nausea, vomiting, diarrhoea; rash, pruritus, fever, bronchospasm, rigors, urticaria, angioedema, anaphylaxis; dizziness, headache; blood disorders including eosinophilia, leucopenia, neutropenia, and thrombocytopenia; disturbances in liver enzymes, transient increase of serum creatinine, renal failure; tinnitus, mild hearing loss, and vestibular disorders also reported; rarely exfoliative dermatitis, Stevens-Johnson syndrome, toxic epidermal necrolysis; local reactions include erythema, pain, thrombophlebitis, injection site abscess and rarely flushing with infusion

Dose: *by intramuscular injection or by intravenous injection or infusion*, initially 400 mg (for severe infections, *by intravenous injection or infusion*, initially 400 mg every 12 hours for 3 doses), then 200 mg daily (400 mg daily for severe infections); higher doses may be required in patients of over 85 kg and in severe burns or endocarditis (consult product literature)
CHILD over 2 months *by intravenous injection or*

infusion, initially 10 mg/kg every 12 hours for 3 doses, subsequently 6 mg/kg daily (severe infections or in neutropenia, 10 mg/kg daily); subsequent doses can be given *by intramuscular injection* (but intravenous administration preferred in children); NEONATE *by intravenous infusion*, initially a single dose of 16 mg/kg, subsequently 8 mg/kg daily

Orthopaedic surgery prophylaxis, *by intravenous injection*, 400 mg at induction of anaesthesia

Endocarditis prophylaxis [unlicensed indication], section 5.1, table 2

Targocid® (Aventis Pharma) PoM
Injection, powder for reconstitution, teicoplanin, net price 200-mg vial (with diluent) = £18.90; 400-mg vial (with diluent) = £38.30
Electrolytes: Na⁺ < 0.5 mmol/200- and 400-mg vial

Linezolid

Linezolid, an oxazolidinone antibacterial, is active against Gram-positive bacteria including methicillin-resistant *Staphylococcus aureus* (MRSA), and vancomycin-resistant enterococci. Resistance to linezolid can develop with prolonged treatment or if the dose is less than that recommended. Linezolid should be reserved for infections resistant to other antibacterials or when other antibacterials are not tolerated. Linezolid is not sufficiently active against common Gram-negative organisms.

LINEZOLID

Indications: pneumonia, complicated skin and soft-tissue infections caused by Gram-positive bacteria (initiated under expert supervision)

Cautions: hepatic impairment (Appendix 2); renal impairment (Appendix 3); pregnancy (Appendix 4); monitor full blood count (including platelet count) weekly (see also CSM Advice below); unless close observation and blood-pressure monitoring possible, avoid in uncontrolled hypertension, phaeochromocytoma, carcinoid tumour, thyrotoxicosis, bipolar depression, schizophrenia, or acute confusional states; **interactions:** Appendix 1 (MAOIs)

CSM ADVICE. Haematopoietic disorders (including thrombocytopenia, anaemia, leucopenia, and pancytopenia) have been reported in patients receiving linezolid. It is recommended that full blood counts are monitored weekly. Close monitoring is recommended in patients who:

- receive treatment for more than 10–14 days;

- have pre-existing myelosuppression;

- are receiving drugs that may have adverse effects on haemoglobin, blood counts, or platelet function;

- have severe renal impairment.

If significant myelosuppression occurs, treatment should be stopped unless it is considered essential, in which case intensive monitoring of blood counts and appropriate management should be implemented.

MONOAMINE OXIDASE INHIBITION. Linezolid is a reversible, non-selective monoamine oxidase inhibitor (MAOI). Patients should avoid consuming large amounts of tyramine-rich foods (such as mature cheese, yeast extracts, undistilled alcoholic beverages, and fermented soya bean products). In addition, linezolid should not be given with another MAOI or within 2 weeks of stopping another MAOI. Unless close observation and blood-pressure monitoring is possible, avoid in those receiving SSRIs, $5HT_1$ agonists ('triptans'), tricyclic antidepressants, sympathomimetics, dopaminergics, buspirone, pethidine and possibly other opioid analgesics. For other **interactions** see Appendix 1 (MAOIs)

Contra-indications: breast-feeding (Appendix 5); see also Monoamine oxidase inhibition above

Side-effects: diarrhoea (antibiotic-associated colitis reported), nausea, vomiting, taste disturbances, headache; less frequently thirst, dry mouth, glossitis, stomatitis, tongue discoloration, abdominal pain, dyspepsia, gastritis, constipation, pancreatitis, hypertension, fever, fatigue, dizziness, insomnia, hypoaesthesia, paraesthesia, tinnitus, polyuria, rash, pruritus, urticaria, diaphoresis, blurred vision, anaemia, leucopenia, thrombocytopenia, pancytopenia, eosinophilia, electrolyte disturbances; injection-site reactions

Dose: *by mouth*, 600 mg every 12 hours for 10–14 days

By intravenous infusion over 30–120 minutes, 600 mg every 12 hours

CHILD under 18 years safety and efficacy not established

Zyvox (Pharmacia) ▼ PoM
Tablets, f/c, linezolid 600 mg, net price 10-tab pack = £335.00. Label: 9, 10 patient information leaflet
Intravenous infusion, linezolid 2 mg/mL, net price 300-mL *Excel®* bag = £33.50
Excipients: include Na+ 5 mmol/300-mL bag, glucose 13.71 g/300-mL bag

Quinupristin and dalfopristin

A combination of the streptogramin antibiotics, **quinupristin** and **dalfopristin** (as *Synercid®*) has recently been licensed for infections due to Gram-positive bacteria. The combination should be reserved for treating infections which have failed to respond to other antibacterials (e.g. methicillin-resistant *Staphylococcus aureus*, MRSA) or for patients who cannot be treated with other antibacterials. Quinupristin and dalfopristin are not active against *Enterococcus faecalis* and they need to be given in combination with other antibacterials for mixed infections which also involve Gram-negative organisms.

QUINUPRISTIN WITH DALFOPRISTIN

A mixture of quinupristin and dalfopristin (both as mesilate salts) in the proportions 3 parts to 7 parts

Indications: serious Gram-positive infections where no alternative antibacterial is suitable including hospital-acquired pneumonia, skin and soft-tissue infections, infections due to vancomycin-resistant *Enterococcus faecium*

Cautions: hepatic impairment (avoid if severe; Appendix 2); renal impairment (Appendix 3); pregnancy (Appendix 4); breast-feeding (Appendix 5); predisposition to cardiac arrhythmias (including congenital QT syndrome, concomitant use of drugs that prolong QT interval, cardiac hypertrophy, dilated cardiomyopathy, hypokalaemia, hypomagnesiaemia, bradycardia); **interactions**: Appendix 1 (Quinupristin/Dalfopristin)

Side-effects: nausea, vomiting, diarrhoea, headache, arthralgia, myalgia, asthenia, rash, pruritus; injection site reactions on peripheral venous administration; less frequently oral candidiasis, stomatitis, constipation, abdominal pain, antibiotic-associated colitis, peripheral oedema, hypotension, chest pain, dyspnoea, anaphylaxis, insomnia, anxiety, confusion, dizziness, paraesthesia, hypertonia, hepatitis, jaundice, pancreatitis, gout; also reported, anaemia, thrombocytopenia, leucopenia, eosinophilia, increased urea and creatinine, electrolyte disturbances

Dose: expressed as a combination of quinupristin and dalfopristin (in a ratio of 3:7)

ADULT over 18 years, by *intravenous infusion* into central vein, 7.5 mg/kg every 8 hours for 7 days in skin and soft-tissue infections; for 10 days in hospital-acquired pneumonia; duration of treatment in *E. faecium* infection depends on site of infection; CHILD under 18 years not recommended

Note. In emergency, first dose may be administered *via* peripheral line until central venous catheter in place

Synercid® (Aventis Pharma) ▼ PoM
Intravenous infusion, powder for reconstitution, quinupristin (as mesilate) 150 mg, dalfopristin (as mesilate) 350 mg, net price 500-mg vial = £37.00
Electrolytes: Na+ approx. 16 mmol/500-mg vial

Polymyxins

The polymyxin antibiotic, **colistin**, is active against Gram-negative organisms, including *Pseudomonas aeruginosa*. It is **not** absorbed by mouth and thus needs to be given by injection to obtain a systemic effect; however, it is toxic and has few, if any, indications for systemic use.

Colistin is used by mouth in bowel sterilisation regimens in neutropenic patients (usually with nystatin); it is **not** recommended for gastro-intestinal infections. It is also given by inhalation of a nebulised solution as an adjunct to standard antibacterial therapy.

Both colistin and polymyxin B are included in some preparations for topical application.

COLISTIN

Indications: see notes above

Cautions: renal impairment; porphyria (section 9.8.2); **interactions:** Appendix 1 (colistin)

Contra-indications: myasthenia gravis; pregnancy; breast-feeding

Side-effects: perioral and peripheral paraesthesia, vertigo, muscle weakness, apnoea, nephrotoxicity; rarely vasomotor instability, slurred speech, visual disturbance, confusion and psychosis; neurotoxicity reported with excessive doses; bronchospasm on inhalation

Dose: *by mouth*, bowel sterilisation, 1.5–3 million units every 8 hours

By intramuscular injection or intravenous injection or infusion, 2 million units every 8 hours (but see notes above)

By inhalation of nebulised solution, patients over 40 kg, 1 million units every 12 hours; patients under 40 kg, 500 000 units every 12 hours

Note. Colistin doses in BNF may differ from those in product literature

Colomycin® (Forest) [PoM]

Tablets, scored, colistin sulphate 1.5 million units. Net price 50 = £62.18

Syrup, colistin sulphate 250 000 units/5 mL when reconstituted with water. Net price 80 mL = £3.71

Injection, powder for reconstitution, colistimethate sodium (colistin sulphomethate sodium). Net price 500 000-unit vial = £1.22; 1 million-unit vial = £1.79

Electrolytes: (before reconstitution) Na+ < 0.5 mmol/500 000- and 1 million-unit vial

---

5.1.8   Sulphonamides and trimethoprim

The importance of the sulphonamides has decreased as a result of increasing bacterial resistance and their replacement by antibacterials which are generally more active and less toxic.

Sulfamethoxazole (sulphamethoxazole) and trimethoprim are used in combination (as **co-trimoxazole**) because of their synergistic activity. However, co-trimoxazole is associated with rare but serious side-effects (e.g. Stevens-Johnson syndrome and blood dyscrasias, notably bone marrow depression and agranulocytosis) especially in the elderly (see CSM recommendations below).

> **CSM recommendations.** Co-trimoxazole should be limited to the role of drug of choice in *Pneumocystis carinii* pneumonia; it is also indicated for *toxoplasmosis* and *nocardiasis*. It should now be considered for use only in *acute exacerbations of chronic bronchitis* and *infections of the urinary tract* when there is good bacteriological evidence of sensitivity to co-trimoxazole and good reason to prefer this combination to a single antibacterial; similarly it should only be used in *acute otitis media in children* when there is good reason to prefer it.

Trimethoprim can be used alone for urinary- and respiratory-tract infections and for prostatitis, shigellosis, and invasive salmonella infections. Trimethoprim has side-effects similar to co-trimoxazole but they are less severe and occur less frequently.

The **longer-acting sulphonamide**, sulfametopyrazine (sulfalene) which is highly bound to plasma proteins, has the advantage of requiring less frequent administration, but toxic effects due to accumulation are more likely to occur.

For *topical preparations* of sulphonamides used in the treatment of burns see section 13.10.1.1.

CO-TRIMOXAZOLE

A mixture of trimethoprim and sulfamethoxazole in the proportions of 1 part to 5 parts

Indications: see CSM recommendations above

Cautions: hepatic impairment (avoid if severe); renal impairment (avoid if severe; Appendix 3); maintain adequate fluid intake; avoid in blood disorders (unless under specialist supervision); monitor blood counts on prolonged treatment; discontinue immediately if blood disorders or rash develop; predisposition to folate deficiency; elderly (see CSM recommendations above); asthma; G6PD deficiency (section 9.1.5); pregnancy (Appendix 4) and breast-feeding (Appendix 5); avoid in infants under 6 weeks (except for treatment or prophylaxis of pneumocystis pneumonia); **interactions:** Appendix 1 (co-trimoxazole)

Contra-indications: porphyria (section 9.8.2)

Side-effects: nausea, vomiting; rash (including Stevens-Johnson syndrome, toxic epidermal necrolysis, photosensitivity)—discontinue immediately; blood disorders (including neutropenia, thrombocytopenia, rarely agranulocytosis and purpura)—discontinue immediately; rarely, allergic reactions, systemic lupus erythematosus, myocarditis, serum sickness, diarrhoea, glossitis, stomatitis, anorexia, arthralgia, myalgia; also reported, liver damage including jaundice and hepatic necrosis, pancreatitis, antibiotic-associated colitis, eosinophilia, cough and shortness of breath, pulmonary infiltrates, aseptic meningitis, headache, depression, convulsions, peripheral neuropathy, ataxia, tinnitus, vertigo, dizziness, hallucinations, megaloblastic anaemia, electrolyte disturbances, crystalluria, renal disorders including interstitial nephritis

Dose: *by mouth*, 960 mg every 12 hours; CHILD, every 12 hours, 6 weeks–5 months, 120 mg; 6 months–5 years, 240 mg; 6–12 years, 480 mg

By intravenous infusion, 960 mg every 12 hours increased to 1.44 g every 12 hours in severe infections; CHILD 36 mg/kg daily in 2 divided doses increased to 54 mg/kg daily in severe infections

Treatment of *Pneumocystis carinii* infections (undertaken where facilities for appropriate monitoring available—consult microbiologist and product literature), *by mouth or by intravenous infusion*, ADULT and CHILD over 4 weeks 120 mg/kg daily in 2–4 divided doses for 14 days

Prophylaxis of *Pneumocystis carinii* infections, *by mouth*, 960 mg once daily (may be reduced to 480 mg once daily to improve tolerance) *or* 960 mg on alternate days (3 times a week) *or* 960 mg twice daily on alternate days (3 times a week); CHILD 6 weeks–5 months 120 mg twice daily on 3 consecutive days *or* 7 days per week; 6 months–5 years 240 mg; 6–12 years 480 mg

Note. 480 mg of co-trimoxazole consists of sulfamethoxazole 400 mg and trimethoprim 80 mg

Co-trimoxazole (Non-proprietary) [PoM]

Tablets, co-trimoxazole 480 mg, net price 28-tab pack = £4.06; 960 mg, 20 = £5.05. Label: 9

Available from Alpharma, DDSA (*Fectrim®*, *Fectrim® Forte*), Hillcross, IVAX, Kent

Paediatric oral suspension, co-trimoxazole 240 mg/5 mL, net price 100 mL = £1.12. Label: 9

Available from IVAX

Oral suspension, co-trimoxazole 480 mg/5 mL. Net price 100 mL = £3.50. Label: 9
Available from Kent
Strong sterile solution, co-trimoxazole 96 mg/mL. For dilution and use as an intravenous infusion. Net price 5-mL amp = £1.58, 10-mL amp = £3.06
Available from Faulding DBL

Septrin® (GlaxoWellcome) PoM
Tablets, co-trimoxazole 480 mg. Net price 20 = £3.34. Label: 9
Forte tablets, scored, co-trimoxazole 960 mg. Net price 20 = £5.05. Label: 9
Adult suspension, vanilla-flavoured, co-trimoxazole 480 mg/5 mL. Net price 100 mL = £4.74. Label: 9
Paediatric suspension, sugar-free, banana- and vanilla-flavoured, co-trimoxazole 240 mg/5 mL. Net price 100 mL = £2.63. Label: 9
Intravenous infusion, co-trimoxazole 96 mg/mL. To be diluted before use. Net price 5-mL amp = £1.59

SULFADIAZINE

(Sulphadiazine)
Indications: prevention of rheumatic fever recurrence, toxoplasmosis [unlicensed]—see section 5.4.7
Cautions: see under Co-trimoxazole; renal impairment (avoid if severe; Appendix 3)
Contra-indications: see under Co-trimoxazole
Side-effects: see under Co-trimoxazole
Dose: prevention of rheumatic fever, *by mouth*, 1 g daily (500 mg daily for patients less than 30kg)

Sulfadiazine (Non-proprietary) PoM
Tablets, sulfadiazine 500 mg, net price 56-tab pack = £17.60. Label: 9, 27
Available from CP
Injection, sulfadiazine (as sodium salt) 250 mg/ mL, net price 4-mL amp = £4.97
Available from Concord

SULFAMETOPYRAZINE ◤

(Sulfalene)
Indications: urinary-tract infections, chronic bronchitis
Cautions: see under Co-trimoxazole
Contra-indications: see under Co-trimoxazole
Side-effects: see under Co-trimoxazole
Dose: 2 g once weekly

Kelfizine W® (Pharmacia) PoM ◤
Tablets, sulfametopyrazine 2 g, net price 5-tab pack = £6.38. Label: 9, 13

◤ denotes preparations that are considered to be less suitable for prescribing (see p. vi)

TRIMETHOPRIM

Indications: urinary-tract infections, acute and chronic bronchitis
Cautions: renal impairment (Appendix 3); pregnancy (Appendix 4); breast-feeding (Appendix 5); predisposition to folate deficiency; elderly; manufacturer recommends blood counts on long-term therapy (but evidence of practical value unsatisfactory); neonates (specialist supervision

required); porphyria (section 9.8.2); **interactions:** Appendix 1 (trimethoprim)
BLOOD DISORDERS. On long-term treatment, patients and their carers should be told how to recognise signs of blood disorders and advised to seek immediate medical attention if symptoms such as fever, sore throat, rash, mouth ulcers, purpura, bruising or bleeding develop
Contra-indications: blood dyscrasias
Side-effects: gastro-intestinal disturbances including nausea and vomiting, pruritus, rashes, hyperkalaemia, depression of haematopoiesis; rarely erythema multiforme, toxic epidermal necrolysis, photosensitivity and other allergic reactions including angioedema and anaphylaxis; aseptic meningitis reported
Dose: *by mouth*, acute infections, 200 mg every 12 hours; CHILD, every 12 hours, 6 weeks–5 months 25 mg, 6 months–5 years 50 mg, 6–12 years 100 mg
Chronic infections and prophylaxis, 100 mg at night; CHILD 1–2 mg/kg at night
By slow intravenous injection or infusion, 200 mg every 12 hours; CHILD under 12 years, 8 mg/kg daily in 2–3 divided doses

Trimethoprim (Non-proprietary) PoM
Tablets, trimethoprim 100 mg, net price 20 = 48p; 200 mg, 20 = 96p. Label: 9
Available from Alpharma, APS, Berk (*Trimopan®*), IVAX, Kent

Monotrim® (Solvay) PoM
Tablets, both scored, trimethoprim 100 mg, net price 20 = 97p; 200 mg, 20 = £1.75. Label: 9
Suspension, sugar-free, trimethoprim 50 mg/5 mL. Net price 100 mL = £1.77. Label: 9
Injection, trimethoprim (as lactate) 20 mg/mL. Net price 5-mL amp = £1.11

Trimopan® (Berk) PoM
Suspension, sugar-free, trimethoprim 50 mg/5 mL. Net price 100 mL = £1.77. Label: 9

5.1.9   Antituberculous drugs

Tuberculosis is treated in two phases—an *initial phase* using at least three drugs and a *continuation phase* using two drugs in fully sensitive cases. Treatment requires specialised knowledge, particularly where the disease involves resistant organisms or non-respiratory organs.

The regimens given below are based on the Joint Tuberculosis Committee of the British Thoracic Society guidelines for the treatment of tuberculosis in the UK; variations occur in other countries. Either the unsupervised regimen or the supervised regimen described below should be used; the two regimens should **not** be used concurrently.

INITIAL PHASE. The concurrent use of at least three drugs during the initial phase is designed to reduce the bacterial population as rapidly as possible and to prevent the emergence of drug-resistant bacteria. The drugs are best given as combination preparations unless one of the components cannot be given because of resistance or intolerance. The treatment of choice for the initial phase is the daily use of isoniazid, rifampicin, pyrazinamide and ethambutol; ethambutol can be omitted from the regimen if the risk of resistance to isoniazid is low (e.g. those who have not been treated previously for tuberculosis, those who are not immunosuppressed, and those who have not been in contact with organisms likely to be drug resistant. Streptomycin is rarely used in the UK although it may be used in the initial phase of treatment if resistance to isoniazid has been established before therapy is commenced. The initial phase drugs should be continued for 2 months. Where a positive culture for *M. tuberculosis* has been obtained, but susceptibility results are not available after 2 months, treatment with pyrazinamide (and ethambutol if appropriate) should be continued until full susceptibility is confirmed, even if this is for longer than 2 months.

CONTINUATION PHASE. After the initial phase, treatment is continued for a further 4 months with isoniazid and rifampicin (preferably given as a combination preparation). Longer treatment is necessary for meningitis and for resistant organisms which may also require modification of the regimen.

UNSUPERVISED TREATMENT. The following regimen should be used for patients who are likely to take antituberculous drugs reliably **without supervision**. Patients who are unlikely to comply with daily administration of antituberculous drugs should be treated with the regimen described under Supervised Treatment.

Recommended dosage for standard unsupervised 6-month treatment
Rifater® [rifampicin, isoniazid, and pyrazinamide] (for 2-month initial phase only)
   ADULT under 40 kg 3 tablets daily, 40–49 kg 4 tablets daily, 50–64 kg 5 tablets daily, over 65 kg 6 tablets daily
¹Ethambutol (for 2-month initial phase only)
   ADULT and CHILD 15 mg/kg daily
Rifinah® or **Rimactazid®** [rifampicin and isoniazid] (for 4-month continuation phase following initial treatment with Rifater®)
   ADULT under 50 kg 3 tablets daily of *Rifinah®-150* or *Rimactazid®-150*, 50 kg and over, 2 tablets daily of *Rifinah®-300* or *Rimactazid®-300*

or (if combination preparations not appropriate):
Isoniazid (for 2-month initial and 4-month continuation phases)
   ADULT 300 mg daily; CHILD 5–10 mg/kg (max. 300 mg) daily
Rifampicin (for 2-month initial and 4-month continuation phases)
   ADULT under 50 kg 450 mg daily, 50 kg and over 600 mg daily; CHILD 10 mg/kg (max. 600 mg) daily
Pyrazinamide (for 2-month initial phase only)
   ADULT under 50 kg 1.5 g daily, 50 kg and over 2 g daily; CHILD 35 mg/kg daily
¹Ethambutol (for 2-month initial phase only)
   ADULT and CHILD 15 mg/kg daily
1. Ethambutol may be omitted from the regimen if the risk of isoniazid resistance is low

PREGNANCY AND BREAST-FEEDING. The standard regimen (above) may be used during pregnancy and breast-feeding. Streptomycin should not be given in pregnancy.

CHILDREN. Children are given isoniazid, rifampicin, and pyrazinamide for the first 2 months followed by isoniazid and rifampicin during the next 4 months. Ethambutol should be included in the first 2 months in children with a high risk of resistant infection (see Initial Phase, above). However, care is needed in young children because of the difficulty in testing eyesight and in obtaining reports of visual symptoms (see below).

SUPERVISED TREATMENT. Drug administration needs to be **fully supervised** (directly observed therapy, DOT) in patients who cannot comply reliably with the treatment regimen. These patients are given isoniazid, rifampicin, pyrazinamide and ethambutol (or streptomycin) 3 times a week under supervision for the first 2 months followed by isoniazid and rifampicin 3 times a week for a further 4 months.

Recommended dosage for intermittent supervised 6-month treatment
Isoniazid (for 2-month initial and 4-month continuation phases)
   ADULT and CHILD 15 mg/kg (max. 900 mg) 3 times a week
Rifampicin (for 2-month initial and 4-month continuation phases)
   ADULT 600–900 mg 3 times a week; CHILD 15 mg/kg (max. 900 mg) 3 times a week
Pyrazinamide (for 2-month initial phase only)
   ADULT under 50 kg 2 g 3 times a week, 50 kg and over 2.5 g 3 times a week; CHILD 50 mg/kg 3 times a week
¹Ethambutol (for 2-month initial phase only)
   ADULT and CHILD 30 mg/kg 3 times a week
1. Ethambutol may be omitted from the regimen if the risk of isoniazid resistance is low

IMMUNOCOMPROMISED PATIENTS. Multiresistant *Mycobacterium tuberculosis* may be present in immunocompromised patients. The organism should always be cultured to confirm its type and drug sensitivity. Confirmed *M. tuberculosis* infection sensitive to first-line drugs should be treated with a standard 6-month regimen; after completing treatment, patients should be closely monitored. The regimen may need to be modified if infection is caused by resistant organisms, and specialist advice is needed.

Specialist advice should be sought about tuberculosis treatment or chemoprophylaxis in a HIV-positive individual; care is required in choosing the regimen and in avoiding potentially hazardous interactions.

Infection may also be caused by other mycobacteria e.g. *M. avium* complex in which case specialist advice on management is needed.

PREVENTION OF TUBERCULOSIS. Some individuals may develop tuberculosis owing to reactivation of previously latent disease. Chemoprophylaxis is required in those who have evidence of previously untreated tuberculosis and are receiving treatment with ciclosporin or with cytotoxics (but not those receiving corticosteroids alone). In these cases, isoniazid chemoprophylaxis may be given for 6 months; longer chemoprophylaxis is not recommended.

For prevention of tuberculosis in susceptible close contacts or those who have become tuberculin-positive, see Table 2, section 5.1. For advice on immunisation against tuberculosis, see section 14.4.

MONITORING. Since isoniazid, rifampicin and pyrazinamide are associated with liver toxicity (see Appendix 2), *hepatic function* should be checked before treatment with these drugs. Those with pre-existing liver disease or alcohol dependence should have frequent checks particularly in the first 2 months. If there is no evidence of liver disease (and pre-treatment liver function is normal), further checks are only necessary if the patient develops fever, malaise, vomiting, jaundice or unexplained deterioration during treatment. In view of the need to comply fully with antituberculous treatment on the one hand and to guard against serious liver damage on the other, patients and their carers should be informed carefully how to recognise signs of liver disorders and advised to discontinue treatment and seek **immediate** medical attention should symptoms of liver disease occur.

Renal function should be checked before treatment with antituberculous drugs and appropriate dosage adjustments made. Streptomycin or ethambutol should preferably be avoided in patients with renal impairment, but if used, the dose should be reduced and the plasma-drug concentration monitored.

Visual acuity should be tested before ethambutol is used (see below).

> Major causes of treatment failure are incorrect prescribing by the physician and inadequate compliance by the patient. Monthly tablet counts and urine examination (rifampicin imparts an orange-red coloration) may be useful indicators of compliance with treatment. Avoid both excessive and inadequate dosage. Treatment should be supervised by a specialist physician.

Isoniazid is cheap and highly effective. Like rifampicin it should always be included in any antituberculous regimen unless there is a specific contra-indication. Its only common side-effect is peripheral neuropathy which is more likely to occur where there are pre-existing risk factors such as diabetes, alcohol dependence, chronic renal failure, malnutrition and HIV infection. In these circumstances pyridoxine 10 mg daily (or 20 mg daily if suitable product not available) (section 9.6.2) should be given prophylactically from the start of treatment. Other side-effects such as hepatitis (important: see Monitoring above) and psychosis are rare.

Rifampicin, a rifamycin, is a key component of any antituberculous regimen. Like isoniazid it should always be included unless there is a specific contra-indication.

During the first two months ('initial phase') of rifampicin administration transient disturbance of liver function with elevated serum transaminases is common but generally does not require interruption of treatment. Occasionally more serious liver toxicity requires a change of treatment particularly in those with pre-existing liver disease (important: see Monitoring above).

On intermittent treatment six toxicity syndromes have been recognised—influenza-like, abdominal, and respiratory symptoms, shock, renal failure, and thrombocytopenic purpura—and can occur in 20 to 30% of patients.

Rifampicin induces hepatic enzymes which accelerate the metabolism of several drugs including oestrogens, corticosteroids, phenytoin, sulphonylureas, and anticoagulants; **interactions:** Appendix 1 (rifamycins). **Important:** the effectiveness of oral contraceptives is reduced and alternative family planning advice should be offered (section 7.3.1).

Rifabutin, a newly introduced rifamycin, is indicated for *prophylaxis* against *M. avium* complex infections in patients with a low CD4 count; it is also licensed for the *treatment* of non-tuberculous mycobacterial disease and pulmonary tuberculosis. As with rifampicin it induces hepatic enzymes and the effectiveness of oral contraceptives is reduced requiring alternative family planning methods.

Pyrazinamide is a bactericidal drug only active against intracellular dividing forms of *Mycobacterium tuberculosis*; it exerts its main effect only in the first two or three months. It is particularly useful in tuberculous meningitis because of good meningeal penetration. It is not active against *M. bovis*. Serious liver toxicity may occasionally occur (important: see Monitoring above).

Ethambutol is included in a treatment regimen if isoniazid resistance is suspected; it can be omitted if the risk of resistance is low.

Side-effects of ethambutol are largely confined to visual disturbances in the form of loss of acuity, colour blindness, and restriction of visual fields. These toxic effects are more common where excessive dosage is used or if the patient's renal function is impaired. The earliest features of ocular toxicity are subjective and patients should be advised to discontinue therapy immediately if they develop deterioration in vision and promptly seek further advice. Early discontinuation of the drug is almost always followed by recovery of eyesight. Patients who cannot understand warnings about visual side-effects should, if possible, be given an alternative drug. In particular, ethambutol should be used with caution in children until they are at least 5 years old and capable of reporting symptomatic visual changes accurately.

Visual acuity should be tested by Snellen chart before treatment with ethambutol.

Streptomycin is now rarely used in the UK except for resistant organisms. It is given intramuscularly in a dose of 15 mg/kg (max. 1 g) daily; the dose is reduced in those under 50 kg, those over 40 years or those with renal impairment. Plasma-drug concentration should be measured in patients with impaired renal function in whom streptomycin must be used with great care. Side-effects increase after a cumulative dose of 100 g, which should only be exceeded in exceptional circumstances.

Drug-resistant tuberculosis should be treated by a specialist physician with experience in such cases, and where appropriate facilities for infection-control exist. Second-line drugs available for infections caused by resistant organisms, or when first-line drugs cause unacceptable side-effects, include amikacin, capreomycin, cycloserine, newer macrolides (e.g. azithromycin and clarithromycin), quinolones (e.g. ciprofloxacin and ofloxacin) and protionamide (prothionamide) (no longer on UK market). Advice on the availability of second-line antituberculous drugs can be obtained from Regional Drug Information Services.

CAPREOMYCIN

Indications: in combination with other drugs, tuberculosis resistant to first-line drugs

Cautions: renal, hepatic, or auditory impairment; monitor renal, hepatic, auditory, and vestibular function and electrolytes; pregnancy (teratogenic in *animals*) and breast-feeding; **interactions:** Appendix 1 (capreomycin)

Side-effects: hypersensitivity reactions including urticaria and rashes; leucocytosis or leucopenia, rarely thrombocytopenia; changes in liver function tests; nephrotoxicity, electrolyte disturbances; hearing loss with tinnitus and vertigo; neuromuscular block after large doses, pain and induration at injection site

Dose: *by deep intramuscular injection*, 1 g daily (not more than 20 mg/kg) for 2–4 months, then 1 g 2–3 times each week

Capastat® (Dista) PoM
Injection, powder for reconstitution, capreomycin sulphate 1 million units (≡ capreomycin approx. 1 g). Net price per vial = £16.47

CYCLOSERINE

Indications: in combination with other drugs, tuberculosis resistant to first-line drugs

Cautions: reduce dose in renal impairment (avoid if severe); monitor haematological, renal, and hepatic function; pregnancy and breast-feeding; **interactions:** Appendix 1 (cycloserine)

Contra-indications: severe renal impairment, epilepsy, depression, severe anxiety, psychotic states, alcohol dependence, porphyria (section 9.8.2)

Side-effects: mainly neurological, including headache, dizziness, vertigo, drowsiness, tremor, convulsions, confusion, psychosis, depression (discontinue or reduce dose if symptoms of CNS toxicity); rashes, allergic dermatitis (discontinue or reduce dose); megaloblastic anaemia; changes in liver function tests; heart failure at high doses reported

Dose: initially 250 mg every 12 hours for 2 weeks increased according to blood concentration and response to max. 500 mg every 12 hours; CHILD initially 10 mg/kg daily adjusted according to blood concentration and response

Note. Blood concentration monitoring required especially in renal impairment or if dose exceeds 500 mg daily or if signs of toxicity; blood concentration should not exceed 30 mg/litre

Cycloserine (King) PoM
Capsules, red/grey cycloserine 250 mg, net price 100-cap pack = £220.69. Label: 2, 8

ETHAMBUTOL HYDROCHLORIDE

Indications: tuberculosis, in combination with other drugs

Cautions: reduce dose in renal impairment and if creatinine clearance less than 30 mL/minute also monitor plasma-ethambutol concentration; elderly; pregnancy; test visual acuity before treatment and warn patients to report visual changes—see notes above; young children (see notes above)—routine ophthalmological monitoring recommended

Contra-indications: optic neuritis, poor vision

Side-effects: optic neuritis, red/green colour blindness, peripheral neuritis, rarely rash, pruritus, urticaria, thrombocytopenia

Dose: see notes above

Note. 'Peak' concentration (2–2.5 hours after dose) should be 2–6 mg/litre (7–22 micromol/litre); 'trough' (pre-dose) concentration should be less than 1 mg/litre (4 micromol/litre)

Ethambutol (Non-proprietary) PoM
Tablets, ethambutol hydrochloride 100 mg (yellow), net price 56-tab pack = £11.50; 400 mg (grey), 56-tab pack = £42.73. Label: 8
Available from Genus

ISONIAZID

Indications: tuberculosis, in combination with other drugs; prophylaxis—Table 2, section 5.1

Cautions: hepatic impairment (monitor hepatic function, see below); renal impairment; slow acetylator status (increased risk of side-effects); epilepsy; history of psychosis; alcohol dependence, malnutrition, diabetes mellitus, HIV infection (risk of peripheral neuritis); pregnancy and breast-feeding; porphyria (section 9.8.2); **interactions:** Appendix 1 (isoniazid)

HEPATIC DISORDERS. Patients or their carers should be told how to recognise signs of liver disorder, and advised to discontinue treatment and seek immediate medical attention if symptoms such as persistent nausea, vomiting, malaise or jaundice develop

Contra-indications: drug-induced liver disease

Side-effects: nausea, vomiting, constipation, dry mouth; peripheral neuritis with high doses (pyridoxine prophylaxis, see notes above), optic neuritis, convulsions, psychotic episodes, vertigo; hypersensitivity reactions including fever, erythema multiforme, purpura; blood disorders including agranulocytosis, haemolytic anaemia, aplastic anaemia; hepatitis (especially over age of 35 years); systemic lupus erythematosus-like syndrome, pellagra, hyperreflexia, difficulty with micturition, hyperglycaemia, and gynaecomastia reported

Dose: *by mouth or by intramuscular or intravenous injection*, see notes above

Isoniazid (Non-proprietary) PoM
Tablets, isoniazid 50 mg, net price 56-tab pack = £5.78; 100 mg, 28-tab pack = £5.77. Label: 8, 22
Available from Celltech

Elixir (BPC), isoniazid 50 mg, citric acid monohydrate 12.5 mg, sodium citrate 60 mg, concentrated anise water 0.05 mL, compound tartrazine solution 0.05 mL, glycerol 1 mL, double-strength chloroform water 2 mL, water to 5 mL. Label: 8, 22

'Special order' [unlicensed] product; contact Martindale, Rosemont, or regional hospital manufacturing unit

Injection, isoniazid 25 mg/mL, net price 2-mL amp = £6.77
Available from Cambridge

PYRAZINAMIDE

Indications: tuberculosis in combination with other drugs

Cautions: pregnancy (Appendix 4); hepatic impairment (monitor hepatic function, see also below); diabetes; gout (avoid in acute attack); **interactions:** Appendix 1 (pyrazinamide)

HEPATIC DISORDERS. Patients or their carers should be told how to recognise signs of liver disorder, and advised to discontinue treatment and seek immediate medical attention if symptoms such as persistent nausea, vomiting, malaise or jaundice develop

Contra-indications: liver damage, porphyria (section 9.8.2)

Side-effects: hepatotoxicity including fever, anorexia, hepatomegaly, splenomegaly, jaundice, liver failure; nausea, vomiting, dysuria, arthralgia, sideroblastic anaemia, rash and occasionally photosensitivity

Dose: see notes above

Zinamide® (MSD) [PoM]
Tablets, scored, pyrazinamide 500 mg. Net price 20 = £1.44. Label: 8

RIFABUTIN

Indications: see under Dose

Cautions: see under Rifampicin; renal impairment (Appendix 3); pregnancy (Appendix 4); breast-feeding (Appendix 5); porphyria (section 9.8.2)

Side-effects: nausea, vomiting; leucopenia, thrombocytopenia, anaemia, rarely haemolysis; raised liver enzymes, jaundice, rarely hepatitis; uveitis following high doses or administration with drugs which raise plasma concentration—see also **interactions:** Appendix 1 (rifamycins); arthralgia, myalgia, influenza-like syndrome, dyspnoea; also hypersensitivity reactions including fever, rash, eosinophilia, bronchospasm, shock; urine, saliva and other body secretions coloured orange-red; asymptomatic corneal opacities reported with long-term use

Dose: prophylaxis of *Mycobacterium avium* complex infections in immunosuppressed patients with low CD4 count (see product literature), 300 mg daily as a single dose

Treatment of non-tuberculous mycobacterial disease, in combination with other drugs, 450–600 mg daily as a single dose for up to 6 months after cultures negative

Treatment of pulmonary tuberculosis, in combination with other drugs, 150–450 mg daily as a single dose for at least 6 months

CHILD not recommended

Mycobutin® (Pharmacia) [PoM]
Capsules, red-brown, rifabutin 150 mg. Net price 30-cap pack = £78.59. Label: 8, 14, counselling, lenses, see under Rifampicin

RIFAMPICIN

Indications: see under Dose

Cautions: hepatic impairment (Appendix 2; liver function tests and blood counts in hepatic disorders, alcohol dependence, and on prolonged therapy, see also below); renal impairment (if above 600 mg daily); pregnancy and breast-feeding (see notes above and Appendixes 4 and 5); porphyria (section 9.8.2); **important:** advise patients on oral contraceptives to use additional means (see also section 7.3.1); discolours soft contact lenses; see also notes above; **interactions:** Appendix 1 (rifamycins)

Note. If treatment interrupted re-introduce with low dosage and increase gradually; discontinue permanently if serious side-effects develop

HEPATIC DISORDERS. Patients or their carers should be told how to recognise signs of liver disorder, and advised to discontinue treatment and seek immediate medical attention if symptoms such as persistent nausea, vomiting, malaise or jaundice develop

Contra-indications: jaundice

Side-effects: gastro-intestinal symptoms including anorexia, nausea, vomiting, diarrhoea (antibiotic-associated colitis reported); headache, drowsiness; those occurring mainly on intermittent therapy include influenza-like symptoms (with chills, fever, dizziness, bone pain), respiratory symptoms (including shortness of breath), collapse and shock, haemolytic anaemia, acute renal failure, and thrombocytopenic purpura; alterations of liver function, jaundice; flushing, urticaria, and rashes; other side-effects reported include oedema, muscular weakness and myopathy, exfoliative dermatitis, toxic epidermal necrolysis, pemphigoid reactions, leucopenia, eosinophilia, menstrual disturbances; urine, saliva, and other body secretions coloured orange-red; thrombophlebitis reported if infusion used for prolonged period

Dose: brucellosis, legionnaires' disease and serious staphylococcal infections, in combination with other drugs, *by mouth or by intravenous infusion*, 0.6–1.2 g daily (in 2–4 divided doses)

Tuberculosis, in combination with other drugs, see notes above

Leprosy, section 5.1.10

Prophylaxis of meningococcal meningitis and *Haemophilus influenzae* (type b) infection, section 5.1, table 2

Rifampicin (Non-proprietary) [PoM]
Capsules, rifampicin 150 mg, net price 20 = £4.07; 300 mg, 20 = £8.13. Label: 8, 14, 22, counselling, see lenses above
Available from Generics

Rifadin® (Aventis Pharma) [PoM]
Capsules, rifampicin 150 mg (blue/red), net price 20 = £4.10; 300 mg (red), 20 = £8.20. Label: 8, 14, 22, counselling, see lenses above

Syrup, red, rifampicin 100 mg/5 mL (raspberry-flavoured). Net price 120 mL = £3.98. Label: 8, 14, 22, counselling, see lenses above

Intravenous infusion, powder for reconstitution, rifampicin. Net price 600-mg vial (with solvent) = £8.58

Electrolytes: Na⁺ < 0.5 mmol/vial

Rimactane® (Swedish Orphan Int AB) [PoM]
Capsules, rifampicin 150 mg (red), net price 56-cap pack = £11.39; 300 mg (red/brown), 56-cap pack = £22.77. Label: 8, 14, 22, counselling, see lenses above

Syrup, red, rifampicin 100 mg/5 mL (raspberry-flavoured). Net price 100 mL = £3.06. Label: 8, 14, 22, counselling, see lenses above

Intravenous infusion, powder for reconstitution, rifampicin (as sodium salt). Net price 300-mg vial (with diluent) = £8.01

Electrolytes: Na⁺ < 0.5 mmol/vial

Note. Owing to risk of contact sensitisation care must be taken to avoid contact during preparation and infusion

■ Combined preparations

Rifater® (Aventis Pharma) [PoM]
Tablets, pink, s/c, rifampicin 120 mg, isoniazid 50 mg, pyrazinamide 300 mg. Net price 20 = £4.72. Label: 8, 14, 22, counselling, see lenses above

Dose: initial treatment of pulmonary tuberculosis, patients up to 40 kg 3 tablets daily preferably before breakfast, 40–49 kg 4 tablets daily, 50–64 kg 5 tablets daily, 65 kg or more, 6 tablets daily; not suitable for use in children

Rifinah 150® (Aventis Pharma) [PoM]
Tablets, pink, s/c, rifampicin 150 mg, isoniazid 100 mg, net price 84-tab pack = £16.18. Label: 8, 14, 22, counselling, see lenses above

Dose: ADULT under 50 kg, 3 tablets daily, preferably before breakfast

Rifinah 300® (Aventis Pharma) [PoM]
Tablets, orange, s/c, rifampicin 300 mg, isoniazid 150 mg, net price 56-tab pack = £23.52. Label: 8, 14, 22, counselling, see lenses above

Dose: ADULT 50 kg and over, 2 tablets daily, preferably before breakfast

Rimactazid 150® (Swedish Orphan Int AB) [PoM]
Tablets, pink, s/c, rifampicin 150 mg, isoniazid 100 mg, net price 84-tab pack = £16.42. Label: 8, 14, 22, counselling, see lenses above

Dose: ADULT under 50 kg, 3 tablets daily, preferably before breakfast

Rimactazid 300® (Swedish Orphan Int AB) [PoM]
Tablets, orange, s/c, rifampicin 300 mg, isoniazid 150 mg, net price 56-tab pack = £21.71. Label: 8, 14, 22, counselling, see lenses above

Dose: ADULT 50 kg and over, 2 tablets daily, preferably before breakfast

STREPTOMYCIN

Indications: tuberculosis, in combination with other drugs; adjunct to doxycycline in brucellosis

Cautions: see under Aminoglycosides, section 5.1.4

Contra-indications: see under Aminoglycosides, section 5.1.4

Side-effects: see under Aminoglycosides, section 5.1.4; also hypersensitivity reactions, paraesthesia of mouth

Dose: *by deep intramuscular injection*, tuberculosis, see notes above; brucellosis, expert advice essential

Note. One-hour ('peak') concentration should be 15–40 mg/litre; pre-dose ('trough') concentration should be less than 5 mg/litre (less than 1 mg/litre in renal impairment or in those over 50 years)

Streptomycin Sulphate (Celltech) [PoM]
Injection, powder for reconstitution, streptomycin (as sulphate), net price 1-g vial = £8.25

5.1.10   Antileprotic drugs

Advice from a member of the Panel of Leprosy Opinion is essential for the treatment of leprosy (Hansen's disease). Details of the Panel can be obtained from the Department of Health telephone (020) 7972 4480.

The World Health Organization has made recommendations to overcome the problem of dapsone resistance and to prevent the emergence of resistance to other antileprotic drugs. Drugs recommended are **dapsone**, **rifampicin** (section 5.1.9), and **clofazimine**. Other drugs with significant activity against *Mycobacterium leprae* include ofloxacin, minocycline and clarithromycin, but none of these are as active as rifampicin; at present they should be reserved as second-line drugs for leprosy.

A three-drug regimen is recommended for *multibacillary leprosy* (lepromatous, borderline-lepromatous, and borderline leprosy) and a two-drug regimen for *paucibacillary leprosy* (borderline-tuberculoid, tuberculoid, and indeterminate). The following regimens are widely used throughout the world (with minor local variations):

Multibacillary leprosy (*3-drug regimen*)

Rifampicin	600 mg once-monthly, supervised (450 mg for adults weighing less than 35 kg)
Dapsone	100 mg daily, self-administered (50 mg daily or 1–2 mg/kg daily for adults weighing less than 35 kg)
Clofazimine	300 mg once-monthly, supervised, *and* 50 mg daily (or 100 mg on alternate days), self-administered

Multibacillary leprosy should be treated for at least 2 years. Treatment should be continued unchanged during both type I (reversal) or type II (erythema nodosum leprosum) reactions. During reversal reactions neuritic pain or weakness can herald the rapid onset of permanent nerve damage. Treatment with prednisolone (initially 40–60 mg daily) should be instituted at once. Mild type II reactions may respond to aspirin or chloroquine. Severe type II reactions may require corticosteroids; thalidomide [unlicensed] is also useful in men and post-menopausal women who have become corticosteroid dependent, but it should be used under **specialist supervision** and it should **never** be used in women of child-bearing potential (significant teratogenic risk—for CSM guidance on prescribing, see *Current Problems in Pharmacovigilance* 1994; **20**, 8). Increased doses of clofazimine 100 mg 3 times daily for the first month with subsequent reductions, are also useful but may take 4–6 weeks to attain full effect.

Paucibacillary leprosy (*2-drug regimen*)

Rifampicin	600 mg once-monthly, supervised (450 mg for those weighing less than 35 kg)
Dapsone	100 mg daily, self-administered (50 mg daily or 1–2 mg/kg daily for adults weighing less than 35 kg)

Paucibacillary leprosy should be treated for 6 months. If treatment is interrupted the regimen should be recommenced where it was left off to complete the full course.

Neither the multibacillary nor the paucibacillary antileprosy regimen is sufficient to treat tuberculosis.

DAPSONE

Indications: leprosy, dermatitis herpetiformis; *Pneumocystis carinii* pneumonia (section 5.4.8)

Cautions: cardiac or pulmonary disease; anaemia (treat severe anaemia before starting); susceptibility to haemolysis including G6PD deficiency (section 9.1.5)—susceptible breast-feeding infants also at risk (Appendix 5); pregnancy (Appendix 4); avoid in porphyria (section 9.8.2); **interactions:** Appendix 1 (dapsone)

BLOOD DISORDERS. On long-term treatment, patients and their carers should be told how to recognise signs of blood disorders and advised to seek immediate medical attention if symptoms such as fever, sore throat, rash, mouth ulcers, purpura, bruising or bleeding develop

Side-effects: (dose-related and uncommon at doses used for leprosy), haemolysis, methaemoglobinaemia, neuropathy, allergic dermatitis (rarely including toxic epidermal necrolysis and Stevens-Johnson syndrome), anorexia, nausea, vomiting, tachycardia, headache, insomnia, psychosis, hepatitis, agranulocytosis; dapsone syndrome (rash with fever and eosinophilia)—discontinue immediately (may progress to exfoliative dermatitis, hepatitis, hypoalbuminaemia, psychosis and death)

Dose: leprosy, 1–2 mg/kg daily, see notes above
Dermatitis herpetiformis, see specialist literature

Dapsone (Non-proprietary) [PoM]
Tablets, dapsone 50 mg, net price 28-tab pack = £2.06; 100 mg, 28-tab pack = £2.95. Label: 8
Available from Alpharma

CLOFAZIMINE

Indications: leprosy

Cautions: hepatic and renal impairment; pregnancy and breast-feeding; may discolour soft contact lenses; avoid if persistent abdominal pain and diarrhoea

Side-effects: nausea, vomiting (hospitalise if persistent), abdominal pain; headache, tiredness; brownish-black discoloration of lesions and skin including areas exposed to light; reversible hair discoloration; dry skin; red discoloration of faeces, urine and other body fluids; also rash, pruritus, photosensitivity, acne-like eruptions, anorexia, eosinophilic enteropathy, bowel obstruction, dry eyes, dimmed vision, macular and subepithelial corneal pigmentation; elevation of blood sugar, weight loss, splenic infarction lymphadenopathy

Dose: leprosy, see notes above
Lepromatous lepra reactions, dosage increased to 300 mg daily for max. of 3 months

Lamprene® (Alliance) [PoM]
Capsules, brown, clofazimine 100 mg, net price 100-cap pack = £23.50. Label: 8, 14, 21

5.1.11   Metronidazole and tinidazole

Metronidazole is an antimicrobial drug with high activity against anaerobic bacteria and protozoa; indications include trichomonal vaginitis (section 5.4.3), bacterial vaginosis (notably *Gardnerella*

vaginalis infections), and *Entamoeba histolytica* and *Giardia lamblia* infections (section 5.4.2). It is also used for surgical and gynaecological sepsis in which its activity against colonic anaerobes, especially *Bacteroides fragilis*, is important. Metronidazole is also effective in the treatment of antibiotic-associated colitis (pseudomembranous colitis, see also section 1.5) in a dose of 400 mg by mouth 3 times daily. Metronidazole by the rectal route is an effective alternative to the intravenous route when oral administration is not possible. Intravenous metronidazole is used for the treatment of established cases of tetanus; diazepam (section 10.2.2) and tetanus immunoglobulin (section 14.5) are also used.

Topical metronidazole (section 13.10.1.2) reduces the odour produced by anaerobic bacteria in fungating tumours; it is also used in the management of rosacea (section 13.6).

Tinidazole is similar to metronidazole but has a longer duration of action.

METRONIDAZOLE

Indications: anaerobic infections (including dental), see under Dose below; protozoal infections (section 5.4.2); *Helicobacter pylori* eradication (section 1.3); skin (section 13.10.1.2)

Cautions: disulfiram-like reaction with alcohol, hepatic impairment and hepatic encephalopathy (Appendix 2); pregnancy and breast-feeding (Appendixes 4 and 5); clinical and laboratory monitoring advised if treatment exceeds 10 days; **interactions:** Appendix 1 (metronidazole)

Side-effects: nausea, vomiting, unpleasant taste, furred tongue, and gastro-intestinal disturbances; rashes; rarely drowsiness, headache, dizziness, ataxia, darkening of urine, erythema multiforme, pruritus, urticaria, angioedema, and anaphylaxis; also reported abnormal liver function tests, hepatitis, jaundice, thrombocytopenia, aplastic anaemia, myalgia, arthralgia; on prolonged or intensive therapy peripheral neuropathy, transient epileptiform seizures, and leucopenia

Dose: anaerobic infections (usually treated for 7 days), *by mouth, either* 800 mg initially then 400 mg every 8 hours *or* 500 mg every 8 hours, CHILD 7.5 mg/kg every 8 hours; *by rectum*, 1 g every 8 hours for 3 days, then 1 g every 12 hours, CHILD every 8 hours for 3 days, then every 12 hours, age up to 1 year 125 mg, 1–5 years 250 mg, 5–10 years 500 mg, over 10 years, adult dose; *by intravenous infusion*, 500 mg every 8 hours; CHILD 7.5 mg/kg every 8 hours

Leg ulcers and pressure sores, *by mouth*, 400 mg every 8 hours for 7 days

Bacterial vaginosis, *by mouth*, 400–500 mg twice daily for 5–7 days *or* 2 g as a single dose

Pelvic inflammatory disease (see also Table 1, section 5.1), *by mouth*, 400 mg twice daily for 14 days

Acute ulcerative gingivitis, *by mouth*, 200–250 mg every 8 hours for 3 days; CHILD 1–3 years 50 mg every 8 hours for 3 days; 3–7 years 100 mg every 12 hours; 7–10 years 100 mg every 8 hours

Acute dental infections, *by mouth*, 200 mg every 8 hours for 3–7 days

Surgical prophylaxis, *by rectum*, 1 g 2 hours before surgery; further doses may be given every 8 hours for high-risk procedures; CHILD 5–10 years 500 mg 2 hours before surgery

By intravenous infusion (if rectal administration inappropriate), 500 mg at induction; further doses may be given every 8 hours for high-risk procedures; CHILD 7.5 mg/kg at induction

Note. Metronidazole doses in BNF may differ from those in product literature

Metronidazole (Non-proprietary) PoM
Tablets, metronidazole 200 mg, net price 20 =40p; 400 mg, 20 =83p. Label: 4, 9, 21, 25, 27
Available from Alpharma, DDSA (*Vaginyl®*), Hillcross, IVAX, Kent, Rosemont
Tablets, metronidazole 500 mg, net price 21-tab pack = £3.50. Label: 4, 9, 21, 25, 27
Available from Alpharma
Suspension, metronidazole (as benzoate) 200 mg/ 5 mL. Net price 100 mL = £7.68. Label: 4, 9, 23
Available from Hillcross, Rosemont
Intravenous infusion, metronidazole 5 mg/mL. Net price 20-mL amp = £1.53, 100-mL container = £3.83
Available from Braun, Galen, Phoenix

Flagyl® (Hawgreen) PoM
Tablets, both f/c, ivory, metronidazole 200 mg, net price 21-tab pack = £3.89; 400 mg, 14-tab pack = £5.50. Label: 4, 9, 21, 25, 27
Suppositories, metronidazole 500 mg, net price 10 = £13.17; 1 g, 10 = £20.00. Label: 4, 9

Flagyl® (Aventis Pharma) PoM
Intravenous infusion, metronidazole 5 mg/mL, net price 100-mL *Viaflex®* bag = £3.41
Electrolytes: Na+ 13.6 mmol/100-mL bag

Flagyl S® (Hawgreen) PoM
Suspension, metronidazole (as benzoate) 200 mg/ 5 mL. Net price 100 mL = £9.69. Label: 4, 9, 23

Metrolyl® (Lagap) PoM
Intravenous infusion, metronidazole 5 mg/mL, net price 100-mL Steriflex® bag = £12.22
Electrolytes: Na+ 14.53 mmol/100-mL bag
Suppositories, metronidazole 500 mg, net price 10 = £13.27; 1 g, 10 = £19.76. Label: 4, 9

■ With antifungal
Flagyl Compak® (Hawgreen) PoM
Treatment pack, tablets, off-white, f/c, metronidazole 400 mg, with pessaries, yellow, nystatin 100 000 units, net price 14 tablets and 14 pessaries (with applicator) = £9.49
Dose: for mixed trichomonal and candidal infections, 1 tablet twice daily for 7 days and 1 pessary inserted twice daily for 7 days *or* 1 pessary at night for 14 nights

TINIDAZOLE

Indications: anaerobic infections, see under Dose below; protozoal infections (section 5.4.2); *Helicobacter pylori* eradication (section 1.3)
Cautions: see under Metronidazole; pregnancy (manufacturer advises avoidance in first trimester); avoid in porphyria (section 9.8.2)
Side-effects: see under Metronidazole
Dose: anaerobic infections *by mouth*, 2 g initially, followed by 1 g daily *or* 500 mg twice daily, usually for 5–6 days
Bacterial vaginosis and acute ulcerative gingivitis, a single 2-g dose

Abdominal surgery prophylaxis, a single 2-g dose approximately 12 hours before surgery
Fasigyn® (Pfizer) PoM
Tablets, f/c, tinidazole 500 mg. Net price 20-tab pack = £11.50. Label: 4, 9, 21, 25

5.1.12   Quinolones

Nalidixic acid and **norfloxacin** are effective in uncomplicated urinary-tract infections.

Ciprofloxacin is active against both Gram-positive and Gram-negative bacteria. It is particularly active against Gram-negative bacteria, including salmonella, shigella, campylobacter, neisseria, *Bacillus anthracis* (see below) and pseudomonas. Ciprofloxacin has only moderate activity against Gram-positive bacteria such as *Streptococcus pneumoniae* and *Enterococcus faecalis*; it is not the drug of first choice for pneumococcal pneumonia. It is active against chlamydia and some mycobacteria. Most anaerobic organisms are not susceptible. Uses for ciprofloxacin include infections of the respiratory tract (but not for pneumococcal pneumonia) and of the urinary tract, and of the gastro-intestinal system (including typhoid fever), and gonorrhoea and septicaemia caused by sensitive organisms.

Ofloxacin is used for urinary-tract infections, lower respiratory-tract infections, gonorrhoea, and non-gonococcal urethritis and cervicitis.

Levofloxacin is active against Gram-positive and Gram-negative organisms. It has greater activity against pneumococci than ciprofloxacin.

Although, ciprofloxacin, levofloxacin and ofloxacin are licensed for skin and soft-tissue infections, many staphylococci are resistant to the quinolones and their use should be avoided in methicillin-resistant *Staphylococcus aureus* (MRSA) infections.

ANTHRAX. **Ciprofloxacin** is recommended as initial therapy for the *treatment* of anthrax. Treatment may be switched to **benzylpenicillin** (section 5.1.1.1), or to **doxycycline** (section 5.1.3), or to **amoxicillin** (section 5.1.1.3) if the infecting strain of *Bacillus anthracis* is susceptible. If meningitis is suspected, the initial use of combination therapy including ciprofloxacin plus benzylpenicillin may be considered. Cutaneous anthrax should be treated for 7 days but in other forms (especially inhalational anthrax), antibacterial treatment should extend to 60 days because of a possible delay in germination.

Ciprofloxacin or doxycycline may be given for *post-exposure prophylaxis*. If exposure is confirmed, antibacterial prophylaxis should continue for 60 days. Antibacterial prophylaxis may be switched to amoxicillin if the strain of *B. anthracis* is susceptible. Vaccination against anthrax (section 14.4) may allow the duration of antibacterial prophylaxis to be shortened.

CAUTIONS. Quinolones should be used with caution in patients with a history of epilepsy or conditions that predispose to seizures, in G6PD deficiency (section 9.1.5), myasthenia gravis (risk of exacerbation), in pregnancy, during breast-feeding, and in children or adolescents (arthropathy has developed in weight-bearing joints in young *ani-*

mals—see below). Exposure to excessive sunlight should be avoided (discontinue if photosensitivity occurs). The CSM has warned that quinolones may induce **convulsions** in patients with or without a history of convulsions; taking NSAIDs at the same time may also induce them. Other **interactions**: Appendix 1 (quinolones).

USE IN CHILDREN. Quinolones cause arthropathy in the weight-bearing joints of immature *animals* and are therefore generally not recommended in children and growing adolescents. However, the significance of this effect in humans is uncertain and in some specific circumstances short-term use of a quinolone in children may be justified. Nalidixic acid is used for urinary-tract infections in children over 3 months of age. Ciprofloxacin is licensed for pseudomonal infections in cystic fibrosis (for children above 5 years of age), and for treatment and prophylaxis of anthrax.

CSM advice (tendon damage)
At the first sign of pain or inflammation, patients taking quinolones should discontinue the treatment and rest the affected limb until tendon symptoms have resolved.

SIDE-EFFECTS. Side-effects of the quinolones include nausea, vomiting, dyspepsia, abdominal pain, diarrhoea (rarely antibiotic-associated colitis), headache, dizziness, sleep disorders, rash (rarely Stevens-Johnson syndrome and toxic epidermal necrolysis), and pruritus. Less frequent side-effects include anorexia, increase in blood urea and creatinine; drowsiness, restlessness, asthenia, depression, confusion, hallucinations, convulsions, paraesthesia; photosensitivity, hypersensitivity reactions including fever, urticaria, angioedema, arthralgia, myalgia, and anaphylaxis; blood disorders (including eosinophilia, leucopenia, thrombocytopenia); disturbances in vision, taste, hearing and smell. Also isolated reports of tendon inflammation and damage (especially in the elderly and in those taking corticosteroids, see also CSM advice above). Other side-effects that have been reported include haemolytic anaemia, renal failure, interstitial nephritis, and hepatic dysfunction (including hepatitis and cholestatic jaundice). The drug should be **discontinued** if psychiatric, neurological or hypersensitivity reactions (including severe rash) occur.

CIPROFLOXACIN

Indications: see notes above and under Dose; eye infections (section 11.3.1)

Cautions: see notes above; renal impairment (Appendix 3); avoid excessive alkalinity of urine and ensure adequate fluid intake (risk of crystalluria); **interactions:** Appendix 1 (quinolones)

DRIVING. May impair performance of skilled tasks (e.g. driving); effects enhanced by alcohol

Side-effects: see notes above; also reported flatulence, dysphagia, tremor, hyperglycaemia, altered prothrombin concentration, vasculitis, erythema nodosum, petechiae, haemorrhagic bullae, tinnitus, tenosynovitis, tachycardia, oedema, syncope, hot flushes and sweating; pain and phlebitis at injection site

Dose: *by mouth*, respiratory-tract infections, 250–750 mg twice daily

Urinary-tract infections, 250–500 mg twice daily (100 mg twice daily for 3 days in acute uncomplicated cystitis in women)

Chronic prostatitis, 500 mg twice daily for 28 days

Gonorrhoea, 500 mg as a single dose

Pseudomonal lower respiratory-tract infection in cystic fibrosis, 750 mg twice daily; CHILD 5–17 years (see Cautions above), up to 20 mg/kg twice daily (max. 1.5 g daily)

Most other infections, 500–750 mg twice daily

Surgical prophylaxis, 750 mg 60–90 minutes before procedure

Prophylaxis of meningococcal meningitis [not licensed], Table 2, section 5.1

By intravenous infusion (over 30–60 minutes; 400 mg over 60 minutes), 200–400 mg twice daily

Pseudomonal lower respiratory-tract infection in cystic fibrosis, 400 mg twice daily; CHILD 5–17 years (see Cautions above), up to 10 mg/kg 3 times daily (max. 1.2 g daily)

Urinary-tract infections, 100 mg twice daily

Gonorrhoea, 100 mg as a single dose

CHILD not recommended (see Cautions above) but where benefit outweighs risk, *by mouth*, 10–30 mg/kg daily in 2 divided doses *or by intravenous infusion*, 8–16 mg/kg daily in 2 divided doses

Anthrax (treatment and post-exposure prophylaxis, see notes above), *by mouth*, 500 mg twice daily; CHILD 30 mg/kg daily in 2 divided doses (max. 1 g daily)

By intravenous infusion, 400 mg twice daily; CHILD 20 mg/kg daily in 2 divided doses (max. 800 mg daily)

Ciproxin® (Bayer) PoM

Tablets, all f/c, ciprofloxacin (as hydrochloride) 100 mg, net price 6-tab pack = £2.80; 250 mg (scored), 10-tab pack = £7.50, 20-tab pack = £15.00; 500 mg (scored), 10-tab pack = £14.20, 20-tab pack = £28.40; 750 mg, 10-tab pack = £20.00. Label: 6, 9, 25, counselling, driving

Suspension, strawberry-flavoured, ciprofloxacin for reconstitution with diluent provided, 250 mg/5 mL, net price 100 mL = £15.00. Label: 6, 9, 25, counselling, driving

Intravenous infusion, ciprofloxacin (as lactate) 2 mg/mL, in sodium chloride 0.9%, net price 50-mL bottle = £8.65

Electrolytes: Na+ 15.4 mmol/100-mL bottle

Intravenous infusion (Flexibag), ciprofloxacin (as lactate) 2 mg/mL, in glucose 5%, net price 100-mL infusion bag = £16.89, 200-mL infusion bag = £25.70

LEVOFLOXACIN

Indications: see under Dose

Cautions: see notes above; renal impairment (Appendix 3); **interactions:** Appendix 1 (quinolones)

DRIVING. May impair performance of skilled tasks (e.g. driving)

Side-effects: see notes above; asthenia; rarely tremor, anxiety, tachycardia, hypotension, hypoglycaemia, pneumonitis, rhabdomyolysis; local reactions and transient hypotension reported with infusion

Dose: *by mouth*, acute sinusitis, 500 mg daily for 10–14 days

Exacerbation of chronic bronchitis, 250–500 mg daily for 7–10 days

Community-acquired pneumonia, 500 mg once or twice daily for 7–14 days

Complicated urinary-tract infections, 250 mg daily for 7–10 days

Skin and soft tissue infections, 250 mg daily *or* 500 mg once or twice daily for 7–14 days

By intravenous infusion (over at least 60 minutes for 500 mg), community-acquired pneumonia, 500 mg once or twice daily

Complicated urinary-tract infections, 250 mg daily, increased in severe infections

Skin and soft tissue infections, 500 mg twice daily

Tavanic® (Hoechst Marion Roussel) ▼ PoM
Tablets, f/c, scored, levofloxacin 250 mg, net price 5-tab pack = £7.77, 10-tab pack = £15.54; 500 mg, 5-tab pack = £13.90, 10-tab pack = £27.80. Label: 6, 9, 25, counselling, driving
Intravenous infusion, levofloxacin 5 mg/mL, net price 100-mL bottle = £28.39

NALIDIXIC ACID

Indications: urinary-tract infections

Cautions: see notes above; avoid in porphyria (section 9.8.2); liver disease; renal impairment (Appendix 3); false positive urinary glucose (if tested for reducing substances); monitor blood counts, renal and liver function if treatment exceeds 2 weeks; **interactions:** Appendix 1 (quinolones)

Side-effects: see notes above; also reported toxic psychosis, weakness, increased intracranial pressure, cranial nerve palsy, metabolic acidosis

Dose: 1 g every 6 hours for 7 days, reduced in chronic infections to 500 mg every 6 hours; CHILD over 3 months max. 50 mg/kg daily in divided doses; reduced in prolonged therapy to 30 mg/kg daily

Mictral® (Sanofi-Synthelabo) PoM
Granules, effervescent, nalidixic acid 660 mg, sodium citrate (as sodium citrate and citric acid) 4.1 g/sachet (Na+ 41 mmol/sachet). Net price 9-sachet pack = £5.48. Label: 9, 11, 13
Dose: 1 sachet in water 3 times daily for 3 days

Negram® (Sanofi-Synthelabo) PoM
Tablets, beige, nalidixic acid 500 mg. Net price 56-tab pack = £12.83. Label: 9, 11, 23
Suspension, pink, sugar-free, nalidixic acid 300 mg/5 mL (raspberry-flavoured), net price 120 mL = £10.28. Label: 9, 11, 23

Uriben® (Rosemont) PoM
Suspension, pink, nalidixic acid 300 mg/5 mL, net price 150 mL = £12.15. Label: 9, 11

NORFLOXACIN

Indications: see under Dose

Cautions: see notes above; renal impairment (Appendix 3); **interactions:** Appendix 1 (quinolones)

DRIVING. May impair performance of skilled tasks (e.g. driving)

Side-effects: see notes above; also reported euphoria, anxiety, tinnitus, polyneuropathy, exfoliative dermatitis, pancreatitis, vasculitis

Dose: urinary-tract infections, 400 mg twice daily for 7–10 days (for 3 days in uncomplicated lower urinary-tract infections)

Chronic relapsing urinary-tract infections, 400 mg twice daily for up to 12 weeks; may be reduced to 400 mg once daily if adequate suppression within first 4 weeks

Chronic prostatitis, 400 mg twice daily for 28 days

Norfloxacin (Non-proprietary) PoM
Tablets, norfloxacin 400 mg, net price 6-tab pack = £2.19, 14-tab pack = £5.11. Label: 7, 9, 23, counselling driving
Available from Genus

Utinor® (MSD) PoM
Tablets, scored, norfloxacin 400 mg. Net price 6-tab pack = £2.19, 14-tab pack = £5.11. Label: 7, 9, 23, counselling, driving

OFLOXACIN

Indications: see under Dose

Cautions: see notes above; hepatic and renal impairment (Appendices 2 and 3); history of psychiatric illness; **interactions:** Appendix 1 (quinolones)

DRIVING. May affect performance of skilled tasks (e.g. driving); effects enhanced by alcohol

Side-effects: see notes above; also reported, tachycardia, transient hypotension, vasculitic reactions, anxiety, unsteady gait and tremor, hypaesthesia, neuropathy, extrapyramidal symptoms, psychotic reactions (discontinue treatment—see notes above); very rarely changes in blood sugar; isolated cases of pneumonitis; on intravenous infusion, hypotension and local reactions (including thrombophlebitis)

Dose: *by mouth*, urinary-tract infections, 200–400 mg daily preferably in the morning, increased if necessary in upper urinary-tract infections to 400 mg twice daily

Chronic prostatitis, 200 mg twice daily for 28 days

Lower respiratory-tract infections, 400 mg daily preferably in the morning, increased if necessary to 400 mg twice daily

Skin and soft-tissue infections, 400 mg twice daily

Uncomplicated gonorrhoea, 400 mg as a single dose

Uncomplicated genital chlamydial infection, nongonococcal urethritis, 400 mg daily in single or divided doses for 7 days

Pelvic inflammatory disease (see also section 5.1, table 1), 400 mg twice daily for 14 days

By intravenous infusion (over at least 30 minutes for each 200 mg), complicated urinary-tract infection, 200 mg daily

Lower respiratory-tract infection, 200 mg twice daily

Septicaemia, 200 mg twice daily

Skin and soft-tissue infections, 400 mg twice daily

Severe or complicated infections, dose may be increased to 400 mg twice daily

Ofloxacin (Non-proprietary) PoM
Tablets, ofloxacin 200 mg, net price 10-tab pack = £10.05; 400 mg, 5-tab pack = £10.03, 10-tab pack = £22.46
Available from Dexcel

Tarivid® (Hoechst Marion Roussel) PoM
Tablets, f/c, scored, ofloxacin 200 mg, net price 10-tab pack = £11.29, 20-tab pack = £22.55; 400 mg (yellow), 5-tab pack = £11.26, 10-tab pack = £22.46. Label: 6, 9, 11, counselling, driving
Intravenous infusion, ofloxacin (as hydrochloride) 2 mg/mL, net price 50-mL bottle = £15.41; 100-mL bottle = £24.21 (both hosp. only)

5.1.13   Urinary-tract infections

Urinary-tract infection is more common in women than in men; when it occurs in men there is frequently an underlying abnormality of the renal tract. Recurrent episodes of infection are an indication for radiological investigation especially in children in whom untreated pyelonephritis may lead to permanent kidney damage.

Escherichia coli is the most common cause of urinary-tract infection; *Staphylococcus saprophyticus* is also common in sexually active young women. Less common causes include Proteus and Klebsiella spp. *Pseudomonas aeruginosa* infections are almost invariably associated with functional or anatomical abnormalities of the renal tract. *Staphylococcus epidermidis* and *Enterococcus faecalis* infection may complicate catheterisation or instrumentation. Whenever possible a specimen of urine should be collected for culture and sensitivity testing before starting antibacterial therapy. The antibacterial chosen should reflect local antibacterial sensitivity, which needs to be reviewed regularly.

Uncomplicated lower urinary-tract infections often respond to amoxicillin, nalidixic acid, nitrofurantoin, or trimethoprim given for 7 days (3 days may be adequate for infections in women); those caused by fully sensitive bacteria respond to two 3-g doses of amoxicillin (section 5.1.1.3). Bacterial resistance, however, especially to ampicillin or amoxicillin (to which approximately 50% of *E. coli* are now resistant), has increased the importance of urine culture prior to therapy. Alternatives for resistant organisms include co-amoxiclav (amoxicillin with clavulanic acid), an oral cephalosporin, pivmecillinam, or a quinolone.

Long-term low dose therapy may be required in selected patients to prevent *recurrence of infection*; indications include frequent relapses and significant kidney damage. Trimethoprim, nitrofurantoin and cefalexin have been recommended for long-term therapy.

Methenamine (hexamine) should **not** generally be used because it requires an acidic urine for its antimicrobial activity and it is ineffective for upper urinary-tract infections; it may, however, have a role in chronic bacteriuria particularly in infection caused by highly resistant Gram-negative bacteria or by yeasts.

Acute pyelonephritis can lead to septicaemia and is best treated initially by injection of a broad-spectrum antibacterial such as cefuroxime or a qui-

nolone especially if the patient is severely ill; gentamicin can also be used.

Prostatitis can be difficult to cure and requires treatment for several weeks with an antibacterial which penetrates prostatic tissue such as trimethoprim, or some quinolones.

Where infection is localised and associated with an indwelling *catheter* a bladder instillation is often effective (section 7.4.4).

Patients with *heart-valve lesions* undergoing instrumentation of the urinary tract should be given a parenteral antibiotic to prevent bacteraemia and endocarditis (section 5.1, table 2).

Urinary-tract infection in *pregnancy* may be asymptomatic and requires prompt treatment to prevent progression to acute pyelonephritis. Penicillins and cephalosporins are suitable for treatment of urinary-tract infection during pregnancy. Nitrofurantoin may also be used but it should be avoided at term. Sulphonamides, quinolones, and tetracyclines should be avoided during pregnancy; trimethoprim should also preferably be avoided particularly in the first trimester.

In *renal failure* antibacterials normally excreted by the kidney accumulate with resultant toxicity unless the dose is reduced. This applies especially to the aminoglycosides which should be used with great caution; tetracyclines, hexamine, and nitrofurantoin should be avoided altogether.

CHILDREN. Urinary-tract infections in children require prompt antibacterial treatment to minimise the risk of renal scarring. For the first infection, treatment may be initiated with trimethoprim or co-amoxiclav and the choice of antibacterial is reviewed when sensitivity results are available; full doses of the antibacterial drug should be given for 5–7 days. Antibacterial prophylaxis with low doses of trimethoprim or nitrofurantoin should then be given until investigations for the infection are complete; long-term prophylaxis may be necessary in some cases (e.g. vesicoureteric reflux or renal scarring).

Seriously ill children should be transferred to hospital and treated initially with intravenous antibacterial drugs such as ampicillin with gentamicin or cefotaxime alone until the infection responds; full doses of oral antibacterials are then given for a further period. Antibacterial prophylaxis should then be given as above.

NITROFURANTOIN

Indications: urinary-tract infections

Cautions: anaemia; diabetes mellitus; electrolyte imbalance; vitamin B and folate deficiency; pulmonary disease; hepatic impairment; monitor lung and liver function on long-term therapy, especially in the elderly (discontinue if deterioration in lung function); susceptibility to peripheral neuropathy; false positive urinary glucose (if tested for reducing substances); urine may be coloured yellow or brown; **interactions:** Appendix 1 (nitrofurantoin)

Contra-indications: impaired renal function, infants less than 3 months old, G6PD deficiency (including pregnancy at term, and breast-feeding of affected infants, see section 9.1.5 and Appendixes 4 and 5), porphyria (section 9.8.2)

Side-effects: anorexia, nausea, vomiting, and diarrhoea; acute and chronic pulmonary reactions (pulmonary fibrosis reported; possible association with lupus erythematosus-like syndrome); peripheral neuropathy; also reported, hypersensitivity reactions (including angioedema, anaphylaxis, sialadenitis, urticaria, rash and pruritus); rarely, cholestatic jaundice, hepatitis, exfoliative dermatitis, erythema multiforme, pancreatitis, arthralgia, blood disorders (including agranulocytosis, thrombocytopenia, and aplastic anaemia), benign intracranial hypertension, and transient alopecia

Dose: acute uncomplicated infection, 50 mg every 6 hours with food for 7 days; CHILD over 3 months, 3 mg/kg daily in 4 divided doses

Severe chronic recurrent infection, 100 mg every 6 hours with food for 7 days (dose reduced or discontinued if severe nausea)

Prophylaxis (but see Cautions), 50–100 mg at night; CHILD over 3 months, 1 mg/kg at night

Nitrofurantoin (Non-proprietary) PoM
Tablets, nitrofurantoin 50 mg and 100 mg. Label: 9, 14, 21
Available from Alpharma, Biorex, Kent

Furadantin® (Goldshield) PoM
Tablets, all yellow, scored, nitrofurantoin 50 mg, net price 20 = £1.96; 100 mg, 20 = £3.62. Label: 9, 14, 21
Suspension, yellow, sugar-free, nitrofurantoin 25 mg/5 mL (lemon-apricot-flavoured), net price 300 mL = £65.00. Label: 9, 14, 21

Macrobid® (Goldshield) PoM
Capsules, m/r, blue/yellow, nitrofurantoin 100 mg (as nitrofurantoin macrocrystals and nitrofurantoin monohydrate). Net price 14-cap pack = £4.89. Label: 9, 14, 21, 25
Dose: uncomplicated urinary-tract infection, 1 capsule twice daily with food
Genito-urinary surgical prophylaxis, 1 capsule daily on day of procedure and for 3 days after

Macrodantin® (Goldshield) PoM
Capsules, nitrofurantoin 50 mg (yellow/white), net price 30-cap pack = £3.05; 100 mg (yellow), 20 = £3.84. Label: 9, 14, 21

METHENAMINE HIPPURATE ◢
(Hexamine hippurate)
Indications: prophylaxis and long-term treatment of recurrent urinary-tract infections
Cautions: pregnancy; avoid concurrent administration with sulphonamides (risk of crystalluria) or urinary alkalinising agents; **interactions:** Appendix 1 (hexamine)
Contra-indications: severe renal impairment, dehydration, metabolic acidosis
Side-effects: gastro-intestinal disturbances, bladder irritation, rash
Dose: 1 g every 12 hours (may be increased in patients with catheters to 1 g every 8 hours); CHILD 6–12 years 500 mg every 12 hours

Hiprex® (3M) ◢
Tablets, scored, methenamine hippurate 1 g. Net price 60-tab pack = £7.07. Label: 9

◢ denotes preparations that are considered to be less suitable for prescribing (see p. vi)

5.2 Antifungal drugs

Treatment of fungal infections

The systemic treatment of common fungal infections is outlined below; specialist treatment is required in most forms of systemic or disseminated fungal infections. For local treatment of fungal infections, see section 7.2.2 (genital), section 7.4.4 (bladder), section 11.3.2 (eye), section 12.1.1 (ear), section 12.3.2 (oropharynx), and section 13.10.2 (skin).

ASPERGILLOSIS. Aspergillosis most commonly affects the respiratory tract although, in severely immunocompromised patients, invasive forms can affect the sinuses, heart, brain, and skin. **Amphotericin** by intravenous infusion is the drug of choice but response can be variable; liposomal amphotericin or **itraconazole** are alternatives in patients in whom initial treatment has failed.

CANDIDIASIS. Many superficial candidal infections are treated locally including infections of the vagina (section 7.2.2) and of the skin (section 13.10.2).
Oropharyngeal candidiasis generally responds to topical therapy (section 12.3.2); an imidazole or triazole antifungal is given by mouth for unresponsive infections. Fluconazole is effective and is reliably absorbed.
For *deep and disseminated candidiasis*, **amphotericin** by intravenous infusion is used alone or with **flucytosine** by intravenous infusion; an alternative is **fluconazole** given alone, particularly in AIDS patients (in whom flucytosine is best avoided because of its bone marrow toxicity).

CRYPTOCOCCOSIS. Cryptococcosis is uncommon but infection in the immunocompromised, especially in AIDS patients, can be life-threatening; cryptococcal meningitis is the most common form of fungal meningitis. The treatment of choice is **amphotericin** by intravenous infusion with or without **flucytosine** by intravenous infusion. **Fluconazole** given alone is an alternative particularly in AIDS patients with no disturbance of consciousness. Following successful treatment, fluconazole can be used for prophylaxis against relapse until immunity recovers.

HISTOPLASMOSIS. Histoplasmosis is rare in temperate climates; it can be life-threatening, particularly in HIV-infected persons. **Itraconazole** or **ketoconazole** can be used for the treatment of immunocompetent patients with indolent non-meningeal infection including chronic pulmonary histoplasmosis. **Amphotericin** by intravenous infusion is preferred in patients with fulminant or severe infections. Intravenous itraconazole is also licensed for histoplasmosis.

SKIN AND NAIL INFECTIONS. Mild localised fungal infections of the skin (including tinea corporis, tinea cruris, and tinea pedis) respond to topical therapy (section 13.10.2). Systemic therapy is appropriate if topical therapy fails, if many areas are affected, or if the site of infection is difficult to treat such as in infections of the nails (onychomycosis) and of the scalp (tinea capitis).

Griseofulvin is used for tinea capitis in adults and children; it was used extensively in tinea of various other sites but it has largely been replaced by newer antifungals. Oral imidazole or triazole antifungals (particularly **itraconazole**) and **terbinafine** are used more commonly because they have a broader spectrum of activity and require a shorter duration of treatment; the role of terbinafine in the management of microsporum species (cat or dog ringworm) is uncertain.

Pityriasis versicolor may be treated with **itraconazole** by mouth if topical therapy is ineffective; **fluconazole** by mouth is an alternative. Oral **terbinafine** is **not** effective for pityriasis versicolor.

Terbinafine and **itraconazole** have largely replaced griseofulvin for the systemic treatment of onychomycosis, particularly of the toenail; terbinafine is considered to be the drug of choice. Itraconazole can be administered as intermittent 'pulse' therapy.

IMMUNOCOMPROMISED PATIENTS. Immunocompromised patients are at particular risk of fungal infections and may receive antifungal drugs prophylactically; oral imidazole or triazole antifungals are the drugs of choice. **Fluconazole** is more reliably absorbed than itraconazole and ketoconazole; fluconazole is considered to be less toxic than ketoconazole on long-term use.

Drugs used in fungal infections

POLYENE ANTIFUNGALS. The polyene antifungals include amphotericin and nystatin; neither drug is absorbed when given by mouth. They are used for oral, oropharyngeal, and perioral infections by local application in the mouth (section 12.3.2).

Amphotericin by intravenous infusion is used for the treatment of systemic fungal infections and is active against most fungi and yeasts. It is highly protein bound and penetrates poorly into body fluids and tissues. When given parenterally amphotericin is toxic and side-effects are common. Lipid formulations of amphotericin (*Abelcet®*, *AmBisome®*, and *Amphocil®*) are significantly less toxic and are recommended when the conventional formulation of amphotericin is contra-indicated because of toxicity, especially nephrotoxicity; lipid formulations are more expensive.

Nystatin is used principally for *Candida albicans* infections of the skin and mucous membranes, including oesophageal and intestinal candidiasis.

IMIDAZOLE ANTIFUNGALS. Clotrimazole, econazole, fenticonazole, sulconazole, and tioconazole are used for the local treatment of vaginal candidiasis (section 7.2.2) and for dermatophyte infections (section 13.10.2).

Ketoconazole is better absorbed by mouth than other imidazoles. It has been associated with fatal hepatotoxicity; the CSM has advised that prescribers should weigh the potential benefits of ketoconazole treatment against the risk of liver damage and should carefully monitor patients both clinically

and biochemically. It should not be used for superficial fungal infections.

Miconazole can be used locally for oral infections; it is also effective in intestinal infections. Systemic absorption may follow use of miconazole oral gel and may result in significant drug interactions.

TRIAZOLE ANTIFUNGALS. **Fluconazole** is very well absorbed after oral administration. It also achieves good penetration into the cerebrospinal fluid to treat fungal meningitis.

Itraconazole is active against a wide range of dermatophytes. Itraconazole capsules require an acid environment in the stomach for optimal absorption.

Itraconazole has been associated with liver damage and should not be given to patients with a history of liver disease; fluconazole is less frequently associated with hepatotoxicity.

OTHER ANTIFUNGALS. **Flucytosine** is often used with amphotericin in a synergistic combination. Bone marrow depression can occur which limits its use, particularly in AIDS patients; weekly blood counts are necessary during prolonged therapy. Resistance to flucytosine can develop during therapy and sensitivity testing is essential before and during treatment.

Griseofulvin is effective for widespread or intractable dermatophyte infections but has been superseded by newer antifungals, particularly for nail infections. It is usually well tolerated and is licensed for use in children. Duration of therapy is dependent on the site of the infection and may be required for a number of months.

Terbinafine is the drug of choice for fungal nail infections and is also used for ringworm infections where oral treatment is considered appropriate.

AMPHOTERICIN

(Amphotericin B)

Indications: See under Dose

Cautions: when given parenterally, toxicity common (close supervision necessary and test dose required); renal impairment (Appendix 3); hepatic and renal-function tests, blood counts, and plasma electrolyte monitoring required; corticosteroids (avoid except to control reactions); pregnancy and breast-feeding; avoid rapid infusion (risk of arrhythmias); **interactions:** Appendix 1 (amphotericin)

ANAPHYLAXIS. The CSM has advised that anaphylaxis occurs rarely with any intravenous amphotericin product and a test dose is advisable before the first infusion; the patient should be carefully observed for about 30 minutes after the test dose. Prophylactic antipyretics or hydrocortisone should only be used in patients who have previously experienced acute adverse reactions (in whom continued treatment with amphotericin is essential)

Side-effects: when given parenterally, anorexia, nausea and vomiting, diarrhoea, epigastric pain; febrile reactions, headache, muscle and joint pain; anaemia; disturbances in renal function (including hypokalaemia and hypomagnesaemia) and renal toxicity; also cardiovascular toxicity (including arrhythmias), blood disorders, neurological disorders (including hearing loss, diplopia, convulsions, peripheral neuropathy), abnormal liver function (discontinue treatment), rash, anaphylactoid reactions (see Anaphylaxis, above); pain and thrombophlebitis at injection site

Dose: *by mouth*, intestinal candidiasis, 100–200 mg every 6 hours; INFANT and CHILD, 100 mg 4 times daily

Prophylaxis NEONATE 100 mg once daily

Oral and perioral infections, see section 12.3.2

By intravenous infusion, see under preparations, below

Fungilin® (Squibb) PoM

Tablets, yellow, scored, amphotericin 100 mg, net price 56-tab pack = £8.32. Label: 9

Suspension, yellow, sugar-free, amphotericin 100 mg/mL, net price 12 mL = £2.31. Label: 9, counselling, use of pipette

Fungizone® (Squibb) PoM

Intravenous infusion, powder for reconstitution, amphotericin (as sodium deoxycholate complex). Net price 50-mg vial = £3.70

Electrolytes: Na⁺ < 0.5 mmol/vial

Dose: by intravenous infusion, systemic fungal infections, initial test dose of 1 mg over 20–30 minutes then 250 micrograms/kg daily, gradually increased if tolerated to 1 mg/kg daily; max. (severe infection) 1.5 mg/kg daily or on alternate days

Note. Prolonged treatment usually necessary; if interrupted for longer than 7 days recommence at 250 micrograms/kg daily and increase gradually

■ Lipid formulations

Abelcet® (Elan) PoM

Intravenous infusion, amphotericin 5 mg/mL as lipid complex with L-α-dimyristoylphosphatidylcholine and L-α-dimyristoylphosphatidylglycerol. Net price 10-mL vial = £50.00, 20-mL vial = £82.13 (hosp. only)

Dose: severe invasive candidiasis; severe systemic fungal infections in patients not responding to conventional amphotericin or to other antifungal drugs or where toxicity or renal impairment precludes conventional amphotericin, including invasive aspergillosis, cryptococcal meningitis and disseminated cryptococcosis in HIV patients, by intravenous infusion, ADULT and CHILD, initial test dose 1 mg over 15 minutes then 5 mg/kg daily for at least 14 days

AmBisome® (Gilead) PoM

Intravenous infusion, powder for reconstitution, amphotericin 50 mg encapsulated in liposomes. Net price 50-mg vial = £138.47

Electrolytes: Na⁺ < 0.5 mmol/vial

Dose: severe systemic or deep mycoses where toxicity (particularly nephrotoxicity) precludes use of conventional amphotericin, by intravenous infusion, ADULT and CHILD initial test dose 1 mg over 10 minutes then 1 mg/kg daily as a single dose increased gradually if necessary to 3 mg/kg daily as a single dose

Infections in febrile neutropenic patients unresponsive to broad-spectrum antibacterials, ADULT and CHILD, initial test dose 1 mg over 10 minutes then 3 mg/kg daily as a single dose until afebrile for 3 consecutive days; max. period of treatment 42 days

Visceral leishmaniasis, see section 5.4.5 and product literature

Amphocil® (Cambridge) PoM

Intravenous infusion, powder for reconstitution, amphotericin as a complex with sodium choles-

teryl sulphate. Net price 50-mg vial = £104.10, 100-mg vial = £190.05

Electrolytes: Na⁺ < 0.5 mmol/vial

Dose: severe systemic or deep mycoses where toxicity or renal failure preclude use of conventional amphotericin, by intravenous infusion, ADULT and CHILD initial test dose 2 mg over 10 minutes then 1 mg/kg daily as a single dose increased gradually if necessary to 3–4 mg/kg daily as a single dose

---

FLUCONAZOLE

Indications: see under Dose

Cautions: renal impairment (Appendix 3); pregnancy (Appendix 4) and breast-feeding (Appendix 5); monitor liver function—discontinue if signs or symptoms of hepatic disease (risk of hepatic necrosis); **interactions:** Appendix 1 (antifungals, imidazole and triazole)

Side-effects: nausea, abdominal discomfort, diarrhoea, flatulence, headache, rash (discontinue treatment or monitor closely if infection invasive or systemic); less frequently dyspepsia, vomiting, taste disturbance, hepatic disorders, angioedema, anaphylaxis, dizziness, seizures, alopecia, pruritus, toxic epidermal necrolysis, Stevens-Johnson syndrome (severe cutaneous reactions more likely in AIDS patients), hyperlipidaemia, leucopenia, thrombocytopenia, and hypokalaemia reported

Dose: vaginal candidiasis and candidal balanitis, *by mouth*, a single dose of 150 mg

Mucosal candidiasis (except genital), *by mouth*, 50 mg daily (100 mg daily in unusually difficult infections) given for 7–14 days in oropharyngeal candidiasis (max. 14 days except in severely immunocompromised patients); for 14 days in atrophic oral candidiasis associated with dentures; for 14–30 days in other mucosal infections (e.g. oesophagitis, candiduria, non-invasive bronchopulmonary infections); CHILD *by mouth or by intravenous infusion*, 3–6 mg/kg on first day then 3 mg/kg daily (every 72 hours in NEONATE up to 2 weeks old, every 48 hours in neonate 2–4 weeks old)

Tinea pedis, corporis, cruris, pityriasis versicolor, and dermal candidiasis, *by mouth*, 50 mg daily for 2–4 weeks (for up to 6 weeks in tinea pedis); max. duration of treatment 6 weeks

Invasive candidal infections (including candidaemia and disseminated candidiasis) and cryptococcal infections (including meningitis), *by mouth or intravenous infusion*, 400 mg initially then 200 mg daily, increased if necessary to 400 mg daily; treatment continued according to response (at least 6–8 weeks for cryptococcal meningitis); CHILD 6–12 mg/kg daily (every 72 hours in NEONATE up to 2 weeks old, every 48 hours in NEONATE 2–4 weeks old); max. 400 mg daily

Prevention of relapse of cryptococcal meningitis in AIDS patients after completion of primary therapy, *by mouth or by intravenous infusion*, 100–200 mg daily

Prevention of fungal infections in immunocompromised patients following cytotoxic chemotherapy or radiotherapy, *by mouth or by intravenous infusion*, 50–400 mg daily adjusted according to risk; 400 mg daily if high risk of systemic infections e.g. following bone-marrow transplantation; commence treatment before anticipated onset of neutropenia and continue for 7 days after neutrophil count in desirable range; CHILD according to extent and duration of neutropenia, 3–12 mg/kg daily (every 72 hours in NEONATE up to 2 weeks old, every 48 hours in NEONATE 2–4 weeks old); max. 400 mg daily

Diflucan® (Pfizer)

¹ *Capsules* [PoM], fluconazole 50 mg (blue/white), net price 7-cap pack = £16.61; 150 mg (blue), single-capsule pack = £7.12; 200 mg (purple/white), 7-cap pack = £66.42. Label: 50 and 200 mg, 9

1. Can be sold to the public for vaginal candidiasis in women aged 16–60 years, in a container or packaging containing not more than 150 mg and labelled to show a max. dose of 150 mg; a proprietary brand (*Diflucan® One*) containing a single 150-mg capsule is on sale to the public

Oral suspension [PoM], orange-flavoured, fluconazole for reconstitution with water, 50 mg/5 mL, net price 35 mL = £16.61; 200 mg/5 mL, 35 mL = £66.42. Label: 9

Intravenous infusion [PoM], fluconazole 2 mg/mL in sodium chloride intravenous infusion 0.9%, net price 25-mL bottle = £7.32; 100-mL bottle = £29.28

Electrolytes: Na⁺ 15 mmol/100-mL bottle

FLUCYTOSINE

Indications: systemic yeast and fungal infections; adjunct to amphotericin (or fluconazole) in cryptococcal meningitis, adjunct to amphotericin in severe systemic candidiasis and in other severe or long-standing infections

Cautions: renal impairment (Appendix 3); elderly; blood disorders; liver- and kidney-function tests and blood counts required (weekly in renal impairment or blood disorders); pregnancy, breast-feeding

Side-effects: nausea, vomiting, diarrhoea, rashes; less frequently confusion, hallucinations, convulsions, headache, sedation, vertigo, alterations in liver function tests (hepatitis and hepatic necrosis reported); blood disorders including thrombocytopenia, leucopenia, and aplastic anaemia reported

Dose: *by intravenous infusion* over 20–40 minutes, ADULT and CHILD, 200 mg/kg daily in 4 divided doses usually for not more than 7 days; extremely sensitive organisms, 100–150 mg/kg daily may be sufficient; treat for at least 4 months in cryptococcal meningitis

Note. For plasma concentration monitoring blood should be taken shortly before starting the next infusion; plasma concentration for optimum response 25–50 mg/litre (200–400 micromol/litre)—should not be allowed to exceed 80 mg/litre (620 micromol/litre)

Ancotil® (ICN) [PoM]

Intravenous infusion, flucytosine 10 mg/mL. Net price 250-mL infusion bottle = £35.69 (hosp. only)

Electrolytes: Na⁺ 34.5 mmol/250-mL bottle

Note. Flucytosine tablets may be available on a named-patient basis from Bell and Croyden; the brand name *Alcobon®* was used formerly for flucytosine infusion

GRISEOFULVIN

Indications: dermatophyte infections of the skin, scalp, hair and nails where topical therapy has failed or is inappropriate

Cautions: rarely aggravation or precipitation of systemic lupus erythematosus; breast-feeding; **interactions:** Appendix 1 (griseofulvin)

DRIVING. May impair performance of skilled tasks (e.g. driving); effects of alcohol enhanced

Contra-indications: severe liver disease, lupus erythematosus and related conditions, porphyria (section 9.8.2); pregnancy (**avoid** pregnancy **during** and for **1 month after** treatment; men should not father children within 6 months of treatment)

Side-effects: headache, nausea, vomiting, rashes, photosensitivity; dizziness, fatigue, agranulocytosis and leucopenia reported; lupus erythematosus, erythema multiforme, toxic epidermal necrolysis, peripheral neuropathy, confusion and impaired co-ordination also reported

Dose: 500 mg daily, in divided doses or as a single dose, in severe infection dose may be doubled, reducing when response occurs; CHILD, 10 mg/kg daily in divided doses or as a single dose

Grisovin® (GlaxoWellcome) [PoM]

Tablets, both f/c, griseofulvin 125 mg, net price 20 = 47p; 500 mg, 20 = £1.75. Label: 9, 21, counselling, driving

ITRACONAZOLE

Indications: see under Dose

Cautions: liver disease (Appendix 2); liver function tests required if history of liver disease or if treatment exceeds 1 month or if anorexia, nausea, vomiting, fatigue, abdominal pain or dark urine develop (discontinue if test abnormal); renal impairment (Appendix 3); absorption reduced in AIDS and neutropenia (monitor plasma-itraconazole concentration and increase dose if necessary); history of congestive heart failure (see also CSM advice, below); pregnancy (Appendix 4) and breast-feeding (Appendix 5); **interactions:** Appendix 1 (antifungals, imidazole and triazole)

> **CSM advice (heart failure)**
>
> Following rare reports of heart failure, the CSM has advised caution when prescribing itraconazole to patients at high risk of heart failure. Those at risk include:
>
> - patients receiving high doses and longer treatment courses;
> - older patients and those with cardiac disease;
> - patients receiving treatment with negative inotropic drugs, e.g. calcium channel blockers.

Side-effects: nausea, abdominal pain, dyspepsia, constipation (vomiting and diarrhoea with oral liquid or intravenous infusion), headache, dizziness, raised liver enzymes, menstrual disorders; allergic reactions (including pruritus, rash, urticaria and angioedema), hepatitis and cholestatic jaundice (especially if treatment exceeds 1 month), heart failure, peripheral neuropathy (discontinue treatment), and Stevens-Johnson syndrome reported; on prolonged use hypokalaemia, oedema and hair loss reported

Dose: *by mouth*, oropharyngeal candidiasis, 100 mg daily (200 mg daily in AIDS or neutropenia) for 15 days; see also under *Sporanox*® oral liquid below

Vulvovaginal candidiasis, 200 mg twice daily for 1 day

Pityriasis versicolor, 200 mg daily for 7 days

Tinea corporis and tinea cruris, *either* 100 mg daily for 15 days *or* 200 mg daily for 7 days

Tinea pedis and tinea manuum, *either* 100 mg daily for 30 days *or* 200 mg twice daily for 7 days

Onychomycosis, *either* 200 mg daily for 3 months *or* course ('pulse') of 200 mg twice daily for 7 days, subsequent courses repeated after 21-day interval; fingernails 2 courses, toenails 3 courses

Histoplasmosis, 200 mg 1–2 times daily

Systemic aspergillosis, candidiasis and cryptococcosis including cryptococcal meningitis where other antifungal drugs inappropriate or ineffective, 200 mg once daily (candidiasis 100–200 mg once daily) increased in invasive or disseminated disease and in cryptococcal meningitis to 200 mg twice daily

Maintenance in AIDS patients to prevent relapse of underlying fungal infection and prophylaxis in neutropenia when standard therapy inappropriate, 200 mg once daily, increased to 200 mg twice daily if low plasma-itraconazole concentration (see Cautions)

Prophylaxis in patients with haematological malignancy or undergoing bone-marrow transplant, see under *Sporanox*® oral liquid below

CHILD and ELDERLY safety and efficacy not established

By intravenous infusion, systemic aspergillosis, candidiasis and cryptococcosis including cryptococcal meningitis where other antifungal drugs inappropriate or ineffective, histoplasmosis, 200 mg every 12 hours for 2 days, then 200 mg once daily for max. 12 days; CHILD and ELDERLY safety and efficacy not established

Sporanox® (Janssen-Cilag) PoM

Capsules, blue/pink, enclosing coated beads, itraconazole 100 mg, net price 4-cap pack = £4.19; 15-cap pack = £15.72; 28-cap pack (*Sporanox*®-*Pulse*) = £29.35; 60-cap pack = £62.89. Label: 5, 9, 21, 25

Oral liquid, sugar-free, itraconazole 10 mg/mL, net price 150 mL (with 10-mL measuring cup) = £52.28. Label: 9, 23, counselling, administration

Dose: oral or oesophageal candidiasis in HIV-positive or other immunocompromised patients, 20 mL (2 measuring cups) daily in 1–2 divided doses for 1 week (continue for another week if no response)

Fluconazole-resistant oral or oesophageal candidiasis, 10–20 mL (1–2 measuring cups) twice daily for 2 weeks (continue for another 2 weeks if no response; the higher dose should not be used for longer than 2 weeks if no signs of improvement)

Prophylaxis of deep fungal infections (when standard therapy is inappropriate) in patients with haematological malignancy or undergoing bone-marrow transplantation who are expected to become neutropenic, 5 mg/kg daily in 2 divided doses; start 1 week before transplantation or immediately before chemotherapy and continue until neutrophil count recovers; CHILD and ELDERLY safety and efficacy not established

COUNSELLING. Do not take with food; swish around mouth and swallow, do not rinse afterwards

Concentrate for intravenous infusion ▼, itraconazole 10 mg/mL. For dilution before use. Net price 25-mL amp (with infusion bag and filter) = £71.43

Excipients: include propylene glycol

KETOCONAZOLE

Indications: systemic mycoses, serious chronic resistant mucocutaneous candidiasis, serious resistant gastro-intestinal mycoses, chronic resistant vaginal candidiasis, resistant dermatophyte infections of skin or finger nails (not toe nails); prophylaxis of mycoses in immunosuppressed patients

Cautions: monitor liver function clinically and biochemically—for treatment lasting longer than 14 days perform liver function tests before starting, 14 days after starting, then at monthly intervals (for details consult product literature)—for CSM advice see p. 294; avoid in porphyria (section 9.8.2); **interactions:** Appendix 1 (antifungals, imidazole and triazole)

Contra-indications: hepatic impairment; pregnancy (Appendix 4) and breast-feeding

Side-effects: nausea, vomiting, abdominal pain; headache; rashes, urticaria, pruritus; rarely angioedema, thrombocytopenia, paraesthesia, photophobia, dizziness, alopecia, gynaecomastia and oligospermia; fatal liver damage—see also under Cautions, risk of developing hepatitis greater if given for longer than 14 days

Dose: 200 mg once daily with food, usually for 14 days; if response inadequate after 14 days continue until at least 1 week after symptoms have cleared and cultures negative; max. 400 mg (ELDERLY 200 mg) daily

CHILD 3 mg/kg daily

Chronic resistant vaginal candidiasis, 400 mg once daily with food for 5 days

Prophylaxis and maintenance treatment in immunosuppressed patients, 200 mg daily

Nizoral® (Janssen-Cilag) PoM

Tablets, scored, ketoconazole 200 mg. Net price 30-tab pack = £15.69. Label: 5, 9, 21

MICONAZOLE

Indications: see under Dose

Cautions: pregnancy and breast-feeding; avoid in porphyria (section 9.8.2); **interactions:** Appendix 1 (antifungals, imidazole and triazole)

Contra-indications: hepatic impairment

Side-effects: nausea and vomiting, diarrhoea (usually on long-term treatment); rarely allergic reactions; isolated reports of hepatitis

Dose: prevention and treatment of oral and intestinal fungal infections, 5–10 mL in the mouth after food 4 times daily; retain near lesions before swallowing; CHILD under 2 years, 2.5 mL twice daily, 2–6 years, 5 mL twice daily, over 6 years, 5 mL 4 times daily

Localised lesions, smear on affected area with clean finger (dental prostheses should be removed at night and brushed with gel); treatment continued for 48 hours after lesions have resolved

¹ **Daktarin®** (Janssen-Cilag) PoM
Oral gel, sugar-free, orange-flavoured, miconazole
24 mg/mL (20 mg/g). Net price 15-g tube = £2.27,
80-g tube = £5.00. Label: 9, counselling advised,
hold in mouth, after food
1. 15-g tube can be sold to public

NYSTATIN

Indications: candidiasis; vaginal infection (section
7.2.2); oral infection (section 12.3.2); skin infection (section 13.10.2)

Side-effects: nausea, vomiting, diarrhoea at high
doses; oral irritation and sensitisation; rash
(including urticaria) and rarely Stevens-Johnson
syndrome reported

Dose: *by mouth*, intestinal candidiasis
500 000 units every 6 hours, doubled in severe
infections; CHILD over 1 month, 100 000 units 4
times daily
Prophylaxis, 1 million units once daily; NEONATE
100 000 units once daily

Nystatin (Non-proprietary) PoM
Oral suspension, nystatin 100 000 units/mL. Net
price 30 mL = £2.05. Label: 9, counselling use of
pipette
Available from Hillcross, Kent, Rosemont (sugar-free,
Nystamont®)

Nystan® (Squibb) PoM
Tablets, brown, s/c, nystatin 500 000 units, net
price 56-tab pack = £4.70. Label: 9
Suspension, yellow, nystatin 100 000 units/mL, net
price 30 mL with pipette = £2.05. Label: 9, counselling, use of pipette

TERBINAFINE

Indications: dermatophyte infections of the nails,
ringworm infections (including tinea pedis, cruris, and corporis) where oral therapy appropriate
(due to site, severity or extent)

Cautions: hepatic and renal impairment (Appendixes 2 and 3); pregnancy, breast-feeding (Appendix 5); psoriasis (risk of exacerbation);
interactions: Appendix 1 (terbinafine)

Side-effects: abdominal discomfort, anorexia,
nausea, diarrhoea; headache; rash and urticaria
occasionally with arthralgia or myalgia; less frequently taste disturbance; rarely liver toxicity
(including jaundice, cholestasis, and hepatitis)—
discontinue treatment, angioedema, dizziness,
malaise, paraesthesia, hypoaesthesia, photosensitivity, skin reactions (including Stevens-Johnson
syndrome and toxic epidermal necrolysis)—discontinue treatment if progressive skin rash; also
reported, psychiatric disturbances, blood disorders (including leucopenia and thrombocytopenia)

Dose: 250 mg daily usually for 2–6 weeks in tinea
pedis, 2–4 weeks in tinea cruris, 4 weeks in tinea
corporis, 6 weeks–3 months in nail infections
(occasionally longer in toenail infections); CHILD
[unlicensed] usually for 2 weeks, tinea capitis,
over 1 year, body-weight 10–20 kg, 62.5 mg once
daily; body-weight 20–40 kg, 125 mg once daily;
body-weight over 40 kg, 250 mg once daily

Lamisil® (Novartis) PoM
Tablets, off-white, scored, terbinafine 250 mg (as
hydrochloride), net price 14-tab pack = £23.16,
28-tab pack = £44.66. Label: 9

5.3　Antiviral drugs

The majority of virus infections resolve spontaneously in immunocompetent subjects. A number of
specific treatments for viral infections are available,
particularly for the immunocompromised. This section includes notes on herpes simplex and varicella-
zoster, human immunodeficiency virus, cytomegalovirus, respiratory syncytial virus, viral
hepatitis and influenza.

Herpes simplex and varicella–zoster

Aciclovir is active against herpes viruses but does
not eradicate them. It is effective only if started at
the onset of the episode. Uses of aciclovir include
the systemic treatment of varicella–zoster (chickenpox–shingles) and the systemic and topical treatment of herpes simplex infections of the skin and
mucous membranes (including initial and recurrent
genital herpes); it is also used topically in the eye. It
can be life-saving in herpes simplex and varicella–
zoster infections in the immunocompromised, and
is also used for prevention of recurrence and for
herpes simplex prophylaxis in the immunocompromised. Aciclovir may also be given by mouth to
immunocompetent adults and older adolescents
with chickenpox; it is not generally indicated for
immunocompetent children in whom the disease is
milder. See also section 11.3.3 (eye) and section
13.10.3 (skin, including herpes labialis).

Famciclovir, a prodrug of penciclovir, is similar
to aciclovir and it is recommended for herpes zoster
and initial and recurrent genital herpes. Penciclovir
itself is used as a cream for herpes simplex labialis
(section 13.10.3). **Valaciclovir** is an ester of aciclovir which is licensed for herpes zoster and for
herpes simplex infections of the skin and mucous
membranes (including initial and recurrent genital
herpes).

Idoxuridine (section 13.10.3) is also only effective if started at the onset of infection; it is too toxic
for systemic use. It has been used topically in the
treatment of herpes simplex lesions of the skin and
external genitalia with variable results; it has also
been used topically in the treatment of zoster, but
evidence of its value is dubious.

Inosine pranobex has been used by mouth for
herpes simplex infections; its effectiveness has not
been established.

ACICLOVIR
(Acyclovir)
Indications: herpes simplex and varicella–zoster
(see also under Dose)
Cautions: maintain adequate hydration (especially
with infusion or high doses); renal impairment
(Appendix 3); pregnancy and breast-feeding;
interactions: Appendix 1 (aciclovir and famciclovir)
Side-effects: nausea, vomiting, abdominal pain,
diarrhoea, headache, fatigue, rash, urticaria, pru-

ritus, photosensitivity; rarely hepatitis, jaundice, dyspnoea, angioedema, anaphylaxis, neurological reactions (including dizziness, confusion, hallucinations and drowsiness), acute renal failure, decreases in haematological indices; on *intravenous infusion*, severe local inflammation (sometimes leading to ulceration), fever, and rarely agitation, tremors, psychosis and convulsions

Dose: *by mouth*,

Herpes simplex, treatment, 200 mg (400 mg in the immunocompromised or if absorption impaired) 5 times daily, usually for 5 days; CHILD under 2 years, half adult dose, over 2 years, adult dose

Herpes simplex, prevention of recurrence, 200 mg 4 times daily *or* 400 mg twice daily possibly reduced to 200 mg 2 or 3 times daily and interrupted every 6–12 months

Herpes simplex, prophylaxis in the immunocompromised, 200–400 mg 4 times daily; CHILD under 2 years, half adult dose, over 2 years, adult dose

Varicella and herpes zoster, treatment, 800 mg 5 times daily for 7 days; CHILD, varicella, 20 mg/kg (max. 800 mg) 4 times daily for 5 days *or* under 2 years 200 mg 4 times daily, 2–5 years 400 mg 4 times daily, over 6 years 800 mg 4 times daily

By intravenous infusion, treatment of herpes simplex in the immunocompromised, severe initial genital herpes, and varicella–zoster, 5 mg/kg every 8 hours usually for 5 days, doubled to 10 mg/kg every 8 hours in varicella–zoster in the immunocompromised and in simplex encephalitis (usually given for 10 days in encephalitis); prophylaxis of herpes simplex in the immunocompromised, 5 mg/kg every 8 hours

NEONATE up to 3 months, herpes simplex, 10 mg/kg every 8 hours usually for 10 days; CHILD 3 months–12 years, herpes simplex or varicella–zoster, 250 mg/m[2] every 8 hours usually for 5 days, doubled to 500 mg/m[2] every 8 hours for varicella–zoster in the immunocompromised and in simplex encephalitis (usually given for 10 days in encephalitis)

By topical application, see sections 13.10.3 (skin) and 11.3.3 (eye)

Aciclovir (Non-proprietary) PoM

Tablets, aciclovir 200 mg, net price 25-tab pack = £4.96; 400 mg, 56-tab pack = £12.05; 800 mg, 35-tab pack = £48.40. Label:9

Available from Alpharma, CP, Opus (*Virovir*®), Sovereign, Sterwin, Zurich

Dispersible tablets, aciclovir 200 mg, net price 25-tab pack = £6.02; 400 mg, 56-tab pack = £21.83; 800 mg, 35-tab pack = £21.88. Label: 9

Available from Genus, Hillcross, IVAX, Pharmacia, Ranbaxy, Sanofi-Synthelabo, Sterwin

Intravenous infusion, powder for reconstitution, aciclovir (as sodium salt). Net price 250-mg vial = £8.06; 500-mg vial = £18.71

Electrolytes: Na⁺ 1.1 mmol/250-mg vial

Available from Genus, Sovereign, Zurich

Intravenous infusion, aciclovir (as sodium salt), 25 mg/mL, net price 10-mL (250-mg) vial = £10.37; 20-mL (500-mg) vial = £19.21; 40-mL (1-g) vial = £40.44

Electrolytes: Na⁺ 1.16 mmol/250-mg vial

Available from Faulding DBL

Zovirax® (GlaxoWellcome) PoM

Tablets, all dispersible, aciclovir 200 mg (blue), net price 25-tab pack = £20.22; 400 mg (pink), 56-tab pack = £74.17; 800 mg (scored, *Shingles Treatment Pack*), 35-tab pack = £75.11. Label: 9

Suspension, both off-white, sugar-free, aciclovir 200 mg/5 mL (banana-flavoured), net price 125 mL = £28.89; 400 mg/5 mL (*Chickenpox Treatment*, orange-flavoured) 50 mL = £16.14. Label: 9

Intravenous infusion, powder for reconstitution, aciclovir (as sodium salt). Net price 250-mg vial = £10.91; 500-mg vial = £20.22

Electrolytes: Na⁺ 1.1 mmol/250-mg vial

FAMCICLOVIR

Note. Famciclovir is a pro-drug of penciclovir

Indications: treatment of herpes zoster, acute genital herpes simplex and suppression of recurrent genital herpes

Cautions: renal impairment (Appendix 3); pregnancy and breast-feeding; **interactions:** Appendix 1 (aciclovir and famciclovir)

Side-effects: nausea, vomiting; headache; rarely dizziness, confusion, hallucinations, rash; abdominal pain and fever have been reported in immunocompromised patients

Dose: herpes zoster, 250 mg 3 times daily for 7 days *or* 750 mg once daily for 7 days (in immunocompromised, 500 mg 3 times daily for 10 days)

Genital herpes, first episode, 250 mg 3 times daily for 5 days; recurrent infection, 125 mg twice daily for 5 days (in immunocompromised, all episodes, 500 mg twice daily for 7 days)

Genital herpes, suppression, 250 mg twice daily (in HIV patients, 500 mg twice daily) interrupted every 6–12 months

CHILD not recommended

Famvir® (Novartis) PoM

Tablets, all f/c, famciclovir 125 mg, net price 10-tab pack = £28.12; 250 mg, 15-tab pack = £84.35, 21-tab pack = £118.08; 56-tab pack = £314.90; 500 mg, 14-tab pack = £157.47, 30-tab pack = £337.34, 56-tab pack = £629.89; 750 mg, 7-tab pack = £112.72. Label: 9

INOSINE PRANOBEX ▰◣

Indications: see under Dose

Cautions: avoid in renal impairment; history of gout or hyperuricaemia

Side-effects: reversible increase in serum and urinary uric acid

Dose: mucocutaneous herpes simplex, 1 g 4 times daily for 7–14 days

Adjunctive treatment of genital warts, 1 g 3 times daily for 14–28 days

Subacute sclerosing panencephalitis, 50–100 mg/kg daily in 6 divided doses

Imunovir® (Ardern) PoM ▰◣

Tablets, inosine pranobex 500 mg. Net price 100 = £39.50. Label: 9

▰◣ denotes preparations that are considered to be less suitable for prescribing (see p. vi)

VALACICLOVIR

Note. Valaciclovir is a pro-drug of aciclovir

Indications: treatment of herpes zoster; treatment of initial and suppression of recurrent herpes simplex infections of skin and mucous membranes including initial and recurrent genital herpes

Cautions: see under Aciclovir

Side-effects: see under Aciclovir

Dose: herpes zoster, 1 g 3 times daily for 7 days
Herpes simplex, first episode, 500 mg twice daily for 5 days (up to 10 days if severe); recurrent infection, 500 mg twice daily for 5 days
Herpes simplex, suppression, 500 mg daily in 1–2 divided doses (in immunocompromised, 500 mg twice daily)
CHILD not recommended

Valtrex® (GlaxoWellcome) [PoM]
Tablets, f/c, valaciclovir (as hydrochloride) 500 mg, net price 10-tab (*HS Treatment*) pack = £23.50, 42-tab (*Shingles Treatment*) pack = £98.50. Label: 9

Human immunodeficiency virus

There is no cure for infection caused by the human immunodeficiency virus (HIV) but a number of drugs slow or halt disease progression. Drugs for HIV infection are toxic and expensive but they increase life expectancy. Treatment should be undertaken only by those experienced in their use. Advice on the management of HIV infection changes rapidly.

PRINCIPLES OF TREATMENT. Treatment is aimed at reducing the plasma viral load as much as possible and for as long as possible; it should be started before the immune system is irreversibly damaged. The need for early drug treatment should, however, be balanced against the development of toxicity. Commitment to treatment and strict adherence over many years are required; the regimen chosen should take into account convenience and patient tolerance. The development of drug resistance is reduced by using a combination of drugs; such combinations should have synergistic or additive activity while ensuring that their toxicity is not additive. Testing for resistance to antiviral drugs particularly in therapeutic failure should be considered.

INITIATION OF TREATMENT. The optimum time for initiation of antiviral treatment will depend primarily on the CD4 cell count; the plasma viral load and clinical symptoms may also help. Initiating treatment with a combination of drugs ('highly active antiretroviral therapy' which includes 2 nucleoside reverse transcriptase inhibitors with *either* a non-nucleoside reverse transcriptase inhibitor *or* 1 or 2 protease inhibitors) is recommended.

SWITCHING THERAPY. Deterioration of the condition (including clinical and virological changes) may require either switching therapy or adding another antiviral drug. The choice of an alternative regimen depends on factors such as the response to previous treatment, tolerance and the possibility of cross-resistance.

PREGNANCY AND BREAST-FEEDING. Treatment of HIV infection in pregnancy aims to reduce the risk of toxicity to the fetus (although the teratogenic potential of most antiretroviral drugs is unknown), to minimise the viral load and disease progression in the mother, and to prevent transmission of infection to the neonate. **All treatment options require careful assessment by a specialist.** Zidovudine monotherapy reduces transmission of infection to the neonate. However, combination antiretroviral therapy maximises the chance of preventing transmission and represents optimal therapy for the mother.

Breast-feeding by HIV-positive mothers may cause HIV infection in the infant and should be avoided.

POST-EXPOSURE PROPHYLAXIS. Treatment with antiviral drugs may be appropriate following occupational exposure to HIV-contaminated material. Immediate expert advice should be sought in such cases; national guidelines on post-exposure prophylaxis for healthcare workers have been developed (by the Chief Medical Officer's Expert Advisory Group on AIDS) and local ones may also be available.

DRUGS USED FOR HIV INFECTION. **Zidovudine,** a nucleoside reverse transcriptase inhibitor (or 'nucleoside analogue'), was the first anti-HIV drug to be introduced. High doses of zidovudine alone have been used to prevent the AIDS dementia complex but combination therapy using standard doses of zidovudine is now preferred. Other nucleoside reverse transcriptase inhibitors include **abacavir, didanosine, lamivudine, stavudine,** and **zalcitabine.**

The protease inhibitors include **amprenavir, indinavir, lopinavir, nelfinavir, ritonavir** and **saquinavir.** A combination of lopinavir and ritonavir has been introduced recently; the small amount of ritonavir in the combination has no intrinsic antiviral activity but it increases the antiviral activity of lopinavir by reducing its metabolism. The protease inhibitors are metabolised by cytochrome P450 enzyme system and therefore have a potential for significant drug interactions. Protease inhibitors are associated with lipodystrophy and metabolic effects (see below).

The non-nucleoside reverse transcriptase inhibitors **efavirenz** and **nevirapine** may interact with a number of drugs metabolised in the liver. Nevirapine is associated with a high incidence of rash (including Stevens-Johnson syndrome) and occasionally fatal hepatitis. Rash is also associated with efavirenz but it is usually milder. Efavirenz treatment has also been associated with an increased plasma cholesterol concentration.

LIPODYSTROPHY AND METABOLIC EFFECTS. The MCA has advised that combination antiretroviral therapy, including regimens containing a protease inhibitor, is associated with redistribution of body fat in some patients (e.g. decreased fat under the skin, increased abdominal fat, 'buffalo humps' and breast enlargement). Protease inhibitors are also associated with metabolic abnormalities such as hyperlipidaemia, insulin resistance, and hyperglycaemia. Clinical examination should include an evaluation of fat distribution; measurement of serum lipids and blood glucose should be considered.

Nucleoside reverse transcriptase inhibitors

ABACAVIR

Indications: HIV infection in combination with other antiretroviral drugs

Cautions: hepatic impairment (see below and Appendix 2); renal impairment (Appendix 3); **interactions:** Appendix 1 (abacavir)

HYPERSENSITIVITY REACTIONS. Life-threatening hypersensitivity reactions reported—characterised by fever or rash and possibly nausea, vomiting, diarrhoea, abdominal pain, lethargy, malaise, headache, myalgia and renal failure; less frequently mouth ulceration, oedema, hypotension, dyspnoea, sore throat, cough, paraesthesia, arthralgia, conjunctivitis, lymphadenopathy, lymphocytopenia and anaphylaxis (CSM has identified hypersensitivity reactions presenting as sore throat, influenza-like illness, cough and breathlessness); rarely myolysis; laboratory abnormalities may include raised liver function tests (see below) and creatine phosphokinase; symptoms usually appear in the first 6 weeks, but may occur at any time; monitor for symptoms every 2 weeks for 2 months; discontinue immediately if any symptom of hypersensitivity develops and do not rechallenge (risk of more severe hypersensitivity reaction); discontinue if hypersensitivity cannot be ruled out, even when other diagnoses possible—if rechallenge necessary it must be carried out in hospital setting; if abacavir is stopped for any reason other than hypersensitivity, exclude hypersensitivity reaction as the cause and rechallenge only if medical assistance is readily available; care needed with concomitant use of drugs which cause skin toxicity

COUNSELLING. Patients should be told the importance of regular dosing (intermittent therapy may increase the risk of sensitisation), how to recognise signs of hypersensitivity, and advised to seek immediate medical attention if symptoms develop or before re-starting treatment; patients should be advised to keep Alert card with them at all times

HEPATIC DISEASE. Potentially life-threatening lactic acidosis and severe hepatomegaly with steatosis reported therefore caution in liver disease, liver enzyme abnormalities, or risk factors for liver disease (particularly in obese women); suspend or discontinue if deterioration in liver function tests, hepatic steatosis, progressive hepatomegaly or unexplained lactic acidosis

Contra-indications: pregnancy (Appendix 4); breast-feeding

Side-effects: hypersensitivity reactions (see above), nausea, vomiting, diarrhoea, anorexia lethargy, fatigue, fever, headache, pancreatitis, lactic acidosis (see above)

Dose: 300 mg every 12 hours; CHILD safety and efficacy not established

Ziagen® (GlaxoWellcome) ▼ PoM

Tablets, yellow, f/c, abacavir (as sulphate) 300 mg, net price 60-tab pack = £238.50. Counselling, hypersensitivity reactions

Oral solution, sugar-free, banana and strawberry-flavoured, abacavir (as sulphate) 20 mg/ml, net price 240-mL = £63.60. Counselling, hypersensitivity reactions

■ With lamivudine and zidovudine

Trizivir® (GlaxoWellcome) ▼ PoM

Tablets, blue-green, f/c, abacavir (as sulphate) 300 mg, lamivudine 150 mg, zidovudine 300 mg, net price 60-tab pack = £581.08. Counselling, hypersensitivity reactions

Dose: ADULT over 18 years, 1 tablet twice daily

Note. For patients stabilised (for 6–8 weeks) on the individual components in the same proportions. For cautions, contra-indications and side-effects of individual drugs see Abacavir, Lamivudine and Zidovudine

DIDANOSINE

(ddI, DDI)

Indications: HIV infection in combination with other antiretroviral drugs

Cautions: history of pancreatitis (preferably avoid, otherwise extreme caution, see also below); peripheral neuropathy or hyperuricaemia (see under Side-effects); history of liver disease (see below); hepatic and renal impairment (see Appendixes 2 and 3); pregnancy; dilated retinal examinations recommended (especially in children) every 6 months, or if visual changes occur; **interactions:** Appendix 1 (didanosine)

PANCREATITIS. If symptoms of pancreatitis develop or if serum amylase or lipase is raised (even if asymptomatic) suspend treatment until diagnosis of pancreatitis excluded; on return to normal values re-initiate treatment only if essential (using low dose increased gradually if appropriate). Whenever possible avoid concomitant treatment with other drugs known to cause pancreatic toxicity (e.g. intravenous pentamidine isetionate); monitor closely if concomitant therapy unavoidable. Since significant elevations of triglycerides cause pancreatitis monitor closely if elevated

HEPATIC DISEASE. Potentially life-threatening lactic acidosis and severe hepatomegaly with steatosis reported therefore caution in liver disease, excessive alcohol intake, liver enzyme abnormalities, or risk factors for liver disease (particularly in obese women); suspend or discontinue if deterioration in liver function tests, hepatic steatosis, progressive hepatomegaly or unexplained lactic acidosis

Contra-indications: breast-feeding

Side-effects: pancreatitis (see also under Cautions); peripheral neuropathy especially in advanced HIV infection—suspend (reduced dose may be tolerated when symptoms resolve); hyperuricaemia (suspend treatment if significant elevation); diarrhoea (occasionally serious); also reported, nausea, vomiting, dry mouth, asthenia, headache, hypersensitivity reactions, retinal and optic nerve changes (especially in children), diabetes mellitus, raised liver function tests (see also under Cautions) liver failure

Dose: ADULT under 60 kg 250 mg daily in 1–2 divided doses, 60 kg and over 400 mg daily in 1–2 divided doses; CHILD over 3 months (under 6 years *Videx®* tablets only), 240 mg/m² daily (180 mg/m² daily in combination with zidovudine) in 1–2 divided doses

Videx® (Bristol-Myers Squibb) PoM

Tablets, both with calcium and magnesium antacids, didanosine 25 mg, net price 60-tab pack = £28.60; 100 mg, 60-tab pack = £88.00; 150 mg, 60-tab pack = £132.00; 200 mg, 60-tab pack =

£176.00. Label: 23, counselling, administration, see below

Excipients: include aspartame equivalent to phenylalanine 36.5 mg per tablet (section 9.4.1)

Note. Antacids in formulation may affect absorption of other drugs—see **interactions:** Appendix 1 (antacids)

COUNSELLING. To ensure sufficient antacid, each dose to be taken as 2 tablets (CHILD under 1 year 1 tablet) chewed thoroughly, crushed or dispersed in water; clear apple juice may be added for flavouring

Videx® *EC capsules,* enclosing e/c granules, didanosine 125 mg, net price 30-cap pack = £55.00; 200 mg, 30-cap pack = £88.00; 250 mg, 30-cap pack = £110.00; 400 mg, 30-cap pack = £176.00. Label 25, counselling, administration, see below

COUNSELLING. Capsules to be taken at least 2 hours after food

LAMIVUDINE

(3TC)

Indications: see preparations below

Cautions: renal impairment (Appendix 3), hepatic disease (see below); pregnancy (Appendix 4); **interactions:** Appendix 1 (lamivudine)

HEPATIC DISEASE. Potentially life-threatening lactic acidosis and severe hepatomegaly with steatosis reported therefore caution (particularly in obese women) in liver disease, liver enzyme abnormalities, or risk factors for liver disease; suspend or discontinue if deterioration in liver function tests, hepatic steatosis, progressive hepatomegaly or unexplained lactic acidosis. Recurrent hepatitis in patients with chronic hepatitis B may occur on discontinuation of lamivudine. When treating chronic hepatitis B with lamivudine, monitor liver function tests at least every 3 months and serological markers of hepatitis B every 6 months, more frequently in patients with advanced liver disease or following transplantation (monitoring to continue after discontinuation)—consult product literature

Contra-indications: breast-feeding

Side-effects: nausea, vomiting, diarrhoea, abdominal pain; cough; headache, insomnia; malaise, fever, rash, alopecia, muscle disorders; nasal symptoms; peripheral neuropathy reported; rarely pancreatitis (discontinue); neutropenia, anaemia and thrombocytopenia; lactic acidosis; raised liver enzymes and serum amylase reported

Dose: see preparations below

Epivir® (GlaxoWellcome) [PoM]

Tablets, f/c, lamivudine 150 mg, net price 60-tab pack = £163.59; 300 mg, 30-tab pack = £179.80

Oral solution, banana- and strawberry-flavoured, lamivudine 50 mg/5 mL, net price 240-mL pack = £44.53

Excipients: include sucrose 1 g/5 mL

Dose: HIV infection in combination with other antiretroviral drugs, 150 mg every 12 hours *or* 300 mg once daily; CHILD 3 months–12 years, 4 mg/kg every 12 hours; max. 300 mg daily

Zeffix® (GlaxoWellcome) [PoM]

Tablets, brown, f/c, lamivudine 100 mg, net price 28-tab pack = £76.34

Oral solution, banana and strawberry-flavoured, lamivudine 25 mg/5 mL, net price 240-mL pack = £22.27

Excipients: include sucrose 1 g/5 mL

Dose: chronic hepatitis B infection (with evidence of viral replication and *either* decompensated liver disease *or* histologically documented active liver inflammation or fibrosis), ADULT over 16 years, 100 mg daily; patients receiving lamivudine for concomitant HIV infection should continue to receive lamivudine in a dose appropriate for HIV infection

■ **With zidovudine**
See under Zidovudine

■ **With abacavir and zidovudine**
See under Abacavir

STAVUDINE

(d4T)

Indications: HIV infection in combination with other antiretroviral drugs

Cautions: history of peripheral neuropathy (see below); history of pancreatitis or concomitant use with other drugs associated with pancreatitis; hepatic disease (see below); renal impairment (Appendix 3); pregnancy; **interactions:** Appendix 1 (stavudine)

PERIPHERAL NEUROPATHY. Suspend if peripheral neuropathy develops—characterised by persistent numbness, tingling or pain in feet or hands; if symptoms resolve satisfactorily on withdrawal, resume treatment at half previous dose

HEPATIC DISEASE. Potentially life-threatening lactic acidosis and severe hepatomegaly with steatosis reported therefore caution in liver disease, liver enzyme abnormalities, or risk factors for liver disease (particularly in obese women); suspend or discontinue if deterioration in liver function tests, hepatic steatosis, progressive hepatomegaly or unexplained lactic acidosis

Contra-indications: breast-feeding

Side-effects: peripheral neuropathy (dose-related, see above); pancreatitis; nausea, vomiting, diarrhoea, constipation, anorexia, abdominal discomfort; chest pain; dyspnoea; headache, dizziness, insomnia, mood changes; asthenia, musculoskeletal pain; influenza-like symptoms, rash and other allergic reactions; lymphadenopathy; neoplasms; elevated liver enzymes and serum amylase; neutropenia, thrombocytopenia

Dose: ADULT under 60 kg, 30 mg every 12 hours preferably at least 1 hour before food; 60 kg and over, 40 mg every 12 hours; CHILD over 3 months, under 30 kg, 1 mg/kg every 12 hours; 30 kg and over, adult dose

Zerit® (Bristol-Myers Squibb) [PoM]

Capsules, stavudine 15 mg (yellow/red), net price 56-cap pack = £153.87; 20 mg (brown), 56-cap pack = £159.19; 30 mg (light orange/dark orange), 56-cap pack = £166.94; 40 mg (dark orange), 56-cap pack = £171.98 (all hosp. only)

Oral solution, cherry-flavoured, stavudine for reconstitution with water, 1 mg/mL, net price 200 mL = £24.35

ZALCITABINE

(ddC, DDC)

Indications: HIV infection in combination with other antiretroviral drugs

Cautions: patients at risk of developing peripheral neuropathy (see below); pancreatitis (see also below)—monitor serum amylase in those with history of elevated serum amylase, pancreatitis, alcohol abuse, or receiving parenteral nutrition; cardiomyopathy, history of congestive cardiac failure; hepatotoxicity (see below); pregnancy (women of childbearing age should use effective contraception during treatment); renal impairment (Appendix 3); **interactions:** Appendix 1 (zalcitabine)

PERIPHERAL NEUROPATHY. Discontinue immediately if peripheral neuropathy develops—characterised by numbness and burning dysaesthesia possibly followed by sharp shooting pains or severe continuous burning and potentially irreversible pain; extreme caution and close monitoring required in those at risk of peripheral neuropathy (especially those with low CD4 cell count for whom risk is greater and those receiving another drug known to cause peripheral neuropathy)

PANCREATITIS. Discontinue permanently if clinical pancreatitis develops; suspend if raised serum amylase associated with dysglycaemia, rising triglyceride, decreasing serum calcium or other signs of impending pancreatitis until pancreatitis excluded; suspend if treatment required with another drug known to cause pancreatic toxicity (e.g. intravenous pentamidine isetionate); caution and close monitoring if history of pancreatitis (or of elevated serum amylase) or if at risk of pancreatitis

HEPATIC DISEASE. Potentially life-threatening lactic acidosis and severe hepatomegaly with steatosis reported therefore caution in liver disease, liver enzyme abnormalities, or history of alcohol abuse or hepatitis; suspend or discontinue if deterioration in liver function tests, hepatic steatosis, progressive hepatomegaly or unexplained lactic acidosis

Contra-indications: peripheral neuropathy (see also above); breast-feeding

Side-effects: peripheral neuropathy (discontinue immediately, see also above); oral ulcers, nausea, vomiting, dysphagia, anorexia, diarrhoea, abdominal pain, constipation; pharyngitis; headache, dizziness; myalgia, arthralgia; rash, pruritus, sweating, weight loss, fatigue, fever, rigors, chest pain, anaemia, leucopenia, neutropenia, thrombocytopenia, disorders of liver function; less frequently pancreatitis (see also above), oesophageal ulcers (suspend treatment if no response to treatment for specific organisms), rectal ulcers, jaundice and hepatocellular damage (see also under Cautions); other less frequent side-effects include taste, hearing and visual disturbances, tachycardia, cardiomyopathy, congestive heart failure, dyspnoea, seizures, tremor, movement disorders, mood changes, sleep disturbances, alopecia, hyperuricaemia and renal disorders

Dose: 750 micrograms every 8 hours; CHILD under 13 years safety and efficacy not established

---

Hivid® (Roche) PoM

Tablets, both f/c, zalcitabine 375 micrograms (beige), net price 100-tab pack = £99.51; 750 micrograms (grey), 100-tab pack = £151.57

ZIDOVUDINE

(Azidothymidine, AZT)

Note. The abbreviation AZT which has sometimes been used for zidovudine has also been used for another drug

Indications: HIV infection in combination with other antiretroviral drugs; monotherapy for prevention of maternal-fetal HIV transmission (but see notes above under Pregnancy and breast-feeding)

Cautions: haematological toxicity (blood tests at least every 2 weeks for first 3 months then at least once a month, early disease with good bone marrow reserves may require less frequent tests e.g. every 1–3 months); vitamin B_{12} deficiency (increased risk of neutropenia); reduce dose or interrupt treatment according to product literature

if anaemia or myelosuppression; renal impairment (Appendix 3); hepatic impairment (see below and Appendix 2); risk of lactic acidosis, (see below); elderly; pregnancy; **interactions:** Appendix 1 (zidovudine)

HEPATIC DISEASE. Potentially life threatening lactic acidosis and severe hepatomegaly with steatosis reported therefore caution in liver disease, liver enzyme abnormalities, or risk factors for liver disease (particularly in obese women), suspend or discontinue if deterioration in liver function tests, hepatic steatosis, progressive hepatomegaly or unexplained lactic acidosis

Contra-indications: abnormally low neutrophil counts or haemoglobin values (consult product literature); neonates with hyperbilirubinaemia requiring treatment other than phototherapy, or with raised transaminase (consult product literature); breast-feeding

Side-effects: anaemia (may require transfusion), neutropenia, and leucopenia (all more frequent with high dose and advanced disease); also include, nausea and vomiting, abdominal pain, dyspepsia, diarrhoea, flatulence, taste disturbance, pancreatitis, liver disorders including fatty change and raised bilirubin and liver enzymes (see also under Cautions); chest pain, dyspnoea, cough; influenza-like symptoms, headache, fever, paraesthesia, neuropathy, convulsions, dizziness, somnolence, insomnia, anxiety, depression, loss of mental acuity, malaise, anorexia, asthenia, myopathy, myalgia; pancytopenia, thrombocytopenia; gynaecomastia; urinary frequency; rash, pruritus, pigmentation of nail, skin and oral mucosa

Dose: *by mouth,* 500–600 mg daily in 2–3 divided doses; CHILD over 3 months 360–480 mg/m² daily in 3–4 divided doses; max. 200 mg every 6 hours

Prevention of maternal-fetal HIV transmission, seek specialist advice (combination therapy preferred)

Patients temporarily unable to take zidovudine by mouth, *by intravenous infusion* over 1 hour, 1–2 mg/kg every 4 hours (approximating to 1.5–3 mg/kg every 4 hours by mouth) usually for no more than 2 weeks; CHILD 80–160 mg/m² every 6 hours (120 mg/m² every 6 hours approximates to 180 mg/m² every 6 hours by mouth)

Retrovir® (GlaxoWellcome) PoM

Capsules, zidovudine 100 mg (white/blue band), net price 100-cap pack = £119.33; 250 mg (blue/white/dark blue band), 40-cap pack = £119.33

Syrup, sugar-free, strawberry-flavoured, zidovudine 50 mg/5 mL, net price 200-mL pack with 10-mL oral syringe = £23.87

Injection, zidovudine 10 mg/mL. For dilution and use as an intravenous infusion. Net price 20-mL vial = £11.98

■ With lamivudine
For cautions, contra-indications, and side-effects of lamivudine, see Lamivudine

Combivir® (GlaxoWellcome) PoM

Tablets, f/c, zidovudine 300 mg, lamivudine 150 mg, net price 60-tab pack = £342.58

Dose: 1 tablet twice daily

■ With abacavir and lamivudine
See under Abacavir

Protease inhibitors

AMPRENAVIR

Indications: HIV infection in combination with other antiretroviral drugs in patients previously treated with other protease inhibitors

Cautions: hepatic impairment (Appendix 2); pregnancy (Appendix 4); diabetes; haemophilia; avoid vitamin E supplements (vitamin E included in formulation); oral solution contains propylene glycol—avoid in hepatic impairment, in severe renal impairment (Appendix 3), and in pregnancy; increased susceptibility to propylene glycol toxicity in slow metabolisers; **interactions:** Appendix 1 (amprenavir)

RASH. Rash may occur, usually in the second week of therapy; discontinue permanently if severe rash with systemic or allergic symptoms or, mucosal involvement; if rash mild or moderate, may continue without interruption—rash usually resolves within 2 weeks and may respond to antihistamines

Contra-indications: breast-feeding

Side-effects: rash including rarely Stevens-Johnson syndrome (see also above); nausea, vomiting, diarrhoea, flatulence, abdominal discomfort, dyspepsia; headache, sleep disturbances, tremors, oral or perioral paraesthesia, fatigue, mood disorders including depression; reports of elevated amylase; lipodystrophy and metabolic effects, see notes above

Dose: see preparations below

Agenerase® (GlaxoWellcome) ▼ PoM

Capsules, both ivory, amprenavir 50 mg, net price 480-cap pack = £150.00; 150 mg, 240-cap pack = £225.00. Label: 5

Excipients: include vitamin E 36 units/50 mg amprenavir

Dose: ADULT over 12 years, body-weight over 50 kg, 1.2 g every 12 hours; ADULT over 12 years, body-weight under 50 kg and CHILD over 4 years, 20 mg/kg every 12 hours (max. 2.4 g daily), CHILD under 4 years safety and efficacy not established

Oral solution, grape-bubblegum- and peppermint-flavoured, amprenavir 15 mg/mL, net price 240-mL pack = £36.00. Label: 4, 5

Excipients: include vitamin E 46 units/mL, propylene glycol 550 mg/mL

Dose: ADULT and CHILD over 4 years, 17 mg/kg every 8 hours (max. 2.8 g daily); CHILD under 4 years not recommended

Note. The bioavailability of *Agenerase®* oral solution is lower than that of capsules; the two formulations are **not** interchangeable on a milligram-for-milligram basis

INDINAVIR

Indications: HIV infection in combination with nucleoside reverse transcriptase inhibitors

Cautions: hepatic impairment (Appendix 2); ensure adequate hydration to reduce risk of nephrolithiasis; diabetes; haemophilia; pregnancy (Appendix 4); metabolism of many drugs inhibited if administered concomitantly, **interactions:** Appendix 1 (indinavir)

Contra-indications: breast-feeding

Side-effects: nausea, vomiting, diarrhoea, abdominal discomfort, dyspepsia, flatulence, pancreatitis, dry mouth, taste disturbances; headache, dizziness, insomnia; myalgia, myositis, rhabdomyolysis, asthenia, hypoaesthesia, paraesthesia; anaphylactoid reactions, rash (including Stevens-Johnson syndrome), pruritus, dry skin, hyperpigmentation, alopecia, paronychia; interstitial nephritis, nephrolithiasis (may require interruption or discontinuation; more frequent in children), dysuria, haematuria, crystalluria, proteinuria, pyuria (in children); hepatitis, transient hyperbilirubinaemia; blood disorders including neutropenia, haemolytic anaemia; lipodystrophy and metabolic effects, see notes above

Dose: 800 mg every 8 hours; CHILD and ADOLESCENT 4–17 years, 500 mg/m² every 8 hours (max. 800 mg every 8 hours); CHILD under 4 years, safety and efficacy not established

Crixivan® (MSD) PoM

Capsules, indinavir (as sulphate) 100 mg, net price 180-cap pack = £51.43; 200 mg, 360-cap pack = £205.71; 333 mg, 135-cap pack = £128.45; 400 mg, 90-cap pack = £102.86, 180-cap pack = £205.71. Counselling, administration

COUNSELLING. Administer 1 hour before or 2 hours after a meal; may be administered with a low-fat, light meal; in combination with didanosine, allow 1 hour between each drug (antacids in didanosine tablets reduce absorption of indinavir)

Note. Bottles include desiccant canisters

LOPINAVIR WITH RITONAVIR

Indications: HIV infection in combination with other antiretroviral drugs

Cautions: hepatic impairment—avoid if severe (Appendix 2, *Kaletra®*); renal impairment (Appendix 3, *Kaletra®*); oral solution contains propylene glycol—avoid in severe hepatic and renal impairment and in pregnancy, increased susceptibility to propylene glycol toxicity in slow metabolisers; haemophilia; pregnancy (Appendix 4, *Kaletra®*); diabetes; **interactions:** Appendix 1 (*Kaletra®*)

PANCREATITIS. Signs and symptoms suggestive of pancreatitis (including raised serum amylase and lipase) should be evaluated—discontinue if pancreatitis diagnosed

Contra-indications: breast-feeding (Appendix 5, *Kaletra®*)

Side-effects: diarrhoea, nausea, vomiting, colitis, abdominal discomfort, asthenia, headache, insomnia; rash; less frequently, dry mouth, pancreatitis (see also Cautions), dyspepsia, dysphagia, oesophagitis, influenza-like syndrome, appetite changes; hypertension, palpitations, thrombophlebitis, vasculitis, chest pain, dyspnoea, agitation, anxiety, ataxia, hypertonia, confusion, depression, dizziness, dyskinesia, paraesthesia, peripheral neuritis, somnolence; Cushing's syndrome, hypothyroidism, sexual dysfunction, anaemia, leucopenia, dehydration, oedema, lactic acidosis; arthralgia, myalgia, abnormal vision, otitis media, taste disturbances, tinnitus; acne, alopecia, dry skin, pruritus, skin discoloration, nail disorders, sweating; lipodystrophy and metabolic effects, see notes above;

raised bilirubin and lowered sodium, low platelet and low neutrophil counts also reported in children

Dose: see preparations below

Kaletra® (Abbott) ▼ [PoM]

Capsules, orange, lopinavir 133.3 mg, ritonavir 33.3 mg, net price 180-cap pack = £332.31. Label: 21

Dose: ADULT and ADOLESCENT with body surface area of 1.3 m² or greater, 3 capsules twice daily with food; CHILD with body surface area less than 1.3 m², see under Oral Solution

Oral solution, lopinavir 400 mg, ritonavir 100 mg/ 5 mL, net price 5×60-mL packs = £332.31. Label: 21

Excipients: include propylene glycol, alcohol 42%

Dose: ADULT and ADOLESCENT with body surface area of 1.3 m² or greater, 5 mL twice daily with food; CHILD over 2 years 2.9 mL/m² twice daily with food, max. 5 mL twice daily; CHILD under 2 years, safety and efficacy not established

Note. 5 mL oral solution ≡ 3 capsules; where appropriate, capsules may be used instead of oral solution

NELFINAVIR

Indications: HIV infection in combination with other antiretroviral drugs

Cautions: hepatic and renal impairment; diabetes; haemophilia; pregnancy; **interactions:** Appendix 1 (nelfinavir)

Contra-indications: breast-feeding

Side-effects: diarrhoea, nausea, vomiting, flatulence, abdominal pain; rash; reports of elevated creatine kinase, hepatitis, pancreatitis, neutropenia, hypersensitivity reactions including bronchospasm, fever, pruritus and facial oedema, lipodystrophy and metabolic effects, see notes above

Dose: 1.25 g twice daily *or* 750 mg 3 times daily; CHILD 3–13 years, initially 25–30 mg/kg 3 times daily, under 3 years safety and efficacy not established

Viracept® (Roche) [PoM]

Tablets, f/c, nelfinavir (as mesilate) 250 mg, net price 270-tab pack = £289.23. Label: 21

Oral powder, nelfinavir (as mesilate) 50 mg/g. Net price 144 g (with 1-g and 5-g scoop) = £30.88. Label: 21, counselling, administration

Excipients: include aspartame (section 9.4.1)

COUNSELLING. Powder may be mixed with water, milk, formula feeds or pudding; it should **not** be mixed with acidic foods or juices owing to its taste

RITONAVIR

Indications: progressive or advanced HIV infection in combination with nucleoside reverse transcriptase inhibitors

Cautions: hepatic impairment; diabetes; haemophilia; pregnancy; **interactions:** Appendix 1 (ritonavir)

PANCREATITIS. Signs and symptoms suggestive of pancreatitis (including raised serum amylase and lipase) should be evaluated—discontinue if pancreatitis diagnosed

Contra-indications: severe hepatic impairment; breast-feeding

Side-effects: nausea, vomiting, diarrhoea (may impair absorption—close monitoring required), abdominal pain, taste disturbances, dyspepsia, anorexia, throat irritation; vasodilatation; headache, circumoral and peripheral paraesthesia, hyperaesthesia, dizziness, sleep disturbances, asthenia, rash, leucopenia; raised liver enzymes, bilirubin, and uric acid; occasionally flatulence, eructation, dry mouth and ulceration, cough, anxiety, fever, pain, myalgia, weight loss, decreased thyroxine, sweating, pruritus, electrolyte disturbances, anaemia, neutropenia, increased prothrombin time; pancreatitis (see also under Cautions); lipodystrophy and metabolic effects, see notes above

Dose: 600 mg every 12 hours; CHILD over 2 years initially 250 mg/m² every 12 hours, increased by 50 mg/m² at intervals of 2–3 days to 350 mg/m² every 12 hours (max. 600 mg every 12 hours)

Norvir® (Abbott) [PoM]

Capsules, ritonavir 100 mg, net price 336-cap pack = £377.39. Label 21

Excipients: include alcohol 12%

Oral solution, sugar-free, ritonavir 400 mg/5 mL, net price 5 × 90-mL packs (with measuring cup) = £403.20. Label: 21, counselling

COUNSELLING. Oral solution contains 43% alcohol; bitter taste can be masked by mixing with chocolate milk; do not mix with water, measuring cup must be dry

■ With lopinavir
See under Lopinavir with ritonavir

SAQUINAVIR

Indications: HIV infection in combination with other antiretroviral drugs

Cautions: hepatic impairment (Appendix 2); renal impairment (Appendix 3); diabetes; haemophilia; pregnancy (Appendix 4); **interactions:** Appendix 1 (saquinavir)

Contra-indications: severe hepatic impairment (Appendix 2), breast-feeding

Side-effects: diarrhoea, buccal and mucosal ulceration, abdominal discomfort, nausea, vomiting; headache, peripheral neuropathy, paraesthesia, dizziness, insomnia, mood changes, ataxia, musculoskeletal pain, asthenia; fever, pruritus, rash and other skin eruptions, rarely Stevens-Johnson syndrome; other rare side-effects include thrombocytopenia and other blood disorders, seizures, liver damage, pancreatitis and nephrolithiasis; reports of elevated creatine kinase, raised liver enzymes and neutropenia when used in combination therapy; lipodystrophy and metabolic effects, see notes above

Dose: see preparations below

Note. To avoid confusion between the different formulations of saquinavir, prescribers should specify the brand to be dispensed; absorption from *Fortovase*® is much greater than from *Invirase*®. Treatment should generally be initiated with *Fortovase*®

Fortovase® (Roche) [PoM]

Capsules (gel-filled), beige, saquinavir 200 mg, net price 180-cap pack = £104.34. Label: 21

Dose: 1.2 g every 8 hours (within 2 hours after a meal); CHILD under 16 years, safety and efficacy not established

Invirase® (Roche) ‖PoM‖

Capsules, brown/green, saquinavir (as mesilate) 200 mg, net price 270-cap pack = £289.23. Label: 21

Dose: 600 mg every 8 hours (within 2 hours after a meal); CHILD under 16 years, safety and efficacy not established

Non-nucleoside reverse transcriptase inhibitors

EFAVIRENZ

Indications: HIV infection in combination with other antiretroviral drugs

Cautions: hepatic impairment (avoid if severe; Appendix 2); severe renal impairment; pregnancy; elderly; history of mental illness or substance abuse; **interactions:** Appendix 1 (efavirenz)

RASH. Rash, usually in the first 2 weeks, is the most common side-effect; discontinue if severe rash with blistering, desquamation, mucosal involvement or fever; if rash mild or moderate, may continue without interruption—rash usually resolves within 1 month

Contra-indications: breast-feeding

Side-effects: rash including Stevens-Johnson syndrome (see also above); dizziness, headache, insomnia, somnolence, abnormal dreams, fatigue, impaired concentration (administration at bedtime especially in the first 2–4 weeks reduces CNS effects); nausea; less frequently vomiting, diarrhoea, hepatitis, depression, anxiety, psychosis, amnesia, ataxia, stupor, vertigo; also reported raised serum cholesterol, elevated liver enzymes (especially if seropositive for hepatitis B or C), pancreatitis

Dose: 600 mg once daily; CHILD over 3 years, body-weight 13–14 kg, 200 mg daily; body-weight 15–19 kg, 250 mg once daily; body-weight 20–24 kg, 300 mg once daily; body-weight 25–32.4 kg, 350 mg once daily; body-weight 32.5–39 kg, 400 mg once daily; body-weight 40 kg and over, adult dose

Sustiva (Bristol-Myers Squibb) ▼ ‖PoM‖

Capsules, efavirenz 50 mg (yellow/white), net price 30-cap pack = £18.72; 100 mg (white), 30-cap pack = £37.39; 200 mg (yellow), 90-cap pack = £224.09

NEVIRAPINE

Indications: progressive or advanced HIV infection, in combination with at least two other antiretroviral drugs

Cautions: hepatic impairment (see below and Appendix 2); renal impairment; pregnancy; **interactions:** Appendix 1 (nevirapine)

HEPATIC DISEASE. Potentially life-threatening hepatotoxicity including fatal fulminant hepatitis reported usually occurring in first 8 weeks; monitor liver function before treatment then every 2 weeks for 2 months then after 1 month and then every 3–6 months; discontinue permanently if abnormalities in liver function tests accompanied by hypersensitivity reaction (rash, fever, arthralgia, myalgia, lymphadenopathy, hepatitis, renal impairment, eosinophilia, granulocytopenia); suspend if severe abnormalities in liver function tests but no hyper-

sensitivity reaction—discontinue permanently if significant liver function abnormalities recur; monitor patient closely if mild to moderate abnormalities in liver function tests with no hypersensitivity reaction

Note. If treatment interrupted for more than 7 days reintroduce with 200 mg daily (CHILD 4 mg/kg daily) and increase dose cautiously

RASH. Rash, usually occurring in first 8 weeks, is most common side-effect; incidence reduced if introduced at low dose and dose increased gradually; discontinue permanently if severe rash or if rash accompanied by blistering, oral lesions, conjunctivitis, swelling, general malaise or hypersensitivity reactions; if rash mild or moderate may continue without interruption but dose should not be increased until rash resolves

COUNSELLING. Patients should be told how to recognise hypersensitivity reactions and advised to seek immediate medical attention if symptoms develop

Contra-indications: breast-feeding

Side-effects: rash including Stevens-Johnson syndrome and rarely, toxic epidermal necrolysis (see also Cautions above); hepatitis or jaundice reported (see also Cautions above); nausea, vomiting, abdominal pain, diarrhoea, headache, drowsiness, fatigue, fever; hypersensitivity reactions (may involve hepatic reactions and rash, see Cautions above); anaphylaxis, angioedema, urticaria also reported

Dose: 200 mg once daily for first 14 days then (if no rash present) 200 mg twice daily; CHILD 2 months–8 years, 4 mg/kg once daily for first 14 days then (if no rash present) 7 mg/kg twice daily (max. 400 mg daily); 8–16 years (but under 50 kg), 4 mg/kg once daily for first 14 days then (if no rash present) 4 mg/kg twice daily (max. 400 mg daily); over 50 kg, adult dose

Viramune® (Boehringer Ingelheim) ▼ ‖PoM‖

Tablets, nevirapine 200 mg, net price 60-tab pack = £168.00. Counselling, hypersensitivity reactions

Suspension, nevirapine 50 mg/5 mL, net price 240-mL pack = £50.40. Counselling, hypersensitivity reactions

Cytomegalovirus (CMV)

Recommendations for the optimum maintenance therapy of cytomegalovirus (CMV) infections and the duration of treatment are subject to rapid change.

Ganciclovir is related to aciclovir but it is more active against cytomegalovirus; it is also much more toxic than aciclovir and should therefore be prescribed only when the potential benefit outweighs the risks. Ganciclovir is administered by intravenous infusion for the *initial treatment* of CMV retinitis. Capsules are available for *maintenance treatment* of CMV retinitis in AIDS patients following intravenous therapy and for *prevention* of cytomegalovirus disease in liver and kidney transplant patients. Ganciclovir causes profound myelosuppression when given with zidovudine; the two should not normally be given together particularly during initial ganciclovir therapy. The likelihood of ganciclovir resistance increases in patients with a high viral load or in those who receive the drug over a long duration; cross-resistance to cidofovir is common.

Foscarnet is also active against cytomegalovirus; it is toxic and can cause renal impairment.

Cidofovir is a DNA polymerase chain inhibitor which is given for CMV retinitis in AIDS patients when ganciclovir and foscarnet are contra-indicated; it is given in combination with probenecid. It is nephrotoxic.

For local treatment of CMV retinitis, see section 11.3.3.

CIDOFOVIR

Indications: cytomegalovirus retinitis in AIDS patients for whom other drugs are inappropriate

Cautions: monitor renal function (serum creatinine and urinary protein) and neutrophil count within 24 hours before each dose; co-treatment with probenecid and prior hydration with intravenous fluids necessary to minimise potential nephrotoxicity (see below); diabetes mellitus (increased risk of ocular hypotony)

NEPHROTOXICITY. Do not initiate treatment in renal impairment (assess creatinine clearance and proteinuria—consult product literature); discontinue treatment and hydrate with intravenous fluids if deterioration of renal function occurs—consult product literature

OCULAR DISORDERS. Regular ophthalmological examinations recommended; iritis and uveitis have been reported which may respond to a topical corticosteroid with or without a cycloplegic drug—discontinue cidofovir if no response to topical corticosteroid or if condition worsens, or if iritis or uveitis recurs after successful treatment

Contra-indications: renal impairment (creatinine clearance 55 mL/minute or less); concomitant administration of potentially nephrotoxic drugs (discontinue potentially nephrotoxic drugs at least 7 days before starting cidofovir); pregnancy (avoid pregnancy during and for 1 month after treatment, men should not father a child during or within 3 months of treatment), breast-feeding

Side-effects: nephrotoxicity (see Cautions above); neutropenia, fever, asthenia, alopecia, nausea, vomiting, decreased intra-ocular pressure, iritis, uveitis (see Cautions above)

Dose: by intravenous infusion over 1 hour, initial (induction) treatment, 5 mg/kg once weekly for 2 weeks (give probenecid and intravenous fluids with each dose, see below); CHILD not recommended

Maintenance treatment, beginning 2 weeks after completion of induction, by intravenous infusion over 1 hour, 5 mg/kg once every 2 weeks (give probenecid and intravenous fluids with each dose, see below)

PROBENECID CO-TREATMENT, by mouth (preferably after food), probenecid 2 g 3 hours before cidofovir infusion followed by probenecid 1 g at 2 hours and 1 g at 8 hours after the end of cidofovir infusion (total probenecid 4 g); for cautions, contra-indications and side-effects of probenecid see section 10.1.4

PRIOR HYDRATION, sodium chloride 0.9%, by intravenous infusion, 1 litre over 1 hour immediately before cidofovir infusion (if tolerated an additional 1 litre may be given over 1–3 hours, starting at the same time as the cidofovir infusion or immediately afterwards

Vistide® (Pharmacia) ▒PoM▒
Intravenous infusion, cidofovir 75 mg/mL, net price 5-mL vial = £544.35
CAUTION IN HANDLING. Cidofovir is toxic and personnel should be adequately protected during handling and administration; if solution comes into contact with skin or mucosa, wash off immediately with water

GANCICLOVIR

Indications: life-threatening or sight-threatening cytomegalovirus infections in immunocompromised patients only; prevention of cytomegalovirus disease during immunosuppressive therapy following organ transplantation; local treatment of CMV retinitis (section 11.3.3)

Cautions: close monitoring of blood counts (dose adjustment or interruption may be required—consult product literature); history of cytopenia; low platelet count; potential carcinogen and teratogen; renal impairment (consult product literature); ensure adequate hydration during intravenous administration; vesicant—infuse into vein with adequate flow preferably using a plastic cannula; limited experience in children (possible risk of long-term carcinogenic or reproductive toxicity—not for neonatal or congenital cytomegalovirus disease); **interactions:** Appendix 1 (ganciclovir)

Contra-indications: pregnancy (ensure effective contraception during treatment and barrier contraception for men during and for at least 90 days after treatment); breast-feeding (until 72 hours after last dose); hypersensitivity to ganciclovir or aciclovir; abnormally low neutrophil or platelet counts (see product literature)

Side-effects: nausea, diarrhoea, abdominal pain, asthenia, leucopenia, anaemia; less frequently, vomiting, dyspepsia, flatulence, anorexia, headache, paraesthesia, fever, rash, pruritus, alopecia, injection site reactions, thrombocytopenia; rarely, mouth ulcers, dry mouth, dysphagia, oesophagitis, gastritis, gastro-intestinal haemorrhage, faecal incontinence, constipation, pancreatitis, hepatitis, jaundice, chest pain, arrhythmias, hypertension, hypotension, oedema, thrombophlebitis, dyspnoea, migraine, dizziness, sleep disturbances, abnormal dreams, anxiety, amnesia, ataxia, emotional lability, psychosis, abnormal gait, seizures, tremor, neuropathy, hyperkinesia, hypertonia, coma, breast pain, urinary frequency, haematuria, impotence, aspermatogenesis, decreased libido, renal impairment, arthralgia, myalgia, myasthenia, urticaria, dry skin, acne, photosensitivity, sweating, disturbances in taste, hearing, and vision, eye or ear pain, changes in blood glucose, hypokalaemia, eosinophilia, pancytopenia, splenomegaly

Dose: by intravenous infusion, initial (induction) treatment, 5 mg/kg every 12 hours for 14–21 days for treatment or for 7–14 days for prevention; maintenance (for patients at risk of relapse of retinitis) 6 mg/kg daily on 5 days per week or 5 mg/kg daily every day until adequate recovery of immunity; if retinitis progresses initial induction treatment may be repeated

Maintenance treatment in AIDS patients where retinitis stable (following at least 3 weeks of intravenous ganciclovir), by mouth, 1 g 3 times daily with food or 500 mg 6 times daily with food

Prevention of cytomegalovirus disease in liver and kidney transplant patients, by mouth, 1 g 3 times daily with food

Cymevene® (Roche) ▒PoM▒
Capsules, ganciclovir 250 mg (green), net price 84-cap pack = £253.70; 500 mg (green/yellow), 90-cap pack = £543.64. Label: 21

Intravenous infusion, powder for reconstitution, ganciclovir (as sodium salt). Net price 500-mg vial = £33.98

Electrolytes: Na⁺ 2 mmol/500-mg vial

CAUTION IN HANDLING. Ganciclovir is toxic and personnel should be adequately protected during handling and administration; if solution comes into contact with skin or mucosa, wash off immediately with soap and water

FOSCARNET SODIUM

Indications: cytomegalovirus retinitis in AIDS patients; mucocutaneous herpes simplex virus infections unresponsive to aciclovir in immuno-compromised patients

Cautions: renal impairment (reduce dose or avoid if severe); monitor electrolytes, particularly calcium and magnesium; monitor serum creatinine every second day during induction and every week during maintenance; ensure adequate hydration; avoid rapid infusion

Contra-indications: pregnancy, breast-feeding

Side-effects: nausea, vomiting, diarrhoea (occasionally constipation and dyspepsia), abdominal pain, anorexia; changes in blood pressure and ECG; headache, fatigue, mood disturbances (including psychosis), asthenia, paraesthesia, convulsions, tremor, dizziness, and other neurological disorders; rash; impairment of renal function including acute renal failure; hypocalcaemia (sometimes symptomatic) and other electrolyte disturbances; abnormal liver function tests; decreased haemoglobin concentration, leucopenia, granulocytopenia, thrombocytopenia; thrombophlebitis if given undiluted by peripheral vein; genital irritation and ulceration (due to high concentrations excreted in urine); isolated reports of pancreatitis

Dose: CMV retinitis induction, *by intravenous infusion*, 60 mg/kg every 8 hours for 2–3 weeks then maintenance, 60 mg/kg daily, increased to 90–120 mg/kg if tolerated; if retinitis progresses on maintenance dose, repeat induction regimen

Mucocutaneous herpes simplex infection, *by intravenous infusion*, 40 mg/kg every 8 hours for 2–3 weeks or until lesions heal

Foscavir® (AstraZeneca) PoM

Intravenous infusion, foscarnet sodium hexahydrate 24 mg/mL, net price 250-mL bottle = £31.35

Viral hepatitis

The management of uncomplicated acute viral hepatitis is largely symptomatic. Early treatment of acute hepatitis C with interferon alfa [unlicensed indication] may reduce the risk of chronic infection. Hepatitis B and hepatitis C viruses are major causes of chronic hepatitis. For details on immunisation against hepatitis A and B infections, see section 14.4 (active immunisation) and section 14.5 (passive immunisation).

CHRONIC HEPATITIS B. **Interferon alfa** (section 8.2.4) is used in the treatment of chronic hepatitis B but its use is limited by a response rate of less than 50%, and relapse is frequent. If no improvement occurs after 3–4 months of treatment, interferon alfa should be discontinued. Interferon alfa is contra-indicated in patients receiving immunosuppressant treatment (or who have received it recently). The manufacturers of interferon alfa contra-indicate its use in decompensated liver disease but low doses can be used with great caution in these patients.

Lamivudine (see p. 302) is licensed for the treatment of chronic hepatitis B. It is usually reserved for patients in whom interferon alfa cannot be used or if seroconversion is unlikely; it can be used in patients with decompensated liver disease. Treatment should be continued if there is no loss of efficacy and until adequate seroconversion is achieved (consult product literature); it is continued long-term in decompensated liver disease. Hepatitis B viruses with reduced susceptibility to lamivudine have emerged following extended therapy. In patients infected with HIV and hepatitis B, lamivudine should be given only as part of combination antiretroviral therapy and in a dose appropriate for treating HIV; the use of lamivudine alone is likely to result in lamivudine-resistant HIV.

CHRONIC HEPATITIS C. **Ribavirin** (tribavirin) (*Rebetol®*, see p. 310) can be used in combination with either **peginterferon alfa-2b** or **interferon alfa** (section 8.2.4) for the treatment of chronic hepatitis C; ribavirin monotherapy is ineffective. The combination should usually be continued for at least 6 months but in some cases it may be necessary to extend treatment by a further 6 months according to viral genotype (consult product literature). Combination therapy can also be used in patients with chronic hepatitis C who have not responded to interferon alfa or to peginterferon alfa monotherapy.

Peginterferon alfa-2b alone may be used in the treatment of chronic hepatitis C if ribavirin is not tolerated or is contra-indicated but monotherapy is less effective and relapse is more common. Interferon alfa alone has also been used but it is less effective than peginterferon alfa-2b.

NICE guidance (ribavirin and interferon alfa for hepatitis C). The National Institute for Clinical Excellence has recommended that the combination of interferon alfa and ribavirin should be used for the treatment of moderate to severe hepatitis C (as determined by liver histology or, if biopsy too risky, determined on clinical grounds) in patients aged over 18 years who have:

- not previously been treated with combination therapy;
- previously responded to interferon alfa mono-therapy, but have since relapsed.

Combination therapy with interferon alfa and ribavirin should be continued for 6 months. Extension of treatment by a further 6 months is recommended only in patients infected with hepatitis C virus of genotype I and who have responded to treatment during the first 6 months (as judged by clearance of circulating viral RNA).

Interferon alfa monotherapy should be considered when ribavirin is contra-indicated or not tolerated. Treatment with interferon alfa alone or in combination with ribavirin is not recommended in patients who continue to abuse intravenous drugs and are at risk of reinfection or who are heavy users of alcohol (risk of exacerbating liver damage).

Influenza

For advice on immunisation against influenza, see section 14.4.

Amantadine may be used for prophylaxis during an outbreak of influenza A **only** in:

- unimmunised patients in 'at risk' groups (see under Influenza vaccine, section 14.4), for 2 weeks while the vaccine takes effect

- patients in 'at risk' groups for whom immunisation is contra-indicated, for the duration of the outbreak

- health care workers and other key personnel (to prevent disruption of service), during an epidemic

The Joint Committee on Vaccination and Immunisation has advised that amantadine should not be used for both prophylaxis and treatment of influenza in the same household (risk of resistance). Amantadine has also been used by mouth for herpes zoster, but its effectiveness has not been established.

Zanamivir is licensed for the treatment of influenza A or B within 48 hours after the onset of symptoms. In otherwise healthy adults it reduces the duration of symptoms by about 1 day. No reliable data are available on the impact of zanamivir on hospitalisation or on mortalitiy in those considered to be at risk of serious complications from influenza. The cautions under Zanamivir should also be noted.

NICE guidance (zanamivir for treatment of influenza). The National Institute for Clinical Excellence has recommended that:

- zanamivir should **not** be used to treat otherwise healthy adults with influenza;

- zanamivir should be used to treat at-risk adults when influenza is circulating in the community if they are able to commence treatment within 48 hours after the onset of symptoms.

At-risk patients are defined as those aged over 65 years *or* those who have one or more of the following conditions:

- chronic respiratory disease (including chronic obstructive pulmonary disease and asthma) requiring regular medication [but see cautions under Zanamivir below];

- significant cardiovascular disease (excluding hypertension);

- immunosuppression;

- diabetes mellitus.

Community-based virological surveillance schemes including those ran by the Public Health Laboratory Service and the Royal College of General Practitioners should be used to indicate when influenza is circulating in the community.

AMANTADINE HYDROCHLORIDE

Indications: see under Dose; parkinsonism (section 4.9.1)

Cautions: see section 4.9.1

Contra-indications: see section 4.9.1

Side-effects: see section 4.9.1

Dose: herpes zoster (but see notes above), 100 mg twice daily for 14 days, if necessary extended for a further 14 days for post-herpetic pain
Influenza A (see also notes above), ADULT and CHILD over 10 years, treatment, 100 mg daily for 4–5 days; prophylaxis, 100 mg daily usually for 6 weeks *or* with influenza vaccination for 2–3 weeks after vaccination
ELDERLY 100 mg daily

Lysovir® (Alliance) PoM
Capsules, red-brown, amantadine hydrochloride 100 mg, net price 5-cap pack = £2.40, 14-cap pack = £4.80. Counselling, driving

---

ZANAMIVIR

Indications: treatment of influenza A or B within 48 hours after onset of symptoms when influenza is endemic in the community

Cautions: asthma and chronic pulmonary disease (risk of bronchospasm—short-acting bronchodilator should be available; avoid in severe asthma unless close monitoring possible and appropriate facilities available to treat bronchospasm; uncontrolled chronic illness; other inhaled drugs should be administered before zanamivir; pregnancy (Appendix 4)

Contra-indications: breast-feeding

Side-effects: gastro-intestinal disturbances; reported rarely, bronchospasm, respiratory impairment, and rash

Dose: *by inhalation of powder*, 10 mg twice daily for 5 days, CHILD under 12 years not recommended

Relenza® (GlaxoWellcome) ▼ PoM
Dry powder for inhalation, disks containing 4 blisters of zanamivir 5mg/blister, net price 5 disks with *Diskhaler®* device = £24.00

Respiratory syncytial virus

Ribavirin (tribavirin) inhibits a wide range of DNA and RNA viruses. It is licensed for administration by inhalation for the treatment of severe bronchiolitis caused by the respiratory syncytial virus (RSV) in infants, especially when they have other serious diseases. However, there is no clear evidence that ribavirin produces clinically relevant benefit in RSV bronchiolitis. Ribavirin is given by mouth with peginterferon alfa-2b or interferon alfa for the treatment of chronic hepatitis C infection (see Viral Hepatitis, p. 308). It is also effective in Lassa fever [unlicensed indication].

Palivizumab is a monoclonal antibody indicated for the prevention of respiratory syncytial virus infection in infants at high risk of infection. It is licensed for monthly use during the RSV season; the first dose should be administered before the start of the RSV season.

PALIVIZUMAB

Indications: prevention of serious lower respiratory-tract infection caused by respiratory syncytial virus (RSV) requiring hospitalisation in children born at 35 weeks gestation or less and who are less than 6 months old at onset of RSV season, or in children less than 2 years old who have received treatment for bronchopulmonary dysplasia within the last 6 months

Cautions: moderate to severe acute infection or febrile illness; congenital heart disease; thrombocytopenia; facilities for cardiopulmonary resuscitation must be at hand

Contra-indications: hypersensitivity to humanised monoclonal antibodies

Side-effects: fever, injection site reactions, nervousness; less frequently diarrhoea, vomiting, rhinitis, cough, wheeze, pain, rash, leucopenia, abnormal liver function tests

Dose: *by intramuscular injection* (preferably in anterolateral thigh), 15 mg/kg once a month during season of RSV risk; injection volume over 1 mL should be divided between more than one site

Synagis® (Abbott) ▼ PoM
Injection, powder for reconstitution, palivizumab, net price 50-mg vial = £424.00; 100-mg vial = £706.00

RIBAVIRIN
(Tribavirin)

Indications: severe respiratory syncytial virus bronchiolitis in infants and children; in combination with peginterferon alfa-2b or interferon alfa for chronic hepatitis C not previously treated in patients without liver decompensation and who have fibrosis or high inflammatory activity or for relapse following previous response to interferon alfa

Cautions:
SPECIFIC CAUTIONS FOR INHALED TREATMENT. Maintain standard supportive respiratory and fluid management therapy; monitor electrolytes closely; monitor equipment for precipitation; pregnant women (and those planning pregnancy) should avoid exposure to aerosol
SPECIFIC CAUTIONS FOR ORAL TREATMENT. Exclude pregnancy before treatment; effective contraception essential during treatment and for 4 months after treatment in women and for 7 months after treatment in men; routine monthly pregnancy tests recommended; condoms must be used if partner of male patient is pregnant (ribavirin excreted in semen); cardiac disease (assessment including ECG recommended before and during treatment—discontinue if deterioration); gout; determine full blood count, platelets, electrolytes, serum creatinine, liver function tests and uric acid before starting treatment and then on weeks 2 and 4 of treatment, then as indicated clinically—adjust dose if adverse reactions or laboratory abnormalities develop (consult product literature)

Contra-indications: pregnancy (**important teratogenic risk**: see Cautions and Appendix 4); breast-feeding
SPECIFIC CONTRA-INDICATIONS FOR ORAL TREATMENT. Severe cardiac disease, including unstable or uncontrolled cardiac disease in previous 6 months; haemoglobinopathies; severe debilitating medical conditions; renal impairment (Appendix 3); severe hepatic dysfunction or decompensated cirrhosis (Appendix 2); autoimmune disease (including autoimmune hepatitis); history of severe psychiatric condition

Side-effects:
SPECIFIC SIDE-EFFECTS FOR INHALED TREATMENT. Worsening respiration, bacterial pneumonia, and pneumotho-

rax reported; rarely non-specific anaemia and haemolysis
SPECIFIC SIDE-EFFECTS FOR ORAL TREATMENT. Haemolytic anaemia; also reported (in combination with peginterferon alfa-2b or interferon alfa-2b) nausea, vomiting, dry mouth, stomatitis, glossitis, dyspepsia, abdominal pain, diarrhoea, constipation, pancreatitis, anorexia, weight loss; chest pain, tachycardia, syncope, flushing; dyspnoea, cough, rhinitis, pharyngitis; sleep disturbances, asthenia, impaired concentration, irritability, aggression, anxiety, depression, dizziness, tremor, hypertonia, myalgia, arthralgia, paraesthesia, influenza-like symptoms, headache; thyroid disorders, menstrual disturbances, reduced libido; rash, pruritus, photosensitivity, alopecia, dry skin; taste disturbance, blurred vision, tinnitus; neutropenia, thrombocytopenia, aplastic anaemia, lymphadenopathy, hyperuricaemia

Dose: bronchiolitis, *by aerosol inhalation or nebulisation* (via small particle aerosol generator) of solution containing 20 mg/mL for 12–18 hours for at least 3 days; max. 7 days
Chronic hepatitis C, *by mouth*, ADULT over 18 years, body-weight under 65 kg, 400 mg twice daily; body-weight 65–85 kg, 400 mg in the morning and 600 mg in the evening; body-weight over 85 kg, 600 mg twice daily

Rebetol® (Schering-Plough) ▼ PoM
Capsules, ribavirin 200 mg, net price 84-cap pack = £296.40, 140-cap pack = £494.00, 168-cap pack = £592.80. Label 21

Virazole® (ICN) PoM
Inhalation, ribavirin 6 g for reconstitution with 300 mL water for injections. Net price 3 × 6-g vials = £349.00
Note. The brand name *Virazid®* was used formerly for ribavirin inhalation

5.4 Antiprotozoal drugs

Advice on specific problems available from:

Malaria Reference Laboratory   (020) 7636 3924
(for healthcare professionals   (prophylaxis only)
only)
Scottish Centre for Infection   (0141) 300 1130
and Environmental Health   (weekdays 2–4 p.m.
(registered users of Travax   only)
only)
Birmingham   (0121) 424 0357
Liverpool   (0151) 708 9393
London   020) 7387 9300 (treatment)
    (020) 7388 9600 (travel
    prophylaxis)
    (020) 8200 6868
Oxford   (01865) 225 214
Recorded advice
for Travellers   09065 508 908
(£1.00/minute standard rate)
Hospital for Tropical Diseases
Travel Healthline   09061 337 733
(50p/minute)
WHO advice on international travel and health
    www.who.int/ith/english/index.htm
NHS advice for travellers
    www.fitfortravel.scot.nhs.uk

5.4.1 Antimalarials

Recommendations on the prophylaxis and treatment of malaria reflect guidelines agreed by UK malaria specialists.

The centres listed above should be consulted for advice on special problems.

Treatment of malaria

If the infective species is **not known**, or if the infection is **mixed**, initial treatment should be with quinine or mefloquine or *Malarone®* (proguanil with atovaquone) as for *falciparum malaria*. Falciparum malaria can progress rapidly in unprotected individuals and antimalarial treatment should be considered in those with features of severe malaria and possible exposure, even if the initial blood tests for the organism are negative.

Falciparum malaria (treatment)

Falciparum malaria (malignant malaria) is caused by *Plasmodium falciparum*. In most parts of the world *P. falciparum* is now resistant to chloroquine which should not therefore be given for treatment[1].

Quinine, **mefloquine** or *Malarone®* (proguanil with atovaquone) can be given *by mouth* if the patient can swallow and retain tablets and there are no serious manifestations (e.g. impaired consciousness); quinine should be given *by intravenous infusion* (see below) if the patient is seriously ill or unable to take tablets. Specialist advice should be sought in difficult cases since other drugs such as **artesunate** (given intravenously) and **artemether** (given intramuscularly) may be available for 'named-patient use'.

Oral. The adult dosage regimen for **quinine** *by mouth* is:

600 mg (of quinine salt[2]) every 8 hours for 7 days *and* (if quinine resistance known or suspected) *followed by*

either Fansidar® 3 tablets as a single dose *or* (if *Fansidar®*-resistant) **doxycycline** 200 mg daily for at least 7 days.

Alternatively **mefloquine** or *Malarone®* may be given instead of quinine but resistance to mefloquine has been reported in several countries. It is not necessary to give *Fansidar®* or doxycycline after mefloquine or *Malarone®* treatment.

The adult dosage regimen for **mefloquine** *by mouth* is:

20–25 mg/kg (of mefloquine base) as a single dose (up to maximum 1.5 g) *or preferably* as 2–3 divided doses 6–8 hours apart.

The adult dose of *Malarone®* *by mouth* is:
4 tablets once daily for 3 days.

Parenteral. If the patient is seriously ill, **quinine** should be given *by intravenous infusion.* The adult dosage regimen for quinine *by infusion* is:

loading dose[3] of 20 mg/kg[4] (up to maximum 1.4 g) of quinine salt[2] infused over 4 hours *then after 8–12 hours* maintenance dose of 10 mg/kg[5] (up to maximum 700 mg) of quinine salt[2] infused over 4 hours every 8–12 hours (until patient can swallow tablets to complete the 7-day course) *followed by either Fansidar®* or doxycycline as above. Alternatively, after at least 2–3 days' treatment with a parenteral quinine salt, treatment may be completed with mefloquine by mouth started at least 12 hours after parenteral quinine salt has been administered.

CHILDREN.

Oral. **Quinine** is well tolerated by children although the salts are bitter. The dosage regimen for quinine *by mouth* for children is:

10 mg/kg (of quinine salt[2]) every 8 hours for 7 days *then* (if quinine resistance known or suspected)

Fansidar® as a single dose: up to 4 years ½ tablet, 5–6 years 1 tablet, 7–9 years 1½ tablets, 10–14 years 2 tablets.

Alternatively **mefloquine** or *Malarone®* may be given instead of quinine; it is not necessary to give *Fansidar®* after mefloquine or *Malarone®* treatment. The dosage regimen for mefloquine *by mouth* for children is calculated on a mg/kg basis as for adults (see above). The dosage regimen for *Malarone®* *by mouth* for children over 40 kg is the same as for adults (see above); the dosage regimen for *Malarone®* for smaller children is reduced as follows:

weight under 11 kg, no suitable dose form
weight 11–20 kg, 1 tablet daily for 3 days
weight 21–30 kg, 2 tablets daily for 3 days
weight 31–40kg, 3 tablets daily for 3 days.

Parenteral. The dosage regimen for quinine *by intravenous infusion* for children is calculated on a mg/kg basis as for adults (see above).

PREGNANCY. Falciparum malaria is particularly dangerous in pregnancy, especially in the last trimester. The adult treatment doses of oral and intravenous quinine given above (including the loading dose) can safely be given to pregnant women. Doxycycline should be avoided in pregnancy (causes dental discoloration); *Fansidar®*, mefloquine, and *Malarone®* are also best avoided until more information is available.

1. For chloroquine-sensitive strains of falciparum malaria chloroquine is effective *by mouth* in the dosage schedule outlined under benign malarias but it should **not** be used unless there is an **unambiguous exposure history** in one of the few remaining areas of chloroquine sensitivity.
If the patient with a *chloroquine-sensitive infection* is seriously ill, chloroquine is given *by continuous intravenous infusion.* The dosage (for adults and children) is chloroquine 10 mg/kg (of base) infused over 8 hours, followed by three 8-hour infusions of 5 mg/kg (of base) each. *Oral therapy* is started as soon as possible to complete the course; the total cumulative dose for the course should be 25 mg/kg of base.
2. Valid for quinine hydrochloride, dihydrochloride, and sulphate; not valid for quinine bisulphate which contains a correspondingly smaller amount of quinine.
3. In intensive care units the loading dose can alternatively be given as quinine salt[2] 7 mg/kg infused over 30 minutes followed immediately by 10 mg/kg over 4 hours then (after 8 hours) maintenance dose as described.
4. **Important:** the loading dose of 20 mg/kg should **not** be used if the patient has received quinine (or quinidine) or mefloquine during the previous 24 hours
5. Maintenance dose should be reduced to 5–7 mg/kg of salt in patients with renal impairment or if parenteral treatment is required for more than 48 hours.

Benign malarias (treatment)

Benign malaria is usually caused by *Plasmodium vivax* and less commonly by *P. ovale* and *P. malariae*. **Chloroquine**[6] is the drug of choice for the treatment of benign malarias (but chloroquine-resistant *P. vivax* infection has been reported from New Guinea and some adjacent islands).

The adult dosage regimen for **chloroquine** *by mouth* is:

initial dose of 600 mg (of base) *then*
a single dose of 300 mg after 6 to 8 hours *then*
a single dose of 300 mg daily for 2 days
(approximate total cumulative dose of 25 mg/kg of base)

Chloroquine alone is adequate for *P. malariae* infections but in the case of *P. vivax* and *P. ovale*, a *radical cure* (to destroy parasites in the liver and thus prevent relapses) is required. This is achieved with **primaquine**[7] in an adult dosage of 15 mg daily for 14 to 21 days given after the chloroquine; a 21-day (or even longer) course may be needed for Chesson-type strains of *P. vivax* from south-east Asia and western Pacific.

CHILDREN. The dosage regimen of chloroquine for benign malaria in children is:

initial dose of 10 mg/kg (of base) *then*
a single dose of 5 mg/kg after 6–8 hours *then*
a single dose of 5 mg/kg daily for 2 days

For a *radical cure* children are then given primaquine[7] in a dose of 250 micrograms/kg daily.

PREGNANCY. The adult treatment doses of chloroquine can be given for benign malaria. In the case of *P. vivax* or *P. ovale*, however, the radical cure with primaquine should be **postponed** until the pregnancy is over; instead chloroquine should be continued at a dose of 600 mg each week during the pregnancy.

Prophylaxis against malaria

The recommendations on prophylaxis reflect guidelines agreed by UK malaria specialists; the advice is aimed at residents of the UK who travel to endemic areas. The choice of drug for a particular individual should take into account:

risk of exposure to malaria;
extent of drug resistance;
efficacy of the recommended drugs;
side-effects of the drugs;
patient-related factors (e.g. age, pregnancy, renal or hepatic impairment).

PROTECTION AGAINST BITES. **Prophylaxis is not absolute**, and breakthrough infection can occur with any of the drugs recommended. Personal protection against being bitten is very important. Mosquito nets impregnated with permethrin provide the most effective barrier protection against insects; coils, mats and vaporised insecticides are also useful. Diethyltoluolamide (DEET) in lotions, sprays or roll-on formulations is safe and effective when applied to the skin but the protective effect only lasts for a few hours. Long sleeves and trousers worn after dusk also provide protection.

LENGTH OF PROPHYLAXIS. In order to determine tolerance and to establish habit, prophylaxis should generally be started one week (preferably 2–3 weeks in the case of mefloquine) before travel into an endemic area (or if not possible at earliest opportunity up to 1 or 2 days before travel); *Malarone*® prophylaxis should be started 1–2 days before travel. Prophylaxis should be continued for **4 weeks after leaving** (except for *Malarone*® prophylaxis which should be stopped 1 week after leaving).

In those requiring long-term prophylaxis, chloroquine and proguanil may be used for periods of over 5 years (although it has been used for up to 2 years without undue problems). Doxycycline can be used for up to 6 months while *Malarone*® is licensed for up to 28 days but can probably be used for up to 3 months. Specialist advice should be sought for long-term prophylaxis.

RETURN FROM MALARIAL REGION. It is important to be aware that **any illness** that occurs within 1 year and **especially within 3 months of return might be malaria** even if all recommended precautions against malaria were taken. Travellers should be **warned** of this and told that if they develop any illness **particularly within 3 months** of their return they should go **immediately** to a doctor and specifically mention their exposure to malaria.

CHILDREN. Prophylactic doses in the table (next page) are based on guidelines agreed by UK malaria experts and may differ from advice in product literature. If in doubt telephone centres listed on p. 310.

EPILEPSY. Both chloroquine and mefloquine are unsuitable for malaria prophylaxis in individuals with a history of epilepsy. In areas *without chloroquine resistance* proguanil 200 mg daily alone is recommended; in areas *with chloroquine resistance*, doxycycline or *Malarone*® may be considered; the metabolism of doxycycline may be influenced by antiepileptics (see **interactions**: Appendix 1 (tetracyclines)). *Maloprim*® may be another alternative; it should be supplemented with folic acid (5 mg daily) in those taking phenytoin or phenobarbital.

RENAL IMPAIRMENT. Avoidance (or dosage reduction) of proguanil is recommended since it is excreted by the kidneys. *Malarone*® may not be suitable for use in moderate to severe renal impairment. Chloroquine is only partially excreted by the kidneys and reduction of the dose for prophylaxis is not required except in severe impairment. Mefloquine is considered to be appropriate for use in renal impairment and does not require dosage reduction. Doxycycline is also considered to be appropriate.

---

6. Mefloquine is also active in benign malarias (but is not required since chloroquine is usually effective); as with chloroquine a radical cure is required for *P. vivax* and *P. ovale* infections.
7. Before starting primaquine blood should be tested for glucose-6-phosphate dehydrogenase (G6PD) activity since the drug can cause haemolysis in G6PD-deficient patients. In G6PD deficiency primaquine, in a dose for adults of 30 mg once a week (children 500–750 micrograms/kg once a week) for 8 weeks, has been found useful and without undue harmful effects.

Doses for malaria prophylaxis in children

Age	Weight	Dose and frequency				
		[1]Chloroquine base once weekly	Proguanil hydrochloride once daily	Mefloquine once weekly	Doxycycline once daily	*Maloprim®* once weekly
0–12 weeks	under 6 kg	37.5 mg	25 mg	—	—	—
12 weeks–11 months	6–9.9 kg	75 mg	50 mg	62.5 mg	—	¼ tablet
1–3 years	10–15.9 kg	112.5 mg	75 mg	62.5 mg	—	¼ tablet
4–7 years	16–24.9 kg	150 mg	100 mg	125 mg	—	½ tablet
8–12 years	25–44.9 kg	225 mg	150 mg	187.5 mg	over 12 years, adult dose (100mg)	¾ tablet
over 13 years	over 45 kg	adult dose (300 mg)	adult dose (200 mg)	adult dose (250 mg)	adult dose (100 mg)	adult dose (1 tablet)

Note. Weight is a better guide than age. Specialist advice should be obtained for use of *Maloprim®* in children under 1 year of age. *Malarone®* is not licensed for use in children.
Prophylaxis is required in **breast-fed infants**; although antimalarials are present in milk, the amounts are too variable to give reliable protection.

PREGNANCY. Travel to malarious areas should be avoided during pregnancy; if travel is unavoidable, effective prophylaxis must be used. Chloroquine and proguanil may be given in usual doses in areas where *P. falciparum* strains are sensitive; in the case of proguanil, folic acid 5 mg daily should be given. The manufacturer advises that prophylaxis with mefloquine should be avoided as a matter of principle but studies of mefloquine in pregnancy (including use in the first trimester) have revealed no evidence of harm; it may therefore be considered for travel to chloroquine-resistant areas. *Maloprim®* should not be used in pregnancy. Doxycycline is contra-indicated during pregnancy. *Malarone®* should be avoided during pregnancy unless there is no suitable alternative. The centres listed on p. 310 should be consulted for advice on prophylaxis in resistant areas.

Specific recommendations

Where a journey requires two regimens, the regimen for the higher risk area should be used for the whole journey. Those travelling to remote or little-visited areas may require expert advice.

> Risk may vary in different parts of a country—check under all risk levels

> WARNING. Settled immigrants (or long-term visitors) to the UK may be unaware that they will have **lost some of their immunity** and also that the areas where they previously lived **may now be malarious**

North Africa and the Middle East

VERY LOW RISK. Risk *very low* in Abu Dhabi, Algeria, tourist areas of Egypt, Libya, Morocco, Tunisia, most tourist areas of Turkey:

> no prophylaxis recommended but consider malaria if fever presents

1. Chloroquine can alternatively be given as an oral syrup. For doses see under *Nivaquine®* syrup

LOW RISK. Risk *low* in Armenia (June–October; no risk in tourist areas), Azerbaijan (southern border areas and Khachmas, June–October), Egypt (El Fayoum only, June–October), Georgia (July–October), rural north Iraq and Basrah Province (May–November), north border of Syria (May–October), Tajikistan (June–October), Turkey (plain around Adana, Side, south-east Anatolia, May–October), Turkmenistan (June–October):

preferably

> chloroquine 300 mg (as base) once weekly

or
(if chloroquine not appropriate)

> proguanil hydrochloride 200 mg once daily

RISK. Risk *present* and *chloroquine resistance present* in Afghanistan (below 2000 m, May–November), Iran, Oman (rural areas only), Saudi Arabia (except Northern, Eastern and Central Provinces, Asir plateau, and western border cities where very little risk), northern rural United Arab Emirates, Yemen:

> chloroquine 300 mg (as base) once weekly
> **plus**
> proguanil hydrochloride 200 mg once daily

Sub-Saharan Africa

No prophylaxis recommended for Cape Verde and non-rural areas of Mauritius (but consider malaria if fever presents); *chloroquine prophylaxis* appropriate for rural areas of **Mauritius**

SEASONAL RISK. Risk *present* (in *parts of country*) and *some chloroquine resistance* in northern half of Botswana (November–June), Mauritania (all year in south; July–October in north), Namibia (all year along Kavango and Kunene rivers; November–June in northern third), areas below 1200 m in Zimbabwe (November–June; all year in Zambezi valley where prophylaxis as for *Very High Risk*, below; risk negligible in Harare and Bulawayo):

preferably

chloroquine 300 mg (as base) once weekly
plus
proguanil hydrochloride 200 mg once daily

or
(if chloroquine plus proguanil not appropriate)

mefloquine 250 mg once weekly

or

doxycycline 100 mg once daily

or

Malarone® 1 tablet daily

Note. In Zimbabwe and neighbouring countries, *Maloprim®* (also known as *Deltaprim®*) prophylaxis is used by local residents (sometimes with chloroquine).

VERY HIGH RISK. Risk *very high* (or *locally very high*) and *chloroquine resistance very widespread* in Angola, Benin, Burkina Faso, Burundi, Cameroon, Central African Republic, Chad, Comoros, Congo, Democratic Republic of the Congo (formely Zaïre), Djibouti, Equatorial Guinea, Eritrea, Ethiopia (below 2200m; no risk in Addis Ababa), Gabon, Gambia, Ghana, Guinea, Guinea-Bissau, Ivory Coast, Kenya, Liberia, Madagascar, Malawi, Mali, Mozambique, Niger, Nigeria, Principe, Rwanda, São Tomé, Senegal, Sierra Leone, Somalia, South Africa (Kruger Park, north-east, low-altitude areas of Northern Province and Mpumalanga, and eastern KwaZulu-Natal down to 100 km north of Durban), Sudan, Swaziland, Tanzania, Togo, Uganda, Zambia, Zimbabwe (Zambezi valley, see also above):

preferably

mefloquine 250 mg once weekly

or

doxycycline 100 mg once daily

or

Malarone® 1 tablet daily

or
(if mefloquine, or doxycycline, or *Malarone®* not appropriate)

chloroquine 300 mg (as base) once weekly
plus
proguanil hydrochloride 200 mg once daily
Note. This regimen does not give optimal protection

South Asia

VARIABLE RISK. Risk *variable* and *chloroquine resistance usually moderate* in Bangladesh (except in Chittagong Hill Tracts, see below; no risk in Dhaka city), southern districts of Bhutan, India (no risk in mountain states of north), Nepal (below 1300 m; no risk in Kathmandu), Pakistan (below 2000 m), Sri Lanka (no risk in and just south of Colombo):

chloroquine 300 mg (as base) once weekly
plus
proguanil hydrochloride 200 mg once daily

HIGH RISK. Risk *high* and *chloroquine resistance high* in Bangladesh (only in Chittagong Hill Tracts):

mefloquine 250 mg once weekly

or

doxycycline 100 mg once daily

or

Malarone® 1 tablet daily

South-East Asia

VERY LOW RISK. Risk *very low* in Bali, Brunei (no risk), main tourist areas of China (but *substantial risk* in Yunnan and Hainan, see below; *chloroquine prophylaxis* appropriate for other remote areas), Hong Kong, Java, Korea (both Democratic People's Republic and Republic), Malaysia (but *substantial risk* in Sabah, and *variable risk* in deep forests, see below), Sarawak (but *variable risk* in deep forests, see below), Singapore (no risk), Thailand (Bangkok, main tourist centres and rural areas away from borders—**important:** regional risk exists, see under *Great risk*, below):

no prophylaxis recommended but consider malaria if fever presents

VARIABLE RISK. Risk *variable* and *some chloroquine resistance* in Indonesia (low risk in Bali, Java, and cities but *substantial risk* in Irian Jaya, Lombok and East Timor, see below), rural Philippines below 600 m (no risk in Cebu, Leyte, Bohol, Catanduanes, metropolitan Manila), deep forests of peninsular Malaysia and Sarawak (but *Substantial risk* in Sabah, see below):

chloroquine 300 mg (as base) once weekly
plus
proguanil hydrochloride 200 mg once daily

SUBSTANTIAL RISK. Risk *substantial* and *drug resistance common* in Cambodia (no risk in Phnom Penh; **important:** specialist advice needed for western provinces, see below), China (Yunnan and Hainan; *chloroquine prophylaxis* appropriate for other remote areas), East Timor, Irian Jaya, Laos (no risk in Vientiane), Lombok, Malaysia (Sabah[1]; see also *Very low risk* and *Variable risk* above), Myanmar (formerly Burma), Vietnam (no risk in cities, Red River delta area, coastal plain north of Nha Trang):

mefloquine 250 mg once weekly

or

doxycycline 100 mg once daily

or

Malarone® 1 tablet daily

1. Prophylaxis with chloroquine plus proguanil also acceptable for short visits to Sabah

GREAT RISK and drug resistance present. Risk *great and mefloquine resistance present* in western provinces of Cambodia, borders of Thailand with Cambodia and Myanmar, and Ko Chang:

doxycycline 100 mg once daily

or

Malarone® 1 tablet daily

Oceania

RISK. Risk *high* and *chloroquine resistance high* in Papua New Guinea (below 1800 m), Solomon Islands, Vanuatu:

doxycycline 100 mg once daily

or

mefloquine 250 mg once weekly

or

Malarone® 1 tablet daily

Central and South America and the Caribbean

VARIABLE TO LOW RISK. Risk *variable to low* in Argentina (small area in north-west only), rural Belize (except Belize district), rural Costa Rica (below 500 m), Dominican Republic, El Salvador, Guatemala (below 1500 m), Haiti, Honduras, some rural areas of Mexico (not regularly visited by tourists), Nicaragua, Panama (west of Panama Canal but *variable to high risk* east of Panama Canal, see below), rural Paraguay:

preferably

chloroquine 300 mg (as base) once weekly

or
(if chloroquine not appropriate)

proguanil hydrochloride 200 mg once daily

VARIABLE TO HIGH RISK. Risk *variable to high* and *chloroquine resistance present* in rural areas of Bolivia (below 2500 m), Ecuador (below 1500 m; no malaria in Quito; see below for Esmeraldas Province), Panama (east of Panama Canal), rural areas of Peru (below 1500 m; see below for Amazon basin area), rural areas of Venezuela (except on coast, Caracas free of malaria):

preferably

chloroquine 300 mg (as base) once weekly

plus

proguanil hydrochloride 200 mg once daily

or
(if chloroquine plus proguanil not appropriate)

mefloquine 250 mg once weekly

or

doxycycline 100 mg once daily

or

Malarone® 1 tablet daily

HIGH RISK. Risk *high* and *marked chloroquine resistance* in Bolivia (Amazon basin area), Brazil (throughout 'Legal Amazon' area which includes the Amazon basin region, Mato Grosso and Maranhao only; elsewhere *very low risk*—no prophylaxis), Colombia (most areas below 800 m), Ecuador (Esmeraldas Province), French Guiana, all interior regions of Guyana (sporadic cases on coast), Peru (Amazon basin area), Surinam (except Paramaribo and coast), Venezuela (Amazon basin area):

mefloquine 250 mg once weekly

or

doxycycline 100 mg once daily

or

Malarone® 1 tablet daily

STANDBY TREATMENT. Adults travelling for prolonged periods to areas of chloroquine-resistance who are unlikely to have easy access to medical care should carry a standby treatment course. Self-medication should be **avoided** if medical help is accessible; prophylaxis should be continued during and after the attack.

In order to avoid excessive self-medication, the traveller should be provided with **written instructions** that urgent medical attention should be sought if fever (38°C or more) develops 7 days (or more) after arriving in a malarious area and that self-treatment is indicated if medical help is not immediately available or the condition is worsening.

In view of the continuing emergence of resistant strains and of the different regimens required for different areas expert advice should be sought on the best treatment course for an individual traveller. A drug used for chemoprophylaxis should not be considered for standby treatment.

Chloroquine

Chloroquine is used for the *prophylaxis of malaria* in areas of the world where the *risk of chloroquine-resistant falciparum malaria is still low*. It is also used with proguanil when chloroquine-resistant falciparum malaria is present but this regimen may not give optimal protection (see specific recommendations by country, pp. 313–15).

Chloroquine is **no longer recommended** for the *treatment of falciparum malaria* owing to widespread resistance, nor is it recommended if the infective species is *not known* or if the infection is *mixed*; in these cases treatment should be with quinine, mefloquine, or *Malarone*® (for details, see p. 311). It is still recommended for the *treatment of benign malarias* (for details, see p. 312).

CHLOROQUINE

Indications: chemoprophylaxis and treatment of malaria, see notes above; rheumatoid arthritis and lupus erythematosus (section 10.1.3)

Cautions: hepatic impairment, renal impairment (see notes above), pregnancy (but for malaria benefit outweighs risk, see Appendix 4, Antimalarials), may exacerbate psoriasis, neurological disorders (avoid for prophylaxis if history of epilepsy, see notes above), may aggravate myasthenia gravis, severe gastro-intestinal disorders,

G6PD deficiency (see section 9.1.5); ophthalmic examination and long-term therapy, see under Chloroquine, section 10.1.3; avoid concurrent therapy with hepatotoxic drugs—other **interactions**: Appendix 1 (chloroquine)

Side-effects: gastro-intestinal disturbances, headache; also convulsions, visual disturbances, depigmentation or loss of hair, skin reactions (rashes, pruritus); rarely, bone-marrow suppression, hypersensitivity reactions such as urticaria and angioedema; other side-effects (not usually associated with malaria prophylaxis or treatment), see under Chloroquine, section 10.1.3; very toxic in **overdosage**—immediate advice from poisons centres essential (see also p. 25)

Dose: see notes above

COUNSELLING. Warn travellers about **importance** of avoiding mosquito bites, **importance** of taking prophylaxis regularly, and **importance** of immediate visit to doctor if ill within 1 year and **especially** within 3 months of return. For details, see notes above

*Avloclor® (AstraZeneca) PoM
Tablets, scored, chloroquine phosphate 250 mg (≡ chloroquine base 155 mg). Net price 20-tab pack = £1.11. Label: 5, counselling, prophylaxis, see above
* Can be sold to the public provided it is licensed and labelled for the prophylaxis of malaria

Nivaquine® (Rhône-Poulenc Rorer)
* *Tablets* PoM, f/c, yellow, chloroquine sulphate 200 mg (≡ chloroquine base 150 mg), net price 28-tab pack = £1.34. Label: 5, counselling, prophylaxis, see above
* *Syrup* PoM, golden, chloroquine sulphate 68 mg/5 mL (≡ chloroquine base 50 mg/5 mL), net price 100 mL = £2.82. Label: 5, counselling, prophylaxis, see above
Dose: chemoprophylaxis, NEONATE and INFANT under 4.5 kg, 2.5 mL once weekly; 4.5–7.9 kg, 5 mL once weekly; 8–10.9 kg, 7.5 mL once weekly; CHILD 11–14.9 kg, 10 mL once weekly; 15–16.5 kg, 12.5 mL once weekly; over 16.5 kg, see notes above
* Can be sold to the public provided it is licensed and labelled for the prophylaxis of malaria

Injection PoM, chloroquine sulphate 54.5 mg/mL (≡ chloroquine base 40 mg/mL), net price 5-mL amp = 76p

■ With proguanil
For cautions and side-effects of proguanil see Proguanil; for dose see notes above

Paludrine/Avloclor® (AstraZeneca)
Travel Pack, 14 tablets of chloroquine phosphate 250 mg (≡ chloroquine base 155 mg) and 98 tablets of proguanil hydrochloride 100 mg, net price 112-tab pack = £8.79. Label 5, 21, counselling, prophylaxis, see above
Available as a generic from Boots

Mefloquine

Mefloquine is used for the *prophylaxis of malaria* in areas of the world where there is a *high risk of chloroquine-resistant falciparum malaria* (for details, see specific recommendations by country, p. 313–15).

Mefloquine is used for the *treatment of falciparum malaria* or if the infective species is *not*

known or if the infection is *mixed* (for details, see p. 311). It is also effective for the *treatment of benign malarias*, but is not required because chloroquine is usually effective. Mefloquine should not be used for treatment if it has been used for prophylaxis.

CSM recommendation. The CSM has advised that:

• Patients should be informed about adverse reactions associated with mefloquine and, if they occur, advised to seek medical advice on alternative antimalarials before the next dose is due
• When possible mefloquine prophylaxis should be started 2–3 weeks before travel to enable any adverse reactions to be identified before departure [over three-quarters of adverse reactions occur by the third dose]
• Mefloquine is contra-indicated in patients with a history of neuropsychiatric disease including convulsions and depression
• The patient information leaflet, which describes adverse reactions should always be provided when dispensing mefloquine

MEFLOQUINE

Indications: chemoprophylaxis of malaria, treatment of uncomplicated falciparum malaria and chloroquine-resistant vivax malaria, see notes above

Cautions: pregnancy (see notes under Treatment of malaria and under Prophylaxis against malaria)—manufacturer advises **avoid** pregnancy during and for 3 months after; breast-feeding (Appendix 5); avoid for chemoprophylaxis in severe hepatic impairment; cardiac conduction disorders; epilepsy (avoid for prophylaxis); not recommended in infants under 3 months (5 kg); other **interactions**: Appendix 1 (mefloquine)

DRIVING. Dizziness or a disturbed sense of balance may affect performance of skilled tasks (e.g. driving); effects may persist for up to 3 weeks

Contra-indications: history of neuropsychiatric disorders, including depression, or convulsions; hypersensitivity to quinine

Side-effects: nausea, vomiting, diarrhoea, abdominal pain; dizziness, loss of balance, headache, sleep disorders (insomnia, drowsiness, abnormal dreams); also neuropsychiatric reactions (including sensory and motor neuropathies, tremor, ataxia, anxiety, depression, panic attacks, agitation, hallucinations, psychosis, convulsions), tinnitus and vestibular disorders, visual disturbances, circulatory disorders (hypotension and hypertension), chest pain, tachycardia, bradycardia, cardiac conduction disorders, dyspnoea, muscle weakness, myalgia, arthralgia, rash, urticaria, pruritus, alopecia, asthenia, malaise, fatigue, fever, loss of appetite, leucopenia or leucocytosis, thrombocytopenia; rarely Stevens-Johnson syndrome, AV block, encephalopathy and anaphylaxis

Dose: chemoprophylaxis, starting 1–3 weeks before departure (see p. 312) and continued for 4 weeks after leaving malarious area, see notes above

LONG-TERM CHEMOPROPHYLAXIS. Mefloquine prophylaxis can be taken for up to 1 year
Treatment, see notes above

COUNSELLING. See CSM recommendation in notes above. Also warn travellers about **importance** of avoiding mosquito bites, **importance** of taking prophylaxis regularly, and **importance** of immediate visit to doctor if ill within 1 year and **especially** within 3 months of return. For details, see notes above

¹ **Lariam®** (Roche) PoM
Tablets, scored, mefloquine (as hydrochloride) 250 mg. Net price 8-tab pack = £14.53. Label: 21, 25, 27, counselling, driving, prophylaxis, see above
1. Prescriptions may be referred to Health Authorities to investigate circumstances under which written since prescriptions for chemoprophylaxis of malaria may not be reimbursable

Primaquine

Primaquine is used to eliminate the liver stages of *P. vivax* or *P. ovale following chloroquine treatment* (for details, see p. 312).

PRIMAQUINE

Indications: adjunct in the treatment of *Plasmodium vivax* and *P. ovale* malaria (eradication of liver stages)
Cautions: G6PD deficiency (see notes above); systemic diseases associated with granulocytopenia (e.g. rheumatoid arthritis, lupus erythematosus); pregnancy and breast-feeding; **interactions:** Appendix 1 (primaquine)
Side-effects: nausea, vomiting, anorexia, abdominal pain; less commonly methaemoglobinaemia, haemolytic anaemia especially in G6PD deficiency, leucopenia
Dose: see notes above

Primaquine (Non-proprietary)
Tablets, primaquine (as phosphate) 7.5 mg
Available from Durbin [unlicensed—special order]

Proguanil

Proguanil is used (usually *with chloroquine*, but occasionally *alone*) for the *prophylaxis of malaria*, (for details, see specific recommendations by country, pp. 313–15).

Proguanil used alone is not suitable for the *treatment of malaria*; Malarone® (a combination of atovaquone with proguanil) is, however, licensed for the treatment of acute uncomplicated falciparum malaria. *Malarone®* is also used for the *prophylaxis of falciparum malaria* in areas of *widespread mefloquine or chloroquine resistance. Malarone®* is also used as an alternative to mefloquine or doxycycline. *Malarone®* is particularly suitable for short trips to highly chloroquine-resistant areas because it needs to be taken only for 7 days after leaving an endemic area.

PROGUANIL HYDROCHLORIDE

Indications: chemoprophylaxis of malaria
Cautions: renal impairment (see notes under Prophylaxis against malaria and Appendix 3); pregnancy (folate supplements needed); **interactions:** Appendix 1 (proguanil)
Side-effects: mild gastric intolerance and diarrhoea; occasionally mouth ulcers and stomatitis; skin reactions and hair loss reported; rarely hypersensitivity reactions such as urticaria and angioedema
Dose: see notes above
COUNSELLING. Warn travellers about **importance** of avoiding mosquito bites, **importance** of taking prophylaxis regularly, and **importance** of immediate visit to doctor if ill within 1 year and **especially** within 3 months of return. For details, see notes above

Paludrine® (AstraZeneca)
Tablets, scored, proguanil hydrochloride 100 mg. Net price 98-tab pack = £7.43. Label: 21, counselling, prophylaxis, see above

■ **With chloroquine**
See under Chloroquine

PROGUANIL HYDROCHLORIDE WITH ATOVAQUONE

Indications: treatment of acute uncomplicated falciparum malaria and prophylaxis of falciparum malaria, particularly where resistance to other antimalarial drugs suspected
Cautions: renal impairment (Appendix 3), diarrhoea or vomiting (reduced absorption of atovaquone), pregnancy (Appendix 4) and breast-feeding (Appendix 5); efficacy not evaluated in cerebral or complicated malaria (including hyperparasitaemia, pulmonary oedema or renal failure); **interactions:** see Appendix 1 (proguanil, atovaquone)
Side-effects: nausea, vomiting, mouth ulcers and stomatitis, diarrhoea, abdominal pain, anorexia; headache, dizziness, abnormal dreams, insomnia, cough, visual disturbances, pruritus, rash, urticaria; blood disorders and hair loss reported
Dose: see under preparation
COUNSELLING. Warn travellers about **importance** of avoiding mosquito bites, **importance** of taking prophylaxis regularly, and **importance** of immediate visit to doctor if ill within 1 year and **especially** within 3 months of return. For details, see notes above

Malarone® (GlaxoWellcome) ▼ PoM
Tablets, pink, f/c, proguanil hydrochloride 100 mg, atovaquone 250 mg. Net price 12-tab pack = £22.92. Label: 21, counselling, prophylaxis, see above
Dose: treatment of falciparum malaria, ADULT and CHILD over 40 kg, 4 tablets once daily for 3 days; CHILD 11–20 kg 1 tablet daily for 3 days; 21–30 kg 2 tablets once daily for 3 days; 31–40 kg 3 tablets once daily for 3 days
Prophylaxis of malaria in adults over 40 kg, see pp. 312–15

Pyrimethamine

Pyrimethamine should not be used alone, but is used with sulfadoxine (in *Fansidar®*) and with dapsone (in *Maloprim®*).

Fansidar® is not recommended for the *prophylaxis of malaria*, but it is used in the treatment of *falciparum malaria* and can be used *with (or following) quinine*.

Maloprim® (used with *chloroquine*) is an option for the *prophylaxis of malaria* in certain areas (e.g. Oceania) where there is a *high risk of chloroquine-resistant falciparum malaria* (but for details of preferred regimens, see specific recommendations by country, p. 313–15). *Maloprim®* is not suitable for the *treatment of malaria*.

PYRIMETHAMINE

Indications: malaria (but used only in combined preparations incorporating dapsone or sulfadoxine); toxoplasmosis [not licensed]—section 5.4.7

Cautions: hepatic or renal impairment, folate supplements in pregnancy, breast-feeding, blood counts required with prolonged treatment; **interactions:** Appendix 1 (pyrimethamine)

Side-effects: depression of haematopoiesis with high doses, rashes, insomnia

Dose: malaria, no dose stated because not recommended

Toxoplasmosis, section 5.4.7

Daraprim® (GlaxoWellcome) PoM ◤▬
Tablets, scored, pyrimethamine 25 mg. Net price 30-tab pack = £2.12

◤▬ denotes preparations that are considered to be less suitable for prescribing (see p. vi)

PYRIMETHAMINE WITH SULFADOXINE

Indications: adjunct to quinine in treatment of *Plasmodium falciparum* malaria (see notes above); **not** recommended for prophylaxis

Cautions: see under Pyrimethamine and under Co-trimoxazole (section 5.1.8); pregnancy and breast-feeding (Appendixes 4 and 5); not recommended for prophylaxis (severe side-effects on long-term use)

Contra-indications: see under Pyrimethamine and under Co-trimoxazole (section 5.1.8); sulphonamide allergy

Side-effects: see under Pyrimethamine and under Co-trimoxazole (section 5.1.8); pulmonary infiltrates (e.g. eosinophilic or allergic alveolitis) reported—discontinue if cough or shortness of breath

Dose: treatment, see notes above
Prophylaxis, not recommended by UK malaria experts

Fansidar® (Roche) PoM
Tablets, scored, pyrimethamine 25 mg, sulfadoxine 500 mg, net price 3-tab pack = 80p

PYRIMETHAMINE WITH DAPSONE

Indications: prophylaxis of *Plasmodium falciparum* malaria (limited use, see notes above)

Cautions: see under Pyrimethamine and under Dapsone (section 5.1.10); G6PD deficiency (section 9.1.5); pregnancy (see notes under Prophylaxis against Malaria and Appendix 4) and breast-feeding (Appendix 5)

Contra-indications: see under Pyrimethamine and under Dapsone (section 5.1.10); sulphonamide allergy

Side-effects: see under Pyrimethamine and under Dapsone (section 5.1.10); including methaemoglobinaemia, thrombocytopenia, mononucleosis-like syndrome, psychosis, jaundice, pneumonia with eosinophilic pulmonary infiltration, and on prolonged treatment hypoalbuminaemia reported

Dose: malaria prophylaxis, see notes above

COUNSELLING. Warn travellers about **importance** of avoiding mosquito bites, **importance** of taking prophylaxis regularly, and **importance** of immediate visit to doctor if ill within 1 year and **especially** within 3 months of return. For details, see notes above

Maloprim® (GlaxoWellcome) PoM
Tablets, scored, pyrimethamine 12.5 mg, dapsone 100 mg. Net price 30-tab pack = £2.64. Counselling, prophylaxis, see above

Quinine

Quinine is not suitable for the *prophylaxis of malaria*.

Quinine is used for the *treatment of falciparum malaria* or if the infective species is *not known* or if the infection is *mixed* (for details see p. 311–12).

QUININE

Indications: falciparum malaria; nocturnal leg cramps, see section 10.2.2

Cautions: atrial fibrillation, conduction defects, heart block, pregnancy (but appropriate for treatment of malaria); monitor blood glucose concentration during parenteral treatment; G6PD deficiency (see section 9.1.5); **interactions:** Appendix 1 (quinine)

Contra-indications: haemoglobinuria, optic neuritis

Side-effects: cinchonism, including tinnitus, headache, hot and flushed skin, nausea, abdominal pain, rashes, visual disturbances (including temporary blindness), confusion; hypersensitivity reactions including angioedema, blood disorders (including thrombocytopenia and intravascular coagulation), and acute renal failure; hypoglycaemia (especially after parenteral administration); cardiovascular effects (see Cautions); very toxic in **overdosage**—immediate advice from poisons centres essential (see also p. 25)

Dose: see notes above

Note. Quinine (anhydrous base) 100 mg ≡ quinine bisulphate 169 mg ≡ quinine dihydrochloride 122 mg ≡ quinine hydrochloride 122 mg ≡ quinine sulphate 121 mg. Quinine bisulphate 300-mg tablets are available but provide less quinine than 300 mg of the dihydrochloride, hydrochloride, or sulphate

Quinine Sulphate (Non-proprietary) PoM
Tablets, coated, quinine sulphate 200 mg, net price 28-tab pack = £1.46; 300 mg, 28-tab pack = £1.36
Available from Alpharma, APS, CP, Generics, Hillcross, Kent

Quinine Dihydrochloride (Non-proprietary) PoM
Injection, quinine dihydrochloride 300 mg/mL. For dilution and use as an infusion. 1- and 2-mL amps
Available from Martindale (special order) or from specialist centres (see p. 310)

Note. Intravenous injection of quinine is so hazardous that it has been superseded by infusion

Tetracyclines

Doxycycline (section 5.1.3) is used for the *prophylaxis of malaria* in areas of *widespread mefloquine or chloroquine resistance*. Doxycycline is also used as an alternative to mefloquine or *Malarone®* (for details, see specific recommendations by country, pp. 313–15).

Doxycycline is also used as an *adjunct to quinine in the treatment of falciparum malaria* (for details see p. 311).

5.4.2   Amoebicides

Metronidazole is the drug of choice for *acute invasive amoebic dysentery* since it is very effective against vegetative forms of *Entamoeba histolytica* in ulcers; it is given in an adult dose of 800 mg three times daily for 5 days. **Tinidazole** is also effective. Metronidazole and tinidazole are also active against amoebae which may have migrated to the liver. Treatment with metronidazole (or tinidazole) is followed by a 10-day course of diloxanide furoate.

Diloxanide furoate is the drug of choice for asymptomatic patients with *E. histolytica* cysts in the faeces; metronidazole and tinidazole are relatively ineffective. Diloxanide furoate is relatively free from toxic effects and the usual course is of 10 days, given alone for chronic infections or following metronidazole or tinidazole treatment.

For *amoebic abscesses* of the liver **metronidazole** is effective in doses of 400 mg 3 times daily for 5–10 days; tinidazole is an alternative. The course may be repeated after 2 weeks if necessary. Aspiration of the abscess is indicated where it is suspected that it may rupture or where there is no improvement after 72 hours of metronidazole; the aspiration may need to be repeated. Aspiration aids penetration of metronidazole and, for abscesses with more than 100 mL of pus, if carried out in conjunction with drug therapy, may reduce the period of disability.

Diloxanide furoate is not effective against hepatic amoebiasis, but a 10-day course should be given at the completion of metronidazole or tinidazole treatment to destroy any amoebae in the gut.

DILOXANIDE FUROATE

Indications: see notes above; chronic amoebiasis and as adjunct to metronidazole or tinidazole in acute amoebiasis
Contra-indications: pregnancy (Appendix 4), breast-feeding (Appendix 5)
Side-effects: flatulence, vomiting, urticaria, pruritus
Dose: 500 mg every 8 hours for 10 days; CHILD over 25 kg, 20 mg/kg daily in 3 divided doses for 10 days
See also notes above

Diloxanide (Non-proprietary) PoM
Tablets, diloxanide furoate 500 mg, net price 30-tab pack = £32.95. Label: 9
Available from Sovereign

METRONIDAZOLE

Indications: see under Dose below; anaerobic infections, section 5.1.11
Cautions: section 5.1.11
Side-effects: section 5.1.11
Dose: *by mouth,* invasive intestinal amoebiasis, 800 mg every 8 hours for 5 days; CHILD 1–3 years 200 mg every 8 hours; 3–7 years 200 mg every 6 hours; 7–10 years 400 mg every 8 hours
Extra-intestinal amoebiasis (including liver abscess) and symptomless amoebic cyst passers, 400–800 mg every 8 hours for 5–10 days; CHILD 1–3 years 100–200 mg every 8 hours; 3–7 years 100–200 mg every 6 hours; 7–10 years 200–400 mg every 8 hours
Urogenital trichomoniasis, 200 mg every 8 hours for 7 days *or* 400–500 mg every 12 hours for 5–7 days, *or* 2 g as a single dose; CHILD 1–3 years 50 mg every 8 hours for 7 days; 3–7 years 100 mg every 12 hours; 7–10 years 100 mg every 8 hours
Giardiasis, 2 g daily for 3 days *or* 400 mg 3 times daily for 5 days *or* 500 mg twice daily for 7–10 days; CHILD 1–3 years 500 mg daily for 3 days; 3–7 years 600–800 mg daily; 7–10 years 1 g daily

Preparations
Section 5.1.11

TINIDAZOLE

Indications: see under Dose below; anaerobic infections, section 5.1.11
Cautions: section 5.1.11
Side-effects: section 5.1.11
Dose: intestinal amoebiasis, 2 g daily for 2–3 days; CHILD 50–60 mg/kg daily for 3 days
Amoebic involvement of liver, 1.5–2 g daily for 3–6 days; CHILD 50–60 mg/kg daily for 5 days
Urogenital trichomoniasis and giardiasis, single 2-g dose; CHILD single dose of 50–75 mg/kg (repeated once if necessary)

Preparations
Section 5.1.11

5.4.3   Trichomonacides

Metronidazole (section 5.4.2) is the treatment of choice for *Trichomonas vaginalis* infection. Contact tracing is recommended and sexual contacts should be treated simultaneously.

If metronidazole is ineffective, **tinidazole** may be tried; it is usually given as a single 2-g dose, with food. A further 2-g dose may be given if there is no clinical improvement.

5.4.4   Antigiardial drugs

Metronidazole (section 5.4.2) is the treatment of choice for *Giardia lamblia* infections, given by mouth in a dosage of 2 g daily for 3 days or 400 mg every 8 hours for 5 days.

Alternative treatments are **tinidazole** (section 5.4.2) 2 g as a single dose or **mepacrine hydrochloride** 100 mg every 8 hours for 5–7 days [unlicensed indication].

MEPACRINE HYDROCHLORIDE
Indications: giardiasis; discoid lupus erythematosus—section 10.1.3
Cautions: hepatic impairment, elderly, history of psychosis; avoid in psoriasis; **interactions:** Appendix 1 (mepacrine)
Side-effects: gastro-intestinal disturbances; dizziness, headache; with large doses nausea, vomiting and occasionally transient acute toxic psychosis and CNS stimulation; on prolonged treatment yellow discoloration of skin and urine, chronic dermatoses (including severe exfoliative dermatitis), hepatitis, aplastic anaemia; also reported blue/black discoloration of palate and nails and corneal deposits with visual disturbances
Dose: giardiasis, 100 mg every 8 hours for 5–7 days; CHILD 2 mg/kg every 8 hours

Mepacrine Hydrochloride
Tablets, mepacrine hydrochloride 100 mg. Label: 4, 9, 14, 21
Available from BCM Specials [unlicensed—special order]

5.4.5   Leishmaniacides

Cutaneous leishmaniasis frequently heals spontaneously but if skin lesions are extensive or unsightly, treatment is indicated, as it is in visceral leishmaniasis (kala-azar).

Sodium stibogluconate, an organic pentavalent antimony compound, is the treatment of choice for visceral leishmaniasis. The dose is 20 mg/kg daily (max. 850 mg) for at least 20 days by intramuscular or intravenous injection; the dosage varies with different geographical regions and expert advice should be obtained. Skin lesions are treated for 10 days.

Amphotericin is used with or after an antimony compound for visceral leishmaniasis unresponsive to the antimonial alone; side-effects may be reduced by using liposomal amphotericin (*AmBisome®*—section 5.2) at a dose of 1–3 mg/kg daily for 10–21 days to a cumulative dose of 21–30 mg/kg. Other lipid formulations of amphotericin (*Abelcet®* and *Amphocil®*) are also likely to be effective but less information is available.

Pentamidine isetionate (pentamidine isethionate) (section 5.4.8) has been used in antimony-resistant visceral leishmaniasis, but although the initial response is often good, the relapse rate is high; it is associated with serious side-effects. Other treatments include paromomycin (available on named-patient basis from IDIS).

SODIUM STIBOGLUCONATE
Indications: leishmaniasis
Cautions: hepatic impairment; pregnancy; intravenous injections must be given slowly over 5 minutes (to reduce risk of local thrombosis) and stopped if coughing or substernal pain; mucocutaneous disease (see below); heart disease (withdraw if conduction disturbances occur); treat intercurrent infection (e.g. pneumonia)
MUCOCUTANEOUS DISEASE. Successful treatment of mucocutaneous leishmaniasis may induce severe inflammation around the lesions (may be life-threatening if pharyngeal or tracheal involvement)—may require corticosteroid

Contra-indications: significant renal impairment; breast-feeding
Side-effects: anorexia, nausea, vomiting, abdominal pain; ECG changes; headache, lethargy, myalgia; raised liver enzymes; coughing and substernal pain (see Cautions); rarely anaphylaxis; also reported, fever, sweating, flushing, vertigo, bleeding from nose or gum, jaundice, rash; pain and thrombosis on intravenous administration, intramuscular injection also painful
Dose: see notes above

Pentostam® (GlaxoWellcome) [PoM]
Injection, sodium stibogluconate equivalent to pentavalent antimony 100 mg/mL. Net price 100-mL bottle = £64.94

5.4.6   Trypanocides

The prophylaxis and treatment of trypanosomiasis is difficult and differs according to the strain of organism. Expert advice should therefore be obtained.

5.4.7   Drugs for toxoplasmosis

Most infections caused by *Toxoplasma gondii* are self-limiting, and treatment is not necessary. Exceptions are patients with eye involvement (toxoplasma choroidoretinitis), and those who are immunosuppressed. Toxoplasmic encephalitis is a common complication of AIDS. The treatment of choice is a combination of pyrimethamine and sulfadiazine (sulphadiazine), given for several weeks (expert advice **essential**). Pyrimethamine is a folate antagonist, and adverse reactions to this combination are relatively common (folinic acid supplements and weekly blood counts needed). Alternative regimens use combinations of pyrimethamine with clindamycin or clarithromycin or azithromycin. Long-term secondary prophylaxis is required after treatment of toxoplasmosis in AIDS.

If toxoplasmosis is acquired in pregnancy, transplacental infection may lead to severe disease in the fetus. Spiramycin (available on named-patient basis from IDIS) may reduce the risk of transmission of maternal infection to the fetus.

5.4.8   Drugs for pneumocystis pneumonia

Pneumonia caused by *Pneumocystis carinii* occurs in immunosuppressed patients; it is a common cause of pneumonia in AIDS. Pneumocystis pneumonia should generally be treated by those experienced in its management. Blood gas measurement is used to assess disease severity.

Treatment
MILD TO MODERATE DISEASE. **Co-trimoxazole** (section 5.1.8) in high dosage is the drug of choice for the treatment of mild to moderate pneumocystis pneumonia.

Atovaquone is licensed for mild to moderate disease in patients who cannot tolerate co-trimoxazole. A combination of **dapsone** 100 mg daily (section

5.1.10) with **trimethoprim** 5 mg/kg every 6–8 hours (section 5.1.8) is given by mouth for the treatment of mild to moderate disease [unlicensed indication].

A combination of **clindamycin** 600 mg by mouth every 6 hours (section 5.1.6) and **primaquine** 15 mg daily by mouth (section 5.4.1) is used in the treatment of mild to moderate disease [unlicensed indication]; this combination is associated with considerable toxicity.

Trimetrexate is an alternative in AIDS patients with moderate disease, who are intolerant of standard therapy or who do not respond to it. Trimetrexate is a potent dihydrofolate reductase inhibitor and must be given with calcium folinate. The relapse rate with trimetrexate is high.

Inhaled **pentamidine isetionate** is sometimes used for mild disease. It is better tolerated than parenteral pentamidine but systemic absorption may still occur.

SEVERE DISEASE. **Co-trimoxazole** (section 5.1.8) in high dosage, given by mouth or by intravenous infusion, is the drug of choice for the treatment of severe pneumocystis pneumonia. **Pentamidine isetionate** given by intravenous infusion is an alternative for patients who cannot tolerate co-trimoxazole, or who have not responded to it. Pentamidine isetionate is a potentially toxic drug that can cause severe hypotension during or immediately after infusion. **Trimetrexate** may be used in AIDS patients who are intolerant of co-trimoxazole and pentamidine isetionate or who do not respond to these drugs.

Corticosteroid treatment can be lifesaving in those with severe pneumocystis pneumonia (see Adjunctive Therapy below).

ADJUNCTIVE THERAPY. In moderate to severe infections associated with HIV infection, prednisolone 50–80 mg daily is given by mouth for 5 days (alternatively, hydrocortisone may be given parenterally); the dose is then reduced to complete 21 days of treatment. Corticosteroid treatment should ideally be started at the same time as the anti-pneumocystis therapy and certainly no later than 24–72 hours afterwards. The corticosteroid should be withdrawn before anti-pneumocystis treatment is complete.

Prophylaxis
Prophylaxis against pneumocystis pneumonia should be given to all patients with a history of the infection. Prophylaxis against pneumocystis pneumonia should also be considered for severely immunocompromised patients. Prophylaxis should continue until immunity recovers sufficiently. It should not be discontinued if the patient has oral candidiasis, continues to lose weight, or is receiving cytotoxic therapy or long-term immunosuppressant therapy.

Co-trimoxazole by mouth is the drug of choice for prophylaxis. It is given in a dose of 960 mg daily or 960 mg on alternate days (3 times a week); the dose may be reduced to co-trimoxazole 480 mg daily to improve tolerance.

Intermittent inhalation of **pentamidine isetionate** is used in patients unable to tolerate co-trimoxazole.

It is effective but patients may be prone to extrapulmonary infection. Alternatively, **dapsone** 100 mg daily (section 5.1.10) can be used. **Atovaquone** 750 mg twice daily has also been used for prophylaxis [unlicensed indication].

ATOVAQUONE

Indications: treatment of mild to moderate *Pneumocystis carinii* pneumonia in patients intolerant of co-trimoxazole

Cautions: initial diarrhoea and difficulty in taking with food may reduce absorption (and require alternative therapy); other causes of pulmonary disease should be sought and treated; elderly; hepatic and renal impairment; pregnancy; avoid breast-feeding; **interactions:** Appendix 1 (atovaquone)

Side-effects: diarrhoea, nausea, vomiting; headache, insomnia; rash, fever; elevated liver enzymes and amylase; anaemia, neutropenia; hyponatraemia

Dose: 750 mg twice daily with food (particularly high fat) for 21 days; CHILD not recommended

Wellvone® (GlaxoWellcome) PoM
Suspension, sugar-free, fruit-flavoured, atovaquone 750 mg/5 mL, net price 226 mL = £360.18. Label: 21

∎ With proguanil hydrochloride
See section 5.4.1

PENTAMIDINE ISETIONATE

Indications: see under Dose (should only be given by specialists)

Cautions: risk of severe hypotension following administration (establish baseline blood pressure and administer with patient lying down; monitor blood pressure closely during administration, and at regular intervals, until treatment concluded); hepatic and renal impairment; hypertension or hypotension; hyperglycaemia or hypoglycaemia; leucopenia, thrombocytopenia, or anaemia; pregnancy and breast-feeding; carry out laboratory monitoring according to product literature; care required to protect personnel during handling and administration

Side-effects: severe reactions, sometimes fatal, due to hypotension, hypoglycaemia, pancreatitis, and arrhythmias; also leucopenia, thrombocytopenia, acute renal failure, hypocalcaemia; also reported: azotaemia, abnormal liver-function tests, anaemia, hyperkalaemia, nausea and vomiting, dizziness, syncope, flushing, hyperglycaemia, rash, and taste disturbances; Stevens-Johnson syndrome reported; on inhalation, bronchoconstriction (may be prevented by prior use of bronchodilators), cough, shortness of breath, and wheezing; discomfort, pain, induration, abscess formation, and muscle necrosis at injection site

Dose: *Pneumocystis carinii* pneumonia, *by intravenous infusion*, 4 mg/kg daily for at least 14 days (reduced according to product literature in renal impairment)

By inhalation of nebulised solution (using suitable equipment—consult product literature) 600 mg pentamidine isetionate daily for 3 weeks;

secondary prevention, 300 mg every 4 weeks *or* 150 mg every 2 weeks

Visceral leishmaniasis (kala-azar, section 5.4.5), *by deep intramuscular injection*, 3–4 mg/kg on alternate days to max. total of 10 injections; course may be repeated if necessary

Cutaneous leishmaniasis, *by deep intramuscular injection*, 3–4 mg/kg once or twice weekly until condition resolves (but see also section 5.4.5)

Trypanosomiasis, *by deep intramuscular injection or intravenous infusion*, 4 mg/kg daily or on alternate days to total of 7–10 injections

Note. Direct bolus intravenous injection should be avoided whenever possible and **never** given rapidly; intramuscular injections should be deep and preferably given into the buttock

Pentacarinat® (JHC) PoM

Injection, powder for reconstitution, pentamidine isetionate, net price 300-mg vial = £32.74

Nebuliser solution, pentamidine isetionate, net price 300-mg bottle = £34.57

CAUTION IN HANDLING. Pentamidine isetionate is toxic and personnel should be adequately protected during handling and administration—consult product literature

---

TRIMETREXATE

Indications: treatment of moderate to severe *Pneumocystis carinii* pneumonia in AIDS patients intolerant of, or refractory to, standard therapy or for whom standard therapy is contra-indicated (specialist use only)

Cautions: administer calcium folinate during treatment and for 72 hours after last dose (to avoid potentially serious or life-threatening bone-marrow suppression, oral and gastro-intestinal ulceration, and renal and hepatic dysfunction); suspend myelosupressive drugs (e.g. zidovudine) to administer therapeutic doses of trimetrexate; hepatic and renal impairment; **interactions:** Appendix 1 (trimetrexate)

MONITORING. Monitor at least twice weekly full blood count, renal and hepatic function; interrupt treatment if significant change in renal or hepatic function (see product literature); adjust dose of trimetrexate and calcium folinate if significant haematological toxicity (see product literature)

Contra-indications: pregnancy (following administration to woman or man, avoid conception for **at least 6 months** after treatment), breastfeeding

Side-effects: blood disorders including thrombocytopenia, granulocytopenia and anaemia (dose modification may be necessary, see also monitoring, above); vomiting, diarrhoea, oral and gastro-intestinal mucosal ulceration (discontinue if interfering with eating and drinking); fever (discontinue if uncontrolled by antipyretics); confusion, rarely seizures; disturbances in liver enzymes; disturbances in plasma calcium, potassium and magnesium reported; rash, anaphylaxis very rarely reported; rarely local irritation at injection site

Dose: *by intravenous infusion*, 45 mg/m^2 daily for 21 days together with calcium folinate *by mouth* or *by intravenous injection* (over 5–10 minutes), 20 mg/m^2 every 6 hours for 24 days; CHILD safety and efficacy not established

Note. Calcium folinate must not be given with trimetrexate in the same intravenous line (administer either before or after trimetrexate infusion)

Neutrexin® (Ipsen) ▼ PoM

Injection, powder for reconstitution, trimetrexate (as glucuronate). Net price 25-mg vial = £32.34

CAUTION IN HANDLING. Trimetrexate is toxic and personnel should be adequately protected during handling and administration; if solution comes into contact with skin or mucosa, wash off immediately with soap and water

---

5.5   Anthelmintics

5.5.1   Drugs for threadworms
5.5.2   Ascaricides
5.5.3   Drugs for tapeworm infections
5.5.4   Drugs for hookworms
5.5.5   Schistosomicides
5.5.6   Filaricides
5.5.7   Drugs for cutaneous larva migrans
5.5.8   Drugs for strongyloidiasis

Advice on prophylaxis and treatment of helminth infections is available from:

Birmingham	(0121) 424 0357
Scottish Centre for Infection and Environmental Health (registered users of Travax only)	(0141) 300 1130 (weekdays 2–4 p.m. only)
Liverpool	(0151) 708 9393
London	(020) 7387 9300 (treatment)

5.5.1   Drugs for threadworms
(pinworms, *Enterobius vermicularis*)

Anthelmintics are effective in threadworm infections, but their use needs to be combined with hygienic measures to break the cycle of auto-infection. All members of the family require treatment.

Adult threadworms do not live for longer than 6 weeks and for development of fresh worms, ova must be swallowed and exposed to the action of digestive juices in the upper intestinal tract. Direct multiplication of worms does not take place in the large bowel. Adult female worms lay ova on the perianal skin which causes pruritus; scratching the area then leads to ova being transmitted on fingers to the mouth, often via food eaten with unwashed hands. Washing hands and scrubbing nails before each meal and after each visit to the toilet is essential. A bath taken immediately after rising will remove ova laid during the night.

Mebendazole is the drug of choice for patients of all ages over 2 years. It is given as a single dose; as reinfection is very common, a second dose may be given after 2–3 weeks.

Piperazine is available in combination with sennosides as a single-dose preparation.

MEBENDAZOLE

Indications: threadworm, roundworm, whipworm, and hookworm infections

Cautions: pregnancy (toxicity in *rats*), breast-feeding; **interactions:** Appendix 1 (mebendazole)

Note. The package insert in the *Vermox®* pack includes the statement that it is not suitable for women known to be pregnant or children under 2 years

Side-effects: rarely abdominal pain, diarrhoea; hypersensitivity reactions (including exanthema, rash, urticaria, and angioedema) reported

Dose: threadworms, ADULT and CHILD over 2 years, 100 mg as a single dose; if reinfection occurs second dose may be needed after 2–3 weeks; CHILD under 2 years, not yet recommended

Whipworms, ADULT and CHILD over 2 years, 100 mg twice daily for 3 days; CHILD under 2 years, not yet recommended

Roundworms—section 5.5.2

Hookworms—section 5.5.4

▏**Mebendazole** (Non-proprietary) PoM
Tablets, chewable, mebendazole 100 mg
1. Can be sold to the public if supplied for oral use in the treatment of enterobiasis in adults and children over 2 years provided its container or package is labelled to show a max. single dose of 100 mg and it is supplied in a container or package containing not more than 800 mg; proprietary brands on sale to the public include *Boots Threadworm Treatment®*, *Ovex®* and *Pripsen® Mebendazole*.

Vermox® (Janssen-Cilag) PoM
Tablets, orange, scored, chewable, mebendazole 100 mg. Net price 6-tab pack = £1.53
Suspension, mebendazole 100 mg/5 mL. Net price 30 mL = £1.77

PIPERAZINE

Indications: threadworm and roundworm infections

Cautions: renal impairment (avoid if severe), liver disease, neurological disease; epilepsy, pregnancy (see also Appendix 4—packs on sale to the general public carry a warning to avoid in epilepsy and pregnancy)

Side-effects: nausea, vomiting, colic, diarrhoea, allergic reactions including urticaria, bronchospasm, and rare reports of Stevens-Johnson syndrome and angioedema; rarely dizziness, muscular incoordination ('worm wobble'); drowsiness, confusion and clonic contractions in patients with neurological or renal abnormalities

Dose: see under Preparation, below

Pripsen® (SSL)
Oral powder, piperazine phosphate 4 g and sennosides 15.3 mg/sachet. Net price two-dose sachet pack = £1.31. Label: 13
Dose: threadworms, stirred into a small glass of milk or water and drunk immediately, ADULT and CHILD over 6 years, 1 sachet, repeated after 14 days; INFANT 3 months–1 year (on doctor's advice only), 1 level 2.5-mL spoonful, repeated after 14 days; CHILD 1–6 years, 1 level 5-mL spoonful, repeated after 14 days
Roundworms, first dose as for threadworms; repeat at monthly intervals for up to 3 months if reinfection risk

Ascaricides
(common roundworm infections)

Levamisole (available on named-patient basis from IDIS) is very effective against *Ascaris lumbricoides* and is generally considered to be the drug of choice. It is very well tolerated; mild nausea or vomiting has been reported in about 1% of treated patients; it is given as a single dose of 120–150 mg in adults.

Mebendazole (section 5.5.1) is also active against ascaris; the usual dose is 100 mg twice daily for 3 days. **Piperazine** may be given in a single adult dose, see Piperazine, above.

Drugs for tapeworm infections

Taenicides

Niclosamide (available on named-patient basis from IDIS) is the most widely used drug for tapeworm infections and side-effects are limited to occasional gastro-intestinal upset, lightheadedness, and pruritus; it is not effective against larval worms. Fears of developing cysticercosis in *Taenia solium* infections have proved unfounded. All the same, it is wise to anticipate this possibility by using an anti-emetic on wakening.

Praziquantel (available on named-patient basis from Merck (*Cysticide®*)) is as effective as niclosamide and is given as a single dose of 10–20 mg/kg after a light breakfast (a single dose of 25 mg/kg for *Hymenolepis nana*).

Hydatid disease

Cysts caused by *Echinococcus granulosus* grow slowly and asymptomatic patients do not always require treatment. Surgical treatment remains the method of choice in many situations. **Albendazole** (available on named-patient basis from IDIS (*Zentel®*)) is used in conjunction with surgery to reduce the risk of recurrence or as primary treatment in inoperable cases. Alveolar echinococcosis due to *E. multilocularis* is usually fatal if untreated. Surgical removal with albendazole cover is the treatment of choice, but where effective surgery is impossible, repeated cycles of albendazole (for a year or more) may help. Careful monitoring of liver function is particularly important during drug treatment.

Drugs for hookworms
(ancylostomiasis, necatoriasis)

Hookworms live in the upper small intestine and draw blood from the point of their attachment to their host. An iron-deficiency anaemia may thereby be produced and, if present, effective treatment of the infection requires not only expulsion of the worms but treatment of the anaemia.

Mebendazole (section 5.5.1) has a useful broad-spectrum activity, and is effective against hookworms; the usual dose is 100 mg twice daily for 3 days.

5.5.5 Schistosomicides
(bilharziasis)

Adult *Schistosoma haematobium* worms live in the genito-urinary veins and adult *S. mansoni* in those of the colon and mesentery. *S. japonicum* is more widely distributed in veins of the alimentary tract and portal system.

Praziquantel (available on named-patient basis from Merck (*Cysticide*®)) is effective against all human schistosomes. The dose is 40 mg/kg in 2 divided doses 4–6 hours apart on one day (60 mg/kg in 3 divided doses on one day for *S. japonicum* infections). No serious toxic effects have been reported. Of all the available schistosomicides, it has the most attractive combination of effectiveness, broad-spectrum activity, and low toxicity.

Hycanthone, lucanthone, niridazole, oxamniquine, and sodium stibocaptate have now been superseded.

5.5.6 Filaricides

Diethylcarbamazine (not on UK market) is effective against microfilariae and adults of *Loa loa*, *Wuchereria bancrofti*, and *Brugia malayi*. To minimise reactions treatment is commenced with a dose of diethylcarbamazine citrate 1 mg/kg on the first day and increased gradually over 3 days to 6 mg/kg daily in divided doses; this dosage is maintained for 21 days and usually gives a radical cure for these infections. Close medical supervision is necessary particularly in the early phase of treatment.

In heavy infections there may be a febrile reaction, and in heavy *Loa loa* infection there is a small risk of encephalopathy. In such cases treatment must be given under careful in-patient supervision and stopped at the first sign of cerebral involvement (and specialist advice sought).

Ivermectin (*Mectizan*®, MSD, available on named-patient basis) is very effective in *onchocerciasis* and it is now the drug of choice. A single dose of 150 micrograms/kg by mouth produces a prolonged reduction in microfilarial levels. Retreatment at intervals of 6 to 12 months depending on symptoms must be given until the adult worms die out. Reactions are usually slight and most commonly take the form of temporary aggravation of itching and rash. Diethylcarbamazine or suramin should no longer be used for onchocerciasis because of their toxicity.

5.5.7 Drugs for cutaneous larva migrans
(creeping eruption)

Dog and cat hookworm larvae may enter human skin where they produce slowly extending itching tracks usually on the foot. Single tracks can be treated with topical tiabendazole (no commercial preparation available). Multiple infections respond to **ivermectin** (*Mectizan*®, MSD, available on named-patient basis), **albendazole** (available on named-patient basis from IDIS (*Zentel*®)) or **tiabendazole** (thiabendazole) (available on a named-patient basis from IDIS (*Mintezol*®, *Triasox*®)) by mouth.

5.5.8 Drugs for strongyloidiasis

Adult *Strongyloides stercoralis* live in the gut and produce larvae which penetrate the gut wall and invade the tissues, setting up a cycle of auto-infection. **Tiabendazole** (thiabendazole) (available on a named-patient basis from IDIS (*Mintezol*®, *Triasox*®)) is the drug of choice for adults (but side-effects are much more marked in the elderly); it is given at a dosage of 25 mg/kg (max. 1.5 g) every 12 hours for 3 days. **Albendazole** is an alternative (available on named-patient basis from IDIS (*Zentel*®)) with fewer side-effects; it is given in a dose of 400 mg twice daily for 3 days, repeated after 3 weeks if necessary. **Ivermectin** (*Mectizan*®, MSD, available on named-patient basis) in a dose of 200 micrograms/kg daily for 2 days may be the most effective drug for chronic *Strongyloides* infection.

6: Endocrine system

6.1 Drugs used in diabetes

6.1.1   Insulins
6.1.2   Oral antidiabetic drugs
6.1.3   Diabetic ketoacidosis
6.1.4   Treatment of hypoglycaemia
6.1.5   Treatment of diabetic nephropathy and neuropathy
6.1.6   Diagnostic and monitoring agents for diabetes mellitus

Diabetes mellitus occurs because of a lack of insulin or resistance to its action. Diabetes is clinically defined by measurement of fasting or random blood-glucose concentration (and occasionally by glucose tolerance test). There are two principal classes of diabetes (and many subtypes not listed here):

TYPE 1 DIABETES. Type 1 diabetes, also referred to as insulin-dependent diabetes mellitus (IDDM), is due to a deficiency of insulin following autoimmune destruction of pancreatic beta cells. Patients with type 1 diabetes require administration of insulin.

TYPE 2 DIABETES. Type 2 diabetes, also referred to as non-insulin-dependent diabetes (NIDDM), is due to reduced secretion of insulin or to peripheral resistance to the action of insulin. Although patients may be controlled on diet alone, many require administration of oral antidiabetic drugs or insulin to maintain satisfactory control.

Treatment should be aimed at alleviating symptoms and minimising the risk of long-term complications by appropriate control of diabetes. Other risk factors for cardiovascular disease (smoking, hypertension, obesity and hyperlipidaemia) should be addressed.

Diabetes is a strong risk factor for cardiovascular disease. There is evidence that the use of an ACE inhibitor (section 2.5.5.1) may be beneficial in patients with diabetes and a high cardiovascular risk. For reference to the use of an ACE inhibitor in the management of diabetic nephropathy, see section 6.1.5.

PREVENTION OF DIABETIC COMPLICATIONS. Optimal glycaemic control in both type 1 diabetes and type 2 diabetes reduces, in the long term, the risk of microvascular complications including retinopathy, development of albuminuria and to some extent neuropathy. However, a temporary deterioration in established diabetic retinopathy may occur when normalising blood-glucose concentration.

A measure of the total glycated (or glycosylated) haemoglobin (HbA_1) or a specific fraction (HbA_{1c}) provides a good indication of long-term glycaemic control. The ideal HbA_{1c} level is around 7% although this cannot always be achieved, and for those on insulin there are significantly increased risks of severe hypoglycaemia. Tight control of blood pressure in hypertensive patients with type 2 diabetes reduces mortality significantly and protects visual acuity (by reducing considerably the risks of maculopathy and retinal photocoagulation) (see also section 2.5).

6.1.1   Insulins

6.1.1.1	Short-acting insulins
6.1.1.2	Intermediate- and long-acting insulins
6.1.1.3	Hypodermic equipment

Insulin plays a key role in the regulation of carbohydrate, fat, and protein metabolism. It is a polypeptide hormone of complex structure. There are differences in the amino-acid sequence of animal insulins, human insulins and the human insulin analogues. Insulin may be extracted from pork pancreas and purified by crystallisation; it may also be extracted from beef pancreas, but beef insulins are now rarely used. Human sequence insulin may be produced semisynthetically by enzymatic modification of porcine insulin (emp) or biosynthetically by recombinant DNA technology using bacteria (crb, prb) or yeast (pyr).

All insulin preparations are to a greater or lesser extent immunogenic in man but immunological resistance to insulin action is uncommon. Preparations of human sequence insulin should theoretically be less immunogenic, but no real advantage has been shown in trials.

Insulin is inactivated by gastro-intestinal enzymes, and must therefore be given by injection; the subcutaneous route is ideal in most circumstances. It is usually injected into the upper arms, thighs, buttocks, or abdomen; there may be increased absorption from a limb site if the limb is used in strenuous exercise following the injection. Generally subcutaneous insulin injections cause few problems; fat hypertrophy does however occur but can be minimised by rotating the injection sites. Local allergic reactions are now rare.

Insulin is needed by all patients who present with ketoacidosis, and most of those with rapid onset of symptoms, weight loss, weakness and sometimes vomiting often associated with ketonuria. It is required by almost all children with diabetes. Insulin is also needed for type 2 diabetes when other methods have failed to achieve good control, and temporarily in the presence of intercurrent illness or perioperatively. Pregnant women with type 2 diabetes should be treated with insulin when diet alone fails. The majority of those who are obese can be managed by dietary changes or, if diet alone fails to achieve adequate control, by also administering oral hypoglycaemic drugs (section 6.1.2).

MANAGEMENT OF DIABETES WITH INSULIN. The aim of treatment is to achieve the best possible control of blood-glucose concentration without making the patient obsessional and to avoid disabling hypoglycaemia; close co-operation is needed between the patient and the medical team since good control reduces the risk of complications. Mixtures of insulin preparations may be required and appropriate combinations have to be determined for the individual patient. For patients with acute-onset diabetes, treatment should be started with soluble insulin given 3 times daily with medium-acting insulin at bedtime. For those less severely ill, treatment is usually started with a mixture of premixed short- and medium-acting insulins (most commonly in a proportion of 30% soluble insulin and 70% isophane insulin) given twice daily; 8 units twice daily is a suitable initial dose for most ambulant patients. The proportion of the short-acting soluble component can be increased in those with excessive post-prandial hyperglycaemia.

The dose of insulin is adjusted on an individual basis, by gradually increasing the dose but avoiding troublesome hypoglycaemic reactions.

There are 3 main types of insulin preparations:

- those of **short** duration which have a relatively rapid onset of action, namely soluble insulin, insulin lispro and insulin aspart;
- those with an **intermediate** action, e.g. isophane insulin and insulin zinc suspension; and
- those whose action is slower in onset and lasts for **long** periods, e.g. crystalline insulin zinc suspension

The duration of action of a particular type of insulin varies considerably from one patient to another, and needs to be assessed individually.

Examples of recommended insulin regimens

- Short-acting insulin mixed with intermediate-acting insulin: twice daily (before meals)
- Short-acting insulin mixed with intermediate-acting insulin: before breakfast
  Short-acting insulin: before evening meal
  Intermediate-acting insulin: at bedtime
- Short-acting insulin: three times daily (before breakfast, midday and evening meal)
  Intermediate-acting insulin: at bedtime
- Intermediate-acting insulin with or without short-acting insulin: once daily either before breakfast or at bedtime suffices for some patients with type 2 diabetes who need insulin, sometimes in combination with oral hypoglycaemic drugs

Insulin requirements may be increased by infection, stress, accidental or surgical trauma, puberty and, during the second and third trimesters of pregnancy. Requirements may be decreased in patients with renal or hepatic impairment and in those with some endocrine disorders (e.g. Addison's disease, hypopituitrism) or coeliac disease. In pregnancy insulin requirements should be assessed frequently by an experienced diabetes physician.

INSULIN ADMINISTRATION. Injection devices ('pens') (section 6.1.1.3) which hold the insulin in a cartridge and meter the required dose are convenient to use. The conventional syringe and needle is still the preferred method of insulin administration by many and is also required for insulins not available in cartridge form.

For intensive insulin regimens multiple injections (3 to 4 times daily) are usually recommended; soluble insulin can also be given by continuous subcutaneous infusion using an infusion pump. This delivers a continuous basal insulin infusion with preprandial boosts provided by patient-activated bolus doses. This technique has a limited place in the treatment of diabetes, and patients using it must be well motivated, reliable, able to monitor their own blood-glucose, and with access to expert advice at all times. Continuous subcutaneous insulin infusion is sometimes valuable for patients with serious problems from recurrent hypoglycaemia.

UNITS. The word 'unit' should **not** be abbreviated.

MONITORING. Many patients monitor their own blood-glucose concentrations (section 6.1.6). Since blood-glucose concentrations vary substantially throughout the day, 'normoglycaemia' cannot always be achieved throughout a 24-hour period without causing damaging hypoglycaemia. It is therefore best to recommend that patients should maintain a blood-glucose concentration of between 4 and 10 mmol/litre for most of the time, while accepting that on occasions, for brief periods, it will be above these values; strenuous efforts should be made to prevent the blood-glucose concentration from falling below 4 mmol/litre. Patients should be advised to look for 'peaks' and 'troughs' of blood glucose, and to adjust their insulin dosage only once or twice weekly. Overall it is ideal to aim for an HbA_{1c} concentration of 7% or less (normal range 4–6%) or an HbA_1 of less than 8.8% (normal range 5–7.5%) although this is not always possible without causing disabling hypoglycaemia. Fructosamine can also be used for assessment of control; this is simpler and cheaper but the measurement of HbA_{1c} is generally a more reliable method.

The intake of energy and of simple and complex carbohydrates should be adequate to allow normal growth and development but obesity must be avoided. The carbohydrate intake needs to be regulated and should be distributed throughout the day. Fine control of plasma glucose can be achieved by moving portions of carbohydrate from one meal to another without altering the total intake.

HYPOGLYCAEMIA. Hypoglycaemia is a potential problem for all patients receiving insulin and careful instruction to the patient must be directed towards avoiding it.

Loss of warning of hypoglycaemia is common among insulin-treated patients and can be a serious hazard, especially for drivers and those in dangerous occupations. Very tight control of diabetes lowers the blood-glucose concentration needed to trigger hypoglycaemic symptoms; increase in the frequency of hypoglycaemic episodes reduces the warning symptoms experienced by the patient. Beta-blockers can also blunt hypoglycaemic awareness (and also delay recovery).

To restore the warning signs, episodes of hypoglycaemia must be reduced to a minimum; this involves appropriate adjustment of insulin type, dose and frequency together with suitable timing and quantity of meals and snacks.

Some patients have reported loss of hypoglycaemia warning after transfer to human insulin. If a patient believes that human insulin is responsible for the loss of warning it is reasonable to revert to animal insulin and essential to educate the patient about avoiding hypoglycaemia. Great care should be taken to specify whether a human or an animal preparation is required.

Few patients are now treated with beef insulins; when undertaking conversion from beef to human insulin, the total dose should be reduced by about 10% with careful monitoring for the first few days. When changing between pork and human sequence insulins, a dose change is not usually needed, but careful monitoring is still advised.

DRIVING. Drivers treated with insulin or oral anti-diabetic drugs are required to notify the Driver and Vehicle Licensing Agency of their condition, as are drivers of Group 2 vehicles (heavy goods vehicles or public service vehicles) whose diabetes is controlled by diet alone; the Agency's Drivers Medical Unit provides guidance on eligibility to drive.

Drivers need to be particularly careful to avoid hypoglycaemia (see also above) and should be warned of the problems. They should normally check their blood-glucose concentration before driving and, on long journeys, at 2-hour intervals and they should ensure that a supply of sugar is always available in the car. If hypoglycaemia occurs a car driver should switch off the ignition until recovery is complete, which may take up to 15 minutes or longer. Driving is not permitted when hypoglycaemic awareness is impaired.

DIABETES AND SURGERY. The following regimen is suitable when surgery in a patient with type 1 diabetes requires intravenous infusion of insulin for 12 hours or longer.

- Give an injection of the patient's usual insulin on the night before the operation.
- Early on the day of the operation, start an intravenous infusion of glucose 5% or 10% containing potassium chloride 10 mmol/litre (provided that the patient is not hyperkalaemic) and infuse at a constant rate appropriate to the patient's fluid requirements (usually 125 mL per hour); make up a solution of soluble insulin 1 unit/mL in sodium chloride 0.9% and infuse intravenously using a syringe pump piggy-backed to the intravenous infusion.
- The rate of the insulin infusion should normally be:
  Blood glucose < 4 mmol/litre, give 0.5 units/hour
  Blood glucose 4–15 mmol/litre, give 2 units/hour
  Blood glucose 15–20 mmol/litre, give 4 units/hour
  Blood glucose > 20 mmol/litre, review.

In resistant cases (such as patients who are in shock or severely ill or those receiving corticosteroids or sympathomimetics) 2–4 times these rates or even more may be needed.

If a syringe pump is not available soluble insulin 16 units/litre should be added to the intravenous infusion of glucose 5% or 10% containing potassium chloride 10 mmol per litre (provided the patient is not hyperkalaemic) and the infusion run at the rate appropriate to the patient's fluid requirements (usually 125 mL per hour) with the insulin dose adjusted as follows:

  Blood glucose < 4 mmol/litre, give 8 units/litre
  Blood glucose 4–15 mmol/litre, give 16 units/litre
  Blood glucose 15–20 mmol/litre, give 32 units/litre
  Blood glucose > 20 mmol/litre, review.

The rate of intravenous infusion depends on the volume depletion, cardiac function, age, and other factors. Blood-glucose concentration should be measured pre-operatively and then hourly until stable, thereafter every 2 hours. The duration of action of intravenous insulin is only a few minutes and the infusion must not be stopped unless the patient becomes overtly hypoglycaemic (blood glucose < 3 mmol/litre) in which case it should be stopped for up to 30 minutes. The amount of potassium chloride required in the infusion needs to be assessed by regular measurement of plasma electrolytes. Sodium chloride 0.9% infusion should replace glucose 5% or 10% if the blood glucose is persistently above 15 mmol/litre.

Once the patient starts to eat and drink, give subcutaneous insulin before breakfast and stop intravenous insulin 30 minutes later; the dose may need to be 10–20% more than usual if the patient is still in bed or unwell. If the patient was not previously receiving insulin, an appropriate initial dose is 30–40 units daily in four divided doses using soluble insulin before meals and intermediate-acting insulin at bedtime and the dose adjusted from day to day. Patients with hyperglycaemia often relapse after conversion back to subcutaneous insulin calling for one of the following approaches:

- additional doses of soluble insulin at any of the four injection times (before meals or bedtime) or
- temporary addition of intravenous insulin infusion (while continuing the subcutaneous regimen) until blood-glucose concentration is satisfactory or
- complete reversion to the intravenous regimen (especially if the patient is unwell).

6.1.1.1   Short-acting insulins

Soluble insulin is a short-acting form of insulin. For maintenance regimens it is usual to inject it 15 to 30 minutes before meals.

Soluble insulin is the only appropriate form of insulin for use in diabetic emergencies and at the time of surgery. It can be given intravenously and intramuscularly, as well as subcutaneously.

When injected subcutaneously, soluble insulin has a rapid onset of action (after 30 to 60 minutes), a peak action between 2 and 4 hours, and a duration of action of up to 8 hours. Human sequence preparations tend to have a more rapid onset and a shorter overall duration.

When injected intravenously, soluble insulin has a very short half-life of only about 5 minutes and its effect disappears within 30 minutes.

The human insulin analogues, **insulin lispro** and **insulin aspart**, have a faster onset and shorter duration of action than soluble insulin; as a result, compared to soluble insulin, fasting and preprandial blood-glucose concentration is a little higher, postprandial blood-glucose concentration is a little lower, and hypoglycaemia occurs slightly less frequently. Subcutaneous injection of insulin lispro or of insulin aspart may prove convenient to those who wish to inject shortly before or, when necessary, shortly after a meal. They may also help those prone to pre-lunch hypoglycaemia and those who eat late in the evening and are prone to early nocturnal hypoglycaemia. Insulin aspart and insulin lispro may also be administered by subcutaneous infusion.

SOLUBLE INSULIN

(Insulin Injection; Neutral Insulin)

A sterile solution of insulin (i.e. bovine or porcine) or of human insulin; pH 6.6–8.0

Indications: diabetes mellitus; diabetic ketoacidosis (section 6.1.3)

Cautions: see notes above; reduce dose in renal impairment; **interactions:** Appendix 1 (antidiabetics)

Side-effects: see notes above; local reactions and fat hypertrophy at injection site; overdose causes hypoglycaemia

Dose: *by subcutaneous, intramuscular, or intravenous injection or intravenous infusion*, according to requirements

COUNSELLING. Show container to patient and confirm that patient is expecting the version dispensed

■ Highly purified animal

Hypurin® Bovine Neutral (CP) PoM

Injection, soluble insulin (bovine, highly purified) 100 units/mL. Net price 10-mL vial = £18.48; 5 × 1.5-mL cartridge (for *Autopen®* device) = £13.86

Hypurin® Porcine Neutral (CP) PoM

Injection, soluble insulin (porcine, highly purified) 100 units/mL. Net price 10-mL vial = £16.80; 5 × 1.5-mL cartridge (for *Autopen®* device) = £12.60

Pork Actrapid® (Novo Nordisk) PoM

Injection, soluble insulin (porcine, highly purified) 100 units/mL. Net price 10-mL vial = £6.58

Note. Not recommended for use in subcutaneous insulin infusion pumps—may precipitate in catheter or needle

■ Human sequence

Human Actrapid® (Novo Nordisk) PoM

Injection, soluble insulin (human, pyr) 100 units/mL. Net price 10-mL vial = £10.50; *Penfill®* cartridge (for *Innovo®* and *NovoPen®* devices) 5 × 1.5-mL = £11.44, 5 × 3-mL = £22.87; 5 × 3-mL *Actrapid®* prefilled disposable injection devices (range 2–78 units, allowing 2-unit dosage adjustment) = £26.50

Note. Not recommended for use in subcutaneous insulin infusion pumps—may precipitate in catheter or needle

Human Velosulin® (Novo Nordisk) PoM

Injection, soluble insulin (human, pyr) 100 units/mL. Net price 10-mL vial = £10.50

Humulin S® (Lilly) PoM

Injection, soluble insulin (human, prb) 100 units/mL. Net price 10-mL vial = £12.50; 5 × 3-mL cartridge (for *Autopen® 3ml* or *HumaPen®* NHS) = £21.30; 5 × 3-mL *Humaject S®* prefilled disposable injection devices (range 2–96 units, allowing 2-unit dosage adjustment) = £22.68

Insuman® Rapid (Aventis Pharma) PoM

Injection, soluble insulin (human, crb) 100 units/mL, net price 5-mL vial = £5.31; 5 × 3-mL cartridge (for *OptiPen® Pro* NHS) = £21.30; 5 × 3-mL *Insuman® Rapid OptiSet®* prefilled disposable injection devices (range 2–40 units, allowing 2-unit dosage adjustment) = £25.37

Note. Not recommended for use in subcutaneous insulin infusion pumps

■ Mixed preparations, see Biphasic Isophane Insulin (section 6.1.1.2)

INSULIN ASPART

(Recombinant human insulin analogue)

Indications: diabetes mellitus

Cautions: see under Soluble Insulin; children (use only if benefit likely compared to soluble insulin)

Side-effects: see under Soluble Insulin

Dose: *by subcutaneous injection,* immediately before meals or when necessary shortly after meals according to requirements

By subcutaneous infusion, according to requirements

COUNSELLING. Show container to patient and confirm that patient is expecting the version dispensed

NovoRapid® (Novo Nordisk) ▼ PoM

Injection, insulin aspart (recombinant human insulin analogue) 100 units/mL, net price 10-mL vial = £15.71; *Penfill®* cartridge (for *Innovo®* and *NovoPen®* devices) 5 × 3-mL = £26.78; 5 × 3-mL *NovoLet®* prefilled disposable injection devices (range 2–78 units, allowing 2-unit dosage adjustment) = £28.31

INSULIN LISPRO

(Recombinant human insulin analogue)
Indications: diabetes mellitus
Cautions: see under Soluble Insulin; children (use only if benefit likely compared to soluble insulin)
Side-effects: see under Soluble Insulin
Dose: *by subcutaneous injection,* shortly before meals or when necessary shortly after meals, according to requirements
By subcutaneous infusion, according to requirements
COUNSELLING. Show container to patient and confirm that patient is expecting the version dispensed

Humalog® (Lilly) PoM

Injection, insulin lispro (recombinant human insulin analogue) 100 units/mL. Net price 10-mL vial = £15.71; 5 × 1.5-mL cartridge (for *Autopen®*) = £13.39; 5 × 3-mL cartridge (for *Autopen® 3ml* or *HumaPen®* NHS) = £26.78; 5 × 3-mL *Humalog®-Pen* prefilled disposable injection devices (range 1–60 units, allowing 1-unit dosage adjustment) = £28.16

6.1.1.2   Intermediate- and long-acting insulins

When given by subcutaneous injection, intermediate- and long-acting insulins have an onset of action of approximately 1–2 hours, a maximal effect at 4–12 hours, and a duration of 16–35 hours. Some are given twice daily in conjunction with short-acting (soluble) insulin, and others are given once daily, particularly in elderly patients. They can be mixed with soluble insulin in the syringe, essentially retaining the properties of the two components, although there may be some blunting of the initial effect of the soluble insulin component (especially on mixing with protamine zinc insulin, see below).

Isophane insulin is a suspension of insulin with protamine which is of particular value for initiation of twice-daily insulin regimens. Patients usually mix isophane with soluble insulin but ready-mixed preparations may be appropriate (**biphasic isophane insulin** or **biphasic insulin lispro**).

Insulin zinc suspension (crystalline) has a more prolonged duration of action; it may be used independently or in **insulin zinc suspension** (30% amorphous, 70% crystalline).

Protamine zinc insulin is usually given once daily with short-acting (soluble) insulin. It has the drawback of binding with the soluble insulin when mixed in the same syringe, and is now rarely used.

INSULIN ZINC SUSPENSION

(Insulin Zinc Suspension (Mixed); I. Z. S.)
A sterile neutral suspension of bovine and/or porcine insulin or of human insulin in the form of a complex obtained by the addition of a suitable zinc salt; consists of rhombohedral crystals (10–40 microns) and of particles of no uniform shape (not exceeding 2 microns)
Indications: diabetes mellitus (long acting)
Cautions: see under Soluble Insulin (section 6.1.1.1)
Side-effects: see under Soluble Insulin (section 6.1.1.1)
Dose: *by subcutaneous injection,* according to requirements
COUNSELLING. Show container to patient and confirm that patient is expecting the version dispensed

■ Highly purified animal
Hypurin® Bovine Lente (CP) PoM
Injection, insulin zinc suspension (bovine, highly purified) 100 units/mL. Net price 10-mL vial = £18.48

■ Human sequence
Human Monotard® (Novo Nordisk) PoM
Injection, insulin zinc suspension (human, pyr) 100 units/mL. Net price 10-mL vial = £10.50
Humulin Lente® (Lilly) PoM
Injection, insulin zinc suspension (human, prb) 100 units/mL. Net price 10-mL vial = £12.50

INSULIN ZINC SUSPENSION (CRYSTALLINE)

(Cryst. I. Z. S.)
A sterile neutral suspension of bovine insulin or of human insulin in the form of a complex obtained by the addition of a suitable zinc salt; consists of rhombohedral crystals (10–40 microns)
Indications: diabetes mellitus (long acting)
Cautions: see under Soluble Insulin (section 6.1.1.1)
Side-effects: see under Soluble Insulin (section 6.1.1.1)
Dose: *by subcutaneous injection,* according to requirements
COUNSELLING. Show container to patient and confirm that patient is expecting the version dispensed

■ Human sequence
Human Ultratard® (Novo Nordisk) PoM
Injection, insulin zinc suspension, crystalline (human, pyr) 100 units/mL. Net price 10-mL vial = £10.50
Humulin Zn® (Lilly) PoM
Injection, insulin zinc suspension, crystalline (human, prb) 100 units/mL. Net price 10-mL vial = £12.50

ISOPHANE INSULIN

(Isophane Insulin Injection; Isophane Protamine Insulin Injection; Isophane Insulin (NPH))
A sterile suspension of bovine or porcine insulin or of human insulin in the form of a complex obtained by the addition of protamine sulphate or another suitable protamine
Indications: diabetes mellitus (intermediate acting)
Cautions: see under Soluble Insulin (section 6.1.1.1)
Side-effects: see under Soluble Insulin (section 6.1.1.1); protamine may cause allergic reactions
Dose: *by subcutaneous injection,* according to requirements
COUNSELLING. Show container to patient and confirm that patient is expecting the version dispensed

- Highly purified animal

Hypurin® Bovine Isophane (CP) PoM
Injection, isophane insulin (bovine, highly purified) 100 units/mL. Net price 10-mL vial = £18.48; 5 × 1.5-mL cartridge (for *Autopen®* device) = £13.86

Hypurin® Porcine Isophane (CP) PoM
Injection, isophane insulin (porcine, highly purified) 100 units/mL. Net price 10-mL vial = £16.80; 5 × 1.5-mL cartridge (for *Autopen®* device) = £12.60

Pork Insulatard® (Novo Nordisk) PoM
Injection, isophane insulin (porcine, highly purified) 100 units/mL. Net price 10-mL vial = £6.58

- Human sequence

Human Insulatard® ge (Novo Nordisk) PoM
Injection, isophane insulin (human, pyr) 100 units/mL. Net price 10-mL vial = £10.50; *Penfill®* cartridge (for *Autopen®* (1.5mL only), *Innovo®*, or *Novopen®* devices) 5 × 1.5-mL = £11.44, 5 × 3-mL = £22.87; 5 × 3-mL prefilled disposable injection devices (range 2–78 units allowing 2-unit dosage adjustment) = £26.50; 5 × 3-mL *Insulatard InnoLet®* prefilled disposable injection devices (range 1–50 units allowing 1-unit dosage adjustment) = £26.84

Humulin I® (Lilly) PoM
Injection, isophane insulin (human, prb) 100 units/mL. Net price 10-mL vial = £12.50; 5 × 3-mL cartridge (for *Autopen® 3ml* or *HumaPen®* NHS) = £21.30; 5 × 3-mL *Humulin I-Pen®* prefilled disposable injection devices (range 1–60 units, allowing 1-unit dosage adjustment) = £22.68

Insuman® Basal (Aventis Pharma) PoM
Injection, isophane insulin (human, crb) 100 units/mL, net price 5-mL vial = £5.31; 5 × 3-mL cartridge (for *OptiPen® Pro* NHS) = £21.30; 5 × 3-mL *Insuman® Basal OptiSet®* prefilled disposable injection devices (range 2–40 units, allowing 2-unit dosage adjustment) = £25.37

- Mixed preparations, see Biphasic Isophane Insulin (below)

PROTAMINE ZINC INSULIN

(Protamine Zinc Insulin Injection)
A sterile suspension of insulin in the form of a complex obtained by the addition of a suitable protamine and zinc chloride; this preparation was included in BP 1980 but is not included in BP 1988

Indications: diabetes mellitus (long acting)
Cautions: see under Soluble Insulin (section 6.1.1.1); see also notes above
Side-effects: see under Soluble Insulin (section 6.1.1.1); protamine may cause allergic reactions
Dose: *by subcutaneous injection*, according to requirements
COUNSELLING. Show container to patient and confirm that patient is expecting the version dispensed

Hypurin® Bovine Protamine Zinc (CP) PoM
Injection, protamine zinc insulin (bovine, highly purified) 100 units/mL. Net price 10-mL vial = £18.48

Biphasic insulins

BIPHASIC INSULIN LISPRO

Indications: diabetes mellitus (intermediate acting)
Cautions: see under Soluble Insulin (section 6.1.1.1)
Side-effects: see under Soluble Insulin (section 6.1.1.1); protamine may cause allergic reactions
Dose: *by subcutaneous injection*, according to requirements
COUNSELLING. Show container to patient and confirm that patient is expecting the version dispensed

Humalog® Mix25 (Lilly) PoM
Injection, biphasic insulin lispro (recombinant human insulin analogue), 25% insulin lispro, 75% insulin lispro protamine, 100 units/mL, net price 5 × 3-mL cartridge (for *Autopen® 3ml* or *HumaPen®* NHS) = £26.78; 5 × 3-mL prefilled disposable injection devices = £28.16

Humalog® Mix50 (Lilly) PoM
Injection, biphasic insulin lispro (recombinant human insulin analogue), 50% insulin lispro, 50% insulin lispro protamine, 100 units/mL, net price 5 × 3-mL prefilled disposable injection devices = £28.16

BIPHASIC ISOPHANE INSULIN

(Biphasic Isophane Insulin Injection)
A sterile buffered suspension of either porcine or human insulin complexed with protamine sulphate (or another suitable protamine) in a solution of insulin of the same species
Indications: diabetes mellitus (intermediate acting)
Cautions: see under Soluble Insulin (section 6.1.1.1)
Side-effects: see under Soluble Insulin (section 6.1.1.1); protamine may cause allergic reactions
Dose: *by subcutaneous injection*, according to requirements
COUNSELLING. Show container to patient and confirm that patient is expecting the version dispensed

- Highly purified animal

Hypurin® Porcine 30/70 Mix (CP) PoM
Injection, biphasic isophane insulin (porcine, highly purified), 30% soluble, 70% isophane, 100 units/mL. Net price 10-mL vial = £16.80; 5 × 1.5-ml cartridge (for *Autopen®* device) = £12.60

Pork Mixtard 30® (Novo Nordisk) PoM
Injection, biphasic isophane insulin (porcine, highly purified), 30% soluble, 70% isophane, 100 units/mL. Net price 10-mL vial = £6.58

- Human sequence

Human Mixtard® 10 (Novo Nordisk) PoM
Injection, biphasic isophane insulin (human, pyr), 10% soluble, 90% isophane, 100 units/mL. Net price *Penfill®* cartridge (for *Autopen®* (1.5mL only), *Innovo®* or *Novopen®* devices) 5 × 1.5-mL = £11.44, 5 × 3-mL = £22.87; 5 × 3-mL prefilled disposable injection devices (range 2–78 units, allowing 2-unit dosage adjustment) = £26.50

Human Mixtard® 20 (Novo Nordisk) PoM
Injection, biphasic isophane insulin (human, pyr), 20% soluble, 80% isophane, 100 units/mL. Net price *Penfill®* cartridge (for *Autopen®* (1.5mL only), *Innovo®* or *Novopen®* devices) 5 × 1.5-ml = £11.44, 5 × 3-mL = £22.87; 5 × 3-mL prefilled disposable injection devices (range 2–78 units, allowing 2-unit dosage adjustment) = £26.50

Human Mixtard® 30 (Novo Nordisk) PoM
Injection, biphasic isophane insulin (human, pyr), 30% soluble, 70% isophane, 100 units/mL. Net price *Penfill®* cartridge (for *Autopen®* (1.5mL only), *Innovo®* or *Novopen®* devices) 5 × 1.5-mL = £11.44, 5 × 3-mL = £22.87; 5 × 3-mL prefilled disposable injection devices (range 2–78 units, allowing 2-unit dosage adjustment) = £26.50; 5 × 3-mL *Mixtard 30 InnoLet®* prefilled disposable injection devices (range 1–50 units allowing 1-unit dosage adjustment) = £26.84

Human Mixtard® 30 ge (Novo Nordisk) PoM
Injection, biphasic isophane insulin (human, pyr), 30% soluble, 70% isophane, 100 units/mL. Net price 10-mL vial = £10.50

Human Mixtard® 40 (Novo Nordisk) PoM
Injection, biphasic isophane insulin (human, pyr), 40% soluble, 60% isophane, 100 units/mL. Net price *Penfill®* cartridge (for *Autopen®* (1.5mL only), *Innovo®* or *Novopen®* devices) 5 × 1.5-ml = £11.44, 5 × 3-mL = £22.87; 5 × 3-mL prefilled disposable injection devices (range 2–78 units, allowing 2-unit dosage adjustment) = £26.50

Human Mixtard® 50 (Novo Nordisk) PoM
Injection, biphasic isophane insulin (human, pyr), 50% soluble, 50% isophane, 100 units/mL. Net price 10-mL vial = £10.50; *Penfill®* cartridge (for *Autopen®* (1.5mL only), *Innovo®* or *Novopen®* devices) 5 × 1.5-mL = £11.44, 5 × 3-mL = £22.87; 5 × 3-mL prefilled disposable injection devices (range 2–78 units, allowing 2-unit dosage adjustment) = £26.50

Humulin M2® (Lilly) PoM
Injection, biphasic isophane insulin (human, prb), 20% soluble, 80% isophane, 100 units/mL. Net price 5 × 3-mL cartridge (for *Autopen®* *3ml* or *HumaPen®* NHS) = £21.30

Humulin M3® (Lilly) PoM
Injection, biphasic isophane insulin (human, prb), 30% soluble, 70% isophane, 100 units/mL. Net price 10-mL vial = £12.50; 5 × 3-mL cartridge (for *Autopen®* *3ml* or *HumaPen®* NHS) = £21.30; 5 × 3-mL *Humaject M3®* prefilled disposable injection devices (range 2–96 units, allowing 2-unit dosage adjustment) = £22.68

Humulin M5® (Lilly) PoM
Injection, biphasic isophane insulin (human, prb), 50% soluble, 50% isophane, 100 units/mL. Net price 10-mL vial = £12.50

Insuman® Comb 15 (Aventis Pharma) PoM
Injection, biphasic isophane insulin (human, crb), 15% soluble, 85% isophane, 100 units/mL, net price 5-mL vial = £5.31; 5 × 3-mL cartridge (for *OptiPen® Pro* NHS) = £21.30; 5 × 3-mL *Insuman® Comb 15 OptiSet®* prefilled disposable injection devices (range 2–40 units, allowing 2-unit dosage adjustment) = £25.37

Insuman® Comb 25 (Aventis Pharma) PoM
Injection, biphasic isophane insulin (human, crb), 25% soluble, 75% isophane, 100 units/mL, net price 5-mL vial = £5.31; 5 × 3-mL cartridge (for *OptiPen® Pro* NHS) = £21.30; 5 × 3-mL *Insuman® Comb 25 OptiSet®* prefilled disposable injection devices (range 2–40 units, allowing 2-unit dosage adjustment) = £25.37

Insuman® Comb 50 (Aventis Pharma) PoM
Injection, biphasic isophane insulin (human, crb), 50% soluble, 50% isophane, 100 units/mL, net price 5-mL vial = £5.31; 5 × 3-mL cartridge (for *OptiPen® Pro* NHS) = £21.30; 5 × 3-mL *Insuman® Comb 50 OptiSet®* prefilled disposable injection devices (range 2–40 units, allowing 2-unit dosage adjustment) = £25.37

6.1.1.3 Hypodermic equipment

Patients should be advised on the safe disposal of lancets, single-use syringes, and needles. Suitable arrangements for the safe disposal of contaminated waste must be made before these products are prescribed for patients who are carriers of infectious diseases.

■ Injection devices

Autopen® (Owen Mumford)
Injection device; *Autopen® 1.5 mL* (for use with CP, Lilly and Novo Nordisk 1.5-mL insulin cartridges), allows adjustment of dosage in multiples of 1 unit, max. 16 units (single-unit version) *or* 2 units, max. 32 units (2-unit version), net price (both) = £14.20; *Autopen® 3 mL* and *Autopen® Junior* (for use with Lilly 3-mL insulin cartridges), allows adjustment of dosage in multiples of 1 unit, max. 21 units (single-unit version) *or* 2 units, max. 42 units (2-unit version), net price (both) = £14.20

HumaPen® (Lilly) NHS
Injection device for use with *Humulin®* and *Humalog®* 3-mL cartridges; allows adjustment of dosage in multiples of 1 unit, max. 60 units (available free of charge from Lilly)

Innovo® (Novo Nordisk)
Injection device for use with 3-mL *Penfill®* insulin cartridges; allows adjustment of dosage in multiples of 1 unit, max. 70 units, net price = £25.00 (available in green or orange)

NovoPen® (Novo Nordisk)
Injection device for use with *Penfill®* insulin cartridges; *NovoPen® 3 Demi* or *NovoPen® Junior* (for 3-mL cartridges), allows adjustment of dosage in multiples of 0.5 units, max. 35 units, net price = £22.39; *NovoPen® 3 Classic* or *Fun* (for 3-mL cartridges), allows adjustment of dosage in multiples of 1 unit, max. 70 units, net price = £22.39

OptiPen® Pro (Aventis Pharma) NHS
Injection device for use with *Insuman®* insulin cartridges; allows adjustment of dosage in multiples of 1 unit, max. 60 units (available free of charge from Aventis and clinics)

■ Lancets—sterile, single use

Type A (Drug Tariff). Cylindrical mount fluted longitudinally; compatible with *B-D Lancer®* NHS (Becton Dickinson), *Glucolet®* NHS (Bayer Diagnostics), *Monojector®* NHS (Tyco), *Penlet®* II NHS (Lifescan) and *Soft Touch®* NHS (Roche Diagnostics) finger-pricking devices
Available from Bayer *Microlet®*, net price 100-lancet pack = £3.31, 200-lancet pack = £6.31), Becton Dickinson (*B-D Microfine®* +, net price 200-lancet pack = £6.13), Entaco (*Milward® Steri-Let*, 0.66 mm/23-gauge, net price 100-lancet pack = £3.00, 200-lancet pack = £5.70; 0.36 mm/28-gauge, net price 100-lancet pack = £3.00, 200-lancet pack = £5.70), LifeScan (*Finepoint®*, net price 100-lancet pack = £3.30, Menarini (*GlucoTip® Fine*, net price 100-lancet pack = £3.17), Owen Mum-

ford (*Unilet General Purpose*®, 0.81 mm/21-gauge, net price 100-lancet pack = £3.30; 200-lancet pack = £6.27; 0.38 mm/28-gauge, net price 100-lancet pack = £3.19, 200-lancet pack = £6.13; *Unilet General Purpose*® *Superlite*, net price 100-lancet pack = £3.28; 200-lancet pack = £6.22; *Unilet*® *Universal ComforTouch*, net price 100-lancet pack = £3.28; 200-lancet pack = £6.22), Tyco (*Monolet*®, net price 100-lancet pack = £3.28; 200-lancet pack = £6.24; *Monolet Extra*®, net price 100-lancet pack = £3.28), Vitrex Medical (*Vitrex Soft*®, 0.65 mm/23-gauge, net price 100-lancet pack = £3.00, 200-lancet pack = £5.70; 0.36 mm/28-gauge, net price 100-lancet pack = £3.19, 200-lancet pack = £6.13), Zygo Medica (*Cleanlet*® *25*, net price 100-lancet pack = £3.19, 200-lancet pack = £6.08; *Cleanlet*® *Fine*, net price 100-lancet pack = £3.19, 200-lancet pack = £6.13).

Type B (Drug Tariff). Cylindrical mount with concentric ribs; compatible with *Autolet*® ᴺᴴˢ (Owen Mumford) and *Glucolet*® ᴺᴴˢ (Bayer Diagnostics) finger-pricking device

Available from Bayer Diagnostics (*Ames*®, net price 100-lancet pack = £3.31; 200-lancet pack = £6.31), Owen Mumford (*Unilet*® *Superlite*, net price 100-lancet pack = £3.28; 200-lancet pack = £6.22; *Unilet*® *Universal ComferTouch*, net price 100-lancet pack = £3.28; 200-lancet pack = £6.22), Zygo Medica (*Cleanlet*® *25XL*, net price 100-lancet pack = £3.19; 200-lancet pack = £6.08)

Type C (Drug Tariff). Device specific; compatible with *Softclix*® ᴺᴴˢ (Roche Diagnostics) finger-pricking device

Available from Roche Diagnostics (*Softclix*®, net price 200-lancet pack = £6.45).

◼ Needles

Hypodermic Needle , Sterile single use (Drug Tariff). For use with reusable glass syringe, sizes 0.5 mm (25G), 0.45 mm (26G), 0.4 mm (27G). Net price 100-needle pack = £2.36

Available from Becton Dickinson (*Microlance*®), Tyco (*Monoject*®)

Needles for Prefilled and Reusable Pen Injectors (Drug Tariff). Screw on, needle length 6.1 mm or less, net price 100-needle pack = £11.30; 6.2–9.9 mm, 100-needle pack = £8.01; 10 mm or more, 100-needle pack = £8.01

Available from Becton Dickinson (*BD Microfine*®+), Exelint, Novo Nordisk (*NovoFine*®), Owen Mumford (*Unifine*® *Pentips*)

Snap on, needle length 6.1 mm or less, net price 100-needle pack = £11.06; 6.2–9.9 mm, 100-needle pack = £7.84; 10 mm or more, 100-needle pack = £7.84

Available from Disotronic (*Penfine*®)

Needle Clipping (Chopping) Device (Drug Tariff). Consisting of a clipper to remove needle from its hub and container from which cut-off needles cannot be retrieved; designed to hold 1200 needles, not suitable for use with lancets. Net price = £1.16

Available from Becton Dickinson (*B-D Safe-clip*®)

◼ Syringes

Hypodermic Syringe (Drug Tariff). Calibrated glass with Luer taper conical fitting, for use with U100 insulin. Net price 0.5 mL and 1 mL = £14.19

Available from Rand Rocket (*Abcare*®)

Pre-Set U100 Insulin Syringe (Drug Tariff). Calibrated glass with Luer taper conical fitting, supplied with dosage chart and strong box, for blind patients. Net price 1 mL = £21.61

Available from Rand Rocket

U100 Insulin Syringe with Needle (Drug Tariff). Disposable with fixed or separate needle for single use or single patient-use, colour coded orange. Needle length 8 mm, diameters 0.33 mm (29G), 0.3 mm (30G), net price 10 (with needle), 0.3 mL = £1.19, 0.5 mL = £1.15; needle length 12 mm, diameters 0.45 mm (26G), 0.4 mm (27G), 0.36 mm (28G), 0.33 mm (29G), net price 10 (with needle), 0.3 mL = £1.28; 0.5 mL = £1.24; 1 mL = £1.25

Available from Becton Dickinson (*B-D Micro-Fine*®+, *Plastipak*®), Braun (*Omnikan*®), Codan (*Insupak*®),

Exelint, Owen Mumford (*Unifine*®), Rand Rocket (*Clinipak*®), Tyco (*Monoject*® *Ultra*)

Oral antidiabetic drugs are used for the treatment of type 2 (non-insulin-dependent) diabetes mellitus. They should be prescribed only if the patient fails to respond adequately to at least 3 months' restriction of energy and carbohydrate intake and an increase in physical activity. They should be used to augment the effect of diet and exercise, and not to replace them. For patients not adequately controlled by diet and oral hypoglycaemic drugs, insulin may be added to the treatment regimen or substituted for oral therapy; weight gain and hypoglycaemia may be complications of insulin therapy.

6.1.2.1   Sulphonylureas

The sulphonylureas act mainly by augmenting insulin secretion and consequently are effective only when some residual pancreatic beta-cell activity is present; during long-term administration they also have an extrapancreatic action. All may cause hypoglycaemia but this is uncommon and usually indicates excessive dosage. Sulphonylurea-induced hypoglycaemia may persist for many hours and must always be treated in hospital.

Several sulphonylureas are available and choice is determined by side-effects and the duration of action as well as the patient's age and renal function. The long-acting sulphonylureas **chlorpropamide** and **glibenclamide** are associated with a greater risk of hypoglycaemia; for this reason they should be avoided in the elderly and shorter-acting alternatives, such as **gliclazide** or **tolbutamide**, should be used instead. Chlorpropamide also has more side-effects than the other sulphonylureas (see below) and therefore it is no longer recommended.

CAUTIONS. Sulphonylureas can encourage weight gain and should be prescribed only if poor control and symptoms persist despite adequate attempts at dieting; metformin (section 6.1.2.2) is considered the drug of choice in obese patients. Caution is needed in the elderly and in those with mild to moderate hepatic (Appendix 2) and renal impairment (Appendix 3) because of the hazard of hypoglycaemia. The short-acting tolbutamide may be used in renal impairment, as may gliquidone and gliclazide which are principally metabolised in the liver, but careful monitoring of blood-glucose concentration is essential; care is required to choose the smallest possible dose that produces adequate control of blood glucose.

CONTRA-INDICATIONS. Sulphonylureas should be avoided where possible in severe hepatic (Appendix 2) and renal (Appendix 3) impairment and in porphyria (section 9.8.2). They should not be used while breast-feeding and insulin therapy should be substituted during pregnancy (see also Appendix 4).

Insulin therapy should also be instituted temporarily during intercurrent illness (such as myocardial infarction, coma, infection, and trauma). Oral antidiabetic drugs should be omitted on the morning of surgery; insulin is often required because of the ensuing hyperglycaemia in these circumstances. Sulphonylureas are contra-indicated in the presence of ketoacidosis.

SIDE-EFFECTS. Side-effects of sulphonylureas are generally mild and infrequent and include gastrointestinal disturbances such as nausea, vomiting, diarrhoea and constipation.

Chlorpropamide has appreciably more sideeffects, mainly because of its very prolonged duration of action and the consequent hazard of hypoglycaemia and it should generally no longer be used. It may also cause facial flushing after drinking alcohol; this effect does not normally occur with other sulphonylureas. Chlorpropamide may also enhance antidiuretic hormone secretion and very rarely cause hyponatraemia (hyponatraemia is also reported with glimepiride and glipizide).

Sulphonylureas can occasionally cause a disturbance in liver function, which may rarely lead to cholestatic jaundice, hepatitis and hepatic failure. Hypersensitivity reactions can occur, usually in the first 6–8 weeks of therapy, they consist mainly of allergic skin reactions which progress rarely to erythema multiforme and exfoliative dermatitis, fever and jaundice; photosensitivity has rarely been reported with chlorpropamide and glipizide. Blood disorders are also rare but may include leucopenia, thrombocytopenia, agranulocytosis, pancytopenia, haemolytic anaemia, and aplastic anaemia.

CHLORPROPAMIDE ▨

Indications: type 2 diabetes mellitus (for use in diabetes insipidus, see section 6.5.2)

Cautions: see notes above; **interactions:** Appendix 1 (antidiabetics)

Contra-indications: see notes above

Side-effects: see notes above

Dose: initially 250 mg daily with breakfast (ELDERLY 100–125 mg but avoid—see notes above), adjusted according to response; max. 500 mg daily

Chlorpropamide (Non-proprietary) PoM ▨
Tablets, chlorpropamide 100 mg, net price 20 = £1.70; 250 mg, 20 = £2.00. Label: 4
Available from Sussex

▨ denotes preparations that are considered to be less suitable for prescribing (see p. vi)

GLIBENCLAMIDE

Indications: type 2 diabetes mellitus

Cautions: see notes above; **interactions:** Appendix 1 (antidiabetics)

Contra-indications: see notes above

Side-effects: see notes above

Dose: initially 5 mg daily with or immediately after breakfast (ELDERLY 2.5 mg, but avoid—see notes above), adjusted according to response; max. 15 mg daily

Glibenclamide (Non-proprietary) PoM
Tablets, glibenclamide 2.5 mg, net price 28-tab pack = 96p; 5 mg, 28 = £1.21
Available from Alpharma, APS, Ashbourne (*Diabetamide*®), CP, Generics, Hillcross, IVAX, Kent (*Gliken*®)

Daonil® (Hoechst Marion Roussel) PoM
Tablets, scored, glibenclamide 5 mg. Net price 28-tab pack = £2.63

Semi-Daonil® (Hoechst Marion Roussel) PoM
Tablets, scored, glibenclamide 2.5 mg. Net price 28-tab pack = £1.58

Euglucon® (Aventis Pharma) PoM
Tablets, glibenclamide 2.5 mg, net price 28-tab pack = £1.58; 5 mg (scored), 28-tab pack = £2.63

GLICLAZIDE

Indications: type 2 diabetes mellitus

Cautions: see notes above; **interactions:** Appendix 1 (antidiabetics)

Contra-indications: see notes above

Side-effects: see notes above

Dose: initially, 40–80 mg daily, adjusted according to response; up to 160 mg as a single dose, with breakfast; higher doses divided; max. 320 mg daily

Gliclazide (Non-proprietary) PoM
Tablets, scored, gliclazide 80 mg, net price 28-tab pack = £2.59, 60-tab pack = £6.35
Available from Alpharma, APS, Dominion, Generics (*DIAGLYK*®), Genus, Hillcross, IVAX

Diamicron® (Servier) PoM
Tablets, scored, gliclazide 80 mg, net price 60-tab pack = £7.00

■ Modified release

Diamicron® **MR** (Servier) PoM
Tablets, m/r, scored, gliclazide 30 mg, net price 28-tab pack = £3.76, 56-tab pack = £7.51, 84-tab pack = £11.27, 112-tab pack = £15.02
Dose: initially 30 mg daily with breakfast, adjusted according to response every 4 weeks (after 2 weeks if no decrease in blood glucose); max. 120 mg daily
Note. Diamicron® *MR* 30 mg may be considered to be approximately equivalent in therapeutic effect to standard formulation *Diamicron*® 80 mg

GLIMEPIRIDE

Indications: type 2 diabetes mellitus

Cautions: see notes above; manufacturer recommends regular hepatic and haematological monitoring but limited evidence of clinical value; **interactions:** Appendix 1 (antidiabetics)

Contra-indications: see notes above

Side-effects: see notes above

Dose: initially 1 mg daily, adjusted according to response in 1-mg steps at 1–2 week intervals; usual max. 4 mg daily (exceptionally, up to 6 mg daily may be used); taken shortly before or with first main meal

Amaryl® (Hoechst Marion Roussel) PoM
Tablets, all scored, glimepiride 1 mg (pink), net price 30-tab pack = £4.90; 2 mg (green), 30-tab pack = £8.05; 3 mg (yellow), 30-tab pack = £12.15; 4 mg (blue), 30-tab pack = £16.10

GLIPIZIDE

Indications: type 2 diabetes mellitus
Cautions: see notes above; **interactions:** Appendix 1 (antidiabetics)
Contra-indications: see notes above
Side-effects: see notes above; also dizziness, drowsiness
Dose: initially 2.5–5 mg daily, adjusted according to response; max. 20 mg daily; up to 15 mg may be given as a single dose before breakfast; higher doses divided

Glipizide (Non-proprietary) PoM
Tablets, glipizide 2.5 mg, net price 28-tab pack = £1.48; 5 mg, 56-tab pack = £4.53
Available from Alpharma, Hillcross, IVAX

Glibenese® (Pfizer) PoM
Tablets, scored, glipizide 5 mg. Net price 56-tab pack = £3.63

Minodiab® (Pharmacia) PoM
Tablets, glipizide 2.5 mg, net price 28-tab pack = £1.48; 5 mg (scored), 28-tab pack = £1.26

GLIQUIDONE

Indications: type 2 diabetes mellitus
Cautions: see notes above; **interactions:** Appendix 1 (antidiabetics)
Contra-indications: see notes above
Side-effects: see notes above
Dose: initially 15 mg daily before breakfast, adjusted to 45–60 mg daily in 2 or 3 divided doses; max. single dose 60 mg, max. daily dose 180 mg

Glurenorm® (Sanofi-Synthelabo) PoM
Tablets, scored, gliquidone 30 mg. Net price 100-tab pack = £17.54

TOLBUTAMIDE

Indications: type 2 diabetes mellitus
Cautions: see notes above; **interactions:** Appendix 1 (antidiabetics)
Contra-indications: see notes above
Side-effects: see notes above; also headache, tinnitus
Dose: 0.5–1.5 g (max. 2 g) daily in divided doses (see notes above); with or immediately after breakfast

Tolbutamide (Non-proprietary) PoM
Tablets, tolbutamide 500 mg. Net price 20 = £1.10
Available from Alpharma, APS, Hillcross

6.1.2.2   Biguanides

Metformin, the only available biguanide, has a different mode of action from the sulphonylureas, and is not interchangeable with them. It exerts its effect mainly by decreasing gluconeogenesis and by increasing peripheral utilisation of glucose; since it acts only in the presence of endogenous insulin it is effective only in diabetics with some residual functioning pancreatic islet cells.

Metformin is the drug of first choice in obese patients in whom strict dieting has failed to control diabetes. It is also used when diabetes is inade-

quately controlled with sulphonylurea treatment. When the combination of strict diet and metformin treatment fails other options which may be considered include:

- combining with acarbose (section 6.1.2.3), which may have a small beneficial effect, but flatulence can be a problem;
- combining with insulin (section 6.1.1) but weight gain and hypoglycaemia can be problems;
- combining with a sulphonylurea (section 6.1.2.1) (reports of increased hazard with this combination are at present unconfirmed);
- combining with pioglitazone or rosiglitazone (section 6.1.2.3).

Repaglinide or nateglinide (section 6.1.2.3) may be given with metformin if metformin alone does not control the diabetes adequately.

Insulin treatment is almost always required in medical and surgical emergencies; insulin should also be substituted before elective surgery (omit metformin on morning of surgery and give insulin if required).

Hypoglycaemia is not a problem with metformin; other advantages are the lower incidence of weight gain and lower plasma-insulin concentration. It does not exert a hypoglycaemic action in non-diabetic subjects unless given in overdose.

Gastro-intestinal side-effects are initially common with metformin, and may persist in some patients, particularly when very high doses such as 3 g daily are given.

Metformin may provoke lactic acidosis which is most likely to occur in patients with renal impairment; it should not be used in patients with even mild renal impairment. Metformin should also be avoided (or discontinued) in other situations which might predispose to lactic acidosis, e.g. severe dehydration, infection, shock, heart failure, respiratory failure, recent myocardial infarction, severe peripheral vascular disease, hepatic impairment, alcohol dependency, use of x-ray contrast media (do not restart metformin until renal function returns to normal), pregnancy and breast-feeding.

METFORMIN HYDROCHLORIDE

Indications: diabetes mellitus (see notes above)
Cautions: see notes above; **interactions:** Appendix 1 (antidiabetics)
Contra-indications: hepatic or renal impairment (withdraw if renal impairment suspected), keto-acidosis, predisposition to lactic acidosis—see notes above, heart failure, severe infection or trauma, dehydration, alcohol dependence; pregnancy, breast-feeding
Side-effects: anorexia, nausea, vomiting, diarrhoea (usually transient), abdominal pain, metallic taste; rarely lactic acidosis (withdraw treatment), decreased vitamin-B_{12} absorption
Dose: initially 500 mg with breakfast for 1 week then 500 mg with breakfast and evening meal for 1 week then 500 mg with breakfast, lunch and evening meal; max. 3 g daily in divided doses but most physicians limit this to 2 g daily (see notes above)

Note. Metformin doses in the BNF may differ from those in the product literature

Metformin (Non-proprietary) PoM

Tablets, coated, metformin hydrochloride 500 mg, net price 28 = 74p, 84 = £2.15; 850 mg, 56-tab pack = £2.29. Label: 21

Available from Alpharma, APS, CP, Generics, Hillcross, IVAX, Opus (*Glucamet*®), Sovereign, Sterwin, Taro

Glucophage® (Merck) PoM

Tablets, f/c, metformin hydrochloride 500 mg, net price 84-tab pack = £2.07; 850 mg, 56-tab pack = £2.28. Label: 21

6.1.2.3   Other antidiabetics

Acarbose, an inhibitor of intestinal alpha glucosidases, delays the digestion and absorption of starch and sucrose. It has a small but significant effect in lowering blood glucose and is used either on its own or as an adjunct to metformin or to sulphonylureas when they prove inadequate. Postprandial hyperglycaemia in type 1 (insulin-dependent) diabetes can be reduced by acarbose, but it has been little used for this purpose. Flatulence deters some from using acarbose although this side-effect tends to decrease with time.

Guar gum, if taken in adequate quantities, results in some reduction of postprandial plasma-glucose concentrations in diabetes mellitus, probably by retarding carbohydrate absorption. It is also used to relieve symptoms of the dumping syndrome.

Nateglinide and **repaglinide** stimulate insulin release. Both drugs have a rapid onset of action and short duration of activity, and should be administered shortly before each main meal. Repaglinide is licensed for use in type 2 diabetes either as monotherapy or in combination with metformin; nateglinide is licensed only for use with metformin.

The thiazolidinediones, **pioglitazone** and **rosiglitazone**, reduce peripheral insulin resistance, leading to a reduction of blood-glucose concentration. They should be initiated only by a physician experienced in treating type 2 diabetes and should always be used in combination with metformin or with a sulphonylurea (if metformin inappropriate). Inadequate response to a combination of metformin and sulphonylurea may indicate failing insulin release; the introduction of pioglitazone or rosiglitazone has a limited role in these circumstances and insulin treatment should not be delayed. Long-term benefits of the thiazolidinediones have not yet been demonstrated.

NICE guidance (pioglitazone and rosiglitazone for type 2 diabetes mellitus). The National Institute for Clinical Excellence has recommended that patients who are unable to take metformin and sulphonylurea combination therapy, or those whose blood-glucose concentration remains high despite an adequate trial of this treatment, should be offered thiazolidinedione (pioglitazone *or* rosiglitazone) combination therapy as an alternative to insulin [but see notes above]. The combination of a thiazolidinedione plus metformin is preferred to a thiazolidinedione plus sulphonylurea, particularly for obese patients.

ACARBOSE

Indications: diabetes mellitus inadequately controlled by diet or by diet with oral hypoglycaemic agents

Cautions: monitor hepatic transaminase levels (higher doses); may enhance hypoglycaemic effects of insulin and sulphonylureas (hypoglycaemic episodes may be treated with oral glucose but not with sucrose); **interactions:** Appendix 1 (antidiabetics)

Contra-indications: pregnancy and breast-feeding; inflammatory bowel disease (e.g. ulcerative colitis, Crohn's disease), partial intestinal obstruction (or predisposition); hepatic impairment, severe renal impairment; hernia, history of abdominal surgery

Side-effects: flatulence, soft stools, diarrhoea (may need to reduce dose or withdraw), abdominal distention and pain; rarely abnormal liver function tests and skin reactions; ileus, oedema, jaundice and hepatitis reported
Note. Antacids not recommended for treating side-effects (unlikely to be beneficial)

Dose: 50 mg daily initially (to minimise side-effects) increased to 50 mg 3 times daily, then increased if necessary after 6–8 weeks to 100 mg 3 times daily; max. 200 mg 3 times daily; CHILD under 12 years not recommended

COUNSELLING. The tablets should either be chewed with first mouthful of food or swallowed whole with a little liquid immediately before food. In order to counteract possible hypoglycaemia, patients receiving insulin or a sulphonylurea as well as acarbose need to carry glucose (not sucrose—acarbose interferes with sucrose absorption)

Glucobay® (Bayer) PoM

Tablets, acarbose 50 mg, net price 90-tab pack = £9.68; 100 mg (scored). 90-tab pack = £12.51. Counselling, administration

---

GUAR GUM

Indications: see notes above

Cautions: maintain adequate fluid intake; **interactions:** Appendix 1 (guar gum)

COUNSELLING. Preparations that swell in contact with liquid should always be carefully swallowed with water and should not be taken immediately before going to bed.

Contra-indications: gastro-intestinal obstruction, oesophageal disease, dysphagia

Side-effects: flatulence, diarrhoea, abdominal distension, intestinal obstruction

Dose: 5 g 3 times daily with main meals (either stirred into 200 mL fluid or sprinkled on food and eaten accompanied by 200 mL fluid); CHILD under 12 years not recommended

Guarem® (Rybar)

Granules, ivory, sugar-free, guar gum 5 g/sachet, net price 50 sachets = £8.70; 100 sachets = £15.67. Label: 13, counselling, administration

---

NATEGLINIDE

Indications: type 2 diabetes mellitus in combination with metformin when metformin alone inadequate

Cautions: substitute insulin during intercurrent illness (such as myocardial infarction, coma, infection, and trauma) and during surgery; debilitated and malnourished patients; moderate hepatic impairment (avoid if severe—Appendix 2); **interactions:** Appendix 1 (nateglinide)

Contra-indications: diabetic ketoacidosis; pregnancy (Appendix 4) and breast-feeding (Appendix 5)

Side-effects: hypoglycaemia; hypersensitivity reactions including pruritus, rashes and urticaria

Dose: initially 60 mg 3 times daily within 30 minutes before main meals, adjusted according to response up to max. 180 mg 3 times daily; CHILD and ADOLESCENT under 18 years not recommended

Starlix® (Novartis) ▼ PoM
Tablets, f/c, nateglinide 60 mg (pink), net price 84-tab pack = £19.75; 120 mg (yellow), 84-tab pack = £22.50; 180 mg (red), 84-tab pack = £22.50

PIOGLITAZONE

Indications: see notes above

Cautions: monitor liver function (see below); cardiovascular disease (risk of heart failure)

LIVER TOXICITY. Rare reports of liver dysfunction; monitor liver function before treatment, then every 2 months for 12 months and periodically thereafter; advise patients to seek immediate medical attention if symptoms such as nausea, vomiting, abdominal pain, fatigue and dark urine develop; discontinue if jaundice occurs; **interactions:** Appendix 1 (antidiabetics)

Contra-indications: hepatic impairment, history of heart failure, combination with insulin (risk of heart failure), pregnancy (Appendix 4), breast-feeding (Appendix 5)

Side-effects: gastro-intestinal disturbances, weight gain, oedema, anaemia, headache, visual disturbances, dizziness, arthralgia, haematuria, impotence; less commonly hypoglycaemia, fatigue, sweating, altered blood lipids, proteinuria

Dose: 15–30 mg once daily

Actos® (Takeda) ▼ PoM
Tablets, pioglitazone (as hydrochloride) 15 mg, net price 28-tab pack = £26.60; 30 mg, 28-tab pack = £36.96

REPAGLINIDE

Indications: type 2 diabetes mellitus (as monotherapy or in combination with metformin when metformin alone inadequate)

Cautions: substitute insulin during intercurrent illness (such as myocardial infarction, coma, infection, and trauma) and during surgery; debilitated and malnourished patients; renal impairment; **interactions:** Appendix 1 (repaglinide)

Contra-indications: diabetic ketoacidosis; severe hepatic impairment; pregnancy (Appendix 4) and breast-feeding

Side-effects: abdominal pain, diarrhoea, constipation, nausea, vomiting; hypoglycaemia, hypersensitivity reactions including pruritus, rashes and urticaria

Dose: initially 500 micrograms within 30 minutes before main meals (1 mg if transferring from another oral hypoglycaemic), adjusted according to response at intervals of 1–2 weeks; up to 4 mg may be given as a single dose, max. 16 mg daily

CHILD and ADOLESCENT under 18 years and ELDERLY over 75 years, not recommended

NovoNorm® (Novo Nordisk) ▼ PoM
Tablets, repaglinide 500 micrograms, net price 30-tab pack = £5.86, 90-tab pack = £17.57; 1 mg (yellow), 30-tab pack = £6.33, 90-tab pack = £18.98; 2 mg (peach), 90-tab pack = £20.40

ROSIGLITAZONE

Indications: see notes above

Cautions: monitor liver function (see below); cardiovascular disease (risk of heart failure), renal impairment (avoid if severe); **interactions:** Appendix 1 (rosiglitazone)

LIVER TOXICITY. Rare reports of liver dysfunction reported; monitor liver function before treatment, then every 2 months for 12 months and periodically thereafter; advise patients to seek immediate medical attention if symptoms such as nausea, vomiting, abdominal pain, fatigue and dark urine develop; discontinue if jaundice occurs

Contra-indications: hepatic impairment, history of heart failure, combination with insulin (risk of heart failure), pregnancy (Appendix 4), breast-feeding (Appendix 5)

Side-effects: gastro-intestinal disturbances, headache, anaemia, fatigue, weight gain, oedema, hypoglycaemia; less commonly dizziness, drowsiness, paraesthesia, rash, alopecia, dyspnoea, altered blood lipids, thrombocytopenia; rarely pulmonary oedema

Dose: (in combination with metformin or a sulphonylurea) 4 mg daily; in combination with metformin may increase to 8 mg daily (in 1 or 2 divided doses) after 8 weeks according to response

Avandia® (SmithKline Beecham) ▼ PoM
Tablets, f/c, rosiglitazone (as maleate) 4 mg (orange), net price 28-tab pack = £26.60, 56-tab pack = £53.20; 8 mg (red/brown), 28-tab pack = £54.60.

6.1.3   Diabetic ketoacidosis

Soluble insulin, the only form of insulin that may be given intravenously, is used in the management of diabetic ketoacidotic and hyperosmolar non-ketotic coma. It is preferable to use the type of soluble insulin that the patient has been using previously. It is necessary to achieve and to maintain an adequate plasma-insulin concentration until the metabolic disturbance is brought under control.

Insulin is best given by intravenous infusion, using an infusion pump, and diluted to 1 unit/mL (care in mixing, see Appendix 6). Adequate plasma-insulin concentration can usually be maintained with infusion rates of 6 units/hour for adults and 0.1 units/kg/hour for children. Blood glucose is expected to decrease by about 5 mmol/litre/hour; if the response is inadequate the infusion rate can be doubled or quadrupled. When the plasma glucose has fallen to 10 mmol/litre the infusion rate can be reduced to 3 units/hour for adults (about 0.02 units/kg/hour for children) and continued until the patient is ready to take food by mouth. The insulin infusion should not be stopped before subcutaneous insulin has been started.

No matter how large, a bolus intravenous injection of insulin can provide an adequate plasma concentration for a short time only; therefore if facilities for intravenous infusion are not available the insulin is given by *intramuscular injection*. An initial loading dose of 20 units intramuscularly is followed by 6 units intramuscularly every hour until the plasma-glucose concentration falls to 10 mmol/litre; intramuscular injections are then given every 2 hours. Although absorption of insulin is usually rapid after intramuscular injection, it may be impaired in the presence of hypotension and poor tissue perfusion; moreover insulin may accumulate during treatment and late hypoglycaemia should be watched for and treated appropriately.

Intravenous replacement of fluid and electrolytes (section 9.2.2) with **sodium chloride** intravenous infusion is an essential part of the management of ketoacidosis; **potassium chloride** is included in the infusion as appropriate to prevent the hypokalaemia induced by the insulin. **Sodium bicarbonate** infusion (1.26% or 2.74%) is used only in cases of extreme acidosis and shock since the acid-base disturbance is normally corrected by the insulin. **Glucose** solution (5%) is infused once the blood glucose has decreased below 10 mmol/litre but insulin infusion must continue.

| 6.1.4 | **Treatment of hypoglycaemia** |

Initially glucose 10–20 g is given by mouth either in liquid form or as granulated sugar or sugar lumps. Glucose 10 g is available from 2 teaspoons sugar, 3 sugar lumps, *Hypostop® Gel* (glucose 10 g/23-g oral ampoule, available from Bio Diagnostics), milk 200 mL, and non-diet versions of *Lucozade® Sparkling Glucose Drink* 50–55 mL, *Coca-Cola®* 90 mL, *Ribena® Original* 15 mL (to be diluted). If necessary this may be repeated in 10–15 minutes.

Hypoglycaemia which causes unconsciousness is an emergency. **Glucagon** can be given for acute insulin-induced hypoglycaemia; it is not appropriate for chronic hypoglycaemia. It is a polypeptide hormone produced by the alpha cells of the islets of Langerhans. It increases plasma-glucose concentration by mobilising glycogen stored in the liver. It can be injected by any route (intramuscular, subcutaneous, or intravenous) in a dose of 1 mg (1 unit) in circumstances when an intravenous injection of glucose would be difficult or impossible to administer. It may be issued to close relatives of insulin-treated patients for emergency use in hypoglycaemic attacks. It is often advisable to prescribe on an 'if necessary' basis to hospitalised insulin-treated patients, so that it may be given rapidly by the nurses during an hypoglycaemic emergency. If not effective in 10 minutes intravenous glucose should be given.

Alternatively, 50 mL of **glucose intravenous infusion 20%** (section 9.2.2) may be given intravenously into a large vein through a large-gauge needle; care is required since this concentration is irritant especially if extravasation occurs. Alternatively, 25 mL of glucose intravenous infusion 50% may be given, but this higher concentration is more irritant and viscous making administration difficult. Glucose intravenous infusion 10% may also be used but larger volumes are needed. Close monitor-

ing is necessary in the case of an overdose with a long-acting insulin because further administration of glucose may be required. Patients whose hypoglycaemia is caused by an oral antidiabetic drug should be transferred to hospital because the hypoglycaemic effects of these drugs may persist for many hours.

GLUCAGON

Indications: see notes above and under Dose

Cautions: see notes above, insulinoma, glucagonoma; ineffective in chronic hypoglycaemia, starvation, and adrenal insufficiency

Contra-indications: phaeochromocytoma

Side-effects: nausea, vomiting, diarrhoea, hypokalaemia, rarely hypersensitivity reactions

Dose: *by subcutaneous, intramuscular, or intravenous injection*, ADULT and CHILD over 8 years (or body-weight over 25 kg), 1 mg; CHILD under 8 years (or body-weight under 25 kg), 500 micrograms; if no response within 10 minutes intravenous glucose must be given

Diagnostic aid, consult product literature

Beta-blocker poisoning, see p. 25

Note. 1 unit of glucagon = 1 mg of glucagon

GlucaGen® HypoKit (Novo Nordisk) PoM
Injection, powder for reconstitution, glucagon (rys) as hydrochloride with lactose, net price 1-mg vial with prefilled syringe containing water for injection = £19.95

Chronic hypoglycaemia

Diazoxide, administered by mouth, is useful in the management of patients with chronic hypoglycaemia from excess endogenous insulin secretion, either from an islet cell tumour or islet cell hyperplasia. It has no place in the management of acute hypoglycaemia.

DIAZOXIDE

Indications: chronic intractable hypoglycaemia (for use in hypertensive crisis see section 2.5.1)

Cautions: ischaemic heart disease, pregnancy, labour, impaired renal function; haematological examinations and blood pressure monitoring required during prolonged treatment; growth, bone, and developmental checks in children; **interactions:** Appendix 1 (diazoxide)

Side-effects: anorexia, nausea, vomiting, hyperuricaemia, hypotension, oedema, tachycardia, arrhythmias, extrapyramidal effects; hypertrichosis on prolonged treatment

Dose: *by mouth*, ADULT and CHILD, initially 5 mg/kg daily in 2–3 divided doses

Eudemine® (Celltech) PoM
Tablets, diazoxide 50 mg. Net price 20 = £7.68

6.1.5 Treatment of diabetic nephropathy and neuropathy

Diabetic nephropathy

Regular review of diabetic patients should include an annual test for urinary protein (using *Albustix®*). If this test is negative, the urine should be tested for microalbuminuria (the earliest sign of nephropathy). If reagent strip tests (*Micral-Test®* [NHS]) are used and prove positive, the result should be confirmed by a laboratory analysis of urine sample. All diabetic patients with nephropathy causing albuminuria and all insulin-dependent patients with established microalbuminuria (at least 3 positive tests) should be treated with an ACE inhibitor (section 2.5.5.1) or an angiotensin-II antagonist (section 2.5.5.2) [unlicensed indication] even if the blood pressure is normal; in any case, to minimise the risk of renal deterioration, blood pressure should be carefully controlled (section 2.5).

ACE inhibitors may potentiate the hypoglycaemic effect of insulin and oral antidiabetic drugs; this effect is more likely during the first weeks of combined treatment and in patients with renal impairment.

For the treatment of hypertension in diabetes, see section 2.5.

Diabetic neuropathy

Optimal diabetic control is beneficial for the management of *painful neuropathy* in patients with type 1 diabetes (see also section 4.7.3). **Paracetamol** or a **non-steroidal anti-inflammatory drug** such as ibuprofen (section 10.1.1) may relieve *mild to moderate pain*.

The **tricyclic antidepressants** amitriptyline and nortriptyline (section 4.3.1) are the drugs of choice for painful diabetic neuropathy [unlicensed use]; amitriptyline is given in a dose of 25–75 mg daily (higher doses under specialist supervision). Other classes of antidepressants do not appear to be effective. **Gabapentin** (section 4.8.1) is licensed for the treatment of neuropathic pain and is an effective alternative to a tricyclic antidepressant.

Carbamazepine and **phenytoin** [both unlicensed] (section 4.8.1) may be useful for shooting or stabbing pain, but adverse effects are common; carbamazepine 200–800 mg daily in divided doses has been used.

Capsaicin cream 0.075% (section 10.3.2) is licensed for painful diabetic neuropathy and may have some effect, but it produces an intense burning sensation during the initial treatment period.

Neuropathic pain may respond partially to some **opioid analgesics**, such as dextropropoxyphene, methadone, oxycodone and tramadol, and they may have a role when other treatments have failed.

In *autonomic neuropathy* diabetic diarrhoea can often be managed by 2 or 3 doses of **tetracycline** 250 mg [unlicensed use] (section 5.1.3). Otherwise **codeine phosphate** (section 1.4.2) is the best drug, but other antidiarrhoeal preparations can be tried.

An **antiemetic** which promotes gastric transit, such as metoclopramide or domperidone (section 4.6), is helpful for gastroparesis. In rare cases when an antiemetic does not help, erythromycin (especially when given intravenously) may be beneficial but this needs confirmation.

For the management of erectile dysfunction, see section 7.4.5.

In *neuropathic postural hypotension* increased salt intake and the use of the **mineralocorticoid** fludrocortisone 100 to 400 micrograms daily [unlicensed use] (section 6.3.1) help by increasing plasma volume, but uncomfortable oedema is a common side-effect. Fludrocortisone can also be combined with **flurbiprofen** (section 10.1.1) and **ephedrine hydrochloride** (section 3.1.1.2) [both unlicensed]. **Midodrine** [unlicensed], an alpha agonist, may also be useful in postural hypotension.

Gustatory sweating can be treated with an **antimuscarinic** such as propantheline bromide (section 1.2); side-effects are common. For the management of hyperhidrosis, see section 13.12.

In some patients with *neuropathic oedema*, **ephedrine hydrochloride** [unlicensed use] 30 to 60 mg 3 times daily offers impressive relief.

6.1.6 Diagnostic and monitoring agents for diabetes mellitus

Blood glucose monitoring

Blood glucose monitoring gives a direct measure of the glucose concentration at the time of the test and can detect hypoglycaemia as well as hyperglycaemia. Patients should be properly trained in the use of blood glucose monitoring systems and to take appropriate action on the results obtained. Inadequate understanding of the normal fluctuations in blood glucose may lead to confusion and inappropriate action. It is ideal for patients to observe the 'peaks' and 'troughs' of blood glucose over 24 hours and make adjustments of their insulin no more than once or twice weekly. Daily alterations to the insulin dose are highly undesirable (except during illness).

Blood glucose monitoring is best carried out by means of a meter. Visual colour comparison is sometimes used but is much less satisfactory. Meters give a more precise reading and are useful for patients with poor eyesight or who are colour blind.

Note. In the UK blood-glucose concentration is expressed in mmol/litre and the British Diabetic Association advises that these units should be used for self-monitoring of blood glucose. In other European countries units of mg/100 mL (or mg/dL) are commonly used.

It is advisable to check that the meter is pre-set in the correct units.

■ Test strips
Active® (Roche Diagnostics)
Reagent strips, for blood glucose monitoring, range 0.6–33.3 mmol/litre, for use with *Glucotrend®* [NHS] and *Accu-Chek® Active* [NHS] meters only. Net price 50-strip pack = £15.02

Advantage II® (Roche Diagnostics)
Reagent strips, for blood glucose monitoring, range 0.6–33.3 mmol/litre, for use with *Accu-Chek® Advantage* [NHS] meter only. Net price 50-strip pack = £15.02

BM-Accutest® (Roche Diagnostics)
Reagent strips, for blood glucose monitoring, range 1.1–33.3 mmol/litre, for use with *Accutrend®* [NHS] meters only. Net price 50-strip pack = £14.56

BM-Test 1–44® (Roche Diagnostics)
Reagent strips, for blood glucose monitoring, visual range 1–44 mmol/litre, meter range 0.5–27.7 mmol/litre, suitable for use with *Reflolux® S* [NHS]. Net price 50-strip pack = £15.33

Esprit® Biosensor (Bayer Diagnostics)
Sensor discs, for blood glucose monitoring, range 0.6–33.3 mmol/L, for use with *Esprit®* [NHS] meter only. Net price 5 × 10-disc pack = £14.77

ExacTech® (MediSense)
Biosensor strips, for blood glucose monitoring, range 2.2–25 mmol/litre, for use with *ExacTech®* [NHS] meter only. Net price 50-strip pack = £14.45

GlucoMen® (Menarini Diagnostics)
Sensor strips, for blood glucose monitoring, range 1.1–33.3 mmol/litre, for use with *GlucoMen® Glyco* [NHS] meter only. Net price 50-strip pack = £13.93

Glucostix® (Bayer Diagnostics)
Reagent strips, for blood glucose monitoring, visual range 1–44 mmol/litre, meter range 2–22 mmol/litre, suitable for use with *Glucometer® GX* [NHS]. Net price 50-strip pack = £15.33

Glucotide® (Bayer Diagnostics)
Reagent strips, for blood glucose monitoring, range 0.6–33.3 mmol/litre, for use with *Glucometer® 4* [NHS] meter only. Net price 50-strip pack = £14.58

Hypoguard® Supreme (Hypoguard)
Reagent strips, for blood glucose monitoring, range 2.2–27.7 mmol/litre, for use with all *Hypoguard® Supreme* [NHS] meters. Net price 50-strip pack = £13.41

Hypoguard® Supreme Spectrum (Hypoguard)
Reagent strips, for blood glucose monitoring, visual range 2.2–27.8 mmol/litre. Net price 50-strip pack = £10.16

MediSense G2® (MediSense)
Sensor strips, for blood glucose monitoring, range 1.1–33.3 mmol/litre, for use with *MediSense Card®* [NHS] or *MediSense Pen®* [NHS] meters only. Net price 50-strip pack = £13.89

MediSense® Optium (MediSense)
Sensor strips, for blood glucose monitoring, range 1.1–33.3 mmol/litre, for use with *MediSense® Optium* [NHS] meter only. Net price 50-strip pack = £14.16

Medi-Test® Glycaemie C (BHR)
Reagent strips, for blood glucose monitoring, visual range 1.1–44.4 mmol/litre, meter range 1.1–33.3 mmol/litre, suitable for use with *Glycotronic® C* [NHS] meter. Net price 50-strip pack = £13.44

One Touch® (LifeScan)
Reagent strips, for blood glucose monitoring, range 0–33.3 mmol/litre, for use with *One Touch® II, Profile* and *Basic* [NHS] meters only. Net price 50-strip pack = £14.61

PocketScan® (LifeScan)
Reagent strips, for blood glucose monitoring, range 1.1–33.3 mmol/litre, for use with *PocketScan®* [NHS] meter only. Net price 50-strip pack = £14.42

Prestige® Smart System (DiagnoSys)
Reagent strips, for blood glucose monitoring, range 1.4–33.3 mmol/litre, for use with *Prestige® Smart System* [NHS] meter only. Net price 50-strip pack = £14.50

■ Meters
Accu-Chek® Active (Roche Diagnostics) [NHS]
Meter for blood glucose monitoring (for use with *Active®* test strips). *Accu-Chek® Active* system = £13.00

Accu-Chek® Advantage (Roche Diagnostics) [NHS]
Meter for blood glucose monitoring (for use with *Advantage II®* test strips). *Accu-Chek® Advantage* system = £16.13

Esprit® (Bayer Diagnostics) [NHS]
Meters for blood glucose monitoring for use with *Esprit® Biosensor* test sensor discs. *Glucometer Esprit®* = £17.49, *Glucometer Esprit® 2* = £17.49

ExacTech® (MediSense) [NHS]
Meters (Sensor) for blood glucose monitoring for use with *ExacTech®* test strips. *ExacTech Card* = £51.63, *ExacTech Card* starter pack = £60.38

GlucoMen® Glycó (Menarini Diagnostics) [NHS]
Meter for blood glucose monitoring (for use with *Gluco-Men®* sensor strips)

Glucometer® (Bayer Diagnostics) [NHS]
Meters for blood glucose monitoring, *Glucometer 4* (for use with *Glucotide®* test strips) = £24.50

Glucotrend® (Roche Diagnostics) [NHS]
Meters for blood glucose monitoring (for use with *Glucotrend®* test strips). *Glucotrend® 2 Soft Test System* pack [NHS] = £25.00; *Glucotrend® Premium* pack [NHS] = £49.00

Glycotronic® C (BHR) [NHS]
Meter for blood glucose monitoring (for use with *Medi-Test® Glycaemic C* test strips) = £40.00

Hypoguard® Supreme (Hypoguard) [NHS]
Meters for blood glucose monitoring (for use with *Hypoguard® Supreme* test strips). *Hypoguard® Supreme Plus* meter = £35.00; *Hypoguard® Supreme Extra* meter = £45.00

MediSense® (MediSense) [NHS]
Meters (Sensor) for blood glucose monitoring. *MediSense Card* = £15.31, *Medisense®* card starter pack = £17.50, *MediSense®* Pen = £30.63, *MediSense®* pen starter pack = £39.38, *MediSense® Precision QID* starter pack = £12.00 (all for use with *MediSense G2®* test strips); *MediSense® Optium* starter pack (for use with *MediSense® Optium* test strips) = £17.50

One Touch® (LifeScan) [NHS]
Meters for blood glucose monitoring for use with *One Touch®* test strips. *One Touch® Basic* system pack = £9.38, *One Touch® Profile* system pack = £18.38

PocketScan® (LifeScan) [NHS]
Meter for blood glucose monitoring (for use with *PocketScan®* test strips). *Complete PocketScan® System* = £17.50

Prestige® Smart System (DiagnoSys) [NHS]
Meter for blood glucose monitoring (for use with *Prestige® Smart System* test strips) = £4.92

Urinalysis

Urine testing for glucose is useful in patients who find blood glucose monitoring difficult. Tests for glucose range from reagent strips specific to glucose to reagent tablets which detect all reducing sugars. Few patients still use *Clinitest®*; *Clinistix®* is suitable for screening purposes only. Tests for ketones by patients are rarely required unless they become unwell.

Microalbuminuria can be detected with *Micral-Test®* [NHS] but this should be followed by confirmation in the laboratory, since false positive results are common.

■ Glucose
Clinistix® (Bayer Diagnostics)
Reagent strips, for detection of glucose in urine. Net price 50-strip pack = £3.03

Clinitest® (Bayer Diagnostics)
Reagent tablets, for detection of glucose and other reducing substances in urine. Pocket set (test tube, dropper and 36 tablets), net price = £3.89, 36-tab pack = £1.93, 6-test tube pack = £2.16, 6-dropper pack = £2.16, test tube rack set (6 tubes and 2 droppers) = £5.73

Diabur-Test 5000® (Roche Diagnostics)
Reagent strips, for detection of glucose in urine. Net price 50-strip pack = £2.50

Diastix® (Bayer Diagnostics)
Reagent strips, for detection of glucose in urine. Net price 50-strip pack = £2.58
Medi-Test® Glucose (BHR)
Reagent strips, for detection of glucose in urine. Net price 50-strip pack = £2.10

■ **Ketones**
Acetest® (Bayer Diagnostics)
Reagent tablets, for detection of ketones in urine. Net price 100-tab pack = £3.42
Ketostix® (Bayer Diagnostics)
Reagent strips, for detection of ketones in urine. Net price 50-strip pack = £2.73
Ketur Test® (Roche Diagnostics)
Reagent strips, for detection of ketones in urine. Net price 50-strip pack = £2.40

■ **Protein**
Albustix® (Bayer Diagnostics)
Reagent strips, for detection of protein in urine. Net price 50-strip pack = £3.75
Medi-Test® Protein 2 (BHR)
Reagent strips, for detection of protein in urine. Net price 50-strip pack = £2.94

Other reagent strips available for urinalysis include: *Combur-3 Test®* NHS (glucose and protein—Roche Diagnostics), *Clinitek Microalbumin®* NHS (albumin and creatinine—Bayer Diagnostics), *Ketodiastix®* NHS (glucose and ketones—Bayer Diagnostics), *Medi-Test Combi 2®* NHS (glucose and protein—BHR), *Micral-Test II®* NHS (albumin—Roche Diagnostics), *Microalbustix®* NHS (albumin and creatinine—Bayer Diagnostics), *Microbumintest®* NHS (albumin—Bayer Diagnostics), *Uristix®* NHS (glucose and protein—Bayer Diagnostics)

Glucose tolerance test

The **glucose** tolerance test is now rarely needed for the diagnosis of diabetes when symptoms of hyperglycaemia are present, though it is still required to establish the presence of gestational diabetes. This generally involves giving anhydrous glucose 75 g (equivalent to Glucose BP 82.5 g) by mouth to the fasting patient, and measuring plasma-glucose concentrations at intervals.

The appropriate amount of glucose should be given with at least 300 mL fluid. Anhydrous glucose 75 g may alternatively be given as 113 mL *Polycal®* (Nutricia Clinical) with extra fluid to administer a total volume of at least 300 mL.

6.2   Thyroid and antithyroid drugs

6.2.1   Thyroid hormones
6.2.2   Antithyroid drugs

6.2.1   Thyroid hormones

Thyroid hormones are used in hypothyroidism (myxoedema), and also in diffuse non-toxic goitre, Hashimoto's thyroiditis (lymphadenoid goitre), and thyroid carcinoma. Neonatal hypothyroidism requires prompt treatment for normal development.

Levothyroxine sodium (thyroxine sodium) is the treatment of choice for *maintenance* therapy. The initial dose should not exceed 100 micrograms daily, preferably before breakfast, or 25 to 50 micrograms in elderly patients or those with car-

diac disease, increased by 25 to 50 micrograms at intervals of at least 4 weeks. The usual maintenance dose to relieve hypothyroidism is 100 to 200 micrograms daily which can be administered as a single dose.

In infants and children doses of thyroxine for congenital hypothyroidism and juvenile myxoedema, should be titrated according to clinical response, growth assessment, and measurements of plasma thyroxine and thyroid-stimulating hormone.

Liothyronine sodium has a similar action to levothyroxine but is more rapidly metabolised and has a more rapid effect; 20 micrograms is equivalent to 100 micrograms of levothyroxine. Its effects develop after a few hours and disappear within 24 to 48 hours of discontinuing treatment. It may be used in *severe hypothyroid states* when a rapid response is desired.

Liothyronine by intravenous injection is the treatment of choice in *hypothyroid coma*. Adjunctive therapy includes intravenous fluids, hydrocortisone, and treatment of infection; assisted ventilation is often required.

LEVOTHYROXINE SODIUM/THYROXINE SODIUM

Indications: hypothyroidism

Cautions: panhypopituitarism or predisposition to adrenal insufficiency from other causes (initiate corticosteroid therapy before starting levothyroxine), elderly, cardiovascular disorders (myocardial insufficiency or ECG evidence of myocardial infarction, see Initial Dosage below), long-standing hypothyroidism, diabetes insipidus, diabetes mellitus (dosage increase may be needed for antidiabetic drugs including insulin); pregnancy (Appendix 4) and breast-feeding (Appendix 5); **interactions:** Appendix 1 (thyroid hormones)

INITIAL DOSAGE. A pre-therapy ECG is valuable as changes induced by hypothyroidism may be confused with evidence of ischaemia. If too rapid an increase of metabolism is produced (causing diarrhoea, nervousness, rapid pulse, insomnia, tremors and sometimes anginal pain where there is latent myocardial ischaemia), reduce dose or withhold for 1–2 days and start again at a lower dose

Contra-indications: thyrotoxicosis

Side-effects: usually at excessive dosage (see Initial Dosage above) include anginal pain, arrhythmias, palpitation, skeletal muscle cramps, tachycardia, diarrhoea, vomiting, tremors, restlessness, excitability, insomnia, headache, flushing, sweating, fever, heat intolerance, excessive loss of weight and muscular weakness

Dose: ADULT, initially 50–100 micrograms (50 micrograms for those over 50 years) daily, preferably before breakfast, adjusted in steps of 50 micrograms every 3–4 weeks until normal metabolism maintained (usually 100–200 micrograms daily); where there is cardiac disease, initially 25 micrograms daily *or* 50 micrograms on alternate days, adjusted in steps of 25 micrograms every 4 weeks; Congenital hypothyroidism and juvenile myxoedema, CHILD up to 1 month initially 5–10 micrograms/kg daily, over 1 month initially 5 micrograms/kg daily adjusted in steps of 25 micrograms every 2–4 weeks until mild toxic symptoms appear then reduce dose slightly

Levothyroxine/Thyroxine (Non-proprietary) PoM

Tablets, levothyroxine sodium 25 micrograms, net price 28-tab pack = 84p; 50 micrograms, 28-tab pack = 56p; 100 micrograms, 28-tab pack = 86p

Available from Alpharma, APS, CP, Goldshield (*Eltroxin®*), Hillcross, IVAX, Kent

LIOTHYRONINE SODIUM

(L-Tri-iodothyronine sodium)

Indications: see notes above

Cautions: see under Levothyroxine Sodium; **interactions:** Appendix 1 (thyroid hormones)

Contra-indications: see under Levothyroxine Sodium

Side-effects: see under Levothyroxine Sodium

Dose: *by mouth,* initially 10–20 micrograms daily gradually increased to 60 micrograms daily in 2–3 divided doses; elderly patients should receive smaller initial doses; CHILD, adult dose reduced in proportion to body-weight

By slow intravenous injection, hypothyroid coma, 5–20 micrograms repeated every 12 hours or as often as every 4 hours if necessary; alternatively 50 micrograms initially then 25 micrograms every 8 hours reducing to 25 micrograms twice daily

Tertroxin® (Goldshield) PoM

Tablets, scored, liothyronine sodium 20 micrograms, net price 28-tab pack = £4.18

Triiodothyronine (Goldshield) PoM

Injection, powder for reconstitution, liothyronine sodium (with dextran). Net price 20-microgram amp = £37.92

6.2.2   Antithyroid drugs

Antithyroid drugs are used for hyperthyroidism either to prepare patients for thyroidectomy or for long-term management. In the UK carbimazole is the most commonly used drug. Propylthiouracil may be used in patients who suffer sensitivity reactions to carbimazole as sensitivity is not necessarily displayed to both drugs. Both drugs act primarily by interfering with the synthesis of thyroid hormones.

CSM warning (neutropenia and agranulocytosis)

Doctors are reminded of the importance of recognising bone marrow suppression induced by carbimazole and the need to stop treatment promptly.

1. Patient should be asked to report symptoms and signs suggestive of infection, especially sore throat.

2. A white blood cell count should be performed if there is any clinical evidence of infection.

3. Carbimazole should be stopped promptly if there is clinical or laboratory evidence of neutropenia.

Carbimazole is given in a dose of 15 to 40 mg daily; occasionally a larger dose may be required. This dose is continued until the patient becomes euthyroid, usually after 4 to 8 weeks and the dose is then gradually reduced to a maintenance dose of 5 to 15 mg. Therapy is usually given for 12 to 18 months. Children may be given carbimazole in an initial dose of 250 micrograms/kg three times daily, adjusted according to response; treatment in chil-

dren should be undertaken by a specialist. Rashes and pruritus are common but they can be treated with antihistamines without discontinuing therapy; alternatively propylthiouracil may be substituted. All patients should be advised to report any sore throat immediately because of the rare complication of agranulocytosis (see CSM warning, above).

Propylthiouracil is given in a dose of 200 to 400 mg daily in adults and this dose is maintained until the patient becomes euthyroid; the dose may then be gradually reduced to a maintenance dose of 50 to 150 mg daily.

Antithyroid drugs only need to be given once daily because of their prolonged effect on the thyroid. Over-treatment with the rapid development of hypothyroidism is not uncommon and should be avoided particularly during pregnancy because it can cause fetal goitre.

A combination of carbimazole, 40 to 60 mg daily with levothyroxine, 50 to 150 micrograms daily, may be used in a *blocking-replacement regimen*; therapy is usually given for 18 months. The blocking-replacement regimen is **not** suitable during pregnancy.

Iodine has been used as an adjunct to antithyroid drugs for 10 to 14 days before partial thyroidectomy; however, there is little evidence of a beneficial effect. Iodine should not be used for long-term treatment because its antithyroid action tends to diminish.

Radioactive sodium iodide (^{131}I) solution is used increasingly for the treatment of thyrotoxicosis at all ages, particularly where medical therapy or compliance is a problem, in patients with cardiac disease, and in patients who relapse after thyroidectomy.

Propranolol is useful for rapid relief of thyrotoxic symptoms and may be used in conjunction with antithyroid drugs or as an adjunct to radioactive iodine. Beta-blockers are also useful in neonatal thyrotoxicosis and in supraventricular arrhythmias due to hyperthyroidism. Propranolol has been used in conjunction with iodine to prepare mildly thyrotoxic patients for surgery but it is preferable to make the patient euthyroid with carbimazole. Laboratory tests of thyroid function are not altered by beta-blockers. Most experience in treating thyrotoxicosis has been gained with propranolol but **nadolol** is also used. For doses and preparations of beta-blockers see section 2.4.

Thyrotoxic crisis ('thyroid storm') requires emergency treatment with intravenous administration of fluids, propranolol (5 mg) and hydrocortisone (100 mg every 6 hours, as sodium succinate), as well as oral iodine solution and carbimazole or propylthiouracil which may need to be administered by nasogastric tube.

PREGNANCY AND BREAST-FEEDING. Radioactive iodine therapy is contra-indicated during pregnancy. Propylthiouracil and carbimazole can be given but the blocking-replacement regimen (see above) is **not** suitable. Both propylthiouracil and carbimazole cross the placenta and in high doses may cause fetal goitre and hypothyroidism—the lowest dose that will control the hyperthyroid state should be used (requirements in Graves' disease tend to fall during pregnancy). Rarely, carbimazole has been associated with aplasia cutis of the neonate.

Carbimazole and propylthiouracil appear in breast milk but this does not preclude breast-feeding as long as neonatal development is closely monitored and the lowest effective dose is used.

CARBIMAZOLE

Indications: hyperthyroidism

Cautions: liver disorders, pregnancy, breast-feeding (see notes above)

Side-effects: nausea, mild gastrointestinal disturbances, headache, rashes and pruritus, arthralgia; rarely alopecia, bone marrow suppression (including pancytopenia and agranulocytosis, see **CSM warning** above), jaundice

Dose: see notes above

COUNSELLING. Warn patient to tell doctor **immediately** if sore throat, mouth ulcers, bruising, fever, malaise, or non-specific illness develops

Neo-Mercazole® (Roche) PoM

Tablets, both pink, carbimazole 5 mg, net price 100-tab pack = £2.87; 20 mg, 100-tab pack = £10.65. Counselling, blood disorder symptoms

IODINE AND IODIDE

Indications: thyrotoxicosis (pre-operative)

Cautions: pregnancy, children; not for long-term treatment

Contra-indications: breast-feeding

Side-effects: hypersensitivity reactions including coryza-like symptoms, headache, lacrimation, conjunctivitis, pain in salivary glands, laryngitis, bronchitis, rashes; on prolonged treatment depression, insomnia, impotence; goitre in infants of mothers taking iodides

Aqueous Iodine Oral Solution (Lugol's Solution), iodine 5%, potassium iodide 10% in purified water, freshly boiled and cooled, total iodine 130 mg/mL. Net price 100 mL = £1.80. Label: 27

Dose: 0.1–0.3 mL 3 times daily well diluted with milk or water

PROPYLTHIOURACIL

Indications: hyperthyroidism

Cautions: see under Carbimazole; reduce dose in renal impairment (Appendix 3)

Side-effects: see under Carbimazole; urticaria, leucopenia; rarely cutaneous vasculitis, thrombocytopenia, aplastic anaemia, hepatitis, lupus erythematous-like syndromes

Dose: see notes above

Propylthiouracil (Non-proprietary) PoM

Tablets, propylthiouracil 50 mg. Net price 20 = £8.74

Available from CP, Hillcross, IVAX

6.3   Corticosteroids

6.3.1   Replacement therapy
6.3.2   Glucocorticoid therapy

6.3.1   Replacement therapy

The adrenal cortex normally secretes hydrocortisone (cortisol) which has glucocorticoid activity and weak mineralocorticoid activity. It also secretes the mineralocorticoid aldosterone.

In deficiency states, physiological replacement is best achieved with a combination of **hydrocortisone** (section 6.3.2) and the mineralocorticoid **fludrocortisone**; hydrocortisone alone does not usually provide sufficient mineralocorticoid activity for complete replacement.

In *Addison's disease* or following adrenalectomy, **hydrocortisone** 20 to 30 mg daily by mouth is usually required. This is given in 2 doses, the larger in the morning and the smaller in the evening, mimicking the normal diurnal rhythm of cortisol secretion. The optimum daily dose is determined on the basis of clinical response. Glucocorticoid therapy is supplemented by fludrocortisone 50 to 300 micrograms daily.

In *acute adrenocortical insufficiency*, **hydrocortisone** is given intravenously (preferably as sodium succinate) in doses of 100 mg every 6 to 8 hours in sodium chloride intravenous infusion 0.9%.

In *hypopituitarism* glucocorticoids should be given as in adrenocortical insufficiency, but since the production of aldosterone is also regulated by the renin-angiotensin system a mineralocorticoid is not usually required. Additional replacement therapy with levothyroxine (section 6.2.1) and sex hormones (section 6.4) should be given as indicated by the pattern of hormone deficiency.

FLUDROCORTISONE ACETATE

Indications: mineralocorticoid replacement in adrenocortical insufficiency

Cautions: section 6.3.2

Contra-indications: section 6.3.2

Side-effects: section 6.3.2

Dose: 50–300 micrograms daily; CHILD 5 micrograms/kg daily

Florinef® (Squibb) PoM

Tablets, pink, scored, fludrocortisone acetate 100 micrograms. Net price 56-tab pack = £2.69. Label: 10 steroid card

6.3.2   Glucocorticoid therapy

In comparing the relative potencies of corticosteroids in terms of their anti-inflammatory (glucocorticoid) effects it should be borne in mind that high glucocorticoid activity in itself is of no advantage unless it occurs in conjunction with relatively low mineralocorticoid activity so that the effect on water and electrolytes is not also increased. The mineralocorticoid activity of **fludrocortisone** (section 6.3.1) is so high that its anti-inflammatory activity is of no clinical relevance. The table below shows equivalent anti-inflammatory doses.

Equivalent Anti-inflammatory Doses of Corticosteroids

This table takes no account of mineralocorticoid effects, nor does it take account of variations in duration of action

Prednisolone 5 mg
≡ Betamethasone 750 micrograms
≡ Cortisone acetate 25 mg
≡ Deflazacort 6 mg
≡ Dexamethasone 750 micrograms
≡ Hydrocortisone 20 mg
≡ Methylprednisolone 4 mg
≡ Triamcinolone 4 mg

The relatively high mineralocorticoid activity of **cortisone** and **hydrocortisone**, and the resulting fluid retention, make them unsuitable for disease suppression on a long-term basis. However, they can be used for adrenal replacement therapy (section 6.3.1); hydrocortisone is preferred because cortisone requires conversion in the liver to hydrocortisone. Hydrocortisone is used on a short-term basis by intravenous injection for the emergency management of some conditions. The relatively moderate anti-inflammatory potency of hydrocortisone also makes it a useful topical corticosteroid for the management of inflammatory skin conditions because side-effects (both topical and systemic) are less marked (section 13.4); cortisone is not active topically.

Prednisolone has predominantly glucocorticoid activity and is the corticosteroid most commonly used by mouth for long-term disease suppression.

Betamethasone and **dexamethasone** have very high glucocorticoid activity in conjunction with insignificant mineralocorticoid activity. This makes them particularly suitable for high-dose therapy in conditions where fluid retention would be a disadvantage (e.g. cerebral oedema).

Betamethasone and dexamethasone also have a long duration of action and this, coupled with their lack of mineralocorticoid action makes them particularly suitable for conditions which require suppression of corticotropin (corticotrophin) secretion (e.g. congenital adrenal hyperplasia). Some esters of betamethasone and of **beclometasone** (beclomethasone) exert a considerably more marked topical effect (e.g. on the skin or the lungs) than when given by mouth; use is made of this to obtain topical effects whilst minimising systemic side-effects (e.g. for skin applications and asthma inhalations).

Deflazacort is a newly introduced corticosteroid with high glucocorticoid activity; it is derived from prednisolone.

Disadvantages of corticosteroids

Overdosage or prolonged use may exaggerate some of the normal physiological actions of corticosteroids leading to mineralocorticoid and glucocorticoid side-effects.

Mineralocorticoid side-effects include hypertension, sodium and water retention and potassium loss. They are most marked with fludrocortisone, but are significant with cortisone, hydrocortisone,

corticotropin, and tetracosactide (tetracosactrin). Mineralocorticoid actions are negligible with the high potency glucocorticoids, betamethasone and dexamethasone, and occur only slightly with methylprednisolone, prednisolone, and triamcinolone.

Glucocorticoid side-effects include diabetes and osteoporosis (section 6.6), which is a danger, particularly in the elderly, as it may result in osteoporotic fractures for example of the hip or vertebrae; in addition high doses are associated with avascular necrosis of the femoral head. Mental disturbances may occur; a serious paranoid state or depression with risk of suicide may be induced, particularly in patients with a history of mental disorder. Euphoria is frequently observed. Muscle wasting (proximal myopathy) may also occur. Corticosteroid therapy is also weakly linked with peptic ulceration (the potential advantage of soluble or enteric-coated preparations to reduce the risk is speculative only).

High doses of corticosteroids may cause Cushing's syndrome, with moon face, striae, and acne; it is usually reversible on withdrawal of treatment, but this must always be gradually tapered to avoid symptoms of acute adrenal insufficiency (**important:** see also Adrenal Suppression below).

In children, administration of corticosteroids may result in suppression of growth. For the effect of corticosteroids given in pregnancy, see Pregnancy and breast-feeding, below.

Adrenal Suppression

During prolonged therapy with corticosteroids, adrenal atrophy may develop and persist for years after stopping. Abrupt withdrawal after a prolonged period may lead to adrenal insufficiency, hypotension or death (see also notes below on withdrawal). Withdrawal may also be associated with fever, myalgia, arthralgia, rhinitis, conjunctivitis, painful itchy skin nodules and weight loss.

To compensate for a diminished adrenocortical response following prolonged corticosteroid treatment, any significant intercurrent illness, trauma, or surgical procedure requires a temporary increase in corticosteroid dose, or if already stopped, a temporary re-introduction of corticosteroid treatment. Anaesthetists **must** therefore know whether a patient is taking or has been taking a corticosteroid, to avoid a precipitous fall in blood pressure during anaesthesia or in the immediate postoperative period. A suitable regimen for corticosteroid replacement, in patients taking more than 10 mg prednisolone daily (or equivalent) within 3 months of surgery, is:

- *Minor surgery under general anaesthesia*—usual oral corticosteroid dose on the morning of surgery or hydrocortisone 25–50 mg (usually the sodium succinate) intravenously at induction; the usual oral corticosteroid dose is recommenced after surgery
- *Moderate or major surgery*—usual oral corticosteroid dose on the morning of surgery and hydrocortisone 25–50 mg intravenously at induction, followed by hydrocortisone 25–50 mg 3 times a day by intravenous injection for 24 hours after moderate surgery or for 48–72 hours after major surgery; the usual preoperative oral corticosteroid dose is recommenced on stopping hydrocortisone injections

Patients on long-term corticosteroid treatment should carry a Steroid Treatment Card (see below) which gives guidance on minimising risk and provides details of prescriber, drug, dosage and duration of treatment.

Infections

Prolonged courses of corticosteroids increase susceptibility to infections and severity of infections; clinical presentation of infections may also be atypical. Serious infections e.g. *septicaemia* and *tuberculosis* may reach an advanced stage before being recognised, and *amoebiasis* or *strongyloidiasis* may be activated or exacerbated (exclude before initiating corticosteroid in those at risk or with suggestive symptoms). Fungal or viral *ocular infections* may also be exacerbated (see also section 11.4.1).

CHICKENPOX. Unless they have had chickenpox, patients receiving oral or parenteral corticosteroids for purposes other than replacement should be regarded as being *at risk of severe chickenpox* (see Steroid Treatment Card). Manifestations of fulminant illness include pneumonia, hepatitis and disseminated intravascular coagulation; rash is not necessarily a prominent feature.

Passive immunisation with varicella–zoster immunoglobulin (section 14.5) is needed for exposed non-immune patients receiving systemic corticosteroids or for those who have used them within the previous 3 months; varicella–zoster immunoglobulin should preferably be given within 3 days of exposure and no later than 10 days. Confirmed chickenpox warrants specialist care and urgent treatment (section 5.3). Corticosteroids should not be stopped and dosage may need to be increased.

Topical, inhaled or rectal corticosteroids are less likely to be associated with an increased risk of severe chickenpox.

MEASLES. Patients taking corticosteroids should be advised to take particular care to avoid exposure to measles and to seek immediate medical advice if exposure occurs. Prophylaxis with intramuscular normal immunoglobulin (section 14.5) may be needed.

Following concern about severe chickenpox associated with systemic corticosteroids, the CSM has issued a notice that **every** patient prescribed a *systemic* corticosteroid should receive the patient information leaflet supplied by the manufacturer.

Steroid treatment cards should also be issued where appropriate. Doctors and pharmacists can obtain supplies of the card from:

England and Wales

Department of Health, PO Box 777, London, SE1 6XH (Tel (08701) 555 455)

Scotland

Banner Business Supplies, 20 South Gyle Crescent, Edinburgh, EH12 9EB (Tel (0131) 479 3279)

For other references to the adverse effects of corticosteroids see section 11.4 (eye) and section 13.4 (skin).

STEROID TREATMENT CARD

I am a patient on STEROID treatment which must not be stopped suddenly

- If you have been taking this medicine for more than three weeks, the dose should be reduced gradually when you stop taking steroids unless your doctor says otherwise.

- Read the patient information leaflet given with the medicine.

- Always carry this card with you and show it to anyone who treats you (for example a doctor, nurse, pharmacist or dentist). For one year after you stop the treatment, you must mention that you have taken steroids.

- If you become ill, or if you come into contact with anyone who has an infectious disease, consult your doctor promptly. If you have never had chickenpox, you should avoid close contact with people who have chickenpox or shingles. If you do come into contact with chickenpox, see your doctor urgently.

- Make sure that the information on the card is kept up to date.

Clinical management

Dosage of corticosteroids varies widely in different diseases and in different patients. If the use of a corticosteroid can save or prolong life, as in exfoliative dermatitis, pemphigus, acute leukaemia or acute transplant rejection, high doses may need to be given, because the complications of therapy are likely to be less serious than the effects of the disease itself.

When long-term corticosteroid therapy is used in some chronic diseases, the danger of treatment may become greater than the disabilities produced by the disease. To minimise side-effects the maintenance dose should be kept as low as possible.

When potentially less harmful measures are ineffective corticosteroids are used topically for the treatment of inflammatory conditions of the skin (section 13.4). Corticosteroids should be avoided or used only under specialist supervision in psoriasis (section 13.5).

Corticosteroids are used both topically (by rectum) and systemically (by mouth or intravenously) in the management of ulcerative colitis and Crohn's disease (section 1.5 and section 1.7.2).

Use can be made of the mineralocorticoid activity of fludrocortisone to treat postural hypotension in autonomic neuropathy (section 6.1.5).

Very high doses of corticosteroids have been given by intravenous injection in septic shock. However a study of high-dose methylprednisolone sodium succinate did not demonstrate efficacy and, moreover, suggested a higher mortality in some subsets of patients given the high-dose corticosteroid therapy.

Dexamethasone and betamethasone have little if any mineralocorticoid action and their long duration of action makes them particularly suitable for suppressing corticotropin secretion in congenital adrenal hyperplasia where the dose should be tailored to clinical response and by measurement of adrenal androgens and 17-hydroxyprogesterone. In common with all glucocorticoids their suppressive action on the hypothalamic-pituitary-adrenal axis is greatest and most prolonged when they are given at night. In most normal subjects a single dose of 1 mg of dexamethasone at night, depending on weight, is sufficient to inhibit corticotropin secretion for 24 hours. This is the basis of the 'overnight dexamethasone suppression test' for diagnosing Cushing's syndrome.

Betamethasone and dexamethasone are also appropriate for conditions where water retention would be a disadvantage, as for example in treating traumatic cerebral oedema with doses of 12 to 20 mg daily.

In acute hypersensitivity reactions such as angioedema of the upper respiratory tract and anaphylactic shock, corticosteroids are indicated as an adjunct to emergency treatment with adrenaline (epinephrine) (section 3.4.3). In such cases hydrocortisone (as sodium succinate) by intravenous injection in a dose of 100 to 300 mg may be required.

Corticosteroids are preferably used by inhalation in the management of asthma (section 3.2) but systemic therapy in association with bronchodilators is required for the emergency treatment of severe acute asthma (section 3.1.1).

Corticosteroids may also be useful in conditions such as rheumatic fever, chronic active hepatitis, and sarcoidosis; they may also lead to remissions of acquired haemolytic anaemia (section 9.1.3), and some cases of the nephrotic syndrome (particularly in children) and thrombocytopenic purpura (section 9.1.4).

Corticosteroids can improve the prognosis of serious conditions such as systemic lupus erythematosus, temporal arteritis, and polyarteritis nodosa; the effects of the disease process may be suppressed and symptoms relieved, but the underlying condition is not cured, although it may ultimately remit. It is usual to begin therapy in these conditions at fairly high dose, such as 40 to 60 mg prednisolone daily, and then to reduce the dose to the lowest commensurate with disease control.

For other references to the use of corticosteroids see Prescribing in palliative care, section 8.2.2 (immunosuppresion), section 11.4 (eye), section 12.1.1 (otitis externa), section 12.2.1 (allergic rhinitis), and section 12.3.1 (aphthous ulcers).

Pregnancy and breast-feeding

Following a review of the data on the safety of systemic corticosteroids used in pregnancy and breast-feeding the CSM has concluded:

- corticosteroids vary in their ability to cross the placenta; betamethasone and dexamethasone cross the placenta readily while 88% of prednisolone is inactivated as it crosses the placenta;
- there is no convincing evidence that systemic corticosteroids increase the incidence of congenital abnormalities such as cleft palate or lip;
- when administration is prolonged or repeated during pregnancy, systemic corticosteroids increase the risk of intra-uterine growth retardation; there is no evidence of intra-uterine growth retardation following short-term treatment (e.g. prophylactic treatment for neonatal respiratory distress syndrome);
- any adrenal suppression in the neonate following prenatal exposure usually resolves spontaneously after birth and is rarely clinically important;
- prednisolone appears in small amounts in breast milk but doses of up to 40 mg daily are unlikely to cause systemic effects in the infant; infants should be monitored for adrenal suppression if the mothers are taking a higher dose.

See also Appendix 4.

Administration

Whenever possible *local treatment* with creams, intra-articular injections, inhalations, eye-drops, or enemas should be used in preference to *systemic treatment*. The suppressive action of a corticosteroid on cortisol secretion is least when it is given in the morning, therefore in an attempt to reduce pituitary-adrenal suppression a corticosteroid (usually prednisolone) should normally be taken as a single dose in the morning. In an attempt to reduce pituitary-adrenal suppression further, the total dose for two days can sometimes be taken as a single dose on alternate days; alternate-day administration has not been very successful in the management of asthma (section 3.2). Pituitary-adrenal suppression can also be reduced by means of intermittent therapy with short courses. In some conditions it may be possible to reduce the dose of corticosteroid by adding a small dose of an immunosuppressive drug (section 8.2.1).

Withdrawal of corticosteroids

The CSM has recommended that *gradual* withdrawal of systemic corticosteroids should be considered in those whose disease is unlikely to relapse and have

- recently received repeated courses (particularly if taken for longer than 3 weeks)
- taken a short course within 1 year of stopping long-term therapy
- other possible causes of adrenal suppression
- received more than 40 mg daily prednisolone (or equivalent)
- been given repeat doses in the evening
- received more than 3 weeks' treatment

Systemic corticosteroids may be stopped abruptly in those whose disease is unlikely to relapse *and* who have received treatment for 3 weeks or less *and* who are not included in the patient groups described above.

During corticosteroid withdrawal the dose may be reduced rapidly down to physiological doses (equivalent to prednisolone 7.5 mg daily) and then reduced more slowly. Assessment of the disease may be needed during withdrawal to ensure that relapse does not occur.

PREDNISOLONE

Indications: suppression of inflammatory and allergic disorders; see also notes above; inflammatory bowel disease, section 1.5; asthma, section 3.2; immunosuppression, section 8.2.2; rheumatic disease, section 10.1.2

Cautions: adrenal suppression and infection (see notes above), children and adolescents (growth retardation possibly irreversible), elderly (close supervision required particularly on long-term treatment); frequent monitoring required if history of tuberculosis (or X-ray changes), hypertension, recent myocardial infarction (rupture reported), congestive heart failure, liver failure, renal impairment, diabetes mellitus including family history, osteoporosis (post-menopausal women at special risk), glaucoma (including family history), severe affective disorders (particularly if history of steroid-induced psychosis), epilepsy, peptic ulcer, hypothyroidism, history of steroid myopathy; pregnancy and breast-feeding (see notes above); **interactions:** Appendix 1 (corticosteroids)

Contra-indications: systemic infection (unless specific antimicrobial therapy given); avoid live virus vaccines in those receiving immunosuppressive doses (serum antibody response diminished)

Side-effects: minimised by using lowest effective dose for minimum period possible; *gastro-intestinal effects* include dyspepsia, peptic ulceration (with perforation), abdominal distension, acute pancreatitis, oesophageal ulceration and candidiasis; *musculoskeletal effects* include proximal myopathy, osteoporosis, vertebral and long bone fractures, avascular osteonecrosis, tendon rupture; *endocrine effects* include adrenal suppression, menstrual irregularities and amenorrhoea, Cushing's syndrome (with high doses, usually reversible on withdrawal), hirsutism, weight gain, negative nitrogen and calcium balance, increased appetite; increased susceptibility to and severity of infection; *neuropsychiatric effects* include euphoria, psychological dependence, depression, insomnia, increased intracranial pressure with papilloedema in children (usually after withdrawal), psychosis and aggravation of schizophrenia, aggravation of epilepsy; *ophthalmic effects* include glaucoma, papilloedema, posterior subcapsular cataracts, corneal or scleral thinning and exacerbation of ophthalmic viral or fungal disease; *other side-effects* include impaired healing, skin atrophy, bruising, striae, telangiectasia, acne, myocardial rupture following recent myocardial infarction, fluid and electrolyte disturbance, leucocytosis, hypersensitivity reactions (including anaphylaxis), thromboembolism, nausea, malaise, hiccups

Dose: *by mouth*, initially, up to 10–20 mg daily (severe disease, up to 60 mg daily), preferably taken in the morning after breakfast; can often be reduced within a few days but may need to be continued for several weeks or months

Maintenance, usual range, 2.5–15 mg daily, but higher doses may be needed; cushingoid side-effects increasingly likely with doses above 7.5 mg daily

By intramuscular injection, prednisolone acetate, 25–100 mg once or twice weekly (for preparation see section 10.1.2.2)

Prednisolone (Non-proprietary) [PoM]
Tablets, prednisolone 1 mg, net price 28-tab pack = 53p; 5 mg, 28-tab pack = 67p. Label: 10 steroid card, 21
Available from Alpharma, APS, CP, Hillcross, Hoechst Marion Roussel (Precortisyl®), IVAX
Tablets, both e/c, prednisolone 2.5 mg (brown), net price 30-tab pack = 26p; 5 mg (red), 30-tab pack = 43p. Label: 5, 10 steroid card, 25
Available from Alpharma, Biorex, IVAX (2.5 mg), Pfizer (Deltacortril Enteric®)
Soluble tablets, prednisolone 5 mg (as sodium phosphate), net price 30-tab pack = £2.20. Label: 10 steroid card, 13, 21
Available from Sovereign
Injection, see section 10.1.2.2

Precortisyl Forte® (Hoechst Marion Roussel) [PoM]
Tablets, scored, prednisolone 25 mg. Net price 56-tab pack = £4.69. Label: 10 steroid card, 21

BETAMETHASONE

Indications: suppression of inflammatory and allergic disorders; congenital adrenal hyperplasia; cerebral oedema; see also notes above; ear (section 12.1.1); eye (section 11.4.1); nose (section 12.2.1)

Cautions: see notes above and under Prednisolone

Contra-indications: see notes above and under Prednisolone

Side-effects: see notes above and under Prednisolone

Dose: *by mouth,* usual range 0.5–5 mg daily; see also Administration (above)

By intramuscular injection or slow intravenous injection or infusion, 4–20 mg, repeated up to 4 times in 24 hours; CHILD, *by slow intravenous injection,* up to 1 year 1 mg, 1–5 years 2 mg, 6–12 years 4 mg

Betnelan® (Celltech) [PoM]
Tablets, scored, betamethasone 500 micrograms. Net price 100-tab pack = £3.63. Label: 10 steroid card, 21

Betnesol® (Celltech) [PoM]
Tablets, pink, scored, soluble, betamethasone 500 micrograms (as sodium phosphate). Net price 100-tab pack = £4.10. Label: 10 steroid card, 13, 21

Injection, betamethasone 4 mg (as sodium phosphate)/mL. Net price 1-mL amp = 97p. Label: 10 steroid card

CORTISONE ACETATE ▭

Indications: see under Dose but now superseded, see also notes above

Cautions: see notes above and under Prednisolone

Contra-indications: see notes above and under Prednisolone

Side-effects: see notes above and under Prednisolone

Dose: for replacement therapy, 25–37.5 mg daily in divided doses

Cortisyl® (Hoechst Marion Roussel) PoM ▰
Tablets, scored, cortisone acetate 25 mg. Net price 56-tab pack = £3.24. Label: 10 steroid card, 21

▰ denotes preparations that are considered to be less suitable for prescribing (see p. vi)

DEFLAZACORT

Indications: suppression of inflammatory and allergic disorders

Cautions: see notes above and under Prednisolone

Contra-indications: see notes above and under Prednisolone

Side-effects: see notes above and under Prednisolone

Dose: usual maintenance 3–18 mg daily (acute disorders, initially up to 120 mg daily); see also Administration (above)
CHILD 0.25–1.5 mg/kg daily (or on alternate days); see also Administration (above)

Calcort® (Shire) ▼ PoM
Tablets, deflazacort 1 mg, net price 100-tab pack = £8.00; 6 mg, 60-tab pack = £16.46; 30 mg, 30-tab pack = £22.80. Label: 5, 10 steroid card

DEXAMETHASONE

Indications: suppression of inflammatory and allergic disorders; shock; diagnosis of Cushing's disease, congenital adrenal hyperplasia; cerebral oedema; nausea and vomiting with chemotherapy (section 8.1); rheumatic disease (section 10.1.2); eye (section 11.4.1); see also notes above

Cautions: see notes above and under Prednisolone

Contra-indications: see notes above and under Prednisolone

Side-effects: see notes above and under Prednisolone; perineal irritation may follow intravenous administration of the phosphate ester

Dose: *by mouth*, usual range 0.5–10 mg daily; see also Administration (above)

By intramuscular injection or slow intravenous injection or infusion (as dexamethasone phosphate), initially 0.5–20 mg; CHILD 200–500 micrograms/kg daily
Cerebral oedema (as dexamethasone phosphate), *by intravenous injection*, 10 mg initially, then 4 mg *by intramuscular injection* every 6 hours as required for 2–10 days
Shock (as dexamethasone phosphate), *by intravenous injection or infusion*, 2–6 mg/kg, repeated if necessary after 2–6 hours (but see notes above)
Note. Dexamethasone 1 mg ≡ dexamethasone phosphate 1.2 mg ≡ dexamethasone sodium phosphate 1.3 mg

Dexamethasone (Non-proprietary) PoM
Tablets, dexamethasone 500 micrograms, net price 20 = 64p; 2 mg, 20 = £1.73. Label: 10 steroid card, 21
Available from Organon

Oral solution, sugar-free, dexamethasone (as dexamethasone sodium phosphate) 2 mg/5 mL, net price 150-mL = £45.00
Available from Rosemont (*Dexsol®*)

Injection, dexamethasone phosphate (as dexamethasone sodium phosphate) 4 mg/mL, net price 1-mL amp = £1.00, 2-mL vial = £1.98; 24 mg/mL, 5-mL vial = £16.66. Label: 10 steroid card
Available from Faulding DBL

Injection, dexamethasone sodium phosphate 5 mg/mL, net price 1-mL amp = 83p, 2-mL vial = £1.27. Label: 10 steroid card
Available from Organon

Decadron® (MSD) PoM
Tablets, scored, dexamethasone 500 micrograms, net price 30-tab pack = 96p. Label: 10 steroid card, 21

HYDROCORTISONE

Indications: adrenocortical insufficiency (section 6.3.1); shock; see also notes above; hypersensitivity reactions e.g. anaphylactic shock and angioedema (section 3.4.3); inflammatory bowel disease (section 1.5); haemorrhoids (section 1.7.2); rheumatic disease (section 10.1.2); eye (section 11.4.1); skin (section 13.4)

Cautions: see notes above and under Prednisolone

Contra-indications: see notes above and under Prednisolone

Side-effects: see notes above and under Prednisolone; phosphate ester associated with paraesthesia and pain (particularly in the perineal region)

Dose: *by mouth*, replacement therapy, 20–30 mg daily in divided doses—see section 6.3.1; CHILD 10–30 mg

By intramuscular injection or slow intravenous injection or infusion, 100–500 mg, 3–4 times in 24 hours or as required; CHILD *by slow intravenous injection* up to 1 year 25 mg, 1–5 years 50 mg, 6–12 years 100 mg

Efcortesol® (Sovereign) PoM ▰
Injection, hydrocortisone 100 mg (as sodium phosphate)/mL. Net price 1-mL amp = 75p; 5-mL amp = £3.40. Label: 10 steroid card
Note. Paraesthesia and pain (particularly in the perineal region) may follow intravenous injection of the phosphate ester

Hydrocortone® (MSD) PoM
Tablets, scored, hydrocortisone 10 mg, net price 30-tab pack = 70p; 20 mg, 30-tab pack = £1.07. Label: 10 steroid card, 21

Solu-Cortef® (Pharmacia) PoM
Injection, powder for reconstitution, hydrocortisone (as sodium succinate). Net price 100-mg vial = 92p, 100-mg vial with 2-mL amp water for injections = 97p. Label: 10 steroid card

▰ denotes preparations that are considered to be less suitable for prescribing (see p. vi)

METHYLPREDNISOLONE

Indications: suppression of inflammatory and allergic disorders; cerebral oedema; see also notes above; rheumatic disease (section 10.1.2); skin (section 13.4)

Cautions: see notes above and under Predniso-lone; rapid intravenous administration of large doses associated with cardiovascular collapse

Contra-indications: see notes above and under Prednisolone

Side-effects: see notes above and under Predniso-lone

Dose: *by mouth*, usual range 2–40 mg daily; see also Administration (above)

By intramuscular injection or slow intravenous injection or infusion, initially 10–500 mg; graft rejection, up to 1 g daily *by intravenous infusion* for up to 3 days

Medrone® (Pharmacia) PoM

Tablets, scored, methylprednisolone 2 mg (pink), net price 30-tab pack = £2.57; 4 mg, 30-tab pack = £4.93; 16 mg, 30-tab pack = £13.67; 100 mg (blue), 20-tab pack = £38.46. Label: 10 steroid card, 21

Solu-Medrone® (Pharmacia) PoM

Injection, powder for reconstitution, methyl-prednisolone (as sodium succinate) (all with solvent). Net price 40-mg vial = £1.26; 125-mg vial = £3.78; 500-mg vial = £7.64; 1-g vial = £13.77; 2-g vial = £26.15. Label: 10 steroid card

■ Intramuscular depot

Depo-Medrone® (Pharmacia) PoM

Injection (aqueous suspension), methylprednisolone acetate 40 mg/mL. Net price 1-mL vial = £2.87; 2-mL vial = £5.15; 3-mL vial = £7.47. Label: 10 steroid card

Dose: by deep intramuscular injection into gluteal muscle, 40–120 mg, a second injection may be given after 2–3 weeks if required

TRIAMCINOLONE

Indications: suppression of inflammatory and allergic disorders; see also notes above; rheumatic disease, section 10.1.2; mouth, section 12.3.1; skin, section 13.4

Cautions: see notes above and under Predniso-lone; high dosage may cause proximal myopathy, avoid in chronic therapy

Contra-indications: see notes above and under Prednisolone

Side-effects: see notes above and under Predniso-lone

Dose: *by deep intramuscular injection*, into gluteal muscle, 40 mg of acetonide for depot effect, repeated at intervals according to the patient's response; max. single dose 100 mg

Kenalog® (Squibb) PoM

Injection (aqueous suspension), triamcinolone acetonide 40 mg/mL. Net price 1-mL vial (intra-muscular/intra-articular) = £1.70; 1-mL syringe (intramuscular only) = £2.11; 2-mL syringe (intramuscular only) = £3.66. Label: 10 steroid card

6.4 Sex hormones

Sex hormones are described under the following section headings:

6.4.1   Female sex hormones
6.4.2   Male sex hormones and antagonists
6.4.3   Anabolic steroids

6.4.1 Female sex hormones

6.4.1.1   Oestrogens and HRT
6.4.1.2   Progestogens

6.4.1.1 Oestrogens and HRT

Oestrogens are necessary for the development of female secondary sexual characteristics; they also stimulate myometrial hypertrophy with endometrial hyperplasia.

In terms of oestrogenic activity *natural oestrogens* (estradiol (oestradiol), estrone (oestrone), and estriol (oestriol)) have a more appropriate profile for hormone replacement therapy (HRT) than *synthetic oestrogens* (ethinylestradiol (ethinyloestradiol) and mestranol); the profile of *conjugated oestrogens* resembles that of natural oestrogens.

Oestrogen therapy is given cyclically or continuously for a number of gynaecological conditions. If long-term therapy is required a progestogen should be added to reduce the risk of cystic hyperplasia of the endometrium and possible transformation to cancer. This addition of a progestogen is not necessary if the patient has had a hysterectomy or in the case of tibolone.

Oestrogens are no longer used to *suppress lactation* because of their association with thrombo-embolism.

Hormone replacement therapy

Menopausal *vasomotor symptoms* and menopausal *vaginitis* are alleviated by administration of small doses of oestrogen. There is also good evidence that small doses of oestrogen given for several years starting in the perimenopausal period will diminish postmenopausal *osteoporosis*. HRT should not be prescribed primarily to reduce the incidence of stroke and myocardial infarction because the evidence of benefit is not clear. There is an increased risk of *endometrial cancer* (reduced by a progestogen) and, after some years of use, possibly an increased risk of *breast cancer* (see below).

Hormone replacement therapy (HRT) is indicated for menopausal women whose lives are inconvenienced by *vaginal atrophy* or *vasomotor instability*. Vaginal atrophy may respond to a short course of vaginal oestrogen preparation (section 7.2.1) given for a few weeks and repeated if necessary. Systemic therapy is needed for vasomotor symptoms and should be given for at least a year; in a woman with a uterus a progestogen should be added to reduce the risk of endometrial cancer. Clonidine (section 4.7.4.2) may be used to reduce vasomotor symptoms in women who cannot take an oestrogen, but clonidine may cause unacceptable side-effects. HRT is also indicated for women with *early natural or surgical menopause (before age 45)*, since they are at high risk of osteoporosis; HRT should be given for at least 5–10 years (for risk of breast cancer, see below).

Long-term HRT is almost certainly favourable in risk-benefit terms for menopausal women *without a uterus* because they do not require progestogen therapy; it should probably be continued for about 10 years (for risk of breast cancer, see below). The picture is less clear for menopausal women *with a uterus* because the need for administration of progestogen may blunt the protective effect of low-dose oestrogen against myocardial infarction and stroke; any effect of the progestogen (favourable or otherwise) on breast cancer is not yet known. Nevertheless, risk factors for osteoporosis should be borne in mind and, if there are several, consideration given to HRT. Risk factors include recent corticosteroid therapy or any disease predisposing to osteoporosis, family history, thinness, lack of exercise, alcoholism or smoking, and fracture of a hip or forearm before the age of 65; women of Afro-Caribbean origin appear to be less susceptible than those who are white or of Asian origin.

RISK OF BREAST CANCER. Following publication of an analysis of pooled original data, the CSM has advised that the increased risk of breast cancer is related to the duration of HRT use and that this excess risk disappears within about 5 years of stopping. Women who use HRT for a short time around the menopause have a very low excess risk. Breast cancers in HRT users were less likely to have spread beyond the breast than those in non-users.

About 45 in every 1000 women aged 50 years not using HRT will have breast cancer diagnosed over the next 20 years; in those using HRT for 5 years, this figure rises by 2 extra cases in 1000, in those using HRT for 10 years 6 extra cases in 1000 and in those using HRT for 15 years 12 extra cases in 1000.

The CSM's view is that these results do not provide a reason for women to stop their treatment but the results do emphasise the importance of breast awareness and regular mammograms.

RISK OF VENOUS THROMBOEMBOLISM. Recent studies show an increased risk of deep vein thrombosis and of pulmonary embolism in women currently taking HRT. The view of the CSM is that the new data do not change the overall positive balance between benefits and risks of treatment for most women. The CSM has advised that there is no need for *women without predisposing factors* for venous thromboembolism to stop taking HRT. In *women who have predisposing factors* (such as a personal or family history of deep vein thrombosis or pulmonary embolism, severe varicose veins, obesity, surgery, trauma or prolonged bed-rest) it may be prudent to review the need for HRT as in some cases the risks of HRT may be expected to exceed the benefits.

CHOICE. The choice of HRT for an individual depends on an overall balance of indication, risk, and convenience. An oestrogen alone is suitable for long-term continuous use in women without a uterus. A woman with an intact uterus requires oestrogen with cyclical progestogen for the last 10 to

13 days of the cycle *or* a preparation which involves continuous administration of an oestrogen and a progestogen (*or* one which provides both oestrogenic and progestogenic activity in a single preparation). Continuous combined preparations are not suitable for use in the perimenopause or within 12 months of the last menstrual period; women who use such preparations may experience irregular bleeding in the early stages of treatment—if bleeding continues endometrial abnormality should be ruled out and consideration given to changing to cyclical HRT.

An oestrogen may be given by mouth or it may be given by subcutaneous or transdermal administration, which avoids first-pass metabolism. In the case of subcutaneous implants, recurrence of vasomotor symptoms at supraphysiological plasma concentrations may occur; moreover, there is evidence of prolonged endometrial stimulation after discontinuation (calling for continued cyclical progestogen). For the use of topical HRT preparations see section 7.2.1.

Provided that calcium intake is adequate calcium supplements (section 9.5.1) do not confer additional benefit (see also Osteoporosis, section 6.6).

CONTRACEPTION. HRT does **not** provide contraception and a woman is considered potentially fertile for *2 years after her last menstrual period* if she is *under 50 years*, and for *1 year* if she is *over 50 years*. A woman who is under 50 years and free of all risk factors for venous and arterial disease can use a low-oestrogen combined oral contraceptive pill (section 7.3.1) to provide both *relief of menopausal symptoms* and *contraception*; it is recommended that the oral contraceptive be stopped at 50 years of age since there are more suitable alternatives. If any potentially fertile woman needs to use HRT, *non-hormonal contraceptive measures* (such as condoms, or by this age, contraceptive foam, section 7.3.3) are necessary.

Although follicle-stimulating hormone measurements can be used as a guide to determine fertility, high measurements alone (particularly in women under the age of 50 years) do not necessarily preclude the possibility of pregnancy.

SURGERY. Major surgery under general anaesthesia, including orthopaedic and vascular leg surgery, is a predisposing factor for venous thromboembolism and it may be prudent to stop HRT a month before surgery (see Risk of Venous Thromboembolism, above). If HRT is continued or discontinuation is not possible (e.g. in non-elective surgery), prophylaxis with heparin and graduated compression hosiery is advised. Oestrogenic activity may persist after discontinuation of estradiol implants (see above).

REASONS TO STOP HRT. For circumstances in which HRT should be stopped, see p. 388.

OESTROGENS FOR HRT

Note. Relates only to small amounts of oestrogens given for hormone replacement therapy

Indications: see notes above and under preparations

Cautions: prolonged exposure to unopposed oestrogens may increase risk of development of endometrial cancer (see notes above); migraine (or migraine-like headaches); history of breast nodules or fibrocystic disease—closely monitor breast status (risk of breast cancer, see notes above); pre-existing uterine fibroids may increase in size, symptoms of endometriosis may be exacerbated; factors predisposing to thromboembolism (see notes above); presence of antiphospholipid antibodies (increased risk of thrombotic events); increased risk of gall bladder disease reported; hypophyseal tumours; porphyria (see section 9.8.2); **interactions:** Appendix 1 (oestrogens)

OTHER CONDITIONS. The product literature advises caution in other conditions including hypertension, cardiac or renal disease, diabetes, asthma, epilepsy, sickle-cell disease, melanoma, otosclerosis, multiple sclerosis, systemic lupus erythematosus (but care required if antiphospholipid antibodies present, see above) and history of stroke and of myocardial infarction. Evidence for caution in these conditions is unsatisfactory and many women with these conditions may stand to benefit from HRT.

Contra-indications: pregnancy; oestrogen-dependent cancer, active thrombophlebitis, thromboembolic disorders or history of recurrent venous thromboembolism (unless already on anticoagulant treatment), liver disease (where liver function tests have failed to return to normal), Dubin-Johnson and Rotor syndromes (or monitor closely), undiagnosed vaginal bleeding, breast-feeding

Side-effects: nausea and vomiting, abdominal cramps and bloating, weight changes, breast enlargement and tenderness, premenstrual-like syndrome, sodium and fluid retention, changes in liver function, cholestatic jaundice, altered blood lipids, rashes and chloasma, changes in libido, depression, headache, migraine, dizziness, leg cramps (rule out venous thrombosis), contact lenses may irritate; transdermal delivery systems may cause contact sensitisation (possible severe hypersensitivity reaction on continued exposure), and headache has been reported on vigorous exercise; nasal spray may cause local irritation, rhinorrhoea and epistaxis

WITHDRAWAL BLEEDING. Cyclical HRT (where a progestogen is taken for 10–14 days of each 28-day oestrogen treatment cycle) usually results in *regular withdrawal bleeding* towards the end of the progestogen. The aim of continuous combined HRT (where a combination of oestrogen and progestogen is taken, usually in a single tablet, throughout each 28-day treatment cycle) is to avoid bleeding, but *irregular bleeding* may occur during the early treatment stages (if it continues endometrial abnormality should be excluded and consideration given to cyclical HRT instead)

Dose: see under preparations

COUNSELLING ON PATCHES. Patch should be removed after 3–4 days (or once a week in case of 7-day patch) and replaced with fresh patch on slightly different site; recommended sites: clean, dry, unbroken areas of skin on trunk below waistline; not to be applied on or near breasts or under waistband. If patch falls off in bath allow skin to cool before applying new patch

Women with uterus

The following preparations contain a **progestogen** as well as an **oestrogen** and are therefore suitable for a woman with an **intact uterus**; they are **not** suitable for use as (or with) hormonal contraceptives.

■ Conjugated oestrogens with progestogen

Premique® (Wyeth) [PoM]

Premique® tablets, s/c, blue, conjugated oestrogen (equine) 625 micrograms and medroxyprogesterone acetate 5 mg. Net price 3 × 28-tab pack = £24.87

Dose: menopausal symptoms and osteoporosis prophylaxis, in women with intact uterus, 1 tablet daily continuously (starting on day 1 of menstruation, if cycles have not ceased)

Premique® Cycle Calendar pack, all s/c, 14 white tablets, conjugated oestrogens (equine) 625 micrograms; 14 green tablets, conjugated oestrogens (equine) 625 micrograms and medroxyprogesterone acetate 10 mg, net price 3 × 28-tab pack = £22.62

Dose: menopausal symptoms and osteoporosis prophylaxis, 1 white tablet daily for 14 days, starting on day 1 of menstruation (or at any time if cycles have ceased or are infrequent) then 1 green tablet daily for 14 days; subsequent courses are repeated without interval

Prempak-C® (Wyeth) [PoM]

Prempak C® 0.625 Calendar pack, s/c, 28 maroon tablets, conjugated oestrogens (equine) 625 micrograms; 12 light brown tablets, nor-gestrel 150 micrograms (≡ levonorgestrel 75 micrograms). Net price 3 × 40-tab pack = £16.20

Dose: menopausal symptoms and osteoporosis prophylaxis, in women with intact uterus, 1 maroon tablet daily continuously, starting on day 1 of menstruation (or at any time if cycles have ceased or are infrequent), and 1 brown tablet daily on days 17–28 of each 28-day treatment cycle; subsequent courses are repeated without interval

Prempak C® 1.25 Calendar pack, s/c, 28 yellow tablets, conjugated oestrogens (equine) 1.25 mg; 12 light brown tablets, norgestrel 150 micrograms (≡ levonorgestrel 75 micrograms). Net price 3 × 40-tab pack = £16.20

Dose: see under 0.625 Calendar pack, but taking 1 yellow tablet daily continuously, (instead of 1 maroon tablet) if symptoms not fully controlled with lower strength

■ Estradiol with progestogen

Adgyn Combi® (Strakan) [PoM]

Tablets, 16 white, estradiol 2 mg; 12 pink, estradiol 2 mg, norethisterone 1 mg, net price 28-tab pack = £2.84

Dose: menopausal symptoms, 1 white tablet daily for 16 days, starting on day 5 of menstruation (or at any time if cycles have ceased or are infrequent) then 1 pink tablet daily for 12 days; subsequent courses are repeated without interval

Climagest® (Novartis) [PoM]

Climagest® 1-mg tablets, 16 grey-blue, estradiol valerate 1 mg; 12 white, estradiol valerate 1 mg and norethisterone 1 mg. Net price 28-tab pack = £4.78; 3 × 28-tab pack = £13.92

Dose: menopausal symptoms, 1 grey-blue tablet daily for 16 days, starting on day 1 of menstruation (or at any time if cycles have ceased or are infrequent) then 1 white tablet for 12 days; subsequent courses are repeated without interval

Climagest® 2-mg tablets, 16 blue, estradiol valerate 2 mg; 12 yellow, estradiol valerate 2 mg and norethisterone 1 mg. Net price 28-tab pack = £4.78; 3 × 28-tab pack = £13.92

Dose: see *Climagest® 1-mg*, but starting with 1 blue tablet daily (instead of 1 grey-blue tablet) if symptoms not controlled with lower strength

Climesse® (Novartis) PoM

Tablets, pink, estradiol valerate 2 mg, norethisterone 700 micrograms. Net price 1 × 28-tab pack = £8.62; 3 × 28-tab pack = £25.86

Dose: menopausal symptoms and osteoporosis prophylaxis, in women with intact uterus, 1 tablet daily continuously

Note. Unsuitable for use in perimenopausal women or within 12 months of last menstrual period—see Choice above

Cyclo-Progynova® (ASTA Medica) PoM

Cyclo-Progynova® 1-mg Tablets, all s/c, 11 beige, estradiol valerate 1 mg; 10 brown, estradiol valerate 1 mg and levonorgestrel 250 micrograms. Net price per pack = £3.34

Dose: menopausal symptoms, in women with intact uterus, 1 beige tablet daily for 11 days, starting on day 5 of menstruation (or at any time if cycles have ceased or are infrequent), then 1 brown tablet daily for 10 days, followed by a 7-day interval

Cyclo-Progynova® 2-mg Tablets, all s/c, 11 white, estradiol valerate 2 mg; 10 brown, estradiol valerate 2 mg and norgestrel 500 micrograms (≡ levonorgestrel 250 micrograms). Net price per pack = £3.34

Dose: menopausal symptoms and osteoporosis prophylaxis as *Cyclo-Progynova® 1-mg*, but starting with 1 white tablet daily for 11 days, then 1 brown tablet daily for 10 days, followed by a 7-day interval

Elleste-Duet® (Pharmacia) PoM

Elleste-Duet® 1-mg tablets, 16 white, estradiol 1 mg; 12 green, estradiol 1 mg and norethisterone acetate 1 mg. Net price 3 × 28-tab pack = £9.72

Dose: menopausal symptoms, 1 white tablet daily for 16 days starting on day 1 of menstruation (or at any time if cycles have ceased or are infrequent), then 1 green tablet daily for 12 days; subsequent courses are repeated without interval

Elleste-Duet® 2-mg tablets, 16 orange, estradiol 2 mg; 12 grey, estradiol 2 mg, norethisterone acetate 1 mg. Net price 3 × 28-tab pack = £9.72

Dose: menopausal symptoms and osteoporosis prophylaxis, 1 orange tablet daily for 16 days, starting on day 1 of menstruation (or at any time if cycles have ceased or are infrequent) then 1 grey tablet daily for 12 days; subsequent courses are repeated without interval

Elleste-Duet Conti® tablets, f/c, grey, estradiol 2 mg, norethisterone acetate 1 mg. Net price 3 × 28–tab pack = £17.97.

Dose: menopausal symptoms and osteoporosis prophylaxis, in women with intact uterus, 1 tablet daily on a continuous basis (if changing from cyclical HRT begin treatment at the end of scheduled bleed)

Note. Unsuitable for use in perimenopausal women or within 12 months of last menstrual period—see Choice above

Estracombi® (Novartis) PoM

Combination pack, self-adhesive patches of *Estraderm TTS® 50* (releasing estradiol approx. 50 micrograms/24 hours) and of *Estragest TTS®* (releasing estradiol approx. 50 micrograms/24 hours and norethisterone acetate 250 micrograms/24 hours); net price 1-month pack (4 of each) =

£11.14, 3-month pack (12 of each) = £33.42. Counselling, administration

Dose: menopausal symptoms and osteoporosis prophylaxis, in women with intact uterus, starting within 5 days of onset of menstruation (or any time if cycles have ceased or are infrequent), 1 *Estraderm TTS® 50* patch to be applied twice weekly for 2 weeks followed by 1 *Estragest TTS®* patch twice weekly for 2 weeks; subsequent courses are repeated without interval

Estrapak 50® (Novartis) PoM

Combination pack, self-adhesive patches of *Estraderm TTS® 50* (releasing estradiol approx. 50 micrograms/24 hours) and tablets, red, norethisterone acetate 1 mg; net price 1-month pack (8 patches plus 12 tablets) = £10.34, 3-month pack (24 patches plus 36 tablets) = £31.03. Counselling, administration

Dose: menopausal symptoms and osteoporosis prophylaxis, in women with intact uterus, starting within 5 days of onset of menstruation (or at any time if cycles have ceased or are infrequent), apply 1 patch twice weekly continuously, and take 1 tablet daily on days 15–26 of each 28-day treatment cycle

Evorel® (Janssen-Cilag) PoM

Evorel® Conti patches, self-adhesive, (releasing estradiol approx. 50 micrograms/24 hours and norethisterone acetate approx. 170 micrograms/24 hours), net price 8-patch pack = £12.90, 24-patch pack = £38.70. Counselling, administration

Dose: menopausal symptoms and osteoporosis prophylaxis, in women with intact uterus, 1 patch to be applied twice weekly continuously

Evorel® Pak calendar pack, 8 self-adhesive patches (releasing estradiol approx. 50 micrograms/24 hours) and 12 tablets, norethisterone 1 mg, net price per pack = £8.45. Counselling, administration

Dose: menopausal symptoms and osteoporosis prophylaxis, in women with intact uterus, apply 1 patch twice weekly continuously (increased if necessary for menopausal symptoms to 2 patches twice weekly after first month) and take 1 tablet daily on days 15–26 of each 28-day treatment cycle

Evorel® Sequi combination pack, 4 self-adhesive patches of *Evorel® 50* (releasing estradiol approx. 50 micrograms/24 hours) and 4 self-adhesive patches of *Evorel® Conti* (releasing estradiol approx. 50 micrograms/24 hours and norethisterone acetate approx. 170 micrograms/24 hours), net price 8-patch pack = £11.00. Counselling, administration

Dose: menopausal symptoms and osteoporosis prophylaxis, in women with intact uterus, 1 *Evorel® 50* patch to be applied twice weekly for 2 weeks followed by 1 *Evorel® Conti* patch twice weekly for 2 weeks; subsequent courses are repeated without interval

Femapak® (Solvay) PoM

Femapak® 40 combination pack of 8 self-adhesive patches of *Fematrix® 40* (releasing estradiol approx. 40 micrograms/24 hours) and 14 tablets of *Duphaston®* (dydrogesterone 10 mg). Net price per pack = £8.45. Counselling, administration

Dose: see under *Femapak® 80*

Femapak® 80 combination pack of 8 self-adhesive patches of *Fematrix® 80* (releasing estradiol approx. 80 micrograms/24 hours) and 14 tablets

of *Duphaston®* (dydrogesterone 10 mg). Net price
per pack = £8.95. Counselling, administration
Dose: menopausal symptoms (and osteoporosis prophylaxis in case of *Femapak® 80* **only**), in women with
intact uterus, starting within 5 days of onset of menstruation (or any time if cycles have ceased or are infrequent),
apply 1 patch twice weekly continuously and take 1 tablet daily on days 15–28 of each 28-day treatment cycle;
therapy should be initiated with *Femapak® 40* in those
with menopausal symptoms, prolonged oestrogen deficiency or anticipated intolerance to higher strengths,
subsequently adjusted to lowest effective dose

Femoston® (Solvay) PoM

Femoston® 1/10 tablets, both f/c, 14 white, estradiol 1 mg; 14 grey, estradiol 1 mg, dydrogesterone
10 mg. Net price 3 × 28-tab pack = £14.97
Dose: menopausal symptoms and osteoporosis prophylaxis, in women with intact uterus, 1 white tablet daily
for 14 days, starting within 5 days of onset of menstruation (or any time if cycles have ceased or are infrequent)
then 1 grey tablet for 14 days; subsequent courses are
repeated without interval; for osteoporosis prophylaxis
Femoston® 2/10 is given first—*Femoston® 1/10* is substituted only if the higher dose is not tolerated
Femoston® 2/10 tablets, both f/c, 14 red, estradiol
2 mg; 14 yellow, estradiol 2 mg, dydrogesterone
10 mg. Net price 3 × 28-tab pack = £14.97
Dose: menopausal symptoms and osteoporosis prophylaxis, in women with intact uterus, 1 orange tablet daily
for 14 days, starting within 5 days of onset of menstruation (or any time if cycles have ceased or are infrequent)
then 1 yellow tablet daily for 14 days; subsequent
courses are repeated without interval; where therapy is
required for control of menopausal symptoms alone,
Femoston® 1/10 is given initially and *Femoston® 2/10*
substituted if symptom control is not achieved
Femoston® 2/20 tablets, both f/c, 14 red, estradiol
2 mg; 14 blue, estradiol 2 mg, dydrogesterone
20 mg. Net price 3 × 28-tab pack = £22.44
Dose: see *Femoston® 2/10*, but taking 1 blue tablet
(instead of 1 yellow tablet) if withdrawal bleed is early
or endometrial biopsy shows inadequate progestational
response
Femoston®-conti tablets, f/c, salmon, estradiol
1 mg, dydrogesterone 5 mg, net price 3 × 28-tab
pack = £22.62
Dose: menopausal symptoms and osteoporosis prophylaxis, in women with intact uterus, 1 tablet daily continuously (if changing from cyclical HRT begin treatment
the day after finishing oestrogen plus progestogen
phase)
Note. Unsuitable for use in perimenopausal women or
within 12 months of last menstrual period—see Choice
above

Indivina® (Orion) PoM

Indivina® 1 mg/2.5 mg tablets, estradiol valerate
1 mg, medroxyprogesterone acetate 2.5 mg, net
price 3 × 28-tab pack = £22.62
Indivina® 1 mg/5 mg tablets, estradiol valerate
1 mg, medroxyprogesterone acetate 5 mg, net
price 3 × 28-tab pack = £22.62
Indivina® 2 mg/5 mg tablets, estradiol valerate
2 mg, medroxyprogesterone acetate 5 mg, net
price 3 × 28-tab pack = £22.62
Dose: menopausal symptoms and osteoporosis prophylaxis, in women with intact uterus, 1 tablet daily continuously; initiate therapy with *Indivina® 1 mg/2.5 mg*
tablets and adjust according to response; start at end of
scheduled bleed if changing from cyclical HRT
Note. Less suitable for use in perimenopausal women or
within 3 years of last menstrual period—see Choice
above

Kliofem® (Novo Nordisk) PoM

Tablets, yellow, estradiol 2 mg, norethisterone
acetate 1 mg. Net price 3 × 28-tab pack = £25.95
Dose: menopausal symptoms and osteoporosis prophylaxis, in women with intact uterus, 1 tablet daily continuously; start at end of scheduled bleed if changing from
cyclical HRT
Note. Unsuitable for use in perimenopausal women or
within 12 months of last menstrual period—see Choice
above

Kliovance® (Novo Nordisk) PoM

Tablets, f/c, estradiol 1mg, norethisterone acetate
500 micrograms, net price 3 × 28-tab pack =
£25.95
Dose: menopausal symptoms and osteoporosis prophylaxis, in women with intact uterus, 1 tablet daily continuously; start at end of scheduled bleed if changing from
cyclical HRT
Note. Unsuitable for use in perimenopausal women or
within 12 months of last menstrual period—see Choice
above

Nuvelle® (Schering Health) PoM

Nuvelle® tablets, all s/c, 16 white, estradiol valerate 2 mg; 12 pink, estradiol valerate 2 mg and
levonorgestrel 75 micrograms. Net price 3 × 28-
tab pack = £15.15
Dose: menopausal symptoms and osteoporosis prophylaxis, in women with intact uterus, 1 white tablet daily
for 16 days, starting on day 5 of menstruation (or any
time if cycles have ceased or are infrequent) then 1 pink
tablet daily for 12 days; subsequent courses are repeated
without interval
Nuvelle® Continuous tablets, f/c, pink, estradiol
2 mg, norethisterone acetate 1 mg, net price 3 x
28-tab pack = £18.02
Dose: menopausal symptoms and osteoporosis prophylaxis, in women with intact uterus, 1 tablet daily continuously; start at end of scheduled bleed if changing from
cyclical HRT
Note. Unsuitable for use in perimenopausal women or
within 12 months of last menstrual period—see Choice
above
Nuvelle® TS, combination pack of self-adhesive
patches of *Nuvelle® TS Phase I* (releasing estradiol approx. 80 micrograms/24 hours) and of *Nuv-
elle® TS Phase II* (releasing estradiol approx.
50 micrograms/24 hours and levonorgestrel
approx. 20 micrograms/24 hours); net price 1-
month pack (4 of each) = £10.51. Counselling,
administration
Dose: menopausal symptoms, in women with intact
uterus, starting within 5 days of onset of menstruation
(or any time if cycles have ceased or are infrequent) 1
Phase I patch to be applied twice weekly for 2 weeks
followed by 1 *Phase II* patch twice weekly for 2 weeks;
subsequent courses are repeated without interval

Tridestra® (Orion) PoM

Tablets, 70 white, estradiol valerate 2 mg; 14 blue,
estradiol valerate 2 mg and medroxyprogesterone
acetate 20 mg; 7 yellow, inactive. Net price 91-tab
pack = £23.78
Dose: menopausal symptoms and osteoporosis prophylaxis, in women with intact uterus, 1 white tablet daily
for 70 days, then 1 blue tablet daily for 14 days, then 1
yellow tablet daily for 7 days; subsequent courses are
repeated without interval

Trisequens® (Novo Nordisk) PoM

Trisequens® tablets, 12 blue, estradiol 2 mg; 10
white, estradiol 2 mg, norethisterone acetate

1 mg; 6 red, estradiol 1 mg, net price 3 × 28-tab pack = £14.40

Dose: menopausal symptoms and osteoporosis prophylaxis, in women with intact uterus, 1 blue tablet daily, starting on day 5 of menstruation (or at any time if cycles have ceased or are infrequent), then 1 tablet daily in sequence (without interruption)

Trisequens Forte® tablets, 12 yellow, estradiol 4 mg; 10 white, estradiol 4 mg, norethisterone acetate 1 mg; 6 red, estradiol 1 mg, net price 3 × 28-tab pack = £14.40

Dose: menopausal symptoms, see under *Trisequens®*, starting with 1 yellow tablet daily (instead of 1 blue tablet) if symptoms not fully controlled with lower strength

Women without uterus

The following preparations do **not** contain a **progestogen**; if the uterus is intact they need to be given with a progestogen in which case packs incorporating a suitable progestogen tablet are preferred (see above).

■ Conjugated oestrogens only

Premarin® (Wyeth) PoM

Tablets, all s/c, conjugated oestrogens (equine) 625 micrograms (maroon), net price 3 × 28-tab pack = £8.91; 1.25 mg (yellow), 3 × 28-tab pack = £12.09

Dose: menopausal symptoms and osteoporosis prophylaxis, (with progestogen for 12–14 days per cycle in women with intact uterus), 0.625–1.25 mg daily

■ Estradiol only

Estradiol Implants (Organon) PoM

Implant, estradiol 25 mg, net price each = £9.59; 50 mg, each = £19.16; 100 mg, each = £33.40

Dose: by implantation, oestrogen replacement, and osteoporosis prophylaxis (with cyclical progestogen for 10–13 days of each cycle in women with intact uterus, see notes above), 25–100 mg as required (usually every 4–8 months) according to oestrogen levels—check before each implant

Note. On removing implant for the last time from those with intact uterus, cyclical progesterone should be continued until withdrawal bleed stops

Adgyn Estro® (Strakan) PoM

Tablets, estradiol 2 mg, net price 28-tab pack = £1.56

Dose: menopausal symptoms, with cyclical progestogen for 10–14 days of each cycle in women with intact uterus, 1 tablet daily starting on day 5 of menstruation (or at any time if cycles have ceased or are infrequent)

Aerodiol® (Servier) ▼ PoM

Nasal spray, estradiol 150 micrograms/metered spray, net price 4.2-mL unit (60 metered sprays) = £6.77

Dose: menopausal symptoms, initially 1 spray into each nostril daily at the same time each day *either* continuously *or* for 21–28 days followed by a 2–7 day treatment-free interval; daily dose adjusted according to response to 1–4 sprays daily in divided doses; with cyclical progestogen for at least 12 days of each cycle in women with intact uterus; not to be used immediately after nasal corticosteroid or nasal vasoconstrictor

Note. If patient has a severely blocked nose, *Aerodiol®* may be temporarily administered into the mouth between the cheek and the gum above the upper teeth; in this situation the normal dose should be doubled

Climaval® (Novartis) PoM

Tablets, estradiol valerate 1 mg (grey-blue), net price 1 × 28-tab pack = £2.55, 3 × 28-tab pack = £7.66; 2 mg (blue), 1 × 28-tab pack = £2.55, 3 × 28-tab pack = £7.66

Dose: menopausal symptoms (if patient has had a hysterectomy), 1–2 mg daily

Dermestril® (Strakan) PoM

Patches, self-adhesive, estradiol, '*25' patch* (releasing approx. 25 micrograms/24 hours), net price 8-patch pack = £4.55; '*50' patch* (releasing approx. 50 micrograms/24 hours), 8-patch pack = £4.56; '*100' patch* (releasing approx. 100 micrograms/24 hours), 8-patch pack = £5.52. Counselling, administration

Dose: menopausal symptoms, 1 patch to be applied every 3–4 days continuously; (with cyclical progestogen for 10–12 days of each cycle in women with intact uterus); therapy should be initiated with '*50' patch* for first month, subsequently adjusted to lowest effective dose

Dermestril®-Septem (Strakan) PoM

Patches, self-adhesive, estradiol, '*25' patch* (releasing approx. 25 micrograms/24 hours), net price 4-patch pack = £4.55; '*50' patch* (releasing approx. 50 micrograms/24 hours), 4-patch pack = £4.56; '*75' patch* (releasing approx. 75 micrograms/24 hours), 4-patch pack = £5.29. Counselling, administration

Dose: menopausal symptoms, 1 patch to be applied once weekly *either* continuously *or* on a cyclical basis (1 patch weekly for 3–4 weeks, followed by a 2–7 day treatment-free interval); with cyclical progestogen for at least 12 days of each cycle in women with intact uterus; therapy should be initiated with '*50' patch* for the first 4–8 weeks, subsequently adjusted to lowest effective dose

Elleste-Solo® (Pharmacia) PoM

Elleste-Solo® 1-mg tablets, estradiol 1 mg. Net price 3 × 28-tab pack = £5.34

Dose: menopausal symptoms, with cyclical progestogen for 12–14 days of each cycle in women with intact uterus, 1 mg daily starting on day 1 of menstruation (or at any time if cycles have ceased or are infrequent)

Elleste-Solo® 2-mg tablets, orange, estradiol 2 mg. Net price 3 × 28-tab pack = £5.34

Dose: menopausal symptoms not controlled with lower strength and osteoporosis prophylaxis, with cyclical progestogen for 12–14 days of each cycle in women with intact uterus, 2 mg daily starting on day 1 of menstruation (or at any time if cycles have ceased or are infrequent)

Elleste Solo® MX (Pharmacia) PoM

Patches, self-adhesive, estradiol, *MX 40 patch* (releasing approx. 40 micrograms/24 hours), net price 8-patch pack = £5.19; *MX 80 patch* (releasing approx. 80 micrograms/24 hours), 8-patch pack = £5.99. Counselling, administration.

Dose: menopausal symptoms (and osteoporosis prophylaxis in case of *Elleste Solo MX 80®* **only**), 1 patch to be applied twice weekly continuously starting within 5 days of onset of menstruation (or at any time if cycles have ceased or are infrequent); with cyclical progestogen for 12–14 days of each cycle in women with intact uterus; therapy should be initiated with *MX 40* in those with menopausal symptoms, prolonged oestrogen deficiency or anticipated intolerance to higher strength, dosage may be increased if required, subsequently adjusted to lowest effective dose

Estraderm MX® (Novartis) PoM

Patches, self-adhesive, estradiol, *MX 25 patch* (releasing approx. 25 micrograms/24 hours), net price 8-patch pack = £5.20, 24-patch pack = £15.59; *MX 50 patch* (releasing approx. 50 micrograms/24 hours), 8-patch pack = £5.22, 24-patch pack = £15.65, 20-patch pack (hosp. only) = £13.04; *MX 75 patch* (releasing approx. 75 micrograms/24 hours), 8-patch pack = £6.08, 24-patch pack = £18.25; *MX 100 patch* (releasing approx. 100 micrograms/24 hours), 8-patch pack = £6.31, 24-patch pack = £18.94. Counselling, administration

Dose: menopausal symptoms (and osteoporosis prophylaxis in case of *Estraderm MX® 50* and *75* **only**), 1 patch to be applied twice weekly continuously, with cyclical progestogen for 12 days of each cycle in women with intact uterus; therapy should be initiated with *MX 50* for first month, subsequently adjusted to lowest effective dose

Estraderm TTS® (Novartis) PoM

Patches, self-adhesive, estradiol, *TTS 25 patch* (releasing approx. 25 micrograms/24 hours), net price, 8-patch pack = £6.21, 24-patch pack = £18.63; *TTS 50 patch* (releasing approx. 50 micrograms/24 hours), 8-patch pack = £6.23, 24-patch pack = £18.69; *TTS 100 patch* (releasing approx. 100 micrograms/24 hours), 8-patch pack = £7.52, 24-patch pack = £22.63, 20-patch pack (hosp. only) = £16.76 . Counselling, administration

Dose: menopausal symptoms (and osteoporosis prophylaxis in case of *Estraderm TTS® 50* **only**), 1 patch to be applied twice weekly continuously, with cyclical progestogen for 12 days of each cycle in women with intact uterus; therapy should be initiated with *TTS 50* for first month, subsequently adjusted to lowest effective dose

Evorel® (Janssen-Cilag) PoM

Patches, self-adhesive, estradiol, *'25' patch* (releasing approx. 25 micrograms/24 hours), net price 8-patch pack = £4.39; *'50' patch* (releasing approx. 50 micrograms/24 hours), 8-patch pack = £4.84, 24-patch pack = £14.52; *'75' patch* (releasing approx. 75 micrograms/24 hours), 8-patch pack = £5.14; *'100' patch* (releasing approx. 100 micrograms/24 hours), 8-patch pack = £5.33. Counselling, administration

Dose: menopausal symptoms and osteoporosis prophylaxis (except *Evorel® 25*), 1 patch to be applied twice weekly continuously, with cyclical progestogen for at least 12 days of each cycle in women with intact uterus; therapy should be initiated with *'50' patch* for first month, subsequently adjusted to lowest effective dose

Fematrix® (Solvay) PoM

Fematrix® 40 patch, self-adhesive, estradiol, *'40' patch* (releasing approx. 40 micrograms/24 hours). Net price 8-patch pack = £5.50. Counselling, administration

Dose: menopausal symptoms, 1 patch to be applied twice weekly continuously starting within 5 days of onset of menstruation (or at any time if cycles have ceased or are infrequent), with cyclical progestogen for 12–14 days of each cycle in women with intact uterus; *'80' patch* may be used if required (subsequently adjusted to lowest effective dose)

Fematrix® 80 patch, self-adhesive, estradiol (releasing approx. 80 micrograms/24 hours). Net price 8-patch pack = £6.00. Counselling, administration

Dose: menopausal symptoms and osteoporosis prophylaxis, as for *Fematrix® 40*; therapy should be initiated

with *Fematrix® 40* in those with menopausal symptoms, prolonged oestrogen deficiency or anticipated intolerance to higher strength

FemSeven® (Merck) PoM

Patches, self-adhesive, estradiol, *'50' patch* (releasing approx. 50 micrograms/24 hours), net price 4-patch pack = £4.57, 12-patch pack = £13.65; *'75' patch* (releasing approx. 75 micrograms/24 hours), net price 4-patch pack = £5.29; *'100' patch* (releasing approx.100 micrograms/24 hours), net price 4-patch pack = £5.52. Counselling, administration

Dose: menopausal symptoms and osteoporosis prophylaxis, 1 patch to be applied once a week continuously, with cyclical progestogen for at least 10 days of each cycle in women with intact uterus; therapy should be initiated with *FemSeven® 50* patches for the first few months, subsequently adjusted according to response

Menorest® (Novartis) PoM

Patches, self-adhesive, estradiol, *'37.5' patch* (releasing approx. 37.5 micrograms/24 hours), net price 8-patch pack = £7.57; *'50' patch* (releasing approx. 50 micrograms/24 hours), 8-patch pack = £7.69; *'75' patch* (releasing approx. 75 micrograms/24 hours), 8-patch pack = £8.95. Counselling administration

Dose: menopausal symptoms and osteoporosis prophylaxis (except *Menorest® 37.5*), 1 patch to be applied twice weekly continuously, with cyclical progestogen for at least 12 days of each cycle in women with intact uterus; therapy should be initiated with *'50' patch* for first month, subsequently adjusted to lowest effective dose

Oestrogel® (Hoechst Marion Roussel) PoM

Gel, estradiol 0.06%, net price 64-dose pump pack = £7.95. Counselling, administration

Dose: menopausal symptoms and osteoporosis prophylaxis, 2 measures (estradiol 1.5 mg) to be applied over an area twice that of the template provided once daily continuously , starting within 5 days of menstruation (or anytime if cycles have ceased or are infrequent), with cyclical progestogen for 12 days of each cycle in women with intact uterus; for menopausal symptoms may be increased if necessary after 1 month to max. 4 measures daily

COUNSELLING. Apply gel to clean, dry, intact skin such as arms, shoulders or inner thighs and allow to dry for 5 minutes before covering with clothing. Not to be applied on or near breasts or on vulval region. Avoid skin contact with another person (particularly male) and avoid other skin products or washing the area for at least 1 hour after application

Progynova® (Schering Health) PoM

Tablets, both s/c, estradiol valerate 1 mg (beige), net price 3 × 28-tab pack = £7.72; 2 mg (blue), 3 × 28-tab pack = £7.72

Dose: menopausal symptoms, 1–2 mg daily continuously; osteoporosis prophylaxis, 2 mg daily continuously; with cyclical progestogen for 12 days of each cycle in women with intact uterus

Progynova® TS (Schering Health) PoM

Patches, self-adhesive, *Progynova®* TS (releasing estradiol approx. 50 micrograms/24 hours), net price 12-patch pack = £17.88; *Progynova® TS forte* (releasing estradiol approx. 100 micrograms/24 hours), 12-patch pack = £19.68. Counselling, administration

Dose: menopausal symptoms, 1 patch to be applied once a week on a continuous or cyclical basis (1 patch per week for three weeks followed by a 7-day patch-free interval), with cyclical progestogen for 12 days of each cycle in women with intact uterus; therapy should be initiated with *Progynova® TS* and subsequently adjusted to lowest effective dose

Sandrena® (Organon) PoM

Gel, estradiol (0.1%), 500 microgram/500 mg sachet, net price 28-sachet pack = £5.68, 1 mg/1 g sachet, 28-sachet pack = £6.54. Counselling, administration

Dose: menopausal symptoms, estradiol 1 mg (1 g gel) to be applied once daily over area 1–2 times size of hand; with cyclical progestogen for 10–12 days of each cycle in women with intact uterus; dose may be adjusted after 2–3 cycles to a usual dose of estradiol 0.5–1.5 mg (0.5–1.5 g gel) daily

COUNSELLING. Apply gel to intact areas of skin such as lower trunk or thighs, using right and left sides on alternate days. Wash hands after application. Not to be applied on the breasts or face and avoid contact with eyes. Allow area of application to dry for 5 minutes and do not wash area for at least 1 hour

Zumenon® (Solvay) PoM

Tablets, f/c, estradiol 1 mg, net price 84-tab pack = £7.65; 2 mg (red), 84-tab pack = £7.65

Dose: menopausal symptoms, initially 1 mg daily starting on day 5 of menstruation (or any time if cycles have ceased or are infrequent) adjusted to 1–4 mg daily according to response; osteoporosis prophylaxis, 2 mg daily; with cyclical progestogen for 10–14 days of each cycle in women with intact uterus

■ Estradiol, estriol and estrone only

Hormonin® (Shire) PoM

Tablets, pink, estradiol 600 micrograms, estriol 270 micrograms, estrone 1.4 mg. Net price 90-tab pack = £7.08

Dose: menopausal symptoms and osteoporosis prophylaxis, 1–2 tablets daily, with cyclical progestogen for 12–14 days of each cycle in women with intact uterus

Note. *Hormonin®* tablets can be given continuously or cyclically (21 days out of 28)

■ Estriol only

Ovestin® (Organon) PoM

Tablets, scored, estriol 1 mg. Net price 30-tab pack = £4.20. Label: 25

Dose: genito-urinary symptoms associated with oestrogen-deficiency states, 0.5–3 mg daily, as single dose, for up to 1 month, then 0.5–1 mg daily until restoration of epithelial integrity (short-term use)

■ Estropipate only

Harmogen® (Pharmacia) PoM

Tablets, peach, scored, estropipate 1.5 mg. Net price 28-tab pack = £3.00

Dose: menopausal symptoms and osteoporosis prophylaxis, 1.5 mg daily continuously (with cyclical progestogen for 10–13 days of each cycle in women with intact uterus); up to 3 mg daily (in single or divided doses) for vasomotor symptoms and menopausal vaginitis

Raloxifene

Raloxifene is licensed for the treatment and prevention of postmenopausal osteoporosis; unlike hormone replacement therapy, raloxifene does not reduce menopausal vasomotor symptoms.

Raloxifene may reduce the incidence of oestrogen-receptor-positive breast cancer but its role in established breast cancer is not yet clear. The manufacturer advises avoiding its use in breast cancer.

RALOXIFENE HYDROCHLORIDE

Indications: treatment and prevention of postmenopausal osteoporosis

Cautions: risk factors for venous thromboembolism (discontinue if prolonged immobilisation); breast cancer (see notes above); **interactions:** Appendix 1 (raloxifene)

Contra-indications: history of venous thromboembolism, undiagnosed uterine bleeding, endometrial cancer, hepatic impairment, cholestasis, severe renal impairment; pregnancy and breast-feeding

Side-effects: venous thromboembolism, thrombophlebitis, hot flushes, leg cramps, peripheral oedema, influenza-like symptoms; rarely rashes and gastro-intestinal disturbances

Dose: 60 mg once daily

Evista® (Lilly) ▼ PoM

Tablets, f/c, raloxifene hydrochloride 60 mg, net price 28-tab pack = £19.76; 84-tab pack = £59.28

Tibolone

Tibolone combines oestrogenic and progestogenic activity with weak androgenic activity. It is indicated for the treatment of vasomotor symptoms of the menopause and osteoporosis prophylaxis. Tibolone is given continuously, without cyclical progestogen.

TIBOLONE

Indications: vasomotor symptoms in oestrogen deficiency (including women being treated with gonadotrophin releasing hormone analogues), osteoporosis prophylaxis

Cautions: renal impairment, history of liver disease, epilepsy, migraine, diabetes mellitus, hypercholesterolaemia; withdraw if signs of thromboembolic disease, abnormal liver function tests or cholestatic jaundice; see also Note below; **interactions:** Appendix 1 (tibolone)

Contra-indications: hormone-dependent tumours, history of cardiovascular or cerebrovascular disease (e.g. thrombophlebitis, thromboembolism), uninvestigated vaginal bleeding, severe liver disease, pregnancy, breast-feeding

Side-effects: weight changes, oedema, dizziness, seborrhoeic dermatitis, vaginal bleeding, headache, abdominal pain, gastro-intestinal disturbances, increased facial hair; depression, arthralgia, myalgia, migraine, visual disturbances, liver-function changes, rash and pruritus also reported

Dose: 2.5 mg daily

Note. Unsuitable for use in the premenopause (unless being treated with gonadotrophin-releasing hormone analogue) and as (or with) an oral contraceptive; also unsuitable for use within 12 months of last menstrual period (may cause irregular bleeding); induce withdrawal bleed with progestogen if transferring from another form of HRT

Livial® (Organon) PoM

Tablets, tibolone 2.5 mg. Net price 28-tab pack = £13.05; 3 × 28-tab pack = £39.14

Ethinylestradiol

Ethinylestradiol (ethinyloestradiol) has been used as hormone replacement for menopausal symptoms in a dose of 10–20 micrograms daily. This has now been largely replaced by more appropriate forms of oestrogen.

Ethinylestradiol is occasionally used, under **specialist supervision**, for the management of *hereditary haemorrhagic telangiectasia* (but evidence of any beneficial effect is uncertain). Side-effects include nausea, fluid retention, and thrombosis. Impotence and gynaecomastia occur in men.

For use in breast cancer, see section 8.3.1.

ETHINYLESTRADIOL

(Ethinyloestradiol)

Indications: see notes above

Cautions: cardiovascular disease (sodium retention with oedema, thromboembolism), hepatic impairment (jaundice); see also under Combined Oral Contraceptives (section 7.3.1) and under Oestrogen for HRT (above)

Contra-indications: see under Combined Oral Contraceptives (section 7.3.1) and under Oestrogen for HRT (above)

Side-effects: feminising effects in men; see also under Combined Oral Contraceptives (section 7.3.1) and under Oestrogen for HRT (above)

Dose: see notes above

Ethinylestradiol (Non-proprietary) PoM
Tablets, ethinylestradiol 10 micrograms, net price 21-tab pack = £12.99; 50 micrograms, 21-tab pack = £15.49; 1 mg, 28-tab pack = £28.85
Available from Celltech

6.4.1.2 Progestogens

There are two main groups of progestogen, *progesterone and its analogues* (dydrogesterone, hydroxyprogesterone, and medroxyprogesterone) and *testosterone analogues* (norethisterone and norgestrel). The newer progestogens (desogestrel, norgestimate, and gestodene) are all derivatives of norgestrel; levonorgestrel is the active isomer of norgestrel and has twice its potency. Progesterone and its analogues are less androgenic than the testosterone derivatives and neither progesterone nor dydrogesterone causes virilisation.

Where *endometriosis* requires drug treatment, it may respond to a progestogen, e.g. norethisterone, administered on a continuous basis. Danazol, gestrinone, and gonadorelin analogues are also available (section 6.7.2).

Although oral progestogens have been used widely for *menorrhagia* they are relatively ineffective compared with tranexamic acid (section 2.11) or, particularly where dysmenorrhoea is also a factor, mefenamic acid (section 10.1.1); the levonorgestrel-releasing intra-uterine system (section 7.3.2.3) may be particularly useful for women also requiring contraception. Oral progestogens have also been used for *severe dysmenorrhoea*, but where contraception is also required in younger

women the best choice is a combined oral contraceptive (section 7.3.1).

Progestogens have also been advocated for the alleviation of *premenstrual symptoms*, but no convincing physiological basis for such treatment has been shown.

Progestogens have been used for the prevention of spontaneous abortion in women with a history of *recurrent miscarriage* (habitual abortion) but there is no evidence of benefit and they are **not** recommended for this purpose. In pregnant women with antiphospholipid antibody syndrome who have suffered recurrent miscarriage, administration of low-dose aspirin (section 2.9) and a prophylactic dose of a low molecular weight heparin (section 2.8.1) may decrease the risk of fetal loss (use under specialist supervision only).

HORMONE REPLACEMENT THERAPY. In women with a uterus a progestogen needs to be added to *long-term oestrogen therapy for hormone replacement*, to prevent cystic hyperplasia of the endometrium and possible transformation to cancer; it can be added on a cyclical or a continuous basis. Combined packs incorporating suitable progestogen tablets are available, see p. 350.

ORAL CONTRACEPTION. Desogestrel, etynodiol (ethynodiol), gestodene, levonorgestrel, norethisterone, and norgestimate are used in *combined oral contraceptives* and in *progestogen-only contraceptives* (section 7.3.1 and section 7.3.2).

CANCER. Progestogens also have a role in *neoplastic disease* (section 8.3.2).

CAUTIONS. Progestogens should be used with caution in conditions that may worsen with fluid retention e.g. epilepsy, hypertension, migraine, asthma, cardiac or renal dysfunction, and in those susceptible to thromboembolism (particular caution with high dose). Care is also required in liver impairment (avoid if severe), and in those with a history of depression. Progestogens can decrease glucose tolerance and diabetes should be monitored closely. For **interactions** see Appendix 1 (progestogens).

CONTRA-INDICATIONS. Progestogens should be avoided in patients with a history of liver tumours, and in severe liver impairment. They are also contra-indicated in those with genital or breast cancer (unless progestogens are being used in the management of these conditions), severe arterial disease, undiagnosed vaginal bleeding and porphyria (section 9.8.2). Progestogens should not be used if there is a history during pregnancy of idiopathic jaundice, severe pruritus, or pemphigoid gestationis.

SIDE-EFFECTS. Side-effects of progestogens include menstrual disturbances, premenstrual-like syndrome (including bloating, fluid retention, breast tenderness), weight gain, nausea, headache, dizziness, insomnia, drowsiness, depression; also skin reactions (including urticaria, pruritus, rash, and acne), hirsutism and alopecia. Jaundice and anaphylactoid reactions have also been reported.

DYDROGESTERONE

Indications: see under Dose and notes above

Cautions: see notes above; breast-feeding (Appendix 5)

Contra-indications: see notes above

Side-effects: see notes above

Dose: endometriosis, 10 mg 2–3 times daily from day 5 to 25 of cycle or continuously

Infertility, irregular cycles, 10 mg twice daily from day 11 to 25 for at least 6 cycles (but not recommended)

Recurrent miscarriage, 10 mg twice daily from day 11 to 25 of cycle until conception, then continuously until week 20 of pregnancy and then gradually reduced (but not recommended, see notes above)

Dysfunctional uterine bleeding, 10 mg twice daily (together with an oestrogen) for 5–7 days to arrest bleeding; 10 mg twice daily (together with an oestrogen) from day 11 to 25 of cycle to prevent bleeding

Dysmenorrhoea (but see notes above), 10 mg twice daily from day 5 to 25 of cycle

Amenorrhoea, 10 mg twice daily from day 11 to 25 of cycle with oestrogen therapy from day 1 to 25 of cycle

Premenstrual syndrome, 10 mg twice daily from day 12 to 26 of cycle increased if necessary (but not recommended, see notes above)

Hormone replacement therapy, with continuous oestrogen therapy, see under *Duphaston® HRT* below

Duphaston® (Solvay) PoM
Tablets, scored, dydrogesterone 10 mg. Net price 60-tab pack = £4.49

Duphaston® HRT (Solvay) PoM
Tablets, scored, dydrogesterone 10 mg. Net price 42-tab pack = £3.14
> *Dose:* 10 mg daily on days 15–28 of each 28-day oestrogen HRT cycle, increased to 10 mg twice daily if withdrawal bleed is early or endometrial biopsy shows inadequate progestational response

HYDROXYPROGESTERONE CAPROATE ◣▬

(Hydroxyprogesterone Hexanoate)

Indications: recurrent miscarriage but see notes above

Cautions: see notes above; monitor pregnancy regularly (Appendix 4), breast-feeding

Contra-indications: see notes above

Side-effects: see notes above; cough, dyspnoea and circulatory irregularities; rarely local reactions at injection site

Dose: *by slow intramuscular injection*, 250–500 mg weekly during first half of pregnancy

Proluton Depot® (Schering Health) PoM ◣▬
Injection (oily), hydroxyprogesterone caproate 250 mg/mL. Net price 1-mL amp = £2.35

> ◣▬ denotes preparations that are considered to be less suitable for prescribing (see p. vi)

MEDROXYPROGESTERONE ACETATE

Indications: see under Dose; contraception (section 7.3.2.2); malignant disease (section 8.3.2)

Cautions: see notes above; breast-feeding (Appendix 5)

Contra-indications: see notes above; pregnancy (Appendix 4)

Side-effects: see notes above; indigestion

Dose: *by mouth*, 2.5–10 mg daily for 5–10 days beginning on day 16 to 21 of cycle, repeated for 2 cycles in dysfunctional uterine bleeding and 3 cycles in secondary amenorrhoea

Mild to moderate endometriosis, 10 mg 3 times daily for 90 consecutive days, beginning on day 1 of cycle

Progestogenic opposition of oestrogen HRT, 10 mg daily for the last 14 days of each 28-day oestrogen HRT cycle

Adgyn Medro® (Strakan) PoM
Tablets, medroxyprogesterone acetate 5 mg, net price 14-tab pack = £1.50, 28-tab pack = £3.01

Provera® (Pharmacia) PoM
Tablets, all scored, medroxyprogesterone acetate 2.5 mg (orange), net price 30-tab pack = £1.84; 5 mg (blue), 10-tab pack = £1.23; 10 mg (white), 10-tab pack = £2.47, 90-tab pack = £22.16

■ Combined preparations
Section 6.4.1.1

NORETHISTERONE

Indications: see under Dose; HRT (section 6.4.1.1); contraception (section 7.3.1 and section 7.3.2); malignant disease (section 8.3.2)

Cautions: see notes above; breast-feeding (Appendix 5)

Contra-indications: see notes above; pregnancy (Appendix 4)

Side-effects: see notes above

Dose: endometriosis, 10–15 mg daily for 4–6 months or longer, starting on day 5 of cycle (if spotting occurs increase dose to 20–25 mg daily, reduced once bleeding has stopped)

Dysfunctional uterine bleeding, menorrhagia (but see notes above), 5 mg 3 times daily for 10 days to arrest bleeding; to prevent bleeding 5 mg twice daily from day 19 to 26

Dysmenorrhoea (but see notes above), 5 mg 3 times daily from day 5 to 24 for 3–4 cycles

Premenstrual syndrome, 5 mg 2–3 times daily from day 19 to 26 for several cycles (but not recommended, see notes above)

Postponement of menstruation, 5 mg 3 times daily starting 3 days before anticipated onset (menstruation occurs 2–3 days after stopping)

Progestogenic opposition of menopausal oestrogen HRT, see under *Micronor® HRT*, below

■ Tablets of 5 mg

Norethisterone (Non-proprietary) PoM
Tablets, norethisterone 5 mg, net price 30-tab pack = £2.15; 100-tab pack = £7.20
Available from Alpharma, CP, Lagap

Primolut N® (Schering Health) [PoM]

Tablets, norethisterone 5 mg. Net price 30-tab pack = £2.16

Utovlan® (Pharmacia) [PoM]

Tablets, scored, norethisterone 5 mg, net price 30-tab pack = £2.16, 90-tab pack = £6.48

■ Tablets of 1 mg for HRT

Micronor® HRT (Janssen-Cilag) [PoM]

Tablets, norethisterone 1 mg. Net price 3 × 12-tab pack = £3.75

Dose: 1 tablet daily on days 15–26 of each 28-day oestrogen HRT cycle

■ Combined preparations
Section 6.4.1.1

PROGESTERONE

Indications: see under preparations

Cautions: see notes above; breast-feeding (Appendix 5)

Contra-indications: see notes above; missed or incomplete abortion

Side-effects: see notes above; injection-site reactions; pain, diarrhoea and flatulence can occur with rectal administration

Crinone® (Serono) [PoM]

Vaginal gel, progesterone 45 mg/application (4%), net price 6 = £11.08; 90 mg/application (8%), 15 = £38.51

Note. 4% vaginal gel may be difficult to obtain

Dose: by vagina, progesterone deficiency, insert 1 applicatorful of 4% gel on alternate mornings from day 15 to day 25 of cycle

Menopausal symptoms, insert 1 applicatorful of 4% gel on alternate days for the last 12 days of oestrogen therapy in each cycle (section 6.4.1.1)

Infertility due to inadequate luteal phase, insert 1 applicatorful of 8% gel daily starting either after documented ovulation or on day 18–21 of cycle

In vitro fertilisation, daily application of 8% gel, continued for 30 days after laboratory evidence of pregnancy

Cyclogest® (Shire) [PoM] ▭

Pessaries, progesterone 200 mg, net price 15 = £5.22; 400 mg, 15 = £7.55

Dose: by vagina or rectum, premenstrual syndrome and post-natal depression, 200 mg daily to 400 mg twice daily; for premenstrual syndrome start on day 12–14 and continue until onset of menstruation (but not recommended, see notes above); rectally if barrier methods of contraception are used, in patients who have recently given birth or in those who suffer from vaginal infection or recurrent cystitis

Gestone® (Ferring) [PoM]

Injection, progesterone 25 mg/mL, net price 1-mL amp = 34p; 50 mg/mL, 1-mL amp = 44p, 2-mL amp = 58p

Dose: by deep intramuscular injection into buttock, Dysfunctional uterine bleeding, 5–10 mg daily for 5–10 days until 2 days before expected onset of menstruation

Recurrent miscarriage due to inadequate luteal phase (but not recommended, see notes above) or following *in vitro* fertilisation *or* gamete intra-fallopian transfer, 25–100 mg 2–7 times a week from day 15, or day of embryo *or* gamete transfer, until 8–16 weeks of pregnancy; max. 200 mg daily

6.4.2 Male sex hormones and antagonists

Androgens cause masculinisation; they may be used as replacement therapy in castrated adults and in those who are hypogonadal due to either pituitary or testicular disease. In the normal male they inhibit pituitary gonadotrophin secretion and depress spermatogenesis. Androgens also have an anabolic action which led to the development of anabolic steroids (section 6.4.3).

Androgens are useless as a treatment of impotence and impaired spermatogenesis unless there is associated hypogonadism; they should not be given until the hypogonadism has been properly investigated. Treatment should be under expert supervision.

When given to patients with hypopituitarism they can lead to normal sexual development and potency but not to fertility. If fertility is desired, the usual treatment is with gonadotrophins or pulsatile gonadotrophin-releasing hormone (section 6.5.1) which will stimulate spermatogenesis as well as androgen production.

Caution should be used when androgens or chorionic gonadotrophin are used in treating boys with delayed puberty since the fusion of epiphyses is hastened and may result in short stature.

Intramuscular depot preparations of **testosterone esters** are preferred for replacement therapy. Testosterone enantate or propionate or alternatively *Sustanon®*, which consists of a mixture of testosterone esters and has a longer duration of action, may be used. Satisfactory replacement therapy can sometimes be obtained with 1 mL of *Sustanon 250®*, given by intramuscular injection once a month, although more frequent dose intervals are often necessary. Implants of testosterone can be used for hypogonadism; the implants are replaced every 4 to 5 months. Menopausal women are also sometimes given implants of testosterone (in a dose of 50–100 mg every 4–8 months) as an adjunct to hormone replacement therapy.

Of the orally active preparations, **testosterone undecanoate** and **mesterolone** are available. Testosterone patches are now also available.

TESTOSTERONE AND ESTERS

Indications: see under preparations

Cautions: cardiac, renal, or hepatic impairment (Appendix 2), elderly, ischaemic heart disease, hypertension, epilepsy, migraine, diabetes mellitus, skeletal metastases (risk of hypercalcaemia), undertake regular examination of the prostate during treatment; pre-pubertal boys (see notes above and under Side-effects); **interactions:** Appendix 1 (testosterone)

Contra-indications: breast cancer in men, prostate cancer, history of primary liver tumours, hypercalcaemia, pregnancy, breast-feeding, nephrosis

Side-effects: prostate abnormalities and prostate cancer, headache, depression, gastro-intestinal bleeding, nausea, cholestatic jaundice, changes in libido, gynaecomastia, polycythaemia, anxiety, asthenia, generalised paraesthesia, electrolyte disturbances including sodium retention with oedema and hypercalcaemia; increased bone growth; androgenic effects such as hirsutism, male-pattern baldness, seborrhoea, acne, excessive frequency and duration of penile erections, precocious sexual development and premature closure of epiphyses in pre-pubertal males, suppression of spermatogenesis in men and virilism in women; rarely liver tumours; *with patches*, local irritation and allergic reactions

■ Oral

Restandol® (Organon) ▣PoM
Capsules, red-brown, testosterone undecanoate 40 mg in oily solution. Net price 28-cap pack = £8.30; 56-cap pack = £16.60. Label: 21, 25
Dose: androgen deficiency, 120–160 mg daily for 2–3 weeks; maintenance 40–120 mg daily

■ Intramuscular

Testosterone Enantate (Non-proprietary) ▣PoM
Injection (oily), testosterone enantate 250 mg/mL. Net price 1-mL amp = £8.33
Available from Cambridge
The brand name *Primoteston Depot®* was formerly used for testosterone enantate injection
Dose: by slow intramuscular injection, hypogonadism, initially 250 mg every 2–3 weeks; maintenance 250 mg every 3–6 weeks
Breast cancer, 250 mg every 2–3 weeks

Sustanon 100® (Organon) ▣PoM
Injection (oily), testosterone propionate 20 mg, testosterone phenylpropionate 40 mg, and testosterone isocaproate 40 mg/mL. Net price 1-mL amp = £1.17
Note. Contains arachis (peanut) oil
Dose: by deep intramuscular injection, androgen deficiency, 1 mL every 2 weeks

Sustanon 250® (Organon) ▣PoM
Injection (oily), testosterone propionate 30 mg, testosterone phenylpropionate 60 mg, testosterone isocaproate 60 mg, and testosterone decanoate 100 mg/mL. Net price 1-mL amp = £2.74
Note. Contains arachis (peanut) oil
Dose: by deep intramuscular injection, androgen deficiency, 1 mL usually every 3 weeks

Virormone® (Ferring) ▣PoM
Injection, testosterone propionate 50 mg/mL. Net price 2-mL amp = 46p
Dose: by intramuscular injection, androgen deficiency, 50 mg 2–3 times weekly
Delayed puberty, 50 mg weekly
Breast cancer in women, 100 mg 2–3 times weekly

■ Implant

Testosterone (Organon) ▣PoM
Implant, testosterone 100 mg, net price = £7.40; 200 mg = £13.79
Dose: by implantation, male hypogonadism, 100–600 mg; 600 mg usually maintains plasma-testosterone concentration within the normal range for 4–5 months
Menopausal women, see notes above

■ Transdermal preparations

Andropatch® (SmithKline Beecham) ▣PoM
Patches, self-adhesive, releasing testosterone approx. 2.5 mg/24 hours, net price 60-patch pack = £52.80; releasing testosterone approx. 5 mg/24 hours, net price 30-patch pack = £52.80. Counselling, administration
Dose: androgen deficiency in men associated with primary or secondary hypogonadism, apply to clean, dry, unbroken skin on back, abdomen, upper arms or thighs, removing after 24 hours and siting replacement patch on a different area (with an interval of 7 days before using the same site); initially apply patches equivalent to testosterone 5 mg/24 hours (2.5 mg/24 hours in non-virilised patients) at night (approx. 10 p.m.), then adjust to 2.5 mg to 7.5 mg every 24 hours according to plasma-testosterone concentration (those with a body-weight over 130 kg may require 7.5 mg every 24 hours)

MESTEROLONE

Indications: see under Dose
Cautions: see under Testosterone and Esters
Contra-indications: see under Testosterone and Esters
Side-effects: see under Testosterone and Esters but spermatogenesis unimpaired
Dose: androgen deficiency and male infertility associated with hypogonadism, 25 mg 3–4 times daily for several months, reduced to 50–75 mg daily in divided doses for maintenance; CHILD not recommended

Pro-Viron® (Schering Health) ▣PoM
Tablets, scored, mesterolone 25 mg. Net price 30-tab pack = £4.75

Anti-androgens

Cyproterone acetate is an anti-androgen used in the treatment of severe hypersexuality and sexual deviation in the male. It inhibits spermatogenesis and produces reversible infertility (but is not a male contraceptive); abnormal sperm forms are produced. Fully informed consent is recommended and an initial spermatogram. As hepatic tumours have been produced in *animal* studies, careful consideration should be given to the risk/benefit ratio before treatment. Cyproterone acetate is also used as an adjunct in prostatic cancer (section 8.3.4.2) and in the treatment of acne and hirsutism in women (section 13.6.2).

Finasteride is a specific inhibitor of the enzyme 5α-reductase which metabolises testosterone into the more potent androgen, dihydrotestosterone. This inhibition of testosterone metabolism leads to reduction in prostate size, with improvement in urinary flow rate and in obstructive symptoms. It is an alternative to alpha-blockers (section 7.4.1) particularly in men with a significantly enlarged prostate.

CYPROTERONE ACETATE

Indications: see notes above; prostate cancer (section 8.3.4.2)
Cautions: ineffective for male hypersexuality in chronic alcoholism (relevance to prostate cancer not known); blood counts initially and throughout treatment; monitor hepatic function regularly (liver function tests should be performed before treatment, see also under Side-effects below);

monitor adrenocortical function regularly; diabetes mellitus (see also Contra-indications)

DRIVING. Fatigue and lassitude may impair performance of skilled tasks (e.g. driving)

Contra-indications: (do not apply in prostate cancer) hepatic disease, severe diabetes, severe cardiac changes); sickle-cell anaemia, malignant or wasting disease, severe depression, history of thrombo-embolic disorders; youths under 18 years (may arrest bone maturation and testicular development)

Side-effects: fatigue and lassitude, breathlessness, weight changes, reduced sebum production (may clear acne), changes in hair pattern, gynaecomastia (rarely leading to galactorrhoea and benign breast nodules); rarely osteoporosis; inhibition of spermatogenesis (see notes above); hepatotoxicity reported (including jaundice, hepatitis and hepatic failure usually in men given 200–300 mg daily for prostatic cancer, see section 8.3.4.2 for details and warnings)

Dose: male hypersexuality, 50 mg twice daily after food

Cyproterone Acetate (Non-proprietary) [PoM]
Tablets, cyproterone acetate 50 mg, net price 56-tab pack = £31.54. Label 21
Available from Generics

Androcur® (Schering Health) [PoM]
Tablets, scored, cyproterone acetate 50 mg. Net price 56-tab pack = £33.84. Label: 21

FINASTERIDE

Indications: benign prostatic hyperplasia

Cautions: obstructive uropathy, prostate cancer (may decrease markers such as prostate specific antigen); use of condoms recommended if sexual partner is pregnant or is likely to become pregnant (finasteride excreted in semen); women of child-bearing potential should avoid handling crushed or broken tablets

Side-effects: impotence, decreased libido, ejaculation disorders, testicular pain, breast tenderness and enlargement, hypersensitivity reactions (including lip and face swelling, pruritus and rash)

Dose: 5 mg daily, review treatment after 6 months (may require several months treatment before benefit is obtained)

Proscar® (MSD) [PoM]
Tablets, blue, f/c, finasteride 5 mg. Net price 28-tab pack = £24.90

6.4.3   Anabolic steroids

All the anabolic steroids have some androgenic activity but they cause less virilisation than androgens in women. Their protein-building property led to the hope that they might be widely useful in medicine but this hope has not been realised. Their use as body builders or tonics is quite unjustified; they are abused by some athletes.

Anabolic steroids have also been given for osteoporosis in women but are no longer advocated for this purpose.

Anabolic steroids are used in the treatment of some *aplastic anaemias* (section 9.1.3) and to reduce the itching of *chronic biliary obstruction* (see Prescribing in Palliative Care p. 15).

NANDROLONE

Indications: osteoporosis in postmenopausal women (but not recommended, see notes above); aplastic anaemia (section 9.1.3)

Cautions: cardiac and renal impairment, hepatic impairment (see Appendix 2), hypertension, diabetes mellitus, epilepsy, migraine; monitor skeletal maturation in young patients; skeletal metastases (risk of hypercalcaemia); **interactions:** Appendix 1 (anabolic steroids)

Contra-indications: severe hepatic impairment, prostate cancer, male breast cancer, pregnancy and breast-feeding, porphyria (section 9.8.2)

Side-effects: acne, sodium retention with oedema, virilisation with high doses including voice changes (sometimes irreversible), amenorrhoea, inhibition of spermatogenesis, premature epiphyseal closure; abnormal liver-function tests reported with high doses; liver tumours reported occasionally on prolonged treatment with anabolic steroids

Dose: see below

Deca-Durabolin® (Organon) [PoM] [▭]
Injection (oily), nandrolone decanoate 50 mg/mL, net price 1-mL amp = £3.54
Note. Contains arachis (peanut) oil
Dose: by deep intramuscular injection, 50 mg every 3 weeks

> ▬ denotes preparations that are considered to be less suitable for prescribing (see p. vi)

STANOZOLOL

Indications: see under Dose

Cautions: cardiac or renal impairment; premature closure of epiphyses in children; peliosis hepatis and hepatic tumours reported on long-term treatment; breast cancer (possibility of hypercalcaemia); monitor liver function, haematocrit and haemoglobin; diabetes mellitus (possible dosage adjustments for oral hypoglycaemic drugs and avoid in insulin-dependent diabetes); **interactions:** Appendix 1 (anabolic steroids)

Contra-indications: pregnancy, breast-feeding, established liver disease (if history of jaundice—liver function tests before starting treatment); prostate cancer, insulin-dependent diabetes mellitus; not indicated for treatment of loss of appetite, unexplained weight loss, or failure to thrive in children; porphyria (section 9.8.2)

Side-effects: androgenic effects (generally mild and reversible on stopping treatment) include acne, hirsutism, amenorrhoea, sodium retention with oedema; voice change—usually at higher dosage (discontinue); menstrual irregularity, headache, muscle cramp, dyspepsia, rash, hair loss, euphoria, depression, increased haematocrit and haemoglobin; cholestatic jaundice and rarely peliosis hepatis and hepatic tumours also reported; changes in liver enzymes, in lipoproteins, and in thyroid hormones; also premature epiphyseal closure (on prolonged treatment)

Dose: *by mouth,* vascular manifestations of Behçet's disease, 10 mg daily

Hereditary angioedema, 2.5–10 mg daily to control attacks, reduced for maintenance (2.5 mg 3 times weekly may be sufficient); CHILD 1–6 years initially 2.5 mg daily, 6–12 years initially 2.5–5 mg daily, reduced for maintenance

Note. In hereditary angioedema restricted to well-established cases who have experienced serious attacks (and not for premenopausal women except in life-threatening situations)

Stromba® (Sanofi-Synthelabo) PoM

Tablets—product discontinued

6.5 Hypothalamic and pituitary hormones and anti-oestrogens

Hypothalamic and pituitary hormones are described under the following section headings:

6.5.1 Hypothalamic and anterior pituitary hormones and anti-oestrogens

6.5.2 Posterior pituitary hormones and antagonists

Use of preparations in these sections requires detailed prior investigation of the patient and *should be reserved for specialist centres.*

6.5.1 Hypothalamic and anterior pituitary hormones and anti-oestrogens

Anti-oestrogens

The anti-oestrogens **clomifene** (clomiphene) and **tamoxifen** (section 8.3.4.1) are used in the treatment of female infertility due to oligomenorrhoea or secondary amenorrhoea (e.g. associated with polycystic ovarian disease). They induce gonadotrophin release by occupying oestrogen receptors in the hypothalamus, thereby interfering with feedback mechanisms; chorionic gonadotrophin is sometimes used as an adjunct. Patients should be warned that there is a risk of multiple pregnancy (*rarely* more than twins).

CLOMIFENE CITRATE

(Clomiphene Citrate)

Indications: anovulatory infertility—see notes above

Cautions: see notes above; polycystic ovary syndrome (cysts may enlarge during treatment), ovarian hyperstimulation syndrome, uterine fibroids, ectopic pregnancy, incidence of multiple births increased (consider ultrasound monitoring), visual symptoms (discontinue and initiate ophthalmological examination); breast-feeding (Appendix 5)

CSM Advice. The CSM has recommended that clomifene should not normally be used for longer than 6 cycles (possibly increased risk of ovarian cancer)

Contra-indications: hepatic disease, ovarian cysts, hormone dependent tumours or abnormal uterine bleeding of undetermined cause, pregnancy (exclude before treatment)

Side-effects: visual disturbances (withdraw), ovarian hyperstimulation (withdraw), hot flushes, abdominal discomfort, occasionally nausea, vomiting, depression, insomnia, breast tenderness, headache, intermenstrual spotting, menorrhagia, endometriosis, convulsions, weight gain, rashes, dizziness, hair loss

Dose: 50 mg daily for 5 days, starting within about 5 days of onset of menstruation (preferably on 2nd day) or at any time (normally preceded by a progestogen-induced withdrawal bleed) if cycles have ceased; second course of 100 mg daily for 5 days may be given in absence of ovulation; most patients who are going to respond will do so in first course; 3 courses should constitute adequate therapeutic trial; long-term cyclical therapy not recommended—see CSM advice, above

Clomifene (Non-proprietary) PoM

Tablets, clomifene citrate 50 mg, net price 30-tab pack = £11.25

Available from Kent

Clomid® (Aventis Pharma) PoM

Tablets, yellow, scored, clomifene citrate 50 mg. Net price 30-tab pack = £11.27; 100-tab pack = £32.80

Anterior pituitary hormones

Corticotrophins

Tetracosactide (tetracosactrin), an analogue of corticotropin (ACTH), is used to test adrenocortical function; failure of the plasma cortisol concentration to rise after administration of tetracosactide indicates adrenocortical insufficiency.

Both corticotropin and tetracosactide were formerly used as alternatives to corticosteroids in conditions such as Crohn's disease or rheumatoid arthritis; their value was limited by the variable and unpredictable therapeutic response and by the waning of their effect with time.

TETRACOSACTIDE

(Tetracosactrin)

Indications: see notes above

Cautions: as for corticosteroids, section 6.3.2; **important:** risk of anaphylaxis (medical supervision; consult product literature)

Contra-indications: as for corticosteroids, section 6.3.2; avoid injections containing benzyl alcohol in neonates (see under preparations)

Side-effects: as for corticosteroids, section 6.3.2

Dose: see under preparations below

Synacthen® (Alliance) [PoM]

Injection, tetracosactide 250 micrograms (as acetate)/mL. Net price 1-mL amp = £3.00

Dose: diagnostic (30-minute test), *by intramuscular or intravenous injection,* 250 micrograms as a single dose

Synacthen Depot® (Alliance) [PoM]

Injection (aqueous suspension), tetracosactide 1 mg (as acetate)/mL, with zinc phosphate complex. Net price 1-mL amp = £4.29

Excipients: include benzyl alcohol (avoid in neonates, see Excipients p. 2)

Dose: diagnostic (5-hour test), *by intramuscular injection,* 1 mg as a single dose

Note. Formerly used therapeutically by intramuscular injection, in an initial dose of 1 mg daily (or every 12 hours in acute cases); reduced to 1 mg every 2–3 days, then 1 mg weekly (or 500 micrograms every 2–3 days) but value was limited (see notes above)

Gonadotrophins

Follicle-stimulating hormone (FSH) and luteinising hormone (LH) together (as in **human menopausal gonadotrophin**), follicle-stimulating hormone alone (as in **urofollitropin** (urofollitrophin) or **follitropin**), or chorionic gonadotrophin, are used in the treatment of infertility in women with proven hypopituitarism or who have not responded to clomifene, or in superovulation treatment for assisted conception (such as *in vitro* fertilisation).

The gonadotrophins are also occasionally used in the treatment of hypogonadotrophic hypogonadism and associated oligospermia. There is no justification for their use in primary gonadal failure.

Chorionic gonadotrophin has also been used in delayed puberty in the male to stimulate endogenous testosterone production, but has little advantage over testosterone (section 6.4.2).

CHORIONIC GONADOTROPHIN

(Human Chorionic Gonadotrophin; HCG)

A preparation of a glycoprotein fraction secreted by the placenta and obtained from the urine of pregnant women having the action of the pituitary luteinising hormone

Indications: see notes above

Cautions: cardiac or renal impairment, asthma, epilepsy, migraine; prepubertal boys (risk of premature epiphyseal closure or precocious puberty)

Contra-indications: androgen-dependent tumours

Side-effects: oedema (particularly in males—reduce dose), headache, tiredness, mood changes, gynaecomastia, local reactions; may aggravate ovarian hyperstimulation, multiple pregnancy

Dose: *by subcutaneous or intramuscular injection,* according to patient's response

Choragon® (Ferring) [PoM]

Injection, powder for reconstitution, chorionic gonadotrophin. Net price 5000-unit amp (with solvent) = £3.50. For intramuscular injection

Pregnyl® (Organon) [PoM]

Injection, powder for reconstitution, chorionic gonadotrophin. Net price 1500-unit amp = £2.37; 5000-unit amp = £3.52 (both with solvent). For subcutaneous or intramuscular injection

Profasi® (Serono) [PoM]

Injection, powder for reconstitution, chorionic gonadotrophin. Net price 2000-unit amp = £2.01; 5000-unit amp = £3.53; 10 000-unit amp = £7.06 (all with solvent). For subcutaneous or intramuscular injection

---

CHORIOGONADOTROPIN ALFA

(Human chorionic gonadotropin)

Indications: see notes above

Cautions: rule out infertility caused by hypothyroidism, adrenocortical deficiency, hyperprolactinemia, tumours of the pituitary or hypothalamus

Contra-indications: ovarian enlargement or cyst (unless caused by polycystic ovarian disease); ectopic pregnancy in previous 3 months; active thromboembolic disorders; hypothalamus, pituitary, ovarian, uterine or mammary malignancy

Side-effects: nausea, vomiting, abdominal pain; headache, tiredness; injection site reactions; ovarian hyperstimulation syndrome; rarely diarrhoea, depression, irritability, breast pain; ectopic pregnancy and ovarian torsion reported

Dose: *by subcutaneous injection,* according to patient's response

Ovitrelle® (Serono) ▼ [PoM]

Injection, powder for reconstitution, choriogonadotropin alfa, net price 6500-unit (250-micrograms) vial = £39.19 (with solvent)

FOLLITROPIN ALFA and BETA

(Recombinant human follicle stimulating hormone)

Indications: see notes above

Cautions: see under Human Menopausal Gonadotrophins

Contra-indications: see under Human Menopausal Gonadotrophins

Side-effects: see under Human Menopausal Gonadotrophins

Dose: *by subcutaneous or intramuscular injection,* according to patient's response

■ Follitropin alfa

Gonal-F® (Serono) [PoM]

Injection, powder for reconstitution, follitropin alfa. Net price 37.5-unit amp = £13.13; 75-unit amp = £26.25; 150-unit amp = £52.50; 600-unit multidose vial = £367.50 (all with diluent). For subcutaneous injection

■ Follitropin beta

Puregon® (Organon) [PoM]

Injection, follitropin beta 100 units/mL, net price 0.5-mL (50-unit) vial = £20.15; 200 units/mL, 0.5-mL (100-unit) vial = £40.30; 300 units/mL, 0.5-mL (150-unit) vial = £54.43; 400 units/mL, 0.5-mL (200-unit) vial = £72.57. For subcutaneous or intramuscular injection

HUMAN MENOPAUSAL GONADOTROPHINS

Purified extract of human post-menopausal urine containing follicle-stimulating hormone (FSH) and luteinising hormone (LH); the relative *in vivo* activity is designated as a ratio; the 1:1 ratio is also known as menotrophin

Indications: see notes above

Cautions: rule out infertility caused by adrenal or thyroid disorders, hyperprolactinaemia or tumours of the pituitary or hypothalamus

Contra-indications: ovarian cysts (not caused by polycystic ovarian syndrome); tumours of breast, uterus, ovaries, testes or prostate; vaginal bleeding of unknown cause; pregnancy and breast-feeding

Side-effects: ovarian hyperstimulation, increased risk of multiple pregnancy and miscarriage, hypersensitivity reactions, nausea, vomiting, joint pain, fever, injection site reactions; gynaecomastia, acne, and weight gain reported in men

Dose: *by deep intramuscular or subcutaneous injection*, according to patient's response

Menogon® (Ferring) PoM
Injection, powder for reconstitution, menotrophin as follicle-stimulating hormone 75 units, luteinising hormone 75 units, net price per amp (with solvent) = £10.64. For intramuscular injection

Menopur® (Ferring) PoM
Injection, powder for reconstitution, menotrophin as follicle-stimulating hormone 75 units, luteinising hormone 75 units, net price per amp (with solvent) = £14.00. For intramuscular or subcutaneous injection

LUTROPIN ALFA

(Recombinant human luteinising hormone)

Indications: see notes above

Cautions: rule out infertility caused by hypothyroidism, adrenocorticol deficiency, hyperprolactinemia, tumours of the pituitary or hypothalamus

Contra-indications: ovarian enlargement or cyst (unless caused by polycystic ovarian disease); undiagnosed vaginal bleeding; tumours of hypothalamus and pituitary; ovarian, uterine or mammary carcinoma

Side-effects: nausea, vomiting, abdominal and pelvic pain; headache, somnolence; injection site reactions; ovarian hyperstimulation syndrome, ovarian cyst, breast pain, ectopic pregnancy; thromboembolism, adnexal torsion, and haemoperitoneum

Dose: *by subcutaneous injection*, in conjunction with follicle stimulating hormone, according to response

Luveris® (Serono) ▼ PoM
Injection, powder for reconstitution, lutropin alfa, net price 75-unit vial = £39.19 (with solvent)

UROFOLLITROPIN

(Urofollitropin)

Extract of the urine of postmenopausal women containing follicle-stimulating hormone

Indications: see notes above

Cautions: see under Human Menopausal Gonadotrophins

Contra-indications: see under Human Menopausal Gonadotrophins

Side-effects: see under Human Menopausal Gonadotrophins

Dose: *by subcutaneous or intramuscular injection*, according to patient's response

Metrodin High Purity® (Serono) PoM
Injection, powder for reconstitution, urofollitropin as follicle-stimulating hormone, net price 75-unit amp = £18.62; 150-unit amp = £37.24 (both with solvent). For subcutaneous or intramuscular injection

Growth hormone

Growth hormone is used to treat deficiency of the hormone and in chronic renal insufficiency in children (see under Somatropin for specific indications). Growth hormone of human origin (HGH; somatotrophin) has been replaced by a growth hormone of human sequence, **somatropin**, produced using recombinant DNA technology.

SOMATROPIN

(Synthetic Human Growth Hormone)

Indications: see under Dose

Cautions: diabetes mellitus (adjustment of antidiabetic therapy may be necessary), papilloedema (see under Side-effects), relative deficiencies of other pituitary hormones (notably hypothyroidism—manufacturers recommend periodic thyroid function tests but limited evidence of clinical value), history of malignant disease, disorders of the epiphysis of the hip (monitor for limping), resolved intracranial hypertension (monitor closely), rotate subcutaneous injection sites to prevent lipoatrophy; breast-feeding; **interactions:** Appendix 1 (somatropin)

Contra-indications: evidence of tumour activity (complete antitumour therapy and ensure intracranial lesions inactive before starting); not to be used after renal transplantation in seriously ill patients or for growth promotion in children with closed epiphyses (or near closure in Prader-Willi syndrome); pregnancy (interrupt treatment if pregnancy occurs)

Side-effects: headache, funduscopy for papilloedema recommended if severe or recurrent headache, visual problems, nausea and vomiting occur—if papilloedema confirmed consider benign intracranial hypertension (rare cases reported); fluid retention (peripheral oedema), arthralgia, myalgia, carpal tunnel syndrome, paraesthesia, antibody formation, hypothyroidism, hyperglycaemia, hypoglycaemia, reactions at injection site; leukaemia in children with growth hormone deficiency also reported

Dose: Gonadal dysgenesis (Turner syndrome), *by subcutaneous injection*, 45–50 micrograms/kg daily *or* 1.4 mg/m^2 daily

Deficiency of growth hormone in children, *by subcutaneous or intramuscular injection*, 23–39 micrograms/kg daily *or* 0.7–1 mg/m^2 daily

Prader-Willi syndrome, *by subcutaneous injection* in children with growth velocity greater than 1 cm/year, in combination with energy-restricted

diet, 35 micrograms/kg daily *or* 1 mg/m² daily;
max. 2.7 mg daily

Chronic renal insufficiency in children (renal function decreased to less than 50%), *by subcutaneous injection*, 45–50 micrograms/kg daily *or* 1.4 mg/m² daily (higher doses may be needed) adjusted if necessary after 6 months

Adult growth hormone deficiency, *by subcutaneous injection*, initially 150–300 micrograms daily, gradually increased if required to max. 1 mg daily; use minimum effective dose (requirements may decrease with age)

Note. Dose formerly expressed in units; somatropin 1 mg ≡ 3 units

Genotropin® (Pharmacia) PoM
Injection, two-compartment cartridge containing powder for reconstitution, somatropin (rbe) and diluent, net price 5.3-mg (16-unit) cartridge = £121.39, 12-mg (36-unit) cartridge = £273.13. For use with *Genotropin® Pen* NHS device (available free of charge from clinics). For subcutaneous injection

KabiVial injection, two-compartment cartridge containing powder for reconstitution, somatropin (rbe) and diluent, net price 5.3-mg (16-unit) vial = £121.39. For subcutaneous injection

MiniQuick injection, two-compartment single-dose syringe containing powder for reconstitution, somatropin (rbe) and diluent, net price 0.2-mg (0.6-unit) syringe = £4.55; 0.4-mg (1.2-unit) syringe = £9.11; 0.6-mg (1.8-unit) syringe = £13.66; 0.8-mg (2.4-unit) syringe = £18.21; 1-mg (3-unit) syringe = £22.77; 1.2-mg (3.6-unit) syringe = £27.32; 1.4-mg (4.2-unit) syringe = £31.87; 1.6-mg (4.8-unit) syringe = £36.42; 1.8-mg (5.4-unit) syringe = £40.98; 2-mg (6-unit) syringe = £45.53. For subcutaneous injection

Humatrope® (Lilly) PoM
Injection, powder for reconstitution, somatropin (rbe), net price 1.33-mg (4-unit) vial (with diluent) = £30.50; 5.33-mg (16-unit) vial (with diluent) = £122.00; 6-mg (18-unit) cartridge = £137.25; 12-mg (36-unit) cartridge = £274.50; 24-mg (72-unit) cartridge = £549.00; all supplied with diluent. For subcutaneous or intramuscular injection; cartridges for subcutaneous injection

Norditropin® (Novo Nordisk) PoM
SimpleXx injection, somatropin (epr) 3.3 mg (10 units)/mL, net price 1.5-mL (5-mg, 15-unit) cartridge = £117.10; 6.7 mg (20 units)/mL, 1.5-mL (10-mg, 30-unit) cartridge = £234.20; 10 mg (30 units)/mL, 1.5-mL (15-mg, 45-unit) cartridge = £351.30. For use with appropriate *NordiPen®* NHS device (available free of charge from clinics). For subcutaneous injection

Saizen® (Serono) PoM
Injection, powder for reconstitution, somatropin (rmc), net price 1.33-mg (4-unit) vial (with diluent) = £30.50; 3.33-mg (10-unit) vial (with diluent) = £76.25. For subcutaneous or intramuscular injection

Click.easy®, powder for reconstitution, somatropin (rmc), net price 8-mg (24-unit) vial (in *Click.easy®* device with diluent) = £183.00. For use with *One.click®* autoinjector device NHS (available free of charge from clinics). For subcutaneous injection

Easyject®, powder for reconstitution, somatropin (rmc), net price 8-mg (24-unit) vial (with diluent) = £183.00. For use with *Easyject®* NHS device (available free of charge from clinics). For subcutaneous injection

Zomacton® (Ferring) PoM
Injection, powder for reconstitution, somatropin (rbe), net price 4-mg (12-unit) vial (with diluent) = £87.44. For use with *ZomaJet® 2* NHS needle-free device or with *Auto-Jector®* NHS (both available free of charge from clinics) or with needles and syringes. For subcutaneous injection

Hypothalamic hormones

Gonadorelin when injected intravenously in normal subjects leads to a rapid rise in plasma concentrations of both luteinising hormone (LH) and follicle-stimulating hormone (FSH). It has not proved to be very helpful, however, in distinguishing hypothalamic from pituitary lesions. **Gonadorelin analogues** are indicated in endometriosis and infertility (section 6.7.2) and in breast and prostate cancer (section 8.3.4).

Protirelin is a hypothalamic releasing hormone which stimulates the release of thyrotrophin from the pituitary. It is indicated for the diagnosis of mild hyperthyroidism or hypothyroidism, but its use has been superseded by immunoassays for thyroid-stimulating hormone.

Sermorelin, an analogue of growth hormone releasing hormone (somatorelin, GHRH), is licensed as a diagnostic test for secretion of growth hormone.

GONADORELIN

(Gonadotrophin-releasing hormone; GnRH; LH–RH)

Indications: see preparations below

Cautions: pituitary adenoma

Side-effects: rarely, nausea, headache, abdominal pain, increased menstrual bleeding; rarely, hypersensitivity reaction on repeated administration of large doses; irritation at injection site

Dose: see under preparations

HRF® (Intrapharm) PoM
Injection, powder for reconstitution, gonadorelin. Net price 100-microgram vial (with diluent) = £13.45 (hosp. only)
For assessment of pituitary function (adults), *by subcutaneous or intravenous injection*, 100 micrograms

PROTIRELIN

(Thyrotrophin-releasing hormone; TRH)

Indications: assessment of thyroid function and thyroid stimulating hormone reserve

Cautions: severe hypopituitarism, myocardial ischaemia, bronchial asthma and obstructive airways disease, pregnancy, breast-feeding (Appendix 5)

Side-effects: after rapid intravenous administration desire to micturate, flushing, dizziness, nausea, strange taste; transient increase in pulse rate and blood pressure; rarely bronchospasm

Dose: *by intravenous injection*, 200 micrograms; CHILD 1 microgram/kg

Protirelin (Non-proprietary) [PoM]
Injection, protirelin 100 micrograms/mL. Net price
2-mL amp = £7.89 (hosp. only)
Available from Cambridge
The brand name *TRH-Cambridge®* was formerly used
for protirelin injection

SERMORELIN

Indications: see notes above
Cautions: epilepsy; discontinue growth hormone
therapy 1–2 weeks before test; untreated hypothyroidism, antithyroid drugs; elevated plasma fatty acids; avoid
preparations which affect release of growth horm-
one (includes those affecting release of somatostatin, insulin or glucocorticoids and cyclo-
oxygenase inhibitors such as aspirin and indometacin)
Contra-indications: pregnancy and breast-feeding
Side-effects: occasional facial flushing and pain at
injection site
Dose: *by intravenous injection*, 1 microgram/kg in
the morning after an overnight fast

Geref 50® (Serono) [PoM]
Injection, powder for reconstitution, sermorelin
50 micrograms (as acetate). Net price per amp
(with solvent) = £52.53

6.5.2 **Posterior pituitary
hormones and
antagonists**

Posterior pituitary hormones

DIABETES INSIPIDUS. **Vasopressin** (antidiuretic
hormone, ADH) is used in the treatment of *pituitary*
('cranial') *diabetes insipidus* as is its analogue
desmopressin. Dosage is tailored to produce a
slight diuresis every 24 hours to avoid water intoxication. Treatment may be required for a limited
period only in diabetes insipidus following trauma
or pituitary surgery.

Desmopressin has a longer duration of action than
vasopressin; unlike vasopressin it has no vasoconstrictor effect. It is given by mouth or intranasally
for maintenance therapy, and by injection in the
postoperative period or in unconscious patients.
Desmopressin is also used in the differential diagnosis of diabetes insipidus. Following a dose of
2 micrograms intramuscularly or 20 micrograms
intranasally, restoration of the ability to concentrate
urine after water deprivation confirms a diagnosis
of cranial diabetes insipidus. Failure to respond
occurs in nephrogenic diabetes insipidus.

In *nephrogenic* and *partial pituitary diabetes insipidus* benefit may be gained from the paradoxical
antidiuretic effect of thiazides (section 2.2.1) e.g.
chlortalidone 100 mg twice daily reduced to maintenance dose of 50 mg daily.

Chlorpropamide (section 6.1.2.1) is also useful in
partial pituitary diabetes insipidus, and probably
acts by sensitising the renal tubules to the action of
remaining endogenous vasopressin; it is given in

doses of up to 350 mg daily in adults and 200 mg
daily in children, care being taken to avoid hypoglycaemia. Carbamazepine (section 4.8.1) is also
sometimes useful (in a dose of 200 mg once or
twice daily) [unlicensed]; its mode of action may be
similar to that of chlorpropamide.

OTHER USES. Desmopressin injection is also used
to boost factor VIII concentrations in mild to moderate haemophilia. For a comment on the use of desmopressin in nocturnal enuresis see section 7.4.2.

Vasopressin infusion is used to control variceal
bleeding in portal hypertension, prior to more definitive treatment and with variable results. Terlipressin, a derivative of vasopressin, is used
similarly.

Oxytocin, another posterior pituitary hormone, is
indicated in obstetrics (section 7.1.1).

VASOPRESSIN

Indications: pituitary diabetes insipidus; bleeding
from oesophageal varices
Cautions: heart failure, hypertension, asthma, epilepsy, migraine or other conditions which might
be aggravated by water retention; renal impairment (see also Contra-indications); pregnancy
(Appendix 4); avoid fluid overload
Contra-indications: vascular disease (especially
disease of coronary arteries) unless extreme caution, chronic nephritis (until reasonable blood
nitrogen concentrations attained)
Side-effects: fluid retention, pallor, tremor, sweating, vertigo, headache, nausea, vomiting, belching, abdominal cramps, desire to defaecate,
hypersensitivity reactions (including anaphylaxis), constriction of coronary arteries (may
cause anginal attacks and myocardial ischaemia),
peripheral ischaemia and rarely gangrene
Dose: *by subcutaneous or intramuscular injection*,
diabetes insipidus, 5–20 units every four hours
By intravenous infusion, initial control of variceal
bleeding, 20 units over 15 minutes

■ Synthetic vasopressin
Pitressin® (Goldshield) [PoM]
Injection, argipressin (synthetic vasopressin)
20 units/mL. Net price 1-mL amp = £14.29 (hosp.
only)

DESMOPRESSIN

Indications: see under Dose
Cautions: see under Vasopressin; less pressor
activity, but still considerable caution in renal
impairment, in cardiovascular disease and in
hypertension (not indicated for nocturnal enuresis
or nocturia in these circumstances); elderly (avoid
for nocturnal enuresis and nocturia in those over
65 years); also considerable caution in cystic
fibrosis; in nocturia and nocturnal enuresis limit
fluid intake to minimum from 1 hour before dose
until 8 hours afterwards; in nocturia periodic
blood pressure and weight checks needed to monitor for fluid overload; **interactions:** Appendix 1
(desmopressin)
HYPONATRAEMIC CONVULSIONS. The CSM has advised
that patients being treated for primary nocturnal enuresis

should be warned to avoid fluid overload (including during swimming) and to stop taking desmopressin during an episode of vomiting or diarrhoea (until fluid balance normal). The risk of hyponatraemic convulsions can also be minimised by keeping to the recommended starting doses and by avoiding concomitant use of drugs which increase secretion of vasopressin (e.g. tricyclic antidepressants)

Contra-indications: cardiac insufficiency and other conditions treated with diuretics

Side-effects: fluid retention, and hyponatraemia (in more serious cases with convulsions) on administration without restricting fluid intake; stomach pain, headache, nausea, and vomiting also reported; epistaxis, nasal congestion, rhinitis with nasal spray

Dose: *by mouth*

Diabetes insipidus, treatment, ADULT and CHILD initially 300 micrograms daily (in 3 divided doses); maintenance, 300–600 micrograms daily in 3 divided doses; range 0.2–1.2 mg daily

Primary nocturnal enuresis (if urine concentrating ability normal), ADULT (under 65 years) and CHILD over 5 years (preferably over 7 years) 200 micrograms at bedtime, only increased to 400 micrograms if lower dose not effective (**important:** see also Cautions); withdraw for at least 1 week for reassessment after 3 months

Postoperative polyuria or polydipsia, adjust dose according to urine osmolality

Intranasally

Diabetes insipidus, diagnosis, ADULT and CHILD 20 micrograms (limit fluid intake to 500 mL from 1 hour before to 8 hours after administration)

Diabetes insipidus, treatment, ADULT 10–40 micrograms daily (in 1–2 divided doses); CHILD 5–20 micrograms daily; infants may require lower doses

Primary nocturnal enuresis (if urine concentrating ability normal), ADULT (under 65 years) and CHILD over 5 years (preferably over 7 years) initially 20 micrograms at bedtime, only increased to 40 micrograms if lower dose not effective (**important:** see also Cautions); withdraw for at least 1 week for reassessment after 3 months

Nocturia associated with multiple sclerosis (when other treatments have failed), ADULT (under 65 years) 10–20 micrograms at bedtime (**important:** see also Cautions), dose not to be repeated within 24 hours

Renal function testing (empty bladder at time of administration and limit fluid intake to 500 mL from 1 hour before until 8 hours after administration), ADULT 40 micrograms; INFANT under 1 year 10 micrograms (restrict fluid intake to 50% at next 2 feeds to avoid fluid overload), CHILD 1–15 years 20 micrograms

By injection

Diabetes insipidus, diagnosis (*subcutaneous or intramuscular*), ADULT and CHILD 2 micrograms (limit fluid intake to 500 mL from 1 hour before to 8 hours after administration)

Diabetes insipidus, treatment (*subcutaneous, intramuscular or intravenous*), ADULT 1–4 micrograms daily; CHILD 400 nanograms

Renal function testing (empty bladder at time of administration and limit fluid intake to 500 mL from 1 hour before until 8 hours after administration) (*subcutaneous or intramuscular*), ADULT and CHILD 2 micrograms; INFANT 400 nanograms

(restrict fluid intake to 50% at next 2 feeds)

Mild to moderate haemophilia and von Willebrands disease, post lumbar puncture headache, fibrinolytic response testing, consult product literature

Desmopressin acetate (Non-proprietary) PoM
Nasal spray, desmopressin acetate 10 micrograms/metered spray, net price 6-mL unit (60 metered sprays) = £28.00. Counselling, fluid intake, see above
Available from Alpharma
Note. Children requiring dose of less than 10 micrograms should be given *DDAVP®* intranasal solution

DDAVP® (Ferring) PoM
Tablets, both scored, desmopressin acetate 100 micrograms, net price 90-tab pack = £46.57; 200 micrograms, 90-tab pack = £93.15. Counselling, fluid intake, see above
Intranasal solution, desmopressin acetate 100 micrograms/mL. Net price 2.5-mL dropper bottle and catheter = £10.45. Counselling, fluid intake, see above
Injection, desmopressin acetate 4 micrograms/mL. Net price 1-mL amp = £1.18

Desmotabs® (Ferring) PoM
Tablets, scored, desmopressin acetate 200 micrograms, net price 30-tab pack = £31.07. Counselling, fluid intake, see above

Desmospray® (Ferring) PoM
Nasal spray, desmopressin acetate 10 micrograms/metered spray. Net price 6-mL unit (60 metered sprays) = £28.00. Counselling, fluid intake, see above
Note. Children requiring dose of less than 10 micrograms should be given *DDAVP®* intranasal solution

Nocutil® (Norgine) PoM
Nasal spray, desmopressin acetate 10 micrograms/metered spray, net price 5-mL unit (50 metered sprays) = £17.50. Counselling, fluid intake, see above

TERLIPRESSIN

Indications: bleeding from oesophageal varices
Cautions: see under Vasopressin
Contra-indications: see under Vasopressin
Side-effects: see under Vasopressin, but effects milder
Dose: *by intravenous injection*, 2 mg followed by 1 or 2 mg every 4 to 6 hours until bleeding is controlled, for up to 72 hours

Glypressin® (Ferring) PoM
Injection, terlipressin, powder for reconstitution. Net price 1-mg vial with 5 mL diluent = £20.90 (hosp. only)

Antidiuretic hormone antagonists

Demeclocycline (section 5.1.3) may be used in the treatment of hyponatraemia resulting from inappropriate secretion of antidiuretic hormone. It is thought to act by directly blocking the renal tubular effect of antidiuretic hormone. Initially 0.9 to 1.2 g is given daily in divided doses, reduced to 600–900 mg daily for maintenance.

should be assessed and where necessary given prophylactic treatment; those aged over 65 years are at greater risk. Patients taking oral corticosteroids who have sustained a low-trauma fracture should receive treatment for osteoporosis. The therapeutic options for *prophylaxis* and *treatment* of corticosteroid-induced osteoporosis are the same:

- hormone replacement (HRT in women, testosterone in men) in those who are deficient;
- a bisphosphonate such as alendronate, etidronate or risedronate;
- calcitriol.

Calcitonin is involved with parathyroid hormone in the regulation of bone turnover and hence in the maintenance of calcium balance and homoeostasis. **Calcitonin (salmon) (salcatonin**, synthetic or recombinant salmon calcitonin) is used to lower the plasma-calcium concentration in some patients with hypercalcaemia (notably when associated with malignant disease). In the treatment of severe Paget's disease of bone it is used mainly for relief of pain but it is also effective in relieving some of the neurological complications, for example deafness. Calcitonin can also be used in the prevention and treatment of postmenopausal osteoporosis (see section 6.6).

CALCITONIN (SALMON)/ SALCATONIN

Indications: see under Dose

Cautions: history of allergy (skin test advised); renal impairment; heart failure; children—use for short periods only and monitor bone growth; pregnancy (Appendix 4), breast-feeding (Appendix 5)

Side-effects: nausea, vomiting, diarrhoea, flushing, dizziness, tingling of hands, unpleasant taste, rash, abdominal pain; allergic reactions including anaphylaxis reported; inflammatory reactions at injection site; nasal spray may cause local irritation and ulceration, rhinitis, sinusitis, epistaxis

Dose: hypercalcaemia, *by subcutaneous or intramuscular injection*, range from 5–10 units/kg daily (in 1–2 divided doses) *to* 400 units every 6–8 hours adjusted according to clinical and biochemical response (no additional benefit with over 8 units/kg every 6 hours); *by slow intravenous infusion* (*Forcaltonin*® and *Miacalcic*® ampoules only), 5–10 units/kg over at least 6 hours

Paget's disease of bone, *by subcutaneous or intramuscular injection*, dose range 50 units 3 times weekly to 100 units daily, in single or divided doses

Bone pain in neoplastic disease, *by subcutaneous or intramuscular injection*, 200 units every 6 hours *or* 400 units every 12 hours for 48 hours; may be repeated at discretion of physician

Postmenopausal osteoporosis, *by subcutaneous or intramuscular injection*, 100 units daily with dietary calcium and vitamin D supplements (see section 9.5.1.1 and section 9.6.4)
Intranasally, 200 units (1 spray) into one nostril daily, with dietary calcium and vitamin D supplements (see section 9.5.1.1 and section 9.6.4)

6.6 Drugs affecting bone metabolism

6.6.1 Calcitonin
6.6.2 Bisphosphonates

See also calcium (section 9.5.1.1), phosphorus (section 9.5.2), vitamin D (section 9.6.4), and oestrogens in postmenopausal osteoporosis (section 6.4.1.1).

Osteoporosis

Osteoporosis occurs most commonly in postmenopausal women and in those taking long-term oral corticosteroids. Other risk factors for osteoporosis include low body weight, cigarette smoking, excess alcohol intake, lack of physical activity, family history of osteoporosis, and early menopause.

> Those at risk of osteoporosis should maintain an adequate intake of **calcium and vitamin D** and any deficiency should be corrected by increasing dietary intake or taking supplements.

Elderly patients, especially those who are housebound or live in residential or nursing homes, are at increased risk of calcium and vitamin D deficiency and may benefit from supplements (section 9.5.1.1 and section 9.6.4). Reversible secondary causes of osteoporosis such as hyperthyroidism, hyperparathyroidism, osteomalacia or hypogonadism should be excluded, in both men and women, before treatment for osteoporosis is initiated.

POSTMENOPAUSAL OSTEOPOROSIS. **Hormone replacement therapy** (HRT, section 6.4.1.1) is recommended for *prophylaxis* of postmenopausal osteoporosis but it needs to be continued for at least 5–10 years to be beneficial. The **bisphosphonates** (such as alendronate, etidronate and risedronate, section 6.6.2) or **calcitonin** (section 6.6.1) may be considered for those at high risk of osteoporosis for whom HRT is unsuitable.

HRT or a bisphosphonate (section 6.6.2) may be used for the *treatment* of postmenopausal osteoporosis. The **bisphosphonates** (such as alendronate, etidronate and risedronate) decrease the risk of vertebral fracture; alendronate and risedronate have also been shown to reduce non-vertebral fractures. If HRT and bisphosphonates are unsuitable **calcitriol** (section 9.6.4) or **calcitonin** may be considered. Calcitonin may also be useful for pain relief for up to 3 months after a vertebral fracture if other analgesics are ineffective.

Raloxifene (section 6.4.1.1) has been introduced for the *prophylaxis* and *treatment* of vertebral fractures in postmenopausal women.

CORTICOSTEROID-INDUCED OSTEOPOROSIS. To reduce the risk of osteoporosis doses of oral corticosteroids should be as low as possible and courses of treatment as short as possible. The greatest rate of bone loss occurs during the first 6–12 months of corticosteroid use and so early steps to prevent the development of osteoporosis are important. Long-term use of inhaled corticosteroids may reduce bone mineral density (section 3.2).

Patients taking the equivalent of prednisolone 7.5 mg or more each day for 3 months or longer

Calsynar® (Rhône-Poulenc Rorer) PoM

Injection, calcitonin (salmon) 100 units/mL, net price 1-mL amp = £7.92; 200 units/mL, 2-mL vial = £28.47

For subcutaneous or intramuscular injection only

Forcaltonin® (Strakan) PoM

Injection, calcitonin (salmon) (recombinant) 100 units/mL, net price 1-mL amp = £3.56

For subcutaneous or intramuscular injection and for dilution and use as an intravenous infusion

Miacalcic® (Novartis) PoM

Nasal spray ▼, calcitonin (salmon) 200 units/metered spray, net price 2-mL unit (approx. 14 metered sprays) = £20.99

Injection, calcitonin (salmon) 50 units/mL, net price 1-mL amp = £4.27; 100 units/mL, 1-mL amp = £8.55; 200 units/mL, 2-mL vial = £30.75

For subcutaneous or intramuscular injection and for dilution and use as an intravenous infusion

---

6.6.2   Bisphosphonates

Bisphosphonates are adsorbed onto hydroxyapatite crystals in bone, slowing both their rate of growth and dissolution, and therefore reducing the rate of bone turnover. Bisphosphonates have an important role in the prophylaxis and treatment of osteoporosis and corticosteroid-induced osteoporosis; **alendronic acid** or **risedronate sodium** are considered the drugs of choice for these conditions, but **disodium etidronate** may be considered if these drugs are unsuitable or not tolerated (see also section 6.6).

Bisphosphonates are also used in the treatment of *Paget's disease* and hypercalcaemia of malignancy (section 9.5.1.2). Disodium etidronate can impair bone mineralisation when used continuously or in high doses (such as in the treatment of *Paget's disease*).

ALENDRONIC ACID

Indications: see under Dose

Cautions: upper gastro-intestinal disorders (dysphagia, symptomatic oesophageal disease, gastritis, duodenitis, or ulcers—see also under Contra-indications and Side-effects); history (within 1 year) of ulcers, active gastro-intestinal bleeding, or surgery of the upper gastro-intestinal tract; renal impairment (manufacturer advises avoid if creatinine clearance is less than 35 mL/minute); correct disturbances of calcium and mineral metabolism (e.g. vitamin-D deficiency, hypocalcaemia) before starting; exclude other causes of osteoporosis; **interactions:** Appendix 1 (bisphosphonates)

Contra-indications: abnormalities of oesophagus and other factors which delay emptying (e.g. stricture or achalasia), hypocalcaemia, pregnancy and breast-feeding

Side-effects: oesophageal reactions (see below), abdominal pain and distension, diarrhoea or constipation, flatulence, musculoskeletal pain, headache; rarely rash, erythema, photosensitivity, uveitis, transient decrease in serum phosphate; nausea, vomiting, peptic ulceration and hyper-

sensitivity reactions (including urticaria and angioedema) also reported

OESOPHAGEAL REACTIONS. Severe oesophageal reactions (oesophagitis, oesophageal ulcers, oesophageal stricture and oesophageal erosions) have been reported; patients should be advised to stop taking the tablets and to seek medical attention if they develop symptoms of oesophageal irritation such as dysphagia, new or worsening heartburn, pain on swallowing or retrosternal pain

Dose: treatment of postmenopausal osteoporosis and osteoporosis in men, 10 mg daily *or* (in postmenopausal osteoporosis) 70 mg once weekly

Prevention of postmenopausal osteoporosis, 5 mg daily

Prevention and treatment of corticosteroid-induced osteoporosis, 5 mg daily (postmenopausal women not receiving hormone replacement therapy, 10 mg daily)

COUNSELLING. Swallow the tablets whole with a full glass of water on an empty stomach at least 30 minutes before breakfast (and any other oral medication); stand or sit upright for at least 30 minutes and do not lie down until after eating breakfast. Do not take the tablets at bedtime or before rising.

Fosamax® (MSD) PoM

Tablets, alendronic acid (as alendronate sodium) 5 mg, net price 28-tab pack = £25.43; 10 mg, 28-tab pack = £23.12. Counselling, administration

Fosamax® Once Weekly (MSD) ▼ PoM

Tablets, alendronic acid (as alendronate sodium) 70 mg, net price 4-tab pack = £23.12. Counselling, administration

---

DISODIUM ETIDRONATE

Indications: see under Dose

Cautions: reduce dose in mild renal impairment (avoid if moderate to severe); **interactions:** Appendix 1 (bisphosphonates)

Contra-indications: moderate to severe renal impairment; pregnancy and breast-feeding; not indicated for osteoporosis in presence of hypercalcaemia or hypercalciuria or for osteomalacia

Side-effects: nausea, diarrhoea or constipation, abdominal pain; increased bone pain in Paget's disease, also increased risk of fractures with high doses in Paget's disease (discontinue if fractures occur); rarely skin reactions (including angioedema, urticaria, and pruritus), transient hyperphosphataemia, headache, paraesthesia, peripheral neuropathy reported; blood disorders (including leucopenia, agranulocytosis and pancytopenia) also reported

Dose: Paget's disease of bone, *by mouth*, 5 mg/kg as a single daily dose for up to 6 months; doses above 10 mg/kg daily for up to 3 months may be used with caution but doses above 20 mg/kg daily are not recommended; after interval of not less than 3 months may be repeated where evidence of reactivation—including biochemical indices (avoid premature retreatment)

MONITORING. Serum phosphate, serum alkaline phosphatase and (if possible) urinary hydroxyproline should be measured before starting and at intervals of 3 months—consult product literature for further details

Osteoporosis, see under *Didronel PMO®*

COUNSELLING. Avoid food for at least 2 hours before and after oral treatment, particularly calcium-containing products e.g. milk; also avoid iron and mineral supplements and antacids

Didronel® (Procter & Gamble Pharm.) PoM
Tablets, disodium etidronate 200 mg. Net price 60-tab pack = £37.30. Counselling, food and calcium (see above)

■ With calcium carbonate
For cautions and side-effects of calcium carbonate see section 9.5.1.1

Didronel PMO® (Procter & Gamble Pharm.) PoM
Tablets, 14 white, disodium etidronate 400 mg; 76 pink, effervescent, calcium carbonate 1.25 g (*Cacit®*). Net price per pack = £40.20. Label: 10 patient information leaflet, counselling, food and calcium (see above)
Dose: treatment of osteoporosis, prevention of bone loss in postmenopausal women (particularly if hormone replacement therapy inappropriate), and prevention and treatment of corticosteroid-induced osteoporosis, given in 90-day cycles, 1 *Didronel®* tablet daily for 14 days, then 1 *Cacit®* tablet daily for 76 days

DISODIUM PAMIDRONATE

Disodium pamidronate was formerly called aminohydroxypropylidenediphosphonate disodium (APD)
Indications: see under Dose
Cautions: renal impairment—monitor renal function in those with pre-existing renal disease or predisposition to renal impairment (e.g. in multiple myeloma or tumour-induced hypercalcaemia); cardiac disease (especially in elderly); previous thyroid surgery (risk of hypocalcaemia); monitor serum electrolytes, calcium and phosphate—possibility of convulsions due to electrolyte changes; avoid concurrent use with other bisphosphonates; **interactions:** Appendix 1 (bisphosphonates)
DRIVING. Patients should be warned against driving or operating machinery immediately after treatment (somnolence or dizziness may occur)
Contra-indications: pregnancy and breast-feeding
Side-effects: hypophosphataemia, transient rise in body temperature, fever and influenza-like symptoms (sometimes accompanied by malaise, rigors, fatigue and flushes); occasionally transient bone pain, arthralgia, myalgia, nausea, vomiting, headache, lymphocytopenia, hypomagnesaemia; rarely muscle cramps, anorexia, abdominal pain, diarrhoea, constipation, dyspepsia, agitation, confusion, dizziness, insomnia, somnolence, lethargy, anaemia, leucopenia, hypotension or hypertension, rash, pruritus, hyperkalaemia or hypokalaemia, hypernatraemia; isolated cases of seizures, hallucinations, thrombocytopenia, haematuria, acute renal failure, deterioration of pre-existing renal disease, conjunctivitis and other ocular symptoms, abnormal liver function tests, reactivation of herpes simplex and zoster also reported; also local reactions at injection site
Dose: *by slow intravenous infusion* (via cannula in a relatively large vein), see also Appendix 6
Hypercalcaemia of malignancy, according to serum calcium concentration 15–60 mg in single infusion or in divided doses over 2–4 days; max. 90 mg per treatment course
Osteolytic lesions and bone pain in bone metastases associated with breast cancer or multiple myeloma, 90 mg every 4 weeks (or every 3 weeks to coincide with chemotherapy in breast cancer)

Paget's disease of bone, 30 mg once a week for 6 weeks (total dose 180 mg) *or* 30 mg in first week then 60 mg every other week (total dose 210 mg); max. total 360 mg (in divided doses of 60 mg) per treatment course; may be repeated every 6 months
CALCIUM AND VITAMIN D SUPPLEMENTS. Oral supplements are advised for those with Paget's disease at risk of calcium or vitamin D deficiency (e.g. through malabsorption or lack of exposure to sunlight) to minimise potential risk of hypocalcaemia

Aredia Dry Powder® (Novartis) PoM
Injection, powder for reconstitution, disodium pamidronate, for use as an infusion. Net price 15-mg vial = £29.82; 30-mg vial = £59.66; 90-mg vial = £170.45 (all with diluent). Counselling, driving, see above

RISEDRONATE SODIUM

Indications: see under Dose
Cautions: oesophageal abnormalities and other factors which delay transit or emptying (e.g. stricture or achalasia—see also under Side-effects); renal impairment (manufacturer advises avoid if creatinine clearance is less than 30 mL/minute); correct hypocalcaemia before starting, correct other disturbances of bone and mineral metabolism (e.g. vitamin-D deficiency) at onset of treatment; **interactions:** Appendix 1 (bisphosphonates)
Contra-indications: hypocalcaemia (see Cautions above), pregnancy and breast-feeding
Side-effects: gastro-intestinal effects (including dyspepsia, nausea, diarrhoea, constipation, oesophageal stricture, and duodenitis); headache; musculoskeletal pain; rarely glossitis, oedema, weight loss, apnoea, bronchitis, sinusitis, rash, nocturia, ambylopia, corneal lesion, dry eye, tinnitus, iritis
Dose: Paget's disease of bone, 30 mg daily for 2 months; may be repeated if necessary after at least 2 months
Treatment and prevention of osteoporosis (including corticosteroid-induced osteoporosis) in postmenopausal women, 5 mg daily
COUNSELLING. Swallow tablets whole with full glass of water; on rising, take on an empty stomach at least 30 minutes before first food or drink of the day **or**, if taking at any other time of the day, avoid food and drink for at least 2 hours before or after risedronate (particularly avoid calcium-containing products e.g. milk, also avoid iron and mineral supplements and antacids); stand or sit upright for at least 30 minutes; do not take tablets at bedtime or before rising

Actonel® (Procter & Gamble Pharm.) ▼ PoM
Tablets, f/c, risedronate sodium 5 mg (yellow), net price 28-tab pack = £21.83; 30 mg (white), 28-tab pack = £152.81. Counselling, administration, food and calcium (see above)

SODIUM CLODRONATE

Indications: see under Dose
Cautions: monitor renal and hepatic function and white cell count; also monitor serum calcium and phosphate periodically; renal dysfunction reported in patients receiving concomitant NSAIDs; maintain adequate fluid intake during

treatment; **interactions:** Appendix 1 (bisphosphonates)

Contra-indications: moderate to severe renal impairment; pregnancy and breast-feeding

Side-effects: nausea, diarrhoea; skin reactions

Dose: osteolytic lesions, hypercalcaemia and bone pain associated with skeletal metastases in patients with breast cancer or multiple myeloma, *by mouth*, 1.6 g daily in single or 2 divided doses increased if necessary to a max. of 3.2 g daily

COUNSELLING. Avoid food for 1 hour before and after treatment, particularly calcium-containing products e.g. milk; also avoid iron and mineral supplements and antacids; maintain adequate fluid intake

Hypercalcaemia of malignancy, *by slow intravenous infusion*, 300 mg daily for max. 7–10 days *or* by single-dose infusion of 1.5 g

Bonefos® (Boehringer Ingelheim) PoM
Capsules, yellow, sodium clodronate 400 mg. Net price 30-cap pack = £43.54, 120-cap pack = £174.16. Counselling, food and calcium
Tablets, f/c, scored, sodium clodronate 800 mg. Net price 10-tab pack = £30.40; 60-tab pack = £182.39. Counselling, food and calcium
Concentrate (= intravenous solution), sodium clodronate 60 mg/mL, for dilution and use as infusion. Net price 5-mL amp = £13.78

Loron® (Roche) PoM
Loron® capsules, sodium clodronate 400 mg. Net price 30-cap pack = £43.54. Label: 10 patient information leaflet, counselling, food and calcium
Loron 520® tablets, f/c, scored, sodium clodronate 520 mg. Net price 10-tab pack = £29.03; 60-tab pack = £174.18. Label: 10 patient information leaflet, counselling, food and calcium
Dose: 2 tablets daily in single or two divided doses; may be increased to max. 4 tablets daily
Note. Due to greater bioavailability one *Loron 520®* tablet (520 mg) is equivalent to two *Loron®* capsules (2 × 400 mg)

TILUDRONIC ACID

Indications: Paget's disease of bone

Cautions: renal impairment (monitor renal function regularly, see under Contra-indications); correct disturbances of calcium metabolism (e.g. vitamin D deficiency, hypocalcaemia) before starting; avoid concomitant use of indometacin; **interactions:** Appendix 1 (bisphosphonates)

Contra-indications: severe renal impairment, juvenile Paget's disease, pregnancy and breast-feeding

Side-effects: stomach pain, nausea, diarrhoea; rarely asthenia, dizziness, headache and skin reactions

Dose: 400 mg daily as a single dose for 12 weeks; may be repeated if necessary after 6 months

COUNSELLING. Avoid food for 2 hours before and after treatment, particularly calcium-containing products e.g. milk; also avoid antacids

Skelid® (Sanofi-Synthelabo) PoM
Tablets, tiludronic acid (as tiludronate disodium) 200 mg. Net price 28-tab pack = £99.00. Counselling, food and calcium

ZOLEDRONIC ACID

Indications: hypercalcaemia of malignancy

Cautions: monitor serum electrolytes, calcium, phosphate and magnesium; renal impairment—monitor renal function (Appendix 3); severe hepatic impairment (Appendix 2); cardiac disease (avoid fluid overload); **interactions:** Appendix 1 (bisphosphonates)

Contra-indications: pregnancy (Appendix 4), breast-feeding

Side-effects: influenza-like symptoms such as fever and bone pain, hypophosphataemia, arthralgia, fatigue, confusion, thirst, taste disturbance, nausea, pancytopenia, bradycardia, elevated creatinine levels; rarely hypomagnesaemia, thrombocytopenia, headache, vomiting, rash, pruritus, conjunctivitis, chest pain; acute renal failure also reported; also local reactions at injection site

Dose: *by intravenous infusion*, 4 mg as a single dose; CHILD not recommended

Zometa® (Novartis) ▼ PoM
Injection, powder for reconstitution, zoledronic acid, for use as an infusion, net price 4-mg vial (with water for injections) = £195.00

6.7   Other endocrine drugs

6.7.1   Bromocriptine and other dopamine-receptor stimulants
6.7.2   Drugs affecting gonadotrophins
6.7.3   Metyrapone and trilostane

6.7.1   Bromocriptine and other dopamine-receptor stimulants

Bromocriptine is a stimulant of dopamine receptors in the brain; it also inhibits release of prolactin by the pituitary. Bromocriptine is used for the treatment of galactorrhoea and cyclical benign breast disease, and for the treatment of prolactinomas (when it reduces both plasma prolactin concentration and tumour size). Bromocriptine also inhibits the release of growth hormone and is sometimes used in the treatment of acromegaly, but somatostatin analogues (such as octreotide, section 8.3.4.3) are more effective.

Cabergoline has actions and uses similar to those of bromocriptine, but its duration of action is longer. Its profile of side-effects appears to differ from that of bromocriptine, which means that patients intolerant of bromocriptine may be able to tolerate cabergoline (and *vice versa*).

Quinagolide has actions and uses similar to those of bromocriptine, but its profile of side-effects differs slightly.

SUPPRESSION OF LACTATION. Although bromocriptine and cabergoline are licensed to suppress lactation, they are **not** recommended for routine suppression (or for the relief of symptoms of postpartum pain and engorgement) that can be adequately treated with simple analgesics and breast support. Quinagolide is not licensed for the suppression of lactation.

BROMOCRIPTINE

Indications: see notes above and under Dose; parkinsonism (section 4.9.1)

Cautions: specialist evaluation—monitor for pituitary enlargement, particularly during pregnancy, annual gynaecological assessment (postmenopausal, every 6 months), monitor for peptic ulceration in acromegalic patients; contraceptive advice if appropriate (oral contraceptives may increase prolactin concentration); caution in patients with history of serious mental disorders (especially psychotic disorders) or with cardiovascular disease or Raynaud's syndrome and monitor for retroperitoneal fibrosis; porphyria (section 9.8.2); **interactions:** Appendix 1 (bromocriptine and cabergoline)

HYPOTENSIVE REACTIONS. Hypotensive reactions may be disturbing in some patients during the first few days of treatment and particular care should be exercised when driving or operating machinery; tolerance may be reduced by alcohol

Contra-indications: hypersensitivity to bromocriptine or other ergot alkaloids; toxaemia of pregnancy and hypertension in postpartum women or in puerperium (see also below); advise women not to breast-feed if lactation prevention fails

POSTPARTUM OR PUERPERIUM. Should not be used postpartum or in puerperium in women with high blood pressure, coronary artery disease or symptoms (or history) of serious mental disorder; monitor blood pressure carefully (especially during first few days) in postpartum women. Very rarely hypertension, myocardial infarction, seizures or stroke (both sometimes preceded by severe headache) and mental disorders have been reported in postpartum women given bromocriptine for lactation suppression—caution with antihypertensive therapy and avoid other ergot alkaloids. Discontinue immediately if hypertension, unremitting headache or signs of CNS toxicity develop

Side-effects: nausea, vomiting, constipation, headache, dizziness, postural hypotension, drowsiness, vasospasm of fingers and toes particularly in patients with Raynaud's syndrome; also, particularly with *high doses*, confusion, psychomotor excitation, hallucinations, dyskinesia, dry mouth, leg cramps, pleural effusions (may necessitate withdrawal of treatment), retroperitoneal fibrosis reported (monitoring required)

Dose: prevention or suppression of lactation (but see notes above and under Contra-indications), 2.5 mg on day 1 (prevention) or daily for 2–3 days (suppression); then 2.5 mg twice daily for 14 days
Hypogonadism, galactorrhoea, infertility, initially 1–1.25 mg at bedtime, increased gradually; usual dose 7.5 mg daily in divided doses, increased if necessary to max. 30 mg daily, usual dose in infertility without hyperprolactinaemia, 2.5 mg twice daily
Cyclical benign breast disease and cyclical menstrual disorders (particularly breast pain), 1–1.25 mg at bedtime, increased gradually; usual dose 2.5 mg twice daily
Acromegaly, initially 1–1.25 mg at bedtime, increase gradually to 5 mg every 6 hours
Prolactinoma, initially 1–1.25 mg at bedtime; increased gradually to 5 mg every 6 hours (occasional patients may require up to 30 mg daily)
CHILD under 15 years, not recommended

Bromocriptine (Non-proprietary) PoM
Tablets, bromocriptine (as mesilate) 2.5 mg, net price 30-tab pack = £5.05. Label: 21, counselling, hypotensive reactions
Available from Alpharma, IVAX, Kent

Parlodel® (Novartis) PoM
Tablets, both scored, bromocriptine (as mesilate) 1 mg, net price 100-tab pack = £9.90; 2.5 mg, 30-tab pack = £5.78. Label: 21, counselling, hypotensive reactions
Capsules, bromocriptine (as mesilate) 5 mg (blue/white), net price 100-cap pack = £37.57; 10 mg (white), 100-cap pack = £69.50. Label: 21, counselling, hypotensive reactions

CABERGOLINE

Indications: see notes above and under Dose

Cautions: see under Bromocriptine; peptic ulcer, gastro-intestinal bleeding; severe hepatic impairment; fibrotic lung disease; monthly pregnancy tests during the amenorrhoeic period; advise non-hormonal contraception if pregnancy not desired (see also Contra-indications); **interactions:** Appendix 1 (bromocriptine and cabergoline)
HYPOTENSIVE REACTIONS. Hypotensive reactions may be disturbing in some patients during the first few days of treatment and particular care should be exercised when driving or operating machinery; tolerance may be reduced by alcohol

Contra-indications: see under Bromocriptine; exclude pregnancy before starting and avoid until at least 1 month after successful treatment (ovulatory cycles persist for 6 months)—discontinue if pregnancy occurs during treatment (specialist advice needed)

Side-effects: see under Bromocriptine (but profile of side-effects may differ, see notes above); dyspepsia, epigastric and abdominal pain, breast pain, palpitations, angina, epistaxis, peripheral oedema, hemianopia, asthenia, erythromelalgia, hot flushes, depression

Dose: prevention of lactation (but see notes above), during first day postpartum, 1 mg as a single dose; suppression of established lactation (but see notes above) 250 micrograms every 12 hours for 2 days
Hyperprolactinaemic disorders, 500 micrograms weekly (as a single dose *or* as 2 divided doses on separate days) increased at monthly intervals in steps of 500 micrograms until optimal therapeutic response (usually 1 mg weekly, range 0.25–2 mg weekly) with monthly monitoring of serum prolactin levels; reduce initial dose and increase more gradually if patient intolerant; over 1 mg weekly give as divided doses; up to 4.5 mg weekly has been used in hyperprolactinaemic patients
Parkinsonism, section 4.9.1
CHILD under 16 years, not recommended

Dostinex® (Pharmacia) ▼ PoM
Tablets, scored, cabergoline 500 micrograms. Net price 8-tab pack = £30.04. Label: 21, counselling, hypotensive reactions

QUINAGOLIDE

Indications: see notes above and under Dose
Cautions: see under Bromocriptine; advise non-hormonal contraception if pregnancy not desired;

discontinue if pregnancy occurs during treatment (specialist advice needed); **interactions:** Appendix 1 (quinagolide)

HYPOTENSIVE REACTIONS. Hypotensive reactions may be disturbing in some patients during the first few days of treatment—monitor blood pressure for a few days after starting treatment and following dosage increases; particular care should be exercised when driving or operating machinery; tolerance may be reduced by alcohol

Contra-indications: see under Bromocriptine; hypersensitivity to quinagolide (but not ergot alkaloids)

Side-effects: see under Bromocriptine (but profile of side-effects may differ, see notes above); also syncope, anorexia, abdominal pain, diarrhoea, insomnia, oedema, flushing and nasal congestion

Dose: hyperprolactinaemia, 25 micrograms at bedtime for 3 days; increased at intervals of 3 days in steps of 25 micrograms to usual maintenance dose of 75–150 micrograms daily; for doses higher than 300 micrograms daily increase in steps of 75–150 micrograms at intervals of not less than 4 weeks

CHILD not recommended

Norprolac® (Novartis) [PoM]
Tablets, quinagolide (as hydrochloride) 75 micrograms (white), net price 30-tab pack = £62.36; starter pack of 3 × 25-microgram tabs (pink) with 3 × 50-microgram tabs (blue) = £5.47.
Label: 21, counselling, hypotensive reactions

6.7.2 Drugs affecting gonadotrophins

Danazol inhibits pituitary gonadotrophins; it combines androgenic activity with antioestrogenic and antiprogestogenic activity. It is used in the treatment of *endometriosis* and has also been used for *mammary dysplasia*, and *gynaecomastia* where other measures have proved unsatisfactory; it has been used for *menorrhagia* and other *menstrual disorders* but in view of its side-effects, treatment with other drugs may be preferable (section 6.4.1.2). It may also be effective in the long-term management of *hereditary angioedema* [unlicensed indication].

Gestrinone has general actions similar to those of danazol and is indicated for the treatment of endometriosis.

Cetrorelix and **ganirelix** are luteinising hormone releasing hormone antagonists, which inhibit the release of gonadotrophins (luteinising hormone and follicle-stimulating hormone). They are used in the treatment of infertility by assisted reproductive techniques.

CETRORELIX

Indications: adjunct in the treatment of female infertility (under specialist supervision)

Contra-indications: pregnancy, breast-feeding, moderate renal impairment, moderate hepatic impairment

Side-effects: nausea, headache, injection site reactions

Dose: by subcutaneous injection into the lower abdominal wall,

either 250 micrograms in the morning, starting on day 5 or 6 of ovarian stimulation with gonadotrophins (or each evening starting on day 5 of ovarian stimulation); continue throughout administration of gonadotrophin including day of ovulation induction (or evening before ovulation induction)

or 3 mg on day 7 of ovarian stimulation with gonadotrophins; if ovulation induction not possible on day 5 after 3-mg dose, additional 250 micrograms once daily until day of ovulation induction

Cetrotide® (Serono) ▼ [PoM]
Injection, powder for reconstitution, cetrorelix (as acetate), net price 250-micrograms vial = £24.00; 3-mg vial = £168.00 (both with solvent)

DANAZOL

Indications: see notes above and under Dose

Cautions: cardiac, hepatic, or renal impairment (avoid if severe), elderly, polycythaemia, epilepsy, diabetes mellitus, hypertension, migraine, lipoprotein disorder, history of thrombosis or thromboembolic disease; withdraw if virilisation (may be irreversible on continued use); non-hormonal contraceptive methods should be used, if appropriate; **interactions:** Appendix 1 (danazol)

Contra-indications: pregnancy (Appendix 4), ensure that patients with amenorrhoea are not pregnant; breast-feeding; severe hepatic, renal or cardiac impairment; thromboembolic disease; undiagnosed genital bleeding; androgen-dependent tumours; porphyria (section 9.8.2)

Side-effects: nausea, dizziness, skin reactions including rashes, photosensitivity and exfoliative dermatitis, fever, backache, nervousness, mood changes, anxiety, changes in libido, vertigo, fatigue, epigastric and pleuritic pain, headache, weight gain; menstrual disturbances, vaginal dryness and irritation, flushing and reduction in breast size; musculo-skeletal spasm, joint pain and swelling, hair loss; androgenic effects including acne, oily skin, oedema, hirsutism, voice changes and rarely clitoral hypertrophy (see also Cautions); temporary alteration in lipoproteins and other metabolic changes, insulin resistance; thrombotic events; leucopenia, thrombocytopenia, eosinophilia, reversible erythrocytosis or polycythaemia reported; headache and visual disturbances may indicate benign intracranial hypertension; rarely cholestatic jaundice, pancreatitis, peliosis hepatis and benign hepatic adenomata

Dose: usually given in up to 4 divided doses; in women of child-bearing potential, treatment should start during menstruation, preferably on day 1

Endometriosis, 200–800 mg daily in up to 4 divided doses, adjusted to achieve amenorrhoea, usually for 6 months (up to 9 months in some cases)

Menorrhagia (but see notes above), 200 mg daily, usually for 3 months

Severe cyclical mastalgia, 100–400 mg daily usually for 3–6 months

Benign breast cysts, 300 mg daily usually for 3–6 months

Gynaecomastia, 400 mg daily in up to 4 divided doses for 6 months (adolescents 200 mg daily, increased to 400 mg daily if no response after 2 months)

For pre-operative thinning of endometrium, 400–800 mg daily in up to 4 divided doses for 3–6 weeks

Danazol (Non-proprietary) PoM
Capsules, danazol 100 mg, net price 60-cap pack = £14.72; 200 mg, net price 56-cap pack = £26.35
Available from Alpharma, Generics, Hillcross, IVAX, Kent, Sterwin

Danol® (Sanofi-Synthelabo) PoM
Capsules, danazol 100 mg (grey/white), net price 60-cap pack = £17.04; 200 mg (pink/white), 60-cap pack = £33.75

GANIRELIX

Indications: adjunct in the treatment of female infertility (under specialist supervision)

Contra-indications: pregnancy, breast-feeding, moderate renal impairment, moderate hepatic impairment

Side-effects: nausea, headache, injection site reactions; dizziness and malaise also reported

Dose: *by subcutaneous injection* preferably into the upper leg (rotate injection sites to prevent lipoatrophy), 250 micrograms in the morning (or each afternoon) starting on day 6 of ovarian stimulation with gonadotrophins; continue throughout administration of gonadotrophins including day of ovulation induction (if administering in afternoon, give last dose in afternoon *before* ovulation induction)

Orgalutran® (Organon) ▼ PoM
Injection, ganirelix, 500 micrograms/mL, net price 0.5-mL prefilled syringe = £24.00

GESTRINONE

Indications: endometriosis

Cautions: cardiac and renal impairment; **interactions:** Appendix 1 (gestrinone)

Contra-indications: pregnancy (use non-hormonal method of contraception) and breast-feeding; severe cardiac, renal or hepatic impairment; metabolic or vascular disorders associated with previous sex hormone treatment

Side-effects: spotting; acne, oily skin, fluid retention, weight gain, hirsutism, voice change; liver enzyme disturbances; headache; gastro-intestinal disturbances; change in libido, flushing, decrease in breast size; nervousness, depression, change in appetite; muscle cramp

Dose: 2.5 mg twice weekly starting on first day of cycle with second dose 3 days later, repeated on same two days preferably at same time each week; duration of treatment usually 6 months
MISSED DOSE. One missed dose—2.5 mg as soon as possible and maintain original sequence; two or more missed doses—discontinue, re-start on first day of new cycle (following negative pregnancy test)

Dimetriose® (Florizel) PoM
Capsules, gestrinone 2.5 mg, net price 8-cap pack = £111.73

Gonadorelin analogues

Administration of **gonadorelin analogues** produces an initial phase of stimulation; continued administration is followed by down-regulation of gonadotrophin-releasing hormone receptors, thereby reducing the release of gonadotrophins (follicle stimulating hormone and luteinising hormone) which in turn leads to inhibition of androgen and oestrogen production.

Gonadorelin analogues are used in the treatment of endometriosis, infertility, anaemia due to uterine fibroids (together with iron supplementation), breast cancer (section 8.3.4.1), prostate cancer (section 8.3.4.2) and before intra-uterine surgery.

CAUTIONS. Non-hormonal, barrier methods of contraception should be used during entire treatment period with gonadorelin analogues; also use with caution in patients with metabolic bone disease because decrease in bone mineral density can occur.

CONTRA-INDICATIONS. Gonadorelin analogues are contra-indicated for use longer than 6 months (do not repeat), where there is undiagnosed vaginal bleeding, in pregnancy (exclude pregnancy—also give first injection during menstruation or shortly afterwards *or* use barrier contraception for 1 month beforehand) and in breast-feeding.

SIDE-EFFECTS. Side-effects of the gonadorelin analogues related to the inhibition of oestrogen production include menopausal-like symptoms (e.g. hot flushes, increased sweating, vaginal dryness, dyspareunia and loss of libido) and a decrease in trabecular bone density; these effects can be reduced by hormone replacement (e.g. with an oestrogen and a progestogen or with tibolone). Side-effects of gonadorelin analogues also include headache (rarely migraine) and hypersensitivity reactions including urticaria, pruritus, skin rashes, asthma and anaphylaxis; when treating uterine fibroids bleeding associated with fibroid degeneration can occur; spray formulations can cause irritation of the nasal mucosa including nose bleeds; local reactions at injection site can occur; other side-effects also reported with some gonadorelin analogues include palpitations, hypertension, ovarian cysts (may require withdrawal), changes in breast size, musculoskeletal pain or weakness, visual disturbances, paraesthesia, changes in scalp and body hair, oedema of the face and extremities, weight changes, and mood changes including depression.

BUSERELIN

Indications: see under Dose; prostate cancer (section 8.3.4.2)

Cautions: see notes above; polycystic ovarian disease, depression, hypertension, diabetes

Contra-indications: see notes above; hormone-dependent tumours

Side-effects: see notes above; initially withdrawal bleeding and subsequently breakthrough bleeding, leucorrhoea; nausea, vomiting, constipation, diarrhoea; anxiety, memory and concentration disturbances, sleep disturbances, nervousness, dizziness, drowsiness; breast tenderness, lactation; abdominal pain; fatigue; increased thirst, changes in appetite; acne, dry skin, splitting nails, dry eyes; altered blood lipids, leucopenia, thrombocytopenia; hearing disturbances; reduced glucose tolerance

Dose: endometriosis, *intranasally*, 300 micrograms (one 150-microgram spray in each nostril) 3 times daily (starting on days 1 or 2 of menstruation); max. duration of treatment 6 months (do not repeat)

Pituitary desensitisation before induction of ovulation by gonadotrophins for *in vitro* fertilisation (under specialist supervision), *by subcutaneous injection*, 200–500 micrograms daily given as a single injection (occasionally up to 500 micrograms twice daily may be needed) starting in early follicular phase (day 1) *or*, after exclusion of pregnancy, in midluteal phase (day 21) and continued until down-regulation achieved (usually about 1–3 weeks) then maintained during gonadotrophin administration (stopping gonadotrophin and buserelin on administration of chorionic gonadotrophin at appropriate stage of follicular development)

Intranasally, 150 micrograms (one spray in one nostril) 4 times daily during waking hours (occasionally up to 300 micrograms 4 times daily may be needed) starting in early follicular phase (day 1) *or*, after exclusion of pregnancy, in midluteal phase (day 21) and continued until down-regulation achieved (usually about 2–3 weeks) then maintained during gonadotrophin administration (stopping gonadotrophin and buserelin on administration of chorionic gonadotrophin at appropriate stage of follicular development)

COUNSELLING. Avoid use of nasal decongestants before and for at least 30 minutes after treatment

Suprecur® (Shire) ▨PoM▨
Nasal spray, buserelin (as acetate)
150 micrograms/metered spray. Net price 2 × 100-dose pack (with metered dose pumps) = £75.43. Counselling, see above
Injection, buserelin (as acetate) 1mg/mL. Net price 5.5-mL vial = £11.85.

GOSERELIN

Indications: see under Dose; prostate cancer (section 8.3.4.2); advanced breast cancer (section 8.3.4.1)

Cautions: see notes above; polycystic ovarian disease

Contra-indications: see notes above

Side-effects: see notes above; withdrawal bleeding

Dose: *by subcutaneous injection* into anterior abdominal wall, endometriosis, 3.6 mg every 28 days; max. duration of treatment 6 months (do not repeat); endometrial thinning before intra-uterine surgery, 3.6 mg (may be repeated after 28 days if uterus is large or to allow flexible surgical timing); before surgery in women who have anaemia due to uterine fibroids, 3.6 mg every 28 days (with supplementary iron); max. duration of treatment 3 months

Pituitary desensitisation before induction of ovulation by gonadotrophins for *in vitro* fertilisation (under specialist supervision), after exclusion of pregnancy, 3.6 mg to achieve pituitary down-regulation (usually 1–3 weeks) then gonadotrophin is administered (stopping gonadotrophin on administration of chorionic gonadotrophin at appropriate stage of follicular development)

Preparation
Section 8.3.4.2

LEUPRORELIN ACETATE

Indications: see under Dose; prostate cancer (section 8.3.4.2)

Cautions: see notes above; family history of osteoporosis; chronic use of other drugs which reduce bone density including alcohol and tobacco; diabetes

Contra-indications: see notes above

Side-effects: see notes above; breast tenderness; nausea, vomiting, diarrhoea, anorexia; fever, chills; sleep disturbances, dizziness, fatigue, leucopenia, thrombocytopenia, altered blood lipids

Dose: *by subcutaneous or intramuscular injection*, endometriosis, 3.75 mg as a single dose in first 5 days of menstrual cycle then every month for max. 6 months (course not to be repeated)

Endometrial thinning before intra-uterine surgery, 3.75 mg as a single dose (given between days 3 and 5 of menstrual cycle) 5–6 weeks before surgery

Reduction of size of uterine fibroids and of associated bleeding before surgery, 3.75 mg as a single dose every month usually for 3–4 months (max. 6 months)

Preparation
Section 8.3.4.2

NAFARELIN

Indications: see under Dose
Cautions: see notes above
Contra-indications: see notes above
Side-effects: see notes above; acne
Dose: women over 18 years, endometriosis, 200 micrograms twice daily as one spray in one nostril in the morning and one spray in the other nostril in the evening (starting on days 2–4 of menstruation), max. duration of treatment 6 months (do not repeat)

Pituitary desensitisation before induction of ovulation by gonadotrophins for *in vitro* fertilisation (under specialist supervision), 400 micrograms (one spray in each nostril) twice daily starting in early follicular phase (day 2) or, after exclusion of pregnancy, in midluteal phase (day 21) and continued until down-regulation achieved (usually within 4 weeks) then maintained (usually for 8–12 days) during gonadotrophin administration (stopping gonadotrophin and nafarelin on administration of chorionic gonadotrophin at follicular maturity); discontinue if down-regulation not achieved within 12 weeks

COUNSELLING. Avoid use of nasal decongestants before and for at least 30 minutes after treatment; repeat dose if sneezing occurs during or immediately after administration

Synarel® (Pharmacia) [PoM]

Nasal spray, nafarelin 200 micrograms (as acetate)/metered spray. Net price 30-dose unit = £30.74; 60-dose unit = £53.01. Label: 10 patient information leaflet, counselling, see above

TRIPTORELIN

Indications: see under dose; prostate cancer (section 8.3.4.2)

Cautions: see notes above

Contra-indications: see notes above

Side-effects: see notes above; asthenia

Dose: *by intramuscular injection*, endometriosis and reduction in size of uterine fibroids, 3 mg every 4 weeks starting during the first 5 days of menstrual cycle; for uterine fibroids continue treatment for at least 3 months; max. duration of treatment 6 months (do not repeat)

Preparations

Section 8.3.4.2

Breast pain (mastalgia)

Once any serious underlying cause for breast pain has been ruled out, most women will respond to reassurance and reduction in dietary fat; withdrawal of an oral contraceptive or of hormone replacement therapy may help to resolve the pain.

Mild, non-cyclical breast pain is treated with simple analgesics (section 4.7.1); moderate to severe pain, cyclical pain or symptoms that persist for longer than 6 months may require specific drug treatment. **Gamolenic acid** can be useful for cyclical pain and, because it lacks anti-oestrogenic side-effects, it may be preferred, particularly in younger women who wish to continue taking an oral contraceptive. Although **danazol** is effective it may be unacceptable owing to its adverse effects (which occur in about one-third of patients). **Bromocriptine** (section 6.7.1) like danazol is associated with unpleasant side-effects. Whereas bromocriptine and danazol act within 2 months, gamolenic acid may require up to 4 months to take effect.

Treatment for breast pain should be reviewed after 6 months and continued if necessary. Symptoms recur in about 50% of women within 2 years of withdrawal of therapy but may be less severe.

GAMOLENIC ACID

Indications: symptom relief of cyclical and non-cyclical mastalgia; atopic eczema (section 13.5.1)

Cautions: history of epilepsy, concomitant treatment with epileptogenic drugs e.g. phenothiazines; pregnancy

Side-effects: occasional nausea, indigestion, headache; rarely hypersensitivity reactions including rash, urticaria, pruritus and abdominal pain

Dose: cyclical and non-cyclical mastalgia, 240–320 mg daily in 1–2 divided doses until response obtained then stopped or dose reduced (may take 8–12 weeks for response in some patients)

Efamast® (Pharmacia) [PoM]

Efamast® 40 capsules, gamolenic acid 40 mg in evening primrose oil, net price 224-cap pack = £22.65
Excipients: include vitamin E

Efamast® 80 capsules, gamolenic acid 80 mg in evening primrose oil , net price 112-cap pack = £22.65
Excipients: include vitamin E

6.7.3 Metyrapone and trilostane

Metyrapone is a competitive inhibitor of 11β-hydroxylation in the adrenal cortex; the resulting inhibition of cortisol (and to a lesser extent aldosterone) production leads to an increase in ACTH production which, in turn, leads to increased synthesis and release of cortisol precursors. It may be used as a test of anterior pituitary function.

Although most types of *Cushing's syndrome* are treated surgically, that which occasionally accompanies carcinoma of the bronchus is not usually amenable to surgery. Metyrapone has been found helpful in controlling the symptoms of the disease; it is also used in other forms of Cushing's syndrome to prepare the patient for surgery. The dosages used are either low, and tailored to cortisol production, or high, in which case corticosteroid replacement therapy is also needed.

Trilostane reversibly inhibits 3β-hydroxysteroid dehydrogenase/delta 5-4 isomerase in the adrenal cortex; the resulting inhibition of the synthesis of mineralocorticoids and glucocorticoids may be useful in *Cushing's syndrome* and *primary hyperaldosteronism*. Trilostane appears to be less effective than metyrapone for Cushing's syndrome (where it is tailored to corticosteroid production). It also has a minor role in post-menopausal breast cancer that has relapsed following initial oestrogen antagonist therapy (corticosteroid replacement therapy is also required). **Ketoconazole** (section 5.2) is also used by specialists for the management of *Cushing's syndrome* [unlicensed indication].

See also aminoglutethimide (section 8.3.4)

METYRAPONE

Indications: see notes above and under Dose (specialist supervision in hospital)

Cautions: gross hypopituitarism (risk of precipitating acute adrenal failure); hypertension on long-term administration; hypothyroidism or hepatic impairment (delayed response); many drugs interfere with diagnostic estimation of steroids; avoid in porphyria (section 9.8.2)
DRIVING. Drowsiness may affect the performance of skilled tasks (e.g. driving)

Contra-indications: adrenocortical insufficiency (see Cautions); pregnancy (Appendix 4), breast-feeding (Appendix 5)

Side-effects: occasional nausea, vomiting, dizziness, headache, hypotension, sedation; rarely abdominal pain, allergic skin reactions, hypoadrenalism, hirsutism

Dose: differential diagnosis of ACTH-dependent Cushing's syndrome, 750 mg every 4 hours for 6 doses; CHILD 15 mg/kg (minimum 250 mg) every 4 hours for 6 doses

Management of Cushing's syndrome, range 0.25–6 g daily, tailored to cortisol production; see notes above

Resistant oedema due to increased aldosterone secretion in cirrhosis, nephrosis, and congestive heart failure (with glucocorticoid replacement therapy) 3 g daily in divided doses

Metopirone® (Alliance) PoM
Capsules, ivory, metyrapone 250 mg. Net price 100-tab pack = £42.50. Label: 21, counselling, driving
Note. May be difficult to obtain

TRILOSTANE

Indications: see notes above and under Dose (specialist supervision)

Cautions: breast cancer (concurrent corticosteroid replacement therapy needed, see under Dose), adrenal cortical hyperfunction (tailored to cortisol and electrolytes, concurrent corticosteroid therapy may be needed, see under Dose); hepatic and renal impairment; **interactions:** Appendix 1 (trilostane)

Contra-indications: pregnancy (use non-hormonal method of contraception) and breast-feeding; children

Side-effects: flushing, tingling and swelling of mouth, rhinorrhoea, nausea, vomiting, diarrhoea, and rashes reported; rarely granulocytopenia

Dose: adrenal cortical hyperfunction, 240 mg daily in divided doses for at least 3 days then tailored according to response with regular monitoring of plasma electrolytes and circulating corticosteroids (both mineralocorticoid and glucocorticoid replacement therapy may be needed); usual dose: 120–480 mg daily (may be increased to 960 mg)

Postmenopausal breast cancer (with glucocorticoid replacement therapy) following relapse to initial oestrogen receptor antagonist therapy, initially 240 mg daily increased every 3 days in steps of 240 mg to a maintenance dose of 960 mg daily (720 mg daily if not tolerated)

Modrenal® (Wanskerne) PoM
Capsules, trilostane 60 mg (pink/black), net price 100-cap pack = £49.50; 120 mg (pink/yellow), 100-cap pack = £98.50. Label: 21

7: Obstetrics, gynaecology, and urinary-tract disorders

For hormonal therapy of gynaecological disorders see section 6.4.1, section 6.5.1 and section 6.7.2.

7.1 Drugs used in obstetrics

7.1.1 Prostaglandins and oxytocics
7.1.2 Mifepristone
7.1.3 Myometrial relaxants

Because of the complexity of dosage regimens in obstetrics, in all cases **detailed specialist literature** should be consulted.

7.1.1 Prostaglandins and oxytocics

Prostaglandins and oxytocics are used to induce abortion or induce or augment labour and to minimise blood loss from the placental site. They include oxytocin, ergometrine, and the prostaglandins. All induce uterine contractions with varying degrees of pain according to the strength of contractions induced.

INDUCTION OF ABORTION. **Gemeprost**, administered vaginally as pessaries is the preferred prostaglandin for the medical induction of late therapeutic abortion. Gemeprost ripens and softens the cervix before surgical abortion, particularly in primigravida. The prostaglandin **misoprostol** is given by mouth or by vaginal administration to induce medical abortion [unlicensed indication]; intravaginal use ripens the cervix before surgical abortion [unlicensed indication]. Extra-amniotic **dinoprostone** is rarely used nowadays.

Pre-treatment with **mifepristone** (section 7.1.2) can facilitate the process of medical abortion. It sensitises the uterus to subsequent administration of a prostaglandin and, therefore, abortion occurs in a shorter time and with a lower dose of prostaglandin.

INDUCTION AND AUGMENTATION OF LABOUR. **Dinoprostone** is available as vaginal tablets, pessaries and vaginal gels for the induction of labour. The intravenous solution and oral tablets are rarely used since oral tablets are less effective than vaginal preparations and both are associated with more side-effects.

Oxytocin (*Syntocinon®*) is administered by slow intravenous infusion, using an infusion pump, to induce or augment labour, usually in conjunction with amniotomy. Uterine activity must be monitored carefully and hyperstimulation avoided. Large doses of oxytocin may result in excessive fluid retention.

Misoprostol is given orally or vaginally for the induction of labour [unlicensed indication].

PREVENTION AND TREATMENT OF HAEMORRHAGE. Bleeding due to incomplete abortion can be controlled with **ergometrine** and **oxytocin** (*Syntometrine®*) given intramuscularly; the dose is adjusted according to the patient's condition and blood loss. This is commonly used before surgical evacuation of the uterus, particularly when surgery is delayed. Oxytocin and ergometrine combined are more effective in early pregnancy than either drug alone.

For the routine management of the third stage of labour ergometrine 500 micrograms with oxytocin 5 units (*Syntometrine®* 1 mL) is given by intramuscular injection on delivery of the anterior shoulder or, at the latest, immediately after the baby is delivered. If ergometrine is inappropriate (e.g. in pre-eclampsia), oxytocin alone may be given by intramuscular injection [unlicensed indication].

In excessive uterine bleeding, any placental products remaining in the uterus should be removed. In bleeding caused by uterine atony oxytocic drugs are used in turn as follows:

- oxytocin 5–10 units by intravenous injection
- ergometrine 250–500 micrograms by intravenous injection
- oxytocin 5–30 units in 500 mL infusion fluid given by intravenous infusion at a rate that controls uterine atony

Carboprost has an important role in severe postpartum haemorrhage unresponsive to ergometrine and oxytocin.

Mild secondary postpartum haemorrhage has been treated in domiciliary practice with ergometrine by mouth, but it is rarely used now.

CARBOPROST

Indications: postpartum haemorrhage due to uterine atony in patients unresponsive to ergometrine and oxytocin

Cautions: history of glaucoma or raised intra-ocular pressure, asthma, hypertension, hypotension, anaemia, jaundice, diabetes, epilepsy; uterine scars; excessive dosage may cause uterine rupture

Contra-indications: untreated pelvic infection; cardiac, renal, pulmonary, or hepatic disease

Side-effects: nausea, vomiting and diarrhoea, hyperthermia and flushing, bronchospasm; less frequent effects include raised blood pressure, dyspnoea, and pulmonary oedema; chills, headache, diaphoresis, dizziness; cardiovascular collapse also reported; erythema and pain at injection site reported

Dose: *by deep intramuscular injection,* 250 micrograms repeated if necessary at intervals of 1½ hours (in severe cases the interval may be reduced but should not be less than 15 minutes); total dose should not exceed 2 mg (8 doses)

Hemabate® (Pharmacia) PoM

Injection, carboprost as trometamol salt (tromethamine salt) 250 micrograms/mL, net price 1-mL amp = £15.76 (hosp. only)

DINOPROSTONE

Indications: see notes above and under preparations below

Cautions: history of asthma, glaucoma and raised intra-ocular pressure; cardiac, hepatic or renal impairment; hypertension; history of epilepsy; uterine scarring; monitor uterine activity and fetal status (particular care if history of uterine hypertony); uterine rupture; see also notes above; effect of oxytocin enhanced (care needed in monitoring uterine activity when used in sequence)—see also under *Propess®* and Appendix 1 (oxytocin)

Contra-indications: active cardiac, pulmonary, renal or hepatic disease; placenta praevia or unexplained vaginal bleeding during pregnancy, ruptured membranes, major cephalopelvic disproportion or fetal malpresentation, history of caesarean section or major uterine surgery, untreated pelvic infection, fetal distress, grand multiparas and multiple pregnancy, history of difficult or traumatic delivery; avoid extra-amniotic route in cervicitis or vaginitis

Side-effects: nausea, vomiting, diarrhoea; other side-effects include uterine hypertonus, severe uterine contractions, pulmonary or amniotic fluid embolism, abruptio placenta, fetal distress, maternal hypertension, bronchospasm, rapid cervical dilation, fever, backache; uterine hypercontractility with or without fetal bradycardia, low Apgar scores; cardiac arrest, uterine rupture, stillbirth or neonatal death also reported; vaginal symptoms (warmth, irritation, pain); after intravenous administration—flushing, shivering, headache, dizziness, temporary pyrexia and raised white blood cell count; also local tissue reaction and erythema after intravenous administration and possibility of infection after extra-amniotic administration

Dose: see under Preparations, below

IMPORTANT. Do not confuse dose of *Prostin E2®* vaginal **gel** with that of *Prostin E2®* vaginal **tablets**—not bioequivalent.

Propess® (Ferring) [PoM]
Pessaries (within retrieval system), releasing dinoprostone approx. 5 mg over 12 hours. Net price 1-
pessary pack = £43.43
Dose: by vagina, cervical ripening and induction of
labour at term, 1 pessary inserted high into posterior fornix; if cervical ripening insufficient, remove pessary 8–
12 hours later and replace with a second pessary (which
should also be removed not more than 12 hours later);
max. 2 consecutive pessaries
IMPORTANT. Effect of oxytocin enhanced—particular
care needed to monitor uterine activity when oxytocin
used in sequence (remove pessary beforehand)

Prostin E2® (Pharmacia) [PoM]
Tablets ▬, dinoprostone 500 micrograms. Net
price 10-tab pack = £14.93 (hosp. only)
Dose: by mouth, induction of labour, 500 micrograms,
followed by 0.5–1 mg (max. 1.5 mg) at hourly intervals
Intravenous solution ▬, for dilution and use as
an infusion, dinoprostone 1 mg/mL, net price
0.75-mL amp = £7.43; 10 mg/mL, 0.5-mL amp =
£16.05 (both hosp. only; rarely used, consult
product literature for dose and indications)
Extra-amniotic solution ▬, dinoprostone
10 mg/mL. Net price 0.5-mL amp (with diluent) =
£15.33 (hosp. only; less commonly used nowadays, consult product literature for dose and indications)
Vaginal gel, dinoprostone 400 micrograms/mL, net
price 2.5 mL (1 mg) = £14.52; 800 micrograms/
mL, 2.5 mL (2 mg) = £16.00
Dose: by vagina, induction of labour, inserted high into
posterior fornix (avoid administration into cervical
canal), 1 mg (unfavourable primigravida 2 mg), followed after 6 hours by 1–2 mg if required; max. [gel]
3 mg (unfavourable primigravida 4 mg)
Vaginal tablets, dinoprostone 3 mg. Net price 8-
vaginal tab pack = £65.04
Dose: by vagina, induction of labour, inserted high into
posterior fornix, 3 mg, followed after 6–8 hours by 3 mg
if labour is not established; max. 6 mg [vaginal tablets]
Note. Prostin E2 Vaginal Gel and Vaginal Tablets are **not**
bioequivalent

ERGOMETRINE MALEATE
Indications: see notes above
Cautions: cardiac disease, hypertension, hepatic,
and renal impairment, multiple pregnancy; porphyria (section 9.8.2); **interactions:** Appendix 1
(ergometrine)
Contra-indications: induction of labour, first and
second stages of labour, vascular disease, severe
cardiac disease, impaired pulmonary function,
severe hepatic and renal impairment, sepsis,
severe hypertension, eclampsia
Side-effects: nausea, vomiting, headache, dizziness, tinnitus, abdominal pain, chest pain, palpitation, dyspnoea, bradycardia, transient
hypertension, vasoconstriction; stroke, myocardial
infarction and pulmonary oedema also reported
Dose: see notes above

Ergometrine (Non-proprietary) [PoM]
Tablets ▬, ergometrine maleate
500 micrograms, net price 21-tab pack = £22.20
Available from IVAX
Injection, ergometrine maleate 500 micrograms/
mL. Net price 1-mL amp = 60p
Available from Antigen, Phoenix

■ With oxytocin
Syntometrine® (Alliance) [PoM]
Injection, ergometrine maleate 500 micrograms,
oxytocin 5 units/mL. Net price 1-mL amp = £1.38
Dose: by intramuscular injection, 1 mL; by intravenous
injection, no longer recommended

▬ denotes preparations that are considered to
be less suitable for prescribing (see p. vi)

GEMEPROST
Indications: see under Dose
Cautions: obstructive airways disease, cardiovascular insufficiency, raised intra-ocular pressure,
cervicitis or vaginitis
IMPORTANT. For warnings relating to use of gemeprost
in a patient undergoing induction of abortion with mifepristone, see under Mifepristone
Contra-indications: renal impairment, unexplained vaginal bleeding
Side-effects: vaginal bleeding and uterine pain;
nausea, vomiting, or diarrhoea; headache, muscle
weakness, dizziness, flushing, chills, backache,
dyspnoea, chest pain, palpitations and mild
pyrexia; uterine rupture reported (most commonly in multiparas or if history of uterine surgery or if given with intravenous oxytocics); also
reported severe hypotension, coronary artery
spasm and myocardial infarction
Dose: *by vagina* in pessaries, softening and dilation of the cervix to facilitate transcervical operative procedures in first trimester, inserted into
posterior fornix, 1 mg 3 hours before surgery
Second trimester abortion, inserted into posterior
fornix, 1 mg every 3 hours for max. of 5 administrations; second course may begin 24 hours after
start of treatment (if treatment fails pregnancy
should be terminated by another method)
Second trimester intra-uterine death, inserted into
posterior fornix, 1 mg every 3 hours for max. of 5
administrations only; monitor for coagulopathy

Gemeprost (Non-proprietary) [PoM]
Pessaries, gemeprost 1 mg. Net price 5-pessary
pack = £190.00
Available from Beacon

OXYTOCIN
Indications: see under Dose and notes above
Cautions: particular caution needed when given
for *induction or enhancement of labour* in presence of borderline cephalopelvic disproportion
(avoid if significant), mild or moderate
pregnancy-induced hypertension or cardiac disease, women over 35 years or with history of
lower-uterine segment caesarean section (see also
under Contra-indications below); if fetal death *in
utero* or meconium-stained amniotic fluid avoid
tumultuous labour (may cause amniotic fluid
embolism); water intoxication and hyponatraemia—avoid large infusion volumes and restrict
fluid intake by mouth (see also Appendix 6);
effects enhanced by concomitant prostaglandins
(very careful monitoring); caudal block anaesthesia (may enhance hypertensive effects of sympathomimetic vasopressors), see also
interactions: Appendix 1 (oxytocin)

Contra-indications: hypertonic uterine contractions, mechanical obstruction to delivery, fetal distress; any condition where spontaneous labour or vaginal delivery inadvisable (e.g. significant cephalopelvic disproportion, malpresentation, placenta praevia, vasa praevia, placental abruption, cord presentation or prolapse, predisposition to uterine rupture as in multiple pregnancy, polyhydramnios, grand multiparity and presence of uterine scar from major surgery—including caesarean section); avoid prolonged administration in oxytocin-resistant uterine inertia, severe pre-eclamptic toxaemia or severe cardiovascular disease

Side-effects: uterine spasm (may occur at low doses), uterine hyperstimulation (usually with excessive doses—may cause fetal distress, asphyxia and death, or may lead to hypertonicity, tetanic contractions, soft-tissue damage or uterine rupture); water intoxication and hyponatraemia associated with high doses with large infusion volumes of electrolyte-free fluid (see also under Dose below); also nausea, vomiting, arrhythmias; rashes and anaphylactoid reactions (with dyspnoea, hypotension or shock) also reported; placental abruption and amniotic fluid embolism also reported on overdose

Dose: induction of labour for medical reasons or stimulation of labour in hypotonic uterine inertia, *by intravenous infusion*, see NICE guidance above; do not use total of more than 5 units in any one day (may be repeated the following day starting again at 0.001–0.002 units/minute)

IMPORTANT. Careful monitoring of fetal heart rate and uterine motility essential for dose titration (never give intravenous bolus injection during labour); discontinue immediately in uterine hyperactivity or fetal distress

Caesarean section, *by slow intravenous injection* immediately after delivery, 5 units

Prevention of postpartum haemorrhage, after delivery of placenta, *by slow intravenous injection*, 5 units (if infusion used for induction or enhancement of labour, increase rate during third stage and for next few hours)

Note. May be given in a dose of 10 units by intramuscular injection [unlicensed route] instead of oxytocin with ergometrine (*Syntometrine®*), see notes above

Treatment of postpartum haemorrhage, *by slow intravenous injection*, 5–10 units, followed in severe cases *by intravenous infusion* of 5–30 units in 500 mL infusion fluid at a rate sufficient to control uterine atony

IMPORTANT. Avoid rapid intravenous injection (may cause short-lasting drop in blood pressure); prolonged administration, see warning below

Incomplete, inevitable or missed abortion, *by slow intravenous injection*, 5 units followed if necessary *by intravenous infusion*, 0.02–0.04 units/minute or faster

IMPORTANT. Prolonged intravenous administration at high doses with large volume of fluid (as possible in inevitable or missed abortion or postpartum haemorrhage) may cause water intoxication with hyponatraemia. To avoid: use electrolyte-containing diluent (i.e. not glucose), increase oxytocin concentration to reduce fluid, restrict fluid intake by mouth; monitor fluid and electrolytes

Note. Oxytocin doses in the BNF may differ from those in the product literature

Syntocinon® (Alliance) [PoM]
Injection, oxytocin, net price 5 units/mL, 1-mL amp = £1.23; 10 units/mL, 1-mL amp = £1.40

■ With ergometrine, see Syntometrine® p. 379

Maintenance of patency

Alprostadil (prostaglandin E_1) is used to maintain patency of the ductus arteriosus in neonates with congenital heart defects, prior to corrective surgery in centres where intensive care is immediately available.

ALPROSTADIL

Indications: congenital heart defects in neonates prior to corrective surgery; erectile dysfunction (section 7.4.5)

Cautions: see notes above; history of haemorrhage, avoid in hyaline membrane disease, monitor arterial pressure

Side-effects: apnoea (particularly in infants under 2 kg), flushing, bradycardia, hypotension, tachycardia, cardiac arrest, oedema, diarrhoea, fever, convulsions, disseminated intravascular coagulation, hypokalaemia; cortical proliferation of long bones, weakening of the wall of the ductus arteriosus and pulmonary artery may follow prolonged use; gastric-outlet obstruction reported

Dose: *by intravenous infusion,* initially 50–100 nanograms/kg/minute, then decreased to lowest effective dose

Prostin VR® (Pharmacia) [PoM]
Intravenous solution, alprostadil 500 micrograms/mL in alcohol. For dilution and use as an infusion. Net price 1-mL amp = £59.84 (hosp. only)

Closure of ductus arteriosus

Indometacin (indomethacin) is used to close a patent ductus arteriosus in premature babies, probably by inhibiting prostaglandin synthesis.

INDOMETACIN
(Indomethacin)

Indications: patent ductus arteriosus in premature babies (under specialist supervision in neonatal intensive care unit); rheumatoid disease (section 10.1.1)

Cautions: may mask symptoms of infection; may reduce urine output by 50% or more (monitor carefully—see also under Anuria or Oliguria, below) and precipitate renal impairment especially if extracellular volume depleted, heart failure, sepsis, or hepatic impairment, or if receiving nephrotoxic drugs; may induce hyponatraemia; monitor renal function and electrolytes; inhibition of platelet aggregation (monitor for bleeding); **interactions:** Appendix 1 (NSAIDs)

ANURIA OR OLIGURIA. If anuria or marked oliguria (urinary output less than 0.6 mL/kg/hour) at time of scheduled second or third dose, delay until renal function returns to normal

Contra-indications: untreated infection, bleeding (especially with active intracranial haemorrhage or gastro-intestinal bleeding); thrombocytopenia, coagulation defects, necrotising enterocolitis, renal impairment

Side-effects: include haemorrhagic, renal, gastro-intestinal, metabolic, and coagulation disorders; pulmonary hypertension, intracranial bleeding, fluid retention, and exacerbation of infection

Dose: *by intravenous injection,* over 20–30 minutes (using a suitable syringe driver), 3 doses at intervals of 12–24 hours (provided urine output remains adequate), age less than 48 hours, 200 micrograms/kg then 100 micrograms/kg then 100 micrograms/kg; age 2–7 days, 200 micrograms/kg then 200 micrograms/kg then 200 micrograms/kg; age over 7 days, 200 micrograms/kg then 250 micrograms/kg then 250 micrograms/kg; solution prepared with 1–2 mL sodium chloride 0.9% or water for injections (not glucose and no preservatives)

If ductus arteriosus reopens a second course of 3 injections may be given 48 hours after first course

Indocid PDA® (MSD) PoM
Injection, powder for reconstitution, indometacin (as sodium trihydrate). Net price 3 × 1-mg vials = £22.50 (hosp. only)

7.1.2 Mifepristone

Mifepristone, an antiprogestogenic steroid, sensitises the myometrium to prostaglandin-induced contractions and it softens and dilates the cervix. For the termination of pregnancy, a single dose of mifepristone is followed by vaginal administration of the prostaglandin gemeprost. Although the licensed dose of mifepristone is 600 mg, there is evidence that lower doses are effective for medical abortion in pregnancy of up to 20 weeks' gestation. The Royal College of Obstetricians and Gynaecologists' guidelines for both early and mid-trimester medical abortions include the following [unlicensed] regimens:

- For gestation up to 7 weeks (and as an option for gestation of 7–9 weeks), mifepristone 200 mg by mouth followed 36 hours later by gemeprost 500 micrograms by vagina
- For mid-trimester medical abortion (gestation up to 20 weeks), mifepristone 200 mg by mouth followed 36 hours later by gemeprost 1 mg every 6 hours by vagina

MIFEPRISTONE

Indications: see under dose

Cautions: asthma (avoid if severe); haemorrhagic disorders and anticoagulant therapy; prosthetic heart valve or history of endocarditis (prophylaxis recommended, see section 5.1 table 2); smokers aged over 35 years (increased risk of cardiovascular events); adrenal suppression (may require corticosteroid); not recommended in hepatic or renal impairment; breast-feeding (Appendix 5); avoid aspirin and NSAIDs for analgesia; **interactions:** Appendix 1 (mifepristone)

IMPORTANT. For warnings relating to use of gemeprost in a patient undergoing induction of abortion with mifepristone, see under Gemeprost.

Contra-indications: uncontrolled severe asthma; suspected ectopic pregnancy; chronic adrenal failure, porphyria (section 9.8.2)

Side-effects: vaginal bleeding (sometimes severe) may occur between administration of mifepristone and surgery, and rarely abortion may occur before surgery; malaise, faintness, headache, nausea, vomiting, rashes; uterine pain after gemeprost (may be severe and require parenteral opioids)

Dose: medical termination of intra-uterine pregnancy of up to 63 days gestation, *by mouth,* mifepristone 600 mg as a single dose under medical supervision, followed 36–48 hours later (unless abortion already complete) by gemeprost 1 mg *by vagina* and observed for at least 6 hours (or until bleeding or pain at acceptable level) with follow-up visit 10–14 days later to verify complete expulsion (if treatment fails essential that pregnancy be terminated by another method)

Softening and dilatation of cervix before mechanical cervical dilatation for termination of pregnancy, 36–48 hours before procedure, *by mouth,* mifepristone 600 mg as a single dose under medical supervision

Termination of pregnancy of 13–24 weeks gestation (in combination with gemeprost), *by mouth,* mifepristone 600 mg as a single dose under medical supervision followed 36–48 hours later by gemeprost 1 mg *by vagina* every 3 hours up to max. 5 mg; if abortion does not occur, 24 hours after start of treatment repeat course of gemeprost 1 mg *by vagina* up to max. 5 mg (if treatment fails pregnancy should be terminated by another method); follow-up visit after appropriate interval to assess vaginal bleeding recommended

Note. Careful monitoring essential for 6 hours after administration of gemeprost pessary (risk of profound hypotension)

Labour induction in fetal death in utero, *by mouth,* mifepristone 600 mg as a single daily dose for 2 days under medical supervision; if labour not started within 72 hours of first dose, another method should be used

Mifegyne® (Exelgyn) PoM
Tablets, yellow, mifepristone 200 mg. Net price 3-tab pack = £41.83 (supplied to NHS hospitals and premises approved under Abortion Act 1967).
Label: 10 patient information leaflet

7.1.3 Myometrial relaxants

Beta$_2$ agonists (beta$_2$-sympathomimetics, beta$_2$-adrenoceptor stimulants) relax uterine muscle and are used in selected cases to inhibit *premature delivery.*

Beta$_2$ agonists are indicated for the inhibition of *uncomplicated* premature labour *between 24 and 33 weeks* of gestation and they may permit a delay in delivery of at least 48 hours; no statistically significant effect on perinatal mortality has as yet been observed. The greatest benefit is gained by using the delay to administer corticosteroid therapy (with care to avoid fluid overload) or to implement other measures known to improve perinatal health (including transfer to a unit with neonatal intensive care facility). Prolonged therapy should be avoided since risks to the mother (see under Ritodrine

Hydrochloride, below) increase after 48 hours and there is a lack of evidence of benefit from further treatment; oral therapy following initial parenteral treatment is not therefore recommended.

The recently introduced oxytocin receptor antagonist, **atosiban**, is also licensed for the inhibition of *uncomplicated* premature labour *between 24 and 33 weeks* of gestation. Atosiban has fewer side-effects than other licensed myometrial relaxants and may be useful when a beta$_2$ agonist is not appropriate e.g. in cardiac disease.

Indometacin (indomethacin) (section 10.1.1), a cyclo-oxygenase inhibitor, also inhibits labour [unlicensed indication] and it may be useful in situations where a beta$_2$ agonist is not appropriate; however, there are concerns about neonatal complications such as transient impairment of renal function and premature closure of ductus arteriosus.

ATOSIBAN

Indications: uncomplicated premature labour (see notes above)

Cautions: monitor blood loss after delivery; intra-uterine growth retardation; hepatic and renal impairment

Contra-indications: eclampsia and severe pre-eclampsia, intra-uterine infection, intra-uterine fetal death, antepartum haemorrhage (requiring immediate delivery), placenta praevia, abruptio placenta, intra-uterine growth retardation with abnormal fetal heart rate, premature rupture of membranes after 30 weeks' gestation

Side-effects: nausea, vomiting, tachycardia, hypotension, headache, dizziness, hot flushes, hyperglycaemia, injection site reaction; less commonly pruritus, rash, fever, insomnia

Dose: *by intravenous injection*, initially 6.75 mg over 1 minute, then *by intravenous infusion* 18 mg/hour for 3 hours, then 6 mg/hour for up to 45 hours; max. duration of treatment 48 hours

Tractocile® (Ferring) ▼ [PoM]
Injection, atosiban (as acetate) 7.5 mg/mL, net price 0.9-mL (6.75-mg) vial = £20.00
Concentrate for intravenous infusion, atosiban (as acetate) 7.5 mg/mL, net price 5-mL vial = £55.00

RITODRINE HYDROCHLORIDE

Indications: uncomplicated premature labour (see notes above)

Cautions: suspected cardiac disease (physician experienced in cardiology to assess), hypertension, hyperthyroidism, hypokalaemia (special risk with potassium-depleting diuretics), diabetes mellitus (closely monitor blood glucose during intravenous treatment), mild to moderate pre-eclampsia, monitor blood pressure and pulse rate (should not exceed 140 beats per minute) and avoid over-hydration (Appendix 6); **important:** closely monitor state of hydration (discontinue immediately and institute diuretic therapy if pulmonary oedema occurs); concomitant beta-blocker treatment; drugs likely to enhance sympathomimetic side-effects or induce arrhythmias, see also **interactions**, Appendix 1 (sympathomimetics *and* sympathomimetics, beta$_2$)

Contra-indications: cardiac disease, eclampsia and severe pre-eclampsia, intra-uterine infection, intra-uterine fetal death, antepartum haemorrhage (requires immediate delivery), placenta praevia, cord compression

Side-effects: nausea, vomiting, flushing, sweating, tremor; hypokalaemia, tachycardia, palpitations, and hypotension (left lateral position throughout infusion to minimise risk), uterine bleeding (may be reversed with a non-selective beta-blocker); pulmonary oedema (see below and under Cautions); chest pain or tightness (with or without ECG changes) and arrhythmias reported; salivary gland enlargement also reported; on prolonged administration (several weeks) leucopenia and agranulocytosis reported; liver function abnormalities (including increased transaminases and hepatitis) reported

Dose: *by intravenous infusion* (**important:** minimum fluid volume, see below), initially 50 micrograms/minute, increased gradually according to response by 50 micrograms/minute every 10 minutes until contractions stop or maternal heart rate reaches 140 beats per minute; continue for 12–48 hours after contractions cease (usual rate 150–350 micrograms/minute); max. rate 350 micrograms/minute; or *by intramuscular injection*, 10 mg every 3–8 hours continued for 12–48 hours after contractions have ceased; then *by mouth* (but see notes above), 10 mg 30 minutes before termination of intravenous infusion, repeated every 2 hours for 24 hours, followed by 10–20 mg every 4–6 hours, max. oral dose 120 mg daily

IMPORTANT. Manufacturer states that although *fatal pulmonary oedema* associated with ritodrine infusion is almost certainly multifactorial in origin evidence suggests that **fluid overload** may be the most important single factor. The volume of infusion should therefore be kept to a minimum; for further guidance see Appendix 6. For specific guidance on infusion rates, consult product literature

Yutopar® (Solvay) [PoM]
Tablets, yellow, scored, ritodrine hydrochloride 10 mg. Net price 90-tab pack = £19.80 ▱
Injection, ritodrine hydrochloride 10 mg/mL. Net price 5-mL amp = £2.15

▱ denotes preparations that are considered to be less suitable for prescribing (see p. vi)

SALBUTAMOL

Indications: uncomplicated premature labour (see notes above); asthma (section 3.1.1)

Cautions: see under Ritodrine Hydrochloride

Contra-indications: see under Ritodrine Hydrochloride

Side-effects: see under Ritodrine Hydrochloride; headache, rarely muscle cramps; hypersensitivity reactions including bronchospasm, urticaria, and angioedema reported

Dose: *by intravenous infusion*, initially 10 micrograms/minute, rate increased gradually according to response at 10-minute intervals until contractions diminish then increase rate slowly until contractions cease (max. rate 45 micrograms/minute); maintain rate for 1 hour after contractions have stopped, then gradually reduce by 50% every 6 hours; then *by mouth* (but see notes above), 4 mg every 6–8 hours

Preparations
Section 3.1.1.1

TERBUTALINE SULPHATE

Indications: uncomplicated premature labour (see notes above); asthma (section 3.1.1)

Cautions: see under Ritodrine Hydrochloride

Contra-indications: see under Ritodrine Hydrochloride

Side-effects: see under Ritodrine Hydrochloride

Dose: *by intravenous infusion*, 5 micrograms/minute for 20 minutes, increased every 20 minutes in steps of 2.5 micrograms/minute until contractions have ceased (more than 10 micrograms/minute should **seldom** be given—20 micrograms/minute should **not** be exceeded), continue for 1 hour then decrease every 20 minutes in steps of 2.5 micrograms/minute to lowest dose that maintains suppression, continue at this level for 12 hours then *by mouth* (but see notes above), 5 mg every 8 hours for as long as is desirable to prolong pregnancy (or alternatively follow the *intravenous infusion* by *subcutaneous injection* 250 micrograms every 6 hours for a few days then *by mouth* as above)

Preparations
Section 3.1.1.1

7.2   Treatment of vaginal and vulval conditions

| 7.2.1 | Preparations for vaginal atrophy |
| 7.2.2 | Anti-infective drugs |

Symptoms are primarily referable to the vulva, but infections almost invariably involve the vagina which should also be treated. Applications to the vulva alone are likely to give only symptomatic relief without cure.

Aqueous medicated douches may disturb normal vaginal acidity and bacterial flora.

Topical anaesthetic agents give only symptomatic relief and may cause sensitivity reactions. They are indicated only in cases of pruritus where specific local causes have been excluded.

Systemic drugs are required in the treatment of infections such as gonorrhoea and syphilis (section 5.1).

7.2.1   Preparations for vaginal atrophy

Topical HRT

Application of cream containing an oestrogen may be used on a short-term basis to improve the quality of the vaginal epithelium in *menopausal atrophic vaginitis*. It is **important** to bear in mind that topical oestrogens should be used in the **minimum effective amount** to minimise absorption of the oestrogen; if they are used on a long-term basis, some require **oral progestogen** for 10–14 days of each month to combat endometrial hyperplasia (for details see under preparations below). Modified-release vaginal tablets and an impregnated vaginal ring are now also available.

Topical oestrogens are also used before vaginal surgery in postmenopausal women for prolapse when there is epithelial atrophy.

For a general comment on hormone replacement therapy, including the role of topical oestrogens, see section 6.4.1.1.

OESTROGENS, TOPICAL

Indications: see notes above

Cautions: see Oestrogens for HRT (section 6.4.1.1); interrupt treatment periodically to assess need for continued treatment

Contra-indications: see Oestrogens for HRT (section 6.4.1.1); pregnancy and breast-feeding

Side-effects: see Oestrogens for HRT (section 6.4.1.1); local irritation

Ortho-Gynest® (Janssen-Cilag) PoM
Intravaginal cream, estriol 0.01%. Net price 80 g with applicator = £2.72
  Excipients: include arachis (peanut) oil
  Condoms: damages latex condoms and diaphragms
  Insert 1 applicatorful daily, preferably in evening; reduced to 1 applicatorful twice a week; attempts to reduce or discontinue should be made at 3–6 month intervals with re-examination
Pessaries, estriol 500 micrograms. Net price 15 pessaries = £5.29
  Excipients: include butylated hydroxytoluene
  Condoms: damages latex condoms and diaphragms
  Insert 1 pessary daily, preferably in the evening, until improvement occurs; maintenance 1 pessary twice a week; attempts to reduce or discontinue should be made at 3–6 month intervals with re-examination

Ovestin® (Organon) PoM
Intravaginal cream, estriol 0.1%. Net price 15 g with applicator = £4.98
  Excipients: include cetyl alcohol, polysorbates, stearyl alcohol
  Condoms: effect on latex condoms and diaphragms not yet known
  Insert 1 applicator-dose daily for 2–3 weeks, then reduce to twice a week (discontinue every 2–3 months for 4 weeks to assess need for further treatment); vaginal surgery, 1 applicator-dose daily for 2 weeks before surgery, resuming 2 weeks after surgery

Premarin® (Wyeth) PoM
Vaginal cream, conjugated oestrogens (equine) 625 micrograms/g. Net price 42.5 g with calibrated applicator = £2.19
  Excipients: include cetyl alcohol, propylene glycol
  Condoms: effect on latex condoms and diaphragms not yet known
  Insert 1–2 g daily, starting on day 5 of cycle, for 3 weeks, followed by 1-week interval; if therapy long term in women with intact uterus, oral progestogen for 10–14 days at end of each cycle essential

Tampovagan® (Co-Pharma) PoM ◣
Pessaries, diethylstilbestrol 500 micrograms, lactic acid 5%. Net price 10 pessaries = £9.85
  Excipients: none as listed in section 13.1.3
  Condoms: no evidence of damage to latex condoms and diaphragms
  Insert 2 pessaries at night for 2–3 weeks (short-term only, see notes above)

Vagifem® (Novo Nordisk) PoM
Vaginal tablets, f/c, m/r, estradiol 25 micrograms in disposable applicators. Net price 15-applicator pack = £14.62
Excipients: none as listed in section 13.1.3
Condoms: no evidence of damage to latex condoms and diaphragms
Insert 1 tablet daily for 2 weeks then reduce to 1 tablet twice weekly; discontinue after 3 months to assess need for further treatment

■ Vaginal ring
Estring® (Pharmacia) PoM
Vaginal ring, releasing estradiol approx. 7.5 micrograms/24 hours. Net price 1-ring pack = £31.42. Label: 10 patient information leaflet
For postmenopausal urogenital conditions (not suitable for vasomotor symptoms or osteoporosis prophylaxis), to be inserted into upper third of vagina and worn continuously; replace after 3 months; max. duration of continuous treatment 2 years

Menoring® 50 (Galen) PoM
Vaginal ring, releasing estradiol approx. 50 micrograms/24 hours, net price 1-ring pack = £29.50. Label: 10 patient information leaflet
For postmenopausal vasomotor and urogenital symptoms in women without a uterus, to be inserted into upper third of vagina and worn continuously; replace after 3 months

Non-hormonal preparations

Non-hormonal vaginal preparations include *Replens®* NHS which has an acid pH and provides a high moisture content for up to 3 days, and *Senselle®* NHS which is a water-based lubricant.
See section 7.2.2 for the pH-modifying preparation *Aci-jel®*.

7.2.2   Anti-infective drugs

Effective specific treatments are available for the common vaginal infections.

Fungal infections

Candidal vulvitis can be treated locally with cream but is almost invariably associated with vaginal infection which should also be treated. *Vaginal candidiasis* is treated primarily with antifungal pessaries or cream inserted high into the vagina (including during menstruation). Single-dose preparations offer an advantage when compliance is a problem. Local irritation may occur on application of vaginal antifungal products.

Imidazole drugs (clotrimazole, econazole, fenticonazole, and miconazole) are effective in short courses of 3 to 14 days according to the preparation used. Vaginal applications may be supplemented with antifungal cream for vulvitis and to treat other superficial sites of infection.

Nystatin is a well established antifungal drug. One or two pessaries are inserted for 14 to 28 nights; a cream is also used in cases of vulvitis and infection of other superficial sites. Nystatin stains clothing yellow.

Oral treatment of vaginal infection with fluconazole or itraconazole (section 5.2) is also effective;

oral ketoconazole has been associated with fatal hepatotoxicity (see section 5.2 for CSM warning).

Recurrence is particularly likely if there are predisposing factors such as antibacterial therapy, pregnancy, diabetes mellitus and possibly oral contraceptive use. Possible reservoirs of infection may also lead to recontamination and should be treated. These include other skin sites such as the digits, nail beds, and umbilicus as well as the gastro-intestinal tract and the bladder. The partner may also be the source of re-infection and, if symptomatic, should be treated with cream at the same time.

PREPARATIONS FOR VAGINAL AND VULVAL CANDIDIASIS

Side-effects: occasional local irritation

Clotrimazole (Non-proprietary)
Cream (topical), clotrimazole 1%, net price 20 g = £1.77, 50 g = £3.80
Condoms: effect on latex condoms and diaphragms not yet known
Apply to anogenital area 2–3 times daily
Available from Akita (*Candiden®*), Ashbourne (*Abtrim®*), Dominion, Generics, Genus
Pessary, clotrimazole 500 mg, net price 1 pessary with applicator = £3.43
Insert 1 at night as a single dose
Available from Akita (*Candiden®*), Ashbourne (*Abtrim®*), Tillomed

Canesten® (Bayer Consumer Care)
Cream (topical), clotrimazole 1%. Net price 20 g = £2.14; 50 g = £3.80
Excipients: include benzyl alcohol, cetostearyl alcohol, polysorbates
Condoms: damages latex condoms and diaphragms
Apply to anogenital area 2–3 times daily
Thrush Cream (topical), clotrimazole 2%, net price 20 g = £2.73
Excipients: include benzyl alcohol, cetostearyl alcohol, polysorbates
Condoms: damages latex condoms and diaphragms
Apply to anogenital area 2–3 times daily
Vaginal cream (*10% VC®*) PoM, clotrimazole 10%. Net price 5-g applicator pack = £4.50
Excipients: include benzyl alcohol, cetostearyl alcohol, polysorbates
Condoms: damages latex condoms and diaphragms
Insert 5 g at night as a single dose; may be repeated once if necessary
Note. Available for sale to the public as *Canesten® Once*
Pessaries, clotrimazole 100 mg, net price 6 pessaries with applicator = £3.62; 200 mg, 3 pessaries with applicator = £3.62
Excipients: include polysorbates
Condoms: damages latex condoms and diaphragms
Insert 200 mg for 3 nights *or* 100 mg for 6 nights
Pessary , clotrimazole 500 mg. Net price 1 with applicator = £3.48
Excipients: none as listed in section 13.1.3
Condoms: damages latex condoms and diaphragms
Insert 1 at night as a single dose
Combi, clotrimazole 500-mg pessary and cream (topical) 2%. Net price 1 pessary and 10 g cream = £4.50
Condoms: damages latex condoms and diaphragms

Ecostatin® (Squibb)
Cream (topical), econazole nitrate 1%. Net price 15 g = £1.49; 30 g = £2.75
Excipients: include butylated hydroxyanisole, fragrance
Condoms: damages latex condoms and diaphragms
Apply to anogenital area twice daily

Pessaries PoM , econazole nitrate 150 mg. Net price 3 with applicator = £3.35
Excipients: none as listed in section 13.1.3
Condoms: damages latex condoms and diaphragms
Insert 1 pessary for 3 nights

Pessary (Ecostatin 1®) PoM , econazole nitrate 150 mg, formulated for single-dose therapy. Net price 1 pessary with applicator = £3.35
Excipients: none as listed in section 13.1.3
Condoms: damages latex condoms and diaphragms
Insert 1 pessary at night as a single dose

Twinpack PoM , econazole nitrate 150-mg pessaries and cream 1%. Net price 3 pessaries and 15 g cream = £4.35
Condoms: damages latex condoms and diaphragms

Flagyl Compak® PoM see section 5.1.11

Gyno-Daktarin® (Janssen-Cilag) PoM
Intravaginal cream, miconazole nitrate 2%. Net price 78 g with applicators = £4.95
Excipients: include butylated hydroxyanisole
Condoms: damages latex condoms and diaphragms
Insert 5-g applicatorful once daily for 10–14 days *or* twice daily for 7 days; *topical,* apply to anogenital area twice daily

Pessaries, miconazole nitrate 100 mg. Net price 14 = £3.35
Excipients: none as listed in section 13.1.3
Condoms: damages latex condoms and diaphragms
Insert 1 pessary daily for 14 days or 1 pessary twice daily for 7 days

Combipack, miconazole nitrate 100-mg pessaries and cream (topical) 2%. Net price 14 pessaries and 15 g cream = £4.35
Condoms: damages latex condoms and diaphragms

Ovule (= vaginal capsule) *(Gyno-Daktarin®),* miconazole nitrate 1.2 g in a fatty basis. Net price 1 ovule (with finger stall) = £3.35
Excipients: include hydroxybenzoates (parabens)
Condoms: damages latex condoms and diaphragms
Insert 1 ovule at night as a single dose

Gyno-Pevaryl® (Janssen-Cilag)
Cream, econazole nitrate 1%. Net price 15 g = £1.50; 30 g = £3.45
Excipients: none as listed in section 13.1.3
Condoms: damages latex condoms and diaphragms
Insert 5-g applicatorful intravaginally and apply to vulva at night for at least 14 nights

Pessaries, econazole nitrate 150 mg. Net price 3 pessaries = £3.17
Excipients: none as listed in section 13.1.3
Condoms: damages latex condoms and diaphragms
Insert 1 pessary for 3 nights

Pessary (Gyno-Pevaryl 1®), econazole nitrate 150 mg, formulated for single-dose therapy. Net price 1 pessary with applicator = £3.37
Excipients: none as listed in section 13.1.3
Condoms: damages latex condoms and diaphragms
Insert 1 pessary at night as a single dose

Combipack, econazole nitrate 150-mg pessaries, econazole nitrate 1% cream. Net price 3 pessaries and 15 g cream = £4.35
Condoms: damages latex condoms and diaphragms

CP pack (Gyno-Pevaryl 1®), econazole nitrate 150-mg pessary, econazole nitrate 1% cream. Net price 1 pessary and 15 g cream = £4.35
Condoms: damages latex condoms and diaphragms

Lomexin® (Akita) PoM
Pessaries, fenticonazole nitrate 200 mg, net price 3 pessaries = £2.83; 600 mg, 1 pessary = £2.83
Excipients: include hydroxybenzoates (parabens)
Condoms: damages latex condoms and diaphragms
Insert 600 mg for 1 night *or* 200 mg for 3 nights

Nizoral® (Janssen-Cilag) PoM
Cream (topical), ketoconazole 2%. Net price 30 g = £3.81
Excipients: include polysorbates, propylene glycol, stearyl alcohol
Apply to anogenital area once or twice daily

Nystan® (Squibb) PoM
Cream and *Ointment,* see section 13.10.2

Vaginal cream, nystatin 100 000 units/4-g application. Net price 60 g with applicator = £2.77
Excipients: include benzyl alcohol, propylene glycol
Condoms: damages latex condoms and diaphragms
Insert 1–2 applicatorfuls at night for at least 14 nights

Pessaries, yellow, nystatin 100 000 units. Net price 28-pessary pack = £1.96
Excipients: none as listed in section 13.1.3
Condoms: no evidence of damage to latex condoms and diaphragms
Insert 1–2 pessaries at night for at least 14 nights

Pevaryl® (Janssen-Cilag)
Cream, econazole nitrate 1%. Net price 30 g = £2.65
Excipients: include butylated hydroxyanisole, fragrance
Condoms: effect on latex condoms and diaphragms not yet known
Apply to anogenital area twice daily

Other infections

Vaginal preparations intended to restore normal acidity *(Aci-Jel®)* may prevent recurrence of vaginal infections and permit the re-establishment of the normal vaginal flora.

Trichomonal infections commonly involve the lower urinary tract as well as the genital system and need systemic treatment with metronidazole or tinidazole (section 5.1.11).

Bacterial infections with Gram-negative organisms are particularly common in association with gynaecological operations and trauma. Metronidazole is effective against certain Gram-negative organisms, especially *Bacteroides* spp. and may be used prophylactically in gynaecological surgery.

Topical vaginal products containing povidone–iodine can be used to treat vaginitis due to candidal, trichomonal, non-specific or mixed infections; they are also used for the pre-operative preparation of the vagina. Clindamycin cream and metronidazole gel are also indicated for bacterial vaginosis; *Sultrin®* cream is licensed for the treatment of infections due to *Haemophilus vaginalis* only.

The antiviral drugs aciclovir, famciclovir and valaciclovir may be used in the treatment of genital infection due to *herpes simplex virus,* the HSV type 2 being a major cause of genital ulceration. They have a beneficial effect on virus shedding and healing, generally giving relief from pain and other symptoms. See section 5.3 for systemic preparations, and section 13.10.3 for topical preparations.

PREPARATIONS FOR OTHER VAGINAL INFECTIONS

Aci-Jel® (Janssen-Cilag)
Vaginal jelly, glacial acetic acid 0.94% in a buffered (pH 4) basis. Net price 85 g with applicator = £3.37
Excipients: include hydroxybenzoates (parabens), fragrance
Condoms: effect on latex condoms and diaphragms not yet known
Non-specific infections, insert 1 applicatorful once or twice daily for up to 2 weeks to restore vaginal acidity

Betadine® (SSL)

Cautions: avoid in pregnancy (also if planned) and in breast-feeding; renal impairment (see Appendix 3); avoid regular use in thyroid disorders

Side-effects: rarely sensitivity; may interfere with thyroid function

Vaginal Cleansing Kit, solution, povidone-iodine 10%. Net price 250 mL with measuring bottle and applicator = £2.79

Excipients: include fragrance

Condoms: effect on latex condoms and diaphragms not yet known

To be diluted and used once daily, preferably in the morning; may be used with Betadine® pessaries or vaginal gel

Pessaries, brown, povidone-iodine 200 mg. Net price 28 pessaries with applicator = £6.06

Condoms: effect on latex condoms and diaphragms not yet known

Vaginal gel, brown, povidone-iodine 10%. Net price 80 g with applicator = £2.79

Excipients: none as listed in section 13.1.3

Condoms: effect on latex condoms and diaphragms not yet known

Vaginal infections or pre-operatively, insert 1 moistened pessary night and morning for up to 14 days *or* use morning pessary with one applicatorful of gel at night *or* morning douche with pessary (or one applicatorful of gel) at night

Dalacin® (Pharmacia) [PoM]

Side-effects: irritation, cervicitis and vaginitis; poorly absorbed into the blood—very low likelihood of systemic effects (section 5.1.6)

Cream, clindamycin 2% (as phosphate). Net price 40-g pack with 7 applicators = £8.64

Excipients: include benzyl alcohol, cetostearyl alcohol, polysorbates, propylene glycol

Condoms: damages latex condoms and diaphragms

Bacterial vaginosis, insert 5-g applicatorful at night for 3–7 nights

Sultrin® (Janssen-Cilag) [PoM]

Cautions: absorption of sulphonamides may produce systemic effects

Contra-indications: pregnancy and breast-feeding; hypersensitivity to peanuts

Side-effects: sensitivity

Cream, sulfathiazole 3.42%, sulfacetamide 2.86%, sulfabenzamide 3.7%. Net price 80 g with applicator = £3.48

Excipients: include arachis (peanut) oil, cetyl alcohol, hydroxybenzoates (parabens), propylene glycol, wool fat

Condoms: damages latex condoms and diaphragms

Bacterial vaginosis, insert 1 applicatorful of cream twice daily for 10 days, then once daily if necessary (but see also notes above)

Zidoval® (3M) [PoM]

Cautions: not recommended during menstruation; some absorption may occur, see section 5.1.11 for systemic effects

Side-effects: local effects including irritation, candidiasis, abnormal discharge, pelvic discomfort

Vaginal gel, metronidazole 0.75%. Net price 40-g pack with 5 applicators = £4.63

Excipients: include disodium edetate, hydroxybenzoates (parabens), propylene glycol

Bacterial vaginosis, insert 5-g applicatorful at night for 5 nights

 denotes preparations that are considered to be less suitable for prescribing (see p. vi)

7.3   Contraceptives

7.3.1	Combined oral contraceptives
7.3.2	Progestogen-only contraceptives
7.3.3	Spermicidal contraceptives
7.3.4	Contraceptive devices

The criteria by which contraceptive methods should be judged are effectiveness, acceptability, and freedom from side-effects.

Hormonal contraception is the most effective method of fertility control, short of sterilisation, but has unwanted major and minor side-effects, especially for certain groups of women.

Intra-uterine devices have a high use-effectiveness but may produce undesirable local side-effects. They are most suitable for older parous women, but less appropriate for younger nulliparous women and for those with an increased risk of pelvic inflammatory disease.

Barrier methods alone (condoms, diaphragms, and caps) are less effective but can be very reliable for well-motivated couples if used in conjunction with a **spermicide**. Occasionally sensitivity reactions occur. The female condom (*Femidom®*) is now also available; it is prelubricated but does not contain a spermicide.

7.3.1   Combined oral contraceptives

Oral contraceptives containing an oestrogen and a progestogen ('combined oral contraceptives') are the most effective preparations for general use. Advantages of combined oral contraceptives include:

- reliable and reversible;
- reduced dysmenorrhoea and menorrhagia;
- reduced incidence of premenstrual tension;
- less symptomatic fibroids and functional ovarian cysts;
- less benign breast disease;
- reduced risk of ovarian and endometrial cancer;
- reduced risk of pelvic inflammatory disease, which may be a risk with intra-uterine devices.

Combined oral contraceptives containing a fixed amount of an oestrogen and a progestogen in each active tablet are termed 'monophasic'; those with varying amounts of the two hormones according to the stage of the cycle are termed 'biphasic' and 'triphasic'.

CHOICE. The oestrogen content ranges from 20 to 50 micrograms and generally a preparation with the lowest oestrogen and progestogen content which gives good cycle control and minimal side-effects in the individual woman is chosen.

- *Low strength preparations* (containing ethinylestradiol 20 micrograms) are particularly appropriate for women with risk factors for circulatory disease, provided a combined oral contraceptive is otherwise suitable. It is recommended that the combined oral contraceptive is not continued beyond 50 years of age since more suitable alternatives exist.
- *Standard strength preparations* (containing ethinylestradiol 30 or 35 micrograms or in 30/40 microgram *phased* preparations) are appropriate for standard use—but see Risk of

Venous Thromboembolism below. Phased preparations are generally reserved for women who *either* do not have withdrawal bleeding *or* who have breakthrough bleeding with monophasic products.

- *High strength preparations* (containing either ethinylestradiol 50 micrograms or mestranol 50 micrograms) provide greater contraceptive security but increase the possibility of side-effects. These are used mainly in circumstances of reduced bioavailability (e.g. during long-term use of enzyme-inducing antiepileptics, see FPA advice under Interactions below).

The progestogens desogestrel and gestodene (in combination with ethinylestradiol) may be considered for women who experience side-effects (such as acne, headache, depression, weight gain, breast symptoms and breakthrough bleeding) with other progestogens. However, women should be advised that desogestrel and gestodene have also been associated with an increased risk of *venous thromboembolism*.

RISK OF VENOUS THROMBOEMBOLISM. There is an increased risk of venous thromboembolic disease in users of oral contraceptives but this risk is considerably smaller than that associated with pregnancy (about 60 cases of venous thromboembolic disease per 100 000 pregnancies). In all cases the risk of venous thromboembolism increases with age and in the presence of other risk factors for venous thromboembolism (e.g. obesity).

The incidence of venous thromboembolism in healthy, non-pregnant women who are not taking an oral contraceptive is about 5 cases per 100 000 women per year. For those using combined oral contraceptives containing second generation progestogens e.g. levonorgestrel, this incidence is about 15 per 100 000 women per year of use. Some studies have reported a greater risk of venous thromboembolism in women using preparations containing the third generation progestogens desogestrel and gestodene; the incidence in these women is about 25 per 100 000 women per year of use.

The absolute risk of venous thromboembolism in women using combined oral contraceptives containing these third generation progestogens remains very small and well below the risk associated with pregnancy. Provided that women are informed of and accept the relative risks of venous thromboembolism, the choice of oral contraceptive is for the woman together with the prescriber jointly to decide in the light of her individual medical history and any contra-indications.

TRAVEL. Women taking oral contraceptives may be at an increased risk of deep-vein thrombosis during travel involving long periods of immobility (over 5 hours). The risk may be reduced by appropriate exercise during the journey and possibly by wearing elastic hosiery.

MISSED PILL. It is important to bear in mind that the critical time for loss of protection is when a pill is omitted at the *beginning* or *end* of a cycle (which lengthens the pill-free interval). The following is now recommended by family planning organisations:

'If you forget a pill, take it as soon as you remember, and the next one at your normal time. If you are 12 or more hours late with any pill (especially the first in the packet) the pill may not work. As soon as you remember, continue normal pill taking. However, you will not be protected for the next seven days and must either not have sex or use another method such as the condom. If these seven days run beyond the end of your packet, start the next packet at once when you have finished the present one, i.e. do not have a gap between packets. This will mean you may not have a period until the end of two packets but this does you no harm. Nor does it matter if you see some bleeding on tablet-taking days. If you are using everyday (ED) pills—miss out the seven inactive pills. If you are not sure which these are, ask your doctor.'

In addition to these precautions, emergency contraception is recommended if:

- 2 or more combined oral contraceptive tablets are missed from the first 7 tablets in a packet;
- 4 or more consecutive tablets are missed mid-packet.

DIARRHOEA AND VOMITING. Vomiting up to 3 hours after taking an oral contraceptive *or* very severe diarrhoea can interfere with its absorption. Additional precautions should therefore be used during and for 7 days after recovery. If the vomiting and diarrhoea occurs during the last 7 tablets, the next pill-free interval should be omitted (in the case of ED tablets the inactive ones should be omitted).

INTERACTIONS. The effectiveness of both *combined* and *progestogen-only* oral contraceptives may be considerably reduced by interaction with drugs that induce hepatic enzyme activity (e.g. **carbamazepine, griseofulvin, modafinil, nelfinavir, nevirapine, oxcarbazepine, phenytoin, phenobarbital, primidone, ritonavir, topiramate,** and, above all, **rifabutin** and **rifampicin**); advice on the possibility of interaction with newer antiretroviral drugs should be sought from HIV specialists.

Family Planning Association (FPA) advice relating to a *short-term course of an enzyme-inducing drug* (for rifampicin and rifabutin, see also below) is that additional contraceptive precautions should be taken whilst taking the enzyme-inducing drug and for at least 7 days after stopping it; if these 7 days run beyond the end of a packet the new packet should be started immediately without a break (in the case of ED tablets the inactive ones should be omitted). It should be noted that **rifampicin** and **rifabutin** are such potent enzyme-inducing drugs that even if a course lasts for less than 7 days the additional contraceptive precautions should be continued for at least 4 weeks after stopping.

FPA advice relating to a *long-term course of an enzyme-inducing drug* (for rifampicin and rifabutin, see also below) in a woman unable to use an alternative method of contraception is to take an oral contraceptive containing ethinylestradiol 50 micrograms or more; 'tricycling' (i.e. taking 3 or 4 packets of monophasic tablets without a break followed by a short tablet-free interval of 4 days) is recommended [but woman should be warned of uncertainty about the effectiveness of this regimen]. **Rifampicin** and **rifabutin** are such potent enzyme-inducing drugs that an alternative method of contraception (such as an IUD) is **always** recommended. Since the excretory function of the liver does not return to normal for several weeks after stopping an enzyme-inducing drug, FPA advice relating to *withdrawal* is that appropriate contraceptive measures are required for 4 to 8 weeks after stopping.

Some **broad-spectrum antibiotics** (e.g. ampicillin, doxycycline) may reduce the efficacy of *combined* oral contraceptives by impairing the bacterial flora responsible for recycling of ethinylestradiol from the large bowel. FPA advice is that additional contraceptive precautions should be taken whilst taking a *short course of a broad-spectrum antibiotic* and for 7 days after stopping. If these 7 days run beyond the end of a packet the next packet should be started immediately without a break (in the case of ED tablets the inactive ones should be omitted). If the antibiotic course *exceeds 3 weeks*, the bacterial flora develops antibiotic resistance and additional precautions become unnecessary; additional precautions are also unnecessary if a woman starting a *combined* oral contraceptive has been on a course of antibiotics for 3 weeks or more.

SURGERY. Oestrogen-containing oral contraceptives should preferably be discontinued (and adequate alternative contraceptive arrangements made) 4 weeks before major elective surgery and all surgery to the legs; they should normally be recommenced at the first menses occurring at least 2 weeks after full mobilisation. A depot injection of a progestogen-only contraceptive may be offered and the oestrogen-containing contraceptive restarted later—if preferred before the next injection would be due. When discontinuation of an oestrogen-containing contraceptive is not possible, e.g. after trauma or if a patient admitted for an elective procedure is still on an oestrogen-containing oral contraceptive, thromboprophylaxis (with heparin and graduated compression hosiery) is advised. These recommendations do not apply to minor surgery with short duration of anaesthesia, e.g. laparoscopic sterilisation or tooth extraction, or to women taking oestrogen-free hormonal contraceptives (whether by mouth or by injection).

REASON TO STOP IMMEDIATELY. Combined oral contraceptives or hormone replacement therapy (HRT) should be stopped (pending investigation and treatment), if any of the following occur:

- Sudden severe chest pain (even if not radiating to left arm);
- Sudden breathlessness (or cough with blood-stained sputum);
- Severe pain in calf of one leg;
- Severe stomach pain;
- Serious neurological effects including unusual severe, prolonged headache especially if first time or getting progressively worse *or* sudden partial or complete loss of vision *or* sudden disturbance of hearing or other perceptual disorders *or* dysphasia *or* bad fainting attack or collapse *or* first unexplained epileptic seizure *or* weakness, motor disturbances, very marked numbness suddenly affecting one side or one part of body;
- Hepatitis, jaundice, liver enlargement;
- Severe depression;
- Blood pressure above systolic 160 mmHg and diastolic 100 mmHg;
- Detection of a risk factor see Cautions and Contra-indications under Combined Oral Contraceptives.

COMBINED ORAL CONTRACEPTIVES
('COC')

Indications: contraception; menstrual symptoms (section 6.4.1.2)

Cautions: risk factors for venous thromboembolism (see below and also notes above), arterial disease and migraine, see below; hyperprolactinaemia (seek specialist advice); severe depres-

sion, sickle-cell disease, inflammatory bowel disease including Crohn's disease; **interactions:** see above and Appendix 1 (contraceptives, oral)

RISK FACTORS FOR VENOUS THROMBOEMBOLISM (see also notes above). Use with **caution** if any of following factors present but **avoid** if two or more factors present:
- *family history of venous thromboembolism* in first degree relative aged under 45 years (avoid contraceptive containing desogestrel or gestodene, *or* if known prothrombotic coagulation abnormality e.g. factor V Leiden or antiphospholipid antibodies (including lupus anticoagulant));
- *obesity*—body mass index above 30 kg/m^2 (avoid if body mass index above 39 kg/m^2);
- *long-term immobilisation* e.g. in a wheelchair (avoid if confined to bed or leg in plaster cast);
- *varicose veins* (avoid during sclerosing treatment or where definite history of thrombosis).

RISK FACTORS FOR ARTERIAL DISEASE. Use with **caution** if any one of following factors present but **avoid** if two or more factors present:
- *family history of arterial disease* in first degree relative aged under 45 years (avoid if atherogenic lipid profile);
- *diabetes mellitus* (avoid if diabetes complications present);
- *hypertension*—blood pressure above *systolic 140 mmHg and diastolic 90 mmHg* (avoid if blood pressure above *systolic 160 mmHg and diastolic 100 mmHg*);
- *smoking* (avoid if smoking 40 or more cigarettes daily);
- *age* over 35 years (avoid if over 50 years);
- *obesity* (avoid if body mass index above 39 kg/m^2);
- *migraine*—see below.

MIGRAINE. Subject should report any increase in headache frequency or onset of focal symptoms (discontinue immediately and refer urgently to neurology expert if focal neurological symptoms not typical of aura persist for more than 1 hour—see also Reason to stop immediately in notes above); **contra-indicated** in
- migraine with typical focal aura,
- severe migraine regularly lasting over 72 hours despite treatment,
- migraine treated with ergot derivatives;

use with **caution** in
- migraine without focal aura,
- migraine controlled with 5HT$_1$ agonist (section 4.7.4.1).

Contra-indications: pregnancy; personal history of venous or arterial thrombosis, severe or multiple risk factors for arterial disease or for venous thromboembolism (see above), heart disease associated with pulmonary hypertension or risk of embolus; migraine (see above), transient cerebral ischaemic attacks without headaches; liver disease including disorders of hepatic excretion (e.g. Dubin-Johnson or Rotor syndromes), infective hepatitis (until liver function returns to normal); systemic lupus erythematosus; porphyria (section 9.8.2); liver adenoma; gallstones; after evacuation of hydatidiform mole (until return to normal of urine and plasma gonadotrophin concentration); history of haemolytic uraemic syndrome or history during pregnancy of pruritus, cholestatic jaundice, chorea or deterioration of otosclerosis, pemphigoid gestationis; breast or genital-tract carcinoma; undiagnosed vaginal bleeding; breast-feeding (until weaning or for 6 months after birth)

Side-effects: nausea, vomiting, headache, breast tenderness, changes in body weight, fluid retention, thrombosis (more common when factor V Leiden present or in blood groups A, B, and AB; see also notes above), changes in libido, depression, chorea, skin reactions, chloasma, hypertension, contact lenses may irritate, impairment of liver function, hepatic tumours, reduced menstrual loss, 'spotting' in early cycles, absence of withdrawal bleeding; rarely photosensitivity

BREAST CANCER. There is a small increase in the risk of having breast cancer diagnosed in women taking the combined oral contraceptive pill; this relative risk may wholly or partly be due to an earlier diagnosis. In users of combined oral contraceptive pills the cancers are more likely to be localised to the breast. The most important risk factor appears to be the age at which the contraceptive is stopped rather than the duration of use; the risk disappears gradually during the 10 years after stopping and there is no excess risk by 10 years. The CSM has advised that a small increase in the risk of breast cancer should be weighed against the benefits and evidence of the protective effect against cancers of the ovary and endometrium

Dose: each tablet should be taken at approximately same time each day; if delayed by longer than 12 hours contraceptive protection may be lost

21-day combined (monophasic) preparations, 1 tablet daily for 21 days; subsequent courses repeated after a 7-day interval (during which withdrawal bleeding occurs); first course usually started on day 1 of cycle—if starting on day 4 of cycle or later additional precautions (barrier methods) necessary during first 7 days

Every day (ED) combined (monophasic) preparations, 1 *active* tablet starting on day 1 of cycle (see also under preparations below)—if starting on day 4 of cycle or later additional precautions (barrier methods) necessary during first 7 days; if starting with *inactive* tablet on day 1 additional precautions required for 14 days; withdrawal bleeding occurs when *inactive* tablets being taken; subsequent courses repeated without interval

Biphasic and triphasic preparations, see under individual preparations below

CHANGING TO COMBINED PREPARATION CONTAINING DIFFERENT PROGESTOGEN.

21-day combined preparations: continue current pack until last tablet and start first tablet of new brand the next day. If a 7-day break is taken before starting new brand, additional precautions (barrier methods) should be used during first 7 days of taking the new brand.

Every Day (ED) combined preparations: start the new brand (first tablet of a *21-day preparation* or the first *active* tablet of an *ED preparation*) the day after taking the last *active* tablet of previous brand (omitting the *inactive* tablets). If not possible to avoid taking the *inactive* tablets of an *ED preparation*, additional precautions (barrier methods) necessary during first 14 days of taking the new brand

CHANGING FROM PROGESTOGEN-ONLY TABLET: start on day 1 of menstruation or any day if amenorrhoea present and pregnancy has been excluded

SECONDARY AMENORRHOEA (exclude pregnancy): start any day, additional precautions (barrier methods) necessary during first 7 days

AFTER CHILDBIRTH (*not* breast-feeding): start 3 weeks postpartum (increased risk of thrombosis if started earlier); later than 3 weeks postpartum additional precautions (barrier methods) necessary for first 7 days

Not recommended if woman breast-feeding—oral progestogen-only contraceptive preferred

AFTER ABORTION OR MISCARRIAGE: start same day

Low Strength

■ Ethinylestradiol with Norethisterone

Loestrin 20® (Parke-Davis) PoM
Tablets, norethisterone acetate 1 mg, ethinylestradiol 20 micrograms. Net price 3 × 21-tab pack = £2.58
Dose: 1 tablet daily for 21 days; subsequent courses repeated after 7-day tablet-free interval (during which withdrawal bleeding occurs); for 'starting routines' see under Dose above

■ Ethinylestradiol with Desogestrel
See Risk of venous thromboembolism in notes above before prescribing

Mercilon® (Organon) PoM
Tablets, desogestrel 150 micrograms, ethinylestradiol 20 micrograms. Net price 3 × 21-tab pack = £8.57
Dose: 1 tablet daily for 21 days; subsequent courses repeated after 7-day tablet-free interval (during which withdrawal bleeding occurs); for 'starting routines' see under Dose above

■ Ethinylestradiol with Gestodene
See Risk of venous thromboembolism in notes above before prescribing

Femodette® (Schering Health) PoM
Tablets, s/c, gestodene 75 micrograms, ethinylestradiol 20 micrograms, net price 3 × 21-tab pack = £7.50
Dose: 1 tablet daily for 21 days; subsequent courses repeated after 7-day tablet-free interval (during which withdrawal bleeding occurs); for 'starting routines' see under Dose above

Standard Strength

■ Ethinylestradiol with Levonorgestrel

Eugynon 30® (Schering Health) PoM
Tablets, levonorgestrel 250 micrograms, ethinylestradiol 30 micrograms. Net price 3 × 21-tab pack = £2.28
Dose: 1 tablet daily for 21 days; subsequent courses repeated after 7-day tablet-free interval (during which withdrawal bleeding occurs); for 'starting routines' see under Dose above

Logynon® (Schering Health) PoM
6 light brown tablets, ethinylestradiol 30 micrograms, levonorgestrel 50 micrograms;
5 white tablets, ethinylestradiol 40 micrograms, levonorgestrel 75 micrograms;
10 ochre tablets, ethinylestradiol 30 micrograms, levonorgestrel 125 micrograms.
Net price 3 × 21-tab pack = £3.60
Dose: 1 tablet daily for 21 days, starting with light brown tablet marked 1 on day 1 of cycle; repeat after 7-day tablet-free interval

Logynon ED® (Schering Health) PoM
6 light brown tablets, ethinylestradiol 30 micrograms, levonorgestrel 50 micrograms;
5 white tablets, ethinylestradiol 40 micrograms, levonorgestrel 75 micrograms;
10 ochre tablets, ethinylestradiol 30 micrograms, levonorgestrel 125 micrograms;
7 white, inactive tablets.

Net price 3 × 28-tab pack = £3.60

Dose: 1 tablet daily starting in red sector on day 1 of cycle; continue in sequence without interruption; for 'starting routines' see under Dose above

Microgynon 30® (Schering Health) PoM

Tablets, s/c, levonorgestrel 150 micrograms, ethinylestradiol 30 micrograms. Net price 21-tab pack = 78p

Dose: 1 tablet daily for 21 days; subsequent courses repeated after 7-day tablet-free interval (during which withdrawal bleeding occurs); for 'starting routines' see under Dose above

Microgynon 30 ED® (Schering Health) PoM

Tablets, beige, levonorgestrel 150 micrograms, ethinylestradiol 30 micrograms, white inactive tablets. Net price 3 × 28-tab (7 are inactive) pack = £2.34

Dose: 1 tablet daily for 28 days starting on day 1 of cycle with active tablet (withdrawal bleeding occurs when inactive tablets being taken); subsequent courses repeated without interval; for 'starting routines' see under Dose above

Ovran 30® (Wyeth) PoM

Tablets, levonorgestrel 250 micrograms, ethinylestradiol 30 micrograms. Net price 21-tab pack = 69p

Dose: 1 tablet daily for 21 days; subsequent courses repeated after 7-day tablet-free interval (during which withdrawal bleeding occurs); for 'starting routines' see under Dose above

Ovranette® (Wyeth) PoM

Tablets, levonorgestrel 150 micrograms, ethinylestradiol 30 micrograms. Net price 3 × 21-tab pack = £2.26

Dose: 1 tablet daily for 21 days; subsequent courses repeated after 7-day tablet-free interval (during which withdrawal bleeding occurs); for 'starting routines' see under Dose above

Trinordiol® (Wyeth) PoM

6 light brown tablets, ethinylestradiol 30 micrograms, levonorgestrel 50 micrograms;

5 white tablets, ethinylestradiol 40 micrograms, levonorgestrel 75 micrograms;

10 ochre tablets, ethinylestradiol 30 micrograms, levonorgestrel 125 micrograms.

Net price 3 × 21-tab pack = £3.97

Dose: 1 tablet daily for 21 days, starting with light brown tablet marked 1 on day 1 of cycle; repeat after 7-day tablet-free interval

■ Ethinylestradiol with Norethisterone

BiNovum® (Janssen-Cilag) PoM

7 white tablets, ethinylestradiol 35 micrograms, norethisterone 500 micrograms;

14 peach tablets, ethinylestradiol 35 micrograms, norethisterone 1mg.

Net price 3 × 21-tab pack = £2.24

Dose: 1 tablet daily for 21 days, starting with white tablet on day 1 of cycle; repeat after 7-day tablet-free interval

Brevinor® (Pharmacia) PoM

Tablets, blue, norethisterone 500 micrograms, ethinylestradiol 35 micrograms. Net price 3 × 21-tab pack = £1.67

Dose: 1 tablet daily for 21 days; subsequent courses repeated after 7-day tablet-free interval (during which withdrawal bleeding occurs); for 'starting routines' see under Dose above

Loestrin 30® (Parke-Davis) PoM

Tablets, norethisterone acetate 1.5 mg, ethinylestradiol 30 micrograms. Net price 3 × 21-tab pack = £3.78

Dose: 1 tablet daily for 21 days; subsequent courses repeated after 7-day tablet-free interval (during which withdrawal bleeding occurs); for 'starting routines' see under Dose above

Norimin® (Pharmacia) PoM

Tablets, norethisterone 1 mg, ethinylestradiol 35 micrograms. Net price 3 × 21-tab pack = £1.90

Dose: 1 tablet daily for 21 days; subsequent courses repeated after 7-day tablet-free interval (during which withdrawal bleeding occurs); for 'starting routines' see under Dose above

Ovysmen® (Janssen-Cilag) PoM

Tablets, norethisterone 500 micrograms, ethinylestradiol 35 micrograms. Net price 3 × 21-tab pack = £1.70

Dose: 1 tablet daily for 21 days; subsequent courses repeated after 7-day tablet-free interval (during which withdrawal bleeding occurs); for 'starting routines' see under Dose above

Synphase® (Pharmacia) PoM

7 blue tablets, ethinylestradiol 35 micrograms, norethisterone 500 micrograms;

9 white tablets, ethinylestradiol 35 micrograms, norethisterone 1 mg;

5 blue tablets, ethinylestradiol 35 micrograms, norethisterone 500 micrograms.

Net price 21-tab pack = £1.08

Dose: 1 tablet daily for 21 days, starting with blue tablet marked 1 on day 1 of cycle; repeat after 7-day tablet-free interval

TriNovum® (Janssen-Cilag) PoM

7 white tablets, ethinylestradiol 35 micrograms, norethisterone 500 micrograms;

7 light peach tablets, ethinylestradiol 35 micrograms, norethisterone 750 micrograms;

7 peach tablets, ethinylestradiol 35 micrograms, norethisterone 1 mg.

Net price 3 × 21-tab pack = £3.11

Dose: 1 tablet daily for 21 days, starting with white tablet on day 1 of cycle; repeat after 7-day tablet-free interval

■ Ethinylestradiol with Norgestimate

Cilest® (Janssen-Cilag) PoM

Tablets, blue, norgestimate 250 micrograms, ethinylestradiol 35 micrograms. Net price 3 × 21-tab pack = £6.42, 6 × 21-tab pack = £12.84

Dose: 1 tablet daily for 21 days; subsequent courses repeated after 7-day tablet-free interval (during which withdrawal bleeding occurs); for 'starting routines' see under Dose above

■ Ethinylestradiol with Desogestrel

See Risk of venous thromboembolism in notes above before prescribing

Marvelon® (Organon) PoM

Tablets, desogestrel 150 micrograms, ethinylestradiol 30 micrograms. Net price 3 × 21-tab pack = £6.70

Dose: 1 tablet daily for 21 days; subsequent courses repeated after 7-day tablet-free interval (during which withdrawal bleeding occurs); for 'starting routines' see under Dose above

■ Ethinylestradiol with Gestodene

See Risk of venous thromboembolism in notes above before prescribing

Femodene® (Schering Health) [PoM]

Tablets, s/c, gestodene 75 micrograms, ethinylestradiol 30 micrograms. Net price 3 × 21-tab pack = £6.27

> *Dose:* 1 tablet daily for 21 days; subsequent courses repeated after 7-day tablet-free interval (during which withdrawal bleeding occurs); for 'starting routines' see under Dose above

Femodene® ED (Schering Health) [PoM]

Tablets, s/c, gestodene 75 micrograms, ethinylestradiol 30 micrograms. Net price 3 × 28-tab (7 are inactive) pack = £6.27

> *Dose:* 1 tablet daily for 28 days starting in red sector on day 1 of cycle (withdrawal bleeding occurs when inactive tablets are being taken); subsequent courses repeated without interval; for 'starting routines' see under Dose above

Minulet® (Wyeth) [PoM]

Tablets, gestodene 75 micrograms, ethinylestradiol 30 micrograms. Net price 3 × 21-tab pack = £6.27

> *Dose:* 1 tablet daily for 21 days; subsequent courses repeated after 7-day tablet-free interval (during which withdrawal bleeding occurs); for 'starting routines' see under Dose above

Triadene® (Schering Health) [PoM]

6 beige tablets, ethinylestradiol 30 micrograms, gestodene 50 micrograms;

5 dark brown tablets, ethinylestradiol 40 micrograms, gestodene 70 micrograms;

10 white tablets, ethinylestradiol 30 micrograms, gestodene 100 micrograms.

Net price 3 × 21-tab pack = £8.75

> *Dose:* 1 tablet daily for 21 days, starting with beige tablet marked 'start' on day 1 of cycle; repeat after 7-day tablet-free interval

Tri-Minulet® (Wyeth) [PoM]

6 beige tablets, ethinylestradiol 30 micrograms, gestodene 50 micrograms;

5 dark brown tablets, ethinylestradiol 40 micrograms, gestodene 70 micrograms;

10 white tablets, ethinylestradiol 30 micrograms, gestodene 100 micrograms.

Net price 3 × 21-tab pack = £8.75

> *Dose:* 1 tablet daily for 21 days, starting with beige tablet marked 1 on day 1 of the cycle; repeat after 7-day tablet-free interval

■ Ethinylestradiol with cyproterone acetate

See co-cyprindiol (section 13.6.2)

High Strength

■ Ethinylestradiol with Levonorgestrel

Ovran® (Wyeth) [PoM]

Tablets, levonorgestrel 250 micrograms, ethinylestradiol 50 micrograms. Net price 21-tab pack = 45p

> *Dose:* 1 tablet daily for 21 days; subsequent courses repeated after 7-day tablet-free interval (during which withdrawal bleeding occurs); for 'starting routines' see under Dose above

■ Mestranol with Norethisterone

Norinyl-1® (Pharmacia) [PoM]

Tablets, norethisterone 1 mg, mestranol 50 micrograms. Net price 3 × 21-tab pack = £1.83

> *Dose:* 1 tablet daily for 21 days; subsequent courses repeated after 7-day tablet-free interval (during which withdrawal bleeding occurs); for 'starting routines' see under Dose above

Emergency contraception

Hormonal methods

Hormonal emergency contraception involves the use of **levonorgestrel**. It is effective if the first dose is taken within 72 hours (3 days) of unprotected intercourse; taking the first dose as soon as possible increases efficacy. Levonorgestrel may be used between 72 and 120 hours after unprotected intercourse [unlicensed use] but efficacy decreases with time. Hormonal emergency contraception is less effective than insertion of an intra-uterine device (see below).

Levonorgestrel is taken as 1 tablet of 750 micrograms followed 12 hours later (and no later than 16 hours) by a further tablet. It is not suitable for women with active acute porphyria.

If vomiting occurs within 3 hours of taking levonorgestrel, a replacement dose can be given. If an anti-emetic is required domperidone is preferred.

When prescribing hormonal emergency contraception the doctor should explain:

- that the next period may be early or late;
- that a barrier method of contraception needs to be used until the next period;
- the need to return promptly if any lower abdominal pain occurs (and also in 3 to 4 weeks if the subsequent menstrual bleed is abnormally light, heavy or brief, or is absent, or if she is otherwise concerned).

Pregnancy despite treatment: see Appendix 4 (contraceptives, oral).

INTERACTIONS. The effectiveness of the hormonal method of emergency contraception is reduced by enzyme-inducing drugs; a copper intra-uterine device may be offered or, otherwise, the first dose of levonorgestrel should be increased to 1.5 mg followed 12 hours later by the usual dose of 750 micrograms. There is no need to increase the dose for emergency contraception if the patient is taking antibacterials that are not enzyme inducers.

¹ Levonelle®-2 (Schering Health) [PoM]

Tablets, levonorgestrel 750 micrograms, net price 2-tab pack = £5.00

> For post-coital contraception as an occasional emergency measure; should not be administered if menstrual bleeding overdue or if unprotected intercourse occurred more than 72 hours previously
>
> *Dose:* 1 tablet as soon as possible after coitus (up to 72 hours) then 1 further tablet 12 hours later
>
> 1. Can be sold to women over 16 years as *Levonelle®*; when supplying emergency contraception to the public, pharmacists should refer to guidance issued by the Royal Pharmaceutical Society of Great Britain

Intra-uterine device

Insertion of an intra-uterine device is more effective than the hormonal methods of emergency contraception. A copper intra-uterine contraceptive device (section 7.3.4) can be inserted up to 120 hours (5 days) after unprotected intercourse; sexually transmitted diseases should be tested for and insertion of the device should usually be covered by antibacterial prophylaxis (e.g. azithromycin 1 g as a single dose). If intercourse has occurred more than 5 days previously, the device can still be inserted up to 5 days after the earliest likely calculated ovulation (i.e. within the minimum period before implantation).

<table>
<tr><td>**7.3.2**</td><td colspan="2">**Progestogen-only contraceptives**</td></tr>
<tr><td>**7.3.2.1**</td><td>Oral progestogen-only contraceptives</td></tr>
<tr><td>**7.3.2.2**</td><td>Parenteral progestogen-only contraceptives</td></tr>
<tr><td>**7.3.2.3**</td><td>Intra-uterine progestogen-only contraceptive</td></tr>
</table>

7.3.2.1 Oral progestogen-only contraceptives

Oral progestogen-only preparations may offer a suitable alternative when oestrogens are contra-indicated (including those patients with venous thrombosis or a past history or predisposition to venous thrombosis), but have a higher failure rate than combined preparations. They are suitable for older women, for heavy smokers, and for those with hypertension, valvular heart disease, diabetes mellitus, and migraine. Menstrual irregularities (oligomenorrhoea, menorrhagia) are more common but tend to resolve on long-term treatment.

INTERACTIONS. Effectiveness of oral progestogen-only preparations is not affected by broad-spectrum antibiotics but is reduced by enzyme-inducing drugs—see p. 387 and Appendix 1 (progestogens).

SURGERY. All progestogen-only contraceptives (including those given by injection) are suitable for use as an alternative to combined oral contraceptives before major elective surgery.

STARTING ROUTINE. One tablet daily, on a continuous basis, starting on day 1 of cycle and taken at the same time each day (if delayed by longer than 3 hours contraceptive protection may be lost). Additional contraceptive precautions are not necessary when initiating treatment.
   Changing from a combined oral contraceptive: start on the day following completion of the combined oral contraceptive course without a break (or in the case of ED tablets omitting the inactive ones).
   After childbirth: start any time after 3 weeks postpartum (increased risk of breakthrough bleeding if started earlier)—lactation is not affected.

MISSED PILL. The following advice is now recommended by family planning organisations:
   'If you forget a pill, take it as soon as you remember and carry on with the next pill at the right time. If the pill was more than three hours overdue you are not protected. Continue normal pill-taking but you must also use another method, such as the condom, for the next 7 days'.
The Faculty of Family Planning and Reproductive Health Care recommends emergency contraception

(see p. 391) if one or more progestogen-only contraceptive tablets are missed or taken more than 3 hours late.

DIARRHOEA AND VOMITING. Vomiting up to 3 hours after taking an oral contraceptive *or* very severe diarrhoea can interfere with its absorption. Additional precautions should be used during and for 7 days after recovery.

ORAL PROGESTOGEN-ONLY CONTRACEPTIVES

(Progestogen-only pill, 'POP')
Indications: contraception
Cautions: heart disease, sex-steroid dependent cancer, past ectopic pregnancy, malabsorption syndromes, functional ovarian cysts, active liver disease, recurrent cholestatic jaundice, history of jaundice in pregnancy; **interactions:** p. 387 and Appendix 1 (progestogens)
   OTHER CONDITIONS. The product literature advises caution in patients with history of thromboembolism, hypertension, diabetes mellitus and migraine; evidence for caution in these conditions is unsatisfactory
Contra-indications: pregnancy, undiagnosed vaginal bleeding; severe arterial disease; liver adenoma, porphyria (section 9.8.2); after evacuation of hydatidiform mole (until return to normal of urine and plasma gonadotrophin values)
Side-effects: menstrual irregularities (see also notes above); nausea, vomiting, headache, dizziness, breast discomfort, depression, skin disorders, disturbance of appetite, weight changes, changes in libido
   BREAST CANCER. There is a small increase in the risk of having breast cancer diagnosed in women using, or who have recently used, a progestogen-only contraceptive pill; this relative risk may wholly or partly be due to an earlier diagnosis. The most important risk factor appears to be the age at which the contraceptive is stopped rather than the duration of use; the risk disappears gradually during the 10 years after stopping and there is no excess risk by 10 years. The CSM has advised that a small increase in the risk of breast cancer should be weighed against the benefits
Dose: 1 tablet daily at same time each day, starting on day 1 of cycle then continuously; if administration delayed for 3 hours or more it should be regarded as a 'missed pill', see notes above

Femulen® (Pharmacia) PoM
   Tablets, etynodiol diacetate 500 micrograms. Net price 3 × 28-tab pack = £2.76
Micronor® (Janssen-Cilag) PoM
   Tablets, norethisterone 350 micrograms. Net price 3 × 28-tab pack = £1.89
Microval® (Wyeth) PoM
   Tablets, levonorgestrel 30 micrograms. Net price 35-tab pack = 90p
Neogest® (Schering Health) PoM
   Tablets, brown, s/c, norgestrel 75 micrograms (≡ levonorgestrel 37.5 micrograms). Net price 35-tab pack = 90p
Norgeston® (Schering Health) PoM
   Tablets, s/c, levonorgestrel 30 micrograms. Net price 35-tab pack = 90p
Noriday® (Pharmacia) PoM
   Tablets, norethisterone 350 micrograms. Net price 3 × 28-tab pack = £1.75

7.3.2.2 Parenteral progestogen-only contraceptives

Medroxyprogesterone acetate (*Depo-Provera®*) is a long-acting progestogen given by intramuscular injection; it is as effective as the combined oral preparations but because of its prolonged action it should never be given without *full counselling backed by the manufacturer's approved leaflet*. It may be used as a short-term or long-term contraceptive for women who have been counselled about the likelihood of menstrual disturbance and the potential for a delay in return to full fertility. Delayed return of fertility and irregular cycles may occur after discontinuation of treatment but there is no evidence of permanent infertility. Heavy bleeding has been reported in patients given medroxyprogesterone acetate in the immediate puerperium (the first dose is best delayed until 6 weeks after birth). If the woman is not breast-feeding, the first injection may be given within 5 days postpartum (she should be warned that the risk of heavy or prolonged bleeding may be increased). Reduction in bone mineral density has also been reported. **Norethisterone enantate** (*Noristerat®*) is a long-acting progestogen given as an oily injection which provides contraception for 8 weeks; it is used as short-term interim contraception e.g. before vasectomy becomes effective. The **cautions** and **contra-indications** of oral progestogen-only contraceptives apply except that because the injection also reliably inhibits ovulation, it protects against ectopic pregnancy and functional ovarian cysts.

An **etonogestrel-releasing implant** (*Implanon®*), consisting of a single flexible rod, is also available; the rod is inserted subdermally into the lower surface of the upper arm and is effective for up to 3 years. In women with a body mass index greater than 35 kg/m², blood concentrations of etonogestrel are lower and therefore the implant may not provide effective contraception during the third year; earlier replacement should be considered in such patients. Local reactions such as bruising and itching may occur at the insertion site. The **cautions**, **contra-indications** and **side-effects** of oral preparations apply; the contraceptive effect of *Implanon®* is rapidly reversed on removal of the implant. *The doctor or nurse administering (or removing) the system should be fully trained in the technique and should provide full counselling backed by the manufacturer's approved leaflet.*

The **levonorgestrel-releasing implant system** (*Norplant®*, Hoechst Marion Roussel) has been discontinued, but some women may have the system in place until 2004. Unlike the injectable progestogen-only contraceptive method, the effects of *Norplant®* are almost immediately reversible on removal of the implants. *The doctor removing the system should be fully trained in the technique.*

INTERACTIONS. Effectiveness of parenteral progestogen-only contraceptives is not affected by broad-spectrum antibiotics. However, effectiveness may be reduced by enzyme-inducing drugs; another contraceptive method should be considered instead or an additional contraceptive method used while the enzyme-inducing drug is being taken. In long-term users of *Depo-Provera®*, the interval between injections should be reduced from 12 weeks to 10 weeks—see Appendix 1 (progestogens)

PARENTERAL PROGESTOGEN-ONLY CONTRACEPTIVES

Indications: contraception, see also notes above and under preparations (roles vary according to preparation)

Cautions: see notes above and under preparations; possible risk of breast cancer, see also progestogen-only contraceptives (section 7.3.2.1); history during pregnancy of pruritus or of deterioration of otosclerosis, disturbances of lipid metabolism; **interactions:** see notes above and Appendix 1 (progestogens)

COUNSELLING. Full counselling backed by *manufacturer's approved leaflet* required before administration

Contra-indications: see notes above

Side-effects: see notes above

Dose: see under preparations

■ Injectable preparations

Depo-Provera® (Pharmacia) PoM

Injection (aqueous suspension), medroxyprogesterone acetate 150 mg/mL, net price 1-mL prefilled syringe = £4.55. Counselling, see patient information leaflet

Dose: by deep intramuscular injection, 150 mg within first 5 days of cycle or within first 5 days after parturition (delay until 6 weeks after parturition if breast-feeding); for long-term contraception, repeated every 12 weeks (if interval greater than 12 weeks and 5 days, exclude pregnancy before next injection and advise patient to use additional contraceptive measures (e.g. barrier) for 14 days after the injection)

Noristerat® (Schering Health) PoM

Injection (oily), norethisterone enantate 200 mg/mL. Net price 1-mL amp = £3.30. Counselling, see patient information leaflet

Dose: by deep intramuscular injection given very slowly into gluteal muscle, short-term contraception, 200 mg within first 5 days of cycle or immediately after parturition (duration 8 weeks); may be repeated once after 8 weeks (withhold breast-feeding for neonates with severe or persistent jaundice requiring medical treatment)

■ Implants

Implanon® (Organon) ▼ PoM

Implant, containing etonogestrel 68 mg in each flexible rod, net price = £90.00. Counselling, see patient information leaflet

Dose: by subdermal implantation, no previous hormonal contraceptive, 1 implant inserted during first 5 days of cycle; parturition or abortion in second trimester, 1 implant inserted between days 21–28 after delivery or abortion (if inserted after 28 days additional precautions necessary for next 7 days); abortion in first trimester, 1 implant inserted immediately; changing from an oral contraceptive, consult product literature; remove within 3 years of insertion

7.3.2.3 Intra-uterine progestogen-only device

The progestogen-only intra-uterine system, *Mirena®*, releases **levonorgestrel** directly into the uterine cavity. It is licensed for use as a contraceptive and for the treatment of primary menorrhagia. This may therefore be a contraceptive method of choice for women who have excessively heavy menses. The effects of the intra-uterine system are mainly local and hormonal including prevention of endometrial proliferation, thickening of cervical mucus, and suppression of ovulation in some women (in some cycles). In addition to the progestogenic activity, the intra-uterine system itself may contribute slightly to the contraceptive effect. Return of fertility after removal is rapid and appears to be complete. Advantages over copper intra-uterine devices are that there may be an improvement in any dysmenorrhoea and a reduction in blood loss; there is also evidence that the frequency of pelvic inflammatory disease may be reduced (particularly in the youngest age groups who are most at risk).

In primary menorrhagia, menstrual bleeding is reduced significantly within 3–6 months of inserting the levonorgestrel intra-uterine system, probably because it prevents endometrial proliferation. Another treatment should be considered if menorrhagia does not improve within this period (section 6.4.1.2).

Generally the **cautions** and **contra-indications** are as for standard intra-uterine devices (section 7.3.4) but the risk of ectopic pregnancy is considerably smaller. Moreover, since the progestogen is released close to the site of the main contraceptive action (on cervical mucus and endometrium) progestogenic side-effects and interactions are less likely to be a problem—in particular, enzyme-inducing drugs are unlikely to significantly reduce the contraceptive effect. Initially changes in the pattern and duration of menstrual bleeding (spotting or prolonged bleeding) are common and the patient should be fully counselled (and provided with a patient information leaflet) before insertion. Improvement in progestogenic side-effects, such as mastalgia and mood changes, and in the bleeding pattern usually occurs a few months after insertion and bleeding may often become very light or absent. Functional ovarian cysts (usually asymptomatic) may occur and usually resolve spontaneously (ultrasound monitoring recommended).

INTRA-UTERINE PROGESTOGEN-ONLY SYSTEM

Indications: contraception, primary menorrhagia

Cautions: see notes above; in case of pregnancy—remove system (teratogenicity cannot be excluded); not suitable for emergency contraception; **interactions:** see notes above and Appendix 1 (progestogens)

Contra-indications: see notes above

Side-effects: see notes above

Mirena® (Schering Health) [PoM]
  Intra-uterine system, T-shaped plastic frame (impregnated with barium sulphate and with threads attached to base) with polydimethylsiloxane reservoir releasing levonorgestrel 20 micrograms/24 hours. Net price = £89.25. Counselling, see patient information leaflet
  Insert into uterine cavity within 7 days of onset of menstruation (anytime if replacement) or immediately after

first-trimester termination by curettage; postpartum insertions should be delayed until 6 weeks after delivery; effective for 5 years

---

7.3.3   Spermicidal contraceptives

Spermicidal contraceptives are useful additional safeguards but do **not** give adequate protection if used alone except where fertility is already significantly diminished (section 6.4.1.1); they are suitable for use with barrier methods. They have two components: a spermicide and a vehicle which itself may have some inhibiting effect on sperm activity.

> **CSM Advice.** Products such as petroleum jelly (vaseline), baby oil and oil-based vaginal and rectal preparations are likely to damage condoms and contraceptive diaphragms made from latex rubber, and may render them less effective as a barrier method of contraception and as a protection from sexually transmitted diseases (including HIV).

Condoms: no evidence of harm to latex condoms and diaphragms with the products listed below

Delfen® (Janssen-Cilag)
  Foam, nonoxinol '9' 12.5%, pressurised aerosol unit in a water-miscible basis. Net price 20 g (with applicator) = £4.65
  Excipients: include cetyl alcohol, hydroxybenzoates (parabens), propylene glycol, fragrance

Duragel® (SSL)
  Gel, nonoxinol '9' 2% in a water-soluble basis. Net price 100-g tube = £3.45
  Excipients: include propylene glycol

Gynol II® (Janssen-Cilag)
  Jelly, nonoxinol '9' 2% in a water-soluble basis. Net price 81 g = £2.61; applicator = 75p
  Excipients: include hydroxybenzoates (parabens), propylene glycol, sorbic acid

Ortho-Creme® (Janssen-Cilag)
  Cream, nonoxinol '9' 2% in a water-miscible basis. Net price 70 g = £2.44; applicator = 75p
  Excipients: include cetyl alcohol, hydroxybenzoates (parabens), propylene glycol, sorbic acid, fragrance

Orthoforms® (Janssen-Cilag)
  Pessaries, nonoxinol '9' 5% in a water-soluble basis. Net price 15 pessaries = £2.40
  Excipients: none as listed in section 13.1.3

7.3.4   Contraceptive devices

Intra-uterine devices

The intra-uterine device (IUD) is suitable for older parous women and as a second-line contraceptive in young nulliparous women who should be carefully screened because they have an increased background risk of pelvic inflammatory disease.

Smaller devices have been introduced to minimise side-effects; these consist of a plastic carrier wound with copper wire or fitted with copper bands; some also have a central core of silver to prevent fragmentation of the copper. Any copper intra-uterine device licensed currently in the UK, which is fitted in a woman over the age of 40, may remain in the uterus until menopause. The intra-uterine device *Gyne-T 380®* (Janssen-Cilag) is no longer available, but some women may have the device in place until 2009.

A frameless, copper-bearing intra-uterine device (*GyneFix®*) has been introduced recently. It consists of a knotted, polypropylene thread with 6 copper sleeves; the device is anchored in the uterus by inserting the knot into the uterine fundus. *The healthcare professional inserting (or removing) the device should be fully trained in the technique and should provide full counselling backed by the manufacturer's approved leaflet.*

The timing and technique of fitting an intra-uterine device are critical for its subsequent performance and call for proper training and experience. Devices should not be fitted during the heavy days of the period; they are best fitted after the end of menstruation and before the calculated time of implantation. The main excess risk of infection occurs in the first 20 days after insertion and is believed to be related to existing carriage of a sexually transmitted disease, therefore pre-screening (at least for chlamydia) should ideally be performed. The woman should be advised to attend *as an emergency* if she experiences sustained pain during the next 20 days.

An intra-uterine device should not be removed in mid-cycle unless an additional contraceptive was used for the previous 7 days. If removal is essential (e.g. to treat severe pelvic infection) post-coital contraception should be considered.

If an intra-uterine device fails and the woman wishes to continue to full-term the device should be removed in the first trimester if possible.

INTRA-UTERINE CONTRACEPTIVE DEVICES

Indications: see notes above

Cautions: anaemia, heavy menses (progestogen intra-uterine system might be preferable, section 7.3.2.3), endometriosis, severe primary dysmenorrhoea, history of pelvic inflammatory disease, history of ectopic pregnancy or tubal surgery, diabetes, fertility problems, nulliparity and young age, severely scarred uterus (including after endometrial resection) or severe cervical stenosis, valvular heart disease (antibacterial cover needed—section 5.1 table 2)—avoid if prosthetic valve or history of infective endocarditis; drug- or disease-induced immunosuppression (risk of infection—avoid if marked immunosuppression); joint and other prostheses (increased risk of infection); epilepsy; increased risk of expulsion if inserted before uterine involution; gynaecological examination before insertion, 6–8 weeks after then annually but counsel women to see doctor promptly in case of significant symptoms, especially pain; anticoagulant therapy (avoid if possible); remove if pregnancy occurs; if pregnancy occurs, increased likelihood that it may be ectopic

Contra-indications: pregnancy, severe anaemia, recent sexually transmitted infection (if not fully investigated and treated), unexplained uterine bleeding, distorted or small uterine cavity, genital malignancy, active trophoblastic disease, pelvic inflammatory disease, established or marked immunosuppression; *copper devices:* copper allergy, Wilson's disease, medical diathermy

Side-effects: uterine or cervical perforation, displacement, expulsion; pelvic infection may be exacerbated, heavy menses, dysmenorrhoea, allergy; *on insertion:* pain (alleviated by NSAID such as ibuprofen 30 minutes before insertion) and bleeding, occasionally, epileptic seizure, vasovagal attack

Flexi-T® 300 (FP)

Intra-uterine device, copper wire, surface area approx. 300 mm² wound on vertical stem of T-shaped plastic carrier, impregnated with barium sulphate for radio-opacity, monofilament thread attached to base of vertical stem; preloaded in inserter, net price = £8.65

For uterine length over 5 cm; replacement every 5 years (see also notes above)

GyneFix® (FP)

Intra-uterine device, 6 copper sleeves with surface area of 330 mm² on polypropylene thread, net price = £24.75

Suitable for all uterine sizes; replacement every 5 years

Multiload® Cu250 (Organon)

Intra-uterine device, copper wire, surface area approx. 250 mm² wound on vertical stem of plastic carrier, 3.5 cm length, with 2 down-curving flexible arms, monofilament thread attached to base of vertical stem; preloaded in inserter, net price = £7.09

For uterine length 6–9 cm; replacement every 3 years (but see notes above)

Multiload® Cu250 Short (Organon)

Intra-uterine device, as above, with vertical stem length 2.4 cm, net price = £7.09

For uterine length 5–7 cm; replacement every 3 years (but see notes above)

Multiload® Cu375 (Organon)

Intra-uterine device, as above, with copper surface area approx. 375 mm² and vertical stem length 3.5 cm, net price = £9.19

For uterine length 6–9 cm; replacement every 5 years (see notes above)

Nova-T® 380 (Schering Health)

Intra-uterine device, copper wire with silver core, surface area approx. 380 mm² wound on vertical stem of T-shaped plastic carrier, impregnated with barium sulphate for radio-opacity, threads attached to base of vertical stem, net price = £13.50

For uterine length 6.5–9 cm; replacement every 5 years (see notes above)

T-Safe® CU 380 A (FP)

Intra-uterine device, copper wire, wound on vertical stem of T-shaped plastic carrier with copper collar on the distal portion of each arm, total surface area approx. 380 mm², impregnated with barium sulphate for radio-opacity, threads attached to base of vertical stem, net price = £9.40

For uterine length 6.5–9 cm; replacement every 8 years (see notes above)

Other contraceptive devices

■ Contraceptive caps

Type A contraceptive pessary

Opaque rubber, sizes 1 to 5 (55–75 mm rising in steps of 5 mm), net price = £6.07

Available from Lamberts (*Dumas Vault Cap®*)

Type B contraceptive pessary

Opaque rubber, sizes 22 to 31 mm (rising in steps of 3 mm), net price = £7.18

Available from Lamberts (*Prentif Cavity Rim Cervical Cap®*)

Type C contraceptive pessary
Opaque rubber, sizes 1 to 3 (42, 48 and 54 mm),
net price = £6.07
Available from Lamberts (*Vimule Cap®*)

■ Contraceptive diaphragms

Type A Diaphragm with flat metal spring
Transparent rubber with flat metal spring, sizes
55–95 mm (rising in steps of 5 mm), net price =
£5.59
Available from Lamberts (*Reflexions®*)

Type B Diaphragm with coiled metal rim
Opaque rubber with coiled metal rim, sizes 60–
100 mm (rising in steps of 5 mm), net price =
£5.84
Available from Janssen-Cilag (*Ortho®*)

Type C Arcing Spring Diaphragm
Opaque rubber with arcing spring, sizes 60–95 mm
(rising in steps of 5 mm), net price = £6.64
Available from Janssen-Cilag (*All-Flex®*)

■ Fertility thermometer

Fertility (Ovulation) Thermometer (Zeal)
Mercury in glass thermometer, range 35 to 39°C
(graduated in 0.1°C). Net price = £1.68
For monitoring ovulation for the fertility awareness
method of contraception

7.4   Drugs for genito-urinary disorders

7.4.1   Drugs for urinary retention
7.4.2   Drugs for urinary frequency, enuresis, and incontinence
7.4.3   Drugs used in urological pain
7.4.4   Bladder instillations and urological surgery
7.4.5   Drugs for erectile dysfunction

For drugs used in the treatment of urinary-tract
infections see section 5.1.13.

7.4.1   Drugs for urinary retention

Acute retention is painful and is treated by catheterisation.

Chronic retention is painless and often long-
standing. Catheterisation is unnecessary unless
there is deterioration of renal function. After the
cause has initially been established and treated,
drugs may be required to increase detrusor muscle
tone.

Benign prostatic hyperplasia is treated either surgically or medically with alpha-blockers (see
below) or with the anti-androgen finasteride (section 6.4.2).

Alpha-blockers

The selective alpha-blockers, **alfuzosin**, **doxazosin**,
indoramin, **prazosin**, **tamsulosin** and **terazosin**
relax smooth muscle in benign prostatic hyperplasia
producing an increase in urinary flow-rate and an
improvement in obstructive symptoms.

CAUTIONS. Since selective alpha-blockers reduce
blood pressure, patients receiving antihypertensive
treatment may require reduced dosage and specialist supervision. Caution may be required in the elderly and in patients with hepatic impairment
(Appendix 2) and severe renal impairment (Appendix 3). For **interactions** see Appendix 1 (alpha-
blockers).

CONTRA-INDICATIONS. Alpha-blockers should
be avoided in patients with a history of orthostatic
hypotension and micturition syncope.

SIDE-EFFECTS. Side-effects of selective alpha-
blockers include drowsiness, hypotension (notably
postural hypotension), syncope, asthenia, depression, headache, dry mouth, gastro-intestinal disturbances (including nausea, vomiting, diarrhoea,
constipation), oedema, blurred vision, rhinitis, erectile disorders (including priapism), tachycardia, and
palpitations. Hypersensitivity reactions including
rash, pruritus and angioedema have also been
reported.

FIRST DOSE EFFECT. First dose of alfuzosin,
prazosin and terazosin may cause collapse due to
hypotensive effect (see below).

ALFUZOSIN HYDROCHLORIDE

Indications: see notes above
Cautions: see notes above
Contra-indications: see notes above; severe liver
impairment
Side-effects: see notes above; flushes, chest pain
Dose: 2.5 mg 3 times daily, max. 10 mg daily; ELD-
ERLY initially 2.5 mg twice daily
FIRST DOSE EFFECT. First dose may cause collapse due to
hypotensive effect (therefore should be taken on retiring
to bed). Patient should be warned to lie down if symp-
toms such as dizziness, fatigue or sweating develop, and
to remain lying down until they abate completely

Xatral® (Sanofi-Synthelabo) PoM
Tablets, f/c, alfuzosin hydrochloride 2.5 mg, net
price 60-tab pack = £19.00. Label: 3, counselling,
see dose above

■ Modified release

Xatral® XL (Sanofi-Synthelabo) PoM
Tablets, m/r, yellow/white, alfuzosin hydrochloride 10 mg, net price 10-tab pack = £7.93, 30-
tab pack = £23.80. Label: 3, 21, 25, counselling,
see above
Dose: 10 mg once daily

DOXAZOSIN

Indications: see notes above and section 2.5.4
Cautions: see notes above and section 2.5.4
Contra-indications: see notes above
Side-effects: see notes above and section 2.5.4
Dose: initially 1 mg daily; dose may be doubled at
intervals of 1–2 weeks according to response, up
to max. 8 mg daily; usual maintenance 2–4 mg
daily

Preparations
Section 2.5.4

INDORAMIN

Indications: see notes above and section 2.5.4

Cautions: see notes above and section 2.5.4

Contra-indications: see notes above and section 2.5.4

Side-effects: see notes above and section 2.5.4

Dose: 20 mg twice daily; increased if necessary by 20 mg every 2 weeks to max. 100 mg daily in divided doses; ELDERLY, 20 mg at night may be adequate

Doralese® (SmithKline Beecham) PoM
Tablets, yellow, f/c, indoramin 20 mg, net price 60-tab pack = £12.30. Label: 2

PRAZOSIN HYDROCHLORIDE

Indications: see notes above and section 2.5.4

Cautions: see notes above and section 2.5.4

Contra-indications: see notes above and section 2.5.4

Side-effects: see notes above and section 2.5.4; paraesthesia, arthralgia, epistaxis, nervousness, dyspnoea, hallucinations, alopecia

Dose: initially 500 micrograms twice daily for 3–7 days, subsequently adjusted according to response; usual maintenance (and max.) 2 mg twice daily; ELDERLY initiate with lowest possible dose

FIRST DOSE EFFECT. First dose may cause collapse due to hypotensive effect (therefore should be taken on retiring to bed). Patient should be warned to lie down if symptoms such as dizziness, fatigue or sweating develop, and to remain lying down until they abate completely

Hypovase® (Pfizer) PoM
Tablets, prazosin hydrochloride 500 micrograms, net price 56-tab pack = £2.09; 1 mg (orange, scored), 56-tab pack = £2.69; 2 mg (scored), 56-tab pack = £3.66; starter pack of 8 × 500-microgram tabs with 32 × 1-mg tabs = £2.52. Label: 3, counselling, see dose above

TAMSULOSIN HYDROCHLORIDE

Indications: see notes above

Cautions: see notes above

Contra-indications: see notes above; severe liver impairment

Side-effects: see notes above

Dose: 400 micrograms daily as a single dose after food

Flomax® MR (Yamanouchi) PoM
Capsules, m/r, tamsulosin hydrochloride 400 micrograms. Net price 30-cap pack = £23.90. Label: 25

TERAZOSIN

Indications: see notes above and section 2.5.4

Cautions: see notes above and section 2.5.4

Contra-indications: see notes above

Side-effects: see notes above and section 2.5.4; weight gain, paraesthesia, dyspnoea, thrombocytopenia, nervousness, decreased libido, back pain and pain in extremities

Dose: initially 1 mg at bedtime; if necessary dose may be doubled at intervals of 1–2 weeks according to response, up to max. 10 mg once daily; usual maintenance 5–10 mg daily

FIRST DOSE EFFECT. First dose may cause collapse due to hypotensive effect (therefore should be taken on retiring to bed). Patient should be warned to lie down if symptoms such as dizziness, fatigue or sweating develop, and to remain lying down until they abate completely

Hytrin BPH® (Abbott) PoM
Tablets, terazosin (as hydrochloride) 2 mg (yellow), net price 28-tab pack = £8.07; 5 mg (tan), 28-tab pack = £13.07; 10 mg (blue), 28-tab pack = £26.59; starter pack of 7 × 1-mg tab with 14 × 2-mg tab and 7 × 5-mg tab = £10.97. Label: 3, counselling, see dose above

Parasympathomimetics

The parasympathomimetics **carbachol** and **bethanechol** increase detrusor muscle contraction. However, they have only a limited role in the relief of urinary retention; the use of both has been superseded by catheterisation.

Distigmine inhibits the breakdown of acetylcholine. It may help patients with an upper motor neurone neurogenic bladder.

CAUTIONS and CONTRA-INDICATIONS. Parasympathomimetics should be used with caution or avoided in hyperthyroidism or in cardiac disorders including bradycardia, arrhythmias and recent myocardial infarction. They are contra-indicated in intestinal or urinary obstruction or where increased motility of the gastro-intestinal or urinary tract could be harmful. Parasympathomimetics should also be avoided in gastro-intestinal ulceration, asthma, hypotension, epilepsy, parkinsonism, pregnancy, and breast-feeding. **Interactions:** Appendix 1 (parasympathomimetics)

SIDE-EFFECTS. Parasympathomimetic side-effects such as nausea, vomiting, intestinal colic, bradycardia, blurred vision, and sweating may occur, particularly in the elderly.

BETHANECHOL CHLORIDE

Indications: urinary retention, but see notes above

Cautions: see notes above

Contra-indications: see notes above

Side-effects: see notes above

Dose: 10–25 mg 3–4 times daily half an hour before food

Myotonine® (Glenwood) PoM
Tablets, both scored, bethanechol chloride 10 mg, net price 20 = £2.80; 25 mg, 20 = £3.00. Label: 22

CARBACHOL

Indications: urinary retention, but see notes above

Cautions: see notes above

Contra-indications: see notes above

Side-effects: see notes above but side-effects more acute than bethanechol chloride

Dose: *by mouth*, 2 mg 3 times daily half an hour before food

By subcutaneous injection (acute symptoms, post-operative urinary retention) 250 micrograms, repeated twice if necessary at 30-minute intervals

Note. Inadvertent intravenous administration of carbachol is **extremely hazardous** and calls for emergency treatment with atropine

Carbachol (Non-proprietary) [PoM] ▰

Tablets, carbachol 2 mg. Net price 20 = £4.36. Label: 22

Available from IVAX

Injection, carbachol 250 micrograms/mL

▰ denotes preparations that are considered to be less suitable for prescribing (see p. vi)

DISTIGMINE BROMIDE

Indications: postoperative urinary retention (see notes above), neurogenic bladder; myasthenia gravis (section 10.2.1)

Cautions: see notes above; also pregnancy (Appendix 4), breast-feeding

Contra-indications: see notes above; also severe postoperative shock, serious circulatory insufficiency

Side-effects: see notes above, but action slower than bethanecol chloride (therefore side-effects less acute; see also Neostigmine (section 10.2.1); also dyspnoea, muscle twitching, and urinary frequency

Dose: urinary retention, 5 mg daily, half an hour before breakfast

Neurogenic bladder, 5 mg daily or on alternate days, half an hour before breakfast

Ubretid® (Rhône-Poulenc Rorer) [PoM]

Tablets, scored, distigmine bromide 5 mg. Net price 30-tab pack = £31.26. Label: 22

| 7.4.2 | **Drugs for urinary frequency, enuresis, and incontinence** |

Urinary incontinence

Antimuscarinic drugs are used to treat *urinary frequency*; they relax the detrusor muscle and increase bladder capacity by diminishing unstable detrusor contractions. **Oxybutynin** also directly relaxes urinary smooth muscle, but has a high level of side-effects which limits its use; the dosage needs to be determined carefully, particularly in the elderly. **Flavoxate** has less marked side-effects but it is also less effective. **Propiverine, tolterodine** and **trospium** are used for urinary frequency, urgency and incontinence. **Propantheline** was formerly widely used in urinary incontinence but had a low response rate and a high incidence of side-effects; it is now used mainly for adult enuresis. The need for continuing antimuscarinic drug therapy should be reviewed after 6 months.

The **tricyclic antidepressants** imipramine, amitriptyline, and nortriptyline (section 4.3.1) are sometimes useful in the management of urge incontinence [unlicensed use], but they are more effective for nocturnal enuresis (see below).

Conservative methods of managing stress and urge incontinence, such as pelvic floor exercises and behavourial therapy, are effective alternatives.

Purified bovine collagen implant (*Contigen®*, Bard) is indicated for *urinary incontinence* caused by intrinsic sphincter deficiency (poor or non-functioning bladder outlet mechanism). The implant should only be used by surgeons or physicians familiar with the use of a cystoscope and trained in the technique for injection of the implant.

CAUTIONS. Antimuscarinic drugs should be used with caution in the elderly (especially if frail) and in those with autonomic neuropathy. They should also be used with caution in hiatus hernia with reflux oesophagitis, and in hepatic impairment (Appendix 2; avoid propiverine) and renal impairment (Appendix 3). Antimuscarinics may worsen hyperthyroidism, coronary artery disease, congestive heart failure, prostatic hypertrophy, arrhythmias and tachycardia. For **interactions** see Appendix 1 (antimuscarinics).

CONTRA-INDICATIONS. Antimuscarinic drugs should be avoided in patients with myasthenia gravis, glaucoma, significant bladder outflow obstruction or urinary retention, severe ulcerative colitis, toxic megacolon, and in gastro-intestinal obstruction or intestinal atony.

SIDE-EFFECTS. Side-effects of antimuscarinic drugs include dry mouth, constipation, blurred vision, drowsiness, nausea, vomiting, abdominal discomfort, difficulty in micturition (less commonly urinary retention), palpitations, and skin reactions (including dry skin, rash, and photosensitivity); also headache, diarrhoea, angioedema, arrhythmias and tachycardia. Central nervous system stimulation, such as restlessness, disorientation, hallucination and convulsion may occur; children are at higher risk of these effects. Antimuscarinic drugs may reduce sweating leading to heat sensation and fainting in hot environments.

FLAVOXATE HYDROCHLORIDE

Indications: urinary frequency and incontinence, dysuria, urgency; bladder spasms due to catheterisation

Cautions: see notes above; pregnancy (Appendix 4), breast-feeding (Appendix 5)

Contra-indications: see notes above; gastro-intestinal haemorrhage

Side-effects: see notes above; also vertigo, fatigue, eosinophilia

Dose: 200 mg 3 times daily; CHILD under 12 years not recommended

Urispas 200® (Shire) [PoM]

Tablets, f/c, flavoxate hydrochloride 200 mg, net price 90-tab pack = £11.87

OXYBUTYNIN HYDROCHLORIDE

Indications: urinary frequency, urgency and incontinence, neurogenic bladder instability and nocturnal enuresis

Cautions: see notes above; pregnancy (Appendix 4), porphyria (section 9.8.2)

Contra-indications: see notes above; breast-feeding (Appendix 5)

Side-effects: see notes above; also anorexia, facial flushing (more marked in children) and dizziness

Dose: initially 2.5–5 mg 2–3 times daily increased if necessary to max. 5 mg 4 times daily
ELDERLY initially 2.5–3 mg twice daily, increased to 5 mg twice daily according to response and tolerance
CHILD over 5 years, neurogenic bladder instability, 2.5–3 mg twice daily increased to 5 mg twice daily (max. 5 mg 3 times daily); nocturnal enuresis (preferably over 7 years, see notes below), 2.5–3 mg twice daily increased to 5 mg 2–3 times daily (last dose before bedtime)

Oxybutynin Hydrochloride (Non-proprietary) PoM
Tablets, oxybutynin hydrochloride 2.5 mg, net price 56-tab pack = £3.53, 84-tab pack = £10.91; 3 mg, 56-tab pack = £7.84; 5 mg, 56-tab pack = £9.67, 84-tab pack = £19.77. Label: 3
Available from Alpharma, APS, Berk (*Contimin®*), Dominion, Generics, IVAX, Lagap, Pharmacia, Sterwin

Cystrin® (Sanofi-Synthelabo) PoM
Tablets, oxybutynin hydrochloride 3 mg, net price 56-tab pack = £9.15; 5 mg (scored), 84-tab pack = £22.88. Label: 3

Ditropan® (Sanofi-Synthelabo) PoM
Tablets, both blue, scored, oxybutynin hydrochloride 2.5 mg, net price 21-tab pack = £2.93, 84-tab pack = £6.86; 5 mg, 21-tab pack = £5.72, 84-tab pack = £13.34. Label: 3
Elixir, oxybutynin hydrochloride 2.5 mg/5 mL. Net price 150-mL pack = £4.78. Label: 3.

■ Modified release
Ditropan® XL (Sanofi-Synthelabo) PoM
Tablets, m/r, oxybutynin hydrochloride 5 mg (yellow), net price 30-tab pack = £9.49; 10 mg (pink), 30-tab pack = £18.98. Label: 3, 25
Dose: ADULT over 18 years, initially 5 mg daily, adjusted according to response in 5-mg steps at weekly intervals; max. 30 mg daily taken as a single dose
Note. Patients taking immediate-release oxybutynin may be transferred to the nearest equivalent daily dose of *Ditropan® XL*

PROPANTHELINE BROMIDE

Indications: adult enuresis

Cautions: see notes above; ulcerative colitis, pregnancy (Appendix 4) and breast-feeding (Appendix 5)

Contra-indications: see notes above

Side-effects: see notes above; also facial flushing

Dose: initially 15 mg 3 times daily at least one hour before food and 30 mg at bedtime, subsequently adjusted according to response (max. 120 mg daily)

Preparations
Section 1.2

PROPIVERINE HYDROCHLORIDE

Indications: urinary frequency, urgency and incontinence; neurogenic bladder instability

Cautions: see notes above

Contra-indications: see notes above; pregnancy (Appendix 4) and breast-feeding (Appendix 5)

Side-effects: see notes above

Dose: 15 mg 1–3 times daily, increased if necessary to max. 15 mg 4 times daily
CHILD not recommended

Detrunorm® (Schering-Plough) PoM
Tablets, pink, s/c, propiverine hydrochloride 15 mg, net price 28-tab pack = £15.28, 56-tab pack = £32.00. Label: 3

TOLTERODINE TARTRATE

Indications: urinary frequency, urgency and incontinence

Cautions: see notes above

Contra-indications: see notes above; pregnancy (Appendix 4) and breast-feeding (Appendix 5)

Side-effects: see notes above; also dyspepsia, flatulence, dry eyes, paraesthesia and, less commonly, chest pain

Dose: 2 mg twice daily; reduce to 1mg twice daily if necessary to minimise side-effects
CHILD not recommended

Detrusitol® (Pharmacia) PoM
Tablets, f/c, tolterodine tartrate 1 mg, net price 56-tab pack = £27.50; 2mg, 56-tab pack = £30.56

■ Modified release
Detrusitol® XL (Pharmacia) PoM
Capsules, blue, m/r, tolterodine tartrate 4 mg, net price 28-cap pack = £29.03. Label: 25
Dose: 4 mg once daily (dose form not appropriate for hepatic and renal impairment)

TROSPIUM CHLORIDE

Indications: urinary frequency, urgency and incontinence

Cautions: see notes above; pregnancy and breast-feeding

Contra-indications: see notes above

Side-effects: see notes above; also flatulence, chest pain, dyspnoea, rash and asthenia

Dose: 20 mg twice daily before food
CHILD not recommended

Regurin® (Galen) ▼ PoM
Tablets, brown, f/c, trospium chloride 20 mg, net price 60-tab pack = £25.00. Label 23

Nocturnal enuresis

Nocturnal enuresis is a normal occurrence in young children but persists in as many as 5% by 10 years of age. Treatment is not usually needed in those aged under 7 years and in cases where the child and parents are not anxious about the bedwetting; however, children over 10 years usually require prompt treatment. An **enuresis alarm** should be first-line treatment for well-motivated children aged over 7 years, use of an alarm may be combined with drug therapy if either method alone is unsuccessful.

Drug therapy is not usually appropriate for children under 7 years of age and should be reserved for when alternative measures have failed preferably on a short-term basis to cover periods away from home. The possible side-effects of the various drugs should be borne in mind when they are prescribed.

Desmopressin (section 6.5.2), an analogue of vasopressin, is used for nocturnal enuresis; it is best given intranasally but when this route is not appropriate, desmopressin may be given by mouth as tablets. Particular care is needed to avoid fluid overload and treatment should not be continued for longer than 3 months without stopping for a week for full re-assessment.

Tricyclics (section 4.3.1) such as **amitriptyline**, **imipramine**, and less often **nortriptyline** are also used but behaviour disturbances may occur and relapse is common after withdrawal. Treatment should not normally exceed 3 months unless a full physical examination is given and the child is fully re-assessed; toxicity following overdosage with tricyclics is of particular concern.

7.4.3 Drugs used in urological pain

The acute pain of *ureteric colic* may be relieved with **pethidine** (section 4.7.2). **Diclofenac** by injection or as suppositories (section 10.1.1) is also effective and compares favourably with pethidine; other non-steroidal anti-inflammatory drugs are occasionally given by injection.

Lidocaine (lignocaine) gel is a useful topical application in *urethral pain* or to relieve the discomfort of catheterisation (section 15.2).

Alkalinisation of urine

Alkalinisation of urine may be undertaken with **potassium citrate**. The alkalinising action may relieve the discomfort of *cystitis* caused by lower urinary tract infections. **Sodium bicarbonate** is used as a urinary alkalinising agent in some metabolic and renal disorders (section 9.2.1.3).

POTASSIUM CITRATE

Indications: relief of discomfort in mild urinary-tract infections; alkalinisation of urine

Cautions: renal impairment; cardiac disease; elderly; **interactions:** Appendix 1 (potassium salts)

Side-effects: hyperkalaemia on prolonged high dosage, mild diuresis

Potassium Citrate Mixture BP
(Potassium Citrate Oral Solution)
Oral solution, potassium citrate 30%, citric acid monohydrate 5% in a suitable vehicle with a lemon flavour. Extemporaneous preparations should be recently prepared according to the following formula: potassium citrate 3 g, citric acid monohydrate 500 mg, syrup 2.5 mL, quillaia tinc-

ture 0.1 mL, lemon spirit 0.05 mL, double-strength chloroform water 3 mL, water to 10 mL. Contains about 28 mmol K+/10 mL. Label: 27
Dose: 10 mL 3 times daily well diluted with water
Note. Concentrates for preparation of Potassium Citrate Mixture BP are available from Hillcross
Proprietary brands of potassium citrate on sale to the public for the relief of discomfort in mild urinary-tract infections include *Cystopurin®* (Roche Consumer Health) and *Effercitrate®* (Typharm)

SODIUM BICARBONATE

Indications: relief of discomfort in mild urinary-tract infections; alkalinisation of urine

Cautions: hepatic and renal impairment, cardiac disease, pregnancy; patients on sodium-restricted diet; elderly; avoid prolonged use; **interactions:** Appendix 1 (antacids)

Side-effects: belching, alkalosis on prolonged use

Dose: 3 g in water every 2 hours until urinary pH exceeds 7; maintenance of alkaline urine 5–10 g daily

Preparations
Section 9.2.1.3

SODIUM CITRATE

Indications: relief of discomfort in mild urinary-tract infections

Cautions: renal impairment, cardiac disease, hypertension, pregnancy, patients on a sodium-restricted diet; elderly

Side-effects: mild diuresis

Note. Proprietary brands of sodium citrate on sale to the public for the relief of discomfort in mild urinary-tract infections include *Boots Cystitis Relief Sachets* and *Tablets, Canesten® Oasis* (Bayer), *Cymalon®* (SSL), and *Cystemme®* (Abbott)

Acidification of urine

Urine acidification is difficult; it is very occasionally used in the management of recurrent urinary-tract infections and to prevent renal stone formation, especially in patients with paraplegia or with a neurogenic bladder. Methenamine (section 5.1.13) requires acid urine for its antimicrobial activity.

Ammonium chloride may be used for urinary acidification but tolerance can develop rapidly. Vomiting and, with large doses, hypokalaemia and acidosis can also occur. Ammonium chloride oral solution needs to be prepared extemporaneously and may not be readily available. **Ascorbic acid** is less suitable for urine acidification because it is not always reliable and high doses, which can lead to renal stones in those with hyperoxaluria, are required.

For pH-modifying solutions for the maintenance of indwelling urinary catheters, see section 7.4.4.

Other preparations for urinary disorders

A terpene mixture (Rowatinex®) is claimed to be of benefit in *urolithiasis* for the expulsion of calculi.

Rowatinex® (Rowa) [PoM] [⬛]
Capsules, yellow, e/c, anethol 4 mg, borneol 10 mg, camphene 15 mg, cineole 3 mg, fenchone 4 mg, pinene 31 mg. Net price 50 = £7.35. Label: 25
Dose: 1–2 capsules 3–4 times daily before food; CHILD not recommended

▰ denotes preparations that are considered to be less suitable for prescribing (see p. vi)

7.4.4   Bladder installations and urological surgery

BLADDER INFECTION. Various solutions are available as irrigations or washouts.

Aqueous **chlorhexidine** (section 13.11.2) may be used in the management of common infections of the bladder but it is ineffective against most *Pseudomonas* spp. Solutions containing chlorhexidine 1 in 5000 (0.02%) are used but they may irritate the mucosa and cause burning and haematuria (in which case they should be discontinued); sterile **sodium chloride solution 0.9%** (physiological saline) is usually adequate and is preferred as a mechanical irrigant.

Continuous bladder irrigation with **amphotericin** 50 micrograms/mL (section 5.2) may be of value in mycotic infections.

DISSOLUTION OF BLOOD CLOTS. Clot retention is usually treated by irrigation with sterile **sodium chloride solution 0.9%** but sterile **sodium citrate solution for bladder irrigation 3%** may also be helpful. **Streptokinase-streptodornase** (*Varidase Topical®*, section 13.11.7) is an alternative.

BLADDER CANCER. Bladder installations of **doxorubicin** (section 8.1.2), **mitomycin** (section 8.1.2), and **thiotepa** (section 8.1.1) are used for recurrent superficial bladder tumours. Such installations reduce systemic side-effects; adverse effects on the bladder (e.g. micturition disorders and reduction in bladder capacity) may occur.

Installation of **epirubicin** (section 8.1.2) is used for treatment and prophylaxis of certain forms of superficial bladder cancer; installation of **doxorubicin** (section 8.1.2) is also used for some papillary tumours.

Installation of **BCG** (Bacillus Calmette-Guérin), a live attenuated strain derived from *Mycobacterium bovis* (section 8.2.4), has been licensed for the treatment of primary or recurrent bladder carcinoma *in situ* and for the prevention of recurrence following transurethral resection.

INTERSTITIAL CYSTITIS. **Dimethyl sulfoxide** (dimethyl sulphoxide) may be used for symptomatic relief in patients with interstitial cystitis (Hunner's ulcer). 50 mL of a 50% solution (*Rimso-50®*—available on named-patient basis from Britannia) is instilled into the bladder, retained for 15 minutes, and voided by the patient. Treatment is repeated at intervals of 2 weeks. Bladder spasm and hypersensitivity reactions may occur and long-term use requires ophthalmic, renal, and hepatic assessment at intervals of 6 months.

SODIUM CITRATE

Indications: bladder washouts, see notes above

Sterile Sodium Citrate Solution for Bladder Irrigation, sodium citrate 3%, dilute hydrochloric acid 0.2%, in purified water, freshly boiled and cooled, and sterilised

Urological surgery

There is a high risk of fluid absorption from the irrigant used in endoscopic surgery within the urinary tract; if this occurs in excess, hypervolaemia, haemolysis, and renal failure may result. **Glycine irrigation solution 1.5%** is the irrigant of choice for transurethral resection of the prostate gland and bladder tumours; **sterile sodium chloride solution 0.9%** (physiological saline) is used for percutaneous renal surgery.

GLYCINE

Indications: bladder irrigation during urological surgery; see notes above

Cautions: see notes above

Side-effects: see notes above

Glycine Irrigation Solution (Non-proprietary)
Irrigation solution, glycine 1.5% in water for injections
Available from Baxter

Maintenance of indwelling urinary catheters

The deposition which occurs in catheterised patients is usually chiefly composed of phosphate and to minimise this the catheter (if latex) should be changed at least as often as every 6 weeks. If the catheter is to be left for longer periods a silicone catheter should be used together with the appropriate use of catheter maintenance solutions. Repeated blockage usually indicates that the catheter needs to be changed.

CATHETER PATENCY SOLUTIONS

Chlorhexidine 0.02%. Available from Braun (*Uro-Tainer Chlorhexidine®*, 100-mL sachet = £2.60), SSL (*Uriflex C®*, 100-mL sachet = £2.40)

Mandelic acid 1% Available from Braun (*Uro-Tainer Mandelic Acid®*, 100-mL sachet = £2.60)

Sodium chloride 0.9%. Available from Braun (*Uro-Tainer Sodium Chloride®*, 50- and 100-mL sachets = £2.45, *Uro-Tainer M®*, with integral drug additive port, 50- and 100-mL sachets = £2.90), SSL (*Uriflex S®*, 100-mL sachet = £2.40, *Uriflex SP®* with integral drug additive port, 100-mL sachet = £2.24)

Solution G, citric acid 3.23%, magnesium oxide 0.38%, sodium bicarbonate 0.7%, disodium edetate 0.01%. Available from Braun (*Uro-Tainer Suby G®*, 50- and 100-mL sachets = £2.60), SSL (*Uriflex G®*, 100-mL sachet = £2.40)

Solution R, citric acid 6%, gluconolactone 0.6%, magnesium carbonate 2.8%, disodium edetate 0.01%. Available from Braun (*Uro-Tainer Solution R®*, 50- and 100-mL sachets = £2.60), SSL (*Uriflex R®*, 100-mL sachet = £2.40)

Drugs for erectile dysfunction

Reasons for failure to produce a satisfactory erection include *psychogenic, vascular, neurogenic,* and *endocrine abnormalities*; impotence can also be drug-induced. Intracavernosal injection or urethral application of vasoactive drugs under careful medical supervision is used for both diagnostic and therapeutic purposes.

Erectile disorders may also be treated with drugs given by mouth which increase the blood flow to the penis. Drugs should be used with caution if the penis is deformed (e.g. in angulation, cavernosal fibrosis, and Peyronie's disease).

Drug treatments for erectile dysfunction may only be prescribed on the NHS under certain circumstances (see individual preparations). The Department of Health (England) has recommended that treatment should also be available from specialist services (commissioned by Health Authorities and Primary Care Groups, and operating under local agreement) when the condition is causing severe distress; specialist centres should use form FP10(HP) (or form HBP in Scotland) and endorse them 'SLS' if the treatment is to be dispensed in the community. The following criteria should be considered when assessing distress:

* significant disruption to normal social and occupational activities;

* a marked effect on mood, behaviour, social and environmental awareness;

* a marked effect on interpersonal relationships.

Alprostadil

Alprostadil (prostaglandin E_1) is given by intracavernosal injection or intraurethral application for the management of erectile dysfunction (after exclusion of treatable medical causes); it is also used as a diagnostic test.

ALPROSTADIL

Indications: erectile dysfunction (including aid to diagnosis); neonatal congenital heart defects (section 7.1.1.1)

Cautions: priapism—patients should be instructed to report any erection lasting 4 hours or longer—for recommendations, see below; anatomical deformations of penis (painful erection more likely)—follow up regularly to detect signs of penile fibrosis (consider discontinuation if angulation, cavernosal fibrosis or Peyronie's disease develop); **interactions:** Appendix 1 (alprostadil)

Contra-indications: predisposition to prolonged erection (as in sickle cell anaemia, multiple myeloma or leukaemia); not for use with other agents for erectile dysfunction, in patients with penile implants or when sexual activity medically inadvisable; urethral application also contra-indicated in urethral stricture, severe hypospadia, severe curvature, balanitis, urethritis

Side-effects: penile pain, priapism (see below and under Cautions); reactions at injection site include haematoma, haemosiderin deposits, penile rash, penile oedema, penile fibrosis, haemorrhage, inflammation; other local reactions include urethral burning and bleeding, penile warmth, numbness, penile or urinary-tract infection, irritation, sensitivity, phimosis, pruritus, erythema, venous leak, abnormal ejaculation; systemic effects reported include testicular pain and swelling, scrotal disorders, changes in micturition (including haematuria), nausea, dry mouth, fainting, hypotension (very rarely circulatory collapse) or hypertension, rapid pulse, vasodilatation, chest pain, supraventricular extrasystole, peripheral vascular disorder, dizziness, weakness, localised pain (buttocks, legs, genital, perineal, abdominal), headache, pelvic pain, back pain, influenza-like syndrome, swelling of the leg veins
PRIAPISM. If priapism should occur treatment should not be delayed more than 6 hours and is as follows:
Initial therapy by penile aspiration—using aseptic technique a 19–21 gauge butterfly needle inserted into the corpus cavernosum and 20–50 mL of blood aspirated; if necessary the procedure may be repeated on the opposite side.
If aspiration unsuccessful, *cautious* intracavernosal injection of a sympathomimetic with action on alpha-adrenergic receptors, continuously monitoring blood pressure and pulse (*extreme caution:* coronary heart disease, hypertension, cerebral ischaemia or if taking antidepressant) as follows:

* intracavernosal injections of phenylephrine 100–200 micrograms (0.5–1 mL of a 200 microgram/mL solution) every 5–10 minutes; max. total dose 1 mg [unlicensed indication] [*important:* if suitable strength of phenylephrine injection not available may be specially prepared by diluting 0.1 mL of the phenylephrine 1% (10 mg/mL) injection to 5 mL with sodium chloride 0.9%];
alternatively

* intracavernosal injections of adrenaline 10–20 micrograms (0.5–1 mL of a 20 microgram/mL solution) every 5–10 minutes; max. total dose 100 micrograms [*important:* if suitable strength of adrenaline not available may be specially prepared by diluting 0.1 mL of the adrenaline 1 in 1000 (1 mg/mL) injection to 5 mL with sodium chloride 0.9%];
alternatively

* intracavernosal injection of metaraminol (*caution: has been associated with fatal hypertensive crises*); metaraminol 1 mg (0.1 mL of 10 mg/mL metaraminol injection) is diluted to 50 mL with sodium chloride injection 0.9% and given carefully by slow injection into the corpora in 5-mL injections every 15 minutes [unlicensed indication].
If necessary the sympathomimetic injections can be followed by further aspiration of blood through the same butterfly needle.
If sympathomimetics unsuccessful, urgent surgical referral for management (possibly including shunt procedure).

Dose: see under preparations below

■ Intracavernosal injection

¹Caverject® (Pharmacia) ⓃⒽⓈ ⒫Ⓞⓜ
Injection, powder for reconstitution, alprostadil, net price 5-microgram vial = £6.44; 10-microgram vial = £7.70; 20-microgram vial = £9.50; 40-microgram vial = £17.98 (all with diluent-filled syringe, needles and swabs)
Caverject® Dual Chamber, double-chamber cartridges (containing alprostadil and diluent), net

price 10-microgram cartridge (for doses 2.5–10 micrograms) = £7.35; 20-microgram cartridge (for doses 5–20 micrograms) = £9.50 (both with needles)

Dose: by direct intracavernosal injection, erectile dysfunction, first dose 2.5 micrograms, second dose 5 micrograms (if some response to first dose) *or* 7.5 micrograms (if no response to first dose), increasing in steps of 5–10 micrograms to obtain dose suitable for producing erection not lasting more than 1 hour (neurological dysfunction, first dose 1.25 micrograms, second dose 2.5 micrograms, third dose 5 micrograms, increasing in steps of 5 micrograms to obtain suitable dose); if no response to dose then next higher dose can be given within 1 hour, if there is a response the next dose should not be given for at least 24 hours; usual range 5–20 micrograms; max. 60 micrograms (max. frequency of injection not more than once daily and not more than 3 times in any 1 week)

Note. The first dose must be given by medically trained personnel; self-administration may only be undertaken after proper training

Aid to diagnosis, 20 micrograms as a single dose (where evidence of neurological dysfunction, initially 5 micrograms and max. 10 micrograms)—consult product literature for details

¹**Viridal® Duo** (Schwarz) ⓃⒽⓈ PoM

Starter Pack (hosp. only), contents as for *Continuation Pack* below plus *Duoject* applicator, 10-microgram starter pack = £21.65, 20-microgram starter pack = £26.39, 40-microgram starter pack = £32.08; *Continuation Pack*, 2 double-chamber cartridges (containing alprostadil and diluent), 2 needles, swabs, 10-microgram continuation pack = £16.18, 20-microgram continuation pack = £20.91, 40-microgram continuation pack = £26.61; *Duoject®* applicator available free of charge from Schwarz

Dose: by direct intracavernosal injection, erectile dysfunction, initially 2.5 micrograms (1.25 micrograms in neurogenic erectile dysfunction) increasing in steps of 2.5–5 micrograms to obtain dose suitable for producing erection not lasting more than 1 hour; usual range 10–20 micrograms; max. 40 micrograms (max. frequency of injection not more than 2–3 times per week with at least 24-hour interval between injections); erection lasting longer than 2 hours—re-titrate dose; patient should report to doctor erection lasting longer than 4 hours

Note. The first dose must be given by medically trained personnel; self-administration may only be undertaken after proper training

■ Urethral application

COUNSELLING. If partner pregnant barrier contraception should be used

¹**MUSE®** (Abbott) ⓃⒽⓈ PoM

Urethral application, alprostadil, net price 125-microgram single-use applicator = £9.60, 250-microgram single-use applicator = £10.45, 500-microgram single-use applicator = £10.45, 1-mg single-use applicator = £10.69 (all strengths also available in packs of 6 applicators)

Condoms: no evidence of harm to latex condoms and diaphragms

Dose: by direct urethral application, erectile dysfunction, initially 250 micrograms adjusted according to response (usual range 0.125–1 mg); max. 2 doses in 24 hours and 7 doses in 7 days)

Note. The first dose must be given by medically trained personnel; self-administration may only be undertaken after proper training

Aid to diagnosis, 500 micrograms as a single dose

Apomorphine

Apomorphine has been introduced recently for the treatment of erectile dysfunction; it is given as sublingual tablets. Compared to subcutaneous injection, absorption from the sublingual site is limited; vasovagal symptoms (including sweating and syncope) can occur infrequently.

APOMORPHINE HYDROCHLORIDE

Indications: erectile dysfunction; Parkinson's disease (section 4.9.1)

Cautions: hepatic impairment (Appendix 2), renal impairment (Appendix 3); uncontrolled hypertension, hypotension; elderly; anatomical deformation of penis (e.g. angulation, cavernosal fibrosis, Peyronie's disease); not recommended for use in combination with other treatments for erectile dysfunction; **interactions:** Appendix 1 (apomorphine)

DRIVING. May impair performance of skilled tasks (e.g. driving)

Contra-indications: recent myocardial infarction; severe unstable angina, severe heart failure or hypotension; conditions where sexual activity is medically inadvisable

Side-effects: nausea, headache, dizziness, yawning, drowsiness, rhinitis, pharyngitis, cough, flushing, taste disturbance, sweating; rarely transient vasovagal syndrome

Dose: *by sublingual administration*, initially 2 mg approx. 20 minutes before sexual activity, subsequent doses may be increased to 3 mg if necessary; minimum of 8 hours between doses

Uprima® (Abbott) ▼ PoM

Sublingual tablets, both red, apomorphine hydrochloride 2 mg, net price 2-tab pack = £8.20, 4-tab pack = £16.40; 3 mg, 2-tab pack = £9.70, 4-tab pack = £19.40. Counselling, driving

Sildenafil

Sildenafil, is licensed for the treatment of erectile dysfunction; it is given by mouth. Appropriate assessment should be carried out before prescribing sildenafil. Since sildenafil is administered systemically it has a potential for drug interactions; it should be **not** be used in those receiving nitrates.

SILDENAFIL

Indications: erectile dysfunction

Cautions: cardiovascular disease; anatomical deformation of penis (e.g. angulation, cavernosal fibrosis, Peyronie's disease); predisposition to prolonged erection (as in sickle-cell anaemia, multiple myeloma, leukaemia); hepatic impairment (Appendix 2—avoid if severe); renal impairment (Appendix 3); not recommended for use in combination with other treatments for erectile dysfunction; **interactions:** Appendix 1 (sildenafil)

Contra-indications: treatment with nitrates; conditions in which vasodilation or sexual activity inadvisable; manufacturer advises contra-indicated in recent stroke or myocardial infarction, blood pressure below 90/50 mmHg and hereditary degenerative retinal disorders

Side-effects: dyspepsia, vomiting; headache, flushing, dizziness, visual disturbances and increased intra-ocular pressure, nasal congestion; hypersensitivity reactions (including rash), priapism and painful, red eyes reported; serious cardiovascular events also reported

Dose: initially 50 mg (ELDERLY 25 mg) approx. 1 hour before sexual activity, subsequent doses adjusted according to response to 25–100 mg as a single dose as needed; max. 1 dose in 24 hours (max. single dose 100 mg)

Note. Onset of effect may be delayed if taken with food

¹**Viagra**® (Pfizer) ⃞NHS⃞ ⃞PoM⃞
Tablets, all blue, f/c, sildenafil (as citrate), 25 mg, net price 4-tab pack = £16.59, 8-tab pack = £33.19; 50 mg, 4-tab pack = £19.34, 8-tab pack = £38.67; 100 mg, 4-tab pack = £23.50, 8-tab pack = £46.99

1. ⃞NHS⃞ except to treat erectile dysfunction in men who:
   - have diabetes, multiple sclerosis, Parkinson's disease, poliomyelitis, prostate cancer, severe pelvic injury, single gene neurological disease, spina bifida or spinal cord injury;
   - are receiving dialysis for renal failure;
   - have had radical pelvic surgery, prostatectomy, or kidney transplant;
   - were receiving *Caverject*®, *Erecnos*®, *MUSE*®, *Viagra*® or *Viridal*® for erectile dysfunction, at the expense of the NHS, on 14 September 1998;
   - are suffering severe distress as a result of impotence (prescribed by specialist centres only, see notes above.

   The prescription must be endorsed 'SLS'.

Papaverine and phentolamine

Although not licensed the smooth muscle relaxant **papaverine** has also been given by intracavernosal injection for erectile dysfunction. Patients with neurological or psychogenic impotence are more sensitive to the effect of papaverine than those with vascular abnormalities. **Phentolamine** is added if the response is inadequate [unlicensed indication].

Persistence of the erection for longer than 4 hours is an emergency, see advice under Alprostadil, above.

8: Malignant disease and immunosuppression

Malignant disease may be treated by surgery, radiotherapy, and chemotherapy. Certain tumours are highly sensitive to chemotherapy but many are not, and inappropriate drug administration in these circumstances can only increase morbidity or mortality.

8.1   Cytotoxic drugs

8.1.1   Alkylating drugs
8.1.2   Cytotoxic antibiotics
8.1.3   Antimetabolites
8.1.4   Vinca alkaloids and etoposide
8.1.5   Other antineoplastic drugs

The chemotherapy of cancer is complex and should be confined to specialists in oncology. Cytotoxic drugs have both anti-cancer activity and the potential for damage to normal tissue. Chemotherapy may be given with a curative intent or it may aim to prolong life or to palliate symptoms. In an increasing number of cases chemotherapy may be combined with radiotherapy or surgery or both as either neoadjuvant treatment (initial chemotherapy aimed at shrinking the primary tumour, thereby rendering local therapy less destructive or more effective) or as adjuvant treatment (which follows definitive treatment of the primary disease, when the risk of sub-clinical metastatic disease is known to be high). All chemotherapy drugs cause side-effects and a balance has to be struck between likely benefit and acceptable toxicity.

CRM guidelines on handling cytotoxic drugs:

1. Trained personnel should reconstitute cytotoxics;

2. Reconstitution should be carried out in designated areas;

3. Protective clothing (including gloves) should be worn;

4. The eyes should be protected and means of first aid should be specified;

5. Pregnant staff should not handle cytotoxics;

6. Adequate care should be taken in the disposal of waste material, including syringes, containers, and absorbent material.

Intrathecal chemotherapy
A Health Service Circular (HSC 2001/022) provides guidance on the introduction of safe practice in those NHS Trusts where intrathecal chemotherapy is administered.
Copies may be obtained from:
Department of Health
PO Box 777
London SE1 6XH
Fax 01623 724524
www.doh.gov.uk/publications/coinh.html

Cytotoxic drugs may be used either singly, or in combination. In the latter case, the initial letters of the approved or proprietary names of the drugs, identify the regimen used. Drug combinations are frequently more toxic than single drugs but may have the advantage in certain tumours of enhanced response, reduced development of drug resistance and increased survival. However for some tumours, single-agent chemotherapy remains the treatment of choice.

> Most cytotoxic drugs are teratogenic, and all may cause life-threatening toxicity; administration should, where possible, be confined to those experienced in their use.
>
> Because of the complexity of dosage regimens in the treatment of malignant disease, dose statements have been omitted from some of the drug entries in this chapter. *In all cases detailed specialist literature should be consulted.*
>
> Prescriptions should **not** be repeated except on the instructions of a specialist.

Cytotoxic drugs fall naturally into a number of classes, each with characteristic antitumour activity, sites of action, and toxicity. A knowledge of sites of metabolism and excretion is important because impaired drug handling as a result of disease is not uncommon and may result in enhanced toxicity.

Side-effects of cytotoxic drugs

Side-effects commonly encountered with cytotoxic drugs are discussed below whilst side-effects characteristic of a particular drug or class of drugs (e.g. neurotoxicity with vinca alkaloids) are described in the appropriate sections. Manufacturers' product literature should be consulted for full details of side-effects associated with individual drugs.

EXTRAVASATION OF INTRAVENOUS DRUGS. A number of cytotoxic drugs will cause severe local tissue necrosis if leakage into the extravascular compartment occurs. To reduce the risk of extravasation injury it is recommended that cytotoxic drugs are administered by appropriately trained staff. For information on the prevention and management of extravasation injury see section 10.3.

HYPERURICAEMIA. Hyperuricaemia, which can result in uric acid crystal formation in the urinary tract with associated renal dysfunction is a complication of the treatment of non-Hodgkin's lymphoma and leukaemia. Allopurinol (section 10.1.4) should be started 24 hours before treating such tumours; patients should be adequately hydrated. The dose of mercaptopurine or azathioprine should be reduced if allopurinol needs to be given concomitantly (see Appendix 1).

Rasburicase (section 10.1.4) is a recombinant urate oxidase, which has been licensed recently for hyperuricaemia in patients with haematological malignancy, for details, see p. 494.

NAUSEA AND VOMITING. Nausea and vomiting cause considerable distress to many patients who receive chemotherapy, and to a lesser extent abdo-

minal radiotherapy, and may lead to refusal of further treatment. Symptoms may be acute (occurring within 24 hours of treatment), delayed (first occurring more than 24 hours after treatment) or anticipatory (occurring prior to subsequent doses). Delayed and anticipatory symptoms are more difficult to control than acute symptoms and require different management.

Patients vary in their susceptibility to drug-induced nausea and vomiting; those affected more often include women, patients under 50 years of age, anxious patients, and those who experience motion sickness. Susceptibility also increases with repeated exposure to the drug.

Drugs may be divided according to their emetogenic potential and some examples are given below, but the symptoms vary according to the dose, to other drugs administered and to individual susceptibility.

Mildly emetogenic treatment—fluorouracil, etoposide, methotrexate (less than $100 \, mg/m^2$), the vinca alkaloids, and abdominal radiotherapy.

Moderately emetogenic treatment—doxorubicin, intermediate and low doses of cyclophosphamide, mitoxantrone (mitozantrone), and high doses of methotrexate ($0.1–1.2 \, g/m^2$).

Highly emetogenic treatment—cisplatin, dacarbazine, and high doses of cyclophosphamide.

Prevention of acute symptoms. For patients at a low risk of emesis, pretreatment with oral phenothiazines (e.g. prochlorperazine) or with domperidone, continued for up to 24 hours after chemotherapy, is often effective (section 4.6). For patients at a higher risk dexamethasone (6–10 mg by mouth) alone or with lorazepam (1–2 mg by mouth) may be added prior to chemotherapy.

For patients at a high risk of emesis or when other therapies are ineffective, a specific ($5HT_3$) serotonin antagonist (section 4.6) is used, often with dexamethasone. The $5HT_3$ antagonists are highly effective in controlling early emesis and have largely replaced the use of high-dose intravenous metoclopramide (section 4.6).

Prevention of delayed symptoms. Dexamethasone is the drug of choice for the prevention of delayed symptoms; it is used alone or with metoclopramide or prochlorperazine. The $5HT_3$ antagonists may be less effective for delayed symptoms.

Prevention of anticipatory symptoms. Good symptom control is the best way to prevent anticipatory symptoms. The addition of lorazepam to antiemetic therapy is helpful because of its amnesic, sedative and anxiolytic effects.

BONE-MARROW SUPPRESSION. All cytotoxic drugs except vincristine and bleomycin cause bone-marrow depression. This commonly occurs 7 to 10 days after administration, but is delayed for certain drugs, such as carmustine, lomustine, and melphalan. Peripheral blood counts must be checked before each treatment, and doses should be reduced or therapy delayed if bone-marrow has not recovered. Fever in a neutropenic patient (neutrophil count less than $1.0 \times 10^9/litre$) requires immediate broad-spectrum antibacterial therapy. Patients at low risk (those receiving chemotherapy for solid tumours, lymphoma or chronic leukaemia) can be treated with oral ciprofloxacin with or without co-amoxiclav (initially in hospital). All other patients should receive parenteral broad-spectrum antibacterial therapy. Appropriate bacteriological investigations should be conducted as soon as possible.

It is now possible, in selected patients, to lessen both the duration and the severity of neutropenia by the use of parenterally administered bone marrow growth factors known as colony stimulating factors (section 9.1.6) or (in patients with ovarian carcinoma receiving cisplatin and cyclophosphamide) by the use of amifostine (see p. 408).

ALOPECIA. Reversible hair loss is a common complication, although it varies in degree between drugs and individual patients. No pharmacological methods of preventing this are available.

REPRODUCTIVE FUNCTION. Most cytotoxic drugs are teratogenic and should not be administered during pregnancy, especially during the first trimester.

Contraceptive advice should be offered where appropriate before cytotoxic therapy begins (and should cover the duration of contraception required after therapy has ended). Regimens that do not contain an alkylating drug may have less effect on fertility, but those with an alkylating drug carry the risk of causing permanent male sterility (there is no effect on potency). Pre-treatment counselling and consideration of sperm storage may be appropriate. Women are less severely affected, though the span of reproductive life may be shortened by the onset of a premature menopause. No increase in fetal abnormalities or abortion-rate has been recorded in patients who remain fertile after cytotoxic chemotherapy.

Drugs for cytotoxic-induced side-effects

Methotrexate-induced mucositis and myelosuppression

Folinic acid (given as calcium folinate) is used to counteract the folate-antagonist action of methotrexate and thus speed recovery from methotrexate-induced mucositis or myelosuppression. It is generally given 24 hours after the methotrexate, in a dose of 15 mg by mouth every 6 hours, for 2–8 doses (depending on the dose of methotrexate). It does not counteract the antibacterial activity of folate antagonists such as trimethoprim.

When folinic acid and fluorouracil are used together in metastatic colorectal cancer the response-rate improves compared to that with fluorouracil alone.

The calcium salt of **levofolinic acid**, a single isomer of folinic acid, is also used for rescue therapy following methotrexate administration and for use with fluorouracil for colorectal cancer. The dose of calcium levofolinate is generally half that of calcium folinate.

The disodium salt of folinic acid is also licensed for rescue therapy following methotrexate therapy and for use with fluorouracil for colorectal cancer.

CALCIUM FOLINATE

(Calcium leucovorin)

Indications: see notes above

Cautions: avoid simultaneous administration of methotrexate; **not** indicated for pernicious anaemia or other megaloblastic anaemias due to vitamin B_{12} deficiency; pregnancy and breast-feeding; **interactions:** Appendix 1 (folic acid and folinic acid)

IMPORTANT. Intrathecal injection **contra-indicated**

Side-effects: hypersensitivity reactions; rarely pyrexia after parenteral use

Dose: expressed in terms of folinic acid

As an antidote to methotrexate (usually started 24 hours after the beginning of methotrexate infusion), usually up to 120 mg in divided doses over 12–24 hours *by intramuscular or intravenous injection or by intravenous infusion*, followed by 12–15 mg *intramuscularly or* 15 mg *by mouth* every 6 hours for the next 48–72 hours

Suspected methotrexate overdosage, immediate administration of folinic acid at a rate not exceeding 160 mg/minute in a dose equal to (or higher than) the dose of methotrexate

Adjunct to fluorouracil in colorectal cancer, consult product literature

Calcium Folinate (Non-proprietary) PoM

Tablets, scored, folinic acid (as calcium salt) 15 mg, net price 10-tab pack (Faulding DBL) = £37.85, (Hillcross) = £40.95, (Lederle) = £41.22, 30-tab pack (Pharmacia, *Refolinon®*) = £90.25

Injection, folinic acid (as calcium salt) 3 mg/mL, net price 1-mL amp (Faulding DBL) = £2.28, 10-mL amp (Pharmacia, *Refolinon®*) = £5.44

Injection, folinic acid (as calcium salt) 7.5 mg/mL, net price 2-mL amp (Faulding DBL) = £7.80

Injection, folinic acid (as calcium salt) 10 mg/mL, net price 5-mL vial (Faulding DBL) = £19.41, 10-mL vial (Faulding DBL) = £35.09, 30-mL vial (Faulding DBL) = £94.69, 35-mL vial (Lederle, *Lederfolin®*) = £90.98

Injection, powder for reconstitution, folinic acid (as calcium salt), net price 15-mg vial (Lederle) = £4.46; 30-mg vial (Lederle) = £8.36

CALCIUM LEVOFOLINATE

(Calcium levoleucovorin)

Indications: see notes above

Cautions: see Calcium Folinate

Side-effects: see Calcium Folinate

Dose: expressed in terms of levofolinic acid

As an antidote to methotrexate (usually started 24 hours after the beginning of methotrexate infusion), usually 7.5 mg, *by intramuscular injection, or by intravenous injection or by intravenous infusion* every 6 hours for 10 doses

Suspected methotrexate overdosage, immediate administration of levofolinic acid at a rate not exceeding 160 mg/minute in a dose which is at least 50% of the dose of methotrexate

Adjunct to fluorouracil in colorectal cancer, consult product literature

Isovorin® (Wyeth) ▼ |PoM|

Injection, levofolinic acid (as calcium salt) 10 mg/mL, net price 2.5-mL vial = £13.00, 5-mL vial = £26.00, 17.5-mL vial = £91.00

DISODIUM FOLINATE

Indications: see notes above
Cautions: see Calcium Folinate
Side-effects: see Calcium Folinate
Dose: as an antidote to methotrexate, see Calcium Folinate

Adjunct to fluorouracil in colorectal cancer, consult product literature

Sodiofolin® (Medac) |PoM|

Injection, folinic acid (as disodium salt) 50 mg/mL, net price 2-mL vial = £35.09, 8-mL vial = £126.25, 18-mL vial = £284.07

Platinum-induced neutropenic infection and nephrotoxicity

Amifostine is licensed for the reduction of risk of infection associated with the development of neutropenia induced by cisplatin and cyclophosphamide in advanced ovarian carcinoma, and for the reduction of nephrotoxicity caused by cisplatin. Amifostine is also licensed for protection against xerostomia during radiotherapy for head and neck cancer.

Other drugs for the reduction of risk of infection associated with neutropenia include granulocyte-colony stimulating factor and granulocyte macrophage-colony stimulating factor (section 9.1.6).

AMIFOSTINE

Indications: (specialist use only) see under Dose
Cautions: ensure adequate hydration before treatment; infuse with patient supine and monitor arterial blood pressure (interrupt infusion if blood pressure decreases significantly, consult product literature); during chemotherapy interrupt antihypertensive therapy 24 hours before treatment with amifostine and monitor closely, during radiotherapy monitor closely if concomitant antihypertensive therapy; monitor serum calcium in patients at risk of hypocalcaemia; not recommended in renal and hepatic impairment; pregnancy and breast-feeding; **interactions:** Appendix 1 (amifostine)
Side-effects: hypotension (reversed by infusion of physiological saline and postural management), nausea, vomiting, flushing, chills, dizziness, drowsiness, hiccups, sneezing; rarely convulsions, clinical hypocalcaemia; allergic reactions
Dose: reduction of neutropenia-related risk of infection due to cyclophosphamide and cisplatin treatment in patients with advanced ovarian carcinoma, *by intravenous infusion* over 15 minutes, 910 mg/m^2 once daily started within 30 minutes before chemotherapy (reduced to 740 mg/m^2 for subsequent cycles if full dose could not be given first time due to hypotension lasting more than 5

minutes after interruption, consult product literature)

Reduction of cumulative nephrotoxicity due to cisplatin in patients with advanced solid tumours of non-germ cell origin, consult product literature

Prevention of xerostomia during radiotherapy for head and neck cancer, *by intravenous infusion* over 3 minutes, 200 mg/m^2 once daily starting 15–30 minutes before radiotherapy

CHILD and ELDERLY (over 70 years) not recommended

Ethyol® (Schering-Plough) |PoM|

Intravenous infusion, powder for reconstitution, amifostine, net price 375-mg vial = £108.00; 500-mg vial = £144.00

Urothelial toxicity

Haemorrhagic cystitis is a common manifestation of urothelial toxicity which occurs with the oxazaphosphorines, cyclophosphamide and ifosfamide; it is caused by the metabolite acrolein. **Mesna** reacts specifically with this metabolite in the urinary tract, preventing toxicity. Mesna is used routinely (preferably by mouth) in patients receiving ifosfamide, and in patients receiving cyclophosphamide by the intravenous route at a high dose (e.g. more than 2 g) or in those who experienced urothelial toxicity when given cyclophosphamide previously.

MESNA

Indications: see notes above
Contra-indications: hypersensitivity to thiol-containing compounds
Side-effects: nausea, vomiting, colic, diarrhoea, fatigue, headache, limb and joint pains, depression, irritability, rash, hypotension and tachycardia; rarely hypersensitivity reactions (more common in patients with auto-immune disorders)
Dose: calculated according to oxazaphosphorine (cyclophosphamide or ifosfamide) treatment—for details consult product literature; when given *by mouth*, dose is given 2 hours *before* oxazaphosphorine treatment and repeated 2 and 6 hours *after* treatment; when given *by intravenous injection*, dose is given *with* oxazaphosphorine treatment and repeated 4 and 8 hours *after* treatment

Uromitexan® (ASTA Medica) |PoM|
Tablets, f/c, mesna 400 mg, net price 10-tab pack = £17.43; 600 mg, 10-tab pack = £22.63
Injection, mesna 100 mg/mL. Net price 4-mL amp = £1.61; 10-mL amp = £3.62

Note. For oral administration contents of ampoule are taken in a flavoured drink such as orange juice or cola which may be stored in a refrigerator for up to 24 hours in a sealed container

---

8.1.1 Alkylating drugs

Extensive experience is available with these drugs, which are among the most widely used in cancer chemotherapy. They act by damaging DNA, thus interfering with cell replication. In addition to the side-effects common to many cytotoxic drugs (section 8.1), there are two problems associated with prolonged usage. Firstly, gametogenesis is often severely affected (section 8.1). Secondly, prolonged use of these drugs, particularly when combined with extensive irradiation, is associated with a marked increase in the incidence of acute non-lymphocytic leukaemia.

Cyclophosphamide is widely used in the treatment of chronic lymphocytic leukaemia, the lymphomas, and solid tumours. It is given by mouth or intravenously and is inactive until metabolised by the liver. A urinary metabolite of cyclophosphamide, acrolein, may cause haemorrhagic cystitis; this is a rare but very serious complication. An increased fluid intake, for 24–48 hours after intravenous injection, will help avoid this complication. When high-dose therapy (e.g. more than 2 g intravenously) is used or when the patient is considered to be at high risk of cystitis (e.g. previous pelvic irradiation) mesna (given initially intravenously then by mouth) will also help prevent this—see under Urothelial toxicity (section 8.1).

Ifosfamide is related to cyclophosphamide and is given intravenously; mesna (section 8.1) is routinely given with it to reduce urothelial toxicity.

Chlorambucil is commonly used to treat chronic lymphocytic leukaemia, the indolent non-Hodgkin's lymphomas, Hodgkin's disease, and ovarian cancer. It is given by mouth. Side-effects, apart from marrow suppression, are uncommon. However occasional patients develop severe widespread rashes which can progress to Stevens-Johnson syndrome or to toxic epidermal necrolysis. If a rash occurs further chlorambucil is contra-indicated and cyclophosphamide is substituted.

Melphalan is used to treat myeloma and occasionally solid tumours and lymphomas. It is usually given by mouth, but may also be given intravenously. Because bone marrow toxicity is delayed the drug is usually given at intervals of 6 weeks.

Busulfan (busulphan) is used almost exclusively to treat chronic myeloid leukaemia and is given by mouth. Frequent blood counts are necessary because excessive myelosuppression may result in irreversible bone-marrow aplasia. Hyperpigmentation of the skin is a common side-effect and, rarely, progressive pulmonary fibrosis may occur.

Lomustine is a lipid-soluble nitrosourea and is given by mouth. It is mainly used to treat Hodgkin's disease and certain solid tumours. Bone marrow toxicity is delayed, and the drug is therefore given at intervals of 4 to 6 weeks. Permanent bone marrow damage may occur with prolonged use. Nausea and vomiting are common and moderately severe.

Carmustine is given intravenously. It has similar activity and toxicity to lomustine and is most commonly given to patients with myeloma, lymphoma, and brain tumours. Cumulative renal damage and delayed pulmonary fibrosis may occur.

Chlormethine (**mustine**) is now much less commonly used. It is a very toxic drug which causes severe vomiting. The freshly prepared injection must be given into a fast-running intravenous infusion. Local extravasation causes severe tissue necrosis.

Estramustine is a combination of an oestrogen and chlormethine (mustine) used predominantly in prostate cancer. It is given by mouth and has both an antimitotic effect and (by reducing testosterone concentration) a hormonal effect.

Treosulfan is given by mouth or intravenously and is used to treat ovarian cancer. Skin pigmentation is a common side-effect and allergic alveolitis, pulmonary fibrosis and haemorrhagic cystitis occur rarely.

Thiotepa is usually used as an intracavitary drug for the treatment of malignant effusions or bladder cancer (section 7.4.4). It is also occasionally used to treat breast cancer, but requires parenteral administration.

Mitobronitol is occasionally used to treat chronic myeloid leukaemia; it is available on a named-patient basis only (as *Myelobromol*®, Sinclair).

BUSULFAN

(Busulphan)

Indications: chronic myeloid leukaemia

Cautions: see section 8.1 and notes above; avoid in porphyria (section 9.8.2)

Side-effects: see section 8.1 and notes above

Dose: induction of remission, 60 micrograms/kg to max. 4 mg daily; maintenance, 0.5–2 mg daily

Myleran® (GlaxoWellcome) PoM
Tablets, f/c, busulfan 2 mg, net price 25-tab pack = £5.08

CARMUSTINE

Indications: see notes above

Cautions: see section 8.1 and notes above

Side-effects: see section 8.1 and notes above; irritant to tissues

BiCNU® (Bristol-Myers Squibb) PoM
Injection, powder for reconstitution, carmustine. Net price 100-mg vial (with diluent) = £12.50

CHLORAMBUCIL

Indications: see notes above; immunosuppression (section 8.2.1)

Cautions: see section 8.1 and notes above; avoid in porphyria (section 9.8.2)

Side-effects: see section 8.1 and notes above

Dose: used alone, usually 100–200 micrograms/kg daily for 4–8 weeks

Leukeran® (GlaxoWellcome) PoM
Tablets, f/c, brown, chlorambucil 2 mg, net price 25-tab pack = £8.17

CHLORMETHINE HYDROCHLORIDE/ MUSTINE HYDROCHLORIDE

Indications: Hodgkin's disease—see notes above

Cautions: see section 8.1 and notes above; caution in handling

Side-effects: see section 8.1 and notes above; irritant to tissues

Chlormethine Hydrochloride/Mustine Hydrochloride (Sovereign) PoM
Injection, powder for reconstitution, chlormethine hydrochloride, net price 10-mg vial = £43.99

CYCLOPHOSPHAMIDE

Indications: see notes above

Cautions: see section 8.1 and notes above; hepatic and renal impairment (Appendixes 2 and 3); avoid in porphyria (section 9.8.2); **interactions:** Appendix 1 (cyclophosphamide)

Side-effects: see section 8.1 and notes above

Cyclophosphamide (Pharmacia) [PoM]
Tablets, pink, s/c, cyclophosphamide (anhydrous) 50 mg. Net price 20 = £2.12. Label: 27
Injection, powder for reconstitution, cyclophosphamide. Net price 200-mg vial = £1.65; 500-mg vial = £2.88; 1-g vial = £5.04

Endoxana® (ASTA Medica) [PoM]
Tablets, s/c, cyclophosphamide 50 mg, net price 100-tab pack = £10.03. Label: 27
Injection, powder for reconstitution, cyclophosphamide. Net price 200-mg vial = £1.54; 500-mg vial = £2.68; 1-g vial = £4.68

ESTRAMUSTINE PHOSPHATE

Indications: prostate cancer

Cautions: see section 8.1; renal impairment

Contra-indications: peptic ulceration, severe liver disease (Appendix 2), cardiac disease

Side-effects: see section 8.1; also gynaecomastia, altered liver function, cardiovascular disorders (angina and rare reports of myocardial infarction)

Dose: 0.14–1.4 g daily in divided doses (usual initial dose 560 mg daily)

COUNSELLING. Each dose should be taken not less than 1 hour before or 2 hours after meals and should not be taken with dairy products

Estracyt® (Pharmacia) [PoM]
Capsules, estramustine phosphate 140 mg (as disodium salt). Net price 100-cap pack = £142.73. Label: 23, counselling, see above

IFOSFAMIDE

Indications: see notes above

Cautions: see section 8.1 and notes above; renal impairment (Appendix 3); **interactions:** Appendix 1 (cyclophosphamide and ifosfamide)

Contra-indications: hepatic impairment

Side-effects: see section 8.1 and notes above

Mitoxana® (ASTA Medica) [PoM]
Injection, powder for reconstitution, ifosfamide. Net price 1-g vial = £20.31; 2-g vial = £37.59 (hosp. only)

LOMUSTINE

Indications: see notes above

Cautions: see section 8.1 and notes above

Side-effects: see section 8.1 and notes above

Dose: used alone, 120–130 mg/m² body-surface every 6–8 weeks

Lomustine (Medac) [PoM]
Capsules, blue/clear, lomustine 40 mg. Net price 20-cap pack = £171.35
Note. The brand name *CCNU®* has been used for lomustine capsules

MELPHALAN

Indications: multiple myeloma; see also notes above

Cautions: see section 8.1 and notes above; renal impairment (Appendix 3); **interactions:** Appendix 1 (melphalan)

Side-effects: see section 8.1 and notes above

Dose: *by mouth*, multiple myeloma, 150 micrograms/kg daily in divided doses for 4 days, repeated at intervals of 6 weeks

Alkeran® (GlaxoWellcome) [PoM]
Tablets, melphalan 2 mg, net price 25 = £11.20
Injection, powder for reconstitution, melphalan 50 mg (as hydrochloride). Net price 50-mg vial (with solvent-diluent) = £26.99

THIOTEPA

Indications: see notes above and section 7.4.4

Cautions: see section 8.1; **interactions:** Appendix 1 (thiotepa)

Side-effects: see section 8.1

Thiotepa (Lederle) [PoM]
Injection, powder for reconstitution, thiotepa, net price 15-mg vial = £4.73

TREOSULFAN

Indications: see notes above

Cautions: see section 8.1

Side-effects: see section 8.1 and notes above

Dose: *by mouth*, courses of 1–2 g daily in 3–4 divided doses to provide total dose of 21–28 g over initial 8 weeks (with treatment-free intervals during this period—consult product literature)

Treosulfan (Medac) [PoM]
Capsules, treosulfan 250 mg. Net price 20 = £39.30. Label: 25
Injection, powder for reconstitution, treosulfan. Net price 1 g = £24.10; 5 g = £80.98 (both in infusion bottle with transfer needle)

8.1.2   Cytotoxic antibiotics

Drugs in this group are widely used. Many cytotoxic antibiotics act as radiomimetics and simultaneous use of radiotherapy should be **avoided** as it may result in markedly enhanced toxicity.

Aclarubicin, daunorubicin, doxorubicin, epirubicin and idarubicin are anthracycline antibiotics. Mitoxantrone (mitozantrone) is an anthracycline derivative.

Doxorubicin is one of the most successful and widely used antitumour drugs, and it is used to treat the acute leukaemias, lymphomas, and a variety of solid tumours. It is given by fast running infusion, commonly at 21-day intervals. Local extravasation will cause severe tissue necrosis. Common toxic effects include nausea and vomiting, myelosuppression, alopecia, and mucositis. This drug is largely excreted by the biliary tract, and an elevated bilirubin concentration is an indication for reducing the dose. Supraventricular tachycardia related to drug administration is an uncommon complication.

Higher cumulative doses are associated with cardiomyopathy. It is usual to limit total cumulative doses to $450\,mg/m^2$ body-surface area because symptomatic and potentially fatal heart failure is common above this dose. Patients with pre-existing cardiac disease, the elderly, and those who have received myocardial irradiation should be treated cautiously. Cardiac monitoring, for example by sequential radionuclide ejection fraction measurement, may assist in safely limiting total dosage. Some evidence suggests that weekly low-dose administration may be associated with less cardiac damage. Doxorubicin is also given by bladder instillation. Liposomal formulations for intravenous use are also available.

Epirubicin is structurally related to doxorubicin and clinical trials suggest that it is as effective in the treatment of breast cancer. A maximum cumulative dose of $0.9–1\,g/m^2$ is recommended to help avoid cardiotoxicity. Like doxorubicin it is given intravenously and by bladder instillation.

Aclarubicin and **idarubicin** are anthracyclines with general properties similar to those of doxorubicin. They are both given intravenously. Idarubicin may also be given by mouth.

Daunorubicin also has general properties similar to those of doxorubicin. It should be given by intravenous infusion and is indicated for acute leukaemias. A liposomal formulation for intravenous use is licensed for AIDS-related Kaposi's sarcoma.

> **Use with trastuzumab.** Concomitant use of anthracyclines with trastuzumab (section 8.1.5) is associated with cardiotoxicity; for details, see p. 420.

Mitoxantrone (mitozantrone) is structurally related to doxorubicin; it is used in breast cancer. Mitoxantrone is also licensed for use in the treatment of non-Hodgkin's lymphoma and adult non-lymphocytic leukaemia. It is given intravenously and is well tolerated but myelosuppression and dose-related cardiotoxicity occur; cardiac examinations are recommended after a cumulative dose of $160\,mg/m^2$.

Bleomycin is given intravenously or intramuscularly to treat the lymphomas and certain solid tumours; it is given by the intracavitary route for malignant effusions. It causes little bone-marrow suppression but dermatological toxicity is common and increased pigmentation particularly affecting the flexures and subcutaneous sclerotic plaques may occur. Mucositis is also relatively common and an association with Raynaud's phenomenon is reported. Hypersensitivity reactions manifest by chills and fevers commonly occur a few hours after drug administration and may be prevented by simultaneous administration of a corticosteroid, for example hydrocortisone intravenously. The principal problem associated with the use of bleomycin is progressive pulmonary fibrosis. This is dose-related, occurring more commonly at cumulative doses greater than 300 000 units (see Bleomycin, below) and in the elderly. Basal lung crepitations or suspicious chest X-ray changes are an indication to stop therapy with this drug. Patients who have received extensive treatment with bleomycin (e.g. cumulative dose more than 100 000 units—see Bleomycin below) may be at risk of developing respiratory failure if a general anaesthetic is given with high inspired oxygen concentrations. Anaesthetists should be warned of this.

Dactinomycin is principally used to treat paediatric cancers; it is given intravenously. Its side-effects are similar to those of doxorubicin, except that cardiac toxicity is not a problem.

Mitomycin is given intravenously to treat upper gastro-intestinal and breast cancers and by bladder instillation for superficial bladder tumours. It causes delayed bone-marrow toxicity and therefore it is usually administered at 6-weekly intervals. Prolonged use may result in permanent bone-marrow damage. It may also cause lung fibrosis and renal damage.

ACLARUBICIN

Indications: acute non-lymphocytic leukaemia in patients who have relapsed or are resistant or refractory to first-line chemotherapy

Cautions: see section 8.1 and notes above; hepatic and renal impairment; irritant to tissues

Side-effects: see section 8.1 and notes above

Aclarubicin (Medac) [PoM]
Injection, powder for reconstitution, aclarubicin 20 mg (as hydrochloride). Net price 20-mg vial = £98.55
Note. The brand names *Aclacin®* and *Aclaplastin®* have been used for aclarubicin preparations

BLEOMYCIN

Indications: squamous cell carcinoma; see also notes above

Cautions: see section 8.1 and notes above; renal impairment (Appendix 3); caution in handling—irritant to tissues

Side-effects: see section 8.1 and notes above

Bleomycin (Non-proprietary) [PoM]
Injection, powder for reconstitution, bleomycin (as sulphate). Net price 15 000-unit vial = £16.29
Note. To conform to the European Pharmacopoeia vials previously labelled as containing '15 units' of bleomycin are now labelled as containing 15 000 units. The amount of bleomycin in the vial has not changed.
Available from Faulding DBL, Kyowa Hakko (*Bleo-Kyowa®*)

DACTINOMYCIN
(Actinomycin D)
Indications: see notes above
Cautions: see section 8.1 and notes above; caution in handling—irritant to tissues
Side-effects: see section 8.1 and notes above

Cosmegen Lyovac® (MSD) [PoM]
Injection, powder for reconstitution, dactinomycin, net price 500-microgram vial = £1.50

DAUNORUBICIN

Indications: see notes above
Cautions: see section 8.1 and notes above; hepatic impairment (Appendix 2), renal impairment (Appendix 3); caution in handling—irritant to tissues

Side-effects: see section 8.1 and notes above

Daunorubicin (Non-proprietary) PoM
Injection, powder for reconstitution, daunorubicin (as hydrochloride), net price 20-mg vial = £33.00
Available from Beacon
Note. The brand name *Cerubidin®* was formerly used

■ Lipid formulation
DaunoXome® (Gilead) PoM
Concentrate for intravenous infusion, daunorubicin encapsulated in liposomes. For dilution before use. Net price 50-mg vial = £148.03
For advanced AIDS-related Kaposi's sarcoma

DOXORUBICIN HYDROCHLORIDE

Indications: see notes above and section 7.4.4
Cautions: see section 8.1 and notes above; hepatic impairment (Appendix 2); caution in handling—irritant to tissues; **interactions:** Appendix 1 (doxorubicin)
Side-effects: see section 8.1 and notes above

Doxorubicin Rapid Dissolution (Pharmacia) PoM
Injection, powder for reconstitution, doxorubicin hydrochloride, net price 10-mg vial = £18.72; 50-mg vial = £93.60
Note. This preparation has replaced *Adriamycin®*
Various strengths also available from Medac
Doxorubicin Solution for Injection (Pharmacia) PoM
Injection, doxorubicin hydrochloride 2 mg/mL, net price 5-ml vial = £20.60, 25-mL vial = £102.99
Various strengths and sizes also available from Faulding DBL, Medac

■ Lipid formulation
Caelyx® (Schering-Plough) PoM
Concentrate for intravenous infusion, doxorubicin hydrochloride 2 mg/mL encapsulated in liposomes. For dilution before use. Net price 10-mL vial = £411.30, 25-mL vial = £813.49
For AIDS-related Kaposi's sarcoma in patients with low CD4 count and extensive mucocutaneous or visceral disease and for advanced ovarian cancer when platinum-based chemotherapy has failed
Myocet® (Elan) ▼ PoM
Injection, powder for reconstitution, doxorubicin hydrochloride (as doxorubicin–citrate complex) encapsulated in liposomes, net price 50-mg vial (with vials of liposomes and buffer) = £929.00
For use with cyclophosphamide for metastatic breast cancer

EPIRUBICIN HYDROCHLORIDE

Indications: see notes above and section 7.4.4
Cautions: see section 8.1 and notes above; hepatic impairment (Appendix 2); caution in handling—irritant to tissues
Side-effects: see section 8.1 and notes above

Pharmorubicin® Rapid Dissolution (Pharmacia) PoM
Injection, powder for reconstitution, epirubicin hydrochloride. Net price 10-mg vial = £16.09; 20-mg vial = £32.18; 50-mg vial = £80.45

Pharmorubicin® Solution for Injection (Pharmacia) PoM
Injection, epirubicin hydrochloride 2 mg/mL, net price 5-mL vial = £17.71, 25-mL vial = £88.53

IDARUBICIN HYDROCHLORIDE

Indications: advanced breast cancer after failure of first-line chemotherapy (not including anthracyclines); acute leukaemias—see notes above
Cautions: see section 8.1 and notes above; hepatic and renal impairment (Appendixes 2 and 3); caution in handling—irritant to tissues
Side-effects: see section 8.1 and notes above
Dose: *by mouth,* acute non-lymphocytic leukaemia, 30 mg/m^2 daily for 3 days alone *or* 15–30 mg/m^2 daily for 3 days in combination therapy
Advanced breast cancer, 45 mg/m^2 alone, as a single dose *or* divided over 3 consecutive days; repeat every 3–4 weeks
Max. cumulative dose (for all indications) 400 mg/m^2

Zavedos® (Pharmacia) PoM
Capsules, idarubicin hydrochloride, 5 mg (red), net price 1-cap pack = £27.50; 10 mg (red/white), 1-cap pack = £55.01; 25 mg (white), 1-cap pack = £137.52. Label: 25
Injection, powder for reconstitution, idarubicin hydrochloride, net price 5-mg vial = £69.52; 10-mg vial = £139.05

MITOMYCIN

Indications: see notes above and section 7.4.4
Cautions: see section 8.1 and notes above; caution in handling—irritant to tissues
Side-effects: see section 8.1 and notes above

Mitomycin (Non-proprietary) PoM
Injection, powder for reconstitution, mitomycin. Net price 10-mg vial = £22.67; 20-mg vial = £41.70
Available from Faulding DBL
Mitomycin C Kyowa® (Kyowa Hakko) PoM
Injection, powder for reconstitution, mitomycin. Net price 2-mg vial = £5.88; 10-mg vial = £19.37; 20-mg vial = £36.94; 40-mg vial = £73.88 (hosp. only)

MITOXANTRONE/MITOZANTRONE

Indications: see notes above
Cautions: see section 8.1 and notes above; intrathecal administration not recommended
Side-effects: see section 8.1 and notes above

Novantrone® (Lederle) PoM
Concentrate for intravenous infusion, mitoxantrone (as hydrochloride) 2 mg/mL, net price 10-mL vial = £150.43, 12.5-mL vial = £188.05, 15-mL vial = £225.60
Onkotrone® (ASTA Medica) PoM
Concentrate for intravenous infusion, mitoxantrone (as hydrochloride) 2 mg/mL, net price 10-mL vial = £135.39, 12.5-mL vial = £169.25, 15-mL vial = £203.04

8.1.3 Antimetabolites

Antimetabolites are incorporated into new nuclear material or combine irreversibly with vital cellular enzymes, preventing normal cellular division.

Methotrexate inhibits the enzyme dihydrofolate reductase, essential for the synthesis of purines and pyrimidines. It is given by mouth, intravenously, intramuscularly, or intrathecally.

Methotrexate is used as maintenance therapy for childhood acute lymphoblastic leukaemia. Other uses include choriocarcinoma, non-Hodgkin's lymphoma, and a number of solid tumours. Intrathecal methotrexate is used in the CNS prophylaxis of childhood acute lymphoblastic leukaemia, and as a therapy for established meningeal cancer or lymphoma.

Methotrexate causes myelosuppression, mucositis, and rarely pneumonitis. It is **contra-indicated** in significant renal impairment because it is excreted primarily by the kidney. It is also contra-indicated in patients with severe hepatic impairment. It should also be **avoided** if a significant pleural effusion or ascites is present because it tends to accumulate in these fluids, and its subsequent return to the circulation will be associated with myelosuppression. Systemic toxicity may occur following intrathecal administration and blood counts should be carefully monitored.

Folinic acid (section 8.1) following methotrexate administration helps to prevent methotrexate-induced mucositis or myelosuppression.

Capecitabine, which is metabolised to fluorouracil, is given by mouth as monotherapy for metastatic colorectal cancer. It has been shown to be of similar efficacy as a combination of fluorouracil and folinic acid.

Cytarabine acts by interfering with pyrimidine synthesis. It is given subcutaneously, intravenously, or intrathecally. Its predominant use is in the induction of remission of acute myeloblastic leukaemia. It is a potent myelosuppressant and requires careful haematological monitoring.

Fludarabine is recommended for patients with B-cell chronic lymphocytic leukaemia (CLL) after initial treatment with an alkylating agent has failed; it is given daily by mouth for 5 days every 28 days. Fludarabine is generally well tolerated but it does cause myelosuppression, which may be cumulative. Immunosuppression is also common and co-trimoxazole is often used to prevent pneumocystis infection. Immune-mediated haemolytic anaemia, thrombocytopenia, and neutropenia are less common side-effects.

NICE guidance (fludarabine). The National Institute for Clinical Excellence has recommended oral fludarabine as second-line therapy for B-cell chronic lymphocytic leukaemia (CLL) for patients who have either failed, or are intolerant of, first-line chemotherapy.

Cladribine is an effective but potentially toxic drug given by intravenous infusion for the treatment of hairy cell leukaemia. It is also licensed for chronic lymphocytic leukaemia in patients who have failed to respond to standard regimens containing an alkylating agent; it is given by intra-venous infusion. Myelosuppression may be severe and serious neurotoxicity has been reported rarely.

Gemcitabine is used intravenously; it is given alone for palliative treatment or with cisplatin as first-line treatment for locally advanced or metastatic non-small cell lung cancer. It is also used in the treatment of locally advanced or metastatic pancreatic cancer. Combined with cisplatin, gemcitabine is also licensed for the treatment of advanced bladder cancer. It is generally well tolerated but it may cause mild gastro-intestinal side-effects and rashes; renal impairment, pulmonary toxicity and influenza-like symptoms have also been reported. Haemolytic uraemic syndrome has been reported rarely and gemcitabine should be discontinued if signs of microangiopathic haemolytic anaemia occur.

NICE guidance (gemcitabine). The National Institute for Clinical Excellence has recommended that gemcitabine is an option for first-line chemotherapy for patients with advanced or metastatic adenocarcinoma of the pancreas and a Karnofsky score of at least 50 [Karnofsky score is a measure of the ability to perform ordinary tasks].

Gemcitabine is not recommended for patients who can have potentially curative surgery. There is insufficient evidence about its use for second-line treatment of pancreatic adenocarcinoma.

NICE guidance (docetaxel, paclitaxel, gemcitabine and vinorelbine for non-small cell lung cancer). The National Institute for Clinical Excellence has recommended that chemotherapy should be considered for non-small cell lung cancer in patients who are unsuitable for curative treatment or who are unlikely to respond to such treatment.

Gemcitabine, paclitaxel, or vinorelbine should be considered as first-line chemotherapy for advanced non-small cell lung cancer. Combination of each of these drugs with platinum-based chemotherapy, where tolerated, is likely to be most effective.

Docetaxel monotherapy should be considered for locally advanced or metastatic non-small cell lung cancer which relapses after previous chemotherapy.

Fluorouracil is usually given intravenously because absorption following oral administration is unpredictable. It is used to treat a number of solid tumours, including gastro-intestinal tract cancers and breast cancer. It is commonly used with folinic acid in advanced colorectal cancer. It may also be used topically for certain malignant and pre-malignant skin lesions. Toxicity is unusual, but may include myelosuppression, mucositis, and rarely a cerebellar syndrome.

Raltitrexed, a thymidylate synthase inhibitor, is given intravenously for palliation of advanced colorectal cancer when fluorouracil and folinic acid cannot be used. It is probably of similar efficacy to fluorouracil. Raltitrexed is generally well tolerated, but can cause marked myelosuppression and gastro-intestinal side-effects.

Mercaptopurine is used almost exclusively as maintenance therapy for the acute leukaemias. Azathioprine, which is metabolised to mercaptopurine, is generally used as an immunosuppressant (section 8.2.1). The dose of both drugs should be reduced if the patient is receiving allopurinol since it interferes with their metabolism.

Tegafur (in combination with uracil) is given by mouth, together with calcium folinate, in the management of metastatic colorectal cancer. Tegafur is a prodrug of fluorouracil; uracil inhibits the degradation of fluorouracil. Tegafur (with uracil) has been shown to be of similar efficacy as a combination of fluorouracil and folinic acid for metastatic colorectal cancer.

Tioguanine (thioguanine) is given by mouth to induce remission in acute myeloid leukaemia.

CAPECITABINE

Indications: see notes above

Cautions: see section 8.1; **interactions:** Appendix 1 (capecitabine)

Contra-indications: hepatic impairment, renal impairment (Appendix 3)

Side-effects: see section 8.1 and notes above; hand–foot (desquamative) syndrome

Dose: ADULT over 18 years, 1.25 g/m^2 twice daily for 14 days; subsequent courses repeated after a 7-day interval

Xeloda® (Roche) ▼ PoM
Tablets, f/c, peach, capecitabine 150 mg, net price 60-tab pack = £44.47; 500 mg, 120-tab pack = £295.06. Label: 21

CLADRIBINE

Indications: see notes above

Cautions: see section 8.1 and notes above

Side-effects: see section 8.1 and notes above

Leustat® (Janssen-Cilag) PoM
Injection, cladribine 1 mg/mL. For dilution and use as an infusion, net price 10-mL vial = £182.29

CYTARABINE

Indications: acute leukaemias

Cautions: see section 8.1 and notes above; hepatic impairment (Appendix 2)

Side-effects: see section 8.1 and notes above

Cytarabine (Non-proprietary) PoM
Injection (for intravenous, subcutaneous or intrathecal use), cytarabine 20 mg/mL, net price 5-mL vial (Faulding DBL) = £4.00
Injection (for intravenous or subcutaneous use), cytarabine 20 mg/mL, net price 5-mL vial (Pharmacia) = £3.90, 25-mL vial (Pharmacia) = £19.50
Injection (for intravenous or subcutaneous use), cytarabine 100 mg/mL, net price 1-mL vial (Faulding DBL) = £4.00; 5-mL vial (Faulding DBL) = £20.00; 10-mL vial (Faulding DBL) = £40.00, (Pharmacia) = £39.00; 20-mL vial (Faulding DBL) = £79.00, (Pharmacia) = £77.50; 20-mL *Onco-vial®* (Faulding DBL) = £79.00

Cytosar® (Pharmacia) PoM
Injection, powder for reconstitution, cytarabine. Net price 100-mg vial = £2.87, 100-mg vial (with diluent) = £3.03; 500-mg vial = £14.28, 500-mg vial (with diluent) = £14.75. For intravenous injection or infusion and subcutaneous injection only; not recommended for intrathecal use

FLUDARABINE PHOSPHATE

Indications: see notes above

Cautions: see section 8.1 and notes above; renal impairment (Appendix 3); **interactions:** Appendix 1 (fludarabine) ♦

Side-effects: see section 8.1 and notes above

Dose: *by mouth*, ADULT 40 mg/m^2 for 5 days every 28 days usually for 6 cycles

Fludara® (Schering Health) PoM
Tablets ▼, f/c, pink, fludarabine phosphate 10 mg, net price 15-tab pack = £279.00, 20-tab pack = £372.00
Injection, powder for reconstitution, fludarabine phosphate. Net price 50-mg vial = £130.00

FLUOROURACIL

Indications: see notes above

Cautions: see section 8.1 and notes above; caution in handling—irritant to tissues; **interactions:** Appendix 1 (fluorouracil)

Side-effects: see section 8.1 and notes above; also local irritation with topical preparation

Dose: *by mouth*, maintenance 15 mg/kg weekly; max. in one day 1 g

Fluorouracil (Non-proprietary) PoM
Capsules, fluorouracil 250 mg.
Available from Cambridge on a named-patient basis
Injection, fluorouracil (as sodium salt) 25 mg/mL, net price 10-mL vial = £3.20, 20-mL vial = £6.40, 100-mL vial = £32.00; 50 mg/mL, 10-mL vial = £6.40, 20-mL vial = £12.80, 50-mL vial = £32.00, 100-mL vial = £64.00
Available from Faulding DBL, Medac

■ Topical preparations

Efudix® (ICN) PoM
Cream, fluorouracil 5%. Net price 20 g = £18.27
Excipients: include hydroxybenzoates (parabens)
Dose: malignant and pre-malignant skin lesions, apply thinly to the affected area once or twice daily; cover with occlusive dressing in malignant conditions; max. area of skin treated at one time, 500 cm^2; usual duration of initial therapy, 3–4 weeks

GEMCITABINE

Indications: see notes above

Cautions: see section 8.1 and notes above

Side-effects: see section 8.1 and notes above

Gemzar® (Lilly) PoM
Injection, powder for reconstitution, gemcitabine (as hydrochloride), net price 200-mg vial = £32.55; 1-g vial = £162.76 (both hosp. only)

MERCAPTOPURINE

Indications: acute leukaemias; inflammatory bowel disease [unlicensed indication] (section 1.5)

Cautions: see section 8.1 and notes above; renal impairment (Appendix 3); avoid in porphyria (section 9.8.2); **interactions:** Appendix 1 (mercaptopurine)

Side-effects: see section 8.1 and notes above

Dose: initially 2.5 mg/kg daily

Puri-Nethol® (GlaxoWellcome) PoM
Tablets, fawn, scored, mercaptopurine 50 mg. Net
price 25 = £18.35

METHOTREXATE

Indications: see notes above and under Dose;
rheumatoid arthritis (section 10.1.3); psoriasis
(section 13.5.2)
Cautions: see section 8.1, notes above and section
13.5.2; hepatic and renal impairment (Appendixes 2 and 3); porphyria (section 9.8.2); **interactions:** Appendix 1 (methotrexate)
Side-effects: see section 8.1, notes above and section 13.5.2
Dose: *by mouth*, leukaemia in children (maintenance), 15 mg/m² weekly in combination with
other drugs

> IMPORTANT. Note that the above dose is a **weekly**
> dose. The CSM has received reports of prescription
> and dispensing errors including fatalities. Attention
> should be paid to the **strength** of methotrexate
> tablets prescribed and the **frequency** of dosing

Methotrexate (Non-proprietary) PoM
Tablets, yellow, methotrexate 2.5 mg. Net price
100 = £11.40. Counselling, NSAIDs, see section
13.5.2
Available from Faulding DBL, Lederle, Pharmacia
(*Maxtrex®*)
Tablets, yellow, methotrexate 10 mg. Net price 100
(Faulding DBL) = £55.07; (Pharmacia, *Maxtrex®*)
= £45.16. Counselling, NSAIDs, see section
13.5.2
Injection, methotrexate 2.5 mg (as sodium salt)/
mL. Net price 2-mL vial (Faulding DBL) = £1.68
Injection, methotrexate 25 mg (as sodium salt)/
mL. Net price 2-mL vial (Faulding DBL) = £4.58,
(Lederle) = £2.62; 8-mL vial (Lederle) = £10.02;
20-mL vial (Faulding DBL) = £39.09, (Lederle) =
£25.07; 40-mL vial (Lederle) = £44.57; 200-mL
vial (Lederle) = £200.57
Injection, methotrexate 100 mg/mL (not for
intrathecal use). Net price 10-mL vial (Faulding
DBL) = £78.33; 50-mL vial (Faulding DBL) =
£380.07

RALTITREXED

Indications: see notes above
Cautions: see section 8.1 and notes above; hepatic
and renal impairment (Appendixes 2 and 3)
Side-effects: see section 8.1 and notes above

Tomudex® (AstraZeneca) PoM
Injection, powder for reconstitution, raltitrexed.
Net price 2-mg vial = £110.78

TEGAFUR WITH URACIL

Indications: see notes above
Cautions: see section 8.1; cardiac disease; renal
impairment; hepatic impairment (avoid if severe);
interactions: Appendix 1 (*Uftoral®*)
Side-effects: see section 8.1 and notes above
Dose: ADULT, tegafur 300 mg/m² (with uracil
672 mg/m²) daily in 3 divided doses for 28 days;
subsequent courses repeated after 7-day interval;

for dose adjustment due to toxicity, consult product literature
Uftoral® (Bristol-Myers Squibb) ▼ PoM
Capsules, tegafur 100 mg, uracil 224 mg, net price
21-cap pack = £119.91, 28-cap pack = £159.88,
35-cap pack = £199.85, 42-cap pack = £239.82.
Label: 23

TIOGUANINE
(Thioguanine)
Indications: acute leukaemias
Cautions: see section 8.1 and notes above; renal
impairment (Appendix 3)
Side-effects: see section 8.1 and notes above
Dose: initially 2–2.5 mg/kg daily

Lanvis® (GlaxoWellcome) PoM
Tablets, yellow, scored, tioguanine 40 mg. Net
price 25-tab pack = £44.39

8.1.4 Vinca alkaloids and etoposide

The vinca alkaloids, **vinblastine**, **vincristine**, and
vindesine, are used to treat the acute leukaemias,
lymphomas, and some solid tumours (e.g. breast
and lung cancer). **Vinorelbine**, a semi-synthetic
vinca alkaloid, is used for advanced breast cancer
(where anthracycline-containing regimens have
failed) and for advanced non-small cell lung cancer
(see also NICE guidance, p. 413).

Neurological toxicity, usually manifested as
peripheral or autonomic neuropathy, is a feature of
treatment with all vinca alkaloids and is a limiting
side-effect of vincristine; it occurs less often with
vindesine, vinblastine and vinorelbine. Patients
with neurological toxicity commonly experience
peripheral paraesthesia, loss of deep tendon
reflexes, abdominal pain, and constipation. If symptoms of neurotoxicity are severe, doses should be
reduced. Motor weakness can also occur, and
increasing motor weakness calls for discontinuation
of treatment with these drugs. Generally recovery
of the nervous system is slow but complete.

Myelosuppression is the dose-limiting side-effect
of vinblastine, vindesine and vinorelbine; vincristine causes negligible myelosuppression. The vinca
alkaloids may cause reversible alopecia. They cause
severe local irritation and care must be taken to
avoid extravasation.

> Vinblastine, vincristine, vindesine and vinorelbine are
> for **intravenous administration only**. They are
> **not** for intrathecal administration because of severe
> neurotoxicity which is usually fatal.

Etoposide may be given orally or by slow intravenous infusion, the oral dose being double the
intravenous dose. A preparation containing etoposide phosphate can be given by intravenous injection or infusion. Etoposide is usually given daily for
3–5 days and courses should not be repeated more
frequently than at intervals of 21 days. It has particularly useful activity in small cell carcinoma of the
bronchus, the lymphomas, and testicular cancer.
Toxic effects include alopecia, myelosuppression,
nausea, and vomiting.

ETOPOSIDE

Indications: see notes above
Cautions: see section 8.1 and notes above
Contra-indications: see section 8.1 and notes above; severe hepatic impairment
Side-effects: see section 8.1 and notes above; irritant to tissues
Dose: *by mouth*, 120–240 mg/m^2 daily for 5 days

Etoposide (Non-proprietary) PoM
Concentrate for intravenous infusion, etoposide 20 mg/mL, net price 5-mL vial (Faulding DBL; Medac, *Eposin®*) = £13.50, 10-mL vial (APS; Faulding DBL) = £26.24, 25-mL vial (Medac, *Eposin®*) = £67.50

Etopophos® (Bristol-Myers Squibb) PoM
Injection, powder for reconstitution, etoposide (as phosphate), net price 100-mg vial = £29.87 (hosp. only)

Vepesid® (Bristol-Myers Squibb) PoM
Capsules, both pink, etoposide 50 mg, net price 20 = £113.95; 100 mg, 10-cap pack = £99.57 (hosp. only). Label: 23
Concentrate for intravenous infusion, etoposide 20 mg/mL, net price 5-mL vial = £14.58 (hosp. only)

VINBLASTINE SULPHATE

Indications: see notes above
Cautions: see section 8.1 and notes above; hepatic impairment (Appendix 2); caution in handling
Contra-indications: see section 8.1 and notes above
IMPORTANT. Intrathecal injection **contra-indicated**
Side-effects: see section 8.1 and notes above; irritant to tissues

Vinblastine (Non-proprietary) PoM
Injection, vinblastine sulphate 1 mg/mL. Net price 10-mL vial = £13.09
Available from Faulding DBL

Velbe® (Lilly) PoM
Injection, powder for reconstitution, vinblastine sulphate. Net price 10-mg amp = £14.15

VINCRISTINE SULPHATE

Indications: see notes above
Cautions: see section 8.1 and notes above; hepatic impairment (Appendix 2); caution in handling; **interactions:** Appendix 1 (vincristine)
Contra-indications: see section 8.1 and notes above
IMPORTANT. Intrathecal injection **contra-indicated**
Side-effects: see section 8.1 and notes above; irritant to tissues

Vincristine (Non-proprietary) PoM
Injection, vincristine sulphate 1 mg/mL. Net price 1-mL vial = £10.92; 2-mL vial = £21.17; 5-mL vial = £44.16; 1-mL syringe = £13.27; 2-mL syringe = £20.55
Available from Faulding DBL

Oncovin® (Lilly) PoM
Injection, vincristine sulphate 1 mg/mL, net price 1-mL vial = £14.18; 2-mL vial = £28.05

VINDESINE SULPHATE

Indications: see notes above
Cautions: see section 8.1 and notes above; hepatic impairment (Appendix 2); caution in handling
Contra-indications: see section 8.1 and notes above
IMPORTANT. Intrathecal injection **contra-indicated**
Side-effects: see section 8.1 and notes above; irritant to tissues

Eldisine® (Lilly) PoM
Injection, powder for reconstitution, vindesine sulphate, net price 5-mg vial = £78.30 (hosp. only)

VINORELBINE

Indications: see notes above
Cautions: see section 8.1 and notes above; hepatic impairment (Appendix 2); caution in handling
Contra-indications: see section 8.1 and notes above
IMPORTANT. Intrathecal injection **contra-indicated**
Side-effects: see section 8.1 and notes above; irritant to tissues

Navelbine® (Fabre) PoM
Injection concentrate, vinorelbine (as tartrate) 10 mg/mL. Net price 1-mL vial = £31.25; 5-mL vial = £147.06

8.1.5 Other antineoplastic drugs

Amsacrine

Amsacrine has an action and toxic effects similar to those of doxorubicin (section 8.1.2) and is given *intravenously*. It is occasionally used in acute myeloid leukaemia. Side-effects include myelosuppression and mucositis; electrolytes should be monitored as fatal arrhythmias have occurred in association with hypokalaemia.

AMSACRINE

Indications: see notes above
Cautions: see section 8.1 and notes above; reduce dose in renal or hepatic impairment; also caution in handling—irritant to skin and tissues
Side-effects: see section 8.1 and notes above

Amsidine® (Goldshield) PoM
Concentrate for intravenous infusion, amsacrine 5 mg (as lactate)/mL, when reconstituted by mixing two solutions. Net price 1.5-mL (75-mg) amp with 13.5-mL diluent vial = £47.62 (hosp. only)
Note. Use glass apparatus for reconstitution

Altretamine

Altretamine is licensed for the treatment of advanced ovarian cancer where other regimens have failed. It is given by mouth. Prophylactic antiemetic treatment is recommended because nausea and vomiting are common and may not respond to symptomatic management. Peripheral and central neurotoxicity has been reported and regular neurological examination is therefore recommended. Altretamine should be discontinued if dose reduction fails to stabilise symptoms of neurological toxicity. Other side-effects include renal and hepatic toxicity, rash and pruritus.

ALTRETAMINE

Indications: see notes above
Cautions: see section 8.1 and notes above; hepatic and renal impairment (Appendixes 2 and 3); **interactions:** Appendix 1 (altretamine)
Contra-indications: see section 8.1 and notes above
Side-effects: see section 8.1 and notes above
Dose: 260 mg/m² daily in 4 divided doses (after meals and at bedtime) for 14 days of a 28-day cycle; given for up to 12 cycles

Hexalen® (Ipsen) [PoM]
Capsules, altretamine 50 mg. Net price 60-cap pack = £142.77. Label: 21.

Crisantaspase

Crisantaspase is the enzyme asparaginase produced by *Erwinia chrysanthemi*. It is given *intramuscularly* or *subcutaneously* almost exclusively in acute lymphoblastic leukaemia. Facilities for the management of anaphylaxis should be available. Side-effects also include nausea, vomiting, CNS depression, and liver function and blood lipid changes; careful monitoring is therefore necessary and the urine is tested for glucose to exclude hyperglycaemia.

CRISANTASPASE

Indications: see notes above
Cautions: see section 8.1 and notes above
Side-effects: see section 8.1 and notes above

Erwinase® (Ipsen) [PoM]
Injection, powder for reconstitution, crisantaspase. Net price 10 000-unit vial = £39.94

Dacarbazine and temozolomide

Dacarbazine is used to treat metastatic melanoma and, in combination therapy, the soft tissue sarcomas. It is also a component of a commonly used combination for Hodgkin's disease (ABVD—doxorubicin [previously *Adriamycin®*], bleomycin, vinblastine, and dacarbazine). It is given *intravenously*. The predominant side-effects are myelosuppression and intense nausea and vomiting.

Temozolomide is structurally related to dacarbazine and is licensed for second-line treatment of malignant glioma.

NICE guidance (temozolomide). The National Institute for Clinical Excellence has recommended that temozolomide may be considered for the treatment of patients with recurrent malignant glioma who have failed first-line chemotherapy.

DACARBAZINE

Indications: see notes above
Cautions: see section 8.1; hepatic and renal impairment (Appendixes 2 and 3); caution in handling
Side-effects: see section 8.1 and notes above; rarely liver necrosis due to hepatic vein thrombosis; irritant to skin and tissues

Dacarbazine (Non-proprietary) [PoM]
Injection, powder for reconstitution, dacarbazine (as citrate), net price 100-mg vial = £5.11 (Medac); 200-mg vial = £7.24 (Medac) or £7.50 (Faulding DBL); 500-mg vial = £16.50 (Medac); 600-mg vial = £22.50 (Faulding DBL); 1-g vial = £31.80 (Medac)
Available from Faulding DBL, Medac
DTIC-Dome® (Bayer) [PoM]
Injection, powder for reconstitution, dacarbazine. Net price 200-mg vial = £7.40

TEMOZOLOMIDE

Indications: see notes above
Cautions: see section 8.1; severe hepatic impairment and renal impairment; **interactions:** Appendix 1 (temozolomide)
Side-effects: see section 8.1
Dose: 200 mg/m² once daily for 5 days of a 28-day cycle; for patients previously treated with chemotherapy—consult product literature; CHILD under 3 years not recommended

Temodal® (Schering-Plough) ▼ [PoM]
Capsules, temozolomide 5 mg, net price 5-cap pack = £17.30; 20 mg, 5-cap pack = £69.20; 100 mg, 5-cap pack = £346.00; 250 mg, 5-cap pack = £865.00. Label: 23, 25

Hydroxycarbamide/Hydroxyurea

Hydroxycarbamide (hydroxyurea) is an orally active drug used mainly in the treatment of chronic myeloid leukaemia. It is occasionally used for polycythaemia (the usual treatment is venesection). Myelosuppression, nausea, and skin reactions are the most common toxic effects.

HYDROXYCARBAMIDE/ HYDROXYUREA

Indications: see notes above
Cautions: see section 8.1 and notes above
Side-effects: see section 8.1 and notes above
Dose: 20–30 mg/kg daily *or* 80 mg/kg every third day

Hydrea® (Squibb) [PoM]
Capsules, pink/green, hydroxycarbamide 500 mg. Net price 20 = £2.39

Imatinib

Imatinib is a protein–tyrosine kinase inhibitor, which is licensed for the treatment of chronic myeloid leukaemia in chronic phase after failure of interferon alfa, or in accelerated phase, or in blast crisis. The most frequent side-effects of imatinib are nausea, vomiting, diarrhoea, oedema, muscle pain, and headache.

IMATINIB

Indications: see notes above
Cautions: consult product literature; pregnancy (see Appendix 4 and section 8.1)
Contra-indications: breast-feeding
Side-effects: see section 8.1 and notes above
Dose: consult product literature

Glivec® (Novartis) ▼ PoM
Capsules, orange, imatinib (as mesilate) 100 mg, net price 120-cap pack = £1557.36

Pentostatin

Pentostatin is highly active in hairy cell leukaemia. It is given *intravenously* on alternate weeks and is capable of inducing prolonged complete remission. It is potentially toxic, causing myelosuppression, immunosuppression and a number of other side-effects which may be severe. Its use is probably best confined to specialist centres.

PENTOSTATIN

Indications: see notes above
Cautions: see section 8.1 and notes above; **interactions:** Appendix 1 (pentostatin)
Side-effects: see section 8.1 and notes above

Nipent® (Lederle) PoM
Injection, powder for reconstitution, pentostatin. Net price 10-mg vial = £851.40

Platinum compounds

Carboplatin is widely used in the treatment of advanced ovarian cancer and lung cancer (particulary the small cell type). It is given *intravenously*. The dose of carboplatin is determined according to renal function rather than body surface area. Carboplatin can be given on an outpatient basis and is better tolerated than cisplatin; nausea and vomiting are reduced in severity and nephrotoxicity, neurotoxicity, and ototoxicity are much less of a problem than with cisplatin. It is, however, more myelosuppressive than cisplatin.

Cisplatin is of value in patients with metastatic germ cell cancers (seminoma and teratoma). It is also used in the treatment of bladder, lung, upper gastro-intestinal and ovarian cancer (although carboplatin is preferred for ovarian cancer). It is given *intravenously*. Cisplatin requires intensive intravenous hydration and treatment may be complicated by severe nausea and vomiting. Cisplatin is toxic, causing nephrotoxicity (monitoring of renal function is essential), ototoxicity, peripheral neuropathy, hypomagnesaemia and myelosuppression. It is, however, increasingly given in a day-care setting.

Oxaliplatin is given *intravenously* for the treatment of metastatic colorectal cancer in combination with fluorouracil and folinic acid. Neurotoxic side-effects (including sensory peripheral neuropathy) are dose limiting. Other side-effects include gastro-intestinal disturbances, ototoxicity, and myelosuppression. Manufacturers advise renal function monitoring in moderate impairment.

CARBOPLATIN

Indications: see notes above
Cautions: see section 8.1 and notes above; renal impairment (Appendix 3); **interactions:** Appendix 1 (platinum compounds)
Side-effects: see section 8.1 and notes above

Carboplatin (Non-proprietary) PoM
Injection, carboplatin 10 mg/mL, net price 5-mL vial = £22.86 (Faulding DBL), 15-mL vial = £62.83 (APS) or £65.83 (Faulding DBL), 15-mL *Onco-vial®* = £72.41 (Faulding DBL), 45-mL vial = £187.61 (APS) or £197.48 (Faulding DBL), 45-mL *Onco-vial®* = £217.23 (Faulding DBL), 60-mL vial = £260.00 (Faulding DBL)
Available from APS, Faulding DBL

Paraplatin® (Bristol-Myers Squibb) PoM
Injection, carboplatin, net price 5-mL vial = £22.86, 15-mL vial = £65.83, 45-mL vial = £197.48, 60-mL vial = £263.31

CISPLATIN

Indications: see notes above
Cautions: see section 8.1 and notes above; renal impairment (Appendix 3); **interactions:** Appendix 1 (platinum compounds)
Side-effects: see section 8.1 and notes above

Cisplatin (Non-proprietary) PoM
Injection, cisplatin 1 mg/mL. Net price 10-mL vial = £5.85; 50-mL vial = £26.70 (APS) or £28.11 (Bristol-Myers Squibb, Faulding DBL); 100-mL vial = £52.86 (APS) or £55.64 (Bristol-Myers Squibb, Faulding DBL)
Available from Faulding DBL, APS
Injection, powder for reconstitution, cisplatin, net price 50-mg vial = £17.00
Available from Pharmacia

OXALIPLATIN

Indications: metastatic colorectal cancer in combination with fluorouracil and folinic acid
Cautions: see section 8.1 and notes above; renal impairment (Appendix 3); **interactions:** Appendix 1 (platinum compounds)
Contra-indications: see section 8.1; peripheral neuropathy with functional impairment
Side-effects: see section 8.1 and notes above

Eloxatin® (Sanofi-Synthelabo) ▼ PoM
Injection, powder for reconstitution, oxaliplatin, net price 50-mg vial = £165.00, 100-mg vial = £330.00

Porfimer sodium

Porfimer sodium has been licensed for photodynamic therapy of non-small cell lung cancer and obstructing oesophageal cancer. It accumulates in malignant tissue and is activated by laser light to produce its cytotoxic effect.

PORFIMER SODIUM

Indications: non-small cell lung cancer; oeso-phageal cancer; see notes above

Cautions: see section 8.1; avoid exposure of skin and eyes to direct sunlight or bright indoor light for at least 30 days

Contra-indications: see section 8.1; severe hepatic impairment; tracheo-oesophageal or bron-cho-oesophageal fistula; porphyria (section 9.8.2)

Side-effects: see section 8.1; photosensitivity (see Cautions above—sunscreens offer no protection), constipation

Dose: *by intravenous injection* over 3 to 5 minutes, 2 mg/kg

Note. For further information on administration and light activation, consult product literature

Photofrin® (Sinclair) ▼ PoM
Injection, powder for reconstitution, porfimer sodium, net price 15-mg vial = £154.00; 75-mg vial = £770.00

Procarbazine

Procarbazine is most often used in Hodgkin's disease, for example in MOPP (chlormethine (mustine), vincristine [*Oncovin®*], procarbazine, and prednisolone) chemotherapy. It is given *by mouth*. Toxic effects include nausea, myelosuppression, and a hypersensitivity rash preventing further use of this drug. It is a mild monoamine-oxidase inhibitor but dietary restriction is not considered necessary. Alcohol ingestion may cause a disulf-iram-like reaction.

PROCARBAZINE

Indications: see notes above

Cautions: see section 8.1 and notes above; hepatic impairment—avoid if severe; renal impairment—avoid if severe; **interactions:** Appendix 1 (procarbazine)

Side-effects: see section 8.1 and notes above

Dose: used alone, initially 50 mg daily, increased by 50 mg daily to 250–300 mg daily in divided doses; maintenance (on remission) 50–150 mg daily to cumulative total of at least 6 g

Procarbazine (Cambridge) PoM
Capsules, ivory, procarbazine (as hydrochloride) 50 mg, net price 50-cap pack = £37.44. Label: 4

Razoxane

Razoxane has limited activity in the leukaemias, and is little used.

RAZOXANE

Indications: see notes above

Cautions: see section 8.1

Side-effects: see section 8.1

Dose: acute leukaemias, 150–500 mg/m² daily for 3–5 days

Razoxane (Cambridge) PoM
Tablets, scored, razoxane 125 mg. Net price 30-tab pack = £71.01

Taxanes

Paclitaxel is a member of a group of drugs termed the taxanes. It is given by *intravenous infusion*. There is increasing evidence that paclitaxel given with carboplatin or cisplatin is the treatment of choice for ovarian cancer (see NICE guidance below); the combination is also considered appropriate for women whose ovarian cancer is initially considered inoperable. Paclitaxel is also used in the secondary treatment of metastatic breast cancer (see NICE guidance below). There is limited evidence to support its use in non-small cell lung cancer. Routine premedication with a corticosteroid, an antihistamine and a histamine H_2-receptor antagonist is recommended to prevent severe hypersensitivity reactions; hypersensitivity reactions may occur rarely despite premedication, although more commonly only bradycardia or asymptomatic hypotension occur.

Other side-effects of paclitaxel include myelosuppression, peripheral neuropathy, and cardiac conduction defects with arrhythmias (which are nearly always asymptomatic). It also causes alopecia and muscle pain; nausea and vomiting is mild to moderate.

Docetaxel is used in the treatment of advanced or metastatic breast cancer (see NICE guidance below) and non-small cell lung cancer. Docetaxel has also been licensed recently for initial chemotherapy with doxorubicin for advanced breast cancer. Its side-effects are similar to those of paclitaxel but persistent fluid retention (commonly as leg oedema that worsens during treatment) can be resistant to treatment; hypersensitivity reactions also occur. Dexamethasone by mouth for 3 days, starting on the day before each course of docetaxel, is recommended for reducing fluid retention and hypersensitivity reactions.

NICE guidance (breast cancer). The National Institute for Clinical Excellence has recommended that both docetaxel and paclitaxel should be available for the treatment of advanced breast cancer where initial cytotoxic chemotherapy (including an anthracycline) has failed or is inappropriate. The use of taxanes for adjuvant treatment of early breast cancer or for the first-line treatment of advanced breast cancer should be limited to clinical trials [but see notes above].

NICE guidance (ovarian cancer). The National Institute for Clinical Excellence has recommended that paclitaxel in combination with a platinum compound (cisplatin or carboplatin) should be the standard initial therapy for ovarian cancer following surgery [but see notes above]. Treatment of recurrent or resistant ovarian cancer with paclitaxel and platinum combination therapy is only recommended in the context of clinical trials *or* if the patient has not previously received this combination.

NICE guidance (docetaxel, paclitaxel, gemcitabine and vinorelbine for non-small cell lung cancer)—see p. 413

DOCETAXEL

Indications: with doxorubicin for initial chemotherapy of advanced or metastatic breast cancer; advanced or metastatic breast cancer where adjuvant cytotoxic chemotherapy (with anthracycline or alkylating drug) has failed; advanced or metastatic non-small cell lung cancer where first-line chemotherapy has failed

Cautions: see section 8.1 and notes above; hepatic impairment (Appendix 2); **interactions:** Appendix 1 (docetaxel)

Side-effects: see section 8.1 and notes above

Taxotere® (Aventis Pharma) [PoM]

Concentrate for intravenous infusion, docetaxel 40 mg/mL. Net price 0.5-mL vial = £175.00, 2-mL vial = £575.00 (both with diluent) (hosp. only)

PACLITAXEL

Indications: primary ovarian cancer (advanced or residual disease following laparotomy) in combination with cisplatin; metastatic ovarian cancer where standard platinum-containing therapy has failed; metastatic breast carcinoma where standard anthracycline-containing therapy has failed or is inappropriate; non-small cell lung cancer (in combination with cisplatin) when surgery or radiation therapy not appropriate

Cautions: see section 8.1 and notes above; **interactions:** Appendix 1 (paclitaxel)

Contra-indications: see section 8.1 and notes above; severe hepatic impairment

Side-effects: see section 8.1 and notes above

Taxol® (Bristol-Myers Squibb) ▼ [PoM]

Concentrate for intravenous infusion, paclitaxel 6 mg/mL, net price 5-mL vial = £124.79, 16.7-mL vial = £374.00, 50-mL vial = £1122.00 (hosp. only)

Excipients: include polyoxyl castor oil (risk of anaphylaxis, see Excipients, p. 2)

Topoisomerase I inhibitors

Irinotecan and topotecan inhibit topoisomerase I, an enzyme involved in DNA replication.

Irinotecan is given by intravenous infusion in metastatic colorectal cancer in combination with fluorouracil and folinic acid or when treatment containing fluorouracil has failed.

Topotecan is given by intravenous infusion in metastatic ovarian cancer when first-line or subsequent therapy has failed.

In addition to dose-limiting myelosuppression, side-effects of irinotecan and topotecan include gastro-intestinal effects (delayed diarrhoea requiring prompt treatment may follow irinotecan treatment), asthenia, alopecia, and anorexia.

NICE guidance (topotecan). The National Institute for Clinical Excellence has recommended that topotecan be considered as one option for the second-line (or subsequent) treatment of advanced ovarian cancer where the disease is initially refractory to first-line platinum-based combination therapy or it has become resistant after successive courses of platinum-based combination therapy.

Topotecan is not recommended in patients with poor performance status (Eastern Cooperative Oncology Group score 3 or worse), bowel obstruction, or after previous exposure to topotecan or another drug in the same class.

IRINOTECAN HYDROCHLORIDE

Indications: metastatic colorectal cancer in combination with fluorouracil and folinic acid or where treatment containing fluorouracil has failed

Cautions: see section 8.1 and notes above; raised plasma-bilirubin concentration (see under Contra-indications and Appendix 2)

Contra-indications: see section 8.1 and notes above, also chronic inflammatory bowel disease; bowel obstruction; plasma bilirubin concentration more than 1.5 times the upper limit of reference range; avoid conception for at least 3 months after cessation of treatment

Side-effects: see section 8.1 and notes above; also acute cholinergic syndrome (with early diarrhoea) and delayed diarrhoea (consult product literature)

Campto® (Rhône-Poulenc Rorer) [PoM]

Concentrate for intravenous infusion, irinotecan hydrochloride 20 mg/mL, net price 2-mL vial = £53.00; 5-mL vial = £130.00

TOPOTECAN

Indications: metastatic ovarian cancer where first-line or subsequent therapy has failed

Cautions: see section 8.1 and notes above

Contra-indications: see section 8.1 and notes above

Side-effects: see section 8.1 and notes above

Hycamtin® (Merck) ▼ [PoM]

Intravenous infusion, powder for reconstitution, topotecan (as hydrochloride), net price 1-mg vial = £105.00; 4-mg vial = £312.50

Trastuzumab

Trastuzumab is a monoclonal antibody for the treatment of metastatic breast cancer in patients whose tumours overexpress the human epidermal growth factor receptor 2 (HER2). Trastuzumab treatment should be reserved for patients who have previously received appropriate chemotherapy or in whom such treatment is inappropriate. Resuscitation facilities should be available and treatment should be initiated by a specialist.

USE WITH ANTHRACYCLINES. Concomitant use of trastuzumab with anthracyclines (section 8.1.2) is associated with cardiotoxicity. The EMEA has advised that the use of anthracyclines even after stopping trastuzumab may carry a higher risk of cardiotoxicity and if possible should be avoided for up to 22 weeks. If anthracyclines need to be used, cardiac function should be monitored.

TRASTUZUMAB

Indications: see notes above and product literature

Cautions: symptomatic heart failure, history of hypertension, coronary artery disease; pregnancy (Appendix 4)

Contra-indications: severe dyspnoea at rest; breast-feeding (Appendix 5)

Side-effects: infusion-related side-effects including chills, fever, hypersensitivity reactions such as anaphylaxis, urticaria and angioedema, pulmonary events; cardiotoxicity—for details (including monitoring and management of side-effects) consult product literature; gastro-intestinal symptoms, asthenia, headache, chest pains, arthralgia, myalgia, hypotension

Herceptin® (Roche) ▼ PoM

Injection, powder for reconstitution, trastuzumab, net price 150-mg vial = £407.40. For intravenous infusion

Tretinoin

Tretinoin is licensed for the induction of remission in acute promyelocytic leukaemia. It is used in previously untreated patients as well as in those who have relapsed after standard chemotherapy or who are refractory to it.

TRETINOIN

Note. Tretinoin is the acid form of vitamin A

Indications: see notes above; acne (section 13.6.1); photodamage (section 13.8.1)

Cautions: exclude pregnancy before starting treatment and avoid pregnancy during and for at least 1 month after treatment; monitor haematological and coagulation profile, liver function, serum calcium and plasma lipids before and during treatment; increased risk of thrombo-embolism during first month of treatment; hepatic and renal impairment (Appendixes 2 and 3); **interactions:** Appendix 1 (retinoids)

Contra-indications: pregnancy (**important teratogenic risk:** see Cautions and Appendix 4) and breast-feeding

Side-effects: retinoic acid syndrome (fever, dyspnoea, acute respiratory distress, pulmonary infiltrates, pleural effusion, hyperleukocytosis, hypotension, oedema, weight gain, hepatic, renal and multi-organ failure) requires immediate treatment—consult product literature; gastro-intestinal disturbances, pancreatitis; arrhythmias, flushing, oedema; headache, benign intracranial hypertension (mainly in children—consider dose reduction if intractable headache in children), shivering, dizziness, confusion, anxiety, depression, insomnia, paraesthesia, visual and hearing disturbances; raised liver enzymes, serum creatinine and lipids; bone and chest pain, alopecia, erythema, rash, pruritus, sweating, dry skin and mucous membranes, cheilitis; thromboembolism, hypercalcaemia, and genital ulceration reported

Dose: ADULT and CHILD 45 mg/m² daily in 2 divided doses, max. duration of treatment 90 days (consult product literature for details of concomitant chemotherapy)

Vesanoid® (Roche) PoM

Capsules, yellow/brown, tretinoin 10 mg. Net price 100-cap pack = £183.36. Label: 21.

8.2 Drugs affecting the immune response

8.2.1	Antiproliferative immunosuppressants
8.2.2	Corticosteroids and other immunosuppressants
8.2.3	Rituximab and alemtuzumab
8.2.4	Interferons
8.2.5	Aldesleukin

Immunosuppressant therapy

Immunosuppressants are used to suppress rejection in organ transplant recipients and to treat a variety of chronic inflammatory and autoimmune diseases. Solid organ transplant patients are usually maintained on a corticosteroid combined with a calcineurin inhibitor (ciclosporin or tacrolimus), _or_ with an antiproliferative drug (azathioprine or mycophenolate mofetil), _or_ with both. Specialist management is required and other immunomodulators may be used to initiate treatment or to treat rejection.

IMPAIRED IMMUNE RESPONSIVENESS. Modification of tissue reactions caused by corticosteroids and other immunosuppressants may result in the rapid _spread of infection_. Corticosteroids may suppress clinical signs of infection and allow diseases such as septicaemia or tuberculosis to reach an advanced stage before being recognised—**important:** for advice on measles and chickenpox (varicella) exposure, see Immunoglobulins (section 14.5). For general comments and warnings relating to corticosteroids and immunosuppressants see section 6.3.2 (under Prednisolone).

PREGNANCY. Transplant patients immunosuppressed with azathioprine should not discontinue it on becoming pregnant; there is no evidence that azathioprine is teratogenic. There is less experience of ciclosporin in pregnancy but it does not appear to be any more harmful than azathioprine. The use of these drugs during pregnancy needs to be supervised in specialist units.
Any risk to the offspring of azathioprine-treated men is small.
Tacrolimus and mycophenolate are contra-indicated by the manufacturers in pregnancy (Appendix 4).

8.2.1 Antiproliferative immunosuppressants

Azathioprine is widely used for transplant recipients and it is also used to treat a number of autoimmune conditions, usually when corticosteroid therapy alone provides inadequate control. It is metabolised to mercaptopurine, and doses should be reduced when allopurinol is given concurrently. The predominant toxic effect is myelosuppression, although hepatic toxicity is also well recognised. Blood tests and monitoring for signs of myelosuppression are essential in long-term treatment with azathioprine. The enzyme thiopurine methyltransferase (TPMT) metabolises azathioprine; the risk of myelosuppression is increased in those with a low activity of the enzyme, particularly in the very few individuals who are homozygous for low TPMT activity.

Mycophenolate mofetil is metabolised to mycophenolic acid which has a more selective mode of action than azathioprine. It is licensed for the prophylaxis of acute rejection in renal or cardiac transplantation when used in combination with ciclosporin and corticosteroids. There is evidence that compared with similar regimens incorporating azathioprine, mycophenolate mofetil reduces the risk of acute rejection episodes; the risk of opportunistic infections (particularly due to tissue-invasive cytomegalovirus) and the occurrence of blood disorders such as leucopenia may be higher.

Cyclophosphamide and chlorambucil (section 8.1.1) are less commonly prescribed as immunosuppressants.

AZATHIOPRINE

Indications: see notes above

Cautions: monitor for toxicity throughout treatment; monitor full blood count weekly (more frequently with higher doses or if hepatic or renal impairment) for first 4 weeks (manufacturer advises weekly monitoring for 8 weeks but evidence of practical value unsatisfactory), thereafter reduce frequency of monitoring to at least every 3 months; hepatic impairment (Appendix 2); renal impairment (Appendix 3); reduce dose in elderly; pregnancy (see section 8.2)—treatment should not generally be initiated during pregnancy; **interactions:** Appendix 1 (azathioprine)

BONE MARROW SUPPRESSION. Patients should be warned to report immediately any signs or symptoms of bone marrow suppression e.g. inexplicable bruising or bleeding, infection

Contra-indications: hypersensitivity to azathioprine or mercaptopurine

Side-effects: hypersensitivity reactions (including malaise, dizziness, vomiting, diarrhoea, fever, rigors, myalgia, arthralgia, disturbed liver function, cholestatic jaundice, arrhythmias, rash, hypotension and interstitial nephritis—calling for immediate and permanent withdrawal); dose-related bone marrow suppression (see also Cautions); hair loss and increased susceptibility to infections and colitis in patients also receiving corticosteroids; nausea; rarely pancreatitis and pneumonitis

Dose: *by mouth, or* (if oral administration not possible—intravenous solution very irritant, see below) *by intravenous injection* over at least 1 minute (followed by 50 mL sodium chloride intravenous infusion), *or by intravenous infusion*, autoimmune conditions, 1–3 mg/kg daily, adjusted according to response (consider withdrawal if no improvement in 3 months)

Suppression of transplant rejection, initially up to 5 mg/kg then 1–4 mg/kg daily according to response

Note. Intravenous injection is alkaline and very irritant, intravenous route should therefore be used **only** if oral route not feasible, see also Appendix 6

Azathioprine (Non-proprietary) PoM

Tablets, azathioprine 25 mg, net price 28-tab pack = £9.29; 50 mg, 56-tab pack = £9.97. Label: 21

Available from Alpharma, Ashbourne (*Immunoprin®*), Hillcross, IVAX, Kent, Opus (*Oprisine®*), Penn (*Azamune®*)

Imuran® (GlaxoWellcome) PoM

Tablets, both f/c, azathioprine 25 mg (orange), net price 100-tab pack = £39.35; 50 mg (yellow), 100-tab pack = £65.61. Label: 21

Injection, powder for reconstitution, azathioprine (as sodium salt). Net price 50-mg vial = £16.54

MYCOPHENOLATE MOFETIL

Indications: prophylaxis of acute renal, cardiac, or hepatic transplant rejection (in combination with ciclosporin and corticosteroids) under specialist supervision

Cautions: full blood counts every week for 4 weeks then twice a month for 2 months then every month in the first year (possibly interrupt treatment if neutropenia develops); elderly (increased risk of infection, gastro-intestinal haemorrhage and pulmonary oedema); children (higher incidence of side-effects may call for temporary reduction of dose or interruption); active serious gastro-intestinal disease (risk of haemorrhage, ulceration and perforation); delayed graft function; increased susceptibility to skin cancer (avoid exposure to strong sunlight); **interactions:** Appendix 1 (mycophenolate mofetil)

BONE MARROW SUPPRESSION. Patients should be warned to report immediately any signs or symptoms of bone marrow suppression e.g. infection and inexplicable bruising or bleeding

Contra-indications: pregnancy (exclude before starting and avoid for 6 weeks after discontinuation) (Appendix 4); breast-feeding (Appendix 5)

Side-effects: diarrhoea, vomiting, constipation, nausea, dyspepsia, pancreatitis, abdominal pain; hypertension, oedema, chest pain; dyspnoea, cough, rhinitis; dizziness, insomnia, headache, tremor; infection (including cytomegalovirus viraemia, herpes simplex, candidiasis, aspergillosis, sepsis, urinary-tract infection and pneumonia); leucopenia (see also Cautions), anaemia, thrombocytopenia, leucocytosis, polycythaemia; electrolyte disturbances, hyperglycaemia, hypercholesterolaemia; asthenia; renal damage, haematuria; acne; lymphoproliferative disease; less frequently, gastro-intestinal perforation, abnormal liver-function tests, hepatitis, gingivitis, mouth ulceration, haemorrhage, influenza-like syndrome, hypotension, arrhythmias, tachycardia, hypoglycaemia, weight gain; allergic reactions, benign neoplasm of skin and skin carcinoma reported

Dose: renal transplantation, *by mouth*, 1 g twice daily starting within 72 hours of transplantation *or by intravenous infusion*, 1 g twice daily starting within 24 hours of transplantation for up to max. 14 days (then transfer to oral therapy); CHILD and ADOLESCENT 2–18 years (and body-surface area over 1.25 m²) 600 mg/m² twice daily (max. 2 g daily)

Cardiac transplantation, *by mouth*, 1.5 g twice daily starting within 5 days of transplantation

Hepatic transplantation, *by intravenous infusion*, 1 g twice daily starting within 24 hours of transplantation for 4 days (up to max. 14 days), then *by mouth*, 1.5 g twice daily as soon as is tolerated

CellCept® (Roche) ▼ PoM

Capsules, blue/brown, mycophenolate mofetil
250 mg, net price 100-cap pack = £113.41

Tablets, lavender, mycophenolate mofetil 500 mg,
net price 50-tab pack = £113.41

Intravenous infusion, powder for reconstitution,
mycophenolate mofetil (as hydrochloride), net
price 500-mg vial = £9.69

8.2.2 Corticosteroids and other immunosuppressants

Prednisolone (section 6.3.2) is widely used in
oncology. It has a marked antitumour effect in acute
lymphoblastic leukaemia, Hodgkin's disease, and
the non-Hodgkin lymphomas. It is also active in
hormone-sensitive breast cancer and may cause
useful disease regression. Finally, it has a role in the
palliation of symptomatic end-stage malignant disease when it may enhance appetite and produce a
sense of well-being (see also Prescribing in Palliative Care).

The corticosteroids are also powerful immunosuppressants. They are used to prevent organ transplant rejection, and in high dose to treat rejection
episodes.

Ciclosporin (cyclosporin), a calcineurin inhibitor, is a potent immunosuppressant which is virtually non-myelotoxic but markedly nephrotoxic. It
has found particular use in the field of organ and tissue transplantation, for prevention of graft rejection
following bone marrow, kidney, liver, pancreas,
heart, lung, and heart-lung transplantation, and for
prophylaxis and treatment of graft-versus-host disease.

Tacrolimus is also a calcineurin inhibitor.
Although not chemically related to ciclosporin it
has a similar mode of action and side-effects, but
the incidence of neurotoxicity and nephrotoxicity
appears to be greater; cardiomyopathy has also
been reported. Disturbance of glucose metabolism
also appears to be significant; hypertrichosis
appears to be less of a problem than with
ciclosporin.

Sirolimus is a potent non-calcineurin inhibiting
immunosuppressant introduced recently for renal
transplantation. It can cause hyperlipidaemia.

Basiliximab and **daclizumab** are monoclonal
antibodies that prevent T-lymphocyte proliferation;
they are used for prophylaxis of acute rejection in
allogenic renal transplantation. They are given with
ciclosporin and corticosteroid immunosuppression
regimens; their use should be confined to specialist
centres.

BASILIXIMAB

Indications: see notes above

Contra-indications: pregnancy (Appendix 4) and
breast-feeding

Side-effects: severe hypersensitivity reactions
reported rarely; for side-effects of regimen see
under Ciclosporin (below) and Prednisolone (section 6.3.2)

Dose: *by intravenous infusion*, 20 mg within 2
hours before transplant surgery and a further
20 mg 4 days after surgery—withhold second
dose if postoperative complications such as graft
loss occur

Simulect® (Novartis) PoM

Injection, powder for reconstitution, basiliximab,
net price 20-mg vial (with water for injections) =
£842.38. For intravenous infusion

CICLOSPORIN
(Cyclosporin)

Indications: see notes above, and under Dose;
atopic dermatitis and psoriasis (section 13.5.2);
rheumatoid arthritis (section 10.1.3)

Cautions: monitor kidney function—dose dependent increase in serum creatinine and urea during
first few weeks may necessitate dose reduction in
transplant patients (exclude rejection if kidney
transplant) or discontinuation in non-transplant
patients; monitor liver function (dosage adjustment based on bilirubin and liver enzymes may
be needed); monitor blood pressure—discontinue
if hypertension develops that cannot be controlled
by antihypertensives; hyperuricaemia; monitor
serum potassium especially in marked renal dysfunction (and avoid high dietary potassium);
measure blood lipids before treatment and thereafter as appropriate; pregnancy (see p. 421) and
breast-feeding (Appendix 5); porphyria (section
9.8.2); use with tacrolimus specifically contra-
indicated and apart from specialist use in transplant patients preferably avoid other immunosuppressants with the exception of corticosteroids
(increased risk of infection and lymphoma);
interactions: Appendix 1 (ciclosporin)

ADDITIONAL CAUTIONS IN NEPHROTIC SYNDROME.
Contra-indicated in uncontrolled hypertension, uncontrolled infections, and malignancy; reduce dose by 25–
50% if serum creatinine more than 30% above baseline
on more than one measurement; in renal impairment initially 2.5 mg/kg daily; in long-term management, perform renal biopsies at yearly intervals

ADDITIONAL CAUTIONS. Atopic Dermatitis and Psoriasis, section 13.5.2; Rheumatoid Arthritis, section
10.1.3

Side-effects: dose-dependent increase in serum
creatinine and urea during first few weeks (see
also under Cautions); less commonly renal struc-
tural changes on long-term administration; also
hypertrichosis, tremor, hypertension (especially
in heart transplant patients), hepatic dysfunction,
fatigue, gingival hypertrophy, gastro-intestinal
disturbances, burning sensation in hands and feet
(usually during first week); *occasionally* headache, rash (possibly allergic), mild anaemia,
hyperkalaemia, hyperuricaemia, gout, hypomagnesaemia, hypercholesterolaemia, weight
increase, oedema, pancreatitis, neuropathy, confusion, paraesthesia, convulsions, dysmenorrhoea
or amenorrhoea; muscle weakness, cramps,
myopathy, gynaecomastia (in patients receiving
concomitant spironolactone), colitis, and cortical
blindness also reported; thrombocytopenia
(sometimes with haemolytic uraemic syndrome)
also reported; incidence of malignancies and lymphoproliferative disorders similar to that with
conventional immunosuppressive therapy

Dose: organ transplantation, used alone, ADULT
and CHILD over 3 months 10–15 mg/kg *by mouth*
4–12 hours before transplantation followed by
10–15 mg/kg daily for 1–2 weeks postoperatively
then reduced gradually to 2–6 mg/kg daily for
maintenance (dose should be adjusted according
to blood-ciclosporin concentration and renal

function'), dose lower if given concomitantly with other immunosuppressant therapy (e.g. corticosteroids); if necessary one-third corresponding oral dose can be given *by intravenous infusion* over 2–6 hours

Bone-marrow transplantation, prevention and treatment of graft-versus-host disease, ADULT and CHILD over 3 months 3–5 mg/kg daily *by intravenous infusion* over 2–6 hours from day before transplantation to 2 weeks postoperatively (or 12.5–15 mg/kg daily *by mouth*) then 12.5 mg/kg daily *by mouth* for 3–6 months then tailed off (may take up to a year after transplantation)

Nephrotic syndrome, *by mouth*, 5 mg/kg daily in 2 divided doses; CHILD 6 mg/kg daily in 2 divided doses; maintenance treatment reduce to lowest effective dose according to proteinuria and serum creatinine measurements; discontinue after 3 months if no improvement in glomerulonephritis or glomerulosclerosis (after 6 months in membranous glomerulonephritis)

CONVERSION Any conversion between brands should be undertaken very carefully and the manufacturer contacted for further information. Currently only *Neoral®* and *SangCya®* remain available for oral use; *Sandimmun®* capsules and oral solution are available on named-patient basis only for patients who cannot be transferred to another brand of oral ciclosporin

> Because of differences in bioavailability, the brand of ciclosporin to be dispensed should be specified by the prescriber

Neoral® (Novartis) PoM
Capsules, ciclosporin 10 mg (yellow/white), net price 30-cap pack = £8.22; 25 mg (blue/grey), 30-cap pack = £20.54; 50 mg (yellow/white), 30-cap pack = £40.22; 100 mg (blue/grey), 30-cap pack = £76.33. Counselling, administration

Oral solution, yellow, sugar-free, ciclosporin 100 mg/mL, net price 50 mL = £114.38. Counselling, administration

COUNSELLING. Total daily dose should be taken in 2 divided doses. Avoid grapefruit or grapefruit juice for 1 hour before dose.

Mix solution with orange juice (or squash) or apple juice (to improve taste) or with water immediately before taking (and rinse with more to ensure total dose). Do not mix with grapefruit juice. Keep medicine measure away from other liquids (including water)

Sandimmun® (Novartis) PoM
Concentrate for intravenous infusion (oily), ciclosporin 50 mg/mL. To be diluted before use. Net price 1-mL amp = £1.94; 5-mL amp = £9.17

Excipients: include polyoxyl castor oil (risk of anaphylaxis, see Excipients, p. 2)

Note. Observe for at least 30 minutes after starting infusion and at frequent intervals thereafter

SangCya® (Sangstat) PoM
Oral solution, sugar-free, ciclosporin 100 mg/mL, net price 50 mL = £94.36. Counselling, administration

COUNSELLING. Total daily dose should be taken in 2 divided doses. Avoid grapefruit or grapefruit juice for 1 hour before dose.

To mask taste, mix solution with cold milk, cold chocolate drink, cola or orange juice immediately before taking (and rinse with more to ensure total dose). Do not mix with grapefruit juice. Keep medicine measure away from other liquids (including water)

DACLIZUMAB

Indications: see notes above

Contra-indications: pregnancy and breast-feeding

Side-effects: severe hypersensitivity reactions reported rarely; for side-effects of regimen see under Ciclosporin (above) and Prednisolone (section 6.3.2)

Dose: *by intravenous infusion*, 1 mg/kg within the 24-hour period before transplantation, then 1 mg/kg every 14 days for a total of 5 doses

Zenapax® (Roche) ▼ PoM
Concentrate for intravenous infusion, daclizumab 5 mg/mL, net price 5-mL = £240.52

SIROLIMUS

Indications: prophylaxis of organ rejection in kidney allograft recipients (initially in combination with ciclosporin and corticosteroid, then with corticosteroid only); see also under Dose

Cautions: monitor kidney function when given with ciclosporin; Afro-Caribbean patients may require higher doses; hepatic impairment (Appendix 2); **interactions:** Appendix 1 (sirolimus)

Contra-indications: pregnancy (Appendix 4); breast-feeding (Appendix 5)

Side-effects: lymphocele, abdominal pain, diarrhoea, tachycardia, anaemia, thrombocytopenia, hyperlipidaemias (including hypercholesterolaemia, hypertriglyceridaemia), increase in serum creatinine in patients also receiving ciclosporin, hypokalaemia, arthralgia, acne; less commonly, epistaxis, impaired healing, increased susceptibility to infection, stomatitis, leucopenia, thrombotic thrombocytopenic purpura, bone necrosis, rash, pyelonephritis; rarely, pancreatitis, pneumonitis, susceptibility to lymphoma and other malignancies particularly of the skin

Dose: initially 6 mg, after surgery, then 2 mg once daily (dose adjusted according to blood-sirolimus concentration) in combination with ciclosporin and corticosteroid for 2–3 months (sirolimus given 4 hours after ciclosporin); ciclosporin should then be withdrawn over 4–8 weeks (if not possible, sirolimus should be discontinued and an alternate immunosuppressive regimen used)

Note. Pre-dose ('trough') blood-sirolimus concentration (using chromatographic assay) when used with ciclosporin should be 4–12 micrograms/litre; after withdrawal of ciclosporin pre-dose blood-sirolimus concentration should be 12–20 micrograms/litre; close monitoring of blood-sirolimus concentration required in hepatic impairment, during treatment with potent inducers or inhibitors of metabolism and after discontinuing them

Rapamune® (Wyeth) ▼ PoM
Oral solution, sirolimus 1 mg/mL, net price 60 mL = £148.20, 30 × 1-mL sachets = £74.10; 30 × 2-mL sachets = £148.20. Counselling, administration

COUNSELLING. Mix solution with at least 60 mL water or orange juice in a glass or plastic container immediately before taking; refill container with at least 120 mL and drink immediately (to ensure total dose). Do not mix with any other liquids

TACROLIMUS

Indications: primary immunosuppression in liver and kidney allograft recipients and allograft rejection resistant to conventional immunosuppressive regimens; see also notes above

Cautions: see under Ciclosporin; also monitor ECG (**important:** also echocardiography, see CSM warning below), visual status, blood glucose, haematological and neurological parameters; **interactions:** Appendix 1 (tacrolimus)

DRIVING. May affect performance of skilled tasks (e.g. driving)

Contra-indications: hypersensitivity to macrolides; pregnancy (exclude before starting—if contraception needed non-hormonal methods should be used), breast-feeding; avoid concurrent administration with ciclosporin (care if patient has previously received ciclosporin)

Side-effects: include gastro-intestinal disturbances such as nausea, dyspepsia and ulceration; hypertension, angina, tachycardia, pleural and pericardial effusion, less frequently hypotension, arrhythmias, rarely ventricular or septal hypertrophy, cardiomyopathy (**important:** see CSM warning below) and pericarditis; tremor, headache, insomnia, anxiety, depression, encephalopathy and rarely agitation, drowsiness, hallucinations, dizziness, decreased reflexes, migraine, convulsions, confusion, amblyopia, cataract, retinopathy, photophobia, deafness and tinnitus; haematological effects including leucocytosis, leucopenia, aplastic and haemolytic anaemia and rarely thrombocytopaenia; increased serum creatinine and urea, less frequently kidney damage and renal failure; electrolyte disturbances including hypophosphataemia, hypercalcaemia, hyperkalaemia (occasionally hypokalaemia), hyperuricaemia, thyroid disorders, altered acid-base balance and glucose metabolism; pruritus, erythema, alopecia, sweating, hirsutism, photosensitivity; allergic reactions including anaphylaxis; gynaecomastia, oedema, hepatic dysfunction, cirrhosis, pancreatitis, weight and appetite changes, isolated cases of respiratory failure and pulmonary fibrosis

CSM Warning. Cardiomyopathy has been reported in children given tacrolimus after transplantation. Patients using the drug should be monitored carefully by echocardiography for hypertrophic changes; dose reduction or discontinuation should be considered if these occur

Dose: liver transplantation, starting 6 hours after transplantation, *by mouth*, 100–200 micrograms/kg daily in 2 divided doses *or by intravenous infusion* over 24 hours, 10–50 micrograms/kg; CHILD *by mouth*, 300 micrograms/kg daily in 2 divided doses *or by intravenous infusion* over 24 hours, 50 micrograms/kg

Renal transplantation, starting within 24 hours of transplantation, *by mouth*, 150–300 micrograms/kg daily in 2 divided doses *or by intravenous infusion* over 24 hours, 50–100 micrograms/kg; CHILD *by mouth*, 300 micrograms/kg daily in 2 divided doses *or by intravenous infusion* over 24 hours, 100 micrograms/kg

Maintenance treatment, dose adjusted according to response

Prograf® (Fujisawa) PoM

Capsules, tacrolimus 500 micrograms (yellow), net price 50-cap pack = £71.56; 1 mg (white), 50-cap pack = £92.93, 100-cap pack = £185.86; 5 mg (greyish-red), 50-cap pack = £371.85. Label: 23, counselling, driving

Concentrate for intravenous infusion, tacrolimus 5 mg/mL. To be diluted before use. Net price 1-mL amp = £67.67

Excipients: include polyoxyl castor oil (risk of anaphylaxis, see Excipients, p. 2)

8.2.3 Rituximab and alemtuzumab

Rituximab, a monoclonal antibody which causes lysis of B lymphocytes, is licensed for the treatment of chemotherapy-resistant advanced follicular lymphoma. Full resuscitation facilities should be at hand and as with other cytotoxics, treatment should be undertaken under the close supervision of a specialist.

Rituximab should be used with caution in patients receiving cardiotoxic chemotherapy or with a history of cardiovascular disease because exacerbation of angina, arrhythmia, and heart failure have been reported. Transient hypotension occurs frequently during infusion and antihypertensives may need to be withheld for 12 hours before infusion.

Infusion-related side-effects (including cytokine release syndrome) are reported commonly with rituximab and occur predominantly during the first infusion; they include fever and chills, nausea and vomiting, allergic reactions (such as rash, pruritus, angioedema, bronchospasm and dyspnoea), flushing and tumour pain. Patients should be given an analgesic and an antihistamine before each dose of rituximab to reduce the incidence of these effects. Premedication with a corticosteroid should also be considered. The infusion may have to be stopped temporarily and the infusion-related effects treated—consult product literature for appropriate management. Evidence of pulmonary infiltration and features of tumour lysis syndrome should be sought if infusion-related effects occur.

Fatalities following **severe** cytokine release syndrome (characterised by severe dyspnoea) and associated with features of tumour lysis syndrome have occurred 1–2 hours after infusion of rituximab. Patients with a high tumour burden as well as those with pulmonary insufficiency or infiltration are at increased risk and should be monitored **very closely** (and a slower rate of infusion considered).

Alemtuzumab, another monoclonal antibody that causes lysis of B lymphocytes, is licensed for use in patients with chronic lymphocytic leukaemia which has failed to respond completely or partially to treatment with an alkylating drug, or which has remitted for only a short period (less than 6 months) following fludarabine treatment. In common with rituximab, it causes infusion-related side-effects including cytokine release syndrome (see above).

ALEMTUZUMAB

Indications: see notes above

Cautions: see notes above—for full details (including monitoring) consult product literature

Contra-indications: pregnancy (Appendix 4) and

breast-feeding (Appendix 5); for full details consult product literature

Side-effects: see notes above—for full details (including monitoring and management of side-effects) consult product literature

Dose: consult product literature

MabCampath® (Schering Health) ▼ PoM
Concentrate for intravenous infusion, alemtuzumab 10 mg/mL, net price 3-mL amp = £283.33

RITUXIMAB

Indications: see notes above
Cautions: see notes above—but for full details (including monitoring) consult product literature; pregnancy (Appendix 4)
Contra-indications: breast-feeding
Side-effects: see notes above—but for full details (including monitoring and management of side-effects) consult product literature

MabThera® (Roche) ▼ PoM
Concentrate for intravenous infusion, rituximab 10 mg/mL, net price 10-mL vial = £174.63, 50-mL vial = £873.15

8.2.4 Other immunomodulating drugs

Interferon alfa

Interferon alfa (formerly called leucocyte interferon or lymphoblastoid interferon) has shown some antitumour effect in certain lymphomas and solid tumours. Interferon alfa preparations are also used in the treatment of chronic hepatitis B and chronic hepatitis C (section 5.3). Side-effects are dose-related, but commonly include anorexia, nausea, influenza-like symptoms, and lethargy. Ocular side-effects and depression (including suicidal behaviour) have also been reported. Myelosuppression may occur, particularly affecting granulocyte counts. Cardiovascular problems (hypotension, hypertension, and arrhythmias), nephrotoxicity and hepatotoxicity have been reported. Other side-effects include hypersensitivity reactions, thyroid abnormalities, hyperglycaemia, alopecia, psoriasiform rash, confusion, coma and seizures (usually with high doses in the elderly).

A polyethylene glycol-conjugated ('pegylated') derivative of interferon alfa-2b, **peginterferon alfa-2b** has been introduced recently; pegylation prolongs the persistence of the interferon in the blood. It is licensed for use in the treatment of chronic hepatitis C, ideally in combination with ribavirin (see section 5.3)

INTERFERON ALFA

Indications: see under preparations
Cautions: consult product literature; **interactions:** Appendix 1 (interferons)
Contra-indications: consult product literature; avoid injections containing benzyl alcohol in neonates (see under preparations below)
Side-effects: see notes above and consult product literature
Dose: consult product literature

IntronA® (Schering-Plough) PoM
Injection, interferon alfa-2b (rbe) 10 million units/mL, net price 2.5-mL vial = £135.00. For subcutaneous or intravenous injection
Injection, powder for reconstitution, interferon alfa-2b (rbe), net price 1-million unit vial = £5.40; 3-million unit vial = £16.20; 5-million unit vial = £27.00; 10-million unit vial = £53.96 (all with injection equipment and water for injections). For subcutaneous and intravenous injection
Injection pen, interferon alfa-2b (rbe), net price 15 million units/mL, 1.5-mL cartridge = £97.20; 25 million units/mL, 1.5-mL cartridge = £162.00; 50 million units/mL, 1.5-mL cartridge = £324.00. For subcutaneous injection
Note. Each 1.5-mL multidose cartridge delivers 6 doses of 0.2 mL i.e. a total of 1.2 mL
For hairy cell leukaemia, follicular lymphoma, chronic myelogenous leukaemia, lymph or liver metastases of carcinoid tumour, chronic hepatitis B, chronic hepatitis C, adjunct to surgery in malignant melanoma and maintenance of remission in multiple myeloma

Roferon-A® (Roche) PoM
Injection, interferon alfa-2a (rbe). Net price 6 million units/mL, 0.5-mL (3 million-unit) prefilled syringe = £16.20; 9 million units/mL, 0.5-mL (4.5 million-unit) prefilled syringe = £24.30; 12 million units/mL, 0.5-mL (6 million-unit) prefilled syringe = £32.39; 18 million units/mL, 0.5-mL (9 million-unit) prefilled syringe = £48.59, 1-mL (18 million-unit) vial = £97.19; 30 million units/mL, 0.6-mL (18 million-unit) cartridge = £97.19, for use with *Roferon* pen device. For subcutaneous injection (cartridges, vials, and prefilled syringes) and intramuscular injection (cartridges and vials)
Excipients: include benzyl alcohol (avoid in neonates, see Excipients, p. 2)
For AIDS-related Kaposi's sarcoma, hairy cell leukaemia, chronic myelogenous leukaemia, recurrent or metastatic renal cell carcinoma, progressive cutaneous T-cell lymphoma, chronic hepatitis B and chronic hepatitis C, follicular non-Hodgkin's lymphoma, adjunct to surgery in malignant melanoma

Viraferon® (Schering-Plough) PoM
Injection, interferon alfa-2b (rbe) 6 million units/mL, net price 3-mL vial = £97.20. For subcutaneous injection
Injection pen, interferon alfa-2b (rbe), net price 15 million units/mL, 1.5-mL cartridge = £97.20; 25 million units/mL, 1.5-mL cartridge = £162.00. For subcutaneous injection
Note. 1.5-mL multidose cartridge delivers 6 doses of 0.2 mL each
For chronic hepatitis B and chronic hepatitis C

PEGINTERFERON ALFA

Indications: combined with ribavirin for chronic hepatitis C; as monotherapy if ribavirin not tolerated or contra-indicated (see section 5.3)
Cautions: consult product literature; **interactions:** Appendix 1 (interferons)
Contra-indications: consult product literature
Side-effects: see notes above and consult product literature
Dose: consult product literature

PegIntron® (Schering-Plough) ▼ PoM
Injection, powder for reconstitution, peginterferon alfa-2b (rbe), net price 50-microgram vial = £67.50, 80-microgram vial = £108.00, 100-microgram vial = £135.00, 120-microgram vial =

£162.00, 150-microgram vial = £202.50 (all with injection equipment and water for injections). For subcutaneous injection

ViraferonPeg® (Schering-Plough) ▼ [PoM]
Injection, powder for reconstitution, peginterferon alfa-2b (rbe), net price 50-microgram vial = £67.50, 80-microgram vial = £108.00, 100-microgram vial = £135.00, 120-microgram vial = £162.00, 150-microgram vial = £202.50 (all with injection equipment and water for injections). For subcutaneous injection

Interferon beta

Interferon beta (formerly called fibroblast interferon) is licensed for use in patients with *relapsing, remitting multiple sclerosis* (characterised by at least two attacks of neurological dysfunction over the previous two- or three-year period, followed by complete or incomplete recovery) who are able to walk unaided. Not all patients respond and a deterioration in the bouts has been observed in some. Interferon beta-1b is also licensed for use in patients with *secondary progressive multiple sclerosis* but its role in this condition has not been confirmed.

Interferon beta should not be used in those with a history of severe depressive illness (or of suicidal ideation), in those with inadequately controlled epilepsy, or in decompensated hepatic impairment; caution is advised in those with a history of these conditions or with cardiac disorders or myelosuppression. Most frequently reported side-effects include irritation at injection site (including inflammation, hypersensitivity, necrosis) and influenza-like symptoms (fever, chills, myalgia, or malaise) but these decrease over time; nausea and vomiting occur occasionally. Other side-effects include hypersensitivity reactions (including anaphylaxis and urticaria), raised liver enzymes (hepatitis reported rarely with interferon beta-1b), blood disorders, menstrual disorders, mood and personality changes, suicide attempts, confusion and convulsions; alopecia and thyroid dysfunction have been reported rarely with interferon beta-1b.

> **NICE guidance (interferon beta and glatiramer for multiple sclerosis)**. The National Institute for Clinical Excellence does not recommend either interferon beta or glatiramer acetate for the treatment of multiple sclerosis in the NHS in England and Wales.
>
> Patients who are currently receiving interferon beta or glatiramer acetate for multiple sclerosis, whether as routine therapy or as part of a clinical trial, should have the option to continue treatment until they and their consultant consider it appropriate to stop, having regard to the established criteria for withdrawal from treatment.

> **Provision of disease-modifying therapies for multiple sclerosis**. The Department of Health, the National Assembly for Wales, the Scottish Executive, the Northern Ireland Department of Health, Social Services & Public Safety, and the manufacturers have reached agreement on a risk-sharing scheme for the NHS supply of interferon beta and glatiramer acetate for multiple sclerosis. Health Service Circular (HSC 2002/004) explains how patients can participate in the scheme (www.doh.gov.uk/publications/coinh.html).

INTERFERON BETA

Indications: see notes above
Cautions: see notes above and consult product literature
Contra-indications: consult product literature; pregnancy (Appendix 4—advise contraceptive measures if appropriate), breast-feeding (Appendix 5)
Side-effects: see notes above and consult product literature
Dose: consult product literature

■ Interferon beta-1a

Avonex® (Biogen) ▼ [PoM]
Injection, powder for reconstitution, interferon beta-1a. Net price 30-microgram (6 million-unit) vial with diluent = £174.25. For intramuscular injection

Rebif® (Serono) [PoM]
Injection, interferon beta-1a, net price 22-microgram (6 million-unit) prefilled syringe = £58.26; 44-microgram (12 million-unit) prefilled syringe = £77.36. For subcutaneous injection

■ Interferon beta-1b

Betaferon® (Schering Health) [PoM]
Injection, powder for reconstitution, interferon beta-1b. Net price 300-microgram (9.6 million-unit) vial with diluent = £39.78. For subcutaneous injection

Aldesleukin

Aldesleukin (recombinant interleukin-2) is licensed for use by subcutaneous injection in metastatic renal cell carcinoma; it is no longer given by intravenous infusion. Aldesleukin is a very toxic drug which, although responsible for tumour shrinkage in a small proportion of patients, has not been shown to increase survival. Toxicity is universal and often severe. A common acute problem is the development of a capillary leak syndrome causing pulmonary oedema and hypotension. Bone marrow, hepatic, renal, thyroid, and CNS toxicity is also common. It is for use in **specialist units only**.
Interactions: Appendix 1 (aldesleukin)

Proleukin® (Chiron) [PoM]
Injection, powder for reconstitution, aldesleukin. Net price 18-million unit vial = £140.00
For metastatic renal cell carcinoma, **excluding** patients in whom all three of the following prognostic factors are present; performance status of Eastern Co-operative Oncology Group of 1 or greater, more than one organ with metastatic disease sites, and a period of less than 24 months between initial diagnosis of primary tumour and date of evaluation of treatment.

BCG bladder instillation

BCG (Bacillus Calmette-Guérin) is a live attenuated strain derived from *Mycobacterium bovis*. It is licensed as a bladder instillation for the treatment of primary or recurrent bladder carcinoma and for the prevention of recurrence following transurethral resection.

BACILLUS CALMETTE-GUÉRIN

Indications: see notes above; BCG immunisation (section 14.4)

Cautions: screen for active tuberculosis (contra-indicated if tuberculosis confirmed); traumatic catheterisation (delay administration until mucosal damage healed)

Contra-indications: impaired immune response, HIV infection, urinary-tract infection, tuberculosis, fever of unknown origin; pregnancy and breast-feeding

Side-effects: cystitis, dysuria, urinary frequency, haematuria, malaise, fever, influenza-like syndrome; also systemic BCG infection (with fatalities)—consult product literature; rarely hypersensitivity reactions (such as arthralgia and rash), orchitis, transient urethral obstruction, bladder contracture, renal abscess; ocular symptoms reported

Dose: consult product literature

ImmuCyst® (Cambridge) ▼ PoM
Bladder instillation, freeze-dried powder containing attenuated *Mycobacterium bovis* prepared from the Connaught strain of bacillus of Calmette and Guérin, net price 81-mg vial = £89.00

OncoTICE® (Organon) ▼ PoM
Bladder instillation, freeze-dried powder containing attenuated *Mycobacterium bovis* prepared from the TICE strain of bacillus of Calmette and Guérin, net price 12.5-mg vial = £80.00

Glatiramer acetate

Glatiramer is an immunomodulating drug comprising synthetic polypeptides. It is licensed for reducing the frequency of relapses in ambulatory patients with relapsing-remitting multiple sclerosis who have had at least one clinical relapse in the past two years. Initiation of treatment with glatiramer should be supervised by a specialist.

> **NICE guidance (interferon beta and glatiramer for multiple sclerosis)**—see p. 427

> **Provision of disease-modifying therapies for multiple sclerosis**—see p. 427

GLATIRAMER ACETATE

Indications: see notes above

Cautions: cardiac disorders; renal impairment; pregnancy (Appendix 4) and breast-feeding (Appendix 5)

Side-effects: flushing, chest pain, palpitations, tachycardia, and dyspnoea may occur within minutes of injection; injection site reactions; nausea, peripheral and face oedema, syncope, asthenia, headache, tremor, sweating, lymphadenopathy, hypertonia, arthralgia, rash; convulsions, hypersensitivity reactions such as anaphylaxis, bronchospasm and urticaria reported rarely

Dose: *by subcutaneous injection*, ADULT over 18 years, 20 mg daily

Copaxone® (Teva) ▼ PoM
Injection, powder for reconstitution, glatiramer acetate, net price 20-mg vial with diluent = £18.22

Hormonal manipulation has an important role in the treatment of breast, prostate, and endometrial cancer, and a more marginal role in the treatment of hypernephroma. These treatments are not curative, but may provide excellent palliation of symptoms in selected patients, sometimes for a period of years. Tumour response, and treatment toxicity should be carefully monitored and treatment changed if progression occurs or side-effects exceed benefit.

8.3.1 Oestrogens

Diethylstilbestrol (stilboestrol) is rarely used to treat prostate cancer because of its side-effects. It is occasionally used in postmenopausal women with breast cancer. Toxicity is common and dose-related side-effects include nausea, fluid retention, and venous and arterial thrombosis. Impotence and gynaecomastia always occur in men, and withdrawal bleeding may be a problem in women. Hypercalcaemia and bone pain may also occur in breast cancer.

Fosfestrol is also used for prostate cancer; it is activated by the enzyme acid phosphatase to produce diethylstilbestrol. Side-effects are as for diethylstilbestrol; in addition, perineal pain may complicate intravenous use.

Ethinylestradiol (ethinyloestradiol) is the most potent oestrogen available; unlike other oestrogens it is only slowly metabolised in the liver. It is used in breast cancer.

DIETHYLSTILBESTROL
(Stilboestrol)

Indications: see notes above

Cautions: cardiovascular disease; hepatic impairment

Side-effects: sodium retention with oedema, thromboembolism, jaundice, feminising effects in men; see also notes above

Dose: breast cancer, 10–20 mg daily
Prostate cancer, 1–3 mg daily

Diethylstilbestrol (Non-proprietary) PoM
Tablets, diethylstilbestrol 1 mg, net price 56 = £52.79; 5 mg, 28 = £39.60
Available from APS (*Apstil®*)

ETHINYLESTRADIOL

(Ethinyloestradiol)

Indications: see notes above; other indications (section 6.4.1.1)

Cautions: see under Diethylstilbestrol and notes above

Side-effects: see under Diethylstilbestrol and notes above

Dose: breast cancer, 1–3 mg daily

Preparations

Section 6.4.1.1

FOSFESTROL TETRASODIUM

Indications: prostate cancer

Cautions: see under Diethylstilbestrol and notes above

Side-effects: see under Diethylstilbestrol and notes above; also nausea and vomiting; after intravenous injection, perineal irritation and pain in bony metastases

Dose: *by slow intravenous injection*, 0.6–1.2 g daily for at least 5 days; maintenance 300 mg 1–4 times weekly

By mouth, maintenance, initially up to 240 mg 3 times daily for 7 days then reducing over 14 days to 120–360 mg daily in divided doses

Honvan® (ASTA Medica) PoM

Tablets, f/c, fosfestrol tetrasodium 120 mg, net price 100-tab pack = £14.81

Note. Fosfestrol tetrasodium 100 mg tablets have now been replaced by 120 mg tablets

Injection, fosfestrol tetrasodium 60 mg/mL, net price 5-mL amp = £1.43

8.3.2   Progestogens

Progestogens are used largely as second- or third-line therapy in breast cancer. They are also used to treat endometrial cancer and renal cell carcinoma, but are little used for prostate cancer. **Medroxyprogesterone** or **megestrol** are usually chosen and can be given orally; high-dose or parenteral treatment cannot be recommended. Side-effects are mild but may include nausea, fluid retention, and weight gain.

GESTONORONE CAPROATE

(Gestronol Hexanoate)

Indications: see notes above; benign prostatic hypertrophy

Cautions: see section 6.4.1.2 and notes above

Contra-indications: see section 6.4.1.2 and notes above

Side-effects: see section 6.4.1.2 and notes above

Dose: endometrial cancer, *by intramuscular injection*, 200–400 mg every 5–7 days

Benign prostatic hypertrophy, *by intramuscular injection*, 200 mg every week, increased to 300–400 mg every week if necessary

Gestonorone Caproate (Non-proprietary) PoM

Injection (oily), gestonorone caproate 100 mg/mL. Net price 2-mL amp = £12.50

Available from Cambridge

MEDROXYPROGESTERONE ACETATE

Indications: see notes above; other indications (section 6.4.1.2)

Cautions: see section 6.4.1.2 and notes above; **interactions:** Appendix 1 (progestogens)

Contra-indications: see section 6.4.1.2 and notes above

Side-effects: see section 6.4.1.2 and notes above; glucocorticoid effects at high dose may lead to a cushingoid syndrome

Dose: see preparations below

> *Farlutal®* and *Provera®* tablets may **not** be bioequivalent

Farlutal® (Pharmacia) PoM

Tablets, both scored, medroxyprogesterone acetate 100 mg, net price 20 = £7.75; 250 mg, 50 = £48.45

Tablets, scored, medroxyprogesterone acetate 500 mg. Net price 56 = £108.52. Label: 27

Injection, medroxyprogesterone acetate 200 mg/ mL. Net price 2.5-mL vial = £13.26

Dose: by mouth, breast cancer, 1–1.5 g daily, up to 2 g daily has been used; other hormone-dependent cancers, 100–500 mg daily

By deep intramuscular injection into the gluteal muscle, breast carcinoma, initially 0.5–1 g daily for 4 weeks; maintenance, 500 mg twice a week

Endometrial carcinoma, initially 500 mg twice weekly for 3 months; maintenance, 500 mg once weekly

Renal adenocarcinoma, initially 500 mg on alternate days for 30 days; maintenance, 500 mg twice weekly until day 60, then 250 mg once weekly

Prostatic adenocarcinoma, initially 500 mg twice weekly; maintenance, 500 mg once weekly

Provera® (Pharmacia) PoM

Tablets, medroxyprogesterone acetate 100 mg (scored), net price 60-tab pack = £23.86; 200 mg (scored), 30-tab pack = £23.60; 400 mg, 30-tab pack = £46.69

Dose: endometrial and renal cell cancer, 200–400 mg daily; breast cancer, 400–800 mg daily

Tablets, medroxyprogesterone acetate 2.5 mg, 5 mg and 10 mg, see section 6.4.1.2

MEGESTROL ACETATE

Indications: see notes above

Cautions: see under Medroxyprogesterone acetate (section 6.4.1.2) and notes above

Contra-indications: see under Medroxyprogesterone acetate (section 6.4.1.2) and notes above

Side-effects: see under Medroxyprogesterone acetate (section 6.4.1.2) and notes above

Dose: breast cancer, 160 mg daily in single or divided doses; endometrial cancer, 40–320 mg daily in divided doses

Megace® (Bristol-Myers Squibb) PoM

Tablets, both scored, megestrol acetate 40 mg, net price 20 = £5.08; 160 mg (off-white), 30-tab pack = £29.30

NORETHISTERONE

Indications: see notes above; other indications, (section 6.4.1.2)

Cautions: see section 6.4.1.2 and notes above; **interactions:** Appendix 1 (progestogens)

Contra-indications: see section 6.4.1.2 and notes above

Side-effects: see section 6.4.1.2 and notes above

Dose: breast cancer, 40 mg daily, increased to 60 mg daily if required

Preparations
Section 6.4.1.2

8.3.3   Androgens

Testosterone esters (section 6.4.2) are occasionally still used as second- or third-line therapy for metastatic breast cancer.

8.3.4   Hormone antagonists

8.3.4.1   Breast cancer

The management of patients with breast cancer involves surgery, radiotherapy, drug therapy, or a combination of these. All women with invasive breast cancer should be considered for adjuvant therapy, which is determined by an assessment of the risk of recurrence, oestrogen-receptor status of the primary tumour, and menopausal status.

Tamoxifen is an oestrogen-receptor antagonist and at a dose of 20 mg daily is the adjuvant hormonal treatment of choice in women with oestrogen-receptor-positive breast cancer supplemented in selected cases by chemotherapy. Treatment with tamoxifen delays the growth of metastases and increases survival; if tolerated it should be continued for 5 years.

Tamoxifen is also used in women with oestrogen-receptor-positive metastatic breast cancer. Approximately 60% of such patients respond to initial hormonal manipulation, whereas less than 10% of oestrogen-receptor-negative tumours respond.

Severe side-effects are unusual with tamoxifen but patients with bony metastases may experience an exacerbation of pain, sometimes associated with hypercalcaemia; this reaction commonly precedes tumour response. Amenorrhoea commonly develops in premenopausal women. For details of endometrial changes see under Cautions and for CSM advice see under Dose.

Patients with non-life-threatening metastases unresponsive to tamoxifen rarely respond to a secondary hormonal treatment. However, patients who initially respond to tamoxifen may respond to other hormone treatment. For premenopausal women ovarian ablation or a progestogen (section 8.3.2) can be used; for postmenopausal patients a newer aromatase inhibitor (see below) or a progestogen can be used. The newer aromatase inhibitors are well tolerated and are more effective than progestogens. Patients who respond can be given further hormone treatment on relapse; refractory disease is better treated with chemotherapy or managed with palliative therapy.

Toremifene, also an oestrogen-receptor antagonist, is licensed for hormone-dependent metastatic breast cancer in postmenopausal women.

Aminoglutethimide, a non-steroidal aromatase inhibitor, acts predominantly by blocking the conversion of androgens to oestrogens in the peripheral tissues; in breast cancer it has largely been replaced by the newer aromatase inhibitors which are better tolerated. Aminoglutethimide is also used as second-line treatment for prostate cancer (section 8.3.4.2). Aminoglutethimide may cause adrenal hypofunction and corticosteroid replacement therapy is necessary (section 6.3.1). Early toxicity is common and may include drowsiness, drug fever, and a morbilliform eruption; these side-effects generally settle spontaneously. Hepatic enzyme induction occurs, and may require modification of the doses of other drugs (e.g. oral anticoagulants).

Anastrozole and **letrozole** are non-steroidal aromatase inhibitors; **exemestane** is a steroidal aromatase inhibitor. Anastrozole and possibly exemestane and letrozole are now considered alternatives to tamoxifen for the treatment of advanced postmenopausal breast cancer. They are much better tolerated than aminoglutethimide and corticosteroid replacement therapy is not necessary.

Trilostane (section 6.7.3) is also licensed for postmenopausal breast cancer. It is quite well tolerated but diarrhoea and abdominal discomfort may be a problem. Like aminoglutethimide, trilostane may cause adrenal hypofunction and corticosteroid replacement therapy is needed.

Goserelin (section 8.3.4.2), a gonadorelin analogue, is licensed for the management of advanced breast cancer in premenopausal and perimenopausal women and as an alternative to chemotherapy for oestrogen-receptor-positive early breast cancer in premenopausal and perimenopausal women.

TAMOXIFEN

Indications: see under Dose and notes above

Cautions: occasional cystic ovarian swellings in premenopausal women, occasional hypercalcaemia if bony metastases; increased risk of thromboembolic events when used with cytotoxics; breast-feeding (Appendix 5); endometrial changes (**important:** see below); porphyria (section 9.8.2); **interactions:** Appendix 1 (tamoxifen); ENDOMETRIAL CHANGES. Increased endometrial changes, including hyperplasia, polyps, and cancer reported; prompt investigation required if abnormal vaginal bleeding including menstrual irregularities, vaginal discharge, and pelvic pain or pressure in those receiving (or who have received) tamoxifen.

Contra-indications: pregnancy (exclude before commencing and advise non-hormonal contraception if appropriate—Appendix 4)

Side-effects: hot flushes, vaginal bleeding and vaginal discharge (**important:** see also Endometrial Changes under Cautions), suppression of menstruation in some premenopausal women, pruritus vulvae, gastro-intestinal disturbances, headache, light-headedness, tumour flare, decreased platelet counts; occasionally oedema, alopecia, rashes, uterine fibroids; also visual disturbances (including corneal changes, cataracts, retinopathy); leucopenia (sometimes with anaemia and thrombocytopenia), rarely neutropenia; hypertriglyceridaemia reported (sometimes with pancreatitis); thromboembolic events reported; liver enzyme changes (rarely fatty liver, cholestasis, hepatitis); rarely interstitial pneumonitis, hypersensitivity reactions including angioedema, Stevens-Johnson syndrome, bullous pemphigoid; see also notes above

Dose: breast cancer, 20 mg daily

CSM ADVICE. The CSM has advised that tamoxifen in a dose of 20 mg daily substantially increases survival in early breast cancer, and that no further benefit has been demonstrated with higher doses. Patients should be told of the small risk of endometrial cancer (see under Cautions above) and encouraged to report relevant symptoms early. They can, however, be reassured that the benefits of treatment far outweigh the risks

Anovulatory infertility, 20 mg daily on days 2, 3, 4 and 5 of cycle; if necessary the daily dose may be increased to 40 mg then 80 mg for subsequent courses; if cycles irregular, start initial course on any day, with subsequent course starting 45 days later *or* on day 2 of cycle if menstruation occurs

Tamoxifen (Non-proprietary) PoM
Tablets, tamoxifen (as citrate) 10 mg, net price 30-tab pack = £1.96; 20 mg, 30-tab pack = £2.24; 40 mg, 30-tab pack = £8.41
Available from Alpharma, APS, Berk (*Emblon®*), CP, Hillcross, IVAX, Kent, Pharmacia (*Tamofen®*)
Oral solution, tamoxifen (as citrate) 10 mg/5 mL, net price 150 mL = £31.50
Available from Rosemont (*Soltamox®*)

Nolvadex® (AstraZeneca) PoM
Tablets, tamoxifen (as citrate) 10 mg, net price 30-tab pack = £5.78; 20 mg (*Nolvadex-D®*), 30-tab pack = £8.71

AMINOGLUTETHIMIDE

Indications: see notes above and under Dose

Cautions: see notes above; adrenal hypofunction (see below); monitor blood pressure, plasma electrolytes, blood counts, and thyroid function; **interactions:** Appendix 1 (aminoglutethimide)

ADRENAL HYPOFUNCTION. May cause adrenal hypofunction especially under conditions of stress (such as surgery, trauma, or acute illness), therefore corticosteroid replacement therapy is necessary (section 6.3.1). If a synthetic glucocorticoid such as dexamethasone is used instead of hydrocortisone a relatively high dose may be needed (metabolism of synthetic corticosteroids accelerated)

Contra-indications: pregnancy (advise non-hormonal contraceptive methods if appropriate) and breast-feeding; porphyria (section 9.8.2)

Side-effects: see notes above; drowsiness, lethargy, rash (sometimes with fever—usually in first 2 weeks and resolves despite continued administration); occasionally dizziness, nausea; other side-effects reported include ataxia, headache, depression, insomnia, pruritus, urticaria, diarrhoea, vomiting, constipation, anorexia, sweating, hypotension, adrenal insufficiency, hyponatraemia, hypoglycaemia, agranulocytosis, leucopenia, thrombocytopenia, hyperkalaemia, exfoliative dermatitis, Stevens-Johnson syndrome, hypothyroidism, inappropriate ADH-secretion, masculinisation and hirsutism in females, renal impairment, pancytopenia, anae-

mia, allergy, anaphylactic reactions, allergic alveolitis (withdraw immediately if suspected), cholestatic hepatitis, confusion

Dose: advanced breast or prostate cancer, 250 mg daily, increased once a week to max. 250 mg 4 times daily (in breast cancer 250 mg twice daily has proved sufficient in some patients; in prostate cancer up to 750 mg daily is usually satisfactory); given with a glucocorticoid (and sometimes with a mineralocorticoid as well)
Cushing's syndrome due to malignant disease, 250 mg daily, increased gradually to 1 g daily in divided doses (occasionally 1.5–2 g daily); glucocorticoid given only if necessary

Orimeten® (Novartis) PoM
Tablets, scored, aminoglutethimide 250 mg. Net price 56-tab pack = £24.27. Label: 2

ANASTROZOLE

Indications: advanced breast cancer in postmenopausal women

Cautions: laboratory test for menopause if doubt

Contra-indications: pregnancy and breast-feeding; moderate or severe hepatic disease, moderate or severe renal impairment; not for premenopausal women

Side-effects: hot flushes, vaginal dryness, vaginal bleeding, hair thinning, anorexia, nausea, vomiting, diarrhoea, headache, arthralgia, rash (including Stevens-Johnson syndrome); asthenia and drowsiness—may initially affect ability to drive or operate machinery; slight increases in total cholesterol levels reported

Dose: 1 mg daily

Arimidex® (AstraZeneca) PoM
Tablets, f/c, anastrozole 1 mg. Net price 28-tab pack = £83.16

EXEMESTANE

Indications: advanced breast cancer in postmenopausal women in whom anti-oestrogen therapy has failed

Cautions: hepatic and renal impairment

Contra-indications: pregnancy and breast-feeding; not indicated for premenopausal women

Side-effects: hot flushes, nausea, dizziness, fatigue, sweating; less frequently vomiting, dyspepsia, constipation, abdominal pain, anorexia, peripheral oedema, headache, depression, insomnia, alopecia, rash; rarely thrombocytopenia, leucopenia

Dose: 25 mg daily

Aromasin® (Pharmacia) ▼ PoM
Tablets, s/c, exemestane 25 mg, net price 15-tab pack = £51.43, 30-tab pack = £102.86, 90-tab pack = £308.58. Label: 21

LETROZOLE

Indications: advanced breast cancer in postmenopausal women; pre-operative treatment in postmenopausal women with localised hormone-receptor-positive breast cancer to allow subsequent breast conserving surgery

Cautions: severe renal impairment

Contra-indications: severe hepatic impairment; not indicated for premenopausal women; pregnancy and breast-feeding

Side-effects: hot flushes, nausea, vomiting, dyspepsia, constipation, diarrhoea, abdominal pain, anorexia (and weight gain), dyspnoea, chest pain, coughing, dizziness, fatigue, headache, infection, musculoskeletal pain, peripheral oedema, rash, pruritus

Dose: 2.5 mg daily until tumour progression is evident

Femara® (Novartis) [PoM]
Tablets, f/c, letrozole 2.5 mg. Net price 14-tab pack = £41.58, 28-tab pack = £83.16

TOREMIFENE

Indications: hormone-dependent metastatic breast cancer in postmenopausal women

Cautions: hypercalcaemia may occur (especially if bone metastases and usually at beginning of treatment); **interactions:** Appendix 1 (toremifene)

ENDOMETRIAL CHANGES. There is a risk of increased endometrial changes including hyperplasia, polyps and cancer. Abnormal vaginal bleeding including menstrual irregularities, vaginal discharge and symptoms such as pelvic pain or pressure should be promptly investigated

Contra-indications: endometrial hyperplasia, severe hepatic impairment, history of severe thromboembolic disease; pregnancy and breast-feeding

Side-effects: hot flushes, vaginal bleeding or discharge (**important:** see also Cautions), dizziness, oedema, sweating, nausea, vomiting, chest or back pain, fatigue, headache, skin discoloration, weight increase, insomnia, constipation, dyspnoea, paresis, tremor, vertigo, pruritus, anorexia, corneal opacity (reversible), asthenia; thromboembolic events reported; rarely dermatitis, alopecia, emotional lability, depression, jaundice, stiffness

Dose: 60 mg daily

Fareston® (Orion) [PoM]
Tablets, toremifene (as citrate) 60 mg. Net price 30-tab pack = £30.37

8.3.4.2 Prostate cancer and gonadorelin analogues

Metastatic cancer of the prostate usually responds to hormonal treatment aimed at androgen depletion. Standard treatments include bilateral subcapsular orchidectomy or use of a gonadorelin analogue (**buserelin**, **goserelin**, **leuprorelin**, or **triptorelin**). Response in most patients lasts for 12 to 18 months. No entirely satisfactory therapy exists for disease progression despite this treatment (hormone refractory prostate cancer), but occasional patients respond to other hormone manipulation e.g. with an anti-androgen. Bone disease can often be palliated with irradiation or if widespread with strontium, aminoglutethimide (section 8.3.4.1), or prednisolone (section 6.3.2).

Gonadorelin analogues

Gonadorelin analogues are as effective as orchidectomy or **diethylstilbestrol** (section 8.3.1) but are expensive and require parenteral administration, at least initially. They cause initial stimulation then depression of luteinising hormone release by the pituitary. During the initial stage (1–2 weeks) increased production of testosterone may be associated with progression of prostate cancer. In susceptible patients this tumour 'flare' may cause spinal cord compression, ureteric obstruction or increased bone pain. When such problems are anticipated, alternative treatments (e.g. orchidectomy) or concomitant use of an anti-androgen such as cyproterone acetate or flutamide (see below) are recommended; anti-androgen treatment should be started 3 days before the gonadorelin analogue and continued for 3 weeks. Gonadorelin analogues are also used in women for breast cancer (section 8.3.4.1) and other indications (section 6.7.2).

CAUTIONS. Men at risk of tumour 'flare' (see above) should be monitored closely during the first month of therapy. Caution is required in women with metabolic bone disease because decreases in bone mineral density may occur. The injection site should be rotated.

SIDE-EFFECTS. The gonadorelin analogues cause side-effects similar to the menopause in women and orchidectomy in men and include hot flushes and sweating, sexual dysfunction, vaginal dryness or bleeding, and gynaecomastia or changes in breast size. Signs and symptoms of prostate or breast cancer may worsen initially (managed in prostate cancer with anti-androgens, see above). Other side-effects include hypersensitivity reactions (rashes, pruritus, asthma, and rarely anaphylaxis), injection site reactions (see Cautions), headache (rarely migraine), visual disturbances, dizziness, arthralgia and possibly myalgia, hair loss, peripheral oedema, gastro-intestinal disturbances, weight changes, sleep disorders, and mood changes.

Anti-androgens

Cyproterone acetate, flutamide and **bicalutamide** are anti-androgens that inhibit the tumour 'flare' which may occur after commencing gonadorelin analogue administration. Cyproterone acetate and flutamide are also licensed for use alone in patients with metastatic prostate cancer refractory to gonadorelin analogue therapy. Bicalutamide is used for prostate cancer either alone or as an adjunct to other therapy, according to the clinical circumstances.

BICALUTAMIDE

Indications: prostate cancer, see notes above

Cautions: hepatic impairment (Appendix 2), also consider periodic liver function tests; **interactions:** Appendix 1 (bicalutamide)

Side-effects: dyspepsia, nausea, vomiting, diarrhoea, abdominal pain, asthenia, depression, gynaecomastia, breast tenderness, decreased libido, hot flushes, alopecia, hirsutism, pruritus, dry skin, haematuria, cholestasis and jaundice (very rarely hepatic failure); rarely cardiovascular disorders (including angina, heart failure, conduction defects, arrhythmias and ECG changes); also reported, other gastro-intestinal disorders, oedema, chest pain, dyspnoea, dry mouth, headache, dizziness, insomnia, drowsiness, impotence, nocturia, rash, sweating, hyperglycaemia, weight changes, pelvic pain, anaemia, thrombocytopenia

Dose: with orchidectomy or gonadorelin therapy, 50 mg daily (in gonadorelin therapy, started 3 days beforehand, see also notes above)

Prostate cancer, 150 mg once daily

Casodex® (AstraZeneca) PoM
Tablets, f/c, bicalutamide 50 mg, net price 28-tab pack = £128.00; 150 mg, 28-tab pack = £240.00

BUSERELIN

Indications: advanced prostate cancer; other indications (section 6.7.2)

Cautions: depression, see also notes above

Side-effects: see notes above; worsening hypertension, palpitations, glucose intolerance, altered blood lipids, thrombocytopenia, leucopenia, nervousness, fatigue, memory and concentration disturbances, anxiety, increased thirst, hearing disorders, musculoskeletal pain; nasal irritation, nose bleeds and altered sense of taste and smell (spray formulation only)

Dose: *by subcutaneous injection*, 500 micrograms every 8 hours for 7 days, then *intranasally*, 1 spray into each nostril 6 times daily (see also notes above)

COUNSELLING. Avoid use of nasal decongestants before and for at least 30 minutes after treatment.

Suprefact® (Shire) PoM
Injection, buserelin (as acetate) 1 mg/mL. Net price 2 × 5.5-mL vial = £23.69
Nasal spray, buserelin (as acetate) 100 micrograms/metered spray. Net price treatment pack of 4 × 10-g bottle with spray pump = £87.68. Counselling, see above

---

CYPROTERONE ACETATE

Indications: prostate cancer, see under Dose and also notes above; other indications, see section 6.4.2

Cautions: in prostate cancer, blood counts initially and throughout treatment, hepatic impairment (Appendix 2); monitor hepatic function (liver function tests should be performed before treatment, see also under Side-effects below); monitor adrenocortical function regularly; risk of recurrence of thromboembolic disease; diabetes mellitus, sickle-cell anaemia, severe depression (in other indications some of these are contra-indicated, see section 6.4.2)

DRIVING. Fatigue and lassitude may impair performance of skilled tasks (e.g. driving)

Contra-indications: none in prostate cancer; for contra-indications relating to other indications see section 6.4.2

Side-effects: see section 6.4.2
HEPATOTOXICITY. Direct hepatic toxicity including jaundice, hepatitis and hepatic failure have been reported (usually after several months) in patients treated with cyproterone acetate 200–300 mg daily. Liver function tests should be performed before treatment and whenever symptoms suggestive of hepatotoxicity occur—if confirmed cyproterone should normally be withdrawn unless the hepatotoxicity can be explained by another cause such as metastatic disease (in which case cyproterone should be continued only if the perceived benefit exceeds the risk)

Dose: flare with initial gonadorelin therapy, 300 mg daily in 2–3 divided doses, reduced to 200 mg daily in 2–3 divided doses if necesssary
Long-term palliative therapy where gonadorelin analogues or orchidectomy contra-indicated, not tolerated, or where oral therapy preferred, 200–300 mg daily in 2–3 divided doses
Hot flushes with gonadorelin therapy or after orchidectomy, initially 50 mg daily, adjusted according to response to 50–150 mg daily in 1–3 divided doses

Cyproterone Acetate (Non-proprietary) PoM
Tablets, cyproterone acetate 50 mg, net price 56-tab pack = £32.23; 100 mg, 84-tab pack = £96.69. Label: 21
Available from Generics

Cyprostat® (Schering Health) PoM
Tablets, scored, cyproterone acetate 50 mg net price 168-tab pack = £101.54; 100 mg, 84-tab pack = £101.54. Label: 21

FLUTAMIDE

Indications: advanced prostate cancer, see also notes above

Cautions: cardiac disease (oedema reported); hepatic impairment (Appendix 2), also periodic liver function tests on long-term therapy and at the first sign or symptom indicating liver disorder (e.g. pruritus, dark urine, persistent anorexia, jaundice, abdominal pain, unexplained influenza-like symptoms); **interactions:** Appendix 1 (flutamide)

Side-effects: gynaecomastia (sometimes with galactorrhoea); nausea, vomiting, diarrhoea, increased appetite, insomnia, tiredness; other side-effects reported include decreased libido, inhibition of spermatogenesis, gastric and chest pain, headache, dizziness, oedema, blurred vision, thirst, rashes, pruritus, haemolytic anaemia, systemic lupus erythematosus-like syndrome, and lymphoedema; hepatic injury (with transaminase abnormalities, cholestatic jaundice, hepatic necrosis, encephalopathy and occasional fatality) reported

Dose: 250 mg 3 times daily (see also notes above)

Flutamide (Non-proprietary) PoM
Tablets, flutamide 250 mg. Net price 84-tab pack = £65.00
Available from Alpharma, Chiron (*Chimax®*), Generics, Hillcross, Orion, Tillomed

Drogenil® (Schering-Plough) PoM
Tablets, yellow, scored, flutamide 250 mg, net price 84-tab pack = £70.00

GOSERELIN

Indications: prostate cancer; advanced breast cancer; oestrogen-receptor positive early breast cancer (section 8.3.4.1); other indications (section 6.7.2)

Cautions: see notes above; breast-feeding (Appendix 5)

Contra-indications: pregnancy (Appendix 4); undiagnosed vaginal bleeding

Side-effects: see notes above; also transient changes in blood pressure, paraesthesia, rarely hypercalcaemia (in patients with metastatic breast cancer)

Dose: see under preparations below

Zoladex® (AstraZeneca) [PoM]
Implant, goserelin 3.6 mg (as acetate) in syringe applicator. Net price each = £122.27
Dose: breast cancer and prostate cancer *by subcutaneous injection* into anterior abdominal wall, 3.6 mg every 28 days (see also notes above)

Zoladex® LA (AstraZeneca) [PoM]
Implant, goserelin 10.8 mg (as acetate) in syringe applicator. Net price each = £366.81
Dose: prostate cancer, *by subcutaneous injection* into anterior abdominal wall, 10.8 mg every 12 weeks (see also notes above)

LEUPRORELIN ACETATE

Indications: advanced prostate cancer; other indications (section 6.7.2)

Cautions: see notes above

Side-effects: see notes above; also fatigue, muscle weakness, paraesthesia, hypertension, palpitations, alteration of glucose tolerance and of blood lipids; thrombocytopenia and leucopenia reported

Dose: see under preparations below

Prostap® SR (Wyeth) [PoM]
Injection (microsphere powder for reconstitution), leuprorelin acetate, net price 3.75-mg vial with 1-mL vehicle-filled syringe = £125.40
Dose: advanced prostate cancer, *by subcutaneous or by intramuscular injection*, 3.75 mg every 4 weeks (see also notes above)

Prostap® 3 (Wyeth) [PoM]
Injection (microsphere powder for reconstitution), leuprorelin acetate, net price 11.25-mg vial with 2-mL vehicle-filled syringe = £376.20
Dose: advanced prostate cancer, *by subcutaneous injection*, 11.25 mg every three months (see also notes above)

TRIPTORELIN

Indications: advanced prostate cancer; endometriosis (section 6.7.2)

Cautions: see notes above

Side-effects: see notes above; transient hypertension, dry mouth, excessive salivation, paraesthesia, increased dysuria

Dose: *by intramuscular injection*, 3 mg every 4 weeks (see also notes above)

De-capeptyl® sr (Ipsen) [PoM]
Injection (copolymer microsphere powder for aqueous suspension), triptorelin. Net price 4.2-mg vial (with diluent) = £105.05

8.3.4.3   Somatostatin analogues

Octreotide and **lanreotide** are analogues of the hypothalamic release-inhibiting hormone somatostatin. They are indicated for the relief of symptoms associated with neuroendocrine (particularly carcinoid) tumours and acromegaly. Octreotide is also licensed for the prevention of complications following pancreatic surgery; it may also be valuable in reducing vomiting in palliative care (see p. 16) and in stopping variceal bleeding [unlicensed indication]—see also vasopressin and terlipressin (section 6.5.2).

CAUTIONS. Growth hormone-secreting pituitary tumours can expand causing serious complications; during treatment with somatostatin analogues patients should be monitored for signs of tumour expansion (e.g. visual field defects). Ultrasound examination of the gallbladder is recommended before treatment and at intervals of 6–12 months during treatment (avoid abrupt withdrawal of short-acting octreotide—see Side-effects below). In insulinoma an increase in the depth and duration of hypoglycaemia may occur (observe patients when initiating treatment and changing doses); in diabetes mellitus, insulin or oral antidiabetic requirements may be reduced. Thyroid function should be monitored on long-term therapy.

SIDE-EFFECTS. Gastro-intestinal disturbances including anorexia, nausea, vomiting, abdominal pain and bloating, flatulence, diarrhoea, and steatorrhoea may occur. Postprandial glucose tolerance may be impaired and rarely persistent hyperglycaemia occurs with chronic administration; hypoglycaemia has also been reported. Gallstones have been reported after long-term treatment (abrupt withdrawal of subcutaneous octreotide is associated with biliary colic and pancreatitis). Pain and irritation may occur at the injection site and sites should be rotated.

OCTREOTIDE

Indications: see under Dose

Cautions: see notes above; hepatic impairment (Appendix 2); pregnancy and breast-feeding (Appendixes 4 and 5); **interactions:** Appendix 1 (octreotide)

Side-effects: see notes above; rarely altered liver function tests, hepatitis, pancreatitis and transient alopecia

Dose: symptoms associated with carcinoid tumours with features of carcinoid syndrome, VIPomas, glucagonomas, *by subcutaneous injection*, initially 50 micrograms once or twice daily, gradually increased according to response to 200 micrograms 3 times daily (higher doses required exceptionally); maintenance doses variable; in carcinoid tumours discontinue after 1 week if no effect; if rapid response required, initial dose *by intravenous injection* (with ECG monitoring and after dilution to a concentration of 10–50% with sodium chloride 0.9% injection)
Acromegaly, short-term treatment before pituitary surgery *or* long-term treatment in those inadequately controlled by other treatment *or* until

radiotherapy becomes fully effective *by subcutaneous injection*, 100–200 micrograms 3 times daily; discontinue if no improvement within 3 months

Prevention of complications following pancreatic surgery, consult product literature

Sandostatin® (Novartis) PoM

Injection, octreotide (as acetate) 50 micrograms/ mL, net price 1-mL amp = £3.47; 100 micrograms/mL, 1-mL amp = £6.53; 200 micrograms/mL 5-mL vial = £65.10; 500 micrograms/mL, 1-mL amp = £31.65

■ Depot preparation

Sandostatin LAR® (Novartis) ▼ PoM

Injection (microsphere powder for aqueous suspension), octreotide (as acetate) 10-mg vial = £637.50; 20-mg vial = £850.00; 30-mg vial = £1062.50 (all supplied with diluent and syringe)

Dose: acromegaly and neuroendocrine tumours in patients adequately controlled on subcutaneous octreotide, *by deep intramuscular injection* (into the gluteal muscle), initially 20 mg every 4 weeks for 3 months, then adjusted according to symptoms and laboratory tests; max. 30 mg every 4 weeks

For acromegaly, start depot octreotide 1 day after the last dose of subcutaneous octreotide; for neuroendocrine tumours, continue subcutaneous octreotide for 2 weeks after first dose of depot octreotide

LANREOTIDE

Indications: see notes above

Cautions: see notes above; pregnancy and breast-feeding (Appendixes 4 and 5); **interactions:** Appendix 1 (lanreotide)

Side-effects: see notes above

Dose: acromegaly, *by intramuscular injection*, initially 30 mg every 14 days for 3 months; at 3 months increase dose if necessary to 30 mg every 7–10 days; if poor initial response before third fortnightly injection increase dose to 30 mg every 7–10 days

Neuroendocrine tumours, as for acromegaly; adjust dose interval according to symptoms

Somatuline® LA (Ipsen) ▼ PoM

Injection (copolymer microparticles for aqueous suspension), lanreotide (as acetate) 30-mg vial (with vehicle) = £334.25.

9: Nutrition and blood

9.1   Anaemias and some other blood disorders

9.1.1   Iron-deficiency anaemias
9.1.2   Drugs used in megaloblastic anaemias
9.1.3   Drugs used in hypoplastic, haemolytic, and renal anaemias
9.1.4   Drugs used in autoimmune thrombocytopenic purpura
9.1.5   G6PD deficiency
9.1.6   Drugs used in neutropenia

Before initiating treatment for anaemia it is essential to determine which type is present. Iron salts may be harmful and result in iron overload if given alone to patients with anaemias other than those due to iron deficiency.

9.1.1   Iron-deficiency anaemias

9.1.1.1   Oral iron
9.1.1.2   Parenteral iron

Treatment is only justified in the presence of a demonstrable iron-deficiency state. Before starting treatment, it is important to exclude any serious underlying cause of the anaemia (e.g. gastric erosion, colonic carcinoma).

Prophylaxis is justifiable in pregnancy only for women who have additional risk factors for iron deficiency (e.g. poor diet), menorrhagia, after subtotal or total gastrectomy, and in the management of low birth-weight infants such as premature babies, twins, and in infants delivered by caesarean section.

9.1.1.1   Oral iron

Iron salts should be given by mouth unless there are good reasons for using another route.

Ferrous salts show only marginal differences between one another in efficiency of absorption of iron, but ferric salts are much less well absorbed. Haemoglobin regeneration rate is little affected by the type of salt used provided sufficient iron is given, and in most patients the speed of response is not critical. Choice of preparation is thus usually decided by incidence of side-effects and cost.

The oral dose of elemental iron for deficiency should be 100 to 200 mg daily. It is customary to give this as dried **ferrous sulphate**, 200 mg ($\equiv$ 65 mg elemental iron) three times daily; a dose of ferrous sulphate 200 mg once or twice daily may be effective for prophylaxis or for mild iron deficiency. Ferrous sulphate 200–300 mg 3 times daily may be required to produce an optimum response to epoetin in iron-deficient patients with chronic renal failure. If side-effects occur, the dose may be reduced; alternatively, another iron salt may be used but an improvement in tolerance may simply be a result of a lower content of elemental iron. The incidence of side-effects due to ferrous sulphate is no greater than with other iron salts when compared on the basis of equivalent amounts of elemental iron.

Iron content of different iron salts

Iron salt	Amount	Content of ferrous iron
Ferrous fumarate	200 mg	65 mg
Ferrous gluconate	300 mg	35 mg
Ferrous succinate	100 mg	35 mg
Ferrous sulphate	300 mg	60 mg
Ferrous sulphate, dried	200 mg	65 mg

THERAPEUTIC RESPONSE. The haemoglobin concentration should rise by about 100–200 mg/100 mL (1–2 g/litre) per day *or* 2 g/100 mL (20 g/litre) over 3–4 weeks. When the haemoglobin is in the normal range, treatment should be continued for a further 3 months to replenish the iron stores. Epithelial tissue changes such as atrophic glossitis and koilonychia are usually improved, but the response is often slow.

COMPOUND PREPARATIONS. Some oral preparations contain ascorbic acid to aid absorption of the iron but the therapeutic advantage of such preparations is minimal and cost may be increased.

There is no justification for the inclusion of other ingredients, such as the B group of vitamins (except folic acid for pregnant women, see Iron and Folic Acid below and p. 438).

MODIFIED-RELEASE PREPARATIONS. Modified-release preparations are designed to release iron gradually so that a smaller amount of iron is present in the gastro-intestinal tract at any one time. These preparations are licensed for once-daily dosage.

However, modified-release preparations are likely to carry the iron past the first part of the duodenum into an area of the gut where iron absorption may be poor. The low incidence of side-effects may reflect the small amounts of iron available for absorption under these conditions and so the preparations have no therapeutic advantage and should not be used.

SIDE-EFFECTS. Gastro-intestinal irritation may occur with iron salts. Nausea and epigastric pain are dose-related but the relationship between dose and altered bowel habit (constipation or diarrhoea) is less clear. Oral iron, particularly modified-release preparations, may exacerbate diarrhoea in patients with inflammatory bowel disease; care is also needed in patients with intestinal strictures and diverticula.

Iron preparations taken orally may be constipating, particularly in older patients, occasionally leading to faecal impaction.

Iron preparations are an important cause of accidental overdose in children. For the treatment of **iron overdose**, see Emergency Treatment of Poisoning p. 25.

FERROUS SULPHATE

Indications: iron-deficiency anaemia
Cautions: pregnancy (see section 9.1.1); **interactions:** Appendix 1 (iron)
Side-effects: see notes above
Dose: see under preparations below and notes above

> COUNSELLING. Although iron preparations are best absorbed on an empty stomach they may be taken after food to reduce gastro-intestinal side-effects; they may discolour stools

Ferrous Sulphate (Non-proprietary)
Tablets, coated, dried ferrous sulphate 200 mg (65 mg iron), net price 20 = 64p
Dose: prophylactic, 1 tablet daily; therapeutic, 1 tablet 2–3 times daily

■ Modified-release preparations

Feospan® (Celltech) [NHS] ▭
Spansule® (= capsules m/r), clear/red, enclosing green and brown pellets, dried ferrous sulphate 150 mg (47 mg iron). Net price 30-cap pack = £1.11. Label: 25
Dose: 1–2 capsules daily; CHILD over 1 year 1 capsule daily; can be opened and sprinkled on food

Ferrograd® (Abbott) ▭
Filmtabs® (= tablets f/c), m/r, red, dried ferrous sulphate 325 mg (105 mg iron). Net price 30-tab pack = 54p. Label: 25
Dose: 1 tablet daily before food

Slow-Fe® (Novartis) ▭
Tablets, m/r, dried ferrous sulphate 160 mg (50 mg iron). Net price 28-tab pack = 24p. Label: 25
Dose: prophylactic, 1 tablet daily; therapeutic, 2 tablets daily; CHILD over 6 years, 1 tablet daily

FERROUS FUMARATE

Indications: iron-deficiency anaemia
Cautions: pregnancy (see section 9.1.1); **interactions:** Appendix 1 (iron)
Side-effects: see notes above
Dose: see under preparations below and notes above

Fersaday® (Goldshield)
Tablets, brown, f/c, ferrous fumarate 322 mg (100 mg iron). Net price 28-tab pack = 50p
Dose: prophylactic, 1 tablet daily; therapeutic, 1 tablet twice daily

Fersamal® (Goldshield)
Tablets, brown, ferrous fumarate 210 mg (68 mg iron). Net price 20 = 24p
Dose: 1–2 tablets 3 times daily
Syrup, brown, ferrous fumarate approx. 140 mg (45 mg iron)/5 mL. Net price 200 mL = £2.35
Dose: 10–20 mL twice daily; PREMATURE INFANT 0.6–2.4 mL/kg daily; CHILD up to 6 years 2.5–5 mL twice daily

Galfer® (Galen)
Capsules, red/green, ferrous fumarate 305 mg (100 mg iron). Net price 20 = 36p
Dose: 1 capsule 1–2 times daily before food
Syrup, brown, sugar-free ferrous fumarate 140 mg (45 mg iron)/5 mL. Net price 300 mL = £4.86
Dose: 10 mL 1–2 times daily before food; CHILD (full-term infant and young child) 2.5–5 mL 1–2 times daily

FERROUS GLUCONATE

Indications: iron-deficiency anaemia
Cautions: pregnancy (see section 9.1.1); **interactions:** Appendix 1 (iron)
Side-effects: see notes above
Dose: see under preparation below and notes above

Ferrous Gluconate (Non-proprietary)
Tablets, red, coated, ferrous gluconate 300 mg (35 mg iron). Net price 20 = 73p
Dose: prophylactic, 2 tablets daily before food; therapeutic, 4–6 tablets daily in divided doses before food; CHILD 6–12 years, prophylactic and therapeutic, 1–3 tablets daily

FERROUS GLYCINE SULPHATE

Indications: iron-deficiency anaemia
Cautions: pregnancy (see section 9.1.1); **interactions:** Appendix 1 (iron)
Side-effects: see notes above
Dose: see under preparation below and notes above

Plesmet® (Link)
Syrup, ferrous glycine sulphate equivalent to 25 mg iron/5 mL. Net price 100 mL = 62p
Dose: 5–10 mL 3 times daily; CHILD 2.5–5 mL 1–3 times daily, according to age

POLYSACCHARIDE-IRON COMPLEX

Indications: iron-deficiency anaemia
Cautions: pregnancy (see section 9.1.1); **interactions:** Appendix 1 (iron)
Side-effects: see notes above
Dose: see under preparation below and notes above

Niferex® (Tillomed)
Elixir, brown, sugar-free, polysaccharide-iron complex equivalent to 100 mg of iron/5 mL. Net price 240-mL pack = £6.06; [NHS]* 30-mL dropper bottle for paediatric use = £2.16. Counselling, use of dropper
Dose: prophylactic, 2.5 mL daily; therapeutic, 5 mL 1–2 times daily (once daily if required during second and third trimester of pregnancy); PREMATURE INFANT and INFANT, (from dropper bottle) 1 drop (approx. 500 micrograms iron) per 450 g body-weight 3 times daily; CHILD 2–6 years 2.5 mL daily, 6–12 years 5 mL daily
* except 30 mL paediatric dropper bottle for prophylaxis and treatment of iron deficiency in infants born prematurely and endorsed 'SLS'

SODIUM FEREDETATE

(Sodium ironedetate)
Indications: iron-deficiency anaemia
Cautions: pregnancy (see section 9.1.1); **interactions:** Appendix 1 (iron)
Side-effects: see notes above
Dose: see under preparation below and notes above

Sytron® (Link)
Elixir, sugar-free, sodium feredetate 190 mg equivalent to 27.5 mg of iron/5 mL. Net price 100 mL = 94p
Dose: 5 mL increasing gradually to 10 mL 3 times daily; INFANT and PREMATURE INFANT 2.5 mL twice daily (smaller doses should be used initially); CHILD 1–5 years 2.5 mL 3 times daily, 6–12 years 5 mL 3 times daily

Iron and folic acid

These preparations are used during pregnancy in women who are at high risk of developing iron and folic acid deficiency; they should be distinguished from those used for the prevention of neural tube defects in women planning a pregnancy (see p. 440).

It is important to note that the small doses of folic acid contained in these preparations are inadequate for the treatment of megaloblastic anaemias.

Fefol® (Celltech) [NHS] [▱]
Spansule® (= capsules m/r), clear/green, enclosing brown, yellow, and white pellets, dried ferrous sulphate 150 mg (47 mg iron), folic acid 500 micrograms. Net price 30-cap pack = £1.18. Label: 25
Dose: 1 capsule daily

Ferrograd Folic® (Abbott) [▱]
Filmtabs® (= tablets f/c), red/yellow, dried ferrous sulphate 325 mg (105 mg iron) for sustained release, folic acid 350 micrograms. Net price 30-tab pack = 60p. Label: 25
Dose: 1 tablet daily before food

Galfer FA® (Galen)
Capsules, red/yellow, ferrous fumarate 305 mg (100 mg iron), folic acid 350 micrograms. Net price 20 = 40p
Dose: 1 capsule daily before food

Lexpec with Iron-M® (Rosemont) [PoM]
Syrup, brown, sugar-free, ferric ammonium citrate equivalent to 80 mg iron, folic acid 500 micrograms/5 mL. Net price 125 mL = £3.63
Dose: 5–10 mL daily before food
Note. Lexpec with Iron-M® contains five times less folic acid than *Lexpec with Iron®*

Pregaday® (Celltech)
Tablets, brown, f/c, ferrous fumarate equivalent to 100 mg iron, folic acid 350 micrograms. Net price 28-tab pack = 51p
Dose: 1 tablet daily

Slow-Fe Folic® (Novartis) [PoM] [▱]
Tablets, m/r, ivory, f/c, dried ferrous sulphate 160 mg (50 mg iron), folic acid 400 micrograms. Net price 28-tab pack = 27p. Label: 25
Dose: 1–2 tablets daily

> [▱] denotes preparations that are considered to be less suitable for prescribing (see p. vi)

■ **Higher folic acid content**

Appropriate in context of prevention of *recurrence of neural tube defects*, see recommendations on p. 440. *Cautions:* theoretical possibility of masking anaemia due to vitamin-B_{12} deficiency (which could allow vitamin-B_{12} neuropathy to develop).

Ferfolic SV® (Durbin) [NHS] [PoM]
Tablets, pink, ferrous gluconate 250 mg (30 mg iron), folic acid 4 mg, ascorbic acid 10 mg. Net price 20 = 40p
Dose: anaemia, 1–3 tablets daily after food
Prophylaxis of neural tube defects in women known to be at risk, 1 tablet daily started before conception and continued for at least first trimester; see also recommendations on p. 440

Lexpec with Iron® (Rosemont) [PoM]
Syrup, brown, sugar-free, ferric ammonium citrate equivalent to 80 mg iron, folic acid 2.5 mg/5 mL. Net price 150 mL = £4.35
Dose: 5–10 mL daily before food
Note. Lexpec with Iron® contains five times as much folic acid as *Lexpec with Iron-M®*

Compound iron preparations

There is no justification for prescribing compound iron preparations, except for preparations of iron and folic acid for prophylactic use in pregnancy (see above).

Ferrograd C® (Abbott) [NHS] ◣▬
Filmtabs® (= tablets f/c), red, dried ferrous sulphate 325 mg (105 mg iron) for sustained release, ascorbic acid 500 mg (as sodium salt). Net price 30-tab pack = £1.71. Label: 25
Dose: 1 tablet daily before food

Givitol® (Galen) [NHS] ◣▬
Capsules, red/maroon, ferrous fumarate 305 mg (100 mg iron) with vitamins B group and C. Net price 20 = 88p
Dose: 1 capsule daily before food

◣▬ denotes preparations that are considered to be less suitable for prescribing (see p. vi)

9.1.1.2   Parenteral iron

Iron may be administered parenterally as iron dextran, iron sorbitol, or iron sucrose. Parenteral iron is generally reserved for use when oral therapy is unsuccessful because the patient cannot tolerate oral iron, or does not take it reliably, or if there is continuing blood loss, or in malabsorption.

Also, many patients with chronic renal failure who are receiving haemodialysis (and some who are receiving peritoneal dialysis) require iron by the intravenous route on a regular basis (see Erythropoietin, section 9.1.3).

With the exception of patients with severe renal failure receiving haemodialysis, parenteral iron does not produce a faster haemoglobin response than oral iron provided that the oral iron preparation is taken reliably and is absorbed adequately.

Iron dextran, a complex of ferric hydroxide with dextrans, and **iron sucrose**, a complex of ferric hydroxide with sucrose, are given either by *slow intravenous injection* or by *intravenous infusion*. Anaphylactoid reactions can occur and patients should be given a small test dose initially. A complex of iron, sorbitol and citric acid as **iron sorbitol injection** is given by *deep intramuscular injection* and is **not** suitable for intravenous injection; the low mean molecular weight allows rapid absorption from the injection site, but excretion in the saliva and substantial urinary losses occur. To prevent leakage along the needle track with subsequent staining of the skin, intramuscular injections should be deep with suitable technique.

IRON DEXTRAN

A complex of ferric hydroxide with dextrans containing 5% (50 mg/mL) of iron
Indications: iron-deficiency anaemia, see notes above
Cautions: facilities for cardiopulmonary resuscitation must be at hand; increased risk of allergic reaction in immune or inflammatory conditions; hepatic impairment (Appendix 2); renal impairment; oral iron not to be given until 5 days after last injection; pregnancy (Appendix 4)
Contra-indications: history of allergic disorders including asthma and eczema; infection; active rheumatoid arthritis

Side-effects: nausea, dyspepsia, diarrhoea, chest pains, hypotension, dyspnoea, arthralgia, myalgia, pruritus, urticaria, rash, fever, shivering, flushing, headache; rarely anaphylactoid reactions; injection site reactions including phlebitis reported
Dose: *by slow intravenous injection* or *by intravenous infusion*, calculated according to body-weight and iron deficit, consult product literature
CHILD under 14 years, not recommended

CosmoFer® (Vitaline) ▼ [PoM]
Injection, iron (as iron dextran) 50 mg/mL, net price 2-mL amp = £7.97

IRON SORBITOL

Colloidal solution of a complex of iron, sorbitol and citric acid, stabilised with dextrin and sorbitol; contains 5% (50 mg/mL) of iron
Indications: iron-deficiency anaemia, see notes above
Cautions: oral iron should be stopped at least 24 hours before; history of allergic disorders including asthma; elderly, underweight or debilitated; pregnancy (Appendix 4)
Contra-indications: liver disease, kidney disease, untreated urinary-tract infections; preferably avoid in patients with pre-existing cardiac abnormalities (e.g. angina or arrhythmias)
Side-effects: nausea, vomiting, diarrhoea, haematuria, taste disturbances, dizziness, flushing, myalgia; hypersensitivity reactions including urticaria and hypotension; occasionally severe arrhythmias; rarely anaphylactoid reactions; injection site reactions
Dose: *by deep intramuscular injection,* calculated according to body-weight and iron deficit, consult product literature

Jectofer® (AstraZeneca) [PoM]
Injection, iron sorbitol (iron 50 mg/mL). Net price 2-mL amp = 45p

IRON SUCROSE

A complex of ferric hydroxide with sucrose containing 2% (20 mg/mL) of iron
Indications: iron-deficiency anaemia, see notes above
Cautions: oral iron therapy should not be given until 5 days after last injection; facilities for cardiopulmonary resuscitation must be at hand; pregnancy (Appendix 4)
Contra-indications: history of allergic disorders including asthma, eczema and anaphylaxis; liver disease; infection
Side-effects: nausea, vomiting, taste disturbances, headache, hypotension; less frequently paraesthesia, abdominal disorders, myalgia, fever, flushing, urticaria, peripheral oedema; rarely anaphylactoid reactions; injection site reactions including phlebitis reported
Dose: *by slow intravenous injection* or *by intravenous infusion,* calculated according to body-weight and iron deficit, consult product literature
CHILD not recommended

Venofer® (Syner-Med) [PoM]
Injection, iron (as iron sucrose) 20 mg/mL, net price 5-mL amp = £8.98

9.1.2 Drugs used in megaloblastic anaemias

Most megaloblastic anaemias result from a lack of either vitamin B_{12} or folate, and it is essential to establish in every case which deficiency is present and the underlying cause. In emergencies, where delay might be dangerous, it is sometimes necessary to administer both substances after the bone marrow test while plasma assay results are awaited. Normally, however, appropriate treatment should be instituted only when the results of tests are available.

One cause of megaloblastic anaemia in the UK is *pernicious anaemia* in which lack of gastric intrinsic factor resulting from an auto-immune gastritis causes malabsorption of vitamin B_{12}.

Vitamin B_{12} is also needed in the treatment of megaloblastosis caused by *prolonged nitrous oxide anaesthesia*, which inactivates the vitamin, and in the rare syndrome of *congenital transcobalamin II deficiency*.

Vitamin B_{12} should be given prophylactically after *total gastrectomy* or *total ileal resection* (or after *partial gastrectomy* if a vitamin B_{12} absorption test shows vitamin B_{12} malabsorption).

Apart from dietary deficiency, all other causes of vitamin-B_{12} deficiency are attributable to malabsorption. There is little place for the use of low-dose vitamin B_{12} orally and none for vitamin B_{12} intrinsic factor complexes given by mouth. Vitamin B_{12} in larger oral doses of 1–2 mg daily [unlicensed] may be effective.

Hydroxocobalamin has completely replaced cyanocobalamin as the form of vitamin B_{12} of choice for therapy; it is retained in the body longer than cyanocobalamin and thus for maintenance therapy can be given at intervals of up to 3 months. Treatment is generally initiated with frequent administration of intramuscular injections to replenish the depleted body stores. Thereafter, maintenance treatment, which is usually for life, can be instituted. There is no evidence that doses larger than those recommended provide any additional benefit in vitamin-B_{12} neuropathy.

Folic acid has few indications for long-term therapy since most causes of folate deficiency are self-limiting and will yield to a short course of treatment. It should not be used in undiagnosed megaloblastic anaemia unless vitamin B_{12} is administered concurrently otherwise neuropathy may be precipitated (see above).

In *folate-deficient megaloblastic anaemia* (e.g. due to poor nutrition, pregnancy, or antiepileptics), standard treatment to bring about a haematological remission and replenish body stores, is oral administration of folic acid 5 mg daily for 4 months; up to 15 mg daily may be necessary in malabsorption states.

For *prophylaxis in chronic haemolytic states or in renal dialysis*, it is sufficient to give folic acid 5 mg daily or even weekly, depending on the diet and the rate of haemolysis.

For *prophylaxis in pregnancy* the dose of folic acid is 200–500 micrograms daily (see Iron and Folic Acid, section 9.1.1.1). See also Prevention of Neural Tube Defects below.

Folinic acid is also effective in the treatment of folate-deficient megaloblastic anaemia but it is generally used in association with cytotoxic drugs (see section 8.1); it is given as calcium folinate.

PREVENTION OF NEURAL TUBE DEFECTS. Recommendations of an expert advisory group of the Department of Health include the advice that:

> To prevent *recurrence of neural tube defect* (in a child of a man or woman with spina bifida or if there is a history of neural tube defect in a previous child) women who wish to become pregnant (or who are at risk of becoming pregnant) should be advised to take folic acid supplements at a dose of 5 mg daily (reduced to 4 mg daily if a suitable preparation becomes available); supplementation should continue until week 12 of pregnancy. Women receiving antiepileptic therapy need individual counselling from their doctor before starting folic acid.
>
> To prevent *first occurrence of neural tube defect* women who are planning a pregnancy should be advised to take folic acid as a medicinal or food supplement at a dose of 400 micrograms daily before conception and during the first 12 weeks of pregnancy. Women who have not been taking supplements and who suspect they are pregnant should start at once and continue until week 12 of pregnancy.

There is **no** justification for prescribing multiple-ingredient vitamin preparations containing vitamin B_{12} or folic acid.

HYDROXOCOBALAMIN

Indications: see under dose below

Cautions: should not be given before diagnosis fully established but see also notes above

Side-effects: itching, exanthema; fever, chills, hot flushes; nausea, dizziness; initial hypokalaemia; rarely acneiform and bullous eruptions; anaphylaxis

Dose: *by intramuscular injection*, pernicious anaemia and other macrocytic anaemias without neurological involvement, initially 1 mg 3 times a week for 2 weeks then 1 mg every 3 months

Pernicious anaemia and other macrocytic anaemias with neurological involvement, initially 1 mg on alternate days until no further improvement, then 1 mg every 2 months

Prophylaxis of macrocytic anaemias associated with vitamin-B_{12} deficiency, 1 mg every 2–3 months

Tobacco amblyopia and Leber's optic atrophy, initially 1 mg daily for 2 weeks, then 1 mg twice weekly until no further improvement, thereafter 1 mg every 1–3 months

CHILD, doses as for adult

Hydroxocobalamin (Non-proprietary) PoM
Injection, hydroxocobalamin 1 mg/mL. Net price 1-mL amp = £2.50

Note. The BP directs that when vitamin B_{12} injection is prescribed or demanded hydroxocobalamin injection shall be dispensed or supplied

Available from Celltech (*Neo-Cytamen®* NHS), Goldshield, Link (*Cobalin-H®* NHS)

CYANOCOBALAMIN

Indications: see notes above

Dose: *by mouth*, vitamin-B$_{12}$ deficiency of dietary origin, 50–150 micrograms or more daily taken between meals; CHILD 50–105 micrograms daily in 1–3 divided doses

By intramuscular injection, initially 1 mg repeated 10 times at intervals of 2–3 days, maintenance 1 mg every month, but see notes above

Cyanocobalamin (Non-proprietary)
Tablets NHS, cyanocobalamin 50 micrograms.
Net price 50-tab pack = £3.04
* NHS except to treat or prevent vitamin-B$_{12}$ deficiency in a patient who is a vegan or who has a proven vitamin-B$_{12}$ deficiency of dietary origin and endorsed 'SLS'
Available from Goldshield (*Cytacon®* NHS)
Liquid NHS, cyanocobalamin 35 micrograms/5 mL. Net price 200 mL = £2.77
Available from Goldshield (*Cytacon®* NHS)
Injection PoM, cyanocobalamin 1 mg/mL. Net price 1-mL amp = £1.67
Note. The BP directs that when vitamin B$_{12}$ injection is prescribed or demanded hydroxocobalamin injection shall be dispensed or supplied
Available from Celltech (*Cytamen®* NHS)

FOLIC ACID

Indications: see notes above

Cautions: should never be given alone for pernicious anaemia and other vitamin B$_{12}$-deficiency states (may precipitate subacute combined degeneration of the spinal cord); **interactions:** Appendix 1 (folic acid and folinic acid)

Dose: *by mouth*, initially, 5 mg daily for 4 months (see notes above); maintenance, 5 mg every 1–7 days depending on underlying disease; CHILD up to 1 year, 500 micrograms/kg daily; over 1 year, as adult dose

Prevention of neural tube defects, see notes above

Folic Acid (Non-proprietary) PoM
Tablets, folic acid 400 micrograms, net price = 90-tab pack = £2.19; 5 mg, 20 = 49p
Note. 400-microgram tablets available from Lane (*Preconceive®*), 5-mg tablets available from various suppliers
1. Can be sold to the public provided daily doses do not exceed 500 micrograms
Syrup, folic acid 2.5 mg/5 mL, net price 150 mL = £9.74; 400 micrograms/5 mL, 150 mL = £2.45
Note. 2.5 mg/5 mL syrup available from Hillcross and Rosemont (*Lexpec®*, sugar-free); 400 micrograms/5 mL oral solution available from Rosemont (*Folicare®*)
Injection, folic acid 15 mg/mL, net price 1-mL amp = £1.24
Available from BCM Specials [unlicensed—special order]

9.1.3 Drugs used in hypoplastic, haemolytic, and renal anaemias

Anabolic steroids, pyridoxine, antilymphocyte immunoglobulin, and various corticosteroids are used in hypoplastic and haemolytic anaemias.

The appropriate use of **anabolic steroids** in the therapy of *aplastic anaemia* remains unclear. There is a wide variation in the reported successful responses. Occasional patients, however, do seem to derive benefit. Since nandrolone decanoate (section 6.4.3) requires intramuscular injection it is unsuitable in aplastic anaemia or cytotoxic aplasia because of the low platelet count. Oxymetholone tablets (available only on named-patient basis) may alternatively be used in aplastic anaemia. Controlled trials have shown that antilymphocyte globulin given by intravenous infusion produces a response in 50% of acquired cases; higher response rates have been reported when ciclosporin is given as well.

It is unlikely that dietary deprivation of **pyridoxine** (section 9.6.2) produces clinically relevant haematological effects. However, certain forms of *sideroblastic anaemia* respond to pharmacological doses, possibly reflecting its role as a co-enzyme during haemoglobin synthesis. Pyridoxine is indicated in both *idiopathic acquired* and *hereditary sideroblastic anaemias*. Although complete cures have not been reported, some increase in haemoglobin may occur; the dose required is usually high, up to 400 mg daily. *Reversible sideroblastic anaemias* respond to treatment of the underlying cause but in pregnancy, haemolytic anaemias, and alcohol dependence, or during isoniazid treatment, pyridoxine is also indicated.

Corticosteroids (see section 6.3) have an important place in the management of a wide variety of haematological disorders. They include conditions with an immune basis such as *autoimmune haemolytic anaemia*, *immune thrombocytopenias* and *neutropenias*, and *major transfusion reactions*. They are also used in chemotherapy schedules for many types of *lymphoma*, *lymphoid leukaemias*, and *paraproteinaemias*, including *multiple myeloma*.

Erythropoietin

Epoetin (recombinant human erythropoietin) is used for the anaemia associated with erythropoietin deficiency in chronic renal failure, to increase the yield of autologous blood in normal individuals and to shorten the period of anaemia in patients receiving platinum-containing chemotherapy. The clinical efficacy of epoetin alfa and epoetin beta is similar. Epoetin beta is also used for the prevention of anaemia in premature infants of low birth-weight.

Darbepoetin, is a hyperglycosylated derivative of epoetin which has a longer half-life and may be administered less frequently than epoetin.

Other factors which contribute to the anaemia of chronic renal failure such as iron or folate deficiency should be corrected before treatment and monitored during therapy. Supplemental iron may improve the response in resistant patients. Aluminium toxicity, concurrent infection or other inflammatory disease may impair the response to erythropoietin.

DARBEPOETIN ALFA

Indications: anaemia associated with chronic renal failure

Cautions: see Epoetin; hepatic disease (Appendix 2); pregnancy (Appendix 4) and breast-feeding (Appendix 5)

Contra-indications: see Epoetin

Side-effects: see Epoetin

Dose: *by intravenous* or *subcutaneous injection*, ADULT and CHILD over 11 years, initially 450 nanograms/kg once weekly adjusted according to response by approx. 25% of initial dose at intervals of at least 4 weeks; reduce dose by 25–50% if haemoglobin rise exceeds 2.5 g/100 mL per month; suspend if haemoglobin exceeds 14 g/100 mL until it falls below 13 g/100 mL and then restart with dose at 25% below previous dose

Note. When changing route give same dose then adjust according to weekly or fortnightly haemoglobin measurements

Aranesp® (Amgen) ▼ PoM
Injection, prefilled syringe, darbepoetin alfa, net price 10 micrograms = £16.76; 15 micrograms = £25.14; 20 micrograms = £33.52; 30 micrograms = £50.28; 40 micrograms = £67.04; 50 micrograms = £83.80; 60 micrograms = £100.56; 80 micrograms = £134.08; 100 micrograms = £167.60; 150 micrograms = £251.40.

EPOETIN ALFA and BETA

(Recombinant human erythropoietins)
Note. Although epoetin alfa and beta are clinically indistinguishable the prescriber must specify which is required

Indications: see under preparations, below

Cautions: inadequately treated or poorly controlled blood pressure (monitor closely blood pressure, haemoglobin, and electrolytes), interrupt treatment if blood pressure uncontrolled; sudden stabbing migraine-like pain is warning of hypertensive crisis; exclude other causes of anaemia (e.g. folic acid or vitamin B$_{12}$ deficiency) and give iron supplements if necessary (see also notes above); ischaemic vascular disease; thrombocytosis (monitor platelet count for first 8 weeks); epilepsy; malignant disease; chronic liver failure; increase in heparin dose may be needed; risk of thrombosis may be increased when used for anaemia before orthopaedic surgery—avoid in cardiovascular disease including recent myocardial infarction or cerebrovascular accident; pregnancy (Appendix 4) and breast-feeding (Appendix 5); **interactions:** Appendix 1 (epoetin)

Contra-indications: uncontrolled hypertension; avoid injections containing benzyl alcohol in neonates (see under preparations, below)

Side-effects: dose-dependent increase in blood pressure or aggravation of hypertension; in isolated patients with normal or low blood pressure, hypertensive crisis with encephalopathy-like symptoms and generalised tonic-clonic seizures requiring immediate medical attention; dose-dependent increase in platelet count (but thrombocytosis rare) regressing during treatment; influenza-like symptoms (may be reduced if intravenous injection given over 5 minutes); shunt thrombosis especially if tendency to hypotension or arteriovenous shunt complications; isolated reports of hyperkalaemia, skin reactions; very rarely sudden loss of response because of pure red cell aplasia (discontinue erythropoietin therapy)

Dose: aimed at increasing haemoglobin concentration at rate not exceeding 2 g/100 mL/month to stable level of 10–12 g/100 mL (9.5–11 g/100 mL in children); see under preparations, below

■ Epoetin alfa

Eprex® (Janssen-Cilag) PoM
Injection, epoetin alfa 40 000 units/mL, net price 1-mL (40 000-unit) vial = £335.20

Injection, prefilled syringe, epoetin alfa, net price 1000 units = £8.38; 2000 units = £16.76; 3000 units = £25.14; 4000 units = £33.52; 10 000 units = £83.80. An auto-injector device is available for use with 10 000-units prefilled syringes

Dose: anaemia associated with chronic renal failure in patients on haemodialysis, *by subcutaneous injection* (preferred route; max. 1 mL per injection site) or *by intravenous injection* over 1–5 minutes, initially 50 units/kg 3 times weekly adjusted according to response in steps of 25 units/kg 3 times weekly at intervals of at least 4 weeks; maintenance dose (when haemoglobin concentration of 10–12 g/100 mL achieved), usually 25–100 units/kg 3 times weekly; CHILD (intravenous route only) initially as for adults; maintenance dose (when haemoglobin concentration of 9.5–11 g/100 mL achieved), under 10 kg usually 75–150 units/kg 3 times weekly, 10–30 kg usually 60–150 units/kg 3 times weekly, over 30 kg usually 30–100 units/kg 3 times weekly

Note. Subcutaneous dose generally about 20–30% lower than intravenous dose; when changing route give same dose then adjust according to weekly haemoglobin measurements

Anaemia associated with chronic renal failure in adults on peritoneal dialysis, *by subcutaneous injection* (max. 1 mL per injection site), initially 50 units/kg twice weekly; maintenance dose (when haemoglobin concentration of 10–12 g/100 mL achieved), 25–50 units/kg twice weekly

Severe symptomatic anaemia of renal origin in adults with renal insufficiency not yet on dialysis, preferably *by subcutaneous injection* (max. 1 mL per injection site), initially 50 units/kg 3 times weekly increased according to response in steps of 25 units/kg 3 times weekly at intervals of at least 4 weeks; maintenance dose (when haemoglobin concentration of 10–12 g/100 mL achieved), 17–33 units/kg 3 times weekly; max. 600 units/kg weekly in 3 divided doses;

Anaemia in adults receiving cancer chemotherapy, *by subcutaneous injection* (max. 1 mL per injection site), initially 150 units/kg 3 times weekly, increased if appropriate rise in haemoglobin (or reticulocyte count) not achieved after 4 weeks to 300 units/kg 3 times weekly; discontinue if inadequate response after 4 weeks at higher dose; reduce dose by 25–50% if haemoglobin rise exceeds 2 g/100 mL per month; suspend if haemoglobin exceeds 14 g/100 mL until it falls below 12 g/100 mL and reinstate with dose at 25% below previous dose; continue epoetin for 1 month after end of chemotherapy

To increase yield of autologous blood (to avoid homologous blood) in predonation programme in moderate anaemia *either* when large volume of blood required for elective major surgery *or* if insufficient period to obtain required volume of blood, *by intravenous injection* over 1–5 minutes, 600 units/kg twice weekly for 3 weeks before surgery; consult product literature for details and advice on ensuring high iron stores

Moderate anaemia (haemoglobin concentration 10–13 g/100 mL) before elective orthopaedic surgery in adults with expected moderate blood loss to reduce exposure to homologous transfusion or if autologous transfusion unavailable, *by subcutaneous injection* (max. 1 mL per injection site), 600 units/kg every week for 3 weeks before surgery and on day of surgery *or* 300 units/kg daily for 15 days starting 10 days before surgery; consult product literature for details

■ **Epoetin beta**

NeoRecormon® (Roche) PoM

Injection, powder for reconstitution, epoetin beta, net price 500-unit vial = £4.19 (with water for injection)

Excipients: include phenylalanine up to 1 mg/vial (section 9.4.1)

Note. Avoid contact of reconstituted injection with glass; use only plastic materials

Injection, prefilled syringe, epoetin beta, net price 500 units = £4.19; 1000 units = £8.38; 2000 units = £16.76; 3000 units = £25.14; 4000 units = £33.52; 5000 units = £41.90; 6000 units = £50.28; 10 000 units = £83.80

Excipients: include phenylalanine up to 300 micrograms/syringe (section 9.4.1)

Multidose injection, powder for reconstitution, epoetin beta, net price 50 000-unit vial = £419.01; 100 000-unit vial = £838.01 (both with solvent)

Excipients: include phenylalanine up to 5 mg/vial (section 9.4.1), benzyl alcohol (avoid in neonates, see Excipients p. 2)

Note. Avoid contact of reconstituted injection with glass; use only plastic materials

Reco-Pen, (for subcutaneous use), double-chamber cartridges (containing epoetin beta and solvent), net price 10 000-unit cartridge = £83.80; 20 000-unit cartridge = £167.60; 60 000-unit cartridge = £502.81; for use with *Reco-Pen* injection device and needles (both available free from Roche)

Excipients: include phenylalanine up to 500 micrograms/cartridge (section 9.4.1), benzyl alcohol (avoid in neonates, see Excipients p. 2)

Dose: anaemia associated with chronic renal failure in dialysis patients, symptomatic anaemia of renal origin in patients not yet on dialysis, ADULT and CHILD

By subcutaneous injection, initially 60 units/kg weekly (in 1–7 divided doses) for 4 weeks, increased according to response at intervals of 4 weeks in steps of 60 units/kg; maintenance dose (when haemoglobin concentration of 10–12 g/100 mL achieved), initially reduce dose by half then adjust according to response at intervals of 1–2 weeks; max. 720 units/kg weekly

By intravenous injection over 2 minutes, initially 40 units/kg 3 times weekly for 4 weeks, increased according to response to 80 units/kg 3 times weekly with further increases if needed at intervals of 4 weeks in steps of 20 units/kg 3 times weekly; maintenance dose (when haemoglobin concentration of 10–12 g/100 mL achieved), initially reduce dose by half then adjust according to response at intervals of 1–2 weeks; max. 720 units/kg weekly

Prevention of anaemias of prematurity in infants with birth-weight of 0.75–1.5 kg and gestational age of less than 34 weeks, *by subcutaneous injection* (of single-dose, unpreserved injection), 250 units/kg 3 times weekly preferably starting within 3 days of birth and continued for 6 weeks

Anaemia in adults with solid tumours receiving platinum-containing chemotherapy, *by subcutaneous injection*, initially 450 units/kg weekly (in 3–7 divided doses), increased if appropriate rise in haemoglobin not achieved after 4 weeks to 900 units/kg weekly (in 3–7 divided doses); reduce dose by half if haemoglobin rise exceeds 2 g/100 mL per month; suspend if haemoglobin exceeds 14 g/100 mL until concentration falls below 12 g/100 mL and reinstate at 50% of the previous weekly dose; continue for up to 3 weeks after end of chemotherapy

Note. If haemoglobin concentration falls by more than 1 g/100 mL in the first cycle of chemotherapy despite treatment with epoetin beta, further treatment may not be effective

To increase yield of autologous blood (to avoid homologous blood) in predonation programme in moderate anaemia when blood conserving procedures are insufficient or unavailable, consult product literature

Anaemia in adults with multiple myeloma, low-grade non-Hodgkin's lymphoma or chronic lymphocytic leukaemia receiving chemotherapy, *by subcutaneous injection*, initially 450 units/kg weekly (in 3–7 divided doses), increased if rise in haemoglobin of at least 1 g/100 mL not achieved after 4 weeks to 900 units/kg weekly (in 3–7 divided doses); reduce dose by half if haemoglobin rise exceeds 2 g/100 mL per month; suspend if haemoglobin exceeds 14 g/100 mL until concentration falls below 13 g/100 mL and reinstate at 50% of previous dose; max. 900 units/kg weekly; continue for up to 4 weeks after end of chemotherapy in chronic lymphocytic leukaemia

Note. Discontinue treatment if haemoglobin concentration does not increase by at least 1 g/100 mL after 8 weeks of therapy

Iron overload

Severe tissue iron overload may occur in aplastic and other refractory anaemias, mainly as the result of repeated blood transfusions. It is a particular problem in refractory anaemias with hyperplastic bone marrow, especially *thalassaemia major*, where excessive iron absorption from the gut and inappropriate iron therapy may add to the tissue siderosis.

Iron overload associated with haemochromatosis may be treated with repeated venesection. Venesection may also be used for patients who have received multiple transfusions and whose bone marrow has recovered. Where venesection is contra-indicated, the long-term administration of the iron chelating compound **desferrioxamine mesilate** is useful. Subcutaneous infusions of desferrioxamine are given over 8–12 hours, 3–7 times a week. The dose should reflect the degree of iron overload. For children starting therapy (and who have low iron overload) the dose should not exceed 30 mg/kg. For established overload the dose is usually between 20 and 50 mg/kg daily. Desferrioxamine (up to 2 g per unit of blood) may also be given at the time of blood transfusion, provided that the desferrioxamine is **not** added to the blood and is **not** given through the same line as the blood (but the two may be given through the same cannula).

Iron excretion induced by desferrioxamine is enhanced by administration of ascorbic acid (vitamin C, section 9.6.3) in a dose of 200 mg daily (100 mg in infants); it should be given separately from food since it also enhances iron absorption. Ascorbic acid should not be given to patients with cardiac dysfunction; in patients with normal cardiac function ascorbic acid should be introduced 1 month after starting desferrioxamine.

Infusion of desferrioxamine may be used to treat *aluminium overload* in dialysis patients; theoretically 100 mg of desferrioxamine binds with 4.1 mg of aluminium.

Deferiprone, an oral iron chelator, is licensed for the treatment of iron overload in patients with thalassaemia major in whom desferrioxamine is contra-indicated or is not tolerated. Blood dyscrasias, particularly agranulocytosis, have been reported with deferiprone.

DEFERIPRONE

Indications: see notes above

Cautions: neutropenia (monitor neutrophil count weekly and discontinue treatment if neutropenia develops); hepatic and renal impairment; limited experience in children 6–10 years

BLOOD DISORDERS. Patients or their carers should be told how to recognise signs of neutropenia and advised to seek immediate medical attention if symptoms such as fever or sore throat develop

Contra-indications: pregnancy (Appendix 4) and breast-feeding

Side-effects: gastro-intestinal disturbances; red-brown urine discoloration; arthropathy; neutropenia, agranulocytosis

Dose: ADULT and CHILD over 6 years 25 mg/kg (to the nearest 250 mg) 3 times daily (max. 100 mg/kg daily); CHILD under 6 years not recommended

Ferriprox® (Swedish Orphan Int AB) ▼ PoM

Tablets, f/c, scored, deferiprone 500 mg, net price 100-tab pack = £152.39. Label: 14, counselling, blood disorders

DESFERRIOXAMINE MESILATE

(Deferoxamine Mesilate)

Indications: see notes above; iron poisoning, see Emergency Treatment of Poisoning

Cautions: renal impairment; eye and ear examinations before treatment and at 3-month intervals during treatment; aluminium-related encephalopathy (may exacerbate neurological dysfunction); pregnancy (Appendix 4), breast-feeding; **interactions:** Appendix 1 (desferrioxamine)

Side-effects: hypotension (especially when given too rapidly by intravenous injection), disturbances of hearing and vision (including lens opacity and retinopathy); injection site reactions, gastro-intestinal disturbances, asthma, fever, headache, arthralgia and myalgia; very rarely anaphylaxis, acute respiratory distress syndrome, neurological disturbances (including dizziness, neuropathy and paraesthesia), Yersinia and mucormycosis infections, rash, renal impairment, and blood dyscrasias

Dose: see notes above; iron poisoning, see Emergency Treatment of Poisoning

Note. For full details and warnings relating to administration, consult product literature

Desferal® (Novartis) PoM

Injection, powder for reconstitution, desferrioxamine mesilate, net price 500-mg vial = £4.44, 2-g vial = £17.77

9.1.4 Drugs used in autoimmune thrombocytopenic purpura

It is usual to commence the treatment of autoimmune (idiopathic) thrombocytopenic purpura with corticosteroids, e.g. prednisolone 1 mg/kg daily, gradually reducing the dosage over the subsequent weeks. In patients who fail to achieve a satisfactory platelet count or relapse when corticosteroid dosage is reduced or withdrawn, splenectomy is considered.

Other therapy that has been tried in refractory cases includes azathioprine (section 8.2.1), cyclophosphamide (section 8.1.1), vincristine (section 8.1.4), ciclosporin (section 8.2.2), and danazol (section 6.7.2). Intravenous immunoglobulins (section 14.5), have also been used in refractory cases or where a temporary rapid rise in platelets is needed, as in pregnancy or pre-operatively. For patients with chronic severe thrombocytopenia refractory to other therapy, tranexamic acid (section 2.11) may be given to reduce the severity of haemorrhage.

9.1.5 G6PD deficiency

Glucose 6-phosphate dehydrogenase (G6PD) deficiency is highly prevalent in individuals originating from most parts of Africa, from most parts of Asia, from Oceania, and from Southern Europe; it can also occur, rarely, in any other individuals.

Individuals with G6PD deficiency are susceptible to developing acute haemolytic anaemia on taking a number of common drugs. They are also susceptible to developing acute haemolytic anaemia upon ingestion of fava beans (broad beans, *Vicia faba*); this is termed *favism* and can be more severe in children or when the fresh fava beans are eaten raw.

When prescribing drugs for patients with G6PD deficiency, the following points should be kept in mind:

1. G6PD deficiency is genetically heterogeneous; susceptibility to the haemolytic risk from drugs varies; thus, a drug found to be safe in some G6PD-deficient individuals may not be equally safe in others;

2. manufacturers do not routinely test drugs for their effects in G6PD-deficient individuals;

3. the risk and severity of haemolysis is almost always dose-related.

The lists below should be read with these points in mind. Ideally, information about G6PD deficiency should be available before prescribing a drug listed below. However, in the absence of this information, the possibility of haemolysis should be considered, especially if the patient belongs to a group in which G6PD deficiency is common.

A very few G6PD-deficient individuals with chronic non-spherocytic haemolytic anaemia have haemolysis even in the absence of an exogenous trigger. These patients must be regarded as being at high risk of severe exacerbation of haemolysis following administration of any of the drugs listed below.

Drugs with definite risk of haemolysis in most G6PD-deficient individuals
Dapsone and other sulphones (higher doses for dermatitis herpetiformis more likely to cause problems)
Methylthioninium chloride (methylene blue)
Niridazole [not on UK market]
Nitrofurantoin
Pamaquin [not on UK market]
Primaquine (30 mg weekly for 8 weeks has been found to be without undue harmful effects in African and Asian people, see section 5.4.1)
Quinolones (including ciprofloxacin, nalidixic acid, norfloxacin, and ofloxacin)
Sulphonamides (including co-trimoxazole; some sulphonamides, e.g. sulfadiazine, have been tested and found not to be haemolytic in many G6PD-deficient individuals)

Drugs with possible risk of haemolysis in some G6PD-deficient individuals
Aspirin (acceptable up to a dose of at least 1 g daily in most G6PD-deficient individuals)
Chloroquine (acceptable in acute malaria)
Menadione, water-soluble derivatives (e.g. menadiol sodium phosphate)
Probenecid [not on UK market]
Quinidine (acceptable in acute malaria)
Quinine (acceptable in acute malaria)

Note. Mothballs may contain naphthalene which also causes haemolysis in individuals with G6PD-deficiency.

9.1.6 Drugs used in neutropenia

Recombinant human granulocyte-colony stimulating factor (rhG-CSF) stimulates the production of neutrophils and may reduce the duration of chemotherapy-induced neutropenia and thereby reduce the incidence of associated sepsis; there is as yet no evidence that it improves overall survival. **Filgrastim** (unglycosylated rhG-CSF) and **lenograstim** (glycosylated rhG-CSF) have similar effects; both have been used in a variety of clinical settings but they do not have any clear-cut routine indications. In congenital neutropenia filgrastim usually elevates the neutrophil count with appropriate clinical response. Prolonged use may be associated with an increased risk of myeloid malignancy.

Molgramostim (recombinant human granulocyte macrophage-colony stimulating factor) stimulates the production of all granulocytes and monocytes. It has more side-effects than granulocyte-colony stimulating factor and is ineffective in congenital neutropenia.

Treatment with recombinant human growth factors should only be prescribed by those experienced in their use.

For the use of **amifostine** in cytotoxic-induced neutropenic infection, see section 8.1.

FILGRASTIM

(Recombinant human granulocyte-colony stimulating factor, G-CSF)

Indications: (specialist use only) reduction in duration of neutropenia and incidence of febrile neutropenia in cytotoxic chemotherapy for malignancy (except chronic myeloid leukaemia and myelodysplastic syndromes); reduction in duration of neutropenia (and associated sequelae) in myeloablative therapy followed by bone-marrow transplantation; mobilisation of peripheral blood progenitor cells for harvesting and subsequent autologous or allogeneic infusion; severe congenital neutropenia, cyclic neutropenia, or idiopathic neutropenia and history of severe or recurrent infections (distinguish carefully from other haematological disorders, consult product literature); persistent neutropenia in advanced HIV infection

Cautions: reduced myeloid precursors; monitor leucocyte count (discontinue treatment if leucocytosis, consult product literature); monitor platelet count and haemoglobin; regular morphological and cytogenetic bone-marrow examinations recommended in severe congenital neutropenia (possible risk of myelodysplastic syndromes or leukaemia); secondary acute myeloid leukaemia, sickle cell disease; monitor spleen size; osteoporotic bone disease (monitor bone density if given for more than 6 months); does not prevent other toxic effects of high-dose chemotherapy; pregnancy (Appendix 4), breast-feeding (Appendix 5); **interactions:** Appendix 1 (filgrastim)

Contra-indications: severe congenital neutropenia (Kostman's syndrome) with abnormal cytogenetics

Side-effects: musculoskeletal pain, transient hypotension, disturbances in liver enzymes and serum uric acid; thrombocytopenia; urinary abnormalities including dysuria; allergic reactions (more common after intravenous infusion), proteinuria, haematuria, and transient decrease in blood glucose reported; cutaneous vasculitis also reported, also splenic enlargement, hepatomegaly, headache, diarrhoea, anaemia, epistaxis, alopecia, osteoporosis, and rash, reactions at injection site; rarely reported, exacerbation of rheumatoid arthritis, adult respiratory distress syndrome

Dose: cytotoxic-induced neutropenia, preferably *by subcutaneous injection or by intravenous infusion* (over 30 minutes), ADULT and CHILD, 500 000 units/kg daily started not less than 24 hours after cytotoxic chemotherapy, continued until neutrophil count in normal range, usually for up to 14 days (up to 38 days in acute myeloid leukaemia)

Myeloablative therapy followed by bone-marrow transplantation, *by intravenous infusion* over 30 minutes or over 24 hours *or by subcutaneous infusion* over 24 hours, 1 million units/kg daily, started not less than 24 hours following cytotoxic chemotherapy (and within 24 hours of bone-marrow infusion), then adjusted according to absolute neutrophil count (consult product literature)

Mobilisation of peripheral blood progenitor cells for autologous infusion, used alone, *by subcutaneous injection or by subcutaneous infusion* over 24 hours, 1 million units/kg daily for 5–7 days;

used following adjunctive myelosuppressive chemotherapy (to improve yield), *by subcutaneous injection*, 500 000 units/kg daily, started the day after completion of chemotherapy and continued until neutrophil count in normal range; for timing of leukapheresis consult product literature

Mobilisation of peripheral blood progenitor cells in normal donors for allogeneic infusion, *by subcutaneous injection*, ADULT under 60 years and ADOLESCENT over 16 years, 1 million units/kg daily for 4–5 days; for timing of leukapheresis consult product literature

Severe chronic neutropenia, *by subcutaneous injection*, ADULT and CHILD, in severe congenital neutropenia, initially 1.2 million units/kg daily in single or divided doses (initially 500 000 units/kg daily in idiopathic or cyclic neutropenia), adjusted according to response (consult product literature)

Persistent neutropenia in HIV infection, *by subcutaneous injection*, initially 100 000 units/kg daily, increased as necessary until absolute neutrophil count in normal range (usual max. 400 000 units/kg daily), then adjusted to maintain absolute neutrophil count in normal range (consult product literature)

Neupogen® (Amgen) PoM
Injection, filgrastim 30 million units (300 micrograms)/mL; net price 1-mL vial = £73.56, 1.6-mL (48 million-unit) vial = £117.32
Injection (*Singleject®*), filgrastim 60 million units (600 micrograms)/mL, net price 0.5-mL prefilled syringe = £73.56; 96 million units (960 micrograms)/mL, 0.5-mL prefilled syringe = £117.32

LENOGRASTIM

(Recombinant human granulocyte-colony stimulating factor, rHuG-CSF)

Indications: (specialist use only) reduction in the duration of neutropenia and associated complications following bone-marrow transplantation for non-myeloid malignancy or following treatment with cytotoxic chemotherapy associated with a significant incidence of febrile neutropenia; mobilisation of peripheral blood progenitor cells for harvesting and subsequent infusion

Cautions: see under Filgrastim; pre-malignant myeloid conditions; **interactions:** Appendix 1 (lenograstim)

Side-effects: see under Filgrastim; asthenia, abdominal pain and generalised pain reported in healthy donors

Dose: following bone-marrow transplantation, *by intravenous infusion*, ADULT and CHILD over 2 years 19.2 million units/m² daily started the day after transplantation, continued until neutrophil count stable in acceptable range (max. 28 days)

Cytotoxic-induced neutropenia, *by subcutaneous injection*, ADULT 19.2 million units/m² daily started the day after completion of chemotherapy, continued until neutrophil count stable in acceptable range (max. 28 days)

Mobilisation of peripheral blood progenitor cells, used alone, *by subcutaneous injection*, ADULT 1.28 million units/kg daily for 4–6 days (5–6 days in healthy donors); used following adjunctive

myelosuppressive chemotherapy (to improve yield), *by subcutaneous injection*, 19.2 million units/m² daily, started the day after completion of chemotherapy and continued until neutrophil count in acceptable range; for timing of leukapheresis consult product literature

Granocyte® (Chugai) PoM
Injection, powder for reconstitution, lenograstim, net price 13.4 million-unit (105-microgram) vial = £42.00; 33.6 million-unit (263-microgram) vial = £77.03 (both with 1-mL amp or 1-mL prefilled syringe water for injections)

MOLGRAMOSTIM

(Recombinant human granulocyte macrophage-colony stimulating factor, GM-CSF)

Indications: (specialist use only) reduction of severity of neutropenia (and risk of infection) in cytotoxic chemotherapy; acceleration of myeloid recovery following bone-marrow transplantation; neutropenia in patients treated with ganciclovir in AIDS-related cytomegalovirus retinitis

Cautions: monitor serum albumin concentration and full blood count including differential white cell, platelet and haemoglobin; monitor closely patients with pulmonary disease; history of or predisposition to autoimmune disease; pregnancy and breast-feeding; not yet recommended for patients under 18 years

Contra-indications: myeloid malignancies

Side-effects: nausea, diarrhoea, vomiting, anorexia; dyspnoea; asthenia, fatigue; rash, fever, rigors, flushing, musculoskeletal pain; local reaction following subcutaneous injection; also reported, non-specific chest pain, stomatitis, headache, increased sweating, abdominal pain, pruritus, peripheral oedema, dizziness, paraesthesia, and myalgia; serious reactions reported include anaphylaxis, cardiac failure, capillary leak syndrome, cerebrovascular disorders, confusion, convulsions, hypotension, cardiac rhythm abnormalities, intracranial hypertension, pericardial effusion, pericarditis, pleural effusion, pulmonary oedema, syncope

Dose: (first dose under medical supervision)
Cytotoxic chemotherapy, *by subcutaneous injection*, 60 000–110 000 units/kg daily, starting 24 hours after last dose of chemotherapy, continued for 7–10 days

Bone-marrow transplantation, *by intravenous infusion*, 110 000 units/kg daily, starting day after transplantation, continued until absolute neutrophil count in desirable range (see product literature); max. duration of treatment 30 days

Adjunct in ganciclovir treatment, *by subcutaneous injection*, 60 000 units/kg daily for 5 days then adjusted to maintain desirable absolute neutrophil count and white blood cell count

Leucomax® (Novartis, Schering-Plough) PoM
Injection, powder for reconstitution, molgramostim, net price 1.67 million-unit (150-microgram) vial = £42.13; 3.33 million-unit (300-microgram) vial = £84.26; 4.44 million-unit (400 microgram) vial = £112.34

9.2 Fluids and electrolytes

9.2.1 Oral preparations for fluid and electrolyte imbalance

9.2.2 Parenteral preparations for fluid and electrolyte imbalance

The following tables give a selection of useful electrolyte values:

Electrolyte concentrations—intravenous fluids

Intravenous infusion	Millimoles per litre				
	Na$^+$	K$^+$	HCO$_3^-$	Cl$^-$	Ca^{2+}
Normal Plasma Values	142	4.5	26	103	2.5
Sodium Chloride 0.9%	150	—	—	150	—
Compound Sodium Lactate (Hartmann's)	131	5	29	111	2
Sodium Chloride 0.18% and Glucose 4%	30	—	—	30	—
Potassium Chloride 0.3% and Glucose 5%	—	40	—	40	—
Potassium Chloride 0.3% and Sodium Chloride 0.9%	150	40	—	190	—
To correct metabolic acidosis					
Sodium Bicarbonate 1.26%	150	—	150	—	—
Sodium Bicarbonate 8.4% for cardiac arrest	1000	—	1000	—	—
Sodium Lactate (m/6)	167	—	167	—	—

Electrolyte content—gastro-intestinal secretions

Type of fluid	Millimoles per litre				
	H$^+$	Na$^+$	K$^+$	HCO$_3^-$	Cl$^-$
Gastric	40–60	20–80	5–20	—	100–150
Biliary	—	120–140	5–15	30–50	80–120
Pancreatic	—	120–140	5–15	70–110	40–80
Small bowel	—	120–140	5–15	20–40	90–130

Faeces, vomit, or aspiration should be saved and analysed where possible if abnormal losses are suspected; where this is impracticable the approximations above may be helpful in planning replacement therapy

9.2.1 Oral preparations for fluid and electrolyte imbalance

9.2.1.1 Oral potassium
9.2.1.2 Oral sodium and water
9.2.1.3 Oral bicarbonate

Sodium and potassium salts, which may be given by mouth to prevent deficiencies or to treat established deficiencies of mild or moderate degree, are discussed in this section. Oral preparations for removing excess potassium and preparations for oral rehydration therapy are also included here. Oral bicarbonate, for metabolic acidosis, is also described in this section.

For reference to calcium, magnesium, and phosphate, see section 9.5.

9.2.1.1 Oral potassium

Compensation for potassium loss is especially necessary:

1. in those taking digoxin or anti-arrhythmic drugs, where potassium depletion may induce arrhythmias;
2. in patients in whom secondary hyperaldosteronism occurs, e.g. renal artery stenosis, cirrhosis of the liver, the nephrotic syndrome, and severe heart failure;
3. in patients with excessive losses of potassium in the faeces, e.g. chronic diarrhoea associated with intestinal malabsorption or laxative abuse.

Measures to compensate for potassium loss may also be required in the elderly since they frequently take inadequate amounts of potassium in the diet (but see below for **warning** on **renal insufficiency**). Measures may also be required during long-term administration of drugs known to induce potassium loss (e.g. corticosteroids). Potassium supplements are **seldom required** with the small doses of diuretics given to treat hypertension; **potassium-sparing diuretics** (rather than potassium supplements) are recommended for prevention of hypokalaemia due to diuretics such as furosemide (frusemide) or the thiazides when these are given to eliminate oedema.

DOSAGE. If potassium salts are used for the *prevention of hypokalaemia*, then doses of potassium chloride 2 to 4 g (approx. 25 to 50 mmol) daily by mouth are suitable in patients taking a normal diet. *Smaller doses* must be used if there is *renal insufficiency (common in the elderly)* otherwise there is **danger of hyperkalaemia**. Potassium salts cause nausea and vomiting therefore poor compliance is a major limitation to their effectiveness; where appropriate, potassium-sparing diuretics are preferable (see also above). When there is *established potassium depletion* larger doses may be necessary, the quantity depending on the severity of any continuing potassium loss (monitoring of plasma-potassium concentration and specialist advice would be required). Potassium depletion is frequently associated with chloride depletion and with metabolic alkalosis, and these disorders require correction.

ADMINISTRATION. Potassium salts are preferably given as a liquid (or effervescent) preparation, rather than modified-release tablets; they should be given as the chloride (the use of effervescent potassium tablets BPC 1968 should be restricted to *hyperchloraemic states*, section 9.2.1.3).

Salt substitutes. A number of salt substitutes which contain significant amounts of potassium chloride are readily available as health food products (e.g. *Losalt®* and *Ruthmol®*). These should not be used by patients with renal failure as potassium intoxication may result.

POTASSIUM CHLORIDE

Indications: potassium depletion (see notes above)
Cautions: elderly, mild to moderate renal impairment (close monitoring required), intestinal stricture, history of peptic ulcer, hiatus hernia (for sustained-release preparations); **important:** special hazard if given with drugs liable to raise plasma potassium concentration such as potassium-sparing diuretics, ACE inhibitors, or ciclosporin, for other **interactions:** Appendix 1 (potassium salts)

Contra-indications: severe renal impairment, plasma potassium concentrations above 5 mmol/litre

Side-effects: nausea and vomiting (severe symptoms may indicate obstruction), oesophageal or small bowel ulceration

Dose: see notes above

Note. Do not confuse Effervescent Potassium Tablets BPC 1968 (section 9.2.1.3) with effervescent potassium chloride tablets. Effervescent Potassium Tablets BPC 1968 do not contain chloride ions and their use should be restricted to hyperchloraemic states (section 9.2.1.3). Effervescent Potassium Chloride Tablets BP are usually available in two strengths, one containing 6.7 mmol each of K⁺ and Cl⁻ (corresponding to *Kloref®*), the other containing 12 mmol K⁺ and 8 mmol Cl⁻ (corresponding to *Sando-K®*). Generic prescriptions must specify the strength required.

Kay-Cee-L® (Geistlich)
Syrup, red, sugar-free, potassium chloride 7.5% (1 mmol/mL each of K⁺ and Cl⁻). Net price 500 mL = £2.86. Label: 21

Kloref® (Alpharma)
Tablets, effervescent, betaine hydrochloride, potassium benzoate, bicarbonate, and chloride, equivalent to potassium chloride 500 mg (6.7 mmol each of K⁺ and Cl⁻). Net price 50 = £1.90. Label: 13, 21
Note. May be difficult to obtain

Sando-K® (HK Pharma)
Tablets, effervescent, potassium bicarbonate and chloride equivalent to potassium 470 mg (12 mmol of K⁺) and chloride 285 mg (8 mmol of Cl⁻). Net price 20 = £1.53. Label: 13, 21

■ Modified-release preparations
Avoid unless effervescent tablets or liquid preparations inappropriate

Slow-K® (Alliance) ▭
Tablets, m/r, orange, s/c, potassium chloride 600 mg (8 mmol each of K⁺ and Cl⁻). Net price 20 = 55p. Label: 25, 27, counselling, swallow whole with fluid during meals while sitting or standing

▭ denotes preparations that are considered to be less suitable for prescribing (see p. vi)

Potassium removal

Ion-exchange resins may be used to remove excess potassium in *mild hyperkalaemia* or in *moderate hyperkalaemia* when there are not ECG changes; intravenous therapy is required in emergencies (section 9.2.2).

POLYSTYRENE SULPHONATE RESINS

Indications: hyperkalaemia associated with anuria or severe oliguria, and in dialysis patients

Cautions: children (impaction of resin with excessive dosage or inadequate dilution); monitor for electrolyte disturbances (stop if plasma-potassium concentration below 5 mmol/litre); pregnancy and breast-feeding; sodium-containing resin in congestive heart failure, hypertension, renal impairment, and oedema

Contra-indications: obstructive bowel disease; oral administration or reduced gut motility in neonates; avoid calcium-containing resin in hyperparathyroidism, multiple myeloma, sarcoidosis, or metastatic carcinoma

Side-effects: rectal ulceration following rectal administration; colonic necrosis reported following enemas containing sorbitol; sodium retention, hypercalcaemia, gastric irritation, anorexia, nausea and vomiting, constipation (discontinue treatment—avoid magnesium-containing laxatives), diarrhoea; calcium-containing resin may cause hypercalcaemia (in dialysed patients and occasionally in those with renal impairment), hypomagnesaemia

Dose: *by mouth*, 15 g 3–4 times daily in water (not fruit squash which has a high potassium content) or as a paste; CHILD 0.5–1 g/kg daily in divided doses

By rectum, as an enema, 30 g in methylcellulose solution, retained for 9 hours followed by irrigation to remove resin from colon; NEONATE and CHILD, 0.5–1 g/kg daily

Calcium Resonium® (Sanofi-Synthelabo)
Powder, buff, calcium polystyrene sulphonate. Net price 300 g = £43.23. Label: 13

Resonium A® (Sanofi-Synthelabo)
Powder, buff, sodium polystyrene sulphonate. Net price 454 g = £58.53. Label: 13

9.2.1.2   Oral sodium and water

Sodium chloride is indicated in states of sodium depletion and usually needs to be given intravenously (section 9.2.2). In chronic conditions associated with mild or moderate degrees of sodium depletion, e.g. in salt-losing bowel or renal disease, oral supplements of sodium chloride or sodium bicarbonate (section 9.2.1.3), according to the acid-base status of the patient, may be sufficient.

SODIUM CHLORIDE

Indications: sodium depletion; see also section 9.2.2.

Slow Sodium® (HK Pharma)
Tablets, m/r, sodium chloride 600 mg (approx. 10 mmol each of Na⁺ and Cl⁻). Net price 100-tab pack = £6.05. Label: 25
Dose: prophylaxis of sodium chloride deficiency 4–8 tablets daily with water (in severe depletion up to max. 20 tablets daily)
Chronic renal salt wasting, up to 20 tablets daily with appropriate fluid intake
CHILD, according to requirements

Oral rehydration therapy (ORT)

As a worldwide problem *diarrhoea* is by far the most important indication for fluid and electrolyte replacement. Intestinal absorption of sodium and water is enhanced by glucose (and other carbohydrates). Replacement of fluid and electrolytes lost through diarrhoea can therefore be achieved by giving solutions containing sodium, potassium, and glucose or another carbohydrate such as rice starch.

Oral rehydration solutions should:

- enhance the absorption of water and electrolytes;
- replace the electrolyte deficit adequately and safely;
- contain an alkalinising agent to counter acidosis;
- be slightly hypo-osmolar (about 250 mmol/litre) to prevent the possible induction of osmotic diarrhoea;
- be simple to use in hospital and at home;
- be palatable and acceptable, especially to children;
- be readily available.

It is the policy of the World Health Organization (WHO) to promote a single oral rehydration solution but to use it flexibly (e.g. by giving extra water between drinks of oral rehydration solution to moderately dehydrated infants).

Oral rehydration solutions used in the UK are lower in sodium (50–60 mmol/litre) than the WHO formulation since, in general, patients suffer less severe sodium loss.

Rehydration should be rapid over 3 to 4 hours (except in hypernatraemic dehydration in which case rehydration should occur more slowly over 12 hours). The patient should be reassessed after initial rehydration and if still dehydrated rapid fluid replacement should continue.

Once rehydration is complete further dehydration is prevented by encouraging the patient to drink normal volumes of an appropriate fluid and by replacing continuing losses with an oral rehydration solution; in infants, breast-feeding or formula feeds should be offered between oral rehydration drinks.

For intravenous rehydration see section 9.2.2.

ORAL REHYDRATION SALTS (ORS)

Indications: fluid and electrolyte loss in diarrhoea, see notes above

Dose: according to fluid loss, usually 200–400 mL solution after every loose motion; INFANT 1–1½ times usual feed volume; CHILD 200 mL after every loose motion

■ UK formulations

Note. After reconstitution any unused solution should be discarded no later than 1 hour after preparation unless stored in a refrigerator when it may be kept for up to 24 hours.

Proprietary brands of oral rehydration salts on sale to the public include *Boots Diareze Oral rehydration treatment.*

Dioralyte® (Rhône-Poulenc Rorer)

Effervescent tablets, sodium chloride 117 mg, sodium bicarbonate 336 mg, potassium chloride 186 mg, citric acid anhydrous 384 mg, anhydrous glucose 1.62 g. Net price 10-tab pack (blackcurrant- or citrus-flavoured) = £1.42

Reconstitute 2 tablets with 200 mL of water (only for adults and for children over 1 year)

Note. Ten tablets when reconstituted with 1 litre of water provide Na+ 60 mmol, K+ 25 mmol, Cl- 45 mmol, citrate 20 mmol, and glucose 90 mmol

Oral powder, sodium chloride 470 mg, potassium chloride 300 mg, disodium hydrogen citrate 530 mg/sachet, glucose 3.56 g/sachet, net price 6-sachet pack = £1.90, 20-sachet pack (blackcurrant- or citrus-flavoured or natural) = £5.16

Reconstitute one sachet with 200 mL of water (freshly boiled and cooled for infants).

Note. Five sachets reconstituted with 1 litre of water provide Na+ 60 mmol, K+ 20 mmol, Cl- 60 mmol, citrate 10 mmol, and glucose 90 mmol

Dioralyte® Relief (Rhône-Poulenc Rorer)

Oral powder, sodium chloride 350 mg, potassium chloride 300 mg, sodium citrate 580 mg, cooked rice powder 6 g/sachet, net price 6-sachet pack (apricot-, blackcurrant- or raspberry-flavoured) = £2.14, 20-sachet pack (apricot-flavoured) = £6.81

Reconstitute one sachet with 200 mL of water (freshly boiled and cooled for infants)

Note. 5 sachets when reconstituted with 1 litre of water provide Na+ 60 mmol, K+ 20 mmol, Cl- 50 mmol and citrate 10 mmol; contains aspartame (section 9.4.1)

Electrolade® (Eastern)

Oral powder, sodium chloride 236 mg, potassium chloride 300 mg, sodium bicarbonate 500 mg, anhydrous glucose 4 g/sachet, (banana-, blackcurrant-, melon-, or orange-flavoured). Net price 6-sachet (plain or multiflavoured) pack = £1.33, 20-sachet (single- or multiflavoured) pack = £4.99

Reconstitute one sachet with 200 mL of water (freshly boiled and cooled for infants)

Note. Five sachets when reconstituted with 1 litre of water provide Na+ 50 mmol, K+ 20 mmol, Cl- 40 mmol, HCO3- 30 mmol, and glucose 111 mmol

Rehidrat® (Pharmacia)

Oral powder, sodium chloride 440 mg, potassium chloride 380 mg, sodium bicarbonate 420 mg, citric acid 440 mg, glucose 4.09 g, sucrose 8.07 g, fructose 70 mg/sachet. Net price 24-sachet pack (orange, blackcurrant or lemon and lime flavour) = £6.44; 16-sachet pack (mixed flavours) = £4.29

Note. Lemon and lime version stains vomit green; blackcurrant version contains greater amounts of glucose (4.13 g) and sucrose (8.17 g), and less fructose (10 mg)

Reconstitute one sachet with 250 mL of water (freshly boiled and cooled for infants)

Note. Four sachets when reconstituted with 1 litre of water provide Na+ 50 mmol, K+ 20 mmol, Cl- 50 mmol, HCO3- 20 mmol, citrate 9 mmol, glucose approx. 91 mmol, sucrose approx. 94 mmol, and fructose approx. 1–2 mmol

■ WHO formulation

Oral Rehydration Salts (Non-proprietary)

Oral powder, sodium chloride 3.5 g, potassium chloride 1.5 g, sodium citrate 2.9 g, anhydrous glucose 20 g. To be dissolved in sufficient water to produce 1 litre (providing Na+ 90 mmol, K+ 20 mmol, Cl- 80 mmol, citrate 10 mmol, glucose 111 mmol/litre)

Note. Recommended by the WHO and the United Nations Childrens Fund but not commonly used in the UK.

9.2.1.3   Oral bicarbonate

Sodium bicarbonate is given by mouth for *chronic acidotic states* such as uraemic acidosis or renal tubular acidosis. The dose for correction of metabolic acidosis is not predictable and the response must be assessed; 4.8 g daily (57 mmol each of Na+ and HCO3-) or more may be required. For severe metabolic acidosis, sodium bicarbonate can be given intravenously (section 9.2.2).

Sodium bicarbonate may also be used to make the pH of the urine alkaline (see section 7.4.3); for use in dyspepsia see section 1.1.1.

Sodium supplements may increase blood pressure or cause fluid retention and pulmonary oedema in those at risk; hypokalaemia may be exacerbated.

Where *hyperchloraemic acidosis* is associated with potassium deficiency, as in some renal tubular and gastro-intestinal disorders it may be appropriate to give oral **potassium bicarbonate**, although acute or severe deficiency should be managed by intravenous therapy.

SODIUM BICARBONATE

Indications: see notes above
Cautions: see notes above; avoid in respiratory acidosis; **interactions:** Appendix 1 (antacids)
Dose: see notes above

Sodium Bicarbonate (Non-proprietary)
Capsules, sodium bicarbonate 500 mg (approx. 6 mmol each of Na$^+$ and HCO$_3^-$). Net price 20 = £6.11
Available from Generics, IVAX
Tablets, sodium bicarbonate 600 mg, net price 20 tabs = 50p
IMPORTANT. Oral solutions of sodium bicarbonate are required occasionally; these need to be obtained on special order and the strength of sodium bicarbonate should be stated on the prescription

POTASSIUM BICARBONATE

Indications: see notes above
Cautions: cardiac disease, renal impairment; **interactions:** Appendix 1 (potassium salts)
Contra-indications: hypochloraemia; plasma potassium concentration above 5 mmol/litre
Side-effects: nausea and vomiting
Dose: see notes above

Potassium Tablets, Effervescent (Non-proprietary)
Effervescent tablets, potassium bicarbonate 500 mg, potassium acid tartrate 300 mg, each tablet providing 6.5 mmol of K$^+$. To be dissolved in water before administration. Net price 100 = £4.29. Label: 13, 21
Available from Alpharma, Hillcross
Note. These tablets do not contain chloride; for effervescent tablets containing potassium and chloride, see under Potassium Chloride, section 9.2.1.1

| 9.2.2 | **Parenteral preparations for fluid and electrolyte imbalance** |

9.2.2.1 Electrolytes and water
9.2.2.2 Plasma and plasma substitutes

9.2.2.1 Electrolytes and water

Solutions of electrolytes are given intravenously, to meet normal fluid and electrolyte requirements or to replenish substantial deficits or continuing losses, when the patient is nauseated or vomiting and is unable to take adequate amounts by mouth. When intravenous administration is not possible large volumes of fluid can also be given subcutaneously by hypodermoclysis.

In an individual patient the nature and severity of the electrolyte imbalance must be assessed from the history and clinical and biochemical examination. Sodium, potassium, chloride, magnesium, phosphate, and water depletion can occur singly and in combination with or without disturbances of acid-base balance; for reference to the use of magnesium and phosphates, see section 9.5.

Isotonic solutions may be infused safely into a peripheral vein. Solutions more concentrated than plasma, for example 20% glucose are best given through an indwelling catheter positioned in a large vein.

Intravenous sodium

Sodium chloride in isotonic solution provides the most important extracellular ions in near physiological concentration and is indicated in *sodium depletion* which may arise from such conditions as gastro-enteritis, diabetic ketoacidosis, ileus, and ascites. In a severe deficit of from 4 to 8 litres, 2 to 3 litres of isotonic sodium chloride may be given over 2 to 3 hours; thereafter infusion can usually be at a slower rate. Excessive administration should be avoided; the jugular venous pressure should be assessed, the bases of the lungs should be examined for crepitations, and in elderly or seriously ill patients it is often helpful to monitor the right atrial (central) venous pressure.

Chronic hyponatraemia should ideally be corrected by fluid restriction. However, if sodium chloride is required, the deficit should be corrected slowly to avoid the risk of osmotic demyelination syndrome; the rise in plasma-sodium concentration should be limited to no more than 10 mmol/litre in 24 hours.

Compound sodium lactate (Hartmann's solution) can be used instead of isotonic sodium chloride solution during surgery or in the initial management of the injured or wounded.

Sodium chloride and glucose solutions are indicated when there is combined *water and sodium depletion*. A 1:1 mixture of isotonic sodium chloride and 5% glucose allows some of the water (free of sodium) to enter body cells which suffer most from dehydration while the sodium salt with a volume of water determined by the normal plasma Na$^+$ remains extracellular. Combined sodium, potassium, chloride, and water depletion may occur, for example, with severe diarrhoea or persistent vomiting; replacement is carried out with sodium chloride intravenous infusion 0.9% and glucose intravenous infusion 5% with potassium as appropriate.

SODIUM CHLORIDE

Indications: electrolyte imbalance, also section 9.2.1.2
Cautions: restrict intake in impaired renal function, cardiac failure, hypertension, peripheral and pulmonary oedema, toxaemia of pregnancy
Side-effects: administration of large doses may give rise to sodium accumulation and oedema
Dose: see notes above

Sodium Chloride Intravenous Infusion (Non-proprietary) [PoM]

Intravenous infusion, usual strength sodium chloride 0.9% (9 g, 150 mmol each of Na^+ and Cl^-/litre), this strength being supplied when normal saline for injection is requested. Net price 2-mL amp = 23p; 5-mL amp = 30p; 10-mL amp = 33p; 20-mL amp = 97p; 50-mL amp = £2.01

In hospitals, 500- and 1000-mL packs, and sometimes other sizes, are available

Note. The term 'normal saline' should **not** be used to describe sodium chloride intravenous infusion 0.9%; the term 'physiological saline' is acceptable but it is preferable to give the composition (i.e. sodium chloride intravenous infusion 0.9%).

■ With other ingredients

Sodium Chloride and Glucose Intravenous Infusion (Non-proprietary) [PoM]

Intravenous infusion, usual strength sodium chloride 0.18% (1.8 g, 30 mmol each of Na^+ and Cl^-/litre) and 4% of anhydrous glucose

In hospitals, 500- and 1000-mL packs, and sometimes other sizes are available

Ringer's Solution for Injection [PoM] calcium chloride (dihydrate) 322 micrograms, potassium chloride 300 micrograms, sodium chloride 8.6 mg/mL, providing the following ions (in mmol/litre), Ca^{2+} 2.2, K^+ 4, Na^+ 147, Cl^- 156

In hospitals, 500- and 1000-mL packs, and sometimes other sizes, are available

Sodium Lactate Intravenous Infusion, Compound (Non-proprietary) [PoM]

(Hartmann's Solution for Injection; Ringer-Lactate Solution for Injection),

Intravenous infusion, sodium chloride 0.6%, sodium lactate 0.25%, potassium chloride 0.04%, calcium chloride 0.027% (containing Na^+ 131 mmol, K^+ 5 mmol, Ca^{2+} 2 mmol, HCO_3^- (as lactate) 29 mmol, Cl^- 111 mmol/litre)

In hospitals, 500- and 1000-mL packs, and sometimes other sizes, are available

---

Intravenous glucose

Glucose solutions (5%) are mainly used to replace water deficits and should be given alone when there is no significant loss of electrolytes. Average water requirements in a healthy adult are 1.5 to 2.5 litres daily and this is needed to balance unavoidable losses of water through the skin and lungs and to provide sufficient for urinary excretion. Water depletion (dehydration) tends to occur when these losses are not matched by a comparable intake, as for example may occur in coma or dysphagia or in the aged or apathetic who may not drink water in sufficient amount on their own initiative.

Excessive loss of water without loss of electrolytes is uncommon, occurring in fevers, hyperthyroidism, and in uncommon water-losing renal states such as diabetes insipidus or hypercalcaemia. The volume of glucose solution needed to replace deficits varies with the severity of the disorder, but usually lies within the range of 2 to 6 litres.

Glucose solutions are also given in regimens with calcium, bicarbonate, and insulin for the emergency management of *hyperkalaemia.* They are also given, after correction of hyperglycaemia, during treatment of diabetic ketoacidosis, when they must be accompanied by continuing insulin infusion.

GLUCOSE

(Dextrose Monohydrate)

Note. Glucose BP is the monohydrate but Glucose Intravenous Infusion BP is a sterile solution of anhydrous glucose or glucose monohydrate, potency being expressed in terms of anhydrous glucose

Indications: fluid replacement (see notes above), provision of energy (section 9.3)

Side-effects: glucose injections especially if hypertonic may have a low pH and may cause venous irritation and thrombophlebitis

Dose: water replacement, see notes above; energy source, 1–3 litres daily of 20–50% solution

Glucose Intravenous Infusion (Non-proprietary) [PoM]

Intravenous infusion, glucose or anhydrous glucose (potency expressed in terms of anhydrous glucose), usual strength 5% (50 mg/mL). 25% solution, net price 25-mL amp = £2.21; 50% solution, 25-mL amp = £3.11, 50-mL amp = £1.63

In hospitals, 500- and 1000-mL packs, and sometimes other sizes and strengths, are available; also available from Celltech (*Min-I-Jet® Glucose,* 50% in 50-mL disposable syringe).

Intravenous potassium

Potassium chloride and sodium chloride intravenous infusion is the initial treatment for the correction of *severe hypokalaemia* and when sufficient potassium cannot be taken by mouth. Ready-mixed infusion solutions should be used when possible; alternatively, potassium chloride concentrate, as ampoules containing 1.5 g (K^+ 20 mmol) in 10 mL, is **thoroughly mixed** with 500 mL of sodium chloride 0.9% intravenous infusion and given slowly over 2 to 3 hours, with specialist advice and ECG monitoring in difficult cases. Higher concentrations of potassium chloride may be given in very severe depletion, but require specialist advice.

Repeated measurements of plasma-potassium concentration are necessary to determine whether further infusions are required and to avoid the development of hyperkalaemia, which is especially likely in renal impairment.

Initial potassium replacement therapy should **not** involve glucose infusions, because glucose may cause a further decrease in the plasma-potassium concentration.

POTASSIUM CHLORIDE

Indications: electrolyte imbalance; see also oral potassium supplements, section 9.2.1.1

Cautions: for intravenous infusion the concentration of solution should not usually exceed 3.2 g (43 mmol)/litre; specialist advice and ECG monitoring (see notes above)

Side-effects: rapid infusion toxic to heart

Dose: *by slow intravenous infusion,* depending on the deficit or the daily maintenance requirements, see also notes above

Potassium Chloride and Glucose Intravenous Infusion (Non-proprietary) [PoM]

Intravenous infusion, usual strength potassium chloride 0.3% (3 g, 40 mmol each of K^+ and Cl^-/litre) with 5% of anhydrous glucose

In hospitals, 500- and 1000-mL packs, and sometimes other sizes, are available

Potassium Chloride and Sodium Chloride Intravenous Infusion (Non-proprietary) PoM

Intravenous infusion, usual strength potassium chloride 0.3% (3 g/litre) and sodium chloride 0.9% (9 g/litre), containing K$^+$ 40 mmol, Na$^+$ 150 mmol, and Cl$^-$ 190 mmol/litre

In hospitals, 500- and 1000-mL packs, and sometimes other sizes, are available

Potassium Chloride, Sodium Chloride, and Glucose Intravenous Infusion (Non-proprietary) PoM

Intravenous infusion, sodium chloride 0.18% (1.8 g, Na$^+$ 30 mmol/litre) with 4% of anhydrous glucose and usually sufficient potassium chloride to provide K$^+$ 10–40 mmol/litre (to be specified by the prescriber)

In hospitals, 500- and 1000-mL packs, and sometimes other sizes, are available

Potassium Chloride Concentrate, Sterile (Non-proprietary) PoM

Sterile concentrate, potassium chloride 15% (150 mg, approximately 2 mmol each of K$^+$ and Cl$^-$/mL). Net price 10-mL amp = 58p

IMPORTANT. Must be diluted with **not less** than 50 times its volume of sodium chloride intravenous infusion 0.9% or other suitable diluent and **mixed well**

Solutions containing 10 and 20% of potassium chloride are also available in both 5- and 10-mL ampoules

---

Bicarbonate and lactate

Sodium bicarbonate is used to control severe *metabolic acidosis* (as in renal failure). Since this condition is usually attended by sodium depletion, it is reasonable to correct this first by the administration of isotonic sodium chloride intravenous infusion, provided the kidneys are not primarily affected and the degree of acidosis is not so severe as to impair renal function. In these circumstances, isotonic sodium chloride alone is usually effective as it restores the ability of the kidneys to generate bicarbonate. In renal acidosis or in severe metabolic acidosis of any origin (for example blood pH < 7.1) sodium bicarbonate (1.26%) may be infused with isotonic sodium chloride when the acidosis remains unresponsive to correction of anoxia or fluid depletion; a total volume of up to 6 litres (4 litres of sodium chloride and 2 litres of sodium bicarbonate) may be necessary in the adult. In severe shock due for example to cardiac arrest (see section 2.7), metabolic acidosis may develop without sodium depletion; in these circumstances sodium bicarbonate is best given in a small volume of hypertonic solution, such as 50 mL of 8.4% solution intravenously; plasma pH should be monitored.

Sodium bicarbonate infusion is also used in the emergency management of *hyperkalaemia* (see also under Glucose).

Sodium lactate intravenous infusion is obsolete in metabolic acidosis, and carries the risk of producing lactic acidosis, particularly in seriously ill patients with poor tissue perfusion or impaired hepatic function.

SODIUM BICARBONATE

Indications: metabolic acidosis

Dose: *by slow intravenous injection*, a strong solution (up to 8.4%), or *by continuous intravenous infusion*, a weaker solution (usually 1.26%), an amount appropriate to the body base deficit (see notes above)

Sodium Bicarbonate Intravenous Infusion PoM usual strength sodium bicarbonate 1.26% (12.6 g, 150 mmol each of Na$^+$ and HCO$_3^-$/litre); various other strengths available

In hospitals, 500- and 1000-mL packs, and sometimes other sizes, are available

Min-I-Jet® Sodium Bicarbonate (Celltech) PoM

Intravenous injection, sodium bicarbonate in disposable syringe, net price 4.2%, 10 mL = £5.29; 8.4%, 10 mL = £5.71, 50 mL = £8.53

SODIUM LACTATE �

Indications: see notes above

Sodium Lactate (Non-proprietary) PoM ▰

Intravenous infusion, sodium lactate M/6, contains the following ions (in mmol/litre), Na$^+$ 167, HCO$_3^-$ (as lactate) 167

▰ denotes preparations that are considered to be less suitable for prescribing (see p. vi)

Water

Water for Injections PoM Net price 1-mL amp = 18p; 2-mL amp = 15p; 5-mL amp = 26p; 10-mL amp = 29p; 20-mL amp = 53p; 50-mL amp = £1.91

9.2.2.2 Plasma and plasma substitutes

Albumin solutions, prepared from whole blood, contain soluble proteins and electrolytes but no clotting factors, blood group antibodies, or plasma cholinesterases; they may be given without regard to the recipient's blood group.

Albumin solutions are used for the treatment of severe hypoproteinaemia, particularly when associated with a low plasma volume. Concentrated albumin solutions may also be used to obtain a diuresis in hypoalbuminaemic patients (e.g. in hepatic cirrhosis). The use of albumin solutions in acute plasma or blood loss may be wasteful; plasma substitutes are more appropriate. Albumin solutions have been linked with increased mortality in patients with hypovolaemia or hypoalbuminaemia such as those with acute blood loss or burns; it is uncertain whether albumin is responsible for the extra deaths.

Plasma and plasma substitutes are often used in very ill patients whose condition is unstable. Therefore, close monitoring is required and fluid and electrolyte therapy should be adjusted according to the patient's condition at all times.

CSM advice. Following the publication of a meta-analysis in July 1998 concerning the safety of human albumin solution, the CSM has asked that product literature for albumin products should reflect the following:

- indications should focus on the use of albumin to replace lost fluids rather than the underlying cause of hypovolaemia; hypoalbuminaemia itself is not an appropriate indication;
- warnings should be added about the risks of hypervolaemia and cardiovascular overload, and the importance of monitoring patients receiving albumin to avoid these complications;
- special care is needed when administering albumin in conditions where capillary integrity is affected.

ALBUMIN SOLUTION

(Human Albumin Solution)

A solution containing protein derived from plasma, serum, or normal placentas; at least 95% of the protein is albumin. The solution may be isotonic (containing 4–5% protein) or concentrated (containing 15–25% protein).

Indications: see under preparations, below and also CSM advice above

Cautions: history of cardiac or circulatory disease (administer slowly to avoid rapid rise in blood pressure and cardiac failure, and monitor cardiovascular and respiratory function); correct dehydration when administering concentrated solution

Contra-indications: cardiac failure; severe anaemia

Side-effects: hypersensitivity reactions (including anaphylaxis) with nausea, vomiting, increased salivation, fever, tachycardia, hypotension and chills reported

■ Isotonic solutions

Indications: acute or sub-acute loss of plasma volume e.g. in burns, pancreatitis, trauma, and complications of surgery; plasma exchange

Available as: *Human Albumin Solution 4.5%* (50-, 100-, 250- and 400-mL bottles—Baxter Bioscience); *Human Albumin Solution 5%* (100-, 250- and 500-mL bottles—Grifols); *ALBA® 4.5%* (100- and 400-mL bottles—SNBTS); *Albutein® 5%* (250- and 500-mL bottles—Alpha); *Zenalb® 4.5* (50-, 100-, 250-, and 500-mL bottles—BPL)

■ Concentrated solutions (20–25%)

Indications: severe hypoalbuminaemia associated with low plasma volume and generalised oedema where salt and water restriction with plasma volume expansion are required; adjunct in the treatment of hyperbilirubinaemia by exchange transfusion in the newborn

Available as: *Human Albumin Solution 20%* (50- and 100-mL vials—Baxter Bioscience); *Human Albumin Solution 20%* (50- and 100-mL bottles—Grifols); *ALBA® 20%* (100-mL vials—SNBTS); *Albutein® 20%* (50-, and 100-mL bottles—Alpha); *Albutein® 25%* (20-, 50-, and 100-mL vials—Alpha); *Zenalb® 20* (50- and 100-mL bottles—BPL)

Plasma substitutes

Dextrans, **gelatin**, and the etherified starches, **hexastarch**, **hydroxyethyl starch** and **pentastarch** are macromolecular substances which are metabolised slowly; they may be used at the outset to expand and maintain blood volume in shock arising from

conditions such as burns or septicaemia. Plasma substitutes may be used as an immediate short-term measure to treat haemorrhage until blood is available. They are rarely needed when shock is due to sodium and water depletion because, in these circumstances, the shock responds to water and electrolyte repletion. See also section 2.7.1 for the management of shock.

Plasma substitutes should **not** be used to maintain plasma volume in conditions such as burns or peritonitis where there is loss of plasma protein, water and electrolytes over periods of several days or weeks. In these situations, plasma or plasma protein fractions containing large amounts of albumin should be given.

Large volumes of *some* plasma substitutes can increase the risk of bleeding through depletion of coagulation factors; however, the risk is reduced if 1–2 litres of a substitute such as hexastarch are used.

Dextran 70 by intravenous infusion is used predominantly for volume expansion. Dextran 40 intravenous infusion is used in an attempt to improve peripheral blood flow in ischaemic disease of the limbs. Dextrans 40 and 70 have also been used in the prophylaxis of thromboembolism but are now rarely used for this purpose.

Dextrans may interfere with blood group crossmatching or biochemical measurements and these should be carried out before infusion is begun.

CAUTIONS. Plasma substitutes should be used with caution in patients with cardiac disease or renal impairment; urine output should be monitored. Care should be taken to avoid haematocrit concentration from falling below 25–30% and the patient should be monitored for hypersensitivity reactions.

SIDE-EFFECTS. Hypersensitivity reactions may occur including, rarely, severe anaphylactoid reactions. Transient increase in bleeding time may occur.

DEXTRAN 40

Dextrans of weight average molecular weight about '40 000'

Indications: conditions associated with peripheral local slowing of the blood flow; prophylaxis of post-surgical thromboembolic disease (but see notes above)

Cautions: see notes above; can interfere with some laboratory tests (see also above); correct dehydration beforehand, give adequate fluids during therapy and, where possible, monitor central venous pressure; pregnancy (Appendix 4)

Side-effects: see notes above

Dose: *by intravenous infusion*, initially 500–1000 mL; further doses are given according to the patient's condition (see notes above)

Gentran 40® (Baxter) PoM

Intravenous infusion, dextran 40 intravenous infusion in glucose intravenous infusion 5% or in sodium chloride intravenous infusion 0.9%. Net price 500-mL bottle (both) = £4.56

DEXTRAN 70

Dextrans of weight average molecular weight about '70 000'

Indications: short-term blood volume expansion; prophylaxis of post-surgical thromboembolic disease (but see notes above)

Cautions: see notes above; can interfere with some laboratory tests (see also above); where possible, monitor central venous pressure; pregnancy (Appendix 4)

Side-effects: see notes above

Dose: *by intravenous infusion*, after moderate to severe haemorrhage or in the shock phase of burn injury (initial 48 hours), 500–1000 mL rapidly initially followed by 500 mL later if necessary (see also notes above); total dosage should not exceed 20 mL/kg during initial 24 hours; CHILD total dosage should not exceed 20 mL/kg

Gentran 70® (Baxter) PoM
Intravenous infusion, dextran 70 intravenous infusion in glucose intravenous infusion 5% or in sodium chloride intravenous infusion 0.9%. Net price 500-mL bottle (both) = £4.78

■ Hypertonic solution

RescueFlow® (Horizon) PoM
Intravenous infusion, dextran 70 intravenous infusion 6% in sodium chloride intravenous infusion 7.5%. Net price 250-mL bottle = £28.50
Indications: initial treatment of hypovolaemia with hypotension induced by traumatic injury
Cautions: see notes above; severe hyperglycaemia and hyperosmolality
Dose: by intravenous infusion over 2–5 minutes, 250 mL, followed immediately by administration of isotonic fluids

GELATIN

Note. The gelatin is partially degraded

Indications: low blood volume

Cautions: see notes above

Side-effects: see notes above

Dose: *by intravenous infusion*, initially 500–1000 mL of a 3.5–4% solution (see notes above)

Gelofusine® (Braun) PoM
Intravenous infusion, succinylated gelatin (modified fluid gelatin, average molecular weight 30 000) 40 g (4%), Na^+ 154 mmol, Cl^- 120 mmol/litre, net price 500-mL *Ecobag®* = £4.63, 1-litre *Ecobag®* = £9.45

Haemaccel® (Beacon) PoM
Intravenous infusion, polygeline (degraded and modified gelatin, average molecular weight 30 000) 35 g (3.5%), Na^+ 145 mmol, K^+ 5.1 mmol, Ca^{2+} 6.25 mmol, Cl^- 145 mmol/litre, net price 500-mL bottle = £3.71

> Plasma and plasma substitutes are often used in very ill patients whose condition is unstable. Therefore, close monitoring is required and fluid and electrolyte therapy should be adjusted according to the patient's condition at all times.

ETHERIFIED STARCH

A starch composed of more than 90% of amylopectin that has been etherified with hydroxyethyl groups; hetastarch has a higher degree of etherification than pentastarch

Indications: low blood volume

Cautions: see notes above; children

Side-effects: see notes above

Dose: see under preparations below

Voluven® (Fresenius Kabi) PoM
Intravenous infusion, hydroxyethyl starch (weight average molecular weight 130 000) 6% in sodium chloride intravenous infusion 0.9%, net price 500-mL bag = £14.00
Dose: by intravenous infusion, up to 33 mL/kg daily (see notes above)

■ Hexastarch

eloHAES® (Fresenius Kabi) PoM
Intravenous infusion, hexastarch (weight average molecular weight 200 000) 6% in sodium chloride intravenous infusion 0.9%. Net price 500-mL *Steriflex®* bag = £12.50
Dose: by intravenous infusion, 500–1000 mL; usual daily max. 1500 mL (see notes above)

■ Pentastarch

HAES-steril® (Fresenius Kabi) PoM
Intravenous infusion, pentastarch (weight average molecular weight 200 000), net price (both in sodium chloride intravenous infusion 0.9%) 6%, 500 mL = £10.50; 10%, 500 mL = £16.50
Dose: by intravenous infusion, pentastarch 6%, up to 2500 mL daily; pentastarch 10%, up to 1500 mL daily (see notes above)

Hemohes® (Braun) PoM
Intravenous infusion, pentastarch (weight average molecular weight 200 000), net price (both in sodium chloride intravenous infusion 0.9%) 6%, 500 mL = £12.50; 10%, 500 mL = £16.50
Dose: by intravenous infusion, pentastarch 6%, up to 2500 mL daily; pentastarch 10%, up to 1500 mL daily (see notes above)

9.3 Intravenous nutrition

When adequate feeding through the alimentary tract is not possible, nutrients may be given by intravenous infusion. This may be in addition to ordinary oral or tube feeding—**supplemental parenteral nutrition**, or may be the sole source of nutrition—**total parenteral nutrition** (TPN). Indications for this method include preparation of undernourished patients for surgery, chemotherapy, or radiation therapy; severe or prolonged disorders of the gastro-intestinal tract; major surgery, trauma, or burns; prolonged coma or refusal to eat; and some patients with renal or hepatic failure. The composition of proprietary preparations available is given in the table below.

Total parenteral nutrition requires the use of a solution containing amino acids, glucose, fat, electrolytes, trace elements, and vitamins. This is now commonly provided by the pharmacy in the form of a 3-litre bag. A single dose of vitamin B_{12}, as hydroxocobalamin, is given by intramuscular injection; regular vitamin B_{12} injections are not usually required unless total parenteral nutrition continues for many months. Folic acid is given in a dose of 15 mg once or twice each week, usually in the nutrition solution. Other vitamins are usually given daily; they are generally introduced in the parenteral nutrition solution. Alternatively, if the patient is able to take small amounts by mouth, vitamins may be given orally.

The nutrition solution is infused through a central venous catheter inserted under full surgical precautions. Alternatively infusion through a peripheral vein is used for supplementary as well as total parenteral nutrition for periods of up to a month, depending on the availability of peripheral veins; factors prolonging cannula life and preventing thrombophlebitis include the use of soft polyurethane paediatric cannulae and use of feeds of low osmolality and neutral pH. Only nutritional fluids should be given by the dedicated intravenous line.

Before starting, the patient should be well oxygenated with a near normal circulating blood volume and attention should be given to renal function and acid-base status. Appropriate biochemical tests should have been carried out beforehand and serious deficits corrected. Nutritional and electrolyte status must be monitored throughout treatment.

Complications of long-term TPN include gall bladder sludging, gall stones, cholestasis and abnormal liver function tests. For details of the prevention and management of TPN complications, specialist literature should be consulted.

Protein is given as mixtures of essential and non-essential synthetic L-amino acids. Ideally, all essential amino acids should be included with a wide variety of non-essential ones to provide sufficient nitrogen together with electrolytes (see also section 9.2.2). Solutions vary in their composition of amino acids; they often contain an energy source (usually glucose) and electrolytes.

Energy is provided in a ratio of 0.6 to 1.1 megajoules (150–250 kcals) per gram of protein nitrogen. Energy requirements must be met if amino acids are to be utilised for tissue maintenance. A mixture of carbohydrate and fat energy sources (usually 30–50% as fat) gives better utilisation of amino acids than glucose alone.

Glucose is the preferred source of carbohydrate, but if more than 180 g is given per day frequent monitoring of blood glucose is required, and insulin may be necessary. Glucose in various strengths from 10 to 50% must be infused through a central venous catheter to avoid thrombosis.

In total parenteral nutrition regimens, it is necessary to provide adequate phosphate in order to allow phosphorylation of the glucose; between 20 and 30 mmol of phosphate is required daily.

Fructose and sorbitol have been used in an attempt to avoid the problem of hyperosmolar hyperglycaemic non-ketotic acidosis but other metabolic problems may occur, as with xylitol and ethanol which are now rarely used.

Fat emulsions have the advantages of a high energy to fluid volume ratio, neutral pH, and iso-osmolarity with plasma, and provide essential fatty acids. Several days of adaptation may be required to attain maximal utilisation. Reactions include occasional febrile episodes (usually only with 20% emulsions) and rare anaphylactic responses. Interference with biochemical measurements such as those for blood gases and calcium may occur if samples are taken before fat has been cleared. Daily checks are necessary to ensure complete clearance from the plasma in conditions where fat metabolism may be disturbed. **Additives may only be mixed with fat emulsions where compatibility is known**.

Administration. Because of the complex requirements relating to parenteral nutrition full details relating to administration have been omitted. In all cases *product literature and other specialist literature should be consulted.*

Supplementary preparations

Compatibility with the infusion solution must be ascertained before adding supplementary preparations.

Addiphos® (Fresenius Kabi) PoM
Solution, sterile, phosphate 40 mmol, K^+ 30 mmol, Na^+ 30 mmol/20 mL. For addition to *Vamin®* solutions and glucose intravenous infusions. Net price 20-mL vial = £1.15

Additrace® (Fresenius Kabi) PoM
Solution, trace elements for addition to *Vamin®* solutions and glucose intravenous infusions, traces of Fe^{3+}, Zn^{2+}, Mn^{2+}, Cu^{2+}, Cr^{3+}, Se^{4+}, Mo^{6+}, F^-, I^-. For adults and children over 40 kg. Net price 10-mL amp = £1.75

Cernevit® (Baxter) PoM
Solution, *dl*-alpha tocopherol 11.2 units, ascorbic acid 125 mg, biotin 69 micrograms, colecalciferol 220 units, cyanocobalamin 6 micrograms, folic acid 414 micrograms, glycine 250 mg, nicotinamide 46 mg, pantothenic acid (as dexpanthenol) 17.25 mg, pyridoxine hydrochloride 5.5 mg, retinol (as palmitate) 3500 units, riboflavin (as dihydrated sodium phosphate) 4.14 mg, thiamine (as cocarboxylase tetrahydrate) 3.51 mg. Dissolve in 5 mL water for injections. Net price per vial = £2.90

Decan® (Baxter) PoM
Solution, trace elements for addition to infusion solutions, Fe^{2+}, Zn^{2+}, Cu^{2+}, Mn^{2+}, F^-, Co^{2+}, I^-, Se^{4+}, Mo^{6+}, Cr^{3+}. For adults and children over 40 kg. Net price 40-mL vial = £2.00

Dipeptiven® (Fresenius Kabi) PoM
Solution, *N*(2)-L-alanyl-L-glutamine 200 mg/mL (providing L-alanine 82 mg, L-glutamine 134.6 mg). For addition to infusion solutions containing amino acids. Net price 50 mL = £25.00, 100 mL = £29.60
Dose: amino acid supplement for hypercatabolic or hypermetabolic states, 300–400 mg/kg daily; max. 400 mg/kg daily, dose not to exceed 20% of total amino acid intake

Multibionta® (Merck) PoM
Solution, ascorbic acid 500 mg, dexpanthenol 25 mg, nicotinamide 100 mg, pyridoxine hydrochloride 15 mg, riboflavin sodium phosphate 10 mg, thiamine hydrochloride 50 mg, tocopheryl acetate 5 mg, vitamin A 10 000 units. For addition to infusion solutions. Net price 10-mL amp = £1.61
Excipients: include benzyl alcohol (avoid in neonates, see Excipients p. 2)

Proprietary Infusion Fluids for Parenteral Feeding

Preparation	Nitrogen g/litre	[1]Energy kJ/litre	K+	Mg2+	Na+	Acet-	Cl-	Other components/litre
Aminoplasmal 5% E (Braun) Net price 500 mL = £9.02	8		25	2.6	43	59	29	dihydrogen phosphate 9 mmol, malic acid 1.01 g
Aminoplasmal 10% (Braun) Net price 500 mL = £17.06	16					57		
Aminoplex 12 (Geistlich) Net price 250 mL = £5.41; 500 mL = £10.80; 1000 mL = £19.07	12.44		30	2.5	35	5	67	malic acid 4.6 g
Aminoplex 24 (Geistlich) Net price 250 mL = £9.35; 500 mL = £16.50	24.9		30	2.5	35	5	67	malic acid 4.5 g
Aminoplex 24 Electrolyte-Free (Geistlich) Net price 250 mL = £9.79; 500 mL = £17.28	24.9							malic acid 9.5 g
Clinimix N9G20E (Baxter) Net price (dual compartment bag of amino acids with electrolytes 1000 mL and glucose 20% with calcium 1000 mL) = £29.00	4.55	1680	30	2.5	35	50	40	Ca2+ 2.25 mmol, phosphate 15 mmol, anhydrous glucose 100 g
Clinimix N14G30E (Baxter) Net price (dual compartment bag of amino acids with electrolytes 1000 mL and glucose 30% with calcium 1000 mL) = £33.00	7	2520	30	2.5	35	70	40	Ca2+ 2.25 mmol, phosphate 15 mmol, anhydrous glucose 150 g
ClinOleic 20% (Baxter) Net price 100 mL = £6.28; 250 mL = £10.08; 500 mL = £13.88		8360						purified olive and soya oil 200 g, glycerol 22.5 g, egg phosphatides 12 g
Clinomel N4-550 (Baxter) Net price (triple compartment bag of amino acids 800 mL or 1000 mL; glucose 20% with calcium 800 mL or 1000 mL; lipid emulsion 10% 400 mL or 500 mL) 2000 mL = £58.00, 2500 mL = £63.00	3.65	2268	24	2	28	40	32	Ca2+ 1.8 mmol, phosphate 12 mmol, anhydrous glucose 80 g, soya oil 20 g
Clinomel N5-800 (Baxter) Net price (2000-mL triple compartment bag of amino acids with electrolytes 800 mL, glucose 25% with calcium 800 mL, lipid emulsion 20% 400 mL) = £61.00; 2500 mL = £66.00	4.6	3360	24	2	28	50	32	Ca2+ 1.8 mmol, phosphate 12 mmol, glycerol 5 g, soya oil 40 g, purified egg phospholipids 2.4 g, anhydrous glucose 100 g
Clinomel N6-900 (Baxter) Net price (triple compartment bag of amino acids 800 mL or 1000 mL; glucose 30% with calcium 800 mL or 1000 mL; lipid emulsion 20% 400 mL or 500 mL) 2000 mL = £64.00, 2500 mL = £69.00	5.6	3696	24	2	28	56	32	Ca2+ 1.8 mmol, phosphate 12 mmol, glycerol 5 g, soya oil 40 g, purified egg phospholipids 2.4 g, anhydrous glucose 120 g
Clinomel N7-1000 (Baxter) Net price (triple compartment bag of amino acids 400 mL, 600 mL or 800 mL; glucose 40% with calcium 400 mL, 600 mL or 800 mL; lipid emulsion 20% 200 mL, 300 mL or 400 mL) 1000 mL = £34.38, 1500 mL = £38.00, 2000 mL = £67.00	6.6	4368	24	2	28	60	32	Ca2+ 1.8 mmol, phosphate 12 mmol, glycerol 5 g, soya oil 40 g, purified egg phospholipids 2.4 g, anhydrous glucose 160 g
Compleven (Fresenius Kabi) Net price (2500-mL triple compartment bag of amino acids 1000 mL, glucose 1000 mL, lipid emulsion 500 mL) = £67.00	4.8	3275	20	2	32		32.4	Ca2+ 2 mmol, Zn2+ 0.04 mmol, glycerophosphate 8 mmol, anhydrous glucose 96 g, soya oil 40 g, egg lecithin 2.4 g, glycerol 2.4 g
Glamin (Fresenius Kabi) Net price 250 mL = £14.16; 500 mL = £26.38	22.4				62			
Hepanutrin (Geistlich) Net price 500 mL = £15.74	15.6							
Hyperamine 30 (Braun) Net price 500 mL = £23.67	30				5			
Intrafusin 11 (Fresenius Kabi) Net price 1000 mL = £14.24	11.4		40	5	80		76	Ca2+ 3 mmol, phosphate 20 mmol, citrate 6 mmol
Intrafusin 22 (Fresenius Kabi) Net price 500 mL = £14.24	22.8							
Intralipid 10% (Fresenius Kabi) Net price 100 mL = £3.90; 500 mL = £8.58		4600						soya oil 100 g, glycerol 22 g, purified egg phospholipids 12 g, phosphate 15 mmol
Intralipid 20% (Fresenius Kabi) Net price 100 mL = £5.85; 250 mL = £9.65; 500 mL = £12.87		8400						soya oil 200 g, glycerol 22 g, purified egg phospholipids 12 g, phosphate 15 mmol
Intralipid 30% (Fresenius Kabi) Net price 333 mL = £14.40		12600						soya oil 300 g, glycerol 16.7 g, purified egg phospholipids 12 g, phosphate 15 mmol

1. Excludes protein- or amino acid-derived energy

Note. 1000 kcal = 4200 kJ; 1000 kJ = 238.8 kcal. All entries are PoM

Proprietary Infusion Fluids for Parenteral Feeding

Preparation	Nitrogen g/litre	¹Energy kJ/litre	Electrolytes mmol/litre					Other components/litre
			K⁺	Mg²⁺	Na⁺	Acet⁻	Cl⁻	
Ivelip 10% (Baxter) Net price 100 mL = £4.78; 500 mL = £9.08		4600						soya oil 100 g, glycerol 25 g
Ivelip 20% (Baxter) Net price 100 mL = £6.28; 500 mL = £13.88; 1000 mL = £24.68		8400						soya oil 200 g, glycerol 25 g
KabiMix 9 (Fresenius Kabi) Net price 2580 mL = £64.00	3.49	2600	23	1.9	31	21.3	31	Ca²⁺ 1.9 mmol, anhydrous glucose 58.14 g, phosphate 10.9 mmol, soya oil 38.76 g, glycerol 4.26 g, purified egg phospholipids 2.33 g
KabiMix 11 (Fresenius Kabi) Net price 2000 mL = £67.00	5.3	3500	23	2	31	34.9	31	Ca²⁺ 1.9 mmol, anhydrous glucose 116.28 g, phosphate 10.9 mmol, soya oil 38.76 g, glycerol 4.26 g, purified egg phospholipids 2.33 g
KabiMix 14 (Fresenius Kabi) Net price 2580 mL = £70.00	5.23	3570	23	1.9	31	34.9	31	Ca²⁺ 1.9 mmol, anhydrous glucose 116.28 g, phosphate 10.9 mmol, soya oil 38.76 g, glycerol 4.26 g, purified egg phospholipids 2.33 g
Kabiven (Fresenius Kabi) Net price (triple compartment bag of amino acids and electrolytes 300 mL, 450 mL, 600 mL, or 750 mL; glucose 526 mL, 790 mL, 1053 mL, or 1316 mL; lipid emulsion 200 mL, 300 mL, 400 mL, or 500 mL) 1026 mL = £8.75, 1540 mL = £12.50, 2053 mL = £33.50, 2566 mL = £35.00	5.3	3275	23	4	31	38	45	Ca²⁺ 2 mmol, phosphate 9.7 mmol, anhydrous glucose 97 g, soya oil 39 g
Kabiven Peripheral (Fresenius Kabi) Net price (triple compartment bag of amino acids and electrolytes 300 mL, 400 mL, or 500 mL; glucose 885 mL, 1180 mL, or 1475 mL; lipid emulsion 255 mL, 340 mL, or 425 mL) 1440 mL = £8.75, 1920 mL = £25.00, 2400 mL = £32.00	3.75	2625	17	2.8	22	27	33	Ca²⁺ 1.4 mmol, phosphate 7.5 mmol, anhydrous glucose 67.5 g, soya oil 35.4 g
Lipofundin MCT/LCT 10% (Braun) Net price 100 mL = £7.70; 500 mL = £12.90		4430						soya oil 50 g, medium chain triglycerides 50 g
Lipofundin MCT/LCT 20% (Braun) Net price 100 mL = £8.79; 250 mL = £11.30; 500 mL = £19.18		8000						soya oil 100 g, medium chain triglycerides 100 g
Lipofundin N 10% (Braun) Net price 100 mL = £7.10; 250 mL = £9.50; 500 mL = £11.76		4470						soya oil 100 g, glycerol 25 g, egg lethicin 8 g
Lipofundin N 20% (Braun) Net price 100 mL = £8.10; 250 mL = £9.99; 500 mL = £15.38		8520						soya oil 200 g, glycerol 25 g, egg lethicin 12 g
Nutracel 400 (Baxter) Net price 500 mL = £2.43		3400			18	0.16	66	Ca²⁺ 15 mmol, Mn²⁺ 0.01 mmol, Zn²⁺ 0.08 mmol, anhydrous glucose 200 g
Nutracel 800 (Baxter) Net price 1000 mL = £4.19		3400			9	0.08	33	Ca²⁺ 7.5 mmol, Mn²⁺ 0.005 mmol, Zn²⁺ 0.04 mmol, anhydrous glucose 200 g
NuTRIflex Lipid peri (Braun) Net price (triple compartment bag of amino acids 500 mL or 1000 mL; glucose 500 mL or 1000 mL; lipid emulsion 20% 250 mL or 500 mL) 1250 mL = £43.38, 2500 mL = £65.05	4.56	2664	24	2.4	40	32	38.4	Ca²⁺ 2.4 mmol, Zn²⁺ 0.024 mmol, phosphate 6 mmol, anhydrous glucose 64 g, soya oil 20 g, medium chain triglycerides 20 g
NuTRIflex Lipid plus (Braun) Net price (triple compartment bag of amino acids 500 mL, 750 mL or 1000 mL; glucose 500 mL, 750 mL or 1000 mL; lipid emulsion 20% 250 mL, 375 mL or 500 mL) 1250 mL = £47.17, 1875 mL = £60.23, 2500 mL = £69.27	5.44	3600	28	3.2	40	36	36	Ca²⁺ 3.2 mmol, Zn²⁺ 0.024 mmol, phosphate 12 mmol, anhydrous glucose 120 g, soya oil 20 g, medium chain triglycerides 20 g
NuTRIflex Lipid plus without Electrolytes (Braun) Net price (triple compartment bag of amino acids 500 mL, 750 mL or 1000 mL; glucose 500 mL, 750 mL or 1000 mL; lipid emulsion 20% 250 mL, 375 mL or 500 mL) 1250 mL = £47.17, 1875 mL = £60.23, 2500 mL = £69.27	5.44	3600						anhydrous glucose 120 g, soya oil 20 g, medium chain triglycerides 20 g

1. Excludes protein- or amino acid-derived energy

Note. 1000 kcal = 4200 kJ; 1000 kJ = 238.8 kcal. All entries are PoM

Proprietary Infusion Fluids for Parenteral Feeding

Preparation	Nitrogen g/litre	¹Energy kJ/litre	K⁺	Mg²⁺	Na⁺	Acet⁻	Cl⁻	Other components/litre
NuTRIflex Lipid special (Braun) Net price (triple compartment bag of amino acids 500 mL, 750 mL or 1000 mL; glucose 500 mL, 750 mL or 1000 mL; lipid emulsion 20% 250 mL, 375 mL or 500 mL) 1250 mL = £57.69, 1875 mL = £75.58, 2500 mL = £89.21	8	4004	37.6	4.24	53.6	48	48	Ca^{2+} 4.24 mmol, Zn^{2+} 0.032 mmol, phosphate 16 mmol, anhydrous glucose 144 g, soya oil 20 g, medium chain triglycerides 20 g
NuTRIflex Lipid special without Electrolytes (Braun) Net price (triple compartment bag of amino acids 500 mL, 750 mL or 1000 mL; glucose 500 mL, 750 mL or 1000 mL; lipid emulsion 20% 250 mL, 375 mL or 500 mL) 1250 mL = £57.69, 1875 mL = £75.58, 2500 mL = £89.21	8	4004						anhydrous glucose 144 g, soya oil 20 g, medium chain triglycerides 20 g
Nutriflex Basal (Braun) Net price (dual compartment bag of 800 mL and 1200 mL) = £28.35	4.6	2095	30	5.7	49.9	35	50	Ca^{2+} 3.6 mmol, phosphate 12.8 mmol, anhydrous glucose 125 g
Nutriflex Peri (Braun) Net price (dual compartment bag of 800 mL and 1200 mL) = £33.00	5.7	1340	15	4	27	19.5	31.6	Ca^{2+} 2.5 mmol, phosphate 5.7 mmol, anhydrous glucose 80 g
Nutriflex Plus (Braun) Net price (dual compartment bag of 800 mL and 1200 mL) = £39.18	6.8	2510	25	5.7	37.2	22.9	35.5	Ca^{2+} 3.6 mmol, phosphate 20 mmol, anhydrous glucose 150 g
Nutriflex Special (Braun) Net price (dual compartment bag of 750 mL and 750 mL) = £43.30	10	4020	25.7	5	40.5	22	49.5	Ca^{2+} 4.1 mmol, phosphate 15 mmol, anhydrous glucose 240 g
Plasma-Lyte 148 (water) (Baxter) Net price 1000 mL = £1.59			5	1.5	140	27	98	gluconate 23 mmol
Plasma-Lyte 148 (dextrose 5%) (Baxter) Net price 1000 mL = £1.59		840	5	1.5	140	27	98	gluconate 23 mmol, anhydrous glucose 50 g
Plasma-Lyte M (dextrose 5%) (Baxter) Net price 1000 mL = £1.33		840	16	1.5	40	12	40	Ca^{2+} 2.5 mmol, lactate 12 mmol, anhydrous glucose 50 g
²Primene 10% (Baxter) Net price 100 mL = £5.78; 250 mL = £7.92	15						19	
Structolipid 20% (Fresenius Kabi) Net price 500 mL = £16.09		8200						Purified structured triglyceride 200 g (contains coconut oil, palm kernel oil, and soya oil triglycerides)
Synthamin 9 (Baxter) Net price 500 mL = £6.66; 1000 mL = £12.34	9.1		60	5		70	100	acid phosphate 30 mmol
Synthamin 9 EF (electrolyte-free) (Baxter) Net price 500 mL = £6.66; 1000 mL = £12.34	9.1					44	22	
Synthamin 14 (Baxter) Net price 500 mL = £9.64; 1000 mL = £17.13; 3000 mL = £48.98	14.0		60	5		70	140	acid phosphate 30 mmol
Synthamin 14 EF (electrolyte-free) (Baxter) Net price 500 mL = £9.87; 1000 mL = £17.51	14.0					68	34	
Synthamin 17 (Baxter) Net price 500 mL = £12.66; 1000 mL = £23.00	16.5		60	5		70	150	acid phosphate 30 mmol
Synthamin 17 EF (electrolyte-free) (Baxter) Net price 500 mL = £12.66	16.5					82	40	
Vamin 9 (Fresenius Kabi) Net price 500 mL = £5.85; 1000 mL = £10.04	9.4		20	1.5	50		50	Ca^{2+} 2.5 mmol
Vamin 9 Glucose (Fresenius Kabi) Net price 100 mL = £3.02; 500 mL = £6.14; 1000 mL = £11.02	9.4	1700	20	1.5	50		50	Ca^{2+} 2.5 mmol, anhydrous glucose 100 g
Vamin 14 (Fresenius Kabi) Net price 500 mL = £8.63; 1000 mL = £14.67	13.5		50	8	100	135	100	Ca^{2+} 5 mmol, SO_4^{2-} 8 mmol
Vamin 14 (Electrolyte-Free) (Fresenius Kabi) Net price 500 mL = £8.29; 1000 mL = £14.67	13.5					90		
Vamin 18 (Electrolyte-Free) (Fresenius Kabi) Net price 500 mL = £10.97; 1000 mL = £19.74	18					110		
Vaminolact (Fresenius Kabi) Net price 100 mL = £3.36; 500 mL = £7.75	9.3							
Vitrimix KV (Fresenius Kabi) Net price (combined pack of Intralipid 20% 250 mL and Vamin 9 glucose 750 mL) = £19.40	7.0	3340	15	1.1	38		38	Ca^{2+} 1.9 mmol, anhydrous glucose 75 g, soya oil 50 g, purified egg phospholipids 3 g, glycerol 5.5 g, phosphate 3.75 mmol

1. Excludes protein- or amino acid-derived energy
2. For use in neonates and children only

Note. 1000 kcal = 4200 kJ; 1000 kJ = 238.8 kcal. All entries are PoM

Peditrace® (Fresenius Kabi) PoM

Solution, trace elements for addition to *Vaminol-act®*, *Vamin® 14 Electrolyte-Free* solutions and glucose intravenous infusions, traces of Zn^{2+}, Cu^{2+}, Mn^{2+}, Se^{4+}, F^-, I^-. For use in infants (when kidney function established, usually second day of life) and children. Net price 10-mL vial = £3.10

Cautions: reduced biliary excretion especially in cholestatic liver disease or in markedly reduced urinary excretion (careful biochemical monitoring required); total parenteral nutrition exceeding 1 month (measure serum manganese concentration and check liver function before commencing treatment and regularly during treatment)—discontinue if manganese concentration raised or if cholestasis develops

Solivito N® (Fresenius Kabi) PoM

Solution, powder for reconstitution, biotin 60 micrograms, cyanocobalamin 5 micrograms, folic acid 400 micrograms, glycine 300 mg, nicotinamide 40 mg, pyridoxine hydrochloride 4.9 mg, riboflavin sodium phosphate 4.9 mg, sodium ascorbate 113 mg, sodium pantothenate 16.5 mg, thiamine mononitrate 3.1 mg. Dissolve in water for injections or glucose intravenous infusion for adding to glucose intravenous infusion or *Intralipid®*; dissolve in *Vitlipid N®* or *Intralipid®* for adding to *Intralipid®* only. Net price per vial = £1.75

Vitlipid N® (Fresenius Kabi) PoM

Emulsion, adult, vitamin A 330 units, ergocalciferol 20 units, *dl*-alpha tocopherol 1 unit, phytomenadione 15 micrograms/mL. For addition to *Intralipid®*. For adults and children over 11 years. Net price 10-mL amp = £1.71

Emulsion, infant, vitamin A 230 units, ergocalciferol 40 units, *dl*-alpha tocopherol 0.7 unit, phytomenadione 20 micrograms/mL. For addition to *Intralipid®*. Net price 10-mL amp = £1.71

9.4 Oral nutrition

9.4.1 Foods for special diets
9.4.2 Enteral nutrition

9.4.1 Foods for special diets

These are preparations that have been modified to eliminate a particular constituent from a food or are nutrient mixtures formulated as substitutes for the food. They are for patients who either cannot tolerate or cannot metabolise certain common constituents of food.

PHENYLKETONURIA. Phenylketonuria (phenylalaninaemia), which results from the inability to metabolise phenylalanine, is managed by restricting its dietary intake to a small amount sufficient for tissue building and repair. Aspartame (as a sweetener in some foods and medicines) contributes to the phenylalanine intake and may affect control of phenylketonuria. Where the presence of aspartame is specified in the product literature this is indicated in the BNF against the preparation.

COELIAC DISEASE. Coeliac disease, which results from an intolerance to gluten, is managed by completely eliminating gluten from the diet.

ACBS. In certain clinical conditions some foods may have the characteristics of drugs and the Advisory Committee on Borderline Substances advises as to the circumstances in which such foods may be regarded as drugs and so can be prescribed in the NHS. Prescriptions for these foods issued in accordance with the advice of this committee and endorsed 'ACBS' will normally not be investigated. See Appendix 7 for details of these foods and a listing by clinical condition (consult Drug Tariff for late amendments).

■ Preparations
For preparations on the ACBS list see Appendix 7

Forceval Protein Powder® (Unigreg)

Powder, strawberry, vanilla and natural flavours, protein (calcium caseinate, providing all essential amino acids) 55%, carbohydrate 30%, with vitamins, minerals, trace elements, fat and low electrolytes (lactose- and gluten-free), net price 14 × 30-g sachets = £17.11; chocolate flavour (as above but protein content is 45%), 14 × 36-g sachets = £17.11. For hypoproteinaemia, malabsorption states and as an adjunct to nutritional support. Not to be prescribed for any CHILD under 2 years or for those with renal or hepatic failure; unsuitable as a sole source of nutrition

9.4.2 Enteral nutrition

The body's reserves of protein rapidly become exhausted in severely ill patients, especially during chronic illness or in those with severe burns, extensive trauma, pancreatitis, or intestinal fistula. Much can be achieved by frequent meals and by persuading the patient to take supplementary snacks of ordinary food between the meals.

However, extra calories, protein, other nutrients, and vitamins are often best given by supplementing ordinary meals with sip or tube feeds of one of the nutritionally complete foods.

When patients cannot feed normally at all, for example patients with severe facial injury, oesophageal obstruction, or coma, a diet composed solely of nutritionally complete foods must be given. This is planned by a dietitian who will take into account the protein and total energy requirement of the patient and decide on the form and relative contribution of carbohydrate and fat to the energy requirements.

There are a number of nutritionally complete foods available and their use reduces an otherwise heavy workload in hospital or in the home. Most contain protein derived from milk or soya. Some contain protein hydrolysates or free amino acids and are only appropriate for patients who have diminished ability to break down protein, as may be the case in inflammatory bowel disease or pancreatic insufficiency.

Even when nutritionally complete feeds are being given it may be important to monitor water and electrolyte balance. Extra minerals (e.g. magnesium and zinc) may be needed in patients where gastrointestinal secretions are being lost. Additional vitamins may also be needed. Regular haematological and biochemical tests may be needed particularly in the unstable patient.

Some feeds are supplemented with vitamin K; for drug interactions of vitamin K see Appendix 1 (vitamins).

CHILDREN. Infants and young children have special requirements and in most situations liquid feeds prepared for adults are totally unsuitable and should not be given. Expert advice should be sought.

■ Preparations
See Appendix 7

9.5   Minerals

9.5.1	Calcium and magnesium
9.5.2	Phosphorus
9.5.3	Fluoride
9.5.4	Zinc

See section 9.1.1 for iron salts.

9.5.1   Calcium and magnesium

9.5.1.1	Calcium supplements
9.5.1.2	Hypercalcaemia and hypercalciuria
9.5.1.3	Magnesium

9.5.1.1   Calcium supplements

Calcium supplements are usually only required where dietary calcium intake is deficient. This dietary requirement varies with age and is relatively greater in childhood, pregnancy, and lactation, due to an increased demand, and in old age, due to impaired absorption. In osteoporosis, a calcium intake which is double the recommended daily amount (RDA) reduces the rate of bone loss. If the actual dietary intake is less than the RDA, a supplement of as much as 40 mmol is appropriate.

In hypocalcaemic tetany an initial intravenous injection of 10 mL (2.25 mmol) of calcium gluconate injection 10% should be followed by the continuous infusion of about 40 mL (9 mmol) daily, but plasma calcium should be monitored. This regimen can also be used, immediately but temporarily, to reduce the toxic effects of hyperkalaemia.

CALCIUM SALTS

Indications: see notes above; calcium deficiency
Cautions: renal impairment; sarcoidosis; **interactions:** Appendix 1 (calcium salts)
Contra-indications: conditions associated with hypercalcaemia and hypercalciuria (eg. some forms of malignant disease)
Side-effects: mild gastro-intestinal disturbances; bradycardia, arrhythmias, and irritation after intravenous injection
Dose: *by mouth,* daily in divided doses, see notes above
By slow intravenous injection, acute hypocalcaemia, calcium gluconate 1–2 g (Ca^{2+} 2.25–4.5 mmol)
CHILD obtain paediatric advice

■ Oral preparations

Calcium Gluconate (Non-proprietary)
Tablets, calcium gluconate 600 mg (calcium 53.4 mg or Ca^{2+} 1.35 mmol), net price 20 = 78p. Label: 24

Effervescent tablets, calcium gluconate 1 g (calcium 89 mg or Ca^{2+} 2.25 mmol), net price 28-tab pack = £4.62. Label: 13
Note. Each tablet usually contains 4.46 mmol Na$^+$

Calcium Lactate (Non-proprietary)
Tablets, calcium lactate 300 mg (calcium 39 mg or Ca^{2+} 1 mmol), net price 20 = 63p

Adcal® (Strakan)
Chewable tablets, calcium carbonate 1.5 g (calcium 600 mg or Ca^{2+} 15 mmol), net price 100-tab pack = £7.25. Label: 24

Cacit® (Procter & Gamble Pharm.)
Tablets, effervescent, pink, calcium carbonate 1.25 g, providing calcium citrate when dispersed in water (calcium 500 mg or Ca^{2+} 12.6 mmol), net price 76-tab pack = £10.92. Label: 13

Calcichew® (Shire)
Tablets (chewable), calcium carbonate 1.25 g (calcium 500 mg or Ca^{2+} 12.6 mmol), net price 100-tab pack = £9.33

Forte tablets (chewable), scored, calcium carbonate 2.5 g (calcium 1 g or Ca^{2+} 25 mmol), net price 100-tab pack = £21.94. Label: 24
Excipients: include aspartame

Calcidrink® (Shire)
Granules, effervescent, calcium carbonate 2.52 g (calcium 1 g or Ca^{2+} 25 mmol). Net price 30-sachet pack = £8.48. Label: 13

Calcium-500 (Martindale)
Tablets, pink, f/c, calcium carbonate 1.25 g (calcium 500 mg or Ca^{2+} 12.5 mmol). Net price 100-tab pack = £10.17. Label: 25

Calcium-Sandoz® (Alliance)
Syrup, calcium glubionate 1.09 g, calcium lactobionate 727 mg (calcium 108.3 mg or Ca^{2+} 2.7 mmol)/5 mL. Net price 300 mL = £3.48

Ossopan® (Sanofi-Synthelabo)
Tablets, buff, f/c, hydroxyapatite 830 mg (calcium 178 mg or Ca^{2+} 4.4 mmol). Net price 50 = £9.64
Granules, brown, hydroxyapatite 3.32 g (calcium 712 mg or Ca^{2+} 17.8 mmol)/sachet, net price 28-sachet pack = £17.23

Ostram® (Merck)
Powder, calcium phosphate 3.3 g (calcium 1.2 g or Ca^{2+} 29.9 mmol)/sachet. Net price 30-sachet pack = £5.95. Label: 13

Sandocal® (Novartis)
Sandocal-400 tablets, effervescent, calcium lactate gluconate 930 mg, calcium carbonate 700 mg, anhydrous citric acid 1.189 g, providing calcium 400 mg (Ca^{2+} 10 mmol). Net price 5 × 20-tab pack = £6.85. Label: 13

Sandocal-1000 tablets, effervescent, calcium lactate gluconate 2.327 g, calcium carbonate 1.75 g, anhydrous citric acid 2.973 g providing 1 g calcium (Ca^{2+} 25 mmol). Net price 3 × 10-tab pack = £6.18. Label: 13

Titralac®, section 9.5.2.2

■ Parenteral preparations

Calcium Gluconate (Non-proprietary) PoM

Injection, calcium gluconate 10% (calcium 8.9 mg or Ca²⁺ 220 micromol)/mL. Net price 10-mL amp = 60p

Available from Phoenix

Calcium Chloride (Non-proprietary) PoM

Injection, calcium chloride 100 mg/mL (calcium 27.3 mg or Ca²⁺ 680 micromol/mL). Net price 10-mL disposable syringe = £4.32

Available from Aurum, Celltech (*Min-I-Jet® Calcium Chloride 10%*)

■ With vitamin D

Section 9.6.4

9.5.1.2 Hypercalcaemia and hypercalciuria

SEVERE HYPERCALCAEMIA. Severe hypercalcaemia calls for urgent treatment before detailed investigation of the cause. Dehydration should be corrected first with intravenous infusion of **sodium chloride 0.9%**. Drugs (such as thiazides and vitamin D compounds) which promote hypercalcaemia, should be discontinued and dietary calcium should be restricted.

If *severe hypercalcaemia persists* drugs which inhibit mobilisation of calcium from the skeleton may be required. The **bisphosphonates** are useful and disodium pamidronate (section 6.6.2) is probably the most effective.

Corticosteroids (section 6.3) are widely given, but may only be useful where hypercalcaemia is due to sarcoidosis or vitamin D intoxication; they often take several days to achieve the desired effect.

Calcitonin (section 6.6.1) is relatively non-toxic but is expensive and its effect can wear off after a few days despite continued use; it is rarely effective where bisphosphonates have failed to reduce serum calcium adequately.

Intravenous chelating drugs such as **trisodium edetate** are rarely used; they usually cause pain in the limb receiving the infusion and may cause renal damage.

After treatment of severe hypercalcaemia the underlying cause must be established. *Further treatment* is governed by the same principles as for initial therapy. Salt and water depletion and drugs promoting hypercalcaemia should be avoided; oral administration of a bisphosphonate may be useful. Parathyroidectomy may be indicated for hyperparathyroidism.

HYPERCALCIURIA. Hypercalciuria should be investigated for an underlying cause, which should be treated. Where a cause is not identified (idiopathic hypercalciuria), the condition is managed by increasing fluid intake and giving bendroflumethiazide in a dose of 2.5 mg daily (a higher dose is not usually necessary). Reducing dietary calcium intake may be beneficial but severe restriction of calcium intake has not proved beneficial and may even be harmful.

TRISODIUM EDETATE

Indications: hypercalcaemia (but see notes above); lime burns in the eye (see under Preparations)

Cautions: repeated plasma-calcium determinations important; caution in tuberculosis; avoid rapid infusion, see under Dose

Contra-indications: impaired renal function

Side-effects: nausea, diarrhoea, cramp; in overdosage renal damage

Dose: hypercalcaemia, *by intravenous infusion* over 2–3 hours, up to 70 mg/kg daily; CHILD up to 60 mg/kg daily

IMPORTANT. Ensure rate of infusion and concentration correct (see Appendix 6); too rapid a rate or too high a concentration is extremely hazardous and repeated measurements of plasma calcium concentrations are important for control and maintenance of near normal ionised calcium concentrations. Decrease infusion rate on signs of increased muscle reactivity; discontinue if tetany occurs and restart cautiously only after plasma ionised and total calcium concentrations indicate need for further treatment (and tetany has stopped)

Limclair® (Sinclair) PoM

Injection, trisodium edetate 200 mg/mL. For dilution and use as an intravenous infusion. Net price 5-mL amp = £4.76

Note. For topical use in the eye, dilute 1 mL to 50 mL with sterile purified water

9.5.1.3 Magnesium

Magnesium is an essential constituent of many enzyme systems, particularly those involved in energy generation; the largest stores are in the skeleton.

Magnesium salts are not well absorbed from the gastro-intestinal tract which explains the use of magnesium sulphate (section 1.6.4) as an osmotic laxative.

Magnesium is mainly excreted by the kidneys and is therefore retained in renal failure although significant *hypermagnesaemia* (causing muscle weakness and arrhythmias) is rare.

HYPOMAGNESAEMIA. Since magnesium is secreted in large amounts in the gastro-intestinal fluid, excessive losses in diarrhoea, stoma or fistula are the most common causes of *hypomagnesaemia*; deficiency may also occur in alcoholism or diuretic therapy and it has been reported after prolonged treatment with aminoglycosides. Hypomagnesaemia often causes secondary hypocalcaemia (with which it may be confused) and also hypokalaemia and hyponatraemia.

Symptomatic *hypomagnesaemia* is associated with a deficit of 0.5–1 mmol/kg; up to 160 mmol Mg²⁺ over up to 5 days may be required to replace the deficit (allowing for urinary losses). Magnesium is given initially by intravenous infusion or by intramuscular injection of **magnesium sulphate**; the intramuscular injection is painful. Plasma magnesium concentrations should be measured to determine the rate and duration of infusion and the dose should be reduced in renal impairment. To prevent *recurrence of the deficit*, magnesium may be given by mouth in a dose of 24 mmol Mg²⁺ daily in divided doses; a suitable preparation is magnesium glycerophosphate tablets [not licensed, available from IDIS]. For maintenance (e.g. in intravenous nutrition), parenteral doses of magnesium are of the order of 10–20 mmol Mg^{2+} daily (often about 12 mmol Mg^{2+} daily).

ARRHYTHMIAS. Magnesium sulphate has also been recommended for the emergency treatment of *serious arrhythmias*, especially in the presence of hypokalaemia (when hypomagnesaemia may also be present) and when salvos of rapid ventricular tachycardia show the characteristic twisting wave front known as *torsades de pointes*. The usual dose of magnesium sulphate is intravenous injection of 8 mmol Mg^{2+} over 10–15 minutes (repeated once if necessary).

MYOCARDIAL INFARCTION. Evidence suggesting a substantial reduction in mortality in patients with *suspected myocardial infarction* given an initial intravenous injection of magnesium sulphate 8 mmol Mg^{2+} over 20 minutes followed by an intravenous infusion of 65–72 mmol Mg^{2+} over the following 24 hours, has not been borne out by a larger study. Some workers, however, continue to hold the view that magnesium is beneficial if given immediately (and for as long as there is a likelihood of reperfusion taking place).

ECLAMPSIA. Magnesium sulphate has been shown to have a major role in *eclampsia* for the prevention of recurrent seizures. Regimens in the UK may vary between hospitals but typically involve initial intravenous administration of magnesium sulphate 4 g (approx. 16 mmol Mg^{2+}) over 5–10 minutes followed by intravenous infusion at a rate of 1 g (approx. 4 mmol Mg^{2+}) every hour for at least 24 hours after the last seizure; recurrence of seizures may require an additional intravenous bolus of 2 g (approx. 8 mmol Mg^{2+}). Monitoring of blood pressure, respiratory rate and urinary output is carried out, as is monitoring for clinical signs of overdosage (loss of patellar reflexes, weakness, nausea, sensation of warmth, flushing, drowsiness, double vision, and slurred speech. Calcium gluconate injection is used for the management of magnesium toxicity).

MAGNESIUM SULPHATE

Indications: see notes above; constipation (section 1.6.4); paste for boils (section 13.10.5)

Cautions: see notes above; hepatic impairment (Appendix 2); renal impairment (risk of accumulation); in severe hypomagnesaemia administer initially via controlled infusion device (preferably syringe pump); **interactions:** Appendix 1 (magnesium salts)

Side-effects: generally associated with hypermagnesaemia, nausea, vomiting, thirst, flushing of skin, hypotension, arrhythmias, coma, respiratory depression, drowsiness, confusion, loss of tendon reflexes, muscle weakness; colic and diarrhoea following oral administration

Dose: see notes above

Magnesium Sulphate (Non-proprietary) PoM
Injection, magnesium sulphate 50% (approx. 2 mmol Mg^{2+}/mL), net price 2-mL (1-g) amp = £2.69, 5-mL (2.5-g) amp = £2.28, 10-mL (5-g) amp = £3.05; prefilled 10-mL (5-g) syringe = £4.50
Available from Aurum, Celltech

9.5.2   Phosphorus

9.5.2.1   Phosphate supplements
9.5.2.2   Phosphate-binding agents

9.5.2.1   Phosphate supplements

Oral phosphate supplements may be required in addition to vitamin D in a small minority of patients with hypophosphataemic vitamin D-resistant rickets. Diarrhoea is a common side-effect and should prompt a reduction in dosage.

Phosphate infusion is occasionally needed in alcohol dependence or in phosphate deficiency arising from use of parenteral nutrition deficient in phosphate supplements; phosphate depletion also occurs in severe diabetic ketoacidosis. For *established hypophosphataemia*, monobasic potassium phosphate may be infused at a maximum rate of 9 mmol every 12 hours. Excessive doses of phosphates may cause hypocalcaemia and metastatic calcification; it is **essential** to monitor closely plasma concentrations of calcium, phosphate, potassium, and other electrolytes.

For phosphate requirements in *total parenteral nutrition* regimens, see section 9.3.

Phosphate-Sandoz® (HK Pharma)
Tablets, effervescent, anhydrous sodium acid phosphate 1.936 g, sodium bicarbonate 350 mg, potassium bicarbonate 315 mg, equivalent to phosphorus 500 mg (phosphate 16.1 mmol), sodium 468.8 mg (Na^+ 20.4 mmol), potassium 123 mg (K^+ 3.1 mmol). Net price 20 = £3.29. Label: 13
Dose: hypercalcaemia, up to 6 tablets daily adjusted according to response; CHILD under 5 years up to 3 tablets daily
Vitamin D-resistant hypophosphataemic osteomalacia, 4–6 tablets daily; CHILD under 5 years 2–3 tablets daily

9.5.2.2   Phosphate-binding agents

Aluminium-containing and calcium-containing preparations are used as phosphate-binding agents in the management of hyperphosphataemia complicating renal failure. Calcium-containing phosphate-binding agents are contra-indicated in hypercalcaemia or hypercalciuria. Phosphate-binding agents which contain aluminium may increase plasma aluminium in dialysis patients.

Sevelamer is licensed for the treatment of hyperphosphataemia in patients on haemodialysis.

ALUMINIUM HYDROXIDE

Indications: hyperphosphataemia; dyspepsia (section 1.1)

Cautions: hyperaluminaemia; porphyria (section 9.8.2); see also notes above; **interactions:** Appendix 1 (antacids)

Side-effects: see section 1.1.1

Aluminium Hydroxide (Non-proprietary)
Mixture (gel), about 4% w/w Al_2O_3 in water. Net price 200 mL = 41p
Dose: hyperphosphataemia, 20–100 mL according to requirements of patient
Note. The brand name *Aludrox®* NHS (Pfizer Consumer) is used for aluminium hydroxide mixture, net price 200 mL = £1.42

Alu-Cap® (3M)
Capsules, green/red, dried aluminium hydroxide 475 mg (low Na^+). Net price 120-cap pack = £4.03
Dose: phosphate-binding agent in renal failure, 4–20 capsules daily in divided doses with meals

CALCIUM SALTS

Indications: hyperphosphataemia
Cautions: see notes above; **interactions:** Appendix 1 (calcium salts)
Side-effects: hypercalcaemia

Adcal®, section 9.5.1.1
Calcichew®, section 9.5.1.1
Calcium-500, section 9.5.1.1

Phosex® (Vitaline)
Tablets, yellow, calcium acetate 1 g (calcium 250 mg or Ca^{2+} 6.2 mmol), net price 180-tab pack = £19.79. Label: 25
Dose: phosphate-binding agent (with meals) in renal failure, according to the requirements of the patient

Titralac® (3M)
Tablets, calcium carbonate 420 mg (calcium 168 mg or Ca^{2+} 4.2 mmol), glycine 180 mg. Net price 180-tab pack = £2.81
COUNSELLING. May be chewed, crushed or swallowed whole
Dose: calcium supplement, or phosphate-binding agent (with meals) in renal failure, according to the requirements of the patient

SEVELAMER

Indications: hyperphosphataemia in patients on haemodialysis
Cautions: pregnancy and breast-feeding; gastrointestinal disorders
Contra-indications: bowel obstruction
Dose: initially 2.4–4.836 g (as 6–12 403-mg capsules *or* 3–6 800-mg tablets) daily in 3 divided doses with meals, then adjusted according to plasma-phosphate concentration

Renagel® (Genzyme) ▼ PoM
Capsules, sevelamer 403 mg, net price 200-cap pack = £73.00. Label: 21
Tablets, f/c, sevelamer 800 mg, net price 180-tab pack = £132.00. Label: 21

9.5.3   Fluoride

Availability of adequate fluoride confers significant resistance to dental caries. It is now considered that the topical action of fluoride on enamel and plaque is more important than the systemic effect.

Where the natural fluoride content of the drinking water is significantly less than 1 mg per litre (one part per million) artificial fluoridation is the most economical method of supplementing fluoride intake.

Daily administration of tablets or drops is a suitable alternative, but systemic fluoride supplements should not be prescribed without reference to the fluoride content of the local water supply; they are not advisable when the water contains more than 700 micrograms per litre (0.7 parts per million). In addition, infants need not receive fluoride supplements until the age of 6 months.

Dentifrices which incorporate sodium fluoride or monofluorophosphate are also a convenient source of fluoride.

Individuals who are either particularly caries prone or medically compromised may be given additional protection by use of fluoride rinses or by application of fluoride gels. Rinses may be used daily or weekly; daily use of a less concentrated rinse is more effective than weekly use of a more concentrated one. High-strength gels must be applied on a regular basis under professional supervision; extreme caution is necessary to prevent the child from swallowing any excess. Less concentrated gels are available for home use. Varnishes are also available and are particularly valuable for young or handicapped children since they adhere to the teeth and set in the presence of moisture.

FLUORIDES

Note. Sodium fluoride 2.2 mg provides approx. 1 mg fluoride ion
Indications: prophylaxis of dental caries—see notes above
Contra-indications: not for areas where drinking water is fluoridated
Side-effects: occasional white flecks on teeth with recommended doses; rarely yellowish-brown discoloration if recommended doses are exceeded
Dose: expressed as fluoride ion (F^-):
Water content less than F^- 300 micrograms/litre (0.3 parts per million), CHILD up to 6 months none; 6 months–3 years F^- 250 micrograms daily, 3–6 years F^- 500 micrograms daily, over 6 years F^- 1 mg daily
Water content between F^- 300 and 700 micrograms/litre (0.3–0.7 parts per million), CHILD up to 3 years none, 3–6 years F^- 250 micrograms daily, over 6 years F^- 500 micrograms daily
Water content above F^- 700 micrograms/litre (0.7 parts per million), supplements not advised
Note. These doses reflect the recommendations of the British Dental Association, the British Society of Paediatric Dentistry and the British Association for the Study of Community Dentistry (*Br Dent J* 1997; **182:** 6–7)

■ Tablets
COUNSELLING. Tablets should be sucked or dissolved in the mouth and taken preferably in the evening
There are arrangements for health authorities to supply fluoride tablets in the course of pre-school dental schemes, and they may also be supplied in school dental schemes.

En-De-Kay® (Manx)
Fluotabs 3–6 years, orange-flavoured, scored, sodium fluoride 1.1 mg (F^- 500 micrograms). Net price 200-tab pack = £1.83
Fluotabs 6+ years, orange-flavoured, scored, sodium fluoride 2.2 mg (F^- 1 mg). Net price 200-tab pack = £1.83

Fluor-a-day® (Dental Health)
Tablets, buff, sodium fluoride 1.1 mg (F^- 500 micrograms), net price 200-tab pack = £1.77; 2.2 mg (F^- 1 mg), 200-tab pack = £1.77

FluoriGard® (Colgate-Palmolive)
Tablets 0.5, purple, grape-flavoured, scored, sodium fluoride 1.1 mg (F⁻ 500 micrograms). Net price 200-tab pack = £1.91
Tablets 1.0, orange, orange-flavoured, scored, sodium fluoride 2.2 mg (F⁻ 1 mg). Net price 200-tab pack = £1.91

■ Oral drops
Note. Fluoride supplements not considered necessary below 6 months of age (see notes above)
En-De-Kay® (Manx)
Fluodrops® (= paediatric drops), sugar-free, sodium fluoride 550 micrograms (F⁻ 250 micrograms)/0.15 mL. Net price 60 mL = £1.62
Note. Corresponds to Sodium Fluoride Oral Drops DPF 0.37% equivalent to sodium fluoride 80 micrograms (F⁻ 36 micrograms)/drop

■ Mouthwashes
Rinse mouth for 1 minute and spit out
COUNSELLING. Avoid eating, drinking, or rinsing mouth for 15 minutes after use
Duraphat® (Colgate-Palmolive)
Weekly dental rinse (= mouthwash), blue, sodium fluoride 0.2%. Net price 150 mL = £2.22. Counselling, see above
CHILD 6 years and over, for *weekly* use, rinse with 10 mL
En-De-Kay® (Manx)
Daily fluoride mouthrinse (= mouthwash), blue, sodium fluoride 0.05%. Net price 250 mL = £1.81
CHILD 6 years and over, for *daily* use, rinse with 10 mL
PoM *Fluorinse* (= mouthwash), red, sodium fluoride 2%. Net price 100 mL = £3.97. Counselling, see above
CHILD 8 years and over, for *daily* use, dilute 5 drops to 10 mL of water; for *weekly* use, dilute 20 drops to 10 mL
FluoriGard® (Colgate-Palmolive)
Daily dental rinse (= mouthwash), blue, sodium fluoride 0.05%. Net price 500 mL = £3.11. Counselling, see above
CHILD 6 years and over, for *daily* use, rinse with 10 mL

■ Gels
FluoriGard® (Colgate-Palmolive)
Gel-Kam (= gel), stannous fluoride 0.4% in glycerol basis. Net price 100 mL = £3.05. Counselling, see below
ADULT and CHILD 3 years and over, for *daily* use, using a toothbrush, apply onto all tooth surfaces
COUNSELLING. Swish between teeth for 1 minute before spitting out. Avoid eating, drinking, or rinsing mouth for at least 30 minutes after use

9.5.4   Zinc

Oral zinc therapy should only be given when there is good evidence of deficiency (hypoproteinaemia spuriously lowers plasma-zinc concentrations). Zinc deficiency can occur in individuals on inadequate diets, in malabsorption, with increased body loss due to trauma, burns and protein-losing conditions, and during intravenous feeding. Therapy should continue until clinical improvement occurs and be replaced by dietary measures unless there is severe malabsorption, metabolic disease, or continuing zinc loss. Side-effects of zinc salts are abdominal pain and dyspepsia.

ZINC SALTS

Indications: see notes above
Cautions: see notes above; **interactions:** Appendix 1 (zinc)
Side-effects: see notes above

Solvazinc® (Thames)
Effervescent tablets, yellow-white, zinc sulphate monohydrate 125 mg (45 mg zinc). Net price 30 = £4.32. Label: 13, 21
Dose: ADULT and CHILD over 30 kg, 1 tablet in water 1–3 times daily after food; CHILD under 10 kg, ½ tablet daily; 10–30 kg, ½ tablet 1–3 times daily

9.6   Vitamins

9.6.1	Vitamin A
9.6.2	Vitamin B group
9.6.3	Vitamin C
9.6.4	Vitamin D
9.6.5	Vitamin E
9.6.6	Vitamin K
9.6.7	Multivitamin preparations

Vitamins are used for the prevention and treatment of specific deficiency states or where the diet is known to be inadequate; they may be prescribed in the NHS to prevent or treat deficiency but not as dietary supplements.

Their use as general 'pick-me-ups' is of unproven value and, in the case of preparations containing vitamin A or D, may actually be harmful if patients take more than the prescribed dose. The 'fad' for mega-vitamin therapy with water-soluble vitamins, such as ascorbic acid and pyridoxine, is unscientific and can be harmful.

Dietary reference values for vitamins are available in the Department of Health publication:

Dietary Reference Values for Food Energy and Nutrients for the United Kingdom: Report of the Panel on Dietary Reference Values of the Committee on Medical Aspects of Food Policy. *Report on Health and Social Subjects 41.* London: HMSO, 1991

9.6.1   Vitamin A

Deficiency of vitamin A (retinol) is associated with ocular defects (particularly xerophthalmia) and an increased susceptibility to infections, but deficiency is rare in the UK (even in disorders of fat absorption). Despite initial epidemiological evidence suggesting that vitamin A or carotene may have a protective effect against some epithelial cancers, the claims have not been substantiated.

Massive overdose can cause rough skin, dry hair, an enlarged liver, and a raised erythrocyte sedimentation rate and raised serum calcium and serum alkaline phosphatase concentrations.

In view of evidence suggesting that high levels of vitamin A may cause birth defects, women who are (or may become) pregnant are advised not to take vitamin A supplements (including tablets and fish-liver oil drops), except on the advice of a doctor or an antenatal clinic; nor should they eat liver or products such as liver paté or liver sausage.

VITAMIN A

(Retinol)

Indications: see notes above

Cautions: see notes above

Side-effects: see notes above

Dose: see notes above and under preparations

■ Vitamins A and D

Halibut-liver Oil (Non-proprietary)

Capsules, vitamin A 4000 units [also contains vitamin D]. Net price 20 = 22p

Available from Thornton & Ross

Vitamins A and D (Non-proprietary)

Capsules, vitamin A 4000 units, vitamin D 400 units. Net price 20 = 60p

Available from CP

Halycitrol® (LAB) NHS

Emulsion, vitamin A 4600 units, vitamin D 380 units/5 mL. Net price 114 mL = £1.61

Dose: 5 mL daily but see notes above

■ Vitamins A, C and D

Mothers' and Children's Vitamin Drops (Cupal)

Oral drops, vitamin A 5000 units, vitamin D 2000 units, ascorbic acid 150 mg/mL

Available free of charge to pregnant women and children aged under 5 years in families receiving Income Support or an income-based Jobseeker's Allowance under the Welfare Food Scheme. If prescribed, prescription needs to be endorsed 'ACBS'. Otherwise available direct to the public from maternity and child health clinics

Dose: pregnant and nursing mothers and CHILD 1 month–5 years, 5 drops daily (5 drops contain vitamin A approx. 700 units, ascorbic acid approx. 20 mg, vitamin D approx. 300 units)

Note. Recommended by the Department of Health for routine supplementation in all pregnant women (but see notes above) and children from 1 year to 5 years. For breast-fed baby whose mother was in good vitamin status during pregnancy, supplementation may begin at 6 months of age; where there is doubt about the mother's vitamin status during pregnancy, supplementation should begin at 1 month of age; a baby consuming 500 mL infant formula feed or follow-on formula feed daily does not need vitamin supplementation because the formula feeds are fortified with vitamin D

Vitamin Tablets (with Calcium and Iodine) for Nursing Mothers (Sussex)

Tablets, orange, s/c, vitamin A (as retinyl acetate) 8 mg, ascorbic acid 60 mg, ergocalciferol 400 units, calcium hydrogen phosphate 190 mg (40 mg calcium or 1 mmol Ca^{2+}), potassium iodide 130 micrograms

Recommended by the Department of Health for routine supplementation in nursing mothers. Free of charge to nursing mothers with children aged under 1 year in families receiving Income Support or an income-based Jobseeker's Allowance under the Welfare Food Scheme. If prescribed, prescription needs to be endorsed 'ACBS'. Otherwise available direct to the public from maternity and child health clinics

Dose: one tablet daily

Note. Women who are (or may become) pregnant are advised not to take this supplement except on the advice of a doctor or antenatal clinic

■ Vitamin A injection

Vitamin A Palmitate (Cambridge) PoM

Injection, vitamin A (retinol) 50 000 units (as palmitate)/mL. Net price 2-mL amp = £3.45

Dose: by deep intramuscular injection, deficiency, 100 000 units monthly, increased to weekly in acute deficiency states; courses no longer than 6 weeks with 2-week interval

Liver disease, 100 000 units every 2–4 months

INFANT under 1 year and CHILD 50 000 units monthly

Excipients: include polyoxyl castor oil (risk of anaphylaxis, see Excipients p. 2)

Note. Do **not** mix or dilute

Cautions: children, liver disease (specialist use), see also notes above

9.6.2 Vitamin B group

Deficiency of the B vitamins, other than deficiency of vitamin B_{12} (section 9.1.2) is rare in the UK and is usually treated by preparations containing thiamine (B_1), riboflavin (B_2), and nicotinamide, which is used in preference to nicotinic acid, as it does not cause vasodilatation. Other members (or substances traditionally classified as members) of the vitamin B complex such as aminobenzoic acid, biotin, choline, inositol, and pantothenic acid or panthenol may be included in vitamin B preparations but there is no evidence of their value.

The severe deficiency states Wernicke's encephalopathy and Korsakoff's psychosis, especially as seen in chronic alcoholism, are best treated initially by the parenteral administration of B vitamins (*Pabrinex®*), followed by oral administration of thiamine in the longer term. Anaphylaxis has been reported with parenteral B vitamins (see CSM advice, below).

As with other vitamins of the B group, pyridoxine (B_6) deficiency is rare, but it may occur during isoniazid therapy (section 5.1.9) and is characterised by peripheral neuritis. High doses of pyridoxine are given in some metabolic disorders, such as hyperoxaluria, and it is also used in sideroblastic anaemia (section 9.1.3). There is evidence to suggest that pyridoxine in a dose not exceeding 100 mg daily may provide some benefit in premenstrual syndrome. It has been tried for a wide variety of other disorders, but there is little sound evidence to support the claims of efficacy, and overdosage induces toxic effects.

Nicotinic acid inhibits the synthesis of cholesterol and triglyceride (see section 2.12). Folic acid and vitamin B_{12} are used in the treatment of megaloblastic anaemia (section 9.1.2). Folinic acid (available as calcium folinate) is used in association with cytotoxic therapy (section 8.1).

RIBOFLAVIN

(Riboflavine, vitamin B_2)

Indications: see notes above

Preparations

Injections of vitamins B and C, see under Thiamine

■ Oral vitamin B complex preparations, see below

THIAMINE
(Vitamin B₁)

Indications: see notes above
Cautions: anaphylactic shock may occasionally follow injection (see CSM advice below)
Dose: mild chronic deficiency, 10–25 mg daily; severe deficiency, 200–300 mg daily

Thiamine (Non-proprietary)
Tablets, thiamine hydrochloride 50 mg, net price 20 = 53p; 100 mg, 20 = 84p
Available from Roche Consumer Health (*Benerva*® ⓃⒽⓈ)

Pabrinex® (Link) ⓅⓞⓂ
Parenteral vitamins B and C for rapid correction of severe depletion or malabsorption (e.g in alcoholism, after acute infections, postoperatively, or in psychiatric states), maintenance of vitamins B and C in chronic intermittent haemodialysis
Dose: see CSM advice above
Coma or delirium from alcohol, from opioids, or from barbiturates, collapse following narcosis, by intravenous injection or infusion of *I/V High potency*, 2-3 pairs every 8 hours
Psychosis following narcosis or electroconvulsive therapy, toxicity from acute infections, by intravenous injection or infusion of *I/V High potency* or by deep intramuscular injection into the gluteal muscle of *I/M High potency*, 1 pair twice daily for up to 7 days
Haemodialysis, by intravenous infusion of *I/V High potency* (in sodium chloride intravenous infusion 0.9%) 1 pair every 2 weeks
I/M High potency injection, for intramuscular use only, ascorbic acid 500 mg, nicotinamide 160 mg, pyridoxine hydrochloride 50 mg, riboflavin 4 mg, thiamine hydrochloride 250 mg/7 mL. Net price 7 mL (in 2 amps) = £1.86
I/V High potency injection, for intravenous use only, ascorbic acid 500 mg, anhydrous glucose 1 g, nicotinamide 160 mg, pyridoxine hydrochloride 50 mg, riboflavin 4 mg, thiamine hydrochloride 250 mg/10 mL. Net price 10 mL (in 2 amps) = £1.66

CSM advice

Since potentially serious allergic adverse reactions may occur during, or shortly after, administration, the CSM has recommended that:

1. Use be restricted to patients in whom parenteral treatment is essential;

2. Intravenous injections should be administered slowly (over 10 minutes);

3. Facilities for treating anaphylaxis should be available when administered.

■ Oral vitamin B complex preparations, see below

PYRIDOXINE HYDROCHLORIDE
(Vitamin B₆)
Indications: see under Dose
Cautions: interactions: Appendix 1 (vitamins)
Dose: deficiency states, 20–50 mg up to 3 times daily
Isoniazid neuropathy, prophylaxis 10 mg daily [or

20 mg daily if suitable product not available]; therapeutic, 50 mg three times daily
Idiopathic sideroblastic anaemia, 100–400 mg daily in divided doses
Premenstrual syndrome, 50–100 mg daily (see notes above)

Important. Concerns about possible toxicity resulting from prolonged use of pyridoxine (vitamin B₆) at high dosage have not yet been resolved. The Royal Pharmaceutical Society of Great Britain has advised that pharmacists should consider how to advise customers requesting preparations containing higher doses and that they should decide their own policy on the display of products containing more than 10 mg per daily dose of pyridoxine.

Pyridoxine (Non-proprietary)
Tablets, pyridoxine hydrochloride 10 mg, net price 20 = 34p; 20 mg, 20 = 34p; 50 mg, 20 = 38p
Available from BR, CP, Hillcross

Orovite Complement B6® (SSL) ⓃⒽⓈ
Tablets, m/r, yellow, pyridoxine hydrochloride 100 mg. Net price 28-tab pack = £2.39. Label: 25

■ Injections of vitamins B and C, see under Thiamine

NICOTINAMIDE
Indications: see notes above; acne vulgaris, see section 13.6.1

Nicotinamide (Non-proprietary)
Tablets, nicotinamide 50 mg. Net price 20 = £1.37

■ Injections of vitamins B and C, see under Thiamine

Oral vitamin B complex preparations

Note. Other multivitamin preparations are in section 9.6.7.
Vitamin B Tablets, Compound ▰ nicotinamide 15 mg, riboflavin 1 mg, thiamine hydrochloride 1 mg. Net price 20 = 7p
Dose: prophylactic, 1–2 tablets daily
Vitamin B Tablets, Compound, Strong ▰ brown, f/c or s/c, nicotinamide 20 mg, pyridoxine hydrochloride 2 mg, riboflavin 2 mg, thiamine hydrochloride 5 mg. Net price 28-tab pack = 41p
Dose: treatment of vitamin-B deficiency, 1–2 tablets 3 times daily
Vigranon B® (Wallace Mfg) ⓃⒽⓈ ▰
Syrup, thiamine hydrochloride 5 mg, riboflavin 2 mg, nicotinamide 20 mg, pyridoxine hydrochloride 2 mg, panthenol 3 mg/5 mL. Net price 150 mL = £2.02

▰ denotes preparations that are considered to be less suitable for prescribing (see p. vi)

Other compounds

Potassium aminobenzoate has been used in the treatment of various disorders associated with excessive fibrosis such as scleroderma but its therapeutic value is **doubtful**.

Potaba® (Glenwood) ▰
Capsules, potassium aminobenzoate 500 mg. Net price 20 = £1.42. Label: 21

Tablets, potassium aminobenzoate 500 mg. Net price 20 = £1.00. Label: 21
Envules® (= powder in sachets), potassium amino-benzoate 3 g. Net price 40 sachets = £15.37.
Label: 13, 21

Dose: Peyronie's disease, scleroderma, 12 g daily in divided doses after food

9.6.3 Vitamin C
(Ascorbic acid)

Vitamin C therapy is essential in scurvy, but less florid manifestations of vitamin C deficiency are commonly found, especially in the elderly. It is rarely necessary to prescribe more than 100 mg daily except early in the treatment of scurvy.

Claims that vitamin C ameliorates colds or promotes wound healing have not been proved.

ASCORBIC ACID

Indications: prevention and treatment of scurvy
Dose: prophylactic, 25–75 mg daily; therapeutic, not less than 250 mg daily in divided doses

Ascorbic Acid (Non-proprietary)
Tablets, ascorbic acid 50 mg, net price 20 = 80p; 100 mg, 20 = 18p; 200 mg, 20 = 22p; 500 mg (label: 24), 20 = 40p
Available from Alpharma, Roche Consumer Health (Redoxon® [NHS])
Tablets [NHS], effervescent, ascorbic acid 1 g. Net price 10-tab pack = £1.23. Label: 13
Available from Roche Consumer Health (Redoxon® [NHS])
Injection, ascorbic acid 100 mg/mL. Net price 5-mL amp = £2.51

■ For children's welfare vitamin drops containing vitamin C with A and D, see vitamin A

9.6.4 Vitamin D

Note. The term Vitamin D is used for a range of compounds which possess the property of preventing or curing rickets. They include ergocalciferol (calciferol, vitamin D_2), colecalciferol (vitamin D_3), dihydrotachysterol, alfacalcidol (1α-hydroxycholecalciferol), and calcitriol (1,25-dihydroxycholecalciferol).

Simple vitamin D deficiency can be prevented by taking an oral supplement of only 10 micrograms (400 units) of ergocalciferol (calciferol, vitamin D_2) daily. Vitamin D deficiency is not uncommon in Asians consuming unleavened bread and in the elderly living alone and can be prevented by taking an oral supplement of 20 micrograms (800 units) of ergocalciferol daily. Since there is no plain tablet of this strength available **calcium and ergocalciferol tablets** can be given (although the calcium is unnecessary).

Vitamin D deficiency caused by *intestinal malabsorption* or *chronic liver disease* usually requires vitamin D in pharmacological doses, such as **calciferol tablets** up to 1 mg (40 000 units) daily; the hypocalcaemia of *hypoparathyroidism* often requires doses of up to 2.5 mg (100 000 units) daily in order to achieve normocalcaemia. The newer vitamin D derivatives, **alfacalcidol** and **calcitriol**, have a shorter duration of action, and therefore have

the advantage that problems associated with hyper-calcaemia due to excessive dosage are shorter lasting and easier to treat.

Vitamin D requires hydroxylation by the kidney to its active form therefore the hydroxylated derivatives **alfacalcidol** or **calcitriol** should be prescribed if patients with *severe renal impairment* require vitamin D therapy. Calcitriol is also licensed for the management of postmenopausal osteoporosis.

Important. All patients receiving pharmacological doses of vitamin D should have the plasma-calcium concentration checked at intervals (initially weekly) and whenever nausea or vomiting are present. Breast milk from women taking pharmacological doses of vitamin D may cause hypercalcaemia if given to an infant.

ERGOCALCIFEROL
(Calciferol, Vitamin D_2)

Indications: see notes above
Cautions: take care to ensure correct dose in infants; monitor plasma calcium in patients receiving high doses and in renal impairment; **interactions**: Appendix 1 (vitamins)
Contra-indications: hypercalcaemia; metastatic calcification
Side-effects: symptoms of overdosage include anorexia, lassitude, nausea and vomiting, diarrhoea, weight loss, polyuria, sweating, headache, thirst, vertigo, and raised concentrations of calcium and phosphate in plasma and urine
Dose: see notes above

■ Daily supplements

Note. There is no plain vitamin D tablet available for treating simple deficiency (see notes above). Alternatives include vitamins capsules (see 9.6.7), preparations of vitamins A and D (see 9.6.1), and calcium and ergocalciferol tablets (see below).

Calcium and Ergocalciferol (Non-proprietary)
(Calcium and Vitamin D)
Tablets, calcium lactate 300 mg, calcium phosphate 150 mg (calcium 97 mg or Ca^{2+} 2.4 mmol), ergocalciferol 10 micrograms (400 units). Net price 28-tab pack = 69p. Counselling, crush before administration or may be chewed

Adcal-D$_3$® (Strakan)
Tablets (chewable), calcium carbonate 1.5 g (calcium 600 mg or Ca^{2+} 15.1 mmol), colecalciferol 10 micrograms (400 units), net price 100-tab pack = £7.50. Label: 24

Cacit® D3 (Procter & Gamble Pharm.)
Granules, effervescent, calcium carbonate 1.25 g (calcium 500 mg or Ca^{2+} 12.6 mmol), colecalciferol 11 micrograms (440 units)/sachet. Net price 30-sachet pack = £3.91. Label: 13

Calceos® (Thames)
Tablets (chewable), calcium carbonate 1.25 g (calcium 500 mg or Ca^{2+} 12.6 mmol), colecalciferol 10 micrograms (400 units). Net price 60-tab pack = £8.00. Label: 24

Calcichew® D3 (Shire)

Tablets (chewable), calcium carbonate 1.25 g (calcium 500 mg or Ca^{2+} 12.6 mmol), colecalciferol 5 micrograms (200 units). Net price 100-tab pack = £15.02. Label: 24

Excipients: include aspartame

Calcichew® D3 Forte (Shire)

Tablets (chewable), calcium carbonate 1.25 g (calcium 500 mg or Ca^{2+} 12.6 mmol), colecalciferol 10 micrograms (400 units). Net price 100-tab pack = £9.50. Label: 24.

Excipients: include aspartame

■ Pharmacological strengths (see notes above)

Calciferol (Non-proprietary)

Tablets, colecalciferol or ergocalciferol 250 micrograms (10 000 units), net price 20 = £4.40; 1.25 mg (50 000 units) may also be available

Available from Celltech

Note. The BP directs that when calciferol tablets qualified by a descriptor relating to strength (such as 'high strength') are prescribed or demanded, the intention of the prescriber or purchaser with respect to the strength expressed in micrograms or milligrams per tablet should be ascertained. To avoid **errors** arising from the use of such titles prescribers are required to **abandon** them and **specify strength required**

Injection PoM, colecalciferol or ergocalciferol, 7.5 mg (300 000 units)/mL in oil. Net price 1-mL amp = £5.92, 2-mL amp = £7.07

Available from Celltech

ALFACALCIDOL

(1α-Hydroxycholecalciferol)

Indications: see notes above

Cautions: see under Ergocalciferol

Contra-indications: see under Ergocalciferol

Side-effects: see under Ergocalciferol

Dose: *by mouth or by intravenous injection* over 30 seconds, ADULT and CHILD over 20 kg, initially 1 microgram daily (elderly 500 nanograms), adjusted to avoid hypercalcaemia; maintenance, usually 0.25–1 microgram daily; NEONATE and PREMATURE INFANT initially 50–100 nanograms/kg daily, CHILD under 20 kg initially 50 nanograms/kg daily

AlfaD® (Berk) PoM

Capsules, alfacalcidol 250 nanograms (pink), net price 30-cap pack = £3.37; 1 microgram (orange), 30-cap pack = £10.06

Excipients: include arachis (peanut) oil

One-Alpha® (Leo) PoM

Capsules, alfacalcidol 250 nanograms (white), net price 30-cap pack = £3.37; 500 nanograms (red), 30-cap pack = £6.74; 1 microgram (brown), 30-cap pack = £10.06

Excipients: include sesame oil

Oral drops, sugar-free, alfacalcidol 2 micrograms/mL (1 drop contains approx. 100 nanograms), net price 10 mL = £24.18

Excipients: include alcohol

Note. The concentration of alfacalcidol in *One-Alpha®* drops is **10 times greater** than that of the former presentation *One-Alpha®* solution.

Injection, alfacalcidol 2 micrograms/mL, net price 0.5-mL amp = £2.32, 1-mL amp = £4.42

Note. Contains propylene glycol and should be used with caution in small premature infants

CALCITRIOL

(1,25-Dihydroxycholecalciferol)

Indications: see notes above

Cautions: see under Ergocalciferol; monitor plasma calcium and creatinine during dosage titration

Contra-indications: see under Ergocalciferol

Side-effects: see under Ergocalciferol

Dose: see under preparations below

Calcijex® (Abbott) PoM

Injection, calcitriol 1 microgram/mL, net price 1-mL amp = £5.14; 2 micrograms/mL, 1-mL amp = £10.28

Dose: hypocalcaemia in dialysis patients with chronic renal failure, by intravenous injection (or injection through catheter) after haemodialysis, initially 500 nanograms (approx. 10 nanograms/kg) 3 times a week, increased if necessary in steps of 250–500 nanograms at intervals of 2–4 weeks; usual dose 0.5–3 micrograms 3 times a week; CHILD not established

Rocaltrol® (Roche) PoM

Capsules, calcitriol 250 nanograms (red/white), net price 20 = £4.12; 500 nanograms (red), 20 = £7.36

Dose: renal osteodystrophy, ADULT, initially 250 nanograms daily, or on alternate days (in patients with normal or only slightly reduced plasma calcium), increased if necessary within 2–4 weeks in steps of 250 nanograms at intervals of 2–4 weeks; usual dose 0.5–1 microgram daily; CHILD not established

Established postmenopausal osteoporosis, 250 nanograms twice daily (monitor plasma calcium and creatinine, consult product literature)

COLECALCIFEROL

(Cholecalciferol, vitamin D_3)

Indications: see under Ergocalciferol—alternative to ergocalciferol in calciferol tablets and injection

Cautions: see under Ergocalciferol

Contra-indications: see under Ergocalciferol

Side-effects: see under Ergocalciferol

DIHYDROTACHYSTEROL

Indications: see under Ergocalciferol

Cautions: see under Ergocalciferol

Contra-indications: see under Ergocalciferol

Side-effects: see under Ergocalciferol

AT 10® (Intrapharm)

Oral solution, dihydrotachysterol 250 micrograms/mL. Net price 15-mL dropper bottle = £22.87

Note. Contains arachis (peanut) oil

Dose: acute, chronic, and latent forms of hypocalcaemic tetany due to hypoparathyroidism, consult product literature

9.6.5   Vitamin E

(Tocopherols)

The daily requirement of vitamin E has not been well defined but is probably about 3 to 15 mg daily. There is little evidence that oral supplements of vitamin E are essential in adults, even where there is fat malabsorption secondary to cholestasis. In young children with congenital cholestasis, abnormally low vitamin E concentrations may be found in association with neuromuscular abnormalities, which usually respond only to the parenteral administration of vitamin E.

Vitamin E has been tried for various other conditions but there is little scientific evidence of its value.

ALPHA TOCOPHERYL ACETATE

Indications: see notes above

Cautions: predisposition to thrombosis; increased risk of necrotising enterocolitis in premature infants weighing less than 1.5 kg

Side-effects: diarrhoea and abdominal pain with doses more than 1 g daily

Vitamin E Suspension (Cambridge)
Suspension, alpha tocopheryl acetate 500 mg/5 mL. Net price 100 mL = £14.79
Dose: malabsorption in cystic fibrosis, 100–200 mg daily; CHILD under 1 year 50 mg daily; 1 year and over, 100 mg daily
Malabsorption in abetalipoproteinaemia, ADULT and CHILD 50–100 mg/kg daily
Malabsorption in chronic cholestasis, INFANT 150–200 mg/kg daily
Note. Tablets containing tocopheryl acetate 50 mg and 200 mg available from Roche Consumer Health (*Ephynal®*)

9.6.6   Vitamin K

Vitamin K is necessary for the production of blood clotting factors and proteins necessary for the normal calcification of bone.

Because vitamin K is fat soluble, patients with fat malabsorption, especially in biliary obstruction or hepatic disease, may become deficient. For oral administration to prevent vitamin-K deficiency in malabsorption syndromes, a water-soluble preparation, **menadiol sodium phosphate** must be used; the usual dose is about 10 mg daily.

Oral coumarin anticoagulants act by interfering with vitamin K metabolism in the hepatic cells and their effects can be antagonised by giving vitamin K; for British Society for Haematology Guidelines, see section 2.8.2.

VITAMIN K DEFICIENCY BLEEDING Infants are relatively deficient in vitamin K and those who do not receive supplements of vitamin K are at risk of serious bleeds including intracranial bleeding. The Chief Medical Officer and the Chief Nursing Officer have recommended that all newborn babies should receive vitamin K to prevent vitamin K deficiency bleeding (haemorrhagic disease of the newborn). An appropriate regimen should be selected after discussion with parents in the antenatal period.

Vitamin K (as **phytomenadione**) 1 mg may be given by a single intramuscular injection at birth; this prevents vitamin K deficiency bleeding in virtually all babies. Fears about the safety of parenteral vitamin K appear to be unfounded.

Alternatively, vitamin K may be given by mouth, and arrangements must be in place to ensure the appropriate regimen is followed. Two doses of a colloidal (mixed micelle) preparation of phytomenadione 2 mg should be given in the first week. For breast-fed babies, a third dose of phytomenadione 2 mg is given at 1 month of age; the third dose is omitted in formula-fed babies because formula feeds contain vitamin K.

MENADIOL SODIUM PHOSPHATE

Indications: see notes above

Cautions: G6PD deficiency (section 9.1.5) and vitamin E deficiency (risk of haemolysis); **interactions:** Appendix 1 (vitamins)

Contra-indications: neonates and infants, late pregnancy

Dose: see notes above

Menadiol Phosphate (Non-proprietary)
Tablets, menadiol sodium phosphate equivalent to 10 mg of menadiol phosphate. Net price 100-tab pack = £32.33
Available from Cambridge

PHYTOMENADIONE

(Vitamin K_1)

Indications: see notes above

Cautions: intravenous injections should be given very slowly (see also below); pregnancy (Appendix 4); **interactions:** Appendix 1 (vitamins)

Dose: see notes above and section 2.8.2

Konakion® (Roche) PoM
Tablets, s/c, phytomenadione 10 mg, net price 10-tab pack = £1.77. To be chewed or allowed to dissolve slowly in the mouth (Label: 24)
Injection (*Konakion® Neonatal*), phytomenadione 2 mg/mL, net price 0.5-mL amp = 23p
Excipients: include polyoxyl castor oil (risk of anaphylaxis, see Excipients p. 2)
Note. Konakion® Neonatal is for use in healthy neonates of over 36 weeks gestation; for intramuscular injection only

■ Colloidal formulation

Konakion® MM (Roche) PoM
Injection, phytomenadione 10 mg/mL in a mixed micelles vehicle. Net price 1-mL amp = 43p
Excipients: include glycocholic acid 54.6 mg/amp, lecithin
Cautions: reduce dose in elderly; liver impairment (glycocholic acid may displace bilirubin); reports of anaphylactoid reactions
Note. Konakion® MM may be administered by slow intravenous injection or by intravenous infusion in glucose 5% (see Appendix 6); **not** for intramuscular injection

Konakion® MM Paediatric (Roche) PoM
Injection, phytomenadione 10 mg/mL in a mixed micelles vehicle. Net price 0.2-mL amp = £1.55
Excipients: include glycocholic acid 10.9 mg/amp, lecithin
Cautions: parenteral administration in premature infants of less than 2.5 kg (increased risk of kernicterus)
Note. Konakion® MM Paediatric may be administered *by mouth* or *by intramuscular injection* or *by intravenous injection*

9.6.7 Multivitamin preparations

Vitamins Capsules, ascorbic acid 15 mg, nicotinamide 7.5 mg, riboflavin 500 micrograms, thiamine hydrochloride 1 mg, vitamin A 2500 units, vitamin D 300 units. Net price 20 = 21p

Abidec® (W-L)
Drops, vitamins A, B group, C, and D. Net price 25 mL (with dropper) = £1.84

Dalivit® (Eastern)
Oral drops, vitamins A, B group, C, and D, net price 25 mL = £1.60, 50 mL = £2.85

Vitamin and mineral supplements and adjuncts to synthetic diets

Forceval® (Unigreg)
Capsules, brown/red, vitamins (ascorbic acid 60 mg, biotin 100 micrograms, cyanocobalamin 3 micrograms, folic acid 400 micrograms, nicotinamide 18 mg, pantothenic acid 4 mg, pyridoxine 2 mg, riboflavin 1.6 mg, thiamine 1.2 mg, vitamin A 2500 units, vitamin D_2 400 units, vitamin E 10 mg, minerals and trace elements (calcium 100 mg, chromium 200 micrograms, copper 2 mg, iodine 140 micrograms, iron 12 mg, magnesium 30 mg, manganese 3 mg, molybdenum 250 micrograms, phosphorus 77 mg, potassium 4 mg, selenium 50 micrograms, zinc 15 mg). Net price 30-cap pack = £5.15, 45-cap pack = £7.35; 90-cap pack = £14.04
Dose: vitamin and mineral deficiency and as adjunct in synthetic diets, 1 capsule daily
Junior capsules, brown, vitamins (ascorbic acid 25 mg, biotin 50 micrograms, cyanocobalamin 2 micrograms, folic acid 100 micrograms, nicotinamide 7.5 mg, pantothenic acid 2 mg, pyridoxine 1 mg, riboflavin 1 mg, thiamine 1.5 mg, vitamin A 1250 units, vitamin D_2 200 units, vitamin E 5 mg, vitamin K_1 25 micrograms), minerals and trace elements (chromium 50 micrograms, copper 1 mg, iodine 75 micrograms, iron 5 mg, magnesium 1 mg, manganese 1.25 mg, molybdenum 50 micrograms, selenium 25 micrograms, zinc 5 mg). Net price 30-cap pack = £3.87, 60-cap pack = £7.35
Dose: vitamin and mineral deficiency and as adjunct in synthetic diets, CHILD over 5 years, 2 capsules daily

Ketovite® (Paines & Byrne)
Tablets [PoM], yellow, ascorbic acid 16.6 mg, riboflavin 1 mg, thiamine hydrochloride 1 mg, pyridoxine hydrochloride 330 micrograms, nicotinamide 3.3 mg, calcium pantothenate 1.16 mg, alpha tocopheryl acetate 5 mg, inositol 50 mg, biotin 170 micrograms, folic acid 250 micrograms, acetomenaphthone 500 micrograms. Net price 100-tab pack = £4.17
Dose: prevention of deficiency in disorders of carbohydrate or amino acid metabolism, 1 tablet 3 times daily; with Ketovite® Liquid as vitamin supplement with synthetic diets
Liquid, pink, sugar-free, vitamin A 2500 units, ergocalciferol 400 units, choline chloride 150 mg, cyanocobalamin 12.5 micrograms/5 mL. Net price 150-mL pack = £2.70
Dose: prevention of deficiency in disorders of carbohydrate or amino acid metabolism, 5 mL daily; with Ketovite® Tablets as vitamin supplement with synthetic diets

Vivioptal® (Pharma-Global)
Capsules, brown, vitamins (biotin 50 micrograms, calcium ascorbate 60 mg, colecalciferol 400 units, cyanocobalamin 3 micrograms, dexpanthenol 10 mg, folic acid 400 micrograms, inositol 30 mg, nicotinamide 25 mg, pyridoxine 6.08 mg, riboflavin 3 mg, rutoside 20 mg, thiamine nitrate 5 mg, vitamin A 5000 units, vitamin E 10 mg), minerals and trace elements (calcium hydrogen phosphate 35 mg, cobalt sulphate 100 micrograms, copper sulphate 500 micrograms, iron 3.25 mg, magnesium glycerophosphate 40 mg, manganese sulphate 500 micrograms, potassium sulphate 8 mg, sodium molybdate 80 micrograms, zinc oxide 500 micrograms); also contains adenosine, choline hydrogen tartrate, ethyl linoleate, lecithin, lysine hydrochloride, and orotic acid, net price 30-cap pack = £5.35, 90-cap pack = £13.60
Dose: vitamin and mineral deficiency and as an adjunct in synthetic diets, 1 capsule daily
Excipients: include arachis (peanut) oil

9.7 Bitters and tonics

Mixtures containing simple and aromatic bitters, such as alkaline gentian mixture, are traditional remedies for loss of appetite. All depend on suggestion.

Gentian Mixture, Acid, BP
Mixture, concentrated compound gentian infusion 10%, dilute hydrochloric acid 5% in a suitable vehicle. Extemporaneous preparations should be recently prepared according to the following formula: concentrated compound gentian infusion 1 mL, dilute hydrochloric acid 0.5 mL, double-strength chloroform water 5 mL, water to 10 mL
Dose: 10 mL 3 times daily in water before meals

Gentian Mixture, Alkaline, BP
(Alkaline Gentian Oral Solution)
Mixture, concentrated compound gentian infusion 10%, sodium bicarbonate 5% in a suitable vehicle. Extemporaneous preparations should be recently prepared according to the following formula: concentrated compound gentian infusion 1 mL, sodium bicarbonate 500 mg, double-strength chloroform water 5 mL, water to 10 mL
Dose: 10 mL 3 times daily in water before meals

Effico® (Forest) [NHS] [▨]
Tonic, orange-red, thiamine hydrochloride 180 micrograms, nicotinamide 2.1 mg, caffeine 20.2 mg, compound gentian infusion 0.31 mL/5 mL. Net price 300-mL pack = £2.28, 500-mL pack = £2.93

Labiton® (LAB) [NHS] [▨]
Tonic, brown, thiamine hydrochloride 375 micrograms, caffeine 3.5 mg, kola nut dried extract 3.025 mg, alcohol 1.4 mL/5 mL. Net price 200 mL = £2.38

Metatone® (W-L) [NHS] [▨]
Tonic, thiamine hydrochloride 500 micrograms, calcium glycerophosphate 45.6 mg, manganese glycerophosphate 5.7 mg, potassium glycerophosphate 45.6 mg, sodium glycerophosphate 22.8 mg/5 mL. Net price 300 mL = £2.79

> [▨] denotes preparations that are considered to be less suitable for prescribing (see p. vi)

9.8   Metabolic disorders

9.8.1   Drugs used in metabolic disorders
9.8.2   Acute porphyrias

This section covers drugs used in metabolic disorders and not readily classified elsewhere.

9.8.1   Drugs used in metabolic disorders

Wilson's disease

Penicillamine (see also section 10.1.3) is used in Wilson's disease (hepatolenticular degeneration) to aid the elimination of copper ions. See below for other indications.

Trientine is used for the treatment of Wilson's disease only, in patients intolerant of penicillamine; it is **not** an alternative to penicillamine for rheumatoid arthritis or cystinuria. Penicillamine-induced systemic lupus erythematosus may not resolve on transfer to trientine.

PENICILLAMINE

Indications: see under Dose below
Cautions: see section 10.1.3
Contra-indications: see section 10.1.3
Side-effects: see section 10.1.3
Dose: Wilson's disease, 1.5–2 g daily in divided doses before food; max. 2 g daily for 1 year; maintenance 0.75–1 g daily; ELDERLY 20 mg/kg daily in divided doses, adjusted according to response; CHILD up to 20 mg/kg daily in divided doses, minimum 500 mg daily
Autoimmune hepatitis (used rarely; after disease controlled with corticosteroids), initially 500 mg daily in divided doses increased slowly over 3 months; usual maintenance dose 1.25 g daily; ELDERLY not recommended
Cystinuria, therapeutic, 1–3 g daily in divided doses before food, adjusted to maintain urinary cystine below 200 mg/litre; prophylactic (maintain urinary cystine below 300 mg/litre) 0.5–1 g at bedtime; maintain adequate fluid intake (at least 3 litres daily); CHILD and ELDERLY minimum dose to maintain urinary cystine below 200 mg/litre
Severe active rheumatoid arthritis, section 10.1.3
Copper and lead poisoning, see Emergency Treatment of Poisoning

Preparations
Section 10.1.3

TRIENTINE DIHYDROCHLORIDE

Indications: Wilson's disease in patients intolerant of penicillamine
Cautions: see notes above; pregnancy; **interactions:** Appendix 1 (trientine)
Side-effects: nausea, rash; rarely anaemia
Dose: 1.2–2.4 g daily in 2–4 divided doses before food; CHILD initially 0.6–1.5 g daily in 2–4 divided doses before food, adjusted according to response

Trientine Dihydrochloride Capsules,▼ PoM
trientine dihydrochloride 300 mg. Label: 6, 22
Available from Anstead
Note. The CSM has requested that in addition to the usual CSM reporting request special records should also be kept by the pharmacist

Carnitine deficiency

Carnitine is available for the management of primary carnitine deficiency due to inborn errors of metabolism or of secondary deficiency in haemodialysis patients.

CARNITINE

Indications: primary and secondary carnitine deficiency
Cautions: renal impairment; monitoring of free and acyl carnitine in blood and urine recommended; pregnancy (but appropriate to use) and breast-feeding
Side-effects: nausea, vomiting, abdominal pain, diarrhoea, body odour; side-effects may be dose-related—monitor tolerance during first week and after any dose increase
Dose: primary deficiency, *by mouth*, up to 200 mg/kg daily in 2–4 divided doses; higher doses of up to 400 mg/kg daily occasionally required; *by intravenous injection*, up to 100 mg/kg daily in 3–4 divided doses
Secondary deficiency, *by intravenous injection*, 20 mg/kg after each dialysis session (dosage adjusted according to carnitine concentration); maintenance, *by mouth*, 1 g daily

Carnitor® (Shire) PoM
Oral liquid, L-carnitine 1 g/10-mL single-dose bottle. Net price 10 × 10-mL single-dose bottle = £35.00
Paediatric solution, L-carnitine 30%. Net price 20 mL = £21.00
Injection, L-carnitine 200 mg/mL. Net price 5-mL amp = £11.90

Gaucher's disease

Imiglucerase, an enzyme produced by recombinant DNA technology, is administered as enzyme replacement therapy in Gaucher's disease, a familial disorder affecting principally the liver, spleen, bone marrow, and lymph nodes.

IMIGLUCERASE

Indications: (specialist use only) type I Gaucher's disease
Cautions: pregnancy and breast-feeding; monitor for imiglucerase antibodies; when stabilised monitor all parameters and response to treatment at intervals of 6–12 months
Side-effects: pruritus, pain, swelling or sterile abscess at injection site; hypersensitivity reactions; also reported nausea, vomiting, diarrhoea, abdominal pain, fatigue, headache, dizziness, fever, rash

Dose: *by intravenous infusion*, initially 60 units/kg once every 2 weeks (2.5 units/kg 3 times a week or 15 units/kg once every 2 weeks may improve haematological parameters and organomegaly, but not bone parameters); maintenance, adjust dose according to response

Cerezyme® (Genzyme) PoM

Intravenous infusion, powder for reconstitution, imiglucerase, net price 200-unit vial = £595.00; 400-unit vial = £1190.00

Nephropathic cystinosis

Mercapatamine (Cysteamine) is available for the treatment of nephropathic cystinosis.

MERCAPTAMINE
(Cysteamine)

Indications: (specialist use only) nephropathic cystinosis

Cautions: leucocyte-cystine concentration and haematological monitoring required—consult product literature; dose of phosphate supplement may need to be adjusted

Contra-indications: pregnancy and breast-feeding; hypersensitivity to mercaptamine or penicillamine

Side-effects: breath and body odour, nausea, vomiting, diarrhoea, anorexia, lethargy, fever, rash; also reported dehydration, hypertension, abdominal discomfort, gastroenteritis, drowsiness, encephalopathy, headache, nervousness, depression; anaemia, leucopenia, increases in liver enzymes; rarely gastro-intestinal ulceration and bleeding, seizures, hallucinations, urticaria, interstitial nephritis

Dose: initial doses should be one-sixth to one-quarter of the expected maintenance dose, increased gradually over 4–6 weeks

Maintenance, ADULT and CHILD over 50 kg body-weight, 2 g daily in 4 divided doses

CHILD up to 12 years, 1.3 g/m² (approx. 50 mg/kg) daily in 4 divided doses

Cystagon® (Orphan Europe) ▼ PoM

Capsules, mercaptamine (as bitartrate) 50 mg, net price 100-cap pack = £44.00; 150 mg, 100-cap pack = £125.00

Note. CHILD under 6 years at risk of aspiration, capsules can be opened and contents sprinkled on food (at a temperature suitable for eating); avoid adding to acidic drinks (e.g. orange juice)

Urea cycle disorders

Sodium phenylbutyrate has recently become available for the management of urea cycle disorders. It is indicated as adjunctive therapy in all patients with neonatal-onset disease and in those with late-onset disease who have a history of hyperammonaemic encephalopathy.

SODIUM PHENYLBUTYRATE

Indications: adjunct in long-term treatment of urea cycle disorders (under specialist supervision)

Cautions: congestive heart failure, hepatic and renal impairment

Contra-indications: pregnancy (Appendix 4) and breast-feeding

Side-effects: amenorrhoea and irregular menstrual cycles, decreased appetite, body odour, taste disturbances; less commonly nausea, vomiting, abdominal pain, peptic ulcer, pancreatitis, rectal bleeding, arrhythmia, oedema, syncope, depression, headache, rash, weight gain, renal tubular acidosis, aplastic anaemia, ecchymoses

Dose: ADULT and CHILD over 20 kg, 9.9–13 g/m² daily in divided doses with meals (max. 20 g daily); CHILD less than 20 kg, 450–600 mg/kg daily in divided doses with meals

Ammonaps® (Orphan Europe) ▼ PoM

Tablets, sodium phenylbutyrate 500 mg. Contains Na⁺ 2.7 mmol/tablet. Net price 250-tab pack = £493.00

Granules, sodium phenylbutyrate 940 mg/g. Contains Na⁺ 5.4 mmol/g. Net price 266-g pack = £860.00

Note. Granules should be mixed with food before taking

9.8.2   Acute porphyrias

The acute porphyrias (acute intermittent porphyria, variegate porphyria, hereditary coproporphyria and 5-aminolaevulinic acid dehydratase deficiency porphyria) are hereditary disorders of haem biosynthesis; they have a prevalence of about 1 in 10 000 of the population.

Great care must be taken when prescribing for patients with acute porphyria since many drugs can induce acute porphyric crises. Since acute porphyrias are hereditary, relatives of affected individuals should be screened and advised about the potential danger of certain drugs.

Haem arginate is administered by short intravenous infusion as haem replacement in moderate, severe or unremitting acute porphyria crises.

Supplies of haem arginate may be obtained outside office hours from the on-call pharmacist at:

St. James's University Hospital,
Leeds   (0113) 243 3144
                      or   (0113) 283 7010

St Thomas's Hospital,
London   (020) 7928 9292

HAEM ARGINATE
(Human hemin)

Indications: acute porphyrias (acute intermittent porphyria, porphyria variegata, hereditary coproporphyria)

Cautions: pregnancy and breast feeding

Side-effects: rarely hypersensitivity reactions and fever; pain and thrombophlebitis at injection site

Dose: *by intravenous infusion*, ADULT and CHILD 3 mg/kg once daily (max. 250 mg daily) for 4 days; if response inadequate, repeat 4-day course with close biochemical monitoring

Normosang® (Orphan Europe) ▼ PoM

Concentrate for intravenous infusion, haem arginate 25 mg/mL, net price 10-mL amp = £281.25

Drugs unsafe for use in acute porphyrias

The following list contains drugs on the UK market
that have been classified as 'unsafe' in porphyria
because they have been shown to be porphyrinogenic in animals or *in vitro*, or have been associated
with acute attacks in patients.

Further information may be obtained from:

Welsh Medicines Information Centre
University Hospital of Wales
Cardiff CF14 4XW
Telephone (029) 2074 2979

Note. Quite modest changes in chemical structure can lead
to changes in porphyrinogenicity but where possible general statements have been made about groups of drugs;
these should be checked first

Drug groups (please check first)

Amphetamines	Ergot Derivatives[7]
Anabolic Steroids	Gold Salts
Antidepressants[1]	Hormone Replacement
Antihistamines[2]	Therapy[5]
Barbiturates[3]	Menopausal Steroids[5]
Benzodiazepines[4]	Progestogens[5]
Cephalosporins	Sulphonamides[8]
Contraceptives, steroid[5]	Sulphonylureas[9]
Diuretics[6]	

Individual Drugs (please check groups above first)

Alcohol	Lidocaine (lignocaine)[14]
Aluminium-containing	Loxapine
Antacids[10]	Mebeverine
Aminoglutethimide	Mefenamic Acid
Amiodarone	Meprobamate
Azapropazone	Methotrexate
Baclofen	Methyldopa
Bromocriptine	Metoclopramide[15]
Busulfan	Metyrapone
Captopril	Miconazole
Carbamazepine	Mifepristone
Carisoprodol	Minoxidil[15]
Chloral Hydrate[11]	Nalidixic Acid
Chlorambucil	Nifedipine
Chloramphenicol	Nitrofurantoin
Chloroform[12]	Orphenadrine
Ciclosporin	Oxybutynin
Clonidine	Oxycodone
Cocaine	Oxymetazoline
Colistin	Oxytetracycline
Cyclophosphamide	Pentazocine[13]
Cycloserine	Pentoxifylline (oxenti-
Danazol	fylline)
Dapsone	Phenoxybenzamine
Dexfenfluramine	Phenylbutazone
Dextropropoxyphene[13]	Phenytoin
Diclofenac	Piroxicam
Doxycycline	Prilocaine
Econazole	Probenecid
Enflurane	Pyrazinamide
Erythromycin	Ranitidine
Etamsylate	Rifabutin[16]
Ethionamide	Rifampicin[16]
Ethosuximide	Simvastatin
Etomidate	Sulfinpyrazone
Fenfluramine	Sulpiride
Flucloxacillin	Tamoxifen
Flupentixol	Theophylline[17]
Griseofulvin	Thioridazine
Halothane	Tinidazole
Hydralazine	Triclofos[11]
Hyoscine	Trimethoprim
Isometheptene Mucate	Valproate[4]
Isoniazid	Verapamil
Ketoconazole	Zuclopenthixol
Ketorolac	

---

1. Includes tricyclic (and related) and MAOIs; fluoxetine thought to be safe.

2. Cetirizine, chlorphenamine, cyclizine, diphenhydramine, doxylamine, ketotifen, loratadine, and alimemazine (tri-meprazine) thought to be safe.

3. Includes methohexital, primidone, and thiopental.

4. Status epilepticus has been treated successfully with intravenous diazepam; temazepam is thought to be safe; where essential, seizure prophylaxis has been undertaken with clonazepam or valproate. Clobazam, lorazepam, and mid-azolam probably safe.

5. Progestogens are more porphyrinogenic than oestrogens; oestrogens may be safe at least in replacement doses. Pro-gestogens should be avoided whenever possible by all women susceptible to acute porphyria; however, where non-hor-monal contraception is inappropriate, progestogens may be used with extreme caution if the potential benefit outweighs risk. The risk of an acute attack is greatest in women who have had a previous attack or are aged under 30 years. Long-acting progestogen preparations should never be used in those at risk of acute porphyria.

6. Acetazolamide, amiloride, bumetanide, cyclopenthiazide and triamterene have been used.

7. Includes ergometrine (oxytocin probably safe), lisuride and pergolide.

8. Includes co-trimoxazole and sulfasalazine.

9. Glipizide is thought to be safe

10. Absorption limited but magnesium-containing antacids preferable.

11. Although evidence of hazard is uncertain, manufacturer advises avoid

12. Small amounts in medicines probably safe.

13. Buprenorphine, codeine, diamorphine, dihydrocodeine, fentanyl, morphine, and pethidine are thought to be safe.

14. Bupivacaine is thought to be safe; lidocaine (lignocaine) and prilocaine may be used with caution.

15. May be used with caution if safer alternative not available.

16. Rifamycins have been used in a few patients without evidence of harm—use with caution if safer alternative not available.

17. Includes aminophylline.

10: Musculoskeletal and joint diseases

For treatment of septic arthritis see section 5.1, table 1.

10.1 Drugs used in rheumatic diseases and gout

10.1.1	Non-steroidal anti-inflammatory drugs
10.1.2	Corticosteroids
10.1.3	Drugs which suppress the rheumatic disease process
10.1.4	Gout and cytotoxic-induced hyperuricaemia

Rheumatoid arthritis and other inflammatory disorders

Most rheumatic diseases require symptomatic treatment to relieve pain. A non-steroidal anti-inflammatory drug (NSAID) is indicated when pain and stiffness are due to inflammatory rheumatic disease. Drugs are also used to influence the disease process itself (section 10.1.3). For rheumatoid arthritis these include penicillamine, gold salts, antimalarials (chloroquine and hydroxychloroquine), immunosuppressants (azathioprine, ciclosporin, cyclophosphamide, etanercept, infliximab, leflunomide, and methotrexate), and sulfasalazine—they are known as disease-modifying antirheumatic drugs; corticosteroids may also reduce the rate of joint destruction (section 10.1.2.1). Drugs which may affect the disease process in psoriatic arthritis include gold salts, azathioprine, and methotrexate (section 10.1.3) and for gout they include uricosuric drugs and allopurinol (section 10.1.4).

Osteoarthritis and soft-tissue disorders

In osteoarthritis (sometimes called degenerative joint disease or osteoarthrosis) non-drug measures such as weight reduction and exercise should be encouraged. For pain relief in osteoarthritis and soft-tissue disorders, paracetamol (section 4.7.1) is often adequate and should be used first. Alternatively a low-dose NSAID (e.g. ibuprofen up to 1.2 g daily) may be used. If pain relief with either drug is inadequate, both paracetamol (in a full dose of 4 g daily) and a low-dose NSAID may be required; if necessary the dose of the NSAID may need to be increased or a low dose of an opioid analgesic given with paracetamol (as co-codamol 8/500 or co-dydramol 10/500).

Topical treatment including application of an NSAID or capsaicin 0.025% (section 10.3.2) may provide some pain relief in osteoarthritis.

Intra-articular corticosteroid injections (section 10.1.2.2) may produce temporary benefit in osteoarthritis, especially if associated with soft-tissue inflammation.

Hyaluronic acid and its derivatives are available for osteoarthritis of the knee. Sodium hyaluronate (*Fermathron*®, Biomet Merck; *Hyalgan*®, Shire; *Orthovisc*®, Zimmer; *Supartz*®, S&N Hlth.; *Suplasyn*®, Dominion) or hylan G-F 20 (*Synvisc*®,

Biomatrix) is injected intra-articularly to supplement natural hyaluronic acid in the synovial fluid. These injections may reduce pain over 1–6 months but they are associated with a short-term increase in knee inflammation.

10.1.1 Non-steroidal anti-inflammatory drugs

In *single doses* non-steroidal anti-inflammatory drugs (NSAIDs) have analgesic activity comparable to that of paracetamol (section 4.7.1), but paracetamol is preferred, particularly in the elderly (see also Prescribing for the elderly, p. 18).

In regular *full dosage* NSAIDs have both a lasting analgesic and an anti-inflammatory effect which makes them particularly useful for the treatment of continuous or regular pain associated with inflammation. Therefore, although paracetamol often gives adequate pain control in osteoarthritis, NSAIDs are more appropriate than paracetamol or the opioid analgesics in the *inflammatory arthritides* (e.g. rheumatoid arthritis) and in some cases of *advanced osteoarthritis*. They may also be of benefit in the less well defined conditions of *back pain* and *soft-tissue disorders*.

CHOICE. Differences in anti-inflammatory activity between different NSAIDs are small, but there is considerable variation in individual patient tolerance and response. About 60% of patients will respond to any NSAID; of the others, those who do not respond to one may well respond to another. A full analgesic effect should normally be obtained within a week, whereas an anti-inflammatory effect may not be achieved (or may not be clinically assessable) for up to 3 weeks. If appropriate responses are not obtained within these times, another NSAID should be tried.

The main differences between NSAIDs are in the incidence and type of side-effects. Before treatment is started the prescriber should weigh efficacy against possible side-effects.

NSAIDs vary in their selectivity for inhibiting different types of cyclo-oxygenase; selective inhibition of cyclo-oxygenase-2 improves gastro-intestinal tolerance. A number of other factors also determine susceptibility to gastro-intestinal effects and an NSAID should be chosen on the basis of the incidence of gastro-intestinal and other side-effects.

Ibuprofen is a propionic acid derivative with anti-inflammatory, analgesic, and antipyretic properties. It has fewer side-effects than other NSAIDs but its anti-inflammatory properties are weaker. Doses of 1.6 to 2.4 g daily are needed for rheumatoid arthritis and it is unsuitable for conditions where inflammation is prominent such as acute gout.

Other propionic acid derivatives:

Naproxen has emerged as one of the first choices as it combines good efficacy with a low incidence of side-effects (but more than ibuprofen, see CSM comment below) and administration is only twice daily.

Fenbufen is claimed to be associated with less gastro-intestinal bleeding, but there is a high risk of rashes (see p. 480).

Fenoprofen is as effective as naproxen, and **flurbiprofen** may be slightly more effective. Both are associated with slightly more gastro-intestinal side-effects than ibuprofen.

Ketoprofen has anti-inflammatory properties similar to ibuprofen and has more side-effects (see also CSM comment below). **Dexketoprofen**, an isomer of ketoprofen, has been introduced for the short-term relief of mild to moderate pain.

Tiaprofenic acid is as effective as naproxen; it has more side-effects than ibuprofen (**important:** reports of severe cystitis, see CSM advice on p. 484).

Drugs with properties similar to those of propionic acid derivatives:

Azapropazone is similar in effect to naproxen; it has a tendency to cause rashes and is associated with an increased risk of severe gastro-intestinal toxicity (**important:** see CSM restrictions on p. 478).

Diclofenac and **aceclofenac** have actions similar to that of naproxen; their side-effects are also similar to naproxen.

Diflunisal is an aspirin derivative but its clinical effect more closely resembles that of the propionic acid derivatives than that of its parent compound. Its long duration of action allows twice-daily administration.

Etodolac is a selective inhibitor of cyclo-oxygenase-2; it is comparable in effect to naproxen. Side-effects of etodolac appear to be comparable to those of ibuprofen.

Indometacin (indomethacin) has an action equal to or superior to that of naproxen, but with a high incidence of side-effects including headaches, dizziness, and gastro-intestinal disturbances (see also CSM comment below).

Ketorolac is used in the short-term management of moderate to severe postoperative pain (section 15.1.4.2)

Lornoxicam is licensed for relieving pain and inflammation in osteoarthritis and rheumatoid arthritis, pain of acute lumbo-sciatica, and management of moderate postoperative pain.

Mefenamic acid has minor anti-inflammatory properties. Occasionally, it has been associated with diarrhoea and haemolytic anaemia which require discontinuation of treatment.

Meloxicam is licensed for the short-term treatment of osteoarthritis and long-term treatment of rheumatoid arthritis. It is a selective inhibitor of cyclo-oxygenase-2.

Nabumetone is comparable in effect to naproxen.

Phenylbutazone is a potent anti-inflammatory drug but because of occasional serious side-effects its use is limited to the hospital treatment of ankylosing spondylitis; prolonged administration may be necessary but it should not be used unless other drugs have failed.

Piroxicam is as effective as naproxen and has a prolonged duration of action which permits once-daily administration. It has more gastro-intestinal side-effects than ibuprofen, especially in the elderly (see also CSM comment below).

Rofecoxib and **celecoxib** are selective inhibitors of cyclo-oxygenase-2 ; they are similar in effect to diclofenac. Rofecoxib is also licensed for the relief of acute pain. Rofecoxib and celecoxib share the side-effects of other NSAIDs. The risk of serious upper gastro-intestinal events is lower but this advantage may be lost in patients who require concomitant low-dose aspirin. The CSM has issued a reminder that rofecoxib and celecoxib do not provide protection against ischaemic cardiovascular events.

NICE guidance (cyclo-oxygenase-2 selective inhibitors). The National Institute for Clinical Excellence has recommended that cyclo-oxygenase-2 selective inhibitors (celecoxib, etodolac, meloxicam and rofecoxib) should:

- **not** be used routinely in the management of patients with rheumatoid arthritis or osteoarthritis;

- be used in preference to standard NSAIDs **only** when clearly indicated (and in accordance with UK licensing), for patients with a history of gastroduodenal ulcer or perforation or gastro-intestinal bleeding—in these patients even the use of cyclo-oxygenase-2 selective inhibitors should be considered very carefully; they should also be used in preference to standard NSAIDs for other patients at **high risk** of developing serious gastro-intestinal side-effects (e.g. those aged over 65 years, those who are taking other medicines which increase the risk of gastro-intestinal effects, those who are debilitated or those receiving long-term treatment with maximal doses of standard NSAIDs);

- **not** be used routinely in preference to standard NSAIDs for patients with cardiovascular disease; the benefit of cyclo-oxygenase-2 selective inhibitors is reduced in patients taking concomitant low-dose aspirin and this combination is **not justified**.

There is no evidence to justify the simultaneous use of gastro-protective drugs with cyclo-oxygenase-2 selective inhibitors as a means of further reducing potential gastro-intestinal side-effects.

CSM advice (rofecoxib)

The CSM has reminded prescribers that rofecoxib is contra-indicated in patients with:

- active peptic ulceration or gastro-intestinal bleeding;

- severe congestive heart failure and caution should be exercised in patients with a history of cardiac failure, left ventricular dysfunction, or hypertension and in patients with oedema for any other reason.

Sulindac is similar in tolerance to naproxen.

Tenoxicam is similar in activity and tolerance to naproxen. Its long half-life allows once-daily administration.

Tolfenamic acid is indicated for the treatment of migraine (section 4.7.4.1)

CAUTIONS AND CONTRA-INDICATIONS. NSAIDs should be used with caution in the elderly (risk of serious side-effects and fatalities, see also Prescribing for the elderly p. 18), in allergic disorders (they are **contra-indicated** in patients with a history of hypersensitivity to aspirin or any other NSAID—which includes those in whom attacks of asthma, angioedema, urticaria or rhinitis have been precipitated by aspirin or any other NSAID), during pregnancy and breast-feeding (see Appendixes 4 and 5), and in coagulation defects. Long-term use of some NSAIDs is associated with reduced female fertility which is reversible on stopping treatment.

In patients with renal, cardiac, or hepatic impairment caution is required since the use of NSAIDs may result in deterioration of renal function (see also under Side-effects, below and Appendixes 2 and 3); the dose should be kept as **low as possible** and renal function should be **monitored**.

NSAIDs should not be given to patients with active peptic ulceration (see also **CSM advice** below). While it is preferable to avoid them in patients with current or previous gastro-intestinal ulceration or bleeding, and to withdraw them if gastro-intestinal lesions develop, nevertheless patients with serious rheumatic diseases (e.g. rheumatoid arthritis) are usually dependent on NSAIDs for effective relief of pain and stiffness. For advice on the prophylaxis and treatment of NSAID-associated peptic ulcers, see section 1.3.

For **interactions** of NSAIDs, see Appendix 1 (NSAIDs)

SIDE-EFFECTS. The side-effects of NSAIDs vary in severity and frequency. Gastro-intestinal discomfort, nausea, diarrhoea, and occasionally bleeding and ulceration occur (see also CSM advice below). Systemic as well as local effects of NSAIDs contribute to gastro-intestinal damage; taking oral formulations with milk or food, or using enteric-coated formulations or changing the route of administration may only partially reduce symptoms such as dyspepsia. Those at risk of duodenal or gastric ulceration (including the elderly) who need to continue NSAID treatment should receive either a selective inhibitor of cyclo-oxygenase-2 alone, or a standard NSAID with gastroprotective treatment (section 1.3). Other side-effects include hypersensitivity reactions (particularly rashes, angioedema, and bronchospasm—see CSM advice below), headache, dizziness, nervousness, depression, drowsiness, insomnia, vertigo, hearing disturbances such as tinnitus, photosensitivity, and haematuria. Blood disorders have also occurred. Fluid retention may occur (rarely precipitating congestive heart failure in elderly patients). Renal failure may be provoked by NSAIDs especially in patients with pre-existing renal impairment (**important**, see also under Cautions above). Rarely, papillary necrosis or interstitial fibrosis associated with NSAIDs may lead to renal failure. Hepatic damage, alveolitis, pulmonary eosinophilia, pancreatitis, eye changes, Stevens-Johnson syndrome and toxic epidermal necrolysis are other rare side-effects. Induction of or exacerbation of colitis has been reported. Aseptic meningitis has been reported rarely with NSAIDs; patients with connective tissue disorders such as systemic lupus erythematosus may be especially susceptible.

Overdosage: see Emergency Treatment of Poisoning, p. 22.

CSM advice (gastro-intestinal side-effects)

Recent evidence on the relative safety of 7 oral NSAIDs has indicated differences in the risks of serious upper gastro-intestinal side-effects. **Azapropazone** is associated with the *highest risk* (**important:** see also restrictions on p. 478) and **ibuprofen** with the *lowest*; **piroxicam, ketoprofen, indometacin, naproxen** and **diclofenac** are associated with *intermediate risks* (possibly higher in the case of piroxicam). There are insufficient data to reach clear conclusions on other available oral NSAIDs.

Recommendations are that NSAIDs associated with low risk should *generally be preferred*, to start at the *lowest recommended dose*, *not to use more than one* oral NSAID at a time, and to remember that all NSAIDs are *contra-indicated* in patients with peptic ulceration.

Previous recommendations of the CSM have included the advice that in patients with a history of peptic ulcer disease and in the elderly, NSAIDs should be given only after other forms of treatment have been carefully considered.

CSM warning (asthma)

Any degree of worsening of asthma may be related to the ingestion of NSAIDs, either prescribed or (in the case of ibuprofen and others) purchased over the counter.

IBUPROFEN

Indications: pain and inflammation in rheumatic disease (including juvenile arthritis) and other musculoskeletal disorders; mild to moderate pain including dysmenorrhoea; postoperative analgesia; migraine; fever and pain in children

Cautions: see notes above; **interactions:** Appendix 1 (NSAIDs)

Contra-indications: see notes above;

Side-effects: see notes above; **overdosage:** see Emergency Treatment of Poisoning, p. 22

Dose: initially 1.2–1.8 g daily in 3–4 divided doses preferably after food; increased if necessary to max. 2.4 g daily; maintenance dose of 0.6–1.2 g daily may be adequate

Juvenile rheumatoid arthritis, CHILD over 7 kg bodyweight 30–40 mg/kg daily in 3–4 divided doses

Fever and pain in children, CHILD over 7 kg bodyweight 20–30 mg/kg daily in divided doses *or* 1–2 years 50 mg 3–4 times daily, 3–7 years 100 mg 3–4 times daily, 8–12 years 200 mg 3–4 times daily

Ibuprofen (Non-proprietary) PoM

Tablets, coated, ibuprofen 200 mg, net price 84-tab pack = £1.69; 400 mg, 84-tab pack = £2.46; 600 mg, 84-tab pack = £3.38. Label: 21

Various strengths available from Alpharma, APS, Ashbourne (*Arthrofen*®), Berk (*Lidifen*®), CP, DDSA (*Ebufac*®), IVAX, Kent, Ranbaxy (*Rimafen*®), Pharmacia (*Motrin*®, including an 800-mg strength), Sovereign, Sterwin

Oral suspension, ibuprofen 100 mg/5 mL, net price 100 mL = £1.82, 150 mL = £2.73. Label: 21

Note. Sugar-free versions are available and can be ordered by specifying 'sugar-free' on the prescription

Available from Crookes (*Nurofen*® *for Children*), Galpharm (*Galprofen*®), Orbis (*Orbifen*® *for Children*)

Note. Proprietary brands of ibuprofen preparations are on sale to the public; brand names include, Advil®, Anadin Ibuprofen®, Anadin Ultra®, Arthrofen®, Boots Children's 6 years Plus Fever & Pain Relief®, Cuprofen®, Galprofen®, Hedex® Ibuprofen, Ibrufhalal®, Ibufem®, Inoven®, Librofem®, Migrafen®, Novaprin®, Nurofen®, Nurofen® Advance, Nurofen® Long Lasting, Nurofen® Meltlets, Obifen®, Pacifene®, PhorPain®, Relcofen®; compound proprietary preparations containing ibuprofen include Nurofen® Plus (ibuprofen, codeine), Solpaflex® (ibuprofen, codeine)

Brufen® (Abbott) PoM

Tablets, all magenta, ibuprofen 200 mg (s/c), net price 20 = 82p; 400 mg (s/c), 20 = £1.54; 600 mg (f/c), 20 = £2.45. Label: 21

Syrup, orange, ibuprofen 100 mg/5 mL. Net price 500 mL = £8.07. Label: 21

Granules, effervescent, ibuprofen 600 mg/sachet. Net price 20-sachet pack = £6.80. Label: 13, 21

Note. Contains sodium approx. 9 mmol/sachet

Topical preparations: section 10.3.2

■ Modified release

Brufen Retard® (Abbott) PoM

Tablets, m/r, f/c, ibuprofen 800 mg, net price 56-tab pack = £7.24. Label: 25, 27

Dose: 2 tablets daily as a single dose, preferably in the early evening, increased in severe cases to 3 tablets daily in 2 divided doses; CHILD not recommended

Fenbid® (Goldshield) PoM

Spansule® (= capsule m/r), maroon/pink, enclosing off-white pellets, ibuprofen 300 mg. Net price 120-cap pack = £9.64. Label: 25

Dose: 1–3 capsules every 12 hours; CHILD not recommended

■ With codeine

For an adverse comment on compound analgesic preparations, see p. 208. For details of the **side-effects, cautions,** and **contra-indications** of opioid analgesics, see p. 214 (**important:** the elderly are particularly susceptible to opioid side-effects).

Codafen Continus® (Napp) PoM ▄▄▄

Tablets, white/pink, ibuprofen 300 mg (m/r), codeine phosphate 20 mg. Net price 56-tab pack = £6.40; 112-tab pack = £12.78. Label: 2, 21, 25

Dose: 1–2 tablets every 12 hours; max. 3 tablets every 12 hours; CHILD not recommended

▄▄▄ denotes preparations that are considered to be less suitable for prescribing (see p. vi)

ACECLOFENAC

Indications: pain and inflammation in rheumatoid arthritis, osteoarthritis and ankylosing spondylitis

Cautions: see notes above; avoid in porphyria (section 9.8.2); **interactions:** Appendix 1 (NSAIDs)

Contra-indications: see notes above

Side-effects: see notes above

Dose: 100 mg twice daily (reduce to 100 mg daily initially in hepatic impairment); CHILD not recommended

Preservex® (UCB Pharma) PoM

Tablets, f/c, aceclofenac 100 mg, net price 60-tab pack = £16.44. Label: 21

ACEMETACIN

(Glycolic acid ester of indometacin)

Indications: pain and inflammation in rheumatic disease and other musculoskeletal disorders; post-operative analgesia

Cautions: see under Indometacin and notes above

DRIVING. Dizziness may affect performance of skilled tasks (e.g. driving)

Contra-indications: see under Indometacin and notes above

Side-effects: see under Indometacin and notes above

Dose: 120 mg daily in divided doses with food, increased if necessary to 180 mg daily; CHILD not recommended

Emflex® (Merck) PoM
Capsules, yellow/orange, acemetacin 60 mg, net price 90-cap pack = £21.36. Label: 21, counselling, driving

AZAPROPAZONE

Indications: see under CSM restrictions, below

CSM RESTRICTIONS. CSM *has restricted* azapropazone to use in rheumatoid arthritis, ankylosing spondylitis and acute gout only when other NSAIDs have been tried and failed, *has* **contra-indicated** it in patients with a history of peptic ulceration, and *has reduced* the maximum daily dose to 600 mg for rheumatoid arthritis and ankylosing spondylitis in patients over 60 years

Cautions: see notes above; **interactions:** Appendix 1 (NSAIDs)

Contra-indications: see notes above; porphyria (section 9.8.2); history of peptic ulceration, inflammatory bowel disease or blood disorder; for specific restrictions and contra-indications relating to renal impairment see under Dose

Side-effects: see notes above; photosensitivity, see CSM advice below

PHOTOSENSITIVITY. CSM has reminded of need to advise patients taking azapropazone to avoid direct exposure to sunlight (or to use sunblock preparations)

Dose:

Rheumatoid arthritis and ankylosing spondylitis, 1.2 g daily in 2 or 4 divided doses; in renal impairment or in elderly 300 mg twice daily, avoid altogether in severe renal impairment; CHILD not recommended

Acute gout (always ensure increased fluid intake), 1.8 g daily in divided doses until acute symptoms subside (usually by day 4) *then* 1.2 g daily in divided doses until symptoms resolve—consider appropriate alternative therapy if they persist; in mild renal impairment or in elderly, 1.8 g daily for first 24 hours *then* 1.2 g daily in divided doses reducing to max. 600 mg daily in divided doses as soon as possible (preferably by day 4) *then* continuing only until acute symptoms resolve—consider appropriate alternative therapy if they persist, and *avoid altogether for gout* in moderate to severe renal impairment and *avoid for gout in elderly* even in mild renal impairment; CHILD not recommended

Rheumox® (Goldshield) PoM
Capsules, orange, azapropazone 300 mg. Net price 100-cap pack = £14.32. Label: 11 (also photosensitivity counselling, see above), 21

Tablets, orange, f/c, scored, azapropazone 600 mg. Net price 100-tab pack = £24.88. Label: 11 (also photosensitivity counselling, see above), 21

CELECOXIB

Indications: pain and inflammation in osteoarthritis or rheumatoid arthritis

Cautions: see notes above; **interactions:** Appendix 1 (NSAIDs)

Contra-indications: see notes above; sulphonamide sensitivity; renal impairment (creatinine clearance less than 30 mL/minute); inflammatory bowel disease; severe congestive heart failure

Side-effects: see notes above; flatulence, insomnia, pharyngitis, sinusitis; less frequently stomatitis, constipation, palpitations, anxiety, depression, fatigue, paraesthesia, muscle cramps; rarely taste alteration, alopecia

Dose: osteoarthritis, 200 mg daily in 1–2 divided doses, increased if necessary to max. 200 mg twice daily; CHILD not recommended

Rheumatoid arthritis, 200–400 mg daily in 2 divided doses; ELDERLY or Afro-Caribbean patient, initially 200 mg daily in 2 divided doses; max. 200 mg twice daily; CHILD not recommended

Celebrex® (Searle) ▼ PoM
Capsules, celecoxib 100 mg (white/blue), net price 60-cap pack = £18.34; 200 mg (white/gold), 30-cap pack = £18.34

DEXKETOPROFEN

Indications: short-term treatment of mild to moderate pain including dysmenorrhoea

Cautions: see notes above; **interactions:** Appendix 1 (NSAIDs)

Contra-indications: see notes above

Side-effects: see notes above

Dose: 12.5 mg every 4–6 hours *or* 25 mg every 8 hours; max. 75 mg daily; ELDERLY initially max. 50 mg daily; CHILD not recommended

Keral® (Menarini) PoM
Tablets, f/c, scored, dexketoprofen (as trometamol) 25 mg, net price 10-tab pack = £1.95 (hosp. only), 20-tab pack = £3.90, 50-tab pack = £9.75. Label: 22

DICLOFENAC SODIUM

Indications: pain and inflammation in rheumatic disease (including juvenile arthritis) and other musculoskeletal disorders; acute gout; postoperative pain

Cautions: see notes above; **interactions:** Appendix 1 (NSAIDs)

Contra-indications: see notes above; porphyria (section 9.8.2)

INTRAVENOUS USE. Additional contra-indications include concomitant NSAID or anticoagulant use (including low-dose heparin), history of haemorrhagic diathesis, history of confirmed or suspected cerebrovascular bleeding, operations with high risk of haemorrhage, history of asthma, moderate or severe renal impairment, hypovolaemia, dehydration

Side-effects: see notes above; suppositories may cause rectal irritation; injection site reactions

Dose: *by mouth*, 75–150 mg daily in 2–3 divided doses

By deep intramuscular injection into the gluteal muscle, acute exacerbation of pain and postoperative pain, 75 mg once daily (twice daily in severe cases) for max. of 2 days

Ureteric colic, 75 mg then a further 75 mg after 30 minutes if necessary

By intravenous infusion (in hospital setting), 75 mg repeated if necessary after 4–6 hours for max. 2 days

Prevention of postoperative pain, initially after surgery 25–50 mg over 15–60 minutes then 5 mg/hour for max. 2 days

By rectum in suppositories, 75–150 mg daily in divided doses

Max. total daily dose by any route 150 mg

CHILD 1–12 years, juvenile arthritis, *by mouth or by rectum*, 1–3 mg/kg daily in divided doses (25 mg e/c tablets, 12.5 mg and 25 mg suppositories only)

Diclofenac Sodium (Non-proprietary) [PoM]
Tablets, both e/c, diclofenac sodium 25 mg, net price 84-tab pack = £2.37; 50 mg, 84-tab pack = £3.67. Label: 5, 25
Available from Alpharma, Arun (*Diclovol®*), Ashbourne (*Diclozip®*), Berk (*Flamrase®*), Dexcel Pharma (*Dicloflex®*), Eastern (*Volraman®*), Goldshield (*Acoflam®*), IVAX, Kent (*Enzed®*), Lagap, Sterwin, Trinity (*Lofensaid®*)
Suppositories, diclofenac sodium 100 mg, net price 10 = £3.70
Available from Goldshield (*Econac®*)
Injection, diclofenac sodium 25 mg/mL. Net price 3-mL amp = 80p
Available from Antigen
Note. Licensed for intramuscular use

Voltarol® (Novartis) [PoM]
Tablets, both e/c, diclofenac sodium 25 mg (yellow), net price 84-tab pack = £3.94; 50 mg (brown), 84-tab pack = £6.13. Label: 5, 25
Dispersible tablets, sugar-free, pink, diclofenac, equivalent to diclofenac sodium 50 mg, net price 21-tab pack = £5.63. Label: 13, 21
Note. Voltarol Dispersible tablets are more suitable for **short-term** use in acute conditions for which treatment required for no more than 3 months (no information on use beyond 3 months)
Injection, diclofenac sodium 25 mg/mL. Net price 3-mL amp = 83p
Excipients: include benzyl alcohol (see Excipients, p. 2)
Suppositories, diclofenac sodium 12.5 mg, net price 10 = 71p; 25 mg, 10 = £1.26; 50 mg, 10 = £2.07; 100 mg, 10 = £3.70
Emulgel® gel, section 10.3.2

■ Diclofenac potassium

Voltarol® Rapid (Novartis) [PoM]
Tablets, s/c, diclofenac potassium 25 mg (red), net price 28-tab pack = £3.36; 50 mg (brown), 28-tab pack = £6.44
Dose: rheumatic disease, musculoskeletal disorders, acute gout, post-operative pain, 75–150 mg daily in 2–3 divided doses; CHILD over 14 years, 75–100 mg daily in 2–3 divided doses
Migraine, 50 mg at onset, repeated after 2 hours if necessary then after 4–6 hours; max. 200 mg in 24 hours; CHILD not recommended

■ Modified release

Diclomax SR® (Parke-Davis) [PoM]
Capsules, m/r, yellow, diclofenac sodium 75 mg. Net price 56-cap pack = £13.01. Label: 21, 25
Dose: 1 capsule 1–2 times daily *or* 2 capsules once daily, preferably with food; CHILD not recommended

Diclomax Retard® (Parke-Davis) [PoM]
Capsules, m/r, diclofenac sodium 100 mg. Net price 28-tab pack = £9.36. Label: 21, 25
Dose: 1 capsule daily preferably with food; CHILD not recommended

Motifene® 75 mg (Sankyo) [PoM]
Capsules, e/c, m/r, diclofenac sodium 75 mg (enclosing e/c pellets containing diclofenac sodium 25 mg and m/r pellets containing diclofenac sodium 50 mg). Net price 56-cap pack = £14.99. Label: 25
Dose: 1 capsule 1–2 times daily; CHILD not recommended

Voltarol® 75 mg SR (Novartis) [PoM]
Tablets, m/r, pink, diclofenac sodium 75 mg. Net price 28-tab pack = £8.68; 56-tab pack = £17.35. Label: 21, 25
Dose: 75 mg 1–2 times daily preferably with food; CHILD not recommended
Note. Modified-release tablets containing diclofenac sodium 75 mg available from Alpharma (*Flamatak® 75 MR*), Arun (*Diclovol®SR, Flamrase®SR*), Dexcel Pharma (*Dicloflex® 75 SR*), Galen (*Diclotard® 75 MR*), Goldshield (*Acoflam® 75 SR*), Hillcross (*Dexomon® 75 SR*), IVAX, Lagap (*Rhumalgan® CR*), Pharmacia (*Flexotard® MR 75*), Sovereign (*Rheumatac® Retard 75*), Sterwin (*Slofenac® SR*), Trinity (*Lofensaid® Retard 75, Volsaid® Retard 75*)

Voltarol® Retard (Novartis) [PoM]
Tablets, m/r, red, diclofenac sodium 100 mg. Net price 28-tab pack = £12.72. Label: 21, 25
Dose: 1 tablet daily preferably with food; CHILD not recommended
Note. Modified-release tablets containing diclofenac sodium 100 mg available from Alpharma (*Flamatak® 100 MR*), APS, Arun (*Diclovol®Retard*), Berk (*Flamrase® SR*[1]), Dexcel Pharma (*Dicloflex® Retard*), Genus (*Digenac® XL*[1]), Goldshield (*Acoflam® Retard*), Hillcross (*Dexomon® Retard 100*), IVAX, Lagap (*Rhumalgan® CR*), Pharmacia (*Flexotard® MR 100*), Sterwin (*Slofenac® Retard 100*), Trinity (*Lofensaid® Retard 100, Volsaid® Retard 100*)
1. Also licensed for dysmenorrhoea and associated menorrhagia

■ With misoprostol

For **cautions, contra-indications**, and **side-effects** of misoprostol, see section 1.3.4

Arthrotec® (Searle) [PoM]
Arthrotec® 50 tablets, diclofenac sodium (in e/c core) 50 mg, misoprostol 200 micrograms. Net price 60-tab pack = £13.31. Label: 21, 25
Dose: prophylaxis against NSAID-induced gastroduodenal ulceration in patients requiring diclofenac for rheumatoid arthritis or osteoarthritis, 1 tablet 2–3 times daily with food; CHILD not recommended

Arthrotec® 75 tablets, diclofenac sodium (in e/c core) 75 mg, misoprostol 200 micrograms. Net price 60-tab pack = £17.59. Label: 21, 25
Dose: prophylaxis against NSAID-induced gastroduodenal ulceration in patients requiring diclofenac for rheumatoid arthritis or osteoarthritis, 1 tablet twice daily with food; CHILD not recommended

DIFLUNISAL

Indications: pain and inflammation in rheumatic disease and other musculoskeletal disorders; mild to moderate pain including dysmenorrhoea

Cautions: see notes above; **interactions:** Appendix 1 (NSAIDs)

Contra-indications: see notes above

Side-effects: see notes above

Dose: mild to moderate pain, initially 1 g, then 500 mg every 12 hours (increased to max. 500 mg every 8 hours if necessary)

Osteoarthritis, rheumatoid arthritis, 0.5–1 g daily as a single daily dose *or* in 2 divided doses

Dysmenorrhoea, initially 1 g, then 500 mg every 12 hours

CHILD not recommended

Dolobid® (MSD) PoM

Tablets, both f/c, diflunisal 250 mg (peach), net price 60-tab pack = £5.41; 500 mg (orange), 60-tab pack = £10.82. Label: 21, 25, counselling, avoid aluminium hydroxide

ETODOLAC

Indications: pain and inflammation in rheumatoid arthritis and osteoarthritis

Cautions: see notes above; **interactions:** Appendix 1 (NSAIDs)

Contra-indications: see notes above

Side-effects: see notes above

Dose: 600 mg daily; CHILD not recommended

Lodine SR® (Shire) PoM

Tablets, m/r, light-grey, etodolac 600 mg. Net price 30-tab pack = £15.50. Label: 25

FENBUFEN

Indications: pain and inflammation in rheumatic disease and other musculoskeletal disorders

Cautions: see notes above; **interactions:** Appendix 1 (NSAIDs)

Contra-indications: see notes above

Side-effects: see notes above, but also high risk of rashes especially in seronegative rheumatoid arthritis, psoriatic arthritis and in women (discontinue immediately); erythema multiforme and Stevens-Johnson syndrome reported; also allergic interstitial lung disorders (may follow rashes)

Dose: 300 mg in the morning and 600 mg at bedtime *or* 450 mg twice daily; CHILD under 14 years not recommended

Fenbufen (Non-proprietary) PoM

Capsules, fenbufen 300 mg, net price 84-cap pack = £15.26. Label: 21

Available from Genus, Hillcross, IVAX, Kent

Tablets, fenbufen 300 mg, net price 84-tab pack = £14.56; 450 mg, 56-tab pack = £13.17. Label: 21

Available from Cox, Generics, Genus, Hillcross, IVAX, Kent, Sterwin

Lederfen® (Wyeth) PoM

Capsules, dark blue, fenbufen 300 mg. Net price 84-cap pack = £20.71. Label: 21

Tablets, both light blue, f/c, fenbufen 300 mg, net price 84-tab pack = £20.71; 450 mg, 56-tab pack = £20.11. Label: 21

FENOPROFEN

Indications: pain and inflammation in rheumatic disease and other musculoskeletal disorders; mild to moderate pain

Cautions: see notes above; **interactions:** Appendix 1 (NSAIDs)

Contra-indications: see notes above

Side-effects: see notes above; upper respiratory-tract infection, nasopharyngitis, and cystitis also reported

Dose: 300–600 mg 3–4 times daily with food; max. 3 g daily; CHILD not recommended

Fenopron® (Typharm) PoM

Tablets, both orange, fenoprofen (as calcium salt) 300 mg (*Fenopron®* 300), net price 100-tab pack = £9.45; 600 mg (*Fenopron®* 600, scored), 100-tab pack = £18.29. Label: 21

FLURBIPROFEN

Indications: pain and inflammation in rheumatic disease and other musculoskeletal disorders; mild to moderate pain including dysmenorrhoea; migraine; postoperative analgesia; relief of sore throat (section 12.3.1)

Cautions: see notes above; **interactions:** Appendix 1 (NSAIDs)

Contra-indications: see notes above

Side-effects: see notes above; suppositories may cause rectal irritation

Dose: *by mouth or by rectum* in suppositories, 150–200 mg, daily in divided doses, increased in acute conditions to 300 mg daily

Dysmenorrhoea, initially 100 mg, then 50–100 mg every 4–6 hours; max. 300 mg daily

CHILD not recommended

Froben® (Abbott) PoM

Tablets, both yellow, s/c, flurbiprofen 50 mg, net price 20 = £2.00; 100 mg, 20 = £3.79. Label: 21

Note. Flurbiprofen tablets also available from Alpharma, IVAX, Kent

Suppositories, flurbiprofen 100 mg. Net price 12 = £2.90

■ Modified release

Froben SR® (Abbott) PoM

Capsules, m/r, yellow, enclosing off-white beads, flurbiprofen 200 mg. Net price 30-cap pack = £10.88. Label: 21, 25

Dose: rheumatic disease, 1 capsule daily, preferably in the evening; CHILD not recommended

INDOMETACIN

(Indomethacin)

Indications: pain and moderate to severe inflammation in rheumatic disease and other acute musculoskeletal disorders; acute gout; dysmenorrhoea; closure of ductus arteriosus (section 7.1.1.1)

Cautions: see notes above; also epilepsy, parkinsonism, psychiatric disturbances; during prolonged therapy ophthalmic and blood examinations particularly advisable; avoid rectal administration in proctitis and haemorrhoids; **interactions:** Appendix 1 (NSAIDs)

DRIVING. Dizziness may affect performance of skilled tasks (e.g. driving)

Contra-indications: see notes above

Side-effects: see notes above; frequently gastro-intestinal disturbances (including diarrhoea), headache, dizziness, and light-headedness; also gastro-intestinal ulceration and bleeding; rarely, drowsiness, confusion, insomnia, convulsions, psychiatric disturbances, depression, syncope, blood disorders (particularly thrombocytopenia), hypertension, hyperglycaemia, blurred vision, corneal deposits, peripheral neuropathy, and intestinal strictures; suppositories may cause rectal irritation and occasional bleeding

Dose: *by mouth*, rheumatic disease, 50–200 mg daily in divided doses, with food; CHILD not recommended

Acute gout, 150–200 mg daily in divided doses

Dysmenorrhoea, up to 75 mg daily

By rectum in suppositories, 100 mg at night and in the morning if required; CHILD not recommended

Combined oral and rectal treatment, max. total daily dose 150–200 mg

Indometacin (Non-proprietary) PoM

Capsules, indometacin 25 mg, net price 20 = 51p; 50 mg, 20 = 40p. Label: 21, counselling, driving, see above

Available from Alpharma, Kent, MSD (*Indocid®*), Ranbaxy (*Rimacid®*)

Suppositories, indometacin 100 mg. Net price 10 = £1.27. Counselling, driving, see above

Available from Alpharma, IVAX, MSD (*Indocid®*)

■ Modified release

Indometacin m/r preparations PoM

Capsules, m/r, indometacin 75 mg. Label: 21, 25, counselling, driving, see above

Dose: 1 capsule 1–2 times daily; CHILD not recommended

Available from Alpharma (*Pardelprin®*),Ashbourne (*Indomax 75 SR®*), Generics (*Slo-Indo®*), Hillcross (*Rheumacin LA®*), Lagap (*Indolar SR®*), MSD (*Indocid-R®*), Pharmacia (*Indomod®*; also 25-mg strength)

Tablets, m/r, indometacin 25 mg (*Flexin-25 Continus®*, green), net price 56-tab pack = £7.27; 50 mg (*Flexin-50 Continus®*, red), 28-tab pack = £7.27; 75 mg (*Flexin-75 Continus®*, yellow), 28-tab pack = £10.38. Label: 21, 25, counselling, driving, see above

Dose: initially 75 mg daily, adjusted in steps of 25–50 mg; range 25–200 mg daily in 1–2 divided doses; dysmenorrhoea, up to 75 mg daily; CHILD not recommended

Available from Napp

KETOPROFEN

Indications: pain and mild inflammation in rheumatic disease and other musculoskeletal disorders, and after orthopaedic surgery; acute gout; dysmenorrhoea

Cautions: see notes above; **interactions:** Appendix 1 (NSAIDs)

Contra-indications: see notes above

Side-effects: see notes above; pain may occur at injection site (occasionally tissue damage); suppositories may cause rectal irritation

Dose: *by mouth*, rheumatic disease, 100–200 mg daily in 2–4 divided doses with food; CHILD not recommended

Pain and dysmenorrhoea, 50 mg up to 3 times daily; CHILD not recommended

By rectum in suppositories, rheumatic disease, 100 mg at bedtime; CHILD not recommended

Combined oral and rectal treatment, max. total daily dose 200 mg

By deep intramuscular injection into the gluteal muscle, 50–100 mg every 4 hours (max. 200 mg in 24 hours) for up to 3 days; CHILD not recommended

Ketoprofen (Non-proprietary) PoM

Capsules, ketoprofen 50 mg, net price 28-cap pack = £4.48; 100 mg, 100-cap pack = £13.48. Label: 21

Available from Lagap

Orudis® (Hawgreen) PoM

Capsules, ketoprofen 50 mg (green/purple), net price 112-cap pack = £17.28; 100 mg (pink), 56-cap pack = £17.33. Label: 21

Suppositories, ketoprofen 100 mg. Net price 10 = £7.44

Oruvail® (Hawgreen) PoM

Injection, ketoprofen 50 mg /mL. Net price 2-mL amp = £1.20

Gel, section 10.3.2

■ Modified release

Oruvail® (Hawgreen) PoM

Capsules, all m/r, enclosing white pellets, ketoprofen 100 mg (pink/purple), net price 56-cap pack = £26.77; 150 mg (pink), 28-cap pack = £15.28; 200 mg (pink/white), 28-cap pack = £26.69. Label: 21, 25

Dose: 100–200 mg once daily with food; CHILD not recommended

Note. Modified-release capsules containing ketoprofen 100 mg and 200 mg also available from Alpharma (*Jomethid XL®*-200 mg), APS (*Ketovail®*), Ashbourne (*Ketozip XL®*-200 mg), Galen (*Ketotard® 200XL*), Goldshield (*Ketpron XL®* 100 mg, *Ketpron®* 200 mg) Lagap (*Larafen CR®*-200 mg), Tillomed (*Ketil CR*), Trinity (*Fenoket®*-200 mg, *Ketocid®*-200 mg)

LORNOXICAM

Indications: pain and inflammation in osteoarthritis and rheumatoid arthritis; pain in acute lumbo-sciatica; moderate postoperative pain

Cautions: see notes above; **interactions:** Appendix 1 (NSAIDs)

Contra-indications: see notes above

INTRAMUSCULAR OR INTRAVENOUS USE. Additional contra-indications include severe cardiac insufficiency, moderate or severe renal impairment, hypovolaemia, dehydration, confirmed or suspected cerebrovascular bleeding, haemorrhagic diathesis, operations with risk of haemorrhage or incomplete haemostasis

Side-effects: see notes above; also flatulence, dry mouth, stomatitis, taste disturbance, dysphagia, tachycardia, appetite changes, weight changes, malaise, agitation, tremor, paraesthesia, micturition disorder, myalgia, sweating, alopecia; injection site reactions

Dose: *by mouth*, osteoarthritis, rheumatoid arthritis, 4 mg 3 times daily *or* 8 mg in the morning and 4 mg in the evening; CHILD and ADOLESCENT under 18 years not recommended

Postoperative pain, acute lumbo-sciatica, 8 mg 1–2 times daily; CHILD and ADOLESCENT under 18 years not recommended

By intramuscular injection or by intravenous injection, postoperative pain, 8 mg up to twice daily for max. 2 days (increased to max. 8 mg 3 times daily on first day if necessary); CHILD and ADOLESCENT under 18 years, and ELDERLY over 65 years not recommended

Acute lumbo-sciatica, 8 mg twice daily for 1–2 days; CHILD and ADOLESCENT under 18 years, and ELDERLY over 65 years not recommended

Xefo® (CeNeS) ▼ PoM
Tablets, f/c, lornoxicam 4 mg, net price 30-tab pack = £8.85; 8 mg, 30-tab pack = £8.85
Injection, powder for reconstitution, lornoxicam 8.6 mg (= lornoxicam 8 mg/2 mL when reconstituted with 2.15 mL water for injections), net price 8.6-mg vial = £2.25

MEFENAMIC ACID

Indications: mild to moderate pain in rheumatoid arthritis (including juvenile arthritis), osteoarthritis, and related conditions; dysmenorrhoea and menorrhagia

Cautions: see notes above; porphyria (section 9.8.2); **interactions:** Appendix 1 (NSAIDs)

Contra-indications: see notes above; inflammatory bowel disease

Side-effects: see notes above; drowsiness; diarrhoea or rashes (withdraw treatment); thrombocytopenia, haemolytic anaemia (positive Coombs' test), and aplastic anaemia reported; convulsions in overdosage

Dose: 500 mg 3 times daily preferably after food; CHILD over 6 months, 25 mg/kg daily in divided doses for not longer than 7 days, except in juvenile arthritis

Mefenamic Acid (Non-proprietary) PoM
Capsules, mefenamic acid 250 mg. Net price 20 = 50p. Label: 21
Available from Alpharma, Ashbourne (*Dysman 250®*), Chemidex (*Ponstan®*), IVAX, Kent, Sanofi-Synthelabo, Sterwin
Tablets, mefenamic acid 500 mg, net price 28-tab pack = £2.54. Label: 21
Available from Alpharma, APS, Ashbourne (*Dysman 500®*), Chemidex (*Ponstan Forte®*), IVAX, Sanofi-Synthelabo
Paediatric oral suspension, mefenamic acid 50 mg/5 mL. Net price 125 mL = £19.98. Label: 21
Available from Chemidex

MELOXICAM

Indications: pain and inflammation in rheumatic disease; exacerbation of osteoarthritis (short-term); ankylosing spondylitis

Cautions: see notes above; avoid rectal administration in proctitis or haemorrhoids; **interactions:** Appendix 1 (NSAIDs)

Contra-indications: see notes above; renal failure (unless receiving dialysis)

Side-effects: see notes above

Dose: *by mouth*, osteoarthritis, 7.5 mg daily with food, increased if necessary to max. 15 mg once daily

Rheumatoid arthritis and ankylosing spondylitis, 15 mg once daily with food (7.5 mg daily in elderly)

By rectum, in suppositories, osteoarthritis, 7.5 mg daily; rheumatoid arthritis, 15 mg once daily (7.5 mg daily in elderly); ankylosing spondylitis, 15 mg once daily

CHILD under 15 years not recommended

Mobic® (Boehringer Ingelheim) PoM
Tablets, both yellow, scored, meloxicam 7.5 mg, net price 30-tab pack = £10.00; 15 mg, 30-tab pack = £13.90. Label: 21
Suppositories, meloxicam 7.5 mg, net price 12 = £4.00; 15 mg, 12 = £6.00

NABUMETONE

Indications: pain and inflammation in osteoarthritis and rheumatoid arthritis

Cautions: see notes above; **interactions:** Appendix 1 (NSAIDs)

Contra-indications: see notes above

Side-effects: see notes above

Dose: 1 g at night, in severe conditions 0.5–1 g in morning as well; elderly 0.5–1 g daily; CHILD not recommended

Nabumetone (Non-proprietary) PoM
Tablets, 500 mg, net price 56-tab pack = £17.84
Available from Alpharma, APS, Generics
Relifex® (SmithKline Beecham) PoM
Tablets, red, f/c, nabumetone 500 mg. Net price 56-tab pack = £18.11. Label: 21, 25
Suspension, sugar-free, nabumetone 500 mg/5 mL. Net price 300-mL pack = £25.22. Label: 21

NAPROXEN

Indications: pain and inflammation in rheumatic disease (including juvenile arthritis) and other musculoskeletal disorders; dysmenorrhoea; acute gout

Cautions: see notes above; **interactions:** Appendix 1 (NSAIDs)

Contra-indications: see notes above

Side-effects: see notes above

Dose: 0.5–1 g daily in 1–2 divided doses; CHILD (over 5 years), juvenile arthritis, 10 mg/kg daily in 2 divided doses

Acute musculoskeletal disorders and dysmenorrhoea, 500 mg initially, then 250 mg every 6–8 hours as required; max. dose after first day 1.25 g daily; CHILD under 16 years not recommended

Acute gout, 750 mg initially, then 250 mg every 8 hours until attack has passed; CHILD under 16 years not recommended

Naproxen (Non-proprietary) PoM
Tablets, naproxen 250 mg, net price 28-tab pack = £1.57; 500 mg, 28-tab pack = £3.08. Label: 21
Available from Alpharma, APS, Ashbourne (*Arthrosin®*), Berk (*Timpron®*), CP (*Arthroxen®*), Hillcross, IVAX, Sterwin

Tablets, e/c, naproxen 250 mg, net price 56-tab pack = £4.44; 375 mg, 56-tab pack = £6.96; 500 mg, 56-tab pack = £8.14. Label: 21
Available from Alpharma, Ardern (*Nycopren®*), APS, Ashbourne (*Arthrosin® EC*), Berk (*Timpron® EC*), Galen, Generics, IVAX

Naprosyn® (Roche) `PoM`
Tablets, all scored, naproxen 250 mg (buff), net price 56-tab pack = £4.89; 500 mg (buff), 56-tab pack = £9.77. Label: 21
Tablets, e/c, (*Naprosyn EC®*), naproxen 250 mg, net price 56-tab pack = £4.89; 375 mg, 56-tab pack = £7.33; 500 mg, 56-tab pack = £9.77. Label: 5, 25
Suspension, orange-flavoured, naproxen 125 mg/5 mL. Contains about 1.7 mmol Na$^+$/5 mL. Net price 240 mL = £3.65. Label: 21

Synflex® (Roche) `PoM`
Tablets, blue, naproxen sodium 275 mg. Net price 60-tab pack = £8.11. Label: 21
Note. 275 mg naproxen sodium ≅ 250 mg naproxen
Dose: musculoskeletal disorders, postoperative analgesia, 550 mg twice daily when necessary, preferably after food; max. 1.1 g daily; CHILD under 16 years not recommended
Dysmenorrhoea and acute gout, initially 550 mg then 275 mg every 6–8 hours as required; max. of 1.375 g on first day and 1.1 g daily thereafter; CHILD under 16 years not recommended
Migraine, 825 mg at onset, then 275–550 mg at least 30 minutes after initial dose; max 1.375 g in 24 hours; CHILD under 16 years not recommended

■ Modified release

Naprosyn® S/R (Roche) `PoM`
Tablets, m/r, f/c, scored, naproxen 500 mg (as sodium salt), net price 56-tab pack = £14.60. Label: 25
Dose: rheumatic and musculoskeletal disorders, 1–2 tablets once daily; CHILD under 16 years not recommended

■ With misoprostol
For **cautions**, **contra-indications**, and **side-effects** of misoprostol, see section 1.3.4

Napratec® (Searle) `PoM`
Combination pack, 56 yellow scored tablets, naproxen 500 mg; 56 white scored tablets, misoprostol 200 micrograms. Net price = £19.80. Label: 21
Dose: patients requiring naproxen for rheumatoid arthritis, osteoarthritis, or ankylosing spondylitis, with prophylaxis against NSAID-induced gastroduodenal ulceration, 1 naproxen 500-mg tablet and 1 misoprostol 200-microgram tablet taken together twice daily with food; CHILD not recommended

PHENYLBUTAZONE ▄▄▄

Indications: ankylosing spondylitis when other therapy unsuitable
Cautions: blood counts before and during treatment if for more than 7 days; elderly (reduce dose); breast-feeding; allergic disorders (see also under Contra-indications), withdraw if acute pulmonary syndrome including fever and dyspnoea; see also notes above; **interactions:** Appendix 1 (NSAIDs)
COUNSELLING. Warn patient to tell doctor immediately if sore throat, mouth ulcers, bruising, fever, malaise, rash, or non-specific illness develops

Contra-indications: cardiovascular disease, pulmonary, renal and hepatic impairment; pregnancy; history of peptic ulceration, of gastrointestinal haemorrhage, inflammatory bowel disease, or of blood disorders (including coagulation defects); history of hypersensitivity precipitated by aspirin or other NSAIDs (see also below); porphyria (section 9.8.2); Sjögren's syndrome; thyroid disease; children under 14 years
HYPERSENSITIVITY. NSAIDs are **contra-indicated** in history of hypersensitivity to aspirin or to any other NSAID—*which includes those* in whom attacks of *asthma, angioedema, urticaria or rhinitis* have been precipitated by aspirin or any other NSAID

Side-effects: see notes above; also parotitis, stomatitis, goitre, pancreatitis, hepatitis, nephritis, visual disturbances; rarely leucopenia, thrombocytopenia, agranulocytosis, aplastic anaemia, Stevens-Johnson syndrome, toxic epidermal necrolysis, pulmonary toxicity

Dose: initially 200 mg 2–3 times daily for 2 days, with or after food, then reduced to minimum effective, usually 100 mg 2–3 times daily; CHILD under 14 years not recommended

Butacote® (Novartis) `PoM` ▄▄▄
Tablets, light blue, e/c, s/c, phenylbutazone 100 mg, net price 20 = 48p (hosp. only). Label: 5, 21, 25, counselling, blood disorder symptoms (see above)

▄▄▄ **denotes preparations that are considered to be less suitable for prescribing (see p. vi)**

PIROXICAM

Indications: pain and inflammation in rheumatic disease (including juvenile arthritis) and other musculoskeletal disorders; acute gout
Cautions: see notes above; avoid in porphyria (section 9.8.2); **interactions:** Appendix 1 (NSAIDs)
Contra-indications: see notes above
Side-effects: see notes above; pain at injection site (occasionally tissue damage); suppositories may cause rectal irritation and occasional bleeding
Dose: *by mouth or by rectum*, rheumatic disease, initially 20 mg daily, maintenance 10–30 mg daily, in single or divided doses
CHILD (over 6 years) *by mouth*, juvenile arthritis, less than 15 kg, 5 mg daily; 16–25 kg, 10 mg; 26–45 kg, 15 mg; over 46 kg, 20 mg
Acute musculoskeletal disorders, 40 mg daily in single or divided doses for 2 days, then 20 mg daily for 7–14 days; CHILD not recommended
Acute gout, 40 mg initially, then 40 mg daily in single or divided doses for 4–6 days; CHILD not recommended
By deep intramuscular injection into gluteal muscle, for initial treatment of acute conditions, as dose by mouth (on short-term basis); CHILD not recommended

Piroxicam (Non-proprietary) `PoM`
Capsules, piroxicam 10 mg, net price 56-cap pack = £2.83; 20 mg, 28-cap pack = £3.16. Label: 21
Available from Alpharma, APS, Ashbourne (*Pirozip®*), Berk (*Flamatrol®*), Hillcross, IVAX, Kent (*Kentene®*)

Feldene® (Pfizer) [PoM]

Capsules, piroxicam 10 mg (maroon/blue), net price 56-cap pack = £6.00; 20 mg (maroon), 28-cap pack = £6.00. Label: 21

Tablets, (Feldene Melt®), piroxicam 20 mg, net price 28-tab pack = £9.83. Label: 10 patient information leaflet, 21

Excipients: include aspartame equivalent to phenylalanine 140 micrograms/tablet (section 9.4.1)

Note. Feldene Melt® tablets can be taken by placing on tongue or by swallowing

Dispersible tablets, piroxicam 10 mg (scored), net price 56-tab pack = £9.75; 20 mg, 28-tab pack = £9.75. Label: 13, 21

Note. Piroxicam dispersible tablets also available from Hillcross

Injection, piroxicam 20 mg/mL. Net price 1-mL amp = 70p

Suppositories, piroxicam 20 mg. Net price 10 = £5.20

Gel, section 10.3.2

Brexidol® (Trinity) [PoM]

Tablets, yellow, scored, piroxicam (as betadex) 20 mg, net price 30-tab pack = £12.22. Label: 21

Dose: osteoarthritis, rheumatic disease and acute musculoskeletal disorders, 1 tablet daily (may be halved in elderly); CHILD not recommended

ROFECOXIB

Indications: pain and inflammation in osteoarthritis and rheumatoid arthritis; acute pain (including postoperative pain, dysmenorrhoea)

Cautions: see notes above; **interactions**: Appendix 1 (NSAIDs)

Contra-indications: see notes above; also renal impairment (creatinine clearance less than 30 mL/minute); inflammatory bowel disease; severe congestive heart failure

Side-effects: see notes above; also mouth ulcers, chest pain, weight gain, sleep disturbance, atopic eczema, sweating, alopecia, and muscle cramps reported; raised liver enzymes (discontinue if persistently high)

Dose: osteoarthritis, 12.5 mg daily, increased if necessary to max. 25 mg once daily; CHILD not recommended

Rheumatoid arthritis, 25 mg once daily; CHILD not recommended

Acute pain, 50 mg initially then 25–50 mg once daily; CHILD not recommended

Vioxx® (MSD) ▼ [PoM]

Tablets, rofecoxib 12.5 mg (ivory), net price 28-tab pack = £21.58; 25 mg (yellow), 28-tab pack = £21.58

Suspension, sugar-free, yellow, strawberry-flavoured, rofecoxib 12.5 mg/5 mL, net price 150 mL = £23.12; 25 mg/5 mL, 150 mL = £23.12

Vioxx® Acute tablets, rofecoxib 25 mg (yellow), net price 14-tab pack = £10.79; 50 mg (orange), 7-tab pack = £5.39

SULINDAC

Indications: pain and inflammation in rheumatic disease and other musculoskeletal disorders; acute gout

Cautions: see notes above; also history of renal stones and ensure adequate hydration; **interactions:** Appendix 1 (NSAIDs)

Contra-indications: see notes above

Side-effects: see notes above; also urine discoloration occasionally reported

Dose: 200 mg twice daily with food (may be reduced according to response); max. 400 mg daily; acute gout should respond within 7 days; limit treatment of peri-articular disorders to 7–10 days; CHILD not recommended

Sulindac (Non-proprietary) [PoM]

Tablets, sulindac 100 mg, net price 56-tab pack = £7.43; 200 mg, 56-tab pack = £13.00. Label: 21

Available from Generics

Clinoril® (MSD) [PoM]

Tablets, both yellow, scored, sulindac 100 mg, net price 60-tab pack = £6.73; 200 mg, 60-tab pack = £12.96. Label: 21

TENOXICAM

Indications: pain and inflammation in rheumatic disease and other musculoskeletal disorders

Cautions: see notes above; **interactions:** Appendix 1 (NSAIDs)

Contra-indications: see notes above

Side-effects: see notes above

Dose: *by mouth*, rheumatic disease, 20 mg daily; CHILD not recommended

Acute musculoskeletal disorders, 20 mg daily for 7 days; max. 14 days; CHILD not recommended

By intravenous or intramuscular injection, for initial treatment for 1–2 days, as dose by mouth; CHILD not recommended

Mobiflex® (Roche) [PoM]

Tablets, red-brown, f/c, tenoxicam 20 mg. Net price 28-tab pack = £13.47. Label: 21

Injection, powder for reconstitution, tenoxicam 20 mg. Net price per amp (with solvent) = 89p

TIAPROFENIC ACID

Indications: pain and inflammation in rheumatic disease and other musculoskeletal disorders

Cautions: see notes above; **interactions:** Appendix 1 (NSAIDs)

Contra-indications: see notes above; also active bladder or prostate disease (or symptoms) and history of recurrent urinary-tract disorders—if urinary symptoms develop discontinue immediately and perform urine tests and culture; see also CSM advice below

> CSM ADVICE. Following reports of **severe cystitis** CSM has recommended that tiaprofenic acid should not be given to patients with urinary-tract disorders and should be stopped if urinary symptoms develop. Patients should be advised to stop taking tiaprofenic acid and to report to their doctor promptly if they develop urinary-tract symptoms (such as increased frequency, nocturia, urgency, pain on urinating, or blood in urine)

Side-effects: see notes above

Dose: 600 mg daily in 2–3 divided doses; CHILD not recommended

Tiaprofenic Acid (Non-proprietary) [PoM]

Tablets, tiaprofenic acid 200 mg, net price 84-tab pack = £19.45; 300 mg, 56-tab pack = £19.45. Label: 21

Available from Alpharma

Surgam® (Florizel) PoM
Tablets, tiaprofenic acid 200 mg, net price 84-tab
pack = £20.48; 300 mg, 56-tab pack = £20.48.
Label: 21

■ Modified release

Surgam SA® (Florizel) PoM
Capsules, m/r, maroon/pink enclosing white pellets, tiaprofenic acid 300 mg. Net price 56-cap
pack = £20.48. Label: 25
Dose: 2 capsules once daily; CHILD not recommended

Aspirin and the salicylates

Aspirin was the traditional first choice anti-
inflammatory analgesic but most physicians now
prefer to start treatment with another NSAID which
may be better tolerated and more convenient for the
patient.

In regular high dosage aspirin has about the same
anti-inflammatory effect as other NSAIDs. The
required dose for active inflammatory joint disease
is at least 3.6 g daily. There is little anti-inflammatory effect with less than 3 g daily. Gastro-intestinal side-effects such as nausea, dyspepsia, and
gastro-intestinal bleeding may occur with any dosage of aspirin but anti-inflammatory doses are associated with a much higher incidence of side-effects.
Anti-inflammatory doses of aspirin may also cause
mild chronic salicylate intoxication (salicylism)
characterised by dizziness, tinnitus, and deafness;
these symptoms may be controlled by reducing the
dosage.

ASPIRIN

(Acetylsalicylic Acid)
Indications: pain and inflammation in rheumatic
disease and other musculoskeletal disorders
(including juvenile arthritis); see also section
4.7.1; antiplatelet (section 2.9)
Cautions: asthma, allergic disease, uncontrolled
hypertension, hepatic or renal impairment (avoid
if severe), dehydration, pregnancy (particularly at
term; see also Appendix 4), elderly; preferably
avoid during fever or viral infection in adolescents (risk of Reye's syndrome, see below);
G6PD-deficiency (section 9.1.5); **interactions:**
Appendix 1 (aspirin)
REYE'S SYNDROME. Owing to an association with Reye's
syndrome aspirin-containing preparations should not be
given to children under 12 years, unless specifically
indicated, e.g. for juvenile arthritis (Still's disease).
Aspirin should also preferably be avoided during fever
or viral infection in children and adolescents over 12
years. Families should be advised that aspirin should not
be given to children under 12 years except when prescribed by a doctor and it is best avoided in adolescents
with feverish conditions.
Contra-indications: gastro-intestinal ulceration;
children under 12 years (except for juvenile arthritis) and breast-feeding (association with Reye's
syndrome, see above); haemophilia and other
bleeding disorders; not for treatment of gout
HYPERSENSITIVITY. Aspirin and other NSAIDs **contra-
indicated** in history of hypersensitivity to aspirin or any
other NSAID—which includes those in whom attacks of
asthma, angioedema, urticaria or rhinitis have been precipitated by aspirin or any other NSAID

Side-effects: common with anti-inflammatory
doses; gastro-intestinal discomfort or nausea,
ulceration with occult bleeding (but occasionally
major haemorrhage); also other haemorrhage
(e.g. subconjunctival); hearing disturbances such
as tinnitus (leading rarely to deafness), vertigo,
confusion, hypersensitivity reactions (angioedema, bronchospasm and rashes); increased
bleeding time; rarely oedema, myocarditis, blood
disorders, particularly thrombocytopenia; **overdosage:** see Emergency Treatment of Poisoning,
p. 22
Dose: 0.3–1 g every 4 hours after food; max. in
acute conditions 8 g daily; CHILD, juvenile arthritis, up to 80 mg/kg daily in 5–6 divided doses
after food, increased in acute exacerbations to
130 mg/kg
Note. High doses of aspirin are very rarely required and
are now given under specialist supervision only, and
with plasma monitoring (especially in children)

Preparations
Section 4.7.1

BENORILATE

(Benorylate)
(Aspirin-paracetamol ester; 2 g benorilate is equivalent to
approximately 1.15 g aspirin and 970 mg paracetamol)
Indications: pain and inflammation in rheumatic
disease and other musculoskeletal disorders; mild
to moderate pyrexia
Cautions: see under Aspirin (above) and Paracetamol (section 4.7.1)
Contra-indications: see under Aspirin (above)
and Paracetamol (section 4.7.1)
Side-effects: see under Aspirin (above) and Paracetamol (section 4.7.1)
Dose: rheumatic disease, 4–8 g daily divided into
2–3 doses; max. 6 g daily for elderly; CHILD not
recommended
Mild to moderate pain, 2 g twice daily preferably
after food; CHILD not recommended

Benorilate (Non-proprietary)
Tablets, benorilate 750 mg. Net price 100-tab pack
= £8.67. Label: 21, 31
Granules, benorilate 2 g/sachet. Net price 60
sachet-pack = £13.77. Label: 13, 21, 31
Suspension, sugar-free, benorilate 2 g/5 mL. Net
price 300 mL = £10.96. Label: 21, 31
Available from Sanofi-Synthelabo (*Benoral®*), Sterwin

10.1.2 Corticosteroids

10.1.2.1 Systemic corticosteroids

The general actions and uses of the corticosteroids
are described in section 6.3. Treatment with corticosteroids in rheumatic diseases should be reserved
for specific indications, e.g. when other anti-
inflammatory drugs are unsuccessful. Corticosteroids can induce osteoporosis, and prophylaxis
should be considered on long-term treatment (section 6.6).

In severe, possibly life-threatening, situations a
high initial dose of corticosteroid is given to induce
remission and the dose then gradually reduced to

the lowest maintenance dose that will control the disease or, if possible, discontinued altogether. A major problem is that relapse may occur as the dose is reduced, particularly if the reduction is too rapid. The tendency is therefore to increase and maintain dosage and consequently the patient becomes dependent on corticosteroids. For this reason pulse doses of corticosteroids (e.g. methylprednisolone (as sodium succinate) up to 1 g intravenously on three consecutive days) are used to suppress highly active inflammatory disease while long-term and slower-acting medication is being commenced.

Prednisolone is used for most purposes; it has the advantage over the more potent corticosteroids (see section 6.3.2) of permitting finer dosage adjustments. To minimise side-effects the maintenance dose of prednisolone should be kept as low as possible, usually 7.5 mg daily. Recent evidence has suggested that prednisolone 7.5 mg daily may substantially reduce the rate of joint destruction in moderate to severe *rheumatoid arthritis* of less than 2 years duration. The reduction in joint destruction must be distinguished from mere symptomatic improvement (which lasts only 6 to 12 months at this dose) and care should be taken to avoid increasing the dosage beyond 7.5 mg daily. Current evidence supports maintenance of this anti-erosive dose for 2–4 years only, after which, treatment should be tapered off to reduce long-term adverse effects.

Polymyalgia rheumatica and *giant cell (temporal) arteritis* are always treated with corticosteroids. The usual initial dose of prednisolone in polymyalgia rheumatica is 10 to 15 mg daily and in giant cell arteritis 40 to 60 mg daily (the higher dose being used if visual symptoms occur). Treatment should be continued until remission of disease activity and doses are then reduced gradually to about 7.5–10 mg daily for maintenance. Relapse is common if therapy is stopped prematurely. Many patients require treatment for at least 2 years and in some patients it may be necessary to continue long-term low-dose corticosteroid treatment.

Polyarteritis nodosa and *polymyositis* are usually treated with corticosteroids. An initial dose of 60 mg of prednisolone daily is often used and reduced to a maintenance dose of 10 to 15 mg daily.

Systemic lupus erythematosus is treated with corticosteroids when necessary using a similar dosage regimen to that for polyarteritis nodosa and polymyositis (above). Patients with pleurisy, pericarditis, or other systemic manifestations will respond to corticosteroids. It may then be possible to reduce the dosage; alternate-day treatment is sometimes adequate, and the drug may be gradually withdrawn. In some mild cases corticosteroid treatment may be stopped after a few months. Many mild cases of systemic lupus erythematosus do not require corticosteroid treatment. Alternative treatment with anti-inflammatory analgesics, and possibly chloroquine or hydroxychloroquine, should be considered.

Ankylosing spondylitis should not be treated with long-term corticosteroids; rarely, pulse doses may be needed and may be useful in extremely active disease that does not respond to conventional treatment.

10.1.2.2 Local corticosteroid injections

Corticosteroids are injected locally for an anti-inflammatory effect. In inflammatory conditions of the joints, particularly in rheumatoid arthritis, they are given by *intra-articular injection* to relieve pain, increase mobility, and reduce deformity in one or a few joints. Full aseptic precautions are essential; infected areas should be avoided. Occasionally an acute inflammatory reaction develops after an intra-articular or soft-tissue injection of a corticosteroid. This may be a reaction to the microcrystalline suspension of the corticosteroid used, but must be distinguished from sepsis introduced into the injection site. An almost insoluble compound such as triamcinolone hexacetonide has a long-acting (depot) effect and is preferred for intra-articular injection.

Smaller amounts of corticosteroids may also be injected directly into soft tissues for the relief of inflammation in conditions such as *tennis* or *golfer's elbow* or *compression neuropathies.* In *tendinitis*, injections should be made into the tendon sheath and not directly into the tendon (due to the absence of a true tendon sheath, the Achilles tendon should not be injected). A soluble preparation (e.g. containing betamethasone or dexamethasone sodium phosphate) is preferred for injection into the carpal tunnel.

Hydrocortisone acetate or one of the synthetic analogues such as triamcinolone hexacetonide is generally used for local injection. The risk of necrosis and muscle wasting in small areas may be slightly increased with triamcinolone; flushing has been reported with intra-articular corticosteroid injections. Charcot-like arthropathies have also been reported (particularly following repeated intra-articular injections). Intra-articular injections may affect the hyaline cartilage and each joint should not usually be treated more than 3 times in one year.

Corticosteroid injections are also injected into soft tissues for the treatment of skin lesions (see section 13.4).

LOCAL CORTICOSTEROID INJECTIONS

Indications: local inflammation of joints and soft tissues (for details, consult product literature)

Cautions: see notes above and consult product literature; see also section 6.3.2

Contra-indications: see notes above and consult product literature

Side-effects: see notes above and consult product literature

Dose: see under preparations

■ Dose calculated as dexamethasone sodium phosphate

Dexamethasone (Organon) PoM

Injection, dexamethasone sodium phosphate 5 mg/mL (≡ dexamethasone 3.8 mg/mL ≡ dexamethasone phosphate 4.6 mg/mL). Net price 1-mL amp = 83p; 2-mL vial = £1.27

> *Dose: by intra-articular or intrasynovial injection* (for details consult product literature), 0.4–4 mg (calculated as dexamethasone sodium phosphate) according to size; where appropriate may be repeated at intervals of 3–21 days according to response

■ Dose calculated as dexamethasone phosphate

Dexamethasone (Faulding DBL) PoM

Injection, dexamethasone phosphate 4 mg/mL (as sodium phosphate) (≡ dexamethasone 3.3 mg/mL ≡ dexamethasone sodium phosphate 4.4 mg/mL), net price 1-mL amp = £1.00; 2-mL vial = £1.98

> *Dose: by intra-articular or intrasynovial injection* (for details consult product literature), 0.4–4 mg (calculated as dexamethasone phosphate) according to size (*soft-tissue infiltration* 2–6 mg); where appropriate may be repeated at intervals of 3–21 days

■ Hydrocortisone acetate

Hydrocortistab® (Sovereign) PoM

Injection, (aqueous suspension), hydrocortisone acetate 25 mg/mL. Net price 1-mL amp = £4.77

> *Dose: by intra-articular or intrasynovial injection* (for details consult product literature), 5–50 mg according to size; where appropriate may be repeated at intervals of 21 days; not more than 3 joints should be treated on any one day; CHILD 5–30 mg (divided)

■ Methylprednisolone acetate

Depo-Medrone® (Pharmacia) PoM

Injection (aqueous suspension), methylprednisolone acetate 40 mg/mL. Net price 1-mL vial = £2.87; 2-mL vial = £5.15; 3-mL vial = £7.47

> *Dose: by intra-articular or intrasynovial injection* (for details consult product literature), 4–80 mg, according to size; where appropriate may be repeated at intervals of 7–35 days; also for *intralesional injection*

Depo-Medrone® with Lidocaine (Pharmacia) PoM

Injection (aqueous suspension), methylprednisolone acetate 40 mg, lidocaine hydrochloride 10 mg/mL. Net price 1-mL vial = £2.87; 2-mL vial = £5.15

> *Dose: by intra-articular or intrasynovial injection* (for details consult product literature), 4–80 mg, according to size; where appropriate may be repeated at intervals of 7–35 days

■ Prednisolone acetate

Deltastab® (Sovereign) PoM

Injection (aqueous suspension), prednisolone acetate 25 mg/mL. Net price 1-mL amp = £4.77

> *Dose: by intra-articular or intrasynovial injection* (for details consult product literature), 5–25 mg according to size; not more than 3 joints should be treated on any one day; where appropriate may be repeated when relapse occurs

For *intramuscular injection*, see section 6.3.2

■ Triamcinolone acetonide

Adcortyl® Intra-articular/Intradermal (Squibb) PoM

Injection (aqueous suspension), triamcinolone acetonide 10 mg/mL. Net price 1-mL amp = £1.02; 5-mL vial = £4.14

> *Dose: by intra-articular injection or intrasynovial injection* (for details consult product literature), 2.5–15 mg according to size (for larger doses use *Kenalog®*); where appropriate may be repeated when relapse occurs
> *By intradermal injection*, (for details consult product literature): 2–3 mg; max. 5 mg at any one site (total max. 30 mg); where appropriate may be repeated at intervals of 1–2 weeks
> CHILD under 6 years not recommended

Kenalog® Intra-articular/Intramuscular (Squibb) PoM

Injection (aqueous suspension), triamcinolone acetonide 40 mg/mL. Net price 1-mL vial = £1.70

> *Dose: by intra-articular or intrasynovial injection* (for details consult product literature), 5–40 mg according to size; total max. 80 mg (for doses below 5 mg use *Adcortyl® Intra-articular/Intradermal*); where appropriate may be repeated when relapse occurs; CHILD under 6 years not recommended
> For *intramuscular injection*, see section 6.3.2

10.1.3   Drugs which suppress the rheumatic disease process

Certain drugs such as gold, penicillamine, hydroxychloroquine, chloroquine, immunosuppressants, and sulfasalazine may suppress the disease process in *rheumatoid arthritis*, as may gold and immunosuppressants in *psoriatic arthritis*. They are sometimes known as second-line or disease-modifying antirheumatic drugs (DMARDs). Unlike NSAIDs they do not produce an immediate therapeutic effect but require 4 to 6 months of treatment for a full response. If one of these drugs does not lead to objective benefit within 6 months, it should be discontinued. Response to a disease-modifying antirheumatic drug may allow the dose of the NSAID to be reduced.

Disease-modifying antirheumatic drugs may improve not only the symptoms and signs of inflammatory joint disease but also extra-articular manifestations such as vasculitis. They reduce the erythrocyte sedimentation rate, C-reactive protein, and sometimes the titre of rheumatoid factor. Some (e.g. methotrexate and ciclosporin) are believed to retard erosive damage as judged radiologically.

Since in the first few months, the course of rheumatoid arthritis is unpredictable and the diagnosis uncertain, it is usual to start treatment with an NSAID alone. Disease-modifying antirheumatic drugs are however instituted by specialists as soon as diagnosis, progression, and severity of the disease have been confirmed. The choice of a disease-modifying antirheumatic drug should take into account co-morbidity and patient preference. Sulfasalazine, methotrexate, intramuscular gold and penicillamine are similar in efficacy. However, sulfasalazine or methotrexate are often used first because they may be better tolerated.

Penicillamine and immunosuppressants are also sometimes used in rheumatoid arthritis where there are troublesome extra-articular features such as vasculitis, and in patients who are taking excessive doses of corticosteroids. Where the response is satisfactory there is often a striking reduction in requirements of both corticosteroids and other drugs. Gold and penicillamine are effective in *palindromic rheumatism*. *Systemic* and *discoid lupus erythematosus* are sometimes treated with chloroquine or hydroxychloroquine.

JUVENILE IDIOPATHIC ARTHRITIS. Gold, penicillamine, and related drugs may also be used to treat *juvenile idiopathic arthritis* (juvenile chronic arthritis) when indications are similar.

Gold

Gold may be given by intramuscular injection as sodium aurothiomalate or by mouth as auranofin.

Sodium aurothiomalate must be given by deep intramuscular injection and the area gently massaged. A test dose of 10 mg must be given followed by doses of 50 mg at weekly intervals until there is definite evidence of remission. Benefit is not to be expected until about 300 to 500 mg has been given; if there is no remission after 1 g has been given it should be discontinued. In patients who do respond, the interval between injections is then gradually increased to 4 weeks and treatment is continued for up to 5 years after complete remission. If relapse occurs the dosage frequency may be immediately increased to 50 mg weekly and only once control has been obtained again should the dosage frequency be decreased; if no response is seen within 2 months, alternative treatment should be sought. It is important to avoid complete relapse since second courses of gold are not usually effective. Children may be given 1 mg/kg weekly to a maximum of 50 mg weekly, the intervals being gradually increased to 4 weeks according to response; an initial test dose is given corresponding to one-tenth to one-fifth of the calculated dose.

Auranofin is given by mouth. If there is no response after 6 months treatment should be discontinued. Auranofin is less effective than parenteral gold.

Gold therapy should be discontinued in the presence of blood disorders or proteinuria (associated with immune complex nephritis) which is repeatedly above 300 mg/litre without other cause (such as urinary-tract infection). Urine tests and full blood counts (including total and differential white cell and platelet counts) must therefore be performed before starting treatment with gold and before each intramuscular injection; in the case of oral treatment the urine and blood tests should be carried out monthly. Rashes with pruritus often occur after 2 to 6 months of intramuscular treatment and may necessitate discontinuation of treatment; the most common side-effect of oral therapy, diarrhoea with or without nausea or abdominal pain, may respond to bulking agents (such as bran) or temporary reduction in dosage.

SODIUM AUROTHIOMALATE

Indications: active progressive rheumatoid arthritis, juvenile arthritis

Cautions: see notes above; renal and hepatic impairment, elderly, history of urticaria, eczema, colitis, drugs which cause blood disorders; annual chest X-ray; **interactions:** Appendix 1 (gold)

Contra-indications: severe renal and hepatic disease (see notes above); history of blood disorders or bone marrow aplasia, exfoliative dermatitis, systemic lupus erythematosus, necrotising enterocolitis, pulmonary fibrosis; pregnancy and breastfeeding (Appendixes 4 and 5); porphyria (section 9.8.2)

Side-effects: severe reactions (occasionally fatal) in up to 5% of patients; mouth ulcers, skin reactions (including, on prolonged parenteral treatment, irreversible pigmentation in sun-exposed areas), proteinuria, blood disorders (sometimes sudden and fatal); rarely colitis, peripheral neuritis, pulmonary fibrosis, hepatotoxicity with cholestatic jaundice, nephrotic syndrome, alopecia

Dose: *by deep intramuscular injection*, administered on expert advice, see notes above

COUNSELLING. Warn patient to tell doctor immediately if sore throat, fever, infection, non-specific illness, unexplained bleeding and bruising, purpura, mouth ulcers, metallic taste, or rashes develop; also ask patients to report immediately any breathlessness or cough

Myocrisin® (JHC) [PoM]
Injection, sodium aurothiomalate 20 mg/mL, net price 0.5-mL (10-mg) amp = £3.16; 40 mg/mL, 0.5-mL (20-mg) amp = £4.60; 100 mg/mL, 0.5-mL (50-mg) amp = £9.36. Counselling, blood disorder symptoms

AURANOFIN

Indications: active progressive rheumatoid arthritis

Cautions: see under Sodium Aurothiomalate; also caution in inflammatory bowel disease

BLOOD COUNTS. Withdraw if platelet count falls below 100 000/mm³ or if signs and symptoms suggestive of thrombocytopenia occur, see also notes above

Contra-indications: see under Sodium Aurothiomalate

Side-effects: diarrhoea most common (reduced by bulking agents such as bran); see also under Sodium Aurothiomalate

Dose: administered on expert advice, 6 mg daily (initially in 2 divided doses then if tolerated as single dose), if response inadequate after 6 months, increase to 9 mg daily (in 3 divided doses), discontinue if no response after a further 3 months; CHILD not recommended

COUNSELLING. Warn patient to tell doctor immediately if sore throat, fever, infection, non-specific illness, unexplained bleeding and bruising, purpura, mouth ulcers, metallic taste, or rashes develop; also ask patients to report immediately any breathlessness or cough

Note. The package insert for *Ridaura®* also advises that patients must also report immediately if conjunctivitis or hair loss develops

Ridaura® (Yamanouchi) [PoM]
Tablets, pale yellow, f/c, auranofin 3 mg. Net price 60-tab pack = £22.40. Label: 21, counselling, blood disorder symptoms (see above)

Penicillamine

Penicillamine has a similar action to gold, and more patients are able to continue treatment than with gold but side-effects occur frequently. Penicillamine should be discontinued if there is no improvement in 1 year.

Patients should be warned not to expect improvement for at least 6 to 12 weeks after treatment is initiated. If remission has been sustained for 6 months, reduction of dosage by 125 to 250 mg every 12 weeks may be attempted.

Blood counts, including platelets, and urine examinations should be carried out before starting treatment and then every 1 or 2 weeks for the first 2 months then every 4 weeks to detect blood disorders and proteinuria (they should also be carried out in the week after any dose increase). A reduction in platelet count calls for discontinuation with subsequent re-introduction at a lower dosage and then, if possible, gradual increase. Proteinuria, associated with immune complex nephritis, occurs in up to 30% of patients, but may resolve despite continuation of treatment; treatment may be continued provided that renal function tests remain normal, oedema is absent, and the 24-hour urinary excretion of protein does not exceed 2 g.

Nausea may occur but is not usually a problem provided that penicillamine is taken before food or on retiring and that low initial doses are used and only gradually increased. Loss of taste may occur about 6 weeks after treatment is started but usually returns 6 weeks later irrespective of whether or not treatment is discontinued; mineral supplements are not recommended. Rashes are a common side-effect. Those which occur in the first few months of treatment disappear when the drug is stopped and treatment may then be re-introduced at a lower dose level and gradually increased. Late rashes are more resistant and often necessitate discontinuation of treatment.

Patients who are hypersensitive to penicillin may react rarely to penicillamine.

PENICILLAMINE

Indications: see notes above and under Dose

Cautions: see notes above; renal impairment (Appendix 3), pregnancy (Appendix 4); avoid concurrent gold, chloroquine, hydroxychloroquine, or immunosuppressive treatment; avoid oral iron within 2 hours of a dose; interactions: Appendix 1 (penicillamine)

BLOOD COUNTS and URINE TESTS. See notes above. Longer intervals may be adequate in cystinuria and Wilson's disease. Consider withdrawal if platelet count falls below 120 000/mm³ or white blood cells below 2500/mm³ or if 3 successive falls within reference range (can restart at reduced dose when counts return to within reference range but permanent withdrawal necessary if recurrence of neutropenia or thrombocytopenia)

COUNSELLING. Warn patient to tell doctor immediately if sore throat, fever, infection, non-specific illness, unexplained bleeding and bruising, purpura, mouth ulcers, or rashes develop

Contra-indications: hypersensitivity (except in life-threatening situation when desensitisation may be attempted—consult product literature); lupus erythematosus

Side-effects: (see also notes above) initially nausea, anorexia, fever, and skin reactions; taste loss (mineral supplements not recommended); blood disorders including thrombocytopenia, neutropenia, agranulocytosis and aplastic anaemia; proteinuria, rarely haematuria (withdraw immediately); haemolytic anaemia, nephrotic syndrome, lupus erythematosus-like syndrome, myasthenia gravis-like syndrome, polymyositis (rarely with cardiac involvement), dermatomyositis, mouth ulcers, stomatitis, alopecia, bronchiolitis and pneumonitis, pemphigus, Goodpasture's syndrome, and Stevens-Johnson syndrome also reported; male and female breast enlargement reported; in non-rheumatoid conditions rheumatoid arthritis-like syndrome also reported; late rashes (reduce dose or withdraw treatment)

Dose: severe active rheumatoid arthritis, administered on expert advice, ADULT initially 125–250 mg daily before food for 1 month increased by similar amounts at intervals of not less than 4 weeks to usual maintenance of 500–750 mg daily in divided doses; max. 1.5 g daily; ELDERLY initially up to 125 mg daily before food for 1 month increased by similar amounts at intervals of not less than 4 weeks; max. 1 g daily; CHILD maintenance of 15–20 mg/kg daily (initial dose lower and increased at intervals of 4 weeks over a period of 3-6 months)

Wilson's disease, chronic active hepatitis, and cystinuria, section 9.8.1

Copper and lead poisoning, see Emergency Treatment of Poisoning, p. 27

Penicillamine (Non-proprietary) PoM
Tablets, penicillamine 125 mg, net price 20 = £1.97; 250 mg, 20 = £3.41. Label: 6, 22, counselling, blood disorder symptoms (see above)
Available from Alpharma, APS, Hillcross, IVAX

Distamine® (Alliance) PoM
Tablets, all f/c, penicillamine 125 mg, net price 20 = £2.17; 250 mg, 20 = £3.74. Label: 6, 22, counselling, blood disorder symptoms (see above)

Antimalarials

The antimalarials chloroquine and hydroxychloroquine are used to treat rheumatoid arthritis of moderate inflammatory activity. The antimalarials should not be used for psoriatic arthritis.

Chloroquine and hydroxychloroquine are better tolerated than gold or penicillamine. Retinopathy (see below) occurs rarely provided that the recommended doses are not exceeded; in the elderly it is difficult to distinguish drug-induced retinopathy from ageing changes.

Mepacrine (section 5.4.4) is sometimes used in discoid lupus erythematosus [unlicensed].

CAUTIONS. Chloroquine and hydroxychloroquine should be used with caution in hepatic impairment and in renal impairment (Appendix 3). Manufacturers recommend regular ophthalmological examination but the evidence of practical value is unsatisfactory (see advice of Royal College of Ophthalmologists, below). Hydroxychloroquine should be avoided in pregnancy and breast-feeding; chloroquine can, however, be used for malaria during pregnancy and breast-feeding. Both should be used with caution in neurological disorders (especially in those with a history of epilepsy), in severe gastro-intestinal disorders, in G6PD deficiency (section 9.1.5), in porphyria, and in the elderly (see also above). Chloroquine and hydroxychloroquine may exacerbate psoriasis and aggravate myasthenia gravis. Concurrent use of hepatotoxic drugs should be avoided; other **interactions**: Appendix 1 (chloroquine and hydroxychloroquine).

Advice of Royal College of Ophthalmologists
The Royal College of Ophthalmologists has advised that a screening protocol for chloroquine should be negotiated with local ophthalmologists; no screening is recommended for mepacrine because it is not thought to be associated with ophthalmological effects. The following recommendations relate to hydroxychloroquine.

Before treatment:
- Assess renal and liver function (adjust dose if impaired)
- Ask patient about visual impairment (not corrected by glasses). If impairment or eye disease present, assessment by an optometrist is advised and any abnormality should be referred to an ophthalmologist
- Record near visual acuity of each eye (with glasses where appropriate) using a standard reading chart
- Initiate hydroxychloroquine treatment if no abnormality detected (at a dose not exceeding hydroxychloroquine sulphate 6.5 mg/kg daily)

During treatment:
- Ask patient about visual symptoms and monitor visual acuity annually using the standard reading chart
- Refer to ophthalmologist if visual acuity changes or if vision blurred and warn patient to stop treatment and seek prescribing doctor's advice
- A child treated for juvenile arthritis should receive slit-lamp examination routinely to check for uveitis
- If long-term treatment is required (more than 5 years), individual arrangement should be agreed with the local ophthalmologist

Note. To avoid excessive dosage in obese patients, the dose of hydroxychloroquine and chloroquine should be calculated on the basis of lean body weight. Ocular toxicity is unlikely with chloroquine phosphate not exceeding 4 mg/kg daily (equivalent to chloroquine base approx. 2.5 mg/kg daily)

SIDE-EFFECTS. The side-effects of chloroquine and hydroxychloroquine include gastro-intestinal disturbances, headache and skin reactions (rashes, pruritus); those occurring less frequently include ECG changes, convulsions, visual changes, retinal damage (see above), keratopathy, ototoxicity, hair depigmentation, hair loss, and discoloration of skin, nails, and mucous membranes. Side-effects that occur rarely include blood disorders (including thrombocytopenia, agranulocytosis, and aplastic anaemia), mental changes (including emotional disturbances and psychosis), myopathy (including cardiomyopathy and neuromyopathy), acute generalised exanthematous pustulosis, exfoliative dermatitis, Stevens-Johnson syndrome, and hepatic damage. **Important**: very toxic in overdosage—immediate advice from poisons centres essential (see also p. 25).

CHLOROQUINE

Indications: active rheumatoid arthritis (including juvenile arthritis), systemic and discoid lupus erythematosus; malaria (section 5.4.1)
Cautions: see notes above

Side-effects: see notes above
Dose: administered on expert advice, chloroquine (base) 150 mg daily; max. 2.5 mg/kg daily, see recommendations above; CHILD, up to 3 mg/kg daily
Note. Chloroquine base 150 mg ≡ chloroquine sulphate 200 mg ≡ chloroquine phosphate 250 mg (approx.).

Preparations
See section 5.4.1

HYDROXYCHLOROQUINE SULPHATE

Indications: active rheumatoid arthritis (including juvenile arthritis), systemic and discoid lupus erythematosus; dermatological conditions caused or aggravated by sunlight
Cautions: see notes above
Side-effects: see notes above
Dose: administered on expert advice, initially 400 mg daily in divided doses; maintenance 200–400 mg daily; max. 6.5 mg/kg daily (but not exceeding 400 mg daily), see recommendations above; CHILD, up to 6.5 mg/kg daily (max. 400 mg daily)

Plaquenil® (Sanofi-Synthelabo) **PoM**
Tablets, f/c, hydroxychloroquine sulphate 200 mg. Net price 60-tab pack = £4.55. Label: 5, 21

Immunosuppressants

Methotrexate is a disease-modifying antirheumatic drug suitable for moderate to severe rheumatoid arthritis. **Azathioprine, ciclosporin, cyclophosphamide,** and **leflunomide** are considered more toxic and they are used in cases that have not responded to other disease-modifying drugs.

Methotrexate is usually given in an initial dose of 7.5 mg by mouth once a week, adjusted according to response to a maximum of 15 mg once a week (occasionally 20 mg once a week). Regular full blood counts (including differential white cell count and platelet count), renal and liver-function tests are required. In patients who experience mucosal or gastro-intestinal side-effects with methotrexate, folic acid 5 mg every week may help to reduce the frequency of such side-effects.

Azathioprine is usually given in a dose of 1.5 to 2.5 mg/kg daily in divided doses. Blood counts are needed to detect possible neutropenia or thrombocytopenia (usually resolved by reducing the dose). Nausea, vomiting, and diarrhoea may occur, usually starting early during the course of treatment, and may necessitate withdrawal of the drug; herpes zoster infection may also occur.

Leflunomide acts on the immune system as a disease-modifying antirheumatic drug. Its therapeutic effect starts after 4–6 weeks and improvement may continue for a further 4–6 months. Leflunomide, which is similar in efficacy to sulfasalazine and methotrexate, may be chosen when these drugs cannot be used. The active metabolite of leflunomide persists for a long period; active procedures to wash the drug out are required in case of serious adverse effects, or before starting treatment with another disease-modifying antirheumatic drug, or, in men or women, before conception. Side-effects of leflunomide include bone-marrow toxicity; its immunosuppressive effects increase the risk of infection and malignancy.

Ciclosporin (cyclosporin) is licensed for severe active rheumatoid arthritis when conventional second-line therapy is inappropriate or ineffective. There is some evidence that ciclosporin may retard the rate of erosive progression and improve symptom control in those who respond only partially to methotrexate.

Cyclophosphamide (section 8.1.1) may be used at a dose of 1 to 1.5 mg/kg daily by mouth for rheumatoid arthritis with severe systemic manifestations [unlicensed indication]; it is toxic and regular blood counts (including platelet count) should be carried out. Cyclophosphamide may also be given intravenously in a dose of 0.5 to 1 g (with prophylactic mesna) for *severe systemic rheumatoid arthritis* and for other connective tissue diseases (especially with active vasculitis), repeated initially at fortnightly then at monthly intervals (according to clinical response and haematological monitoring).

Etanercept (*Enbrel* ® ▼, Wyeth) and **infliximab** (*Remicade* ® ▼, Schering-Plough) inhibit the activity of tumour necrosis factor. They are used for the treatment of highly active rheumatoid arthritis in adults who have failed to respond to at least two standard disease-modifying antirheumatic drugs; they should be used under specialist supervision only. Etanercept or infliximab should be withdrawn if there is no response after 3 months. Infliximab must be given concomitantly with methotrexate. Etanercept is also licensed for polyarticular-course juvenile idiopathic arthritis in children over 4 years who have responded inadequately to methotrexate or who are intolerant of it. Etanercept has been associated with serious blood disorders and demyelinating disorders of the central nervous system. Severe infections have been reported with etanercept and infliximab. Infliximab has been associated with the development of tuberculosis (often in extrapulmonary sites) and with worsening heart failure.

Immunosuppressants are also used in the management of severe cases of *systemic lupus erythematosus* and other connective tissue disorders. They are often given in conjunction with corticosteroids for patients with severe or progressive renal disease though the evidence for their benefit is doubtful. They may be used in cases of *polymyositis* which are resistant to corticosteroids. They are used for their corticosteroid-sparing effect in patients whose corticosteroid requirements are excessive. **Azathioprine** is usually used.

Azathioprine and methotrexate are used in the treatment of *psoriatic arthropathy* [unlicensed indication] for severe or progressive cases which are not controlled with anti-inflammatory drugs.

AZATHIOPRINE

Indications: see notes above; transplantation rejection, see section 8.2.1

Cautions: see section 8.2.1

Contra-indications: see section 8.2.1

Side-effects: see section 8.2.1

Dose: *by mouth*, initially, rarely more than 3 mg/kg daily, reduced according to response; maintenance 1–3 mg/kg daily; consider withdrawal if no improvement within 3 months

Preparations
Section 8.2.1

CICLOSPORIN

(Cyclosporin)

Indications: severe active rheumatoid arthritis when conventional second-line therapy inappropriate or ineffective; graft-versus-host disease (section 8.2.2); atopic dermatitis and psoriasis (section 13.5.2).

Cautions: see section 8.2.2

ADDITIONAL CAUTIONS IN RHEUMATOID ARTHRITIS. **Contra-indicated** in abnormal renal function, uncontrolled hypertension (see also below), uncontrolled infections, and malignancy. Measure serum creatinine at least twice before treatment and monitor every 2 weeks for first 3 months, then every 4 weeks (or more frequently if dose increased or concomitant NSAIDs introduced or increased (see also **interactions:** Appendix 1 (ciclosporin)), reduce dose if serum creatinine increases more than 30% above baseline in more than 1 measurement; if above 50%, reduce dose by 50% (even if within normal range) and discontinue if reduction not successful within 1 month; monitor blood pressure (discontinue if hypertension develops that cannot be controlled by antihypertensive therapy); monitor hepatic function if concomitant NSAIDs given.

Side-effects: see section 8.2.2

Dose: *by mouth*, administered in accordance with expert advice, initially 2.5 mg/kg daily in 2 divided doses, if necessary increased gradually after 6 weeks; max. 4 mg/kg daily (discontinue if response insufficient after 3 months); dose adjusted according to response for maintenance and treatment reviewed after 6 months (continue only if benefits outweigh risks); CHILD and under 18 years, not recommended

IMPORTANT. For preparations and counselling and for advice on conversion between the preparations, see section 8.2.2

Preparations
Section 8.2.2

LEFLUNOMIDE

Indications: moderate to severe active rheumatoid arthritis

Cautions: renal impairment (Appendix 3); impaired bone-marrow function including anaemia, leucopenia or thrombocytopenia (avoid if significant and due to causes other than rheumatoid arthritis); recent treatment with other hepatotoxic or myelotoxic disease-modifying antirheumatic drugs (avoid concomitant use); history of tuberculosis; exclude pregnancy before treatment; effective contraception **essential** during treatment and for at least 2 years after treatment in women and at least 3 months after treatment in men (plasma concentration monitoring required; waiting time before conception may be reduced with washout procedures—consult product literature and see Washout Procedure below); monitor full blood count (including differential white cell count and platelet count) before treatment and every 2 weeks for 6 months then every 8 weeks; monitor liver function—(see Hepatotoxicity below); monitor blood pressure; washout procedures recommended for serious adverse effects and before transferring to other disease modifying antirheumatic drugs (consult product literature and see below); **interactions:** Appendix 1 (leflunomide)

HEPATOTOXICITY. Potentially life-threatening hepatotoxicity reported usually in the first 6 months; monitor liver function before treatment and at least monthly for first 6 months then every 2 months. Discontinue treatment (and institute washout procedure—consult product literature and see Washout Procedure below) or reduce dose according to liver-function abnormality; if liver-function abnormality persists after dose reduction, discontinue treatment and institute washout procedure

WASHOUT PROCEDURE. To aid drug elimination in case of serious adverse-effect, before starting another disease-modifying antirheumatic drug, or before conception (see also Appendix 4), stop treatment and give *either* colestyramine 8 g 3 times daily for 11 days *or* activated charcoal 50 g 4 times daily for 11 days; the concentration of the active metabolite after washout should be less than 20 micrograms/litre (measured on 2 occasions 14 days apart) in men or women before conception—consult product literature

Contra-indications: severe immunodeficiency; serious infection; hepatic impairment; severe hypoproteinaemia; pregnancy (**important teratogenic risk:** see Cautions and Appendix 4); breast-feeding (Appendix 5)

Side-effects: diarrhoea, nausea, vomiting, anorexia, oral mucosal disorders, abdominal pain, weight loss; increase in blood pressure; headache, dizziness, asthenia, paraesthesia; tenosynovitis; alopecia, eczema, dry skin, rash, pruritus; leucopenia; rarely taste disturbances, anxiety, tendon rupture, urticaria, anaemia, thrombocytopenia, eosinophilia, hyperlipidaemia, hypokalaemia, hypophosphataemia, hepatic dysfunction (see Hepatotoxicty above); also reported, anaphylaxis, pancytopenia, Stevens-Johnson syndrome, toxic epidermal necrolysis (discontinue and initiate washout procedure—consult product literature)

Dose: initially 100 mg once daily for 3 days then maintenance, 10–20 mg once daily; CHILD under 18 years safety and efficacy not established

Arava® (Aventis Pharma) ▼ PoM
Tablets, f/c, leflunomide 10 mg, net price 30-tab pack = £46.50; 20 mg (ochre), 30-tab pack = £46.50; 100 mg, 3-tab pack = £23.25. Label: 4

METHOTREXATE

Indications: moderate to severe active rheumatoid arthritis; malignant disease (section 8.1.3); psoriasis (section 13.5.2)

Cautions: see section 13.5.2

PULMONARY TOXICITY. Pulmonary toxicity may be a special problem in rheumatoid arthritis (patient to contact doctor immediately if dyspnoea or cough). For other special warnings, including CSM advice and counselling advice relating to interaction with aspirin and NSAIDs, see Methotrexate, section 13.5.2.

Contra-indications: see section 13.5.2

Side-effects: see section 13.5.2

Dose: *by mouth*, 7.5 mg once weekly (as a single dose *or* divided into 3 doses of 2.5 mg given at intervals of 12 hours), adjusted according to response; max. total weekly dose 20 mg

IMPORTANT. Note that the above dose is a **weekly** dose. The CSM has received reports of prescription and dispensing errors including fatalities. Attention should be paid to the **strength** of methotrexate tablets prescribed and the **frequency** of dosing.

Preparations
Section 8.1.3

Sulfasalazine

Sulfasalazine (sulphasalazine) has a beneficial effect in suppressing the inflammatory activity of rheumatoid arthritis. Side-effects include rashes, gastro-intestinal intolerance and, especially in patients with rheumatoid arthritis, occasional leucopenia, neutropenia, and thrombocytopenia. These haematological abnormalities occur usually in the first 3 to 6 months of treatment and are reversible on cessation of treatment. Close monitoring of full blood counts (including differential white cell count and platelet count) is necessary initially, and at monthly intervals during the first 3 months (liver function tests also being performed at monthly intervals for the first 3 months). Although the manufacturer recommends renal function tests, evidence of practical value is unsatisfactory.

SULFASALAZINE

(Sulphasalazine)

Indications: active rheumatoid arthritis; ulcerative colitis, see section 1.5 and notes above

Cautions: see section 1.5 and notes above

The CSM has recommended that patients should be advised to report any unexplained bleeding, bruising, purpura, sore throat, fever or malaise. A blood count should be performed and the drug stopped immediately if there is suspicion of a blood dyscrasia.

Contra-indications: see section 1.5 and notes above

Side-effects: see section 1.5 and notes above

Dose: *by mouth*, administered on expert advice, as enteric-coated tablets, initially 500 mg daily, increased by 500 mg at intervals of 1 week to a max. of 2–3 g daily in divided doses

Sulfasalazine (Non-proprietary) PoM
Tablets, e/c, sulfasalazine 500 mg. Net price 112-tab pack = £9.69. Label: 5, 14, 25, counselling, blood disorder symptoms (see CSM recommendation above), contact lenses may be stained

Available from Alpharma (*Sulazine EC®*)

Salazopyrin EN-Tabs® (Pharmacia) PoM
Tablets, e/c, yellow, f/c, sulfasalazine 500 mg. Net price 112-tab pack = £8.43. Label: 5, 14, 25, counselling, blood disorder symptoms (see CSM recommendation above), contact lenses may be stained

Gout and cytotoxic-induced hyperuricaemia

It is important to distinguish drugs used for the treatment of acute attacks of gout from those used in the long-term control of the disease. The latter exacerbate and prolong the acute manifestations if started during an attack.

Acute attacks of gout

Acute attacks of gout are usually treated with high doses of **NSAIDs** such as diclofenac, indometacin, ketoprofen, naproxen, piroxicam, or sulindac (section 10.1.1). The use of azapropazone should be restricted to patients in whom less toxic drugs have been ineffective (**important:** see CSM restrictions on p. 478). Colchicine is an alternative. Aspirin is *not* indicated in gout. Allopurinol and uricosurics are not effective in treating an acute attack and may prolong it indefinitely if started during the acute episode.

Colchicine is probably as effective as NSAIDs. Its use is limited by the development of toxicity at higher doses, but it is of value in patients with heart failure since, unlike NSAIDs, it does not induce fluid retention; moreover it can be given to patients receiving anticoagulants.

Intra-articular injection of a **corticosteroid** may be used in acute monoarticular gout [unlicensed indication].

COLCHICINE

Indications: acute gout, short-term prophylaxis during initial therapy with allopurinol and uricosuric drugs; prophylaxis of familial Mediterranean fever (recurrent polyserositis) [unlicensed]

Cautions: breast-feeding (Appendix 5), elderly, gastro-intestinal disease, cardiac, hepatic and renal impairment; **interactions:** Appendix 1 (colchicine)

Contra-indications: pregnancy

Side-effects: most common are nausea, vomiting, and abdominal pain; excessive doses may also cause profuse diarrhoea, gastro-intestinal haemorrhage, rashes, renal and hepatic damage. Rarely peripheral neuritis, myopathy, alopecia, and with prolonged treatment blood disorders

Dose: treatment of gout, 1 mg initially, followed by 500 micrograms every 2–3 hours until relief of pain is obtained or vomiting or diarrhoea occurs, or until a total dose of 6 mg has been reached; the course should not be repeated within 3 days

Prevention of gout attacks during initial treatment with allopurinol or uricosuric drugs, 500 micrograms 2–3 times daily

Prophylaxis of familial Mediterranean fever [unlicensed], 0.5–2 mg daily

Colchicine (Non-proprietary) [PoM]

Tablets, colchicine 500 micrograms, net price 20 = £3.32

Available from CP, IVAX

Long-term control of gout

Frequent recurrence of acute attacks of gout may call for the initiation of long-term ('interval') treatment. For long-term control of gout the formation of uric acid from purines may be reduced with the xanthine-oxidase inhibitor allopurinol, or the uricosuric drug sulfinpyrazone may be used to increase the excretion of uric acid in the urine. Treatment should be continued indefinitely to prevent further attacks of gout by correcting the hyperuricaemia. These drugs should never be started during an acute attack. The initiation of treatment may precipitate an acute attack therefore colchicine or an anti-inflammatory analgesic should be used as a prophylactic and continued for at least one month after the hyperuricaemia has been corrected (usually about 3 months of prophylaxis). However, if an acute attack develops during treatment, then the treatment should continue at the same dosage and the acute attack treated in its own right.

Allopurinol is a well tolerated drug which is widely used. It is especially useful in patients with renal impairment or urate stones where uricosuric drugs cannot be used; it is *not* indicated for the treatment of asymptomatic hyperuricaemia. It is usually given once daily, since the active metabolite of allopurinol has a long half-life, but doses over 300 mg daily should be divided. It may occasionally cause rashes.

Sulfinpyrazone (sulphinpyrazone) can be used instead of allopurinol, or in conjunction with it in cases that are resistant to treatment.

Probenecid (available on a named-patient basis) is a uricosuric drug used to prevent nephrotoxicity associated with cidofovir (section 5.3).

Crystallisation of urate in the urine may occur with the uricosuric drugs and it is important to ensure an adequate urine output especially in the first few weeks of treatment. As an additional precaution the urine may be rendered alkaline.

Aspirin and salicylates antagonise the uricosuric drugs; they do not antagonise allopurinol but are nevertheless *not* indicated in gout.

ALLOPURINOL

Indications: prophylaxis of gout and of uric acid and calcium oxalate renal stones; prophylaxis of hyperuricaemia associated with cancer chemotherapy

Cautions: administer prophylactic colchicine or NSAID (*not* aspirin or salicylates) until at least 1 month after hyperuricaemia corrected; ensure adequate fluid intake (2–3 litres/day); hepatic impairment (Appendix 2), renal impairment (monitor liver function; Appendix 3); for hyperuricaemia associated with cancer therapy, allopurinol treatment should be started before cancer therapy; pregnancy and breast-feeding; **interactions:** Appendix 1 (allopurinol)

Contra-indications: not a treatment for acute gout but continue if attack develops when already receiving allopurinol, and treat attack separately (see notes above)

Side-effects: rashes (**withdraw** therapy; if rash mild re-introduce cautiously but **discontinue** immediately if recurrence—hypersensitivity reactions occur rarely and include exfoliation, fever, lymphadenopathy, arthralgia, and eosinophilia resembling Stevens-Johnson or Lyell's syndrome, vasculitis, hepatitis, renal impairment, and very rarely epilepsy); gastro-intestinal disorders; rarely malaise, headache, vertigo, drowsiness, visual and taste disturbances, hypertension, alopecia, hepatotoxicity, paraesthesia and neuropathy, gynaecomastia, blood disorders (including leucopenia, thrombocytopenia, haemoytic anaemia and aplastic anaemia)

Dose: initially 100 mg daily, preferably after food, then adjusted according to plasma or urinary uric acid concentration; usual maintenance dose in mild conditions 100–200 mg daily, in moderately severe conditions 300–600 mg daily, in severe conditions 700–900 mg daily; doses over 300 mg daily given in divided doses; CHILD under 15 years, (in neoplastic conditions, enzyme disorders) 10–20 mg/kg daily (max. 400 mg daily)

Allopurinol (Non-proprietary) PoM
Tablets, allopurinol 100 mg, net price 28-tab pack = 91p; 300 mg, 28-tab pack = £2.17. Label: 8, 21, 27
Available from Alpharma, APS, Ashbourne (*Xanthomax®*), Berk (*Caplenal®*), CP, DDSA (*Cosuric®*), Generics, Hillcross, IVAX, Kent, Ranbaxy (*Rimapurinol®*), Sovereign

Zyloric® (GlaxoWellcome) PoM
Tablets, allopurinol 100 mg, net price 100-tab pack = £10.96; 300 mg, 28-tab pack = £7.86. Label: 8, 21, 27

PROBENECID

Indications: prevention of nephrotoxicity associated with cidofovir (section 5.3)

Cautions: ensure adequate fluid intake (about 2–3 litres daily) and render urine alkaline if uric acid overload is high; peptic ulceration, renal impairment (avoid if severe); transient false-positive Benedict's test; G6PD deficiency (section 9.1.5); **interactions:** Appendix 1 (probenecid)

Contra-indications: history of blood disorders, nephrolithiasis, porphyria (section 9.8.2), acute gout attack; avoid aspirin and salicylates

Side-effects: gastro-intestinal disturbances, urinary frequency, headache, flushing, dizziness, alopecia, anaemia, haemolytic anaemia, sore gums; hypersensitivity reactions including anaphylaxis, dermatitis, pruritus, urticaria, fever and Stevens-Johnson syndrome; rarely nephrotic syndrome, hepatic necrosis, leucopenia, aplastic anaemia; toxic epidermal necrolysis reported with concurrent colchicine

Dose: used with cidofovir, see section 5.3

Probenecid (Non-proprietary) PoM
Tablets, probenecid 500 mg. Label: 12, 21, 27
Available on named-patient basis from IDIS (*Benuryl®*, *Probecid®*)

SULFINPYRAZONE
(Sulphinpyrazone)

Indications: gout prophylaxis, hyperuricaemia

Cautions: see under Probenecid; regular blood counts advisable; cardiac disease (may cause salt and water retention); **interactions:** Appendix 1 (sulfinpyrazone)

Contra-indications: see under Probenecid; avoid in hypersensitivity to NSAIDs

Side-effects: gastro-intestinal disturbances, occasionally allergic skin reactions, salt and water retention; rarely blood disorders, gastro-intestinal ulceration and bleeding, acute renal failure, raised liver enzymes, jaundice and hepatitis

Dose: initially 100–200 mg daily with food (or milk) increasing over 2–3 weeks to 600 mg daily (rarely 800 mg daily), continued until serum uric acid concentration normal then reduced for maintenance (maintenance dose may be as low as 200 mg daily)

Anturan® (Novartis) PoM
Tablets, both yellow, s/c, sulfinpyrazone 100 mg, net price 84-tab pack = £4.72; 200 mg, 84-tab pack = £9.38. Label: 12, 21

Hyperuricaemia associated with cytotoxic drugs

Allopurinol is used to prevent hyperuricaemia associated with cytotoxic drugs—see section 8.1 (Hyperuricaemia) and Allopurinol above.

Rasburicase is licensed for the prophylaxis and treatment of acute hyperuricaemia, before and during initiation of chemotherapy, in patients with haematological malignancy and a high tumour burden at risk of rapid lysis.

RASBURICASE

Indications: prophylaxis and treatment of acute hyperuricaemia with initial chemotherapy for haematological malignancy

Cautions: monitor closely for hypersensitivity; atopic allergies; may interfere with test for uric acid—consult product literature

Contra-indications: susceptibility to haemolytic anaemia including G6PD deficiency; pregnancy; breast-feeding

Side-effects: fever; nausea, vomiting; less frequently diarrhoea, headache, hypersensitivity reactions (including rash and bronchospasm); haemolytic anaemia

Dose: *by intravenous infusion*, 200 micrograms/kg once daily for 5–7 days

Fasturtec® (Sanofi-Synthelabo) ▼ PoM
Intravenous infusion, powder for reconstitution, rasburicase, net price 1.5-mg vial (with solvent) = £40.20

Anticholinesterases are used as first-line treatment in *ocular myasthenia gravis* and as an adjunct to immunosuppressant therapy for *generalised myasthenia gravis*.

Corticosteroids are used unless anticholinesterases control symptoms completely. A second-line immunosuppressant such as azathioprine is frequently used to reduce the dose of corticosteroid.

Plasmapheresis or infusion of intravenous immunoglobulin [unlicensed indication] may induce temporary remission in severe relapses, particularly where bulbar or respiratory function is compromised or before thymectomy.

Anticholinesterases

Anticholinesterase drugs enhance neuromuscular transmission in voluntary and involuntary muscle in myasthenia gravis. They prolong the action of acetylcholine by inhibiting the action of the enzyme acetylcholinesterase. Excessive dosage of these drugs may impair neuromuscular transmission and precipitate 'cholinergic crises' by causing a depolarising block. This may be difficult to distinguish from a worsening myasthenic state.

Muscarinic side-effects of anticholinesterases include increased sweating, salivary, and gastric secretion, also increased gastro-intestinal and uterine motility, and bradycardia. These parasympathomimetic effects are antagonised by atropine.

Edrophonium has a very brief action and is therefore used mainly for the diagnosis of myasthenia gravis. A single test-dose usually causes substantial improvement in muscle power (lasting about 5 minutes) in patients with the disease (if respiration already impaired, *only* in conjunction with someone skilled at intubation).

Edrophonium can also be used to determine whether a patient with myasthenia is receiving inadequate or excessive treatment with cholinergic drugs. If treatment is excessive an injection of edrophonium will either have no effect or will intensify symptoms (if respiration already impaired, *only* in conjunction with someone skilled at intubation). Conversely, transient improvement may be seen if the patient is being inadequately treated. The test is best performed just before the next dose of anticholinesterase.

Neostigmine produces a therapeutic effect for up to 4 hours. Its pronounced muscarinic action is a disadvantage, and simultaneous administration of an antimuscarinic drug such as atropine or propantheline may be required to prevent colic, excessive salivation, or diarrhoea. In severe disease neostigmine may be given every 2 hours. The maximum that most patients can tolerate is 180 mg daily.

Pyridostigmine is less powerful and slower in action than neostigmine but it has a longer duration of action. It is preferable to neostigmine because of its smoother action and the need for less frequent dosage. It is particularly preferred in patients whose muscles are weak on wakening. It has a comparatively mild gastro-intestinal effect but an antimuscarinic drug may still be required. It is inadvisable to exceed a total daily dose of 450 mg in order to avoid acetylcholine receptor downregulation. Immunosuppressant therapy may be required if the dose of pyridostigmine exceeds 360 mg daily.

Distigmine has the longest action but the danger of a 'cholinergic crisis' caused by accumulation of the drug is greater than with shorter-acting drugs; it is rarely used in the management of myasthenia gravis.

Neostigmine and edrophonium are also used to reverse the actions of the non-depolarising muscle relaxants (see section 15.1.6).

NEOSTIGMINE

Indications: myasthenia gravis; other indications (section 15.1.6)

Cautions: asthma (*extreme* caution), bradycardia, recent myocardial infarction, epilepsy, hypotension, parkinsonism, vagotonia, peptic ulceration, renal impairment, pregnancy and breastfeeding; atropine or other antidote to muscarinic effects may be necessary (particularly when neostigmine is given by injection), but not given routinely because it may mask signs of overdosage; **interactions:** Appendix 1 (parasympathomimetics)

Contra-indications: intestinal or urinary obstruction

Side-effects: nausea, vomiting, increased salivation, diarrhoea, abdominal cramps (more marked with higher doses); signs of overdosage include bronchoconstriction, increased bronchial secretions, lacrimation, excessive sweating, involuntary defaecation and micturition, miosis, nystagmus, bradycardia, heart block, arrhythmias, hypotension, agitation, excessive dreaming, and weakness eventually leading to fasciculation and paralysis

Dose: *by mouth*, neostigmine bromide 15–30 mg at suitable intervals throughout day, total daily dose 75–300 mg (but see also notes above); NEONATE 1–5 mg every 4 hours, half an hour before feeds; CHILD up to 6 years initially 7.5 mg, 6–12 years initially 15 mg, usual total daily dose 15–90 mg

By subcutaneous or intramuscular injection, neostigmine metilsulfate 1–2.5 mg at suitable intervals throughout day (usual total daily dose 5–20 mg); NEONATE 50–250 micrograms every 4 hours half an hour before feeds; CHILD 200–500 micrograms as required

Neostigmine (Non-proprietary) PoM
Tablets, scored, neostigmine bromide 15 mg. Net price 20 = £3.57
Available from Cambridge
Injection, neostigmine metilsulfate 2.5 mg/mL.
Net price 1-mL amp = 58p
Available from Antigen, Phoenix

DISTIGMINE BROMIDE

Indications: myasthenia gravis (but rarely used); urinary retention and other indications (section 7.4.1)

Cautions: see under Neostigmine; also oesophagitis

Contra-indications: see under Neostigmine; also severe constipation, severe postoperative shock, serious circulatory insufficiency

Side-effects: see under Neostigmine

Dose: initially 5 mg daily half an hour before breakfast, increased at intervals of 3–4 days if necessary to a max. of 20 mg daily; CHILD up to 10 mg daily according to age

Preparations
Section 7.4.1

EDROPHONIUM CHLORIDE

Indications: see under Dose and notes above; reversal of non-depolarising neuromuscular blockade and diagnosis of dual block (section 15.1.6)

Cautions: see under Neostigmine; have resuscitation facilities; *extreme* caution in respiratory distress (see notes above) and in asthma

Note. Severe cholinergic reactions can be counteracted by injection of atropine sulphate (which should always be available)

Contra-indications: see under Neostigmine

Side-effects: see under Neostigmine

Dose: diagnosis of myasthenia gravis, *by intravenous injection*, 2 mg followed after 30 seconds (if no adverse reaction has occurred) by 8 mg; in adults without suitable veins, *by intramuscular injection*, 10 mg

Detection of overdosage or underdosage of cholinergic drugs, *by intravenous injection*, 2 mg (best before next dose of anticholinesterase, see notes above)

CHILD *by intravenous injection*, 20 micrograms/kg followed after 30 seconds (if no adverse reaction has occurred) by 80 micrograms/kg

Edrophonium (Non-proprietary) PoM
Injection, edrophonium chloride 10 mg/mL. Net price 1-mL amp = £4.58
Available from Cambridge

PYRIDOSTIGMINE BROMIDE

Indications: myasthenia gravis

Cautions: see under Neostigmine; weaker muscarinic action

Contra-indications: see under Neostigmine

Side-effects: see under Neostigmine

Dose: *by mouth*, 30–120 mg at suitable intervals throughout day, total daily dose 0.3–1.2 g (but see also notes above); NEONATE 5–10 mg every 4 hours, 30–60 minutes before feeds; CHILD up to 6 years initially 30 mg, 6–12 years initially 60 mg, usual total daily dose 30–360 mg

Mestinon® (ICN) PoM
Tablets, scored, pyridostigmine bromide 60 mg. Net price 20 = £5.02

Immunosuppressant therapy

Corticosteroids (section 6.3) are established as treatment for myasthenia gravis; although they are commonly given on alternative days there is little evidence of benefit over daily administration. Corticosteroid treatment is usually initiated under in-patient supervision and all patients should receive osteoporosis prophylaxis.

In *generalised myasthenia gravis* small initial doses of prednisolone (10 mg on alternate days) are increased in steps of 10 mg on alternate days to 1–1.5 mg/kg on alternate days. About 10% of patients experience a transient but very serious worsening of symptoms in the first 2–3 weeks, especially if the corticosteroid is started at a high dose. However, ventilated patients may be started on 1.5 mg/kg on alternate days. Smaller doses of corticosteroid are usually required in *ocular myasthenia*. Once clini-

cal remission has occurred (usually after 2–6 months), the dose of prednisolone should be reduced slowly to the minimum effective dose (usually 10–40 mg on alternate days).

The use of **azathioprine** (section 8.2.1) allows the maintenance dose of the corticosteroid to be reduced; azathioprine is initiated at a low dose which is increased over 3–4 weeks to 2–2.5 mg/kg daily. **Ciclosporin** (section 8.2.2), **methotrexate** (section 8.1.3), or **mycophenolate mofetil** (section 8.2.1) may be used in patients unresponsive or intolerant to other treatments [unlicensed indications].

10.2.2 Skeletal muscle relaxants

Drugs described below are used for the relief of chronic muscle spasm or spasticity associated with multiple sclerosis or other neurological damage; they are not indicated for spasm associated with minor injuries. They act principally on the central nervous system with the exception of dantrolene which has a peripheral site of action. They differ in action from the muscle relaxants used in anaesthesia (section 15.1.5) which block transmission at the neuromuscular junction.

The underlying cause of spasticity should be treated and any aggravating factors (e.g. pressure sores, infection) remedied. Skeletal muscle relaxants are effective in most forms of spasticity except the rare alpha variety. The major disadvantage of treatment with these drugs is that reduction in muscle tone can cause a loss of splinting action of the spastic leg and trunk muscles and sometimes lead to an increase in disability.

Dantrolene acts directly on skeletal muscle and produces fewer central adverse effects making it a drug of choice. The dose should be increased slowly.

Baclofen inhibits transmission at spinal level and also depresses the central nervous system. The dose should be increased slowly to avoid the major side-effects of sedation and muscular hypotonia (other adverse events are uncommon).

Diazepam may also be used. Sedation and, occasionally, extensor hypotonus are disadvantages. Other benzodiazepines also have muscle-relaxant properties. Muscle-relaxant doses of benzodiazepines are similar to anxiolytic doses (section 4.1.2).

Tizanidine is a newly introduced alpha$_2$-adrenoceptor agonist indicated for spasticity associated with multiple sclerosis or spinal cord injury.

BACLOFEN

Indications: chronic severe spasticity resulting from disorders such as multiple sclerosis or traumatic partial section of spinal cord

Cautions: renal impairment (Appendix 3); psychiatric illness, cerebrovascular disease, elderly; respiratory impairment, epilepsy; history of peptic ulcer; diabetes; hypertonic bladder sphincter; pregnancy (Appendix 4); avoid abrupt withdrawal (risk of hyperactive state, may exacerbate spasticity, and precipitate autonomic dysfunction including hyperthermia, psychiatric reactions and convulsions, see also under Withdrawal below); porphyria (section 9.8.2); **interactions:** Appendix 1 (muscle relaxants)

WITHDRAWAL. CSM has advised that serious side-effects can occur on abrupt withdrawal; to minimise risk, discontinue by gradual dose reduction over at least 1–2 weeks (longer if symptoms occur)

DRIVING. Drowsiness may affect performance of skilled tasks (e.g. driving); effects of alcohol enhanced

Contra-indications: peptic ulceration

Side-effects: frequently sedation, drowsiness, muscular hypotonia, nausea, urinary disturbances; occasionally lassitude, confusion, speech disturbance, dizziness, ataxia, hallucinations, nightmares, headache, euphoria, insomnia, depression, anxiety, agitation, tremor, nystagmus, paraesthesias, convulsions, myalgia, fever, respiratory or cardiovascular depression, hypotension, dry mouth, gastro-intestinal disturbances, sexual dysfunction, visual disorders, rash, pruritus, urticaria, hyperhidrosis, angioedema; rarely taste alterations, blood sugar changes, and paradoxical increase in spasticity

Dose: *by mouth*, 5 mg 3 times daily, preferably with or after food, gradually increased; max. 100 mg daily (discontinue if no benefit within 6 weeks); CHILD 0.75–2 mg/kg daily (over 10 years, max. 2.5 mg/kg daily) *or* 2.5 mg 4 times daily increased gradually according to age to maintenance: 1–2 years 10–20 mg daily, 2–6 years 20–30 mg daily, 6–10 years 30–60 mg daily

By intrathecal injection, see preparation below

Baclofen (Non-proprietary) PoM
Tablets, baclofen 10 mg, net price 28-tab pack = £1.02, 84-tab pack = £3.05. Label: 2, 8
Available from Alpharma, APS, Ashbourne (*Baclospas*®), Berk (*Balgifen*®), Hillcross, IVAX, Lagap

Lioresal® (Cephalon) PoM
Tablets, scored, baclofen 10 mg. Net price 84-tab pack = £10.84. Label: 2, 8
Excipients: include gluten
Liquid, sugar-free, raspberry-flavoured, baclofen 5 mg/5 mL. Net price 300 mL = £8.95. Label: 2, 8

■ By intrathecal injection

Lioresal® (Novartis) PoM
Intrathecal injection, baclofen, 50 micrograms/mL, net price 1-mL amp (for test dose) = £2.74; 500 micrograms/mL, 20-mL amp (for use with implantable pump) = £60.77; 2 mg/mL, 5-mL amp (for use with implantable pump) = £60.77
Important: consult product literature for details on dose testing and titration—important to monitor patients closely in appropriately equipped and staffed environment during screening and immediately after pump implantation, and to have resuscitation equipment available for immediate use
Dose: by intrathecal injection, specialist use only, severe chronic spasticity unresponsive to oral antispastic drugs (or where side-effects of oral therapy unacceptable) *or* as alternative to ablative neurosurgical procedures, initial *test dose* 25–50 micrograms over at least 1 minute via catheter or lumbar puncture, increased in 25-microgram steps (not more often than every 24 hours) to max. 100 micrograms to determine appropriate dose *then dose-titration phase*, most often using infusion pump (implanted into chest wall or abdominal wall tissues) to establish *appropriate maintenance dose* (ranging from 12 micrograms to 2 mg daily for spasticity of spinal origin *or* 22 micrograms to 1.4 mg daily for

spasticity of cerebral origin) retaining some spasticity to avoid sensation of paralysis; CHILD 4–18 years (spasticity of cerebral origin only), initial *test dose* 25 micrograms then titrated as for ADULT to *appropriate maintenance dose* (ranging from 24 micrograms to 1.2 mg daily in children under 12 years)

DANTROLENE SODIUM

Indications: chronic severe spasticity of voluntary muscle; malignant hyperthermia (section 15.1.8)

Cautions: impaired cardiac and pulmonary function; test liver function before and at intervals during therapy; therapeutic effect may take a few weeks to develop but if treatment is ineffective it should be discontinued after 4–6 weeks. Avoid when spasticity is useful, for example, locomotion; **interactions:** Appendix 1 (muscle relaxants).

DRIVING. Drowsiness may affect performance of skilled tasks (e.g. driving); effects of alcohol enhanced

Contra-indications: hepatic impairment (may cause severe liver damage); acute muscle spasm

Side-effects: transient drowsiness, dizziness, weakness, malaise, fatigue, diarrhoea (withdraw if severe, discontinue treatment if recurs on reintroduction), anorexia, nausea, headache, rash; less frequently constipation, dysphagia, speech and visual disturbances, confusion, nervousness, insomnia, depression, seizures, chills, fever, increased urinary frequency; rarely, tachycardia, erratic blood pressure, dyspnoea, haematuria, possible crystalluria, urinary incontinence or retention, pleural effusion, pericarditis, dose-related hepatotoxicity (occasionally fatal) may be more common in women over 30 especially those taking oestrogens

Dose: initially 25 mg daily, may be increased at weekly intervals to max. of 100 mg 4 times daily; usual dose 75 mg 3 times daily; CHILD not recommended

Dantrium® (Procter & Gamble Pharm.) PoM
Capsules, both orange/brown, dantrolene sodium 25 mg, net price 20 = £2.53; 100 mg, 20 = £8.85. Label: 2

DIAZEPAM

Indications: muscle spasm of varied aetiology, including tetanus; other indications (section 4.1.2, section 4.8, section 15.1.4.1)

Cautions: see section 4.1.2; special precautions for intravenous injection (section 4.8.2)

Contra-indications: see section 4.1.2

Side-effects: see section 4.1.2; also hypotonia

Dose: *by mouth*, 2–15 mg daily in divided doses, increased if necessary in spastic conditions to 60 mg daily according to response
Cerebral spasticity in selected cases, CHILD 2–40 mg daily in divided doses

By intramuscular or by slow intravenous injection (into a large vein at a rate of not more than 5 mg/minute), in acute muscle spasm, 10 mg repeated if necessary after 4 hours
Note. Only use intramuscular route when oral and intravenous routes not possible; special precautions for intravenous injection see section 4.8.2

Tetanus, ADULT and CHILD, *by intravenous injection*, 100–300 micrograms/kg repeated every 1–4 hours; *by intravenous infusion* (*or by nasoduodenal tube*), 3–10 mg/kg over 24 hours, adjusted according to response

Preparations

Section 4.1.2

TIZANIDINE

Indications: spasticity associated with multiple sclerosis or spinal cord injury or disease

Cautions: elderly, renal impairment (Appendix 3), pregnancy and breast-feeding, monitor liver function monthly for first 4 months and in those who develop unexplained nausea, anorexia or fatigue; concomitant administration of drugs that prolong QT interval; **interactions:** Appendix 1 (muscle relaxants)

DRIVING Drowsiness may affect performance of skilled tasks (e.g. driving); effects of alcohol enhanced

Contra-indications: severe hepatic impairment

Side-effects: drowsiness, fatigue, dizziness, dry mouth, nausea, gastro-intestinal disturbances, hypotension; also reported, bradycardia, insomnia, hallucinations and altered liver enzymes (discontinue if persistently raised—consult product literature); rarely acute hepatitis

Dose: initially 2 mg daily as a single dose increased according to response at intervals of at least 3–4 days in steps of 2 mg daily (and given in divided doses) usually up to 24 mg daily in 3–4 divided doses; max. 36 mg daily; CHILD not recommended

Zanaflex® (Elan) [PoM]

Tablets, scored, tizanidine (as hydrochloride) 2 mg, net price 120-tab pack = £71.76; 4 mg, 120-tab pack = £89.70. Label: 2

Other muscle relaxants

The clinical efficacy of carisoprodol, meprobamate (section 4.1.2), and methocarbamol as muscle relaxants is **not** well established although they have been included in compound analgesic preparations.

CARISOPRODOL [image]

Indications: short-term symptomatic relief of muscle spasm (but see notes above)

Cautions: see under Meprobamate (section 4.1.2)

Contra-indications: see under Meprobamate (section 4.1.2); porphyria (section 9.8.2)

Side-effects: see under Meprobamate (section 4.1.2); drowsiness is common

Dose: 350 mg 3 times daily; ELDERLY half adult dose or less

Carisoma® (Forest) [PoM] [image]

Tablets, carisoprodol 125 mg, net price 100 = £7.10; 350 mg, 100 = £7.95. Label: 2

METHOCARBAMOL [image]

Indications: short-term symptomatic relief of muscle spasm (but see notes above)

Cautions: hepatic and renal impairment; pregnancy; **interactions:** Appendix 1 (muscle relaxants)

DRIVING. Drowsiness may affect performance of skilled tasks (e.g. driving); effects of alcohol enhanced

Contra-indications: coma or pre-coma, brain damage, epilepsy, myasthenia gravis

Side-effects: lassitude, light-headedness, dizziness, restlessness, confusion, drowsiness, nausea, allergic rash or angioedema, convulsions

Dose: 1.5 g 4 times daily; may be reduced to 750 mg 3 times daily; ELDERLY up to 750 mg 4 times daily may be sufficient; CHILD not recommended

Robaxin® (Shire) [PoM] [image]

750 Tablets, f/c, scored, methocarbamol 750 mg, net price 20 = £2.53. Label: 2

> [image] denotes preparations that are considered to be less suitable for prescribing (see p. vi)

Nocturnal leg cramps

Quinine salts (section 5.4.1) 200–300 mg at bedtime are effective in reducing the frequency of nocturnal leg cramps by about 25% in ambulatory patients. It may take up to 4 weeks for improvement to become apparent and it is then given on a continuous basis if there is benefit. Patients should be monitored closely during the early stages for adverse effects as well as for benefit. Treatment should be interrupted at intervals of approximately 3 months to assess the need for further quinine treatment. Quinine is very toxic in overdosage and accidental fatalities have occurred in children (see also below).

QUININE

Indications: see notes above; malaria (section 5.4.1)

Cautions: see section 5.4.1

Contra-indications: see section 5.4.1

Side-effects: see section 5.4.1; **important:** very toxic in **overdosage**—immediate advice from poison centres essential (see also p. 25)

Dose: see notes above

Preparations

Section 5.4.1

10.3	**Drugs for the relief of soft-tissue inflammation**
10.3.1	Enzymes
10.3.2	Rubefacients and other topical antirheumatics

Extravasation

> Local guidelines for the management of extravasation should be followed where they exist or specialist advice sought.

Extravasation injury follows leakage of drugs or intravenous fluids from the veins or inadvertent administration into the subcutaneous or subdermal tissue. It must be dealt with **promptly** to prevent tissue necrosis.

Acidic or alkaline preparations and those with an osmolarity greater than that of plasma can cause extravasation injury and excipients including alcohol and polyethylene glycol have also been implicated. Cytotoxic drugs commonly cause extravasation injury. In addition, certain patients such as the very young and the elderly are at increased risk. Those receiving anticoagulants are more likely to lose blood into surrounding tissues if extravasation occurs whilst those receiving sedatives or analgesics may not notice the early signs or symptoms of extravasation.

PREVENTION OF EXTRAVASATION. Precautions should be taken to avoid extravasation; ideally, drugs liable to cause extravasation injury should be given through a central line and patients receiving repeated doses of hazardous drugs peripherally should have the cannula resited at regular intervals. Attention should be paid to the manufacturers' recommendations for administration. Placing a glyceryl trinitrate patch (section 2.6.1) distal to the cannula may improve the patency of the vessel in patients with small veins or in those whose veins are prone to collapse.

Patients should be asked to report any pain or burning at the site of injection immediately.

MANAGEMENT OF EXTRAVASATION. If extravasation is suspected the infusion should be stopped immediately but the cannula should not be removed until after an attempt has been made to aspirate the area (through the cannula) in order to remove as much of the drug as possible. Aspiration is sometimes possible if the extravasation presents with a raised bleb or blister at the injection site and is surrounded by hardened tissue, but it is often unsuccessful if the tissue is soft or soggy. Corticosteroids are usually given to treat inflammation, although there is little evidence to support their use in extravasation. Hydrocortisone or dexamethasone (section 6.3.2) may be given either locally by subcutaneous injection or intravenously at a site distant from the injury. Antihistamines (section 3.4.1) and analgesics (section 4.7) may be required for symptom relief.

The management of extravasation beyond these measures is not well standardised and calls for specialist advice. Treatment depends on the nature of the offending substance; one approach is to localise and neutralise the substance whereas another is to spread and dilute it. The first method may be appropriate following extravasation of vesicant drugs and involves administration of an antidote (if available) and the application of cold compresses 3–4 times a day (consult specialist literature for details of specific antidotes). Spreading and diluting the offending substance involves infiltrating the area with physiological saline, applying warm compresses, elevating the affected limb, and administering hyaluronidase (section 10.3.1). A saline flush-out technique (involving flushing the subcutaneous tissue with physiological saline) may be effective but requires specialist advice. Hyaluronidase should **not** be administered following extravasation of vesicant drugs (unless it is either specifically indicated or used in the saline flush-out technique).

Hyaluronidase is used to render the tissues more easily permeable to injected fluids, e.g. for introduction of fluids by subcutaneous infusion (termed hypodermoclysis).

HYALURONIDASE

Indications: enhance permeation of subcutaneous or intramuscular injections, local anaesthetics and subcutaneous infusions; promote resorption of excess fluids and blood

Cautions: infants or elderly (control speed and total volume and avoid overhydration especially in renal impairment)

Contra-indications: do not apply direct to cornea; avoid sites where infection or malignancy; not for anaesthesia in unexplained premature labour; not to be used to reduce swelling of bites or stings; not for intravenous administration

Side-effects: occasional severe allergy

Dose: With subcutaneous or intramuscular injection, 1500 units dissolved directly in solution to be injected (ensure compatibility)

With local anaesthetics, 1500 units mixed with local anaesthetic solution (ophthalmology, 15 units/mL)

Hypodermoclysis, 1500 units dissolved in 1 mL water for injections or 0.9% sodium chloride injection, administered before start of 500–1000 mL infusion fluid

Extravasation (see notes above) or haematoma, 1500 units dissolved in 1 mL water for injections or 0.9% sodium chloride injection, infiltrated into affected area (as soon as possible after extravasation)

Hyalase® (CP) PoM

Injection, powder for reconstitution, hyaluronidase (ovine). Net price 1500-unit amp = £7.60

10.3.2 Rubefacients and other topical antirheumatics

Rubefacients act by counter-irritation. Pain, whether superficial or deep-seated, is relieved by any method which itself produces irritation of the skin. Counter-irritation is comforting in painful lesions of the muscles, tendons, and joints, and in non-articular rheumatism. Rubefacients probably all act through the same essential mechanism and differ mainly in intensity and duration of action.

Topical **NSAIDs** (e.g. felbinac, ibuprofen, ketoprofen and piroxicam) may provide some slight relief of pain in musculoskeletal conditions.

Topical NSAIDs and counter-irritants

CAUTIONS. Apply with gentle massage only. Avoid contact with eyes, mucous membranes, and inflamed or broken skin; discontinue if rash develops. Hands should be washed immediately after use. Not for use with occlusive dressings. Topical application of large amounts may result in systemic effects including hypersensitivity and asthma (renal disease has also been reported). Not generally suitable for children. Patient packs carry a **warning** to avoid during **pregnancy** or **breast-feeding**.

HYPERSENSITIVITY. For NSAID hypersensitivity and asthma warning, see p. 476–7

PHOTOSENSITIVITY. Patients should be advised against excessive exposure to sunlight of area treated in order to avoid possibility of photosensitivity

Piroxicam (Non-proprietary) PoM
Gel, piroxicam 0.5%, net price 60 g = £5.00; 112 g = £7.84
Apply 3–4 times daily
Excipients: include propylene glycol
Available from Sovereign

■ Proprietary preparations
Feldene® (Pfizer) PoM
Gel, piroxicam 0.5%. Net price 60 g = £5.00; 112 g = £7.84 (also 7.5 g starter pack, hosp. only)
Apply 3–4 times daily; therapy should be reviewed after 4 weeks
Excipients: include benzyl alcohol, propylene glycol

Fenbid® Forte Gel (Goldshield) PoM
Gel, ibuprofen 10%, net price 100 g = £6.50
Apply up to 4 times daily; therapy should be reviewed after 14 days
Excipients: include benzyl alcohol

Ibugel® (Dermal)
Forte gel PoM, ibuprofen 10%, net price 100 g = £6.50
Apply up to 3 times daily
Excipients: none as listed in section 13.1.3

Oruvail® (Rhône-Poulenc Rorer) PoM
Gel, ketoprofen 2.5%. Net price 100 g = £7.46
Apply 2–4 times daily for up to 7 days (usual recommended dose 15 g daily)
Excipients: include fragrance

Pennsaid® (Provalis) PoM
Topical solution, diclofenac sodium 1.5%, net price 60-mL = £16.00
Pain in osteoarthritis of superficial medium to large joints, apply 0.5–1 mL 4 times daily
Excipients: include propylene glycol

Powergel® (Menarini) PoM
Gel, ketoprofen 2.5%. Net price 50 g = £3.25; 100 g = £6.25
Apply 2–3 times daily for up to max. 10 days
Excipients: include hydroxybenzoates (parabens), fragrance

Traxam® (Goldshield) PoM
Foam, felbinac 3.17%. Net price 100 g = £7.00. Label:15
Excipients: include cetostearyl alcohol
Gel, felbinac 3%. Net price 100 g = £7.00
Apply 2–4 times daily; max. 25 g daily; therapy should be reviewed after 14 days
Excipients: none as listed in section 13.1.3
Note. Felbinac is an active metabolite of the NSAID fenbufen

Voltarol Emulgel® (Novartis) PoM
Gel, diclofenac diethylammonium salt 1.16% (equivalent to diclofenac sodium 1%). Net price 20 g (hosp. only) = £1.55; 100 g = £7.00
Apply 3–4 times daily; therapy should be reviewed after 14 days (or after 28 days for osteoarthritis)
Excipients: include propylene glycol, fragrance

Topical NSAIDs and counter-irritants on sale to the public together with their significant ingredients include:

Algesal® (diethylamine salicylate), **Algipan Rub®** (capsicum oleoresin, glycol salicylate, methyl nicotinate), **Balmosa®** (camphor, capsicum oleoresin, menthol, methyl salicylate), **Boots Pain Relief Balm®** (ethyl nicotinate, glycol monosalicylate, nonylic acid vanillylamide), **Boots Pain Relief Embrocation®** (camphor, turpentine oil), **Boots Pain Relief Warming Spray®** (camphor, ethyl nicotinate, methyl salicylate), **Cremalgin®** (capsicin, glycol salicylate, methyl nicotinate), **Cuprofen® Ibutop® Gel** (ibuprofen) **Deep Freeze Cold Gel®** (menthol), **Deep Freeze Spray®** (levomenthol), **Deep Heat Massage Liniment®**, **Deep Heat Maximum®** (menthol, methyl salicylate), **Deep Heat Rub®** (eucalyptus oil, menthol, methyl salicylate, turpentine oil), **Deep Heat Spray®** (glycol salicylate, ethyl salicylate, methyl salicylate, methyl nicotinate), **Deep Relief®** (ibuprofen, menthol), **Difflam® Cream** (benzydamine), **Difflam®-P Cream** (benzydamine), **Dubam Cream®** (methyl salicylate, menthol, cineole), **Dubam Spray®** (ethyl salicylate, methyl salicylate, glycol salicylate, methyl nicotinate) **Elliman's Universal Embrocation®** (acetic acid, turpentine oil) **Feldene P® Gel** (piroxicam), **Fenbid® Gel** (ibuprofen), **Fiery Jack Cream®** (capsicum oleoresin, diethylamine salicylate, glycol salicylate, methyl nicotinate), **Fiery Jack Ointment®** (capsicum oleoresin) **Goddard's White Oil Embrocation®** (dilute acetic acid, dilute ammonia solution, turpentine oil) **Hansaplast® Thermo Plaster** (capsaicinoids, colophony) **Ibuderm®** (ibuprofen), **Ibugel®** (ibuprofen), **Ibuleve®**, **Ibuleve Mousse®**, **Ibuleve Sports Gel®** (ibuprofen), **Ibumousse®** (ibuprofen), **Ibuspray®** (ibuprofen), **Intralgin®** (benzocaine, salicylamide) **Lloyds Cream®** (diethyl salicylate) **Mentholatum® Ibuprofen Gel** (ibuprofen), **Movelat® Cream** (mucopolysaccharide polysulphate, salicylic acid, thymol), **Movelat® Gel** (mucopolysaccharide polysulphate, salicylic acid), **Movelat® Relief Cream** (mucopolysaccharide polysulphate, salicylic acid, thymol), **Movelat® Relief Gel** (mucopolysaccharide polysulphate, salicylic acid) **Nasciodine®** (camphor, iodine, menthol, methyl salicylate, turpentine oil), **Nella Red Oil®** (arachis oil, clove oil, mustard oil, methyl nicotinate) **Nurofen® Gel Maximum Strength** (ibuprofen), **Nurofen® Muscular Pain Relief Gel** (ibuprofen), **Oruvail® Gel** (ketoprofen 30-g tube; 100-g tube prescribable on NHS (PoM)) **PR Heat Spray®** (ethyl nicotinate, methyl salicylate, camphor); **Proflex® Cream** (ibuprofen), **Proflex Pain Relief Gel®** (ibuprofen) **Radian®-B Ibuprofen Gel** (ibuprofen), **Radian®-B Muscle Lotion**, **Radian®-B Heat Spray** (ammonium salicylate, camphor, menthol, salicylic acid), **Radian®-B Muscle Rub** (camphor, capsicin, menthol, methyl salicylate), **Ralgex Cream®** (capsicin, glycol monosalicylate, methyl nicotinate), **Ralgex Freeze Spray®** (dimethyl ether, glycol monosalicylate, isopentane), **Ralgex® Ibutop® Gel** (ibuprofen), **Ralgex Low Odour Spray®** (glycol monosalicylate, methyl nicotinate), **Ralgex Spray®** (ethyl salicylate, methyl salicylate, glycol monosalicylate, methyl nicotinate), **Ralgex Stick®** (capsicin, ethyl salicylate, methyl salicylate, glycol salicylate, menthol)

Salonair® (benzyl nicotinate, camphor, glycol salicylate, menthol, methyl salicylate, squalane), **Salonpas Plasters**® (glycol salicylate, methyl salicylate), **Solpaflex® Gel** (ketoprofen)

Tiger Balm Red® (camphor, clove oil, cajuput oil, menthol), **Tiger Balm White**® (cajuput oil, camphor, clove oil, menthol), **Transvasin Cream**® (ethyl nicotinate, hexyl nicotinate, thurfyl salicylate), **Transvasin Spray**® (diethylamine salicylate, hydroxyethyl salicylate, methyl nicotinate), **Traxam Pain Relief**® (felbinac)

Capsaicin

CAUTIONS. See under Topical NSAIDs and Counter-irritants, above; avoid taking a hot shower or bath just before or after applying capsaicin—burning sensation enhanced.

SIDE-EFFECTS. Transient burning sensation may occur during initial treatment, particularly if too much cream is used, or if the frequency of administration is less than 3–4 times daily.

Axsain® (Elan) PoM
 Cream, capsaicin 0.075%. Net price 45 g = £15.04. For post-herpetic neuralgia (**important: after** lesions have healed), apply a small amount up to 3–4 times daily; for painful diabetic neuropathy, under supervision of hospital consultant, apply 3–4 times daily for 8 weeks then review
 Excipients: include benzyl alcohol, cetyl alcohol

Zacin® (Elan) PoM
 Cream, capsaicin 0.025%. Net price 45 g = £15.04. Symptomatic relief in osteoarthritis, apply a small amount 4 times daily
 Excipients: include benzyl alcohol, cetyl alcohol

Poultices

Kaolin Poultice ◢◣ , heavy kaolin 52.7%, thymol 0.05%, boric acid 4.5%, peppermint oil 0.05%, methyl salicylate 0.2%, glycerol 42.5%. Net price 200 g = £1.91
 Warm and apply directly or between layers of muslin; avoid application of overheated poultice
Kaolin Poultice K/L Pack® (K/L) ◢◣
 Kaolin poultice. Net price 4 × 100-g pouches = £5.72

◢◣ denotes preparations that are considered to be less suitable for prescribing (see p. vi)

11: Eye

11.1   Administration of drugs to the eye

EYE DROPS AND EYE OINTMENTS. When administered in the form of eye drops, drugs penetrate the globe, probably through the cornea. However, systemic effects, which are usually undesirable, may well arise from absorption of drugs into the general circulation via conjunctival vessels or from the nasal mucosa after the excess of the preparation has drained down through the tear ducts; nasal drainage of drugs is much more often associated with eye drops than with eye ointments. For example, a beta-blocker administered as eye drops may induce bronchospasm or bradycardia in susceptible individuals. The extent of systemic absorption following ocular administration is highly variable.

Eye drops are generally instilled into the pocket formed by gently pulling down the lower eyelid and keeping the eye closed for as long as possible after application, preferably 1–2 minutes; one drop is all that is needed. A small amount of eye ointment is applied similarly; the ointment melts rapidly and blinking helps to spread it.

When two different preparations in the form of eye drops are required at the same time of day, for example pilocarpine and timolol in glaucoma, dilution and overflow may occur when one immediately follows the other. The patient should therefore leave an interval of 5 minutes.

Generally it is inadvisable for patients to continue to wear contact lenses, particularly hydrophilic (soft) contact lenses when receiving eye drops. For warnings relating to eye drops and contact lenses, see section 11.9.

EYE LOTIONS. These are solutions for the irrigation of the conjunctival sac. They act mechanically to flush out irritants or foreign bodies as a first-aid treatment. Sterile sodium chloride 0.9% solution (section 11.8.1) is usually used. Clean water will suffice in an emergency.

OTHER PREPARATIONS. Subconjunctival injection may be used to administer anti-infective drugs, mydriatics, or corticosteroids for conditions not responding to topical therapy. The drug diffuses through the cornea and sclera to the anterior and posterior chambers and vitreous humour. However, because the dose-volume is limited (usually not more than 1 mL), this route is suitable only for drugs which are readily soluble.

Drugs such as antimicrobials and corticosteroids may be administered systemically to treat an eye condition. Implants which gradually release a drug over a prolonged period are also available (e.g. *Vitrasert*®).

PRESERVATIVES AND SENSITISERS. Information on preservatives and on substances identified as skin sensitisers (see section 13.1.3) is provided under preparation entries.

11.2 Control of microbial contamination

Preparations for the eye should be sterile when issued. Eye drops in multiple-application containers include a preservative but care should nevertheless be taken to avoid contamination of the contents during use.

Eye drops in multiple-application containers for *domiciliary use* should not be used for more than 4 weeks after first opening (unless otherwise stated).

Eye drops for use in *hospital wards* are normally discarded 1 week after first opening. Individual containers should be provided for each patient. Containers used before an operation should be discarded at the time of the operation and fresh containers supplied. A fresh supply should also be provided upon discharge from hospital; it may be acceptable in specialist ophthalmology units to issue on discharge eye drop bottles that have been in use for the patient for less than 36 hours.

Eye drops used in *out-patient departments* should be discarded at the end of each day. In clinics for eye diseases and in accident and emergency departments, where the dangers of infection are high, single-application packs should be used; if a multiple-application pack is used, it should be discarded after single use.

Diagnostic dyes (e.g. fluorescein) should be used only from single-application packs.

In *eye surgery* it is wise to use single-application containers. Preparations used during intra-ocular procedures and others that may penetrate into the anterior chamber must be isotonic and without preservatives and buffered if necessary to a neutral pH. Large volume intravenous infusion preparations are not suitable for this purpose. For all surgical procedures, a previously unopened container is used for each patient.

11.3 Anti-infective eye preparations

11.3.1	Antibacterials
11.3.2	Antifungals
11.3.3	Antivirals

EYE INFECTIONS. Most acute superficial eye infections can be treated topically. Blepharitis and conjunctivitis are often caused by staphylococci; keratitis and endophthalmitis may be bacterial, viral, or fungal.

Bacterial *blepharitis* is treated by application of an antibacterial eye ointment to the conjunctival sac or to the lid margins. Systemic treatment may occasionally be required and is usually undertaken after culturing organisms from the lid margin and determining their antimicrobial sensitivity; antibiotics such as the tetracyclines given for 3 months or longer may be appropriate.

Acute *infective conjunctivitis* is treated with antibacterial eye drops and eye ointment. A poor response might indicate viral or allergic conjunctivitis. *Gonococcal conjunctivitis* is treated with systemic and topical antibacterials.

Corneal ulcer and *keratitis* require specialist treatment and may call for subconjunctival or systemic administration of antimicrobials.

Endophthalmitis is a medical emergency which also calls for specialist management and often requires parenteral, subconjunctival, or intra-ocular administration of antimicrobials.

For reference to the treatment of *crab lice of the eyelashes*, see section 13.10.4

11.3.1 Antibacterials

Bacterial infections are generally treated topically with eye drops and eye ointments. Systemic administration is sometimes appropriate in blepharitis. In intra-ocular infection, a variety of routes (intracorneal, intravitreal and systemic) may be used.

Chloramphenicol has a broad spectrum of activity and is the drug of choice for *superficial eye infections*. Chloramphenicol eye drops are well tolerated and the recommendation that chloramphenicol eye drops should be avoided because of an increased risk of aplastic anaemia is not well founded.

Other antibiotics with a broad spectrum of activity include **framycetin**, **gentamicin**, and **neomycin**, and also **ciprofloxacin**, **ofloxacin** and the recently introduced **lomefloxacin**. Gentamicin, ciprofloxacin and ofloxacin are effective for infections caused by *Pseudomonas aeruginosa*.

Ciprofloxacin eye drops are licensed for *corneal ulcers*; intensive application (especially in the first 2 days) is required throughout the day and night.

Chlortetracycline is used in the treatment of *chlamydial infections* including *trachoma* (consult World Health Organization guidelines).

Fusidic acid is useful for staphylococcal infections.

Propamidine isetionate is of little value in bacterial infections but is specific for the rare but potentially devastating condition of *acanthamoeba keratitis* (see also section 11.9).

WITH CORTICOSTEROIDS. Many antibacterial preparations also incorporate a corticosteroid but such mixtures should **not** be used unless a patient is under close specialist supervision. In particular they should not be prescribed for undiagnosed 'red eye' which is sometimes caused by the herpes simplex virus and may be difficult to diagnose (section 11.4).

ADMINISTRATION
Eye drops. Apply 1 drop at least every 2 hours then reduce frequency as infection is controlled and continue for 48 hours after healing.
Eye ointment. Apply *either* at night (if eye drops used during the day) *or* 3–4 times daily (if eye ointment used alone).

CHLORAMPHENICOL

Indications: see notes above
Side-effects: transient stinging; see also notes above
Administration: see notes above

Chloramphenicol (Non-proprietary) PoM

Eye drops, chloramphenicol 0.5%. Net price
10 mL = £1.17

Eye ointment, chloramphenicol 1%. Net price 4 g =
£1.04

Chloromycetin® (Goldshield) PoM

Redidrops (= eye drops), chloramphenicol 0.5%.
Net price 5 mL = £1.65; 10 mL = £2.01
Excipients: include phenylmercuric acetate

Ophthalmic ointment (= eye ointment), chloramphenicol 1%. Net price 4 g = £2.01

Sno Phenicol® (Chauvin) PoM

Eye drops, chloramphenicol 0.5%, in a viscous
vehicle. Net price 10 mL = £1.08
Excipients: include chlorhexidine acetate

■ Single use

Minims® Chloramphenicol (Chauvin) PoM

Eye drops, chloramphenicol 0.5%. Net price 20 ×
0.5 mL = £4.92

CHLORTETRACYCLINE

Indications: local treatment of infections, including trachoma (see notes above)

Administration: see notes above

Aureomycin® (Lederle) PoM

Ophthalmic ointment (= eye ointment), chlortetracycline hydrochloride 1%. Net price 3.5 g = 92p

CIPROFLOXACIN

Indications: superficial bacterial infections, see
notes above; corneal ulcers

Cautions: not recommended for children under 1
year; pregnancy and breast-feeding

Side-effects: local burning and itching; lid margin
crusting; hyperaemia; taste disturbance; corneal
staining, keratitis, lid oedema, lacrimation, photophobia, corneal infiltrates; nausea and visual disturbances reported

Administration: superficial bacterial infection,
see notes above
Corneal ulcer, apply throughout day and night,
day 1 apply every 15 minutes for 6 hours then
every 30 minutes, then on day 2 apply every hour,
days 3–14 apply every 4 hours; if longer treatment required physician to decide frequency
(max. duration of treatment 21 days)

Ciloxan® (Alcon) PoM

Ophthalmic solution (= eye drops), ciprofloxacin
(as hydrochloride) 0.3%. Net price 5 mL = £4.94
Excipients: include benzalkonium chloride

FRAMYCETIN SULPHATE

Indications: see notes above
Administration: see notes above

Soframycin® (Florizel) PoM

Eye drops, framycetin sulphate 0.5%. Net price
10 mL = £4.62
Excipients: include benzalkonium chloride

Eye ointment, framycetin sulphate 0.5%. Net price
5 g = £2.52

FUSIDIC ACID

Indications: see notes above
Administration: see under preparation below

Fucithalmic® (Leo) PoM

Eye drops, m/r, fusidic acid 1% in gel basis (liqui-
fies on contact with eye). Net price 5 g = £2.09
Excipients: include benzalkonium chloride, disodium edetate
Apply twice daily

GENTAMICIN

Indications: see notes above
Administration: see notes above

Garamycin® (Schering-Plough) PoM

Drops (for ear or eye), gentamicin 0.3% (as sulphate). Net price 10 mL = £1.79
Excipients: include benzalkonium chloride

Genticin® (Roche) PoM

Drops (for ear or eye), gentamicin 0.3% (as sulphate). Net price 10 mL = £1.91
Excipients: include benzalkonium chloride

■ Single use

Minims® Gentamicin Sulphate (Chauvin) PoM

Eye drops, gentamicin 0.3% (as sulphate). Net
price 20 × 0.5 mL = £5.75

LOMEFLOXACIN

Indications: see notes above
Cautions: pregnancy and breast-feeding
Side-effects: local irritation; rarely hypersensitivity reactions
Administration: initially apply every 5 minutes
for 20 minutes (5 doses), then twice daily for 7–9
days

Okacyn® (Novartis Ophthalmics) ▼ PoM

Eye drops, lomefloxacin (as hydrochloride) 0.3%,
net price 5 mL = £2.05
Excipients: include benzalkonium chloride, disodium edetate

NEOMYCIN SULPHATE

Indications: see notes above
Administration: see notes above

Neomycin (Non-proprietary) PoM

Eye drops, neomycin sulphate 0.5% (3500 units/
mL). Net price 10 mL = £2.96
Available from Martindale

Eye ointment, neomycin sulphate 0.5%
(3500 units/g). Net price 3 g = £2.32
Available from Martindale

■ Single use

Minims® Neomycin Sulphate (Chauvin) PoM

Eye drops, neomycin sulphate 0.5%. Net price 20
× 0.5 mL = £5.75
Excipients: include disodium edetate

■ With antibacterials

Neosporin® (Dominion) [PoM]
Eye drops, gramicidin 25 units, neomycin sulphate
1700 units, polymyxin B sulphate 5000 units/mL.
Net price 5 mL = £5.12
Excipients: include thiomersal
Apply 2–4 times daily or more frequently if required

■ With hydrocortisone
Section 12.1.1

OFLOXACIN

Indications: see notes above
Cautions: pregnancy and breast-feeding; not to be
used for more than 10 days
Side-effects: local irritation including photophobia; dizziness, numbness, nausea and headache
reported
Administration: see notes above

Exocin® (Allergan) [PoM]
Ophthalmic solution (= eye drops), ofloxacin
0.3%. Net price 5 mL = £2.17
Excipients: include benzalkonium chloride

POLYMYXIN B SULPHATE

Indications: see notes above
Administration: see notes above

■ With antibacterials

Polyfax® (Dominion) [PoM]
Eye ointment, polymyxin B sulphate 10 000 units,
bacitracin zinc 500 units/g. Net price 4 g = £3.26

Polytrim® (Dominion) [PoM]
Eye drops, trimethoprim 0.1%, polymyxin B sul-
phate 10 000 units/mL. Net price 5 mL = £3.05
Excipients: include thiomersal
Eye ointment, trimethoprim 0.5%, polymyxin B
sulphate 10 000 units/g. Net price 4 g = £3.05

PROPAMIDINE ISETIONATE

Indications: local treatment of infections (but see
notes above)

Brolene® (Rhône-Poulenc Rorer)
Eye drops, propamidine isetionate 0.1%. Net price
10 mL = £2.55
Apply 4 times daily
Excipients: include benzalkonium chloride
Note. Eye drops containing propamidine isetionate 0.1%
also available from Typharm (*Golden Eye Drops*)
Eye ointment, dibromopropamidine isetionate
0.15%. Net price 5 g = £2.67
Apply 1–2 times daily
Note. Eye ointment containing dibromopropamidine ise-
tionate 0.15% also available from Typharm (*Golden Eye
Ointment*)

11.3.2 Antifungals

Fungal infections of the cornea are rare but can
occur after agricultural injuries, especially in hot
and humid climates. Orbital mycosis is rarer, and
when it occurs it is usually because of a direct
spread of infection from the paranasal sinuses.
Increasing age, debility, or immunosuppression

may encourage fungal proliferation. The spread of
infection via the bloodstream occasionally produces
a metastatic endophthalmitis.

Many different fungi are capable of producing
ocular infection; they may be identified by appropriate laboratory procedures.

Antifungal preparations for the eye are not generally available. Treatment will normally be carried
out at specialist centres, but requests for information about supplies of preparations not available
commercially should be addressed to the local
Health Authority (or equivalent in Scotland or
Northern Ireland), or to the nearest hospital ophthalmology unit, or to Moorfields Eye Hospital,
City Road, London EC1V 2PD (tel. (020) 7253
3411).

11.3.3 Antivirals

Herpes simplex infections producing, for example,
dendritic corneal ulcer can be treated with **aciclovir**.
Ganciclovir eye drops are licensed for the treatment of acute herpetic keratitis.

Fomivirsen is licensed for the local treatment of
cytomegalovirus (CMV) retinitis in patients with
AIDS. Slow-release ocular implants containing
ganciclovir (*Vitrasert®*, available from Bausch &
Lomb) may be inserted surgically to treat immediate sight-threatening CMV retinitis. Local treatments do not protect against systemic infection or
infection in the other eye. For systemic treatment of
CMV retinitis, see section 5.3.

ACICLOVIR

(Acyclovir)
Indications: local treatment of herpes simplex
infections
Side-effects: local irritation and inflammation
reported
Administration: apply 5 times daily (continue for
at least 3 days after complete healing)

Zovirax® (GlaxoWellcome) [PoM]
Eye ointment, aciclovir 3%. Net price 4.5 g =
£10.67
Tablets and *injection*, see section 5.3
Cream, see section 13.10.3

FOMIVIRSEN SODIUM

Indications: local treatment of cytomegalovirus
retinitis in patients with AIDS when other therapy
is ineffective or unsuitable
Cautions: monitor intra-ocular pressure and visual
field regularly; recent (2–4 weeks) cidofovir
treatment
Side-effects: local irritation and inflammation (if
severe intra-ocular inflammation occurs suspend
therapy until it improves), conjunctival haemorrhage, visual disturbances, cataract, intra-ocular
pressure increase, retinal disorders (including retinal detachment, haemorrhage and oedema), vitreous disorders (including vitritis and vitreous
haemorrhage); less commonly conjunctivitis,
corneal oedema, cystoid macular oedema, HIV
ocular microangiopathy, photophobia, keratitis,
lens pigment deposits, orbital cellulitis, photopsia
Dose: *by intravitreal injection*, newly diagnosed
disease, 165 micrograms weekly for 3 weeks fol-

lowcd by 165 micrograms every 2 weeks; previously treated disease, 330 micrograms every other week for 2 doses followed by 330 micrograms every 4 weeks

Vitravene® (Novartis Ophthalmics) ▼ PoM
Injection, fomivirsen sodium 6.6 mg/mL (165 micrograms/0.025 mL), net price 0.25-mL vial = £500.00

GANCICLOVIR

Indications: acute herpetic keratitis
Cautions: pregnancy and breast-feeding
Side-effects: ocular irritation, visual disturbances; superficial punctate keratitis
Administration: apply 5 times daily until complete corneal re-epithelialisation, then 3 times daily for 7 days (usual duration of treatment 21 days)

Virgan® (Chauvin) ▼ PoM
Eye drops, ganciclovir 0.15 % in gel basis, net price 5 g = £10.64
Excipients: include benzalkonium chloride

11.4 Corticosteroids and other anti-inflammatory preparations

11.4.1 Corticosteroids
11.4.2 Other anti-inflammatory preparations

11.4.1 Corticosteroids

Corticosteroids administered locally (as eye drops, eye ointments or subconjunctival injection) or by mouth have an important place in treating anterior segment inflammation, including that which results from surgery.

Topical corticosteroids should normally only be used under expert supervision; three main dangers are associated with their use:

- a 'red eye', where the diagnosis is unconfirmed, may be due to herpes simplex virus, and a corticosteroid may aggravate the condition, leading to corneal ulceration, with possible damage to vision and even loss of the eye. Bacterial, fungal and amoebic infections pose a similar hazard;
- 'steroid glaucoma' may follow the use of corticosteroid eye preparations in susceptible individuals;
- a 'steroid cataract' may follow prolonged use.

Other side-effects include thinning of the cornea and sclera.

Use of a combination product containing a corticosteroid with an anti-infective is rarely justified.

Systemic corticosteroids (section 6.3.2) may be useful for ocular conditions. The risk of producing a 'steroid cataract' is very high (75%) if the equivalent of more than 15 mg prednisolone is given daily for several years.

BETAMETHASONE

Indications: local treatment of inflammation (short-term)
Cautions: see notes above
Side-effects: see notes above
Administration: apply eye drops every 1–2 hours until controlled then reduce frequency, eye ointment 2–4 times daily or at night when used with eye drops

Betnesol® (Celltech) PoM
Drops (for ear, eye, or nose), betamethasone sodium phosphate 0.1%. Net price 10 mL = £1.31
Excipients: include benzalkonium chloride, disodium edetate
Eye ointment, betamethasone sodium phosphate 0.1%. Net price 3 g = 56p
Note. May be difficult to obtain

Vista-Methasone® (Martindale) PoM
Drops (for ear, eye, or nose), betamethasone sodium phosphate 0.1%. Net price 5 mL = £1.10; 10 mL = £1.25
Excipients: include benzalkonium chloride

■ With neomycin

Betnesol-N® (Celltech) PoM ▭
Drops (for ear, eye, or nose), see section 12.1.1
Eye ointment, betamethasone sodium phosphate 0.1%, neomycin sulphate 0.5%. Net price 3 g = 64p
Note. May be difficult to obtain

Vista-Methasone N® (Martindale) PoM ▭
Drops (for ear, eye, or nose), see section 12.1.1

CLOBETASONE BUTYRATE

Indications: local treatment of inflammation (short-term)
Cautions: see notes above
Side-effects: see notes above
Administration: apply eye drops 4 times daily; severe conditions every 1–2 hours until controlled then reduce frequency

Cloburate® (Dominion) PoM
Eye drops, clobetasone butyrate 0.1%. Net price 10 mL = £2.72
Excipients: include benzalkonium chloride

DEXAMETHASONE

Indications: local treatment of inflammation (short-term)
Cautions: see notes above
Side-effects: see notes above
Administration: apply eye drops 4–6 times daily; severe conditions every 30–60 minutes until controlled then reduce frequency

Maxidex® (Alcon) PoM
Eye drops, dexamethasone 0.1%, hypromellose 0.5%. Net price 5 mL = £1.49; 10 mL = £2.95
Excipients: include benzalkonium chloride, disodium edetate, polysorbate 80

■ Single use

Minims® Dexamethasone (Chauvin) PoM
Eye drops, dexamethasone sodium phosphate 0.1%. Net price 20 × 0.5 mL = £6.95
Excipients: include disodium edetate

■ With antibacterials

Maxitrol® (Alcon) [PoM] [▨]

Eye drops, dexamethasone 0.1%, hypromellose 0.5%, neomycin 0.35% (as sulphate), polymyxin B sulphate 6000 units/mL. Net price 5 mL = £1.77

Excipients: include benzalkonium chloride, polysorbate 20

Eye ointment, dexamethasone 0.1%, neomycin 0.35% (as sulphate), polymyxin B sulphate 6000 units/g. Net price 3.5 g = £1.52

Excipients: include hydroxybenzoates (parabens), wool fat

Sofradex® (Florizel) [PoM] [▨]

Drops and ointment (for ear or eye), see section 12.1.1

Tobradex® (Alcon) [PoM] [▨]

Eye drops, dexamethasone 0.1%, tobramycin 0.3%. Net price 5 mL = £5.65

Excipients: include benzalkonium chloride, disodium edetate

> [▨] denotes preparations that are considered to be less suitable for prescribing (see p. vi)

FLUOROMETHOLONE

Indications: local treatment of inflammation (short-term)

Cautions: see notes above

Side-effects: see notes above

Administration: apply eye drops 2–4 times daily (initially every hour for 24–48 hours then reduce frequency)

FML® (Allergan) [PoM]

Ophthalmic suspension (= eye drops), fluoro- metholone 0.1%, polyvinyl alcohol (*Liquifilm®*) 1.4%. Net price 5 mL = £1.71; 10 mL = £2.95

Excipients: include benzalkonium chloride, disodium edetate, polysorbate 80

HYDROCORTISONE ACETATE

Indications: local treatment of inflammation (short-term)

Cautions: see notes above

Side-effects: see notes above

Hydrocortisone (Non-proprietary) [PoM]

Eye drops, hydrocortisone acetate 1%. Net price 10 mL = £3.21

Available from Martindale

Eye ointment, hydrocortisone acetate 0.5%, net price 3 g = £2.17; 1%, 3 g = £2.19; 2.5%, 3 g = £2.22

Available from Martindale

■ With neomycin

Neo-Cortef® (Dominion) [PoM] [▨]

Drops and *ointment* (for ear or eye), see section 12.1.1

Note. May be difficult to obtain

PREDNISOLONE

Indications: local treatment of inflammation (short-term)

Cautions: see notes above

Side-effects: see notes above

Administration: apply eye drops every 1–2 hours until controlled then reduce frequency

Pred Forte® (Allergan) [PoM]

Eye drops, prednisolone acetate 1%. Net price 5 mL = £1.52; 10 mL = £3.05

Excipients: include benzalkonium chloride, disodium edetate, polysorbate 80

Apply 2–4 times daily

Predsol® (Celltech) [PoM]

Drops (for ear or eye), prednisolone sodium phos- phate 0.5%. Net price 10 mL = £1.31

Excipients: include benzalkonium chloride, disodium edetate

■ Single use

Minims® Prednisolone Sodium Phosphate (Chauvin) [PoM]

Eye drops, prednisolone sodium phosphate 0.5%. Net price 20 × 0.5 mL = £5.75

Excipients: include disodium edetate

■ With neomycin

Predsol-N® (Celltech) [PoM] [▨]

Drops (for ear or eye), see section 12.1.1

RIMEXOLONE

Indications: local treatment of inflammation (short-term)

Cautions: see notes above

Side-effects: see notes above

Administration: postoperative inflammation, apply 4 times daily for 2 weeks, beginning 24 hours after surgery

Steroid-responsive inflammation, apply at least 4 times daily for up to 4 weeks

Uveitis, apply every hour during daytime in week 1, then every 2 hours in week 2, then 4 times daily in week 3, then twice daily for first 4 days of week 4, then once daily for remaining 3 days of week 4

Vexol® (Alcon) ▼ [PoM]

Eye drops, rimexolone 1%, net price 5 mL = £5.95

Excipients: include benzalkonium chloride, disodium edetate, polysorbate 80

11.4.2 Other anti-inflammatory preparations

Other preparations used for the topical treatment of inflammation and allergic conjunctivitis include antihistamines, lodoxamide, and sodium cromogli- cate.

Topical preparations of **antihistamines** such as eye drops containing **antazoline** (with xylomet- azoline as *Otrivine-Antistin®*), **azelastine** and **levo- cabastine** may be used for allergic conjunctivitis.

Sodium cromoglicate (sodium cromoglycate) and **nedocromil sodium** eye drops may be useful for vernal keratoconjunctivitis and other allergic forms of conjunctivitis.

Lodoxamide eye drops are used for allergic con- junctival conditions including seasonal allergic con- junctivitis.

Emedastine eye drops have been introduced recently for seasonal allergic conjunctivitis.

ANTAZOLINE SULPHATE

Indications: allergic conjunctivitis

Otrivine-Antistin® (Novartis Ophthalmics)
Eye drops, antazoline sulphate 0.5%, xylometazoline hydrochloride 0.05%. Net price 10 mL = £2.35

Excipients: include benzalkonium chloride, disodium edetate

ADULT and CHILD over 5 years, apply 2–3 times daily

Note. Xylometazoline is a sympathomimetic; it should be avoided in angle-closure glaucoma; absorption of antazoline and xylometazoline may result in systemic side-effects and the possibility of interaction with other drugs

AZELASTINE HYDROCHLORIDE

Indications: allergic conjunctivitis

Side-effects: mild transient irritation; bitter taste reported

Administration: Seasonal allergic conjunctivitis, ADULT and CHILD over 4 years, apply twice daily, increased if necessary to 4 times daily

Perennial conjunctivitis, ADULT and ADOLESCENT over 12 years, apply twice daily, increased if necessary to 4 times daily; max. duration of treatment 6 weeks

Optilast® (ASTA Medica) PoM
Eye drops, azelastine hydrochloride 0.05%. Net price 6 mL = £6.88

Excipients: include benzalkonium chloride, disodium edetate

EMEDASTINE

Indications: seasonal allergic conjunctivitis

Side-effects: transient burning or stinging; blurred vision, local oedema, keratitis, irritation, dry eye, lacrimation, corneal infiltrates (discontinue) and staining; photophobia; headache, and rhinitis occasionally reported

Administration: ADULT and CHILD over 3 years, apply twice daily

Emadine® (Alcon) ▼ PoM
Eye drops, emedastine 0.05% (as difumarate), net price 5 mL = £7.69

Excipients: include benzalkonium chloride

LEVOCABASTINE

Indications: seasonal allergic conjunctivitis

Side-effects: local irritation, blurred vision, local oedema, urticaria; dyspnoea, headache

Administration: ADULT and CHILD over 9 years, apply twice daily, increased if necessary to 3–4 times daily, discontinue if no improvement within 3 days

¹**Livostin®** (Novartis Ophthalmics) PoM
Eye drops, levocabastine 0.05% (as hydrochloride). Net price 4 mL = £9.29

Excipients: include benzalkonium chloride, disodium edetate, polysorbate 80, propylene glycol

1. Levocabastine 0.05% eye drops can be sold to the public (in max. pack size of 4 mL) for treatment of seasonal allergic conjunctivitis in adults and children over 12 years; proprietary brands on sale to the public include *Livostin®Direct* eye drops

LODOXAMIDE

Indications: allergic conjunctivitis

Side-effects: mild transient burning, stinging, itching, and lacrimation; flushing and dizziness reported

Administration: ADULT and CHILD over 4 years, apply eye drops 4 times daily

Alomide® (Alcon) PoM
Ophthalmic solution (= eye drops), lodoxamide 0.1% (as trometamol). Net price 10 mL = £5.48

Excipients: include benzalkonium chloride, disodium edetate

NEDOCROMIL SODIUM

Indications: allergic conjunctivitis; vernal keratoconjunctivitis

Side-effects: transient burning and stinging; distinctive taste reported

Administration: seasonal and perennial conjunctivitis, ADULT and CHILD over 6 years, apply twice daily increased if necessary to 4 times daily; max. 12 weeks treatment for seasonal allergic conjunctivitis

Vernal keratoconjunctivitis, ADULT and CHILD over 6 years, apply 4 times daily

Rapitil® (Rhône-Poulenc Rorer) PoM
Eye drops, nedocromil sodium 2%. Net price 5 mL = £9.75

Excipients: include benzalkonium chloride, disodium edetate

SODIUM CROMOGLICATE

(Sodium cromoglycate)

Indications: allergic conjunctivitis; vernal keratoconjunctivitis

Side-effects: transient burning and stinging

Administration: apply eye drops 4 times daily, eye ointment 2–3 times daily

¹**Sodium Cromoglicate** (Non-proprietary) PoM
Eye drops, sodium cromoglicate 2%. Net price 13.5 mL = £1.96

Available from Alpharma, Dominion, IVAX (*Hay-Crom® Aqueous*), Rhône-Poulenc Rorer (*Opticrom® Aqueous*), Opus (*Viz-on®*), Pharma-Global (*Vividrin®*)

1. Sodium cromoglicate 2% eye drops can be sold to the public (in max. pack size of 10 mL) for treatment of acute seasonal and perennial allergic conjunctivitis; proprietary brands on sale to the public include *Boots Hayfever Relief*, *Clariteyes®*, *Opticrom® Allergy*, and *Optrex® Allergy*

11.5   Mydriatics and cycloplegics

Antimuscarinics dilate the pupil and paralyse the ciliary muscle; they vary in potency and duration of action.

Short-acting, relatively weak mydriatics, such as **tropicamide** 0.5%, facilitate the examination of the fundus of the eye. **Cyclopentolate** 1% or **atropine** are preferable for producing cycloplegia for refraction in young children. Atropine 1% (in ointment form) is sometimes preferred for children under 5 years of age. Atropine, which has a longer duration of action, is also used for the treatment of anterior uveitis mainly to prevent posterior synechiae, often with phenylephrine 10% eye drops (2.5% in children, the elderly, and those with cardiac disease). **Homatropine** 1% is also used in the treatment of anterior segment inflammation, and may be preferred for its shorter duration of action.

CAUTIONS. Darkly pigmented iris is more resistant to pupillary dilatation and caution should be exercised to avoid overdosage. Mydriasis may precipitate acute angle-closure glaucoma in a very few patients, usually aged over 60 years and hypermetropic (long-sighted), who are predisposed to the condition because of a shallow anterior chamber. Phenylephrine may interact with systemically administered monoamine-oxidase inhibitors; other **interactions**: Appendix 1 (sympathomimetics).

DRIVING. Patients should be warned not to drive for 1–2 hours after mydriasis.

SIDE-EFFECTS. Ocular side-effects of mydriatics and cycloplegics include transient stinging and raised intra-ocular pressure; on prolonged administration, local irritation, hyperaemia, oedema and conjunctivitis may occur. Contact dermatitis (conjunctivitis) is not uncommon with the antimuscarinic mydriatic drugs, especially atropine.

Toxic systemic reactions to atropine and cyclopentolate may occur in the very young and the very old; see under Atropine Sulphate (section 1.2) for systemic side-effects of antimuscarinic drugs.

Antimuscarinics

ATROPINE SULPHATE

Indications: refraction procedures in young children; anterior uveitis—see also notes above
Cautions: risk of systemic effects with eye drops in infants under 3 months—eye ointment preferred; see also notes above
Side-effects: see notes above

Atropine (Non-proprietary) PoM
Eye drops, atropine sulphate 0.5%, net price 10 mL = £2.21; 1%, 10 mL = 84p
Available from Martindale
Eye ointment, atropine sulphate 1%. Net price 3 g = £2.59
Available from Martindale

Isopto Atropine® (Alcon) PoM
Eye drops, atropine sulphate 1%, hypromellose 0.5%. Net price 5 mL = 99p
Excipients: include benzalkonium chloride

■ Single use

Minims® Atropine Sulphate (Chauvin) PoM
Eye drops, atropine sulphate 1%. Net price 20 × 0.5 mL = £4.92

CYCLOPENTOLATE HYDROCHLORIDE

Indications: see notes above
Cautions: see notes above
Side-effects: see notes above

Mydrilate® (Intrapharm) PoM
Eye drops, cyclopentolate hydrochloride 0.5%, net price 5 mL = 73p; 1%, 5 mL = 98p
Excipients: include benzalkonium chloride

■ Single use

Minims® Cyclopentolate Hydrochloride (Chauvin) PoM
Eye drops, cyclopentolate hydrochloride 0.5 and 1%. Net price 20 × 0.5 mL (both) = £4.92

HOMATROPINE HYDROBROMIDE

Indications: see notes above
Cautions: see notes above
Side-effects: see notes above

Homatropine (Non-proprietary) PoM
Eye drops, homatropine hydrobromide 1%, net price 10 mL = £1.98; 2%, 10 mL = £2.10
Available from Martindale

■ Single use

Minims® Homatropine Hydrobromide (Chauvin) PoM
Eye drops, homatropine hydrobromide 2%. Net price 20 × 0.5 mL = £5.75

TROPICAMIDE

Indications: see notes above
Cautions: see notes above
Side-effects: see notes above

Mydriacyl® (Alcon) PoM
Eye drops, tropicamide 0.5%, net price 5 mL = £1.36; 1%, 5 mL = £1.68
Excipients: include benzalkonium chloride, disodium edetate

■ Single use

Minims® Tropicamide (Chauvin) PoM
Eye drops, tropicamide 0.5 and 1%. Net price 20 × 0.5 mL (both) = £5.75

Sympathomimetics

PHENYLEPHRINE HYDROCHLORIDE

Indications: mydriasis; see also notes above
Cautions: children and elderly (avoid 10% strength); cardiovascular disease (avoid or use 2.5% strength only); tachycardia; hyperthyroidism; diabetes; see also notes above
Contra-indications: angle-closure glaucoma
Side-effects: eye pain and stinging; blurred vision, photophobia; systemic effects include arrhythmias, hypertension, coronary artery spasm

Phenylephrine (Non-proprietary)
Eye drops, phenylephrine hydrochloride 10%. Net price 10 mL = £3.11
Available from Martindale
See also under Hypromellose (section 11.8.1)

■ Single use

Minims® Phenylephrine Hydrochloride (Chauvin)

Eye drops, phenylephrine hydrochloride 2.5%, net price 20 × 0.5 mL = £5.75; 10%, 20 × 0.5 mL = £5.75

Excipients: include disodium edetate, sodium metabisulphite

11.6 Treatment of glaucoma

Glaucoma is usually (but not always) associated with an abnormally high intra-ocular pressure; it may result in blindness. The rise in pressure is almost always due to reduced outflow of aqueous humour, the inflow remaining constant. Treatment is aimed at reducing intra-ocular pressure.

Probably the commonest condition is *chronic simple glaucoma* where the obstruction is in the trabecular meshwork. It is commonly first treated with a topical beta-blocker and other drugs added as necessary to control the intra-ocular pressure e.g. adrenaline or pilocarpine.

Dorzolamide and brinzolamide are topical carbonic anhydrase inhibitors that can be used as an alternative to topical beta-blockers or as an adjunct to them. Acetazolamide is a carbonic anhydrase inhibitor which is given by mouth.

Brimonidine, a selective alpha$_2$-adrenoceptor stimulant, is licensed for open-angle glaucoma and ocular hypertension when other drugs are inappropriate.

Apraclonidine (section 11.8.2) is an alpha$_2$-adrenoceptor stimulant which reduces the rate of production of aqueous humour.

Latanoprost is a prostaglandin analogue which increases the uveoscleral outflow of aqueous humour. It is indicated for open-angle glaucoma and ocular hypertension in patients for whom other drugs are inappropriate.

In emergency or before surgery, mannitol 20% (up to max. of 500 mL) should be given by slow intravenous infusion until the intra-ocular pressure has been satisfactorily reduced. Acetazolamide by intravenous injection may also be used for the emergency management of raised intra-ocular pressure.

If supplementary topical treatment is required after *iridectomy* or a drainage operation in either open-angle or angle-closure glaucoma, a beta-blocker is preferred to pilocarpine. This is because of the risk that posterior synechiae will be formed as a result of the miotic effect of pilocarpine, especially in angle-closure glaucoma.

Miotics

The small pupil is an unfortunate side-effect of these drugs (except when pilocarpine is used temporarily before an operation for *angle-closure glaucoma*). They act by opening up the inefficient drainage channels in the trabecular meshwork resulting from contraction or spasm of the ciliary muscle.

Miotics used in the management of raised intra-ocular pressure include carbachol and pilocarpine; ecothiopate iodide (as *Phospholine Iodide®*,

Dominion) is no longer on the UK market but is still available on a named-patient basis for use under expert supervision.

CAUTIONS. A darkly pigmented iris may require higher concentration of the miotic or more frequent administration and care should be taken to avoid overdosage. Retinal detachment has occurred in susceptible individuals and those with retinal disease; therefore fundus examination is advised before starting treatment with a miotic. Care is also required in conjunctival or corneal damage. Intra-ocular pressure and visual fields should be monitored in those with chronic simple glaucoma and those receiving long-term treatment with a miotic. Miotics should be used with caution in cardiac disease, hypertension, asthma, peptic ulceration, urinary-tract obstruction, and Parkinson's disease.
COUNSELLING. Blurred vision may affect performance of skilled tasks (e.g. driving) particularly at night or in reduced lighting

CONTRA-INDICATIONS. Miotics are contra-indicated in conditions where pupillary constriction is undesirable such as acute iritis, anterior uveitis and some forms of secondary glaucoma. They should be avoided in acute inflammatory disease of the anterior segment.

SIDE-EFFECTS. Ciliary spasm leads to headache and browache which may be more severe in the initial 2–4 weeks of treatment (a particular disadvantage in patients under 40 years of age). Ocular side-effects include burning, itching, smarting, blurred vision, conjunctival vascular congestion, myopia, lens changes with chronic use, vitreous haemorrhage, and pupillary block. Systemic side-effects (see under Parasympathomimetics, section 7.4.1) are rare following application to the eye.

CARBACHOL

Indications: see notes above
Cautions: see notes above
Contra-indications: see notes above
Side-effects: see notes above
Administration: apply up to 4 times daily

Isopto Carbachol® (Alcon) PoM
Eye drops, carbachol 3%, hypromellose 1%. Net price 10 mL = £1.76
Excipients: include benzalkonium chloride

PILOCARPINE

Indications: see notes above; dry mouth (section 12.3.5)
Cautions: see notes above
Contra-indications: see notes above
Side-effects: see notes above
Administration: apply up to 4 times daily; long-acting preparations, see under preparations below

Pilocarpine Hydrochloride (Non-proprietary) PoM
Eye drops, pilocarpine hydrochloride 0.5%, net price 10 mL = £1.36; 1%, 10 mL = £1.05; 2%, 10 mL = £1.19; 3%, 10 mL = £1.41; 4%, 10 mL = £1.58
Available from Alpharma, Cusi, Hillcross, Martindale

■ Single use

Minims® Pilocarpine Nitrate (Chauvin) PoM
Eye drops, pilocarpine nitrate 1, 2, and 4%, net
price 20 × 0.5 mL (all) = £4.92

■ Long acting

Pilogel® (Alcon) PoM
Ophthalmic gel, pilocarpine hydrochloride 4%,
carbomer 940 (polyacrylic acid) 3.5%, net price
5 g = £6.86
Excipients: include benzalkonium chloride, disodium edetate
Apply 1–1.5 cm gel once daily at bedtime

Sympathomimetics

Adrenaline (epinephrine) probably acts both by
reducing the rate of production of aqueous humour
and by increasing the outflow through the trabecular meshwork. It is contra-indicated in angle-closure glaucoma because it is a mydriatic, unless an
iridectomy has been carried out. Side-effects
include severe smarting and redness of the eye; adrenaline should be used with caution in patients with
hypertension and heart disease.

Dipivefrine is a pro-drug of adrenaline. It is
claimed to pass more rapidly through the cornea
and is then converted to the active form.

Guanethidine enhances and prolongs the effects
of adrenaline. Prolonged use, particularly of the
higher strength, may result in conjunctival fibrosis
with secondary corneal changes; the conjunctiva
and cornea should be examined at least every six
months.

Brimonidine, a selective alpha₂-adrenoceptor
stimulant, is licensed for the reduction of intra-ocular pressure in open-angle glaucoma or ocular
hypertension in patients for whom beta-blockers are
inappropriate; it may also be used as adjunctive
therapy when intra-ocular pressure is inadequately
controlled by a beta-blocker alone.

Apraclonidine (section 11.8.2) is another alpha₂-
adrenoceptor stimulant. Eye drops containing apraclonidine 0.5% are used for a short term to delay
laser treatment or surgery for glaucoma in patients
not adequately controlled by another drug; eye
drops containing 1% are used for control of intra-
ocular pressure after anterior segment laser surgery.

ADRENALINE/EPINEPHRINE

Indications: see notes above
Contra-indications: see notes above
Side-effects: see notes above
Administration: apply eye drops 1–2 times daily

Eppy® (Chauvin) PoM
Eye drops, adrenaline 1%, net price 7.5 mL =
£4.06
Excipients: include benzalkonium chloride, also acetylcysteine as
antioxidant

BRIMONIDINE TARTRATE

Indications: adjunct to beta-blockers or used alone
in raised intra-ocular pressure in ocular hypertension or open-angle glaucoma in patients unresponsive to beta-blockers or if beta-blockers
contra-indicated
Cautions: severe cardiovascular disease; cerebral
or coronary insufficiency, Raynaud's syndrome,

postural hypotension, depression, hepatic or renal
impairment; pregnancy, breast-feeding; **interactions:** Appendix 1 (alpha₂-adrenoceptor
stimulants)
DRIVING. Drowsiness may affect performance of skilled
tasks (e.g. driving)
Side-effects: ocular reactions include hyperaemia, burning, stinging, blurring, pruritus, allergy,
and conjunctival follicles; occasionally corneal
erosion and staining, photophobia, eyelid inflammation, conjunctivitis; headache, dry mouth, taste
alteration, fatigue, dizziness, drowsiness reported;
rarely depression, nasal dryness, palpitations, and
hypersensitivity reactions
Administration: apply one drop twice daily

Alphagan® (Allergan) ▼ PoM
Eye drops, brimonidine tartrate 0.2%, net price
5 mL = £10.31
Excipients: include benzalkonium chloride

DIPIVEFRINE HYDROCHLORIDE

Indications: as for Adrenaline/Epinephrine, see
notes above
Contra-indications: see notes above
Side-effects: see notes above
Administration: apply 1 drop twice daily

Propine® (Allergan) PoM
Eye drops, dipivefrine hydrochloride 0.1%, net
price 5 mL = £3.81, 10 mL = £4.77
Excipients: include benzalkonium chloride, disodium edetate

GUANETHIDINE MONOSULPHATE

Indications: see notes above
Cautions: see notes above
Administration: apply eye drops 1–2 times daily

■ With adrenaline

Ganda® (Chauvin) PoM
Eye drops '1 + 0.2', guanethidine monosulphate
1%, adrenaline 0.2% in a viscous vehicle, net
price 7.5 mL = £4.49
Excipients: include benzalkonium chloride
Eye drops '3 + 0.5', guanethidine monosulphate
3%, adrenaline 0.5% in a viscous vehicle, net
price 7.5 mL = £5.86
Excipients: include benzalkonium chloride

Beta-blockers

Topical application of a beta-blocker to the eye
reduces intra-ocular pressure effectively in *chronic
simple glaucoma*, probably by reducing the rate of
production of aqueous humour. Administration by
mouth also reduces intra-ocular pressure but this
route is not used since side-effects may be troublesome.

Beta-blockers used as eye drops include **betaxolol, carteolol, levobunolol, metipranolol**, and
timolol.

CAUTIONS, CONTRA-INDICATIONS AND SIDE-
EFFECTS. Systemic absorption may follow topical
application therefore eye drops containing a beta-
blocker are contra-indicated in patients with brady-

cardia, heart block, or uncontrolled heart failure. **Important:** for a warning to avoid in asthma see CSM advice below. Consider also other cautions, contra-indications and side-effects of beta-blockers (pp. 76–7). Local side-effects of eye drops include ocular stinging, burning, pain, itching, erythema, dry eyes and allergic blepharoconjunctivitis; occasionally corneal disorders have been reported.

CSM advice. The CSM has advised that beta-blockers, even those with apparent cardioselectivity, should not be used in patients with asthma or a history of obstructive airways disease, unless no alternative treatment is available. In such cases the risk of inducing bronchospasm should be appreciated and appropriate precautions taken.

INTERACTIONS. Since systemic absorption may follow topical application the possibility of interactions, in particular, with drugs such as verapamil should be borne in mind. See also Appendix 1 (beta-blockers).

BETAXOLOL HYDROCHLORIDE

Indications: see notes above
Cautions: see notes above
Contra-indications: see notes above
Side-effects: see notes above
Administration: apply twice daily

Betoptic® (Alcon) [PoM]
Ophthalmic solution (= eye drops), betaxolol (as hydrochloride) 0.5%, net price 5 mL = £3.81
Excipients: include benzalkonium chloride, disodium edetate
Ophthalmic suspension (= eye drops), m/r, betaxolol (as hydrochloride) 0.25%, net price 5 mL = £4.77
Excipients: include benzalkonium chloride, disodium edetate
Unit dose eye drop suspension, m/r, betaxolol (as hydrochloride) 0.25%, net price 50 × 0.25 mL = £14.49

CARTEOLOL HYDROCHLORIDE

Indications: see notes above
Cautions: see notes above
Contra-indications: see notes above
Side-effects: see notes above
Administration: apply twice daily

Teoptic® (Novartis Ophthalmics) [PoM]
Eye drops, carteolol hydrochloride 1%, net price 5 mL = £4.60; 2%, 5 mL = £5.40
Excipients: include benzalkonium chloride

LEVOBUNOLOL HYDROCHLORIDE

Indications: see notes above
Cautions: see notes above
Contra-indications: see notes above
Side-effects: see notes above; anterior uveitis occasionally reported
Administration: apply once or twice daily

Levobunolol (Non-proprietary) [PoM]
Eye drops, levobunolol hydrochloride 0.5%. Net price 5 mL = £4.66
Available from Cusi

Betagan® (Allergan) [PoM]
Eye drops, levobunolol hydrochloride 0.5%, polyvinyl alcohol (*Liquifilm®*) 1.4%. Net price 5-mL= £4.66, triple pack (3 × 5 mL) = £11.89
Excipients: include benzalkonium chloride, disodium edetate, sodium metabisulphite
Unit dose eye drops, levobunolol hydrochloride 0.5%, polyvinyl alcohol (*Liquifilm®*) 1.4%. Net price 30 × 0.4 mL = £9.98
Excipients: include disodium edetate

METIPRANOLOL

Indications: see notes above but in chronic open-angle glaucoma **restricted** to patients allergic to preservatives or to those wearing soft contact lenses (in whom benzalkonium chloride should be avoided)
Cautions: see notes above
Contra-indications: see notes above
Side-effects: see notes above; granulomatous anterior uveitis reported (discontinue treatment)
Administration: apply twice daily

Minims® Metipranolol (Chauvin) [PoM]
Eye drops, metipranolol 0.1%, net price 20 × 0.5 mL = £10.19; 0.3%, 20 × 0.5 mL = £11.09

TIMOLOL MALEATE

Indications: see notes above
Cautions: see notes above
Contra-indications: see notes above
Side-effects: see notes above
Administration: apply twice daily; long-acting preparations, see under preparations below

Timolol (Non-proprietary) [PoM]
Eye drops, timolol (as maleate) 0.25%, net price 5 mL = £3.65; 0.5%, 5 mL = £3.92
Available from Alpharma, APS, Bioglan, Hillcross, IVAX, Lagap, Martindale, Opus (*Glau-opt®*)
Timoptol® (MSD) [PoM]
Eye drops, in Ocumeter® metered-dose unit, timolol (as maleate) 0.25%, net price 5 mL = £3.12; 0.5%, 5 mL = £3.12
Excipients: include benzalkonium chloride
Unit dose eye drops, timolol (as maleate) 0.25%, net price 30 × 0.2 mL = £8.45; 0.5%, 30 × 0.2 mL = £9.65

■ Long acting
Timoptol®-LA (MSD) [PoM]
Ophthalmic gel-forming solution (= eye drops), timolol (as maleate) 0.25%, net price 2.5 mL = £3.12; 0.5%, 2.5 mL = £3.12
Excipients: include benzododecinium bromide
Apply eye drops once daily

■ With dorzolamide
See under Dorzolamide

Carbonic anhydrase inhibitors and systemic drugs

The **carbonic anhydrase inhibitors**, acetazolamide and dorzolamide, reduce intra-ocular pressure by reducing aqueous humour production. Systemic use also produces weak diuresis.

Acetazolamide is given by mouth or by intravenous injection (intramuscular injections are painful because of the alkaline pH of the solution). Acetazolamide is a sulphonamide; blood disorders, rashes and other sulphonamide-related side-effects occur occasionally. It is not generally recommended for long-term use but electrolyte disturbances and metabolic acidosis that occur may be corrected by administering potassium bicarbonate (as effervescent potassium tablets, section 9.2.1.3).

Dorzolamide and brinzolamide are topical carbonic anhydrase inhibitors. They are licensed for use in patients resistant to beta-blockers or those in whom beta-blockers are contra-indicated. They are used alone or as an adjunct to a topical beta-blocker. Systemic absorption may rarely give rise to sulphonamide-like side-effects and may require discontinuation if severe.

The osmotic diuretics, intravenous hypertonic mannitol (section 2.2.5), or glycerol by mouth, are useful short-term ocular hypotensive drugs.

ACETAZOLAMIDE

Indications: reduction of intra-ocular pressure in open-angle glaucoma, secondary glaucoma, and peri-operatively in angle-closure glaucoma; diuresis (section 2.2.7); epilepsy

Cautions: not generally recommended for prolonged use but if given monitor blood count and plasma electrolyte concentration; pulmonary obstruction (risk of acidosis); elderly; pregnancy and breast-feeding; avoid extravasation at injection site (risk of necrosis); **interactions:** Appendix 1 (diuretics)

Contra-indications: hypokalaemia, hyponatraemia, hyperchloraemic acidosis; severe hepatic impairment; renal impairment; sulphonamide hypersensitivity

Side-effects: nausea, vomiting, diarrhoea, taste disturbance; loss of appetite, paraesthesia, flushing, headache, dizziness, fatigue, irritability, depression; thirst, polyuria; reduced libido; metabolic acidosis and electrolyte disturbances on long-term therapy; occasionally, drowsiness, confusion, hearing disturbances, urticaria, malaena, glycosuria, haematuria, abnormal liver function, renal calculi, blood disorders including agranulocytosis and thrombocytopenia, rashes including Stevens-Johnson syndrome and toxic epidermal necrolysis; rarely, photosensitivity, liver damage, flaccid paralysis, convulsions; transient myopia reported

Dose: glaucoma, *by mouth or by intravenous injection*, 0.25–1 g daily in divided doses
Epilepsy, 0.25–1 g daily in divided doses; CHILD 8–30 mg/kg daily, max. 750 mg daily
By intramuscular injection, as for intravenous injection but preferably avoided because of alkalinity

Diamox® (Wyeth) [PoM]
Tablets, acetazolamide 250 mg. Net price 112-tab pack = £12.68. Label: 3
Sodium Parenteral (= injection), powder for reconstitution, acetazolamide (as sodium salt). Net price 500-mg vial = £14.76

Diamox® SR (Wyeth) [PoM]
Capsules, m/r, two-tone orange, enclosing orange f/c pellets, acetazolamide 250 mg. Net price 28-cap pack = £11.55. Label: 3, 25
Dose: glaucoma, 1–2 capsules daily

BRINZOLAMIDE

Indications: adjunct to beta-blockers or used alone in raised intra-ocular pressure in ocular hypertension and in open-angle glaucoma if beta-blocker alone inadequate or inappropriate

Cautions: hepatic impairment; pregnancy (Appendix 4); **interactions:** Appendix 1 (brinzolamide)

Contra-indications: renal impairment (creatinine clearance less than 30 mL/minute), hyperchloraemic acidosis; breast-feeding

Side-effects: local irritation, taste disturbance; less commonly nausea, dyspepsia, dry mouth, chest pain, epistaxis, haemoptysis, dyspnoea, rhinitis, pharyngitis, bronchitis, paraesthesia, depression, dizziness, headache, dermatitis, alopecia, corneal erosion

Administration: apply twice daily increased to 3 times daily if necessary

Azopt® (Alcon) ▼ [PoM]
Eye drops, brinzolamide 10 mg/mL, net price 5 mL = £7.17
Excipients: include benzalkonium chloride, disodium edetate

DORZOLAMIDE

Indications: raised intra-ocular pressure in ocular hypertension, open-angle glaucoma, pseudo-exfoliative glaucoma *either* as adjunct to beta-blocker *or* used alone in patients unresponsive to beta-blockers or if beta-blockers contra-indicated

Cautions: hepatic impairment; systemic absorption follows topical application; history of renal calculi; chronic corneal defects, history of intra-ocular surgery; **interactions:** Appendix 1 (dorzolamide)

Contra-indications: severe renal impairment or hyperchloraemic acidosis; pregnancy and breast-feeding

Side-effects: ocular burning, stinging and itching, blurred vision, lacrimation, conjunctivitis, superficial punctate keratitis, eyelid inflammation and crusting, anterior uveitis, transient myopia, corneal oedema, iridocyclitis; headache, dizziness, paraesthesia, asthenia, nausea; hypersensitivity reactions (including urticaria, angioedema, bronchosopasm); bitter taste, epistaxis, urolithiasis

Administration: used alone, apply 3 times daily; with topical beta-blocker, apply twice daily

Trusopt® (MSD) [PoM]
Ophthalmic solution (= eye drops), dorzolamide (as hydrochloride) 2%, net price 5 mL = £9.31
Excipients: include benzalkonium chloride

■ With timolol
For cautions, contra-indications, and side-effects of timolol, see section 11.6, Beta-blockers

Cosopt® (MSD) PoM

Ophthalmic solution (= eye drops), dorzolamide (as hydrochloride) 2%, timolol (as maleate) 0.5%, net price 5 mL = £13.50

Excipients: include benzalkonium chloride

For raised intra-ocular pressure in open-angle glaucoma, or pseudoexfoliative glaucoma when beta-blockers alone not adequate, apply twice daily

Prostaglandin analogue

Latanoprost and **travoprost** are prostaglandin analogues which increase uveoscleral outflow. They are used to reduce intra-ocular pressure in ocular hypertension or in open-angle glaucoma if other drugs cannot control the condition adequately or are not tolerated. Patients receiving latanoprost or travoprost should be monitored for any changes to eye coloration since an increase in the brown pigment in the iris may occur; particular care is required in those with mixed coloured irides and those receiving treatment to one eye only.

LATANOPROST

Indications: raised intra-ocular pressure in open-angle glaucoma and ocular hypertension in patients intolerant or unresponsive to other drugs

Cautions: before initiating treatment, advise patients of possible change in eye colour; monitor for eye colour change; aphakia, or pseudophakia with torn posterior lens capsule or anterior chamber lenses; risk factors for cystoid macular oedema; brittle or severe asthma; not to be used within 5 minutes of use of thiomersal-containing preparations; manufacturer advises avoid in pregnancy and breast-feeding

Side-effects: brown pigmentation particularly in those with mixed-colour irides (withdraw treatment if possible); ocular irritation; darkening, thickening and lengthening of eye lashes; periorbital oedema; conjunctival hyperaemia; transient punctate epithelial erosions; dyspnoea, exacerbation of asthma; macular oedema, iritis and uveitis reported rarely; darkening of palpebral skin reported very rarely

Administration: apply 1 drop once daily, preferably in the evening

Xalatan® (Pharmacia) PoM

Eye drops, latanoprost 50 micrograms/mL, net price 2.5 mL = £15.28

Excipients: include benzalkonium chloride

■ With timolol

For cautions, contra-indications, and side-effects of timolol, see section 11.6, Beta-blockers

Xalacom® (Pharmacia) ▼ PoM

Eye drops, latanoprost 50 micrograms, timolol (as maleate) 5 mg/mL, net price 2.5 mL = £17.15

Excipients: include benzalkonium chloride

For raised intra-ocular pressure in patients with open-angle glaucoma and ocular hypertension when beta-blocker alone not adequate; apply once daily, in the morning

TRAVOPROST

Indications: monotherapy or adjunctive therapy for raised intra-ocular pressure in open-angle glaucoma and ocular hypertension in patients intolerant or insufficiently responsive to other drugs

Cautions: see under Latanoprost and notes above

Side-effects: see under Latanoprost; also headache, ocular pruritus, ocular pain, photophobia, and keratitis reported; rarely, hypotension, bradycardia, conjunctivitis, lid oedema, blepharitis, browache

Administration: apply once daily, preferably in the evening; CHILD and ADOLESCENT under 18 years, not recommended

Travatan® (Alcon) ▼ PoM

Eye drops, travoprost 40 micrograms/mL, net price 2.5mL = £11.46

Excipients: include benzalkonium chloride

11.7 Local anaesthetics

Oxybuprocaine and tetracaine (amethocaine) are probably the most widely used topical local anaesthetics. Proxymetacaine causes less initial stinging and is useful for children. Oxybuprocaine or a combined preparation of lidocaine (lignocaine) and fluorescein is used for tonometry. Tetracaine produces a more profound anaesthesia and is suitable for use before minor surgical procedures, such as the removal of corneal sutures. It has a temporary disruptive effect on the corneal epithelium. Lidocaine, with or without adrenaline (epinephrine), is injected into the eyelids for minor surgery, while retrobulbar or peribulbar injections are used for surgery of the globe itself. Local anaesthetics should never be used for the management of ocular symptoms.

LIDOCAINE HYDROCHLORIDE/ LIGNOCAINE HYDROCHLORIDE

Indications: local anaesthetic

Minims® Lignocaine and Fluorescein (Chauvin) PoM

Eye drops, lidocaine hydrochloride 4%, fluorescein sodium 0.25%. Net price 20 × 0.5 mL = £6.93

OXYBUPROCAINE HYDROCHLORIDE

Indications: local anaesthetic

Minims® Benoxinate (Oxybuprocaine) Hydrochloride (Chauvin) PoM

Eye drops, oxybuprocaine hydrochloride 0.4%. Net price 20 × 0.5 mL = £4.92

PROXYMETACAINE HYDROCHLORIDE

Indications: local anaesthetic

Minims® Proxymetacaine (Chauvin) PoM

Eye drops, proxymetacaine hydrochloride 0.5%. Net price 20 × 0.5 mL = £6.95

■ With fluorescein

Minims® Proxymetacaine and Fluorescein
(Chauvin) [PoM]
Eye drops, proxymetacaine hydrochloride 0.5%,
fluorescein sodium 0.25%. Net price 20 × 0.5 mL
= £7.95

TETRACAINE HYDROCHLORIDE/
AMETHOCAINE HYDROCHLORIDE

Indications: local anaesthetic

Minims® Amethocaine Hydrochloride
(Chauvin) [PoM]
Eye drops, tetracaine hydrochloride 0.5 and 1%.
Net price 20 × 0.5 mL (both) = £5.75

11.8   Miscellaneous
ophthalmic
preparations

11.8.1   Tear deficiency, ocular lubricants and
          astringents
11.8.2   Ocular diagnostic and peri-operative
          preparations and photodynamic
          treatment

Certain eye drops, e.g. amphotericin, ceftazidime,
cefuroxime,   colistin,   desferrioxamine,
dexamethasone, gentamicin and vancomycin may
be prepared aseptically from material supplied for
injection; for details on preparation of trisodium
edetate eye drops see under *Limclair®* section
9.5.1.2.

11.8.1   Tear deficiency, ocular
lubricants, and
astringents

Chronic soreness of the eyes associated with
reduced or abnormal tear secretion (e.g. in Sjögren's syndrome) often responds to tear replacement therapy or pilocarpine given by mouth
(section 12.3.5). The severity of the condition and
patient preference will often guide the choice of
preparation.

Hypromellose is the traditional choice of treatment for tear deficiency. It may need to be instilled
frequently (e.g. hourly) for adequate relief. Ocular
surface mucin is often abnormal in tear deficiency
and the combination of hypromellose with a muco-
lytic such as **acetylcysteine** can be helpful.

The ability of **carbomers** to cling to the eye surface may help reduce frequency of application to 4
times daily.

Polyvinyl alcohol increases the persistence of the
tear film and is useful when the ocular surface
mucin is reduced.

Povidone eye drops are also used in the management of tear deficiency.

Sodium chloride 0.9% drops are sometimes useful in tear deficiency, and can be used as 'comfort
drops' by contact lens wearers, and to facilitate lens
removal.

Eye ointments containing a **paraffin** may be used
to lubricate the eye surface, especially in cases of

recurrent corneal epithelial erosion. They may
cause temporary visual disturbance and are best
suited for application before sleep. Ointments
should not be used during contact lens wear.

Zinc sulphate is a traditional astringent that is
now little used.

ACETYLCYSTEINE

Indications: tear deficiency, impaired or abnormal
mucus production
Administration: apply eye drops 3–4 times daily

Ilube® (Alcon) [PoM]
Eye drops, acetylcysteine 5%, hypromellose
0.35%. Net price 10 mL = £4.63
Excipients: include benzalkonium chloride, disodium edetate

CARBOMERS

(Polyacrylic acid)
Synthetic high molecular weight polymers of acrylic acid
cross-linked with either allyl ethers of sucrose or allyl
ethers of pentaerithrityl
Indications: dry eyes including keratoconjunctivitis sicca, unstable tear film
Administration: apply 3–4 times daily or as
required

GelTears® (Chauvin)
Gel (= eye drops), carbomer 980 (polyacrylic acid)
0.2%, net price 10 g = £2.80
Excipients: include benzalkonium chloride
Viscotears® (Novartis Ophthalmics)
Liquid gel (= eye drops), carbomer 980 (poly-
acrylic acid) 0.2%, net price 10 g = £3.12
Excipients: include cetrimide, disodium edetate
Liquid gel (= eye drops), carbomer 980 (poly-
acrylic acid) 0.2%, net price 15 × 0.6-mL single-
dose units = £3.90

CARMELLOSE SODIUM

Indications: dry eye conditions
Administration: apply as required

Celluvisc® (Allergan) ▼
Eye drops, carmellose sodium 1%, net price 30 ×
0.4 mL = £5.75

HYDROXYETHYLCELLULOSE

Indications: tear deficiency

Minims® Artificial Tears (Chauvin)
Eye drops, hydroxyethylcellulose 0.44%, sodium
chloride 0.35%. Net price 20 × 0.5 mL = £5.75

HYPROMELLOSE

Indications: tear deficiency
Note. The Royal Pharmaceutical Society of Great Britain has stated that where it is not possible to ascertain
the strength of hypromellose prescribed, the prescriber
should be contacted to clarify the strength intended.

Hypromellose (Non-proprietary)
Eye drops, hypromellose 0.3%, net price 10 mL =
75p
Available from Alpharma, IVAX, Martindale

Isopto Alkaline® (Alcon)
Eye drops, hypromellose 1%, net price 10 mL = 99p
Excipients: include benzalkonium chloride

Isopto Plain® (Alcon)
Eye drops, hypromellose 0.5%, net price 10 mL = 85p
Excipients: include benzalkonium chloride

Moisture-eyes® (Co-Pharma)
Eye drops, hypromellose 0.3% (buffered), net price 10 mL = £1.13
Excipients: include benzalkonium chloride

Tears Naturale® (Alcon)
Eye drops, dextran '70' 0.1%, hypromellose 0.3%, net price 15 mL = £1.68
Excipients: include benzalkonium chloride, disodium edetate

■ Single use
Artelac® SDU (Pharma-Global)
Eye drops, hypromellose 0.32%, net price 30 × 0.5 mL = £9.95

■ With phenylephrine
Note. Phenylephrine (section 11.5) acts to constrict conjunctival vessels, thus producing a whiter eye; it is not recommended for prolonged use
Isopto Frin® (Alcon) ▱
Eye drops, phenylephrine hydrochloride 0.12%, hypromellose 0.5%, net price 10 mL = £1.14
Excipients: include benzethonium chloride
Temporary relief of redness due to minor irritation, apply up to 4 times daily

LIQUID PARAFFIN

Indications: dry eye conditions

Lacri-Lube® (Allergan)
Eye ointment, white soft paraffin 57.3%, liquid paraffin 42.5%, wool alcohols 0.2%. Net price 3.5 g = £1.90, 5 g = £2.47

Lubri-Tears® (Alcon)
Eye ointment, white soft paraffin 60%, liquid paraffin 30%, wool fat 10%. Net price 5 g = £2.29

PARAFFIN, YELLOW, SOFT

Indications: see notes above

Simple Eye Ointment, liquid paraffin 10%, wool fat 10%, in yellow soft paraffin. Net price 4 g = £2.67
Available from Martindale

POLYVINYL ALCOHOL

Indications: tear deficiency

Hypotears® (Novartis Ophthalmics)
Eye drops, macrogol '8000' 2%, polyvinyl alcohol 1%. Net price 15 mL = £1.09
Excipients: include benzalkonium chloride, disodium edetate

Liquifilm Tears® (Allergan)
Ophthalmic solution (= eye drops), polyvinyl alcohol 1.4%. Net price 15 mL = £1.61
Excipients: include benzalkonium chloride, disodium edetate
Ophthalmic solution (= eye drops), polyvinyl alcohol 1.4%, povidone 0.6%. Net price 30 × 0.4 mL = £5.35

Sno Tears® (Chauvin)
Eye drops, polyvinyl alcohol 1.4%. Net price 10 mL = £1.06
Excipients: include benzalkonium chloride, disodium edetate

POVIDONE

Indications: dry eye conditions
Administration: apply 4 times daily or as required

Oculotect® (Novartis Ophthalmics)
Eye drops, povidone 5%. Net price 20 × 0.4 mL = £3.40

SODIUM CHLORIDE

Indications: irrigation, including first-aid removal of harmful substances

Sodium Chloride 0.9% Solutions
See section 13.11.1
Balanced Salt Solution
Solution (sterile), sodium chloride 0.64%, sodium acetate 0.39%, sodium citrate 0.17%, calcium chloride 0.048%, magnesium chloride 0.03%, potassium chloride 0.075%
For intra-ocular or topical irrigation during surgical procedures
Available from Alcon (15 mL, 250 mL and 500 mL) and from Novartis Ophthalmics (*Iocare®*, 15 mL and 500 mL)

■ Single use
Minims® Saline (Chauvin)
Eye drops, sodium chloride 0.9%. Net price 20 × 0.5 mL = £4.92

ZINC SULPHATE

Indications: see notes above
Cautions: see notes above

Zinc Sulphate (Non-proprietary)
Eye drops, zinc sulphate 0.25%. Net price 10 mL = £2.91
Available from Martindale

11.8.2	**Ocular diagnostic and peri-operative preparations and photodynamic treatment**

Ocular diagnostic preparations

Fluorescein sodium and **rose bengal** are used in diagnostic procedures and for locating damaged areas of the cornea due to injury or disease. Rose bengal is more efficient for the diagnosis of conjunctival epithelial damage but it stings excessively unless a local anaesthetic is instilled beforehand.

FLUORESCEIN SODIUM

Indications: detection of lesions and foreign bodies

Minims® Fluorescein Sodium (Chauvin)
Eye drops, fluorescein sodium 1 or 2%. Net price 20 × 0.5 mL (both) = £4.92

■ With local anaesthetic
Section 11.7

ROSE BENGAL

Indications: detection of lesions and foreign bodies

Minims® Rose Bengal (Chauvin)
Eye drops, rose bengal 1%. Net price 20 × 0.5 mL = £5.75

Ocular peri-operative drugs

Drugs used to prepare the eye for surgery and drugs that are injected into the anterior chamber at the time of surgery are included here.

Sodium hyaluronate preparations (*Healonid®*, Pharmacia; *Ophthalin®*, Novartis Ophthalmics) are used during surgical procedures on the eye.

Apraclonidine, an alpha$_2$ adrenoceptor stimulant, reduces intra-ocular pressure possibly by reducing the production of aqueous humour. It is used for short-term treatment only.

Special presentations of **sodium chloride 0.9%** solution are used routinely in intra-ocular surgery (section 11.8.1).

ACETYLCHOLINE CHLORIDE

Indications: cataract surgery, penetrating keratoplasty, iridectomy, and other anterior segment surgery requiring rapid complete miosis

Miochol-E® (Novartis Ophthalmics) [PoM]
Solution for intra-ocular irrigation, acetylcholine chloride 1%, mannitol 3% when reconstituted. Net price 2 mL-vial = £9.10

APRACLONIDINE

Note. Apraclonidine is a derivative of clonidine
Indications: control of intra-ocular pressure
Cautions: history of angina, severe coronary insufficiency, recent myocardial infarction, cardiac failure, cerebrovascular disease, vasovagal attack, chronic renal failure; depression; pregnancy and breast-feeding; monitor intra-ocular pressure and visual fields; loss of effect may occur over time; suspend treatment if reduction in vision occurs in end-stage glaucoma; exaggerated reduction in intra-ocular pressure following perioperative use should be closely monitored; **interactions:** Appendix 1 (alpha$_2$-adrenoceptor stimulants)
DRIVING. Drowsiness may affect performance of skilled tasks (e.g. driving)
Contra-indications: history of severe or unstable and uncontrolled cardiovascular disease

Side-effects: dry mouth, taste disturbance; hyperaemia, ocular pruritus, discomfort and lacrimation (withdraw if ocular intolerance including oedema of lids and conjunctiva); headache, asthenia, dry nose; lid retraction, conjunctival blanching and mydriasis reported after peri-operative use; since absorption may follow topical application systemic effects (see Clonidine Hydrochloride, section 2.5.2) may occur
Administration: see under preparations below

Iopidine® (Alcon) [PoM]
Ophthalmic solution (= eye drops), apraclonidine 1% (as hydrochloride). Net price 12 × 2 single use 0.25-mL units = £81.90
Administration: control or prevention of postoperative elevation of intra-ocular pressure after anterior segment laser surgery, apply 1 drop 1 hour before laser procedure then 1 drop immediately after completion of procedure; CHILD not recommended
Iopidine 0.5% ophthalmic solution (= eye drops), apraclonidine 0.5% (as hydrochloride). Net price 5 mL = £11.45
Excipients: include benzalkonium chloride
Administration: short-term adjunctive treatment of chronic glaucoma in patients not adequately controlled by another drug (see note below), apply 1 drop 3 times daily usually for max. 1 month; CHILD not recommended
Note. May not provide additional benefit if patient already using two drugs that suppress the production of aqueous humour

DICLOFENAC SODIUM

Indications: inhibition of intraoperative miosis during cataract surgery (but does not possess intrinsic mydriatic properties); postoperative inflammation in cataract surgery; pain in corneal epithelial defects after photorefractive keratectomy or accidental trauma

Voltarol® Ophtha (Novartis Ophthalmics) [PoM]
Eye drops, diclofenac sodium 0.1%. Net price pack of 5 single-dose units = £4.00, 40 single-dose units = £32.00

FLURBIPROFEN SODIUM

Indications: inhibition of intraoperative miosis (but does not possess intrinsic mydriatic properties); anterior segment inflammation following postoperative and post-laser trabeculoplasty when corticosteroids contra-indicated

Ocufen® (Allergan) [PoM]
Ophthalmic solution (= eye drops), flurbiprofen sodium 0.03%, polyvinyl alcohol (Liquifilm®) 1.4%. Net price 40 × 0.4 mL = £37.15

KETOROLAC TROMETAMOL

Indications: prophylaxis and reduction of inflammation and associated symptoms following ocular surgery

Acular® (Allergan) [PoM]
Eye drops, ketorolac trometamol 0.5%. Net price 5 mL = £6.68
Excipients: include benzalkonium chloride, disodium edetate

Subfoveal choroidal neovascularisation

Verteporfin is licensed for use in the photodynamic treatment of subfoveal choroidal neovascularisation associated with age-related macular degeneration *or* with pathological myopia. Following intravenous infusion, verteporfin is activated by local irradiation using non-thermal red light to produce cytotoxic derivatives. Only specialists experienced in the management of these conditions should use it.

VERTEPORFIN

Indications: see notes above—specialist use only

Cautions: photosensitivity—avoid exposure of unprotected skin and eyes to bright light during infusion and for 48 hours afterwards; hepatic impairment (avoid if severe), biliary obstruction; avoid extravasation; pregnancy (Appendix 4)

Contra-indications: porphyria; breast-feeding (Appendix 5)

Side-effects: visual disturbances (including blurred vision, flashing lights, visual-field defects), nausea, back pain, asthenia, pruritus, hypercholesterolaemia, hypertension, chest pain, syncope, fever; rarely lacrimation disorder, subretinal or vitreous haemorrhage; injection site reactions including pain, oedema, inflammation, haemorrhage, discoloration

Dose: *by intravenous infusion* over 10 minutes, 6 mg/m^2

Note. For information on administration and light activation, consult product literature

Visudyne® (Novartis Ophthalmics) ▼ [PoM]
Injection, powder for reconstitution, verteporfin, net price 15-mg vial = £850.00

11.9   Contact lenses

Note. Some recommendations in this section involve non-licensed indications.

For cosmetic reasons many people prefer to wear contact lenses rather than spectacles; contact lenses are also sometimes required for medical indications. Visual defects are corrected by either rigid ('hard' or gas permeable) lenses or soft (hydrogel) lenses; soft lenses are the most popular type, because they are the most comfortable, though they may not give the best vision. Lenses should usually be worn for a specified number of hours each day. Continuous (extended) wear involves much greater risks to eye health and is not recommended except where medically indicated.

Contact lenses require meticulous care. Poor compliance with directions for use, and with daily cleaning and disinfection, may result in complications which include ulcerative keratitis, conjunctival problems (such as purulent or papillary conjunctivitis). One-day disposable lenses, which are worn only once and therefore require no maintenance or storage, are becoming increasingly popular.

Acanthamoeba keratitis, a sight-threatening condition, is associated with ineffective lens cleaning and disinfection or the use of contaminated lens cases. The condition is especially associated with the use of soft lenses (including frequently replaced lenses). Acanthamoeba keratitis is treated by specialists with intensive use of polihexanide (polyhexamethylene biguanide), propamidine isetionate, chlorhexidine and neomycin drops, sometimes in combination.

CONTACT LENSES AND DRUG TREATMENT. Special care is required in prescribing eye preparations for contact lens users. Some drugs and preservatives in eye preparations can accumulate in hydrogel lenses and may induce toxic reactions. Therefore, unless medically indicated, the lenses should be removed before instillation and not worn during the period of treatment. Alternatively, unpreserved drops can be used. Eye drops may, however, be instilled over rigid corneal contact lenses. Ointment preparations should never be used in conjunction with contact lens wear.

Many drugs given systemically can also have adverse effects on contact lens wear. These include oral contraceptives (particularly those with a higher oestrogen content), drugs which reduce blink rate (e.g. anxiolytics, hypnotics, antihistamines, and muscle relaxants), drugs which reduce lacrimation (e.g. antihistamines, antimuscarinics, phenothiazines and related drugs, some beta-blockers, diuretics, and tricyclic antidepressants), and drugs which increase lacrimation (including ephedrine and hydralazine). Other drugs that may affect contact lens wear are isotretinoin (may cause conjunctival inflammation), primidone (may cause ocular or eyelid oedema), aspirin (salicylic acid appears in tears and may be absorbed by contact lenses—leading to irritation), and rifampicin and sulfasalazine (may discolour lenses).

12: Ear, nose, and oropharynx

12.1 Drugs acting on the ear

12.1.1 Otitis externa
12.1.2 Otitis media
12.1.3 Removal of ear wax

12.1.1 Otitis externa

Otitis externa is an inflammatory reaction of the meatal skin. It is important to exclude an underlying chronic otitis media before treatment is commenced. Many cases recover after thorough cleansing of the external ear canal by suction, dry mopping, or gentle syringing. A frequent problem in resistant cases is the difficulty in applying lotions and ointments satisfactorily to the relatively inaccessible affected skin. The most effective method is to introduce a ribbon gauze dressing soaked with **corticosteroid** ear drops or with an astringent such as **aluminium acetate** solution. When this is not practical, the ear should be gently cleansed with a probe covered in cotton wool and the patient encouraged to lie with the affected ear uppermost for ten minutes after the canal has been filled with a liberal quantity of the appropriate solution.

If infection is present, a topical anti-infective which is not used systemically (such as **neomycin** or **clioquinol**) may be used, but for only about a week as excessive use may result in fungal infections; these may be difficult to treat and require expert advice. Sensitivity to the anti-infective or solvent may occur and resistance to antibacterials is a possibility with prolonged use. **Chloramphenicol** may also be used but the ear drops contain propylene glycol and cause sensitivity in about 10% of patients (the eye ointment can be used instead [unlicensed indication]). Solutions containing an anti-infective and a corticosteroid (such as *Locorten-Vioform®*) are used for treating cases where infection is present with inflammation and eczema. In view of reports of ototoxicity in patients with a perforated tympanic membrane (eardrum), the CSM has issued a reminder that treatment with a topical aminoglycoside antibiotic is contra-indicated in those with a tympanic perforation. However, many specialists do use these drops cautiously in the presence of a perforation in patients with otitis media (section 12.1.2).

A solution of **acetic acid** 2% acts as an antifungal and antibacterial in the external ear canal. It may be used to treat mild otitis externa but in severe cases an anti-inflammatory preparation with or without an anti-infective drug is required. A proprietary preparation containing acetic acid 2% (*EarCalm®* spray) is on sale to the public.

An acute infection may cause severe pain and a systemic antibacterial is required with a simple analgesic such as paracetamol. When a resistant staphylococcal infection (a boil) is present in the external auditory meatus, **flucloxacillin** is the drug of choice (section 5.1, table 1); **ciprofloxacin** (or an aminoglycoside) may be needed in pseudomonal infections which may occur if the patient has diabetes or is immunocompromised.

The skin of the pinna adjacent to the ear canal is often affected by eczema. Topical corticosteroid creams and ointments (see section 13.4) are then required, but prolonged use should be avoided.

Astringent preparations

ALUMINIUM ACETATE

Indications: inflammation in otitis externa (see notes above)

Administration: insert into meatus or apply on a gauze wick which should be kept saturated with the ear drops

Aluminium Acetate (Non-proprietary)
Ear drops 13%, aluminium sulphate 2.25 g, calcium carbonate 1 g, tartaric acid 450 mg, acetic acid (33%) 2.5 mL, purified water 7.5 mL
Available from manufacturers of 'special order' products
Ear drops 8%, dilute 8 parts aluminium acetate ear drops (13%) with 5 parts purified water. Must be freshly prepared

Anti-inflammatory preparations

BETAMETHASONE SODIUM PHOSPHATE

Indications: eczematous inflammation in otitis externa (see notes above)

Cautions: avoid prolonged use

Contra-indications: untreated infection

Side-effects: local sensitivity reactions

Betnesol® (Celltech) [PoM]
Drops (for ear, eye, or nose), betamethasone sodium phosphate 0.1%. Net price 10 mL = £1.84
Excipients: include benzalkonium chloride, disodium edetate
Ear, apply 2–3 drops every 2–3 hours; reduce frequency when relief obtained; *eye*, see section 11.4.1; *nose*, see section 12.2.1

Vista-Methasone® (Martindale) [PoM]
Drops (for ear, eye, or nose), betamethasone sodium phosphate 0.1%. Net price 5 mL = £1.10; 10 mL = £1.25
Excipients: include benzalkonium chloride, disodium edetate
Ear, apply 2–3 drops every 3–4 hours; reduce frequency when relief obtained; *eye*, see section 11.4.1; *nose*, see section 12.2.1

■ With antibacterial

Betnesol-N® (Celltech) [PoM]
Drops (for ear, eye, or nose), betamethasone sodium phosphate 0.1%, neomycin sulphate 0.5%. Net price 10 mL = £1.89
Excipients: include benzalkonium chloride, disodium edetate
Ear, apply 2–3 drops 3–4 times daily; *eye*, see section 11.4.1; *nose*, section 12.2.3

Vista-Methasone N® (Martindale) [PoM]
Drops (for ear, eye, or nose), betamethasone sodium phosphate 0.1%, neomycin sulphate 0.5%. Net price 5 mL = £1.17; 10 mL = £1.29
Excipients: include thiomersal
Ear, apply 2–3 drops every 3–4 hours; reduce frequency when relief obtained; *eye*, see section 11.4.1; *nose*, section 12.2.3

DEXAMETHASONE

Indications: eczematous inflammation in otitis externa (see notes above)

Cautions: avoid prolonged use

Contra-indications: untreated infection

Side-effects: local sensitivity reactions

■ With antibacterial

Otomize® (Stafford-Miller) [PoM]
Ear spray, dexamethasone 0.1%, neomycin sulphate 3250 units/mL, glacial acetic acid 2%. Net price 5-mL pump-action aerosol unit = £3.85
Excipients: include hydroxybenzoates (parabens)
Apply 1 metered spray into the ear 3 times daily

Sofradex® (Florizel) [PoM]
Drops (for ear or eye), dexamethasone (as sodium metasulphobenzoate) 0.05%, framycetin sulphate 0.5%, gramicidin 0.005%. Net price 10 mL = £5.21
Excipients: include polysorbate 80
Ear, apply 2–3 drops 3–4 times daily; *eye*, see section 11.4.1
Ointment (for ear or eye), dexamethasone 0.05%, framycetin sulphate 0.5%, gramicidin 0.005%. Net price 5 g = £3.72
Ear, apply 1–2 times daily; *eye*, see section 11.4.1

FLUMETASONE PIVALATE
(Flumethasone Pivalate)

Indications: eczematous inflammation in otitis externa (see notes above)

Cautions: avoid prolonged use

Contra-indications: untreated infection

Side-effects: local sensitivity reactions

■ With antibacterial

Locorten-Vioform® (Novartis Consumer Health) [PoM]
Ear drops, flumetasone pivalate 0.02%, clioquinol 1%. Net price 7.5 mL = 97p
Apply 2–3 drops into the ear twice daily for up to 7–10 days; not recommended for child under 2 years

HYDROCORTISONE

Indications: eczematous inflammation in otitis externa (see notes above)

Cautions: avoid prolonged use

Contra-indications: untreated infection

Side-effects: local sensitivity reactions

■ With antibacterial

Gentisone HC® (Roche) [PoM]
Ear drops, hydrocortisone acetate 1%, gentamicin 0.3% (as sulphate). Net price 10 mL = £3.97
Excipients: include benzalkonium chloride, disodium edetate
Apply 2–4 drops into the ear 3–4 times daily and at night

Neo-Cortef® (Dominion) [PoM]
Drops (for ear or eye), hydrocortisone acetate 1.5%, neomycin sulphate 0.5%. Net price 10 mL = £4.11
Excipients: include miripirium chloride (myristyl-gamma-picolinium chloride)
Ear, apply 2–3 drops 3–4 times daily; *eye*, see section 11.4.1
Note. May be difficult to obtain
Ointment (for ear or eye), hydrocortisone acetate 1.5%, neomycin sulphate 0.5%. Net price 3.9 g = £1.53
Excipients: include wool fat
Ear, apply 1–2 times daily; *eye*, see section 11.4.1
Note. May be difficult to obtain

Otosporin® (GlaxoWellcome) [PoM] [▃▃]
Ear drops, hydrocortisone 1%, neomycin sulphate 3400 units, polymyxin B sulphate 10 000 units/mL. Net price 5 mL = £2.15; 10 mL = £4.30
Excipients: include cetostearyl alcohol, hydroxybenzoates (parabens), polysorbate 20
Apply 3 drops into the ear 3–4 times daily

PREDNISOLONE SODIUM PHOSPHATE

Indications: eczematous inflammation in otitis externa (see notes above)
Cautions: avoid prolonged use
Contra-indications: untreated infection
Side-effects: local sensitivity reactions

Predsol® (Celltech) [PoM]
Drops (for ear or eye), prednisolone sodium phosphate 0.5%. Net price 10 mL = £1.83
Excipients: include benzalkonium chloride, disodium edetate
Ear, apply 2–3 drops every 2–3 hours; reduce frequency when relief obtained; *eye*, see section 11.4.1

■ With antibacterial
Predsol-N® (Celltech) [PoM]
Drops (for ear or eye), prednisolone sodium phosphate 0.5%, neomycin sulphate 0.5%. Net price 10 mL = £1.95
Excipients: include benzalkonium chloride, disodium edetate
Ear, apply 2–3 drops 3–4 times daily; *eye*, see section 11.4.1

TRIAMCINOLONE ACETONIDE

Indications: eczematous inflammation in otitis externa (see notes above)
Cautions: avoid prolonged use
Contra-indications: untreated infection
Side-effects: local sensitivity reactions

■ With antibacterial
Audicort® (Wyeth) [PoM]
Ear drops, triamcinolone acetonide 0.1%, neomycin (as neomycin undecenoate) 0.35%. Net price 10 mL = £5.20
Excipients: include disodium edetate, propylene glycol, sodium metabisulphite
Apply 2–5 drops into the ear 3–4 times daily; CHILD not recommended

Tri-Adcortyl Otic® (Squibb) [PoM] [▃▃]
Ear ointment, triamcinolone acetonide 0.1%, gramicidin 0.025%, neomycin 0.25% (as sulphate), nystatin 100 000 units/g in *Plastibase®*. Net price 10 g = £1.58
Apply into the ear 2–4 times daily

Anti-infective preparations

CHLORAMPHENICOL [▃▃]

Indications: bacterial infection in otitis externa (but see notes above)
Cautions: avoid prolonged use (see notes above)
Side-effects: high incidence of sensitivity reactions to vehicle

Chloramphenicol (Non-proprietary) [PoM] [▃▃]
Ear drops, chloramphenicol in propylene glycol, net price 5%, 10 mL = £1.40; 10%, 10 mL = £1.40
Available from Martindale
Apply 2–3 drops into the ear 2–3 times daily

> [▃▃] denotes preparations that are considered to be less suitable for prescribing (see p. vi)

CLIOQUINOL

Indications: mild bacterial or fungal infections in otitis externa (see notes above)
Cautions: avoid prolonged use (see notes above)
Contra-indications: perforated tympanic membrane
Side-effects: local sensitivity; stains skin and clothing

■ With corticosteroid
Locorten-Vioform®, [PoM] see Flumetasone

CLOTRIMAZOLE

Indications: fungal infection in otitis externa (see notes above)
Side-effects: occasional local irritation or sensitivity

Canesten® (Bayer Consumer Care)
Solution, clotrimazole 1% in polyethylene glycol (macrogol 400). Net price 20 mL = £2.43
Ear, apply 2–3 times daily continuing for at least 14 days after disappearance of infection; *skin*, see section 13.10.2

FRAMYCETIN SULPHATE

Indications: see under Gentamicin
Cautions: see under Gentamicin
Contra-indications: perforated tympanic membrane (see notes above)
Side-effects: local sensitivity

■ With corticosteroid
Sofradex®, [PoM] see Dexamethasone

GENTAMICIN

Indications: bacterial infection in otitis externa (see notes above)
Cautions: avoid prolonged use (see notes above)
Contra-indications: perforated tympanic membrane (but see also notes above and section 12.1.2)
Side-effects: local sensitivity

Garamycin® (Schering-Plough) PoM
Drops (for ear or eye), gentamicin 0.3% (as sulphate). Net price 10 mL = £1.79
Excipients: include benzalkonium chloride
Ear, apply 3–4 drops 3–4 times daily; reduce frequency when relief obtained; *eye*, see section 11.3.1

Genticin® (Roche) PoM
Drops (for ear or eye), gentamicin 0.3% (as sulphate). Net price 10 mL = £1.91
Excipients: include benzalkonium chloride
Ear, apply 2–3 drops 3–4 times daily and at night; *eye*, see section 11.3.1

■ With corticosteroid
Gentisone HC®, PoM see Hydrocortisone

NEOMYCIN SULPHATE

Indications: bacterial infection in otitis externa (see notes above)
Cautions: avoid prolonged use (see notes above)
Contra-indications: perforated tympanic membrane (see notes above)
Side-effects: local sensitivity

■ With corticosteroid
Audicort® PoM see Triamcinolone
Betnesol-N® PoM see Betamethasone
Neo-Cortef® PoM see Hydrocortisone
Otomize® PoM see Dexamethasone
Otosporin® PoM see Hydrocortisone
Predsol-N® PoM see Prednisolone
Tri-Adcortyl Otic® PoM see Triamcinolone
Vista-Methasone N® PoM see Betamethasone

Other aural preparations

Choline salicylate is a mild analgesic but it is of doubtful value when applied topically.

Audax® (SSL) NHS ▭
Ear drops, choline salicylate 21.6%, glycerol 12.6%. Net price 10 mL = £2.56
Excipients: include propylene glycol

▭ denotes preparations that are considered to be less suitable for prescribing (see p. vi)

12.1.2   Otitis media

Acute otitis media is the commonest cause of severe pain in small children. Many infections are viral, especially those accompanying coryza, and they only need treatment with a **simple analgesic** such as paracetamol. Acute bacterial otitis media requires treatment with a **systemic antibacterial** in addition to an analgesic. Topical treatment of acute otitis media is ineffective and there is no place for drops containing a local anaesthetic. If the tympanic membrane has perforated, bacterial examination of any discharge is helpful in selecting an appropriate systemic antibacterial (Table 1, section 5.1).

In *recurrent acute otitis media* prophylaxis with an antibacterial (trimethoprim or erythromycin) during the winter months can be tried. A full course of a systemic antibacterial is required if otitis media recurs.

Otitis media with effusion ('glue ear') is present in about 10% of children and in 90% of children with cleft palates. Systemic antibacterials are not usually required for otitis media with effusion. If 'glue ear' persists for more than a month or two, the child should be referred to hospital for assessment and follow up because of the risk of long-term hearing impairment which can delay language development. Untreated or resistant glue ear may be responsible for some types of *chronic otitis media*.

The organisms recovered from patients with *chronic otitis media* are often opportunists living in the debris, keratin, and necrotic bone present in the middle ear and mastoid. Thorough cleansing with an aural suction tube may completely resolve infection of many years duration. Acute exacerbations of chronic infection may require systemic antibiotics (section 5.1, table 1). A swab should be taken to determine the organism present and its antibiotic sensitivity. Presence of *Pseudomonas aeruginosa* and *Proteus* spp, requires treatment with parenteral antibiotics. Local debridement of the meatal and middle ear contents may then be followed by topical treatment with ribbon gauze dressings as for otitis externa (section 12.1.1). This is particularly true with infections in mastoid cavities when dusting powders can also be tried.

The CSM has issued a reminder (section 12.1.1) that topical treatment with ototoxic antibiotics is contra-indicated in the presence of a perforation. However, many specialists use ear drops containing **aminoglycosides** (e.g. neomycin) or **polymyxins** if the otitis media has failed to settle with systemic antibiotics; it is considered that the pus in the middle ear associated with otitis media carries a higher risk of ototoxicity than the drops themselves.

12.1.3   Removal of ear wax

Wax is a normal bodily secretion which provides a protective film on the meatal skin and need only be removed if it causes deafness or interferes with a proper view of the ear drum. Syringing is generally best avoided in patients with a history of recurring otitis externa, a history of ear drum perforation, or previous ear surgery. A person who has hearing in one ear only should not have that ear syringed because even a very slight risk of damage is unacceptable in this situation.

Wax may be removed by syringing with water (warmed to body temperature). If necessary, wax can be softened before syringing with simple remedies such as **sodium bicarbonate** ear drops, **olive oil** ear drops or **almond oil** ear drops, which are safe, effective and inexpensive. If the wax is hard and impacted the drops may be used twice daily for a few days before syringing; otherwise the wax may be softened on the day of syringing. The patient should lie with the affected ear uppermost for 5 to 10 minutes after a generous amount of the softening remedy has been introduced into the ear. Some proprietary preparations containing organic solvents can cause irritation of the meatal skin, and in most cases the simple remedies indicated above are just as effective and less likely to cause irritation. Docusate sodium or urea–hydrogen peroxide are ingredients in a number of proprietary preparations.

Almond Oil (Non-proprietary)
Ear drops, almond oil in a suitable container
Allow to warm to room temperature before use

Olive Oil (Non-proprietary)
Ear drops, olive oil in a suitable container
Allow to warm to room temperature before use

Sodium Bicarbonate (Non-proprietary)
Ear drops, sodium bicarbonate 5%, net price 10 mL = £1.18
Available from Thornton & Ross

Cerumol® (LAB) ▱
Ear drops, chlorobutanol 5%, paradichlorobenzene 2%, arachis (peanut) oil 57.3%. Net price 11 mL = £1.45

Exterol® (Dermal) ▱
Ear drops, urea–hydrogen peroxide complex 5% in glycerol. Net price 8 mL = £1.97

Molcer® (Wallace Mfg) ▱
Ear drops, docusate sodium 5%. Net price 15 mL = £1.32

Otex® (DDD) ▱
Ear drops, urea–hydrogen peroxide 5%. Net price 8 mL = £2.64

Waxsol® (Norgine) ▱
Ear drops, docusate sodium 0.5%. Net price 10 mL = £1.24

▱ denotes preparations that are considered to be less suitable for prescribing (see p. vi)

12.2 Drugs acting on the nose

12.2.1	Drugs used in nasal allergy
12.2.2	Topical nasal decongestants
12.2.3	Nasal preparations for infection and epistaxis

Rhinitis may be self-limiting and sinusitis is best treated with systemic antibiotics (section 5.1, table 1). There are few indications for nasal sprays and drops except in allergic rhinitis and perennial rhinitis (section 12.2.1). Many nasal preparations contain sympathomimetic drugs which may damage the nasal cilia (section 12.2.2). Some specialists use saline sniffs for a short period after endonasal surgery.

NASAL POLYPS. Short-term use of corticosteroid nasal drops helps to produce significant shrinkage of nasal polyps; to be effective, the drops must be administered with the patient in the 'head down' position. The reduction in swelling can be maintained by continuing treatment with a corticosteroid nasal spray. A short course of a systemic corticosteroid may be required initially to shrink large polyps.

12.2.1 Drugs used in nasal allergy

Mild cases of allergic rhinitis are controlled by topical **nasal corticosteroids** or **oral antihistamines** (section 3.4.1); **systemic nasal decongestants** are of doubtful value (section 3.10).

More persistent symptoms and nasal congestion can be relieved by topical nasal **corticosteroids** and **cromoglicate** (cromoglycate); topical antihistamines (azelastine and levocabastine) are also used in allergic rhinitis. In seasonal allergic rhinitis (e.g. hay fever), treatment should begin 2 to 3 weeks before the season commences and may have to be continued for several months; treatment may be required for years in perennial rhinitis.

In allergic rhinitis, topical preparations of corticosteroids and cromoglicate have a well-established role; although it may be less effective, cromoglicate is often the first choice in children. Topical antihistamines are considered less effective than topical corticosteroids but probably more effective than cromoglicate.

Sometimes allergic rhinitis is accompanied by vasomotor rhinitis. In this situation, the addition of topical nasal ipratropium bromide (section 12.2.2) can reduce watery rhinorrhoea.

Very disabling symptoms occasionally justify the use of **systemic corticosteroids** for short periods (section 6.3), for example in students taking important examinations. They may also be used at the beginning of a course of treatment with a corticosteroid spray to relieve severe mucosal oedema and allow the spray to penetrate the nasal cavity.

Antihistamines

AZELASTINE HYDROCHLORIDE

Indications: allergic rhinitis
Side-effects: irritation of nasal mucosa; bitter taste (if applied incorrectly)

[1]**Rhinolast®** (ASTA Medica) PoM
Aqueous nasal spray, azelastine hydrochloride 140 micrograms (0.14 mL)/metered spray. Net price 20 mL (with metered pump) = £11.92
Excipients: include benzalkonium chloride, sodium edetate
ADULT and CHILD over 5 years, apply 140 micrograms (1 spray) into each nostril twice daily
1. Can be sold to the public for nasal administration in aqueous form (other than by aerosol) if supplied for the treatment of seasonal allergic rhinitis or perennial allergic rhinitis in adults and children over 5 years, subject to max. single dose of 140 micrograms per nostril, max. daily dose of 280 micrograms per nostril, and a pack size limit of 36 doses; a proprietary brand (*Rhinolast® Allergy*) is on sale to the public

LEVOCABASTINE

Indications: treatment of allergic rhinitis
Cautions: renal impairment (see Appendix 3)
Side-effects: nasal irritation; hypersensitivity reactions, headache, fatigue, drowsiness reported

¹Livostin® (Novartis) [PoM]

Aqueous nasal spray, levocabastine (as hydrochloride) 0.05%. Net price 10-mL spray pump = £9.74

Excipients: include disodium edetate, propylene glycol, polysorbate 80 and benzalkonium chloride

ADULT and CHILD over 9 years, apply 2 sprays into each nostril twice daily, increased if necessary to 3–4 times daily

1. Can be sold to the public for nasal administration if supplied for symptomatic treatment of seasonal allergic rhinitis in adults and children over 12 years subject to max. strength of levocabastine 0.05% and max. pack size 10 mL; proprietary brands on sale to the public include *Livostin® Direct Nasal Spray*

Corticosteroids

Nasal preparations containing corticosteroids (beclometasone, betamethasone, budesonide, flunisolide, fluticasone, mometasone, and triamcinolone) have a useful role in the prophylaxis and treatment of allergic rhinitis (see notes above).

CAUTIONS. Corticosteroid nasal preparations should be avoided in the presence of untreated nasal infections, and also after nasal surgery (until healing has occurred); they should also be avoided in pulmonary tuberculosis. Patients transferred from systemic corticosteroids may experience exacerbation of some symptoms. Systemic absorption may follow nasal administration particularly if high doses are used or if treatment is prolonged; for cautions and side-effects of systemic corticosteroids, see section 6.3.2. The risk of systemic effects may be greater with nasal drops than with nasal sprays; drops are administered incorrectly more often than sprays. The CSM recommends that the height of children receiving prolonged treatment with nasal corticosteroids is monitored; if growth is slowed, referral to a paediatrician should be considered.

SIDE-EFFECTS. Local side-effects include dryness, irritation of nose and throat, epistaxis and rarely ulceration; nasal septal perforation (usually following nasal surgery) and raised intra-ocular pressure or glaucoma may also occur rarely. Smell and taste disturbances may also occur. Hypersensitivity reactions, including bronchospasm, have been reported.

BECLOMETASONE DIPROPIONATE
(Beclomethasone Dipropionate)

Indications: prophylaxis and treatment of allergic and vasomotor rhinitis

Cautions: see notes above

Side-effects: see notes above

Dose: ADULT and CHILD over 6 years, apply 100 micrograms (2 sprays) into each nostril twice daily *or* 50 micrograms (1 spray) into each nostril 3–4 times daily; max. total 400 micrograms (8 sprays) daily; when symptoms controlled, dose reduced to 50 micrograms (1 spray) into each nostril twice daily

¹Beclometasone (Non-proprietary) [PoM]

Nasal spray, beclometasone dipropionate 50 micrograms/metered spray. Net price 200-spray unit = £3.44

Available from Alpharma, Galen (*Beclo-aqua® 50*), Generics, IVAX (*Nasobec Aqueous®*)

1. Can be sold to the public for nasal administration (other than by aerosol) if supplied for the prevention and

treatment of allergic rhinitis in adults over 18 years subject to max. single dose of 100 micrograms per nostril, max. daily dose of 200 micrograms per nostril for max. period of 3 months, and a pack size of 20 mg; proprietary brands on sale to the public include *Beconase® Allergy, Boots Hayfever Relief®, Care Hayfever Relief®, Nasobec® Hayfever*

Beconase® (A&H) [PoM]

Nasal spray (aqueous suspension), beclometasone dipropionate 50 micrograms/metered spray. Net price 200-spray unit with applicator = £4.01

Excipients: include benzalkonium chloride, polysorbate 80

BETAMETHASONE SODIUM PHOSPHATE

Indications: non-infected inflammatory conditions of nose

Cautions: see notes above

Side-effects: see notes above

Betnesol® (Celltech) [PoM]

Drops (for ear, eye, or nose), betamethasone sodium phosphate 0.1%. Net price 10 mL = £1.35

Excipients: include benzalkonium chloride, disodium edetate

Nose, apply 2–3 drops into each nostril 2–3 times daily; *ear,* section 12.1.1; *eye,* see section 11.4.1

Vista-Methasone® (Martindale) [PoM]

Drops (for ear, eye, or nose), betamethasone sodium phosphate 0.1%. Net price 5 mL = £1.10, 10 mL = £1.25

Excipients: include benzalkonium chloride, disodium edetate

Nose, apply 2–3 drops into each nostril twice daily; *ear,* section 12.1.1; *eye,* see section 11.4.1

BUDESONIDE

Indications: prophylaxis and treatment of allergic and vasomotor rhinitis; nasal polyps

Cautions: see notes above

Side-effects: see notes above

Dose: rhinitis, ADULT and CHILD over 12 years, apply 200 micrograms (2 sprays) into each nostril once daily in the morning *or* 100 micrograms (1 spray) into each nostril twice daily; when control achieved reduce to 100 micrograms (1 spray) into each nostril once daily

Nasal polyps, ADULT and CHILD over 12 years, 100 micrograms (1 spray) into each nostril twice daily for up to 3 months

¹Budesonide (Non-proprietary) [PoM]

Nasal spray, budesonide 100 micrograms/metered spray, net price 100-spray unit = £5.85

Available from Generics

1. Can be sold to the public for nasal administration (other than by aerosol) if supplied for the prevention and treatment of seasonal allergic rhinitis in adults over 18 years subject to max. single dose of 200 micrograms per nostril, max. daily dose of 200 micrograms per nostril for max. period of 3 months, and a pack size of 10 mg

Rhinocort Aqua® (AstraZeneca) [PoM]

Nasal spray, budesonide 100 micrograms/metered spray. Net price 100-spray unit = £5.85

Excipients: include disodium edetate, polysorbate 80, potassium sorbate

DEXAMETHASONE ISONICOTINATE

Indications: treatment of allergic rhinitis
Cautions: see notes above; avoid contact with eyes
Side-effects: see notes above

■ With sympathomimetic
For cautions and side-effects of sympathomimetics see Ephedrine Hydrochloride, section 12.2.2

Dexa-Rhinaspray Duo® (Boehringer Ingelheim) PoM

Nasal spray, dexamethasone isonicotinate 20 micrograms, tramazoline hydrochloride 120 micrograms/metered spray. Net price 110-dose unit = £2.15
Excipients: include benzalkonium chloride, polysorbate 80
Allergic rhinitis, ADULT and CHILD over 12 years, apply 1 spray into each nostril 2–3 times daily, max. 6 times daily; max. duration 14 days; CHILD 5–12 years 1 spray into each nostril up to twice daily; under 5 years not recommended

FLUNISOLIDE

Indications: prophylaxis and treatment of allergic rhinitis
Cautions: see notes above
Side-effects: see notes above

Syntaris® (Roche) PoM

Aqueous nasal spray, flunisolide 25 micrograms/metered spray. Net price 240-spray unit with pump and applicator = £5.25
Excipients: include benzalkonium chloride, butylated hydroxytoluene, disodium edetate, polysorbates, propylene glycol
ADULT, apply 50 micrograms (2 sprays) into each nostril twice daily, increased if necessary to max. 3 times daily then reduced for maintenance; CHILD 5–14 years initially 25 micrograms (1 spray) into each nostril up to 3 times daily

FLUTICASONE PROPIONATE

Indications: see under preparations below
Cautions: see notes above
Side-effects: see notes above

Flixonase® (A&H) PoM

Aqueous nasal spray, fluticasone propionate 50 micrograms/metered spray. Net price 150-spray unit with applicator = £11.43
Excipients: include benzalkonium chloride, polysorbate 80
Prophylaxis and treatment of allergic rhinitis, ADULT and CHILD over 12 years, apply 100 micrograms (2 sprays) into each nostril once daily, preferably in the morning, increased to max. twice daily if required; when control achieved reduce to 50 micrograms (1 spray) into each nostril once daily; CHILD 4–11 years, 50 micrograms (1 spray) into each nostril once daily, increased to max. twice daily if required

Flixonase Nasule® (A&H) ▼ PoM

Nasal drops, fluticasone propionate 400 micrograms/unit dose, net price 28 × 0.4-mL units = £13.48
Excipients: include polysorbate 20
Nasal polyps, apply approx. 6 drops into each nostril once or twice daily, consider alternative treatment if no improvement after 4–6 weeks; CHILD not recommended

MOMETASONE FUROATE

Indications: prophylaxis and treatment of allergic rhinitis
Cautions: see notes above
Side-effects: see notes above

Nasonex® (Schering-Plough) PoM

Aqueous nasal spray, mometasone furoate 50 micrograms/metered spray. Net price 140-spray unit = £10.92
Excipients: include benzalkonium chloride, polysorbate 80
ADULT and CHILD over 12 years, apply 100 micrograms (2 sprays) into each nostril once daily, increased if necessary to max. 200 micrograms (4 sprays) into each nostril once daily; when control achieved reduce to 50 micrograms (1 spray) into each nostril once daily; CHILD 6–11 years, 50 micrograms (1 spray) into each nostril once daily

TRIAMCINOLONE ACETONIDE

Indications: prophylaxis and treatment of allergic rhinitis
Cautions: see notes above
Side-effects: see notes above

¹Nasacort® (Rhône-Poulenc Rorer) PoM

Aqueous nasal spray, triamcinolone acetonide 55 micrograms/metered spray. Net price 120-spray unit = £9.60
Excipients: include benzalkonium chloride, disodium edetate, polysorbate 80
ADULT and CHILD over 12 years apply 110 micrograms (2 sprays) into each nostril once daily; when control achieved, reduce to 55 micrograms (1 spray) into each nostril once daily; CHILD 6–12 years, 55 micrograms (1 spray) into each nostril once daily

1. Can be sold to the public for nasal administration as a non-pressurised nasal spray if supplied for the symptomatic treatment of seasonal allergic rhinitis in adults over 18 years, subject to max. daily dose of 110 micrograms per nostril for max. 3 months, and a pack size of 3.575 mg

Cromoglicate

SODIUM CROMOGLICATE

(Sodium Cromoglycate)
Indications: prophylaxis of allergic rhinitis
Side-effects: local irritation; rarely transient bronchospasm

Rynacrom® (Pantheon)

4% aqueous nasal spray, sodium cromoglicate 4% (5.2 mg/squeeze). Net price 22 mL with pump = £19.10
Excipients: include benzalkonium chloride
ADULT and CHILD, apply 1 squeeze into each nostril 2–4 times daily

Vividrin® (Pharma-Global)

Nasal spray, sodium cromoglicate 2%. Net price 15 mL = £8.15
Excipients: include benzalkonium chloride, edetic acid, polysorbate 80
ADULT and CHILD, apply 1 spray into each nostril 4–6 times daily

■ With sympathomimetic

Rynacrom Compound® (Pantheon)
Nasal spray, sodium cromoglicate 2% (2.6 mg/metered spray) and xylometazoline hydrochloride 0.025% (32.5 micrograms/metered spray). Net price 26 mL with pump = £14.33
Excipients: include benzalkonium chloride, disodium edetate
Apply 1 spray into each nostril 4 times daily
Note. A proprietary brand of sodium cromoglicate 2% and xylometazoline hydrochloride 0.025% (*Rynacrom Allergy®*) is on sale to the public

12.2.2 Topical nasal decongestants

The nasal mucosa is sensitive to changes in atmospheric temperature and humidity and these alone may cause slight nasal congestion. The nose and nasal sinuses produce a litre of mucus in 24 hours and much of this finds its way silently into the stomach via the nasopharynx. Slight changes in the nasal airway, accompanied by an awareness of mucus passing along the nasopharynx causes some patients to be inaccurately diagnosed as suffering from chronic sinusitis. These symptoms are particularly noticeable in the later stages of the common cold. **Sodium chloride** 0.9% given as nasal drops may relieve nasal congestion by helping to liquefy mucous secretions. Corticosteroid nasal drops produce shrinkage of nasal polyps (section 12.2).

Symptoms of nasal congestion associated with vasomotor rhinitis and the common cold can be relieved by the short-term use (usually not longer than 7 days) of decongestant nasal drops and sprays. These all contain sympathomimetic drugs which exert their effect by vasoconstriction of the mucosal blood vessels which in turn reduces oedema of the nasal mucosa. They are of limited value because they can give rise to a rebound congestion (rhinitis medicamentosa) on withdrawal, due to a secondary vasodilation with a subsequent temporary increase in nasal congestion. This in turn tempts the further use of the decongestant, leading to a vicious cycle of events. **Ephedrine nasal drops** is the safest sympathomimetic preparation and can give relief for several hours. The more potent sympathomimetic drugs oxymetazoline, and xylometazoline are more likely to cause a rebound effect. **All** of these preparations may cause a hypertensive crisis if used during treatment with a monoamine-oxidase inhibitor.

Non-allergic watery rhinorrhoea often responds well to treatment with the antimuscarinic **ipratropium bromide**.

Inhalation of **warm moist air** is useful in the treatment of symptoms of acute infective conditions, and the use of compounds containing volatile substances such as menthol and eucalyptus may encourage their use (section 3.8).

Systemic nasal decongestants—see section 3.10.

Sympathomimetics

EPHEDRINE HYDROCHLORIDE

Indications: nasal congestion
Cautions: avoid excessive or prolonged use; caution in infants under 3 months (no good evidence of value—if irritation occurs might narrow nasal

passage); **interactions:** Appendix 1 (sympathomimetics)
Side-effects: local irritation, nausea, headache; after excessive use tolerance with diminished effect, rebound congestion; cardiovascular effects also reported
Administration: see below

Ephedrine (Non-proprietary)
Nasal drops, ephedrine hydrochloride 0.5%, net price 10 mL = £1.09; 1%, 10 mL = £1.15
Note. The BP directs that if no strength is specified 0.5% drops should be supplied
Instil 1–2 drops into each nostril up to 3 or 4 times daily when required

XYLOMETAZOLINE HYDROCHLORIDE

Indications: nasal congestion
Cautions: see under Ephedrine Hydrochloride and notes above
Side-effects: see under Ephedrine Hydrochloride and notes above
Administration: see below

Xylometazoline (Non-proprietary)
Nasal drops, xylometazoline hydrochloride 0.1%, net price 10 mL = £1.69
Instil 2–3 drops into each nostril 2–3 times daily when required; max. duration 7 days; not recommended for children under 12 years
Available from Manx (*Otradrops®*), Novartis Consumer Health (*Otrivine®* [NHS])
Paediatric nasal drops, xylometazoline hydrochloride 0.05%, net price 10 mL = £1.59
CHILD over 3 months instil 1–2 drops into each nostril 1–2 times daily when required (not recommended for infants under 3 months of age, doctor's advice only under 2 years); max. duration 7 days
Available from Manx (*Otradrops®*), Novartis Consumer Health (*Otrivine®* [NHS], *Tixycolds®*)
Nasal spray, xylometazoline hydrochloride 0.1%, net price 10 mL = £1.78
Apply 1 spray into each nostril 2–3 times daily when required; max. duration 7 days; not recommended for children under 12 years
Available from Manx (*Otraspray®*), Novartis Consumer Health (*Otrivine®* [NHS])

Sympathomimetic nasal preparations on sale to the public (not prescribable on the NHS) include:

Afrazine® (oxymetazoline), **Dristan®** (oxymetazoline), **Fenox®** (phenylephrine), **Sudafed®** nasal spray (oxymetazoline), **Vicks Sinex®** (oxymetazoline)

Antimuscarinic

IPRATROPIUM BROMIDE

Indications: rhinorrhoea associated with allergic and non-allergic rhinitis
Cautions: see section 3.1.2; avoid spraying near eyes
Side-effects: nasal dryness and epistaxis
Administration: apply 42 micrograms (2 sprays) into each nostril 2–3 times daily; CHILD under 12 years not recommended

Rinatec® (Boehringer Ingelheim) [PoM]
Nasal spray 0.03%, ipratropium bromide 21 micrograms/metered spray. Net price 180-dose unit = £4.55
Excipients: include benzalkonium chloride

12.2.3 Nasal preparations for infection and epistaxis

There is **no** evidence that topical anti-infective nasal preparations have any therapeutic value in rhinitis or sinusitis; for elimination of nasal staphylococci, see below.

Systemic treatment of sinusitis—see section 5.1, table 1.

Betnesol-N® (Celltech) PoM ◢

Drops (for ear, eye, or nose), betamethasone sodium phosphate 0.1%, neomycin sulphate 0.5%. Net price 10 mL = £1.35

Excipients: include benzalkonium chloride

Nose, apply 2–3 drops into nostril 2–3 times daily; *eye*, see section 11.4.1; *ear*, see section 12.1.1

¹ **Locabiotal®** (Servier) NHS   PoM ◢

Spray, fusafungine 500 micrograms/metered spray. Net price 50-spray unit with nasal (yellow) and oral (white) adapters = £1.55

Excipients: include alcohol

1. NHS Except for treatment of infections and inflammation of the oropharynx and endorsed 'SLS'

Infection and inflammation of upper respiratory tract (but not recommended, see notes above), 1 spray into each nostril or into mouth every 4 hours; CHILD 1 spray into each nostril or into mouth every 6 hours; withdraw if no improvement after 7 days

Vista-Methasone N® (Martindale) PoM ◢

Drops (for ear, eye, or nose), betamethasone sodium phosphate 0.1%, neomycin sulphate 0.5%. Net price 5 mL = £1.17, 10 mL = £1.29

Excipients: include thiomersal

Nose, apply 2–3 drops into each nostril twice daily; *eye*, see section 11.4.1; *ear*, see section 12.1.1

◢ denotes preparations that are considered to be less suitable for prescribing (see p. vi)

Nasal staphylococci

Elimination of organisms such as staphylococci from the nasal vestibule can be achieved by the use of a cream containing **chlorhexidine and neomycin** (*Naseptin®*), but re-colonisation frequently occurs. Coagulase-positive staphylococci are present in the noses of 40% of the population.

A nasal ointment containing **mupirocin** is also available; it should probably be held in reserve for resistant cases. In hospital, mupirocin nasal ointment should be reserved for the eradication (in both patients and staff) of nasal carriage of methicillin-resistant *Staphylococcus aureus* (MRSA). The ointment should be applied 3 times daily for 5 days and a sample taken 2 days after treatment to confirm eradication. The course may be repeated if the sample is positive (and the throat is not colonised). To avoid the development of resistance, the treatment course should not exceed 7 days and the course should not be repeated on more than one occasion. If the MRSA strain is mupirocin-resistant or does not respond after 2 courses, consider alternative products such as chlorhexidine and neomycin cream.

Bactroban Nasal® (Beecham) PoM

Nasal ointment, mupirocin 2% (as calcium salt) in white soft paraffin basis. Net price 3 g = £6.24

For eradication of nasal carriage of staphylococci, including methicillin-resistant *Staphylococcus aureus* (MRSA), apply 2–3 times daily to the inner surface of each nostril

Naseptin® (Alliance) PoM

Cream, chlorhexidine hydrochloride 0.1%, neomycin sulphate 3250 units/g. Net price 15 g = £1.48

Excipients: include arachis (peanut) oil

For eradication of nasal carriage of staphylococci, apply to nostrils 4 times daily for 10 days; for preventing nasal carriage of staphylococci apply to nostrils twice daily

---

Epistaxis

Bismuth iodoform paraffin paste (BIPP) is used for packing cavities after ear, nose and oropharyngeal surgery as a mild disinfectant and astringent; it is also used to pack nasal cavities in acute epistaxis. It is available either as a paste, to be applied to ribbon gauze packing, or as BIPP-impregnated ribbon gauze.

BISMUTH SUBNITRATE AND IODOFORM

Indications: packing cavities after ear, nose or oropharyngeal surgery; epistaxis

Cautions: hyperthyroidism

Side-effects: erythematous rash (discontinue use); encephalopathy reported only with large packs or when placed directly on neural tissue

Bismuth Subnitrate and Iodoform (Non-proprietary)

Paste, 30-g sachet, net price = £9.50; 30-g tube = £9.50

Available from Aurum

Impregnated gauze, sterile, net price 1.25 cm × 100 cm, 10 = £89.70; 1.25 cm × 125 cm, 5 = £44.85; 1.25 cm × 200 cm, 5 = £62.05; 1.25 cm × 300 cm, 5 = £81.15; 2.5 cm × 100 cm, 10 = £97.20; 2.5 cm × 125 cm, 5 = £48.60; 2.5 cm × 200 cm, 5 = £70.35; 2.5 cm × 300 cm, 5 = £92.55

Available from Aurum

12.3 Drugs acting on the oropharynx

12.3.1 Drugs for oral ulceration and inflammation
12.3.2 Oropharyngeal anti-infective drugs
12.3.3 Lozenges and sprays
12.3.4 Mouthwashes, gargles, and dentifrices
12.3.5 Treatment of dry mouth

12.3.1 Drugs for oral ulceration and inflammation

Ulceration of the oral mucosa may be caused by trauma (physical or chemical), recurrent aphthae, infections, carcinoma, dermatological disorders, nutritional deficiencies, gastro-intestinal disease, haematopoietic disorders, and drug therapy. It is important to establish the diagnosis in each case as the majority of these lesions require specific management in addition to local treatment. Patients with an unexplained mouth ulcer of more than 3 weeks' duration require urgent referral to hospital to exclude oral cancer. Local treatment aims at protecting the ulcerated area, or at relieving pain or reducing inflammation.

SIMPLE MOUTHWASHES. A **saline** or **compound thymol glycerin** mouthwash (section 12.3.4) may relieve the pain of traumatic ulceration. The mouthwash is made up with warm water and used at frequent intervals until the discomfort and swelling subsides.

ANTISEPTIC MOUTHWASHES. Secondary bacterial infection may be a feature of any mucosal ulceration; it can increase discomfort and delay healing. Use of a **chlorhexidine** or **povidone–iodine** mouthwash (section 12.3.4) is often beneficial and may accelerate healing of recurrent aphthae.

MECHANICAL PROTECTION. **Carmellose gelatin paste** may relieve some discomfort arising from ulceration by protecting the ulcer site. The paste adheres to the mucosa, but is difficult to apply effectively to some parts of the mouth.

CORTICOSTEROIDS. Topical corticosteroid therapy may be used for some forms of oral ulceration. In the case of aphthous ulcers it is most effective if applied in the 'prodromal' phase.

Thrush or other types of candidiasis are recognised complications of corticosteroid treatment.

Hydrocortisone lozenges are allowed to dissolve next to an ulcer and are useful in recurrent aphthae and erosive lichenoid lesions (mucositis).

Triamcinolone dental paste is designed to keep the corticosteroid in contact with the mucosa for long enough to permit penetration of the lesion, but is difficult for patients to apply properly.

Systemic corticosteroid therapy is reserved for severe conditions such as pemphigus vulgaris (section 6.3.4).

LOCAL ANALGESICS. Local analgesics have a limited role in the management of oral ulceration. When applied topically their action is of a relatively short duration so that analgesia cannot be maintained continuously throughout the day. The main indication for a topical local analgesic is to relieve the pain of otherwise intractable oral ulceration particularly when it is due to major aphthae. For this purpose lidocaine (lignocaine) 5% ointment or lozenges containing a local anaesthetic are applied to the ulcer. When local anaesthetics are used in the mouth care must be taken not to produce anaesthesia of the pharynx before meals as this might lead to choking.

Benzydamine mouthwash or spray may be useful in palliating the discomfort associated with a variety of ulcerative conditions. It has also been found to be effective in reducing the discomfort of post-irradiation mucositis. Some patients find the full-strength mouthwash causes some stinging and, for them, it should be diluted with an equal volume of water. **Flurbiprofen** lozenges are licensed for the relief of sore throat.

Choline salicylate dental gel has some analgesic action and may provide relief for recurrent aphthae, but excessive application or confinement under a denture irritates the mucosa and can itself cause ulceration. Benefit in teething may merely be due to pressure of application (comparable with biting a teething ring); excessive use can lead to salicylate poisoning.

OTHER PREPARATIONS. **Carbenoxolone** gel or mouthwash may be of some value. **Tetracycline** rinsed in the mouth may also be of value.

BENZYDAMINE HYDROCHLORIDE

Indications: painful inflammatory conditions of oropharynx

Side-effects: occasional numbness or stinging; rarely hypersensitivity reactions

Difflam® (3M)
Oral rinse, green, benzydamine hydrochloride 0.15%, net price 200 mL (*Difflam® Sore Throat Rinse*) = £2.83; 300 mL = £3.92
Rinse or gargle, using 15 mL (diluted with water if stinging occurs) every 1½–3 hours as required, usually for not more than 7 days; not suitable for children aged 12 years or under
Spray, benzydamine hydrochloride 0.15%. Net price 30-mL unit = £3.41
ADULT, 4–8 puffs onto affected area every 1½–3 hours; CHILD under 6 years 1 puff per 4 kg body-weight to max. 4 puffs every 1½–3 hours; 6–12 years 4 puffs every 1½–3 hours

---

CARBENOXOLONE SODIUM

Indications: mild oral and perioral lesions

Bioral Gel® (Merck Consumer Health)
Gel, carbenoxolone sodium 2% in adhesive basis. Net price 5 g = £2.38
Apply after meals and at bedtime

Bioplex® (Provalis) [PoM]
Mouthwash granules, carbenoxolone sodium 1% (20 mg/sachet). Net price 24 × 2-g sachets = £7.23
For mouth ulcers, rinse with 1 sachet in 30–50 mL of warm water 3 times daily and at bedtime

---

CARMELLOSE SODIUM

Indications: mechanical protection of oral and perioral lesions

Orabase® (ConvaTec)
Protective paste (= oral paste), carmellose sodium 16.7%, pectin 16.7%, gelatin 16.7%, in *Plastibase®*. Net price 30 g = £1.84; 100 g = £4.10
Apply a thin layer when necessary after meals

Orahesive® (ConvaTec)
Powder, carmellose sodium, pectin, gelatin, equal parts. Net price 25 g = £2.09
Sprinkle on the affected area

CORTICOSTEROIDS

Indications: oral and perioral lesions
Contra-indications: untreated oral infection; manufacturer of triamcinolone contra-indicates use on tuberculous and viral lesions
Side-effects: occasional exacerbation of local infection

¹**Adcortyl in Orabase®** (Squibb) [PoM]
Oral paste, triamcinolone acetonide 0.1% in adhesive basis. Net price 10 g = £1.27
ADULT and CHILD, apply a thin layer 2–4 times daily; do not rub in; use limited to 5 days for children and short-term use also advised for elderly
1. A 5-g tube (*Adcortyl in Orabase® for Mouth Ulcers*) is on sale to the public for the treatment of common mouth ulcers for max. 5 days

Corlan® (Celltech)
Pellets (= lozenges), hydrocortisone 2.5 mg (as sodium succinate). Net price 20 = £2.10
Note. Supplies may be difficult to obtain
ADULT and CHILD, 1 lozenge 4 times daily, allowed to dissolve slowly in the mouth in contact with the ulcer

FLURBIPROFEN

Indications: relief of sore throat
Cautions: see section 10.1.1
Contra-indications: see section 10.1.1
Side-effects: taste disturbance, mouth ulcers (move lozenge around mouth); see also section 10.1.1

Strefen® (Crookes) [PoM]
Lozenges, flurbiprofen 8.75 mg, net price 16 = £2.00
Allow 1 lozenge to dissolve slowly in the mouth every 3–6 hours, max. 5 lozenges in 24 hours, for max. 3 days; CHILD under 12 years not recommended

LOCAL ANAESTHETICS

Indications: relief of pain in oral lesions
Cautions: avoid prolonged use; hypersensitivity

Preparations
Local anaesthetics are included in some mouth ulcer preparations, for details see below
Local anaesthetics are also included in some throat lozenges and sprays, see section 12.3.3

SALICYLATES

Indications: mild oral and perioral lesions
Cautions: frequent application, especially in children, may give rise to salicylate poisoning
Note. CSM warning on aspirin and Reye's syndrome does not apply to non-aspirin salicylates or to topical preparations such as teething gels

■ Choline salicylate
Choline Salicylate Dental Gel, BP
Oral gel, choline salicylate 8.7% in a flavoured gel basis
Available as *Bonjela®* (R&C), net price 15 g (sugar-free) = £1.70; *Dinnefords Teejel®* (SSL), 10 g = £1.36
Apply ½-inch of gel with gentle massage not more often than every 3 hours; CHILD over 4 months ¼-inch of gel not more often than every 3 hours; max. 6 applications daily

■ Salicylic acid
Pyralvex® (Norgine)
Oral paint, brown, rhubarb extract (anthraquinone glycosides 0.5%), salicylic acid 1%. Net price 10 mL with brush = £1.41
Apply 3–4 times daily; CHILD under 12 years not recommended

TETRACYCLINE

Indications: severe recurrent aphthous ulceration; oral herpes (section 12.3.2)
Side-effects: fungal superinfection
For side-effects, cautions and contra-indications relating to systemic administration of tetracyclines see section 5.1.3

Local application
For preparation of a mouthwash, the contents of a 250–mg tetracycline capsule (see section 5.1.3) can be stirred into a small amount of water, then held in the mouth for 2–3 minutes 3-4 times daily usually for 3 days; longer courses are sometimes used (but precautions may be required to avoid oral thrush, section 12.3.2); it should preferably not be swallowed [unlicensed indication]
Note. Tetracycline stains teeth; avoid in children under 12 years of age

The following list includes topical treatments for mouth ulcers and for teething on sale to the public, together with their significant ingredients:

Anbesol Liquid® and **Anbesol Teething gel®** (cetylpyridinium, chlorocresol, lidocaine (lignocaine)), **Bansor®** (cetrimide), **Bioral Gel®** (carbenoxolone), **Bonjela gel®** (choline salicylate), **Calgel®** (cetylpyridinium, lidocaine (lignocaine)), **Dentinox Teething gel®** (cetylpyridinium, lidocaine (lignocaine)), **Dinnefords Teejel®** (choline salicylate, chlorobutanol, menthol), **Medijel®** (aminoacridine (aminacrine), lidocaine (lignocaine)), **Pyralvex®** (anthraquinone glycoside, salicylic acid), **Rinstead Adult gel®** (benzocaine, chloroxylenol), **Rinstead Contact pastilles®** (lidocaine (lignocaine)), **Rinstead pastilles®** (cetylpyridinium, menthol), **Rinstead Teething gel®** (cetylpyridinium, lidocaine (lignocaine)), **Woodward's Teething gel®** (cetylpyridinium, lidocaine (lignocaine))

Drugs for periodontitis

Low-dose doxycycline (*Periostat®*) is licensed as an adjunct to scaling and root planing for the treatment of periodontitis; doxycycline reduces collagenase activity at a low dose without inhibiting bacteria associated with periodontitis. For anti-infectives used in the treatment of periodontal disease, see section 12.3.2. For mouthwashes used for oral hygiene and plaque inhibition, see section 12.3.4.

DOXYCYCLINE

Indications: periodontitis (as an adjunct to gingival scaling and root planing)
Cautions: see section 5.1.3; monitor for superficial fungal infection, particularly, if predisposition to oral candidiasis
Contra-indications: see section 5.1.3

Side-effects: see section 5.1.3

Dose: 20 mg twice daily for 3 months; CHILD under 12 years not recommended

COUNSELLING. Tablets should be swallowed whole with plenty of fluid, while sitting or standing

Periostat® (CollaGenex) PoM

Tablets, f/c, doxycycline (as hyclate) 20 mg, net price 56-tab pack = £16.50. Label: 6, 11, 27, counselling, posture, see above

12.3.2 Oropharyngeal anti-infective drugs

The most common cause of a sore throat is a viral infection which does not benefit from anti-infective treatment. Streptococcal sore throats require systemic **penicillin** therapy (section 5.1, table 1). Acute ulcerative gingivitis (Vincent's infection) responds to systemic **metronidazole** 200 mg 3 times daily for 3 days (section 5.1.11).

Preparations administered in the dental surgery for the local treatment of periodontal disease include gels of metronidazole (*Elyzol®*, Alpharma) and of minocycline (*Dentomycin®*, Blackwell).

Fungal infections

Candida albicans may cause thrush and other forms of stomatitis which are sometimes associated with the use of broad-spectrum antibiotics or of cytotoxics; withdrawing the causative drug may lead to rapid resolution. Otherwise, an antifungal drug may be effective.

Of the antifungal drugs used for mouth infections, **amphotericin** and **nystatin** are not absorbed from the gastro-intestinal tract and are used by local application in the mouth. **Miconazole** occupies an intermediate position since it is used by local application in the mouth but is also absorbed to the extent that potential interactions need to be considered. **Fluconazole** and **itraconazole** are absorbed when taken by mouth and are available for administration by mouth for oropharyngeal candidiasis (section 5.2). For advice on prevention of fungal infections in immunocompromised patients see p. 294.

AMPHOTERICIN

Indications: oral and perioral fungal infections

Side-effects: mild gastro-intestinal disturbances reported

Fungilin® (Squibb) PoM

Lozenges, yellow, amphotericin 10 mg. Net price 60-lozenge pack = £3.95. Label: 9, 24, counselling, after food

Allow 1 lozenge to dissolve slowly in the mouth 4 times daily for 10–15 days (continued for 48 hours after lesions have resolved); increase to 8 daily if infection severe

Oral suspension, yellow, sugar-free, amphotericin 100 mg/mL. Net price 12 mL with pipette =

£2.31. Label: 9, counselling, use of pipette, hold in mouth, after food

Place 1 mL in the mouth after food and retain near lesions 4 times daily for 14 days (continued for 48 hours after lesions have resolved)

MICONAZOLE

Indications: see under Preparations; intestinal fungal infections (section 5.2)

Cautions: pregnancy and breast-feeding; avoid in porphyria (section 9.8.2); **interactions:** Appendix 1 (antifungals, imidazole and triazole)

Contra-indications: hepatic impairment

Side-effects: nausea and vomiting, diarrhoea (with long-term treatment); rarely allergic reactions; isolated reports of hepatitis

¹**Daktarin®** (Janssen-Cilag) PoM

Oral gel, sugar-free, orange-flavoured, miconazole 24 mg/mL (20 mg/g). Net price 15-g tube = £2.27, 80-g tube = £5.00. Label: 9, counselling, hold in mouth, after food

Prevention and treatment of oral fungal infections, place 5–10 mL in the mouth after food and retain near lesions 4 times daily; CHILD under 2 years 2.5 mL twice daily, 2–6 years 5 mL twice daily, over 6 years 5 mL 4 times daily; treatment continued for 48 hours after lesions have resolved

Localised lesions, smear small amount of gel on affected area with clean finger (dental prostheses should be removed at night and brushed with gel)

1. 15-g tube can be sold to the public

NYSTATIN

Indications: oral and perioral fungal infections

Side-effects: oral irritation and sensitisation, nausea reported; see also section 5.2

Dose: (as pastilles or as suspension) ADULT and CHILD over 1 month, 100 000 units 4 times daily after food, usually for 7 days (continued for 48 hours after lesions have resolved)

Note. Immunosuppressed patients may require higher doses (e.g. 500 000 units 4 times daily)

Nystatin (Non-proprietary) PoM

Oral suspension, nystatin 100 000 units/mL. Net price 30 mL = £1.96. Label: 9, counselling, hold in mouth, after food

Available from Hillcross, Rosemont (*Nystamont®*, sugar-free)

Nystan® (Squibb) PoM

Pastilles, yellow/brown, nystatin 100 000 units. Net price 28-pastille pack = £3.24. Label: 9, 24, counselling, after food

Oral suspension, yellow, nystatin 100 000 units/mL. Net price 30 mL with pipette = £2.05. Label: 9, counselling, use of pipette, hold in mouth, after food

Viral infections

The management of herpes infections of the mouth is a soft diet, adequate fluid intake, analgesics as required, and the use of **chlorhexidine** mouthwash (section 12.3.4) to control plaque accumulation if toothbrushing is painful. In the case of severe herpetic stomatitis, systemic **aciclovir** is required (section 5.3).

Herpes infections of the mouth may also respond to **tetracycline** (section 12.3.1) rinsed in the mouth.

Idoxuridine 0.1% paint has been superseded by more effective preparations.

12.3.3 Lozenges and sprays

There is no convincing evidence that antiseptic lozenges and sprays have a beneficial action and they sometimes irritate and cause sore tongue and sore lips. Some of these preparations also contain local anaesthetics which relieve pain but may cause sensitisation.

The following list includes throat lozenges and sprays on sale to the public, together with their significant ingredients.

AAA® (benzocaine), **Beechams Throat Plus®** (benzalkonium, hexylresorcinol), **Bradosol®** (benzalkonium), **Bradosol Plus®** (domiphen, lidocaine (lignocaine)), **Dequacaine®** (benzocaine, dequalinium), **Dequadin®** (dequalinium), **Eludril®** spray (tetracaine (amethocaine), chlorhexidine), **Labosept®** (dequalinium), **Meggezones®** (menthol), **Mentholatum®** lozenges (amylmetacresol, menthol), **Merocaine®** (benzocaine, cetylpyridinium), **Merocets®** lozenges (cetylpyridinium), **Merocets Plus®** lozenges (cetylpyridinium, menthol), **Strepsils®** lozenges (amylmetacresol, dichlorobenzyl alcohol), **Strepsils Extra®** lozenges (hexylresorcinol), **Strepsils Pain Relief Plus®** lozenges (amylmetacresol, dichlorobenzyl alcohol, lidocaine (lignocaine)), **Strepsils Pain Relief Spray®** (lidocaine (lignocaine)), **TCP®** pastilles (phenols), **Tyrozets®** (benzocaine, tyrothricin), **Vicks Ultra Chloraseptic®** (benzocaine)

12.3.4 Mouthwashes, gargles, and dentifrices

Mouthwashes have a mechanical cleansing action and freshen the mouth. Warm **compound sodium chloride mouthwash** or **compound thymol glycerin** is as useful as any.

Mouthwashes containing an oxidising agent, such as **hydrogen peroxide**, may be useful in the treatment of acute ulcerative gingivitis (Vincent's infection) since the organisms involved are anaerobes. It also has a mechanical cleansing effect due to frothing when in contact with oral debris. **Sodium perborate** is similar in effect to hydrogen peroxide.

There is evidence that **chlorhexidine** has a specific effect in inhibiting the formation of plaque on teeth. A chlorhexidine mouthwash may be useful as an adjunct to other oral hygiene measures for oral infection or when toothbrushing is not possible.

Povidone–iodine mouthwash is useful for mucosal infections but does not inhibit plaque accumulation. It should not be used for periods longer than 14 days because a significant amount of iodine is absorbed.

There is no convincing evidence that gargles are effective.

CHLORHEXIDINE GLUCONATE

Indications: see under preparations below

Side-effects: mucosal irritation (discontinue if desquamation); reversible brown staining of teeth, parotid gland swelling reported

Note. Chlorhexidine gluconate may be incompatible with some ingredients in toothpaste; leave an interval of at least 30 minutes between using mouthwash and toothpaste

Chlorhexidine (Non-proprietary)
Mouthwash, chlorhexidine gluconate 0.2%, net price 300 mL = £1.93
Oral hygiene and plaque inhibition, rinse mouth with 10 mL for about 1 minute twice daily
Denture stomatitis, cleanse and soak dentures in mouthwash solution for 15 minutes twice daily
Available from Blackwell (original, aniseed-, or mint-flavoured)

Chlorohex® (Colgate-Palmolive)
Chlorohex 1200® mouthwash, chlorhexidine gluconate 0.12% (mint-flavoured). Net price 300 mL = £2.20
Oral hygiene and plaque inhibition, rinse mouth with 15 mL for about 30 seconds twice daily
Chlorohex 2000® mouthwash, chlorhexidine gluconate 0.2% (mint-flavoured). Net price 300 mL = £2.20
Oral hygiene and plaque inhibition, rinse mouth with 10 mL for about 1 minute twice daily
Denture stomatitis, cleanse and soak dentures in mouthwash solution for 15 minutes twice daily

Corsodyl® (GSK Consumer Healthcare)
Dental gel, chlorhexidine gluconate 1%. Net price 50 g = £1.21
Oral hygiene and plaque inhibition, brush on the teeth once or twice daily
Mouthwash, chlorhexidine gluconate 0.2%. Net price 300 mL (original or mint) = £1.93, 600 mL (mint) = £3.85
Oral hygiene and plaque inhibition, rinse mouth with 10 mL for about 1 minute twice daily
Oral spray, chlorhexidine gluconate 0.2% (mint-flavoured). Net price 60 mL = £4.10
Oral hygiene and plaque inhibition, apply as required to tooth and gingival surfaces using up to max. 12 actuations (approx. 0.14 mL/actutation) twice daily

■ With chlorobutanol

Eludril® (Ceuta)
Mouthwash or gargle, chlorhexidine gluconate 0.1%, chlorobutanol 0.5% (mint-flavoured), net price 90 mL = £1.22; 250 mL = £2.56; 500 mL = £4.64
Oral hygiene, plaque inhibition, minor throat infections, use 10–15 mL (diluted with warm water in measuring cup provided) 2–3 times daily
Denture disinfection, soak previously cleansed dentures in mouthwash (diluted with 2 volumes of water) for 60 minutes

HEXETIDINE

Indications: oral hygiene

Oraldene® (Warner Lambert)
Mouthwash or gargle, red, hexetidine 0.1%. Net price 100 mL = £1.31; 200 mL = £2.02
Use 15 mL undiluted 2–3 times daily

OXIDISING AGENTS

Indications: oral hygiene, see notes above

Hydrogen Peroxide Mouthwash, BP
Mouthwash, consists of Hydrogen Peroxide Solution 6% (≡ approx. 20 volume) BP
Rinse the mouth for 2–3 minutes with 15 mL in half a tumblerful of warm water 2–3 times daily

Peroxyl ® (Colgate-Palmolive)

Mouthwash, hydrogen peroxide 1.5%, net price 250 mL = £2.05

Rinse the mouth with 10 mL for about 1 minute up to 4 times daily (after meals and at bedtime)

Bocasan® (Oral B Labs)

Mouthwash, sodium perborate 68.6% (buffered). Net price 20 × 1.7-g sachet pack = £1.77

Use 1 sachet in 30 mL of water 3 times daily after meals

Cautions: do not use for longer than 7 days because of possible absorption of borate; not recommended in renal impairment or for children under 5 years

POVIDONE–IODINE

Indications: oral hygiene

Cautions: pregnancy (Appendix 4); breast-feeding (Appendix 5); see also notes above

Contra-indications: avoid regular use in patients with thyroid disorders or those receiving lithium therapy

Side-effects: idiosyncratic mucosal irritation and hypersensitivity reactions; may interfere with thyroid-function tests and with tests for occult blood

Betadine® (SSL)

Mouthwash or gargle, amber, povidone-iodine 1%. Net price 250 mL = £1.12

Adults and children over 6 years, up to 10 mL undiluted or diluted with an equal quantity of warm water for up to 30 seconds up to 4 times daily for up to 14 days

SODIUM CHLORIDE

Indications: oral hygiene, see notes above

Sodium Chloride Mouthwash, Compound, BP

Mouthwash, sodium bicarbonate 1%, sodium chloride 1.5% in a suitable vehicle with a peppermint flavour.

Extemporaneous preparations should be prepared according to the following formula: sodium chloride 1.5 g, sodium bicarbonate 1 g, concentrated peppermint emulsion 2.5 mL, double-strength chloroform water 50 mL, water to 100 mL
To be diluted with an equal volume of warm water

THYMOL

Indications: oral hygiene, see notes above

Compound Thymol Glycerin, BP 1988

Mouthwash, glycerol 10%, thymol 0.05% with colouring and flavouring, net price 100 mL = 40p

To be used undiluted or diluted with 3 volumes of warm water

Available from William Ransom, Thornton & Ross

Mouthwash Solution-tablets

Consist of tablets which may contain antimicrobial, colouring, and flavouring agents in a suitable soluble effervescent basis to make a mouthwash suitable for dental purposes.

Dissolve 1 tablet in a tumblerful of warm water

12.3.5 Treatment of dry mouth

Dry mouth (xerostomia) may be caused by drugs with antimuscarinic (anticholinergic) side-effects (e.g. antispasmodics, tricyclic antidepressants, and some antipsychotics), by irradiation of the head and neck region or by damage to or disease of the salivary glands. Patients with a persistently dry mouth may develop a burning or scalded sensation and have poor oral hygiene; they may develop increased dental caries, periodontal disease, intolerance of dentures, and oral infections (particularly candidiasis). Dry mouth may be relieved in many patients by simple measures such as frequent sips of cool drinks or sucking pieces of ice or sugar-free fruit pastilles. Sugar-free chewing gum stimulates salivation in patients with residual salivary function.

An **artificial saliva** can provide useful relief of dry mouth. A properly balanced artificial saliva should be of a neutral pH and contain electrolytes (including fluoride) to correspond approximately to the composition of saliva. Of the proprietary preparations available, *Luborant®* is licensed for any condition giving rise to a dry mouth; *Saliva Orthana®*, *Salivace®*, *Saliveze®*, *Glandosane®* and *Oralbalance®* have ACBS approval for dry mouth associated only with radiotherapy or sicca syndrome. *Salivix®* pastilles, which act locally as salivary stimulants, are also available and have similar ACBS approval. *SST* tablets may be prescribed for dry mouth in patients with salivary gland impairment (and patent salivary ducts).

Pilocarpine tablets are licensed for the treatment of xerostomia following irradiation for head and neck cancer and for dry mouth and dry eyes (xerophthalmia) in Sjögren's syndrome. They are effective only in patients who have some residual salivary gland function, and therefore should be withdrawn if there is no response.

Local treatment

AS Saliva Orthana® (AS Pharma)

Oral spray, gastric mucin 3.5%, xylitol 2%, sodium fluoride 4.2 mg/litre, with preservatives and flavouring agents. Net price 50-mL bottle = £3.95; 450-mL refill = £23.47

Lozenges, mucin 65 mg, xylitol 59 mg, in a sorbitol basis. Net price 45-lozenge pack = £3.03

ACBS: patients suffering from dry mouth as a result of having (or having undergone) radiotherapy, or sicca syndrome, spray 2–3 times onto oral and pharyngeal mucosa, when required

Note. AS Saliva Orthana® lozenges do not contain fluoride

Glandosane® (Fresenius Kabi)

Aerosol spray, carmellose sodium 500 mg, sorbitol 1.5 g, potassium chloride 60 mg, sodium chloride 42.2 mg, magnesium chloride 2.6 mg, calcium chloride 7.3 mg, and dipotassium hydrogen phosphate 17.1 mg/50 g. Net price 50-mL unit (neutral, lemon or peppermint flavoured) = £4.15

ACBS: patients suffering from dry mouth as a result of having (or having undergone) radiotherapy, or sicca syndrome, spray onto oral and pharyngeal mucosa as required

Luborant® (Antigen)

Oral spray, pink, sorbitol 1.8 g, carmellose sodium (sodium carboxymethylcellulose) 390 mg, dibasic potassium phosphate 48.23 mg, potassium chloride 37.5 mg, monobasic potassium phosphate 21.97 mg, calcium chloride 9.972 mg, magnesium chloride 3.528 mg, sodium fluoride 258 micrograms/60 mL, with preservatives and colouring agents. Net price 60-mL unit = £3.96

Saliva deficiency, 2–3 sprays onto oral mucosa up to 4 times daily, or as directed

Note. May be difficult to obtain

Oralbalance® (Anglian)

Saliva replacement gel, lactoperoxidase, glucose oxidase, xylitol in a gel basis. Net price 50-g tube = £3.69

ACBS: patients suffering from dry mouth as a result of having (or having undergone) radiotherapy, or sicca syndrome, apply to gums and tongue as required

Salivace® (Penn)

Oral spray, carmellose sodium (sodium carboxymethylcellulose), xylitol, calcium chloride, dibasic potassium phosphate, sodium chloride, potassium chloride, and methyl hydroxybenzoate. Net price 100 mL = £4.95

ACBS: patients suffering from dry mouth as a result of having (or having undergone) radiotherapy, or sicca syndrome, 1–2 sprays onto oral mucosa as required

Saliveze® (Wyvern)

Oral spray, carmellose sodium (sodium carboxymethylcellulose), calcium chloride, magnesium chloride, potassium chloride, sodium chloride, and dibasic sodium phosphate. Net price 50-mL bottle (mint-flavoured) = £3.50

ACBS: patients suffering from dry mouth as a result of having (or having undergone) radiotherapy, or sicca syndrome, 1 spray onto oral mucosa as required

Salivix® (Provalis)

Pastilles, sugar-free, reddish-amber, acacia, malic acid and other ingredients. Net price 50-pastille pack = £2.86

ACBS: patients suffering from dry mouth as a result of having (or having undergone) radiotherapy, or sicca syndrome, suck 1 pastille when required

SST (Sinclair)

Tablets, sugar-free, citric acid, malic acid and other ingredients in a sorbitol base, net price 100-tab pack = £4.86

Symptomatic treatment of dry mouth in patients with impaired salivary gland function and patent salivary ducts, allow 1 tablet to dissolve slowly in the mouth when required

Systemic treatment

PILOCARPINE HYDROCHLORIDE

Indications: xerostomia following irradiation for head and neck cancer (see also notes above); dry mouth and dry eyes in Sjögren's syndrome

Cautions: asthma and chronic obstructive pulmonary disease (avoid if uncontrolled, see Contra-indications), cardiovascular disease (avoid if significant); cholelithiasis or biliary-tract disease, peptic ulcer, hepatic impairment (Appendix 2), renal impairment; risk of increased urethral smooth muscle tone and renal colic; maintain adequate fluid intake to avoid dehydration associated with excessive sweating; cognitive or psychiatric disturbances; **interactions:** Appendix 1 (parasympathomimetics)

COUNSELLING. Blurred vision may affect ability to drive, particularly at night, and to perform hazardous activities in reduced lighting

Contra-indications: uncontrolled asthma and chronic obstructive pulmonary disease (increased bronchial secretions and increased airways resistance); significant cardiovascular disease; acute iritis, angle-closure glaucoma; pregnancy and breast-feeding

Side-effects: sweating; also nausea, diarrhoea, dyspepsia, abdominal pain, flushing, headache, dizziness, rhinitis, increased urinary frequency, lacrimation, influenza-like syndrome; less frequently vomiting, flatulence, constipation, palpitations, hypertension, urinary urgency, blurred and abnormal vision

Dose: xerostomia following irradiation for head and neck cancer, 5 mg 3 times daily with or immediately after meals (last dose always with evening meal); if tolerated but response insufficient after 4 weeks, may be increased to max. 30 mg daily in divided doses; max. therapeutic effect normally within 4–8 weeks; discontinue if no improvement after 2–3 months; CHILD not recommended

Dry mouth and dry eyes in Sjögren's syndrome, 5 mg 4 times daily (with meals and at bedtime); if tolerated but response insufficient, may be increased to max. 30 mg daily in divided doses; discontinue if no improvement after 2–3 months; CHILD not recommended

Salagen® (Novartis Ophthalmics) PoM

Tablets, f/c, pilocarpine hydrochloride 5 mg. Net price 84-tab pack = £51.43. Label: 21, 27, counselling, driving

13: Skin

13.1 Management of skin conditions

13.1.1 Vehicles

Both vehicle and active ingredients are important in the treatment of skin conditions; the vehicle alone may have more than a mere placebo effect. The vehicle affects the degree of hydration of the skin, has a mild anti-inflammatory effect, and aids the penetration of active drug.

Applications are usually viscous solutions, emulsions, or suspensions for application to the skin (including the scalp) or nails.

Collodions are painted on the skin and allowed to dry to leave a flexible film over the site of application.

Creams are emulsions of oil and water and are generally well absorbed into the skin. They may contain an antimicrobial preservative unless the active ingredient or basis is intrinsically bactericidal and fungicidal. Generally, creams are cosmetically more acceptable than ointments because they are less greasy and easier to apply.

Gels consist of active ingredients in suitable hydrophilic or hydrophobic bases; they generally have a high water content. Gels are particularly suitable for application to the face and scalp.

Lotions have a cooling effect and may be preferred to ointments or creams for application over a hairy area. Lotions in alcoholic basis can sting if used on broken skin. *Shake lotions* (such as calamine lotion) contain insoluble powders which leave a deposit on the skin surface.

Ointments are greasy preparations which are normally anhydrous and insoluble in water, and are more occlusive than creams. They are particularly suitable for chronic, dry lesions. The most commonly used ointment bases consist of soft paraffin or a combination of soft, liquid and hard paraffin. Some ointment bases have both *hydrophilic and lipophilic* properties; they may have occlusive properties on the skin surface, encourage hydration, and also be miscible with water; they often have a mild anti-inflammatory effect. *Water-soluble ointments* contain macrogols which are freely soluble in water and are therefore readily washed off; they have a limited but useful role where ready removal is desirable.

Pastes are stiff preparations containing a high proportion of finely powdered solids such as zinc oxide and starch suspended in an ointment. They are used for circumscribed lesions such as those which occur in lichen simplex, chronic eczema, or psoriasis. They are less occlusive than ointments and can be used to protect inflamed, lichenified, or excoriated skin.

Dusting powders are used only rarely. They reduce friction between opposing skin surfaces. Dusting powders should not be applied to moist areas because they can cake and abrade the skin. Talc is a lubricant but it does not absorb moisture whereas starch is less lubricant but absorbs water.

DILUTION. The BP directs that creams and ointments should **not** normally be diluted but that should dilution be necessary care should be taken, in particular, to prevent microbial contamination. The appropriate diluent should be used and heating should be avoided during mixing; excessive dilution may affect the stability of some creams. Diluted creams should normally be used within 2 weeks of their preparation.

13.1.2 Suitable quantities for prescribing

Suitable quantities of dermatological preparations to be prescribed for specific areas of the body are:

	Creams and Ointments	Lotions
Face	15 to 30 g	100 mL
Both hands	25 to 50 g	200 mL
Scalp	50 to 100 g	200 mL
Both arms or both legs	100 to 200 g	200 mL
Trunk	400 g	500 mL
Groins and genitalia	15 to 25 g	100 mL

These amounts are usually suitable for an adult for twice daily application for 1 week. The recommendations do not apply to corticosteroid preparations—for suitable quantities of corticosteroid preparations see section 13.4

13.1.3 Excipients and sensitisation

Excipients in topical products rarely cause problems. If a patch test indicates allergy to an excipient, then products containing the substance should be avoided. The following excipients in topical preparations may rarely be associated with sensitisation; the presence of these excipients is indicated in the entries for topical products.

Beeswax	Imidurea
Benzyl alcohol	Isopropyl palmitate
Butylated hydroxyanisole	N-(3-Chloroallyl)hexaminium chloride (quaternium 15)
Butylated hydroxytoluene	Polysorbates
Cetostearyl alcohol (including cetyl and stearyl alcohol)	Propylene glycol
Chlorocresol	Sodium metabisulphite
Edetic acid (EDTA)	Sorbic acid
Ethylenediamine	Wool fat and related substances including lanolin[1]
Fragrances	
Hydroxybenzoates (parabens)	

---

1. Purified versions of wool fat have reduced the problem

13.2 Emollient and barrier preparations

13.2.1   Emollients
13.2.2   Barrier preparations

BORDERLINE SUBSTANCES.   The preparations marked 'ACBS' are regarded as drugs when prescribed in accordance with the advice of the Advisory Committee on Borderline Substances for the clinical conditions listed. Prescriptions issued in accordance with this advice and endorsed 'ACBS' will normally not be investigated. See Appendix 7 for listing by clinical condition.

13.2.1 Emollients

Emollients soothe, smooth and hydrate the skin and are indicated for all dry or scaling disorders. Their effects are short-lived and they should be applied frequently even after improvement occurs. They are useful in dry and eczematous disorders, and to a lesser extent in psoriasis (section 13.5.2). Light emollients such as **aqueous cream** are suitable for many patients with dry skin but a wide range of more greasy preparations including **white soft paraffin**, **emulsifying ointment**, and **liquid and white soft paraffin ointment** are available; the severity of the condition, patient preference and site of application will often guide the choice of emollient; emollients should be applied in the direction of hair growth. Some ingredients may rarely cause sensitisation (section 13.1.3) and this should be suspected if an eczematous reaction occurs.

Preparations such as **aqueous cream** and **emulsifying ointment** can be used as soap substitutes for hand washing and in the bath; the preparation is rubbed on the skin before rinsing off completely. The addition of a bath oil may also be helpful.

Preparations containing an antibacterial should be avoided unless infection is present (section 13.10) or is a frequent complication.

Urea is employed as a hydrating agent. It is used in scaling conditions and may be useful in elderly patients. It is occasionally used with other topical agents such as corticosteroids to enhance penetration.

Aqueous Cream, BP, emulsifying ointment 30%, [1]phenoxyethanol 1% in freshly boiled and cooled purified water. Net price 100 g = 21p
1. The BP permits use of alternative antimicrobials provided their identity and concentration are stated on the label
Excipients: include cetostearyl alcohol
Emulsifying Ointment, BP, emulsifying wax 30%, white soft paraffin 50%, liquid paraffin 20%. Net price 100 g = 30p
Excipients: include cetostearyl alcohol
Hydrous Ointment, BP (oily cream), dried magnesium sulphate 0.5%, phenoxyethanol 1%, wool alcohols ointment 50%, in freshly boiled and cooled purified water. Net price 100 g = 40p
Liquid and White Soft Paraffin Ointment, NPF
Ointment, liquid paraffin 50%, white soft paraffin 50%. Net price 250 g = 88p, 500 g = £1.75
Paraffin, White Soft, BP (white petroleum jelly). Net price 100 g = 32p
Paraffin, Yellow Soft, BP (yellow petroleum jelly). Net price 100 g = 32p

Alcoderm® (Galderma)

Cream, containing liquid paraffin, cetyl alcohol, stearyl alcohol, sodium lauryl sulphate, carbomer, triethanolamine, sorbitan stearate, sorbitol, spermaceti, silicone fluid. Net price 60 g = £2.40

For dry skin conditions

Excipients: include cetyl alcohol, hydroxybenzoates (parabens), isopropyl palmitate, stearyl alcohol

Lotion, water-miscible, ingredients as above. Net price 200 mL = £4.77

For dry skin conditions

Excipients: include cetostearyl alcohol, fragrance, hydroxybenzoates (parabens)

Aveeno® (Bioglan)

Cream, colloidal oatmeal in emollient basis, net price 100 mL = £3.78

Excipients: include benzyl alcohol, cetyl alcohol, isopropyl palmitate

ACBS: For endogenous and exogenous eczema, xeroderma, ichthyosis, and senile pruritus (pruritus of the elderly) associated with dry skin

Lotion, colloidal oatmeal in emollient basis, net price 400-mL pump pack = £6.02

Excipients: include benzyl alcohol, cetyl alcohol, isopropyl palmitate

ACBS: as for *Aveeno®* Cream

Cetraben® Emollient Cream (Sankyo)

Cream, white soft paraffin 13.2 %, light liquid paraffin 10.5 %, net price 50 g = £1.14; 125 g = £2.31; 500-g pump pack = £5.61

For inflamed, damaged, dry or chapped skin including eczema

Excipients: include cetostearyl alcohol, hydroxybenzoates (parabens)

Decubal® Clinic (Alpharma)

Cream, isopropyl myristate 17%, glycerol 8.5%, wool fat 6%, dimeticone 5%, net price 50 g = £1.53, 100 g = £1.98

For dry skin conditions including ichthyosis, psoriasis, dermatitis and hyperkeratosis

Excipients: include cetyl alcohol, polysorbates, sorbic acid, wool fat

Dermamist® (Yamanouchi)

Spray application, white soft paraffin 10% in a basis containing liquid paraffin, fractionated coconut oil. Net price 250-mL pressurised aerosol unit = £9.17

For dry skin conditions including eczema, ichthyosis, pruritus of the elderly

Caution: flammable

Excipients: none as listed in section 13.1.3

Diprobase® (Schering-Plough)

Cream, cetomacrogol 2.25%, cetostearyl alcohol 7.2%, liquid paraffin 6%, white soft paraffin 15%, water-miscible basis used for *Diprosone®* cream. Net price 50 g = £1.54; 500-g dispenser = £6.61

For dry skin conditions

Excipients: include cetostearyl alcohol, chlorocresol

Ointment, liquid paraffin 5%, white soft paraffin 95%, basis used for *Diprosone®* ointment. Net price 50 g = £1.54

For dry skin conditions

Excipients: none as listed in section 13.1.3

Doublebase® (Dermal)

Gel, isopropyl myristate 15 %, liquid paraffin 15 %, net price 100 g = £2.98; 500 g = £6.55

For dry chapped or itchy skin conditions

Excipients: none as listed in section 13.1.3

Drapolene® —section 13.2.2

E45® (Crookes)

Cream, light liquid paraffin 12.6%, white soft paraffin 14.5%, hypoallergenic hydrous wool fat (hypoallergenic lanolin) 1% in self-emulsifying

monostearin, net price 50 g = £1.18, 125 g = £2.39, 350 g = £4.14, 500 g = £5.61, 500-g pump pack = £6.20

For dry skin conditions

Excipients: include cetyl alcohol, cetostearyl alcohol, hydroxybenzoates (parabens)

Emollient Wash Cream, soap substitute, zinc oxide 5% in an emollient basis, net price 250-mL pump pack = £2.87

ACBS: for endogenous and exogenous eczema, xeroderma, ichthyosis and senile pruritus (pruritus of the elderly) associated with dry skin

Excipients: none as listed in section 13.1.3

Lotion, light liquid paraffin 4%, cetomacrogol, white soft paraffin 10%, hypoallergenic anhydrous wool fat (hypoallergenic lanolin) 1% in glyceryl monostearate, net price 200 mL = £2.23, 500-mL pump pack = £4.21

ACBS: for symptomatic relief of dry skin conditions, such as those associated with atopic eczema and contact dermatitis

Excipients: include isopropyl palmitate, hydroxybenzoates (parabens), benzyl alcohol

Epaderm® (SSL)

Ointment, emulsifying wax 30%, yellow soft paraffin 30%, liquid paraffin 40%, net price 125 g = £3.67, 500 g = £6.21

For use as an emollient or soap substitute

Excipients: include cetostearyl alcohol

Hewletts Cream® (Kestrel)

Cream, hydrous wool fat 4%, zinc oxide 8%, arachis (peanut) oil, oleic acid, white soft paraffin, net price 35 g = £1.19, 400 g = £4.85

For nursing hygiene and care of skin, and chapped hands

Excipients: include fragrance

Hydromol® (Adams Hlth)

Cream, sodium pidolate 2.5%, net price 50 g = £2.04, 100 g = £3.80, 500 g = £12.60

For dry skin conditions

Excipients: include cetostearyl alcohol, hydroxybenzoates (parabens)

Kamillosan® (Goldshield)

Ointment, chamomile extracts 10.5% in a basis containing wool fat, net price 50 g = £2.50, 100 g = £5.00

For nappy rash, sore nipples and chapped hands

Excipients: include beeswax, cetostearyl alcohol, hydroxybenzoates (parabens)

Keri® (Bristol-Myers Squibb)

Lotion, mineral oil 16%, with lanolin oil, net price 190-mL pump pack = £3.56, 380-mL pump pack = £5.81

For dry skin conditions and nappy rash

Excipients: include hydroxybenzoates (parabens), *N*-(3-chloroallyl)hexaminium chloride (quaternium 15), propylene glycol, fragrance

LactiCare® (Stiefel)

Lotion, lactic acid 5%, sodium pidolate 2.5%. Net price 150 mL = £3.19

For dry skin conditions

Excipients: include cetostearyl alcohol, imidurea, isopropyl palmitate, fragrance

Lipobase® (Yamanouchi)

Cream, fatty cream basis used for *Locoid Lipocream®*. Net price 50 g = £1.85

Excipients: include cetostearyl alcohol, hydroxybenzoates (parabens)

Morhulin® (SSL)

Ointment, cod-liver oil 11.4%, zinc oxide 38%, in a basis containing liquid paraffin and yellow soft paraffin. Net price 50 g = £1.46

For minor wounds, varicose ulcers, pressure sores, eczema and nappy rash

Excipients: include wool fat derivative

Neutrogena® Dermatological Cream (J&J)
Cream, glycerol 40% in an emollient basis. Net price 100 g = £3.79
For dry skin conditions
Excipients: include cetostearyl alcohol, hydroxybenzoates (parabens)

Oilatum® (Stiefel)
Cream, light liquid paraffin 6%, white soft paraffin 15%. Net price 40 g = £1.79, 80 g = £2.78, 150 g = £3.38
For dry skin conditions
Excipients: include benzyl alcohol, cetostearyl alcohol
Shower emollient (gel), light liquid paraffin 70%. Net price 125 g = £4.84
For dry skin conditions including dermatitis
Excipients: include fragrance

Ultrabase® (Schering Health)
Cream, water-miscible, containing liquid paraffin and white soft paraffin. Net price 50 g = £1.05; 500-g dispenser = £6.89
For dry skin conditions
Excipients: include fragrance, hydroxybenzoates (parabens), disodium edetate, stearyl alcohol

Unguentum M® (Crookes)
Cream, cetostearyl alcohol, glyceryl monostearate, saturated neutral oil, liquid paraffin, white soft paraffin, net price 50 g = £1.59, 100 g = £3.13, 200-mL dispenser = £6.19, 500 g = £9.55
For dry skin conditions and nappy rash
Excipients: include cetostearyl alcohol, polysorbate 40, propylene glycol, sorbic acid

Vaseline Dermacare® (Elida Faberge)
Cream, dimeticone 1%, white soft paraffin 15%. Net price 150 mL = £2.11
ACBS: for endogenous and exogenous eczema, xeroderma, ichthyosis and senile pruritus (pruritus of the elderly) associated with dry skin
Excipients: include hydroxybenzoates (parabens)
Lotion, dimeticone 1%, liquid paraffin 4%, white soft paraffin 5% in an emollient basis. Net price 75 mL = £1.18; 200 mL = £2.29
ACBS: as for *Vaseline Dermacare® Cream*
Excipients: include disodium edetate, hydroxybenzoates (parabens), wool fat

■ Preparations containing urea

Aquadrate® (Procter & Gamble Pharm.)
Cream, urea 10%. Net price 30 g = £1.18; 100 g = £3.54
For dry, scaling and itching skin, apply thinly and rub into area when required
Excipients: none as listed in section 13.1.3

Balneum® Plus (Crookes)
Cream, urea 5%, lauromacrogols 3%, net price 100 g = £5.58, 175-g pump pack = £7.81, 500-g pump pack = £19.50
For dry, scaling and itching skin, apply twice daily
Excipients: include benzyl alcohol, polysorbates

Calmurid® (Galderma)
Cream, urea 10%, lactic acid 5%. Diluent aqueous cream, life of diluted cream 14 days. Net price 100 g = £4.75; 500-g dispenser = £21.48
For dry, scaling and itching skin, apply a thick layer for 3–5 minutes, massage into area, and remove excess, usually twice daily. Use half-strength cream for 1 week if stinging occurs
Excipients: none as listed in section 13.1.3

E45® Itch Relief Cream (Crookes)
Cream, urea 5%, lauromacrogols 3%, net price 50 g = £2.10, 100 g = £3.83
For dry, scaling, and itching skin, apply twice a day
Excipients: include benzyl alcohol, polysorbates

Eucerin® (Beiersdorf)
Cream, urea 10%, net price 50 mL = £3.52, 150 mL = £8.57
For dry skin conditions including eczema, ichthyosis, xeroderma, hyperkeratosis, apply thinly and rub into area twice daily
Excipients: include benzyl alcohol, isopropyl palmitate, wool fat
Lotion, urea 10%, net price 150 mL = £3.36, 250 mL = £4.28
For dry skin conditions including eczema, ichthyosis, xeroderma, hyperkeratosis, apply sparingly and rub into area twice daily
Excipients: include benzyl alcohol, isopropyl palmitate

Nutraplus® (Galderma)
Cream, urea 10%. Net price 100 g = £4.37
For dry, scaling and itching skin, apply 2–3 times daily
Excipients: include hydroxybenzoates (parabens), propylene glycol

■ With antimicrobials

Dermol® (Dermal)
Dermol® 500 Lotion, benzalkonium chloride 0.1%, chlorhexidine hydrochloride 0.1%, liquid paraffin 2.5%, isopropyl myristate 2.5%, net price 500-mL dispenser = £6.79
For dry and pruritic skin conditions including eczema and dermatitis, apply to skin or use as soap substitute
Excipients: include cetostearyl alcohol
Dermol® 200 Shower Emollient, benzalkonium chloride 0.1%, chlorhexidine hydrochloride 0.1%, liquid paraffin 2.5%, isopropyl myristate 2.5%, net price 200 mL = £3.99
For dry and pruritic skin conditions including eczema and dermatitis, apply to skin or use as soap substitute
Excipients: include cetostearyl alcohol

13.2.1.1 Emollient bath additives

Alpha Keri Bath® (Bristol-Myers Squibb)
Bath oil, liquid paraffin 91.7%, oil-soluble fraction of wool fat 3%. Net price 240 mL = £3.45; 480 mL = £6.43
For dry skin conditions including ichthyosis and pruritus of the elderly, add 10–20 mL/bath (infants 5 mL)
Excipients: include fragrance

Aveeno® (Bioglan)
Aveeno® Bath oil, colloidal oatmeal, white oat fraction in emollient basis. Net price 250 mL = £4.28
ACBS: for endogenous and exogenous eczema, xeroderma, ichthyosis, and senile pruritus (pruritus of the elderly) associated with dry skin, add 30 mL/bath
Excipients: include beeswax, fragrance
Aveeno Colloidal® Bath additive, oatmeal, white oat fraction in emollient basis. Net price 10 × 50-g sachets = £7.33
ACBS: as for Aveeno® Bath oil; add 1 sachet/bath (infants half sachet)
Excipients: none as listed in section 13.1.3

Balneum® (Crookes)
Balneum® bath oil, soya oil 84.75%, net price 200 mL = £2.79, 500 mL = £6.06, 1 litre = £11.70
For dry skin conditions including those associated with dermatitis and eczema; add 20 mL/bath (infant 5 mL)
Excipients: include butylated hydroxytoluene, propylene glycol, fragrance
Balneum Plus® bath oil, soya oil 82.95%, mixed lauromacrogols 15%, net price 500 mL = £7.50
For dry skin conditions including those associated with dermatitis and eczema where pruritus also experienced; add 20 mL/bath (infant 5 mL)
Excipients: include butylated hydroxytoluene, propylene glycol, fragrance

Dermalo® (Dermal)
Bath emollient, acetylated wool alcohols 5%, liquid paraffin 65%, net price 500 mL = £3.87
For dermatitis, dry skin conditions including ichthyosis and pruritus of the elderly; add 15–20 mL/bath (infant and child 5–10 mL)
Excipients: none as listed in section 13.1.3

Diprobath® (Schering-Plough)
Bath additive, isopropyl myristate 39%, light liquid paraffin 46%. Net price 500 mL = £7.50
For dry skin conditions including dermatitis and eczema; add 25 mL/bath (infant 10 mL)
Excipients: none as listed in section 13.1.3

E45® (Crookes)
Emollient bath oil, cetyl dimeticone 5%, liquid paraffin 91%, net price 250 mL = £2.87, 500 mL = £4.57
ACBS: for endogenous and exogenous eczema, xeroderma, ichthyosis, and senile pruritus (pruritus of the elderly) associated with dry skin; add 15 mL/bath (child 5–10 mL)
Excipients: none as listed in section 13.1.3

Eurax® (Novartis Consumer Health)
Dermatological bath oil, acetylated wool alcohols 5%, light liquid paraffin 65%. Net price 200 mL = £3.38
For dry skin conditions including dermatitis, pruritus of the elderly and ichthyosis; add 15–20 mL/bath (infant and child 5–10 mL)

Hydromol Emollient® (Adams Hlth)
Bath additive, isopropyl myristate 13%, light liquid paraffin 37.8%. Net price 150 mL = £1.87; 350 mL = £3.80; 1 litre = £9.00
For dry skin conditions including eczema, ichthyosis and pruritus of the elderly; add 1–3 capfuls/bath (infant ½–2 capfuls)
Excipients: none as listed in section 13.1.3

Imuderm® (Goldshield)
Bath oil, almond oil 30%, light liquid paraffin 69.6%, net price 250 mL = £3.75
For dry skin conditions including dermatitis, eczema, pruritus of the elderly, and ichthyosis, add 15–30 mL/bath (infant and child 7.5–15 mL)
Excipients: include butylated hydroxyanisole

Oilatum® (Stiefel)
Oilatum® Emollient bath additive (emulsion), acetylated wool alcohols 5%, liquid paraffin 63.4%. Net price 250 mL = £2.75; 500 mL = £4.57
For dry skin conditions including dermatitis, pruritus of the elderly and ichthyosis; add 1–3 capfuls (infant 0.5–2 capfuls)
Excipients: include isopropyl palmitate, fragrance
Oilatum® Fragrance Free bath additive, light liquid paraffin 63.4%, net price 500 mL = £5.75
For dry skin conditions including dermatitis, pruritus of the elderly and ichthyosis; add 1–3 capfuls/bath (infant 0.5–2 capfuls)
Excipients: include wool fat, isopropyl palmitate

■ With antimicrobials

Dermol® (Dermal)
Dermol® 600 Bath Emollient, benzalkonium chloride 0.5%, liquid paraffin 25%, isopropyl myristate 25%, net price 600 mL = £8.49
For dry and pruritic skin conditions including eczema and dermatitis, add up to 30 mL/bath (infant up to 15 mL)
Excipients: include polysorbate 60

Emulsiderm® (Dermal)
Liquid emulsion, liquid paraffin 25%, isopropyl myristate 25%, benzalkonium chloride 0.5%. Net price 300 mL (with 15-mL measure) = £4.33; 1 litre (with 30-mL measure) = £13.49
For dry skin conditions including eczema and ichthyosis; add 7–30 mL/bath
Excipients: include polysorbate 60

Oilatum® (Stiefel)
Oilatum® Plus bath additive, benzalkonium chloride 6%, triclosan 2%, light liquid paraffin 52.5%. Net price 500 mL = £7.86, 1 litre = £15.30
For topical treatment of eczema including eczema at risk from infection; add 1–2 capfuls/bath (infant over 6 months 1 mL)
Excipients: include wool fat, isopropyl palmitate

13.2.2   Barrier preparations

Barrier preparations often contain water-repellent substances such as **dimeticone** (dimethicone) or other silicones. They are used on the skin around stomas, bedsores, and pressure areas in the elderly where the skin is intact. Where the skin has broken down, barrier preparations have a limited role in protecting adjacent skin. They are no substitute for adequate nursing care, and it is doubtful if they are any more effective than the traditional compound **zinc ointments**.

NAPPY RASH. Barrier creams and ointments are used for protection against nappy rash which is usually a local dermatitis. The first line of treatment is to ensure that nappies are changed frequently, and that tightly fitting water-proof pants are avoided. The rash may clear when left exposed to the air and a barrier preparation may be helpful. If the rash is associated with a fungal infection, an antifungal cream such as clotrimazole cream (section 13.10.2) is useful. A mild corticosteroid such as hydrocortisone 1% may be useful but treatment should be limited to a week or less; the occlusive effect of nappies and water-proof pants may increase absorption (for cautions, see Hydrocortisone p. 541).

Zinc Cream, BP, zinc oxide 32%, arachis (peanut) oil 32%, calcium hydroxide 0.045%, oleic acid 0.5%, wool fat 8%, in freshly boiled and cooled purified water. Net price 50 g = 49p
For nappy and urinary rash and eczematous conditions

Zinc Ointment, BP, zinc oxide 15%, in Simple Ointment BP 1988 (which contains wool fat 5%, hard paraffin 5%, cetostearyl alcohol 5%, white soft paraffin 85%). Net price 25 g = 14p
For nappy and urinary rash and eczematous conditions

Zinc and Castor Oil Ointment, BP, zinc oxide 7.5%, castor oil 50%, arachis (peanut) oil 30.5%, white beeswax 10%, cetostearyl alcohol 2%. Net price 25 g = 14p
For nappy and urinary rash

Conotrane® (Yamanouchi)
Cream, benzalkonium chloride 0.1%, dimeticone '350' 22%. Net price 100 g = 66p; 500 g = £3.12
For nappy and urinary rash and pressure sores
Excipients: include cetostearyl alcohol, fragrance

Drapolene® (Warner Lambert)
Cream, benzalkonium chloride 0.01%, cetrimide 0.2% in a basis containing white soft paraffin, cetyl alcohol and wool fat. Net price 100 g = £1.37; 200 g = £2.23; 350 g = £3.66
For nappy and urinary rash; minor wounds
Excipients: include cetyl alcohol, chlorocresol, wool fat

Medicaid® (Eastern)
Cream, cetrimide 0.5% in a basis containing light liquid paraffin, white soft paraffin, cetostearyl alcohol, glyceryl monostearate, net price 50 g = £1.49
For nappy rash, minor burns and abrasions
Excipients: include cetostearyl alcohol, fragrance, hydroxybenzoates (parabens), wool fat

Metanium® (Roche Consumer Health)
Ointment, titanium dioxide 20%, titanium peroxide 5%, titanium salicylate 3% in a basis containing dimeticone, light liquid paraffin, white soft paraffin, and benzoin tincture. Net price 30 g = £1.71
For nappy rash and related disorders
Excipients: none as listed in section 13.1.3

Siopel® (Bioglan)
Barrier cream, dimeticone '1000' 10%, cetrimide 0.3%, arachis (peanut) oil. Net price 50 g = 86p
For protection against water-soluble irritants
Excipients: include butylated hydroxytoluene, cetostearyl alcohol, hydroxybenzoates (parabens)

Sprilon® (S&N Hlth.)
Spray application, dimeticone 1.04%, zinc oxide 12.5%, in a basis containing wool alcohols, cetostearyl alcohol, dextran, white soft paraffin, liquid paraffin, propellants. Net price 115-g pressurised aerosol unit = £3.54
For urinary rash, pressure sores, leg ulcers, moist eczema, fissures, fistulae and ileostomy care
Note. Flammable
Excipients: include cetostearyl alcohol, hydroxybenzoates (parabens), wool fat

Sudocrem® (Forest)
Cream, benzyl alcohol 0.39%, benzyl benzoate 1.01%, benzyl cinnamate 0.15%, hydrous wool fat (hypoallergenic lanolin) 4%, zinc oxide 15.25%. Net price 30 g = 89p, 60 g = £1.01, 125 g = £1.52, 250 g = £2.60, 400 g = £3.76
For nappy rash and pressure sores
Excipients: include beeswax (synthetic), polysorbates, propylene glycol, fragrance

Vasogen® (Forest)
Barrier cream, dimeticone 20%, calamine 1.5%, zinc oxide 7.5%. Net price 50 g = 74p; 100 g = £1.30
For nappy rash, pressure sores, ileostomy and colostomy care
Excipients: include hydroxybenzoates (parabens), wool fat

13.3 Topical local anaesthetics and antipruritics

Pruritus may be caused by systemic disease (such as drug hypersensitivity, obstructive jaundice, endocrine disease, and certain malignant diseases) as well as by skin disease (e.g. psoriasis, eczema, urticaria, and scabies). Where possible the underlying causes should be treated. An **emollient** (section 13.2.1) may be of value where the pruritus is associated with dry skin. Pruritus that occurs in otherwise healthy elderly people can also be treated with an emollient. For advice on the treatment of pruritus in palliative care, see Prescribing in Palliative Care, p. 15.

Preparations containing **crotamiton** are sometimes used but are of uncertain value. Preparations containing **calamine** are often ineffective.

A topical preparation containing **doxepin** 5% is licensed for the relief of pruritus in eczema; it can cause drowsiness and there may be a risk of sensitisation.

Pruritus is common in biliary obstruction, especially in primary biliary cirrhosis and drug-induced cholestasis. Oral administration of **colestyramine** (cholestyramine) is the treatment of choice (section 1.9.2).

Topical antihistamines and local anaesthetics are only marginally effective and may occasionally cause sensitisation. A short course of a topical corticosteroid is appropriate in treating *insect stings*. Insect stings should not be treated with calamine preparations.

A short treatment with a **sedating antihistamine** (section 3.4.1) may help in insect stings and in intractable pruritus where sedation is desirable.

For preparations used in *pruritus ani*, see section 1.7.1.

CALAMINE

Indications: pruritus

Calamine (Non-proprietary)
Aqueous cream, calamine 4%, zinc oxide 3%, liquid paraffin 20%, self-emulsifying glyceryl monostearate 5%, cetomacrogol emulsifying wax 5%, phenoxyethanol 0.5%, freshly boiled and cooled purified water 62.5%. Net price 100 mL = 65p
Lotion (= cutaneous suspension), calamine 15%, zinc oxide 5%, glycerol 5%, bentonite 3%, sodium citrate 0.5%, liquefied phenol 0.5%, in freshly boiled and cooled purified water. Net price 200 mL = 64p
Oily lotion (BP 1980), calamine 5%, arachis (peanut) oil 50%, oleic acid 0.5%, wool fat 1%, in calcium hydroxide solution. Net price 200 mL = £1.06

> ◢ denotes preparations that are considered to be less suitable for prescribing (see p. vi)

CROTAMITON

Indications: pruritus (including pruritus after scabies—section 13.10.4); see notes above
Cautions: avoid use near eyes and broken skin; use on doctor's advice for children under 3 years
Contra-indications: acute exudative dermatoses
Administration: pruritus, apply 2–3 times daily; CHILD below 3 years, apply once daily

Eurax® (Novartis Consumer Health)
Cream, crotamiton 10%, net price 30 g = £2.27; 100 g = £3.95
Excipients: include beeswax, fragrance, hydroxybenzoates (parabens), stearyl alcohol
Lotion, crotamiton 10%, net price 100 mL = £2.99
Excipients: include cetyl alcohol, fragrance, propylene glycol, sorbic acid, stearyl alcohol

---

DOXEPIN HYDROCHLORIDE

Indications: pruritus in eczema; depressive illness (section 4.3.1)
Cautions: glaucoma, urinary retention, severe

liver impairment, mania; avoid application to large areas; pregnancy and breast-feeding; **interactions**: Appendix 1 (antidepressants, tricyclic)

DRIVING. Drowsiness may affect performance of skilled tasks (e.g. driving); effects of alcohol enhanced

Side-effects: drowsiness; local burning, stinging, irritation, tingling and rash; dry mouth and other systemic side-effects reported (section 4.3.1)

Administration: apply thinly 3–4 times daily; usual max. 3 g per application; usual total max. 12 g daily; coverage should be less than 10% of body surface area; CHILD under 12 years not recommended

Xepin® (Bioglan) PoM

Cream, doxepin hydrochloride 5%, net price 30 g = £12.61. Label: 2, 10 patient information leaflet
Excipients: include benzyl alcohol

TOPICAL LOCAL ANAESTHETICS

Indications: relief of local pain, see notes above. See section 15.2 for use in surface anaesthesia

Cautions: occasionally cause hypersensitivity

Note. Topical local anaesthetic preparations may be absorbed, especially through mucosal surfaces, therefore excessive application should be avoided and they should preferably not be used for more than about 3 days; not generally suitable for young children

The following is a list of topical local anaesthetic preparations on sale to the public, together with their significant ingredients:

Anethaine® (tetracaine (amethocaine)), **Anthisan® Plus** (benzocaine, mepyramine), **BurnEze®** (benzocaine), **Dermidex®** (lidocaine (lignocaine), alcloxa, cetrimide, chlorobutanol), **Dettol® Antiseptic Pain Relief spray** (lidocaine (lignocaine)), **Lanacane® cream** (benzocaine, chlorothymol), **Solarcaine®** (benzocaine, triclosan), **Solarcaine® gel** (lidocaine (lignocaine)), **Vagisil® cream** (lidocaine (lignocaine)), **Wasp–Eze® spray** (benzocaine, mepyramine)

TOPICAL ANTIHISTAMINES

Indications: see notes above

Cautions: may cause hypersensitivity; avoid in eczema; photosensitivity (diphenhydramine); not recommended for longer than 3 days

The following is a list of topical antihistamine preparations on sale to the public, together with their significant ingredients:

Anthisan® (mepyramine), **Anthisan® Plus** (mepyramine, benzocaine), **Boots Bite & Sting Relief Antihistamine cream** (mepyramine), **Caladryl®** (diphenhydramine, calamine, camphor), **R.B.C.®** (antazoline, calamine, camphor, cetrimide, menthol), **Wasp–Eze® ointment** (antazoline), **Wasp–Eze® spray** (mepyramine, benzocaine)

denotes preparations that are considered to be less suitable for prescribing (see p. vi)

13.4 Topical corticosteroids

Topical corticosteroids are used for the treatment of inflammatory conditions of the skin other than those due to an infection, in particular the *eczematous disorders* (for further details see section 13.5.1). Corticosteroids suppress various components of the inflammatory reaction while in use; they are in no sense curative, and when treatment is discontinued a rebound exacerbation of the condition may occur. They are indicated for the relief of symptoms and for the suppression of signs of the disorder when potentially less harmful measures are ineffective.

Topical corticosteroids are of no value in the treatment of *urticaria* and they are **contra-indicated** in *rosacea*; they may worsen ulcerated or secondarily infected lesions. They should not be used indiscriminately in *pruritus* (where they will only benefit if inflammation is also causing the itch) and are **not** recommended for *acne vulgaris*.

Systemic or potent topical corticosteroids should be avoided or given only under specialist supervision *in psoriasis* because, although they may suppress the psoriasis in the short term, relapse or vigorous rebound occurs on withdrawal (sometimes precipitating severe pustular psoriasis). Topical use of potent corticosteroids on widespread psoriasis also leads to systemic as well as to local side-effects. It is reasonable, however, to prescribe a weaker corticosteroid (such as hydrocortisone) for short periods (perhaps up to 4 weeks) for *flexural* and *facial psoriasis* (**important:** not more potent than hydrocortisone 1% on the face). In the case of *scalp psoriasis* it is reasonable to use a more potent corticosteroid such as betamethasone or fluocinonide.

In general, the most potent topical corticosteroids should be reserved for recalcitrant dermatoses such as *chronic discoid lupus erythematosus, lichen simplex chronicus, hypertrophic lichen planus*, and *palmoplantar pustulosis*. Topical corticosteroids may cause skin atrophy, especially on thin skin areas such as the face or flexures, and may cause acneform pustules; on the face, they may cause a rosacea-like disorder (perioral dermatitis). Potent corticosteroids should therefore generally be avoided on the face and skin flexures, although specialists occasionally prescribe them in certain circumstances.

Intralesional corticosteroid injections (section 10.1.2.2) are more effective than the less potent topical corticosteroid preparations and they should be reserved for severe cases where there are localised lesions (such as *keloid scars, hypertrophic lichen planus*, or *localised alopecia areata*) and topical treatment has failed. Their effects may last for several weeks or even months. Particular care is needed to inject accurately into the lesion in order to avoid severe skin atrophy and loss of pigmentation.

SIDE-EFFECTS. Unlike the *potent* and *very potent* groups, the *moderate* and *mild* groups are rarely associated with side-effects. The more potent the preparation the more care is required, as absorption through the skin can cause severe pituitary-adrenal-axis suppression and Cushing's syndrome (section 6.3.2), both of which depend on the area of the body treated and the duration of the treatment. Absorption is greatest from areas of thin skin, raw surfaces, and intertriginous areas, and is increased by occlusion.

Local side-effects include:
(a) spread and worsening of untreated infection;
(b) thinning of the skin which may be restored over a period of time after stopping although the original structure may never return;
(c) irreversible striae atrophicae and telangiectasia;
(d) contact dermatitis;
(e) perioral dermatitis, an inflammatory papular disorder on the face of young women;
(f) acne at the site of application in some patients;
(g) mild depigmentation which may be reversible

CHOICE OF FORMULATION. *Water-miscible* creams are suitable for moist or weeping lesions whereas *ointments* are generally chosen for dry, lichenified or scaly lesions or where a more occlusive effect is required. *Lotions* may be useful when minimal application to a large or hair-bearing area is required or for the treatment of exudative lesions. *Occlusive polythene or hydrocolloid dressings* increase absorption, but also increase the risk of side-effects; they are therefore used only under supervision on a short-term basis for very thick areas of skin (such as the palms and soles). The *inclusion of urea* or *salicylic acid* increases the penetration of the corticosteroid.

TOPICAL CORTICOSTEROID POTENCIES

Potency	Examples
Mild	Hydrocortisone 1%
Moderately potent	Clobetasone butyrate 0.05%
Potent	Betamethasone 0.1% (as valerate)
	Hydrocortisone butyrate
Very potent	Clobetasol propionate 0.05%

The preparation containing the **least potent** drug at the lowest strength which is effective is the one of choice; dilution should be avoided whenever possible.

APPLICATION. Corticosteroid preparations should normally be applied once or twice daily. It is not necessary to apply them more frequently.

The length of a corticosteroid cream or ointment expelled from a tube may be used to specify the quantity to be applied to a given area of skin. This length may be measured in terms of a *fingertip unit* (the distance from the tip of the adult index finger to the first crease). One fingertip unit (approximately 500 mg) is sufficient to cover an area that is twice that of the flat adult hand.

Suitable quantities of corticosteroid preparations to be prescribed for specific areas of the body are:

	Creams and Ointments
Face and neck	15 to 30 g
Both hands	15 to 30 g
Scalp	15 to 30 g
Both arms	30 to 60 g
Both legs	100 g
Trunk	100 g
Groins and genitalia	15 to 30 g

These amounts are usually suitable for an adult for twice daily application for 1 week

CHILDREN. Children, especially babies, are particularly susceptible to side-effects. The more potent corticosteroids are **contra-indicated** in infants under 1 year, and in general they should be avoided in children or if necessary used with great care and for short periods. A mild corticosteroid such as hydrocortisone 1% ointment or cream is useful for treating nappy rash (section 13.2.2) or for atopic eczema in childhood (but see caution below). A potent or moderately potent corticosteroid may be appropriate for severe atopic eczema on the limbs, for 1–2 weeks **only**, followed by a weaker preparation as the condition improves; an emollient (section 13.2.1) should be used throughout.

COMPOUND PREPARATIONS. The advantages of including other substances (such as antibacterials or antifungals) with corticosteroids in topical preparations are debatable, but they may have a place where there is associated bacterial or fungal infection.

HYDROCORTISONE

Indications: mild inflammatory skin disorders such as eczemas (but for over-the-counter preparations, see below); nappy rash, see notes above and section 13.2.2

Cautions: see notes above; also avoid prolonged use in infants and children (extreme caution in dermatoses of infancy including nappy rash—where possible treatment should be limited to 5–7 days), avoid prolonged use on the face (and keep away from eyes); more potent corticosteroids **contra-indicated** in infants under 1 year (see also notes above)

PSORIASIS. Risks of more potent corticosteroids in psoriasis include possibility of rebound relapse, development of generalised pustular psoriasis, and local and systemic toxicity; they are specifically **contra-indicated** in widespread plaque psoriasis

Contra-indications: untreated bacterial, fungal, or viral skin lesions; rosacea (acne rosacea), perioral dermatitis; not recommended for acne vulgaris (more potent corticosteroids specifically **contra-indicated**)

Side-effects: see notes above
Administration: apply thinly 1–2 times daily

Hydrocortisone (Non-proprietary) PoM
Cream, hydrocortisone 0.5%, net price, 15 g = 34p; 30 g = 60p; 1%, 15 g = 37p. Label: 28. Potency: mild
Ointment, hydrocortisone 0.5%, net price 15 g = 35p; 30 g = 60p; 1%, 15 g = 36p. Label: 28. Potency: mild
When hydrocortisone cream or ointment is prescribed and no strength is stated, the 1% strength should be supplied

Over–the–counter products. The following is a list of skin creams and ointments that contain hydrocortisone (alone or with other ingredients) that can be sold to the public: **Dermacort®** (hydrocortisone 0.1%, cream), **Eurax Hc®** (hydrocortisone 0.25%; crotamiton 10%, cream), **Hc45®** (hydrocortisone acetate 1%, cream), **Lanacort®** (hydrocortisone acetate 1%, cream and ointment), **Zenoxone®** (hydrocortisone 1%, cream). They can be sold to the public for treatment of allergic contact dermatitis, irritant dermatitis, insect bite reactions and mild to moderate eczema
Cautions: not for children under 10 years or in pregnancy, without medical advice
Contra-indications: eyes/face, anogenital region, broken or infected skin (including cold sores, acne, and athlete's foot)
Administration: apply sparingly over small area 1–2 times daily for max. of 1 week

■ **Proprietary hydrocortisone preparations**

Note. The following preparations are PoM; those on sale to the public (with restrictions) are specified above.

Dioderm® (Dermal) PoM
Cream, hydrocortisone 0.1%. Net price 30 g = £2.69. Label: 28. Potency: mild
Excipients: include cetostearyl alcohol, propylene glycol
Note. Although this contains only 0.1% hydrocortisone, the formulation is designed to provide a clinical activity comparable to that of Hydrocortisone Cream 1% BP

Efcortelan® (GlaxoWellcome) PoM
Cream, hydrocortisone 0.5%, net price, 30 g = 60p; 1%, 30 g = 74p; 2.5%, 30 g = £1.66. Label: 28. Potency: mild
Excipients: include cetostearyl alcohol, chlorocresol
Ointment, hydrocortisone 0.5%, net price, 30 g = 60p; 1%, 30 g = 74p; 2.5%, 30 g = £1.66. Label: 28. Potency: mild
Excipients: none as listed in section 13.1.3

Mildison® (Yamanouchi) PoM
Lipocream, hydrocortisone 1%. Net price 30 g = £2.19. Label: 28. Potency: mild
Excipients: include cetostearyl alcohol, hydroxybenzoates (parabens)

■ Compound preparations
Note. Compound preparations with coal tar, section 13.5.2

Alphaderm® (Procter & Gamble Pharm.) PoM
Cream, hydrocortisone 1%, urea 10%. Net price 30 g = £1.75; 100 g = £5.42. Label: 28. Potency: moderate
Excipients: none as listed in section 13.1.3

Calmurid HC® (Galderma) PoM
Cream, hydrocortisone 1%, urea 10%, lactic acid 5%. Net price 30 g = £2.33; 100 g = £7.30. Label: 28. Potency: moderate
Excipients: none as listed in section 13.1.3
Note. Manufacturer advises dilute to half-strength with aqueous cream for 1 week if stinging occurs then transfer to undiluted preparation (but see section 13.1.1 for advice to avoid dilution where possible)

¹**Eurax-Hydrocortisone®** (Novartis Consumer Health) PoM
Cream, hydrocortisone 0.25%, crotamiton 10%. Net price 30 g = 87p. Label: 28. Potency: mild
Excipients: include fragrance, hydroxybenzoates (parabens), propylene glycol, stearyl alcohol
1. A 15-g tube is on sale to the public for treatment of contact dermatitis and insect bites (*Eurax Hc®*)

■ With antimicrobials
See notes above for comment on compound preparations

¹**Canesten HC®** (Bayer Consumer Care) PoM
Cream, hydrocortisone 1%, clotrimazole 1%, net price 30 g = £2.17. Label: 28. Potency: mild
Excipients: include benzyl alcohol, cetostearyl alcohol
1. A 15-g tube is on sale to the public for the treatment of athlete's foot and fungal infection of skin folds with associated inflammation (*Canesten® Hydrocortisone*)

Daktacort® (Janssen-Cilag) PoM
Cream, hydrocortisone 1%, miconazole nitrate 2%. Net price 30 g = £2.24. Label: 28. Potency: mild
Excipients: include butylated hydroxyanisole, disodium edetate
Ointment, hydrocortisone 1%, miconazole nitrate 2%. Net price 30 g = £2.25. Label: 28. Potency: mild
Excipients: none as listed in section 13.1.3

Econacort® (Squibb) PoM
Cream, hydrocortisone 1%, econazole nitrate 1%. Net price 30 g = £2.25. Label: 28. Potency: mild
Excipients: include butylated hydroxyanisole

Fucidin H® (Leo) PoM
Cream, hydrocortisone acetate 1%, fusidic acid 2%. Net price 30 g = £5.30; 60 g = £10.60. Label: 28. Potency: mild
Excipients: include butylated hydroxyanisole, cetyl alcohol, potassium sorbate
Ointment, hydrocortisone acetate 1%, sodium fusidate 2%. Net price 30 g = £4.35; 60 g = £8.70. Label: 28. Potency: mild
Excipients: include cetyl alcohol, wool fat

Gregoderm® (Unigreg) PoM
Ointment, hydrocortisone 1%, neomycin sulphate 0.4%, nystatin 100 000 units/g, polymyxin B sulphate 7250 units/g. Net price 15 g = £2.40. Label: 28. Potency: mild
Excipients: include cetostearyl alcohol

Nystaform-HC® (Typharm) PoM
Cream, hydrocortisone 0.5%, nystatin 100 000 units/g, chlorhexidine hydrochloride 1%. Net price 30 g = £2.66. Label: 28. Potency: mild
Excipients: include benzyl alcohol, cetostearyl alcohol, polysorbate '60'
Note. May be difficult to obtain
Ointment, hydrocortisone 1%, nystatin 100 000 units/g, chlorhexidine acetate 1%. Net price 30 g = £2.66. Label: 28. Potency: mild
Excipients: none as listed in section 13.1.3
Note. May be difficult to obtain

Quinocort® (Adams Hlth) PoM
Cream, hydrocortisone 1%, potassium hydroxyquinoline sulphate 0.5%. Net price 30 g = £1.56. Label: 28. Potency: mild
Excipients: include cetostearyl alcohol, chlorocresol, edetic acid (EDTA)

Terra-Cortril® (Pfizer) PoM
Topical ointment, hydrocortisone 1%, oxytetracycline 3% (as hydrochloride). Net price 15 g = £1.01; 30 g = £1.82. Label: 28. Potency: mild
Excipients: none as listed in section 13.1.3

Terra-Cortril Nystatin® (Pfizer) PoM
Cream, hydrocortisone 1%, nystatin 100 000 units/g, oxytetracycline 3% (as calcium salt). Net price 30 g = £2.01. Label: 28. Potency: mild
Excipients: include fragrance, hydroxybenzoates (parabens), polysorbate, propylene glycol, sodium metabisulphite, stearyl alcohol

Timodine® (R&C) PoM
Cream, hydrocortisone 0.5%, nystatin 100 000 units/g, benzalkonium chloride solution 0.2%, dimeticone '350' 10%. Net price 30 g = £2.38. Label: 28. Potency: mild
Excipients: include butylated hydroxyanisole, cetostearyl alcohol, hydroxybenzoates (parabens), sodium metabisulphite, sorbic acid

Vioform-Hydrocortisone® (Novartis Consumer Health) PoM
Cream, hydrocortisone 1%, clioquinol 3%. Net price 30 g = £1.46. Label: 28. Potency: mild
Excipients: include cetostearyl alcohol
Ointment, hydrocortisone 1%, clioquinol 3%. Net price 30 g = £1.46. Label:28. Potency: mild
Excipients: none as listed in section 13.1.3
Note. Stains clothing

HYDROCORTISONE BUTYRATE

Indications: severe inflammatory skin disorders such as eczemas unresponsive to less potent corticosteroids; psoriasis, see notes above

Cautions: see under Hydrocortisone and notes above

Contra-indications: see under Hydrocortisone and notes above

Side-effects: see under Hydrocortisone and notes above

Administration: apply thinly 1–2 times daily

Locoid® (Yamanouchi) [PoM]
Cream, hydrocortisone butyrate 0.1%. Net price 30 g = £2.04; 100 g = £6.26. Label: 28. Potency: potent
Excipients: include cetostearyl alcohol, hydroxybenzoates (parabens)

Lipocream, hydrocortisone butyrate 0.1%, net price 30 g = £2.14, 100 g = £6.56. Label: 28. Potency: potent
Excipients: include cetostearyl alcohol, hydroxybenzoates (parabens)
Note. For bland cream basis see *Lipobase®,* section 13.2.1

Ointment, hydrocortisone butyrate 0.1%, net price 30 g = £2.04, 100 g = £6.26. Label: 28. Potency: potent
Excipients: none as listed in section 13.1.3

Scalp lotion, hydrocortisone butyrate 0.1%, in an aqueous isopropyl alcohol basis, net price 100 mL = £8.83. Label: 15, 28. Potency: potent
Excipients: none as listed in section 13.1.3

Locoid Crelo® (Yamanouchi) [PoM]
Lotion (topical emulsion), hydrocortisone butyrate 0.1% in a water-miscible basis. Net price 100 g (with applicator nozzle) = £7.50. Label: 28. Potency: potent
Excipients: include cetostearyl alcohol, hydroxybenzoates (parabens), propylene glycol

■ With antimicrobials
See notes above for comment on compound preparations

Locoid C® (Yamanouchi) [PoM]
Cream, hydrocortisone butyrate 0.1%, chlorquinaldol 3%. Net price 30 g = £2.67. Label: 28. Potency: potent
Excipients: include cetostearyl alcohol
Note. Causes staining

Ointment, ingredients as for cream, in a greasy basis. Net price 30 g = £2.67. Label: 28. Potency: potent
Excipients: none as listed in section 13.1.3
Note. Causes staining

ALCLOMETASONE DIPROPIONATE

Indications: inflammatory skin disorders such as eczemas

Cautions: see under Hydrocortisone and notes above

Contra-indications: see under Hydrocortisone and notes above

Side-effects: see under Hydrocortisone and notes above

Administration: apply thinly 1–2 times daily

Modrasone® (Dominion) [PoM]
Cream, alclometasone dipropionate 0.05%. Net price 50 g = £2.82. Label: 28. Potency: moderate
Excipients: include cetostearyl alcohol, chlorocresol, propylene glycol

Ointment, alclometasone dipropionate 0.05%. Net price 50 g = £2.82. Label: 28. Potency: moderate
Excipients: include beeswax, propylene glycol

BECLOMETASONE DIPROPIONATE
(Beclomethasone dipropionate)

Indications: severe inflammatory skin disorders such as eczemas unresponsive to less potent corticosteroids; psoriasis, see notes above

Cautions: see under Hydrocortisone and notes above

Contra-indications: see under Hydrocortisone and notes above

Side-effects: see under Hydrocortisone and notes above

Administration: apply thinly 1–2 times daily

Propaderm® (GlaxoWellcome) [PoM]
Cream, beclometasone dipropionate 0.025%. Net price 30 g = £1.58. Label: 28. Potency: potent
Excipients: include cetostearyl alcohol, chlorocresol
Ointment, beclometasone dipropionate 0.025%. Net price 30 g = £1.58. Label: 28. Potency: potent
Excipients: include propylene glycol

BETAMETHASONE ESTERS

Indications: severe inflammatory skin disorders such as eczemas unresponsive to less potent corticosteroids; psoriasis, see notes above

Cautions: see under Hydrocortisone and notes above; use of more than 100 g per week of 0.1% preparation likely to cause adrenal suppression

Contra-indications: see under Hydrocortisone and notes above

Side-effects: see under Hydrocortisone and notes above

Administration: apply thinly 1–2 times daily

Betamethasone Valerate (Non-proprietary) [PoM]
Cream, betamethasone 0.1% (as valerate). Net price 30 g = £1.40. Label: 28. Potency: potent
Ointment, betamethasone 0.1% (as valerate). Net price 30 g = £1.40. Label: 28. Potency: potent
Available from Dowelhurst, Futuna

Betacap® (Dermal) [PoM]
Scalp application, betamethasone 0.1% (as valerate) in a water-miscible basis containing coconut oil derivative. Net price 100 mL = £4.22. Label: 15, 28. Potency: potent
Excipients: none as listed in section 13.1.3

Betnovate® (GlaxoWellcome) [PoM]
Cream, betamethasone 0.1% (as valerate), in a water-miscible basis. Net price 30 g = £1.40; 100 g = £3.95. Label: 28. Potency: potent
Excipients: include cetostearyl alcohol, chlorocresol
Ointment, betamethasone 0.1% (as valerate), in an anhydrous paraffin basis. Net price 30 g = £1.40; 100 g = £3.95. Label: 28. Potency: potent
Excipients: none as listed in section 13.1.3
Lotion, betamethasone 0.1% (as valerate). Net price 100 mL = £4.75. Label: 28. Potency: potent
Excipients: include cetostearyl alcohol, hydroxybenzoates (parabens)
Scalp application, betamethasone 0.1% (as valerate) in a water-miscible basis. Net price 100 mL = £5.18. Label: 15, 28. Potency: potent
Excipients: none as listed in section 13.1.3

Betnovate-RD® (GlaxoWellcome) [PoM]
Cream, betamethasone 0.025% (as valerate) in a water-miscible basis (1 in 4 dilution of Betnovate® cream). Net price 100 g = £3.26. Label: 28. Potency: moderate
Excipients: include cetostearyl alcohol, chlorocresol

Ointment, betamethasone 0.025% (as valerate) in an anhydrous paraffin basis (1 in 4 dilution of Betnovate® ointment). Net price 100 g = £3.26. Label: 28. Potency: moderate
Excipients: none as listed in section 13.1.3

Bettamousse® (Celltech) PoM
Foam (= scalp application), betamethasone valerate 0.12% (≡ betamethasone 0.1%). Net price 100 g = £7.50. Label: 28. Potency: potent
Excipients: include cetyl alcohol, polysorbate 60, propylene glycol, stearyl alcohol
Note. Flammable

Diprosone® (Schering-Plough) PoM
Cream, betamethasone 0.05% (as dipropionate). Net price 30 g = £2.41; 100 g = £6.84. Label: 28. Potency: potent
Excipients: include cetostearyl alcohol, chlorocresol
Ointment, betamethasone 0.05% (as dipropionate). Net price 30 g = £2.41; 100 g = £6.84. Label: 28. Potency: potent
Excipients: none as listed in section 13.1.3
Lotion, betamethasone 0.05% (as dipropionate). Net price 30 mL = £3.04; 100 mL = £8.71. Label: 28. Potency: potent
Excipients: none as listed in section 13.1.3

■ With salicylic acid
See notes above for comment on compound preparations

Diprosalic® (Schering-Plough) PoM
Ointment, betamethasone 0.05% (as dipropionate), salicylic acid 3%. Net price 30 g = £3.30; 100 g = £9.50. Label: 28. Potency: potent
Excipients: none as listed in section 13.1.3
Apply thinly 1–2 times daily; max. 60 g per week
Scalp application, betamethasone 0.05% (as dipropionate), salicylic acid 2%, in an alcoholic basis. Net price 100 mL = £10.50. Label: 28. Potency: potent
Excipients: include disodium edetate
Apply a few drops 1–2 times daily

■ With antimicrobials
See notes above for comment on compound preparations

Betnovate-C® (GlaxoWellcome) PoM
Cream, betamethasone 0.1% (as valerate), clioquinol 3%. Net price 30 g = £1.72. Label: 28. Potency: potent
Excipients: include cetostearyl alcohol, chlorocresol
Note. Stains clothing
Ointment, betamethasone 0.1% (as valerate), clioquinol 3%. Net price 30 g = £1.72. Label: 28. Potency: potent
Excipients: none as listed in section 13.1.3
Note. Stains clothing

Betnovate-N® (GlaxoWellcome) PoM
Cream, betamethasone 0.1% (as valerate), neomycin sulphate 0.5%. Net price 30 g = £1.72; 100 g = £4.77. Label: 28. Potency: potent
Excipients: include cetostearyl alcohol, chlorocresol
Ointment, betamethasone 0.1% (as valerate), neomycin sulphate 0.5%. Net price 30 g = £1.72; 100 g = £4.77. Label: 28. Potency: potent
Excipients: none as listed in section 13.1.3

FuciBET® (Leo) PoM
Cream, betamethasone 0.1% (as valerate), fusidic acid 2%. Net price 30 g = £6.04; 60 g = £12.07. Label: 28. Potency: potent
Excipients: include cetostearyl alcohol, chlorocresol

Lotriderm® (Dominion) PoM
Cream, betamethasone dipropionate 0.064% (≡ betamethasone 0.05%), clotrimazole 1%. Net price 30 g = £6.34. Label: 28. Potency: potent
Excipients: include benzyl alcohol, cetostearyl alcohol, propylene glycol

CLOBETASOL PROPIONATE

Indications: short-term treatment only of severe resistant inflammatory skin disorders such as recalcitrant eczemas unresponsive to less potent corticosteroids; psoriasis, see notes above
Cautions: see under Hydrocortisone and notes above
Contra-indications: see under Hydrocortisone and notes above
Side-effects: see under Hydrocortisone and notes above
Administration: apply thinly 1–2 times daily for up to 4 weeks; max. 50 g of 0.05% preparation per week

Dermovate® (GlaxoWellcome) PoM
Cream, clobetasol propionate 0.05%. Net price 30 g = £2.56; 100 g = £7.52. Label: 28. Potency: very potent
Excipients: include beeswax (or beeswax substitute), cetostearyl alcohol, chlorocresol, propylene glycol
Ointment, clobetasol propionate 0.05%. Net price 30 g = £2.56; 100 g = £7.52. Label: 28. Potency: very potent
Excipients: include propylene glycol
Scalp application, clobetasol propionate 0.05%, in a thickened alcoholic basis. Net price 30 mL = £2.93; 100 mL = £9.91. Label: 15, 28. Potency: very potent
Excipients: none as listed in section 13.1.3

■ With antimicrobials
See notes above for comment on compound preparations

Dermovate-NN® (GlaxoWellcome) PoM
Cream, clobetasol propionate 0.05%, neomycin sulphate 0.5%, nystatin 100 000 units/g, net price 30 g = £3.50. Label: 28. Potency: very potent
Excipients: include arachis (peanut) oil, beeswax substitute
Ointment, ingredients as for cream, in a paraffin basis, net price 30 g = £3.50. Label: 28. Potency: very potent
Excipients: none as listed in section 13.1.3

CLOBETASONE BUTYRATE

Indications: eczemas and dermatitis of all types; maintenance treatment and control of patches of more potent corticosteroids
Cautions: see under Hydrocortisone and notes above
Contra-indications: see under Hydrocortisone and notes above
Side-effects: see under Hydrocortisone and notes above
Administration: apply thinly 1–2 times daily

¹**Eumovate®** (GlaxoWellcome) PoM
Cream, clobetasone butyrate 0.05%. Net price 30 g = £1.76; 100 g = £5.16. Label: 28. Potency: moderate
Excipients: include beeswax substitute, cetostearyl alcohol, chlorocresol
1. Cream can be sold to the public for short-term symptomatic treatment and control of patches of eczema and dermatitis (but not seborrhoeic dermatitis) in adults and children over 12 years provided pack does not contain more than 15 g.

Ointment, clobetasone butyrate 0.05%. Net price 30 g = £1.76; 100 g = £5.16. Label: 28. Potency: moderate
Excipients: none as listed in section 13.1.3

■ With antimicrobials
See notes above for comment on compound preparations

Trimovate® (GlaxoWellcome) PoM
Cream, clobetasone butyrate 0.05%, oxytetracycline 3% (as calcium salt), nystatin 100 000 units/g, net price 30 g = £3.13. Label: 28. Potency: moderate
Excipients: include cetostearyl alcohol, chlorocresol, sodium metabisulphite
Note. Stains clothing

DESOXIMETASONE

(Desoxymethasone)

Indications: severe acute inflammatory, allergic, and chronic skin disorders; psoriasis, see notes above

Cautions: see under Hydrocortisone and notes above

Contra-indications: see under Hydrocortisone and notes above

Side-effects: see under Hydrocortisone and notes above

Administration: apply thinly 1–2 times daily

Stiedex® (Stiefel) PoM
LP Oily cream, desoximetasone 0.05%. Net price 30 g = £2.73; 100 g = £8.19. Label:28. Potency: moderate
Excipients: include edetic acid (EDTA), wool fat
Lotion, desoximetasone 0.25%, salicylic acid 1%. Net price 50 mL = £7.69. Label: 28. Potency: potent
Excipients: include disodium edetate, propylene glycol

DIFLUCORTOLONE VALERATE

Indications: severe inflammatory skin disorders such as eczemas unresponsive to less potent corticosteroids; high strength (0.3%), short-term treatment of severe exacerbations; psoriasis, see notes above

Cautions: see under Hydrocortisone and notes above

Contra-indications: see under Hydrocortisone and notes above

Side-effects: see under Hydrocortisone and notes above

Administration: apply thinly 1–2 times daily for up to 4 weeks (0.1% preparations) or 2 weeks (0.3% preparations), reducing strength as condition responds; max. 60 g of 0.3% per week

Nerisone® (Schering Health) PoM
Cream, diflucortolone valerate 0.1%. Net price 30 g = £1.59. Label: 28. Potency: potent
Excipients: include disodium edetate, hydroxybenzoates (parabens), stearyl alcohol
Oily cream, diflucortolone valerate 0.1%. Net price 30 g = £2.56. Label: 28. Potency: potent
Excipients: include beeswax
Ointment, diflucortolone valerate 0.1%. Net price 30 g = £1.59. Label: 28. Potency: potent
Excipients: none as listed in section 13.1.3

Nerisone Forte® (Schering Health) PoM
Oily cream, diflucortolone valerate 0.3%. Net price 15 g = £2.09. Label: 28. Potency: very potent
Excipients: include beeswax
Ointment, diflucortolone valerate 0.3%. Net price 15 g = £2.09. Label: 28. Potency: very potent
Excipients: none as listed in section 13.1.3

FLUDROXYCORTIDE/ FLURANDRENOLONE

Indications: inflammatory skin disorders such as eczemas

Cautions: see under Hydrocortisone and notes above

Contra-indications: see under Hydrocortisone and notes above

Side-effects: see under Hydrocortisone and notes above

Administration: apply thinly 1–2 times daily, reducing strength as condition responds

Haelan® (Typharm) PoM
Cream, fludroxycortide 0.0125%. Net price 60 g = £3.26. Label: 28. Potency: moderate
Excipients: include cetyl alcohol, propylene glycol
Ointment, fludroxycortide 0.0125%. Net price 60 g = £3.26. Label: 28. Potency: moderate
Excipients: include beeswax, cetyl alcohol, polysorbate
Tape, polythene adhesive film impregnated with fludroxycortide 4 micrograms /cm^2. Net price 7.5 cm × 50 cm = £5.67; 7.5 cm × 200 cm = £19.07
For chronic localised recalcitrant dermatoses (but not acute or weeping), cut tape to fit lesion, apply to clean, dry skin shorn of hair, usually for 12 of each 24 hours
Note. Haelan® *Tape* cannot be prescribed on form FP10 (GP10 in Scotland) since it is not reimbursable

FLUOCINOLONE ACETONIDE

Indications: inflammatory skin disorders such as eczemas; psoriasis, see notes above

Cautions: see under Hydrocortisone and notes above

Contra-indications: see under Hydrocortisone and notes above

Side-effects: see under Hydrocortisone and notes above

Administration: apply thinly 1–2 times daily, reducing strength as condition responds

Synalar® (Bioglan) PoM
Cream, fluocinolone acetonide 0.025%. Net price 30 g = £1.34. Label: 28. Potency: potent
Excipients: include benzyl alcohol, cetostearyl alcohol, polysorbates, propylene glycol
Gel, fluocinolone acetonide 0.025%. Net price 30 g = £1.98. For use on scalp and other hairy areas. Label: 28. Potency: potent
Excipients: include hydroxybenzoates (parabens), propylene glycol
Ointment, fluocinolone acetonide 0.025%. Net price 30 g = £1.34. Label: 28. Potency: potent
Excipients: include propylene glycol, wool fat

Synalar 1 in 4 Dilution® (Bioglan) PoM
Cream, fluocinolone acetonide 0.00625%. Net price 50 g = £1.56. Label: 28. Potency: moderate
Excipients: include benzyl alcohol, cetostearyl alcohol, polysorbates, propylene glycol

Ointment, fluocinolone acetonide 0.00625%. Net price 50 g = £1.56. Label: 28. Potency: moderate
Excipients: include propylene glycol, wool fat

Synalar 1 in 10 Dilution® (Bioglan) [PoM]
Cream, fluocinolone acetonide 0.0025%. Net price 50 g = £1.48. Label: 28. Potency: mild
Excipients: include benzyl alcohol, cetostearyl alcohol, polysorbates, propylene glycol

■ With antibacterials
See notes above for comment on compound preparations

Synalar C® (Bioglan) [PoM]
Cream, fluocinolone acetonide 0.025%, clioquinol 3%, net price 15 g = 86p. Label: 28. Potency: potent
Excipients: include cetostearyl alcohol, disodium edetate, hydroxybenzoates (parabens), polysorbates, propylene glycol
Ointment, ingredients as for cream, net price 15 g = 86p. Label: 28. Potency: potent.
Note. Stains clothing
Excipients: include propylene glycol, wool fat

Synalar N® (Bioglan) [PoM]
Cream, fluocinolone acetonide 0.025%, neomycin sulphate 0.5%. Net price 30 g = £1.41. Label: 28. Potency: potent
Excipients: include cetostearyl alcohol, hydroxybenzoates (parabens), polysorbates, propylene glycol
Ointment, ingredients as for cream, in a greasy basis. Net price 30 g = £1.41. Label: 28. Potency: potent
Excipients: include propylene glycol, wool fat

FLUOCINONIDE

Indications: severe inflammatory skin disorders such as eczemas unresponsive to less potent corticosteroids; psoriasis, see notes above
Cautions: see under Hydrocortisone and notes above
Contra-indications: see under Hydrocortisone and notes above
Side-effects: see under Hydrocortisone and notes above
Administration: apply thinly 1–2 times daily

Metosyn® (Bioglan) [PoM]
FAPG cream, fluocinonide 0.05%. Net price 25 g = £1.17; 100 g = £3.95. Label: 28. Potency: potent
Excipients: include propylene glycol
Ointment, fluocinonide 0.05%. Net price 25 g = £1.04; 100 g = £3.90. Label: 28. Potency: potent
Excipients: include propylene glycol, wool fat

FLUOCORTOLONE

Indications: severe inflammatory skin disorders such as eczemas unresponsive to less potent corticosteroids; psoriasis, see notes above
Cautions: see under Hydrocortisone and notes above
Contra-indications: see under Hydrocortisone and notes above
Side-effects: see under Hydrocortisone and notes above
Administration: apply thinly 1–2 times daily, reducing strength as condition responds

Ultralanum Plain® (Schering Health) [PoM]
Cream, fluocortolone hexanoate 0.25%, fluocortolone pivalate 0.25%. Net price 50 g = £2.95. Label: 28. Potency: moderate
Excipients: include disodium edetate, fragrance, hydroxybenzoates (parabens), stearyl alcohol

Ointment, fluocortolone 0.25%, fluocortolone hexanoate 0.25%. Net price 50 g = £2.95. Label: 28. Potency: moderate
Excipients: include wool fat, fragrance

FLUTICASONE PROPIONATE

Indications: inflammatory skin disorders such as dermatitis and eczemas unresponsive to less potent corticosteroids
Cautions: see under Hydrocortisone and notes above
Contra-indications: see under Hydrocortisone and notes above
Side-effects: see under Hydrocortisone and notes above
Administration: apply cream thinly once daily *or* ointment twice daily

Cutivate® (GlaxoWellcome) [PoM]
Cream, fluticasone propionate 0.05%, net price 15 g = £2.35; 50 g = £6.95. Label: 28. Potency: potent
Excipients: include cetostearyl alcohol, imidurea, propylene glycol
Ointment, fluticasone propionate 0.005%, net price 15 g = £2.35, 50 g = £6.95. Label: 28. Potency: potent
Excipients: include propylene glycol

HALCINONIDE

Indications: short-term treatment only of severe resistant inflammatory skin disorders such as recalcitrant eczemas unresponsive to less potent corticosteroids; psoriasis, see notes above
Cautions: see under Hydrocortisone and notes above
Contra-indications: see under Hydrocortisone and notes above
Side-effects: see under Hydrocortisone and notes above
Administration: apply thinly 1–2 times daily

Halciderm Topical® (Squibb) [PoM]
Cream, halcinonide 0.1%. Net price 30 g = £3.40. Label: 28. Potency: very potent
Excipients: include propylene glycol

MOMETASONE FUROATE

Indications: severe inflammatory skin disorders such as eczemas unresponsive to less potent corticosteroids; psoriasis, see notes above
Cautions: see under Hydrocortisone and notes above
Contra-indications: see under Hydrocortisone and notes above
Side-effects: see under Hydrocortisone and notes above
Administration: apply thinly once daily (to scalp in case of lotion)

Elocon® (Schering-Plough) [PoM]
Cream, mometasone furoate 0.1%. Net price 30 g = £4.88; 100 g = £14.05. Label: 28. Potency: potent
Excipients: include stearyl alcohol

Ointment, mometasone furoate 0.1%. Net price
30 g = £4.88; 100 g = £14.05. Label: 28. Potency:
potent
Excipients: none as listed in section 13.1.3
Scalp lotion, mometasone furoate 0.1% in an
aqueous isopropyl alcohol basis. Net price 30 mL
= £4.88. Label: 28. Potency: potent
Excipients: include propylene glycol

TRIAMCINOLONE ACETONIDE

Indications: severe inflammatory skin disorders
such as eczemas unresponsive to less potent corticosteroids; psoriasis, see notes above
Cautions: see under Hydrocortisone and notes
above
Contra-indications: see under Hydrocortisone
and notes above
Side-effects: see under Hydrocortisone and notes
above
Administration: apply thinly 1–2 times daily

■ With antimicrobials
See notes above for comment on compound preparations
Aureocort® (Lederle) PoM
Ointment, triamcinolone acetonide 0.1%, chlor-
tetracycline hydrochloride 3%, in an anhydrous
greasy basis containing wool fat and white soft
paraffin. Net price 15 g = £2.70. Label: 28.
Potency: potent
Excipients: include wool fat
Note. Stains clothing
Tri-Adcortyl® (Squibb) PoM ▭
Cream, triamcinolone acetonide 0.1%, gramicidin
0.025%, neomycin (as sulphate) 0.25%, nystatin
100 000 units/g. Net price 30 g = £3.15. Label: 28.
Potency: potent
Excipients: include benzyl alcohol, ethylenediamine, propylene
glycol, fragrance
Ointment, triamcinolone acetonide 0.1%, grami-
cidin 0.025%, neomycin (as sulphate) 0.25%,
nystatin 100 000 units/g. Net price 30 g = £3.15.
Label: 28. Potency: potent
Excipients: none as listed in section 13.1.3
Note. Not recommended owing to presence of ethylenediamine in the cream and also because combination of
antibacterial with antifungal not considered useful in
either the cream or ointment

▭ denotes preparations that are considered to
be less suitable for prescribing (see p. vi)

13.5 Preparations for eczema and psoriasis

13.5.1   Preparations for eczema
13.5.2   Preparations for psoriasis

13.5.1 Preparations for eczema

Eczema (dermatitis) has several causes, which may
influence treatment. The main types of eczema are
irritant, allergic contact, atopic, venous and discoid;
different types may co-exist. Lichenification, due to
scratching and rubbing, may complicate any
chronic eczema. *Atopic eczema* is the most common

type and it usually involves dry skin as well as
infection and lichenification.

Management of eczema involves the removal or
treatment of contributory factors including occupational and domestic irritants. Known or suspected
contact allergens should be avoided. Rarely, ingredients in topical medicinal products may sensitise
the skin; the BNF lists active ingredients together
with excipients that have been associated with skin
sensitisation.

Skin dryness and the consequent irritant eczema
requires **emollients** (section 13.2.1) applied regularly and liberally to the affected area; this may be
supplemented with bath or shower emollients. The
use of emollients should continue even if the eczema improves or if other treatment is being used.

Topical corticosteroids (section 13.4) are also
required in the management of eczema; the potency
of the corticosteroid should be appropriate to the
severity and site of the condition. Mild corticosteroids are generally used on the face and on flexures;
potent corticosteroids are generally required for use
on adults with discoid or lichenified eczema or with
eczema on the scalp, limbs, and trunk. Treatment
should be reviewed regularly, especially if a potent
corticosteroid is required. Bandages (including
those containing **zinc** and **ichthammol**) are sometimes applied over topical corticosteroids to treat
eczema of the limbs.

INFECTION. Bacterial infection (commonly with
Staphylococcus aureus and occasionally with *Streptococcus pyogenes*) can exacerbate eczema and
requires treatment with topical or systemic **antibacterial drugs** (section 13.10.1 and section 5.1). Antibacterial drugs should be used in short courses
(typically 1 week) to reduce the risk of drug resistance or skin sensitisation. Associated eczema is
treated simultaneously with a topical corticosteroid
usually of moderate or high potency.

Eczema which involves widespread or recurrent
infection may be treated with products that combine
an antimicrobial with an emollient application (section 13.2.1) and with a bath emollient (section
13.2.1.1); antiseptic shampoos (section 13.9) may
be used on the scalp.

Intertriginous eczema commonly involves candida and bacteria; it is best treated with a mild or
moderately potent topical corticosteroid and a suitable antimicrobial drug.

Widespread herpes simplex infection may complicate atopic eczema and treatment with a systemic
antiviral drug (section 5.3) is indicated.

The management of *seborrhoeic dermatitis* is
described on p. 548.

MANAGEMENT OF OTHER FEATURES OF ECZEMA.
Lichenification, which results from repeated
scratching is treated initially with a potent corticosteroid. Bandages containing **ichthammol paste** (to
reduce pruritus) and other substances such as **zinc
oxide** may be applied over the corticosteroid. **Coal
tar** (section 13.5.2) and **ichthammol** can be useful
in some cases of *chronic eczema*.

Antihistamines (section 3.4.1) may be of some
value in relieving the itch of eczema, usually
because of their sedating effect.

Exudative ('weeping') eczema requires a potent
corticosteroid initially; infection may also be

present and requires specific treatment (see above). **Potassium permanganate** solution (1 in 10 000) can be used in exudating eczema for its antiseptic and astringent effect; treatment should be stopped when exudation stops.

There is little evidence to support the widespread use of **gamolenic acid** in *atopic eczema* but it may be considered for some cases of severe dryness and itching which have not responded to other treatments. Gamolenic acid should be discontinued if there is no clear benefit after 3 months' use.

Severe refractory eczema is best managed under specialist supervision; it may require phototherapy, systemic corticosteroids (section 6.3.2), or immunosuppressive drugs such as ciclosporin (section 8.2.2 and section 13.5.2), azathioprine (section 8.2.1), or mycophenolate mofetil (section 8.2.1).

ICHTHAMMOL

Indications: chronic lichenified eczema
Side-effects: skin irritation
Administration: apply 1–3 times daily

Ichthammol Ointment, BP 1980, ichthammol 10%, yellow soft paraffin 45%, wool fat 45%. Net price 25 g = 53p
Zinc and Ichthammol Cream, BP, ichthammol 5%, cetostearyl alcohol 3%, wool fat 10%, in zinc cream. Net price 100 g = 77p
Zinc Paste and Ichthammol Bandage, BP
(*Ichthopaste®*, *Icthaband®*), see Appendix 8 (section A8.2.9)

GAMOLENIC ACID

Indications: symptomatic relief of atopic eczema (but see notes above); mastalgia (section 6.7.2)
Cautions: history of epilepsy, concomitant treatment with epileptogenic drugs e.g. phenothiazines; pregnancy
Side-effects: occasional nausea, indigestion, headache; rarely hypersensitivity reactions including rash, urticaria, pruritus and abdominal pain
Dose: 160–240 mg twice daily; CHILD 1–12 years, 80–160 mg twice daily; see notes above

COUNSELLING. Capsules may be swallowed whole (except *Epogam®* paediatric capsules, see below), or cut open and contents swallowed directly or mixed with milk or taken on bread

Gamolenic Acid (Non-proprietary) PoM
Capsules, gamolenic acid 40 mg in evening primrose oil, net price 240-cap pack = £21.70. Counselling, see above.
Excipients: include vitamin E
Available from IVAX

Epogam® (Pharmacia) PoM
Epogam® 40 capsules, gamolenic acid 40 mg in evening primrose oil. Net price 240-cap pack = £23.31. Counselling, see above
Excipients: include vitamin E
Epogam® 80 capsules, gamolenic acid 80 mg in evening primrose oil. Net price 120-cap pack = £23.31. Counselling, see above
Excipients: include vitamin E

Epogam® paediatric capsules, gamolenic acid 80 mg in evening primrose oil. Net price 60-cap pack = £14.72. Counselling, see below
Excipients: include vitamin E
COUNSELLING. *Epogam®* paediatric capsules must *not* be swallowed whole, but cut open at the 'snip-off' neck and contents swallowed directly or mixed with milk or taken on bread

Seborrhoeic dermatitis

Seborrhoeic dermatitis (seborrhoeic eczema) is associated with the yeast *Malassezia furfur* and affects the scalp, paranasal areas, and eyebrows. Shampoos active against the yeast (including those containing ketoconazole and coal tar, section 13.9) and combinations of mild corticosteroids with suitable antimicrobials (section 13.4) are used. **Lithium succinate and zinc sulphate** ointment may be effective.

LITHIUM SUCCINATE

Indications: seborrhoeic dermatitis
Cautions: may exacerbate psoriasis; avoid eyes, mucous membranes
Side-effects: occasional skin irritation
Administration: initially apply thinly twice daily, then reduce; CHILD under 12 years not recommended

Efalith® (Scotia) PoM
Ointment, lithium succinate 8%, zinc sulphate 0.05%. Net price 20 g = £3.00
Excipients: include wool fat derivative

13.5.2 Preparations for psoriasis

Psoriasis is characterised by epidermal thickening and scaling. It commonly affects extensor surfaces and the scalp. Occasionally, psoriasis may be provoked or exacerbated by lithium, chloroquine and hydroxychloroquine, beta-blockers, non-steroidal anti-inflammatory drugs, and ACE inhibitors. For mild conditions, treatment, other than reassurance and an **emollient**, may be unnecessary.

In more troublesome cases of psoriasis, local application of salicylic acid, coal tar, calcipotriol, or dithranol may have a beneficial effect.

Salicylic acid may be used in all hyperkeratotic and scaling conditions to enhance the rate of loss of surface scale. Preparations containing salicylic acid 2% are used initially and then gradually increased to concentrations of 3 to 6%. Side-effects are few but include irritation, or, when large areas are treated, salicylate toxicity.

Coal tar is more active than salicylic acid and has anti-inflammatory and antiscaling properties. It is used in psoriasis and occasionally in *chronic atopic eczema*. The formulation and strength chosen depends on patient acceptability, severity and site of the condition; the 'thicker' the patch of eczema or psoriasis the stronger the concentration of coal tar required. **Coal tar paste** or **zinc and coal tar paste** are generally suitable for most cases but are limited by their unpleasant appearance and smell and they may not be used on the face. Some of the newer preparations are more acceptable. Mild coal tar preparations may be suitable for treating the face. **Tar shampoos** are described in section 13.9. When lesions are extensive coal tar baths are useful. Combinations of coal tar with zinc or salicylic acid have little advantage over the simpler preparations. Preparations containing hydrocortisone and coal tar may be useful in eczemas.

Dithranol is very effective in psoriasis. The preparation is applied carefully to the lesion. Usual concentrations are 0.1–3% and should normally only be applied for short contact periods of 30–60 minutes (**important:** if using above 0.1% the sensitivity of the skin must first be tested—further increases must be gradual). Dithranol must be used with caution as it can cause quite severe skin irritation (especially to perilesional skin). For this reason it must be applied only to the lesions and it is customary to start with low concentrations (e.g. 0.1%) and gradually build up (e.g. every 7 days) to the maximum concentration which produces a therapeutic effect without irritation. It should not be applied to flexural areas since burning may occur. Hands should be washed thoroughly after use. Some patients are intolerant to dithranol even in low concentrations; it is important to recognise them early in treatment because continued use can result in their psoriasis becoming unstable. Fair skin is more sensitive than dark skin. Proprietary preparations may be more convenient as they may cause less staining than dithranol paste. *Ingram's method* of applying dithranol is sometimes used in hospital, which involves the patient soaking in a warm bath containing coal tar solution 1 in 800 and, after drying, exposure to ultraviolet radiation B (UVB) to produce minimal erythema. **Dithranol paste** is applied to the lesions and the normal skin protected by applying talc and stockinette dressings. The procedure is repeated daily.

UVB phototherapy is also effective by itself in mild to moderate, guttate or chronic plaque psoriasis.

Calcipotriol is a vitamin D derivative that is now widely used for topical application for plaque psoriasis; a scalp solution is also used for scalp psoriasis. Advantages are that it does not have an unpleasant smell and does not stain clothing. **Tacalcitol**, another vitamin D analogue, is applied once daily in the treatment of plaque psoriasis.

Tazarotene is a retinoid licensed for topical use in mild to moderate plaque psoriasis affecting up to 10% of skin area.

PUVA, photochemotherapy combining a psoralen with long-wave ultraviolet irradiation (UVA), is effective in some patients with psoriasis; special lamps are required. The psoralen, generally methoxsalen [unlicensed] is used to enhance the therapeutic effect of the irradiation; it may be administered either by mouth or topically. Treatment is available in hospital dermatology centres; it has to be carefully regulated, owing to the short-term hazard of severe burning and the long-term hazards of accelerated ageing of the skin, the development of skin cancer and, unless protected, cataract formation.

Acitretin is a retinoid given by mouth for the treatment of *severe resistant or complicated psoriasis* and some of the *congenital disorders of keratinisation* including Darier's disease (keratosis

follicularis). It is a metabolite of **etretinate** (which it has replaced). It should be prescribed **only** by, or under the supervision of, a consultant dermatologist and is available to hospitals (or specified retail pharmacies) **only**. It is a retinoid (a vitamin A derivative) with marked effects on keratinising epithelia. A therapeutic effect occurs after 2 to 4 weeks with maximum benefit after 4 to 6 weeks. Acitretin treats only manifestations not the ultimate causes of these diseases, but treatment should be limited to a period of 6 to 9 months with a 3- to 4-month rest period before repeating treatment. Most patients suffer from dryness and cracking of the lips. Other side-effects include a mild transient increase in the rate of hair fall (reversible on withdrawal), occasional generalised pruritus, paronychia, and nose bleeds. There is a tendency for the plasma lipids to rise in some patients. Acitretin is **teratogenic** and must be **avoided** in pregnancy. Contraceptive measures must be taken at least **1 month before** and during treatment by women who may become pregnant and for at least **two years after** a course of the drug.

An antimetabolite, usually **methotrexate**, may also be used for *severe resistant psoriasis*, but this must again always be done under hospital supervision, the dose being adjusted according to severity of the condition and in accordance with haematological and biochemical measurements; the usual dose is 10 to 25 mg of methotrexate once weekly, by mouth.

Ciclosporin (cyclosporin) is now also available for *severe resistant psoriasis* and once again its use calls for specialist care in a hospital context.

For comment on the limited role of **corticosteroids** in psoriasis, see section 13.4.

Topical preparations for psoriasis

CALCIPOTRIOL

Indications: plaque psoriasis

Cautions: pregnancy; avoid use on face and inadvertent transfer to other body areas; wash hands thoroughly after application; risk of hypercalcaemia if max. weekly dose exceeded (reported with lower dose in generalised pustular or erythrodermic exfoliative psoriasis); if used with UV treatment apply at least 2 hours before UV exposure

Contra-indications: disorders of calcium metabolism

Side-effects: local irritation; also dermatitis, pruritus, erythema, aggravation of psoriasis, photosensitivity; rarely facial or perioral dermatitis; hypercalcaemia (see Cautions)

Administration: *cream* or *ointment* apply once or twice daily; max. 100 g weekly (less with *scalp solution*, see below); CHILD over 6 years, apply twice daily; 6–12 years max. 50 g weekly; over 12 years max. 75 g weekly

Note. Patient information leaflets for *Dovonex®* cream and ointment advise liberal application (but note max. recommended weekly dose, above)

Dovonex® (Leo) [PoM]

Cream, calcipotriol 50 micrograms/g, net price 120 g = £27.32

Excipients: include cetostearyl alcohol, disodium edetate

Ointment, calcipotriol 50 micrograms/g, net price 120 g = £27.32, 240 g = £54.64

Excipients: include disodium edetate, propylene glycol

Scalp solution, calcipotriol 50 micrograms/mL, net price 60 mL = £20.21, 120 mL = £40.42

Excipients: include propylene glycol

Scalp psoriasis, apply to scalp twice daily; max. 60 mL weekly (less with cream or ointment, see below); CHILD not recommended

MAX. WHEN PREPARATIONS USED TOGETHER. Max. total calcipotriol 5 mg in any one week (e.g. scalp solution 60 mL with cream or ointment 30 g *or* cream or ointment 60 g with scalp solution 30 mL)

TACALCITOL

Indications: plaque psoriasis

Cautions: pregnancy (Appendix 4), breast-feeding (Appendix 5); avoid eyes and inadvertent transfer to other body areas; wash hands thoroughly after application; risk of hypercalcaemia in generalised pustular or erythrodermic exfoliative psoriasis; monitor plasma calcium if risk of hypercalcaemia or in renal impairment; if used in conjunction with UV treatment, UV radiation should be given in the morning and tacalcitol applied at bedtime

Contra-indications: disorders of calcium metabolism

Side-effects: local irritation including itching, erythema, burning, paraesthesia; rarely contact dermatitis, worsening of psoriasis

Administration: apply daily preferably at bedtime; max. 10 g daily; CHILD not recommended

Curatoderm® (Crookes) [PoM]

Ointment, tacalcitol (as monohydrate) 4 micrograms/g, net price 30 g = £15.09, 60 g = £26.06, 100 g = £34.75

Excipients: none as listed in section 13.1.3

TAZAROTENE

Indications: mild to moderate plaque psoriasis affecting up to 10% of skin area

Cautions: wash hands immediately after use, avoid contact with eyes, face, intertriginous areas, hair-covered scalp, eczematous or inflamed skin; avoid excessive exposure to UV light (including sunlight, solariums, PUVA or UVB treatment); do not apply emollients or cosmetics within 1 hour of application

Contra-indications: pregnancy—advise women of child-bearing age to ensure adequate contraceptive protection; breast-feeding (Appendix 5)

Side-effects: local irritation (more common with higher concentration and may require discontinuation), pruritus, burning, erythema, desquamation, non-specific rash, contact dermatitis, and worsening of psoriasis; rarely stinging and inflamed, dry or painful skin

Administration: apply once daily in the evening usually for up to 12 weeks; CHILD under 18 years not recommended

Zorac® (Bioglan) [PoM]

Gel, tazarotene 0.05%, net price 30 g = £14.09, 60 g = £26.26; 0.1%, 30 g = £14.80, 60 g = £27.70

Excipients: include benzyl alcohol, butylated hydroxyanisole, butylated hydroxytoluene, disodium edetate, polysorbate 40

COAL TAR

Indications: psoriasis and occasionally chronic atopic eczema

Cautions: avoid eyes, mucosa, genital or rectal areas, and broken or inflamed skin; use suitable chemical protection gloves for extemporaneous preparation

Contra-indications: not for use in sore, acute, or pustular psoriasis or in presence of infection

Side-effects: skin irritation and acne-like eruptions, photosensitivity; stains skin, hair, and fabric

Administration: apply 1–3 times daily starting with low-strength preparations

Note. For shampoo preparations see section 13.9; impregnated dressings see Appendix 8 (section A8.2.9)

■ Non-proprietary preparations

May be difficult to obtain—moreover some patients may find newer proprietary preparations more acceptable

Calamine and Coal Tar Ointment, BP, calamine 12.5 g, strong coal tar solution 2.5 g, zinc oxide 12.5 g, hydrous wool fat 25 g, white soft paraffin 47.5 g

Apply 1–2 times daily

Excipients: include wool fat

Coal Tar and Salicylic Acid Ointment, BP, coal tar 2 g, salicylic acid 2 g, emulsifying wax 11.4 g, white soft paraffin 19 g, coconut oil 54 g, polysorbate '80' 4 g, liquid paraffin 7.6 g

Apply 1–2 times daily

Excipients: include cetostearyl alcohol

Coal Tar Paste, BP, strong coal tar solution 7.5%, in compound zinc paste

Apply 1–2 times daily

Zinc and Coal Tar Paste, BP, zinc oxide 6%, coal tar 6%, emulsifying wax 5%, starch 38%, yellow soft paraffin 45%

Apply 1–2 times daily

Excipients: include cetostearyl alcohol

■ Proprietary preparations

Alphosyl® (Stafford-Miller)

Cream, coal tar extract 5%, allantoin 2%, in a vanishing-cream basis. Net price 100 g = £1.66

Excipients: include beeswax, cetyl alcohol, hydroxybenzoates (parabens), isopropyl palmitate, propylene glycol, wool fat

Psoriasis, apply to skin 2–4 times daily

Lotion, coal tar extract 5%, allantoin 2%. Net price 250 mL = £1.50

Excipients: include hydroxybenzoates (parabens), isopropyl palmitate, propylene glycol

Psoriasis, apply to skin or scalp 2–4 times daily

Carbo-Dome® (Lagap)

Cream, coal tar solution 10%, in a water-miscible basis. Net price 30 g = £4.77; 100 g = £10.50

Excipients: include beeswax, hydroxybenzoates (parabens)

Psoriasis, apply to skin 2–3 times daily

Clinitar® (CHS)

Cream, coal tar extract 1%. Net price 100 g = £10.99

Excipients: include cetostearyl alcohol, isopropyl palmitate, propylene glycol

Psoriasis and eczema, apply to skin 1–2 times daily

Exorex® (Forest)
Lotion, prepared coal tar 1% in an emollient basis,
net price 100 mL = £8.65; 250 mL = £17.33
Excipients: include hydroxybenzoates (parabens), polysorbate 80
Psoriasis, apply to skin or scalp 2–3 times daily. Dilute
with a few drops of water before application to children
and elderly

Pragmatar® (Alliance)
Cream, cetyl alcohol-coal tar distillate 4%, salicylic acid 3%, sulphur (precipitated) 3%. Net
price 25 g = £3.12; 100 g = £10.07
Excipients: include cetyl alcohol, fragrance
Scaly skin disorders, apply thinly once daily; dandruff
and other seborrhoeic conditions, apply to scalp once
weekly or in severe cases daily. Dilute with a few drops
of water before application to infants

Psoriderm® (Dermal)
Cream, coal tar 6%, lecithin 0.4%, net price
225 mL = £3.55
Excipients: include isopropyl palmitate, propylene glycol
Psoriasis, apply to skin or scalp 1–2 times daily
Scalp lotion—section 13.9

■ Bath preparations

Coal Tar Solution, BP, coal tar 20%, polysorbate
'80' 5%, in alcohol (96%). Net price 100 mL = 80p
Use 100 mL in a bath
Note. Strong Coal Tar Solution BP contains coal tar 40%
Excipients: include polysorbates

Polytar Emollient® (Stiefel)
Bath additive, coal tar solution 2.5%, arachis (peanut) oil extract of coal tar 7.5%, tar 7.5%, cade oil
7.5%, liquid paraffin 35%. Net price 500 mL = £6.50
Excipients: include isopropyl palmitate
Psoriasis, eczema, atopic and pruritic dermatoses, use 2–
4 capfuls (15–30 mL) in bath and soak for 20 minutes

Psoriderm® (Dermal)
Bath emulsion, coal tar 40%. Net price 200 mL =
£3.09
Excipients: include polysorbate 20
Psoriasis, use 30 mL in a bath and soak for 5 minutes

■ With corticosteroids

Alphosyl HC® (Stafford-Miller) [PoM]
Cream, coal tar extract 5%, hydrocortisone 0.5%,
allantoin 2%, net price 100 g = £3.22. Label: 28.
Potency: mild
Excipients: include beeswax, cetyl alcohol, hydroxybenzoates
(parabens), isopropyl palmitate, wool fat
Psoriasis, apply thinly 1–2 times daily; CHILD under 5
years not recommended

DITHRANOL

Indications: subacute and chronic psoriasis, see
notes above
Cautions: avoid use near eyes and sensitive areas
of skin; see also notes above
Contra-indications: hypersensitivity; acute and
pustular psoriasis
Side-effects: local burning sensation and irritation; stains skin, hair, and fabrics
Administration: see notes above and under preparations
Note. Some of these dithranol preparations also contain
coal tar or salicylic acid—for cautions and side-effects
see under Coal Tar (above) or under Salicylic Acid

˟Dithranol Ointment, BP [PoM] dithranol, in
yellow soft paraffin; usual strengths 0.1–2%. Part
of basis may be replaced by hard paraffin if a
stiffer preparation is required. Label: 28
˟ [PoM] if dithranol content more than 1%, otherwise
may be sold to the public

Dithranol Paste, BP, dithranol in zinc and salicylic acid (Lassar's) paste. Usual strengths 0.1–
1% of dithranol. Label: 28

Dithrocream® (Dermal)
Cream, dithranol 0.1%, net price 50 g = £4.24;
0.25%, 50 g = £4.55; 0.5%, 50 g = £5.24; 1%,
50 g = £6.10; [PoM] 2%, 50 g = £7.64. Label: 28.
For application to skin or scalp; 0.1–0.5% suitable for overnight treatment, 1–2% for max. 1 hour
Excipients: include cetostearyl alcohol, chlorocresol, salicylic
acid

Micanol® (Bioglan)
Cream, dithranol 1% in a lipid-stabilised basis, net
price 50 g = £7.98; [PoM] 3%, 50 g = £9.94.
Label: 28
For application to skin, for up to 30 minutes, if
necessary 3% cream may be used under medical
supervision; apply to scalp for up to 30 minutes
Note. At the end of contact time use plenty of lukewarm
(not hot) water to rinse off cream; soap should not be
used
Excipients: none as listed in section 13.1.3

Psorin® (Ayrton Saunders)
Ointment, dithranol 0.11%, crude coal tar 1%, salicylic acid 1.6%, net price 50 g = £6.34, 100 g =
£12.59. Label: 28
For application to skin up to twice daily
Excipients: include beeswax, wool fat
Scalp gel, dithranol 0.25%, salicylic acid 1.6% in
gel basis contaning methyl salicylate, net price
50 g = £4.79. Label: 28
For application to scalp, initially apply on alternate days
for 10–20 minutes; may be increased to daily application
for max. 1 hour and then wash off
Excipients: none as listed in section 13.1.3

SALICYLIC ACID

For coal tar preparations containing salicylic acid,
see under Coal Tar p. 550; for dithranol preparations containing salicylic acid see under Dithranol,
above
Indications: hyperkeratotic skin disorders; acne
(section 13.6.1); warts and calluses (section 13.7);
scalp conditions (section 13.9); fungal nail infections (section 13.10.2)
Cautions: see notes above; avoid broken or
inflamed skin
SALICYLATE TOXICITY. If large areas of skin are treated,
salicylate toxicity may be a hazard
Side-effects: sensitivity, excessive drying, irritation, systemic effects after widespread use (see
under Cautions)

Zinc and Salicylic Acid Paste, BP (Lassar's
Paste), zinc oxide 24%, salicylic acid 2%, starch
24%, white soft paraffin 50%. Net price 25 g =
16p
Apply twice daily

Oral retinoids for psoriasis

ACITRETIN

Note. Acitretin is a metabolite of etretinate
Indications: severe extensive psoriasis resistant to
other forms of therapy; palmoplantar pustular
psoriasis; severe congenital ichthyosis; severe
Darier's disease (keratosis follicularis)
Cautions: exclude pregnancy before starting (perform pregnancy test 2–3 days before expected

menstruation, start treatment on day 2 or 3 of menstrual cycle)—patients should avoid pregnancy at least 1 month before, during, and for at least 2 years after treatment; patients should avoid concomitant tetracycline or methotrexate, high doses of vitamin A (more than 4000–5000 units daily) and use of keratolytics, and should not donate blood during or for at least 1 year after stopping therapy (teratogenic risk); monitor hepatic function and plasma lipids at start, 1 month after initiating treatment, and then at intervals of 3 months; diabetes (can alter glucose tolerance—initial frequent blood glucose checks); radiographic assessment on long-term treatment; investigate atypical musculoskeletal symptoms; not recommended for children except under exceptional circumstances (premature epiphyseal closure reported); avoid excessive exposure to sunlight and unsupervised use of sunlamps; **interactions:** Appendix 1 (retinoids)

Contra-indications: hepatic and renal impairment; hyperlipidaemia, pregnancy (**important teratogenic risk:** see Cautions and Appendix 4); breast-feeding

Side-effects: dryness of mucous membranes (sometimes erosion), of skin (sometimes scaling, thinning, erythema especially of face, and pruritus), and of conjunctiva (sometimes conjunctivitis and decreased tolerance of contact lenses); other side-effects reported include palmoplantar exfoliation, epistaxis, epidermal and nail fragility, paronychia, granulomatous lesions, bullous eruptions, reversible hair thinning and alopecia, myalgia and arthralgia, occasional nausea, headache, malaise, drowsiness, rhinitis, sweating, and gingivitis; benign intracranial hypertension (discontinue if severe headache, vomiting and visual disturbance occur; **avoid** concomitant tetracyclines); photosensitivity, raised liver enzymes, rarely jaundice and hepatitis (**avoid** concomitant methotrexate); raised triglycerides; decreased night vision reported; skeletal hyperostosis and extraosseous calcification reported following long-term administration of etretinate (and premature epiphyseal closure in children, see Cautions)

Dose: under expert supervision, initially 25–30 mg daily (Darier's disease 10 mg daily) for 2–4 weeks, then adjusted according to response, usual range 25–50 mg daily (max. 75 mg daily) for further 6–8 weeks (in Darier's disease and ichthyosis not more than 50 mg daily for up to 6 months); CHILD (**important:** exceptional circumstances only, see Cautions), 500 micrograms/kg daily (occasionally up to 1 mg/kg daily to max. 35 mg daily for limited periods) with careful monitoring of musculoskeletal development

Neotigason® (Roche) PoM

Capsules, acitretin 10 mg (brown/white), net price 56-cap pack = £25.34; 25 mg (brown/yellow), 56-cap pack = £58.80 (**hosp. or specified retail pharmacy only**—consult product literature for details, specialist dermatological supervision). Label: 10 patient information leaflet, 21

Oral immunosuppressants for psoriasis

CICLOSPORIN
(Cyclosporin)

Indications: see under Dose; transplantation and graft-versus-host disease (section 8.2.2)

Cautions: see section 8.2.2

ADDITIONAL CAUTIONS IN ATOPIC DERMATITIS AND PSORIASIS. **Contra-indicated** in abnormal renal function, hypertension not under control (see also below), infections not under control, and malignancy (see also below). Dermatological and physical examination, including blood pressure and renal function measurements required at least twice before starting; discontinue if hypertension develops that cannot be controlled by dose reduction or antihypertensive therapy; avoid excessive exposure to sunlight and use of UVB or PUVA; *in atopic dermatitis,* also allow herpes simplex infections to clear before starting (if they occur during treatment withdraw if severe); *Staphylococcus aureus* skin infections not absolute contra-indication providing controlled (but avoid erythromycin unless no other alternative—see also **interactions:** Appendix 1 (ciclosporin)); monitor serum creatinine every 2 weeks during treatment; *in psoriasis,* also exclude malignancies (including those of skin and cervix) before starting (biopsy any lesions not typical of psoriasis) and treat patients with malignant or pre-malignant conditions of skin only after appropriate treatment (and if no other option); monitor serum creatinine every 2 weeks for first 3 months then every 2 months (monthly if dose more than 2.5 mg/kg daily), reducing dose by 25–50% if increases more than 30% above baseline (even if within normal range) and discontinuing if reduction not successful within 1 month; also discontinue if lymphoproliferative disorder develops

Side-effects: see section 8.2.2

Dose: ADULT over 16 years *by mouth,* administered in accordance with expert advice

Short-term treatment (max. 8 weeks) of severe atopic dermatitis where conventional therapy ineffective or inappropriate, initially 2.5 mg/kg daily in 2 divided doses, if good initial response not achieved within 2 weeks, increase rapidly to max. 5 mg/kg daily; initial dose of 5 mg/kg daily in 2 divided doses if very severe; CHILD under 16 years not recommended

Severe psoriasis where conventional therapy ineffective or inappropriate, initially 2.5 mg/kg daily in 2 divided doses, increased gradually to max. 5 mg/kg daily if no improvement within 1 month (discontinue if response still insufficient after 6 weeks); initial dose of 5 mg/kg daily justified if condition requires rapid improvement; CHILD under 16 years not recommended

IMPORTANT. For preparations and counselling and for advice on conversion between the preparations, see section 8.2.2

Preparations
Section 8.2.2

METHOTREXATE

Indications: severe uncontrolled psoriasis unresponsive to conventional therapy (specialist use only); malignant disease (section 8.1.3); rheumatoid arthritis (section 10.1.3)

Cautions: see also notes above, section 8.1.3, product literature and CSM advice below (blood count, liver and pulmonary toxicity); extreme caution in blood disorders (avoid if severe); renal impairment (avoid in moderate or severe—Appendix 3), peptic ulceration, ulcerative colitis, diarrhoea and ulcerative stomatitis (withdraw if stomatitis develops—may be first sign of gastrointestinal toxicity), photosensitivity—psoriasis lesions aggravated by UV radiation (skin ulceration reported); porphyria (section 9.8.2); **interactions:** see below and Appendix 1 (methotrexate)

CSM ADVICE. In view of reports of blood dyscrasias (including fatalities) and liver cirrhosis with low-dose methotrexate, the CSM has advised:
• full blood count and renal and liver function tests before starting treatment and repeated weekly until therapy stabilised, thereafter patients should be monitored every 2–3 months
• patients should report all symptoms and signs suggestive of infection, especially sore throat
Treatment with folinic acid (as calcium folinate, section 8.1) may be required in acute toxicity

BLOOD COUNT. Haematopoietic suppression may occur abruptly; factors likely to increase toxicity include advanced age, renal impairment and concomitant administration of another anti-folate drug. Any profound drop in white cell or platelet count calls for immediate withdrawal of methotrexate and introduction of supportive therapy

LIVER TOXICITY. Liver cirrhosis reported. Treatment should not be started or should be discontinued if any abnormality of liver function tests or liver biopsy is present or develops during therapy. Abnormalities may return to normal within 2 weeks after which treatment may be recommenced if judged appropriate

PULMONARY TOXICITY. May be special problem in rheumatoid arthritis (patient to contact doctor immediately if dyspnoea or cough)

ASPIRIN and other NSAIDs. If aspirin or other NSAIDs are given concurrently the dose of methotrexate should be carefully monitored. Patients should be advised to avoid self-medication with over-the-counter aspirin or ibuprofen

Contra-indications: see also notes above, section 8.1.3 and product literature; liver impairment (see Appendix 2), pregnancy (following administration to a woman or a man, avoid conception for **at least 6 months** after stopping—Appendix 4), breast-feeding (Cytotoxic drugs, Appendix 5), active infection and immunodeficiency syndromes

Side-effects: see above, section 8.1.3, and product literature

Dose: *by mouth*, 10–25 mg once weekly, adjusted according to response; ELDERLY consider dose reduction (extreme caution); CHILD not recommended

IMPORTANT. Note that the above dose is a **weekly** dose. The CSM has received reports of prescription and dispensing errors including fatalities. Attention should be paid to the **strength** of methotrexate tablets prescribed and the **frequency** of dosing.

Preparations
Section 8.1.3

13.6 Acne and rosacea

13.6.1 Topical preparations for acne
13.6.2 Oral preparations for acne

ACNE. Treatment of acne should be commenced early to prevent scarring. Patients should be counselled that an improvement may not be seen for at least a couple of months. The choice of treatment depends on whether the acne is predominantly inflammatory or comedonal and its severity.

Mild to moderate acne is generally treated with topical preparations (section 13.6.1). Systemic treatment (section 13.6.2) with oral antibiotics is generally used for *moderate to severe acne* or where topical preparations are not tolerated or are ineffective or where application to the site is difficult. Another oral preparation used for acne is the hormone treatment co-cyprindiol (cyproterone acetate with ethinylestradiol); it is for women only.

Severe acne, acne unresponsive to prolonged courses of oral antibiotics, scarring, or acne associated with psychological problems calls for early referral to a consultant dermatologist who may prescribe isotretinoin for administration by mouth.

ROSACEA. Rosacea is not comedonal (but may exist with acne which may be comedonal). The pustules and papules of rosacea respond to topical metronidazole (section 13.10.1.2) or to oral administration of oxytetracycline or tetracycline 500 mg twice daily (section 5.1.3) or of erythromycin 500 mg twice daily (section 5.1.5); courses usually last 6–12 weeks and are repeated intermittently. Alternatively, doxycycline (section 5.1.3) in a dose of 100 mg once daily may be used [unlicensed indication] if oxytetracycline or tetracycline is inappropriate (e.g. in renal impairment). Isotretinoin is occasionally given in refractory cases [unlicensed indication]. Camouflagers (section 13.8.2) may be required for the redness.

13.6.1 Topical preparations for acne

Significant comedonal acne responds well to topical retinoids (see p. 555), whereas both comedones and inflamed lesions respond well to benzoyl peroxide or azelaic acid (see below). Alternatively, topical application of an antibiotic such as erythromycin or clindamycin may be effective for inflammatory acne. If topical preparations prove inadequate oral preparations may be needed (section 13.6.2).

Benzoyl peroxide and azelaic acid

Benzoyl peroxide is effective in mild to moderate acne. Both comedones and inflamed lesions respond well to benzoyl peroxide. The lower concentrations seem to be as effective as higher concentrations in reducing inflammation. It is usual to start with a lower strength and to increase the concentration of benzoyl peroxide gradually. Adverse effects include local skin irritation, particularly when therapy is initiated, but the scaling and redness often subside with treatment continued at a reduced frequency of application. If the acne does not respond after 2 months then use of a topical antibacterial should be considered.

Azelaic acid has antimicrobial and anticomedonal properties. It may be an alternative to benzoyl peroxide or to a topical retinoid for treating mild to moderate comedonal acne, particularly of the face. Some patients prefer it because it is less likely to cause local irritation than benzoyl peroxide.

BENZOYL PEROXIDE

Indications: acne vulgaris

Cautions: avoid contact with eyes, mouth, and mucous membranes; may bleach fabrics and hair; avoid excessive exposure to sunlight

Side-effects: skin irritation (reduce frequency or suspend use until irritation subsides and re-introduce at reduced frequency)

Administration: apply 1–2 times daily preferably after washing with soap and water, start treatment with lower-strength preparations

Note. May bleach clothing

Acnecide® (Galderma)
Gel, benzoyl peroxide 5% in an aqueous gel basis, net price 60 g = £3.00; 10%, 60 g = £3.30
Excipients: include propylene glycol

Brevoxyl® (Stiefel)
Cream, benzoyl peroxide 4% in an aqueous basis, net price 40 g = £3.30
Excipients: include cetyl alcohol, fragrance, stearyl alcohol

PanOxyl® (Stiefel)
Aquagel (= aqueous gel), benzoyl peroxide 2.5%, net price 40 g = £1.76; 5%, 40 g = £1.92; 10%, 40 g = £2.07
Excipients: include propylene glycol
Cream, benzoyl peroxide 5% in a non-greasy basis, net price 40 g = £1.51
Excipients: include isopropyl palmitate, propylene glycol
Gel, benzoyl peroxide 5% in an aqueous alcoholic basis, net price 40 g = £1.51; 10%, 40 g = £1.69
Excipients: include fragrance
Lotion, benzoyl peroxide 5% in a non-greasy basis, net price 30 mL = £1.45; 10%, 30 mL = £1.45
Excipients: include isopropyl palmitate, propylene glycol
Wash, benzoyl peroxide 10% in a detergent basis, net price 150 mL = £4.00
Excipients: include imidurea

■ With antimicrobials

Benzamycin® (Bioglan) [PoM]
Gel, pack for reconstitution, providing erythromycin 3% and benzoyl peroxide 5% in an alcoholic basis. Net price per pack to provide 23.3 g = £7.94, 46.6 g = £15.27
Excipients: none as listed in section 13.1.3
Apply twice daily (very fair skin, initially once daily at night)

Quinoderm® (Adams Hlth)
Cream, benzoyl peroxide 5%, potassium hydroxyquinoline sulphate 0.5%, in an astringent vanishing-cream basis. Net price 50 g = £2.21
Excipients: include cetostearyl alcohol, edetic acid (EDTA)
Cream, benzoyl peroxide 10%, potassium hydroxyquinoline sulphate 0.5%, in an astringent vanishing-cream basis. Net price 25 g = £1.30; 50 g = £2.49
Excipients: include cetostearyl alcohol, edetic acid (EDTA)

Lotio-gel, benzoyl peroxide 5%, potassium hydroxyquinoline sulphate 0.5%, in an astringent creamy basis. Net price 30 mL = £1.47
Excipients: include cetostearyl alcohol, edetic acid (EDTA)

AZELAIC ACID

Indications: acne vulgaris

Cautions: pregnancy, breast-feeding; avoid contact with eyes

Side-effects: local irritation (reduce frequency or discontinue use temporarily); rarely photosensitisation

Skinoren® (Schering Health) [PoM]
Cream, azelaic acid 20%, net price 30 g = £4.00
Excipients: include propylene glycol
Apply twice daily (sensitive skin, once daily for first week). Extended treatment may be required but manufacturer advises period of treatment should not exceed 6 months

Topical antibacterials for acne

For many patients with mild to moderate inflammatory acne, topical antibacterials may be no more effective than topical benzoyl peroxide or tretinoin. Topical antibacterials are probably best reserved for patients who wish to avoid oral antibacterials or who cannot tolerate them. Topical preparations of **erythromycin** and **clindamycin** are effective for inflammatory acne; topical preparations of tetracycline may also be effective. Topical antibacterials can produce mild irritation of the skin, and on rare occasions cause sensitisation.

Antibacterial resistance of *Propionibacterium acnes* is increasing; there is cross-resistance between erythromycin and clindamycin. To avoid development of resistance:

- when possible use non-antibiotic antimicrobials (such as benzoyl peroxide or azelaic acid);
- avoid concomitant treatment with different oral and topical antibiotics;
- if a particular antibiotic is effective, use it for repeat courses if needed (short intervening courses of a topical antibacterial, such as benzoyl peroxide or azelaic acid, may eliminate any resistant propionibacteria);
- do not continue treatment for longer than necessary (however, treatment with a topical preparation should be continued for at least 6 months);

ANTIBIOTICS

Indications: acne vulgaris

Cautions: some manufacturers advise preparations containing alcohol are not suitable for use with benzoyl peroxide

Benzamycin® [PoM] see under Benzoyl Peroxide above

Dalacin T® (Pharmacia) [PoM]
Topical solution, clindamycin (as phosphate) 1%, in an aqueous alcoholic basis. Net price (both with applicator) 30 mL = £4.34; 50 mL = £7.23
Excipients: include propylene glycol
Apply twice daily
Lotion, clindamycin (as phosphate) 1% in an aqueous basis. Net price 30 mL = £5.08; 50 mL = £8.47
Excipients: include cetostearyl alcohol, hydroxybenzoates (parabens)
Apply twice daily

Eryacne® (Galderma) PoM
Gel, erythromycin in an alcoholic basis, 2% (*Eryacne® 2*), net price 30 g = £4.97; 4% (*Eryacne® 4*), 30 g = £4.97
Excipients: include butylated hydroxytoluene
Apply twice daily starting with 4% for 4 weeks then reducing to 2% if condition improves

Stiemycin® (Stiefel) PoM
Solution, erythromycin 2% in an alcoholic basis. Net price 50 mL = £8.60
Excipients: include propylene glycol
Apply twice daily

Topicycline® (Shire) PoM
Solution, powder for reconstitution, tetracycline hydrochloride, 4-epitetracycline hydrochloride, providing tetracycline hydrochloride 2.2 mg/mL when reconstituted with solvent containing *n*-decyl methyl sulphoxide and citric acid in 40% alcohol. Net price per pack of powder and solvent to provide 70 mL = £6.15
Excipients: none as listed in section 13.1.3
Apply twice daily

Zineryt® (Yamanouchi) PoM
Topical solution, powder for reconstitution, erythromycin 40 mg, zinc acetate 12 mg/mL when reconstituted with solvent containing ethanol. Net price per pack of powder and solvent to provide 30 mL = £7.09; 90 mL = £20.62
Excipients: none as listed in section 13.1.3
Apply twice daily

Topical retinoids and related preparations for acne

Tretinoin and its isomer **isotretinoin** are useful in treating comedonal acne but patients should be warned that some redness and skin peeling might occur initially but settles with time. Several months of treatment may be needed to achieve an optimal response and the treatment should be continued until no new lesions develop.

Topical **isotretinoin** is licensed to treat non-inflammatory and inflammatory lesions in patients with mild to moderate acne. Isotretinoin is also given by mouth; see section 13.6.2 for **warnings** relating to use by mouth.

Adapalene, a retinoid-like drug, is licensed for mild to moderate acne. It may be less irritant than other topical retinoids.

CAUTIONS. Topical retinoids should be avoided in severe acne involving large areas. Contact with eyes, nostrils, mouth and mucous membranes, eczematous, broken or sunburned skin should be avoided. These drugs should be used with caution in sensitive areas such as the neck, and accumulation in angles of the nose should be avoided. Exposure to UV light (including sunlight, solariums) should be avoided; if sun exposure is unavoidable, an appropriate sunscreen or protective clothing should be used. Use of retinoids with abrasive cleaners, comedogenic or astringent cosmetics should be avoided. Allow peeling (e.g resulting from use of benzoyl peroxide) to subside before using a topical retinoid; alternating a preparation that causes peeling with a topical retinoid may give rise to contact dermatitis (reduce frequency of retinoid application).

CONTRA-INDICATIONS. Topical retinoids are contra-indicated in pregnancy (Appendix 4); women of child-bearing age should take adequate contraceptive precautions. Tretinoin is contra-indicated in personal or familial history of cutaneous epithelioma.

SIDE-EFFECTS. Local reactions include burning, erythema, stinging, pruritus, dry or peeling skin (discontinue if severe). Increased sensitivity to UVB light or sunlight occurs. Temporary changes of skin pigmentation have been reported. Eye irritation and oedema, and blistering or crusting of skin have been reported rarely.

ADAPALENE

Indications: mild to moderate acne
Cautions: see notes above
Contra-indications: see notes above
Side-effects: see notes above
Administration: apply thinly once daily before retiring

Differin® (Galderma) PoM
Cream, adapalene 0.1%, net price 30 g = £8.00
Excipients: include disodium edetate, hydroxybenzoates (parabens)
Gel, adapalene 0.1%, net price 30 g = £8.00
Excipients: include disodium edetate, hydroxybenzoates (parabens), propylene glycol

---

TRETINOIN

Note. Tretinoin is the acid form of vitamin A
Indications: see under preparations below; photodamage (section 13.8.1); malignant disease (section 8.1.5)
Cautions: see notes above
Contra-indications: see notes above
Side-effects: see notes above
Administration: see under preparations below

Retin-A® (Janssen-Cilag) PoM
Cream, tretinoin 0.025%, net price 60 g = £6.03
Acne vulgaris, for dry or fair skin, apply thinly 1–2 times daily
Excipients: include butylated hydroxytoluene, sorbic acid, stearyl alcohol
Gel, tretinoin 0.01%, net price 60 g = £6.03; 0.025%, 60 g = £6.03
Acne vulgaris and other keratotic conditions, apply thinly 1–2 times daily
Excipients: include butylated hydroxytoluene
Lotion, tretinoin 0.025%. Net price 100 mL = £6.94
Acne vulgaris, apply thinly 1–2 times daily
Excipients: include butylated hydroxytoluene

Acticin® (Strakan) PoM
Cream, tretinoin 0.025%, net price 45 g = £7.50
Acne vulgaris, for dry or fair skin, apply thinly once daily before retiring to bed
Excipients: include butylated hydroxytoluene, propylene glycol, sorbic acid, stearyl alcohol
Gel, tretinoin 0.025% in an alcoholic basis, net price 45 g = £7.50
Acne vulgaris, for oily or dark skin, apply thinly once daily before retiring to bed
Excipients: include butylated hydroxytoluene

■ With antibacterial

Aknemycin® Plus (Crookes) PoM
Solution, tretinoin 0.025%, erythromycin 4% in an alcoholic basis, net price 25 mL = £7.94
Acne, apply thinly 1–2 times daily
Excipients: none as listed in section 13.1.3

ISOTRETINOIN

Note. Isotretinoin is an isomer of tretinoin
IMPORTANT. For **indications, cautions, contra-indications** and **side-effects** of isotretinoin **when given by mouth**, see pp. 557–8
Indications: see notes above; oral treatment (section 13.6.2)
Cautions: (*topical application* only) see notes above
Contra-indications: (*topical application* only) see notes above
Administration: apply thinly 1–2 times daily

Isotrex® (Stiefel) PoM
Gel, isotretinoin 0.05%, net price 30 g = £6.65
Excipients: include butylated hydroxytoluene

■ With antibacterial

Isotrexin® (Stiefel) PoM
Gel, isotretinoin 0.05%, erythromycin 2% in ethanolic basis, net price 30 g = £8.36
Excipients: include butylated hydroxytoluene

Other topical preparations for acne

Salicylic acid is available in various preparations for sale direct to the public for the treatment of mild acne.

Preparations containing **sulphur** and **abrasive agents** are not considered beneficial in acne.

Topical **corticosteroids** should **not** be used in acne.

A topical preparation of **nicotinamide** is available for inflammatory acne.

ABRASIVE AGENTS ▱

Indications: acne vulgaris (but see notes above)
Cautions: avoid contact with eyes; discontinue use temporarily if skin becomes irritated
Contra-indications: superficial venules, telangiectasia

Brasivol® (Stiefel) ▱
Paste No. 1, aluminium oxide 38.09% in fine particles, in a soap-detergent basis; *Paste No. 2*, aluminium oxide 52.2% in medium particles, net price 75 g (both) = £2.49
Excipients: include fragrance, N-(3-Chloroallyl)hexaminium chloride (quaternium 15)
Use instead of soap 1–3 times daily, starting with *No.1*

Ionax Scrub® (Galderma) NHS ▱
Gel, polyethylene granules 21.9%, benzalkonium chloride 0.25% in a foaming aqueous alcoholic basis. Net price 60 g = £3.13
Excipients: include propylene glycol
Use instead of soap 1–2 times daily

▱ denotes preparations that are considered to be less suitable for prescribing (see p. vi)

CORTICOSTEROIDS

Indications: use in acne not recommended (see notes above)
Cautions: see section 13.4 and notes above
Contra-indications: see section 13.4 and notes above
Side-effects: see section 13.4 and notes above

Actinac® (Peckforton) PoM ▱
Lotion (powder for reconstitution with solvent), chloramphenicol 40 mg, hydrocortisone acetate 40 mg, allantoin 24 mg, butoxyethyl nicotinate 24 mg, precipitated sulphur 320 mg/g. Discard 21 days after reconstitution. Net price 2 × 6.25-g bottles powder with 2 × 20-mL bottles solvent = £16.28. Label: 28. Potency: mild
Excipients: none as listed in section 13.1.3

▱ denotes preparations that are considered to be less suitable for prescribing (see p. vi)

NICOTINAMIDE

Indications: see under preparation
Cautions: avoid contact with eyes and mucous membranes (including nose and mouth); reduce frequency of application if excessive dryness, irritation or peeling
Side-effects: dryness of skin; also pruritus, erythema, burning and irritation

Papulex® (Pharmagenix)
Gel, nicotinamide 4%. Net price 60 g = £7.98
Excipients: none as listed in section 13.1.3
Inflammatory acne vulgaris, apply twice daily; reduce to once daily or on alternate days if irritation occurs

SALICYLIC ACID ▱

Indications: acne; psoriasis (section 13.5.2); warts and calluses (section 13.7); fungal nail infections (section 13.10.2)
Cautions: avoid contact with mouth, eyes, mucous membranes; systemic effects after excessive use (see Aspirin and the salicylates, section 10.1.1)
Side-effects: local irritation

Acnisal® (DermaPharm) ▱
Topical solution, salicylic acid 2% in a detergent and emollient basis. Net price 177 mL = £4.13. Use up to 3 times daily
Excipients: include benzyl alcohol

SULPHUR ▱

Cautions: avoid contact with eyes, mouth, and mucous membranes; causes skin irritation

■ With resorcinol
Prolonged application of resorcinol may interfere with thyroid function therefore not recommended

Eskamel® (Goldshield) NHS ▱
Cream, resorcinol 2%, sulphur 8%, in a non-greasy flesh-coloured basis. Net price 25 g = £3.03
Excipients: include propylene glycol, fragrance

13.6.2	**Oral preparations for acne**

Oral antibacterials for acne

Systemic antibacterial treatment is useful for inflammatory acne if topical treatment is not adequately effective or if it is inappropriate. Anticomedonal treatment (e.g. with topical benzoyl peroxide) may also be required.

Either **oxytetracycline** or **tetracycline** (section 5.1.3) is usually given for acne in a dose of 500 mg twice daily. If there is no improvement after the first 3 months another oral antibacterial should be used. Maximum improvement usually occurs after 4 to 6 months but in more severe cases treatment may need to be continued for 2 years or longer.

Doxycycline and **minocycline** (section 5.1.3) are alternatives to tetracycline. Doxycycline may be used in a dose of 100 mg daily. Minocycline offers less likelihood of bacterial resistance but may sometimes cause irreversible pigmentation; it is given in a dose of 100 mg daily (in one or two divided doses).

Erythromycin (section 5.1.5) in a dose of 500 mg twice daily is an alternative for the management of acne but propionibacteria strains resistant to erythromycin are becoming widespread and this may explain poor response.

Trimethoprim (section 5.1.8) in a dose of 300 mg twice daily may be used for acne resistant to other antibacterials [unlicensed indication]. Prolonged treatment with trimethoprim may depress haematopoiesis; it should generally be initiated by specialists.

Concomitant use of different topical and systemic antibacterials is undesirable owing to the increased likelihood of the development of bacterial resistance.

Hormone treatment for acne

Co-cyprindiol (cyproterone acetate with ethinylestradiol) contains an anti-androgen. It is no more effective than an oral broad-spectrum antibacterial but is useful in women who also wish to receive oral contraception.

Improvement of acne with co-cyprindiol probably occurs because of decreased sebum secretion which is under androgen control. Some women with moderately severe hirsutism may also benefit because hair growth is also androgen-dependent. Contra-indications of co-cyprindiol include pregnancy and a predisposition to thrombosis.

CO-CYPRINDIOL

A mixture of cyproterone acetate and ethinylestradiol in the mass proportions 2000 parts to 35 parts, respectively

Indications: severe acne in women refractory to prolonged oral antibacterial therapy (but see notes above)

Cautions: see under Combined Oral Contraceptives, section 7.3.1

Contra-indications: see under Combined Oral Contraceptives, section 7.3.1

Side-effects: see under Combined Oral Contraceptives, section 7.3.1

Dianette® (Schering Health) PoM
Tablets, beige, s/c, co-cyprindiol 2000/35 (cyproterone acetate 2 mg, ethinylestradiol 35 micrograms), net price 21-tab pack = £4.32
Dose: 1 tablet daily for 21 days starting on day 1 of menstrual cycle and repeated after a 7-day interval, usually for several months; withdraw when acne or hirsutism completely resolved (repeat courses may be given if recurrence)

Oral retinoid for acne

The retinoid **isotretinoin** (*Roaccutane®*) reduces sebum secretion. It is used for the systemic treatment of nodulo-cystic and conglobate acne, severe acne, scarring, acne which has not responded to an adequate course of a systemic antibacterial, or acne which is associated with psychological problems. It is also useful in women who develop acne in the third or fourth decades of life, since late onset acne is frequently unresponsive to antibacterials.

Isotretinoin is a toxic drug that should be prescribed **only** by, or under the supervision of, a consultant dermatologist. It is given for at least 16 weeks; repeat courses are not normally required.

Side-effects of isotretinoin include severe dryness of the skin and mucous membranes, nose bleeds, and joint pains. The drug is **teratogenic** and must **not** be given to women of child-bearing age unless they practise effective contraception and then only after detailed assessment and explanation by the physician (see under Cautions below).

ISOTRETINOIN

Note. Isotretinoin is an isomer of tretinoin
Indications: see notes above
Cautions: exclude pregnancy before starting (perform pregnancy test 2–3 days before expected menstruation, start treatment on day 2 or 3 of menstrual cycle)—effective contraception must be practised at least 1 month before, during, and for at least 1 month after treatment; avoid blood donation during treatment and for at least 1 month after treatment; history of depression; measure hepatic function before treatment, 1 month after starting and then every 3 months (reduce dose or discontinue if transaminase raised above normal); measure serum lipids before treatment, 1 month after starting, then at end of treatment (reduce dose or discontinue if raised), discontinue if uncontrolled hypertriglyceridaemia or pancreatitis; diabetes; dry eye syndrome (associated with risk of keratitis); avoid keratolytics; **interactions:** Appendix 1 (retinoids)
WAX EPILATION AND DERMABRASION. Warn patient to avoid wax epilation during treatment and for at least 6 months after stopping (risk of epidermal stripping); avoid dermabrasion during treatment and for at least 6 months after stopping (risk of scarring)
Contra-indications: pregnancy (**important teratogenic risk:** see Cautions and Appendix 4); breast-feeding; renal or hepatic impairment; hypervitaminosis A, hyperlipidaemia

Side-effects: dryness of skin (with scaling, thinning, erythema, pruritus), epidermal fragility (trauma may cause blistering); rarely acne fulminans, facial hyperpigmentation; dryness of nasal mucosa (with mild epistaxis), of pharyngeal mucosa (with hoarseness), of conjunctiva (sometimes conjunctivitis), decreased tolerance to contact lenses and rarely keratitis; visual disturbances (papilloedema, optic neuritis, corneal opacities, cataracts, decreased night vision, photophobia, blurred vision)—expert referral and consider withdrawal; hair thinning (reversible on withdrawal) or (rarely) hirsutism; nausea, headache, malaise, drowsiness, sweating; benign intracranial hypertension (avoid concomitant tetracyclines); myalgia and arthralgia; raised serum creatinine concentrations reported; rarely jaundice and hepatitis; raised plasma triglycerides and cholesterol (risk of pancreatitis if triglycerides above 8 g/litre); allergic vasculitis and granulomatous lesions reported, other side-effects reported include hearing deficiency, mood changes (severe depression), convulsions, menstrual irregularities, hyperuricaemia, inflammatory bowel disease, diarrhoea (discontinue if severe), paronychia and Gram-positive infections, tendinitis, bone changes (including early epiphyseal closure and skeletal hyperostosis following long-term administration), thrombocytopenia, thrombocytosis, neutropenia and anaemia, lymphadenopathy, and haematuria and proteinuria

Dose: initially 500 micrograms/kg daily (in 1–2 divided doses) with food for 4 weeks; if good response continue for further 8–12 weeks; if little response, increase to 1 mg/kg daily for 8–12 weeks; if intolerant, reduce dose to 100–200 micrograms/kg daily

Isotretinoin (Non-proprietary) [PoM]
Capsules, isotretinoin 5 mg, net price 56-cap pack = £18.22; 20 mg, 56-cap pack = £50.21 (**hosp. only**). Label: 10 patient information leaflet, 21
Available from Schering Health

Roaccutane® (Roche) [PoM]
Capsules, isotretinoin 5 mg (red-violet/white), net price 56-cap pack = £18.22; 20 mg (red-violet/white), 56-cap pack = £50.21 (**hosp. or specified retail pharmacy only**). Label: 10 patient information card, 21

13.7 Preparations for warts and calluses

Warts (verrucas) are caused by a human papillomavirus, which most frequently affects the hands, feet (plantar warts), and the anogenital region (see below); treatment usually relies on local tissue destruction. Warts may regress on their own and treatment is required only if the warts are painful, unsightly, persistent, or cause distress.

Preparations of **salicylic acid, formaldehyde, gluteraldehyde** or **silver nitrate** are available for purchase by the public; they are suitable for the removal of warts on hands and feet. **Salicylic acid** is a useful keratolytic which may be considered first; it is also suitable for the removal of *corns and calluses*. Colloidal preparations of salicylic acid are available but some patients may develop an allergy to colophony in the formulation. An ointment combining **salicylic acid** with **podophyllum resin** (*Posalfilin®*) is available for treating plantar warts.

SALICYLIC ACID

Indications: see under preparations; psoriasis (section 13.5.2); acne (section 13.6.1); fungal nail infections (section 13.10.2)

Cautions: protect surrounding skin and avoid broken skin; not suitable for application to face, anogenital region, or large areas

Contra-indications: diabetes or if peripheral blood circulation impaired

Side-effects: skin irritation, see notes above

ADMINISTRATION. Advise patient to apply carefully to wart and to protect surrounding skin (e.g. with soft paraffin or specially designed plaster); rub wart surface gently with file or pumice stone once weekly; treatment may need to be continued for up to 3 months

Cuplex® (S&N Hlth.)
Gel, salicylic acid 11%, lactic acid 4%, in a collodion basis. Net price 5 g = £2.23. Label: 15. For plantar and mosaic warts, corns, and calluses, apply twice daily

Duofilm® (Stiefel)
Paint, salicylic acid 16.7%, lactic acid 16.7%, in flexible collodion. Net price 15 mL (with applicator) = £1.95. Label: 15. For plantar and mosaic warts, apply daily

Occlusal® (DermaPharm)
Application, salicylic acid 26% in polyacrylic solution. Net price 10 mL (with applicator) = £2.98. Label : 15. For common and plantar warts, apply daily

Salactol® (Dermal)
Paint, salicylic acid 16.7%, lactic acid 16.7%, in flexible collodion. Net price 10 mL (with applicator) = £1.93. Label: 15. For warts, particularly plantar warts, verrucas, corns, and calluses, apply daily

Salatac® (Dermal)
Gel, salicylic acid 12%, lactic acid 4%, in a collodion basis. Net price 8 g (with applicator) = £3.36. Label: 15. For warts, verrucas, corns, and calluses, apply daily

Verrugon® (Pickles)
Ointment, salicylic acid 50% in a paraffin basis. Net price 6 g = £2.45. For plantar warts, apply daily

■ With podophyllum

Posalfilin® (Norgine)
Ointment, podophyllum resin 20%, salicylic acid 25%. Net price 10 g = £3.43. For plantar warts apply daily
Note. Owing to the salicylic acid content, not suitable for anogenital warts; owing to the podophyllum content also contra-indicated in pregnancy and breast-feeding

FORMALDEHYDE

Indications: see under preparations
Cautions: see under Salicylic Acid
Contra-indications: see under Salicylic Acid
Side-effects: see under Salicylic Acid

Veracur® (Typharm)

Gel, formaldehyde 0.75% in a water-miscible gel basis. Net price 15 g = £2.41. For warts, particularly plantar warts, apply twice daily

GLUTARALDEHYDE

Indications: warts, particularly plantar warts

Cautions: protect surrounding skin; not for application to face, mucosa, or anogenital areas

Side-effects: rashes, skin irritation (discontinue if severe); stains skin brown

Administration: apply twice daily (see also under Salicylic acid)

Glutarol® (Dermal)

Solution (= application), glutaraldehyde 10%. Net price 10 mL (with applicator) = £2.33

SILVER NITRATE

Indications: see under preparation

Cautions: protect surrounding skin and avoid broken skin; not suitable for application to face, anogenital region, or large areas

Side-effects: stains skin and fabric

Administration: see under preparation; instructions in proprietary packs generally incorporate advice to remove dead skin before use by gentle filing and to cover with adhesive dressing after application

AVOCA® (Bray)

Caustic pencil, tip containing silver nitrate 95%, potassium nitrate 5%, net price, treatment pack (including emery file, 6 adhesive dressings and protector pads) = £1.74. For common warts and verrucas, apply moistened caustic pencil tip for 1–2 minutes; repeat after 24 hours up to max. 3 applications for warts *or* max. 6 applications for verrucas

Anogenital warts

The treatment of anogenital warts (condylomata acuminata) should be accompanied by screening for other sexually transmitted diseases. **Podophyllum** and **podophyllotoxin** (the major active ingredient of podophyllum) may be used for *soft, non-keratinised* external anogenital warts; these preparations can cause considerable irritation of the treated area. They can also cause severe systemic toxicity on excessive application including gastro-intestinal, renal, haematological, and CNS effects. Patients with a limited number of external warts or *keratinised* lesions may be better treated with cryotherapy or other forms of physical ablation.

Imiquimod cream has been introduced for the treatment of external anogenital warts; it may be used for both keratinised and non-keratinised lesions.

Inosine pranobex (section 5.3) is licensed for adjunctive treatment of genital warts but it has been superseded by more effective drugs.

IMIQUIMOD

Indications: external genital and perianal warts

Cautions: avoid normal skin, inflamed skin and open wounds; not suitable for internal genital warts; uncircumcised males (risk of phimosis or stricture of foreskin); pregnancy

Side-effects: local reactions including itching, pain, erythema, erosion, oedema, and excoriation; less commonly local ulceration and scabbing; permanent hypopigmentation or hyperpigmentation reported

Dose: apply thinly 3 times a week at night until lesions resolve (max. 16 weeks); CHILD not recommended

IMPORTANT. Should be rubbed in and allowed to stay on the treated area for 6–10 hours then washed off with mild soap and water (uncircumcised males treating warts under foreskin should wash the area daily). The cream should be washed off before sexual contact

Aldara® (3M) ▼ PoM

Cream, imiquimod 5%, net price 12-sachet pack = £55.18. Label: 10 patient information leaflet

Excipients: include benzyl alcohol, cetyl alcohol, hydroxybenzoates (parabens), polysorbate 60, stearyl alcohol
Condoms: may damage latex condoms and diaphragms

PODOPHYLLUM

Indications: see under preparations

Cautions: avoid normal skin and open wounds; keep away from face; very irritant to eyes; **important:** see also warnings below

Contra-indications: pregnancy and breast-feeding; children

Side-effects: see notes above

Podophyllin Paint, Compound, BP PoM

(podophyllum resin 15% in compound benzoin tincture), podophyllum resin 1.5 g, compound benzoin tincture to 10 mL; 5 mL to be dispensed unless otherwise directed. Label: 15

External genital warts, applied weekly in genitourinary clinic (or at a general practitioner's surgery by trained nurses after screening for other sexually transmitted diseases)

IMPORTANT. Should be allowed to stay on the treated area for not longer than 6 hours and then washed off. Care should be taken to avoid splashing the surrounding skin during application (which must be covered with soft paraffin as a protection). Where there are a large number of warts only a few should be treated at any one time as **severe toxicity** caused by absorption of podophyllin has been reported

■ Podophyllotoxin

Condyline® (Ardern) PoM

Solution, podophyllotoxin 0.5% in alcoholic basis. Net price 3.5 mL (with applicators) = £14.49. Label: 15

Condylomata acuminata affecting the penis or the female external genitalia, apply twice daily for 3 consecutive days; treatment may be repeated at weekly intervals if necessary for a total of five 3-day treatment courses; direct medical supervision for lesions in the female and for lesions greater than 4 cm² in the male; max. 50 single applications ('loops') per session (consult product literature)

Warticon® (Stiefel) [PoM]
Cream, podophyllotoxin 0.15%. Net price 5 g
(with mirror) = £16.62

Excipients: include butylated hydroxyanisole, cetyl alcohol, hydroxybenzoates (parabens), sorbic acid, stearyl alcohol

Condylomata acuminata affecting the penis or the female external genitalia, apply twice daily for 3 consecutive days; treatment may be repeated at weekly intervals if necessary for a total of four 3-day treatment courses; direct medical supervision for lesions greater than 4 cm²

Solution, blue, podophyllotoxin 0.5% in alcoholic basis. Net price 3 mL (with applicators— *Warticon®* [for men]; with applicators and mirror— *Warticon Fem®* [for women]) = £13.85. Label: 15

Condylomata acuminata affecting the penis or the female external genitalia, apply twice daily for 3 consecutive days; treatment may be repeated at weekly intervals if necessary for a total of four 3-day treatment courses; direct medical supervision for lesions greater than 4 cm²; max. 50 single applications ('loops') per session (consult product literature)

13.8   Sunscreens and camouflagers

| 13.8.1 | Sunscreening preparations |
| 13.8.2 | Camouflagers |

13.8.1   Sunscreening preparations

Solar ultraviolet irradiation can be harmful to the skin. It is responsible for disorders such as *polymorphic light eruption, solar urticaria,* and the various *cutaneous porphyrias.* It also provokes (or at least aggravates) disorders such as *rosacea* and *lupus erythematosus.* It may also cause photosensitivity in patients taking some drugs such as demeclocycline, phenothiazines, or amiodarone. All these conditions (as well as *sunburn*) may occur after relatively short periods of exposure to the sun. Exposure over longer periods may cause more serious problems. Both *melanoma* and *non-melanoma skin cancer* are now thought to be caused in many instances by solar ultraviolet irradiation. Exposure to the sun may also cause the skin to wrinkle and develop other signs *associated with ageing.* Solar ultraviolet irradiation also provokes attacks of *recurrent herpes labialis* (although it is not known whether the effect of sunlight exposure is local or systemic).

Solar ultraviolet radiation is approximately 200–400 nm in wavelength. The medium wavelengths (280–310 nm, known as UVB) cause sunburn and contribute to the long-term changes responsible for skin cancer and ageing. The long wavelengths (310–400 nm, known as UVA) do not cause sunburn but are responsible for many *photosensitivity reactions* and *photodermatoses;* they also seem to contribute to long-term damage and to be involved in the pathogenesis of *skin cancer* and *photodamage.*

Sunscreen preparations contain substances that protect the skin against UVB and hence against sunburn. The sun protection factor (SPF, usually indicated in the preparation title) provides guidance on the degree of protection offered against UVB; it indicates the multiples of protection provided against burning, compared with unprotected skin; for example, an SPF of 8 should enable a person to remain 8 times longer in the sun without burning. Such preparations, however, do not prevent long-term damage associated with UVA, which might not become apparent for 10 to 20 years. Preparations that also contain reflective substances, such as titanium dioxide, provide the most effective protection against UVA. Some products now indicate the degree of protection offered against UVA with a star rating system. This system does not refer to an absolute measure but indicates the protection against UVA relative to protection against UVB for the same product. Four stars indicate that the product offers a balanced amount of UVA and UVB protection; products with three, two, or one star rating indicate that the protection offered is greater against UVB than UVA. However the usefulness of the star rating system remains controversial.

Some sunscreens, particularly aminobenzoates, may rarely cause photosensitivity reactions. Bergamot oil (which contains 5-methoxypsoralen) occasionally causes photosensitisation with subsequent pigmentation; it is suspected of increasing the incidence of skin cancers, but this has not been established.

BORDERLINE SUBSTANCES. The preparations marked 'ACBS' are regarded as drugs when prescribed for skin protection against ultraviolet radiation in abnormal cutaneous photosensitivity resulting from genetic disorders or photodermatoses, including vitiligo and those resulting from radiotherapy; chronic or recurrent herpes simplex labialis. Preparations with SPF less than 15 are no longer prescribable. See also Appendix 7.

Ambre Solaire® (Garnier)
Total Screen Sun Intolerant Skin Lotion (UVA and UVB protection; UVB-SPF 60), octocrylene 10%, titanium dioxide 5.3%, drometrizole trisiloxane 2.5%, avobenzone 2.5%, terephthalydene dicamphor sulfonic acid 0.5%, net price 200 mL = £6.64. ACBS

Excipients: include disodium edetate, hydroxybenzoates (parabens), propylene glycol

Delph® (Fenton)
Lotion, (UVA and UVB protection; UVB-SPF 15), ethylhexyl *p*-methoxycinnamate 7.5%, oxybenzone 3%, titanium dioxide 0.6%, net price 200 mL = £1.99. ACBS

Excipients: include cetostearyl alcohol, fragrance, hydroxybenzoates (parabens), imidurea

Lotion, (UVA and UVB protection; UVB-SPF 20), ethylhexyl *p*-methoxycinnamate 7.5%, oxybenzone 3%, titanium dioxide 1.6%, net price 200 mL = £1.99. ACBS

Excipients: include cetostearyl alcohol, fragrance, hydroxybenzoates (parabens), imidurea

Lotion, (UVA and UVB protection; UVB-SPF 25), avobenzone 4%, ethylhexyl *p*-methoxycinnamate 3.5%, titanium dioxide 2.1%, oxybenzone 1.3%, net price 200 mL = £2.85. ACBS

Excipients: include cetostearyl alcohol, fragrance, hydroxybenzoates (parabens), imidurea

Lotion, (UVA and UVB protection; UVB-SPF 30), ethylhexyl *p*-methoxycinnamate 4.8%, avobenzone 4%, titanium dioxide 2.5%, oxybenzone 1.5%, net price 200 mL = £2.85, 400 mL (*Child Sun lotion*) = £5.70. ACBS
Excipients: include cetostearyl alcohol, fragrance, hydroxybenzoates (parabens), imidurea

E45 Sun® (Crookes)
Sunblock lotion (UVA and UVB protection; UVB-SPF 25), waterproof, titanium dioxide 3.6%, zinc oxide 13.9%, net price 150 mL = £6.38. ACBS
Excipients: include hydroxybenzoates (parabens), isopropyl palmitate
Sunblock lotion (UVA and UVB protection; UVB-SPF 50), waterproof, titanium dioxide 6.4%, zinc oxide 16%, net price 150 mL = £6.89. ACBS
Excipients: include hydroxybenzoates (parabens), isopropyl palmitate

RoC Total Sunblock® (J&J)
Cream (UVA and UVB protection; UVB-SPF 25), containing avobenzone 2%, ethylhexyl *p*-methoxycinnamate 7.5%, titanium dioxide 5.5%, net price 50 mL = £4.06. ACBS
Excipients: include beeswax, cetostearyl alcohol, disodium EDTA, hydroxybenzoates (parabens)

SpectraBan® (Stiefel)
Lotion (UVB protection; UVB-SPF 25), aminobenzoic acid 5%, padimate-O 3.2%, in an alcoholic basis, net price 150 mL = £3.45. ACBS
Excipients: include fragrance
Note. Flammable; stains clothing
Ultra lotion (UVA and UVB protection; UVB-SPF 28), water resistant, avobenzone 2%, oxybenzone 3%, padimate-O 8%, titanium dioxide 2%, net price 150 mL = £5.45. ACBS
Excipients: include benzyl alcohol, disodium edetate, sorbic acid, fragrance

Sunsense® Ultra (Lagap)
Lotion (UVA and UVB protection; UVB-SPF 60), ethylhexyl *p*-methoxycinnamate 7.5%, oxybenzone 3%, titanium dioxide 3.5%, net price 50-mL bottle with roll-on applicator = £3.11, 125 mL = £5.10. ACBS
Excipients: include butylated hydroxytoluene, cetyl alcohol, fragrance, hydroxybenzoates (parabens), propylene glycol

Uvistat® (Eastern)
Cream (UVA and UVB protection; UVB-SPF 22 but marketed as 'factor 20'), water-resistant, ethylhexyl *p*-methoxycinnamate 7%, avobenzone 4%, titanium dioxide 4.5%, net price 125 g = £5.10. ACBS
Excipients: include disodium edetate, fragrance, hydroxybenzoates (parabens)
Ultrablock cream (UVA and UVB protection; UVB-SPF 30), water-resistant, ethylhexyl *p*-methoxycinnamate 7.5%, avobenzone 4%, titanium dioxide 6.5%, net price 125 g = £5.61. ACBS
Excipients: include disodium edetate, fragrance, hydroxybenzoates (parabens)

Photodamage

Application of **tretinoin** 0.05% cream is reported to be associated with gradual improvement in *photodamaged skin* (usually within 3–4 months of starting).

Diclofenac gel is licensed for *actinic keratosis*. Treatment should continue for 60 to 90 days (optimal therapeutic effect may not be seen until 30 days after stopping). **Fluorouracil** cream (section 8.1.3) is also licensed for actinic keratosis.

TRETINOIN

Note. Tretinoin is the acid form of vitamin A

Indications: mottled hyperpigmentation, roughness and fine wrinkling of photodamaged skin due to chronic sun exposure; acne vulgaris (section 13.6); malignant disease (section 8.1.5)

Cautions: see section 13.6.1

Contra-indications: see section 13.6.1

Side-effects: see section 13.6.1

Administration: apply thinly at night, then reduce to 1–3 nights weekly

Retinova® (Janssen-Cilag) ⓃⒽⓈ ⓅⓄⓂ
Cream, tretinoin 0.05%, net price 20 g = £13.75.
Excipients: include fragrance

DICLOFENAC SODIUM

Indications: actinic keratosis

Cautions: as for topical NSAIDs, see section 10.3.2

Contra-indications: as for topical NSAIDs, see section 10.3.2

Side-effects: as for topical NSAIDs, see section 10.3.2; also paraesthesia

Administration: apply thinly twice daily for 60–90 days; max. 8 g daily

Solaraze® (Bioglan) ⓅⓄⓂ
Gel, diclofenac sodium 3%, net price 25 g = £17.90
Excipients: include benzyl alcohol

13.8.2 Camouflagers

Disfigurement of the skin can be very distressing to patients and have a marked psychological effect. In skilled hands, or with experience, these preparations can be very effective in concealing scars and birthmarks. The depigmented patches in vitiligo are also very disfiguring and camouflage creams are of great cosmetic value.

BORDERLINE SUBSTANCES. The preparations marked 'ACBS' are regarded as drugs when prescribed for postoperative scars and other deformities and as an adjunctive therapy in the relief of emotional disturbances due to disfiguring skin disease, such as vitiligo. See also Appendix 7.

Covermark® (Epiderm)
Classic foundation (masking cream). Net price 30 mL (10 shades) = £11.23. ACBS
Excipients: include beeswax, hydroxybenzoates (parabens), fragrance
Finishing powder. Net price 60 g = £9.50. ACBS
Excipients: include beeswax, hydroxybenzoates (parabens), fragrance

Dermablend® (Brodie & Stone)
Cover creme. Net price 10.7 g (15 shades) = £7.31; 28.4 g (11 shades) = £11.66. ACBS
Excipients: include beeswax, hydroxybenzoates (parabens)
Leg and body cover, (9 shades). Net price 64 g = £10.67. ACBS
Excipients: include beeswax, hydroxybenzoates (parabens)
Setting powder. Net price 28 g = £10.09. ACBS
Excipients: include hydroxybenzoates (parabens)

Dermacolor® (Fox)

Camouflage creme, (100 shades). Net price 25 g = £7.25. ACBS

Excipients: include beeswax, butylated hydroxytoluene, fragrance, propylene glycol, stearyl alcohol, wool fat

Fixing powder, (7 shades). Net price 60 g = £5.88. ACBS

Excipients: include fragrance

Keromask® (Network)

Masking cream, (2 shades). Net price 15 mL = £5.67. ACBS

Excipients: include butylated hydroxyanisole, hydroxybenzoates (parabens), wool fat, propylene glycol

Finishing powder. Net price 25 g = £5.67. ACBS

Excipients: include butylated hydroxytoluene, hydroxybenzoates (parabens)

Veil® (Blake)

Cover cream, (20 shades), net price 19 g = £7.09, 44 g = £11.63, 70 g = £16.74. ACBS

Excipients: include hydroxybenzoates (parabens), wool fat derivative

Finishing powder, translucent, net price 35 g = £7.09. ACBS

Excipients: include butylated hydroxyanisole, hydroxybenzoates (parabens)

13.9 Shampoos and some other scalp preparations

Dandruff is considered to be a mild form of seborrhoeic dermatitis (see also section 13.5.1). The treatment of choice is the frequent use of a mild detergent shampoo generally once or twice weekly; this rids the scalp of scale but does not have a therapeutic effect in itself. Shampoos containing antimicrobial agents such as **pyrithione zinc** (which are widely available) and **selenium sulphide** may have beneficial effects. Shampoos containing **tar** extracts may be useful and they are also used in *psoriasis*. **Ketoconazole** shampoo is probably the most effective.

For more severe conditions, **ketoconazole** shampoo may be used on the scalp. **Corticosteroid** gels and lotions (section 13.4) can also be used.

Shampoos containing **coal tar** and **salicylic acid** may also be useful. Patients who do not respond to these treatments may need to be referred to exclude the possibility of other skin conditions.

Cradle cap in infants may be treated with **olive oil** or **arachis oil** (ground-nut oil, peanut oil) applications followed by shampooing.

See also section 13.5 (psoriasis and eczema), section 13.10.4 (lice), and section 13.10.2 (ringworm).

Alphosyl 2 in 1® (Stafford-Miller)

Shampoo, alcoholic coal tar extract 5%. Net price 125 mL = £1.81; 250 mL = £3.43

Excipients: include hydroxybenzoates (parabens), fragrance

Dandruff, use once or twice weekly as necessary; psoriasis, seborrhoeic dermatitis, scaling and itching, use every 2–3 days

Betadine® (SSL)

Scalp and skin cleanser—section 13.11.4

Shampoo solution, povidone–iodine 4%, in a surfactant solution. Net price 250 mL = £2.32

Excipients: include fragrance

Seborrhoeic scalp conditions associated with excessive dandruff, pruritus, scaling, exudation and erythema, infected scalp lesions (recurrent furunculosis, infective folliculitis, impetigo), apply 1–2 times weekly; CHILD under 2 years not recommended;

Cautions; Contra-indications; Side-effects: see section 13.11.4, Iodine Compounds

Capasal® (Dermal)

Shampoo, coal tar 1%, coconut oil 1%, salicylic acid 0.5%. Net price 250 mL = £5.28

Excipients: none as listed in section 13.1.3

Scaly scalp disorders including psoriasis, seborrhoeic dermatitis, dandruff, and cradle cap, apply daily as necessary

Ceanel Concentrate® (Adams Hlth)

Shampoo, cetrimide 10%, undecenoic acid 1%, phenylethyl alcohol 7.5%. Net price 50 mL = £1.30; 150 mL = £3.40; 500 mL = £9.80

Excipients: none as listed in section 13.1.3

Scalp psoriasis, seborrhoeic dermatitis, dandruff, apply 3 times in first week then twice weekly

Clinitar® (CHS)

Shampoo solution, coal tar extract 2%. Net price 100 g = £2.50

Excipients: include polysorbates, fragrance

Scalp psoriasis, seborrhoeic dermatitis, and dandruff, apply up to 3 times weekly

Cocois® (Celltech)

Scalp ointment, coal tar solution 12%, salicylic acid 2%, precipitated sulphur 4%, in a coconut oil emollient basis. Net price 40 g (with applicator nozzle) = £5.04; 100 g = £9.46

Excipients: include cetostearyl alcohol

Scalp scalp disorders including psoriasis, eczema, seborrhoeic dermatitis and dandruff, apply to scalp once weekly as necessary (if severe use daily for first 3–7 days), shampoo off after 1 hour; CHILD 6–12 years, medical supervision required (not recommended under 6 years)

Ionil T® (Galderma)

Shampoo application, benzalkonium chloride 0.2%, coal tar solution 4.25%, salicylic acid 2% in an alcoholic basis. Net price 200 mL = £2.56

Excipients: include disodium edetate

Scalp psoriasis, seborrhoeic dermatitis, apply 1–2 times weekly; CHILD under 12 years not recommended

Meted® (DermaPharm)

Shampoo, salicylic acid 3%, sulphur 5%. Net price 120 mL = £3.90

Excipients: include fragrance

Scaly scalp disorders including psoriasis, seborrhoeic dermatitis, and dandruff, apply at least twice weekly

¹Nizoral® (Janssen-Cilag) [PoM]

Shampoo, ketoconazole 2%, net price 120 mL = £4.09

Excipients: include imidurea

For seborrhoeic dermatitis and dandruff apply twice weekly for 2–4 weeks, for pityriasis versicolor once daily for max. 5 days

1. Can be sold to the public for the prevention and treatment of dandruff and seborrhoeic dermatitis of the scalp as a shampoo formulation containing ketoconazole max. 2%, in a pack containing max.120 mL and labelled to show a max. frequency of application of once every 3 days; a brand on sale to the public is *Nizoral® Dandruff Shampoo*; *Neutrogena® Long Lasting Dandruff Control Shampoo* containing ketoconazole 1% is available as a cosmetic.

Pentrax® (DermaPharm)

Shampoo, coal tar 4.3%. Net price 120 mL = £3.90

Excipients: none as listed in section 13.1.3

Scaly scalp disorders including psoriasis, seborrhoeic dermatitis, and dandruff, apply at least twice weekly

Polytar® (Stiefel)

Liquid, arachis (peanut) oil extract of crude coal tar 0.3%, cade oil 0.3%, coal tar solution 0.1%, oleyl alcohol 1%, tar 0.3%, net price 250 mL = £2.23

Excipients: include fragrance, imidurea, polysorbate 80

Scalp disorders including psoriasis, seborrhoea, eczema, pruritus and dandruff, apply 1–2 times weekly

Polytar AF® (Stiefel)

Shampoo, arachis (peanut) oil extract of coal tar 0.3%, cade oil 0.3%, coal tar solution 0.1%, pine tar 0.3%, pyrithione zinc 1%, net price 150 mL = £4.40

Excipients: include fragrance, imidurea

Scaly scalp disorders including psoriasis, seborrhoeic dermatitis, and dandruff, apply 2–3 times weekly for at least 3 weeks

Polytar Plus® (Stiefel)

Liquid, ingredients as *Polytar®* liquid with hydrolysed animal protein 3%, net price 500 mL = £4.40

Excipients: include fragrance, imidurea, polysorbate 80

Scalp disorders including psoriasis, seborrhoea, eczema, pruritus and dandruff, apply 1–2 times weekly

Pragmatar® —section 13.5.2

Psoriderm® (Dermal)

Scalp lotion (= shampoo), coal tar 2.5%, lecithin 0.3%. Net price 250 mL = £5.33

Excipients: include disodium edetate

Scalp psoriasis, use as necessary

Selsun® (Abbott)

Shampoo application, selenium sulphide 2.5%. Net price 50 mL = £1.44; 100 mL = £1.96; 150 mL = £2.75

Excipients: include fragrance

Seborrhoeic dermatitis and dandruff, apply twice weekly for 2 weeks then once weekly for 2 weeks and then as necessary; CHILD under 5 years not recommended; pityriasis versicolor, section 13.10.2 [unlicensed indication]

Caution: avoid using 48 hours before or after applying hair colouring, straightening or waving preparations

T/Gel® (Neutrogena)

Shampoo, coal tar extract 2%. Net price 125 mL = £3.18; 250 mL = £4.78

Excipients: include fragrance, hydroxybenzoates (parabens), imidurea, tetrasodium edetate

Scalp psoriasis, seborrhoeic dermatitis, dandruff, apply as necessary

---

Male-pattern baldness

Topical application of **minoxidil** may stimulate limited hair growth in a small proportion of adults but only for as long as it is used.

MINOXIDIL

Indications: male-pattern baldness (men and women)

Cautions: see section 2.5.1 (only about 1.4–1.7% absorbed); avoid contact with eyes, mouth and mucous membranes, broken, infected, shaved, or inflamed skin; avoid inhalation of spray mist; avoid occlusive dressings and topical drugs which enhance absorption

Contra-indications: see section 2.5.1

Side-effects: see section 2.5.1; irritant dermatitis, allergic contact dermatitis, discontinue if hair loss persists for more than 2 weeks

Administration: apply 1 mL twice daily to dry hair and scalp (discontinue if no improvement after 1 year); 5% strength for use in men only

Regaine® (Pharmacia) NHS

Regaine® Regular Strength topical solution, minoxidil 2% in an aqueous alcoholic basis. Net price 60-mL bottle with applicators = £14.16

Excipients: include propylene glycol

Regaine® Extra Strength topical solution, minoxidil 5% in an aqueous alcoholic basis. Net price 60-mL bottle with applicators = £17.00; 3 × 60-mL bottles = £34.04

Excipients: include propylene glycol

Cautions: flammable; wash hands after application

13.10 Anti-infective skin preparations

13.10.1	Antibacterial preparations
13.10.2	Antifungal preparations
13.10.3	Antiviral preparations
13.10.4	Parasiticidal preparations
13.10.5	Preparations for minor cuts and abrasions

13.10.1 Antibacterial preparations

| 13.10.1.1 | Antibacterial preparations only used topically |
| 13.10.1.2 | Antibacterial preparations also used systemically |

For many skin infections such as *erysipelas* and *cellulitis* systemic antibacterial treatment is more appropriate because the infection is too deeply seated for adequate penetration of topical preparations. For details of suitable treatment see section 5.1, table 1.

Impetigo may be treated by topical application of **fusidic acid** or **mupirocin** or, if widespread, with oral administration of **flucloxacillin** or **erythromycin** (section 5.1, table 1). Mild antiseptics such as **povidone–iodine** (section 13.11.4) are used to soften crusts and exudate.

Although there are a great many antibacterial drugs presented in topical preparations some are potentially hazardous and frequently their use is not necessary if adequate hygienic measures can be taken. Moreover not all skin conditions that are oozing, crusted, or characterised by pustules are actually infected. Topical antibacterials should be **avoided** on *leg ulcers* unless used in short courses for defined infections; treatment of bacterial colonisation is generally inappropriate.

To minimise the development of resistant organisms it is advisable to limit the choice of antibacterials applied topically to those not used systemically. Unfortunately some of these, for example neomycin, may cause sensitisation, and there is cross-sensitivity with other aminoglycoside antibiotics, such as gentamicin. If *large areas of skin* are being treated, ototoxicity may also be a hazard with aminoglycoside antibiotics (and also with polymyxins), particularly in children, in the elderly, and in those with renal impairment. *Resistant organisms* are more common in hospitals, and whenever possible swabs should be taken for bacteriological examination before beginning treatment.

Mupirocin is not related to any other antibacterial in use; it is effective for skin infections, particularly those due to Gram-positive organisms but it is not indicated for pseudomonal infection. Although *Staphylococcus aureus* strains with low-level resistance to mupirocin are emerging, it is particularly useful in infections resistant to other antibacterials. To avoid the development of resistance mupirocin should not be used for longer than 10 days and its use in hospital should be avoided if possible.

Silver sulfadiazine (silver sulphadiazine) is used in the treatment of infected burns.

13.10.1.1 Antibacterial preparations only used topically

FRAMYCETIN SULPHATE

Indications: bacterial skin infections

Cautions: treatment of large areas (risk of ototoxicity particularly in children, elderly, and in renal impairment)

Side-effects: sensitisation (see also notes above)

Sofra-Tulle® *see* Framycetin Gauze Dressing, Appendix 8 (section A8.1.10)

MUPIROCIN

Indications: bacterial skin infections (see also notes above)

Bactroban® (Beecham) [PoM]
Cream, mupirocin (as mupirocin calcium) 2%, net price 15 g = £4.71
Excipients: include benzyl alcohol, cetyl alcohol, stearyl alcohol
Secondarily infected traumatic lesions, apply 3 times daily for up to 10 days; re-evaluate if no response after 3–5 days
Ointment, mupirocin 2%. Net price 15 g = £4.71
Excipients: none as listed in section 13.1.3
Note. Contains macrogol and manufacturer advises caution in renal impairment; may sting
Skin infections, apply up to 3 times daily for up to 10 days
Important: cream and ointment not interchangeable—prescription should specify formulation required
Nasal ointment, see section 12.2.3

NEOMYCIN SULPHATE

Indications: bacterial skin infections

Cautions: large areas, see below
LARGE AREAS. If large areas of skin are being treated ototoxicity may be a hazard, particularly in children, in the elderly, and in those with renal impairment

Contra-indications: neonates

Side-effects: sensitisation (see also notes above)

Neomycin Cream BPC [PoM] [◀▬]
Cream, neomycin sulphate 0.5%, cetomacrogol emulsifying ointment 30%, chlorocresol 0.1%, disodium edetate 0.01%, in freshly boiled and cooled purified water. Net price 15 g = £1.09
Apply up to 3 times daily (short-term use)
Excipients: include cetostearyl alcohol, edetic acid (EDTA)

[▬◀] denotes preparations that are considered to be less suitable for prescribing (see p. vi)

Cicatrin® (GlaxoWellcome) [PoM]
Cream, neomycin sulphate 3300 units, bacitracin zinc 250 units, cysteine 2 mg, glycine 10 mg, threonine 1 mg/g. Net price 15 g = 90p; 30 g = £1.80
Excipients: include wool fat derivative, polysorbates
Superficial bacterial infection of skin, ADULT and CHILD over 2 years, apply up to 3 times daily (short-term use)
Dusting powder, neomycin sulphate 3300 units, bacitracin zinc 250 units, cysteine 2 mg, glycine 10 mg, threonine 1 mg/g. Net price 15 g = 90p; 50 g = £3.00
Excipients: none as listed in section 13.1.3
Superficial bacterial infection of skin, ADULT and CHILD over 2 years, apply up to 3 times daily (short-term use)

Graneodin® (Squibb) [PoM]
Ointment, neomycin sulphate 0.25%, gramicidin 0.025%. Net price 25 g = £1.47
Excipients: none as listed in section 13.1.3
Superficial bacterial infection of skin, apply 2–4 times daily (for max. 7 days—possibly longer for sycosis barbae)

POLYMYXINS
(Includes colistin sulphate and polymyxin B sulphate)

Indications: bacterial skin infections

Cautions: large areas, see below
LARGE AREAS. If large areas of skin are being treated nephrotoxicity and neurotoxicity may be a hazard, particularly in children, in the elderly, and in those with renal impairment

Side-effects: sensitisation (see also notes above)

Polyfax® (Dominion) [PoM]
Ointment, polymyxin B sulphate 10 000 units, bacitracin zinc 500 units/g. Net price 20 g = £4.62
Excipients: none as listed in section 13.1.3
Apply twice daily or more frequently if required

Colomycin® (Forest) [PoM]
Powder, sterile, for making topical preparations (usually 1%), colistin sulphate. Net price 1-g vial = £18.37
Excipients: none as listed in section 13.1.3

SILVER SULFADIAZINE
(Silver sulphadiazine)

Indications: prophylaxis and treatment of infection in burn wounds; as an adjunct to short-term treatment of infection in leg ulcers and pressure sores; as an adjunct to prophylaxis of infection in skin graft donor sites and extensive abrasions; for conservative management of finger-tip injuries

Cautions: hepatic and renal impairment; G6PD deficiency; pregnancy and breast-feeding (avoid in late pregnancy and in neonate—see also Appendix 4); may inactivate enzymatic debriding agents—concomitant use may be inappropriate; for large amounts see also **interactions:** Appendix 1 (co-trimoxazole and sulphonamides)
LARGE AREAS. Plasma-sulfadiazine concentrations may approach therapeutic levels with *side-effects* and *interactions* as for sulphonamides (see section 5.1.8) if large areas of skin are treated. Owing to the association of sulphonamides with severe blood and skin disorders treatment should be stopped immediately if blood disorders or rashes develop—but leucopenia developing 2–3 days after starting treatment of burns patients is reported usually to be self-limiting and silver sulfadiazine need not usually be discontinued provided blood counts are monitored carefully to ensure return to normality within a few days. Argyria may also occur if large areas of skin are treated (or if application is prolonged).

Contra-indications: pregnancy and breast-feeding; sensitivity to sulphonamides; not recommended for neonates (see also Appendix 4)

Side-effects: allergic reactions including burning, itching and rashes; argyria reported following prolonged use; leucopenia reported (monitor blood levels)

Flamazine® (S&N Hlth.) PoM
Cream, silver sulfadiazine 1%, net price 20 g = £3.10, 50 g = £4.11; 250 g = £11.00; 500 g = £19.48
Excipients: include cetyl alcohol, polysorbates, propylene glycol
Apply with sterile applicator; burns, apply daily or more frequently if very exudative; leg ulcers or pressure sores, apply daily or on alternate days (not recommended if ulcer very exudative); finger-tip injuries, apply every 2-3 days; consult product literature for details

13.10.1.2 Antibacterial preparations also used systemically

CHLORTETRACYCLINE HYDROCHLORIDE

Indications: bacterial skin infections (see notes above)

Cautions: see notes above; overgrowth with non-susceptible organisms; stains clothing

Side-effects: rarely hypersensitivity reactions

Administration: apply 1–3 times daily

Aureomycin® (Lederle) PoM
Ointment, chlortetracycline hydrochloride 3%. Net price 30 g = £1.77
Excipients: include wool fat

FUSIDIC ACID

Indications: staphylococcal skin infections

Cautions: see notes above; avoid contact with eyes

Side-effects: rarely hypersensitivity reactions

Administration: apply 3–4 times daily

Fucidin® (Leo) PoM
Cream, fusidic acid 2%. Net price 15 g = £2.74; 30 g = £4.62
Excipients: include butylated hydroxyanisole, cetyl alcohol
Gel, fusidic acid 2%. Net price 15 g = £2.37; 30 g = £4.10
Excipients: include hydroxybenzoates (parabens), polysorbate 80
Ointment, sodium fusidate 2%. Net price 15 g = £2.23; 30 g = £3.79
Excipients: include cetyl alcohol, wool fat

METRONIDAZOLE

Indications: see under preparations

Cautions: avoid exposure to strong sunlight or UV light

Side-effects: skin irritation

Administration: see under preparations

■ Rosacea (see also section 13.6)

Metrogel® (Novartis) PoM
Gel, metronidazole 0.75%, net price 40 g = £19.90. Label: 10 patient information leaflet
Excipients: include hydroxybenzoates (parabens), propylene glycol
Acute inflammatory exacerbations of acne rosacea, apply thinly twice daily for 8–9 weeks

Noritate® (Kestrel) PoM
Cream, metronidazole 1%, net price 30 g = £19.08. Label: 10 patient information leaflet
Excipients: include hydroxybenzoates (parabens)
Acne rosacea, apply once daily for 8 weeks

Rozex® (Galderma) PoM
Cream, metronidazole 0.75%, net price 30 g = £11.46, 40 g = £15.28. Label: 10 patient information leaflet
Excipients: include benzyl alcohol, isopropyl palmitate
Gel, metronidazole 0.75%, net price 30 g = £11.46, 40 g = £15.28. Label: 10 patient information leaflet
Excipients: include disodium edetate, hydroxybenzoates (parabens), propylene glycol
Inflammatory papules, pustules and erythema of acne rosacea, apply twice daily for 3–4 months

Zyomet® (Goldshield) PoM
Gel, metronidazole 0.75%, net price 30 g = £12.00. Label: 10 patient information leaflet
Excipients: include benzyl alcohol, disodium edetate, propylene glycol
Acute inflammatory exacerbations of acne rosacea, apply thinly twice daily for 8–9 weeks

■ Malodorous tumours and skin ulcers

Anabact® (CHS) PoM
Gel, metronidazole 0.75%, net price 15 g = £4.47, 30 g = £7.89
Excipients: include hydroxybenzoates (parabens), propylene glycol
Malodorous fungating tumours and malodorous gravitational and decubitus ulcers, apply to clean wound 1–2 times daily and cover with non-adherent dressing

Metrotop® (SSL) PoM
Gel, metronidazole 0.8%, net price 15 g = £4.73, 30 g = £8.36
Excipients: none as listed in section 13.1.3
Malodorous fungating tumours and malodorous gravitational and decubitus ulcers, apply to clean wound 1–2 times daily and cover (flat wounds, apply liberally; cavities, smear on paraffin gauze and pack loosely)

13.10.2 Antifungal preparations

Most localised fungal infections are treated with topical preparations. Systemic therapy (section 5.2) is necessary for nail or scalp infection or if the skin infection is widespread, disseminated or intractable. Skin scrapings should be examined especially where systemic therapy is being considered or where there is doubt about the diagnosis.

DERMATOPHYTOSES. Ringworm infection can affect the scalp (tinea capitis), body (tinea corporis), groin (tinea cruris), hand (tinea manuum), foot (tinea pedis, athlete's foot), or nail (tinea unguium). Scalp infection requires systemic treatment (section 5.2); additional topical application of an antifungal may reduce the risk of transmission. Most other local ringworm infections can be treated adequately with topical antifungal preparations. The imidazole antifungals clotrimazole, econazole, ketocon-azole, miconazole, and sulconazole are all effec-tive. **Terbinafine** cream is also effective but it is more expensive. Other topical antifungals include **amorolfine** and the **undecenoates**. **Compound benzoic acid ointment** (Whitfield's ointment) has been used for ringworm infections but it is cosmeti-cally less acceptable than proprietary preparations. Topical preparations for athlete's foot containing **tolnaftate** are on sale to the public.

Tinea infection of the nail is almost always treated systemically (section 5.2); topical applica-tion of **amorolfine** or **tioconazole** may be effective for treating early onychomycosis when involve-ment is limited to mild distal disease in up to 2 nails.

PITYRIASIS VERSICOLOR. Pityriasis versicolor may be treated topically with a course of **selenium sulphide** shampoo used as a lotion [unlicensed indication] (section 13.9) repeated after one month. Topical imidazole antifungals **clotrimazole**, **econ-azole**, **ketoconazole**, **miconazole**, and **sulconazole** and topical **terbinafine** are alternatives but large quantities may be required. If topical therapy fails, or if the infection is widespread, pityriasis versi-color is treated systemically with an azole antifun-gal (section 5.2). Relapse is common, especially in the immunocompromised.

CANDIDIASIS. Candidal skin infections may be treated with topical imidazole antifungals, **clotrim-azole**, **econazole**, **ketoconazole**, **miconazole**, and **sulconazole**. Topical application of **nystatin** is also effective for candidiasis but it is ineffective against dermatophytosis. Refractory candidiasis requires systemic treatment (section 5.2).

COMPOUND TOPICAL PREPARATIONS. Combi-nation of an imidazole and a mild corticosteroid (such as hydrocortisone 1%) (section 13.4) may be of value in the treatment of eczematous intertrigo and, in the first few days only, of a severely inflamed patch of ringworm. Combination of a mild corticosteroid with either an imidazole or nystatin may be of use in the treatment of intertrigo associ-ated with candida.

CHOICE OF ANTIFUNGAL FORMULATION. *Lotions* or *sprays* are suitable for application to large and hairy areas. *Ointments* are generally used on dry areas; they are best avoided on moist skin. *Creams* are cosmetically more acceptable than oint-ments and they are suitable for moist areas. *Paints* and *solutions* for application to the nail are occa-sionally effective for early dystrophy in onycho-mycosis (see Dermatophytoses above). *Dusting powders* are of little therapeutic value in the treat-ment of fungal skin infections and may cause skin irritation; they may have some role in preventing re-infection.

CAUTIONS. Contact with eyes and mucous mem-branes should be avoided.

SIDE-EFFECTS. Occasional local irritation and hypersensitivity reactions include mild burning sen-sation, erythema, and itching. Treatment should be discontinued if these are severe.

AMOROLFINE

Indications: see under preparations
Cautions: see notes above; also avoid contact with ears; pregnancy and breast-feeding
Side-effects: see notes above

Loceryl® (Galderma) PoM
Cream, amorolfine (as hydrochloride) 0.25%, net price 20 g = £4.83. Label: 10 patient information leaflet
Excipients: include cetostearyl alcohol, disodium edetate
Fungal skin infections, apply once daily after cleansing in the evening for at least 2–3 weeks (up to 6 weeks for foot infection) continuing for 3–5 days after lesions have healed

Nail lacquer, amorolfine (as hydrochloride) 5%, net price 5-mL pack (with nail files, spatulas and cleansing swabs) = £29.94. Label: 10 patient information leaflet
Excipients: none as listed in 13.1.3
Fungal nail infections, apply to infected nails 1–2 times weekly after filing and cleansing; allow to dry (approx. 3 minutes); treat finger nails for 6 months, toe nails for 9–12 months (review at intervals of 3 months); avoid nail varnish or artificial nails during treatment

BENZOIC ACID

Indications: ringworm (tinea), but see notes above

Benzoic Acid Ointment, Compound, BP
(Whitfield's ointment)
Ointment, benzoic acid 6%, salicylic acid 3%, in emulsifying ointment
Apply twice daily
Excipients: include cetostearyl alcohol

BENZOYL PEROXIDE

Indications: fungal skin infections, particularly tinea pedis; acne vulgaris (section 13.6.1)
Side-effects: see notes above

Quinoped® (Adams Hlth)
Cream, benzoyl peroxide 5%, potassium hydroxy-quinoline sulphate 0.5%, in an astringent basis, net price 25 g = £1.23
Excipients: include cetostearyl alcohol, edetic acid (EDTA)
Apply twice daily
Note. May bleach clothing

CLOTRIMAZOLE

Indications: fungal skin infections
Cautions: see notes above
Side-effects: see notes above
Administration: apply 2–3 times daily

Clotrimazole (Non-proprietary)
Cream, clotrimazole 1%, net price 20 g = £1.77
Available from Akita (*Candiden®*), Alpharma, Ash-bourne (*Abtrim®*), CP, Dominion, Generics, Genus
¹**Canesten®** (Bayer Consumer Care)
Cream, clotrimazole 1%, net price 20 g = £2.14, 50 g = £3.80. On sale to the public as *Canesten® AF* cream
Excipients: include benzyl alcohol, cetostearyl alcohol, polysorb-ate 60
Powder, clotrimazole 1%, net price 30 g = £1.52.
On sale to the public as *Canesten® AF* powder
Excipients: none as listed in section 13.1.3

Solution, clotrimazole 1% in macrogol 400 (poly-ethylene glycol 400), net price 20 mL = £2.43. For hairy areas
Excipients: none as listed in section 13.1.3

Spray, clotrimazole 1%, in 30% isopropyl alcohol, net price 40-mL atomiser = £4.99. Label: 15. For large or hairy areas. On sale to the public as *Canesten® AF* spray
Excipients: include propylene glycol
1. The brand name *Canesten® AF Once Daily* is used for bifonazole

ECONAZOLE NITRATE

Indications: fungal skin infections
Cautions: see notes above
Side-effects: see notes above
Administration: skin infections apply twice daily; nail infections, apply once daily under occlusive dressing

Ecostatin® (Squibb)
Cream, econazole nitrate 1%, net price 15 g = £1.49; 30 g = £2.75
Excipients: include butylated hydroxyanisole, fragrance

Pevaryl® (Janssen-Cilag)
Cream, econazole nitrate 1%, net price 30 g = £2.65
Excipients: include butylated hydroxyanisole, fragrance

KETOCONAZOLE

Indications: fungal skin infections
Cautions: see notes above; do **not** use within 2 weeks of a topical corticosteroid for seborrhoeic dermatitis—risk of skin sensitisation
Side-effects: see notes above
Administration: tinea pedis, apply twice daily; other fungal infections, apply 1–2 times daily

¹**Nizoral®** (Janssen-Cilag) [PoM]
²*Cream*, ketoconazole 2%, net price 30 g = £3.81
Excipients: include cetyl alcohol, polysorbates, propylene glycol, stearyl alcohol
1. A 15-g tube is available for sale to the public for the treatment of tinea pedis, tinea cruris, and candidal intertrigo (*Daktarin® Gold*)
2. [NHS] except for seborrhoeic dermatitis and pityriasis versicolor and endorsed 'SLS'

MICONAZOLE NITRATE

Indications: fungal skin infections
Cautions: see notes above
Side-effects: see notes above
Administration: apply twice daily continuing for 10 days after lesions have healed; nail infections, apply 1–2 times daily

Daktarin® (Janssen-Cilag)
Cream, miconazole nitrate 2%, net price 30 g = £2.07. Also on sale to the public as *Daktarin® Dual Action cream* for athlete's foot
Excipients: include butylated hydroxyanisole
Note. A 15-g tube [NHS] is on sale to the public.

Powder [NHS], miconazole nitrate 2%, net price 20 g = £1.81. Also on sale to the public as *Daktarin® Dual Action powder* for athlete's foot
Excipients: none as listed in section 13.1.3

Dual Action Spray powder, miconazole nitrate 0.16%, in an aerosol basis, net price 100 g = £2.27
Excipients: none as listed in section 13.1.3

NYSTATIN

Indications: skin infections due to *Candida* spp.
Cautions: see notes above
Side-effects: see notes above

Nystaform® (Typharm) [PoM]
Cream, nystatin 100 000 units/g, chlorhexidine hydrochloride 1%, net price 30 g = £2.62
Excipients: include benzyl alcohol, cetostearyl alcohol, polysorbate 60
Apply 2–3 times daily continuing for 7 days after lesions have healed.
Note. May be difficult to obtain

Nystan® (Squibb) [PoM]
Cream, nystatin 100 000 units/g, net price 30 g = £2.18
Excipients: include benzyl alcohol, propylene glycol, fragrance
Apply 2–4 times daily

Ointment, nystatin 100 000 units/g, in *Plastibase®*, net price 30 g = £1.75
Excipients: none as listed in section 13.1.3
Apply 2–4 times daily

Tinaderm-M® (Schering-Plough) [PoM]
Cream, nystatin 100 000 units/g, tolnaftate 1%, net price 20 g = £1.83
Excipients: include butylated hydroxytoluene, cetostearyl alcohol, hydroxybenzoates (parabens), fragrance
Apply 2–3 times daily

SALICYLIC ACID

Indications: fungal nail infections, particularly tinea; hyperkeratotic skin disorders (section 13.5.2); acne vulgaris (section 13.6.1); warts and calluses (section 13.7)
Contra-indications: children under 5 years; pregnancy
Side-effects: see notes above
Administration: apply twice daily

Phytex® (Wynlit) ▰
Paint, salicylic acid 1.46% (total combined), tannic acid 4.89% and boric acid 3.12% (as borotannic complex), in a vehicle containing alcohol and ethyl acetate, net price 25 mL (with brush) = £1.42
Excipients: none as listed in section 13.1.3
Note. Flammable

▰ denotes preparations that are considered to be less suitable for prescribing (see p. vi)

SULCONAZOLE NITRATE

Indications: fungal skin infections
Cautions: see notes above
Side-effects: see notes above; also blistering
Administration: apply 1–2 times daily continuing for 2–3 weeks after lesions have healed

Exelderm® (Bioglan) [PoM]
Cream, sulconazole nitrate 1%, net price 30 g = £2.10
Excipients: include cetyl alcohol, polysorbates, propylene glycol, stearyl alcohol

TERBINAFINE

Indications: fungal skin infections
Cautions: pregnancy, breast-feeding; avoid contact with eyes
Side-effects: redness, itching, or stinging; rarely allergic reactions (discontinue)

¹Lamisil® (Novartis) [PoM]
Cream, terbinafine hydrochloride 1%. Net price 15 g = £4.86; 30 g = £8.76
Apply thinly 1–2 times daily for up to 1 week in tinea pedis, 1–2 weeks in tinea corporis and tinea cruris, 2 weeks in cutaneous candidiasis and pityriasis versicolor; review after 2 weeks; CHILD not recommended
Excipients: include benzyl alcohol, cetyl alcohol, polysorbate 60, stearyl alcohol
1. A 7.5-g tube is available for sale to the public for the treatment of tinea pedis and tinea cruris *(Lamisil® AT)*
Tablets, see section 5.2

TIOCONAZOLE

Indications: fungal nail infections
Cautions: see notes above
Contra-indications: pregnancy (Appendix 4)
Side-effects: see notes above
Administration: apply to nails and surrounding skin twice daily for up to 6 months (may be extended to 12 months)

Trosyl® (Pfizer) [PoM]
Nail solution, tioconazole 28%, net price 12 mL (with applicator brush) = £27.38
Excipients: none as listed in section 13.1.3

UNDECENOATES

Indications: see under preparations below
Side-effects: see notes above
Administration: see under preparations below

Monphytol® (LAB) [icon]
Paint, methyl undecenoate 5%, propyl undecenoate 0.7%, salicylic acid 3%, methyl salicylate 25%, propyl salicylate 5%, chlorobutanol 3%, net price 18 mL (with brush) = £1.61
Excipients: none as listed in section 13.1.3
Fungal skin and nail infections, apply twice daily

Mycota® (SSL)
Cream, zinc undecenoate 20%, undecenoic acid 5%, net price 25 g = £1.17
Excipients: include fragrance
Treatment of athlete's foot, apply twice daily continuing for 7 days after lesions have healed
Prevention of athlete's foot, apply once daily
Powder, zinc undecenoate 20%, undecenoic acid 2%, net price 70 g = £1.74
Excipients: include fragrance
Treatment of athlete's foot, apply twice daily continuing for 7 days after lesions have healed
Prevention of athlete's foot, apply once daily
Spray application, undecenoic acid 2.5%, dichlorophen 0.25% (pressurised aerosol pack), net price 100 mL = £1.88
Excipients: include fragrance
Treatment of athlete's foot, apply twice daily continuing for 7 days after lesions have healed
Prevention of athlete's foot, apply once daily

13.10.3   Antiviral preparations

Aciclovir cream is licensed for the treatment of initial and recurrent labial and genital *herpes simplex infections*; treatment should begin as early as possible. Systemic treatment is necessary for buccal or vaginal infections or if cold sores recur frequently; *herpes zoster (shingles)* also requires systemic treatment (for details of systemic use see section 5.3). **Penciclovir** cream is licensed for the treatment of labial *herpes simplex infection*.

Idoxuridine solution (5% in dimethyl sulfoxide) is of little value.

ACICLOVIR

(Acyclovir)
Indications: see notes above
Cautions: avoid contact with eyes and mucous membranes
Side-effects: transient stinging or burning; occasionally erythema, itching or drying of the skin
Administration: apply to lesions every 4 hours (5 times daily) for 5–10 days, starting at first sign of attack

Aciclovir (Non-proprietary) [PoM]
Cream, aciclovir 5%, net price 2 g = £2.69, 10 g = £7.34
Excipients: include propylene glycol
Available from Alpharma (*excipients* also include sorbic acid), Genus, Pharmacia
¹Zovirax® (GlaxoWellcome) [PoM]
Cream, aciclovir 5%, net price 2 g = £5.29; 10 g = £15.94
Excipients: include cetostearyl alcohol, propylene glycol
1. A 2-g tube and a pump pack are on sale to the public for the treatment of cold sores (*Zovirax® Cold Sore Cream*); other brands on sale to the public include *Boots Avert®*, *Herpetad®*, *Soothelip®*, *Viralief®* and *Virasorb®*
Eye ointment, section 11.3.3
Tablets, section 5.3

PENCICLOVIR

Indications: see notes above
Cautions: avoid contact with eyes and mucous membranes
Side-effects: transient stinging, burning, numbness

Vectavir® (Novartis) [PoM]
Cream, penciclovir 1%, net price 2 g = £4.20
Herpes labialis, apply to lesions every 2 hours during waking hours for 4 days, starting at first sign of attack; CHILD under 12 years, not recommended
Excipients: include cetostearyl alcohol, propylene glycol

IDOXURIDINE IN DIMETHYL SULFOXIDE [icon]

Indications: herpes simplex and herpes zoster infection but of little value
Cautions: avoid contact with the eyes, mucous membranes, and textiles; breast-feeding (may taste unpleasant)
Contra-indications: pregnancy (Appendix 4); **not** to be used in mouth
Side-effects: stinging on application, changes in taste; overuse may cause maceration

Herpid® (Yamanouchi) PoM �1

Application, idoxuridine 5% in dimethyl sulfoxide, net price 5 mL (with applicator) = £5.63

Apply to lesions 4 times daily for 4 days, starting at first sign of attack; CHILD under 12 years, not recommended

---

▙ denotes preparations that are considered to be less suitable for prescribing (see p. vi)

13.10.4 Parasiticidal preparations

Suitable quantities of parasiticidal preparations

	Skin creams	Lotions	Cream rinses
Scalp (headlice)	—	50–100 mL	50-100 mL
Body (scabies)	30–60 g	100 mL	—
Body (crab lice)	30–60 g	100 mL	—

These amounts are usually suitable for an adult for single application.

Scabies

Malathion and **permethrin** are used for *scabies (Sarcoptes scabiei)*.

Aqueous preparations are preferable to alcoholic lotions, which are not recommended owing to irritation of excoriated skin and the genitalia.

Older preparations include **benzyl benzoate**, which is an irritant and should be avoided in children; it is less effective than malathion and permethrin.

Ivermectin (*Mectizan®*, MSD, available on a named patient basis) in a single dose of 200 micrograms/kg by mouth has been used, in combination with topical drugs, for the treatment of hyperkeratotic (crusted or 'Norwegian') scabies that does not respond to topical treatment alone.

APPLICATION. Although acaricides have traditionally been applied after a hot bath, this is **not** necessary and there is even evidence that a hot bath may increase absorption into the blood, removing them from their site of action on the skin.

All members of the affected household should be treated. Treatment should be applied to the whole body, paying particular attention to the webs of the fingers and toes and brushing lotion under the ends of the nails. In infants and young children (up to the age of about 2 years), the elderly, the immunocompromised, and in those whose treatment has failed, application should be extended to the scalp, neck, face, and ears. It is now recommended that malathion and permethrin should be applied twice, one week apart; in the case of benzyl benzoate up to 3 applications on consecutive days may be needed. It is important to warn users **not** to wash their hands since this would require re-application. Patients with hyperkeratotic scabies may require 2 or 3 applications of acaricide on consecutive days to ensure that enough penetrates the skin crusts to kill all the mites.

ITCHING. The *itch of scabies* persists for some weeks after the infestation has been eliminated and antipruritic treatment may be required. Application of **crotamiton** can be used to control itching after treatment with more effective acaricides, but caution is necessary if the skin is excoriated. Oral administration of a **sedating antihistamine** (section 3.4.1) at night may also be useful.

Head lice

Carbaryl, **malathion**, and the **pyrethroids** (permethrin and phenothrin) are effective against *head lice* (*Pediculus humanus capitis*) but lice in some districts have developed resistance; resistance to two or more parasiticidal preparations has also been reported. Benzyl benzoate is licensed for the treatment of head lice but it is less effective than other drugs.

Head lice infestation (pediculosis) should be treated using lotion, liquid or cream rinse formulations. Shampoos are diluted too much in use to be effective. Alcoholic formulations are effective but aqueous formulations are preferred in severe eczema and for asthmatic patients and small children. A contact time of 12 hours or overnight treatment is recommended for lotions and liquids; a 2-hour treatment is not sufficient to kill eggs. Shorter application times are required for permethrin rinse and phenothrin foam application.

In general, a course of treatment for head lice should be 2 applications of product 7 days apart to prevent lice emerging from any eggs that survive the first application.

The policy of rotating insecticides on a district-wide basis is now considered outmoded. To overcome the development of resistance, a mosaic strategy is required whereby, if a course of treatment fails to cure, a different insecticide is used for the next course. If a course of treatment with either permethrin or phenothrin fails, then a non-pyrethyroid parasiticidal product should be used for the next course.

A **head lice repellent** containing piperonal 2% (*Rappell®*) is on sale to the public, but its value is uncertain.

WET COMBING METHODS. Several products are available which require the use of a plastic detection comb and hair conditioner. The methods typically involve meticulous combing with the detection comb (probably for at least 30 minutes each time) over the whole scalp at 4-day intervals for a minimum of 2 weeks. However, recent evidence suggests that treatment with a parasiticidal, such as malathion, is more effective than wet combing.

Crab lice

Carbaryl [unlicensed for crab lice], **permethrin, phenothrin**, and **malathion** are effective for *crab lice* (*Pthirus pubis*). An aqueous preparation should be applied to **all** parts of the body (not merely the groins and axillae) for 12 hours or overnight; a second treatment is needed after 7 days to kill lice emerging from surviving eggs. A different insecticide should be used if a course of treatment fails. Alcoholic lotions are not recommended (owing to irritation of excoriated skin and the genitalia).

Aqueous **malathion** lotion is effective for *crab lice of the eye lashes* [unlicensed use].

Benzyl benzoate

Benzyl benzoate is effective for *scabies* but is not a first-choice for *scabies* (see notes above).

BENZYL BENZOATE ◼

Indications: scabies (but see notes above)

Cautions: children (not recommended, see also under Administration, below), avoid contact with eyes and mucous membranes; do not use on broken or secondarily infected skin; breast-feeding (suspend feeding until product has been washed off)

Side-effects: skin irritation, burning sensation especially on genitalia and excoriations, occasionally rashes

Administration: apply over the whole body; repeat without bathing on the following day and wash off 24 hours later; a third application may be required in some cases

Note. Not recommended for children—dilution to reduce irritant effect also reduces efficacy. Some manufacturers recommend application to the body but to exclude the head and neck, but in the elderly, the immunocompromised and those who have experienced treatment failure, application may need to be extended to the scalp, neck, face, and ears

Benzyl Benzoate Application, BP (Non-proprietary) ◼

Application, benzyl benzoate 25 % in an emulsion basis, net price 500 mL = £2.72

Available from IVAX, Rhône-Poulenc Rorer (*Ascabiol®, excipients: include* triethanolamine)

◼ denotes preparations that are considered to be less suitable for prescribing (see p. vi)

Carbaryl

Carbaryl is recommended for *head lice*; an aqueous solution is recommended for *crab lice* (see notes above) but a suitable product is not currently licensed for this indication. In the light of experimental data in *animals* it would be prudent to consider carbaryl as a potential human carcinogen and it has been restricted to prescription only use. The Department of Health has emphasised that the risk is a theoretical one and that any risk from the intermittent use of head lice preparations is likely to be exceedingly small.

CARBARYL

(Carbaril)

Indications: see notes above and under preparations

Cautions: avoid contact with eyes; do not use on broken or infected skin; do not use more than once a week for 3 consecutive weeks; children under 6 months, medical supervision required; alcoholic lotions **not** recommended for pediculosis in asthma, in severe eczema or in small children

Side-effects: skin irritation

Administration: rub into dry hair and scalp, allow to dry naturally, shampoo after 12 hours, and comb wet hair (see also notes above)

Carylderm® (SSL) PoM

Liquid, carbaryl 1% in an aqueous basis, net price 50 mL = £2.28. For head lice

Excipients: include cetostearyl alcohol, hydroxybenzoates (parabens)

Lotion, carbaryl 0.5%, in an alcoholic basis, net price 50 mL = £2.28. Label: 15. For head lice (alcoholic, see notes above)

Excipients: include fragrance

Malathion

Malathion is recommended for *scabies, head lice* and *crab lice* (for details see notes above).

The risk of systemic effects associated with 1–2 applications of malathion is considered to be very low; however applications repeated at intervals of less than 1 week *or* application for more than 3 consecutive weeks should be **avoided** since the likelihood of eradication of lice is not increased.

MALATHION

Indications: see notes above and under preparations

Cautions: avoid contact with eyes; do not use on broken or infected skin; do not use more than once a week for 3 consecutive weeks; children under 6 months, medical supervision required; alcoholic lotions **not** recommended for head lice in severe eczema, asthma or in small children, or for scabies or crab lice (see notes above)

Side-effects: skin irritation

Administration: head lice, rub 0.5% preparation into dry hair and scalp, allow to dry naturally, remove by washing after 12 hours (see also notes above) *or* apply 1% shampoo to wet hair and rinse after 5 minutes, repeat, comb wet hair; repeat twice at intervals of 3 days

Crab lice, apply 0.5% aqueous preparation over whole body, allow to dry naturally, wash off after 12 hours or overnight

Scabies, apply 0.5% preparation over whole body, and wash off after 24 hours; if hands are washed with soap within 24 hours, they should be retreated; see also notes above

Note. For scabies manufacturer recommends application to the body but not necessarily to the head and neck. In young children, however, application may need to be extended to the scalp, neck, face, and ears; this extended application may also be necessary for the elderly, for the immunocompromised and following treatment failure

Derbac-M® (SSL)

Liquid, malathion 0.5% in an aqueous basis, net price 50 mL = £2.22, 200 mL = £5.42. For crab lice, head lice and scabies

Excipients: include cetostearyl alcohol, fragrance, hydroxybenzoates (parabens)

Prioderm® (SSL)

Lotion, malathion 0.5%, in an alcoholic basis, net price 50 mL = £2.22, 200 mL = £5.42. Label: 15. For head lice (alcoholic, see notes above)

Excipients: include fragrance

Cream shampoo [NHS], malathion 1%. Net price
40 g = £2.77. For crab lice and head lice

Excipients: include cetostearyl alcohol, fragrance, hydroxybenzoates (parabens), sodium edetate, wool fat

Quellada M® (Stafford-Miller)

Liquid, malathion 0.5% in an aqueous basis, net
price 50 mL = £1.85, 200 mL = £4.62. For crab
lice, head lice and scabies

Excipients: include cetostearyl alcohol, fragrance, hydroxybenzoates (parabens)

Cream shampoo, malathion 1%, net price 40 g =
£2.18. For crab lice and head lice

Excipients: include cetostearyl alcohol, fragrance, hydroxybenzoates (parabens), sodium edetate, wool fat

Suleo-M® (SSL)

Lotion, malathion 0.5%, in an alcoholic basis, net
price 50 mL = £2.22, 200 mL = £5.42. Label: 15.
For head lice (alcoholic, see notes above)

Excipients: include fragrance

Permethrin

Permethrin is effective for *scabies, head lice*, and
crab lice (for details see notes above).

PERMETHRIN

Indications: see notes above and under preparations

Cautions: avoid contact with eyes; do not use on
broken or secondarily infected skin; children
under 6 months, medical supervision required for
cream rinse (head lice); children aged 2 months–2
years, medical supervision required for dermal
cream (scabies)

Side-effects: pruritus, erythema, and stinging;
rarely rashes and oedema

Administration: see under preparations

Lyclear® Creme Rinse (Warner Lambert)

Cream rinse, permethrin 1% in basis containing
isopropyl alcohol 20%, net price 59 mL = £2.26, 2
× 59-mL pack = £4.17

Head lice, apply to clean damp hair and rinse after 10
minutes

Note. Not affected by chlorine in swimming pools

Excipients: include cetyl alcohol

Lyclear® Dermal Cream (Kestrel)

Dermal cream, permethrin 5%, net price 30 g =
£5.52. Label: 10 patient information leaflet

Excipients: include butylated hydroxytoluene, wool fat derivative

Scabies, apply over whole body and wash off after 8–12
hours; CHILD (see also Cautions, above) apply over
whole body including face, neck, scalp and ears; if
hands washed with soap within 8 hours of application,
they should be treated again with cream (see notes
above)

Note. Manufacturer recommends application to the body
but to exclude head and neck. In young children, however, application may need to be extended to the scalp,
neck, face, and ears; this extended application may also
be necessary for the elderly, for the immunocompromised and for those who have experienced treatment
failure.

Larger patients may require up to two 30-g packs for
adequate treatment.

Crab lice, ADULT over 18 years, see notes above

Phenothrin

Phenothrin is recommended for *head lice* and *crab
lice* (for details see notes above).

PHENOTHRIN

Indications: see notes above and under preparations

Cautions: avoid contact with eyes; do not use on
broken or secondarily infected skin; do not use
more than once a week for 3 weeks at a time; children under 6 months, medical supervision
required; alcoholic preparations **not** recommended for head lice in severe eczema, in asthma,
in small children, or for scabies or crab lice (see
notes above)

Side-effects: skin irritation

Administration: see under preparations

Full Marks® (SSL)

Liquid, phenothrin 0.5% in an aqueous basis, net
price 50 mL = £2.22, 200 mL = £5.42

Excipients: include cetostearyl alcohol, fragrance, hydroxybenzoates (parabens)

Head lice, apply to dry hair, allow to dry naturally;
shampoo after 12 hours or next day, comb wet hair

Lotion, phenothrin 0.2% in basis containing isopropyl alcohol 69.3%, net price 50 mL = £2.22,
200 mL = £5.42. Label: 15

Excipients: include fragrance

Crab lice and head lice (alcoholic, see above), apply to
dry hair, allow to dry naturally; shampoo after 2 hours,
comb wet hair

Mousse (= foam application), phenothrin 0.5% in
an alcoholic basis, net price 50 g = £2.47, 150 g =
£5.81. Label: 15

Excipients: include cetostearyl alcohol

Head lice (alcoholic, see above), apply to dry hair;
shampoo after 30 minutes, comb wet hair

13.10.5 Preparations for minor cuts and abrasions

Some of the preparations listed are used in minor
burns, and abrasions. They are applied as necessary.
Preparations containing camphor and sulphonamides should be **avoided**. Preparations such as
magnesium sulphate paste are also listed but are
now rarely used to treat carbuncles and boils as
these are best treated with antibiotics (section
5.1.1.2).

Cetrimide Cream, BP, cetrimide 0.5% in a suitable water-miscible basis such as cetostearyl
alcohol 5%, liquid paraffin 50% in freshly boiled
and cooled purified water. Net price 50 g = 76p

Proflavine Cream, BPC, proflavine hemisul-
phate 0.1%, yellow beeswax 2.5%, chlorocresol
0.1%, liquid paraffin 67.3%, freshly boiled and
cooled purified water 25%, wool fat 5%. Net
price 100 mL = 51p

Note. Stains clothing

Excipients: include beeswax, wool fat

■ Preparations for boils

Magnesium Sulphate Paste, BP, dried magnesium sulphate 45 g, glycerol 55 g, phenol 500 mg. Net price 25 g = 56p; 50 g = 67p. Should be stirred before use

Apply under dressing

Collodion

Flexible collodion may be used to seal minor cuts and wounds that have partially healed.

Collodion, Flexible, BP, castor oil 2.5%, colophony 2.5% in a collodion basis, prepared by dissolving pyroxylin (10%) in a mixture of 3 volumes of ether and 1 volume of alcohol (90%). Net price 10 mL = 20p. Label: 15 (**important**: very highly inflammable)

Skin tissue adhesive

Tissue adhesives are used for closure of minor skin wounds and for additional suture support. They should be applied by an appropriately trained healthcare professional.

Dermabond® (Ethicon)
Topical Skin Adhesive, sterile, octylcyanoacrylate, net price 0.5 mL = £10.00
Epiglu® (ICN)
Tissue adhesive, sterile, ethyl-2-cyanoacrylate 954.5 mg/g, polymethylmethacrylate, net price 3-g vial = £14.14, 4 × 3-g vials = £56.54 (all with dispensing pipettes and pallete)
Indermil® (Tyco)
Tissue adhesive, sterile, enbucrilate, net price 5 × 500-mg units = £31.95, 20 × 500-mg units = £127.80
Histoacryl® (Braun)
Tissue adhesive, sterile, enbucrilate, net price 5 × 200-mg unit (blue) = £32.00, 10 × 200-mg unit (blue) = £64.00, 5 × 500-mg unit (clear or blue) = £33.00, 10 × 500-mg unit (blue) = £66.00
LiquiBand® (MedLogic)
Tissue adhesive, sterile, butylcyanoacrylate, net price 0.5-g amp = £5.50

13.11   Disinfectants and cleansers

13.11.1   Alcohols and saline
13.11.2   Chlorhexidine salts
13.11.3   Cationic surfactants and soaps
13.11.4   Chlorine and iodine
13.11.5   Phenolics
13.11.6   Astringents, oxidisers, and dyes
13.11.7   Preparations for promotion of wound healing

The choice of *cleanser* is an important factor in treating skin conditions. For example, scaling disorders are best treated with **emulsifying ointment** (section 13.2.1) or other cleansers that do not irritate the skin.

Sodium chloride solution 0.9% is suitable for general cleansing of skin and wounds.

Useful *disinfectants* for skin cleansing include **cetrimide** (which has useful detergent properties), **chlorhexidine** and **potassium permanganate solution** 1 in 10 000. **Povidone–iodine** is preferred to chlorinated solutions (such as dilute sodium hypochlorite solution) which are too irritant and are no longer recommended. Topical preparations of **hexachlorophene** (hexachlorophane) should be used with caution in neonates and should **not** be used on large raw surfaces.

Astringent preparations, such as **potassium permanganate** solution are useful for oozing eczematous reactions (section 13.5.1). Silver nitrate lotion is now rarely used as it stains the skin black and may cause toxic effects if used for prolonged periods.

13.11.1   Alcohols and saline

ALCOHOL
Indications: skin preparation before injection
Cautions: flammable; avoid broken skin; patients have suffered severe burns when diathermy has been preceded by application of alcoholic skin disinfectants

Industrial Methylated Spirit, BP
Mixture of 19 volumes of ethanol (absolute alcohol) of an appropriate strength with 1 volume of approved wood naphtha and is Industrial Methylated Spirit of the quality known either as '66 OP' or as '74 OP'
Net price 100 mL = 28p. Label: 15
Surgical Spirit, BP, methyl salicylate 0.5 mL, diethyl phthalate 2%, castor oil 2.5%, in industrial methylated spirit. Net price 100 mL = 20p. Label: 15

SODIUM CHLORIDE
Indications: see notes above

Sodium Chloride (Non-proprietary)
Solution (sterile), sodium chloride 0.9%, net price 10 × 10-mL unit = £3.32; 10 × 20-mL unit = £9.68; 10 × 30-mL unit = £3.00
Available from GBM, Generics (20-mL vial only)
Askina® (Braun)
Askina® Spray, solution in aerosol can (sterile), sodium chloride 0.9% (buffered), net price 120-mL can = £2.45, 250-mL can = £2.75, 350-mL can = £3.20
Askina® Jet, solution (sterile), sodium chloride 0.9%, net price 24 × 10-mL unit = £5.62, 24 × 20-mL unit = £6.24, 24 × 30-mL unit = £7.20
Irriclens® (ConvaTec)
Solution in aerosol can, (sterile), sodium chloride 0.9%, net price 240-mL can = £2.85
Normasol® (SSL)
Solution (sterile), sodium chloride 0.9%. Net price 25 × 25-mL sachet = £5.85; 10 × 100-mL sachet = £7.16
See also section 11.8.2
Sterac® Sodium Chloride (Galen)
Solution (sterile), sodium chloride 0.9%. Net price 150 mL = 83p

Steripod® Sodium Chloride (SSL)

Steripod® sodium chloride 0.9% solution (sterile), sodium chloride 0.9%. Net price 25 × 20-mL sachet = £6.83

Saline Steripoules® (Galen)

Solution (sterile), sodium chloride 0.9%. Net price 20 × 2.5-mL units = £5.49, 25 × 20-mL units = £6.83

13.11.2 Chlorhexidine salts

CHLORHEXIDINE

Indications: see under preparations; bladder irrigation and catheter patency solutions (see section 7.4.4)

Cautions: avoid contact with eyes, brain, meninges and middle ear; not for use in body cavities; alcoholic solutions not suitable before diathermy

Side-effects: occasional sensitivity

Chlorhexidine 0.05% (Baxter)

2000 Solution (sterile), pink, chlorhexidine acetate 0.05%. Net price 500 mL = 72p, 1000 mL = 77p

For cleansing and disinfecting wounds and burns

Cepton® (Eastern)

Skin wash (= solution), red, chlorhexidine gluconate 1%, net price 150 mL = £1.99

For use as skin wash in acne

Lotion, blue, chlorhexidine gluconate 0.1%, net price 150 mL = £1.99

For skin disinfection in acne

CX Antiseptic Dusting Powder® (Adams Hlth)

Dusting powder, sterile, chlorhexidine acetate 1%. Net price 15 g = 87p

For skin disinfection

Hibiscrub® (SSL)

Cleansing solution, red, chlorhexidine gluconate solution 20% (≡ 4% chlorhexidine gluconate), perfumed, in a surfactant solution, net price 250 mL = £1.05; 500 mL = £1.54, 5 litres = £12.11

Use instead of soap for pre-operative hand and skin preparation and for general hand and skin disinfection

Hibisol® (SSL)

Solution, chlorhexidine gluconate solution 2.5% (≡ 0.5% chlorhexidine gluconate), in isopropyl alcohol 70% with emollients. Net price 500 mL = £1.60

To be used undiluted for hand and skin disinfection

Hibitane Obstetric® (Bioglan)

Cream, chlorhexidine gluconate solution 5% (≡ 1% chlorhexidine gluconate), in a pourable water-miscible basis. Net price 250 mL = 98p.

For use in obstetrics and gynaecology as an antiseptic and lubricant (for application to skin around vulva and perineum or to hands of midwife or doctor)

Hydrex® (Adams Hlth)

Solution, chlorhexidine gluconate solution 2.5% (≡ chlorhexidine gluconate 0.5%), in an alcoholic solution, net price 600 mL (clear) = £1.40; 600 mL (pink) = £1.40; 600 mL (blue) = £1.50

For pre-operative skin disinfection

Note. Flammable

Surgical scrub, chlorhexidine gluconate 4% in an alcoholic solution, net price 250 mL = 95p, 500 mL = £1.45, 5 litre = £11.60

For pre-operative hand and skin preparation and for general hand disinfection

pHiso-Med® (Sanofi-Synthelabo) [NHS]

Solution, chlorhexidine gluconate 4% in an emulsion basis. Net price 150 mL = £4.64.

For use as a soap substitute in acne and seborrhoeic conditions; for bathing babies in maternity units (as 1 in 10 dilution) to prevent cross-infection and for pre-operative hand and skin preparation

Sterexidine® (Galen)

Solution (sterile), chlorhexidine gluconate 0.02%. Net price 150 mL = 83p

For disinfection and wound cleansing

Steripod® Chlorhexidine (SSL)

Steripod® Chlorhexidine solution, chlorhexidine gluconate solution 0.25% (≡ chlorhexidine gluconate 0.05%). Net price 25 × 20-mL vials = £6.52

For swabbing wounds and burns

Unisept® (SSL)

Solution (sterile), pink, chlorhexidine gluconate 0.05%. Net price 25 × 25-mL sachet = £5.59; 6 × 100-mL sachet = £4.10

For cleansing and disinfecting wounds and burns and swabbing in obstetrics

■ With cetrimide

Steripod® Chlorhexidine/Cetrimide (SSL)

Steripod® Chlorhexidine/Cetrimide solution, chlorhexidine gluconate solution 0.075% (≡ chlorhexidine gluconate 0.015%), cetrimide 0.15%. Net price 25 × 20-mL vials = £6.52

For cleansing and disinfecting wounds and burns

Tisept® (SSL)

Solution (sterile), yellow, chlorhexidine gluconate 0.015%, cetrimide 0.15%. Net price 25 × 25-mL sachet = £5.59; 6 × 100-mL sachet = £4.10

To be used undiluted for general skin disinfection and wound cleansing

Travasept 100® (Baxter)

Solution (sterile), yellow, chlorhexidine acetate 0.015%, cetrimide 0.15%. Net price 500 mL = 72p; 1000 mL = 77p

To be used undiluted in skin disinfection such as wound cleansing and obstetrics

Concentrates

Hibitane 5% Concentrate® (SSL)

Solution, red, chlorhexidine gluconate solution 25% (≡ 5% chlorhexidine gluconate), in a perfumed aqueous solution. Net price 5 litres = £10.94

To be used diluted 1 in 10 (0.5%) with alcohol 70% for pre-operative skin preparation, or 1 in 100 (0.05%) with water for general skin disinfection

Note. Alcoholic solutions not suitable before diathermy (see Alcohol, above)

■ With cetrimide

Hibicet Hospital Concentrate® (SSL)

Solution, orange, chlorhexidine gluconate solution 7.5% (≡ chlorhexidine gluconate 1.5%), cetrimide 15%. Net price 5 litres = £8.16

To be used diluted 1 in 100 (1%) to 1 in 30 with water for skin disinfection and wound cleansing, and diluted 1 in 30 in alcohol 70% for pre-operative skin preparation

Note. Alcoholic solutions not suitable before diathermy (see Alcohol, above)

13.11.3 Cationic surfactants and soaps

CETRIMIDE

Indications: skin disinfection

Cautions: avoid contact with eyes; avoid use in body cavities

Side-effects: skin irritation and occasionally sensitisation

Preparations
Ingredient of *Hibicet Hospital Concentrate®*, *Steripod®*, *Tisept®*, and *Travasept® 100*, see above

SOFT SOAP

Indications: removal of adherent crusts

Soap Spirit, BP, soft soap 65% in alcohol (90%). Net price 100 mL = 41p

13.11.4 Chlorine and iodine

CHLORINATED SOLUTIONS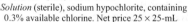

Cautions: bleaches fabric; irritant (protect surrounding tissues with soft paraffin)

Chlorasol® (SSL) NHS ◣

Solution (sterile), sodium hypochlorite, containing 0.3% available chlorine. Net price 25 × 25-mL sachets = £8.49

Irritant therefore no longer recommended

◣ denotes preparations that are considered to be less suitable for prescribing (see p. vi)

IODINE COMPOUNDS

Indications: skin disinfection

Cautions: pregnancy, breast-feeding; broken skin (see below); renal impairment (see Appendix 3)

LARGE OPEN WOUNDS. The application of povidone-iodine to large wounds or severe burns may produce systemic adverse effects such as metabolic acidosis, hypernatraemia and impairment of renal function.

Contra-indications: avoid regular use in patients with thyroid disorders or those receiving lithium therapy

Side-effects: rarely sensitivity; may interfere with thyroid function tests

Betadine® (SSL)

Antiseptic paint, povidone–iodine 10% in an alcoholic solution. Net price 8 mL (with applicator brush) = £1.01

Apply undiluted to minor wounds and infections, twice daily

Alcoholic solution, povidone–iodine 10%. Net price 500 mL = £1.91

To be applied undiluted in pre- and post-operative skin disinfection; CHILD not recommended for regular use in neonates (and contra-indicated in very low birthweight infants)

Note. Flammable—caution in procedures involving hot wire cautery and diathermy

Antiseptic solution, povidone–iodine 10% in aqueous solution. Net price 500 mL = £1.75

To be applied undiluted in pre- and post-operative skin disinfection; CHILD not recommended for regular use in neonates (and contra-indicated in very low birthweight infants)

Note. Not for body cavity irrigation

Dry powder spray, povidone–iodine 2.5% in a pressurised aerosol unit. Net price 150-g unit = £2.79

For skin disinfection, particularly minor wounds and infections; CHILD under 2 years not recommended

Note. Not for use in serous cavities

Ointment, povidone–iodine 10%, in a water-miscible basis, net price 20 g = £1.39; 80 g = £2.79

For skin disinfection, particularly minor wounds and infections; CHILD under 2 years not recommended

Excipients: none as listed in section 13.1.3

Skin cleanser solution, povidone–iodine 4%, in a surfactant basis. Net price 250 mL = £2.14

For infective conditions of the skin. Retain on skin for 3–5 minutes before rinsing; repeat twice daily; CHILD under 2 years not recommended

Surgical scrub, povidone–iodine 7.5%, in a non-ionic surfactant basis. Net price 500 mL = £1.58

To be used as a pre-operative scrub for hands and skin; CHILD not recommended for regular use in neonates (and contra-indicated in very low birthweight infants)

Savlon® Dry Antiseptic (Novartis Consumer Health)

Powder spray, povidone–iodine 1.14% in a pressurised aerosol unit. Net price 50-mL unit = £2.20

For minor wounds

Videne® (Adams Hlth)

Alcoholic tincture, povidone–iodine 10%, net price 500 mL = £1.68

To be applied undiluted in pre-operative skin disinfection

Antiseptic solution, povidone–iodine 10% in aqueous solution, net price 500 mL = £1.54

To be applied undiluted in pre-operative skin disinfection and general antisepsis

Surgical scrub, povidone–iodine 7.5% in aqueous solution, net price 500 mL = £1.45

To be used as a pre-operative scrub for hand and skin disinfection

13.11.5 Phenolics

HEXACHLOROPHENE
(Hexachlorophane)

Indications: see under preparations (below)

Contra-indications: avoid use on badly burned or excoriated skin; pregnancy (Appendix 4); children under 2 years except on medical advice

Side-effects: sensitivity; rarely photosensitivity

Ster-Zac Powder® (SSL)
Dusting-powder, hexachlorophene 0.33%, zinc oxide 3%, talc 88.67%, starch 8% (sterile). Net price 30 g = 83p
Excipients: include fragrance
Prevention of neonatal staphylococcal infection, apply to cord immediately after ligature, and to perineum, buttocks, flexures, and axillae; repeat at each nappy change until stump drops away and wound healed
Adjunct for treatment of recurrent furunculosis and for prevention and treatment of pressure sores, apply to affected area (and surrounding skin) daily

TRICLOSAN

Indications: skin disinfection
Cautions: avoid contact with eyes

Aquasept® (SSL)
Skin cleanser, blue, triclosan 2%. Net price 28.5 mL = 33p; 100 mL = 90p; 250 mL = £1.10; 500 mL = £1.68
For disinfection and pre-operative hand preparation
Excipients: include chlorocresol, edetic acid (EDTA), propylene glycol, fragrance

Manusept® (SSL)
Antibacterial hand rub, triclosan 0.5%, isopropyl alcohol 70%. Net price 100 mL = 59p; 250 mL = £1.07; 500 mL = £1.56
For disinfection and pre-operative hand preparation
Excipients: none as listed in section 13.1.3
Caution: flammable

Ster-Zac Bath Concentrate® (SSL)
Solution, triclosan 2%. Net price 28.5 mL = 40p; 500 mL = £4.47
For prevention of cross-infection use 28.5 mL/bath
Excipients: include edetic acid (EDTA)

13.11.6 **Astringents, oxidisers, and dyes**

ALUMINIUM ACETATE

Indications: exudative eczematous reactions and wounds

Aluminium Acetate Lotion, aluminium acetate solution 5 mL, purified water, freshly boiled and cooled, to 100 mL. It should be freshly prepared.
To be used undiluted as a wet dressing
Note. Aluminium acetate solution (13%) for the preparation of aluminium acetate lotion (0.65%) is available from Martindale (special order)

CRYSTAL VIOLET

(Methylrosanilinium Chloride; Gentian violet)
Indications: see below
Cautions: stains clothes and skin
Side-effects: mucosal ulcerations

Crystal Violet Paint, BP1980, crystal violet 0.5%, in purified water, freshly boiled and cooled.
To be used undiluted
Note. Licensed for topical application on unbroken skin only; no longer recommended for application to mucous membranes or open wounds; restrictions do not apply to use for skin marking prior to surgery

HYDROGEN PEROXIDE

Indications: see under preparations below
Cautions: large or deep wounds; avoid on healthy skin and eyes; bleaches fabric; incompatible with products containing iodine or potassium permanganate

Hydrogen Peroxide Solution, BP
Solution 6% (20 vols). Net price 100 mL = 16p
Solution 3% (10 vols). Net price 100 mL = 19p
For skin disinfection, particularly cleansing and deodorising wounds and ulcers
Note. The BP directs that when hydrogen peroxide is prescribed, hydrogen peroxide solution 6% (20 vols) should be dispensed.
IMPORTANT. Strong solutions of hydrogen peroxide which contain 27% (90 vols) and 30% (100 vols) are only for the preparation of weaker solutions

Crystacide® (Bioglan)
Cream, hydrogen peroxide 1%, net price 10 g = £2.85, 25 g = £4.78
Superficial bacterial skin infection, apply 2-3 times daily for up to 3 weeks
Excipients: include edetic acid (EDTA), propylene glycol
Hioxyl® see section 13.11.7

POTASSIUM PERMANGANATE

Indications: cleansing and deodorising suppurating eczematous reactions and wounds
Cautions: irritant to mucous membranes; stains skin and clothing
Administration: wet dressings or baths, approx. 0.01% solution

Potassium Permanganate Solution, potassium permanganate 0.1% (1 in 1000) in water
To be diluted 1 in 10 to provide a 0.01% (1 in 10 000) solution

Permitabs® (Bioglan)
Solution tablets, for preparation of topical solution, potassium permanganate 400 mg. Net price 30-tab pack = £4.04
1 tablet dissolved in 4 litres of water provides a 0.01% (1 in 10 000) solution

 13.11.7 **Preparations for promotion of wound healing**

Desloughing agents

Desloughing agents for ulcers are second-line treatment and the underlying causes should be treated. The main beneficial effect is removal of slough and clot and the ablation of local infection. Preparations which absorb or help promote the removal of exudate may also help (Appendix 8). It should be noted that substances applied to an open area are easily absorbed and perilesional skin is easily sensitised. Gravitational dermatitis may be complicated by superimposed contact sensitivity to substances such as neomycin or lanolin. Enzyme preparations such as streptokinase-streptodornase or alternatively dextranomer (Appendix 8) are designed for sloughing ulcers. Sterile larvae (maggots) (*LarvE®*, Biosurgical Research Unit) are used in some centres for the management of sloughing wounds.

Aserbine® (Goldshield)
Cream, benzoic acid 0.025%, malic acid 0.375%, propylene glycol 1.75%, salicylic acid 0.006%. Net price 100 g = £2.41
Apply liberally to wound surface (best results with twice daily wound dressing but more frequent changes may be needed)
Excipients: include hydroxybenzoates (parabens)
Solution, benzoic acid 0.15%, malic acid 2.25%, propylene glycol 40%, salicylic acid 0.0375%. Net price 500 mL = £3.61
Use as wash before each application of cream (or use as wet dressing)
Excipients: include fragrance

Hioxyl® (Adams Hlth)
Cream, hydrogen peroxide (stabilised) 1.5%. Net price 25 g = £2.16; 100 g = £6.76
For leg ulcers and pressure sores
Excipients: include cetostearyl alcohol
Apply when necessary and if necessary cover with a dressing

Varidase Topical® (Lederle) [PoM]
Powder, streptokinase 100 000 units, streptodornase 25 000 units. For preparing solutions for topical use. Net price per vial = £9.44; with sterile physiological saline 20 mL (combi-pack) = £9.92
Excipients: none as listed in section 13.1.3
Reconstitute with 20 mL sterile physiological saline (or water for injections) and apply as wet dressing 1–2 times daily; cover with semi-occlusive dressing; irrigate lesion thoroughly with physiological saline and remove loosened material before next application; also used to dissolve clots in the bladder or urinary catheters; *contra-indicated*: active haemorrhage; *side-effects*: infrequent allergic reactions (reduced by careful and frequent removal of exudate and thorough irrigation with physiological saline); transient burning reported

Growth factor

A topical preparation of **becaplermin** (recombinant human platelet-derived growth factor) is licensed as an adjunctive treatment of full-thickness, neuropathic, diabetic ulcers.

Regranex® (Janssen-Cilag) ▼ [PoM]
Gel, becaplermin (recombinant human platelet-derived growth factor) 0.01%, net price 15 g = £275
Excipients: include hydroxybenzoates
Full-thickness, neuropathic, diabetic ulcers (no larger than 5 cm^2), apply thin layer daily and cover with gauze dressing moistened with physiological saline; max. duration of treatment 20 weeks (reassess if no healing after first 10 weeks)
Cautions: malignant disease; avoid on sites with infection, malignancy, peripheral arteriopathy, or osteomyelitis
Side-effects: irritation, rarely bullous eruption, oedema

13.12 Antiperspirants

Aluminium chloride is a potent antiperspirant used in the treatment of severe hyperhidrosis. Aluminium salts are also incorporated in preparations used for minor fungal skin infections associated with hyperhidrosis. **Glycopyrronium bromide** is licensed for use topically, as a 0.05% solution in the iontophoretic treatment of hyperhidrosis of plantar and palmar areas. Botulinum A toxin-haem-agglutinin complex (section 4.9.3) is licensed for use intradermally for severe hyperhidrosis of the axillae unresponsive to topical antiperspirant or antihidrotic treatment.

ALUMINIUM SALTS

Indications: see under Administration below
Cautions: avoid contact with eyes or mucous membranes; avoid use on broken or irritated skin; do not shave axillae or use depilatories within 12 hours of application; avoid contact with clothing
Side-effects: skin irritation
Administration: hyperhidrosis affecting axillae, hands or feet, apply liquid formulation at night to dry skin, wash off the following morning, initially daily then reduce frequency as condition improves—do not bathe immediately before use;
Hyperhidrosis, bromidrosis, intertrigo, and prevention of tinea pedis and related conditions, apply powder to dry skin

Anhydrol Forte® (Dermal)
Solution (= application), aluminium chloride hexahydrate 20% in an alcoholic basis. Net price 60-mL bottle with roll-on applicator = £2.82. Label: 15
Excipients: none as listed in section 13.1.3

¹Driclor® (Stiefel)
Application, aluminium chloride hexahydrate 20% in an alcoholic basis. Net price 60-mL bottle with roll-on applicator = £2.82. Label: 15
1. A 30-mL pack is on sale to the public (*Driclor® Solution*)
Excipients: none as listed in section 13.1.3

ZeaSORB® (Stiefel)
Dusting powder, aldioxa 0.22%, chloroxylenol 0.5%, net price 50 g = £2.15
Excipients: include fragrance

GLYCOPYRRONIUM BROMIDE

Indications: iontophoretic treatment of hyperhidrosis; other indications section 15.1.3
Cautions: see section 15.1.3 (but poorly absorbed and systemic effects unlikely)
Contra-indications: see section 15.1.3 (but poorly absorbed and systemic effects unlikely); infections affecting the treatment site
Side-effects: see section 15.1.3 (but poorly absorbed and systemic effects unlikely), tingling at administration site
Administration: consult product literature; only 1 site to be treated at a time, max. 2 sites treated in any 24 hours, treatment not to be repeated within 7 days

Robinul® (Anpharm) [PoM]
Powder, glycopyrronium bromide, net price 5 g = £132.54

13.13 Wound management products and Elastic Hosiery

Preparations
See Appendix 8

13.14 Topical circulatory preparations

These preparations are used to improve circulation in conditions such as bruising, superficial thrombophlebitis, chilblains and varicose veins but are of little value. Chilblains are best managed by avoidance of exposure to cold; neither systemic nor topical vasodilator therapy is established as being effective. Sclerotherapy of varicose veins is described in section 2.13.

Rubefacients are described in section 10.3.2.

Hirudoid® (Sankyo) ▱
 Cream, heparinoid 0.3% in a vanishing-cream basis. Net price 50 g = £1.35
 Excipients: include cetostearyl alcohol, hydroxybenzoates (parabens)
 Gel, heparinoid 0.3%. Net price 50 g = £1.35
 Excipients: include propylene glycol, fragrance
 Apply up to 4 times daily in superficial soft-tissue injuries and superficial thrombophlebitis

Lasonil® (Bayer Consumer Care) ▱
 Ointment, heparinoid 0.8% in white soft paraffin, net price 40 g = £1.08
 Excipients: include wool fat derivative
 Apply 2–3 times daily in superficial soft-tissue injuries

> ▱ denotes preparations that are considered to be less suitable for prescribing (see p. vi)

14: Immunological products and vaccines

14.1   Active immunity

Vaccines may consist of:
1. a *live attenuated* form of a virus (e.g. rubella or measles vaccine) or bacteria (e.g. BCG vaccine)
2. *inactivated* preparations of the virus (e.g. influenza vaccine) or bacteria, or
3. *extracts of* or *detoxified exotoxins* produced by a micro-organism (e.g. tetanus vaccine).

They stimulate production of antibodies and other components of the immune mechanism.

For **live attenuated** vaccines, immunisation is generally achieved with a single dose (but 3 doses are required with oral poliomyelitis and oral typhoid vaccines). Live attenuated vaccines usually produce a durable immunity but not always as long as that of the natural infection. When two live virus vaccines are required (and are not available as a combined preparation) they should be given either simultaneously at different sites or with an interval of at least 3 weeks.

Inactivated vaccines may require a primary series of injections of vaccine to produce adequate antibody response and in most cases booster (reinforcing) injections are required; the duration of immunity varies from months to many years.

Extracts of or **detoxified exotoxins** are more immunogenic if adsorbed onto an adjuvant (such as aluminium hydroxide). They require a primary series of injections followed by booster doses.

Guidelines in this chapter reflect those in the handbook *Immunisation against Infectious Disease* (1996), which in turn reflects the advice of the Joint Committee on Vaccination and Immunisation (JCVI). Copies can be obtained from:

The Stationery Office
PO Box 29, Norwich NR3 1GN

Telephone orders, 0870 600 5522
Fax: 0870 600 5533
www.thestationeryoffice.com

SIDE-EFFECTS. Some vaccines (e.g. poliomyelitis) produce very few reactions, while others (e.g. measles and rubella) may produce a very mild form of the disease. Some vaccines may produce discomfort at the site of injection and mild fever and malaise. Occasionally there are more serious untoward reactions and these should always be reported to the CSM. Anaphylactic reactions are very rare but can be fatal (see section 3.4.3 for management). For full details of side-effects, the product literature should always be consulted.

CONTRA-INDICATIONS. Most vaccines have some basic contra-indication to their use, and the product literature should always be consulted. In general, vaccination should be postponed if the subject is suffering from an *acute illness*. Minor infections without fever or systemic upset are not contra-indications. A definite severe reaction to a preceding dose is a contra-indication to further doses.

Some viral vaccines contain small quantities of antibacterials such as neomycin or polymyxin B (or both); such vaccines may need to be withheld from individuals who are *sensitive to the antibacterial*. *Hypersensitivity to egg* contra-indicates influenza vaccine (residual egg protein present) and, if evidence of previous anaphylactic reaction, also yellow fever vaccine.

Live vaccines should not be routinely administered to *pregnant women* because of possible harm to the fetus but where there is a significant risk of exposure (e.g. to poliomyelitis or yellow fever), the need for vaccination outweighs any possible risk to the fetus. Live vaccines should not be given to individuals with *impaired immune response*, whether caused by disease (for special reference to *HIV infection*, see below) or as a result of radiotherapy or treatment with high doses of corticosteroids or other immunosuppressive drugs[1,2]. They should not be given to those suffering from *malignant conditions* such as leukaemia and tumours of the reticuloendothelial system[2].

The intramuscular route should not be used in patients with bleeding disorders such as haemophilia or thrombocytopenia.

Note. The Department of Health has advised *against the use of jet guns* for vaccination owing to the risk of transmitting blood-borne infections, such as HIV.

VACCINES AND HIV INFECTION. The Department of Health has advised that HIV-positive subjects with or without symptoms can receive the following live vaccines:
measles[2] (or MMR), mumps, poliomyelitis[3], rubella;
and the following inactivated vaccines:
cholera, diphtheria, haemophilus influenzae type b, hepatitis A, hepatitis B, influenza, meningococcal, pertussis, pneumococcal, poliomyelitis[3], rabies, tetanus, typhoid (injection).
HIV-positive subjects should **not** receive:
BCG, yellow fever[4], typhoid (oral)
Note. The above advice differs from that for other immunocompromised patients.

1. Live vaccines should be postponed until at least 3 months after stopping corticosteroids and 6 months after stopping chemotherapy.
2. Consideration should be given to use of normal immunoglobulin after exposure to measles (see p. 594) and to varicella-zoster immunoglobulin after exposure to chickenpox or herpes zoster (see p. 595).
3. Virus may be excreted for longer periods than in normal subjects; contacts should be warned of this and of need for washing hands after changing a vaccinated infant's nappies; HIV-positive contacts are at greater risk than normal contacts. For HIV-positive symptomatic subjects inactivated poliomyelitis vaccine may be used at discretion of clinician.
4. Because insufficient evidence of safety.

Immunisation schedule

Vaccines for the childhood immunisation schedule should be obtained **via local health authorities** or **direct from Farillon**—not for prescribing on FP10 (GP10 in Scotland) since not available to pharmacies.

During first year of life

Adsorbed Diphtheria, Tetanus and [whole-cell] Pertussis Vaccine [DTwP]

3 doses at intervals of 4 weeks; first dose at 2 months of age

Primary immunisation should continue to be with diphtheria, tetanus and *whole-cell* pertussis [DTwP] vaccine unless whole-cell pertussis is contra-indicated (because of previous reaction to the whole-cell component), in which case adsorbed diphtheria, tetanus and pertussis (acellular component) vaccine may be used

plus

Haemophilus Influenzae type b Vaccine (Hib)

3 doses at intervals of 4 weeks; first dose at 2 months of age

plus

Meningococcal Group C Conjugate Vaccine

3 doses at intervals of 4 weeks; first dose at 2 months of age

plus

Poliomyelitis Vaccine, Live (Oral)

3 doses at intervals of 4 weeks; first dose at 2 months of age

BCG Vaccine (for neonates at risk only)

See section 14.4, BCG Vaccines

During second year of life

Measles, Mumps and Rubella Vaccine, Live (MMR)

Single dose at 12–15 months of age

Haemophilus Influenzae type b Vaccine (Hib) (if not previously immunised)

Single dose at 13 months–4 years of age (over 4 years, see section 14.4, Haemophilus Influenzae type b Vaccine)

Before school or nursery school entry

Adsorbed Diphtheria, Tetanus and Pertussis (Acellular Component) Vaccine [DTaP]

Single booster dose

Pre-school booster should comprise diphtheria, tetanus and *acellular pertussis* [DTaP] vaccine (the vaccine with whole-cell pertussis is **not** recommended because of increased reactions in older children)

Preferably allow interval of at least 3 years after completing basic course; give at same session as MMR Vaccine but use separate syringe and needle, and give in different limb

plus

Poliomyelitis Vaccine, Live (Oral)

Single booster dose

Preferably allow interval of at least 3 years after completing basic course

plus

Measles, Mumps and Rubella Vaccine, Live (MMR)

Single booster dose

Give at same session as Adsorbed Diphtheria and Tetanus Vaccine but use separate syringe and needle; give MMR first (less painful) and use different limb—alternatively, second appointment can be made

Between 10–14 years of age

BCG Vaccine (for tuberculin-negative children)

Single dose

May be given simultaneously with another live vaccine; otherwise an interval of at least 3 weeks should be allowed between the two

Before leaving school or before employment or further education

Adsorbed Diphtheria and Tetanus Vaccine for Adults and Adolescents

Single booster dose

Adsorbed Diphtheria and Tetanus Vaccine, DT/Vac/Ads(Child), **not** to be used for children aged over 10 years and adults

plus

Poliomyelitis Vaccine, Live (Oral)

Single booster dose

During adult life

Poliomyelitis Vaccine, Live (Oral) (if not previously immunised)

3 doses at intervals of 4 weeks

No adult should remain unimmunised; health care workers in possible contact with poliomyelitis, and travellers to areas other than Australia, New Zealand, Northern and Western Europe and The Americas (including the Caribbean) require booster dose if they have not received immunisation within last 10 years

Rubella Vaccine, Live (for susceptible women of child-bearing age)

Single dose

Women of child-bearing age should be tested for rubella antibodies and offered rubella immunisation if sero-negative—exclude pregnancy before immunisation, but see also section 14.4, Rubella Vaccine

Adsorbed Tetanus Vaccine (if not previously immunised)

3 doses at intervals of 4 weeks

Booster dose 10 years after primary course and again 10 years later maintains satisfactory level of protection—if diphtheria cover also needed give Adsorbed Diphtheria and Tetanus Vaccine for Adults and Adolescents

Adsorbed Diphtheria Vaccine for Adults and Adolescents (if not previously immunised)

3 doses at intervals of 4 weeks

Booster dose 10 years after primary course. If tetanus cover also needed give Adsorbed Diphtheria and Tetanus Vaccine for Adults and Adolescents

High-risk groups

For information on high-risk groups, see section 14.4 under individual vaccines

Hepatitis A Vaccine

Hepatitis B Vaccine

Influenza Vaccine

Pneumococcal Vaccine

Post-immunisation pyrexia—Joint Committee on Vaccination and Immunisation recommendation. The doctor should advise the parent that if pyrexia develops after childhood immunisation the child can be given a dose of paracetamol followed, if necessary, by a second dose 4 to 6 hours later. The dose of paracetamol for post-immunisation pyrexia in an infant aged 2–3 months is 60 mg; an oral syringe can be obtained from any pharmacy to give the small dose-volume required. The doctor should warn the parent that if the pyrexia persists after the second dose medical advice should be sought.

For recommendation relating to advice after MMR vaccine, see p. 587

For full range of paracetamol doses, see p. 210

14.2   Passive immunity

Immunity with immediate protection against certain infective organisms can be obtained by injecting preparations made from the plasma of immune individuals with adequate levels of antibody to the disease for which protection is sought (see under Immunoglobulins, section 14.5). This passive immunity lasts only a few weeks; where necessary passive immunisation can be repeated.

Antibodies of human origin are usually termed *immunoglobulins*. The term *antiserum* is applied to material prepared in animals. Because of serum sickness and other allergic-type reactions that may follow injections of antisera, this therapy has been replaced wherever possible by the use of immunoglobulins. Reactions are theoretically possible after injection of human immunoglobulins but reports of such reactions are very rare.

14.3   Storage and use

Care must be taken to store all vaccines and other immunological products under the conditions recommended in the product literature, otherwise the preparation may become ineffective. **Refrigerated storage** is usually necessary; many vaccines need to be stored at 2–8°C and not allowed to freeze. Vaccines should be protected from light. Unused vaccine in multidose vials without preservative (most live virus vaccines) should be discarded within 1 hour of first use; those containing a preservative (including oral poliomyelitis vaccine) should be discarded within 3 hours or at the end of a session. Unused vaccines should be disposed of by incineration at a registered disposal contractor.

Particular attention must be paid to instructions on the use of diluents. Vaccines which are liquid suspensions or are reconstituted before use should be adequately shaken to ensure uniformity of the material to be injected.

14.4   Vaccines and antisera

AVAILABILITY. Anthrax, rabies, and yellow fever vaccines, botulism antitoxin, and snake and spider venom antitoxins are available from local designated holding centres. Details of names, addresses, and telephone numbers of holding centres are given in:
The Health Service Supply Purchasing Guide, section D pp. 1101–1199

For antivenom, see Emergency Treatment of Poisoning, p. 29

Enquiries for vaccines not available commercially can also be made to
Immunisation and Communicable Diseases Branch
Department of Health
Skipton House
80 London Road
London SE1 6LH
Tel (020) 7972 1522

In Scotland information about availability of vaccines can be obtained from the Chief Administrative Pharmaceutical Officer of the local Health Board. In Wales enquiries should be directed to the Welsh Office, Cathays Park, Cardiff CF1 3NQ (Tel (029) 2082 5111, extn 4658) and in Northern Ireland the Regional Pharmacist (procurement co-ordination), United Hospitals Trust, Pharmacy Dept, Whiteabbey Hospital, Doagh Road, Newtownabbey BT37 9RH (Tel (028) 908 65181 ext 2386).

For further details of availability, see under individual vaccines.

Anthrax vaccine

Anthrax immunisation is indicated for individuals who handle infected animals, for those exposed to imported infected animal products, and for laboratory staff who work with *Bacillus anthracis*.

In the event of possible contact with *B. anthracis*, post-exposure immunisation may be indicated, in addition to antimicrobial prophylaxis (section 5.1.12). Advice on the use of anthrax vaccine must be obtained from the Public Health Laboratory Service Communicable Disease Surveillance Centre (PHLS-CDSC) (tel. 020 8200 6868)

The vaccine is the alum precipitate of an antigen from *B. anthracis* and, following the primary course of injections, booster doses should be given at about yearly intervals.

Anthrax Vaccine PoM

Dose: initial course 3 doses of 0.5 mL *by intramuscular injection* at intervals of 3 weeks followed by a 4th dose after an interval of 6 months; a 5th dose 1 year after exposure recommended for post-exposure prophylaxis
Booster doses: 0.5 mL annually
Note. advice on post-exposure prophylaxis must be obtained from PHLS-CDSC
Available from Public Health Laboratory Service

BCG vaccines

BCG (Bacillus Calmette-Guérin) is a live attenuated strain derived from *Mycobacterium bovis* which stimulates the development of hypersensitivity to *M. tuberculosis*. BCG vaccine should be given intradermally by operators skilled in the technique (see below).

Within 2–6 weeks a small swelling appears at the injection site which progresses to a papule or to a benign ulcer about 10 mm in diameter and heals in 6–12 weeks. A dry dressing may be used if the ulcer discharges, but air should **not** be excluded.

> The CSM has reported that serious reactions with BCG are uncommon and most often consist of prolonged ulceration or subcutaneous abscess formation due to faulty injection technique.

BCG is recommended for the following groups if BCG immunisation, as evidenced by a characteristic scar, has not previously been carried out and they are negative for tuberculoprotein hypersensitivity:

- contacts of those with active respiratory tuberculosis;

- immigrants (including infants and children) from countries with a high incidence of tuberculosis should be immunised without delay. Their infants born in the UK should also be immunised within a few days of birth, or at two months of age at the same time as the first dose of routine childhood vaccines;

- health service staff (including medical students, hospital medical staff, nurses, physiotherapists, radiographers, technical staff in pathology departments and any others considered to be at special risk because of the likelihood of contact with infective patients or their sputum; particularly important to test staff in contact with the immunocompromised, e.g. in transplant, oncology and HIV units, and staff in maternity and paediatric departments);

- children between 10 and 14 years of age (see schedule, section 14.1);

- veterinary and other staff who handle animal species known to be susceptible to tuberculosis;

- staff working in prisons, in residential homes and in hostels for refugees and the homeless;

- those intending to stay for more than 1 month in countries with a high incidence of tuberculosis (section 14.6);

- newly-born infants, children or adults where the parents or the adults request immunisation;

Apart from infants of up to 3 months, any person being considered for BCG immunisation must first be given a skin test for hypersensitivity to tuberculoprotein (see under Diagnostic agents, below).

BCG vaccine may be given simultaneously with another live vaccine (see also section 14.1), but if they are not given at the same time, an interval of at least 3 weeks should normally be allowed between them. However, when BCG is given to infants, there is no need to delay the primary immunisations, including poliomyelitis.

See section 14.1 for general contra-indications. BCG is also contra-indicated in subjects with generalised septic skin conditions (in the case of eczema, a vaccination site free from lesions should be chosen).

Bladder instillations of BCG are licensed for the management of bladder carcinoma (section 8.2.4).

For advice on chemoprophylaxis against tuberculosis, see section 5.1.9.

■ Intradermal

Bacillus Calmette-Guérin Vaccine PoM BCG Vaccine, Dried Tub/Vac/BCG. A freeze-dried preparation of live bacteria of a strain derived from the bacillus of Calmette and Guérin.

Dose: by intradermal injection, 0.1 mL (INFANT under 3 months 0.05 mL)

Available from health authorities or direct from Farillon

INTRADERMAL INJECTION TECHNIQUE. After swabbing with spirit and allowing to dry, skin is stretched between thumb and forefinger and needle (size 25G or 26G) inserted (bevel upwards) for about 2 mm into superficial layers of dermis (almost parallel with surface). Needle should be short with short bevel (can usually be seen through epidermis during insertion). Raised blanched bleb showing tips of hair follicles is sign of correct injection; 7 mm bleb ≡ 0.1 mL injection; if considerable resistance not felt, needle is removed and reinserted before giving more vaccine.

Injection site is at insertion of deltoid muscle onto humerus (sites higher on arm more likely to lead to keloid formation); tip of shoulder should be **avoided**; for cosmetic reasons, upper and lateral surface of thigh may be preferred and this is an acceptable alternative.

■ Percutaneous

The percutaneous multiple puncture technique is an acceptable alternative **only** for young infants in whom the technique of intradermal injection may be difficult (18–20 puncture points are required)

Bacillus Calmette-Guérin Vaccine, Percutaneous Tub/Vac/BCG(Perc) PoM A preparation of live bacteria of a strain derived from the bacillus of Calmette and Guérin (**important:** this preparation must **not** be confused with the intradermal preparation)

Dose: by percutaneous administration, about 0.03 mL but only recommended as an alternative for infants, see notes above

Available from health authorities or direct from Farillon

DIAGNOSTIC AGENTS. In the *Mantoux test,* the diagnostic dose is by intradermal injection of Tuberculin Purified Protein Derivative (PPD):

Routine
10 units PPD i.e. 0.1 mL of 100 units/mL (1 in 1000)

Special (hypersensitive or TB suspected)
1 unit PPD i.e. 0.1 mL of 10 units/mL (1 in 10 000)

Special (low sensitivity)
100 units PPD i.e. 0.1 mL of 1000 units/mL (1 in 100)

In the *Heaf test* (multiple puncture) a solution containing Tuberculin Purified Protein Derivative 100 000 units/mL is used; 1 mL is sufficient for up to about 20 tests.

Note. Tuberculin testing should not be carried out within 4 weeks of receiving a live viral vaccine since response to tuberculin may be inhibited.

Tuberculin PPD PoM Prepared from the heat treated products of growth and lysis of the appropriate species of mycobacterium, and containing 100 000 units/mL, net price 1-mL amp = £5.89. Also available diluted 1 in 100 (1000 units/mL), 1 in 1000 (100 units/mL), and 1 in 10 000 (10 units/mL), net price 1 mL (all) = £2.22

Available from health authorities or direct from Farillon

Botulism antitoxin

A trivalent botulism antitoxin is available for the post-exposure prophylaxis of botulism and for the treatment of persons thought to be suffering from botulism. It specifically neutralises the toxins produced by *Clostridium botulinum* types A, B, and E. It is not effective against infantile botulism as the toxin (type A) is seldom, if ever, found in the blood in this type of infection.

Hypersensitivity reactions are a problem. It is essential to read the contra-indications, warnings, and details of sensitivity tests on the package insert. Prior to treatment checks should be made regarding previous administration of any antitoxin and history of any allergic condition, e.g. asthma, hay fever, etc. All patients should be tested for sensitivity (diluting the antitoxin if history of allergy).

Botulism Antitoxin. PoM A preparation containing the specific antitoxic globulins that have the power of neutralising the toxins formed by types A, B, and E of *Clostridium botulinum*.

Note. The BP title Botulinum Antitoxin is not used because the preparation currently available has a higher phenol content (0.45% against 0.25%).

Dose: prophylaxis, *by intramuscular injection*, 20 mL as soon as possible after exposure; treatment, 20 mL (diluted to 100 mL with sodium chloride 0.9%) by slow intravenous infusion followed by 10 mL 2–4 hours later if necessary, and further doses at intervals of 12–24 hours.

Available from local designated centres. For supplies outside working hours apply to other designated centres and, as a last resort, to Department of Health Duty Officer (Tel (020) 7210 3000).

Cholera vaccine

Cholera vaccine contains heat-killed Inaba and Ogawa sub-types of *Vibrio cholerae*, Serovar O1. Cholera vaccine provides little protection and cannot control the spread of the disease; it is no longer available in the UK.

Cholera vaccine is no longer required for international travel. The Department of Health has advised that in the rare circumstance where an unofficial demand may be anticipated, confirmation of non-requirement of cholera vaccine may be given on official notepaper signed and stamped by the medical practitioner.

Travellers to a country where cholera exists should be warned that scrupulous attention to food and water and personal hygiene is **essential**.

Diphtheria vaccines

Protection against diphtheria is essentially due to antitoxin, the production of which is stimulated by vaccines prepared from the toxin of *Corynebacterium diphtheriae*. Adsorbed diphtheria vaccines are recommended for the routine immunisation of babies and are usually given in the form of **adsorbed diphtheria, tetanus, and [whole-cell] pertussis vaccine** (see schedule, section 14.1). Adsorbed diphtheria and tetanus vaccine is used when immunisation against pertussis is contra-indicated.

A booster dose of **adsorbed diphtheria, tetanus and pertussis (acellular component) vaccine** is recommended before school entry (3–5 years of age). This should preferably be given after an interval of at least 3 years from the last dose of the basic course. A further booster dose is now recommended before leaving school; for this purpose **adsorbed diphtheria and tetanus vaccine for adults and adolescents** (a special low-dose version combined in a single injection with tetanus vaccine) is available. For details on booster doses of diphtheria vaccine in a child over 13 years who requires treatment of a tetanus-prone wound, see under Tetanus Vaccines. If there is documented history of a fifth dose of tetanus vaccine having been given when the school-leaving booster dose of adsorbed diphtheria and tetanus vaccine for adults and adolescents is due, then a booster dose of single antigen adsorbed diphtheria vaccine for adults and adolescents should be given instead.

Other booster doses of adsorbed diphtheria vaccine are not recommended as a routine except for staff in contact with diphtheria patients, or handling clinical specimens which may be pathogenic, or working directly with *Corynebacterium diphtheriae;* they should be considered for a booster or for primary immunisation following a risk assessment. A low-dose vaccine, **adsorbed diphtheria vaccine for adults and adolescents**, is available for this purpose; immunity should be checked by antibody testing at least 3 months after completion of immunisation.

Unimmunised contacts of a diphtheria case require a primary course of 3 doses of adsorbed diphtheria vaccine at monthly intervals. *Immunised* contacts require a single booster dose (**important:** adults and children *over 10 years* must be given a **low-dose** vaccine); those also requiring tetanus cover can be given the appropriate strength of adsorbed diphtheria vaccine combined with tetanus vaccine.

Previously immunised travellers to countries where diphtheria is endemic or epidemic require a booster dose if their primary immunisation was more than 10 years ago. *Unimmunised travellers* require a full course of 3 doses at monthly intervals (**important:** adults and children *over 10 years* requiring either a primary course or a booster should be given a **low-dose** vaccine—those also requiring tetanus cover can be given the special low-dose version combined with tetanus vaccine).

See section 14.1 for general contra-indications.

Diphtheria vaccines for children

IMPORTANT. Not recommended for persons *aged 10 years or over* (use diphtheria vaccines for adults and adolescents instead)

■ With tetanus and pertussis (whole-cell)

Adsorbed Diphtheria, Tetanus, and [whole-cell] Pertussis Vaccine DTPer/Vac/Ads, [DTwP] PoM

Injection, suspension of diphtheria formol toxoid, tetanus formol toxoid, and pertussis vaccine adsorbed on a mineral carrier

Dose: primary immunisation of children, *by intramuscu-*

lar or deep subcutaneous injection, 0.5 mL at 2 months followed by second dose after 4 weeks and third dose after another 4 weeks (see schedule, section 14.1)

Available from health authorities or direct from Farillon as Aventis Pasteur brand (excipients include thiomersal)

Note. Adsorbed diphtheria, tetanus and pertussis vaccine is available in combination with Haemophilus influenzae type b vaccine, see under Haemophilus Influenzae type b Vaccine

■ **With tetanus and pertussis (acellular)**

Infanrix® (SmithKline Beecham) ▼ PoM

Injection, suspension of diphtheria toxoid, tetanus toxoid, and acellular pertussis vaccine components adsorbed on a mineral carrier, net price 0.5-mL prefilled syringe = £11.00

Dose: primary immunisation of children, *by deep intramuscular injection* 0.5 mL at 2 months followed by a second dose after 4 weeks and third dose after another 4 weeks (see schedule, section 14.1); booster dose for CHILD up to 6 years previously immunised with 3 doses of diphtheria, tetanus, and pertussis (whole cell or acellular) vaccine, *by deep intramuscular injection*, 0.5 mL

■ **With tetanus**

Adsorbed Diphtheria and Tetanus Vaccine DT/Vac/Ads(Child) PoM

Injection, suspension of diphtheria formol toxoid and tetanus formol toxoid adsorbed on a mineral carrier

Dose: primary immunisation of children omitting pertussis component, *by intramuscular or deep subcutaneous injection*, 0.5 mL at 2 months followed by second dose after 4 weeks and third dose after another 4 weeks (see schedule, section 14.1); booster at school entry (if pertussis not appropriate), 0.5 mL

Available from health authorities or direct from Farillon as Evans Vaccines brand (excipients include thiomersal) or Aventis Pasteur brand (excipients include thiomersal)

Diphtheria vaccines for adolescents and adults

The small quantity of diphtheria toxoid present in the preparations below is sufficient to recall immunity in individuals previously immunised against diphtheria but whose immunity may have diminished with time; it is insufficient to cause the serious reactions that may occur when diphtheria vaccine of conventional formulation is used in an individual who is already immune. The low dose vaccine must be used when immunising adults and children *over 10 years*; may also be given as a booster dose in children under 10 years who have already received a tetanus booster dose [unlicensed indication]. For school leavers a low-dose version combined in a single injection with tetanus vaccine is available (see notes above).

■ **With tetanus**

Adsorbed Diphtheria and Tetanus Vaccine for Adults and Adolescents DT/Vac/Ads(Adult) PoM

Injection, suspension of diphtheria formol toxoid and tetanus formol toxoid adsorbed on a mineral carrier, net price 0.5-mL prefilled syringe = £2.67

Dose: primary immunisation in *patients over 10 years*, *by intramuscular or deep subcutaneous injection*, 3 doses each of 0.5 mL separated by intervals of 4 weeks; booster, 0.5 mL after 10 years

Available from health authorities or direct from Farillon as Aventis Pasteur brand (*Diftavax®*; excipients include thiomersal)

■ **Single antigen**

Adsorbed Diphtheria Vaccine for Adults and Adolescents Dip/Vac/Ads(Adult) PoM

Injection, diphtheria formol toxoid adsorbed on a mineral carrier

Dose: primary immunisation in *patients over 10 years*, *by intramuscular or deep subcutaneous injection*, 3 doses each of 0.5 mL separated by intervals of 1 month; booster, 0.5 mL

Booster in child under 10 years (when tetanus booster already given) [unlicensed use]

Note. Unimmunised adults and children *over 10 years* who are contacts of a diphtheria case or carrier are given the primary immunisation course; immunised adults and children *over 10 years* are given the booster dose.

Available from health authorities or direct from Farillon

Diphtheria antitoxin

Diphtheria antitoxin is used for passive immunisation; it is prepared in horses therefore reactions are common after administration.

It is now only used in suspected cases of diphtheria (without waiting for bacteriological confirmation); tests for hypersensitivity should be first carried out.

It is no longer used for prophylaxis because of the risk of hypersensitivity; unimmunised contacts should be promptly investigated and given erythromycin prophylaxis (section 5.1, table 2) and vaccine (see notes above).

Diphtheria Antitoxin PoM Dip/Ser.

Dose: prophylactic *by intramuscular injection*, 500–2000 units (but **not** used, see notes above); therapeutic 10 000–30 000 units increased to 40 000–100 000 units in severe cases; doses of up to 30 000 units should be given intramuscularly but for those over 40 000 units a portion is given intramuscularly followed by the bulk of the dose intravenously after an interval of ½–2 hours

Note. Children require the same dose as adults, depending on the severity of the case.

Available from Communicable Disease Surveillance Centre (Tel (020) 8200 6868) or in Northern Ireland from Public Health Laboratory, Belfast City Hospital (Tel (028) 9032 9241).

Haemophilus influenzae type B vaccine

Children under the age of 13 months are at high risk of *Haemophilus influenzae* type b infection. **Haemophilus influenzae type b (Hib) vaccine** is a component of the primary course of childhood immunisation (see schedule, section 14.1). The course consists of 3 doses of haemophilus influenzae type b vaccine with an interval of 1 month between each dose. If primary immunisation against diphtheria, tetanus, pertussis and poliomyelitis has already been commenced or completed, children under the age of 13 months should still receive 3 doses of haemophilus influenzae type b vaccine at monthly intervals. Children over the age of 13 months are at a lower risk of infection and, if not previously immunised, need receive only 1 dose of the vaccine. The risk of infection falls sharply after the age of 4 years therefore the vaccine is not normally required for children over 4 years. However, it may be given to those over 4 years who are considered to be at increased risk of invasive *Haemophilus influenzae* type b disease (such as those with sickle cell disease and those receiving treatment for malignancy). Also, asplenic children and adults, irrespective of age or the interval from splenectomy, should receive a single dose of haemophilus influenzae type b vaccine; those under 1 year should be given 3 doses. For elective splenectomy, the vaccine should ideally be given at least 2 weeks before the operation. Side-effects reported include fever, headache, malaise, irritability, prolonged crying, loss of appetite, vomiting, diarrhoea, and rash (including urticaria); convulsions, erythema multiforme, and transient cyanosis of the lower limbs have been reported.

See section 14.1 for general contra-indications

■ Single component

Each single component product may be used to complete a course started with any other single component product listed below

HibTITER® (Wyeth) PoM

Injection, capsular polysaccharide of *Haemophilus influenzae* type b (conjugated to a protein carrier), net price 0.5-mL vial = £10.20

Dose: by intramuscular injection, 0.5 mL; for primary immunisation, 3 doses are required at intervals of 1 month (see schedule, section 14.1)

Note. If required, haemophilus influenzae type b vaccine is available in combination with adsorbed diphtheria, tetanus and pertussis vaccine (see below)

Available, as part of childhood immunisation schedule, from health authorities or Farillon

ACT-HIB® (Aventis Pasteur) PoM

Injection, powder for reconstitution, capsular polysaccharide of *Haemophilus influenzae* type b (conjugated to a protein carrier), net price per vial with diluent (0.5 mL) = £8.83

Dose: by intramuscular or deep subcutaneous injection, 0.5 mL; for primary immunisation, 3 doses are required at intervals of 1 month (see schedule, section 14.1)

Note. If required, haemophilus influenzae type b vaccine is available in combination with adsorbed diphtheria, tetanus and pertussis vaccine (see below); alternatively, *ACT-HIB®* may be reconstituted with 0.5 mL of Aventis Pasteur brand of adsorbed diphtheria, tetanus and pertussis vaccine

Available, as part of childhood immunisation schedule, from health authorities or Farillon

■ With diphtheria, tetanus and pertussis vaccines

Each combined product may be used to complete a course started with any other combined product listed below; **important** see also under Adsorbed Diphtheria, Tetanus and Pertussis Vaccine (p. 582)

ACT-HIB®DTP dc (Aventis Pasteur) ▼ PoM

Injection, powder for reconstitution, capsular polysaccharide of *Haemophilus influenzae* type b (conjugated to a protein carrier) with diluent containing diphtheria toxoid, tetanus toxoid and *Bordetella pertussis* cells, net price per dual-chamber prefilled syringe = £10.41

Excipients: include thiomersal

Dose: CHILD under 4 years, *by intramuscular or deep subcutaneous injection,* 0.5 mL; for primary immunisation, 3 doses are required at intervals of 1 month (see schedule, section 14.1)

Available, as part of childhood immunisation schedule, from health authorities or Farillon

Infanrix®-Hib (SmithKline Beecham) ▼ PoM

Injection, powder for reconstitution, capsular polysaccharide of *Haemophilus influenzae* type b (conjugated to a protein carrier) with diluent con-

taining diphtheria toxoid, tetanus toxoid, and acellular pertussis vaccine adsorbed on a mineral carrier, net price 0.5-mL vial = £19.00.

Dose: primary immunisation of children, 0.5 mL *by deep intramuscular injection* at 2 months followed by a second dose after 4 weeks and third dose after another 4 weeks (see schedule, section 14.1)

Available, as part of childhood immunisation schedule, from health authorities or Farillon

Hepatitis A vaccine

Hepatitis A vaccine is prepared from formaldehyde-inactivated hepatitis A virus grown in human diploid cells.

Immunisation is recommended for:

• laboratory staff who work directly with the virus;
• haemophiliacs treated with Factor VIII or Factor IX concentrates or who have liver disease or who have been infected with hepatitis B or hepatitis C;
• travellers to high-risk areas (see p. 597);
• individuals who are at risk due to their sexual behaviour.

Immunisation should be considered for :

• patients with chronic liver disease;
• staff and residents of homes for those with severe learning difficulties;
• workers at risk of exposure to untreated sewage;
• prevention of secondary cases in close contacts of confirmed cases of hepatitis A, within 7 days of onset of disease in the primary case.

Haemophiliacs and patients with chronic liver disease should be checked for previous exposure before immunisation.

Side-effects of hepatitis A vaccine, usually mild, include transient soreness, erythema, and induration at the injection site. Less common effects include fever, malaise, fatigue, headache, nausea, diarrhoea, and loss of appetite; arthralgia, myalgia, and, generalised rashes are occasionally reported.

See section 14.1 for general contra-indications.

> **Department of Health recommendation (decreased potency of hepatitis A vaccine).** Patients vaccinated with *Vaqta®* Adult or *Vaqta®* Paediatric may not have adequate protection against hepatitis A. The Department of Health has recommended that individuals who remain at risk of hepatitis A and who have been vaccinated with a *Vaqta®* product should be reimmunised with another hepatitis A vaccine; at least 6 months should elapse between doses of hepatitis A vaccine.

■ Single component

Avaxim® (Aventis Pasteur) PoM

Injection, suspension of formaldehyde-inactivated hepatitis A virus (GBM grown in human diploid cells) 320 antigen units/mL adsorbed onto aluminium hydroxide, net price 0.5-mL prefilled syringe = £20.63

Dose: by intramuscular injection (see note below), 0.5 mL as a single dose; booster dose 0.5 mL 6–12 months after initial dose; further booster doses, 0.5 mL every 10 years; CHILD under 16 years, not recommended

Note. The deltoid region is the preferred site of injection. The subcutaneous route may be used for patients with haemophilia

Havrix Monodose® (SmithKline Beecham) PoM
Injection, suspension of formaldehyde-inactivated hepatitis A virus (HM 175 grown in human diploid cells) 1440 ELISA units/mL adsorbed onto aluminium hydroxide, net price 1-mL prefilled syringe = £23.81, 0.5-mL (720 ELISA units) prefilled syringe (*Havrix Junior Monodose®*) = £18.03

Dose: *by intramuscular injection* (see note below), 1 mL as a single dose; booster dose, 1 mL 6–12 months after initial dose; CHILD 1–15 years 0.5 mL; booster dose, 0.5 mL 6–12 months after initial dose

Note. The deltoid region is the preferred site of injection in adults. The subcutaneous route may be used for patients with haemophilia

■ With hepatitis B vaccine
Twinrix® (SmithKline Beecham) PoM
Injection, inactivated hepatitis A virus 720 ELISA units and recombinant (DNA) hepatitis B surface antigen 20 micrograms/mL adsorbed onto aluminium hydroxide and aluminium phosphate, net price 1-mL prefilled syringe (*Twinrix® Adult*) = £29.85, 0.5-mL prefilled syringe (*Twinrix® Paediatric*) = £22.36

Dose: *by intramuscular injection* into deltoid muscle (see note below); primary course of 3 doses of 1 mL, the second 1 month and the third 6 months after the first dose; 1 mL booster dose 5 years after the start of primary course for those at continued risk; CHILD 1–15 years *by intramuscular injection*, 3 doses of 0.5 mL

Note. Primary course should be completed with *Twinrix®* (single component vaccines given at appropriate intervals may be used for booster dose); not to be injected into the buttock (vaccine efficacy reduced); subcutaneous route used for patients with haemophilia (but immune response may be reduced).

IMPORTANT. *Twinrix®* **not** recommended for post-exposure prophylaxis following percutaneous (needle-stick), ocular or mucous membrane exposure to hepatitis B virus.

■ With typhoid vaccine
Hepatyrix® (SmithKline Beecham) ▼ PoM
Injection, suspension of inactivated hepatitis A virus (grown in human diploid cells) 1440 ELISA units/mL adsorbed onto aluminium hydroxide, combined with typhoid vaccine containing 25 micrograms/mL virulence polysaccharide antigen of *Salmonella typhi*, net price 1-mL prefilled syringe = £34.49

Dose: *by intramuscular injection* (see note below) ADULT and ADOLESCENT over 15 years, 1 mL as a single dose; booster doses, see under single component hepatitis A vaccine and under polysaccharide typhoid vaccine

Note. The deltoid region is the preferred site of injection. The subcutaneous route may be used for patients with haemophilia

ViATIM® (Aventis Pasteur) ▼ PoM
Injection, suspension of inactivated hepatitis A virus (grown in human diploid cells) 160 antigen units/mL adsorbed onto aluminium hydroxide, combined with typhoid vaccine containing 25 micrograms/mL virulence polysaccharide antigen of *Salmonella typhi*, net price 1-mL prefilled syringe = £32.49

Dose: *by intramuscular injection* (see note below) ADULT and ADOLESCENT over 16 years, 1 mL as a single dose; booster doses, see under single component hepatitis A vaccine and under polysaccharide typhoid vaccine

Note. The deltoid region is the preferred site of injection. The subcutaneous route may be used for patients with thrombocytopenia or haemophilia

Hepatitis B vaccine

Hepatitis B vaccine contains inactivated hepatitis B virus surface antigen (HBsAg) adsorbed on aluminium hydroxide adjuvant. It is made biosynthetically using recombinant DNA technology. The vaccine is used in individuals at high risk of contracting hepatitis B.

In the UK, high-risk groups include:

• parenteral drug abusers;
• individuals who change sexual partners frequently;
• close family contacts of a case or carrier;
• infants born to mothers who *either* have had hepatitis B during pregnancy, *or* are positive for both hepatitis B surface antigen and hepatitis B e-antigen *or* are surface antigen positive without e markers (or where they have not been determined); active immunisation of the infant is started immediately after delivery and *hepatitis B immunoglobulin* (see p. 595) is given at the same time as the vaccine. Infants born to mothers who are positive for hepatitis B surface antigen and for e-antigen antibody should receive the vaccine but not the immunoglobulin;
• haemophiliacs, those receiving regular blood transfusions or blood products, and carers responsible for the administration of such products;
• patients with chronic renal failure including those on haemodialysis. Haemodialysis patients should be monitored for antibodies annually and re-immunised if necessary;
• health care personnel who have direct contact with blood or blood-stained body fluids or with patients' tissues;
• trainee health care workers;
• other occupational risk groups such as morticians and embalmers;
• staff and patients of day-care or residential accommodation for those with severe learning difficulties;
• inmates of custodial institutions;
• those travelling to areas of high prevalence who are at increased risk or who plan to remain there for lengthy periods (see p. 597);
• families adopting children from countries with a high prevalence of hepatitis B.

Immunisation takes up to 6 months to confer adequate protection; the duration of immunity is not known precisely, but a single booster 5 years after the primary course may be sufficient to maintain immunity for those who continue to be at risk.

More detailed guidance is given in the memorandum *Immunisation against Infectious Disease*. Immunisation does not eliminate the need for commonsense precautions for avoiding the risk of infection from known carriers by the routes of infection which have been clearly established, consult *Guidance for Clinical Health Care Workers: Protection against Infection with HIV and Hepatitis Viruses* and *Protecting Health Care Workers and Patients from Hepatitis B*. Accidental inoculation of hepatitis B virus-infected blood into a wound, incision, needle-prick, or abrasion may lead to infection, whereas it is unlikely that indirect exposure to a carrier will do so.

Specific **hepatitis B immunoglobulin** ('HBIG') is available for use with the vaccine in those accidentally infected and in infants (section 14.5).

A combined hepatitis A and hepatitis B vaccine is also available.

See section 14.1 for general contra-indications.

■ Single component

Engerix B® (SmithKline Beecham) PoM

Injection, suspension of hepatitis B surface antigen (rby, prepared from yeast cells by recombinant DNA technique) 20 micrograms/mL adsorbed onto aluminium hydroxide, net price 0.5-mL (paediatric) vial = £9.85, 1-mL vial = £13.27, 1-mL prefilled syringe = £13.97

Dose: by intramuscular injection (see note below), 3 doses of 1 mL (20 micrograms), the second 1 month and the third 6 months after the first dose; CHILD birth to 15 years 3 doses of 0.5 mL (10 micrograms); if compliance likely to be low in CHILD 10–15 years increase dose to 1 mL (20 micrograms)

Rapid immunisation, third dose 2 months after first dose and a booster dose at 12 months; exceptionally (e.g. for travellers departing within 1 month), ADULT, second dose 7 days after first dose, third dose after a further 14 days and a booster dose after 12 months

INFANT born to hepatitis B surface antigen-positive mothers (see also notes above), 4 doses of 0.5 mL (10 micrograms), first dose at birth with hepatitis B immunoglobulin injection (separate site) the second 1 month, the third 2 months and the fourth 12 months after the first dose

Chronic haemodialysis patients, *by intramuscular injection* (see note below) 4 doses of 2 mL (40 micrograms), the second 1 month, the third 2 months and the fourth 6 months after the first dose; adjustment of immunisation schedule and booster doses may be required in those with low antibody concentration

Note. Deltoid muscle is preferred site of injection in adults and older children; anterolateral thigh is preferred site in infants and young children; not to be injected into the buttock (vaccine efficacy reduced); subcutaneous route used for patients with thrombocytopenia or bleeding disorders

HB-Vax® II (Aventis Pasteur) PoM

Injection, suspension of hepatitis B surface antigen (prepared from yeast cells by recombinant DNA technique) 10 micrograms/mL adsorbed onto aluminium hydroxide, net price 1-mL prefilled syringe = £12.13, 1-mL vial = £11.41, 0.5-mL prefilled syringe (*HB-Vax® II Paediatric*) = £8.99

Excipients: include thiomersal

Dose: ADULT and ADOLESCENT over 16 years, *by intramuscular injection* (see note below) 3 doses of 1 mL (10 micrograms), the second 1 month and the third 6 months after the first dose; more rapid (e.g. for travellers), third dose 2 months after first dose with booster at 12 months; CHILD under 15 years, *by intramuscular injection* (see note below), 3 doses of 0.5 mL (5 micrograms)

INFANT born to hepatitis B surface antigen-positive mothers (see also notes above), 3 doses of 0.5 mL (5 micrograms), first dose at birth with hepatitis B immunoglobulin injection (separate site)

Note. Deltoid muscle is preferred site of injection in adults; anterolateral thigh is preferred site in infants and children; not to be injected into the buttock (vaccine efficacy reduced); subcutaneous route used for patients with haemophilia

■ Single component for dialysis and predialysis patients

HB-Vax® II 40 (Aventis Pasteur) PoM

Injection, suspension of hepatitis B surface antigen (prepared from yeast cells by recombinant DNA technique) 40 micrograms/mL adsorbed onto aluminium hydroxide, net price 1-mL vial = £29.37

Excipients: include thiomersal

Dose: by intramuscular injection (see note below) 3 doses of 1 mL (40 micrograms), the second 1 month and

the third 6 months after the first dose; booster doses may be required in those with low antibody concentration

Note. Deltoid muscle is preferred site of injection in adults; subcutaneous route used for patients with haemophilia

■ With hepatitis A vaccine

See Hepatitis A Vaccine

Influenza vaccines

While most viruses are antigenically stable, the influenza viruses A and B (especially A) are constantly altering their antigenic structure as indicated by changes in the haemagglutinins (H) and neuraminidases (N) on the surface of the viruses. It is essential that influenza vaccines in use contain the H and N components of the prevalent strain or strains. Every year the World Health Organization recommends which strains should be included.

The recommended strains are grown in the allantoic cavity of chick embryos (therefore **contraindicated** in those hypersensitive to eggs).

Since **influenza vaccines** will not control epidemics they are recommended *only for persons at high risk*. Annual immunisation is strongly recommended for those of all ages with the following conditions:

- chronic respiratory disease, including asthma;
- chronic heart disease;
- chronic renal failure;
- diabetes mellitus;
- immunosuppression due to disease or treatment, including asplenia or splenic dysfunction.

Influenza immunisation is also recommended for all persons aged over 65 years and for residents of nursing homes, residential homes for the elderly, and other long-stay facilities.

In non-pandemic years routine immunisation of Health Service Staff is not recommended, except for those at high risk (owing to medical disorders). However, as part of the winter planning, NHS employers should offer vaccination to certain front-line healthcare workers; employers of social care workers should also consider similar action.

Interactions: Appendix 1 (influenza vaccine).

See section 14.1 for general contra-indications.

Inactivated Influenza Vaccine (Split Virion) (Aventis Pasteur) PoM

Injection, suspension of formaldehyde-inactivated influenza virus (split virion) Flu/Vac/Split, net price 0.5-mL prefilled syringe = £5.70

Excipients: include thiomersal

Dose: by deep subcutaneous or by intramuscular injection, 0.5 mL as a single dose; CHILD 6–35 months 0.25–0.5 mL, CHILD 3–12 years 0.5 mL, in children dose repeated after at least 4 weeks if not previously vaccinated

Inactivated Influenza Vaccine (Surface Antigen) (Evans Vaccines) PoM

Injection, suspension of propiolactone-inactivated influenza virus (surface antigen) Flu/Vac/SA, net price 0.5-mL prefilled syringe = £3.98

Excipients: include thiomersal

Dose: by deep subcutaneous or by intramuscular injection, 0.5 mL as a single dose; CHILD 6–35 months 0.25–0.5 mL, CHILD 3–12 years 0.5 mL, in children dose repeated after at least 4 weeks if not previously vaccinated

Agrippal® (Wyeth) [PoM]

Injection, suspension of formaldehyde-inactivated influenza virus (surface antigen) Flu/Vac/SA, net price 0.5-mL prefilled syringe = £5.72

Excipients: include thiomersal

Dose: by deep subcutaneous or by intramuscular injection, 0.5 mL as a single dose; CHILD 6–35 months 0.25–0.5 mL, CHILD 3–12 years 0.5 mL, in children dose repeated after at least 4 weeks if not previously vaccinated

Begrivac® (Wyeth) [PoM]

Injection, suspension of formaldehyde-inactivated influenza virus (split virion) Flu/Vac/Split, net price 0.5-mL prefilled syringe = £6.29

Dose: by deep subcutaneous or by intramuscular injection, 0.5 mL as a single dose; CHILD 6–35 months 0.25–0.5 mL, CHILD 3–12 years 0.5 mL, in children dose repeated after at least 4 weeks if not previously vaccinated

Fluarix® (SmithKline Beecham) [PoM]

Injection, suspension of formaldehyde-inactivated influenza virus (split virion) Flu/Vac/Split, net price 0.5-mL prefilled syringe = £3.99

Excipients: include thiomersal

Dose: by deep subcutaneous or by intramuscular injection, 0.5 mL as a single dose; CHILD 6–35 months 0.25–0.5 mL, CHILD 3–12 years 0.5 mL, in children dose repeated after at least 4 weeks if not previously vaccinated

Fluvirin® (Evans Vaccines) [PoM]

Injection, suspension of propiolactone-inactivated influenza virus (surface antigen) Flu/Vac/SA, net price 0.5-mL prefilled syringe = £5.69

Excipients: include thiomersal

Dose: by deep subcutaneous or by intramuscular injection, 0.5 mL as a single dose; CHILD 6–35 months 0.25–0.5 mL, CHILD 3–12 years 0.5 mL, in children dose repeated after at least 4 weeks if not previously vaccinated

Influvac Sub-unit® (Solvay) [PoM]

Injection, suspension of formaldehyde-inactivated influenza virus (surface antigen) Flu/Vac/SA, net price 0.5-mL prefilled syringe = £5.08

Excipients: include thiomersal

Dose: by deep subcutaneous or by intramuscular injection, 0.5 mL as a single dose; CHILD 6–35 months 0.25–0.5 mL, CHILD 3–12 years 0.5 mL, in children dose repeated after at least 4 weeks if not previously vaccinated

Measles vaccine

Measles vaccine has been replaced by a combined measles/mumps/rubella vaccine (MMR vaccine) for all eligible children.

Administration of a measles-containing vaccine to children may be associated with a mild measles-like syndrome with a measles-like rash and pyrexia about a week after injection. Much less commonly, convulsions and, very rarely, encephalitis have been reported. Convulsions in infants are much less frequently associated with measles vaccines than with other conditions leading to febrile episodes.

MMR vaccine may be used in the control of outbreaks of measles (see under MMR Vaccine).

■ Single antigen vaccine
No longer available in the UK

■ Combined vaccines
See MMR vaccine

MMR vaccine

A combined **measles/mumps/rubella vaccine** (MMR vaccine) aims to eliminate rubella (and congenital rubella syndrome), measles, and mumps. Every child should receive two doses of MMR vaccine by entry to primary school, unless there is a valid contra-indication (see below) or parental refusal. MMR vaccine should be given irrespective of previous measles, mumps or rubella infection.

The first dose of MMR vaccine is given to children aged 12–15 months. A second (booster) dose is given before starting school at 3–5 years of age (see schedule, section 14.1). Children presenting for pre-school booster who have not received the first dose of MMR vaccine should be given a dose of MMR vaccine followed 3 months later by a second dose. At school-leaving age or at entry into further education, individuals of both sexes who have not received either MR or MMR vaccines should be offered MMR immunisation.

MMR vaccine may also be used in the control of outbreaks of measles and should be offered to susceptible children (including babies from 5 months of age) within 3 days of exposure to infection; these children should still receive routine MMR vaccinations. MMR vaccine is **not suitable** for prophylaxis following exposure to mumps and rubella since the antibody response to the mumps and rubella components is too slow for effective prophylaxis.

Children with partially or totally impaired immune response should not receive live vaccines (for advice on AIDS see section 14.1). If they have been exposed to measles infection they should be given normal immunoglobulin (section 14.5).

Malaise, fever or a rash may occur following the first dose of MMR vaccine, most commonly about a week after immunisation and lasting about 2 to 3 days. Leaflets are available to provide parents with advice for reducing fever (including the use of paracetamol). Parotid swelling occasionally occurs, usually in the third week. Adverse reactions are considerably less common after the second dose of MMR vaccine than after the first dose.

Idiopathic thrombocytopenic purpura has occurred rarely following MMR vaccination, usually within 6 weeks of the first dose. The risk of developing idiopathic thrombocytopenic purpura after MMR vaccine is much less than the risk of developing it after infection with wild measles, mumps or rubella virus. The CSM has recommended that children who develop idiopathic thrombocytopenic purpura within 6 weeks of the first dose of MMR should undergo serological testing before the second dose is due; if the results suggest incomplete immunity against measles, mumps and rubella then a second dose of MMR is recommended. The Public Health Laboratory Service offers free serological testing for children developing idiopathic thrombocytopenic purpura *within 6 weeks* of the first dose of MMR.

Post-vaccination meningoencephalitis was reported (rarely and with complete recovery) following immunisation with MMR vaccine containing Urabe mumps vaccine, which has now been discontinued; no cases have been confirmed in association with the currently-used Jeryl Lynn mumps vaccine. Children with post-vaccination symptoms are not infectious.

Following discussions with all major health organisations in January 2001, the Chief Medical Officers have advised that the MMR vaccine is the safest and best way to protect children against measles, mumps, and rubella. Information may be obtained from www.immunisation.org.uk.

An expert group of the Medical Research Council had previously concluded that there was no evidence to indicate any link between MMR vaccination and bowel disease or autism. The Chief Medical Officer had recommended that children should receive MMR vaccine at the appropriate times and should not be given the separate component vaccines since there was no evidence that doing this had any benefit and it may even be harmful.

The CSM has issued an information leaflet stating that neither the CSM's Working Party on MMR vaccine nor an epidemiological study (*Lancet* 1999; **353**: 2026-9) support an association between MMR (or MR) vaccine and autism or Crohn's disease.

Contra-indications to MMR include:
- children with untreated malignant disease or altered immunity (for advice on vaccines and AIDS see section 14.1), and those receiving immunosuppressive drugs or radiotherapy, or high-dose corticosteroids;
- children who have received another live vaccine by injection within 3 weeks;
- children with allergies to gelatin, neomycin, or kanamycin;
- children with acute febrile illness (vaccination should be deferred);
- if given to women, pregnancy should be avoided for 1 month (as for rubella vaccine);
- should not be given within 3 months of an immunoglobulin injection.

It should be noted that:
children with a personal or close family history of convulsions should be given MMR vaccine, provided the parents understand that there may be a febrile response; doctors should seek specialist paediatric advice rather than without vaccination; there is increasing evidence that MMR vaccine can be given safely even when the child has had an anaphylactic reaction to food containing egg (dislike of egg or refusal to eat egg is not a contra-indication).

MMR Vaccine [PoM]

Live measles, mumps, and rubella vaccine
Dose: by deep subcutaneous or by intramuscular injection, 0.5 mL
Available from health authorities or direct from Farillon as *MMR II®* (Aventis Pasteur) or *Priorix®* (SmithKline Beecham)

Meningococcal vaccines

Almost all childhood meningococcal disease in the UK is caused by *Neisseria meningitidis* serogroups B and C. **Meningococcal Group C conjugate vaccine** protects only against infection by serogroup C; it can be given from 2 months of age. After early adult life the risk of meningococcal disease declines, and immunisation is not generally recommended after the age of 25 years.

Travellers to areas where meningococcal infection risk is high require meningococcal polysaccharide A&C vaccine, whilst those travelling to Saudi Arabia for Hajj or Umrah are best protected with quadrivalent ACWY meningococcal polysaccharide vaccine (see below).

CHILDHOOD IMMUNISATION. **Meningococcal Group C conjugate vaccine** provides long-term protection against infection by serogroup C of *Neisseria meningitidis* in children from 2 months of age; it is now a component of the primary course of childhood immunisation. The recommended schedule consists of 3 doses starting at 2 months of age with an interval of 1 month between each dose (see schedule, section 14.1). It is recommended that meningococcal group C conjugate vaccine be given to anyone aged up to and including 24 years who has not been vaccinated previously with this vaccine.

Meningococcal group C conjugate vaccine is also recommended for individuals with a dysfunctional or absent spleen.

IMMUNISATION FOR TRAVELLERS. Individuals travelling abroad (see areas of risk below) should be immunised with a meningococcal polysaccharide vaccine that covers serogroups A and C (or A, C, W135 and Y, see below), even if they have already received meningococcal group C conjugate vaccine.

Meningococcal polysaccharide A&C vaccine is effective against serogroups A and C but children aged under 18 months respond less well than adults. It is indicated for visits of longer than 1 month to areas of the world where the risk of acquiring meningococcal infection is much higher than in the UK, particularly for individuals proposing to travel 'rough' or to live or work with local people. Areas of risk include:

Nepal, Bhutan, Pakistan, Saudi Arabia (but see below), and the meningitis belt of Africa, which encompasses southern sub-Saharan parts of Senegal, Mali, Niger, Chad, and Sudan; all of Burkina Faso, Gambia, Guinea, Togo, and Benin; South-west Ethiopia, northern parts of Sierra Leone, Liberia, Ivory Coast, Nigeria, Cameroon, Central African Republic, Uganda, and Kenya.

A meningococcal polysaccharide vaccine active against meningococci of groups **A, C, W135 and Y** is particularly recommended for travellers to Saudi Arabia during the Hajj and Umrah pilgrimages (because of recent outbreaks of the W135 strain). Saudi Arabia now requires proof of vaccination with the quadrivalent vaccine, for visitors arriving for these pilgrimages. For travel to Saudi Arabia other than for pilgrimage (except seasonal work in the Hajj area) or to other countries, the meningococcal polysaccharide A&C vaccine continues to be recommended.

CONTACTS OF INFECTED INDIVIDUALS AND LABORATORY WORKERS. For advice on the immunisation of *close contacts* of cases of Group A and Group C meningococcal disease in the UK and on the role of the vaccine in the control of *local outbreaks*, consult the replacement chapter for the memorandum *Immunisation against Infectious Disease*. See section 5.1 Table 2 for antibacterial prophylaxis to prevent a secondary case of meningococcal meningitis.

The need for immunisation of laboratory staff who work directly with *Neisseria meningitidis* should be considered.

SIDE-EFFECTS. Side-effects of meningococcal Group C conjugate vaccine include redness and swelling at the site of the injection, dizziness, mild fever, irritability, headache, nausea, vomiting, rash, pruritus, malaise, lymphadenopathy, hypotonia, paraesthesia, hypoaesthesia, and faints. Hypersensitivity reactions (including anaphylaxis, bronchospasm, and angioedema) and seizures have been reported rarely. Symptoms of meningism have also been reported rarely, but there is no evidence that the vaccine causes meningococcal C meningitis. The CSM has advised that vaccination provides clear benefit in terms of lives saved and disabilities prevented.

Meningococcal polysaccharide A&C and ACWY vaccines are associated with injection-site reactions and fever.

See section 14.1 for general contra-indications.

■ Meningococcal Group C conjugate vaccine

Meningitec® (Wyeth) ▼ PoM

Injection, suspension of capsular polysaccharide antigen of *Neisseria meningitidis* group C (conjugated to *Corynebacterium diphtheriae* protein), net price 0.5-mL vial = £17.95

> *Dose: by intramuscular or deep subcutaneous injection*, ADULT and CHILD over 1 year 0.5 mL as a single dose; for routine immunisation in CHILD under 1 year, 3 doses (each of 0.5 mL) are required at intervals of 1 month (see schedule, section 14.1)

Available as part of childhood immunisation schedule from Farillon

Note. Subcutaneous route used for patients with haemophilia

Menjugate® (Chiron) ▼ PoM

Injection, powder for reconstitution, capsular polysaccharide antigen of *Neisseria meningitidis* group C (conjugated to *Corynebacterium diphtheriae* protein), adsorbed onto aluminium hydroxide, single-dose and 10-dose vials

> *Dose: by intramuscular or deep subcutaneous injection*, ADULT and CHILD over 1 year 0.5 mL as a single dose; for routine immunisation in CHILD under 1 year, 3 doses (each of 0.5 mL) are required at intervals of 1 month (see schedule, section 14.1)

Available from Farillon

NeisVac-C® (Baxter) ▼ PoM

Injection, suspension of polysaccharide antigen of *Neisseria meningitidis* group C (conjugated to tetanus toxoid protein), 0.5-mL prefilled syringe

> *Dose: by intramuscular injection* (see also note below), ADULT and CHILD over 1 year 0.5 mL as a single dose; for routine immunisation in CHILD under 1 year, 3 doses (each of 0.5 mL) are required at intervals of 1 month (see schedule, section 14.1)

Available from Farillon

Note. Subcutaneous route used for patients with thrombocytopenia or haemophilia

■ Meningococcal polysaccharide A&C vaccines

AC Vax® (SmithKline Beecham) PoM

Injection, powder for reconstitution, capsular polysaccharide antigens of *Neisseria meningitidis* groups A and C, net price single-dose vial (with diluent) = £7.37

> *Dose: by deep subcutaneous injection or by intramuscular injection*, ADULT and CHILD over 2 years 0.5 mL

Mengivac (A+C)® (Aventis Pasteur) PoM

Injection, powder for reconstitution, capsular polysaccharide antigens of *Neisseria meningitidis* (meningococcus) groups A and C, net price single-dose vial (with syringe containing diluent) = £6.39

> *Dose: by deep subcutaneous injection or by intramuscular injection*, ADULT and CHILD over 18 months 0.5 mL

> *Note.* The lower age range for *AC Vax®* and *Mengivac (A+C)®* differ; in the case of *Mengivac (A+C)®* the product literature states that young children and infants respond less well to the vaccine than older children and adults, with little response to the Group C polysaccharide under 18 months of age and a poor response to Group A polysaccharide under 3 months of age. Additionally, protection in infants under 18 months of age is of shorter duration

■ Meningococcal polysaccharide A, C, W135 and Y vaccine

ACWY Vax® (SmithKline Beecham) PoM

Injection, powder for reconstitution, capsular polysaccharide antigens of Neisseria meningitidis groups A, C, W135 and Y, net price single-dose vial (with diluent) = £17.14

> *Dose: by deep subcutaneous injection*, ADULT and CHILD over 2 years 0.5 mL

Mumps vaccine

▨ Single antigen vaccine
No longer available in the UK

■ Combined vaccine
See MMR Vaccine

Pertussis vaccine

Pertussis vaccine is given combined with diphtheria and tetanus vaccine starting at 2 months of age (see schedule section 14.1).

With some vaccines available in the early 1960s *persistent screaming and collapse* were reported but these reactions are rarely observed with the vaccines now available. *Convulsions and encephalopathy* have been reported as rare complications, but such conditions may arise from other causes and be falsely attributed to the vaccine. Neurological complications *after whooping cough itself* are considerably more common than after the vaccine.

As with any other elective immunisation procedure it is advisable to postpone vaccination if the child is suffering from any acute illness, until fully recovered. Minor infections without fever or systemic upset are not reasons to delay immunisation. Immunisation should not be carried out in children who have a history of severe general reaction to a preceding dose; in these children immunisation should be completed with adsorbed diphtheria and tetanus vaccine. Where there has been a severe local reaction or pyrexia, acellular pertussis vaccine may be used. The following reactions should be regarded as severe:

Local—an extensive area of redness and swelling which becomes indurated and involves most of the antero-lateral surface of the thigh or a major part of the circumference of the upper arm.

General—temperature of 39.5°C or more within 48 hours of vaccine, anaphylaxis, bronchospasm, laryngeal oedema, generalised collapse, prolonged unresponsiveness, prolonged inconsolable screaming, and convulsions occurring within 72 hours.

A personal or family history of allergy is **not** a contra-indication to immunisation against whooping cough; nor are stable neurological conditions such as cerebral palsy or spina bifida.

CHILDREN WITH PROBLEM HISTORIES. When there is a personal or family history of *febrile* convulsions, there is an increased risk of these occurring after pertussis immunisation. In such children, immunisation is *recommended* but advice on the *prevention of fever* (see p. 580) should be given at the time of immunisation.

In a British study, children with a family history of epilepsy were immunised with pertussis vaccine without any significant adverse events. These children's developmental progress has been normal. In children with a close family history (first degree relatives) of *idiopathic epilepsy*, there may be a risk of developing a similar condition, irrespective of vaccine. Immunisation is *recommended* for these children.

Where there is a *still evolving neurological problem*, immunisation should be *deferred* until the condition is stable. Children whose epilepsy is well controlled may receive pertussis vaccine. When there has been a documented history of *cerebral damage in the neonatal period*, immunisation should be *carried out unless there is evidence of an evolving neurological abnormality.* If immunisation is to be deferred, this should be stated on the neonatal discharge summary. Where there is doubt, appropriate advice should be sought from a consultant paediatrician, district immunisation co-ordinator or consultant in communicable disease control *rather than withholding vaccine.*

OLDER CHILDREN. There is no contra-indication to administration of pertussis vaccine to unimmunised older children in order to protect the individuals and siblings under the age of immunisation; however, no suitable vaccine is available for children aged over 7 years.

■ Combined vaccine
Combined vaccine (*pertussis, tetanus,* and *diphtheria*), see under Diphtheria vaccines

Pneumococcal vaccine

A polyvalent (23-valent) unconjugated **pneumococcal polysaccharide vaccine** is used for the immunisation of persons over the age of 2 years (children under 2 years should receive the 7-valent vaccine, see below); it is recommended for any of the following conditions:

• Homozygous sickle cell disease;
• Asplenia or severe dysfunction of the spleen;
• Chronic renal disease or nephrotic syndrome;
• Coeliac syndrome;
• Immunodeficiency or immunosuppression due to disease or treatment, including HIV infection;
• Chronic heart disease;
• Chronic lung disease;
• Chronic liver disease including cirrhosis;
• Diabetes mellitus.

Where possible, the vaccine should be given at least 2 weeks before splenectomy and before chemotherapy; patients should be given advice about increased risk of pneumococcal infection (a patient card and information leaflet for patients with asple-

nia are available from the Department of Health). Prophylactic antibacterial therapy against pneumococcal infection should not be stopped after immunisation. The vaccine is effective in a single dose if the types of pneumonia in the community are reflected in the polysaccharides contained in the vaccine. It should not be given in pregnancy, or when breast-feeding, or when there is infection. Hypersensitivity reactions may occur.

REVACCINATION. Revaccination less than 3 years after the first injection may produce severe reactions in some subjects. Revaccination is therefore not recommended except, after 5–10 years, in individuals in whom the antibody concentration is likely to decline rapidly (e.g. asplenia, splenic dysfunction and nephrotic syndrome). Antibody concentration may decline more rapidly in children and revaccination after 3 years may be considered for children under 10 years. If there is doubt, the need for revaccination should be discussed with a haematologist, immunologist, or microbiologist, and measurement of antibody concentration considered.

A polyvalent (7-valent) **pneumococcal polysaccharide conjugated vaccine** has been introduced recently for the prevention of invasive pneumococcal disease in children aged between 2 months and 2 years who are at special risk because of the conditions shown above; the number of doses required for primary immunisation varies according to age. Children aged over 2 years at high risk of pneumococcal disease who have previously received pneumococcal polysaccharide conjugated vaccine may receive the unconjugated polyvalent (23-valent) pneumococcal polysaccharide vaccine.

See section 14.1 for general contra-indications.
IMPORTANT. Not for intradermal injection which may cause severe local reactions

■ Pneumococcal polysaccharide vaccines
Pneumovax® II (Aventis Pasteur) PoM
Polysaccharide from each of 23 capsular types of pneumococcus, net price 0.5-mL prefilled syringe = £10.00
Dose: by subcutaneous or intramuscular injection, 0.5 mL; revaccination, see notes above; CHILD under 2 years, not recommended (suboptimal response and also safety and efficacy not established)

Pnu-Imune® (Wyeth) PoM
Polysaccharide from each of 23 capsular types of pneumococcus, net price 0.5-mL vial = £9.94
Excipients: include thiomersal
Dose: by subcutaneous or intramuscular injection, 0.5 mL; revaccination, see notes above; CHILD under 2 years, not recommended

■ Pneumococcal polysaccharide conjugated vaccine
Prevenar® (Wyeth) ▼ PoM
Polysaccharide from each of 7 capsular types of pneumococcus adsorbed onto aluminium phosphate, net price 0.5-mL vial = £39.25
Dose: by intramuscular injection, INFANT 2–6 months 3 doses each of 0.5 mL separated by intervals of 1 month and a further dose in second year of life; 7–11 months 2 doses each of 0.5 mL separated by an interval of 1 month and a further dose in second year of life; CHILD 1–2 years 2 doses each of 0.5 mL separated by an interval of 2 months
Note. Deltoid muscle is preferred site of injection in young children; anterolateral thigh is preferred site in infants

Poliomyelitis vaccines

There are two types of poliomyelitis vaccine, poliomyelitis vaccine, live (oral) (Sabin) and poliomyelitis vaccine, inactivated (Salk). The oral vaccine, consisting of a mixture of attenuated strains of virus types 1, 2, and 3 is at present generally used in the UK.

A course of primary immunisation consists of 3 doses of **poliomyelitis vaccine, live (oral)**, starting at two months of age with an interval of 1 month between each dose (see schedule, section 14.1). The initial course of 3 doses should also be given to all unimmunised adults; no adult should remain unimmunised against poliomyelitis.

Two booster doses of poliomyelitis vaccine, live (oral), are recommended, the first before school entry and the second before leaving school (see schedule, section 14.1). Booster doses for adults are not necessary except for those at special risk such as travellers to endemic areas, or laboratory staff likely to be exposed to the viruses, or health care workers in possible contact with cases; booster doses should be given to such individuals every 10 years.

Vaccine-associated poliomyelitis and poliomyelitis in contacts of vaccinees are rare. In England and Wales there is an annual average of 1 recipient and 1 contact case for over 2 million doses of oral vaccine. The need for strict personal hygiene must be stressed; the contacts of a recently vaccinated baby should be advised particularly of the need to wash their hands after changing the baby's nappies.

Contra-indications to the use of oral poliomyelitis vaccine include vomiting and diarrhoea, and immunodeficiency disorders (or household contacts of patients with immunodeficiency disorders). See section 14.1 for further contra-indications.

Poliomyelitis vaccine (inactivated) may be used for those in whom poliomyelitis vaccine (oral) is contra-indicated because of immunosuppressive disorders (for advice on AIDS see section 14.1).

Either live (oral) vaccine or inactivated vaccine may be used to complete a course started with the other, except that live (oral) vaccine must **not** be used for immunosuppressed individuals or their household contacts (see also contra-indications).

TRAVELLERS. Travellers to areas other than Australia, New Zealand, Northern and Western Europe, and North America should be given a full course of oral poliomyelitis vaccine if they have not been immunised in the past. Those who have not received immunisation within the last 10 years should be given a booster dose of oral poliomyelitis vaccine.

■ Live (oral) (Sabin)
Poliomyelitis Vaccine, Live (Oral) PoM Pol/ Vac (Oral)[1]. A suspension of suitable live attenuated strains of poliomyelitis virus, types 1, 2, and 3. Available in single-dose and 10-dose containers

Dose: 3 drops from a multidose container or the total contents of a single-dose container; for primary immunisation 3 doses are required (see schedule, section 14.1). May be given on a lump of sugar; not to be given with foods which contain preservatives

Available from health authorities or direct from Farillon
1. BP permits code OPV for vaccine in single doses provided it also appears on pack.

Note. Poliomyelitis vaccine loses potency once the container has been opened, therefore any vaccine remaining at the end of an immunisation session should be discarded; whenever possible sessions should be arranged to avoid undue wastage.

■ Inactivated (Salk)
Poliomyelitis Vaccine, Inactivated PoM Pol/ Vac (Inact). An inactivated suspension of suitable strains of poliomyelitis virus, types 1, 2, and 3.

Dose: by subcutaneous injection, 0.5 mL or as stated on the label; for primary immunisation 3 doses are required at intervals of 4 weeks

Available direct from Farillon.

Note. Should be ordered one dose at a time (on a named-patient basis) and only when required for use

Rabies vaccine

Pre-exposure, prophylactic immunisation with human diploid cell **rabies vaccine** should be offered to those at high risk—laboratory staff who handle the rabies virus, those working in quarantine stations, animal handlers, veterinary surgeons and field workers who are likely to be exposed to bites of possibly infected wild animals, certain port officials, licensed bat handlers and health workers who are likely to come into close contact with patients with rabies. Pre-exposure immunisation is also recommended for those living or travelling in enzootic areas who may be exposed to unusual risk.

The Department of Health has advised that for *prophylactic use* the vaccine produces a good antibody response when given in a 3-dose schedule on days 0, 7, and 28, with a booster dose every 2–3 years to those at continued risk. For travellers to enzootic areas who are not animal handlers, 2 doses given 4 weeks apart may be acceptable *provided that post-exposure treatment is readily available;* for those who remain at continued risk a booster dose should be given 6–12 months later followed by a booster every 2–3 years.

Post-exposure treatment depends on the level of risk in the country concerned and the individual's immune status. For *post-exposure treatment of fully immunised patients:* countries with no risk, generally no treatment required; countries with low risk and high risk, two booster doses are needed (one on day 0 and one on day 3–7). For *post-exposure treatment of previously unimmunised patients* (or those whose prophylaxis is possibly inadequate): countries with no risk, generally no treatment required; countries with low risk, a course of injections should be started as soon as possible after exposure (days 0, 3, 7, 14 and 30); countries with high risk, as for countries with low risk, **plus** rabies immunoglobulin on day 0 (section 14.5). The course may be discontinued if it is proved that the patient was not at risk.

Staff in attendance on a patient who is highly suspected of, or known to be suffering from, rabies should be offered immunisation. Four intradermal doses of 0.1 mL of human diploid cell vaccine (Aventis Pasteur) given at the same appointment at different sites (ensuring correct intradermal technique) has been suggested for this purpose [unlicensed route].

Advice on up-to-date country-by-country information and on post-exposure immunisation and treatment of rabies is available from the Virus Reference Division, Central Public Health Laboratory, Colindale, London NW9 5HT (Tel (020) 8200 4400) or in Scotland from the Scottish Centre for Infection and Environmental Health (Tel (0141) 946 7120).

There are no specific contra-indications to this diploid cell vaccine and its use should be considered whenever a patient has been attacked by an animal in a country where rabies is endemic, even if there is no direct evidence of rabies in the attacking animal.

Rabies Vaccine (Aventis Pasteur) PoM
Freeze-dried inactivated Wistar rabies virus strain PM/WI 38 1503-3M cultivated in human diploid cells, net price single-dose vial with syringe containing diluent = £22.15
IMPORTANT. Studies have shown that when this vaccine is injected into the gluteal region there is a poor response. Concomitant administration of chloroquine may also affect the antibody response. Because of the potential consequences of inadequately treated rabies exposure and because there is no indication that fetal abnormalities have been associated with rabies vaccination, pregnancy is **not** considered a contra-indication to post-exposure prophylaxis. If there is substantial risk of exposure to rabies, pre-exposure prophylaxis may also be indicated during pregnancy
Dose: prophylactic, *by deep subcutaneous or by intramuscular injection* in the deltoid region, 1 mL on days 0, 7, and 28; also booster doses every 2–3 years to those at continued risk; see above for 2-dose schedule
Post-exposure, *by deep subcutaneous or by intramuscular injection* in the deltoid region, 1 mL, see notes above
Staff in attendance, see notes above
Also available from local designated centres (special workers and post-exposure treatment)

Rabipur® (MASTA) PoM
Freeze-dried inactivated Flury LEP rabies virus strain cultivated in chick embryo cells, net price single-dose vial = £22.15
Dose: prophylactic, *by intramuscular injection* in the deltoid muscle or anterolateral thigh in small children, 1 mL on days 0, 7 and 21 or 28; also booster doses every 2–5 years for those at continued risk
Post-exposure, *by intramuscular injection* in the deltoid muscle or anterolateral thigh in small children, 1 mL, see notes above

Rubella vaccine

The selective policy of protecting women of child-bearing age from the risks of rubella (German measles) in pregnancy has been replaced by a policy of eliminating rubella in children; the single-antigen rubella immunisation programme for 10–14 year old girls has been discontinued. All children should be immunised with rubella-containing vaccine (measles, mumps and rubella) at 12–15 months and at 3–5 years (see MMR vaccine, p. 587). Immigrants who enter the UK after the age of school immunisation are particularly likely to require immunisation.

Every effort must be made to identify and immunise with rubella vaccine all *seronegative women of child-bearing age* (see schedule, section 14.1) as well as those who might put pregnant women at risk of infection (e.g. nurses and doctors in obstetric units).

Rubella vaccine may conveniently be offered to previously *unimmunised and seronegative post-partum women*. Immunising susceptible post-partum women a few days after delivery is important as far as the overall reduction of congenital abnormalities in the UK is concerned, for about 60% of these abnormalities occur in the babies of multiparous women.

PREGNANCY. Rubella immunisation should be avoided in early pregnancy, and women of child-bearing age should be advised not to become pregnant within 1 month of immunisation. However, despite active surveillance in the UK, the USA, and Germany, no case of congenital rubella syndrome has been reported following inadvertent immunisation shortly before or during pregnancy. There is thus no evidence that the vaccine is teratogenic, and routine termination of pregnancy following inadvertent immunisation should **not** be recommended; potential parents should be given this information before making a decision about termination.

See section 14.1 for general contra-indications.

Rubella Vaccine, Live PoM Rub/Vac (Live). Prepared from Wistar RA 27/3 strain propagated in human diploid cells
Dose: *by deep subcutaneous or by intramuscular injection*, 0.5 mL (see schedule, section 14.1 and notes above)
Available from health authorities or direct from Farillon as SmithKline Beecham brand (*Ervevax®*)

■ Combined vaccines
see MMR vaccine

Smallpox vaccine

Smallpox immunisation is no longer required routinely because global eradication has been achieved. Advice on the need for immunisation of workers in laboratories where pox viruses (such as vaccinia) are handled and of others whose work involves an identifiable risk of exposure to pox virus can be obtained from the Viral Zoonosis Reference Unit, Central Public Health Laboratory, Colindale (Tel (020) 8200 4400) who will also supply the vaccine.

Tetanus vaccines

Tetanus vaccines stimulate the production of the protective antitoxin. In general, adsorption on aluminium hydroxide, aluminium phosphate, or calcium phosphate improves antigenicity. Adsorbed tetanus vaccine is offered routinely to babies in combination with adsorbed diphtheria vaccine (DT/Vac/Ads(Child)) and more usually also combined with killed *Bordetella pertussis* organisms as adsorbed diphtheria, tetanus, and pertussis vaccine (DTPer/Vac/Ads), see schedule, section 14.1.

In children, adsorbed diphtheria, tetanus, and pertussis vaccine not only gives protection against tetanus in childhood but also gives the basic immunity for subsequent booster doses at school entry and at school leaving (see schedule, section 14.1) and also for a potentially tetanus-contaminated injury. Normally, booster doses of adsorbed tetanus vaccine should not be given unless more than 10 years have elapsed since the last booster dose because of the possibility that hypersensitivity reactions may develop. If a child over the age of 13 years requires a tetanus booster for a wound then, provided more than 10 years have elapsed since the school-entry booster, adsorbed tetanus vaccine combined with low-dose adsorbed diphtheria vaccine can be given; the routine booster at school-leaving age is omitted.

Active immunisation is important for persons in older age groups who may never have had a routine or complete course of immunisation when younger. In these persons a course of adsorbed tetanus vaccine may be given. Very rarely, tetanus has developed after abdominal surgery; patients awaiting elective surgery should be asked about tetanus immunisation and immunised if necessary. All laboratory staff should be offered a primary course if unimmunised.

Any adult who has received 5 doses is likely to have life-long immunity; booster doses on injury should only be required if more than 10 years have elapsed since the last dose.

WOUNDS. Wounds are considered to be tetanus-prone if they are sustained *either* more than 6 hours before surgical treatment *or* at any interval after injury and are puncture-type or show much devitalised tissue or are septic or are contaminated with soil or manure. All wounds should receive thorough surgical toilet.

- For *clean wounds*, a booster dose of adsorbed tetanus vaccine is given if the primary course (or booster dose) was given more than 10 years previously; non-immunised individuals (or whose immunisation status is not known) should be given a full course of the vaccine.

- For *tetanus-prone wounds,* management is as for clean wounds with the addition of a dose of tetanus immunoglobulin (section 14.5); in an immunised individual who has received a dose of adsorbed tetanus vaccine within the previous 10 years, the immunoglobulin may only be needed if the risk of infection is considered to be especially high (e.g. contamination with manure). Antibacterial prophylaxis (with benzylpenicillin, co-amoxiclav, or metronidazole) may also be required for tetanus-prone wounds.

See section 14.1 for general contra-indications

■ Single antigen vaccines

The BP directs that when Tetanus Vaccine is prescribed or demanded and the form is not stated, Adsorbed Tetanus Vaccine may be dispensed or supplied.

Adsorbed Tetanus Vaccine PoM

Tet/Vac/Ads.

Injection, suspension of tetanus formol toxoid adsorbed on a mineral carrier

Dose: by deep subcutaneous or by intramuscular injection, 3 doses each of 0.5 mL separated by intervals of 1 month

Available from Evans Vaccines as *Clostet*®, net price 0.5-mL single-dose syringe = £1.40) and from Aventis Pasteur (net price 0.5-mL amp = 74p; 0.5-mL single-dose syringe = £1.50; excipients include thiomersal

■ Combined vaccines

see Diphtheria Vaccines

Typhoid vaccines

Typhoid immunisation is advised for travellers to countries where sanitation standards may be poor, although it is not a substitute for scrupulous personal hygiene (see section 14.6). Immunisation is also advised for laboratory workers handling specimens from suspected cases.

Capsular **polysaccharide typhoid vaccine** is given by *intramuscular or deep subcutaneous injection*; further doses are needed every 3 years on continued exposure. Local reactions, including pain, swelling or erythema, may appear 48–72 hours after administration.

An **oral typhoid vaccine** is also available. It is a **live attenuated** vaccine contained in an enteric-coated capsule. It is taken *by mouth* as three doses of one capsule on alternate days, providing protection 7–10 days after the last dose. Protection may persist for up to 3 years in those constantly (or repeatedly) exposed to *Salmonella typhi*, but occasional travellers require a repeat course at intervals of 1 year. Oral typhoid vaccine is **contra-indicated** in individuals who are immunosuppressed (whether due to disease or its treatment) and is inactivated by concomitant administration of *antibacterials*. Oral typhoid vaccine and oral poliomyelitis vaccine should be given at least 3 weeks apart on theoretical grounds. Administration of a dose of oral typhoid vaccine should be coordinated so that *mefloquine* is not taken for at least 12 hours before or after a dose (vaccination with oral typhoid vaccine should preferably be completed at least 3 days before the first dose of mefloquine). Side-effects to oral typhoid vaccine include nausea, vomiting, abdominal cramps, diarrhoea, headache, fever and hypersensitivity reactions including, rarely, anaphylaxis.

For general contra-indications to vaccines, see section 14.1.

■ Polysaccharide vaccine for injection

Typherix® (SmithKline Beecham) PoM

Injection, Vi capsular polysaccharide typhoid vaccine, 50 micrograms/mL virulence polysaccharide antigen of *Salmonella typhi*, net price 0.5-mL prefilled syringe = £10.68

Dose: by intramuscular injection, 0.5 mL; CHILD under 2 years may show suboptimal response

Typhim Vi® (Aventis Pasteur) PoM

Injection, Vi capsular polysaccharide typhoid vaccine, 50 micrograms/mL virulence polysaccharide antigen of *Salmonella typhi*, net price 0.5-mL prefilled syringe = £10.20

Dose: by deep subcutaneous or by intramuscular injection, 0.5 mL; CHILD under 18 months may show suboptimal response

■ Polysaccharide vaccine with hepatitis A vaccine

See Hepatitis A Vaccine

■ Live oral vaccine

Vivotif® (MASTA) PoM

Capsules, e/c, live attenuated *Salmonella typhi* (Ty 21a), net price 3-cap pack = £15.88. Label: 23, 25, C, administration

Dose: ADULT and CHILD over 6 years, 1 capsule on days 1, 3, and 5; under 6 years, not recommended

COUNSELLING. Swallow as soon as possible after placing in mouth with a cold or lukewarm drink; it is important to store capsules in refrigerator

Yellow fever vaccine

Yellow fever vaccine consists of a live attenuated yellow fever virus (17D strain) grown in developing chick embryos. Immunisation is indicated for those travelling or living in areas where infection is endemic (see p. 597) and for laboratory staff who handle the virus or who handle clinical material from suspected cases. Infants under 9 months of age should only be vaccinated if the risk of yellow fever is unavoidable since there is a small risk of encephalitis. The vaccine should not be given to those with impaired immune responsiveness, or who have had an anaphylactic reaction to egg; it should not be given during pregnancy (but where there is a significant risk of exposure the need for immunisation outweighs any risk to the fetus. See section 14.1 for further contra-indications. Reactions are few. The immunity which probably lasts for life is officially accepted for 10 years starting from 10 days after primary immunisation and for a further 10 years immediately after revaccination.

Yellow Fever Vaccine, Live PoM Yel/Vac. A suspension of chick embryo proteins containing attenuated 17D strain virus

Dose: by subcutaneous injection, 0.5 mL

Available (only to designated Yellow Fever Vaccination centres) as *Arilvax®* (Evans Medical) and *Stamaril®* (Aventis Pasteur)

14.5   Immunoglobulins

Human immunoglobulins have replaced immunoglobulins of animal origin (antisera) which were frequently associated with hypersensitivity. Injection of immunoglobulins produces immediate protection lasting for several weeks.

Immunoglobulins are produced from pooled human plasma or serum, and are tested and found non-reactive for hepatitis B surface antigen and for antibodies against hepatitis C virus and human immunodeficiency virus (types 1 and 2)

The two types of human immunoglobulin preparation are **normal immunoglobulin** and **specific immunoglobulins**.

Further information about immunoglobulins is included in *Immunisation against Infectious Disease* (see section 14.1).

AVAILABILITY. **Normal immunoglobulin** is now only available from the *Public Health Laboratory Service* laboratories for contacts and the control of outbreaks. It is available commercially for other purposes.

Specific immunoglobulins are available from the *Public Health Laboratory Service* laboratories and

Blood Centres in England and Wales with the exception of **tetanus immunoglobulin** which is distributed through *BPL* to hospital pharmacies or blood transfusion departments and is also available to general medical practitioners. **Rabies immunoglobulin** is available from the *Central Public Health Laboratory, London*. The large amounts of **hepatitis B immunoglobulin** required by transplant centres should be obtained commercially.

In Scotland all immunoglobulins are available from the *Blood Transfusion Service*. **Tetanus immunoglobulin** is distributed by the *Blood Transfusion Service* to hospitals and general medical practitioners on demand.

Normal immunoglobulin

Human **normal immunoglobulin** ('HNIG') is prepared from pools of at least 1000 donations of human plasma; it contains antibody to measles, mumps, varicella, hepatitis A, and other viruses that are currently prevalent in the general population.

CAUTIONS AND SIDE-EFFECTS. Side-effects of immunoglobulins include malaise, chills, fever, and rarely anaphylaxis. Normal immunoglobulin is **contra-indicated** in patients with known class specific antibody to immunoglobulin A (IgA).

Normal immunoglobulin may **interfere with the immune response to live virus vaccines** which should therefore only be given **at least 3 weeks before or 3 months after** an injection of normal immunoglobulin (this does not apply to yellow fever vaccine since normal immunoglobulin does not contain antibody to this virus). For travellers, if there is insufficient time, the recommended interval may have to be ignored.

Intramuscular immunoglobulins

Normal immunoglobulin is administered by intramuscular injection for the protection of susceptible contacts against **hepatitis A** virus (infectious hepatitis), **measles** and, to a lesser extent, **rubella**.

HEPATITIS A. **Hepatitis A vaccine** is preferred for individuals at risk of infection (see p. 584) including those visiting areas where the disease is highly endemic (all countries excluding Northern and Western Europe, North America, Japan, Australia, and New Zealand). In unimmunised individuals, transmission of hepatitis A is reduced by good hygiene. **Normal immunoglobulin** is no longer recommended for routine prophylaxis in travellers but it may be indicated for immunocompromised patients if their antibody response to vaccine is unlikely to be adequate.

Normal immunoglobulin is of value in the prevention of infection in close contact of confirmed cases of hepatitis A where there has been a delay in identifying cases or for individuals at high risk of severe disease.

MEASLES. Normal immunoglobulin may be given to prevent or attenuate an attack in individuals who do not have adequate immunity against measles. Children and adults with compromised immunity or pregnant women who have come into contact with measles should receive normal immunoglobulin as soon as possible after exposure. MMR vaccination should be considered for infants over 6 months, particularly if the contact is the mother (since the infant will not have maternal antibody). A child over 6 months with normal immunity can be given MMR vaccine within 72 hours of contact with measles, for post-exposure prophylaxis. Infants who have received early MMR should still receive the routine MMR vaccination according to the immunisation schedule.

RUBELLA. Immunoglobulin after exposure does **not** prevent infection in non-immune contacts and is **not** recommended for protection of pregnant women exposed to rubella. It may however reduce the likelihood of a clinical attack which may possibly reduce the risk to the fetus. It should only be used when termination of pregnancy would be unacceptable when it should be given as soon as possible after exposure. Serological follow-up of recipients is essential. For routine prophylaxis, see **Rubella Vaccine** (p. 592).

REPLACEMENT THERAPY. Normal immunoglobulin may also be given intramuscularly for replacement therapy, but intravenous formulations (see below under Intravenous) are normally preferred.

■ For intramuscular use

Normal Immunoglobulin PoM Normal immunoglobulin injection. 250-mg vial; 750-mg vial

Dose: by deep intramuscular injection, to control outbreaks, 500 mg; CHILD under 10 years 250 mg

Measles prophylaxis, CHILD under 1 year 250 mg, 1–2 years 500 mg, 3 years and over 750 mg; to allow attenuated attack, CHILD under 1 year 100 mg, 1 year and over 250 mg

Rubella in pregnancy, prevention of clinical attack, 750 mg

Available from Public Health Laboratory Service (for contacts and control of outbreaks only, see above) and from SNBTS

Gammabulin® (Baxter Bioscience) PoM

Normal immunoglobulin injection, net price 10-mL vial = £10.22

Dose: by intramuscular injection, antibody deficiency syndromes, consult product literature

Kabiglobulin® (Pharmacia) PoM

Normal immunoglobulin injection 16%, net price 2-mL amp = £2.78, 5-mL amp = £6.00

Note. May be difficult to obtain

Intravenous immunoglobulins

Special formulations for intravenous administration are available for replacement therapy for patients with congenital agammaglobulinaemia and hypogammaglobulinaemia, for the treatment of idiopathic thrombocytopenic purpura and Kawasaki syndrome, and for the prophylaxis of infection following bone marrow transplantation.

Intravenous immunoglobulin is also used in the treatment of Guillain-Barré syndrome and is now preferred to plasma exchange.

■ For intravenous use

Normal Immunoglobulin for Intravenous Use PoM

Available as: *Flebogamma®* 5% (0.5 g, 2.5 g, 5 g, 10 g—Grifols); *Gammagard® S/D* (0.5 g, 2.5 g, 5 g, 10 g—Baxter Bioscience); Human Immunoglobulin (3 g, 5 g, 10 g—SNBTS); *Octagam®* (2.5 g, 5 g, 10 g—Octapharma); *Sandoglobulin®* (1 g, 3 g, 6 g, 12 g—Novartis); *Vigam®S* (2.5 g, 5 g—BPL); *Vigam®Liquid* (2.5 g, 5 g, 10 g—BPL)

Dose: consult product literature

Specific immunoglobulins

Specific immunoglobulins are prepared by pooling the plasma of selected donors with high levels of the specific antibody required.

Although a hepatitis B vaccine is now available for those at high risk of infection, specific **hepatitis B immunoglobulin** ('HBIG') is available for use in association with the vaccine for the prevention of infection in laboratory and other personnel who have been accidentally inoculated with hepatitis B virus, and in infants born to mothers who have become infected with this virus in pregnancy or who are high-risk carriers.

Following exposure of an unimmunised individual to an animal in or from a high-risk country, the site of the bite should be washed with soapy water and specific **rabies immunoglobulin** of human origin should be injected at the site of the bite and also given intramuscularly. Rabies vaccine should also be given (for details see Rabies Vaccine, p. 591).

For the management of tetanus-prone wounds, **tetanus immunoglobulin** of human origin ('HTIG') should be used in addition to wound toilet and, where appropriate, antibacterial prophylaxis and adsorbed tetanus vaccine (section 14.4). Tetanus immunoglobulin, together with metronidazole (section 5.1.11) and wound toilet, should also be used for the treatment of established cases of tetanus.

Varicella-zoster immunoglobulin (VZIG) is recommended for individuals who are at increased risk of severe varicella *and* who have no antibodies to varicella-zoster virus *and* who have significant exposure to chickenpox or herpes zoster. Those at increased risk include neonates of women who develop chickenpox in the period 7 days before to 7 days after delivery, women exposed at any stage of pregnancy (but only issued to those exposed in the first 20 weeks' gestation when supplies of VZIG are short), and the immunosuppressed including those who have received corticosteroids in the previous 3 months at the following dose equivalents of prednisolone: *children* 2 mg/kg daily for at least 1 week or 1 mg/kg daily for 1 month; *adults* about 40 mg daily for more than 1 week. (**Important:** for full details consult *Immunisation against Infectious Disease*). **Varicella vaccine** is available on a named-patient basis from SmithKline Beecham.

Cytomegalovirus (CMV) immunoglobulin (available on a named-patient basis from SNBTS) is indicated for prophylaxis in patients receiving immunosuppressive treatment. Also batches of normal immunoglobulin with a high CMV titre are available from Grifols for treatment and prophylaxis of CMV infections [unlicensed indication].

■ Hepatitis B

Hepatitis B Immunoglobulin PoM See notes above

Dose: by intramuscular injection (as soon as possible after exposure), ADULT 500 units; CHILD under 4 years 200 units, 5–9 years 300 units; NEONATE 200 units as soon as possible after birth; for full details consult *Immunisation against Infectious Disease*

Available from Public Health Laboratory Service (except for Transplant Centres, see p. 594), also available from BPL and SNBTS

Note. Hepatitis B immunoglobulin for intravenous use is available from BPL and SNBTS on a named-patient basis.

■ Rabies

Rabies Immunoglobulin PoM (Antirabies Immunoglobulin Injection). See notes above

Dose: 20 units/kg, half *by intramuscular injection* and half *by infiltration* around wound

Available from Public Health Laboratory Service (also from BPL and SNBTS)

■ Tetanus

Tetanus Immunoglobulin PoM (Antitetanus Immunoglobulin Injection). See notes above

Dose: by intramuscular injection, prophylactic 250 units, increased to 500 units if more than 24 hours have elapsed or there is risk of heavy contamination

Therapeutic, 150 units/kg (multiple sites)

Available from BPL and SNBTS

Tetabulin® (Baxter Bioscience) PoM

Tetanus immunoglobulin, net price 250-unit pre-filled syringe = £14.80

Dose: by intramuscular injection, prophylactic, 250 units, increased to 500 units if wound older than 12 hours or if risk of heavy contamination or if patient weighs more than 90 kg; second dose of 250 units given after 3–4 weeks if patient immunosuppressed or if active immunisation with tetanus vaccine contra-indicated

Therapeutic, 30–300 units/kg

Tetanus Immunoglobulin for Intravenous Use PoM Used for proven or suspected clinical tetanus

Dose: by intravenous infusion, 5000–10 000 units

Available from BPL and SNBTS on a named-patient basis

■ Varicella–Zoster

Varicella–Zoster Immunoglobulin PoM (Anti-varicella–zoster Immunoglobulin) See notes above

Dose: by deep intramuscular injection, prophylaxis (as soon as possible—not later than 10 days after exposure), CHILD up to 5 years 250 mg, 6–10 years 500 mg, 11–14 years 750 mg, over 15 years 1 g; give second dose if further exposure occurs after 3 weeks of first dose

Note. No evidence that effective in treatment of severe disease. Normal immunoglobulin for intravenous use may be used to provide an immediate source of antibody.

Available from Public Health Laboratory Service (also from BPL and SNBTS)

Anti-D (Rh₀) immunoglobulin

Anti-D (Rh₀) immunoglobulin is available to prevent a rhesus-negative mother from forming antibodies to fetal rhesus-positive cells which may pass into the maternal circulation. The objective is to protect any subsequent child from the hazard of haemolytic disease of the newborn.

Anti-D immunoglobulin should be administered following any sensitising episode (e.g. abortion, miscarriage and birth); it should be injected within 72 hours of the episode but even if a longer period has elapsed it may still give protection and should be administered. The dose of anti-D immunoglobulin is determined according to the level of exposure to rhesus-positive blood.

Routine antenatal prophylaxis is also recommended by the Royal College of Obstetricians and Gynaecologists for all rhesus-negative women: two doses of at least 500 units of anti-D immunoglobulin should be given, the first at 28 weeks' gestation and the second at 34 weeks.

> *Note. Rubella vaccine* may be administered in the postpartum period simultaneously with anti-D (Rh₀) immunoglobulin injection provided that separate syringes are used and the products are administered into contralateral limbs. If blood is transfused, the antibody response to the vaccine may be inhibited and a test for antibodies should be performed after 8 weeks and the subject revaccinated if necessary.
>
> *MMR vaccine* should not be given within 3 months of an injection of anti-D (Rh₀) immunoglobulin injection.

Anti-D (Rh₀) Immunoglobulin PoM

Dose: by deep intramuscular injection, to rhesus-negative woman for prevention of $Rh_0(D)$ sensitisation:

Following birth of rhesus-positive infant, 500 units immediately or within 72 hours; for transplacental bleed in excess of 4–5 mL fetal red cells, extra 100–125 units per mL fetal red cells

Following any potentially sensitising episode (e.g. still-birth, abortion, amniocentesis) up to 20 weeks' gestation 250 units per episode (after 20 weeks, 500 units) immediately or within 72 hours

Following $Rh_0(D)$ incompatible blood transfusion, 125 units per mL transfused rhesus-positive red cells

Antenatal prophylaxis, 500 units given at weeks 28 and 34 of pregnancy; a further dose is still needed immediately or within 72 hours of delivery

Available from Blood Centres and from BPL and SNBTS

Anti-D (Rh₀) Immunoglobulin (Baxter Bioscience) PoM

Anti-D (Rh₀) immunoglobulin 1250 units/mL, net price 1-mL prefilled syringe = £23.90

Dose: by intramuscular injection, to rhesus-negative woman for prevention of $Rh_0(D)$ sensitisation:

Following abortion, miscarriage or birth of rhesus-positive infant, 1250 units immediately or within 72 hours; for transplacental bleed in excess of 25 mL fetal blood (1% of fetal erythrocytes), 5000 units (*or* 50 units per mL fetal blood)

Following any potentially sensitising episode (e.g. amniocentesis) 1250 units immediately or within 72 hours

Following $Rh_0(D)$ incompatible blood transfusion, at least 50–100 units per mL transfused rhesus-positive blood

Antenatal prophylaxis, 1250 units may be given at weeks 28 and 34 of pregnancy; a further dose is still needed immediately or within 72 hours of delivery

Note. Some UK authorities recommend lower doses for antenatal prophylaxis (see notes above)

WinRho SDF® (Cangene) [PoM]

Injection, powder for reconstitution, anti-D (Rh₀) immunoglobulin, net price 600-unit vial (with sodium chloride 0.9%) = £30.00; 1500-unit vial (with sodium chloride 0.9%) = £39.00

Dose: to rhesus-negative woman for prevention of Rh₀(D) sensitisation:

Following birth of rhesus-positive infant immediately or within 72 hours, *by slow intramuscular injection,* 1500 units *or by intravenous injection,* 600 units; for transplacental bleed in excess of 25 mL fetal blood, *by slow intramuscular injection,* extra 50 units per mL fetal blood

Following any potentially sensitising episode (e.g. miscarriage, abortion, amniocentesis), *by slow intramuscular injection,* up to 12 weeks gestation, 600 units (after 12 weeks, 1500 units) immediately or within 72 hours

Following Rh₀(D) incompatible blood transfusion, *by slow intramuscular injection,* 60 units per mL transfused rhesus-positive blood, in divided doses over several days

Following Rh₀(D) incompatible thrombocyte transfusion, *by intravenous injection,* 1500 units

Antenatal prophylaxis, *by slow intramuscular or intravenous injection,* 1500 units at 28 weeks' gestation; a further dose should be considered after birth if infant rhesus-positive

Note. For antenatal prophylaxis, some UK authorities recommend a lower dose, which is repeated at 34 weeks' gestation (see notes above)

Interferons

Interferon gamma-1b is indicated for chronic granulomatous disease to reduce the frequency of serious infection.

INTERFERON GAMMA-1b

(Immune interferon)

Indications: adjunct to antibacterials to reduce frequency of serious infection in patients with chronic granulomatous disease

Cautions: severe hepatic or renal impairment; seizure disorders or compromised central nervous system function; pre-existing cardiac disease (including ischaemia, congestive heart failure, and arrhythmias); monitor before and during treatment: haematological tests (including full blood count, differential white cell count, and platelet count), blood chemistry tests (including renal and liver function tests) and urinalysis

DRIVING. May impair ability to drive or operate machinery; effects may be enhanced by alcohol

Side-effects: fever, headache, chills, myalgia, fatigue; nausea, vomiting, arthralgia, rashes and injection-site reactions reported

Immukin® (Boehringer Ingelheim) ▼ [PoM]

Injection, recombinant human interferon gamma-1b 200 micrograms/mL, net price 0.5-mL vial = £88.00

Dose: by subcutaneous injection, 50 micrograms/m² 3 times a week; patients with body surface area of 0.5 m² or less, 1.5 micrograms/kg 3 times a week; not yet recommended for children under 6 months

14.6   International travel

Note. For advice on **malaria chemoprophylaxis,** see section 5.4.1.

No particular immunisation is required for travellers to the United States, Europe, Australia, or New Zealand although all travellers should have immunity to tetanus and poliomyelitis (and childhood immunisations should be up to date). In Non-European areas surrounding the Mediterranean, in Africa, the Middle East, Asia, and South America, certain special precautions are required.

Long-term travellers to areas that have a high incidence of **poliomyelitis** or **tuberculosis** should be immunised with the appropriate vaccine; in the case of poliomyelitis previously immunised adults may be given a booster dose of oral poliomyelitis vaccine. BCG immunisation is recommended for travellers proposing to stay for longer than one month (or in close contact with the local population) in Asia, Africa, or Central and South America; it should preferably be given three months or more before departure.

Yellow fever immunisation is recommended for travel to much of Africa and South America. Many countries require an International Certificate of Vaccination from individuals arriving from, or who have been travelling through, endemic areas, whilst other countries require a certificate from all entering travellers (consult the Department of Health Handbook, *Health Information for Overseas Travel).*

Immunisation against **meningococcal meningitis** is recommended for a number of areas of the world (for details, see p. 588).

Protection against **hepatitis A** is recommended for travellers to high-risk areas outside Northern and Western Europe, North America, Japan, Australia and New Zealand. Hepatitis A vaccine (see p. 584) is preferred and it is likely to be effective even if given shortly before departure; normal immunoglobulin is no longer given routinely but may be indicated in the immunocompromised (see p. 594).

Hepatitis B vaccine (see p. 585) is recommended for those travelling to areas of high prevalence who intend to seek employment as health care workers or who plan to remain there for lengthy periods and who may therefore be at increased risk of acquiring infection as the result of medical or dental procedures carried out in those countries. Short-term tourists or business travellers are not generally at increased risk of infection but may place themselves at risk by their sexual behaviour when abroad.

Prophylactic immunisation against **rabies** (see p. 591) is recommended for travellers to enzootic areas on long journeys to remote areas out of reach of immediate medical attention.

Typhoid vaccine is indicated for travellers to those countries where typhoid is endemic but the vaccine is no substitute for personal precautions. Food should be freshly prepared and hot, and uncooked vegetables (including green salads) should be avoided; only fruits which can be peeled should be eaten. Only suitable bottled water, or tap water that has been boiled, or treated with sterilising tablets should be used for drinking. This advice also applies to cholera and other diarrhoeal diseases (including travellers' diarrhoea).

Cholera vaccine has little value in preventing infections and should **not** be given for international travel (see under Cholera Vaccine). It is no longer available.

Advice on **diphtheria**, on **Japanese encephalitis** (vaccine available on named-patient basis from Aventis Pasteur and MASTA) and on **tick-borne encephalitis** (vaccine available on named-patient basis from Baxter Bioscience) is included in *Health Information for Overseas Travel*, see below.

Information on health advice for travellers

The Department of Health booklet, *Health Advice For Travellers* (code: T6) includes information on immunisation requirements (or recommendations) around the world. The booklet can be obtained from travel agents, post-offices or by telephoning 0800 555 777 (24-hour service); also available on the Internet at
http://www.doh.gov.uk/hat/hatcvr.htm

The Department of Health handbook, *Health Information for Overseas Travel* (2001), which draws together essential information *for healthcare professionals* regarding health advice for travellers, can be obtained from
The Stationery Office
PO Box 29, Norwich NR3 1GN
Telephone orders, 0870 600 5522
Fax: 0870 600 5533
www.thestationeryoffice.com

Immunisation requirements change from time to time, and information on the current requirements for any particular country may be obtained from:

Public Health Laboratory Service Communicable Disease Surveillance Centre, Travel Medicine Unit, 61 Colindale Avenue, London NW9 5EQ
Tel (020) 8200 6868 (10.00–12.00 weekdays; for healthcare professionals **only**)

Scottish Centre for Infection and Environmental Health, Clifton House, Clifton Place, Glasgow G3 7LN (Tel (0141) 300 1130 (14.00–16.00 hours weekdays))
http://www.axl.co.uk/scieh (for registered users for the NHS website Travax only)

Scottish Office Department of Health, Public Health Policy Unit, St. Andrew's House, Edinburgh EH1 3DG (Tel (0131) 556 8400)

Welsh Office, Cathays Park, Cardiff CF10 3NQ (Tel (029) 2082 5111)

Department of Health and Social Services, Castle Buildings, Stormont, Belfast BT4 3PP (Tel (028) 9052 0000)

or from the embassy or legation of the appropriate country.

15: Anaesthesia

15.1   General anaesthesia

15.1.1	Intravenous anaesthetics
15.1.2	Inhalational anaesthetics
15.1.3	Antimuscarinic drugs
15.1.4	Sedative and analgesic peri-operative drugs
15.1.5	Muscle relaxants
15.1.6	Anticholinesterases used in anaesthesia
15.1.7	Antagonists for central and respiratory depression
15.1.8	Drugs for malignant hyperthermia

Note. The drugs in section 15.1 should be used only by experienced personnel and where adequate resuscitative equipment is available.

It is now common practice to administer several drugs with different actions to produce a state of surgical anaesthesia with minimal risk of toxic effects. An intravenous anaesthetic is usually used for induction, followed by maintenance with inhalational anaesthetics, perhaps supplemented by other drugs administered intravenously. Specific drugs are often used to produce muscular relaxation. These drugs interfere with spontaneous respiration so intermittent positive-pressure ventilation by manual or mechanical means is commonly employed.

For certain procedures controlled hypotension may be required. Labetalol (section 2.4), sodium nitroprusside (section 2.5.1), and glyceryl trinitrate (section 2.6.1) are used. Glyceryl trinitrate (section 2.6.1) is also used to control hypertension, particularly postoperatively.

Beta-blockers (section 2.4), adenosine, amiodarone (section 2.3.2) or verapamil (section 2.6.2) may be used to control arrhythmias during anaesthesia. Esmolol has a very short duration of action and is particularly suited to the peri- and intra-operative management of arrhythmias, including tachycardia, and hypertension (section 2.4).

SURGERY AND LONG-TERM MEDICATION. The risk of stopping long-term medication before surgery is often greater than the risk of continuing it during surgery; however, surgery itself may alter the need for continued drug therapy of certain conditions. It is vital that the anaesthetist should know of **all** drugs that a patient is (or has been) taking.

Patients with adrenal atrophy resulting from long-term corticosteroid use (section 6.3.2) may experience a precipitous fall in blood pressure unless corticosteroid cover is provided during anaesthesia and in the immediate postoperative period. Anaesthetists must therefore know whether a patient is, or has been, taking corticosteroids.

Other drugs that should normally not be stopped before surgery include antiepileptics, antiparkinsonian drugs, antipsychotics, bronchodilators, cardiovascular drugs, glaucoma drugs, immunosuppressants, drugs of dependence, and thyroid or antithyroid drugs. Expert advice is required for patients receiving antivirals for HIV infection. For general advice on surgery in diabetic patients see section 6.1.1.

Although it is possible to operate on patients taking oral anticoagulants when the INR is close to 2, many surgeons and anaesthetists prefer to stop oral anticoagulants. Individual circumstances will dictate whether it is appropriate to continue prophylaxis in the peri-operative period with heparin and graduated compression hosiery until oral anticoagulation can be re-established; the haematologist should be consulted for further advice.

Drugs that are stopped before surgery include combined oral contraceptives (see Surgery, section 7.3.1 for details); for advice on hormone replacement therapy, see section 6.4.1.1. If antidepressants need to be stopped, they should be withdrawn gradually to avoid withdrawal symptoms. In view of their hazardous interactions MAOIs should normally be stopped 2 weeks before surgery. Tricyclic antidepressants need not be stopped, but there may be an increased risk of arrhythmias and hypotension (and dangerous interaction with vasopressor drugs); the anaesthetist therefore should be informed if they are not stopped. Lithium should be stopped 24 hours before major surgery but the normal dose can be continued for minor surgery (with careful monitoring of fluids and electrolytes). Potassium-sparing diuretics may need to be withheld on the morning of surgery because hyperkalaemia may develop if renal perfusion is impaired or if there is tissue damage.

ANAESTHESIA AND DRIVING. Patients given sedatives and analgesics during minor outpatient procedures should be very carefully warned about the risk of driving afterwards. For intravenous benzodiazepines and for a short general anaesthetic the risk extends to **at least 24 hours** after administration. Responsible persons should be available to take patients home. The dangers of taking **alcohol** should also be emphasised.

PROPHYLAXIS OF ACID ASPIRATION. Regurgitation and aspiration of gastric contents (Mendelson's syndrome) is an important complication of general anaesthesia, particularly in obstetrics and emergency surgery. The damage to the lung is influenced by the pH, the volume of the gastric contents aspirated, and by the presence of food particles.

H_2-receptor antagonists (section 1.3.1) or **omeprazole** (section 1.3.5) may be used before surgery to increase the pH and reduce the volume of gastric fluid. They do not affect the pH of fluid already in the stomach and this limits their value in emergency procedures; oral H_2-receptor antagonists can be given 1–2 hours before the procedure but omeprazole must be given at least 12 hours earlier. Antacids are frequently used to neutralise the acidity of the fluid already in the stomach; 'clear' (non-particulate) antacids such as sodium citrate are preferred.

Gas cylinders

Each gas cylinder bears a label with the name of the gas contained in the cylinder. The name or chemical symbol of the gas appears on the shoulder of the cylinder and is also clearly and indelibly stamped on the cylinder valve.

The colours on the valve end of the cylinder extend down to the shoulder; in the case of mixed gases the colours for the individual gases are applied in four segments, two for each colour.

Gas cylinders should be stored in a cool well-ventilated room, free from flammable materials.

No lubricant of any description should be used on the cylinder valves.

15.1.1 Intravenous anaesthetics

Intravenous anaesthetics may be used either to induce anaesthesia or for maintenance of anaesthesia throughout surgery. Intravenous anaesthetics nearly all produce their effect in one arm-brain circulation time and can cause apnoea and hypotension, and so adequate resuscitative facilities **must** be available. They are **contra-indicated** if the anaesthetist is not confident of being able to maintain the airway (e.g. in the presence of a tumour in the pharynx or larynx). Extreme care is required in surgery of the mouth, pharynx, or larynx and in patients with acute circulatory failure (shock) or fixed cardiac output.

Individual requirements vary considerably and the recommended dosage is only a guide. Smaller dosage is indicated in ill, shocked, or debilitated patients, while robust individuals may require more. To facilitate tracheal intubation, induction is followed by a neuromuscular blocking drug (section 15.1.5).

TOTAL INTRAVENOUS ANAESTHESIA. This is a technique in which major surgery is carried out with all anaesthetic drugs given intravenously. Respiration is controlled, the lungs being inflated with oxygen-enriched air. Muscle relaxants are used to provide relaxation and prevent reflex muscle movements. The main problem to be overcome is the assessment of depth of anaesthesia.

ANAESTHESIA AND DRIVING. See section 15.1.

Barbiturates

Thiopental sodium (thiopentone sodium) is a widely used intravenous anaesthetic, but it has no analgesic properties. Induction is generally smooth and rapid, but owing to its narrow therapeutic margin, overdosage with cardiorespiratory depression may occur. The reconstituted solution is highly alkaline and therefore irritant on misplaced injection outside the vein; arterial injection is particularly dangerous.

Awakening from a moderate dose of thiopental is rapid due to redistribution of the drug in the whole body tissues. Metabolism is, however, slow and some sedative effects may persist for 24 hours. Repeated doses have a cumulative effect.

Thiopental is **contra-indicated** in porphyria (section 9.8.2).

THIOPENTAL SODIUM

(Thiopentone Sodium)

Indications: induction of general anaesthesia; anaesthesia of short duration; reduction of raised intracranial pressure if ventilation controlled

Cautions: see notes above; reduce induction dose in severe liver disease; **interactions:** Appendix 1 (anaesthetics, general)

Contra-indications: see notes above; porphyria (section 9.8.2)

Side-effects: see notes above

Dose: induction of general anaesthesia, *by intravenous injection* as a 2.5% (25 mg/mL) solution, in fit premedicated adults, initially 100–150 mg (reduced in elderly or debilitated) over 10–15 seconds (longer in elderly or debilitated), followed by further quantity if necessary according to response after 30–60 seconds; *or* up to 4 mg/kg; CHILD induction 2–7 mg/kg

Raised intracranial pressure, *by intravenous injection*, 1.5–3 mg/kg, repeated as required

Thiopental (Non-proprietary) PoM
Injection, powder for reconstitution, thiopental sodium, net price 500-mg vial = £3.06
Available from Link

Other intravenous anaesthetics

Etomidate is an induction agent associated with rapid recovery without hangover effect. It causes less hypotension than other drugs used for induction. There is a high incidence of extraneous muscle movement and of pain on injection; these effects can be minimised by premedication with an opioid analgesic and the use of larger veins. Etomidate may suppress adrenocortical function, particularly on continuous administration, and it should not be used for maintenance of anaesthesia.

Propofol is associated with rapid recovery without hangover effect and is very widely used. There is sometimes pain on intravenous injection, but significant extraneous muscle movements do not occur. The CSM has received reports of convulsions, anaphylaxis, and delayed recovery from anaesthesia after propofol administration; since some of the convulsions are delayed the CSM has advised special caution after day surgery. Propofol has been associated with bradycardia, occasionally profound; intravenous administration of an antimuscarinic may be necessary to prevent this.

Ketamine can be given by the intravenous or the intramuscular route, and has good analgesic properties when used in sub-anaesthetic dosage. The maximum effect occurs after more than one arm-brain circulation time. Muscle tone is increased. There is cardiovascular stimulation and arterial pressure may rise with tachycardia. The main disadvantage is the high incidence of hallucinations and other transient psychotic sequelae, though it is believed that these are much less significant in children. The incidence can be reduced when drugs such as diazepam are also used. Ketamine is **contra-indicated** in patients with hypertension and is best avoided in those prone to hallucinations. It is used mainly for

paediatric anaesthesia, particularly when repeated administrations are required. Recovery is relatively slow.

ETOMIDATE

Indications: induction of anaesthesia

Cautions: see notes above; avoid in porphyria (section 9.8.2); **interactions:** Appendix 1 (anaesthetics, general)

Contra-indications: see notes above

Side-effects: see notes above

Dose: *by slow intravenous injection*, 300 micrograms/kg (ELDERLY 150–200 micrograms/kg); CHILD up to 15 years up to 390 micrograms/kg

Hypnomidate® (Janssen-Cilag) PoM
Injection, etomidate 2 mg/mL in propylene glycol 35%. Net price 10-mL amp = £1.58

KETAMINE

Indications: induction and maintenance of anaesthesia

Cautions: see notes above; **interactions:** Appendix 1 (anaesthetics, general)

Contra-indications: see notes above

Side-effects: see notes above

Dose: *by intramuscular injection*, short procedures, initially 6.5–13 mg/kg (10 mg/kg usually produces 12–25 minutes of surgical anaesthesia) Diagnostic manoeuvres and procedures not involving intense pain, initially 4 mg/kg

By intravenous injection over at least 60 seconds, short procedures, initially 1–4.5 mg/kg (2 mg/kg usually produces 5–10 minutes of surgical anaesthesia)

By intravenous infusion of a solution containing 1 mg/mL, longer procedures, induction, total dose of 0.5–2 mg/kg; maintenance (using microdrip infusion), 10–45 micrograms/kg/minute, rate adjusted according to response

Ketalar® (Parke-Davis) PoM
Injection, ketamine (as hydrochloride) 10 mg/mL, net price 20-mL vial = £3.52; 50 mg/mL, 10-mL vial = £7.31; 100 mg/mL, 10-mL vial = £13.42

PROPOFOL

Indications: see under preparations below

Cautions: see notes above; monitor blood-lipid concentration if risk of fat overload or if sedation longer than 3 days; **interactions:** Appendix 1 (anaesthetics, general)

Contra-indications: see notes above; not to be used for sedation of ventilated children and adolescents under 17 years

Side-effects: see notes above; pulmonary oedema, postoperative fever reported

Dose: see under preparations below

Diprivan® (AstraZeneca) [PoM]

1% injection (emulsion), propofol 10 mg/mL, net
price 20-mL amp = £3.88, 50-mL vial = £9.70,
50-mL prefilled syringe (for use with *Diprifusor®*
TCI system) = £10.67, 100-mL vial = £19.40

Note. Diprifusor® TCI ('target controlled infusion') system is for use **only** for induction and maintenance of
general anaesthesia in adults

Dose: induction of anaesthesia, *by intravenous injection*
or infusion, 1.5–2.5 mg/kg (less in those over 55 years)
at a rate of 20–40 mg every 10 seconds; CHILD over 1
month, administer slowly until response (usual dose in
child over 8 years 2.5 mg/kg, may need more in younger
child)

Maintenance of anaesthesia, *by intravenous injection*,
25–50 mg repeated according to response *or by intravenous infusion*, 4–12 mg/kg/hour; CHILD over 3 years,
by intravenous injection or infusion, 9–15 mg/kg/hour

Sedation in intensive care, *by intravenous infusion*,
ADULT over 17 years, 0.3–4 mg/kg/hour

Sedation for surgical and diagnostic procedures, initially
by intravenous injection over 1–5 minutes, 0.5–1 mg/kg;
maintenance, *by intravenous infusion*, 1.5–4.5 mg/
hour (additionally, if rapid increase in sedation required,
by intravenous injection, 10–20 mg); those over 55 years
may require lower dose; CHILD and ADOLESCENT under
17 years not recommended

2% injection (emulsion), propofol 20 mg/mL, net
price 50-mL vial = £19.40, 50-mL prefilled
syringe (for use with *Diprifusor®* *TCI* system) =
£20.37

Note. Diprifusor® TCI ('target controlled infusion') system is for use **only** for induction and maintenance of
general anaesthesia in adults

Dose: induction of anaesthesia, *by intravenous infusion*,
1.5–2.5 mg/kg (less in those over 55 years) at a rate of
20–40 mg every 10 seconds; CHILD over 3 years, administer slowly until response (usual dose in child over 8
years 2.5 mg/kg, may need more in younger child)

Maintenance of anaesthesia, *by intravenous infusion*, 4–
12 mg/kg/hour; CHILD over 3 years, *by intravenous infusion*, 9–15 mg/kg/hour

Sedation in intensive care, *by intravenous infusion*,
ADULT over 17 years, 0.3–4 mg/kg/hour

Note. Propofol injection also available from Baxter (1%,
2%), Braun (*Propofol-Lipuro®* 1%), Fresenius Kabi
(1%, 2%), Zurich (1%, 2%)

15.1.2   Inhalational anaesthetics

Inhalational anaesthetics may be gases or volatile
liquids. They can be used both for induction and
maintenance of anaesthesia and may also be used
following induction with an intravenous anaesthetic
(section 15.1.1).

Gaseous anaesthetics require suitable equipment
for storage and administration. They may be supplied via hospital pipelines or from metal cylinders.
Volatile liquid anaesthetics are administered using
calibrated vaporisers, using air, oxygen, or nitrous
oxide–oxygen mixtures as the carrier gas. It should
be noted that they can all trigger malignant hyperthermia (section 15.1.8).

To prevent hypoxia inhalational anaesthetics must
be given with concentrations of oxygen greater than
in air.

ANAESTHESIA AND DRIVING. See section 15.1.

Volatile liquid anaesthetics

Halothane is a volatile liquid anaesthetic. Its
advantages are that it is potent, induction is smooth,
the vapour is non-irritant, pleasant to inhale, and
seldom induces coughing or breath-holding.
Despite these advantages, however, halothane is
much less widely used than previously owing to its
association with *severe hepatotoxicity* (**important**:
see CSM advice, below).

Halothane causes cardiorespiratory depression.
Respiratory depression results in elevation of arterial carbon dioxide tension and perhaps ventricular
arrhythmias. Halothane also depresses the cardiac
muscle fibres and may cause bradycardia. The
result is diminished cardiac output and fall of arterial pressure. Adrenaline (epinephrine) infiltrations
should be avoided in patients anaesthetised with
halothane as ventricular arrhythmias may result.

Halothane produces moderate muscle relaxation,
but this may be inadequate for major abdominal
surgery and specific muscle relaxants are then used.

> **CSM advice (halothane hepatotoxicity).** In a
> publication on findings confirming that *severe
> hepatotoxicity* can follow halothane anaesthesia the
> CSM has reported that this occurs more frequently
> after repeated exposures to halothane and has a
> high mortality. The risk of severe hepatotoxicity
> appears to be increased by repeated exposures
> within a short time interval, but even after a long
> interval (sometimes of several years) susceptible
> patients have been reported to develop jaundice.
> Since there is no reliable way of identifying suscepti-
> ble patients the CSM recommends the following
> precautions prior to use of halothane:
> 1. a careful anaesthetic history should be taken to
> determine previous exposure and previous reactions
> to halothane;
> 2. repeated exposure to halothane within a period
> of **at least** 3 months should be **avoided** unless
> there are **overriding** clinical circumstances;
> 3. a history of unexplained jaundice or pyrexia in a
> patient following exposure to halothane is an abso-
> lute **contra-indication** to its future use in that
> patient.

Enflurane is a volatile anaesthetic similar to
halothane, but less potent, about twice the concentration being necessary for induction and maintenance.

Enflurane is a powerful cardiorespiratory depressant. Shallow respiration is likely to result in a rise
of arterial carbon dioxide tension, but ventricular
arrhythmias are uncommon and it is probably safe
to use adrenaline (epinephrine) infiltrations. Myocardial depression may result in a fall in cardiac
output and in arterial hypotension. It may cause
EEG changes and should be avoided in those liable
to epileptic seizures. Enflurane may cause hepatotoxicity in those sensitised to halogenated anaesthetics but the risk is smaller than with halothane.

Isoflurane is an isomer of enflurane. It has a
potency intermediate between that of halothane and
enflurane, and even less of an inhaled dose is
metabolised than with enflurane. Heart rhythm is
generally stable during isoflurane anaesthesia, but
heart-rate may rise, particularly in younger patients.
Systemic arterial pressure may fall, owing to a
decrease in systemic vascular resistance and with

less decrease in cardiac output than occurs with halothane. Respiration is depressed. Muscle relaxation is produced and muscle relaxant drugs potentiated. Isoflurane may also cause hepatotoxicity in those sensitised to halogenated anaesthetics but the risk is appreciably smaller than with halothane.

Desflurane is reported to have about one-fifth the potency of isoflurane. Owing to limited experience it is not recommended in neurosurgical patients. It is not recommended for induction in children because cough, breath-holding, apnoea, laryngospasm and increased secretions can occur. The risk of hepatotoxicity with desflurane in those sensitised to halogenated anaesthetics appears to be remote.

Sevoflurane is a rapid acting volatile liquid anaesthetic. Patients may require early postoperative pain relief as emergence and recovery are particularly rapid.

VOLATILE ANAESTHETICS AND CARBOXYHAEMO-GLOBINAEMIA. Carboxyhaemoglobinaemia has been reported during anaesthesia with desflurane, enflurane, or isoflurane used in conjunction with carbon dioxide absorbents in breathing systems in the USA. This phenomenon was very rare and occurred when these absorbents became excessively dried out.
The use of barium hydroxide lime produces significantly more carbon monoxide than soda lime particularly at low water content.
Barium hydroxide lime is not available in the UK. The CSM has advised that no cases of carboxyhaemoglobinaemia have been reported in the UK and it seems unlikely that this problem will arise with the anaesthetic equipment currently in use in the UK.

DESFLURANE

Indications: see notes above

Cautions: see notes above; **interactions:** Appendix 1 (anaesthetics, general)

Contra-indications: see notes above; susceptibility to malignant hyperthermia

Side-effects: see notes above

Dose: using a specifically calibrated vaporiser, *induction*, 4–11%; CHILD not recommended for induction
Maintenance, 2–6% in nitrous oxide; 2.5–8.5% in oxygen or oxygen-enriched air; max. 17%

Suprane® (Baxter Anaesthesia) [PoM]
Desflurane. Net price 240 mL = £44.41

ENFLURANE

Indications: see notes above

Cautions: see notes above; epilepsy; avoid in porphyria (section 9.8.2); **interactions:** Appendix 1 (anaesthetics, general)

Contra-indications: susceptibility to malignant hyperthermia

Side-effects: see notes above

Dose: using a specifically calibrated vaporiser, *induction*, increased gradually from 0.4% to max. of 4.5% in air, oxygen, or nitrous oxide–oxygen, according to response
Maintenance, 0.5–3% in nitrous oxide–oxygen

Enflurane (Abbott)
Enflurane. Net price 250 mL = £24.00

Alyrane® (Baxter Anaesthesia)
Enflurane, net price 250 mL = £20.00

HALOTHANE

Indications: see notes above

Cautions: see notes above (**important:** CSM advice, see notes above); avoid for dental procedures in those under 18 years unless treated in hospital (high risk of arrhythmia); avoid in porphyria (section 9.8.2); **interactions:** Appendix 1 (anaesthetics, general)

Contra-indications: see notes above; susceptibility to malignant hyperthermia

Side-effects: see notes above

Dose: using a specifically calibrated vaporiser, *induction*, increased gradually to 2–4% in oxygen or nitrous oxide–oxygen; CHILD (see cautions) 1.5–2%
Maintenance, 0.5–2%

Halothane (Concord)
Halothane, net price 250 mL = £20.57

ISOFLURANE

Indications: see notes above

Cautions: see notes above; **interactions:** Appendix 1 (anaesthetics, general)

Contra-indications: susceptibility to malignant hyperthermia

Side-effects: see notes above

Dose: using a specifically calibrated vaporiser, *induction*, increased gradually from 0.5% to 3%, in oxygen or nitrous oxide–oxygen
Maintenance, 1–2.5% in nitrous oxide–oxygen; an additional 0.5–1% may be required when given with oxygen alone; caesarean section, 0.5–0.75% in nitrous oxide–oxygen

Isoflurane (Abbott)
Isoflurane. Net price 250 mL = £47.50

Aerrane® (Baxter Anaesthesia)
Isoflurane, net price 100 mL = £7.98, 250 mL = £30.00

SEVOFLURANE

Indications: see notes above

Cautions: see notes above; **interactions:** Appendix 1 (anaesthetics, general)

IMPORTANT. In low-flow anaesthesia systems with standard carbon dioxide absorbents, sevoflurane forms a vinyl ether, compound A, which may cause glucosuria and albuminuria. Sevoflurane should be used with caution in patients with renal insufficiency. To reduce the possibility of Compound A-associated toxicity **avoid** prolonged use in low-flow systems (less than 2 litres/minute) which use standard carbon dioxide absorbents.

Contra-indications: see notes above; susceptibility to malignant hyperthermia

Side-effects: see notes above; also agitation occurs frequently in children

Dose: using a specifically calibrated vaporiser, *induction*, up to 5% in oxygen or nitrous oxide–oxygen; CHILD up to 7%
Maintenance, 0.5–3%

Sevoflurane (Abbott) [PoM]
Sevoflurane, net price 250 mL = £123.00

Nitrous oxide

Nitrous oxide is used for maintenance of anaesthesia and, in sub-anaesthetic concentrations, for analgesia. For anaesthesia it is commonly used in a concentration of 50 to 70% in oxygen as part of a balanced technique in association with other inhalational or intravenous agents. Nitrous oxide is unsatisfactory as a sole anaesthetic owing to lack of potency, but is useful as part of a combination of drugs since it allows a significant reduction in dosage.

A mixture of nitrous oxide and oxygen containing 50% of each gas (*Entonox®, Equanox®*) is used to produce analgesia without loss of consciousness. Self-administration using a demand valve is popular in obstetric practice, for changing painful dressings, as an aid to postoperative physiotherapy, and in emergency ambulances.

Nitrous oxide may have a deleterious effect if used in patients with an air-containing closed space since nitrous oxide diffuses into such a space with a resulting increase in pressure. This effect may be dangerous in the presence of a pneumothorax which may enlarge to compromise respiration.

Exposure of patients to nitrous oxide for prolonged periods, either by continuous or by intermittent administration, may result in megaloblastic anaemia owing to interference with the action of vitamin B_{12}. For the same reason, exposure of theatre staff to nitrous oxide should be minimised. Depression of white cell formation may also occur.

NITROUS OXIDE

Indications: see notes above
Cautions: see notes above; **interactions:** Appendix 1 (anaesthetics, general)
Side-effects: see notes above
Dose: using a suitable anaesthetic apparatus, a mixture with 25–30% oxygen for *maintenance* of light anaesthesia
Analgesic, as a mixture with 50% oxygen, according to the patient's needs

15.1.3   Antimuscarinic drugs

Antimuscarinic drugs are used (less commonly nowadays) as premedicants to dry bronchial and salivary secretions which are increased by intubation, by surgery to the upper airways, and by some inhalational anaesthetics. They are also used before or with neostigmine (section 15.1.6) to prevent bradycardia, excessive salivation, and other muscarinic actions of neostigmine. They are also used to prevent bradycardia and hypotension associated with agents such as halothane, propofol, and suxamethonium.

Atropine is now rarely used for premedication but still has an emergency role in the treatment of vagotonic side-effects. For its role in acute arrhythmias after myocardial infarction, see section 2.3.1; see also cardiopulmonary resuscitation algorithm, section 2.7.3.

Hyoscine effectively reduces secretions and also provides a degree of amnesia, sedation and antiemesis. Unlike atropine it may produce bradycardia rather than tachycardia. In some patients, especially the elderly, hyoscine may cause the central anti-cholinergic syndrome (excitement, ataxia, hallucinations, behavioural abnormalities, and drowsiness).

Glycopyrronium produces good drying of salivary secretions. When given intravenously it produces less tachycardia than atropine. It is widely used with neostigmine for reversal of non-depolarising muscle relaxants (section 15.1.5).

Phenothiazines have too little drying activity to be effective when used alone.

ATROPINE SULPHATE

Indications: drying secretions, reversal of excessive bradycardia; with neostigmine for reversal of non-depolarising neuromuscular block; antispasmodic (section 1.2); bradycardia (section 2.3.1); eye (section 11.5)
Cautions: cardiovascular disease; see also section 1.2; **interactions:** Appendix 1 (antimuscarinics)
DURATION OF ACTION. Since atropine has a shorter duration of action than neostigmine, late unopposed bradycardia may result; close monitoring of the patient is necessary
Side-effects: tachycardia; see also section 1.2
Dose: premedication, *by intravenous injection*, 300–600 micrograms immediately before induction of anaesthesia, and in incremental doses of 100 micrograms for the treatment of bradycardia
By intramuscular injection, 300–600 micrograms 30–60 minutes before induction; CHILD 20 micrograms/kg
For control of muscarinic side-effects of neostigmine in reversal of competitive neuromuscular block, *by intravenous injection*, 0.6–1.2 mg
Arrhythmias after myocardial infarction, see section 2.3.1; see also cardiopulmonary resuscitation algorithm, inside back cover

Atropine (Non-proprietary) PoM
Injection, atropine sulphate 600 micrograms/mL, net price 1-mL amp = 47p
Note. Other strengths also available
Injection, prefilled disposable syringe, atropine sulphate 100 micrograms/mL, net price 5 mL = £4.16, 10 mL = £4.66, 30 mL = £8.52
Available from Celltech (*Min-I-Jet®*)
Injection, prefilled disposable syringe, atropine sulphate 200 micrograms/mL, net price 5 mL = £4.24; 300 micrograms/mL, 10 mL = £4.32
Available from Aurum

■ With morphine
See under Morphine Salts (section 4.7.2)

GLYCOPYRRONIUM BROMIDE

Indications: see under Atropine Sulphate
Cautions: cardiovascular disease; see also Atropine sulphate (section 1.2); **interactions:** Appendix 1 (antimuscarinics)
Side-effects: see under Atropine Sulphate
Dose: premedication, *by intramuscular or intravenous injection*, 200–400 micrograms, *or* 4–5 micrograms/kg to a max. of 400 micrograms; CHILD *by intramuscular or* preferably *by intravenous injection*, 4–8 micrograms/kg to a max. of 200 micrograms
Intra-operative use, *by intravenous injection*, as for premedication, repeated if necessary
Control of muscarinic side-effects of neostigmine in

reversal of non-depolarising neuromuscular block, *by intravenous injection*, 200 micrograms per 1 mg of neostigmine, *or* 10–15 micrograms/kg with neostigmine 50 micrograms/kg; CHILD 10 micrograms/kg with neostigmine 50 micrograms/kg

Robinul® (Anpharm) PoM
Injection, glycopyrronium bromide
200 micrograms/mL, net price 1-mL amp = 60p;
3-mL amp = £1.01
Available as a generic from Antigen

■ With neostigmine metilsulphate
Section 15.1.6

HYOSCINE HYDROBROMIDE
(Scopolamine Hydrobromide)
Indications: drying secretions, amnesia; other indications (section 4.6)
Cautions: see under Atropine Sulphate; avoid in the elderly (see notes above)
Contra-indications: porphyria (section 9.8.2)
Side-effects: see under Atropine Sulphate; bradycardia
Dose: premedication, *by subcutaneous or intramuscular injection*, 200–600 micrograms 30–60 minutes before induction of anaesthesia, usually with papaveretum

Hyoscine (Non-proprietary) PoM
Injection, hyoscine hydrobromide
400 micrograms/mL, net price 1-mL amp = £2.70; 600 micrograms/mL, 1-mL amp = £2.81

■ With papaveretum
See under papaveretum (section 4.7.2)

15.1.4   Sedative and analgesic peri-operative drugs

15.1.4.1	Anxiolytics and neuroleptics
15.1.4.2	Non-opioid analgesics
15.1.4.3	Opioid analgesics

These drugs are given to allay the apprehension of the patient in the pre-operative period (including the night before operation), to relieve pain and discomfort when present, and to augment the action of subsequent anaesthetic agents. A number of the drugs used also provide some degree of pre-operative amnesia. The choice will vary with the individual patient, the nature of the operative procedure, the anaesthetic to be used and other prevailing circumstances such as outpatients, obstetrics, recovery facilities etc. The choice would also vary in elective and emergency operations.

PREMEDICATION IN CHILDREN. Oral administration is preferred to injections where possible but is not altogether satisfactory; the rectal route should only be used in exceptional circumstances. Oral alimemazine (trimeprazine) is still used but when given alone it may cause postoperative restlessness when pain is present.

Atropine or hyoscine is often given orally to children, but may be given intravenously immediately before induction.

The use of a suitable local anaesthetic cream (section 15.2) should be considered to avoid pain at injection site.

ANAESTHESIA AND DRIVING. See section 15.1.

15.1.4.1   Anxiolytics and neuroleptics

Anxiolytic benzodiazepines are widely used whereas neuroleptics such as **chlorpromazine** (section 4.2.1) are rarely used in the UK for premedication although chlorpromazine was used to prevent shivering in induction of hypothermia. **Alimemazine (trimeprazine)** (section 3.4.1) is still occasionally used as a premedicant for children (but see section 15.1.4).

Benzodiazepines

Benzodiazepines possess useful properties for premedication including relief of anxiety, sedation, and amnesia; short-acting benzodiazepines taken by mouth are the most common premedicants. They have no analgesic effect so an opioid analgesic may sometimes be required for pain.

Benzodiazepines can alleviate anxiety at doses that do not necessarily cause excessive sedation and they are of particular value during short procedures or during operations under local anaesthesia (including dentistry). Amnesia reduces the likelihood of any unpleasant memories of the procedure (although benzodiazepines, particularly when used for more profound sedation, can sometimes induce sexual fantasies). Benzodiazepines are also used in intensive care units for sedation, particularly in those receiving assisted ventilation.

Benzodiazepines may occasionally cause marked respiratory depression and facilities for its treatment are essential; flumazenil (section 15.1.7) is used to antagonise the effects of benzodiazepines.

Diazepam is used to produce mild sedation with amnesia. It is a long-acting drug with active metabolites and a second period of drowsiness can occur several hours after its administration. Peri-operative use of diazepam in children is not generally recommended; its effect and timing of response are unreliable and paradoxical effects may occur.

Diazepam is relatively insoluble in water and preparations formulated in organic solvents are painful on intravenous injection and give rise to a high incidence of venous thrombosis (which may not be noticed for several days after the injection). Intramuscular injection of diazepam is painful and absorption is erratic. An emulsion preparation for intravenous injection is less irritant and is followed by a negligible incidence of venous thrombosis; it is not suitable for intramuscular injection. Diazepam is also available as a rectal solution.

Temazepam is given by mouth and has a shorter duration of action and a more rapid onset than diazepam given by mouth. It has been used as a premedicant in inpatient and day-case surgery; anxiolytic and sedative effects last about 90 minutes although there may be residual drowsiness.

Lorazepam produces more prolonged sedation than temazepam and it has marked amnesic effects.

It is used as a premedicant the night before major surgery; a further, smaller dose may be required the following morning if any delay in starting surgery is anticipated. Alternatively the first dose may be given early in the morning on the day of operation.

Midazolam is a water-soluble benzodiazepine which is often used in preference to intravenous diazepam; recovery is faster than from diazepam. Midazolam is associated with profound sedation when high doses are given intravenously or when used with certain other drugs.

DIAZEPAM

Indications: premedication; sedation with amnesia, and in conjunction with local anaesthesia; other indications (section 4.1.2, section 4.8.2, and section 10.2.2)

Cautions: see notes above and section 4.1.2 and section 4.8.2

Contra-indications: see notes above and section 4.1.2 and section 4.8.2

Side-effects: see notes above and section 4.1.2 and section 4.8.2

Dose: *by mouth,* 5 mg on night before minor or dental surgery then 5 mg 2 hours before procedure

By intravenous injection, into a large vein 10–20 mg over 2–4 minutes as sedative cover for minor surgical and medical procedures; premedication 100–200 micrograms/kg

By rectum in solution, 10 mg; ELDERLY 5 mg; CHILD not recommended (see notes above)

Note. Diazepam rectal solution doses in the BNF may differ from those in the product literature

Preparations
Section 4.1.2

LORAZEPAM

Indications: sedation with amnesia; premedication; other indications (section 4.1.2 and section 4.8.2)

Cautions: see notes above and under Diazepam (section 4.1.2 and section 4.8.2)

Contra-indications: see notes above and under Diazepam (section 4.1.2 and section 4.8.2)

Side-effects: see notes above and under Diazepam (section 4.1.2 and section 4.8.2)

Dose: *by mouth,* 2–3 mg the night before operation; 2–4 mg 1–2 hours before operation

By slow intravenous injection, preferably diluted with an equal volume of sodium chloride intravenous infusion 0.9% or water for injections, 50 micrograms/kg 30–45 minutes before operation

By intramuscular injection, diluted as above, 50 micrograms/kg 1–1½ hours before operation

Preparations
Section 4.1.2

MIDAZOLAM

Indications: sedation with amnesia, and in conjunction with local anaesthesia; premedication, induction

Cautions: see notes above and under Diazepam (section 4.1.2 and section 4.8.2); **interactions:** Appendix 1 (anxiolytics and hypnotics)

Contra-indications: see notes above and under Diazepam (section 4.1.2 and section 4.8.2)

Side-effects: see notes above and under Diazepam (section 4.1.2 and section 4.8.2); also respiratory depression and respiratory arrest reported, particularly with high doses or on rapid injection

Dose: sedation, *by intravenous injection* over 30 seconds, 2 mg (elderly 1–1.5 mg) followed after 2 minutes by increments of 0.5–1 mg if sedation not adequate; usual range 2.5–7.5 mg (about 70 micrograms/kg), elderly 1–2 mg

Premedication, *by intramuscular injection,* 70–100 micrograms/kg 30–60 minutes before surgery; usual dose 5 mg (2.5 mg in elderly)

Induction, *by slow intravenous injection,* 200–300 micrograms/kg (elderly 100–200 micrograms/kg); CHILD over 7 years, 150 micrograms/kg

Sedation of patients receiving intensive care, *by intravenous infusion,* initially 30–300 micrograms/kg given over 5 minutes, then 30–200 micrograms/kg/hour; reduce dose (or omit initial dose) in hypovolaemia, vasoconstriction, or hypothermia; low doses may be adequate if opioid analgesic also used; avoid abrupt withdrawal after prolonged administration (safety after more than 14 days not established)

Midazolam (Non-proprietary) PoM
Injection, midazolam (as hydrochloride) 1 mg/mL, net price 50-mL vial = £6.00; 5 mg/mL, 2-mL amp = 78p, 5-mL amp = £2.50, 10-mL amp = £4.86, 18-mL amp = £6.80
Available from Antigen, Aurum, Phoenix

Hypnovel® (Roche) PoM
Injection, midazolam (as hydrochloride) 2 mg/mL, net price 5-mL amp = 96p; 5 mg/mL, 2-mL amp = 81p

TEMAZEPAM

Indications: premedication before surgery; anxiety before investigatory procedures; hypnotic (section 4.1.1)

Cautions: see notes above and under Diazepam (section 4.1.2 and section 4.8.2)

Contra-indications: see notes above and under Diazepam (section 4.1.2 and section 4.8.2)

Side-effects: see notes above and under Diazepam (section 4.1.2 and section 4.8.2)

Dose: *by mouth,* premedication, 20–40 mg (elderly, 10–20 mg) 1 hour before operation; CHILD 1 mg/kg (max. 30 mg)

Preparations
Section 4.1.1

15.1.4.2 Non-opioid analgesics

Since non-steroidal anti-inflammatory drugs (NSAIDs) do not depress respiration, do not impair gastro-intestinal motility, and do not cause dependence, they may be useful alternatives (or adjuncts) to the use of opioids for the relief of postoperative pain. NSAIDs may be inadequate for the relief of severe pain.

Diclofenac, flurbiprofen, ketoprofen (section 10.1.1), and **ketorolac** are licensed for postoperative use. Diclofenac, ketoprofen and ketorolac can be given by injection as well as by mouth. Intramuscular injections of diclofenac and ketoprofen are given deep into the gluteal muscle to minimise pain and tissue damage; diclofenac can also be given by intravenous infusion for the treatment or prevention of postoperative pain. Ketorolac is less irritant on intramuscular injection but pain has been reported; it can also be given by intravenous injection.

Suppositories of diclofenac and ketoprofen may be effective alternatives to the parenteral use of these drugs. Flurbiprofen is also available as suppositories.

KETOROLAC TROMETAMOL

Indications: short-term management of moderate to severe acute postoperative pain

Cautions: see Non-steroidal anti-inflammatory drugs (section 10.1.1); reduce dose in those weighing less than 50 kg; avoid in porphyria (section 9.8.2); **interactions:** Appendix 1 (NSAIDs)

Contra-indications: see Non-steroidal anti-inflammatory drugs (section 10.1.1); also history of asthma, complete or partial syndrome of nasal polyps, angioedema or bronchospasm; history of peptic ulceration or gastro-intestinal bleeding; haemorrhagic diatheses (including coagulation disorders) and operations with high risk of haemorrhage or incomplete haemostasis; confirmed or suspected cerebrovascular bleeding; moderate or severe renal impairment; hypovolaemia or dehydration; pregnancy (including labour and delivery) and breast-feeding

Side-effects: see Non-steroidal anti-inflammatory drugs (section 10.1.1); also anaphylaxis (with rash, bronchospasm, laryngeal oedema and hypotension), dry mouth, excessive thirst, psychotic reactions, convulsions, myalgia, hyponatraemia, hyperkalaemia, raised blood urea and creatinine, urinary symptoms and acute renal failure, flushing or pallor, bradycardia, hypertension, palpitations, chest pain, purpura, postoperative wound haemorrhage, haematoma, epistaxis, liver function changes (discontinue if clinical symptoms); pain at injection site

Dose: *by mouth*, 10 mg every 4–6 hours (ELDERLY every 6–8 hours); max. 40 mg daily; max. duration of treatment 7 days; CHILD under 16 years, not recommended

By intramuscular injection or by intravenous injection over not less than 15 seconds, initially 10 mg, then 10–30 mg every 4–6 hours when required (every 2 hours in initial postoperative period); max. 90 mg daily (ELDERLY and patients weighing less than 50 kg 60 mg daily); max. duration of treatment 2 days by either route; CHILD under 16 years, not recommended

Note. Pain relief may not occur for over 30 minutes after intravenous or intramuscular injection. When converting from parenteral to oral administration, total combined dose on the day of converting should not exceed 90 mg (60 mg in the elderly and patients weighing less than 50 kg) of which the oral component should not exceed 40 mg; patients should be converted to oral route as soon as possible

Toradol® (Roche) [PoM]

Tablets, ivory, f/c, ketorolac trometamol 10 mg, net price 20-tab pack = £6.23. Label: 17, 21

Injection, ketorolac trometamol 10 mg/mL, net price 1-mL amp = £1.02; 30 mg/mL, 1-mL amp = £1.22

15.1.4.3 Opioid analgesics

Opioid analgesics are now rarely used as premedicants; they are more likely to be administered at induction. Pre-operative use of opioid analgesics is generally limited to those patients who require control of existing pain. The main side-effects of opioid analgesics are respiratory depression, cardiovascular depression, nausea, and vomiting; for general notes on opioid analgesics and their use in postoperative pain, see section 4.7.2.

For the management of opioid-induced respiratory depression, see section 15.1.7.

INTRA-OPERATIVE ANALGESIA. Opioid analgesics given in small doses before or with induction reduce the dose requirement of some drugs used during anaesthesia. Pethidine, morphine and papaveretum have been used for this purpose, but shorter-acting and more potent drugs such as alfentanil, fentanyl, and remifentanil are now preferred. Nalbuphine is seldom used.

Alfentanil, **fentanyl** and **remifentanil** are particularly useful because they act within 1–2 minutes. The initial doses of alfentanil or fentanyl are followed either by successive intravenous injections or by an intravenous infusion; prolonged infusions increase the duration of effect. Repeated intra-operative doses of alfentanil or fentanyl should be given with care since the respiratory depression can persist into the postoperative period and occasionally it may become apparent for the first time postoperatively when monitoring of the patient might be less intensive.

In contrast to other opioids which are metabolised in the liver, remifentanil undergoes rapid metabolism by non-specific blood and tissue esterases; its short duration of action allows prolonged administration at high dosage, without accumulation, and with little risk of residual postoperative respiratory depression. Remifentanil should not be given as a bolus injection intra-operatively, but it is well suited to continuous infusion; a supplemental analgesic will often be required after stopping the infusion.

ALFENTANIL

Indications: analgesia especially during short operative procedure and outpatient surgery; enhancement of anaesthesia; analgesia and suppression of respiratory activity in patients receiving intensive care, with assisted ventilation, for up to 4 days

Cautions: see section 4.7.2 and notes above

Contra-indications: see section 4.7.2 and notes above

Side-effects: see section 4.7.2 and notes above

Rapifen® (Janssen-Cilag) |CD|
Injection, alfentanil (as hydrochloride)
500 micrograms/mL. Net price 2-mL amp = 72p;
10-mL amp = £3.31
Intensive care injection, alfentanil (as hydrochloride) 5 mg/mL. To be diluted before use. Net price 1-mL amp = £2.65

FENTANYL

Indications: analgesia during operation, enhancement of anaesthesia; respiratory depressant in assisted respiration; analgesia in other situations (section 4.7.2)

Cautions: see section 4.7.2 and notes above

Contra-indications: see section 4.7.2 and notes above

Side-effects: see section 4.7.2 and notes above

Dose: *by intravenous injection*, with spontaneous respiration,   50–200 micrograms,   then 50 micrograms   as   required;   CHILD   3–5 micrograms/kg,   then   1 microgram/kg   as required
With assisted ventilation, 0.3–3.5 mg, then 100–200 micrograms   as   required;   CHILD 15 micrograms/kg,   then   1–3 micrograms/kg   as required

Sublimaze® (Janssen-Cilag) |CD|
Injection, fentanyl (as citrate) 50 micrograms /mL.
Net price 2-mL amp = 24p; 10-mL amp = £1.17
Available as a generic from Antigen

REMIFENTANIL

Indications: supplementation of general anaesthesia during induction and analgesia during maintenance of anaesthesia (consult product literature for use in patients undergoing cardiac surgery)

Cautions: see section 4.7.2 and notes above

Contra-indications: see section 4.7.2 and notes above

Side-effects: see section 4.7.2 and notes above

Dose: induction, *by intravenous infusion*, 0.5–1 microgram/kg/minute, *with or without* an initial bolus *by intravenous injection* (of a solution containing 20–250 micrograms/mL) over not less than 30 seconds, 1 microgram/kg
Note. If patient is to be intubated more than 8 minutes after start of intravenous infusion, intial intravenous injection dose is unnecessary
Maintenance in ventilated patients, *by intravenous infusion*, 0.05–2 micrograms/kg/minute according to anaesthetic technique and adjusted according to response; supplemental doses in light anaesthesia, *by intravenous injection* every 2–5 minutes
Maintenance in spontaneous respiration anaesthesia, *by   intravenous   infusion*,   initially 40 nanograms/kg/minute adjusted according to response, usual range 25–100 nanograms/kg/minute
CHILD 1–12 years, maintenance, *by intravenous infusion*, 0.05–1.3 micrograms/kg/minute (*with or without* an initial bolus *by intravenous injection* over not less than 30 seconds, 1 microgram/kg/minute) according to anaesthetic technique and adjusted according to response

Ultiva® (Elan) |PoM|
Injection, powder for reconstitution, remifentanil (as hydrochloride), net price 1-mg vial = £5.50; 2-mg vial = £11.00; 5-mg vial = £27.50

15.1.5   Muscle relaxants

Muscle relaxants used in anaesthesia are also known as **neuromuscular blocking drugs**. By specific blockade of the neuromuscular junction they enable light levels of anaesthesia to be employed with adequate relaxation of the muscles of the abdomen and diaphragm. They also relax the vocal cords and allow the passage of a tracheal tube. Their action differs from the muscle relaxants acting on the spinal cord or brain which are used in musculoskeletal disorders (section 10.2.2).

Patients who have received a muscle relaxant should **always** have their respiration assisted or controlled until the drug has been inactivated or antagonised (section 15.1.6).

Non-depolarising muscle relaxants

Non-depolarising muscle relaxants (also known as competitive muscle relaxants) compete with acetylcholine for receptor sites at the neuromuscular junction and their action may be reversed with anticholinesterases such as neostigmine (section 15.1.6). Non-depolarising muscle relaxants may be divided into the **aminosteroid** group which includes pancuronium, rocuronium and vecuronium, and the **benzylisoquinolinium** group which includes atracurium, cisatracurium, gallamine and mivacurium.

Non-depolarising muscle relaxants have a slower onset of action than suxamethonium. These drugs can be classified by their duration of action as short-acting (15–30 minutes), intermediate-acting (30–40 minutes) and long-acting (60–120 minutes), although duration of action is dose-dependent. Drugs with a shorter or intermediate duration of action, such as atracurium and vecuronium, are more widely employed than those with a longer duration of action such as pancuronium.

Non-depolarising muscle relaxants have no sedative or analgesic effects and are not considered to be a triggering factor for malignant hyperthermia.

For patients receiving intensive care and who require tracheal intubation and mechanical ventilation, a non-depolarising muscle relaxant is chosen according to its onset of effect, duration of action and side-effects. Rocuronium, with a rapid onset of effect, may facilitate intubation. Atracurium or cisatracurium may be suitable for long-term muscle relaxation since their duration of action is not dependent on elimination by the liver or the kidneys.

CAUTIONS. Allergic cross-reactivity between neuromuscular blocking agents has been reported; caution is advised in cases of hypersensitivity to these drugs. Their activity is prolonged in patients with myasthenia gravis and in hypothermia, therefore lower doses are required. Resistance may develop in patients with burns who may require increased doses; low plasma cholinesterase activity in these patients requires dose titration for mivacurium. **Interactions:** Appendix 1 (muscle relaxants)

SIDE-EFFECTS. Benzylisoquinolinium non-depolarising muscle relaxants (except cisatracurium) are associated with histamine release which can cause skin flushing, hypotension, tachycardia, bronchospasm and rarely, anaphylactoid reactions. Aminosteroid muscle relaxants are not associated with histamine release. Drugs possessing vagolytic activity can counteract any bradycardia that occurs during surgery.

Atracurium is a mixture of 10 isomers and is a benzylisoquinolinium muscle relaxant with an intermediate duration of action. It undergoes non-enzymatic metabolism which is independent of liver and kidney function, thus allowing its use in patients with hepatic or renal impairment. Cardiovascular effects are associated with significant histamine release.

Cisatracurium is a single isomer of atracurium. It is more potent and has a slightly longer duration of action than atracurium and provides greater cardiovascular stability because cisatracurium lacks histamine-releasing effects.

Mivacurium, a benzylisoquinolinium muscle relaxant, has a short duration of action. It is metabolised by plasma cholinesterase and muscle paralysis is prolonged in individuals deficient in this enzyme. It is not associated with vagolytic activity or ganglionic blockade although histamine release may occur, particularly with rapid injection.

Pancuronium, an aminosteroid muscle relaxant, has a long duration of action and is often used in patients receiving long-term mechanical ventilation in intensive care units. It lacks a histamine-releasing effect, but vagolytic and sympathomimetic effects can cause tachycardia and hypertension.

Rocuronium exerts an effect within 2 minutes and has the most rapid onset of any of the competitive muscle relaxants. It is an aminosteroid muscle relaxant with an intermediate duration of action. It is reported to have minimal histamine-releasing and cardiovascular effects; high doses produce mild vagolytic activity.

Vecuronium, an aminosteroid muscle relaxant, has an intermediate duration of action. It does not generally produce histamine release and lacks cardiovascular effects.

Gallamine has vagolytic and sympathomimetic properties and frequently increases pulse rate and blood pressure. It is rarely used since the other neuromuscular blocking drugs have a more predictable response and it should be avoided in patients with renal impairment.

ATRACURIUM BESILATE

(Atracurium Besylate)

Indications: muscle relaxation for surgery (short to intermediate duration)

Cautions: see notes above

Side-effects: see notes above

Dose: *by intravenous injection*, ADULT and CHILD over 1 month initially 300–600 micrograms/kg, then 100–200 micrograms/kg as required

By intravenous infusion, 5–10 micrograms/kg/minute (300–600 micrograms/kg/hour)

Atracurium (Non-proprietary) PoM
Injection, atracurium besilate 10 mg/mL, net price 2.5-mL amp = £1.85; 5-mL amp = £3.37; 25-mL amp = £14.45
Available from Faulding DBL

Tracrium® (GlaxoWellcome) PoM
Injection, atracurium besilate 10 mg/mL, net price 2.5-mL amp = £1.78; 5-mL amp = £3.23; 25-mL amp = £13.88

CISATRACURIUM

Indications: muscle relaxation for surgery (intermediate duration)

Cautions: see notes above

Side-effects: see notes above

Dose: *by intravenous injection*, intubation, 150 micrograms/kg; maintenance, 30 micrograms/kg approx. every 20 minutes
CHILD over 2 years, initially, 100 micrograms/kg; maintenance, 20 micrograms/kg approx. every 9 minutes

By intravenous infusion, ADULT and CHILD over 2 years, initially, 3 micrograms/kg/minute, *then after stabilisation*, 1–2 micrograms/kg/minute; dose reduced by up to 40% if used with enflurane or isoflurane
CHILD under 2 years not recommended

Nimbex® (GlaxoWellcome) PoM
Injection, cisatracurium (as besilate) 2 mg/mL, net price 2.5-mL amp = £2.20, 10-mL amp = £8.12
Forte injection, cisatracurium (as besilate) 5 mg/mL, net price 30-mL vial = £33.43

GALLAMINE TRIETHIODIDE ◣▬▬

Indications: muscle relaxation for surgery (intermediate duration)

Cautions: see notes above

Contra-indications: renal impairment

Side-effects: see notes above

Dose: *by intravenous injection*, 80–120 mg, then 20–40 mg as required; NEONATE, 600 micrograms/kg; CHILD, 1.5 mg/kg

Flaxedil® (Concord) PoM ◣▬▬
Injection, gallamine triethiodide 40 mg/mL. Net price 2-mL amp = £4.97

◣▬▬ denotes preparations that are considered to be less suitable for prescribing (see p. vi)

MIVACURIUM

Indications: muscle relaxation for surgery (short duration)

Cautions: see notes above; low plasma cholinesterase activity

Side-effects: see notes above

Dose: *by intravenous injection*, 70–250 micrograms/kg; maintenance 100 micrograms/kg every 15 minutes; CHILD 2–6 months initially 150 micrograms/kg, 7 months–12 years initially 200 micrograms/kg; maintenance (CHILD 2 months–12 years) 100 micrograms/kg every 6–9 minutes
Note. Doses up to 150 micrograms/kg may be given over 5–15 seconds, higher doses should be given over 30 seconds. In patients with asthma, cardiovascular disease or

those who are sensitive to falls in arterial blood pressure give over 60 seconds

By intravenous infusion, maintenance of block, 8–10 micrograms/kg/minute, adjusted if necessary every 3 minutes by 1 microgram/kg/minute to usual dose of 6–7 micrograms/kg/minute; CHILD 2 months–12 years, usual dose 11–14 micrograms/kg/minute

Mivacron® (GlaxoWellcome) PoM
Injection, mivacurium (as chloride) 2 mg/mL, net price 5-mL amp = £2.73; 10-mL amp = £4.41

PANCURONIUM BROMIDE

Indications: muscle relaxation for surgery (long duration)

Cautions: see notes above; hepatic impairment Appendix 2) ; renal impairment (Appendix 3); pregnancy (Appendix 4) and breast-feeding (Appendix 5)

Side-effects: see notes above

Dose: *by intravenous injection*, initially for intubation 50–100 micrograms/kg then 10–20 micrograms/kg as required; CHILD initially 60–100 micrograms/kg, then 10–20 micrograms/kg, NEONATE 30–40 micrograms/kg initially then 10–20 micrograms/kg

Intensive care, *by intravenous injection*, 60 micrograms/kg every 60–90 minutes

Pancuronium (Non-proprietary) PoM
Injection, pancuronium bromide 2 mg/mL, net price 2-mL amp = 65p
Available from Antigen, Faulding DBL

Pavulon® (Organon) PoM
Injection, pancuronium bromide 2 mg/mL, net price 2-mL amp = 69p

---

ROCURONIUM BROMIDE

Indications: muscle relaxation for surgery (intermediate duration)

Cautions: see notes above; hepatic (Appendix 2) and renal (Appendix 3) impairment; pregnancy (Appendix 4) and breast-feeding (Appendix 5)

Side-effects: see notes above

Dose: *by intravenous injection*, intubation, 600 micrograms/kg; maintenance, 150 micrograms/kg

By intravenous infusion, 300–600 micrograms/kg/hour (after initial intravenous injection of 600 micrograms/kg)

CHILD similar sensitivity to adults; NEONATE not recommended

Esmeron® (Organon) PoM
Injection, rocuronium bromide 10 mg/mL, net price 5-mL vial = £3.23, 10-mL vial = £6.46

VECURONIUM BROMIDE

Indications: muscle relaxation for surgery (intermediate duration)

Cautions: see notes above; reduce dose in renal impairment

Side-effects: see notes above

Dose: *by intravenous injection*, intubation, 80–100 micrograms/kg; maintenance 20–30 micrograms/kg according to response; NEONATE and INFANT up to 4 months, initially

10–20 micrograms/kg then incremental doses to achieve response; CHILD over 5 months, as adult dose (up to 1 year onset more rapid and high intubation dose may not be required)

By intravenous infusion, 0.8–1.4 micrograms/kg/minute (after initial intravenous injection of 40–100 micrograms/kg)

Norcuron® (Organon) PoM
Injection, powder for reconstitution, vecuronium bromide. Net price 10-mg vial = £4.24 (with water for injections)

Depolarising muscle relaxants

Suxamethonium has the most rapid onset of action of any of the muscle relaxants and is ideal if fast onset and brief duration of action are required e.g. with tracheal intubation. Its duration of action is about 2 to 6 minutes following intravenous doses of about 1 mg/kg; repeated doses can be used for longer procedures.

Suxamethonium acts by mimicking acetylcholine at the neuromuscular junction but hydrolysis is much slower than for acetylcholine; depolarisation is therefore prolonged resulting in neuromuscular blockade. Unlike the non-depolarising muscle relaxants, its action cannot be reversed and recovery is spontaneous; anticholinesterases such as neostigmine potentiate the neuromuscular block.

Suxamethonium should be given after anaesthetic induction because paralysis is usually preceded by painful muscle fasciculations. While tachycardia occurs with single use, bradycardia may occur with repeated doses in adults and with the first dose in children. Premedication with atropine reduces bradycardia as well as the excessive salivation associated with suxamethonium use.

Prolonged paralysis may occur in **dual block**, which occurs with high or repeated doses of suxamethonium and is caused by the development of a non-depolarising block following the initial depolarising block; edrophonium (section 15.1.6) may be used to confirm the diagnosis of dual block. Individuals with myasthenia gravis are resistant to suxamethonium but can develop dual block resulting in delayed recovery. Prolonged paralysis may also occur in those with low or atypical plasma cholinesterase. Assisted ventilation should be continued until muscle function is restored.

SUXAMETHONIUM CHLORIDE

Indications: muscle relaxation (rapid onset, short duration)

Cautions: see notes above; pregnancy (Appendix 4); patients with cardiac, respiratory or neuromuscular disease; raised intra-ocular pressure (avoid in penetrating eye injury); **interactions:** Appendix 1 (muscle relaxants)

Contra-indications: family history of malignant hyperthermia, low plasma cholinesterase activity (including severe liver disease) (Appendix 2), hyperkalaemia

Side-effects: see notes above; also postoperative muscle pain, myoglobinaemia; tachycardia, arrhythmias, hypertension, hypotension; bronchospasm, apnoea, prolonged respiratory depression; hyperkalaemia; hyperthermia

Dose: *by intravenous injection*, ADULT 1 mg/kg (range 0.3–1.1 mg/kg); usual range 20–100 mg; max. 500 mg/hour; INFANT under 1 year, 2 mg/kg; CHILD 1–12 years, 1–2 mg/kg

By intravenous infusion of a solution containing 1–2 mg/mL (0.1–0.2%), 2–5 mg/minute; max. 500 mg/hour

By intramuscular injection, INFANT up to 4–5 mg/kg; CHILD up to 4 mg/kg; max. 150 mg

Suxamethonium Chloride (Non-proprietary) PoM

Injection, suxamethonium chloride 50 mg/mL, net price 2-mL amp = 70p

Available from Antigen

Anectine® (GlaxoWellcome) PoM

Injection, suxamethonium chloride 50 mg/mL, net price 2-mL amp = 70p

---

15.1.6 Anticholinesterases used in anaesthesia

Anticholinesterases reverse the effects of the non-depolarising (competitive) muscle relaxant drugs such as pancuronium but they prolong the action of the depolarising muscle relaxant drug suxamethonium.

Edrophonium has a transient action and may be used in the diagnosis of suspected dual block due to suxamethonium.

Neostigmine has a longer duration of action than edrophonium. It is the specific drug for reversal of non-depolarising (competitive) blockade. It acts within one minute of intravenous injection and lasts for 20 to 30 minutes; a second dose may then be necessary. Atropine or preferably glycopyrronium (section 15.1.3) should be given before or with neostigmine in order to prevent bradycardia, excessive salivation, and other muscarinic actions of neostigmine.

EDROPHONIUM CHLORIDE

Indications: see under Dose; myasthenia gravis (section 10.2.1)

Cautions: see section 10.2.1 and notes above; atropine should also be given

Contra-indications: see section 10.2.1 and notes above

Side-effects: see section 10.2.1 and notes above

Dose: brief reversal of non-depolarising neuromuscular blockade, *by intravenous injection* over several minutes, 500–700 micrograms/kg (after or with atropine sulphate 600 micrograms)
Diagnosis of dual block, *by intravenous injection*, 10 mg

Edrophonium (Non-proprietary) PoM

Injection, edrophonium chloride 10 mg/mL, net price 1-mL amp = £4.58

Available from Cambridge

NEOSTIGMINE METILSULFATE
(Neostigmine Methylsulphate)

Indications: see under Dose

Cautions: see section 10.2.1 and notes above; atropine should also be given

Contra-indications: see section 10.2.1 and notes above

Side-effects: see section 10.2.1 and notes above

Dose: reversal of non-depolarising neuromuscular blockade, *by intravenous injection* over 1 minute, 50–70 micrograms/kg (max. 5 mg) after or with atropine sulphate 0.6–1.2 mg
Myasthenia gravis, see section 10.2.1

Neostigmine (Non-proprietary) PoM

Injection, neostigmine metilsulfate 2.5 mg/mL, net price 1-mL amp = 58p

■ With glycopyrronium

Robinul-Neostigmine® (Anpharm) PoM

Injection, neostigmine metilsulfate 2.5 mg, glycopyrronium bromide 500 micrograms/mL, net price 1-mL amp = £1.01

Dose: reversal of non-depolarising neuromuscular blockade *by intravenous injection* over 10–30 seconds, 1–2 mL *or* 0.02 mL/kg, dose may be repeated if required (total max. 2 mL); CHILD 0.02 mL/kg (*or* 0.2 mL/kg of a 1 in 10 dilution using water for injections or sodium chloride injection 0.9%), dose may be repeated if required (total max. 2 mL)

15.1.7 Antagonists for central and respiratory depression

Respiratory depression is a major concern with opioid analgesics and it may be treated by artificial ventilation or be reversed by **naloxone**. Naloxone will immediately reverse opioid-induced respiratory depression but the dose may have to be repeated because of the short duration of action of naloxone; however, naloxone will also antagonise the analgesic effect.

Flumazenil is a benzodiazepine antagonist for the reversal of the central sedative effects of benzodiazepines after anaesthetic and similar procedures. Flumazenil has a shorter half-life than that of diazepam and midazolam (and there is a risk that patients may become resedated).

Doxapram (section 3.5.1) is a central and respiratory stimulant but is of limited value.

FLUMAZENIL

Indications: reversal of sedative effects of benzodiazepines in anaesthetic, intensive care, and diagnostic procedures

Cautions: short-acting (repeat doses may be necessary—benzodiazepine effects may persist for at least 24 hours); benzodiazepine dependence (may precipitate withdrawal symptoms); epileptics who have received prolonged benzodiazepine therapy (risk of convulsions); ensure neuromuscular blockade cleared before giving; avoid rapid injection in high-risk or anxious patients and following major surgery; hepatic impairment; head injury (rapid reversal of benzodiazepine sedation may cause convulsions); elderly, children, pregnancy and breast-feeding

Contra-indications: life-threatening condition (e.g. raised intracranial pressure, status epilepticus) controlled by benzodiazepines

Side-effects: nausea, vomiting, and flushing; if wakening too rapid, agitation, anxiety, and fear; transient increase in blood pressure and heart-rate in intensive care patients; very rarely convulsions (particularly in epileptics)

Dose: *by intravenous injection,* 200 micrograms over 15 seconds, then 100 micrograms at 60-second intervals if required; usual dose range, 300–600 micrograms; max. total dose 1 mg (2 mg in intensive care); question aetiology if no response to repeated doses

By intravenous infusion, if drowsiness recurs after injection, 100–400 micrograms/hour, adjusted according to level of arousal

Anexate® (Roche) PoM
Injection, flumazenil 100 micrograms/mL. Net price 5-mL amp = £15.59

NALOXONE HYDROCHLORIDE

Indications: reversal of opioid-induced respiratory depression; overdosage with opioids (Emergency treatment of poisoning)

Cautions: cardiovascular disease or those receiving cardiotoxic drugs (serious adverse cardiovascular effects reported); physical dependence on opioids (precipitates withdrawal); pain (see also under Titration of Dose, below); has short duration of action (repeated doses or infusion may be necessary to reverse effects of opioids with longer duration of action)

TITRATION OF DOSE. In postoperative use, the dose should be titrated for each patient in order to obtain sufficient respiratory response; however, naloxone antagonises analgesia

Side-effects: nausea and vomiting reported; tachycardia and fibrillation also reported

Dose: *by intravenous injection,* 100–200 micrograms (1.5–3 micrograms/kg); if response inadequate, increments of 100 micrograms every 2 minutes; further doses *by intramuscular injection* after 1–2 hours if required

CHILD, *by intravenous injection,* 10 micrograms/kg; subsequent dose of 100 micrograms/kg if no response; if intravenous route not possible, may be given in divided doses *by intramuscular or subcutaneous injection*

NEONATE, *by subcutaneous, intramuscular, or intravenous injection,* 10 micrograms/kg, repeated every 2 to 3 minutes *or by intramuscular injection,* 200 micrograms (60 micrograms/kg) as a single dose at birth (onset of action slower)

Naloxone (Non-proprietary) PoM
Injection, naloxone hydrochloride 400 micrograms/mL—see under Emergency Treatment of Poisoning p. 24

Narcan® PoM —see under Emergency Treatment of Poisoning p. 24

Narcan Neonatal® (Bristol-Myers Squibb) PoM
Injection, naloxone hydrochloride 20 micrograms/mL. Net price 2-mL amp = £3.32

Drugs for malignant hyperthermia

Malignant hyperthermia is a rare but potentially lethal complication of anaesthesia. It is characterised by a rapid rise in temperature, increased muscle rigidity, tachycardia, and acidosis. The most common triggers of malignant hyperthermia are the volatile anaesthetics. Suxamethonium has also been implicated, but malignant hyperthermia is more likely if it is given following a volatile anaesthetic. Known trigger agents should be avoided during anaesthesia.

Dantrolene is used in the treatment of malignant hyperthermia. It acts on skeletal muscle cells by interfering with calcium efflux, thereby stopping the contractile process.

DANTROLENE SODIUM

Indications: malignant hyperthermia

Cautions: avoid extravasation; **interactions:** Appendix 1 (muscle relaxants)

Dose: *by rapid intravenous injection,* 1 mg/kg, repeated as required to a cumulative max. of 10 mg/kg

Dantrium Intravenous® (Procter & Gamble Pharm.) PoM
Injection, powder for reconstitution, dantrolene sodium, net price 20-mg vial = £16.67 (hosp. only)

Local anaesthesia

The use of local anaesthetics by injection or by application to mucous membranes to produce local analgesia is discussed in this section.

See also section 1.7 (colon and rectum), section 11.7 (eye), section 12.3 (oropharynx), and section 13.3 (skin).

USE OF LOCAL ANAESTHETICS. Local anaesthetic drugs act by causing a reversible block to conduction along nerve fibres. The drugs used vary widely in their potency, toxicity, duration of action, stability, solubility in water, and ability to penetrate mucous membranes. These variations determine their suitability for use by various routes, e.g. topical (surface), infiltration, plexus, epidural (extradural) or spinal block.

The cold sensation produced by **ethyl chloride** spray is used to test the onset of regional anaesthesia.

ADMINISTRATION. In estimating the safe dosage of these drugs it is important to take account of the rate at which they are absorbed and excreted as well as their potency. The patient's age, weight, physique, and clinical condition, the degree of vascularity of the area to which the drug is to be applied, and the duration of administration are other factors which must be taken into account.

Local anaesthetics do not rely on the circulation to transport them to their sites of action, but uptake into the systemic circulation is important in terminating their action and producing toxicity. Following most regional anaesthetic procedures, maximum arterial plasma concentrations of anaesthetic develop within about 10 to 25 minutes, so **careful surveillance** for toxic effects is necessary during the first 30 minutes after injection. Great care must be taken to avoid accidental intravascular injection.

Epidural anaesthesia is commonly used during surgery, often combined with general anaesthesia, because of its protective effect against the stress response of surgery. It is often used when good postoperative pain relief is essential (e.g. aortic aneurysm surgery or major gut surgery).

TOXICITY. Toxic effects associated with local anaesthetics usually result from excessively high plasma concentrations. Effects initially include a feeling of inebriation and lightheadedness followed by sedation, circumoral paraesthesia and twitching; convulsions can occur in severe reactions. On intravenous injection convulsions and cardiovascular collapse may occur very rapidly. Hypersensitivity reactions occur mainly with the ester-type local anaesthetics such as benzocaine, cocaine, procaine, and tetracaine (amethocaine); reactions are less frequent with the amide types such as lidocaine (lignocaine), bupivacaine, prilocaine, and ropivacaine.

When prolonged analgesia is required, a long-acting local anaesthetic is preferred to minimise the likelihood of cumulative systemic toxicity. Local anaesthetic injections should be given slowly in order to detect inadvertent intravascular administration. Local anaesthetics should **not** be injected into inflamed or infected tissues nor should they be applied to the traumatised urethra. In such cases absorption into the blood may increase the possibility of systemic side-effects. The local anaesthetic effect may also be reduced by the altered local pH.

USE OF VASOCONSTRICTORS. Most local anaesthetics, with the exception of cocaine, cause dilation of blood vessels. The addition of a vasoconstrictor such as **adrenaline (epinephrine)** diminishes local blood flow, slows the rate of absorption of the local anaesthetic, and prolongs its local effect. Adrenaline must be used in a low concentration (e.g. 1 in 200 000) for this purpose and it should **not** be given with a local anaesthetic injection in digits and appendages; it may produce ischaemic necrosis.

When adrenaline is included the final concentration should be 1 in 200 000 (5 micrograms/mL). In dental surgery, up to 1 in 80 000 (12.5 micrograms/mL) of adrenaline is used with local anaesthetics. There is no justification for using higher concentrations.

The total dose of adrenaline should **not** exceed 500 micrograms and it is essential not to exceed a concentration of 1 in 200 000 (5 micrograms/mL) if more than 50 mL of the mixture is to be injected. For general cautions associated with the use of adrenaline, see section 2.7.3. For drug interactions, see Appendix 1 (sympathomimetics).

Lidocaine (Lignocaine)

Lidocaine (lignocaine) is effectively absorbed from mucous membranes and is a useful surface anaesthetic in concentrations of 2 to 4%. Except for surface anaesthesia, solutions should not usually exceed 1% in strength. The duration of the block (with adrenaline) is about 90 minutes.

LIDOCAINE HYDROCHLORIDE/ LIGNOCAINE HYDROCHLORIDE

Indications: see under Dose; also dental anaesthesia (see next page); ventricular arrhythmias (section 2.3.2)

Cautions: epilepsy, hepatic or respiratory impairment, impaired cardiac conduction, bradycardia; porphyria (section 9.8.2); reduce dose in elderly or debilitated; resuscitative equipment should be available; see section 2.3.2 for effects on heart; **interactions:** Appendix 1 (lidocaine)

Contra-indications: hypovolaemia, complete heart block; do not use solutions containing adrenaline for anaesthesia in appendages

Side-effects: CNS effects include confusion, respiratory depression and convulsions; hypotension and bradycardia (may lead to cardiac arrest); hypersensitivity reported; see also notes above

Dose: infiltration anaesthesia, *by injection*, according to patient's weight and nature of procedure, max. 200 mg (or 500 mg if given in solutions containing adrenaline)—see also Administration on p. 612 and see also **important** warning below
Intravenous regional anaesthesia and nerve blocks, seek expert advice
Surface anaesthesia, usual strengths 2–4%, see preparations below

> **Important:** the licensed doses stated above may not be appropriate in some settings and expert advice should be sought

■ Lidocaine hydrochloride injections

Lidocaine/Lignocaine (Non-proprietary) PoM
Injection 0.5%, lidocaine hydrochloride 5 mg/mL, net price 10-mL amp = 35p
Injection 1%, lidocaine hydrochloride 10 mg/mL, net price 2-mL amp = 24p; 5-mL amp = 22p; 10-mL amp = 35p; 20-mL amp = 61p
Injection 2%, lidocaine hydrochloride 20 mg/mL, net price 2-mL amp = 29p; 5-mL amp = 24p

Xylocaine® (AstraZeneca) PoM
Injection 0.5% with adrenaline 1 in 200 000, anhydrous lidocaine hydrochloride 5 mg/mL, adrenaline 1 in 200 000 (5 micrograms/mL). Net price 20-mL vial = 67p
Injection 1% with adrenaline 1 in 200 000, anhydrous lidocaine hydrochloride 10 mg/mL, adrenaline 1 in 200 000 (5 micrograms/mL). Net price 20-mL vial = 69p
Injection 2% with adrenaline 1 in 200 000, anhydrous lidocaine hydrochloride 20 mg/mL, adrenaline 1 in 200 000 (5 micrograms/mL). Net price 20-mL vial = 73p

■ Lidocaine injections for dental use

Note. Consult expert dental sources for specific advice in relation to dose of lidocaine for dental anaesthesia

A large variety of lidocaine injections, plain or with adrenaline or noradrenaline, is also available in dental cartridges under the names *Lignospan®*, *Lignostab A®*, *Rexocaine®*, and *Xylotox®*.

■ Lidocaine for surface anaesthesia

Important. Rapid and extensive absorption may result in systemic side-effects

Emla® (AstraZeneca) [PoM]

Drug Tariff cream, lidocaine 2.5%, prilocaine 2.5%, net price 5-g tube = £1.73

Surgical pack cream, lidocaine 2.5%, prilocaine 2.5%, net price 30-g tube = £10.25

Premedication pack cream, lidocaine 2.5%, prilocaine 2.5%, net price 10 × 5-g tube with 25 occlusive dressings = £19.50

Anaesthesia before minor skin procedures including venepuncture, apply thick layer under occlusive dressing 1–5 hours before procedure (2–5 hours before procedures on large areas e.g. split skin grafting); INFANT under 1 year not recommended
Removal of warts from genital mucosa in adults, apply up to 10 g 5–10 minutes before removal
Cautions: not for wounds, mucous membranes (except genital warts in adults), or atopic dermatitis; avoid use near eyes or middle ear; although systemic absorption low, caution in anaemia, or in congenital or acquired methaemoglobinaemia (see also Prilocaine, p. 615); *side-effects* include transient paleness, redness, and oedema

Instillagel® (CliniMed)

Gel, lidocaine hydrochloride 2%, chlorhexidine gluconate solution 0.25%, in a sterile lubricant basis in disposable syringe. Net price 6-mL syringe = £1.51; 11-mL syringe = £1.70

Excipients: include hydroxybenzoates (parabens)
Dose: 6–11 mL into urethra

Laryng-O-Jet® (Celltech) [PoM]

Jet spray 4% (disposable kit for laryngotracheal anaesthesia), lidocaine hydrochloride 40 mg/mL. Net price per unit (4-mL vial and disposable sterile cannula with cover and vial injector) = £5.01

Dose: usually 160 mg (4 mL) as a single dose instilled as jet spray into lumen of larynx and trachea (reduce dose according to size, age and condition of patient); max. 200 mg (5 mL)
Caution: may be rapidly and almost completely absorbed from respiratory tract and systemic side-effects may occur; extreme caution if mucosa has been traumatised or if sepsis present

Xylocaine® (AstraZeneca)

Spray (= pump spray), lidocaine 10% (100 mg/g) supplying 10 mg lidocaine/dose; 500 spray doses per container. Net price 50-mL bottle = £3.13

Dose: dental practice, 1–5 doses; maxillary sinus puncture, 3 doses; during delivery in obstetrics, up to 20 doses; procedures in pharynx, larynx, and trachea, up to 20 doses

Topical 4%, anhydrous lidocaine hydrochloride 40 mg/mL. Net price 30-mL bottle = £1.21

Excipients: include hydroxybenzoates (parabens)
Dose: bronchoscopy, 1–7.5 mL with suitable spray; biopsy in mouth, 3–4 mL with suitable spray *or* swab (with adrenaline if necessary); max. 7.5 mL

■ Lidocaine for ear, nose, and oropharyngeal use

Lidocaine with Phenylephrine/Lignocaine with Phenylephrine (Non-proprietary)

Topical solution, lidocaine hydrochloride 5%, phenylephrine hydrochloride 0.5%, net price 2.5 mL (with nasal applicator) = £8.00. For cautions, contra-indications and side-effects of phenylephrine, see section 2.7.2

Available from Aurum

Bupivacaine

The advantage of bupivacaine over other local anaesthetics is its longer duration of action. It has a slow onset of action, taking up to 30 minutes for full effect. It is often used in lumbar epidural blockade and is particularly suitable for continuous epidural analgesia in labour. It is the principal drug for spinal anaesthesia in the UK.

BUPIVACAINE HYDROCHLORIDE

Indications: see under Dose

Cautions: see under Lidocaine Hydrochloride and notes above; myocardial depression may be more severe and more resistant to treatment; **interactions:** Appendix 1 (bupivacaine)

Contra-indications: see under Lidocaine Hydrochloride and notes above; intravenous regional anaesthesia (Bier's block)

Side-effects: see under Lidocaine Hydrochloride and notes above

Dose: adjusted according to patient's physical status and nature of procedure—**important**: see also under Administration, above

Local infiltration, 0.25% (up to 60 mL)

Peripheral nerve block, 0.25% (max. 60 mL), 0.5% (max. 30 mL)

Epidural block,
  Surgery, *lumbar*, 0.5% (max. 20 mL)
       caudal, 0.5% (max. 30 mL)
  Labour, *lumbar*, 0.25–0.5% (max. 12 mL)
       caudal, but rarely used, 0.25–0.5% (max. 20 mL)

Sympathetic block, 0.25% (max. 50 mL)

> **Important:** the licensed doses stated above may not be appropriate in some settings and expert advice should be sought.

Bupivacaine (Non-proprietary) [PoM]

Injection, anhydrous bupivacaine hydrochloride 2.5 mg/mL (0.25%), net price 10-mL = £0.80–1.11; 5 mg/mL (0.5%), 10-mL = £0.90–1.27

Note. Bupivacaine injection 0.25% and 0.5% are available in glass or plastic ampoules, and sterile-wrapped glass ampoules

Infusion, anhydrous bupivacaine hydrochloride 1 mg/mL (0.1%), net price 100 mL = £7.75, 250 mL = £9.75; 1.25 mg/mL (0.125%), 250 mL = £9.95

Dose: Continuous lumbar epidural infusion during labour (once epidural block established), 10–15 mg/hour of 0.1% or 0.125% solution; max. 2 mg/kg over 4 hours and total of 400 mg in 24 hours
Continuous thoracic, upper abdominal, or lower abdominal epidural infusion for post-operative pain (once epidural block established), 4–15 mg/hour of 0.1% or 0.125% solution; max. 2 mg/kg over 4 hours and total of 400 mg in 24 hours; not recommended for use in children

Available from Antigen

Marcain® (AstraZeneca) [PoM]
Injection, anhydrous bupivacaine hydrochloride
2.5 mg/mL (*Marcain®* 0.25%), net price 10-mL
Polyamp® = £1.06; 5 mg/mL (*Marcain®* 0.5%),
10-mL *Polyamp®* = £1.21

Marcain Heavy® (AstraZeneca) [PoM]
Injection, anhydrous bupivacaine hydrochloride
5 mg, glucose 80 mg/mL, net price 4-mL amp =
93p

Dose: spinal anaesthesia, 2–4 mL

■ With adrenaline

Bupivacaine and Adrenaline (Non-proprietary)
[PoM]
Injection, anhydrous bupivacaine hydrochloride
2.5 mg/mL (0.25%), adrenaline 1 in 200 000
(5 micrograms/mL), net price 10-mL amp = £1.23
Injection, anhydrous bupivacaine hydrochloride
5 mg/mL (0.5%), adrenaline 1 in 200 000
(5 micrograms/mL), net price 10-mL amp = £1.40
Available from Antigen

Marcain® with Adrenaline (AstraZeneca) [PoM]
Injection 0.25%, bupivacaine hydrochloride
2.5 mg/mL, adrenaline 1 in 200 000
(5 micrograms/mL), net price 10-mL amp = £1.18
Injection 0.5%, bupivacaine hydrochloride 5 mg/
mL, adrenaline 1 in 200 000 (5 micrograms/mL),
net price 10-mL amp = £1.33

Levobupivacaine

Levobupivacaine, an isomer of bupivacaine, has
been introduced recently. It has similar anaesthetic
and analgesic properties to bupivacaine.

LEVOBUPIVACAINE HYDROCHLORIDE

Note. Levobupivacaine is an isomer of bupivacaine
Indications: see under Dose
Cautions: see under Lidocaine Hydrochloride and
notes above; **interactions:** Appendix 1 (levobupivacaine)
Contra-indications: see under Lidocaine Hydrochloride and notes above; intravenous regional
anaesthesia (Bier's block); paracervical block in
obstetrics
Side-effects: see under Lidocaine Hydrochloride
and notes above
Dose: adjusted according to patient's physical
status and nature of procedure—**important:** see
also under Administration, above
Surgical anaesthesia,
lumbar epidural, 10–20 mL (50–150 mg) of 5 or
7.5 mg/mL solution; caesarean section, 15–30 mL
(75–150 mg) of 5 mg/mL solution
intrathecal, 3 mL (15 mg) of 5 mg/mL solution
peripheral nerve block, 1–40 mL of 2.5 mg/mL
solution *or* 1–30 mL of 5 mg/mL solution (max.
150 mg)
ilioinguinal/iliohypogastric block, CHILD 0.25–
0.5 mL/kg (1.25–2.5 mg/kg) of 2.5 or 5 mg/mL
solution
peribulbar block, 5–15 mL (37.5–112.5 mg) of
7.5 mg/mL solution
local infiltration, 1–60 mL (max. 150 mg) of
2.5 mg/mL solution

Acute pain,
lumbar epidural, 6–10 mL (15–25 mg) of 2.5 mg/
mL solution at intervals of at least 15 minutes *or*
4–10 mL/hour (5–12.5 mg/hour) of 1.25 mg/mL
solution as a continuous epidural infusion for
labour pain, *or* 10–15 mL/hour (12.5–18.75 mg/
hour) of 1.25 mg/mL solution or 5–7.5 mL/hour
(12.5–18.75 mg/hour) of 2.5 mg/mL solution as a
continuous epidural infusion for postoperative
pain
Note. 7.5 mg/mL **contra-indicated** for use in obstetrics.

Important: the licensed doses stated above may
not be appropriate in some settings and expert
advice should be sought

Chirocaine® (Abbott) ▼ [PoM]
Injection, levobupivacaine hydrochloride 2.5 mg/
mL, net price 10-mL amp = £1.66; 5 mg/mL, 10-
mL amp = £1.90; 7.5 mg/mL, 10-mL amp = £2.85

Prilocaine

Prilocaine is a local anaesthetic of low toxicity
which is similar to lidocaine (lignocaine). If used in
high doses, methaemoglobinaemia may occur
which can be treated with intravenous injection of
methylthioninium chloride (methylene blue) 1%
using a dose of 1 mg/kg. Infants are particularly
susceptible to methaemoglobinaemia.

PRILOCAINE HYDROCHLORIDE

Indications: infiltration anaesthesia (higher
strengths for dental use only), nerve block
Cautions: see under Lidocaine Hydrochloride and
notes above; renal impairment; **interactions:**
Appendix 1 (prilocaine)
Contra-indications: see under Lidocaine Hydrochloride and notes above; anaemia or congenital
or acquired methaemoglobinaemia
Side-effects: see under Lidocaine Hydrochloride
and notes above; ocular toxicity (including blindness) reported with excessive strengths used for
ophthalmic procedures
Dose: adjusted according to site of operation and
response of patient, to max. 400 mg used alone, or
300 mg if used with felypressin

Citanest® (AstraZeneca) [PoM]
Injection 1%, prilocaine hydrochloride 10 mg/mL,
net price 20-mL multidose vial = 73p

■ For dental use

Citanest® (AstraZeneca) [PoM]
Injection 4%, prilocaine hydrochloride 40 mg/mL,
net price 2-mL cartridge = 15p

Citanest with Octapressin® (AstraZeneca)
[PoM]
Injection 3%, prilocaine hydrochloride 30 mg/mL,
felypressin 0.03 unit/mL, net price 2-mL cartridge
and self-aspirating cartridge (both) = 15p

Procaine

Procaine is now seldom used. It is as potent as lidocaine (lignocaine) but has a shorter duration of
action. It provides less intense analgesia because of
reduced spread through the tissues. It is of no value
as a surface anaesthetic.

PROCAINE HYDROCHLORIDE 🔳

Indications: local anaesthesia by infiltration and regional routes (but see notes above)

Cautions: see notes above

Side-effects: see notes above

Dose: adjusted according to site of operation and patient's response

By injection, up to 1 g (200 mL of 0.5% solution or 100 mL of 1%) with adrenaline 1 in 200 000

Procaine (Non-proprietary) PoM 🔳
Injection, procaine hydrochloride 2% (20 mg/mL) in sodium chloride intravenous infusion, net price 2-mL amp = 86p

Available from Martindale

🔳 denotes preparations that are considered to be less suitable for prescribing (see p. vi)

Ropivacaine

Ropivacaine is an amide-type local anaesthetic agent.

ROPIVACAINE HYDROCHLORIDE

Indications: see under Dose

Cautions: see Lidocaine Hydrochloride and notes above

Contra-indications: see Lidocaine Hydrochloride and notes above; intravenous regional anaesthesia (Bier's block); paracervical block in obstetrics

Side-effects: see Lidocaine Hydrochloride and notes above

Dose: adjust according to patient's physical status and nature of procedure—see also under Administration on p. 612

Surgical anaesthesia,
lumbar epidural, 15–20 mL of 10 mg/mL solution *or* 15–25 mL of 7.5 mg/mL solution; caesarean section, 15–20 mL of 7.5 mg/mL solution
thoracic epidural (to establish block for postoperative pain), 5–15 mL of 7.5 mg/mL solution
major nerve block (brachial plexus block), 30–40 mL of 7.5 mg/mL solution
field block, up to 30 mL of 7.5 mg/mL solution

Acute pain,
lumbar epidural, 10–20 mL of 2 mg/mL solution followed by 10–15 mL of 2 mg/mL solution at intervals of at least 30 minutes *or* 6–10 mL/hour of 2 mg/mL solution as a continuous epidural infusion for labour pain *or* 6–14 mL/hour of 2 mg/mL solution as a continuous epidural infusion for postoperative pain
thoracic epidural, 6–14 mL/hour of 2 mg/mL solution as a continuous infusion
field block, up to 100 mL of 2 mg/mL solution
CHILD over 1 year (body-weight up to 25 kg), *caudal epidural* (for pre- and post-operative pain only), 2 mg/kg of 2 mg/mL solution

Naropin® (AstraZeneca) PoM
Injection, ropivacaine hydrochloride 2 mg/mL, net price 10-mL *Polyamp®* = £1.37; 7.5 mg/mL, 10-mL *Polyamp®* = £2.65; 10 mg/mL, 10-mL *Polyamp®* = £3.20
Epidural infusion, ropivacaine hydrochloride 2 mg/mL, net price 100-mL *Polybag®* = £8.23, 200-mL *Polybag®* = £14.45

Tetracaine (Amethocaine)

Tetracaine (amethocaine) is an effective local anaesthetic for topical application; a 4% gel is indicated for anaesthesia prior to venepuncture or venous cannulation. It is rapidly absorbed from mucous membranes and should **never** be applied to inflamed, traumatised, or highly vascular surfaces. It should **never** be used to provide anaesthesia for bronchoscopy or cystoscopy, as lidocaine (lignocaine) is a safer alternative. It is used in ophthalmology (section 11.7) and in skin preparations (section 13.3). Hypersensitivity to tetracaine has been reported.

TETRACAINE/AMETHOCAINE

Indications: see under preparation below

Cautions: see notes above

Contra-indications: see notes above

Side-effects: see notes above; also erythema, oedema and pruritus; very rarely blistering
Important. Rapid and extensive absorption may result in systemic side-effects (see also notes above)

Ametop® (S&N Hlth.)
Gel, tetracaine 4%, net price 1.5-g tube = £1.50
Dose: apply contents of tube to site of venepuncture or venous cannulation and cover with occlusive dressing; remove gel and dressing after 30 minutes for venepuncture and after 45 minutes for venous cannulation; PREMATURE INFANT and INFANT under 1 month not recommended

---

Other local anaesthetics

Benzocaine is a local anaesthetic of low potency and toxicity. It is an ingredient of some proprietary topical preparations for musculoskeletal conditions (section 10.3.2), mouth-ulcer preparations (section 12.3.1), and throat lozenges (section 12.3.3).

Mepivacaine is a local anaesthetic used in dentistry; it is available in dental cartridges with or without adrenaline (epinephrine) as *Scandonest®*.

Articaine (carticaine) is a newly introduced local anaesthetic for dental use; it is available in cartridges with adrenaline (*Septanest®* ▼).

Cocaine readily penetrates mucous membranes and is an effective surface anaesthetic with an intense vasoconstrictor action. However, apart from its use in otolaryngology (see below), it has now been replaced by less toxic alternatives. It has marked sympathomimetic activity and should **never** be given by injection because of its toxicity. As a result of its intense stimulant effect it is a drug of addiction. In otolaryngology cocaine is applied to the nasal mucosa in concentrations of 4 to 10% (40–100 mg/mL); an oromucosal solution and nasal spray both containing cocaine hydrochloride 10% are available (Aurum). In order to avoid systemic effects, the maximum dose recommended for application to the nasal mucosa in fit adults is a total of 1.5 mg/kg, which is equivalent to a total topical dose of approximately 100 mg for an adult male; this dose relates to direct application of cocaine (application on gauze may reduce systemic absorption). It should be used only by those skilled in the precautions needed to *minimise absorption* and the *consequent risk of arrhythmias*. Although cocaine interacts with other drugs liable to induce arrhythmias, including adrenaline, some otolaryngologists consider that combined use of topical cocaine with topical adrenaline (in the form of a paste or a solution) improves the operative field and may possibly reduce absorption. Cocaine is a mydriatic as well as a local anaesthetic but owing to corneal toxicity it is now little used in ophthalmology. Cocaine should be avoided in porphyria (section 9.8.2).

Appendix 1: Interactions

Two or more drugs given at the same time may exert their effects independently or may interact. The interaction may be potentiation or antagonism of one drug by another, or occasionally some other effect. Adverse drug interactions should be reported to the CSM as for other adverse drug reactions.

Drug interactions may be **pharmacodynamic** or **pharmacokinetic**.

Pharmacodynamic interactions

These are interactions between drugs which have similar or antagonistic pharmacological effects or side-effects. They may be due to competition at receptor sites, or occur between drugs acting on the same physiological system. They are usually predictable from a knowledge of the pharmacology of the interacting drugs; in general, those demonstrated with one drug are likely to occur with related drugs. They occur to a greater or lesser extent in most patients who receive the interacting drugs.

Pharmacokinetic interactions

These occur when one drug alters the absorption, distribution, metabolism, or excretion of another, thus increasing or reducing the amount of drug available to produce its pharmacological effects. They are not easily predicted and many of them affect only a small proportion of patients taking the combination of drugs. Pharmacokinetic interactions occurring with one drug cannot be assumed to occur with related drugs unless their pharmacokinetic properties are known to be similar.

Pharmacokinetic interactions are of several types:

AFFECTING ABSORPTION. The rate of absorption or the total amount absorbed can both be altered by drug interactions. Delayed absorption is rarely of clinical importance unless high peak plasma concentrations are required (e.g. when giving an analgesic). Reduction in the total amount absorbed, however, may result in ineffective therapy.

DUE TO CHANGES IN PROTEIN BINDING. To a variable extent most drugs are loosely bound to plasma proteins. Protein-binding sites are non-specific and one drug can displace another thereby increasing its proportion free to diffuse from plasma to its site of action. This only produces a detectable increase in effect if it is an extensively bound drug (more than 90%) that is not widely distributed throughout the body. Even so displacement rarely produces more than transient potentiation because this increased concentration of free drug results in an increased rate of elimination.

Displacement from protein binding plays a part in the potentiation of warfarin by phenylbutazone, sulphonamides, and tolbutamide but the importance of these interactions is due mainly to the fact that warfarin metabolism is also inhibited.

AFFECTING METABOLISM. Many drugs are metabolised in the liver. Induction of the hepatic microsomal enzyme system by one drug can gradually increase the rate of metabolism of another, resulting in lower plasma concentrations and a reduced effect. On withdrawal of the inducer plasma concentrations increase and toxicity may occur. Barbiturates, griseofulvin, many antiepileptics, and rifampicin are the most important enzyme inducers. Drugs affected include warfarin and the oral contraceptives.

Conversely when one drug inhibits the metabolism of another higher plasma concentrations are produced, rapidly resulting in an increased effect with risk of toxicity. Some drugs which potentiate warfarin and phenytoin do so by this mechanism.

AFFECTING RENAL EXCRETION. Drugs are eliminated through the kidney both by glomerular filtration and by active tubular secretion. Competition occurs between those which share active transport mechanisms in the proximal tubule. For example, salicylates and some other NSAIDs delay the excretion of methotrexate; serious methotrexate toxicity is possible.

Relative importance of interactions

Many drug interactions are harmless and many of those which are potentially harmful only occur in a small proportion of patients; moreover, the severity of an interaction varies from one patient to another. Drugs with a small therapeutic ratio (e.g. phenytoin) and those which require careful control of dosage (e.g. anticoagulants, antihypertensives, and antidiabetics) are most often involved.

Patients at increased risk from drug interactions include the elderly and those with impaired renal or liver function.

HAZARDOUS INTERACTIONS. The symbol • has been placed against interactions that are **potentially hazardous** and where combined administration of the drugs involved should be **avoided** (or only undertaken with caution and appropriate monitoring).

Interactions that have no symbol do not usually have serious consequences.

List of drug interactions

The following is an alphabetical list of drugs and their interactions; to avoid excessive cross-referencing each drug or group is listed twice: in the alphabetical list and also against the drug or group with which it interacts; changes in the interactions lists since BNF No. 42 (September 2001) are <u>underlined</u>.

For explanation of symbol • see previous page

Abacavir
Analgesics: plasma concentration of *methadone* possibly decreased by *abacavir*
Acarbose *see* Antidiabetics
ACE Inhibitors and Angiotensin-II Antagonists
Alcohol: enhanced hypotensive effect
Aldesleukin: enhanced hypotensive effect
Allopurinol: increased risk of toxicity with *captopril*, especially in renal impairment
Alprostadil: enhanced hypotensive effect
• Anaesthetics: enhanced hypotensive effect
• Analgesics: antagonism of hypotensive effect and increased risk of renal impairment with *NSAIDs*; hyperkalaemia with *ketorolac and possibly other NSAIDs*
Antacids: absorption of *captopril, enalapril, fosinopril* and *possibly other ACE inhibitors* reduced
Anti-arrhythmics: *procainamide* increases risk of toxicity with *captopril*, especially in renal impairment
Antibacterials: absorption of *tetracyclines* reduced by *quinapril tablets* (contain magnesium carbonate excipient); *rifampicin* reduces plasma concentration of active metabolite of *imidapril* (reduced antihypertensive effect); *see also* Linezolid
Anticoagulants: increased risk of hyperkalaemia with *heparin*
Antidepressants: possibly enhanced hypotensive effect
Antidiabetics: hypoglycaemic effect possibly enhanced
other Antihypertensives: enhanced hypotensive effect; previous treatment with *clonidine* possibly delays antihypertensive effect of *captopril*
Antipsychotics: severe postural hypotension with *chlorpromazine and possibly other phenothiazines*
Anxiolytics and Hypnotics: enhanced hypotensive effect
Beta-blockers: enhanced hypotensive effect
Calcium-channel Blockers: enhanced hypotensive effect
• Cardiac Glycosides: plasma concentration of *digoxin* increased by *telmisartan* and possibly by *captopril*
• Ciclosporin: increased risk of hyperkalaemia
Corticosteroids: antagonism of hypotensive effect
Cytotoxics: *azathioprine* increases risk of leucopenia with *captopril*
• Diuretics: enhanced hypotensive effect (can be extreme); risk of severe hyperkalaemia with *potassium-sparing diuretics*
Dopaminergics: *levodopa* enhances hypotensive effect
Epoetin: antagonism of hypotensive effect; increased risk of hyperkalaemia
• Lithium: *ACE inhibitors* and *Angiotensin-II antagonists* reduce excretion of *lithium* (increased plasma-lithium concentration)
Moxisylyte: enhanced hypotensive effect
Muscle Relaxants: *baclofen* and *tizanidine* enhance hypotensive effect
Nitrates: enhance hypotensive effect
Oestrogens and Progestogens: *oestrogens* and *combined oral contraceptives* antagonise hypotensive effect
• Potassium Salts: increased risk of hyperkalaemia
Ulcer-healing Drugs: *carbenoxolone* antagonises hypotensive effect
Uricosurics: *probenecid* reduces excretion of *captopril*
Acebutolol *see* Beta-blockers

Aceclofenac *see* NSAIDs
Acemetacin *see* NSAIDs
Acenocoumarol (Nicoumalone) *see* Warfarin and other Coumarins
Acetazolamide *see* Diuretics (carbonic anhydrase inhibitor)
Aciclovir and Famciclovir
Note. Interactions do not apply to topical preparations
Mycophenolate Mofetil: higher plasma concentrations of *aciclovir* and of *mycophenolate mofetil* on concomitant administration
Uricosurics: *probenecid* reduces *aciclovir* and possibly *famciclovir* excretion (increased plasma concentrations)
Acitretin *see* Retinoids
Acrivastine *see* Antihistamines
Adenosine
Note. Possibility of interaction with drugs tending to impair cardiac conduction
• Antiplatelet Drugs: effect enhanced and extended by *dipyridamole* (**important** risk of toxicity)
Theophylline: antagonism of anti-arrhythmic effect
Adrenaline (Epinephrine) *see* Sympathomimetics
Adrenergic Neurone Blockers
ACE inhibitors and Angiotensin-II antagonists: enhanced hypotensive effect
Alcohol: enhanced hypotensive effect
Alprostadil: enhanced hypotensive effect
• Anaesthetics: enhanced hypotensive effect
• Analgesics: *NSAIDs* antagonise hypotensive effect
Anti-arrhythmics: increased risk of myocardial depression with *bretylium*
Antibacterials: *see* Linezolid
Antidepressants: *tricyclics* antagonise hypotensive effect; enhanced hypotensive effect with *MAOIs*
other Antihypertensives: enhanced hypotensive effect
Antipsychotics: *phenothiazines* enhance hypotensive effect (antagonism of hypotensive effect with higher doses of *chlorpromazine*); antagonism of hypotensive effect with *haloperidol*
Anxiolytics and Hypnotics: enhanced hypotensive effect
Beta-blockers: enhanced hypotensive effect
Calcium-channel Blockers: enhanced hypotensive effect
Corticosteroids: antagonism of hypotensive effect
Diuretics: enhanced hypotensive effect
Dopaminergics: *levodopa* enhances hypotensive effect
Moxisylyte: enhanced hypotensive effect
Muscle Relaxants: enhanced hypotensive effect with *tizanidine*
Nitrates: enhance hypotensive effect
Oestrogens and Progestogens: *oestrogens* and *combined oral contraceptives* antagonise hypotensive effect
Pizotifen: antagonism of hypotensive effect
• Sympathomimetics: *some anorectics, some cough and cold remedies (e.g. ephedrine),* and *methylphenidate* antagonise hypotensive effect
Ulcer-healing Drugs: *carbenoxolone* antagonises hypotensive effect
Alcohol
ACE Inhibitors and Angiotensin-II Antagonists: enhanced hypotensive effect
Analgesics: sedative and hypotensive effect of *opioid analgesics* enhanced
• Antibacterials: disulfiram-like reaction with *cefamandole, metronidazole,* and possibly *tinidazole*; increased risk of seizures with *cycloserine*; *see also* Linezolid
• Anticoagulants: *see* Warfarin
• Antidepressants: sedative effect of *tricyclics (and related)* enhanced; *tyramine* (contained in some alcoholic and dealcoholised beverages) interacts with *MAOIs* (hypertensive crisis)—but if no tyramine, enhanced hypotensive effect; effects of alcohol possibly enhanced by *SSRIs*

Alcohol *(continued)*

Antidiabetics: enhanced hypoglycaemic effect; flushing with *chlorpropamide* (in susceptible subjects); increased risk of lactic acidosis with *metformin*

Antiepileptics: CNS side-effects of *carbamazepine* possibly enhanced

Antihistamines: enhanced sedative effect

Antihypertensives: enhanced hypotensive effect; sedative effect of *indoramin* enhanced

Antimuscarinics: sedative effect of *hyoscine* enhanced

Antipsychotics: enhanced sedative effect

Anxiolytics and Hypnotics: enhanced sedative effect

Barbiturates and Primidone: enhanced sedative effect

Beta-blockers: enhanced hypotensive effect

Calcium-channel Blockers: enhanced hypotensive effect; plasma-alcohol concentration possibly increased by *verapamil*

Cytotoxics: disulfiram-like reaction with *procarbazine*

Dopaminergics: reduced tolerance to *bromocriptine*

Lofexidine: enhanced sedative effect

Muscle Relaxants: *baclofen, methocarbamol* and *tizanidine* enhance sedative effect

Nabilone: enhanced sedative effect

Nitrates: enhanced hypotensive effect

• Paraldehyde: enhanced sedative effect

Retinoids: *etretinate* formed from *acitretin* in presence of *alcohol*

Aldesleukin

Antihypertensives: enhanced hypotensive effect

Alendronic Acid *see* Bisphosphonates

Alfentanil *see* Opioid Analgesics

Alfuzosin *see* Alpha-blockers (post-synaptic)

Alimemazine (Trimeprazine) *see* Antihistamines

Almotriptan *see* 5HT$_1$ Agonists

Allopurinol

ACE Inhibitors and Angiotensin-II Antagonists: increased risk of toxicity with *captopril*, especially in renal impairment

Antibacterials: increased risk of rash with concomitant *ampicillin* and *amoxicillin*

Anticoagulants: effects of *acenocoumarol* and *warfarin* possibly enhanced

Ciclosporin: plasma-ciclosporin concentration possibly increased (risk of nephrotoxicity)

• Cytotoxics: effects of *azathioprine* and *mercaptopurine* enhanced with increased toxicity (reduce dose when given with allopurinol); manufacturer of capecitabine advises avoid concomitant use

Theophylline: plasma-theophylline concentration possibly increased

Alpha$_2$-adrenoceptor Stimulants

Antibacterials: *see* Linezolid

Antidepressants: manufacturers of *apraclonidine* and *brimonidine* advise avoid concomitant use with *tricyclics or related antidepressants* or *MAOIs*

Sympathomimetics: possible risk of hypertension with *adrenaline* and *noradrenaline*

Alpha-blockers

ACE Inhibitors and Angiotensin-II Antagonists: enhanced hypotensive effect

Alcohol: enhanced hypotensive effect; sedative effect of *indoramin* enhanced

Aldesleukin: enhanced hypotensive effect

Alprostadil: enhanced hypotensive effect

• Anaesthetics: enhanced hypotensive effect

Analgesics: *NSAIDs* antagonise hypotensive effect

• Antibacterials: *see* Linezolid

• Antidepressants: enhanced hypotensive effect; manufacturer of *indoramin* advises avoid *MAOIs*

other Antihypertensives: additive hypotensive effect

Antipsychotics: enhanced hypotensive effect

Anxiolytics and Hypnotics: enhanced hypotensive and sedative effect

Alpha-blockers *(continued)*

• Beta-blockers: enhanced hypotensive effect; increased risk of first-dose hypotensive effect of *post-synaptic alpha-blockers such as prazosin*

• Calcium-channel Blockers: enhanced hypotensive effect; increased risk of first-dose hypotensive effect of *post-synaptic alpha-blockers such as prazosin*

Corticosteroids : antagonism of hypotensive effect

• Diuretics: enhanced hypotensive effect; increased risk of first-dose hypotensive effect of *post-synaptic alpha-blockers such as prazosin*

Dopaminergics: *levodopa* enhances hypotensive effect

• Moxisylyte: possible severe postural hypotension

Muscle Relaxants: *baclofen* and *tizanidine* enhance hypotensive effect

Nitrates: enhanced hypotensive effect

Oestrogens and Progestogens: *oestrogens and combined oral contraceptives* antagonise hypotensive effect

Ulcer-healing Drugs: *carbenoxolone* antagonises hypotensive effect

Alprazolam *see* Anxiolytics and Hypnotics

Alprostadil

Antihypertensives: enhanced hypotensive effect

Altretamine

• Antibacterials: *see* Linezolid

• Antidepressants: risk of severe postural hypotension with *MAOIs* and *tricyclics*

• Pyridoxine: reduced response to altretamine

Aluminium Hydroxide *see* Antacids

Amantadine

Antihypertensives: *methyldopa* has extrapyramidal side-effects

Antimuscarinics: increased antimuscarinic side-effects

Antipsychotics: all have extrapyramidal side-effects

Metoclopramide and Domperidone: have extrapyramidal side-effects

Tetrabenazine: has extrapyramidal side-effects

Amfebutamone *see* Bupropion

Amifostine

Note. Limited information available—rapid clearance from plasma minimises risk of interactions; possibility of interactions with antihypertensives and other drugs which potentiate hypotension

Amikacin *see* Aminoglycosides

Amiloride *see* Diuretics (potassium-sparing)

Aminoglutethimide

• Anticoagulants: metabolism of *acenocoumarol* and *warfarin* accelerated (reduced anticoagulant effect)

Antidiabetics: manufacturer advises metabolism of *oral antidiabetics* possibly accelerated

Cardiac Glycosides: metabolism of *digitoxin* accelerated (reduced effect)

Corticosteroids: metabolism of *corticosteroids* accelerated (reduced effect)

Diuretics: increased risk of hyponatraemia

other Hormone Antagonists: plasma concentration of *tamoxifen* reduced

Oestrogens and Progestogens: *aminoglutethimide* reduces plasma concentration of *medroxyprogesterone*

Theophylline: metabolism of *theophylline* accelerated (reduced effect)

Aminoglycosides

Analgesics: *indometacin* possibly increases plasma concentration of *gentamicin* and *amikacin* in neonates

other Antibacterials: increased risk of nephrotoxicity with *colistin*; increased risk of ototoxicity and nephrotoxicity with *capreomycin, teicoplanin* and *vancomycin*; *neomycin* reduces absorption of *phenoxymethylpenicillin*

• Anticoagulants: *see* Phenindione and Warfarin

Antidiabetics: *neomycin* possibly enhances hypoglycaemic effect of *acarbose* and increases severity of gastro-intestinal effects

Antifungals: increased risk of nephrotoxicity with *amphotericin*

Aminoglycosides *(continued)*

Bisphosphonates: increased risk of hypocalcaemia

- Botulinum Toxin: neuromuscular block enhanced (risk of toxicity)

Cardiac Glycosides: *neomycin* reduces absorption of *digoxin*

- Ciclosporin: increased risk of nephrotoxicity
- Cytotoxics: increased risk of nephrotoxicity and possibly of ototoxicity with *cisplatin*
- Diuretics: increased risk of ototoxicity with *loop diuretics*
- Muscle Relaxants: effect of *non-depolarising muscle relaxants* enhanced
- Parasympathomimetics: antagonism of effect of *neostigmine and pyridostigmine*

Aminophylline *see* Theophylline

Aminosalicylates

Cardiac Glycosides: absorption of *digoxin* possibly reduced by *sulfasalazine*

Cytotoxics: possible increased risk of leucopenia with *azathioprine* and *mercaptopurine*

Amiodarone

Note. Amiodarone has a long half-life; there is a potential for drug interactions to occur for several weeks (or even months) after treatment with it has been stopped

- *other* Anti-arrhythmics: additive effect with *disopyramide, flecainide, procainamide,* and *quinidine* (increased risk of ventricular arrhythmias—avoid concomitant use); increased plasma concentrations of *flecainide, procainamide* and *quinidine*; increased myocardial depression with any anti-arrhythmic
- Antibacterials: increased risk of ventricular arrhythmias with *erythromycin* (parenteral) and *co-trimoxazole* (avoid concomitant use)
- Anticoagulants: metabolism of *acenocoumarol, phenindione* and *warfarin* inhibited (enhanced anticoagulant effect)
- Antidepressants: increased risk of ventricular arrhythmias with *tricyclics* (avoid concomitant use); manufacturer of *reboxetine* advises caution
- Antiepileptics: metabolism of *phenytoin* inhibited (increased plasma concentration)
- Antihistamines: increased risk of ventricular arrhythmias with *mizolastine* and *terfenadine* (avoid concomitant use)
- Antimalarials: increased risk of ventricular arrhythmias with *chloroquine, hydroxychloroquine, mefloquine* and *quinine* (avoid concomitant use)
- Antipsychotics: increased risk of ventricular arrhythmias with *phenothiazines, haloperidol* and *pimozide* (avoid concomitant use)
- Antivirals: increased risk of ventricular arrhythmias with *nelfinavir* and *ritonavir* (avoid concomitant use)
- Beta-blockers: increased risk of bradycardia, AV block, and myocardial depression; increased risk of ventricular arrhythmias associated with *sotalol* (avoid concomitant use)
- Calcium-channel Blockers: *diltiazem and verapamil* increase risk of bradycardia, AV block, and myocardial depression
- Cardiac Glycosides: increased plasma concentration of *digoxin* (halve digoxin maintenance dose)

Ciclosporin: plasma concentration of *ciclosporin* possibly increased

Diuretics: cardiac toxicity increased if hypokalaemia occurs with *acetazolamide, loop diuretics,* and *thiazides*

Lithium: increased risk of hypothyroidism

- Pentamidine Isetionate: increased risk of ventricular arrhythmias (avoid concomitant use)

Thyroid hormones: for concomitant use see p. 72

Tropisetron: risk of ventricular arrhythmias—manufacturer of tropisetron advises caution

Ulcer-healing Drugs: *cimetidine* increases plasma concentrations of *amiodarone*

Amisulpride *see* Antipsychotics

Amitriptyline *see* Antidepressants, Tricyclic

Amlodipine *see* Calcium-channel Blockers

Amobarbital *see* Barbiturates and Primidone

Amoxapine *see* Antidepressants, Tricyclic

Amoxicillin *see* Penicillins

Amphetamines *see* Sympathomimetics

Amphotericin

Note. Close monitoring required with concomitant administration of nephrotoxic drugs or cytotoxics

Antibacterials: increased risk of nephrotoxicity with *aminoglycosides*

other Antifungals: *imidazoles* and *triazoles* possibly antagonise effect of *amphotericin*; renal excretion of *flucytosine* decreased and cellular uptake increased (flucytosine toxicity possibly increased)

- Cardiac Glycosides: increased toxicity if hypokalaemia occurs
- Ciclosporin: increased risk of nephrotoxicity
- Corticosteroids: increased risk of hypokalaemia (avoid concomitant use unless corticosteroids needed to control reactions)

Diuretics: increased risk of hypokalaemia with *loop diuretics* and *thiazides*

- Tacrolimus: increased risk of nephrotoxicity

Ampicillin *see* Penicillins

Amprenavir

- Antibacterials: concomitant administration with *erythromycin* may increase plasma concentration of both drugs; plasma-amprenavir concentration significantly reduced by *rifampicin* (avoid concomitant use); *amprenavir* increases plasma concentration of *rifabutin* (halve rifabutin dose) and possibly of *dapsone*
- Antidepressants: plasma-amprenavir concentration reduced by *St John's wort* (avoid concomitant use)

Antiepileptics: *amprenavir* possibly increases plasma concentration of *carbamazepine*

Antifungals: *amprenavir* possibly increases plasma concentration of *itraconazole*

- Antihistamines: increased risk of ventricular arrhythmias with *terfenadine* (avoid concomitant use); *amprenavir* possibly increases plasma concentration of *loratadine*
- Antipsychotics: *amprenavir* increases plasma concentration of *pimozide* (risk of ventricular arrhythmias—avoid concomitant use); *amprenavir* possibly increases plasma concentration of *clozapine* and *thioridazine*

other Antivirals: combination with *ritonavir* may increase plasma concentration of both drugs; plasma-amprenavir concentration reduced by *efavirenz* and possibly by *nevirapine*

- Anxiolytics and Hypnotics: increased risk of prolonged sedation and respiratory depression with *alprazolam, clorazepate, diazepam, flurazepam,* and *midazolam*

Calcium-channel Blockers: plasma concentration of *diltiazem, nicardipine, nifedipine* and *nimodipine* possibly increased

- Ergotamine and Ergometrine: increased risk of ergotism—avoid concomitant use
- Lipid-regulating Drugs: plasma concentration of *atorvastatin, fluvastatin, pravastatin,* and *simvastatin* possibly increased (avoid concomitant use with simvastatin)

Oestrogens and Progestogens: contraceptive effect of *combined oral contraceptives* possibly reduced

Sildenafil: *amprenavir* possibly increases plasma concentration of *sildenafil* (reduce initial dose of sildenafil)

Ulcer-healing Drugs: *amprenavir* possibly increases plasma concentration of *cimetidine*

Anabolic Steroids

- Anticoagulants: anticoagulant effect of *acenocoumarol, phenindione, and warfarin* enhanced

Antidiabetics: hypoglycaemic effect possibly enhanced

Anaesthetics, General (*see also* Surgery and Long term Medication, section 15.1)
- ACE Inhibitors and Angiotensin-II Antagonists: enhanced hypotensive effect
  Antibacterials: possible potentiation of *isoniazid* hepatotoxicity; effect of *thiopental* enhanced by *sulphonamides*; hypersensitivity-like reactions can occur with concomitant intravenous *vancomycin*; *see also* Linezolid
  Antidepressants: risk of arrhythmias and hypotension increased with *tricyclics*; *MAOIs, see* section 15.1
- Antihypertensives: enhanced hypotensive effect
- Antipsychotics: enhanced hypotensive effect
  Anxiolytics and Hypnotics: enhanced sedative effect
- Beta-blockers: enhanced hypotensive effect
- Calcium-channel Blockers: enhanced hypotensive effect and AV delay with *verapamil*; hypotensive effect of *dihydropyridines* enhanced by *isoflurane*
- Cytotoxics: antifolate effect of *methotrexate* increased by *nitrous oxide* (avoid concomitant use)
- Dopaminergics: risk of arrhythmias if *volatile liquid anaesthetics such as halothane* given with *levodopa*
  Ergotamine and Ergometrine: *halothane* reduces effect of *ergometrine* on the parturient uterus
  Oxytocin: oxytocic effect possibly reduced by *volatile anaesthetics* (also enhanced hypotensive effect and risk of arrhythmias)
- Sympathomimetics: risk of arrhythmias if *adrenaline or isoprenaline* given with *volatile liquid anaesthetics such as halothane*
  Theophylline: increased risk of arrhythmias with *halothane*; increased risk of convulsions with *ketamine*

Anaesthetics, Local *see* Bupivacaine, Levobupivacaine, Lidocaine, Prilocaine, Ropivacaine

Analgesics *see* Aspirin, Nefopam, NSAIDs, Opioid Analgesics, and Paracetamol

Anion-exchange Resins *see* Colestyramine and Colestipol

Antacids
Note. Antacids should preferably not be taken at the same time as other drugs since they may impair absorption
  ACE Inhibitors and Angiotensin-II Antagonists: reduced absorption of *captopril, enalapril, fosinopril* and *possibly other ACE inhibitors*
  Analgesics: excretion of *aspirin* increased in alkaline urine; absorption of *diflunisal* reduced
  Anti-arrhythmics: excretion of *quinidine* reduced in alkaline urine (may occasionally increase plasma concentrations)
  Antibacterials: reduced absorption of *azithromycin, cefaclor, cefpodoxime, ciprofloxacin, isoniazid, levofloxacin, nitrofurantoin, norfloxacin, ofloxacin, rifampicin,* and *most tetracyclines*
  Antiepileptics: reduced absorption of *gabapentin* and *phenytoin*
  Antifungals: reduced absorption of *itraconazole* and *ketoconazole*
  Antihistamines: reduced absorption of *fexofenadine*
  Antiplatelet Drugs: *dipyridamole* patient information leaflet advises avoidance of *antacids*
  Antimalarials: reduced absorption of *chloroquine and hydroxychloroquine*; *magnesium trisilicate* reduces absorption of *proguanil*
  Antipsychotics: reduced absorption of *phenothiazines* and of *sulpiride*
  Antivirals: reduced absorption of *zalcitabine*
  Bile Acids: possibly reduced absorption of *ursodeoxycholic acid*
  Bisphosphonates: reduced absorption
  Cardiac Glycosides: possibly reduced absorption of *digoxin*
  Corticosteroids: reduced absorption of *deflazacort*
  Iron: *magnesium trisilicate* reduces absorption of *oral iron*

Antacids *(continued)*
  Lithium: *sodium bicarbonate increases excretion* (reduced plasma-lithium concentration)
  Mycophenolate Mofetil: reduced absorption of *mycophenolate mofetil*
  Penicillamine: reduced absorption
  Ulcer-healing Drugs: possibly reduced absorption of *lansoprazole*

Antazoline *see* Antihistamines

Anti-arrhythmics *see* Adenosine; Amiodarone; Disopyramide; Flecainide; Lidocaine; Mexiletine; Procainamide; Propafenone; Quinidine

Anticholinergics *see* Antimuscarinics

Anticholinesterases *see* Parasympathomimetics

Anticoagulants *see* Heparin, Phenindione, and Warfarin

Antidepressants *see* Antidepressants, SSRI; Antidepressants, Tricyclic; MAOIs; Mianserin; Mirtazapine; Moclobemide; Nefazodone; Reboxetine; Trazodone; Tryptophan; Venlafaxine

Antidepressants, SSRI
  Alcohol: effects possibly enhanced
  Anaesthetics: metabolism of *ropivacaine* reduced by *fluvoxamine*—avoid prolonged administration of ropivacaine
- Analgesics: risk of CNS toxicity increased with *tramadol*; plasma concentration of *methadone* possibly increased by *fluvoxamine*
  Anti-arrhythmics: plasma-flecainide concentration increased by *fluoxetine*
- Antibacterials: *see* Linezolid
- Anticoagulants: effect of *acenocoumarol* and *warfarin* possibly enhanced
- *other* Antidepressants: CNS effects of *SSRIs* increased by *MAOIs* (risk of serious toxicity), see also p. 195; *moclobemide see* p. 194; plasma concentrations of some *tricyclics* increased; agitation and nausea with *tryptophan*; manufacturer of *reboxetine* advises avoid concomitant use with *fluvoxamine*; *fluoxetine* increases plasma concentration of *nefazodone*; increased serotonergic effect with *St John's wort* (avoid concomitant use)
- Antiepileptics: antagonism (convulsive threshold lowered); plasma concentration of *carbamazepine* increased by *fluoxetine* and *fluvoxamine*; plasma concentration of *phenytoin* increased by *fluoxetine* and *fluvoxamine*; *phenytoin and possibly other antiepileptics* reduce plasma concentration of *paroxetine*
- Antihistamines: *citalopram, fluoxetine,* and *fluvoxamine* increase risk of arrhythmias with *terfenadine*—avoid concomitant use
  Antimuscarinics: plasma concentration of *procyclidine* increased by *paroxetine*
- Antipsychotics: plasma concentration of *clozapine* increased by *fluoxetine, fluvoxamine, paroxetine, sertraline,* and *venlafaxine*; plasma concentration of *haloperidol* and *zotepine* increased by *fluoxetine*
  Antivirals: plasma concentration possibly increased by *ritonavir*
  Anxiolytics and Hypnotics: plasma concentration of some *benzodiazepines* increased by *fluvoxamine*
- Barbiturates and Primidone: *see under* Antiepileptics, above
  Beta-blockers: plasma concentration of *propranolol* increased by *fluvoxamine*
- Dopaminergics: hypertension and CNS excitation with *fluoxetine, paroxetine* or *sertraline* and *selegiline* (selegiline should not be started until 5 weeks after discontinuation of fluoxetine, avoid fluoxetine for 2 weeks after stopping selegiline; selegiline should not be started until 2 weeks after stopping sertraline, avoid sertraline for 2 weeks after stopping selegiline)

Antidepressants, SSRI *(continued)*
- 5HT$_1$ Agonists: risk of CNS toxicity increased by *sumatriptan* (manufacturer of sertraline advises avoid concomitant use); *fluvoxamine* possibly inhibits metabolism of *zolmitriptan* (reduce dose of zolmitriptan)
- Lithium: increased risk of CNS effects (lithium toxicity reported)
- Sibutramine: increased risk of CNS toxicity (manufacturer of sibutramine recommends avoid concomitant use)
- Theophylline: plasma-theophylline concentration increased by *fluvoxamine* (concomitant use should usually be avoided, but where not possible halve theophylline dose and monitor plasma-theophylline concentration)
  Ulcer-healing Drugs: plasma concentration of *sertraline* increased by *cimetidine*

Antidepressants, Tricyclic
- Alcohol: enhanced sedative effect
  Alpha$_2$-adrenoceptor Stimulants: manufacturers of *apraclonidine* and *brimonidine* advise avoid concomitant use
- Altretamine: risk of severe postural hypotension
  Anaesthetics: risk of arrhythmias and hypotension increased
- Analgesics: possibly increased side-effects with *nefopam*; risk of CNS toxicity increased with *tramadol*; possibly increased sedation with *opioid analgesics*
- Anti-arrhythmics: increased risk of ventricular arrhythmias with drugs which prolong QT interval, including *amiodarone* (avoid concomitant use), *disopyramide*, *procainamide*, *propafenone* and *quinidine*
  Antibacterials: plasma concentrations of some *tricyclics* reduced by *rifampicin* (reduced antidepressant effect); *see also* Linezolid
- *other* Antidepressants: CNS excitation and hypertension with *MAOIs*, see also p. 189; *moclobemide see* p. 194; plasma concentrations of some *tricyclics* increased by *SSRIs*; manufacturer of *reboxetine* advises caution
- Antiepileptics: antagonism (convulsive threshold lowered); plasma concentrations of some *tricyclics* reduced (reduced antidepressant effect)
- Antihistamines: increased antimuscarinic and sedative effects; increased risk of ventricular arrhythmias with *terfenadine* (avoid concomitant use)
- Antihypertensives: in general, hypotensive effect enhanced, but antagonism of effect of *adrenergic neurone blockers* and of *clonidine* (and increased risk of hypertension on clonidine withdrawal)
  Antimuscarinics: increased antimuscarinic side-effects
- Antipsychotics: increased risk of ventricular arrhythmias—avoid concomitant use with *pimozide* or *thioridazine*; increased plasma concentrations of *tricyclic antidepressants* and increased antimuscarinic side-effects with *phenothiazines* and possibly *clozapine*
- Antivirals: plasma concentration possibly increased by *ritonavir*
  Anxiolytics and Hypnotics: enhanced sedative effect
- Barbiturates and Primidone: *see under* Antiepileptics, above
- Beta-blockers: risk of ventricular arrhythmias associated with *sotalol* increased
  Calcium-channel Blockers: *diltiazem* and *verapamil* increase plasma concentration of *imipramine* and possibly *other tricyclics*
  Disulfiram: inhibition of metabolism of *tricyclics* (increased plasma concentrations and increased disulfiram reaction reported with *alcohol with amitriptyline*)
  Diuretics: increased risk of postural hypotension

Antidepressants, Tricyclic *(continued)*
- Dopaminergics: manufacturer advises avoid concomitant use with *entacapone*; CNS toxicity reported with *selegiline*
  Muscle Relaxants: enhanced muscle relaxant effect of *baclofen*
  Nitrates: reduced effect of *sublingual nitrates* (owing to dry mouth)
  Oestrogens and Progestogens: *oral contraceptives* antagonise antidepressant effect (but side-effects may be increased due to increased plasma concentrations of *tricyclics*)
- Sibutramine: increased risk of CNS toxicity (manufacturer of sibutramine recommends avoid concomitant use)
- Sympathomimetics: hypertension and arrhythmias with *adrenaline* (but local anaesthetics with adrenaline appear to be safe); hypertension with *noradrenaline*; *methylphenidate* may inhibit metabolism of *tricyclics*
  Ulcer-healing Drugs: plasma concentrations of *amitriptyline, doxepin, imipramine, nortriptyline, and probably other tricyclics* increased by *cimetidine* (inhibition of metabolism)

Antidiabetics
Note. Includes Acarbose; Insulin; Metformin; Nateglinide; Repaglinide; Sulphonylureas; Thiazolidinediones
  ACE Inhibitors and Angiotensin-II Antagonists: *ACE inhibitors* possibly enhance hypoglycaemic effect
  Alcohol: enhanced hypoglycaemic effect; flushing with *chlorpropamide* (in susceptible subjects); risk of lactic acidosis with *metformin*
  Anabolic Steroids: possibly enhance hypoglycaemic effect
- Analgesics: *azapropazone, phenylbutazone* and possibly *other NSAIDs* enhance effect of *sulphonylureas* (avoid concomitant use with *azapropazone*)
  Anion-exchange Resins: *colestyramine* enhances hypoglycaemic effect of *acarbose*
- Antibacterials: Effect of *sulphonylureas* enhanced by *chloramphenicol* and rarely by *co-trimoxazole* and *sulphonamides*; *ciprofloxacin* possibly enhances effect of *glibenclamide*; *neomycin* possibly enhances hypoglycaemic effect of *acarbose* and increases severity of gastro-intestinal effects; *rifamycins* reduce effect of *chlorpropamide, tolbutamide* and possibly *other sulphonylureas* (accelerate metabolism); *rifampicin* reduces plasma concentration of *repaglinide*; *see also* Linezolid
  Anticoagulants: possibly enhanced hypoglycaemic effects of *sulphonylureas* and changes to anticoagulant effects of *warfarin and other coumarins*
  Antidepressants: *MAOIs* enhance hypoglycaemic effect of *insulin, metformin, sulphonylureas* and possibly other *antidiabetics*
  Antiepileptics: *plasma-phenytoin* concentration transiently increased by *tolbutamide* (possibility of toxicity)
- Antifungals: *fluconazole* and *miconazole* increase plasma concentrations of *sulphonylureas*—avoid concomitant use of *miconazole* with *gliclazide* or *glipizide*
  Antihistamines: depressed thrombocyte count with concomitant use of *biguanides* and *ketotifen*
  Antihypertensives: hypoglycaemic effect antagonised by *diazoxide*
  Antipsychotics: *phenothiazines* possibly antagonise hypoglycaemic effect of *sulphonylureas*
  Antivirals: *ritonavir* possibly increases plasma concentration of *tolbutamide*
  Beta-blockers: enhanced hypoglycaemic effect and masking of warning signs of hypoglycaemia such as tremor
  Calcium-channel Blockers: *nifedipine* may occasionally impair glucose tolerance
  Corticosteroids: antagonism of hypoglycaemic effect

Antidiabetics *(continued)*
Cytotoxics: *paclitaxel* may inhibit metabolism of *rosiglitazone*
Diuretics: hypoglycaemic effect antagonised by *loop and thiazide diuretics*; *chlorpropamide* increases risk of hyponatraemia with *thiazides in combination with potassium-sparing diuretics*
Fibrates: may improve glucose tolerance and have an additive effect
Hormone Antagonists: manufacturer advises metabolism of *oral antidiabetics* possibly accelerated by *aminoglutethimide*; *octreotide* possibly reduces *insulin and antidiabetic drug requirements in diabetes mellitus*
Lithium: may occasionally impair glucose tolerance
Oestrogens and Progestogens: *oral contraceptives* antagonise hypoglycaemic effect
Orlistat: manufacturer advises avoid concomitant use with *acarbose*
Pancreatin: hypoglycaemic effect of *acarbose* reduced by *pancreatin*
Testosterone: hypoglycaemic effect possibly enhanced
Ulcer-healing Drugs: *cimetidine* inhibits renal excretion of *metformin* (increased plasma-metformin concentrations); *cimetidine* enhances hypoglycaemic effect of *sulphonylureas*
• Uricosurics: *sulfinpyrazone* enhances effect of *sulphonylureas*; *probenecid* possibly enhances hypoglycaemic effect of *chlorpropamide*
Antiepileptics see Carbamazepine; Clomethiazole; Clonazepam; Ethosuximide; Gabapentin; Lamotrigine; Levetiracetam; Oxcarbazepine; Phenytoin; Tiagabine; Topiramate; Valproate; Vigabatrin and p. 227
Antifungals see Amphotericin; Antifungals, Imidazole and Triazole; Flucytosine; Griseofulvin; Terbinafine

Antifungals, Imidazole and Triazole
Note. Imidazole antifungals include clotrimazole, ketoconazole and miconazole; triazoles include fluconazole and itraconazole
In general, interactions relate to multiple-dose treatment
Analgesics: metabolism of *alfentanil* inhibited by *ketoconazole* (risk of prolonged or delayed respiratory depression); plasma concentration of *celecoxib* increased by *fluconazole* (halve celecoxib dose)
Antacids: *antacids* reduce absorption of *itraconazole* and *ketoconazole*
• Anti-arrhythmics: plasma concentration of *quinidine* increased by *itraconazole* and *miconazole* (increased risk of ventricular arrhythmias—avoid concomitant use)
• Antibacterials: *rifampicin* accelerates metabolism of *fluconazole, itraconazole* and *ketoconazole* (reduced plasma concentrations); plasma concentration of *rifampicin* may be reduced by *ketoconazole*; plasma concentration of *rifabutin* increased by *fluconazole* and possibly *other triazoles* (risk of uveitis—reduce rifabutin dose); plasma concentration of *ketoconazole* may be reduced by *isoniazid*; plasma concentration of *itraconazole* increased by *clarithromycin*
• Anticoagulants: effect of *acenocoumarol* and *warfarin* enhanced by *fluconazole, itraconazole, ketoconazole,* and *miconazole* (note: oral gel and possibly vaginal formulations absorbed)
• Antidepressants: manufacturer of *reboxetine* advises avoid concomitant use with *imidazoles* and *triazoles*
• Antidiabetics: plasma concentrations of *sulphonylureas* increased by *fluconazole* and *miconazole*—avoid concomitant use of *miconazole* with *gliclazide* or *glipizide*
• Antiepileptics: effect of *phenytoin* enhanced by *fluconazole* and *miconazole*; plasma concentrations of *itraconazole* and *ketoconazole* reduced by *phenytoin* other Antifungals: *imidazoles* and *triazoles* possibly antagonise effect of *amphotericin*

Antifungals, Imidazole and Triazole *(continued)*
• Antihistamines: *imidazoles* and *triazoles* inhibit *terfenadine* metabolism (avoid concomitant use of systemic or topical preparations—risk of hazardous arrhythmias); manufacturer advises possibility of increased plasma-loratadine concentration with *ketoconazole*; metabolism of *mizolastine* inhibited by *itraconazole, ketoconazole* and possibly *other imidazoles* (avoid concomitant use)
Antimuscarinics: reduced absorption of *ketoconazole*; manufacturer of *tolterodine* advises avoid concomitant use of *itraconazole* or *ketoconazole*
• Antipsychotics: risk of ventricular arrhythmias if *imidazoles* or *triazoles* given with *pimozide* (avoid concomitant use)
• Antivirals: *ketoconazole* inhibits metabolism of *indinavir*; plasma-indinavir concentration increased by *itraconazole* (consider reducing dose of indinavir); plasma concentration of *zidovudine* increased by *fluconazole* (increased risk of toxicity); plasma concentration of *ketoconazole* reduced by *nevirapine* (avoid concomitant use); plasma concentration of *ketoconazole* and possibly other *imidazoles* and *triazoles* increased by *ritonavir*; plasma concentration of *saquinavir* increased by *ketoconazole* and possibly by *other imidazoles* and *triazoles*; *amprenavir* possibly increases plasma concentration of *itraconazole*
• Anxiolytics and Hypnotics: plasma concentration of *midazolam* increased by *itraconazole, ketoconazole,* and *fluconazole* (prolonged sedative effect)
• Calcium-channel Blockers: possibly increased negative inotropic effect with *itraconazole*; *itraconazole* and *ketoconazole* inhibit metabolism of *felodipine* and possibly *other dihydropyridines* (increased plasma concentration)
• Cardiac Glycosides: plasma concentration of *digoxin* increased by *itraconazole*
• Ciclosporin: metabolism inhibited by *itraconazole, ketoconazole* and possibly *fluconazole* and *miconazole* (increased plasma-ciclosporin concentration)
Corticosteroids: *ketoconazole* inhibits metabolism of *methylprednisolone* and possibly *other corticosteroids*; *itraconazole* possibly inhibits metabolism of *methylprednisolone*
Cytotoxics: *itraconazole* may inhibit metabolism of *vincristine* (increased risk of neurotoxicity); *in vitro* studies suggest possible interaction between *ketoconazole* and *docetaxel*—consult product literature; plasma concentration of *imatinib* increased by *ketoconazole*
Diuretics: plasma concentration of *fluconazole* increased by *hydrochlorothiazide*
• Lipid-regulating Drugs: *itraconazole, ketoconazole,* and possibly *other imidazoles* and *triazoles* increase risk of myopathy with *simvastatin*—avoid concomitant use of *itraconazole, ketoconazole* or *miconazole* with *simvastatin*; *itraconazole* and possibly *other imidazoles* and *triazoles* may increase risk of myopathy with *atorvastatin*—avoid concomitant use of *itraconazole* with *atorvastatin*
Oestrogens and Progestogens: anecdotal reports of contraceptive failure with *fluconazole, itraconazole, ketoconazole* and possibly others
Sildenafil: *itraconazole* and *ketoconazole* increase plasma-sildenafil concentration (reduce initial dose of sildenafil)
• Sirolimus: plasma concentration increased by *itraconazole, ketoconazole* and *miconazole*
• Tacrolimus: *clotrimazole, fluconazole, ketoconazole* and possibly *other imidazoles* and *triazoles* increase plasma-tacrolimus concentration
• Theophylline: plasma-theophylline concentration possibly increased by *fluconazole* and possibly *ketoconazole*

Antifungals, Imidazole and Triazole *(continued)*
Ulcer-healing Drugs: *histamine H₂- antagonists* reduce absorption of *itraconazole* and *ketoconazole*; *proton-pump inhibitors* reduce absorption of *ketoconazole* and *itraconazole*; *sucralfate* reduces absorption of *ketoconazole*

Antihistamines
Note. Sedative interactions apply to a lesser extent to the non-sedating antihistamines, and they do not appear to potentiate the effects of alcohol.
Interactions do not generally apply to antihistamines used for topical action (including inhalation)
Grapefruit juice increases plasma concentration of ter-fenadine (avoid)
Alcohol: enhanced sedative effect
* Antacids: reduced absorption of *fexofenadine*
* Anti-arrhythmics: increased risk of ventricular arrhythmias with *mizolastine* and *terfenadine* (avoid concomitant use with *amiodarone, disopyramide, procainamide* and *quinidine*)
* Antibacterials: metabolism of *terfenadine* inhibited by *clarithromycin* and *erythromycin* (avoid concomitant use of systemic or topical preparations—risk of hazardous arrhythmias); manufacturer advises possibility of increased plasma-loratadine concentration with *erythromycin*; metabolism of *mizolastine* inhibited by *erythromycin* and possibly *other macrolides* (avoid concomitant use); increased risk of ventricular arrhythmias with *terfenadine* and *quinupristin/dalfopristin* (avoid concomitant use); *see also* Linezolid
* Antidepressants: *MAOIs* and *tricyclics* increase antimuscarinic and sedative effects; *tricyclics* increase risk of ventricular arrhythmias with *terfenadine* (avoid concomitant use); *citalopram, fluoxetine, fluvoxamine,* and *nefazodone* increase risk of arrhythmias with *terfenadine*—avoid concomitant use
Antidiabetics: depressed thrombocyte count with concomitant use of *biguanides* and *ketotifen*
* Antifungals: *imidazoles* and *triazoles* inhibit *terfenadine* metabolism (avoid concomitant use of systemic or topical preparations—risk of hazardous arrhythmias); manufacturer advises possibility of increased plasma-loratadine concentration with *ketoconazole*; metabolism of *mizolastine* inhibited by *itraconazole, ketoconazole* and possibly *other imidazoles* (avoid concomitant use)
* Antimalarials: *quinine* increases risk of ventricular arrhythmias with *terfenadine* (avoid concomitant use)
Antimuscarinics: increased antimuscarinic side-effects
* Antipsychotics: increased risk of ventricular arrhythmias with *terfenadine*—avoid concomitant use with *pimozide, sertindole* or *thioridazine*
* Antivirals: *amprenavir, efavirenz, indinavir, nelfinavir, ritonavir,* and *saquinavir* increase risk of ventricular arrhythmias with *terfenadine*—avoid concomitant use; plasma concentration of *non-sedating antihistamines* possibly increased by *ritonavir*; *amprenavir* possibly increases plasma concentration of *loratadine*
Anxiolytics and Hypnotics: enhanced sedative effect
* Beta-blockers: *sotalol* increases risk of ventricular arrhythmias with *mizolastine* and *terfenadine* (avoid concomitant use)
Betahistine: antagonism (theoretical)
Cytotoxics: *in vitro* studies suggest possible interaction between *docetaxel* and *terfenadine*—consult product literature
* Diuretics: hypokalaemia or other electrolyte imbalance increases risk of ventricular arrhythmias with *terfenadine*
* Hormone Antagonists: manufacturer of *bicalutamide* advises avoid concomitant *terfenadine*
Leukotriene Antagonists: *terfenadine* reduces plasma concentration of *zafirlukast*

Antihistamines *(continued)*
* Pentamidine Isetionate: increased risk of ventricular arrhythmias with *terfenadine* (avoid concomitant use)
Ulcer-healing Drugs: manufacturer advises possibility of increased plasma-loratadine concentration with *cimetidine*

Antihypertensives *see* individual drugs or groups
Antimalarials *see* individual drugs
Antimuscarinics
Note. Many drugs have antimuscarinic effects; concomitant use of two or more such drugs can increase side-effects such as dry mouth, urine retention, and constipation; concomitant use can also lead to confusion in the elderly; interactions do not generally apply to antimuscarinics used by inhalation
Alcohol: sedative effect of *hyoscine* enhanced
Analgesics: increased antimuscarinic effects with *nefopam*
Anti-arrhythmics: increased antimuscarinic effects with *disopyramide; atropine* delays absorption of *mexiletine*
Antibacterials: manufacturer of *tolterodine* advises avoid concomitant use of *clarithromycin* and *erythromycin; see also* Linezolid
Antidepressants: increased antimuscarinic side-effects with *tricyclics and MAOIs*; plasma concentration of *procyclidine* increased by *paroxetine*
Antifungals: reduced absorption of *ketoconazole;* manufacturer of *tolterodine* advises avoid concomitant use with *itraconazole* or *ketoconazole*
Antihistamines: increased antimuscarinic side-effects
Antipsychotics: increased antimuscarinic side-effects of *phenothiazines* (but reduced plasma concentrations); increased antimuscarinic side-effects of *clozapine*
Antivirals: manufacturer of *tolterodine* advises avoid concomitant use of *indinavir, nelfinavir, ritonavir* or *saquinavir*
Dopaminergics: increased antimuscarinic side-effects with *amantadine*; absorption of *levodopa* possibly reduced
Metoclopramide and Domperidone: *antimuscarinics* antagonise gastro-intestinal effects
Nitrates: reduced effect of *sublingual nitrates* (failure to dissolve under tongue owing to dry mouth)
Parasympathomimetics: antagonism of effect
Antiplatelet Drugs *see* Aspirin, Clopidogrel, Dipyridamole, and Ticlopidine
Antipsychotics
Note. Increased risk of toxicity with myelosuppressive drugs—*clozapine* in particular should not be used concurrently with drugs associated with a substantial potential for causing agranulocytosis, such as carbamazepine, co-trimoxazole, chloramphenicol, sulphonamides, pyrazolone analgesics such as azapropazone, penicillamine, or cytotoxics; also avoid clozapine with long-acting depot antipsychotics (have myelosuppressive potential)
ACE Inhibitors and Angiotensin-II Antagonists: severe postural hypotension with *chlorpromazine* and possibly *other phenothiazines*
Alcohol: enhanced sedative effect
* Anaesthetics: enhanced hypotensive effect
* Analgesics: enhanced sedative and hypotensive effect with *opioid analgesics*; severe drowsiness possible if *indometacin* given with *haloperidol*
Antacids and Adsorbents: reduced absorption of *phenothiazines* with *antacids* and possibly with *kaolin;* reduced absorption of *sulpiride* with *antacids*
* Anti-arrhythmics: increased risk of ventricular arrhythmias with drugs which prolong QT interval —avoid concomitant use of *pimozide* or *thioridazine* with *amiodarone, disopyramide, procainamide* or *quinidine* (also avoid haloperidol with amiodarone)

Antipsychotics *(continued)*
- Antibacterials: risk of arrhythmias if *clarithromycin* and possibly *erythromycin* given with *pimozide* (avoid concomitant use); *erythromycin* possibly increases plasma concentration of *clozapine* (possible increased risk of convulsions); *rifampicin* accelerates metabolism of *haloperidol* (reduced plasma-haloperidol concentration); *see also* Linezolid
- Antidepressants: increased risk of arrhythmias with *tricyclic antidepressants*—avoid concomitant use of *pimozide* or *thioridazine* with *tricyclics*; increased plasma concentrations and increased antimuscarinic effects notably on administration of *tricyclics* with *phenothiazines* and possibly *clozapine; fluoxetine, fluvoxamine, paroxetine, sertraline* and *venlafaxine* increase plasma concentration of *clozapine; fluvoxamine* increases plasma concentration of *olanzapine; fluoxetine* increases plasma concentration of *haloperidol* and *zotepine; oxypertine* causes CNS excitation and hypertension with *MAOIs; clozapine* possibly enhances central effects of *MAOIs;* manufacturer of *reboxetine* advises caution with antipsychotics; *nefazodone* increases plasma concentration of *haloperidol*

  Antidiabetics: hypoglycaemic effect of *sulphonylureas* possibly antagonised by *phenothiazines*
- Antiepileptics: antagonism (convulsive threshold lowered); *carbamazepine* accelerates metabolism of *clozapine, haloperidol, olanzapine,* and *risperidone* (reduced plasma concentrations); *phenytoin* accelerates metabolism of *clozapine* and *quetiapine; phenobarbital* accelerates metabolism of *haloperidol* (reduced plasma concentration)
- Antifungals: risk of ventricular arrhythmias if *imidazoles* or *triazoles* given with *pimozide* (avoid concomitant use)
- Antihistamines: increased risk of ventricular arrhythmias with *terfenadine*—avoid concomitant use with *pimozide, sertindole* or *thioridazine*

  Antihypertensives: enhanced hypotensive effect; *haloperidol* and higher doses of *chlorpromazine* antagonise hypotensive effect of *adrenergic neurone blockers;* increased risk of extrapyramidal effects on administration of *methyldopa*

  Antimalarials: avoid concomitant use of *pimozide* with *mefloquine* and *quinine;* avoid concomitant use of *thioridazine* with *quinine*

  Antimuscarinics: antimuscarinic side-effects of *phenothiazines* increased (but reduced plasma concentrations); antimuscarinic side-effects of *clozapine* increased
- *other* Antipsychotics: increased risk of ventricular arrhythmias with *thioridazine* and *other phenothiazines,* with *thioridazine* and *pimozide,* and with *pimozide* and *phenothiazines (*avoid concomitant use)
- Antivirals: *amprenavir, ritonavir* and possibly other *protease inhibitors* increase plasma concentration of *pimozide* (risk of ventricular arrhythmias—avoid concomitant use) and possibly *thioridazine; ritonavir* increases plasma concentration of *clozapine* (risk of toxicity—avoid concomitant use); *amprenavir* possibly increases plasma concentration of *clozapine; ritonavir* possibly increases plasma concentration of *other antipsychotics*

  Anxiolytics and Hypnotics: enhanced sedative effect; *diazepam* increases plasma concentration of *zotepine; buspirone* increases plasma concentration of *haloperidol*

  Barbiturates and Primidone: *see under* Antiepileptics, above
- Beta-blockers: *phenothiazines* and *pimozide* increase risk of ventricular arrhythmias with *sotalol;* concomitant administration of *propranolol* and *chlorpromazine* may increase plasma concentration of both drugs

  Calcium-channel Blockers: enhanced hypotensive effect

Antipsychotics *(continued)*

  Desferrioxamine: manufacturer advises avoid *prochlorperazine* (also *levomepromazine* on theoretical grounds)
- Diuretics: hypokalaemia increases risk of ventricular arrhythmias with *pimozide* or *thioridazine*—avoid concomitant use

  Dopaminergics: antagonism of hypoprolactinaemic and antiparkinsonian effects of *bromocriptine* and *cabergoline;* antagonism of effect of *apomorphine, levodopa, lisuride,* and *pergolide;* manufacturers of *pramipexole* and *ropinirole* advise avoid concomitant use (antagonism of effect)
- Lithium: increased risk of extrapyramidal effects and possibility of neurotoxicity with *clozapine, haloperidol and phenothiazines;* increased risk of extrapyramidal effects with *sulpiride;* increased risk of ventricular arrhythmias with *thioridazine*—avoid concomitant use

  Metoclopramide and Domperidone: increased risk of extrapyramidal effects with *metoclopramide*
- Pentamidine Isetionate: increased risk of ventricular arrhythmias with *thioridazine* (avoid concomitant use)
- Sibutramine: increased risk of CNS toxicity (manufacturer of sibutramine recommends avoid concomitant use)

  Sympathomimetics: antagonise pressor action

  Tetrabenazine: increased risk of extrapyramidal effects

  Ulcer-healing Drugs: *cimetidine* may enhance effects of *chlorpromazine, clozapine,* and possibly *other antipsychotics;* reduced absorption of *sulpiride* with *sucralfate*

Antivirals *see* Abacavir; Aciclovir and Famciclovir; Amprenavir; Didanosine; Efavirenz; Ganciclovir; Indinavir; Lamivudine; Nelfinavir; Nevirapine; Ritonavir; Saquinavir; Stavudine; Valaciclovir; Zalcitabine; Zidovudine

Anxiolytics and Hypnotics

  Alcohol: enhanced sedative effect

  Anaesthetics: enhanced sedative effect

  Analgesics: *opioid analgesics* enhance sedative effect
- Antibacterials: *clarithromycin, erythromycin* and *quinupristin/dalfopristin* inhibit metabolism of *midazolam* (increased plasma-midazolam concentration, with profound sedation); *erythromycin* and *quinupristin/dalfopristin* inhibit metabolism of *zopiclone; isoniazid* inhibits metabolism of *diazepam; rifampicin* increases metabolism of *diazepam* and possibly *other benzodiazepines* and *zaleplon; see also* Linezolid

  Anticoagulants: *chloral hydrate* and *triclofos* may transiently enhance anticoagulant effect of *acenocoumarol* and *warfarin*

  Antidepressants: enhanced sedative effect; manufacturer contra-indicates *buspirone* with *MAOIs;* plasma concentrations of some *benzodiazepines* increased by *fluvoxamine;* plasma concentration of *alprazolam* increased by *nefazodone* (reduce alprazolam dose)

  Antiepileptics: metabolism of *clonazepam* accelerated (reduced effect); plasma-phenytoin concentrations increased or decreased by *diazepam* and possibly *other benzodiazepines*
- Antifungals: *itraconazole, ketoconazole,* and *fluconazole* increase plasma concentration of *midazolam* (prolonged sedative effect)

  Antihistamines: enhanced sedative effect

  Antihypertensives: enhanced hypotensive effect; enhanced sedative effect with *alpha-blockers* and possibly *moxonidine*

  Antipsychotics: enhanced sedative effect; *diazepam* increases plasma concentration of *zotepine; buspirone* increases plasma concentration of *haloperidol*

Anxiolytics and Hypnotics *(continued)*
- Antivirals: *efavirenz, nelfinavir* and *saquinavir* increase risk of prolonged sedation with *midazolam* (avoid concomitant use); *indinavir* increases risk of prolonged sedation with *alprazolam* and *midazolam* (avoid concomitant use); *ritonavir* increases plasma concentration of *alprazolam, clorazepate, diazepam, flurazepam, midazolam* and *zolpidem* (risk of extreme sedation and respiratory depression—avoid concomitant use); *amprenavir* increases plasma concentration of *alprazolam, clorazepate, diazepam, flurazepam* and *midazolam* (increased risk of prolonged sedation and respiratory depression); plasma concentration of *other anxiolytics and hypnotics* possibly increased by *ritonavir*

Calcium-channel Blockers: *diltiazem* and *verapamil* inhibit metabolism of *midazolam* (increased plasma-midazolam concentration, with increased sedation)

Disulfiram: metabolism of *benzodiazepines* inhibited, with enhanced sedative effect (*temazepam* toxicity reported)

Diuretics: concomitant administration of *chloral hydrate* or *triclofos* and parenteral *furosemide* may displace thyroid hormone from binding sites

Dopaminergics: *benzodiazepines* occasionally antagonise effect of *levodopa*

Lofexidine: enhanced sedative effect

Muscle Relaxants: *baclofen* and *tizanidine* enhance sedative effect

Nabilone: enhanced sedative effect

Ulcer-healing Drugs: *cimetidine* inhibits metabolism of *benzodiazepines, clomethiazole* and *zaleplon* (increased plasma concentrations); *omeprazole* and *esomeprazole* possibly inhibit metabolism of *diazepam* (increased plasma concentration)

Apomorphine
Antipsychotics: antagonism of effects
other Dopaminergics: effect possibly enhanced by *entacapone*
Nitrates: enhanced hypotensive effect with sublingual apomorphine

Apraclonidine *see* Alpha$_2$-adrenoceptor Stimulants

Aspirin
- *other* Analgesics: avoid concomitant administration of other *NSAIDs* (increased side-effects)
Antacids and Adsorbents: excretion of *aspirin* increased in alkaline urine; *kaolin* possibly reduces absorption
- Anticoagulants: increased risk of bleeding due to antiplatelet effect
Antiepileptics: enhancement of effect of *phenytoin* and *valproate*
other Antiplatelet Drugs: increased risk of bleeding with *clopidogrel* and *ticlopidine*
Corticosteroids: increased risk of gastro-intestinal bleeding and ulceration; corticosteroids reduce plasma-concentration
- Cytotoxics: reduced excretion of *methotrexate* (increased toxicity)
Diuretics: antagonism of diuretic effect of *spironolactone;* reduced excretion of *acetazolamide* (risk of toxicity)
Leukotriene Antagonists: aspirin increases plasma concentration of *zafirlukast*
Metoclopramide and Domperidone: *metoclopramide* enhances effect of *aspirin* (increased rate of absorption)
Mifepristone: manufacturer of mifepristone recommends avoid *aspirin* on theoretical grounds
Uricosurics: effect of *probenecid* and *sulfinpyrazone* reduced

Atenolol *see* Beta-blockers
Atorvastatin *see* Statins

Atovaquone
- Antibacterials: plasma-atovaquone concentration reduced by *rifampicin* and by *tetracycline* (possible therapeutic failure of *atovaquone*)
Metoclopramide and Domperidone: plasma-atovaquone concentration reduced by *metoclopramide*

Atracurium *see* Muscle Relaxants (non-depolarising)
Atropine *see* Antimuscarinics
Auranofin *see* Gold
Azapropazone *see* NSAIDs
Azatadine *see* Antihistamines
Azathioprine
ACE Inhibitors and Angiotensin-II Antagonists: increased risk of leucopenia with *captopril*
- Allopurinol: enhancement of effect with increased toxicity (reduce dose of azathioprine when given with allopurinol)
Aminosalicylates: possible increased risk of leucopenia
- Antibacterials: manufacturer reports interaction with *rifampicin* (transplants possibly rejected); increased risk of haematological toxicity with *co-trimoxazole* and *trimethoprim*
- Anticoagulants: anticoagulant effect of warfarin possibly reduced
Vaccines: see p. 578

Azelastine *see* Antihistamines
Azithromycin *see* Erythromycin and other Macrolides
Aztreonam
- Anticoagulants: anticoagulant effect of *acenocoumarol* and *warfarin* possibly enhanced

Baclofen *see* Muscle Relaxants
Balsalazide *see* Aminosalicylates
Bambuterol *see* Sympathomimetics, Beta$_2$
Barbiturates and Primidone
Alcohol: enhanced sedative effect
Anti-arrhythmics: metabolism of *disopyramide and quinidine* increased (reduced plasma concentrations)
Antibacterials: metabolism of *chloramphenicol, doxycycline, and metronidazole* accelerated (reduced effect); *sulphonamides* enhance effect of *thiopental; see also* Linezolid
- Anticoagulants: metabolism of *acenocoumarol* and *warfarin* accelerated (reduced anticoagulant effect)
- Antidepressants: antagonism of anticonvulsant effect (convulsive threshold lowered); metabolism of *mianserin* and some *tricyclics* accelerated (reduced plasma concentrations); plasma concentration of *phenobarbital* reduced by *St John's wort* (avoid concomitant use)
Antiepileptics: interactions of *phenobarbital* or *primidone* with other antiepileptics include enhanced effects, increased sedation, and reductions in plasma concentrations; for further details see p. 227
Antifungals: *phenobarbital* reduces absorption of *griseofulvin* (reduced effect)
- Antipsychotics: antagonism of anticonvulsant effect (convulsive threshold lowered); *phenobarbital* accelerates metabolism of *haloperidol* (reduced plasma concentration)
- Antivirals: plasma concentration of *indinavir, lopinavir, nelfinavir* and *saquinavir* possibly reduced
Bupropion (amfebutamone): *phenobarbital* reduces plasma concentration of *bupropion*
- Calcium-channel Blockers: effect of *felodipine, isradipine* and probably *nicardipine, nifedipine* and *other dihydropyridines, diltiazem,* and *verapamil* reduced
Cardiac Glycosides: metabolism of *digitoxin only* accelerated (reduced effect)
- Ciclosporin: metabolism of *ciclosporin* accelerated (reduced effect)

Barbiturates and Primidone *(continued)*
* Corticosteroids: metabolism of *corticosteroids* accelerated (reduced effect)

Folic Acid and Folinic Acid: plasma concentration of *phenobarbital* and *primidone* possibly reduced by *folic acid* and *folinic acid*

Hormone Antagonists: metabolism of *toremifene* possibly accelerated

Leukotriene Antagonists: plasma concentration of *montelukast* reduced by *phenobarbital*
* Oestrogens and Progestogens: metabolism of *gestrinone, tibolone,* and *oral contraceptives* accelerated (reduced contraceptive effect, **important: see pp. 387–8**)

Theophylline: metabolism of *theophylline* accelerated (reduced effect)

Thyroid Hormones: metabolism of levothyroxine and liothyronine accelerated (may increase requirements in hypothyroidism)

Tropisetron: *phenobarbitone* reduces plasma concentration of *tropisetron*

Vitamins: *vitamin D* requirements possibly increased

Beclometasone *see* Corticosteroids

Bendrofluazide (Bendroflumethiazide) *see* Diuretics (thiazide)

Bendroflumethiazide (Bendrofluazide) *see* Diuretics (thiazide)

Benorilate *see* Aspirin *and* Paracetamol

Benperidol *see* Antipsychotics

Benzatropine *see* Antimuscarinics

Benzhexol (Trihexyphenidyl) *see* Antimuscarinics

Benzodiazepines *see* Anxiolytics and Hypnotics

Benzthiazide *see* Diuretics (thiazide)

Benzylpenicillin *see* Penicillins

Beta-blockers
Note. Since systemic absorption may follow topical application of beta-blockers to the eye the possibility of interactions, in particular, with drugs such as verapamil should be borne in mind

ACE Inhibitors and Angiotensin-II Antagonists: enhanced hypotensive effect

Alcohol: enhanced hypotensive effect

Aldesleukin: enhanced hypotensive effect

Alprostadil: enhanced hypotensive effect
* Anaesthetics: enhanced hypotensive effect; increased risk of *bupivacaine* toxicity with *propranolol*
* Analgesics: *NSAIDs* antagonise hypotensive effect; *morphine* possibly increases plasma concentration of *esmolol*
* Anti-arrhythmics: increased risk of myocardial depression and bradycardia; with *amiodarone* increased risk of bradycardia and AV block; increased risk of *lidocaine* toxicity with *propranolol*; *propafenone* increases plasma concentration of *metoprolol* and *propranolol*; risk of ventricular arrhythmias associated with *sotalol* increased by *amiodarone, disopyramide, procainamide,* and *quinidine* (avoid concomitant use)

Antibacterials: *rifampicin* accelerates metabolism of *bisoprolol* and *propranolol* (significantly reduced plasma concentration); *see also* Linezolid
* Antidepressants: enhanced hypotensive effect with *MAOIs; fluvoxamine* increases plasma concentration of *propranolol*; risk of ventricular arrhythmias associated with *sotalol* increased by *tricyclics*

Antidiabetics: enhanced hypoglycaemic effect and masking of warning signs of hypoglycaemia such as tremor
* Antihistamines: risk of ventricular arrhythmias associated with *sotalol* increased by *mizolastine* and *terfenadine* (avoid concomitant use)
* Antihypertensives: enhanced hypotensive effect; increased risk of withdrawal hypertension with *clonidine* (withdraw beta-blocker several days before slowly withdrawing clonidine); increased risk of first-dose hypotensive effect with *post-synaptic alpha-blockers such as prazosin*

Beta-blockers *(continued)*
Antimalarials: increased risk of bradycardia with *mefloquine*
* Antipsychotics: risk of ventricular arrhythmias associated with *sotalol* increased by *phenothiazines* and *pimozide*; concomitant administration of *propranolol* and *chlorpromazine* may increase plasma concentration of both drugs

Anxiolytics and Hypnotics: enhanced hypotensive effect
* Calcium-channel Blockers: increased risk of bradycardia and AV block with *diltiazem*; severe hypotension and heart failure occasionally with *nifedipine* and possibly *nisoldipine*; asystole, severe hypotension, and heart failure with *verapamil* (see p. 107); *lercanidipine* may enhance hypotensive effect of *propranolol* and *metoprolol*

Cardiac Glycosides: increased AV block and bradycardia

Corticosteroids: antagonism of hypotensive effect

Diuretics: enhanced hypotensive effect; risk of ventricular arrhythmias associated with *sotalol* increased by hypokalaemia

Ergotamine and Ergometrine: increased peripheral vasoconstriction

$5HT_1$ Agonists: *propranolol* may increase plasma concentration of *rizatriptan* (reduce rizatriptan dose)
* Moxisylyte: possible severe postural hypotension

Muscle Relaxants: *propranolol* enhances effect; possible enhanced hypotensive effect and bradycardia with *tizanidine*

Oestrogens and Progestogens: *oestrogens* and *combined oral contraceptives* antagonise hypotensive effect

Parasympathomimetics: risk of arrhythmias possibly increased by *pilocarpine*; *propranolol* antagonises effect of *neostigmine* and *pyridostigmine*
* Sympathomimetics: severe hypertension with *adrenaline* and *noradrenaline* and possibly with *dobutamine* (especially with *non-selective beta-blockers*)

Theophylline: *beta-blockers* should be avoided on pharmacological grounds (bronchospasm)

Tropisetron: risk of ventricular arrhythmias—manufacturer of tropisetron advises caution

Ulcer-healing Drugs: plasma concentrations of *labetalol, metoprolol* and *propranolol* increased by *cimetidine*; hypotensive effect antagonised by *carbenoxolone*

Xamoterol: antagonism of effect of *xamoterol* and reduction in beta-blockade

Betahistine
Antihistamines: antagonism (theoretical)

Betamethasone *see* Corticosteroids

Betaxolol *see* Beta-blockers

Bethanechol *see* Parasympathomimetics

Bezafibrate *see* Fibrates

Bicalutamide
Anticoagulants: effect of *warfarin* possibly enhanced
* Antihistamines: manufacturer of *bicalutamide* advises avoid concomitant *terfenadine*

Bile Acids
Antacids: may reduce absorption of bile acids

Ciclosporin: *ursodeoxycholic acid* increases absorption of *ciclosporin*

Colestyramine and Colestipol: may reduce absorption of bile acids

Oestrogens and Progestogens: *oestrogens* increase elimination of cholesterol in bile

Biperiden *see* Antimuscarinics

Bismuth Chelate *see* Tripotassium Dicitratobismuthate

Bisoprolol *see* Beta-blockers

Bisphosphonates
Analgesics: bioavailability of *tiludronic acid* increased by *indometacin*

Antacids: reduced absorption

Antibacterials: increased risk of hypocalcaemia with *aminoglycosides*

Bisphosphonates *(continued)*
  Calcium Salts: reduced absorption
  Iron: reduced absorption
Botulinum Toxin
• Antibacterials: effects enhanced by *aminoglycosides* (risk of toxicity)
• Muscle Relaxants: effects enhanced by *non-depolarising muscle relaxants*
Bretylium *see* Adrenergic Neurone Blockers
Brimonidine *see* Alpha₂-adrenoceptor Stimulants
Brinzolamide *see* Diuretics (carbonic anhydrase inhibitors)
  Note. Since systemic absorption may follow topical application of brinzolamide to the eye, the possibility of interactions should be borne in mind
Bromocriptine and Cabergoline
  Alcohol: reduced tolerance to *bromocriptine*
  Antibacterials: *erythromycin* and possibly *other macrolides* increase plasma concentration (increased risk of toxicity)
  Antipsychotics: antagonism of hypoprolactinaemic and antiparkinsonian effects
  Hormone Antagonists: *octreotide* increases concentration of *bromocriptine*
  Metoclopramide and Domperidone: antagonise hypoprolactinaemic effect
• Sympathomimetics: increased risk of toxicity with *bromocriptine* and *isometheptene* or *phenylpropanolamine*
Brompheniramine *see* Antihistamines
Buclizine *see* Antihistamines
Budesonide *see* Corticosteroids
Bumetanide *see* Diuretics (loop)
Bupivacaine
  Anti-arrhythmics: increased myocardial depression
  Beta-blockers: increased risk of *bupivacaine* toxicity with *propranolol*
Buprenorphine *see* Opioid Analgesics
Bupropion (Amfebutamone)
  Note. Bupropion should be administered with extreme caution to patients receiving other medication known to lower the seizure threshold—see CSM advice, p. 249 and Cautions, Contra-indications and Side-effects of individual drugs
• Antibacterials: *see* Linezolid
• Antidepressants: manufacturer of bupropion advises avoid with or for 2 weeks after *MAOIs* and avoid concomitant use with *moclobemide*
  Antiepileptics: *carbamazepine, phenobarbital* and *phenytoin* reduce plasma concentration of bupropion; *sodium valproate* inhibits metabolism of bupropion
• Antivirals: *ritonavir* increases plasma concentration of *bupropion* (risk of toxicity—avoid concomitant use)
  Barbiturates and primidone: *see under* Antiepileptics, above
  Dopaminergics: increased risk of side-effects with *levodopa*
Buspirone *see* Anxiolytics and Hypnotics
Butobarbital *see* Barbiturates and Primidone
Cabergoline *see* Bromocriptine and Cabergoline
Calcium Salts
  Antibacterials: reduced absorption of *ciprofloxacin* and *tetracyclines*
  Bisphosphonates: reduced absorption
  Cardiac Glycosides: large intravenous doses of *calcium* can precipitate arrhythmias
  Diuretics: increased risk of hypercalcaemia with *thiazides*

Calcium-channel Blockers
  Note. Grapefruit juice significantly increases plasma concentration of dihydropyridine calcium-channel blockers (but amlodipine not affected significantly) and verapamil
  Dihydropyridine calcium-channel blockers include amlodipine, felodipine, isradipine, lacidipine, lercanidipine, nicardipine, nifedipine, nimodipine and nisoldipine
  ACE Inhibitors and Angiotensin-II Antagonists: enhanced hypotensive effect
  Alcohol: enhanced hypotensive effect; plasma-alcohol concentration possibly increased by *verapamil*
  Aldesleukin: enhanced hypotensive effect
  Alprostadil: enhanced hypotensive effect
• Anaesthetics: *verapamil* increases hypotensive effect of *general anaesthetics* and risk of AV delay; *isoflurane* enhances hypotensive effect of *dihydropyridines*
• Anti-arrhythmics: *amiodarone-induced* risk of bradycardia, AV block, and myocardial depression increased by *diltiazem* and *verapamil*; plasma-concentration of *quinidine* reduced by *nifedipine*; increased risk of myocardial depression and asystole if *verapamil* given with *disopyramide* and *flecainide*; with *verapamil* raised plasma concentration of *quinidine* (extreme hypotension may occur)
• Antibacterials: *erythromycin* possibly inhibits metabolism of *felodipine* (increased plasma concentration); *quinupristin/dalfopristin* increases plasma concentration of *nifedipine*; *rifampicin* increases metabolism of *diltiazem, nifedipine, nimodipine, verapamil* and possibly *isradipine, nicardipine* and *nisoldipine* (plasma concentrations significantly reduced); *see also* Linezolid
  Antidepressants: enhanced hypotensive effect with *MAOIs*; *diltiazem* and *verapamil* increase plasma concentration of *imipramine* and *possibly other tricyclics*
  Antidiabetics: *nifedipine* may occasionally impair glucose tolerance
• Antiepileptics: effect of *carbamazepine* enhanced by *diltiazem* and *verapamil; diltiazem* and *verapamil* increase plasma concentration of *phenytoin*; effect of *felodipine* and *isradipine* and probably *nicardipine, nifedipine* and *other dihydropyridines* reduced by *carbamazepine, phenobarbital, phenytoin, and primidone*; effect of *diltiazem* and *verapamil* reduced by *phenobarbital* and *phenytoin*; plasma concentration of *nisoldipine* reduced by *phenytoin*
• Antifungals: possibly increased negative inotropic effect with *itraconazole*; *itraconazole* and *ketoconazole* inhibit metabolism of *felodipine* and possibly other *dihydropyridines* (increased plasma concentration)
• Antihypertensives: enhanced hypotensive effect; increased risk of first-dose hypotensive effect of *post-synaptic alpha-blockers* such as *prazosin*
  Antimalarials: possible increased risk of bradycardia with some *calcium-channel blockers* and *mefloquine*
  Antipsychotics: enhanced hypotensive effect
• Antivirals: *ritonavir* possibly increases plasma concentration of calcium-channel blockers; *amprenavir* possibly increases plasma concentration of *diltiazem, nicardipine, nifedipine,* and *nimodipine*
  Anxiolytics and Hypnotics: *diltiazem* and *verapamil* inhibit metabolism of *midazolam* (increased plasma-midazolam concentration, with increased sedation)
• Barbiturates and Primidone: *see under* Antiepileptics, above
• Beta-blockers: increased risk of bradycardia and AV block with *diltiazem;* occasionally severe hypotension and heart failure with *nifedipine* and possibly *nisoldipine*; asystole, severe hypotension, and heart failure with *verapamil* (see p. 107); *lercanidipine* may enhance hypotensive effect of *propranolol* and *metoprolol*

Calcium-channel Blockers *(continued)*

other Calcium-channel Blockers: clearance of *nifedipine* reduced by *diltiazem* (increased plasma-nifedipine concentration)

- Cardiac Glycosides: plasma concentration of *digoxin* increased by *diltiazem, nicardipine, verapamil* and possibly *nifedipine*; increased AV block and bradycardia with *verapamil*
- Ciclosporin: plasma-ciclosporin concentrations increased by *diltiazem, nicardipine,* and *verapamil*; possibly increases plasma concentration of *nifedipine* (increased risk of side-effects such as gingival hyperplasia)

Diuretics: enhanced hypotensive effect

Lithium: neurotoxicity may occur without increased plasma-lithium concentrations in patients given *diltiazem* and *verapamil*

- Magnesium Salts: profound hypotension reported with *nifedipine* and *intravenous magnesium sulphate* in pre-eclampsia

Moxisylyte: enhanced hypotensive effect

Muscle Relaxants: *nifedipine* and *verapamil* enhance effect of *non-depolarising muscle relaxants*; hypotension, myocardial depression, and hyperkalaemia with *verapamil* and intravenous *dantrolene*; risk of arrhythmias with *diltiazem* and intravenous *dantrolene*; enhanced hypotensive effect with *tizanidine*

Sirolimus: *diltiazem* increases plasma concentrations of *sirolimus*

- Tacrolimus: *nifedipine* and *diltiazem* increase plasma concentration of tacrolimus
- Theophylline: *diltiazem, verapamil* and possibly *other calcium-channel blockers* enhance effect (increased plasma-theophylline concentration)

Ulcer-healing Drugs: *cimetidine* inhibits metabolism of *some calcium-channel blockers* (increased plasma concentrations)

Calcium Levofolinate *see* Folic Acid and Folinic Acid

Candesartan *see* ACE Inhibitors and Angiotensin-II Antagonists

Capecitabine *see* Fluorouracil (prodrug of fluorouracil)

Capreomycin

other Antibacterials: increased risk of nephrotoxicity with *colistin*; increased risk of nephrotoxicity and ototoxicity with *aminoglycosides and vancomycin*

Cytotoxics: increased risk of nephrotoxicity and ototoxicity with *cisplatin*

Captopril *see* ACE Inhibitors and Angiotensin-II Antagonists

Carbachol *see* Parasympathomimetics

Carbamazepine

Alcohol: CNS side-effects of *carbamazepine* possibly enhanced

- Analgesics: *dextropropoxyphene* enhances effect of *carbamazepine;* effect of *methadone* and *tramadol* decreased by *carbamazepine*
- Antibacterials: metabolism of *doxycycline* accelerated (reduced effect); plasma-carbamazepine concentration increased by *clarithromycin, erythromycin* and *isoniazid* (also isoniazid hepatotoxicity possibly increased); plasma-carbamazepine concentration reduced by *rifabutin*; *see also* Linezolid
- Anticoagulants: metabolism of *acenocoumarol* and *warfarin* accelerated (reduced anticoagulant effect)
- Antidepressants: antagonism of anticonvulsant effect (convulsive threshold lowered); plasma concentration of *carbamazepine* increased by *fluoxetine* and *fluvoxamine*; metabolism of *mianserin* and *tricyclics* accelerated (reduced plasma concentrations); plasma concentration increased by *nefazodone* (also plasma-nefazodone concentration reduced); manufacturer advises avoid with *MAOIs* or within 2 weeks of *MAOIs*; plasma concentration of *carbamazepine* reduced by *St John's wort* (avoid concomitant use)

Carbamazepine *(continued)*

other Antiepileptics: interactions include enhanced effects, increased sedation, and reductions in plasma concentrations; for further details, see p. 227

- Antimalarials: *mefloquine* antagonises anticonvulsant effect; *chloroquine* and *hydroxychloroquine* occasionally reduce conulsive threshold
- Antipsychotics: antagonism of anticonvulsant effect (convulsive threshold lowered); metabolism of *clozapine, haloperidol, olanzapine* and *risperidone* accelerated (reduced plasma concentrations)
- Antivirals: plasma concentration of *indinavir, lopinavir, nelfinavir* and *saquinavir* possibly reduced; plasma concentration possibly increased by *amprenavir* and *ritonavir*

Bupropion (amfebutamone): plasma concentration of *bupropion* reduced

- Calcium-channel Blockers: *diltiazem and verapamil* enhance effect of *carbamazepine*; effect of *felodipine, isradipine* and probably *nicardipine, nifedipine* and *other dihydropyridines* reduced

Cardiac Glycosides: metabolism of *digitoxin* accelerated (reduced effect)

- Ciclosporin: metabolism accelerated (reduced plasma-ciclosporin concentration)
- Corticosteroids: metabolism accelerated (reduced effect)
- Diuretics: increased risk of hyponatraemia; *acetazolamide* increases plasma-carbamazepine concentration
- Hormone Antagonists: *danazol* inhibits metabolism of *carbamazepine* (enhanced effect); metabolism of *gestrinone* and possibly *toremifene* accelerated

Lithium: neurotoxicity may occur without increased plasma-lithium concentration

Muscle Relaxants: effect of *non-depolarising muscle relaxants* antagonised (recovery from neuromuscular blockade accelerated)

- Oestrogens and Progestogens: *carbamazepine* accelerates metabolism of *oral contraceptives* (reduced contraceptive effect, **important:** see pp. 387–8) and of *tibolone*

Retinoids: plasma concentration possibly reduced by *isotretinoin*

Theophylline: metabolism of *theophylline* accelerated (reduced effect)

Thyroid Hormones: metabolism of *levothyroxine* and *liothyronine* accelerated (may increase requirements in hypothyroidism)

- Ulcer-healing Drugs: metabolism inhibited by *cimetidine* (increased plasma-carbamazepine concentration)

Vitamins: *carbamazepine* possibly increases *vitamin D* requirements

Carbenoxolone

Note. Interactions do not apply to small amounts used topically on oral mucosa

Antihypertensives: antagonism of hypotensive effect

Cardiac Glycosides: toxicity increased if hypokalaemia occurs

Corticosteroids: increased risk of hypokalaemia

Diuretics: antagonism of diuretic effect; increased risk of hypokalaemia with *acetazolamide, thiazides,* and *loop diuretics*; inhibition of ulcer healing with *amiloride* and *spironolactone*

Carbonic Anhydrase Inhibitors *see* Diuretics

Cardiac Glycosides

- ACE Inhibitors and Angiotensin-II Antagonists: *telmisartan* and possibly *captopril* increase plasma concentration of *digoxin*

Aminosalicylates: absorption of *digoxin* possibly reduced by *sulfasalazine*

Analgesics: *NSAIDs* may exacerbate heart failure, reduce GFR and increase plasma-cardiac glycoside concentrations

Anion-exchange Resins: absorption possibly reduced by *colestyramine and colestipol*

Antacids and Adsorbents: *antacids* and kaolin possibly reduce absorption of *digoxin*

Cardiac Glycosides *(continued)*
* Anti-arrhythmics: plasma concentration of *digoxin* increased by *amiodarone, propafenone, and quinidine* (halve maintenance dose of digoxin)

Antibacterials: *erythromycin* and possibly *other macrolides* enhance effect of *digoxin*; *rifamycins* accelerate metabolism of *digitoxin* (reduced effect); *neomycin* reduces absorption of *digoxin*; *trimethoprim* possibly increases plasma concentration of *digoxin*
* Antidepressants: *nefazodone* increases plasma concentration of *digoxin*; *St John's wort* reduces plasma concentration of *digoxin* (avoid concomitant use)

Antiepileptics: metabolism of *digitoxin* accelerated (reduced effect)
* Antifungals: increased toxicity if hypokalaemia occurs with *amphotericin*; plasma concentration of *digoxin* increased by *itraconazole*
* Antimalarials: *quinine, hydroxychloroquine,* and possibly *chloroquine* raise plasma concentration of *digoxin*; possible increased risk of bradycardia with *mefloquine*

Barbiturates and Primidone: *see under* Antiepileptics, above

Beta-blockers: increased AV block and bradycardia

Calcium Salts: large intravenous doses of *calcium* can precipitate arrhythmias
* Calcium-channel Blockers: plasma concentration of *digoxin* increased by *diltiazem, nicardipine, verapamil* and possibly *nifedipine*; increased AV block and bradycardia with *verapamil*

Corticosteroids: increased risk of hypokalaemia
* Diuretics: increased toxicity if hypokalaemia occurs with *acetazolamide, loop diuretics, and thiazides*; effects of *digoxin* enhanced by *spironolactone*

Hormone Antagonists: *aminoglutethimide* accelerates metabolism of *digitoxin only* (reduced effect)

Lipid-regulating Drugs: plasma concentration of *digoxin* possibly increased by *atorvastatin*

Muscle Relaxants: arrhythmias with *suxamethonium*; possible bradycardia with *tizanidine*

Ulcer-healing Drugs: increased toxicity if hypokalaemia occurs with *carbenoxolone*; plasma concentration of *digoxin* possibly increased by *proton pump inhibitors*; absorption possibly reduced by *sucralfate*

Carisoprodol *see* Anxiolytics and Hypnotics
Carteolol *see* Beta-blockers
Carvedilol *see* Beta-blockers
Cefaclor *see* Cephalosporins
Cefadroxil *see* Cephalosporins
Cefalexin *see* Cephalosporins
Cefamandole *see* Cephalosporins
Cefazolin *see* Cephalosporins
Cefixime *see* Cephalosporins
Cefotaxime *see* Cephalosporins
Cefoxitin *see* Cephalosporins
Cefpirome *see* Cephalosporins
Cefpodoxime *see* Cephalosporins
Cefprozil *see* Cephalosporins
Cefradine *see* Cephalosporins
Ceftazidime *see* Cephalosporins
Ceftriaxone *see* Cephalosporins
Cefuroxime *see* Cephalosporins
Celecoxib *see* NSAIDs
Celiprolol *see* Beta-blockers
Cephalosporins
Alcohol: disulfiram-like reaction with *cefamandole*

Antacids and Adsorbents: *antacids* reduce absorption of *cefaclor* and *cefpodoxime*
* Anticoagulants: anticoagulant effect of *warfarin and acenocoumarol* enhanced by *cefamandole* and possibly others

Diuretics: *loop diuretics* may increase nephrotoxicity of cephalosporins

Cephalosporins *(continued)*
Ulcer-healing Drugs: *histamine H_2-antagonists* reduce absorption of *cefpodoxime*

Uricosurics: excretion of *cephalosporins* reduced by *probenecid* (increased plasma concentrations)
Certoparin *see* Heparin
Cetirizine *see* Antihistamines
Chloral *see* Anxiolytics and Hypnotics
Chloramphenicol
other Antibacterials: *rifampicin* accelerates metabolism (reduced chloramphenicol-plasma concentration)
* Anticoagulants: anticoagulant effect of *acenocoumarol* and *warfarin* enhanced
* Antidiabetics: effect of *sulphonylureas* enhanced
* Antiepileptics: metabolism accelerated by *phenobarbital* (reduced chloramphenicol-plasma concentration); increased plasma concentration of *phenytoin* (risk of toxicity)
* Barbiturates and Primidone: *see under* Antiepileptics, above
* Ciclosporin: plasma-ciclosporin concentration possibly increased
* Tacrolimus: plasma-tacrolimus concentration possibly increased

Chlordiazepoxide *see* Anxiolytics and Hypnotics
Chloroquine and Hydroxychloroquine
Antacids and Adsorbents: *antacids* reduce absorption of *chloroquine* and *hydroxychloroquine*; *kaolin* reduces absorption of *chloroquine*
* Anti-arrhythmics: *chloroquine* and *hydroxychloroquine* increase risk of ventricular arrhythmias with *amiodarone* (avoid concomitant use)

Antiepileptics: *chloroquine* and *hydroxychloroquine* occasionally reduce convulsive threshold
* *other* Antimalarials: increased risk of convulsions with *mefloquine*
* Cardiac Glycosides: *hydroxychloroquine* and possibly *chloroquine* increase plasma concentration of *digoxin*
* Ciclosporin: *chloroquine* increases plasma-ciclosporin concentration (increased risk of toxicity)

Parasympathomimetics: *chloroquine* and *hydroxychloroquine* have potential to increase symptoms of myasthenia gravis and thus diminish effect of *neostigmine* and *pyridostigmine*

Ulcer-healing Drugs: *cimetidine* inhibits metabolism of *chloroquine* (increased plasma concentration)

Vaccines: *see* Rabies Vaccine p. 592
Chlorphenamine (Chlorpheniramine) *see* Antihistamines
Chlorpheniramine (Chlorphenamine) *see* Antihistamines
Chlorpromazine *see* Antipsychotics
Chlorpropamide *see* Antidiabetics (sulphonylurea)
Chlortalidone *see* Diuretics (thiazide-related)
Chlortetracycline *see* Tetracyclines
Cholinergics *see* Parasympathomimetics
Ciclosporin
Note. Grapefruit juice increases plasma-ciclosporin concentration (risk of toxicity)
* ACE Inhibitors and Angiotensin-II Antagonists: increased risk of hyperkalaemia

Allopurinol: possibly increases plasma-ciclosporin concentration (risk of toxicity)
* Analgesics: increased risk of nephrotoxicity with *NSAIDs*; *ciclosporin* increases plasma concentration of *diclofenac* (halve diclofenac dose)

Anti-arrhythmics: *amiodarone* and *propafenone* possibly increase plasma-ciclosporin concentration

Ciclosporin *(continued)*
- Antibacterials: *aminoglycosides, co-trimoxazole* (and *trimethoprim* alone), and *quinolones* increase risk of nephrotoxicity; *chloramphenicol and doxycycline* possibly increase plasma-ciclosporin concentration; *erythromycin, clarithromycin* and possibly *other macrolides* increase plasma-ciclosporin concentration; *quinupristin/dalfopristin* increases plasma-ciclosporin concentration; *rifampicin, intravenous trimethoprim* (and possibly *sulfadiazine*) reduce plasma-ciclosporin concentration
- Antidepressants: manufacturer of *reboxetine* advises caution; plasma concentration reduced by *St John's wort* (avoid concomitant use)
- Antiepileptics: *carbamazepine, phenobarbital, phenytoin,* and *primidone* accelerate metabolism (reduced plasma-ciclosporin concentration)
- Antifungals: *amphotericin* increases risk of nephrotoxicity; *griseofulvin* possibly reduces plasma-ciclosporin concentration; *itraconazole, ketoconazole,* and possibly *fluconazole* and *miconazole* inhibit metabolism (increased plasma-ciclosporin concentration)
- Antimalarials: *chloroquine* increases plasma-ciclosporin concentration (risk of toxicity)
- Antiplatelet Drugs: *ticlopidine* reduces plasma-ciclosporin concentration
- Antivirals: *ritonavir* possibly increases plasma-ciclosporin concentration
- Barbiturates and Primidone: *see under* Antiepileptics, above
- Bile Acids: *ursodeoxycholic acid* increases absorption of *ciclosporin*
- Calcium-channel Blockers: *diltiazem, nicardipine,* and *verapamil* increase plasma-ciclosporin concentration; *ciclosporin* possibly increases plasma concentration of *nifedipine* (increased risk of side-effects such as gingival hyperplasia)
- Colchicine: possibly increases risk of nephrotoxicity and myotoxicity (increased plasma-ciclosporin concentration)
- Corticosteroids: *high-dose methylprednisolone* increases plasma-ciclosporin concentration (risk of convulsions); *ciclosporin* increases plasma concentration of *prednisolone*
- Cytotoxics: increased risk of neurotoxicity with *doxorubicin*; increased risk of nephrotoxicity with *melphalan*; increased toxicity with *methotrexate*; *in vitro* studies suggest possible interaction with *docetaxel*—consult product literature
- Diuretics: *potassium-sparing diuretics* increase risk of hyperkalaemia
- Hormone Antagonists: *danazol* inhibits metabolism (increased plasma-ciclosporin concentration); *lanreotide* and *octreotide* reduce absorption (reduced plasma-ciclosporin concentration)
- Lipid-regulating Drugs: increased risk of myopathy with *statins*; possible increased risk of renal impairment with *fenofibrate*
- Oestrogens and Progestogens: *progestogens* inhibit metabolism (increased plasma-ciclosporin concentration)
- Orlistat: absorption of *ciclosporin* possibly reduced
- Potassium Salts: increased risk of hyperkalaemia Sirolimus: plasma concentration of *sirolimus* possibly increased
- Tacrolimus: plasma-ciclosporin half-life prolonged (increased risk of toxicity—avoid concomitant use)
- Ulcer-healing Drugs: *cimetidine* possibly increases plasma-ciclosporin concentration

Vaccines: *see* p. 578
Cilastatin [ingredient] *see* Primaxin®
Cilazapril *see* ACE Inhibitors and Angiotensin-II Antagonists
Cimetidine *see* Histamine H$_2$-antagonists
Cinnarizine *see* Antihistamines
Ciprofibrate *see* Fibrates

Ciprofloxacin *see* Quinolones
Cisatracurium *see* Muscle Relaxants (non-depolarising)
Cisplatin *see* Platinum Compounds
Citalopram *see* Antidepressants, SSRI
Clarithromycin *see* Erythromycin and other Macrolides
Clemastine *see* Antihistamines
Clindamycin
　Muscle Relaxants: enhancement of effect of *non-depolarising muscle relaxants*
　Parasympathomimetics: antagonism of effect of *neostigmine* and *pyridostigmine*
Clobazam *see* Anxiolytics and Hypnotics
Clodronate Sodium *see* Bisphosphonates
Clomethiazole *see* Anxiolytics and Hypnotics
Clomipramine *see* Antidepressants, Tricyclic
Clonazepam (general sedative interactions *as for* Anxiolytics and Hypnotics)
Clonidine (for general hypotensive interactions *see also* Hydralazine)
　ACE Inhibitors and Angiotensin-II Antagonists: previous treatment with *clonidine* possibly delays antihypertensive effect of *captopril*
　Antibacterials: *see* Linezolid
- Antidepressants: *tricyclics* antagonise hypotensive effect and also increase risk of rebound hypertension on *clonidine* withdrawal; enhanced hypotensive effect with *MAOIs*
- Beta-blockers: increased risk of hypertension on *withdrawal* (withdraw beta-blocker several days before slowly withdrawing clonidine)
Clopamide *see* Diuretics (thiazide)
Clopidogrel
　Analgesics: increased risk of bleeding with *NSAIDs* (including *aspirin*)
- Anticoagulants: enhanced effect due to antiplatelet action of clopidogrel; manufacturer advises avoid concomitant use of *warfarin*
other Antiplatelet Drugs: increased risk of bleeding
Clorazepate *see* Anxiolytics and Hypnotics
Clotrimazole *see* Antifungals, Imidazole and Triazole
Clozapine *see* Antipsychotics
Co-amoxiclav *see* Penicillins
Co-beneldopa *see* Levodopa
Co-careldopa *see* Levodopa
Codeine *see* Opioid Analgesics
Co-fluampicil *see* Penicillins
Colchicine
- Ciclosporin: possibly increases risk of nephrotoxicity and myotoxicity (increased plasma-ciclosporin concentration)
Cold and Cough Remedies *see* Antihistamines and Sympathomimetics
Colestipol *see* Colestyramine and Colestipol
Colestyramine and Colestipol
　Note. Other drugs should be taken at least 1 hour before or 4–6 hours after colestyramine or colestipol to reduce possible interference with absorption
　Analgesics: absorption of *paracetamol* and *phenylbutazone* reduced by *colestyramine*
　Antibacterials: *colestyramine* antagonises effect of oral *vancomycin*
- Anticoagulants: anticoagulant effect of *acenocoumarol, phenindione,* and *warfarin* enhanced or reduced
　Antidiabetics: hypoglycaemic effect of *acarbose* enhanced by *colestyramine*
　Antiepileptics: absorption of *valproate* possibly reduced
　Bile Acids: absorption of *ursodeoxycholic acid* possibly reduced
　Cardiac Glycosides: possibly reduced absorption
　Diuretics: reduced absorption of *thiazides* (give at least 2 hours apart)
　Leflunomide: *colestyramine* significantly decreases effect of *leflunomide* (enhanced elimination)—avoid unless drug elimination desired
　Mycophenolate Mofetil: absorption of *mycophenolate mofetil* reduced

Colestyramine and Colestipol *(continued)*
Raloxifene: absorption reduced by *colestyramine* (manufacturer advises avoid concomitant administration)
Thyroid Hormones: reduced absorption of *levothyroxine* and *liothyronine*
Colistin (other interactions *as for* Aminoglycosides)
Muscle Relaxants: enhanced muscle relaxant effect
Contraceptives, Oral
Note. Also covers oestrogens taken alone; interactions unlikely with low dose hormone replacement therapy
ACE Inhibitors and Angiotensin-II Antagonists: *oestrogens* and *combined oral contraceptives* antagonise hypotensive effect
• Antibacterials: *rifamycins* accelerate metabolism of both *combined* and *progestogen-only oral contraceptives* (reduced effect, **important:** see p. 387); when *broad-spectrum antibacterials such as ampicillin and tetracycline* given with *combined oral contraceptives* possibility of reduced contraceptive effect (risk probably small, but see p. 388)
• Anticoagulants: antagonism of anticoagulant effect of *acenocoumarol, phenindione,* and *warfarin*
• Antidepressants: contraceptive effect reduced by *St John's wort* (avoid concomitant use); antagonism of antidepressant effect has been reported, but side-effects of *tricyclics* may be increased due to higher plasma concentrations
Antidiabetics: antagonism of hypoglycaemic effect
• Antiepileptics: *carbamazepine, oxcarbazepine, phenobarbital, phenytoin, primidone* and *topiramate* accelerate metabolism (reduced effect of both combined and progestogen-only contraceptives, **important:** see p. 387)
• Antifungals: *griseofulvin* accelerates metabolism (reduced contraceptive effect, **important:** see p. 387); anecdotal reports of contraceptive failure with *fluconazole, itraconazole, ketoconazole* and possibly others; occasional reports of breakthrough bleeding with *terbinafine*
Antihypertensives: *combined oral contraceptives* antagonise hypotensive effect
• Antivirals: *nelfinavir, nevirapine* and *ritonavir* accelerate metabolism of *combined oral contraceptives* (reduced contraceptive effect); *amprenavir* and *efavirenz* possibly reduce efficacy of *oral contraceptives*
• Barbiturates and Primidone: *see under* Antiepileptics, above
Beta-blockers: *oestrogens* and *combined oral contraceptives* antagonise hypotensive effect
Bile Acids: *oestrogens* increase elimination of cholesterol in bile
• Ciclosporin: increased plasma-ciclosporin concentration
Corticosteroids: *oral contraceptives* increase plasma concentration of *corticosteroids*
Diuretics: *combined oral contraceptives* antagonise diuretic effect
Dopaminergics: plasma concentration of *ropinirole* increased by *oestrogens*
• Modafinil: accelerates metabolism of *oral contraceptives* (reduced contraceptive effect)
Somatropin: higher doses of *somatropin* may be needed with oral *oestrogen* replacement therapy
Tacrolimus: efficacy of *oral contraceptives* possibly decreased
Theophylline: *combined oral contraceptives* delay excretion (increased plasma-theophylline concentration)
• Tretinoin: oral *tretinoin* reduces contraceptive efficacy of low-dose *progestogens*
Ulcer-healing drugs: manufacturer advises *lansoprazole* possibly accelerates metabolism

Corticosteroids
Note. Do not generally apply to corticosteroids used for topical action (including inhalation)
Analgesics: increased risk of gastro-intestinal bleeding and ulceration with *aspirin* and *NSAIDs;* corticosteroids reduce plasma-*salicylate* concentration
Antacids: reduce absorption of *deflazacort*
• Antibacterials: *rifamycins* accelerate metabolism of *corticosteroids* (reduced effect); *erythromycin* inhibits metabolism of *methylprednisolone* and possibly *other corticosteroids*
• Anticoagulants: anticoagulant effect of *acenocoumarol* and *warfarin* possibly altered
Antidiabetics: antagonism of hypoglycaemic effect
• Antiepileptics: *carbamazepine, phenobarbital, phenytoin, and primidone* accelerate metabolism of *corticosteroids* (reduced effect)
• Antifungals: increased risk of hypokalaemia with *amphotericin* (avoid concomitant use unless corticosteroids required to control reactions); *ketoconazole* inhibits metabolism of *methylprednisolone* and possibly *other corticosteroids*; *itraconazole* possibly inhibits metabolism of *methylprednisolone*
Antihypertensives: antagonism of hypotensive effect
Antivirals: plasma concentration of *indinavir, lopinavir* and *saquinavir* possibly reduced by *dexamethasone*; *ritonavir* possibly increases plasma concentration of *dexamethasone, prednisolone* and possibly *other corticosteroids*
• Barbiturates and Primidone: *see under* Antiepileptics, above
Cardiac Glycosides: increased toxicity if hypokalaemia occurs with *corticosteroids*
• Ciclosporin: plasma-ciclosporin concentration increased by high-dose *methylprednisolone* (risk of convulsions); *ciclosporin* increases plasma concentration of *prednisolone*
Cytotoxics: increased risk of haematological toxicity with *methotrexate*
Diuretics: antagonism of diuretic effect; *acetazolamide, loop diuretics, and thiazides* increase risk of hypokalaemia
Hormone Antagonists: *aminoglutethimide* accelerates metabolism of *corticosteroids* (reduced effect)
Mifepristone: effect of *corticosteroids* (including inhaled corticosteroids) may be reduced for 3–4 days after *mifepristone*
Oestrogens and Progestogens: *oral contraceptives* increase plasma concentration of *corticosteroids*
Somatropin: growth promoting effect may be inhibited
Sympathomimetics: increased risk of hypokalaemia if high doses of *corticosteroids* given with high doses of *bambuterol, fenoterol, formoterol, ritodrine, salbutamol, salmeterol,* and *terbutaline;* see also CSM advice (hypokalaemia), p. 134; *ephedrine* accelerates metabolism of *dexamethasone*
Theophylline: increased risk of hypokalaemia
Ulcer-healing Drugs: *carbenoxolone* increases risk of hypokalaemia
Vaccines: see p. 578
Co-trimoxazole and Sulphonamides
Note. For interactions with co-trimoxazole see also under Trimethoprim
Anaesthetics: effect of *thiopental* enhanced; increased risk of methaemoglobinaemia with *prilocaine*
• Anti-arrhythmics: *co-trimoxazole* increases risk of ventricular arrhythmias with *amiodarone* (avoid concomitant use)
• Anticoagulants: effect of *acenocoumarol* and *warfarin* enhanced
Antidiabetics: effect of *sulphonylureas* rarely enhanced
• Antiepileptics: antifolate effect and plasma concentration of *phenytoin* increased by *co-trimoxazole* and possibly *other sulphonamides*

Co-trimoxazole and Sulphonamides *(continued)*
* Antimalarials: increased risk of antifolate effect with *pyrimethamine* (includes *Fansidar®* and *Maloprim®*)
* Ciclosporin: increased risk of nephrotoxicity; plasma-ciclosporin concentration possibly reduced by *sulfadiazine*
* <u>Cytotoxics</u>: increased risk of haematological toxicity with *azathioprine* and *mercaptopurine*; antifolate effect of *methotrexate* increased by *co-trimoxazole* (avoid concomitant use); risk of *methotrexate* toxicity increased by *sulphonamides*

  Potassium Aminobenzoate: inhibits effect of *sulphonamides*

Cyclizine *see* Antihistamines
Cyclobarbitone *see* Barbiturates
Cyclopenthiazide *see* Diuretics (thiazide)
Cyclopentolate *see* Antimuscarinics
Cyclophosphamide and Ifosfamide
* Anticoagulants: *ifosfamide* possibly enhances effect of *warfarin*
* *other* Cytotoxics: increased toxicity with high-dose cyclophosphamide and *pentostatin* (avoid concomitant use)

  Muscle Relaxants: *cyclophosphamide* enhances effect of *suxamethonium*

Cycloserine
* Alcohol: increased risk of seizures

  other Antibacterials: increased CNS toxicity with *isoniazid*
* Antiepileptics: increased plasma concentration of *phenytoin* (risk of toxicity)

Cyproheptadine *see* Antihistamines
Cytarabine

  Flucytosine: plasma-flucytosine concentration possibly reduced

Cytotoxics *see under* individual drugs
Dalteparin *see* Heparin
Danazol
* Anticoagulants: effect of *acenocoumarol* and *warfarin* enhanced (inhibits metabolism)
* Antiepileptics: inhibits metabolism of *carbamazepine* (increased plasma-carbamazepine concentration)
* Ciclosporin: inhibits metabolism (increased plasma-ciclosporin concentration)

  Tacrolimus: plasma-tacrolimus concentration possibly increased

Dantrolene *see* Muscle Relaxants
Dapsone

  Antibacterials: plasma concentration reduced by *rifamycins*; plasma concentration of both trimethoprim and dapsone possibly increased with concomitant use

  Antivirals: *amprenavir* possibly increases plasma concentration of *dapsone*

  Probenecid: *dapsone* excretion reduced (increased risk of side-effects)

Darbepoetin *see* Epoetin
Debrisoquine *see* Adrenergic Neurone Blockers
Deflazacort *see* Corticosteroids
Demeclocycline *see* Tetracyclines
Desferrioxamine

  Antipsychotics: manufacturer advises avoid *prochlorperazine* (also *levomepromazine* on theoretical grounds)

Desflurane *see* Anaesthetics, General (volatile liquid)
Desmopressin

  Analgesics: effect of *desmopressin* potentiated by *indometacin*

Desogestrel *see* Progestogens
Dexamethasone *see* Corticosteroids
Dexamfetamine *see* Sympathomimetics
Dexketoprofen *see* NSAIDs
Dextromoramide *see* Opioid Analgesics
Dextropropoxyphene *see* Opioid Analgesics
Diamorphine *see* Opioid Analgesics
Diazepam *see* Anxiolytics and Hypnotics

Diazoxide (general hypotensive interactions *as for* Hydralazine)

  Antidiabetics: antagonism of hypoglycaemic effect
Diclofenac *see* NSAIDs
Dicyclomine (Dicycloverine) *see* Antimuscarinics
Dicycloverine (Dicyclomine) *see* Antimuscarinics
Didanosine

  Note. Antacids in **tablet** formulation affect absorption of other drugs, *see also* Antacids, p. 622

  other Antivirals: plasma-didanosine concentration possibly increased by *ganciclovir*

Diflunisal *see* NSAIDs
Digitoxin *see* Cardiac Glycosides
Digoxin *see* Cardiac Glycosides
Dihydrocodeine *see* Opioid Analgesics
Diltiazem *see* Calcium-channel Blockers
Diphenhydramine *see* Antihistamines
Diphenylpyraline *see* Antihistamines
Diphenoxylate *see* Opioid Analgesics
Dipipanone *see* Opioid Analgesics
Dipivefrine *see* Sympathomimetics (*as for* adrenaline)
Dipyridamole

  Antacids: patient information leaflet advises avoidance of *antacids*
* Anti-arrhythmics: effect of *adenosine* enhanced and extended (**important** risk of toxicity)
* Anticoagulants: enhanced effect due to antiplatelet action of *dipyridamole*

  other Antiplatelet Drugs: increased risk of bleeding with *clopidogrel* and *ticlopidine*

  Cytotoxics: efficacy of *fludarabine* possibly reduced

Disodium Etidronate *see* Bisphosphonates
Disodium Pamidronate *see* Bisphosphonates
Disopyramide
* *other* Anti-arrhythmics: *amiodarone* increases risk of ventricular arrhythmias (avoid concomitant use); increased myocardial depression with any *anti-arrhythmic*
* Antibacterials: plasma concentration of *disopyramide* reduced by *rifampicin* but increased by *erythromycin* and possibly *clarithromycin* (risk of toxicity); increased risk of arrhythmias with *quinupristin/dalfopristin* (avoid concomitant use)
* Antidepressants: increased risk of ventricular arrhythmias with *tricyclics*; manufacturer of *reboxetine* advises caution

  Antiepileptics: plasma concentration of *disopyramide* reduced by *phenobarbital, phenytoin, and primidone*
* Antihistamines: increased risk of ventricular arrhythmias with *mizolastine* and *terfenadine* (avoid concomitant use)
* Antimuscarinics: increased antimuscarinic side-effects
* Antipsychotics: increased risk of ventricular arrhythmias—avoid concomitant use with *pimozide* or *thioridazine*
* Antivirals: possibly increased risk of arrhythmias with *ritonavir*

  Barbiturates and Primidone: *see under* Antiepileptics, above
* Beta-blockers: increased myocardial depression; increased risk of ventricular arrhythmias associated with *sotalol* (avoid concomitant use)
* Calcium-channel blockers: increased myocardial depression with *verapamil*
* Diuretics: cardiac toxicity of *disopyramide* increased if hypokalaemia occurs with *acetazolamide, loop diuretics, and thiazides*

  Nitrates: reduced effect of *sublingual nitrates* (failure to dissolve under tongue owing to dry mouth)

  Tropisetron: risk of arrhythmias—manufacturer of tropisetron advises caution

Distigmine *see* Parasympathomimetics

Disulfiram

Alcohol: disulfiram reaction (*see* section 4.10)

Antibacterials: psychotic reaction with *metronidazole* reported

- Anticoagulants: effect of *acenocoumarol* and *warfarin* enhanced

Antidepressants: inhibition of metabolism of *tricyclic antidepressants* (increased plasma concentrations); increased disulfiram reaction with *alcohol* reported if *amitriptyline* also taken

- Antiepileptics: inhibition of metabolism of *phenytoin* (increased risk of toxicity)

Anxiolytics and Hypnotics: inhibition of metabolism of *benzodiazepines*, with enhanced sedative effect (*temazepam* toxicity reported)

- Paraldehyde: increased risk of toxicity with *paraldehyde*

Theophylline: inhibition of metabolism (increased risk of toxicity)

Diuretics

- ACE Inhibitors and Angiotensin-II Antagonists: enhanced hypotensive effect (can be extreme); risk of severe hyperkalaemia with *potassium-sparing diuretics*

Alprostadil: enhanced hypotensive effect

- Analgesics: *diuretics* increase risk of nephrotoxicity of *NSAIDs*; *NSAIDs* notably *indometacin* and *ketorolac* antagonise diuretic effect; *indometacin* and *possibly other NSAIDs* increase risk of hyperkalaemia with *potassium-sparing diuretics*; occasional reports of decreased renal function when *indometacin* given with *triamterene* (avoid concomitant use); diuretic effect of *spironolactone* antagonised by *aspirin*; *aspirin* reduces excretion of *acetazolamide* (risk of toxicity)

Anion-exchange Resins: *colestyramine and colestipol* reduce absorption of *thiazides* (give at least 2 hours apart)

- Anti-arrhythmics: cardiac toxicity of *amiodarone, disopyramide, flecainide, and quinidine* increased if hypokalaemia occurs; action of *lidocaine* and *mexiletine* antagonised by hypokalaemia; *acetazolamide* reduces excretion of *quinidine* (increased plasma concentration)

- Antibacterials: *loop diuretics* increase ototoxicity of *aminoglycosides, colistin,* and *vancomycin; loop diuretics* may increase nephrotoxicity of *cephalosporins; see also* Linezolid

Antidepressants: increased risk of postural hypotension with *tricyclics*; possibly increased risk of hypokalaemia if *loop diuretics* or *thiazides* given with *reboxetine*; enhanced hypotensive effect with *MAOIs*

Antidiabetics: hypoglycaemic effect antagonised by *loop and thiazide diuretics*; *chlorpropamide* increases risk of hyponatraemia associated with *thiazides* in combination with *potassium-sparing diuretics*

- Antiepileptics: increased risk of hyponatraemia with *carbamazepine*; *acetazolamide* increases plasma concentration of *carbamazepine*; *carbonic anhydrase inhibitors* possibly increase risk of osteomalacia with *antiepileptics* such as *phenytoin*

Antifungals: increased risk of hypokalaemia if *loop diuretics* and *thiazides* given with *amphotericin*; *hydrochlorothiazide* increases plasma concentration of *fluconazole*

- Antihistamines: hypokalaemia or other electrolyte imbalance increases risk of ventricular arrhythmias with *terfenadine*

- Antihypertensives: enhanced hypotensive effect; increased risk of first-dose hypotensive effect of post-synaptic *alpha-blockers* such as *prazosin*

- Antipsychotics: hypokalaemia increases risk of ventricular arrhythmias with *pimozide* or *thioridazine* (avoid concomitant use)

Diuretics (continued)

Anxiolytics and Hypnotics: concomitant administration of *chloral hydrate* or *triclofos* and parenteral *furosemide* may displace thyroid hormone from binding sites

Beta-blockers: enhanced hypotensive effect; in hypokalaemia increased risk of ventricular arrhythmias with *sotalol*

Calcium Salts: increased risk of hypercalcaemia with *thiazides*

Calcium-channel Blockers: enhanced hypotensive effect

- Cardiac Glycosides: increased toxicity if hypokalaemia occurs with *acetazolamide, loop diuretics, and thiazides;* effect enhanced by *spironolactone*

- Ciclosporin: increased risk of hyperkalaemia with *potassium-sparing diuretics*

Corticosteroids: increased risk of hypokalaemia with *acetazolamide, loop diuretics, and thiazides;* antagonism of diuretic effect

Cytotoxics: increased risk of nephrotoxicity and ototoxicity with *cisplatin*

other Diuretics: increased risk of hypokalaemia if *acetazolamide, loop diuretics or thiazides* given together; profound diuresis possible if *metolazone* given with *furosemide*

Hormone Antagonists: increased risk of hyponatraemia with *aminoglutethimide*; *thiazides* increase risk of hypercalcaemia with *toremifene*; *trilostane* increases risk of hyperkalaemia with *potassium-sparing diuretics*

- Lithium: *lithium* excretion reduced by *loop diuretics, potassium-sparing diuretics and thiazides* (increased plasma-lithium concentration and risk of toxicity—*loop diuretics* safer than *thiazides*); *lithium* excretion increased by *acetazolamide*

Moxisylyte: enhanced hypotensive effect

Muscle Relaxants: enhanced hypotensive effect with *baclofen* and *tizanidine*

Oestrogens and Progestogens: *oestrogens and combined oral contraceptives* antagonise diuretic effect

- Potassium Salts: hyperkalaemia with *potassium-sparing diuretics*

Sympathomimetics: increased risk of hypokalaemia if *acetazolamide, loop diuretics,* and *thiazides* given with high doses of *bambuterol, fenoterol, formoterol, ritodrine, salbutamol, salmeterol,* and *terbutaline*; see also CSM advice (hypokalaemia), p. 134

- Tacrolimus: increased risk of hyperkalaemia with *potassium-sparing diuretics*

Theophylline: increased risk of hypokalaemia with *acetazolamide, loop diuretics and thiazides*

Ulcer-healing Drugs: increased risk of hypokalaemia if *acetazolamide, loop diuretics,* and *thiazides* given with *carbenoxolone*; *carbenoxolone* antagonises diuretic effect; *amiloride and spironolactone* antagonise ulcer-healing effect of *carbenoxolone*

Vitamins: increased risk of hypercalcaemia if *thiazides* given with *vitamin D*

Dobutamine *see* Sympathomimetics

Docetaxel

Antibacterials: *in-vitro* studies suggest possible interaction with *erythromycin*—consult product literature

Antifungals: *in-vitro* studies suggest possible interaction with *ketoconazole*—consult product literature

Antihistamines: *in-vitro* studies suggest possible interaction with *terfenadine*—consult product literature

Ciclosporin: *in-vitro* studies suggest possible interaction with *ciclosporin*—consult product literature

Domperidone

Analgesics: *opioid analgesics* antagonise effect on gastro-intestinal activity; absorption of *paracetamol* accelerated (enhanced effect)

Antimuscarinics: antagonism of effect on gastro-intestinal activity

Dopaminergics: possible antagonism of hypoprolactinaemic effect of *bromocriptine* and *cabergoline*

Donepezil *see* Parasympathomimetics

Dopamine *see* Sympathomimetics

Dopaminergics *see* Amantadine, Apomorphine, Bromocriptine and Cabergoline, Entacapone, Levodopa, Lisuride, Pramipexole, Quinagolide, Ropinirole

Dopexamine *see* Sympathomimetics

Dorzolamide *see* Diuretics (carbonic anhydrase inhibitor)

Note. Since systemic absorption may follow topical application of dorzolamide to the eye, the possibility of interactions should be borne in mind

Dosulepin (Dothiepin) *see* Antidepressants, Tricyclic

Dothiepin (Dosulepin) *see* Antidepressants, Tricyclic

Doxapram

Antidepressants: *MAOIs* may potentiate *doxapram*

Sympathomimetics: risk of hypertension

Theophylline: increased CNS stimulation

Doxazosin *see* Alpha-blockers (post-synaptic)

Doxepin *see* Antidepressants, Tricyclic

Doxorubicin

Antivirals: may inhibit effect of *stavudine*

• Ciclosporin: increased risk of neurotoxicity

Doxycycline *see* Tetracyclines

Doxylamine *see* Antihistamines

Dydrogesterone *see* Progestogens

Ecothiopate *see* Parasympathomimetics

Edrophonium *see* Parasympathomimetics

Efavirenz

Note. Grapefruit juice may affect plasma-efavirenz concentration

Antibacterials: increased risk of rash with *clarithromycin; rifampicin* reduces plasma concentration of *efavirenz* (increase efavirenz dose)

• Antidepressants: plasma concentration reduced by *St John's wort* (avoid concomitant use)

• Antihistamines: increased risk of ventricular arrhythmias with *terfenadine* (avoid concomitant use)

other Antivirals: *efavirenz* reduces plasma concentration of *amprenavir, indinavir* (increase indinavir dose), and *lopinavir*; increased risk of toxicity with *efavirenz* and *ritonavir* (monitor liver function tests); *efavirenz* significantly reduces plasma concentration of *saquinavir*

• Anxiolytics and Hypnotics: risk of prolonged sedation with *midazolam* (avoid concomitant use)

Oestrogens and Progestogens: possibly reduced efficacy of *oral contraceptives*

Eformoterol (Formoterol) *see* Sympathomimetics, Beta$_2$

Enalapril *see* ACE Inhibitors and Angiotensin-II Antagonists

Enflurane *see* Anaesthetics, General (volatile liquid)

Enoxaparin *see* Heparin

Entacapone

Antibacterials: *see* Linezolid

Antidepressants: manufacturer advises avoid concomitant use with *MAOIs, tricyclics, maprotiline* or *venlafaxine*

Antihypertensives: effect of *methyldopa* possibly enhanced

other Dopaminergics: effect of *apomorphine* possibly enhanced

Iron: absorption of entacapone reduced

Sympathomimetics: effect of *adrenaline, dobutamine, dopamine, isoprenaline* and *noradrenaline* possibly enhanced

Ephedrine *see* Sympathomimetics

Epinephrine (Adrenaline) *see* Sympathomimetics

Epoetin

ACE Inhibitors and Angiotensin-II Antagonists: antagonism of hypotensive effect; increased risk of hyperkalaemia

Eprosartan

• *see* ACE Inhibitors and Angiotensin-II Antagonists

Ergometrine *see* Ergotamine and Ergometrine

Ergotamine and Ergometrine

Anaesthetics: *halothane* reduces effect of *ergometrine* on the parturient uterus

• Antibacterials: increased risk of ergotism with *azithromycin, clarithromycin* and *erythromycin*— avoid concomitant use; increased risk of ergotism with *tetracyclines*

Antidepressants: possibly increased blood pressure with *reboxetine*

• Antivirals: increased risk of ergotism with *amprenavir, indinavir, nelfinavir, ritonavir* and possibly *saquinavir*—avoid concomitant use

Beta-blockers: increased peripheral vasoconstriction

• 5HT$_1$ Agonists: increased risk of vasospasm (avoid ergotamine for 6 hours after almotriptan, rizatriptan, sumatriptan or zolmitriptan; avoid almotriptan, rizatriptan or sumatriptan for 24 hours and zolmitriptan for 6 hours after ergotamine)

Sympathomimetics: increased risk of ergotism

Erythromycin and other Macrolides

Note. Interactions do not apply to small amounts used topically

• Analgesics: plasma concentration of *alfentanil* increased by *erythromycin*

Antacids: *antacids* reduce absorption of *azithromycin*

• Anti-arrhythmics: plasma concentration of *disopyramide* increased by *erythromycin*

• *other* Antibacterials: *clarithromycin* and possibly *other macrolides* increase plasma concentration of *rifabutin* (risk of uveitis—reduce rifabutin dose)

• Anticoagulants: effect of *acenocoumarol* and *warfarin* enhanced by *erythromycin* and possibly enhanced by *clarithromycin* and some *other macrolides*

• Antidepressants: manufacturer of *reboxetine* advises avoid concomitant use

• Antiepileptics: *clarithromycin* and *erythromycin* inhibit metabolism of *carbamazepine* (increased plasma-carbamazepine concentration); *erythromycin* possibly inhibits metabolism of *valproate* (increased plasma-valproate concentration); *clarithromycin* inhibits metabolism of *phenytoin* (increased plasma-phenytoin concentration)

Antifungals: plasma concentration of *itraconazole* increased by *clarithromycin*

• Antihistamines: *clarithromycin* and *erythromycin* inhibit metabolism of *terfenadine* (avoid concomitant use of systemic or topical preparations—risk of hazardous arrhythmias, see p. 153); manufacturer advises possibility of increased plasma-loratadine concentration with *erythromycin;* metabolism of *mizolastine* inhibited by *erythromycin* and possibly *other macrolides* (avoid concomitant use)

• Antimuscarinics: manufacturer of *tolterodine* advises avoid concomitant use with *clarithromycin* or *erythromycin*

• Antipsychotics: risk of arrhythmias if *clarithromycin* and possibly *erythromycin* given with *pimozide* (avoid concomitant use); *erythromycin* possibly increases plasma concentration of *clozapine* (possible increased risk of convulsions)

• Antivirals: *clarithromycin* tablets reduce absorption of *zidovudine; ritonavir* increases plasma concentration of *clarithromycin* and possibly *other macrolides* (reduce clarithromycin dose in those with renal impairment); increased risk of rash when *efavirenz* given with *clarithromycin*; concomitant administration of *amprenavir* and *erythromycin* may increase plasma concentration of both drugs

Erythromycin and other Macrolides *(continued)*
* Anxiolytics and Hypnotics: *clarithromycin* and *erythromycin* inhibit metabolism of *midazolam* (increased plasma-midazolam concentration, with profound sedation); *erythromycin* inhibits metabolism of *zopiclone*

  Calcium-channel Blockers: *erythromycin* possibly inhibits metabolism of *felodipine* (increased plasma concentration)

  Cardiac Glycosides: effect of *digoxin* enhanced by *erythromycin* and possibly enhanced by *other macrolides*
* Ciclosporin: *erythromycin, clarithromycin* and possibly *other macrolides* inhibit metabolism (increased plasma-ciclosporin concentration)

  Corticosteroids: *erythromycin* inhibits metabolism of *methylprednisolone* and possibly *other corticosteroids*

  Cytotoxics: *in vitro* studies suggest possible interaction between *erythromycin* and *docetaxel*—consult product literature

  Dopaminergics: plasma concentration of *bromocriptine* and *cabergoline* increased by *erythromycin* and possibly *other macrolides*
* Ergotamine and Ergometrine: increased risk of ergotism—avoid concomitant use

  Leukotriene Antagonists: *erythromycin* reduces plasma concentration of *zafirlukast*
* Lipid-regulating Drugs: *clarithromycin* and *erythromycin* increase risk of myopathy with *simvastatin* (avoid concomitant use); *erythromycin* possibly increases risk of myopathy with *atorvastatin*; *clarithromycin* increases plasma concentration of *atorvastatin*

  Sildenafil: *erythromycin* increases plasma-sildenafil concentration (reduce initial dose of sildenafil)
* Tacrolimus: *clarithromycin* and *erythromycin* increase plasma-tacrolimus concentration
* Theophylline: *clarithromycin* and *erythromycin* inhibit metabolism (increased plasma-theophylline concentration) (if erythromycin given by mouth, also decreased plasma-erythromycin concentration)

  Ulcer-healing Drugs: *cimetidine* increases plasma-erythromycin concentration (increased risk of toxicity, including deafness)

Erythropoietin *see* Epoetin
Esmolol *see* Beta-blockers
Estropipate *see* Contraceptives, Oral
Ethinylestradiol *see* Contraceptives, Oral
Ethosuximide
* Antibacterials: *isoniazid* increases plasma concentrations (increased risk of toxicity); *see also* Linezolid
* Antidepressants: antagonism (convulsive threshold lowered)

  other Antiepileptics: interactions include enhanced effects, increased sedation, and reductions in plasma concentrations; for further details, see p. 227
* Antimalarials: *mefloquine* antagonises anticonvulsant effect; *chloroquine* and *hydroxychloroquine* occasionally reduce convulsive threshold
* Antipsychotics: antagonism (convulsive threshold lowered)

Etidronate Disodium *see* Bisphosphonates
Etodolac *see* NSAIDs
Etomidate *see* Anaesthetics, General
Etonogestrel *see* Progestogens
Etynodiol *see* Progestogens
Famciclovir *see* Aciclovir and Famciclovir
Famotidine *see* Histamine H_2-antagonists
Fansidar® contains Sulfadoxine and Pyrimethamine
Felodipine *see* Calcium-channel Blockers
Fenbufen *see* NSAIDs
Fenofibrate *see* Fibrates
Fenoprofen *see* NSAIDs

Fenoterol *see* Sympathomimetics, Beta₂
Fentanyl *see* Opioid Analgesics
Ferrous Salts *see* Iron
Fexofenadine *see* Antihistamines
Fibrates
* Anticoagulants: enhancement of effect of *acenocoumarol, phenindione,* and *warfarin*

  Antidiabetics: may improve glucose tolerance and have additive effect
* Ciclosporin: possible increased risk of renal impairment with *fenofibrate*
* *other* Lipid-regulating Drugs: increased risk of myopathy with *statins* (preferably avoid concomitant use of *gemfibrozil* with *statins*)

Filgrastim
  Note. Use not recommended in period from 24 hours before to 24 hours after chemotherapy—for further details consult product literature

  Cytotoxics: possible exacerbation of neutropenia with *fluorouracil*

Finasteride
  Note. No clinically important interactions reported

Flavoxate *see* Antimuscarinics
Flecainide
* *other* Anti-arrhythmics: *amiodarone* increases plasma-flecainide concentration (and increases risk of ventricular arrhythmias—avoid concomitant use); increased myocardial depression with any *anti-arrhythmic*
* Antidepressants: *fluoxetine* increases plasma-flecainide concentration; increased risk of arrhythmias with *tricyclics*; manufacturer of *reboxetine* advises caution
* Antihistamines: increased risk of ventricular arrhythmias with *mizolastine* and *terfenadine* (avoid concomitant use)
* Antimalarials: *quinine* increases plasma concentration of *flecainide*
* Antivirals: plasma concentration increased by *ritonavir* (increased risk of ventricular arrhythmias—avoid concomitant use)
* Beta-blockers: increased myocardial depression and bradycardia
* Calcium-channel Blockers: increased myocardial depression and asystole with *verapamil*
* Diuretics: cardiac toxicity increased if hypokalaemia occurs

  Ulcer-healing Drugs: *cimetidine* inhibits metabolism of *flecainide* (increased plasma-flecainide concentration)

Flucloxacillin *see* Penicillins
Fluconazole *see* Antifungals, Imidazole and Triazole
Flucytosine
  other Antifungals: renal excretion reduced and cellular uptake increased by *amphotericin* (flucytosine toxicity possibly increased)

  Cytotoxics: *cytarabine* possibly reduces plasma-flucytosine concentrations

Fludarabine
  Antiplatelet Drugs: efficacy possibly reduced by *dipyridamole*
* *other* Cytotoxics: increased pulmonary toxicity with *pentostatin* (unacceptably high incidence of fatalities)

Fludrocortisone *see* Corticosteroids
Flunisolide *see* Corticosteroids
Flunitrazepam *see* Anxiolytics and Hypnotics
Fluorouracil
  Allopurinol: manufacturer of *capecitabine* advises avoid concomitant use

  Antibacterials: *metronidazole* inhibits metabolism (increased toxicity)
* Anticoagulants: *fluorouracil* possibly enhances anticoagulant effect of *warfarin* and *other coumarins*

  Filgrastim: possible exacerbation of neutropenia

  Ulcer-healing Drugs: *cimetidine* inhibits metabolism (increased plasma-fluorouracil concentration)

Fluoxetine *see* Antidepressants, SSRI
Flupentixol *see* Antipsychotics
Fluphenazine *see* Antipsychotics
Flurazepam *see* Anxiolytics and Hypnotics
Flurbiprofen *see* NSAIDs
Flutamide
* Anticoagulants: effect of *warfarin* enhanced
Fluticasone *see* Corticosteroids
Fluvastatin *see* Statins
Fluvoxamine *see* Antidepressants, SSRI
Folic Acid and Folinic Acid
   Antiepileptics: plasma concentrations of *phenobarbital, phenytoin* and *primidone* possibly reduced
Formoterol (Eformoterol) *see* Sympathomimetics, Beta$_2$
Fosinopril *see* ACE Inhibitors
Fosphenytoin *see* Phenytoin
Framycetin *see* Aminoglycosides
Frusemide (Furosemide) *see* Diuretics (loop)
Furosemide (Frusemide) *see* Diuretics (loop)
Gabapentin
   Antacids: reduced *gabapentin* absorption
   Antibacterials: *see* Linezolid
* Antidepressants: antagonism of anticonvulsive effect (convulsive threshold lowered)
   other Antiepileptics: none demonstrated with *carbamazepine, phenobarbital, phenytoin,* or *valproate*
* Antimalarials: *mefloquine* antagonises anticonvulsant effect; *chloroquine* and *hydroxychloroquine* occasionally reduces convulsive threshold
Galantamine *see* Parasympathomimetics
Gallamine *see* Muscle Relaxants (non-depolarising)
Ganciclovir
   Note: Increased risk of myelosuppression with other myelosuppressive drugs—consult product literature
* Antibacterials: increased toxicity with *Primaxin*® (convulsions reported)
* *other* Antivirals: plasma concentration of *didanosine* possibly increased; profound myelosuppression with *zidovudine* (if possible avoid concomitant administration particularly during initial ganciclovir therapy)
   Mycophenolate mofetil: possibly increased plasma concentrations of *ganciclovir* and of *mycophenolate mofetil* on concomitant administration
   Uricosurics: *probenecid* reduces renal excretion (increased plasma half-life)
Gemfibrozil *see* Fibrates
Gentamicin *see* Aminoglycosides
Gestodene *see* Progestogens
Gestonorone *see* Progestogens
Gestrinone
   Antibacterials: *rifampicin* accelerates metabolism (reduced plasma concentration)
   Antiepileptics: *carbamazepine, phenobarbital, phenytoin,* and *primidone* accelerate metabolism (reduced plasma concentration)
   Barbiturates and Primidone: *see under* Antiepileptics, above
Glibenclamide *see* Antidiabetics (sulphonylurea)
Gliclazide *see* Antidiabetics (sulphonylurea)
Glimepiride *see* Antidiabetics (sulphonylurea)
Glipizide *see* Antidiabetics (sulphonylurea)
Gliquidone *see* Antidiabetics (sulphonylurea)
Glyceryl Trinitrate *see* Nitrates
Gold
   Note. Increased risk of toxicity with other nephrotoxic and myelosuppressive drugs
Griseofulvin
* Anticoagulants: metabolism of *acenocoumarol* and *warfarin* accelerated (reduced anticoagulant effect)
   Antiepileptics: absorption reduced by *phenobarbital* (reduced effect)
   Barbiturates and Primidone: *see under* Antiepileptics, above

Griseofulvin *(continued)*
   Ciclosporin: plasma-ciclosporin concentration possibly reduced
* Oestrogens and Progestogens: metabolism of *oral contraceptives* accelerated (reduced contraceptive effect, **important**: see p. 387)
Guanethidine *see* Adrenergic Neurone Blockers
Guar Gum
   Antibacterials: absorption of *phenoxymethylpenicillin* reduced
Haloperidol *see* Antipsychotics
Halothane *see* Anaesthetics, General (volatile liquid)
Heparin
   ACE Inhibitors and Angiotensin-II Antagonists: increased risk of hyperkalaemia
* Analgesics: *aspirin* enhances anticoagulant effect; increased risk of haemorrhage with *intravenous diclofenac* and with *ketorolac* (avoid concomitant use, including low-dose heparin); possibly increased risk of bleeding with NSAIDs
   Antiplatelet Drugs: *aspirin, clopidogrel, dipyridamole* and *ticlopidine* enhance anticoagulant effect
* Nitrates: *glyceryl trinitrate infusion* increases excretion (reduced anticoagulant effect)
Histamine H$_1$-antagonists *see* Antihistamines
Histamine H$_2$-antagonists
   Analgesics: *cimetidine* inhibits metabolism of *opioid analgesics notably pethidine* (increased plasma concentrations); *cimetidine* possibly increases plasma concentration of *azapropazone; cimetidine* increases plasma concentration of *lornoxicam*
   Anthelmintics: *cimetidine* possibly inhibits metabolism of *mebendazole* (increased plasma concentration)
* Anti-arrhythmics: *cimetidine* increases plasma concentrations of *amiodarone, flecainide, lidocaine, procainamide, propafenone* and *quinidine*
   Antibacterials: absorption of *cefpodoxime* reduced; *cimetidine* increases plasma-erythromycin concentration (increased risk of toxicity, including deafness); *rifampicin* accelerates metabolism of *cimetidine* (reduced plasma-cimetidine concentration); *cimetidine* inhibits metabolism of *metronidazole* (increased plasma-metronidazole concentration)
* Anticoagulants: *cimetidine* enhances anticoagulant effect of *acenocoumarol* and *warfarin* (inhibits metabolism)
   Antidepressants: *cimetidine* inhibits metabolism of *amitriptyline, doxepin, imipramine, moclobemide, nortriptyline,* and *sertraline* (increased plasma concentrations)
   Antidiabetics: *cimetidine* inhibits renal excretion of *metformin* (increased plasma concentration); *cimetidine* enhances hypoglycaemic effect of *sulphonylureas*
* Antiepileptics: *cimetidine* inhibits metabolism of *carbamazepine, phenytoin, and valproate* (increased plasma concentrations)
   Antifungals: absorption of *itraconazole and ketoconazole* reduced; plasma concentration of *terbinafine* increased by *cimetidine*
   Antihistamines: manufacturer advises possibility of increased plasma-loratadine concentration with *cimetidine*
   Antimalarials: *cimetidine* inhibits metabolism of *chloroquine* and *quinine* (increased plasma concentrations)
   Antipsychotics: *cimetidine* possibly enhances effect of *chlorpromazine, clozapine, and possibly other antipsychotics*
   Antivirals: plasma concentration of *zalcitabine* possibly increased by *cimetidine*; plasma concentration of *saquinavir* increased by *ranitidine*; *amprenavir* possibly increases plasma concentration of *cimetidine*

Histamine H₂-antagonists *(continued)*
Anxiolytics and Hypnotics: *cimetidine* inhibits metabolism of *benzodiazepines, clomethiazole* and *zaleplon* (increased plasma concentrations)
Beta-blockers: *cimetidine* inhibits metabolism of *beta-blockers* such as *labetalol, metoprolol* and *propranolol* (increased plasma concentrations)
Calcium-channel Blockers: *cimetidine* inhibits metabolism of *some calcium-channel blockers* (increased plasma concentrations)
• Ciclosporin: *cimetidine* possibly increases plasma-ciclosporin concentration
Cytotoxics: *cimetidine* increases plasma concentration of *fluorouracil*
Dopaminergics: *cimetidine* inhibits excretion of *pramipexole* (increased plasma-pramipexole concentration)
Hormone Antagonists: *octreotide* possibly delays absorption of *cimetidine*
5HT₁ Agonists: *cimetidine* inhibits metabolism of *zolmitriptan* (reduce dose of zolmitriptan)
Sildenafil: *cimetidine* increases plasma-sildenafil concentration (reduce initial dose of sildenafil)
• Theophylline: *cimetidine* inhibits metabolism (increased plasma-theophylline concentration)
Homatropine *see* Antimuscarinics
Hormone Antagonists *see* Aminoglutethimide; Bicalutamide; Danazol; Finasteride; Flutamide; Gestrinone; Octreotide; Tamoxifen; Toremifene; Trilostane
5HT₁ Agonists
Antibacterials: *quinolones* possibly inhibit metabolism of *zolmitriptan* (reduce dose of zolmitriptan); *see also* Linezolid
• Antidepressants: risk of CNS toxicity with *MAOIs* including *moclobemide* (avoid rizatriptan or sumatriptan for 2 weeks after MAOI, reduce dose of zolmitriptan when given with moclobemide); *sumatriptan* increases risk of CNS toxicity with *SSRIs* (manufacturer of sertraline advises avoid concomitant use); *fluvoxamine* possibly inhibits metabolism of *zolmitriptan* (reduce dose of zolmitriptan); increased serotonergic effects with *St John's wort* (avoid concomitant use)
Beta-blockers: *propranolol* may increase plasma concentration of *rizatriptan* (reduce rizatriptan dose)
• Ergotamine and Ergometrine: increased risk of vasospasm (avoid ergotamine for 6 hours after almotriptan, rizatriptan, sumatriptan or zolmitriptan; avoid almotriptan, rizatriptan or sumatriptan for 24 hours and zolmitriptan for 6 hours after ergotamine)
Ulcer-healing Drugs: *cimetidine* inhibits metabolism of *zolmitriptan* (reduce dose of zolmitriptan)
Hydralazine
ACE Inhibitors and Angiotensin-II Antagonists: enhanced hypotensive effect
Alcohol: enhanced hypotensive effect
Aldesleukin: enhanced hypotensive effect
Alprostadil: enhanced hypotensive effect
• Anaesthetics: enhanced hypotensive effect
Analgesics: *NSAIDs* antagonise hypotensive effect
Antibacterials: *see* Linezolid
Antidepressants: enhanced hypotensive effect
other Antihypertensives: additive hypotensive effect
Antipsychotics: enhanced hypotensive effect
Anxiolytics and Hypnotics: enhanced hypotensive effect
Beta-blockers: enhanced hypotensive effect
Calcium-channel Blockers: enhanced hypotensive effect
Corticosteroids: antagonism of hypotensive effect
Diuretics: enhanced hypotensive effect
Dopaminergics: *levodopa* enhances hypotensive effect
Moxisylyte: enhanced hypotensive effect

Hydralazine *(continued)*
Muscle Relaxants: *baclofen* and *tizanidine* enhance hypotensive effect
Nitrates: enhanced hypotensive effect
Oestrogens and Progestogens: *oestrogens* and *combined oral contraceptives* antagonise hypotensive effect
Ulcer-healing Drugs: *carbenoxolone* antagonises hypotensive effect
Hydrochlorothiazide *see* Diuretics (thiazide)
Hydrocortisone *see* Corticosteroids
Hydroflumethiazide *see* Diuretics (thiazide)
Hydroxychloroquine *see* Chloroquine and Hydroxychloroquine
Hydroxyprogesterone *see* Progestogens
Hydroxyzine *see* Antihistamines
Hyoscine *see* Antimuscarinics (for general sedative interactions *see also* Antihistamines)
Hypericum Perforatum *see* St John's wort
Hypnotics *see* Anxiolytics and Hypnotics
Ibuprofen *see* NSAIDs
Ifosfamide *see* Cyclophosphamide and Ifosfamide
Imatinib
• Analgesics: manufacturer of *imatinib* advises restriction or avoidance of concomitant regular *paracetamol*
Anticoagulants: manufacturer of *imatinib* advises replacement of *warfarin* with a heparin (possibility of enhanced *warfarin* effect)
Antiepileptics: plasma concentration of *imatinib* reduced by *phenytoin*
Antifungals: plasma concentration of *imatinib* increased by *ketoconazole*
Lipid-regulating Drugs: plasma concentration of *simvastatin* increased by *imatinib*
Imidapril *see* ACE Inhibitors and Angiotensin-II Antagonists
Imipenem *see* Primaxin®
Imipramine *see* Antidepressants, Tricyclic
Immunoglobulins
Note. For advice on immunoglobulins and live virus vaccines, see under Normal Immunoglobulin section 14.5
Indapamide *see* Diuretics (thiazide-related)
Indinavir
• Antibacterials: concomitant administration of *indinavir* and *rifabutin* increases plasma-rifabutin concentration and decreases plasma-indinavir concentration (reduce dose of rifabutin and increase dose of indinavir); metabolism enhanced by *rifampicin* (plasma-indinavir concentration significantly reduced—avoid concomitant use)
• Antidepressants: plasma concentration reduced by *St John's wort* (avoid concomitant use)
Antiepileptics: plasma-indinavir concentration possibly reduced by *carbamazepine, phenobarbital* and *phenytoin*
• Antifungals: metabolism inhibited by *ketoconazole*; plasma-indinavir concentration increased by *itraconazole* (consider reducing dose of indinavir)
• Antihistamines: increased risk of arrhythmias with *terfenadine*—avoid concomitant use
Antimuscarinics: manufacturer of *tolterodine* advises avoid concomitant use
• Antipsychotics: possibly increased risk of arrhythmias with *pimozide* (avoid concomitant use); *indinavir* possibly increases plasma concentration of *thioridazine*
other Antivirals: combination with *nelfinavir* may lead to increased plasma concentrations of either drug; *indinavir* increases plasma concentration of *saquinavir*; *ritonavir* increases plasma concentration of *indinavir*; *efavirenz* reduces plasma concentration of *indinavir* (increase indinavir dose); *nevirapine* reduces plasma concentration of *indinavir*
• Anxiolytics and Hypnotics: increased risk of prolonged sedation with *alprazolam* and *midazolam* (avoid concomitant use)

Indinavir (continued)

Barbiturates and Primidone: see under Antiepileptics, above

Corticosteroids: plasma-indinavir concentration possibly reduced by dexamethasone

• Ergotamine and Ergometrine: risk of ergotism—avoid concomitant use

• Lipid-regulating Drugs: increased risk of myopathy with simvastatin (avoid concomitant use), and possibly with atorvastatin

Sildenafil: indinavir possibly increases plasma-sildenafil concentration (reduce initial dose of sildenafil)

Indometacin see NSAIDs

Indoramin see Alpha-blockers

Influenza Vaccine

Anticoagulants: effect of warfarin occasionally enhanced

Antiepileptics: effect of phenytoin enhanced

Theophylline: effect occasionally enhanced

Insulin see Antidiabetics

Interferons

Note. Consult product literature for interactions of interferon beta and gamma

Theophylline: interferon alfa inhibits metabolism of theophylline (enhanced effect)

Ipratropium see Antimuscarinics

Irbesartan see ACE Inhibitors and Angiotensin-II Antagonists

Iron

Antacids: magnesium trisilicate reduces absorption of oral iron

Antibacterials: tetracyclines reduce absorption of oral iron (and vice versa); absorption of ciprofloxacin, levofloxacin, norfloxacin, and ofloxacin reduced by oral iron

Antihypertensives: reduced hypotensive effect of methyldopa

Bisphosphonates: reduced absorption

Dopaminergics: absorption of entacapone and levodopa may be reduced

Penicillamine: reduced absorption of penicillamine

Trientine: reduced absorption of oral iron

Zinc: reduced absorption of oral iron (and vice versa)

Isocarboxazid see MAOIs

Isoflurane see Anaesthetics, General (volatile liquid)

Isometheptene see Sympathomimetics

Isoniazid

Anaesthetics: hepatotoxicity possibly potentiated by isoflurane

Antacids and Adsorbents: antacids reduce absorption

other Antibacterials: increased CNS toxicity with cycloserine

• Antiepileptics: metabolism of carbamazepine, ethosuximide, and phenytoin inhibited (enhanced effect); also, with carbamazepine, isoniazid hepatotoxicity possibly increased

Antifungals: plasma concentration of ketoconazole may be reduced

Anxiolytics and Hypnotics: metabolism of diazepam inhibited

Theophylline: isoniazid possibly increases plasma theophylline concentration

Isoprenaline see Sympathomimetics

Isosorbide Dinitrate see Nitrates

Isosorbide Mononitrate see Nitrates

Isotretinoin see Retinoids

Isradipine see Calcium-channel Blockers

Itraconazole see Antifungals, Imidazole and Triazole

Kaletra® see Lopinavir, Ritonavir

Note. Ritonavir is present to inhibit lopinavir metabolism and increase plasma-lopinavir concentration

Kaolin

Analgesics: absorption of aspirin possibly reduced

Anti-arrhythmics: absorption of quinidine possibly reduced (possibly reduced plasma concentration)

Antibacterials: absorption of tetracyclines possibly reduced

Kaolin (continued)

Antimalarials: absorption of chloroquine reduced

Antipsychotics: absorption of phenothiazines possibly reduced

Cardiac Glycosides: absorption of digoxin possibly reduced

Ketamine see Anaesthetics, General

Ketoconazole see Antifungals, Imidazole and Triazole

Ketoprofen see NSAIDs

Ketorolac see NSAIDs

Ketotifen see Antihistamines

Labetalol see Beta-blockers

Lacidipine see Calcium-channel Blockers

Lamivudine

Antibacterials: trimethoprim increases plasma concentration—avoid concomitant use of high-dose co-trimoxazole

Lamotrigine

Antibacterials: see Linezolid

• Antidepressants: antagonism of anticonvulsive effect (convulsive threshold lowered)

• other Antiepileptics: interactions include enhanced effects, increased sedation, and reductions in plasma concentrations; for further details, see p. 227

• Antimalarials: mefloquine antagonises anticonvulsant effect; chloroquine and hydroxychloroquine occasionally reduce seizure threshold

Lanreotide

Ciclosporin: absorption of ciclosporin reduced (reduced plasma concentration)

Lansoprazole see Proton Pump Inhibitors

Leflunomide

Note. Increased risk of toxicity with other haematotoxic and hepatotoxic drugs

Anion-exchange resin: colestyramine significantly decreases effect of leflunomide (enhanced elimination)—avoid unless drug elimination desired

Vaccines: see p. 578

Lenograstim

Note. Use not recommended from 24 hours before until 24 hours after chemotherapy—for further details consult product literature

Lercanidipine see Calcium-channel Blockers

Leukotriene Antagonists

Analgesics: aspirin increases plasma concentration of zafirlukast

Antibacterials: erythromycin reduces plasma concentration of zafirlukast

Anticoagulants: anticoagulant effect of warfarin enhanced by zafirlukast

Antihistamines: terfenadine reduces plasma concentration of zafirlukast

Barbiturates and Primidone: plasma concentration of montelukast reduced by phenobarbital

Theophylline: zafirlukast possibly increases plasma-theophylline concentration; plasma-zafirlukast concentration reduced

Levetiracetam

• Antidepressants: antagonism of anticonvulsant effect (convulsive threshold lowered)

other Antiepileptics: none demonstrated with carbamazepine, gabapentin, lamotrigine, phenobarbital, phenytoin, primidone, or valproate

• Antimalarials: mefloquine antagonises anticonvulsant effect; chloroquine and hydroxychloroquine occasionally reduce seizure threshold

Levobunolol see Beta-blockers

Levobupivacaine

Anti-arrhythmics: increased myocardial depression

Levocabastine see Antihistamines

Levocetirizine see Antihistamines

Levodopa

• Anaesthetics: risk of arrhythmias with volatile liquid anaesthetics such as halothane

• Antibacterials: see Linezolid

Levodopa *(continued)*
* Antidepressants: hypertensive crisis with *MAOIs* (including moclobemide)—avoid for at least 2 weeks after stopping *MAOI*
  Antihypertensives: enhanced hypotensive effect
  Antimuscarinics: absorption of *levodopa* possibly reduced
  Antipsychotics: antagonism of effect
  Anxiolytics and Hypnotics: occasional antagonism of effect by *chlordiazepoxide, diazepam, lorazepam* and possibly *other benzodiazepines*
* Bupropion (amfebutamone): increased risk of side-effects of levodopa
  Iron: absorption of *levodopa* may be reduced
  Muscle relaxants: agitation, confusion and hallucinations possible with *baclofen*
  Vitamins: effect of *levodopa* antagonised by *pyridoxine* unless a *dopa decarboxylase inhibitor* also given
Levofloxacin *see* Quinolones
Levomepromazine (methotrimeprazine) *see* Antipsychotics
Levonorgestrel *see* Progestogens
Levothyroxine (Thyroxine) *see* Thyroid Hormones
Lidocaine (lignocaine)
  Note. Interactions less likely when lidocaine used topically
  other Anti-arrhythmics: increased myocardial depression
* Antibacterials: increased risk of ventricular arrhythmias with *quinupristin/dalfopristin* (avoid concomitant use)
  Antidepressants: manufacturer of *reboxetine* advises caution
  Beta-blockers: increased risk of myocardial depression; increased risk of *lidocaine* toxicity with *propranolol*
  Diuretics: effect of *lidocaine* antagonised by hypokalaemia with *acetazolamide, loop diuretics, and thiazides*
  Muscle Relaxants: action of *suxamethonium* prolonged
  Ulcer-healing Drugs: *cimetidine* inhibits metabolism of *lidocaine* (increased risk of toxicity)
Lignocaine *see* Lidocaine
Linezolid *see* MAOIs
  Note. Linezolid is a reversible, non-selective MAO inhibitor
Liothyronine *see* Thyroid Hormones
Lipid-regulating Drugs *see* Colestyramine and Colestipol; Fibrates; Nicotinic Acid; Statins
Lisinopril *see* ACE Inhibitors and Angiotensin-II Antagonists
Lisuride
  Antipsychotics: antagonism of effect
Lithium
* ACE Inhibitors and Angiotensin-II Antagonists: *lithium* excretion reduced (increased plasma-lithium concentration)
* Analgesics: excretion of *lithium* reduced by *azapropazone, diclofenac, ibuprofen, indometacin, ketorolac* (avoid concomitant use), *mefenamic acid, naproxen, phenylbutazone, piroxicam, rofecoxib,* and probably *other NSAIDs* (risk of toxicity)
  Antacids: *sodium bicarbonate* increases excretion of *lithium* (reduced plasma-lithium concentrations)
  Anti-arrhythmics: increased risk of hypothyroidism with *amiodarone*
  Antibacterials: *lithium* toxicity reported with *metronidazole*
* Antidepressants: *SSRIs* increase risk of CNS effects (lithium toxicity reported)
  Antidiabetics: *lithium* may occasionally impair glucose tolerance
  Antiepileptics: neurotoxicity may occur with *carbamazepine* and *phenytoin* without increased plasma-lithium concentration

Lithium *(continued)*
* Antihypertensives: neurotoxicity may occur with *methyldopa* without increased plasma-lithium concentration
* Antipsychotics: increased risk of extrapyramidal effects and possibility of neurotoxicity with *clozapine, haloperidol,* and *phenothiazines*; increased risk of extrapyramidal effects with *sulpiride*; increased risk of ventricular arrhythmias with *thioridazine* (avoid concomitant use)
  Calcium-channel Blockers: neurotoxicity may occur with *diltiazem* and *verapamil* without increased plasma-lithium concentration
* Diuretics: *lithium* excretion reduced by *loop diuretics, potassium-sparing diuretics,* and *thiazides* (increased plasma-lithium concentration and risk of toxicity—*loop diuretics* safer than *thiazides*); *lithium* excretion increased by *acetazolamide*
  Muscle Relaxants: muscle relaxant effect enhanced; *baclofen* possibly aggravates hyperkinesis
  Parasympathomimetics: *lithium* antagonises effect of *neostigmine and pyridostigmine*
  Theophylline: *lithium* excretion increased (reduced plasma-lithium concentration)
Lofepramine *see* Antidepressants, Tricyclic
Lofexidine
  Alcohol: enhanced sedative effect
  Anxiolytics and Hypnotics: enhanced sedative effect
Lopinavir
  Note. In combination with Ritonavir as *Kaletra®*—*see also* Ritonavir
* Antibacterials: *rifampicin* reduces plasma-lopinavir concentration (avoid concomitant use)
* *other* Antivirals: *efavirenz* and possibly *nevirapine* reduce plasma-lopinavir concentration
* Antiepileptics: *carbamazepine, phenobarbital,* and *phenytoin* possibly reduce plasma-lopinavir concentration
* Corticosteroids: *dexamethasone* possibly reduces plasma-lopinavir concentration
Loprazolam *see* Anxiolytics and Hypnotics
Loratadine *see* Antihistamines
Lorazepam *see* Anxiolytics and Hypnotics
Lormetazepam *see* Anxiolytics and Hypnotics
Losartan *see* ACE Inhibitors and Angiotensin-II Antagonists
Loxapine *see* Antipsychotics
Lymecycline *see* Tetracyclines
Macrolides *see* Erythromycin and other Macrolides
Magnesium Salts *(see also* Antacids and Adsorbents)
* Calcium-channel Blockers: profound hypotension reported with *nifedipine* and *intravenous magnesium sulphate* in pre-eclampsia
  Muscle Relaxants: effect of *non-depolarising muscle relaxants* enhanced by *parenteral magnesium salts*
Magnesium Trisilicate *see* Antacids
Maloprim® contains Dapsone and Pyrimethamine
MAOIs
  Note. For interactions of reversible MAO-A inhibitors (RIMAs) see Moclobemide, and for interactions of MAO-B inhibitors see Selegiline; the antibacterial linezolid is a reversible, non-selective MAO inhibitor
* Alcohol: some *alcoholic* and *dealcoholised beverages* contain *tyramine* which interacts with *MAOIs* (hypertensive crisis)—but if no tyramine, enhanced hypotensive effect; foods, *see* section 4.3.2
  Alpha$_2$-adrenoceptor Stimulants: manufacturers of *apraclonidine* and *brimonidine* advise avoid concomitant use
* Altretamine: risk of severe postural hypotension
* Analgesics: CNS excitation or depression (hypertension or hypotension) with *pethidine* and possibly *other opioid analgesics*—avoid concomitant use and for 2 weeks after MAOI discontinued; manufacturer advises avoid *nefopam*
  Anaesthetics: *see* section 15.1
* Anorectics: *see* Sympathomimetics, below

MAOIs *(continued)*
- <u>Antibacterials</u>: enhancement of CNS effects and toxicity with *linezolid* (avoid for at least 2 weeks after stopping other MAOI)
- *other* Antidepressants: enhancement of CNS effects and toxicity with *other MAOIs* (avoid for at least 2 weeks after stopping *previous MAOIs* then start with reduced dose); CNS effects of *SSRIs* increased by *MAOIs* (risk of serious toxicity) , see also p. 195; CNS excitation and hypertension with most *tricyclics and related antidepressants*, see p. 189; CNS excitation and confusion with *tryptophan* (reduce tryptophan dose); enhancement of CNS effects and toxicity possible with *nefazodone*, *reboxetine* and *venlafaxine* (avoid for at least 2 weeks after stopping MAOI, and avoid MAOI for at least 1 week after stopping nefazodone, reboxetine or venlafaxine)

  <u>Antidiabetics</u>: effect of *insulin, metformin, sulphonylureas,* and possibly *other antidiabetics* enhanced
- <u>Antiepileptics</u>: antagonism of anticonvulsant effect (convulsive threshold lowered); manufacturer advises avoid *carbamazepine* with or within 2 weeks of *MAOIs*; manufacturer of *oxcarbazepine* advises avoid concomitant use

  Antihistamines: increased antimuscarinic and sedative effects
- Antihypertensives: hypotensive effect enhanced; manufacturer advises avoidance of *indoramin*; manufacturer advises avoid concomitant use with *methyldopa*

  Antimuscarinics: increased side-effects
- Antipsychotics: CNS excitation and hypertension with *oxypertine*; *clozapine* possibly enhances central effects

  Anxiolytics and Hypnotics: manufacturer advises avoidance of *buspirone*
- Barbiturates and Primidone: *see under* Antiepileptics, above
- Bupropion (amfebutamone): manufacturer of bupropion advises avoid with or for 2 weeks after MAOI
- Dopaminergics: hypertensive crisis with *levodopa* (avoid for at least 2 weeks after stopping MAOI); hypotension with *selegiline*; manufacturer advises avoid concomitant use with *entacapone*

  Doxapram: potentiated by *MAOIs*
- 5HT₁ Agonists: risk of CNS toxicity (avoid rizatriptan or sumatriptan for 2 weeks after MAOI)
- Sibutramine: increased risk of CNS toxicity (manufacturer recommends avoid concomitant use); avoid *sibutramine* for 2 weeks after stopping *MAOIs*
- Sympathomimetics: hypertensive crisis with *sympathomimetics* such as *dexamfetamine and other amphetamines, dopamine, dopexamine, ephedrine, isometheptene, methylphenidate, phenylephrine, phenylpropanolamine,* and *pseudoephedrine*
- Tetrabenazine: CNS excitation and hypertension

Maprotiline *see* Antidepressants, Tricyclic

Mebendazole

  Ulcer-healing Drugs: metabolism possibly inhibited by *cimetidine* (increased plasma-mebendazole concentration)

Medroxyprogesterone *see* Progestogens

Mefenamic Acid *see* NSAIDs

Mefloquine
- Anti-arrhythmics: increased risk of ventricular arrhythmias with *amiodarone* (avoid concomitant use) and *quinidine*
- Antiepileptics: antagonism of anticonvulsant effect
- *other* Antimalarials: increased risk of convulsions with *chloroquine* and *quinine*, but should not prevent use of intravenous quinine in severe cases; for full precautions see footnote on p. 311 (also applies to *quinidine*)

Mefloquine *(continued)*
- Antipsychotics: increased risk of ventricular arrhythmias—avoid concomitant use with *pimozide*

  Beta-blockers: possible increased risk of bradycardia

  Calcium-channel Blockers: possible increased risk of bradycardia with some *calcium-channel blockers*

  Cardiac Glycosides: possible increased risk of bradycardia with *digoxin*

  Vaccines: *see* Typhoid Vaccine, p. 593

Megestrol *see* Progestogens

Meloxicam *see* NSAIDs

Melphalan

  Antibacterials: increased toxicity with *nalidixic acid*
- Ciclosporin: increased risk of nephrotoxicity

Mepacrine

  Antimalarials: increased plasma concentration of *primaquine* (risk of toxicity)

Meprobamate *see* Anxiolytics and Hypnotics

Meptazinol *see* Opioid Analgesics

Mercaptopurine
- Allopurinol: enhancement of effect (increased toxicity—reduce dose of mercaptopurine)

  <u>Aminosalicylates</u>: possible increased risk of leucopenia
- Antibacterials: increased risk of haematological toxicity with *co-trimoxazole* and *trimethoprim*

Meropenem

  <u>Antiepileptics</u>: plasma concentration of *valproate* reduced

  <u>Uricosurics</u>: excretion reduced by *probenecid* (concomitant use not recommended by manufacturer)

Mesalazine *see* Aminosalicylates

Mestranol *see* Contraceptives, Oral

Metaraminol *see* Sympathomimetics (*as* noradrenaline)

Metformin *see* Antidiabetics

Methadone *see* Opioid Analgesics

Methenamine

  Potassium Citrate: urine should be acid

Methocarbamol *see* Muscle Relaxants

Methotrexate
- <u>Anaesthetics</u>: antifolate effect increased by nitrous oxide (avoid concomitant use)
- Analgesics: excretion reduced by *aspirin, azapropazone* (avoid concomitant use)*, diclofenac, ibuprofen, indometacin, ketoprofen, meloxicam, naproxen, phenylbutazone,* and probably *other NSAIDs* (increased risk of toxicity)
- Antibacterials: antifolate effect increased by *co-trimoxazole and trimethoprim* (avoid concomitant use); risk of methotrexate toxicity increased by *sulphonamides*; excretion reduced by *penicillins* (increased risk of toxicity)

  Antiepileptics: *phenytoin* increases antifolate effect

  Antimalarials: antifolate effect increased by *pyrimethamine* (ingredient of *Fansidar®* and *Maloprim®*)
- Ciclosporin: increased toxicity
- Corticosteroids: increased risk of haematological toxicity
- Retinoids: plasma concentration of *methotrexate* increased by *acitretin* (also increased risk of hepatotoxicity—avoid concomitant use)
- Uricosurics: excretion reduced by *probenecid* (increased risk of toxicity)

Methotrimeprazine (Levomepromazine) *see* Antipsychotics

Methoxamine *see* Sympathomimetics (*as* noradrenaline)

Methyldopa

  Alcohol: enhanced hypotensive effect

  Alprostadil: enhanced hypotensive effect
- Anaesthetics: enhanced hypotensive effect

  Analgesics: *NSAIDs* antagonise hypotensive effect

  Antibacterials: *see* Linezolid
- <u>Antidepressants</u>: enhanced hypotensive effect; manufacturer advises avoid concomitant use with *MAOIs*

Methyldopa *(continued)*
    other Antihypertensives: enhanced hypotensive effect
    Antipsychotics: increased risk of extrapyramidal
        effects; enhanced hypotensive effect
    Anxiolytics and Hypnotics: enhanced hypotensive
        effect
    Beta-blockers: enhanced hypotensive effect
    Calcium-channel Blockers: enhanced hypotensive
        effect
    Corticosteroids: antagonism of hypotensive effect
    Diuretics: enhanced hypotensive effect
    Dopaminergics: antagonism of antiparkinsonian
        effect; *levodopa* enhances hypotensive effect; effect
        of methyldopa possibly enhanced by *entacapone*
    Iron: reduced hypotensive effect
• Lithium: neurotoxicity may occur without increased
        plasma-lithium concentration
    Moxisylyte: enhanced hypotensive effect
    Muscle Relaxants: enhanced hypotensive effect with
        baclofen and *tizanidine*
    Nitrates: enhance hypotensive effect
    Oestrogens and Progestogens: *oestrogens and
        combined oral contraceptives* antagonise
        hypotensive effect
• Sympathomimetics, Beta₂: acute hypotension
        reported with *salbutamol infusion*
    Ulcer-healing Drugs: *carbenoxolone* antagonises
        hypotensive effect
Methylphenidate *see* Sympathomimetics
Methylprednisolone *see* Corticosteroids
Methysergide *see* Ergotamine
Metipranolol *see* Beta-blockers
Metoclopramide
    Analgesics: increased absorption of *aspirin* and
        paracetamol (enhanced effect); *opioid analgesics*
        antagonise effect on gastro-intestinal activity
    Antimuscarinics: antagonism of effect on gastro-
        intestinal activity
    Antipsychotics: increased risk of extrapyramidal
        effects
    Atovaquone: plasma concentration reduced by
        metoclopramide
    Dopaminergics: antagonism of hypoprolactinaemic
        effect of *bromocriptine*; antagonism of
        antiparkinsonian effects of *pergolide* and *ropinirole*
        (manufacturer of ropinirole advises avoid
        concomitant use)
    Tetrabenazine: increased risk of extrapyramidal effects
Metolazone *see* Diuretics (thiazide-related)
Metoprolol *see* Beta-blockers
Metronidazole
    Alcohol: disulfiram-like reaction
• Anticoagulants: effect of *acenocoumarol* and
        warfarin enhanced
• Antiepileptics: *metronidazole* inhibits metabolism of
        phenytoin (increased plasma-phenytoin
        concentration); *phenobarbital* accelerates
        metabolism of *metronidazole* (reduced plasma-
        metronidazole concentration)
• Barbiturates and Primidone: *see under* Antiepileptics,
        above
    Cytotoxics: *metronidazole* inhibits metabolism of
        fluorouracil (increased toxicity)
    Disulfiram: psychotic reactions reported
    Lithium: increased toxicity reported
    Ulcer-healing Drugs: *cimetidine* inhibits metabolism
        (increased plasma-metronidazole concentration)
Mexiletine
• Analgesics: *opioid analgesics* delay absorption
• *other* Anti-arrhythmics: increased myocardial
        depression with any combination of *anti-
        arrhythmics*
    Antibacterials: *rifampicin* accelerates metabolism
        (reduced plasma-mexiletine concentration)
    Antidepressants: manufacturer of *reboxetine* advises
        caution
    Antiepileptics: *phenytoin* accelerates metabolism
        (reduced plasma-mexiletine concentration)

Mexiletine *(continued)*
• Antihistamines: increased risk of ventricular
        arrhythmias with *mizolastine* and *terfenadine*
        (avoid concomitant use)
    Antimuscarinics: *atropine* delays absorption
• Antivirals: possibly increased risk of arrhythmias with
        ritonavir
    Diuretics: action of *mexiletine* antagonised by
        hypokalaemia due to *acetazolamide, loop diuretics,
        and thiazides*
    Theophylline: plasma-theophylline concentration
        increased
Mianserin
    Alcohol: enhanced effect
    Alpha₂-adrenoceptor Stimulants: manufacturers of
        apraclonidine and *brimonidine* advise avoid
        concomitant use
    other Antidepressants: as for Antidepressants, Tricyclic
• Antiepileptics: antagonism (convulsive threshold
        lowered); metabolism accelerated by
        carbamazepine, phenobarbital, and *phenytoin*
        (reduced plasma-mianserin concentration)
    Anxiolytics and Hypnotics: enhanced effect
• Barbiturates and Primidone: *see* Antiepileptics, above
• Sibutramine: increased risk of CNS toxicity
        (manufacturer of *sibutramine* recommends avoid
        concomitant use)
Miconazole *see* Antifungals, Imidazole and Triazole
Midazolam *see* Anxiolytics and Hypnotics
Mifepristone
    Analgesics: manufacturer recommends avoid *aspirin*
        and *NSAIDs* on theoretical grounds
    Corticosteroids: effect of corticosteroids (including
        inhaled corticosteroids) may be reduced for 3–4
        days after mifepristone
Minocycline *see* Tetracyclines
Minoxidil *see* Hydralazine for general hypotensive
    interactions
Mirtazapine
    Alcohol: enhanced sedative effect
    Alpha₂-adrenoceptor Stimulants: manufacturers of
        apraclonidine and *brimonidine* advise avoid
        concomitant use
• *other* Antidepressants: as for Antidepressants,
        tricyclic
    Anxiolytics and Hypnotics: enhanced sedative effect
• Sibutramine: increased risk of CNS toxicity
        (manufacturer of *sibutramine* recommends avoid
        concomitant use)
Misoprostol
    Analgesics: increased risk of CNS toxicity with
        phenylbutazone
Mivacurium *see* Muscle Relaxants (non-depolarising)
Mizolastine *see* Antihistamines
Moclobemide
    Note. Moclobemide is a reversible MAO-A inhibitor
        (RIMA), see also p. 194
• Analgesics: CNS excitation or depression
        (hypertension or hypotension) with *codeine,
        dextromethorphan, pethidine,* and possibly *fentanyl,
        morphine,* and *other opioid analgesics*; effects of
        ibuprofen and possibly *other NSAIDs* enhanced
• Anorectics: as for MAOIs (see main list)
• *other* Antidepressants: see p. 194
• Bupropion (amfebutamone): manufacturer of
        bupropion advises avoid concomitant use
• Dopaminergics: hypertensive crisis with *levodopa*;
        avoid concomitant use with *selegiline*
• 5HT₁ Agonists: risk of CNS toxicity (reduce dose of
        zolmitriptan)
• Sibutramine: increased risk of CNS toxicity
        (manufacturer of *sibutramine* recommends avoid
        concomitant use); avoid *sibutramine* for 2 weeks
        after stopping *MAOIs*
• Sympathomimetics: as for MAOIs (see main list)
    Ulcer-healing Drugs: *cimetidine* inhibits metabolism
        (increased plasma-moclobemide concentration—
        halve dose of moclobemide)

Moexipril *see* ACE Inhibitors and Angiotensin-II Antagonists

Modafinil
* Oestrogens and Progestogens: modafinil accelerates metabolism of *oral contraceptives* (reduced contraceptive effect)

Monoamine-oxidase Inhibitors *see* MAOIs, Moclobemide, and Selegiline

Montelukast *see* Leukotriene Antagonists

Morphine *see* Opioid Analgesics

Moxisylyte (Thymoxamine)
* Alpha-blockers: possible severe postural hypotension
  other Antihypertensives: enhanced hypotensive effect
* Beta-blockers: possible severe postural hypotension

Moxonidine
  Alprostadil: enhanced hypotensive effect
  other Antihypertensives: enhanced hypotensive effect
  Antibacterials: *see* Linezolid
  Antidepressants: enhanced hypotensive effect with *MAOIs*
  Anxiolytics and Hypnotics: sedative effect of benzodiazepines possibly enhanced
  Moxisylyte: enhanced hypotensive effect
  Muscle Relaxants: enhanced hypotensive effect with *baclofen* and *tizanidine*

Muscle Relaxants
  ACE Inhibitors and Angiotensin-II Antagonists: enhanced hypotensive effect with *baclofen* and *tizanidine*
  Alcohol: enhanced sedative effect with *baclofen*, *methocarbamol* and *tizanidine*
  Analgesics: *ibuprofen* and *possibly other NSAIDs* reduce excretion of *baclofen* (increased risk of toxicity)
* Anti-arrhythmics: *procainamide* and *quinidine* enhance muscle relaxant effect; *lidocaine* prolongs action of *suxamethonium*
* Antibacterials: effect of *non-depolarising muscle relaxants* enhanced by *aminoglycosides, clindamycin, colistin* and *piperacillin*
  Antidepressants: *tricyclics* enhance muscle relaxant effect of *baclofen*
  Antiepileptics: effect of *non-depolarising muscle relaxants* antagonised by *carbamazepine* and *phenytoin* (recovery from neuromuscular blockade accelerated)
  Antihypertensives: enhanced hypotensive effect with *baclofen* and *tizanidine*
  Anxiolytics and Hypnotics: enhanced sedative effect with *baclofen* and *tizanidine*
  Beta-blockers: *propranolol* enhances muscle relaxant effect; possible enhanced hypotensive effect and bradycardia with *tizanidine*
* Botulinum Toxin: neuromuscular block enhanced by *non-depolarising muscle relaxants* (risk of toxicity)
  Calcium-channel Blockers: *nifedipine* and *verapamil* enhance effect of *non-depolarising muscle relaxants*; hypotension, myocardial depression, and hyperkalaemia reported with intravenous *dantrolene* and *verapamil*; risk of arrhythmias with *diltiazem* and intravenous *dantrolene*
  Cardiac Glycosides: arrhythmias if *suxamethonium* given with *digoxin*; possible bradycardia if *tizanidine* given with *digoxin*
  Cytotoxics: *cyclophosphamide* and *thiotepa* enhance effect of *suxamethonium*
  Diuretics: enhanced hypotensive effect with *baclofen* and *tizanidine*
  Dopaminergics: agitation, confusion and, hallucinations possible with *baclofen* and *levodopa*
  Lithium: *lithium* enhances muscle relaxant effect; *baclofen* possibly aggravates hyperkinesis
  Magnesium Salts: *parenteral magnesium* enhances effect of *non-depolarising muscle relaxants*

Muscle Relaxants *(continued)*
  Parasympathomimetics: *ecothiopate* eye-drops, *edrophonium, galantamine, neostigmine, pyridostigmine, rivastigmine* and possibly *donepezil* enhance effect of *suxamethonium* but antagonise effect of *non-depolarising muscle relaxants*
  Sympathomimetics: *bambuterol* enhances effect of *suxamethonium*

Mycophenolate Mofetil
  Anion-exchange Resins: *colestyramine* reduces absorption
  Antacids: reduced absorption of mycophenolate mofetil
  Antivirals: higher plasma concentrations of *mycophenolate mofetil* and of *aciclovir* and possibly *ganciclovir* on concomitant administration

Nabilone
  Alcohol: sedative effect of *nabilone* enhanced
  Anxiolytics and Hypnotics: enhanced sedative effect

Nabumetone *see* NSAIDs

Nadolol *see* Beta-blockers

Nalbuphine *see* Opioid Analgesics

Nalidixic Acid *see* Quinolones

Nandrolone *see* Anabolic Steroids

Naproxen *see* NSAIDs

Naratriptan *see* 5HT$_1$ Agonists

Nateglinide *see* Antidiabetics

Nebivolol *see* Beta-blockers

Nefazodone
  Note. Although interactions with alcohol, and lithium have not been reported, caution should be observed on concomitant use with nefazodone
  Antibacterials: *see* Linezolid
* *other* Antidepressants: increased risk of toxicity with *MAOIs* (nefazodone should not be started until 2 weeks after stopping MAOI, and conversely MAOI should not be started until at least 1 week after stopping nefazodone); *fluoxetine* increases plasma concentration of nefazodone
  Antiepileptics: plasma concentration of *carbamazepine* increased and plasma concentration of *nefazodone* reduced
* Antihistamines: increased risk of arrhythmias with *terfenadine*—avoid concomitant use
  Antihypertensives: hypotensive effect possibly enhanced
  Antipsychotics: plasma concentration of *haloperidol* increased
  Anxiolytics and Hypnotics: possibly enhanced sedative effect with *benzodiazepines*; plasma concentration of *alprazolam* increased (reduce alprazolam dose)
  Cardiac Glycosides: plasma concentration of *digoxin* increased
* Lipid-regulating Drugs: increased risk of myopathy with *simvastatin* (avoid concomitant use)
* Sibutramine: increased risk of CNS toxicity (manufacturer of *sibutramine* recommends avoid concomitant use)
* Tacrolimus: plasma concentration of *tacrolimus* increased

Nefopam
  Antibacterials: *see* Linezolid
* Antidepressants: manufacturer recommends avoid *MAOIs;* possibly increased side-effects with *tricyclics*
  Antimuscarinics: increased side-effects

Nelfinavir
* Anti-arrhythmics: increased risk of arrhythmias with *amiodarone* and *quinidine* (avoid concomitant use)
* Antibacterials: *rifampicin* significantly reduces plasma concentration of *nelfinavir* (avoid concomitant use); *nelfinavir* increases plasma concentration of *rifabutin* (halve rifabutin dose)
* Antidepressants: plasma concentration reduced by *St John's wort* (avoid concomitant use)

Nelfinavir *(continued)*
* Antiepileptics: *carbamazepine* and *phenytoin* possibly reduce plasma concentration of *nelfinavir*
* Antihistamines: increased risk of arrhythmias with *terfenadine* (avoid concomitant use)
* Antimuscarinics: manufacturer of *tolterodine* advises avoid concomitant use
* Antipsychotics: possibly increased risk of arrhythmias with *pimozide* (avoid concomitant use); nelfinavir possibly increases plasma concentration of *thioridazine*
  other Antivirals: combination of *nelfinavir* with *indinavir*, *ritonavir* or *saquinavir* may lead to increased plasma concentrations of either drug (or both)
* Anxiolytics and Hypnotics: risk of prolonged sedation with *midazolam* (avoid concomitant use)
* Barbiturates and Primidone: *phenobarbital* possibly reduces plasma concentration of *nelfinavir*
* Ergotamine and Ergometrine: risk of ergotism—avoid concomitant use
* Lipid-regulating Drugs: increased risk of myopathy with *simvastatin*—avoid concomitant use; *nelfinavir* possibly increases risk of myopathy with *atorvastatin*
* Oestrogens and Progestogens: possibly reduced efficacy of *oral contraceptives*
  Sildenafil: *nelfinavir* possibly increases plasma-sildenafil concentration (reduce initial dose of sildenafil)

Neomycin *see* Aminoglycosides
Neostigmine *see* Parasympathomimetics
Netilmicin *see* Aminoglycosides
Nevirapine
  Analgesics: plasma concentration of *methadone* possibly reduced
  Antibacterials: *rifabutin* and *rifampicin* reduce plasma concentration of *nevirapine*
* Antidepressants: plasma concentration reduced by *St John's wort* (avoid concomitant use)
* Antifungals: plasma concentration of *ketoconazole* reduced (avoid concomitant use)
* *other* Antivirals: plasma concentration of *saquinavir* reduced by *nevirapine* (avoid concomitant use); plasma concentration of *indinavir* and possibly *amprenavir* and *lopinavir* reduced by *nevirapine*
* Oestrogens and Progestogens: accelerated metabolism of *oral contraceptives* and other *hormonal contraceptives* (reduced contraceptive effect)

Nicardipine *see* Calcium-channel Blockers
Nicorandil
  Note. Interactions not observed with acenocoumarol, beta-blockers, digoxin, rifampicin, cimetidine, calcium-channel blockers, or furosemide; possibility of hypotensive interaction with vasodilators, tricyclics, or alcohol
  Antibacterials: *see* Linezolid
  Antidepressants: enhanced hypotensive effect with *MAOIs*
* Sildenafil: hypotensive effect significantly enhanced—avoid concomitant use

Nicotine and Tobacco
  Theophylline: *tobacco smoking* increases metabolism (reduced plasma-theophylline concentration)

Nicotinic Acid
  Note. Interactions apply to lipid-regulating doses of nicotinic acid
* *other* Lipid-regulating Drugs: increased risk of myopathy with *statins*

Nicoumalone (Acenocoumarol) *see* Warfarin and other Coumarins
Nifedipine *see* Calcium-channel Blockers
Nimodipine *see* Calcium-channel Blockers
Nisoldipine *see* Calcium-channel Blockers

Nitrates (general hypotensive interactions *as for* Hydralazine)
  Anti-arrhythmics: *disopyramide* may reduce effect of sublingual nitrates (owing to dry mouth)
* Anticoagulants: excretion of *heparin* increased by *glyceryl trinitrate infusion* (reduced anticoagulant effect)
  Antidepressants: *tricyclics* may reduce effect of sublingual nitrates (owing to dry mouth)
  Antimuscarinics: *antimuscarinics such as atropine and propantheline* may reduce effect of *sublingual nitrates* (owing to dry mouth)
  Apomorphine: enhanced hypotensive effect with sublingual apomorphine
* Sildenafil: hypotensive effect significantly enhanced—avoid concomitant use

Nitrazepam *see* Anxiolytics and Hypnotics
Nitrofurantoin
  Antacids and Adsorbents: *magnesium trisilicate* reduces absorption
  Uricosurics: *probenecid* and *sulfinpyrazone* reduce excretion of *nitrofurantoin* (risk of toxicity)

Nitroprusside as for Hydralazine
Nitrous Oxide *see* Anaesthetics, General
Nizatidine *see* Histamine H_2-antagonists
Noradrenaline (Norepinephrine) *see* Sympathomimetics
Norepinephrine (Noradrenaline) *see* Sympathomimetics
Norethisterone *see* Progestogens
Norfloxacin *see* Quinolones
Norgestimate *see* Progestogens
Norgestrel *see* Progestogens
Nortriptyline *see* Antidepressants, Tricyclic
NSAIDs *(see also* Aspirin)
  Note. Interactions do not generally apply to topical NSAIDs
* ACE Inhibitors and Angiotensin-II Antagonists: antagonism of hypotensive effect; increased risk of renal impairment and increased risk of hyperkalaemia on administration with *ketorolac* and possibly *other NSAIDs*
* *other* Analgesics: avoid concomitant administration of two or more *NSAIDs*, including *aspirin* (increased side-effects)
  Anion-exchange Resins: *colestyramine* reduces absorption of *phenylbutazone*
  Antacids: absorption of *diflunisal* reduced
* Antibacterials: *NSAIDs* possibly increase risk of convulsions with *quinolones; indometacin* possibly increases plasma concentration of *gentamicin* and *amikacin* in neonates; *rifampicin* reduces plasma concentraton of *rofecoxib*
* Anticoagulants: anticoagulant effect of *acenocoumarol, warfarin* (and possibly phenindione) seriously enhanced by *azapropazone* and *phenylbutazone* (avoid concomitant use), and possibly enhanced by *diclofenac, diflunisal, flurbiprofen, ibuprofen, mefenamic acid, meloxicam, piroxicam, sulindac,* and *other NSAIDs*; increased risk of haemorrhage with *intravenous diclofenac* and with *ketorolac* and all *anticoagulants,* including *low-dose heparin* (avoid concomitant use); NSAIDs possibly increase risk of bleeding with *heparin*
  Antidepressants: *moclobemide* enhances effect of *ibuprofen* and possibly *other NSAIDs*
* Antidiabetics: effect of *sulphonylureas* enhanced by *azapropazone* (avoid concomitant use), *phenylbutazone* and possibly *other NSAIDs*
* Antiepileptics: effect of *phenytoin* enhanced by *azapropazone* (avoid concomitant use), *phenylbutazone* and possibly *other NSAIDs*
  Antifungals: plasma concentration of *celecoxib* increased by *fluconazole* (halve celecoxib dose)
  Antihypertensives: antagonism of hypotensive effect
  Antiplatelet Drugs: increased risk of bleeding with *clopidogrel* and *ticlopidine*
  Antipsychotics: severe drowsiness possible if *indometacin* given with *haloperidol*

NSAIDs (*see also* Aspirin) *(continued)*
- Antivirals: increased risk of haematological toxicity with *zidovudine*; plasma concentration of *piroxicam* increased by *ritonavir* (risk of toxicity—avoid concomitant use); plasma concentration of *other NSAIDs* possibly increased by *ritonavir*

  Beta-blockers: antagonism of hypotensive effect

  Bisphosphonates: bioavailability of *tiludronic acid* increased by *indometacin*

  Cardiac Glycosides: *NSAIDs* may exacerbate heart failure, reduce GFR, and increase plasma-cardiac glycoside concentration
- Ciclosporin: increased risk of nephrotoxicity; *ciclosporin* increases plasma concentration of *diclofenac* (halve diclofenac dose)

  Corticosteroids: increased risk of gastro-intestinal bleeding and ulceration
- Cytotoxics: excretion of *methotrexate* reduced by *aspirin, azapropazone* (avoid concomitant use), *diclofenac, ibuprofen, indometacin, ketoprofen, meloxicam, naproxen, phenylbutazone* and probably *other NSAIDs* (increased risk of toxicity)

  Desmopressin: effect potentiated by *indometacin*
- Diuretics: risk of nephrotoxicity of *NSAIDs* increased; *NSAIDs* notably *indometacin* and *ketorolac* antagonise diuretic effect; *indometacin* and possibly *other NSAIDs* increase risk of hyperkalaemia with *potassium-sparing diuretics*; occasional reports of decreased renal function when *indometacin* given with *triamterene* (avoid concomitant use)
- Lithium: excretion of *lithium* reduced by *azapropazone, diclofenac, ibuprofen, indometacin, ketorolac* (avoid concomitant use), *mefenamic acid, naproxen, phenylbutazone, piroxicam, rofecoxib*, and probably *other NSAIDs* (risk of toxicity)

  Mifepristone: manufacturer of mifepristone recommends avoid *aspirin* and *NSAIDs* on theoretical grounds

  Muscle Relaxants: *ibuprofen* and possibly *other NSAIDs* reduce excretion of *baclofen* (increased risk of toxicity)
- Tacrolimus: *ibuprofen* and possibly other NSAIDs increase risk of nephrotoxicity

  Theophylline: *rofecoxib* possibly increases plasma concentration of *theophylline*

  Thyroid Hormones: false low total plasma-thyroxine concentration with *phenylbutazone*

  Ulcer-healing Drugs: plasma concentration of *azapropazone* possibly increased by *cimetidine*; plasma concentration of *lornoxicam* increased by *cimetidine*; risk of CNS toxicity with *phenylbutazone* increased by *misoprostol*
- Uricosurics: *probenecid* delays excretion of *indometacin, ketoprofen, ketorolac* (avoid concomitant use), and *naproxen* and increases plasma-NSAID concentration
- Vasodilators: risk of bleeding associated with *ketorolac* increased by *pentoxifylline* (avoid concomitant use); possibly increased risk of bleeding with *pentoxifylline* and *other NSAIDs*

Octreotide

  Antidiabetics: possibly reduces *insulin* and *antidiabetic drug* requirements in diabetes mellitus

  Ciclosporin: absorption of *ciclosporin* reduced (reduced plasma concentration)

  Dopaminergics: increased concentration of *bromocriptine*

  Ulcer-healing Drugs: absorption of *cimetidine* possibly delayed

Oestrogens *see* Contraceptives, Oral
Ofloxacin *see* Quinolones
Olanzapine *see* Antipsychotics
Olsalazine *see* Aminosalicylates
Omeprazole *see* Proton Pump Inhibitors
Opioid Analgesics

  Alcohol: enhanced sedative and hypotensive effect
- Anti-arrhythmics: delayed absorption of *mexiletine*

Opioid Analgesics *(continued)*

  Antibacterials: *rifampicin* accelerates metabolism of *methadone* (reduced effect); *erythromycin* increases plasma concentration of *alfentanil*; manufacturer of *ciprofloxacin* advises avoid premedication with *opioid analgesics* (reduced plasma-ciprofloxacin concentration); *see also* Linezolid
- Anticoagulants: *dextropropoxyphene* may enhance effect of *acenocoumarol* and *warfarin*
- Antidepressants: CNS excitation or depression (hypertension or hypotension) if *pethidine* and possibly *other opioid analgesics* given to patients receiving *MAOIs* (including *moclobemide*)—avoid concomitant use and for 2 weeks after *MAOI* discontinued; *tramadol* increases risk of CNS toxicity with *SSRIs* and *tricyclics*; possibly increased sedation with *tricyclics*; plasma concentration of *methadone* possibly increased by *fluvoxamine*
- Antiepileptics: *dextropropoxyphene* enhances effect of *carbamazepine*; effect of *methadone* and *tramadol* decreased by *carbamazepine*; *phenytoin* accelerates *methadone* metabolism (reduced effect and risk of withdrawal effects)

  Antifungals: metabolism of *alfentanil* inhibited by *ketoconazole* (risk of prolonged or delayed respiratory depression)
- Antipsychotics: enhanced sedative and hypotensive effect
- Antivirals: *methadone* possibly increases plasma concentration of *zidovudine*; plasma concentration of *dextropropoxyphene* and *pethidine* increased by *ritonavir* (risk of toxicity—avoid concomitant use); plasma concentration of *other opioid analgesics* (except methadone) possibly increased by *ritonavir*; plasma concentration of *methadone* reduced by *ritonavir* and possibly by *abacavir* and *nevirapine*

  Anxiolytics and Hypnotics: enhanced sedative effect
- Beta-blockers: *morphine* possibly increases plasma concentration of *esmolol*
- Dopaminergics: hyperpyrexia and CNS toxicity reported if *pethidine* given to patients receiving *selegiline* (avoid concomitant use)

  Metoclopramide and Domperidone: antagonism of gastro-intestinal effects

  Ulcer-healing Drugs: *cimetidine* inhibits metabolism of opioid analgesics notably *pethidine* (increased plasma concentration)

Orciprenaline *see* Sympathomimetics
Orlistat

  Antidiabetics: manufacturer advises avoid concomitant use with *acarbose*
- Ciclosporin: absorption of *ciclosporin* possibly reduced

Orphenadrine *see* Antimuscarinics
Oxaliplatin *see* Platinum Compounds
Oxazepam *see* Anxiolytics and Hypnotics
Oxcarbazepine

- Antibacterials: *see* Linezolid
- Antidepressants: antagonism of anticonvulsant effect (convulsive threshold lowered); manufacturer advises avoid concomitant use with *MAOIs*

  other Antiepileptics: interactions include enhanced effects, increased sedation, and reductions in plasma concentrations; for further details see p. 227
- Antimalarials: *mefloquine* antagonises anticonvulsant effect; *chloroquine* and *hydroxychloroquine* occasionally reduce seizure threshold
- Oestrogens and Progestogens: *oxcarbazepine* accelerates metabolism of *oral contraceptives* (reduced contraceptive effect)

Oxitropium *see* Antimuscarinics
Oxpentifylline *see* Pentoxifylline
Oxprenolol *see* Beta-blockers
Oxybutynin *see* Antimuscarinics
Oxycodone *see* Opioid Analgesics

Oxymetazoline see Sympathomimetics
Oxypertine see Antipsychotics
Oxytetracycline see Tetracyclines
Oxytocin
Anaesthetics: *inhalational anaesthetics* possibly reduce oxytocic effect (also enhanced hypotensive effect and risk of arrhythmias)
Prostaglandins: uterotonic effect potentiated
Sympathomimetics: enhancement of vasopressor effect of *vasoconstrictor sympathomimetics*
Paclitaxel
Antidiabetics: metabolism of *rosiglitazone* possibly inhibited
Pamidronate Sodium see Bisphosphonates
Pancreatin
Antidiabetics: hypoglycaemic effect of *acarbose* reduced
Pancuronium see Muscle Relaxants (non-depolarising)
Pantoprazole see Proton Pump Inhibitors
Papaveretum see Opioid Analgesics
Paracetamol
Anion-exchange Resins: *colestyramine* reduces absorption of *paracetamol*
Anticoagulants: prolonged regular use of *paracetamol* possibly enhances *warfarin*
Cytotoxics: manufacturer of *imatinib* advises restriction or avoidance of concomitant regular *paracetamol*
Metoclopramide and Domperidone: *metoclopramide* and *domperidone* accelerate absorption of *paracetamol* (enhanced effect)
Paraldehyde
• Alcohol: enhanced sedative effect
• Disulfiram: increased risk of toxicity with *paraldehyde*
Parasympathomimetics
Anti-arrhythmics: *procainamide*, *quinidine* and possibly *propafenone* antagonise effect of *neostigmine* and *pyridostigmine*
• Antibacterials: *aminoglycosides*, *clindamycin* and *colistin* antagonise effect of *neostigmine* and *pyridostigmine*
Antimalarials: *chloroquine* and *hydroxychloroquine* have potential to increase symptoms of myasthenia gravis and thus diminish effect of *neostigmine* and *pyridostigmine*
Antimuscarinics: antagonism of effect
Beta-blockers: risk of arrhythmias possibly increased by *pilocarpine*; *propranolol* antagonises effect of *neostigmine* and *pyridostigmine*
Lithium: antagonism of effect of *neostigmine and pyridostigmine*
Muscle Relaxants: *ecothiopate eye-drops*, *edrophonium*, *galantamine*, *neostigmine*, *pyridostigmine*, *rivastigmine* and possibly *donepezil* enhance effect of *suxamethonium*, but antagonise effect of *non-depolarising muscle relaxants*
Paroxetine see Antidepressants, SSRI
Penicillamine
Antacids: reduced absorption of *penicillamine*
Iron: reduced absorption of *penicillamine*
Zinc: reduced absorption of *penicillamine*
Penicillins
Allopurinol: increased risk of rash with concomitant *ampicillin* and *amoxicillin*
other Antibacterials: *neomycin* reduces absorption of *phenoxymethylpenicillin*
Anticoagulants: *see* Phenindione and Warfarin
Cytotoxics: reduced excretion of *methotrexate* (increased risk of toxicity)
Guar Gum: reduced absorption of *phenoxymethylpenicillin*
Muscle Relaxants: effects of *non-depolarising muscle relaxants* enhanced by *piperacillin*
Oestrogens and Progestogens: *see* Contraceptives, Oral
Uricosurics: excretion of *penicillins* reduced by *probenecid*

Pentamidine Isetionate
• Anti-arrhythmics: increased risk of ventricular arrhythmias with *amiodarone* (avoid concomitant use)
• Antihistamines: increased risk of ventricular arrhythmias with *terfenadine* (avoid concomitant use)
• Antipsychotics: increased risk of ventricular arrhythmias with *thioridazine* (avoid concomitant use)
Pentazocine see Opioid Analgesics
Pentostatin
• *other* Cytotoxics: increases pulmonary toxicity of *fludarabine* (unacceptably high incidence of fatalities); increased toxicity with high-dose *cyclophosphamide* (avoid concomitant use)
Pentoxifylline (Oxpentifylline)
• Analgesics: increased risk of bleeding with *ketorolac* (avoid concomitant use); possibly increased risk of bleeding with *other NSAIDs*
Theophylline: plasma-*theophylline* concentration increased
Pergolide
Antipsychotics: antagonism of effect
Metoclopramide and Domperidone: *metoclopramide* antagonises effect
Pericyazine see Antipsychotics
Perindopril see ACE Inhibitors and Angiotensin-II Antagonists
Perphenazine see Antipsychotics
Pethidine see Opioid Analgesics
Phenazocine see Opioid Analgesics
Phenelzine see MAOIs
Phenindione
Note. Change in patient's clinical condition, particularly associated with liver disease, intercurrent illness, or drug administration, necessitates more frequent testing. Major changes in diet (especially involving salads and vegetables) and in alcohol consumption may also affect anticoagulant control
• Anabolic Steroids: anticoagulant effect enhanced by *oxymetholone, stanozolol and others*
• Analgesics: anticoagulant effect enhanced by *aspirin* and possibly *other NSAIDs*; increased risk of haemorrhage with *intravenous diclofenac* and with *ketorolac* (avoid concomitant use)
Anion-exchange Resins: anticoagulant effect enhanced or reduced by *colestyramine*
• Anti-arrhythmics: metabolism inhibited by *amiodarone* (enhanced anticoagulant effect)
Antibacterials: although studies have failed to demonstrate interaction, common experience in anticoagulant clinics is that INR can be altered by course of *oral broad-spectrum antibacterials* such as *ampicillin* (may also apply to antibacterials given for local action on gut such as *neomycin*)
• Antiplatelet Drugs: anticoagulant effect enhanced by *aspirin, clopidogrel, dipyridamole* and *ticlopidine*
• Antivirals: *ritonavir* possibly increases plasma concentration
• Fibrates: enhanced anticoagulant effect
• Oestrogens and Progestogens: anticoagulant effect antagonised by *oral contraceptives*
• Testosterone: anticoagulant effect enhanced
• Thyroid Hormones: enhanced anticoagulant effect
• Vitamins: anticoagulant effect antagonised by *vitamin K* (present in some enteral feeds)
Phenobarbital see Barbiturates
Phenoperidine see Opioid Analgesics
Phenothiazines see Antipsychotics
Phenoxybenzamine see Alpha-blockers
Phenoxymethylpenicillin see Penicillins
Phentolamine see Alpha-blockers
Phenylbutazone see NSAIDs
Phenylephrine see Sympathomimetics
Phenylpropanolamine see Sympathomimetics

Phenytoin

- Analgesics: plasma-phenytoin concentration increased by *aspirin, azapropazone* (avoid concomitant use), *phenylbutazone* and possibly *other NSAIDs*; metabolism of *methadone* accelerated (reduced effect and risk of withdrawal effects)

  Antacids: reduced *phenytoin* absorption

- Anti-arrhythmics: *amiodarone* increases plasma-phenytoin concentration; *phenytoin* reduces plasma concentrations of *disopyramide, mexiletine,* and *quinidine*

- Antibacterials: plasma-phenytoin concentration increased by *chloramphenicol, clarithromycin, cycloserine, isoniazid,* and *metronidazole*; plasma-phenytoin concentration and antifolate effect increased by *co-trimoxazole* and *trimethoprim* and possibly by *other sulphonamides*; plasma-phenytoin concentration reduced by *rifamycins*; plasma concentration of *doxycycline* reduced by *phenytoin*; plasma-phenytoin concentration possibly altered by *ciprofloxacin; see also* Linezolid

- Anticoagulants: metabolism of *acenocoumarol* and *warfarin* accelerated (possibility of reduced anticoagulant effect, but enhancement also reported)

- Antidepressants: antagonism of anticonvulsant effect (convulsive threshold lowered); *fluoxetine* and *fluvoxamine* increase plasma-phenytoin concentration; *phenytoin* reduces plasma concentrations of *mianserin, paroxetine,* and *tricyclics*; plasma concentration of *phenytoin* reduced by *St John's wort* (avoid concomitant use)

  Antidiabetics: plasma-phenytoin concentration transiently increased by *tolbutamide* (possibility of toxicity)

  other Antiepileptics: interactions include enhanced effects, increased sedation, and reductions in plasma concentrations; for further details see p. 227

- Antifungals: plasma-phenytoin concentration increased by *fluconazole* and *miconazole*; plasma concentration of *itraconazole* and *ketoconazole* reduced

- Antimalarials: *mefloquine* antagonises anticonvulsant effect; *chloroquine* and *hydroxychloroquine* occasionally reduce convulsive threshold; increased risk of antifolate effect with *pyrimethamine* (includes *Fansidar®* and *Maloprim®*)

  Antiplatelet Drugs: plasma-phenytoin concentration increased by *aspirin*

- Antipsychotics: antagonism of anticonvulsant effect (convulsive threshold lowered); *phenytoin* accelerates metabolism of *clozapine* and *quetiapine* (reduced plasma concentrations)

- Antivirals: plasma concentration of *indinavir, lopinavir, nelfinavir* and *saquinavir* possibly reduced; plasma-phenytoin concentrations increased or decreased by *zidovudine*

  Anxiolytics and Hypnotics: *diazepam* and possibly *other benzodiazepines* increase or decrease plasma-phenytoin concentration

  Bupropion (amfebutamone): plasma concentration of bupropion reduced

- Calcium-channel Blockers: *diltiazem* and *nifedipine* increase plasma concentration of *phenytoin*; effect of *felodipine, isradipine, nisoldipine* and probably *nicardipine, nifedipine* and *other dihydropyridines, diltiazem,* and *verapamil* reduced

  Cardiac Glycosides: metabolism of *digitoxin only* accelerated (reduced effect)

- Ciclosporin: metabolism of *ciclosporin* accelerated (reduced plasma concentration)

- Corticosteroids: metabolism of *corticosteroids* accelerated (reduced effect)

  Cytotoxics: reduced absorption of *phenytoin*; increased antifolate effect with *methotrexate*; plasma concentration of *imatinib* reduced by *phenytoin*

- Disulfiram: plasma-phenytoin concentration increased

Phenytoin *(continued)*

  Diuretics: increased risk of osteomalacia with *carbonic anhydrase inhibitors*

  Folic Acid and Folinic Acid: plasma-phenytoin concentration possibly reduced by *folic acid* and *folinic acid*

  Food: some *enteral foods* may interfere with absorption of *phenytoin*

  Hormone Antagonists: metabolism of *toremifene* possibly accelerated

  Lithium: neurotoxicity may occur without increased plasma-lithium concentration

  Muscle Relaxants: effect of *non-depolarising muscle relaxants* antagonised (recovery from neuromuscular blockade accelerated)

- Oestrogens and Progestogens: metabolism of *gestrinone, tibolone,* and *oral contraceptives* accelerated (reduced contraceptive effect, **important:** see p. 387)

  Sympathomimetics: plasma-phenytoin concentration increased by *methylphenidate*

  Theophylline: metabolism of *theophylline* accelerated (reduced plasma-theophylline concentration)

  Thyroid Hormones: metabolism of *levothyroxine* and *liothyronine* accelerated (may increase requirements in hypothyroidism); plasma-*phenytoin* concentration posibly increased by *levothyroxine* and *liothyronine*

- Ulcer-healing Drugs: *cimetidine* inhibits metabolism (increased plasma-phenytoin concentration); *sucralfate* reduces absorption; *esomeprazole* and possibly *omeprazole* enhance effect of *phenytoin* (interaction with *lansoprazole* possibly differs)

- Uricosurics: plasma-phenytoin concentration increased by *sulfinpyrazone*

  Vaccines: effect enhanced by *influenza vaccine*

  Vitamins: *vitamin D* requirements possibly increased

Physostigmine *see* Parasympathomimetics

Phytomenadione *see* Vitamins (Vitamin K)

Pilocarpine *see* Parasympathomimetics

Pimozide *see* Antipsychotics

Pindolol *see* Beta-blockers

Pioglitazone *see* Antidiabetics

Piperacillin *see* Penicillins

Pipotiazine *see* Antipsychotics

Piroxicam *see* NSAIDs

Pivmecillinam *see* Penicillins

Pizotifen

  Antihypertensives: hypotensive effect of *adrenergic neurone blockers* antagonised

Platinum Compounds

- Antibacterials: *aminoglycosides, vancomycin* and *capreomycin* increase risk of nephrotoxicity and possibly of ototoxicity

  Diuretics: increased risk of nephrotoxicity and ototoxicity

Polymyxins *see* Colistin

Polythiazide *see* Diuretics (thiazides)

Potassium Aminobenzoate

  Antibacterials: effect of *sulphonamides* inhibited

Potassium Salts (includes Salt Substitutes)

- ACE Inhibitors and Angiotensin-II Antagonists: increased risk of hyperkalaemia

- Ciclosporin: increased risk of hyperkalaemia

- Diuretics: hyperkalaemia with *potassium-sparing diuretics*

- Tacrolimus: increased risk of hyperkalaemia

Pramipexole

  Antipsychotics: manufacturer of pramipexole advises avoid concomitant use

  Ulcer-healing Drugs: *cimetidine* inhibits excretion (increased plasma-pramipexole concentration)

Pravastatin *see* Statins

Prazosin *see* Alpha-blockers (post-synaptic)

Prednisolone *see* Corticosteroids

Prednisone *see* Corticosteroids

Prilocaine
Antibacterials: increased risk of methaemoglobinaemia with *co-trimoxazole* and *sulphonamides*

Primaquine
Mepacrine: increased plasma concentration of *primaquine* (risk of toxicity)

***Primaxin*®**
• Antivirals: increased toxicity with *ganciclovir* (convulsions reported)

Primidone *see* Barbiturates and Primidone

Probenecid
ACE Inhibitors and Angiotensin-II Antagonists: reduced excretion of *captopril*
• Analgesics: *aspirin* antagonises effect; excretion of *indometacin, ketoprofen, ketorolac* (avoid concomitant use), and *naproxen* delayed and increased plasma-NSAID concentrations
Antibacterials: reduced excretion of *cephalosporins, ciprofloxacin, dapsone, nalidixic acid, nitrofurantoin, norfloxacin,* and *penicillins* (increased plasma-concentrations); reduced excretion of *meropenem* (concomitant use not recommended by manufacturer); antagonism by *pyrazinamide*
Antidiabetics: hypoglycaemic effect of *chlorpropamide* possibly enhanced
Antivirals: reduced excretion of *aciclovir, ganciclovir, zidovudine,* and possibly *famciclovir* and *zalcitabine* (increased plasma concentrations)
• Cytotoxics: reduced excretion of *methotrexate* (increased risk of toxicity)

Procainamide
ACE Inhibitors and Angiotensin-II Antagonists: increased risk of toxicity with *captopril*, especially in renal impairment
• *other* Anti-arrhythmics: *amiodarone* increases procainamide-plasma concentrations (increased risk of ventricular arrhythmias—avoid concomitant use); increased myocardial depression with *any anti-arrhythmic*
Antibacterials: *trimethoprim* increases plasma concentration of *procainamide*
• Antidepressants: increased risk of ventricular arrhythmias with *tricyclics*; manufacturer of *reboxetine* advises caution
• Antihistamines: increased risk of ventricular arrhythmias with *mizolastine* and *terfenadine* (avoid concomitant use)
• Antipsychotics: increased risk of ventricular arrhythmias—avoid concomitant use with *pimozide* or *thioridazine*
• Beta-blockers: increased risk of ventricular arrhythmias associated with *sotalol* (avoid concomitant use)
• Muscle Relaxants: muscle relaxant effect enhanced
Parasympathomimetics: antagonism of effect of *neostigmine* and *pyridostigmine*
Tropisetron: risk of ventricular arrhythmias—manufacturer of tropisetron advises caution
• Ulcer-healing Drugs: *cimetidine* inhibits excretion (increased plasma-procainamide concentration)

Procarbazine
Alcohol: disulfiram-like reaction

Prochlorperazine *see* Antipsychotics

Procyclidine *see* Antimuscarinics

Progestogens (*see also* Contraceptives, Oral)
Antibacterials: metabolism accelerated by *rifamycins* (reduced effect)
• Ciclosporin: increased plasma-ciclosporin concentration (inhibition of metabolism)
Hormone Antagonists: *aminoglutethimide* reduces plasma concentration of *medroxyprogesterone*

Proguanil
Antacids: *magnesium trisilicate* reduces absorption of proguanil
Anticoagulants: isolated report of enhanced effect of warfarin

Promazine *see* Antipsychotics

Promethazine *see* Antihistamines

Propafenone
other Anti-arrhythmics: *quinidine* increases plasma concentration of *propafenone*; increased myocardial depression with any *anti-arrhythmic*
• Antibacterials: *rifampicin* reduces plasma concentration of *propafenone* (reduced effect)
• Anticoagulants: increased plasma concentration of *acenocoumarol* and *warfarin* (enhanced effect)
• Antidepressants: increased risk of arrhythmias with *tricyclics*; manufacturer of *reboxetine* advises caution
• Antihistamines: increased risk of ventricular arrhythmias with *mizolastine* and *terfenadine* (avoid concomitant use)
• Antivirals: plasma concentration increased by *ritonavir* (increased risk of ventricular arrhythmias—avoid concomitant use)
Beta-blockers: increased plasma concentration of *metoprolol* and *propranolol*
• Cardiac Glycosides: increased plasma concentrations of *digoxin* (halve maintenance dose of digoxin)
Ciclosporin: plasma-ciclosporin concentration possibly increased
Parasympathomimetics: possible antagonism of effect of *neostigmine* and *pyridostigmine*
Theophylline: increased plasma-theophylline concentration
Tropisetron: risk of ventricular arrhythmias—manufacturer of tropisetron advises caution
• Ulcer-healing Drugs: *cimetidine* increases plasma-propafenone concentration

Propantheline *see* Antimuscarinics

Propiverine *see* Antimuscarinics

Propofol *see* Anaesthetics, General

Propranolol *see* Beta-blockers

Prostaglandins
Oxytocin: uterotonic effect enhanced

Protease Inhibitors *see* Amprenavir; Indinavir; Nelfinavir; Ritonavir; Saquinavir

Proton Pump Inhibitors
Antacids: possibly reduced absorption of *lansoprazole*
• Anticoagulants: effects of *warfarin* possibly enhanced by *omeprazole*; interaction with *lansoprazole* possibly differs
• Antiepileptics: effects of *phenytoin* enhanced by *esomeprazole* and possibly by *omeprazole*; interaction with *lansoprazole* possibly differs
Antifungals: absorption of *ketoconazole* and *itraconazole* reduced
Anxiolytics and Hypnotics: metabolism of *diazepam* possibly inhibited by *omeprazole* and *esomeprazole* (increased effect possible)
Cardiac Glycosides: plasma concentration of *digoxin* possibly slightly increased
Oestrogens and Progestogens: manufacturer advises that *lansoprazole* possibly accelerates metabolism of *oral contraceptives*
Tacrolimus: *omeprazole* possibly increases plasma-tacrolimus concentration
Ulcer-healing Drugs: *sucralfate* possibly reduces absorption of *lansoprazole*

Pseudoephedrine *see* Sympathomimetics

Pyrazinamide
Uricosurics: antagonism of effect of *probenecid* and *sulfinpyrazone*

Pyridostigmine *see* Parasympathomimetics

Pyridoxine *see* Vitamins

Pyrimethamine
• Antibacterials: increased antifolate effect with *co-trimoxazole* and *trimethoprim*
• Antiepileptics: increased antifolate effect and antagonism of anticonvulsant effect with *phenytoin*
• Cytotoxics: increased antifolate effect with *methotrexate*

Quetiapine *see* Antipsychotics

Quinagolide

Note. No interactions reported; theoretical possibility of reduced effect with dopamine antagonists (eg phenothiazines)

Quinapril *see* ACE Inhibitors and Angiotensin-II Antagonists

Quinidine

Antacids and Adsorbents: reduced excretion in alkaline urine (plasma-quinidine concentration occasionally increased); absorption possibly reduced by *kaolin* (possibly reduced plasma concentration)
* *other* Anti-arrhythmics: *amiodarone* increases plasma-quinidine concentrations (and increases risk of ventricular arrhythmias—avoid concomitant use); plasma concentration of *propafenone* increased; increased myocardial depression with *any anti-arrhythmic*
* Antibacterials: increased risk of arrhythmias with *quinupristin/dalfopristin* (avoid concomitant use); *rifamycins* accelerate metabolism (reduced plasma-quinidine concentration)

Anticoagulants: effect of *acenocoumarol* and *warfarin* may be enhanced
* Antidepressants: increased risk of ventricular arrhythmias with *tricyclics*; manufacturer of *reboxetine* advises caution

Antiepileptics: *phenobarbital, phenytoin,* and *primidone* accelerate metabolism (reduced plasma-quinidine concentration)
* Antifungals: plasma concentration increased by *itraconazole* and *miconazole* (increased risk of ventricular arrhythmias—avoid concomitant use)
* Antihistamines: increased risk of ventricular arrhythmias with *mizolastine* and *terfenadine* (avoid concomitant use)
* Antimalarials: increased risk of ventricular arrhythmias with *mefloquine*
* Antipsychotics: increased risk of ventricular arrhythmias—avoid concomitant use with *pimozide* or *thioridazine*
* Antivirals: increased risk of ventricular arrhythmias with *nelfinavir* and *ritonavir* (avoid concomitant use)

Barbiturates and Primidone: *see under* Antiepileptics, above
* Beta-blockers: increased risk of ventricular arrhythmias associated with *sotalol* (avoid concomitant use)
* Calcium-channel Blockers: *nifedipine* reduces plasma-quinidine concentration; *verapamil* increases plasma-quinidine concentration (possibility of extreme hypotension)
* Cardiac Glycosides: plasma concentration of *digoxin* increased (halve digoxin maintenance dose)
* Diuretics: *acetazolamide* reduces excretion (plasma-quinidine concentration occasionally increased); quinidine toxicity increased if hypokalaemia occurs with *acetazolamide, loop diuretics,* and *thiazides*
* Muscle Relaxants: muscle relaxant effect enhanced

Parasympathomimetics: antagonism of effect of *neostigmine and pyridostigmine*

Tropisetron: risk of ventricular arrhythmias—manufacturer of tropisetron advises caution
* Ulcer-healing Drugs: *cimetidine* inhibits metabolism (increased plasma-quinidine concentration)

Quinine
* Anti-arrhythmics: plasma concentration of *flecainide* increased; increased risk of ventricular arrhythmias with *amiodarone*
* Antihistamines: increased risk of ventricular arrhythmias with *terfenadine*—avoid concomitant use
* Antipsychotics: increased risk of ventricular arrhythmias—avoid concomitant use with *pimozide* or *thioridazine*
* *other* Antimalarials: *see* Mefloquine

Quinine *(continued)*
* Cardiac Glycosides: plasma concentration of *digoxin* increased

Ulcer-healing Drugs: *cimetidine* inhibits metabolism (increased plasma-quinine concentration)

Quinolones
* Analgesics: possible increased risk of convulsions with *NSAIDs*; manufacturer of *ciprofloxacin* advises avoid premedication with *opioid analgesics* (reduced plasma-ciprofloxacin concentration)

Antacids and Adsorbents: *antacids* reduce absorption of *ciprofloxacin, levofloxacin, norfloxacin* and *ofloxacin*
* Anticoagulants: anticoagulant effect of *acenocoumarol* and *warfarin* enhanced by *ciprofloxacin, nalidixic acid, norfloxacin* and *ofloxacin*

Antidiabetics: effect of *glibenclamide* possibly enhanced by *ciprofloxacin*

Antiepileptics: *ciprofloxacin* possibly alters plasma concentration of *phenytoin*

Calcium Salts: reduced absorption of *ciprofloxacin*
* Ciclosporin: increased risk of nephrotoxicity

Cytotoxics: toxicity of *melphalan* increased by *nalidixic acid*

5HT$_1$ Agonists: *quinolones* possibly inhibit metabolism of *zolmitriptan* (reduce dose of zolmitriptan)

Iron: absorption of *ciprofloxacin, levofloxacin, norfloxacin,* and *ofloxacin* reduced by *oral iron*
* Theophylline: possible increased risk of convulsions; *ciprofloxacin* and *norfloxacin* increase plasma-theophylline concentration

Ulcer-healing Drugs: *sucralfate* reduces absorption of *ciprofloxacin, levofloxacin, norfloxacin,* and *ofloxacin*

Uricosurics: *probenecid* reduces excretion of *ciprofloxacin, nalidixic acid* and *norfloxacin*

Zinc Salts: *zinc* reduces absorption of *ciprofloxacin* and *norfloxacin*

Quinupristin/Dalfopristin
* Anti-arrhythmics: increased risk of ventricular arrhythmias with *disopyramide, lidocaine* and *quinidine*—avoid concomitant use
* Antihistamines: increased risk of ventricular arrhythmias with *terfenadine*—avoid concomitant use
* Anxiolytics and Hypnotics: increased plasma concentration of *midazolam* (risk of profound sedation); metabolism of *zopiclone* inhibited
* Calcium-channel Blockers: increased plasma concentration of *nifedipine*
* Ciclosporin: increased plasma concentration of ciclosporin
* Tacrolimus: increased plasma concentration of tacrolimus

Rabeprazole *see* Proton Pump Inhibitors

Rabies Vaccine *see* pp. 578 and 591–2

Raloxifene

Anion-exchange Resins: *colestyramine* reduces absorption of raloxifene (manufacturer advises avoid concomitant administration)

Anticoagulants: antagonism of anticoagulant effect of *warfarin* and *acenocoumarol*

Ramipril *see* ACE Inhibitors and Angiotensin-II Antagonists

Ranitidine *see* Histamine H$_2$-antagonists

Ranitidine Bismuth Citrate *see* Histamine H$_2$-antagonists

Reboxetine

Anti-arrhythmics: manufacturer of reboxetine advises caution
* Antibacterials: manufacturer of reboxetine advises avoid concomitant use with *macrolides*; *see also* Linezolid

Reboxetine *(continued)*
- *other* Antidepressants: risk of increased toxicity with *MAOIs* (reboxetine should not be started until 2 weeks after stopping MAOI, and conversely MAOI should not be started until at least 1 week after stopping reboxetine); manufacturer of reboxetine advises avoid concomitant use with *fluvoxamine* and caution with *tricyclics*
- Antifungals: manufacturer of reboxetine advises avoid concomitant use with *imidazoles* and *triazoles*

Antipsychotics: manufacturer of reboxetine advises caution

Ciclosporin: manufacturer of reboxetine advises caution

Diuretics: possibly increased risk of hypokalaemia with *loop diuretics* or *thiazides*

Ergotamine and Ergometrine: possibly increased blood pressure
- Sibutramine: increased risk of CNS toxicity (manufacturer of sibutramine recommends avoid concomitant use)

Remifentanil *see* Opioid Analgesics
Repaglinide *see* Antidiabetics
Retinoids

Alcohol: etretinate formed from *acitretin* in presence of *alcohol*
- Antibacterials: possible increased risk of benign intracranial hypertension with *tetracyclines* and *acitretin, isotretinoin* and *tretinoin*—avoid concomitant use
- Anticoagulants: *acitretin* possibly reduces anticoagulant effect of *warfarin*

Antiepileptics: plasma concentration of *carbamazepine* possibly reduced by *isotretinoin*
- Cytotoxics: *acitretin* increases plasma concentration of *methotrexate* (also increased risk of hepatotoxicity—avoid concomitant use)
- Oestrogens and Progestogens: oral *tretinoin* reduces contraceptive efficacy of low-dose *progestogens*

Vitamins: risk of hypervitaminosis A with *vitamin A* and *acitretin, isotretinoin* and *tretinoin*

Reviparin *see* Heparin
Rifabutin *see* Rifamycins
Rifampicin *see* Rifamycins
Rifamycins

ACE Inhibitors and Angiotensin-II Antagonists: *rifampicin* reduces plasma concentration of active metabolite of *imidapril* (reduced antihypertensive effect)

Analgesics: metabolism of *methadone* accelerated (reduced effect); *rifampicin* reduces plasma concentration of *rofecoxib*

Antacids: reduced absorption of *rifampicin*
- Anti-arrhythmics: metabolism accelerated—reduced plasma concentrations of *disopyramide, mexiletine, propafenone* and *quinidine*
- *other* Antibacterials: metabolism of *chloramphenicol* accelerated by *rifampicin* (reduced plasma concentration); plasma concentration of *dapsone* reduced; plasma concentration of *rifabutin* increased by *clarithromycin* and possibly *other macrolides* (risk of uveitis—reduce rifabutin dose)
- Anticoagulants: metabolism of *acenocoumarol* and *warfarin* accelerated (reduced anticoagulant effect)

Antidepressants: metabolism of some *tricyclics* accelerated by *rifampicin* (reduced plasma concentration)

Antidiabetics: metabolism of *chlorpropamide, tolbutamide and possibly other sulphonylureas* accelerated (reduced effect); *rifampicin* reduces plasma concentration of *repaglinide*
- Antiepileptics: metabolism of *phenytoin* accelerated (reduced plasma concentration); plasma concentration of *carbamazepine* reduced by *rifabutin*

Rifamycins *(continued)*
- Antifungals: metabolism of *fluconazole, itraconazole* and *ketoconazole* accelerated by *rifampicin* (reduced plasma concentrations); plasma concentration of *rifampicin* may be reduced by *ketoconazole*; plasma concentration of *terbinafine* reduced by *rifampicin*; plasma concentration of *rifabutin* increased by *fluconazole* and possibly *other triazoles* (risk of uveitis—reduce rifabutin dose)

Antipsychotics: metabolism of *haloperidol* accelerated by *rifampicin* (reduced plasma concentration)
- Antivirals: concomitant administration of *indinavir* and *rifabutin* increases plasma-rifabutin concentration and decreases plasma-indinavir concentration (reduce dose of rifabutin and increase dose of indinavir); metabolism of *indinavir* enhanced by *rifampicin* (plasma-indinavir concentration significantly reduced—avoid concomitant use); *rifampicin* reduces plasma concentration of *efavirenz* (increase efavirenz dose); plasma concentration of *amprenavir* and *nelfinavir* significantly reduced by *rifampicin* (avoid concomitant use); plasma concentration of *rifabutin* increased by *amprenavir* and *nelfinavir* (halve rifabutin dose); plasma concentration of *rifabutin* increased by *ritonavir* (risk of uveitis—avoid concomitant use); plasma concentration of *saquinavir* reduced (avoid concomitant use); plasma concentration of *nevirapine* reduced; *rifampicin* reduces plasma-lopinavir concentration (avoid concomitant use)

Anxiolytics and Hypnotics: metabolism of *diazepam* and possibly *other benzodiazepines* and of *zaleplon* accelerated by *rifampicin* (reduced plasma concentration)

Atovaquone: plasma concentration reduced by *rifampicin* (possible therapeutic failure of atovaquone)

Beta-blockers: metabolism of *bisoprolol* and *propranolol* accelerated by *rifampicin* (plasma concentrations significantly reduced)

Calcium-channel Blockers: metabolism of *diltiazem, nifedipine, nimodipine* and *verapamil* and possibly *isradipine, nicardipine* and *nisoldipine* accelerated by *rifampicin* (plasma concentrations significantly reduced)

Cardiac Glycosides: metabolism of *digitoxin only* accelerated (reduced effect)
- Ciclosporin: metabolism accelerated (reduced plasma-ciclosporin concentration)
- Corticosteroids: metabolism of *corticosteroids* accelerated (reduced effect)
- Cytotoxics: manufacturer reports interaction with *azathioprine* (transplants possibly rejected)

Lipid-regulating Drugs: metabolism of *fluvastatin* accelerated (reduced effect)
- Oestrogens and Progestogens: metabolism accelerated (contraceptive effect of *both combined and progestogen-only oral contraceptives* reduced, **important:** see p. 387)
- Sirolimus: plasma concentration reduced by *rifampicin*
- Tacrolimus: *rifampicin* decreases plasma-tacrolimus concentration

Theophylline: metabolism accelerated by *rifampicin* (reduced plasma-theophylline concentration)

Thyroid Hormones: metabolism of *levothyroxine* accelerated by *rifampicin* (may increase requirements in hypothyroidism)

Tropisetron: plasma concentration of *tropisetron* reduced by *rifampicin*

Ulcer-healing Drugs: metabolism of *cimetidine* accelerated by *rifampicin* (reduced plasma concentration)

Riluzole
> *Note.* No clinical data available but since riluzole extensively metabolised by the liver, possibility of interactions with a number of drugs—consult product literature for details

Risedronate sodium *see* Bisphosphonates

Risperidone *see* Antipsychotics

Ritodrine *see* Sympathomimetics, Sympathomimetics, Beta$_2$, and p. 382

Ritonavir
* Analgesics: plasma concentration of *dextropropoxyphene, pethidine* and *piroxicam* increased (risk of toxicity—avoid concomitant use); plasma concentrations of *other opioid analgesics* (except methadone) and *other NSAIDs* possibly increased; plasma concentration of *methadone* reduced
* Anti-arrhythmics: increased plasma concentration of *amiodarone, flecainide, propafenone* and *quinidine* (increased risk of ventricular arrhythmias—avoid concomitant use); possibly increased risk of arrhythmias with *disopyramide* and *mexiletine*
* Antibacterials: plasma concentration of *rifabutin* increased by *ritonavir* (risk of uveitis—avoid concomitant use); plasma concentration of *clarithromycin* and possibly *other macrolides* increased (reduce clarithromycin dose in those with renal impairment)
* Anticoagulants: plasma concentration of *warfarin* and *other anticoagulants* possibly increased
* Antidepressants: plasma concentration of *SSRIs* and *tricyclics* possibly increased; plasma concentration reduced by *St John's wort* (avoid concomitant use)
  Antidiabetics: plasma concentration of *tolbutamide* possibly increased
* Antiepileptics: plasma concentration of *carbamazepine* possibly increased
* Antifungals: plasma concentration of *ketoconazole* and possibly *other imidazoles* and *triazoles* increased
* Antihistamines: increased risk of arrhythmias with *terfenadine*—avoid concomitant use; plasma concentration of *other non-sedating antihistamines* possibly increased
  Antimuscarinics: manufacturer of *tolterodine* advises avoid concomitant use
* Antipsychotics: increased plasma concentration of *pimozide* (risk of ventricular arrhythmias—avoid concomitant use); increased plasma concentration of *clozapine* (risk of toxicity—avoid concomitant use); possibly increased plasma concentration of *other antipsychotics*
* *other* Antivirals: combination with *nelfinavir* may lead to increased plasma concentration of either drug; combination with *amprenavir* may increase plasma concentration of both drugs; *ritonavir* increases plasma concentration of *indinavir* and *saquinavir*; increased risk of toxicity with *efavirenz* (monitor liver function tests)
* Anxiolytics and Hypnotics: plasma concentration of *alprazolam, clorazepate, diazepam, flurazepam, midazolam* and *zolpidem* increased (risk of extreme sedation and respiratory depression—avoid concomitant use); plasma concentration of *other anxiolytics and hypnotics* possibly increased
* Bupropion (amfebutamone): plasma concentration of *bupropion* increased (risk of toxicity—avoid concomitant use)
* Calcium-channel Blockers: plasma concentration of *calcium-channel blocker* possibly increased
* Ciclosporin: plasma-ciclosporin concentration possibly increased
  Corticosteroids: plasma concentration of *dexamethasone* and *prednisolone* (and possibly other corticosteroids) possibly increased
* Ergotamine and Ergometrine: risk of ergotism—avoid concomitant use
* Lipid-regulating Drugs: increased risk of myopathy with simvastatin—avoid concomitant use

Ritonavir *(continued)*
* Oestrogens and Progestogens: metabolism accelerated by *ritonavir* (contraceptive effect of combined oral contraceptives reduced)
* Sildenafil: ritonavir significantly increases plasma-*sildenafil* concentration (avoid concomitant use)
* Tacrolimus: plasma-tacrolimus concentration possibly increased
* Theophylline: metabolism accelerated by *ritonavir* (reduced plasma-theophylline concentration)

Rivastigmine *see* Parasympathomimetics

Rizatriptan *see* 5HT$_1$ Agonists

Rocuronium *see* Muscle Relaxants (non-depolarising)

Rofecoxib *see* NSAIDs

Ropinirole
  Antipsychotics: antagonism of antiparkinsonian effect of ropinirole (manufacturer advises avoid concomitant use)

  Metoclopramide: antagonism of antiparkinsonian effect of ropinirole (manufacturer advises avoid concomitant use)

  Oestrogens and Progestogens: plasma concentration of ropinirole increased by *oestrogens*

Ropivacaine
  Antidepressants: *fluvoxamine* reduces metabolism of ropivacaine—avoid prolonged administration of ropivacaine

Rosiglitazone *see* Antidiabetics

Rowachol®
  Anticoagulants: effect of *acenocoumarol* and *warfarin* possibly reduced

St John's wort
* Anticoagulants: reduced anticoagulant effect of *warfarin* (avoid concomitant use)
* other Antidepressants: increased serotonergic effects with *SSRIs* (avoid concomitant use)
* Antiepileptics: reduced plasma concentration of *carbamazepine, phenobarbital* and *phenytoin* avoid concomitant use)
* Antivirals: reduced plasma concentration of *protease inhibitors, efavirenz* and *nevirapine* (avoid concomitant use)
* Barbiturates and Primidone: *see under* Antiepileptics, above
* Cardiac Glycosides: reduced plasma concentration of *digoxin* (avoid concomitant use)
* Ciclosporin: reduced plasma concentration of *ciclosporin* (avoid concomitant use)
* 5HT$_1$ Agonists: increased serotonergic effects (avoid concomitant use)
* Oestrogens and Progestogens: reduced contraceptive effect of *oral contraceptives* (avoid concomitant use)
* Theophylline: reduced plasma concentration of *theophylline* (avoid concomitant use)

Salbutamol *see* Sympathomimetics, Beta$_2$

Salmeterol *see* Sympathomimetics, Beta$_2$

Salt Substitutes *see* Potassium Salts

Saquinavir
* Antibacterials: metabolism accelerated by *rifamycins* (reduced plasma concentration—avoid concomitant use)
* Antidepressants: plasma concentration reduced by *St John's wort* (avoid concomitant use)
* Antiepileptics: plasma concentration possibly reduced by *carbamazepine, phenobarbital* and *phenytoin*
  Antifungals: plasma concentration increased by *ketoconazole* and possibly by *other imidazoles* and *triazoles*
* Antihistamines: increased risk of arrhythmias with *terfenadine*—avoid concomitant use
  Antimuscarinics: manufacturer of *tolterodine* advises avoid concomitant use
* Antipsychotics: possibly increased risk of arrhythmias with *pimozide* (avoid concomitant use); *saquinavir* possibly increases plasma concentration of *thioridazine*

Saquinavir *(continued)*
* *other* Antivirals: *nevirapine* reduces plasma concentration of *saquinavir* (avoid concomitant use); combination with *nelfinavir* may lead to increased plasma concentration of either drug; *indinavir* and *ritonavir* increase plasma concentration of *saquinavir*; *efavirenz* significantly reduces plasma concentration of *saquinavir*
* Anxiolytics and Hypnotics: plasma concentration of *midazolam* possibly increased (prolonged sedation—avoid concomitant use)
  Barbiturates and Primidone: *see under* Antiepileptics above
  Corticosteroids: plasma concentration possibly reduced by *dexamethasone*
* Ergotamine and Ergometrine: possible risk of ergotism—avoid concomitant use
* Lipid-regulating Drugs: increased risk of myopathy with *simvastatin*—avoid concomitant use
  Sildenafil: *saquinavir* increases plasma-*sildenafil* concentration (reduce initial dose of sildenafil)
  Ulcer-healing Drugs: plasma concentration increased by *ranitidine*

Secobarbital *see* Barbiturates and Primidone
Selegiline
  Note. Selegiline is an MAO-B inhibitor
* Analgesics: hyperpyrexia and CNS toxicity with *pethidine* (avoid concomitant use)
  Antibacterials: *see* Linezolid
* Antidepressants: hypertension and CNS excitation with *fluoxetine, paroxetine* and *sertraline* (selegiline should not be started until 5 weeks after discontinuation of fluoxetine, avoid fluoxetine for 2 weeks after stopping selegiline; selegiline should not be started until 2 weeks after stopping sertraline, avoid sertraline for 2 weeks after stopping selegiline); hypotension with *MAOIs*; CNS toxicity reported with *tricyclic antidepressants*; avoid concomitant use with *moclobemide*

Sermorelin
  Note. Avoid preparations which affect release of growth hormone, see p. 365
Sertraline *see* Antidepressants, SSRI
Sevoflurane *see* Anaesthetics, General
Sibutramine
* Antidepressants: increased risk of CNS toxicity (manufacturer of sibutramine recommends avoid concomitant use); avoid *sibutramine* for 2 weeks after stopping *MAOIs*
* Antipsychotics: increased risk of CNS toxicity (manufacturer of sibutramine recommends avoid concomitant use)

Sildenafil
  Note. Grapefruit juice may increase plasma concentration of sildenafil
  Antibacterials: *erythromycin* increases plasma-sildenafil concentration (reduce initial dose of sildenafil)
  Antifungals: *itraconazole* and *ketoconazole* increase plasma-sildenafil concentration (reduce initial dose of sildenafil)
* Antivirals: *ritonavir* significantly increases plasma-sildenafil concentration (avoid concomitant use); *saquinavir* and possibly *amprenavir, indinavir* and *nelfinavir* increase plasma-sildenafil concentration (reduce initial dose of sildenafil)
* Nicorandil: hypotensive effect significantly enhanced—avoid concomitant use
* Nitrates: hypotensive effect significantly enhanced—avoid concomitant use
  Ulcer-healing Drugs: *cimetidine* increases plasma-sildenafil concentration (reduce initial dose of sildenafil)

Simvastatin *see* Statins

Sirolimus
  Note. Grapefruit juice increases plasma-sirolimus concentration
* Antibacterials: *rifampicin* reduces plasma-sirolimus concentration
* Antifungals: *itraconazole, ketoconazole* and *miconazole* increase plasma-sirolimus concentration
* Calcium-channel blockers: *diltiazem* increases plasma-sirolimus concentration
  Ciclosporin: plasma concentration of *sirolimus* possibly increased
Sodium Aurothiomalate *see* Gold
Sodium Bicarbonate *see* Antacids
Sodium Clodronate *see* Bisphosphonates
Sodium Valproate *see* Valproate
Somatropin
  Corticosteroids: may inhibit growth promoting effect of somatropin
  Oestrogens and Progestogens: higher doses of somatropin may be needed with oral *oestrogen* replacement therapy
Sotalol *see* Beta-blockers
Spironolactone *see* Diuretics (potassium-sparing)
Stanozolol *see* Anabolic Steroids
Statins
  Note. Grapefruit juice increases plasma concentration of *simvastatin*
* Antibacterials: metabolism of *fluvastatin* accelerated by *rifampicin* (reduced effect); *clarithromycin* and *erythromycin* increase risk of myopathy with *simvastatin* (avoid concomitant use); *erythromycin* possibly increases risk of myopathy with *atorvastatin*; *clarithromycin* increases plasma concentration of *atorvastatin*
* Anticoagulants: effect of *acenocoumarol* and *warfarin* enhanced by *simvastatin*
* Antidepressants: *nefazodone* increases risk of myopathy with *simvastatin* (avoid concomitant use)
* Antifungals: *itraconazole, ketoconazole* and possibly other *imidazoles* and *triazoles* increase risk of myopathy with *simvastatin*—avoid concomitant use of *itraconazole, ketoconazole* or *miconazole* with *simvastatin*; *itraconazole* and possibly other *imidazoles* and *triazoles* may increase risk of myopathy with *atorvastatin*—avoid concomitant use of *itraconazole* with *atorvastatin*
* Antivirals: *protease inhibitors* increase risk of myopathy with *simvastatin*—avoid concomitant use; *amprenavir, indinavir,* and *nelfinavir* possibly increase risk of myopathy with *atorvastatin*; *amprenavir* possibly increases risk of myopathy with *fluvastatin* and *pravastatin*
  Cardiac Glycosides: plasma-digoxin concentration possibly increased by *atorvastatin*
* Ciclosporin: increased risk of myopathy
  Cytotoxics: plasma concentration of *simvastatin* increased by *imatinib*
* *other* Lipid-regulating Drugs: increased risk of myopathy with *fibrates* and *nicotinic acid* (preferably avoid concomitant use of *statins* and *gemfibrozil*)

Stavudine
* *other* Antivirals: *zidovudine* may inhibit intracellular activation of *stavudine* (avoid concomitant use)
  Cytotoxics: *doxorubicin* may inhibit effect of *stavudine*
Streptomycin *see* Aminoglycosides
Sucralfate
  Antibacterials: reduced absorption of *ciprofloxacin, levofloxacin, norfloxacin, ofloxacin,* and *tetracycline*
* Anticoagulants: absorption of *warfarin* possibly reduced
* Antiepileptics: reduced absorption of *phenytoin*
  Antifungals: reduced absorption of *ketoconazole*
  Antipsychotics: reduced absorption of *sulpiride*

Sucralfate *(continued)*
Cardiac Glycosides: absorption of *cardiac glycosides* possibly reduced
Thyroid Hormones: reduced absorption of *levothyroxine*
other Ulcer-healing Drugs: possibly reduced absorption of *lansoprazole*

Sulfadiazine *see* Co-trimoxazole and Sulphonamides
Sulfadoxine *see* Co-trimoxazole and Sulphonamides
Sulfametopyrazine *see* Co-trimoxazole and Sulphonamides
Sulfasalazine *see* Aminosalicylates
Sulfinpyrazone
Analgesics: *aspirin* antagonises uricosuric effect
<u>Antibacterials</u>: *pyrazinamide* antagonises effect; sulfinpyrazone reduces excretion of *nitrofurantoin* (risk of toxicity)
• Anticoagulants: anticoagulant effect of *acenocoumarol* and *warfarin* enhanced
• Antidiabetics: effect of *sulphonylureas* enhanced
• Antiepileptics: plasma concentration of *phenytoin* increased
Theophylline: plasma-theophylline concentration reduced

Sulindac *see* NSAIDs
Sulphonamides *see* Co-trimoxazole and Sulphonamides
Sulphonylureas *see* Antidiabetics
Sulpiride *see* Antipsychotics
Sumatriptan *see* 5HT$_1$ Agonists
Suxamethonium *see* Muscle Relaxants
Sympathomimetics (*see below* for Beta$_2$-Sympathomimetics)
Alpha$_2$-adrenoceptor Stimulants: possible risk of hypertension with *adrenaline* and *noradrenaline*
• Anaesthetics: risk of arrhythmias if *adrenaline and isoprenaline* given with *volatile liquid anaesthetics* such as *halothane*
• Antibacterials: *see* Linezolid
• Antidepressants: with *tricyclics* administration of *adrenaline* and *noradrenaline* may cause hypertension and arrhythmias (but local anaesthetics with adrenaline appear to be safe); *methylphenidate* may inhibit metabolism of *tricyclics*; with *MAOIs* administration of inotropics such as *dopamine* and *dopexamine* may cause hypertensive crisis; also with *MAOIs* administration of *dexamfetamine* and other *amphetamines, ephedrine, isometheptene, methylphenidate, phenylephrine, phenylpropanolamine,* and *pseudoephedrine* may cause hypertensive crisis (these drugs are contained in anorectics or cold and cough remedies)
Antiepileptics: *methylphenidate* increases plasma concentration of *phenytoin* and possibly of *phenobarbital* and *primidone*
• Antihypertensives: sympathomimetics in *anorectics* and *cold and cough remedies (see above)* and *methylphenidate* antagonise hypotensive effect of *adrenergic neurone blockers*
Barbiturates and Primidone: *see under* Antiepileptics, above
• Beta-blockers: severe hypertension with *adrenaline* and *noradrenaline* and possibly with *dobutamine* (especially with non-selective beta-blockers)
Corticosteroids: *ephedrine* accelerates metabolism of *dexamethasone*
• Dopaminergics: increased risk of toxicity when *isometheptene* or *phenylpropanolamine* given with *bromocriptine*; effect of *adrenaline, dobutamine, dopamine, isoprenaline* and *noradrenaline* possibly enhanced by *entacapone*
Doxapram: risk of hypertension
Ergotamine and Ergometrine: increased risk of ergotism
Oxytocin: hypertension with vasoconstrictor sympathomimetics
• *other* Sympathomimetics: *dopexamine* possibly potentiates effect of *adrenaline* and *noradrenaline*

Sympathomimetics, Beta$_2$
• Antihypertensives: acute hypotension reported with *salbutamol infusion* and *methyldopa*
Corticosteroids: increased risk of hypokalaemia if high doses of *corticosteroids* given with high doses of *bambuterol, fenoterol, formoterol, ritodrine, salbutamol, salmeterol,* and *terbutaline; see also* CSM advice (hypokalaemia), p. 134
Diuretics: increased risk of hypokalaemia if *acetazolamide, loop diuretics,* and *thiazides* given with high doses of *bambuterol, fenoterol, formoterol, ritodrine, salbutamol, salmeterol, and terbutaline; see also* CSM advice (hypokalaemia), p. 134
Muscle Relaxants: effect of *suxamethonium* enhanced by *bambuterol*
Theophylline: increased risk of hypokalaemia if given with high doses of *bambuterol, fenoterol, formoterol, ritodrine, salbutamol, salmeterol,* and *terbutaline; see also* CSM advice (hypokalaemia), p. 134

Tacrolimus
Note. Grapefruit juice increases the plasma-tacrolimus concentration
• Analgesics: *ibuprofen* and possibly *other NSAIDs* increase risk of nephrotoxicity
• Antibacterials: *clarithromycin, erythromycin, quinupristin/dalfopristin* and possibly *chloramphenicol* increase plasma-tacrolimus concentration; *rifampicin* decreases plasma-tacrolimus concentration
• Antidepressants: *nefazodone* increases plasma-tacrolimus concentration
• Antifungals: *amphotericin* increases risk of nephrotoxicity; *clotrimazole, fluconazole, ketoconazole* and possibly *other imidazoles* and *triazoles* increase plasma-tacrolimus concentration
• Antivirals: *ritonavir* possibly increases plasma-tacrolimus concentration
• Calcium-channel blockers: *nifedipine* and *diltiazem* increase plasma-tacrolimus concentration
• Ciclosporin: plasma-ciclosporin half-life prolonged (increased risk of toxicity—avoid concomitant use)
• Diuretics: *potassium-sparing diuretics* increased risk of hyperkalaemia
Hormone Antagonists: *danazol* possibly increases plasma-tacrolimus concentration
Oestrogens and Progestogens: efficacy of *oral contraceptives* possibly decreased
• Potassium salts: increased risk of hyperkalaemia
Ulcer-healing Drugs: *omeprazole* possibly increases plasma-tacrolimus concentration

Tamoxifen
• Anticoagulants: anticoagulant effect of *acenocoumarol* and *warfarin* enhanced
other Hormone Antagonists: *aminoglutethimide* reduces plasma-tamoxifen concentration
Tamsulosin *see* Alpha-blockers (post-synaptic)
Taxanes *see* Docetaxel, Paclitaxel
Teicoplanin
Antibacterials: increased risk of ototoxicity and nephrotoxicity with *aminoglycosides* and *colistin*
Telmisartan *see* ACE Inhibitors and Angiotensin-II Antagonists
Temazepam *see* Anxiolytics and Hypnotics
Temocillin *see* Penicillins
Temozolomide
Antiepileptics: *valproate* increases plasma concentration of *temozolomide*
Tenoxicam *see* NSAIDs
Terazosin *see* Alpha-blockers (post-synaptic)
Terbinafine
Antibacterials: plasma concentration reduced by *rifampicin*
<u>Oestrogens and Progestogens</u>: occasional reports of breakthrough bleeding with *oral contraceptives*
Ulcer-healing Drugs: plasma concentration increased by *cimetidine*
Terbutaline *see* Sympathomimetics, Beta$_2$

Terfenadine *see* Antihistamines
Testosterone
* Anticoagulants: anticoagulant effect of *warfarin,
  acenocoumarol* and *phenindione* enhanced
  Antidiabetics: hypoglycaemic effect possibly
  enhanced
Tetrabenazine (general extrapyramidal interactions
  as for Antipsychotics)
* Antibacterials: *see* Linezolid
* Antidepressants: CNS excitation and hypertension
  with *MAOIs*
Tetracosactide *see* Corticosteroids
Tetracyclines
  ACE Inhibitors and Angiotensin-II Antagonists:
  quinapril tablets reduce absorption (contain
  magnesium carbonate excipient)
  Antacids and Adsorbents: reduced absorption with
  antacids and possibly with *kaolin*
  Anticoagulants: *see* Phenindione and Warfarin
  Antiepileptics: *carbamazepine, phenobarbital,
  phenytoin,* and *primidone* increase metabolism of
  doxycycline (reduced plasma concentration)
  Atovaquone: plasma-atovaquone concentration
  reduced by *tetracycline*
  Barbiturates and Primidone: *see under* Antiepileptics,
  above
  Calcium Salts: reduced absorption of *tetracyclines*
* Ciclosporin: *doxycycline* possibly increases plasma-
  ciclosporin concentration
  Dairy products: reduced absorption (except
  doxycycline and *minocycline*)
  Ergotamine and Ergometrine: increased risk of
  ergotism
  Iron: absorption of *oral iron* reduced by *tetracyclines*
  and *vice versa*
  Oestrogens and Progestogens: *see* Contraceptives,
  Oral (main list)
* Retinoids: possible increased risk of benign
  intracranial hypertension with *tetracyclines* and
  acitretin, isotretinoin and *tretinoin*—avoid
  concomitant use
  Ulcer-healing Drugs: *tripotassium dicitratobismuthate* and *sucralfate* reduce absorption
  Zinc Salts: reduced absorption (and *vice versa*)
Theophylline
  Allopurinol: possibly increased plasma-theophylline
  concentration
  Anaesthetics: increased risk of arrhythmias with
  halothane; increased risk of convulsions with
  ketamine
  Analgesics: *rofecoxib* possibly increases plasma
  concentration of theophylline
  Anti-arrhythmics: antagonism of anti-arrhythmic
  effect of *adenosine*; plasma-theophylline
  concentration increased by *mexiletine* and
  propafenone
* Antibacterials: possible increased risk of convulsions
  with *quinolones*; plasma-theophylline concentration
  increased by *ciprofloxacin, clarithromycin,
  erythromycin* (if erythromycin given by mouth, also
  decreased plasma-erythromycin concentration), and
  norfloxacin and possibly increased by *isoniazid*;
  plasma-theophylline concentration reduced by
  rifampicin
* Antidepressants: plasma-theophylline concentration
  increased by *fluvoxamine* (concomitant use should
  usually be avoided, but where not possible halve
  theophylline dose and monitor plasma-theophylline
  concentration); plasma-theophylline concentration
  reduced by *St John's wort* (avoid concomitant use)
  Antiepileptics: plasma-theophylline concentration
  reduced by *carbamazepine, phenobarbital,
  phenytoin,* and *primidone*
* Antifungals: plasma-theophylline concentration
  possibly increased by *fluconazole* and *ketoconazole*
* Antiplatelet Drugs: *ticlopidine* increases plasma-
  theophylline concentration (risk of toxicity)

Theophylline *(continued)*
* Antivirals: plasma-theophylline concentration
  reduced by *ritonavir*
  Barbiturates and Primidone: *see under* Antiepileptics,
  above
  Beta-blockers: should be avoided on pharmacological
  grounds (bronchospasm)
* Calcium-channel Blockers: plasma-theophylline
  concentration increased by *diltiazem, verapamil,*
  and possibly *other calcium-channel blockers*
  Corticosteroids: increased risk of hypokalaemia
  Disulfiram: increases plasma-theophylline
  concentration
  Diuretics: increased risk of hypokalaemia with
  acetazolamide, loop diuretics and *thiazides*
  Doxapram: increased CNS stimulation
  Hormone Antagonists: plasma-theophylline
  concentration reduced by *aminoglutethimide*
  Interferons: plasma-theophylline concentration
  increased by *interferon alfa*
  Leukotriene Antagonists: *zafirlukast* possibly
  increases plasma-theophylline concentration;
  plasma-zafirlukast concentration reduced
  Lithium: *lithium* excretion accelerated (reduced
  plasma-lithium concentration)
  Nicotine and Tobacco: plasma-theophylline
  concentration reduced by *tobacco smoking*
  Oestrogens and Progestogens: plasma-theophylline
  concentration increased by *combined oral
  contraceptives*
  Pentoxifylline: plasma-theophylline concentration
  increased
  Sympathomimetics: increased risk of hypokalaemia
  if *theophylline* given with high doses of
  *bambuterol, fenoterol, formoterol, ritodrine,
  salbutamol, salmeterol,* and *terbutaline*; *see also*
  CSM advice (hypokalaemia), p. 134
* Ulcer-healing Drugs: plasma-theophylline
  concentration increased by *cimetidine*
  Uricosurics: plasma-theophylline concentration
  reduced by *sulfinpyrazone*
  Vaccines: plasma-theophylline concentration
  occasionally increased by *influenza vaccine*
Thiopental *see* Anaesthetics, General
Thioridazine *see* Antipsychotics
Thiotepa
  Muscle Relaxants: effect of *suxamethonium* enhanced
Thymoxamine *see* Moxisylyte
Thyroid Hormones
  Analgesics: false low total plasma-thyroxine
  concentration with *phenylbutazone*
  Anion-exchange Resins: *colestyramine* reduces
  absorption of *levothyroxine* and *liothyronine*
  Anti-arrhythmics: for use with *amiodarone*, see p. 72
  Antibacterials: *rifampicin* accelerates metabolism of
  levothyroxine (may increase requirements in
  hypothyroidism)
* Anticoagulants: effect of *acenocoumarol,
  phenindione, and warfarin* enhanced
  Antiepileptics: *carbamazepine, phenobarbital,
  phenytoin,* and *primidone* accelerate metabolism of
  levothyroxine and *liothyronine* (may increase
  requirements in hypothyroidism); plasma
  concentration of *phenytoin* possibly increased by
  levothyroxine and *liothyronine*
  Barbiturates and Primidone: *see under* Antiepileptics,
  above
  Ulcer-healing Drugs: *sucralfate* reduces absorption of
  levothyroxine
Thyroxine *see* Thyroid Hormones
Tiagabine
  Antibacterials: *see* Linezolid
* Antidepressants: antagonism of anticonvulsant effect
  (convulsive threshold lowered)
  other Antiepileptics: interactions include enhanced
  effects, increased sedation, and reductions in
  plasma concentrations; for further details, see
  p. 227

Tiagabine *(continued)*
* Antimalarials: *mefloquine* antagonises anticonvulsant effect; *chloroquine* and *hydroxychloroquine* occasionally reduce convulsive threshold

Tiaprofenic Acid *see* NSAIDs

Tibolone
Antibacterials: *rifampicin* accelerates metabolism (reduced plasma concentration)
Antiepileptics: *carbamazepine, phenobarbital, phenytoin, and primidone* accelerate metabolism (reduced plasma concentration)
Barbiturates and Primidone: *see* Antiepileptics, above

Ticlopidine
Analgesics: increased risk of bleeding with *NSAIDs* (including *aspirin*)
Anticoagulants: increased risk of bleeding
other Antiplatelet Drugs: increased risk of bleeding
* Ciclosporin: reduced plasma concentration of *ciclosporin*
* Theophylline: increased plasma concentration of *theophylline* (risk of toxicity)

Tiludronic Acid *see* Bisphosphonates

Timentin® *see* Penicillins

Timolol *see* Beta-blockers

Tinidazole
Alcohol: possibly disulfiram-like reaction

Tinzaparin *see* Heparin

Tizanidine *see* Muscle Relaxants

Tobramycin *see* Aminoglycosides

Tolbutamide *see* Antidiabetics (sulphonylurea)

Tolfenamic Acid *see* NSAIDs

Tolterodine *see* Antimuscarinics

Topiramate
Antibacterials: *see* Linezolid
* Antidepressants: antagonism of anticonvulsant effect (convulsive threshold lowered)
other Antiepileptics: interactions include enhanced effects, increased sedation, and reductions in plasma concentrations; for further details, see p. 227
* Antimalarials: *mefloquine* antagonises anticonvulsant effect; *chloroquine* and *hydroxychloroquine* occasionally reduce convulsive threshold
Oestrogens and Progestogens: metabolism of *oral contraceptives* accelerated (reduced contraceptive effect, **important:** see p. 387)

Torasemide *see* Diuretics (loop)

Toremifene
* Anticoagulants: anticoagulant effect of *acenocoumarol* and *warfarin* possibly enhanced
Antiepileptics: metabolism possibly accelerated by *carbamazepine, phenobarbital* and *phenytoin* (reduced plasma-toremifene concentration)
Diuretics: increased risk of hypercalcaemia with *thiazides*

Tramadol *see* Opioid Analgesics

Trandolapril *see* ACE Inhibitors and Angiotensin-II Antagonists

Tranylcypromine *see* MAOIs

Trazodone
Alcohol: enhanced sedative effect
Alpha$_2$-adrenoceptor Stimulants: manufacturers of *apraclonidine* and *brimonidine* advise avoid concomitant use
* *other* Antidepressants: as for Antidepressants, Tricyclic
* Antiepileptics: antagonism of anticonvulsant effect
Anxiolytics and Hypnotics: enhanced sedative effect
* Sibutramine: increased risk of CNS toxicity (manufacturer of sibutramine recommends avoid concomitant use)

Tretinoin *see* Retinoids

Triamcinolone *see* Corticosteroids

Triamterene *see* Diuretics (potassium-sparing)

Triclofos *see* Anxiolytics and Hypnotics

Trientine
Iron: absorption of *oral iron* reduced

Trifluoperazine *see* Antipsychotics

Trihexyphenidyl (Benzhexol) *see* Antimuscarinics

Triiodothyroxine (liothyronine) *see* Thyroid Hormones

Trilostane
Diuretics: increased risk of hyperkalaemia with *potassium-sparing diuretics*

Trimeprazine (Alimemazine) *see* Antihistamines

Trimethoprim
Anti-arrhythmics: plasma concentration of *procainamide* increased
Antibacterials: plasma concentration of both *trimethoprim* and *dapsone* possibly increased with concomitant use
Anticoagulants: effect of *acenocoumarol* and *warfarin* possibly enhanced
Antiepileptics: plasma concentration and antifolate effect of *phenytoin* increased
* Antimalarials: increased risk of antifolate effect with *pyrimethamine* (in *Fansidar®* and *Maloprim®*)
Antivirals: plasma concentration of *lamivudine* and possibly *zalcitabine* increased—avoid high-dose co-trimoxazole with *lamivudine*
Cardiac glycosides: plasma concentration of *digoxin* possibly increased
* Ciclosporin: increased risk of nephrotoxicity; plasma-ciclosporin concentration possibly reduced by *intravenous trimethoprim*
* Cytotoxics: increased risk of haematological toxicity with *azathioprine* and *mercaptopurine*; antifolate effect of *methotrexate* increased (avoid concomitant use)

Trimetrexate
Note. Limited clinical data, but potential for serious interactions—consult product literature for details

Trimipramine *see* Antidepressants, Tricyclic

Tripotassium Dicitratobismuthate
Antibacterials: reduced absorption of *tetracyclines*

Triprolidine *see* Antihistamines

Tropicamide *see* Antimuscarinics

Tropisetron
Anti-arrhythmics: risk of ventricular arrhythmias—manufacturer advises caution
Antibacterials: *rifampicin* reduces plasma concentration of *tropisetron*
Barbiturates and Primidone: *phenobarbitone* reduces plasma concentration of *tropisetron*
Beta-blockers: risk of ventricular arrhythmias—manufacturer advises caution

Trospium *see* Antimuscarinics

Tryptophan
* Antibacterials: *see* Linezolid
* *other* Antidepressants: CNS excitation and confusion with *MAOIs* (reduce tryptophan dose); agitation and nausea with *fluoxetine, fluvoxamine, paroxetine, and sertraline*
* Sibutramine: increased risk of CNS toxicity (manufacturer of sibutramine recommends avoid concomitant use)

Typhoid Vaccine *see* p. 593

Uftoral® *see* Fluorouracil

Ulcer-healing Drugs *see* individual drugs

Uricosurics *see* individual drugs

Ursodeoxycholic Acid *see* Bile Acids

Vaccines *see* Influenza Vaccine (p. 586), Rabies Vaccine (pp. 578 and 591–2), Typhoid Vaccine (p. 593)
Note. For a general warning on *live vaccines* and *high doses of corticosteroids* or *other immunosuppressive drugs*, see section 14.1; for advice on *live vaccines* and *immunoglobulins*, see under Normal Immunoglobulin, section 14.5

Valaciclovir *see* Aciclovir and Famciclovir
Note. Interactions as for aciclovir

Valproate
Analgesics: *aspirin* enhances effect
Anion-exchange Resins: *colestyramine* possibly reduces absorption
Antibacterials: *erythromycin* possibly inhibits metabolism (increased plasma-valproate concentration); plasma concentration reduced by *meropenem; see also* Linezolid

Valproate *(continued)*

Anticoagulants: anticoagulant effect of *acenocoumarol* and *warfarin* possibly increased

• Antidepressants: antagonism of anticonvulsant effect (convulsive threshold lowered)

other Antiepileptics: interactions include enhanced effects, increased sedation, and reductions in plasma concentrations; for further details, see p. 227

• Antimalarials: *mefloquine* antagonises anticonvulsant effect; *chloroquine* and *hydroxychloroquine* occasionally reduce convulsive threshold

• Antipsychotics: antagonism of anticonvulsant effect (convulsive threshold lowered)

Antivirals: plasma concentration of *zidovudine* possibly increased (risk of toxicity)

Bupropion (amfebutamone): metabolism of *bupropion* inhibited

Cytotoxics: plasma concentration of *temozolomide* increased

Ulcer-healing Drugs: *cimetidine* inhibits metabolism (increased plasma-valproate concentration)

Valsartan *see* ACE Inhibitors and Angiotensin-II Antagonists

Vancomycin

Anaesthetics: hypersensitivity-like reactions can occur with concomitant vancomycin infusion

Anion-exchange Resins: antagonism of *oral vancomycin* by *colestyramine*

other Antibacterials: increased risk of ototoxicity and nephrotoxicity with *aminoglycosides, colistin* and *capreomycin*

Cytotoxics: increased risk of ototoxicity and nephrotoxicity with *cisplatin*

Diuretics: increased risk of ototoxicity with *loop diuretics*

Vecuronium *see* Muscle Relaxants (non-depolarising)

Venlafaxine

• Antibacterials: *see* Linezolid

• *other* Antidepressants: CNS effects of *MAOIs* increased (risk of toxicity); *venlafaxine* should not be started until 2 weeks after stopping *MAOI*; conversely, *MAOI* should not be started until at least 1 week after stopping *venlafaxine*

Antipsychotics: increased plasma concentration of *clozapine*

Dopaminergics: manufacturer of *entacapone* advises avoid concomitant use

• Sibutramine: increased risk of CNS toxicity (manufacturer of sibutramine recommends avoid concomitant use)

Verapamil *see* Calcium-channel Blockers

Vigabatrin

Antibacterials: *see* Linezolid

other Antiepileptics: interactions include enhanced effects, increased sedation, and reductions in plasma concentrations; for further details, see p. 227

• Antimalarials: *mefloquine* antagonises anticonvulsant effect; *chloroquine* and *hydroxychloroquine* occasionally reduce convulsive threshold

Vincristine

Antifungals: *itraconazole* may inhibit metabolism (increased risk of neurotoxicity)

Vitamins

• Altretamine: *pyridoxine* reduces response to *altretamine*

• Anticoagulants: anticoagulant effect of *acenocoumarol, phenindione, and warfarin* antagonised by *vitamin K* (present in some enteral feeds)

Antiepileptics: *vitamin D* requirements possibly increased by *carbamazepine, phenobarbital, phenytoin,* and *primidone*

Barbiturates and Primidone: *see* Antiepileptics, above

Diuretics: increased risk of hypercalcaemia if *thiazides* given with *vitamin D*

Dopaminergics: effect of *levodopa* antagonised by *pyridoxine* (unless a dopa decarboxylase inhibitor also given)

Vitamins *(continued)*

Retinoids: risk of hypervitaminosis A with *vitamin A* and *acitretin, isotretinoin* and *tretinoin*

Warfarin and other Coumarins

Note. Change in patient's clinical condition, particularly associated with liver disease, intercurrent illness, or drug administration, necessitates more frequent testing. Major changes in diet (especially involving salads and vegetables) and in alcohol consumption may also affect warfarin control

• Alcohol: enhanced anticoagulant effect with large amounts (see also above)

Allopurinol: anticoagulant effect possibly enhanced

• Anabolic Steroids: *oxymetholone, stanozolol and others* enhance anticoagulant effect

• Analgesics: *aspirin* increases risk of bleeding due to antiplatelet effect; anticoagulant effect seriously enhanced by *azapropazone* and *phenylbutazone* (avoid concomitant use), and possibly enhanced by *diclofenac, diflunisal, flurbiprofen, ibuprofen, mefenamic acid, meloxicam, piroxicam, sulindac,* and *other NSAIDs*; anticoagulant effect possibly also enhanced by *dextropropoxyphene* and by prolonged regular use of *paracetamol*; increased risk of haemorrhage with *intravenous diclofenac* and with *ketorolac* (avoid concomitant use)

• Anion-exchange Resins: *colestyramine* may enhance or reduce anticoagulant effect

• Anti-arrhythmics: *amiodarone and propafenone* enhance anticoagulant effect; *quinidine* may enhance anticoagulant effect

• Antibacterials: anticoagulant effect reduced by *rifamycins*; anticoagulant effect enhanced by *cefamandole, chloramphenicol, ciprofloxacin, co-trimoxazole, erythromycin, metronidazole, ofloxacin,* and *sulphonamides*; anticoagulant effect possibly also enhanced by *aztreonam, clarithromycin* and some other *macrolides, nalidixic acid, neomycin, norfloxacin, tetracyclines,* and *trimethoprim*; although studies have failed to demonstrate interaction, common experience in anticoagulant clinics is that INR can be altered following course of oral *broad-spectrum antibacterial, such as ampicillin* (may also apply to antibacterials given for local action on gut such as *neomycin*)

• Antidepressants: *SSRIs* possibly enhance anticoagulant effect; anticoagulant effect of *warfarin* reduced by *St John's wort* (avoid concomitant use)

Antidiabetics: possibly enhanced hypoglycaemic effects of *sulphonylureas* and changes to anticoagulant effect

• Antiepileptics: reduced anticoagulant effect with *carbamazepine, phenobarbital, and primidone*; anticoagulant effect possibly increased by *valproate*; both reduced and enhanced effects reported with *phenytoin*

• Antifungals: anticoagulant effect reduced by *griseofulvin;* anticoagulant effect enhanced by *fluconazole, itraconazole, ketoconazole, and miconazole* (note: oral gel and possibly vaginal formulations absorbed)

Antimalarials: isolated report of enhanced effect of warfarin with *proguanil*

• Antiplatelet Drugs: *aspirin, clopidogrel, dipyridamole* and *ticlopidine* increase risk of bleeding due to antiplatelet effect; manufacturer of *clopidogrel* advises avoid concomitant use with *warfarin*

• Antivirals: *ritonavir* possibly increases plasma concentration

Anxiolytics and Hypnotics: *chloral* and *triclofos* may transiently enhance anticoagulant effect

• Barbiturates and Primidone: anticoagulant effect reduced

• Corticosteroids: anticoagulant effect possibly altered

Warfarin and other Coumarins *(continued)*
* Cytotoxics: anticoagulant effect possibly enhanced by *ifosfamide* and *fluorouracil*; anticoagulant effect of *warfarin* possibly reduced by *azathioprine*; manufacturer of *imatinib* advises replacement of *warfarin* with a heparin (possibility of enhanced warfarin effect)
* Disulfiram: enhanced anticoagulant effect
* Hormone Antagonists: *aminoglutethimide* reduces anticoagulant effect; *danazol, flutamide, tamoxifen* and possibly *bicalutamide* and *toremifene* enhance anticoagulant effect
  Leukotriene Antagonists: *zafirlukast* enhances anticoagulant effect of *warfarin*
* Lipid-regulating Drugs: *fibrates* and *simvastatin* enhance anticoagulant effect
* Oestrogens and Progestogens: *oral contraceptives* reduce anticoagulant effect
  Raloxifene: antagonism of anticoagulant effect
* Retinoids: *acitretin* possibly reduces anticoagulant effect
  Rowachol®: possibly reduced anticoagulant effect
* Testosterone: anticoagulant effect of *warfarin* and *acenocoumarol* enhanced
* Thyroid Hormones: enhanced anticoagulant effect
* Ulcer-healing Drugs: *sucralfate* possibly reduces anticoagulant effect (reduced absorption); *cimetidine* and possibly *omeprazole* enhance anticoagulant effect; interaction with *lansoprazole* possibly differs
* Uricosurics: *sulfinpyrazone* enhances anticoagulant effect
  Vaccines: *influenza vaccine* occasionally enhances anticoagulant effect
* Vitamins: *vitamin K* reduces anticoagulant effect; major changes in diet (especially involving vegetables) may affect control; *vitamin K* also present in some enteral feeds

Xipamide *see* Diuretics (thiazide-related)
Xylometazoline *see* Sympathomimetics
Zafirlukast *see* Leukotriene Antagonists
Zalcitabine
  Note. Clinical data limited. Avoid use with other drugs which have potential to cause peripheral neuropathy or pancreatitis—for further details consult product literature
  Antacids: possibly reduce absorption
  Antibacterials: *trimethoprim* possibly increases plasma concentration of zalcitabine
  Ulcer-healing Drugs: *cimetidine* possibly increases plasma concentration of zalcitabine
  Uricosurics: *probenecid* possibly increases plasma concentration of zalcitabine
Zaleplon *see* Anxiolytics and Hypnotics
Zidovudine
  Note. Increased risk of toxicity with nephrotoxic and myelosuppressive drugs—for further details consult product literature
  Analgesics: increased risk of haematological toxicity with *NSAIDs*; *methadone* possibly increases plasma-zidovudine concentration
  Antibacterials: *clarithromycin tablets* reduce absorption of *zidovudine*
  Antiepileptics: plasma-phenytoin concentrations increased or decreased; plasma-zidovudine concentration possibly increased by *valproate* (risk of toxicity)
  Antifungals: plasma concentration of *zidovudine* increased by *fluconazole* (increased risk of toxicity)
* *other* Antivirals: profound myelosuppression with *ganciclovir* (if possible avoid concomitant administration, particularly during initial ganciclovir therapy); intracellular activation of *stavudine* inhibited (avoid concomitant use)
  Uricosurics: *probenecid* increases plasma-zidovudine concentration and risk of toxicity

Zinc
  Antibacterials: reduced absorption of *ciprofloxacin* and *norfloxacin*; *tetracyclines* reduce absorption of zinc (and *vice versa*)
  Iron: reduced absorption of *oral iron* (and *vice versa*)
  Penicillamine: reduced absorption of *penicillamine*
Zoledronic Acid *see* Bisphosphonates
Zolmitriptan *see* 5HT$_1$ Agonists
Zolpidem *see* Anxiolytics and Hypnotics
Zopiclone *see* Anxiolytics and Hypnotics
Zotepine *see* Antipsychotics
Zuclopenthixol *see* Antipsychotics

Appendix 2: Liver disease

Liver disease may alter the response to drugs in several ways as indicated below, and drug prescribing should be kept to a minimum in all patients with severe liver disease. The main problems occur in patients with jaundice, ascites, or evidence of encephalopathy.

IMPAIRED DRUG METABOLISM. Metabolism by the liver is the main route of elimination for many drugs, but the hepatic reserve appears to be large and liver disease has to be severe before important changes in drug metabolism occur. Routine liver-function tests are a poor guide to the capacity of the liver to metabolise drugs, and in the individual patient it is not possible to predict the extent to which the metabolism of a particular drug may be impaired.

A few drugs, e.g. rifampicin and fusidic acid, are excreted in the bile unchanged and may accumulate in patients with intrahepatic or extrahepatic obstructive jaundice.

HYPOPROTEINAEMIA. The hypoalbuminaemia in severe liver disease is associated with reduced protein binding and increased toxicity of some highly protein-bound drugs such as phenytoin and prednisolone.

REDUCED CLOTTING. Reduced hepatic synthesis of blood-clotting factors, indicated by a prolonged prothrombin time, increases the sensitivity to oral anticoagulants such as warfarin and phenindione.

HEPATIC ENCEPHALOPATHY. In severe liver disease many drugs can further impair cerebral function and may precipitate hepatic encephalopathy. These include all sedative drugs, opioid analgesics, those diuretics that produce hypokalaemia, and drugs that cause constipation.

FLUID OVERLOAD. Oedema and ascites in chronic liver disease may be exacerbated by drugs that give rise to fluid retention, e.g. NSAIDs, corticosteroids, and carbenoxolone.

HEPATOTOXIC DRUGS. Hepatotoxicity is either dose-related or unpredictable (idiosyncratic). Drugs causing dose-related toxicity may do so at lower doses than in patients with normal liver function, and some drugs producing reactions of the idiosyncratic kind do so more frequently in patients with liver disease. These drugs should be avoided or used very carefully.

Table of drugs to be avoided or used with caution in liver disease

The list of drugs given below is not comprehensive and is based on current information concerning the use of these drugs in therapeutic dosage. Products introduced or amended since publication of BNF No. 42 (September 2001) are underlined.

Drug	Comment
Abacavir	No dosage adjustment required in mild hepatic impairment; avoid in moderate or severe hepatic impairment
Abciximab	Avoid in severe liver disease—increased risk of bleeding
Acamprosate	Avoid in severe liver disease
Acarbose	Avoid
ACE Inhibitors	Use of prodrugs such as cilazapril, enalapril, fosinopril, imidapril, moexipril, perindopril, quinapril, ramipril, and trandolapril requires close monitoring in patients with impaired liver function
Aceclofenac	see NSAIDs
Acemetacin	see NSAIDs
Acenocoumarol (nicoumalone)	see Anticoagulants, Oral
Acitretin	Avoid—further impairment of liver function may occur
Aclarubicin	Manufacturer advises caution
Alfentanil	see Opioid Analgesics
Alfuzosin	Reduce dose in mild to moderate liver disease; avoid if severe
Alimemazine (trimeprazine)	Avoid—may precipitate coma in severe liver disease; hepatotoxic
Allopurinol	Reduce dose
Almotriptan	Manufacturer advises caution in mild to moderate liver disease; avoid in severe liver disease
Alprazolam	see Anxiolytics and Hypnotics
Altretamine	Rare reports of hepatotoxicity
Amfebutamone	see Bupropion
Amifostine	Manufacturer advises avoid
Aminophylline	see Theophylline
Amitriptyline	see Antidepressants, Tricyclic
Amlodipine	Half-life prolonged—may need dose reduction
Amoxapine	see Antidepressants, Tricyclic
Amprenavir	Avoid oral solution due to high propylene glycol content; reduce dose of capsules to 450 mg every 12 hours in moderate hepatic impairment and reduce dose to 300 mg every 12 hours in severe impairment
Amsacrine	Reduce dose
Anabolic Steroids	Preferably avoid—dose-related toxicity

Drug	Comment
Analgesics	see Aspirin, NSAIDs, Opioid Analgesics and Paracetamol
Anastrozole	Avoid in moderate to severe liver disease
Androgens	Preferably avoid—dose-related toxicity with some, and produce fluid retention
Antacids	In patients with fluid retention, avoid those containing large amounts of sodium, e.g. magnesium trisilicate mixture, *Gaviscon*® Avoid those causing constipation—can precipitate coma
Anticoagulants, Oral	Avoid in severe liver disease, especially if prothrombin time already prolonged
Antidepressants, MAOI	see MAOIs
Antidepressants, SSRI	Reduce dose or avoid in severe liver disease
Antidepressants, Tricyclic (and related)	Tricyclics preferable to MAOIs but sedative effects increased (avoid in severe liver disease)
Antihistamines	see individual entries
Antipsychotics	All can precipitate coma; phenothiazines are hepatotoxic; see also Clozapine, Olanzapine, Quetiapine, Risperidone and Sertindole
Anxiolytics and Hypnotics	All can precipitate coma; avoid chloral hydrate; small dose of oxazepam or temazepam probably safest; reduce oral dose of clomethiazole; reduce dose of zaleplon to 5mg (avoid if severe); reduce dose of zopiclone (avoid if severe)
Apomorphine	Low sublingual doses may be used with caution
Aspirin	Avoid—increased risk of gastro-intestinal bleeding
Atorvastatin	see Statins
Atosiban	No information available
Atovaquone	Manufacturer advises caution—monitor more closely
Auranofin	see Gold
Aurothiomalate	see Gold
Azapropazone	see NSAIDs
Azatadine	Sedation inappropriate in severe liver disease—avoid
Azathioprine	May need dose reduction
Azithromycin	Avoid; jaundice reported
Bambuterol	Avoid in severe liver disease
Bendrofluazide	see Thiazides
Bendroflumethiazide (bendrofluazide)	see Thiazides
Benorilate [aspirin-paracetamol ester]	see Aspirin
Benperidol	see Antipsychotics
Benzthiazide	see Thiazides
Bezafibrate	Avoid in severe liver disease
Bicalutamide	Increased accumulation possible in moderate to severe hepatic impairment

Drug	Comment
Brompheniramine	Sedation inappropriate in severe liver disease—avoid
Buclizine	Sedation inappropriate in severe liver disease—avoid
Budesonide	Plasma-budesonide concentration may increase on oral administration
Bumetanide	see Loop Diuretics
Bupivacaine	see Lidocaine
Buprenorphine	see Opioid Analgesics
Bupropion	Manufacturer recommends 150mg daily; avoid in severe hepatic cirrhosis
Cabergoline	Reduce dose or avoid in liver disease
Candesartan	Halve initial dose in mild or moderate liver disease; avoid if severe
Capecitabine	Manufacturer advises avoid in severe hepatic impairment
Carbamazepine	Metabolism impaired in advanced liver disease
Carbenoxolone	Produces sodium and water retention and hypokalaemia
Carvedilol	Avoid
Ceftriaxone	Reduce dose and monitor plasma concentration if both hepatic and severe renal impairment
Celecoxib	see NSAIDs
Certoparin	see Heparin
Cetrorelix	Manufacturer advises avoid in moderate liver impairment
Chloral Hydrate	see Anxiolytics and Hypnotics
Chloramphenicol	Avoid if possible—increased risk of bone-marrow depression; reduce dose and monitor plasma-chloramphenicol concentration
Chlordiazepoxide	see Anxiolytics and Hypnotics
Chlorphenamine (chlorpheniramine)	Sedation inappropriate in severe liver disease—avoid
Chlorpheniramine	see Chlorphenamine
Chlorpromazine	see Antipsychotics
Chlorpropamide	see Sulphonylureas
Chlortetracycline	see Tetracyclines
Chlortalidone	see Thiazides
Ciclosporin	May need dose adjustment
Cilazapril	see ACE Inhibitors
Cimetidine	Increased risk of confusion; reduce dose
Cinnarizine	Sedation inappropriate in severe liver disease—avoid
Ciprofibrate	see Bezafibrate
Ciprofloxacin	see Quinolones
Citalopram	Use doses at lower end of range
Cladribine	Regular monitoring recommended
Clarithromycin	Hepatic dysfunction including jaundice reported
Clavulanic Acid [ingredient]	see Co-amoxiclav and *Timentin*®
Clemastine	Sedation inappropriate in severe liver disease—avoid
Clindamycin	Reduce dose

Drug	Comment
Clobazam	*see* Anxiolytics and Hypnotics
Clomethiazole	*see* Anxiolytics and Hypnotics
Clomifene	Avoid in severe liver disease
Clomipramine	*see* Antidepressants, Tricyclic
Clopamide	*see* Thiazides
Clopidogrel	Manufacturer advises caution (risk of bleeding); avoid in severe hepatic impairment
Clorazepate	*see* Anxiolytics and Hypnotics
Clozapine	Initial dose 12.5 mg daily increased slowly with regular monitoring of liver function; avoid in symptomatic or progressive liver disease or hepatic failure
Co-amoxiclav	Monitor liver function in liver disease. Cholestatic jaundice, see p. 263
Codeine	*see* Opioid Analgesics
Colestyramine	Interferes with absorption of fat-soluble vitamins and may aggravate malabsorption in primary biliary cirrhosis; likely to be ineffective in complete biliary obstruction
Contraceptives, Oral	Avoid in active liver disease and if history of pruritus or cholestasis during pregnancy
Co-trimoxazole	Manufacturer advises avoid in severe liver disease
Cyclizine	Sedation inappropriate in severe liver disease—avoid
Cyclopenthiazide	*see* Thiazides
Cyclophosphamide	Reduce dose
Cyclosporin	*see* Ciclosporin
Cyproheptadine	Sedation inappropriate in severe liver disease—avoid
Cyproterone Acetate	Dose-related toxicity; *see also* side-effects of cyproterone, section 8.3.4.2
Cytarabine	Reduce dose
Dacarbazine	Dose reduction may be required in mild to moderate liver disease; avoid if severe
Dalfopristin [ingredient]	*see* Synercid ®
Dalteparin	*see* Heparin
Danaparoid	*see* Heparin
Dantrolene	Avoid—may cause severe liver damage
Darbepoetin	Manufacturer advises caution
Daunorubicin	Reduce dose
Debrisoquine	May need dose reduction
Demeclocycline	*see* Tetracyclines
Desflurane	Reduce dose
Desogestrel	*see* Progestogens
Dexketoprofen	*see* NSAIDs
Dextromethorphan	*see* Opioid Analgesics
Dextromoramide	*see* Opioid Analgesics
Dextropropoxyphene	*see* Opioid Analgesics
Diamorphine	*see* Opioid Analgesics
Diazepam	*see* Anxiolytics and Hypnotics
Diclofenac	*see* NSAIDs

Drug	Comment
Didanosine	Insufficient information but consider dose reduction
Diethylstilbestrol	*see* Oestrogens
Diflunisal	*see* NSAIDs
Dihydrocodeine	*see* Opioid Analgesics
Diltiazem	Reduce dose
Diphenhydramine	Caution in mild to moderate liver disease; avoid in severe disease if sedation is inappropriate
Diphenoxylate	*see* Opioid Analgesics
Diphenylpyraline	Caution in mild to moderate liver disease; avoid in severe disease if sedation is inappropriate
Dipipanone	*see* Opioid Analgesics
Disopyramide	Half-life prolonged—may need dose reduction
Docetaxel	Monitor liver function—reduce dose according to liver enzymes; avoid in severe hepatic impairment
Dosulepin (dothiepin)	*see* Antidepressants, Tricyclic
Dothiepin (dosulepin)	*see* Antidepressants, Tricyclic
Doxazosin	No information—manufacturer advises caution
Doxepin	*see* Antidepressants, Tricyclic
Doxorubicin	Reduce dose according to bilirubin concentration
Doxycycline	*see* Tetracyclines
Doxylamine	Caution in mild to moderate liver disease; avoid in severe disease if sedation is inappropriate
Dydrogesterone	*see* Progestogens
Efavirenz	In mild to moderate liver disease, monitor liver function: avoid in severe hepatic impairment
Eformoterol	*see* Formoterol
Enalapril	*see* ACE Inhibitors
Enoxaparin	*see* Heparin
Entacapone	Avoid
Epirubicin	Reduce dose according to bilirubin concentration
Epoetin	Manufacurers advise caution in chronic hepatic failure
Eprosartan	Halve initial dose in mild or moderate liver disease; avoid if severe
Eptifibatide	Avoid in severe liver disease—increased risk of bleeding
Ergometrine	Avoid in severe liver disease
Ergotamine	Avoid in severe liver disease—risk of toxicity increased
Erythromycin	May cause idiosyncratic hepatotoxicity
Esomeprazole	In severe liver disease dose should not exceed 20 mg daily
Estradiol	*see* Oestrogens
Estramustine	Manufacturer advises caution and regular liver function tests; avoid in severe liver disease
Estriol	*see* Oestrogens

Drug	Comment
Estropipate	*see* Oestrogens
Ethinylestradiol	*see* Oestrogens
Etodolac	*see* NSAIDs
Etoposide	Avoid in severe hepatic impairment
Etynodiol Diacetate	*see* Progestogens
Exemestane	Manufacturer advises caution
Famciclovir	Usual dose in well compensated liver disease (information not available on decompensated)
Felodipine	Reduce dose
Fenbufen	*see* NSAIDs
Fenofibrate	*see* Bezafibrate
Fenoprofen	*see* NSAIDs
Fentanyl	*see* Opioid Analgesics
Flecainide	Avoid (or reduce dose) in severe liver disease
Flucloxacillin	Cholestatic jaundice, see p. 260
Fluconazole	Toxicity with related drugs
Flunitrazepam	*see* Anxiolytics and Hypnotics
Fluoxetine	*see* Antidepressants, SSRI
Flupentixol	*see* Antipsychotics
Fluphenazine	*see* Antipsychotics
Flurazepam	*see* Anxiolytics and Hypnotics
Flurbiprofen	*see* NSAIDs
Flutamide	Use with caution (hepatotoxic)
Fluvastatin	*see* Statins
Fluvoxamine	*see* Antidepressants, SSRI
Formoterol (eformoterol)	Metabolism possibly reduced in severe cirrhosis
Fosfestrol	*see* Oestrogens
Fosinopril	*see* ACE Inhibitors
Fosphenytoin	Consider 10–25% reduction in dose or infusion rate (except initial dose for status epilepticus)
Frusemide	*see* Loop Diuretics
Furosemide (frusemide)	*see* Loop Diuretics
Fusidic Acid	Impaired biliary excretion; possibly increased risk of hepatotoxicity; avoid or reduce dose
Galantamine	Reduce dose in moderate hepatic impairment; avoid in severe impairment
Ganirelix	Manufacturer advises avoid in moderate or severe hepatic impairment
Gemcitabine	Manufacturer advises caution
Gemfibrozil	Avoid in liver disease
Gestodene	*see* Progestogens
Gestrinone	Avoid in severe liver disease
Gestronol	*see* Progestogens
Glibenclamide	*see* Sulphonylureas
Gliclazide	*see* Sulphonylureas
Glimepiride	Manufacturer advises avoid in severe hepatic impairment
Glipizide	*see* Sulphonylureas
Gliquidone	*see* Sulphonylureas
Gold (auranofin, aurothiomalate)	Avoid in severe liver disease—hepatotoxicity may occur
Griseofulvin	Avoid in severe liver disease
Haloperidol	*see* Antipsychotics

Drug	Comment
Halothane	Avoid if history of unexplained pyrexia or jaundice following previous exposure to halothane
Heparin	Reduce dose in severe liver disease
Hydralazine	Reduce dose
Hydrochlorothiazide	*see* Thiazides
Hydroflumethiazide	*see* Thiazides
Hydromorphone	*see* Opioid Analgesics
Hydroxyprogesterone Caproate	*see* Progestogens
Hydroxyzine	Sedation inappropriate in severe liver disease—avoid
Hypnotics	*see* Anxiolytics and Hypnotics
Ibuprofen	*see* NSAIDs
Idarubicin	Reduce dose according to bilirubin concentration
Ifosfamide	Avoid
Imidapril	*see* ACE Inhibitors
Imipramine	*see* Antidepressants, Tricyclic
Indapamide	*see* Thiazides
Indinavir	Reduce dose to 600 mg every 8 hours in mild to moderate hepatic impairment; not studied in severe impairment
Indometacin	*see* NSAIDs
Indoramin	Manufacturer advises caution
Interferon alfa	Close monitoring in mild to moderate hepatic impairment; avoid if severe
Interferon beta	Avoid in decompensated liver disease
Irinotecan	Monitor closely for neutropenia if plasma-bilirubin concentration up to 1.5 times upper limit of normal range; avoid if plasma-bilirubin concentration greater than 1.5 times upper limit of normal range
Iron dextran	Avoid in severe hepatic impairment
Iron sorbitol	Avoid
Iron sucrose	Avoid
Isocarboxazid	*see* MAOIs
Isoniazid	Use with caution; monitor liver function regularly and particularly frequently in the first 2 months; *see also* p. 285
Isotretinoin	Avoid—further impairment of liver function may occur
Isradipine	Reduce dose
Itraconazole	Half-life prolonged—dose reduction may be necessary
Kaletra®	Avoid oral solution because of propylene glycol content; use capsules with caution in mild to moderate hepatic impairment and avoid in severe impairment
Ketoconazole	Avoid
Ketoprofen	*see* NSAIDs
Ketorolac	*see* NSAIDs
Ketotifen	Sedation inappropriate in severe liver disease—avoid
Labetalol	Avoid—severe hepatocellular injury reported

Drug	Comment
Lacidipine	Antihypertensive effect possibly increased
Lamotrigine	Halve dose in moderate liver disease; quarter dose in severe liver disease
Lansoprazole	In severe liver disease dose should not exceed 30 mg daily
Leflunomide	Avoid—active metabolite may accumulate
Lepirudin	No information—manufacturer advises that cirrhosis may affect renal excretion
Lercanidipine	Avoid in severe liver disease
Levetiracetam	Halve dose in severe hepatic impairment (due to concomitant renal impairment)
Levobupivacaine	Manufacturer advises caution in liver disease
Levomepromazine (methotrimeprazine)	*see* Antipsychotics
Levonorgestrel	*see* Progestogens
Lidocaine (lignocaine)	Avoid (or reduce dose) in severe liver disease
Lignocaine	*see* Lidocaine
Linezolid	In severe hepatic impairment manufacturer advises use only if potential benefit outweighs risk
Lofepramine	*see* Antidepressants, Tricyclic
Loop Diuretics	Hypokalaemia may precipitate coma (use potassium-sparing diuretic to prevent this); increased risk of hypomagnesaemia in alcoholic cirrhosis
Lopinavir [ingredinet]	*see* Kaletra®
Loprazolam	*see* Anxiolytics and Hypnotics
Lorazepam	*see* Anxiolytics and Hypnotics
Lormetazepam	*see* Anxiolytics and Hypnotics
Lornoxicam	*see* NSAIDs
Losartan	Consider lower dose
Loxapine	*see* Antipsychotics
Lymecycline	*see* Tetracyclines
Magnesium Salts	Avoid in hepatic coma if risk of renal failure
MAOIs	May cause idiosyncratic hepatotoxicity
Maprotiline	*see* Antidepressants, Tricyclic (and related)
Meclozine	Sedation inappropriate in severe liver disease—avoid
Medroxyprogesterone Acetate	*see* Progestogens
Mefenamic Acid	see NSAIDs
Mefloquine	Avoid for prophylaxis in severe liver disease
Megestrol Acetate	*see* Progestogens
Meloxicam	*see* NSAIDs
Meprobamate	*see* Anxiolytics and Hypnotics
Meptazinol	*see* Opioid Analgesics
Meropenem	Monitor transaminase and bilirubin concentrations
Mesterolone	*see* Androgens
Mestranol	*see* Oestrogens

Drug	Comment
Metformin	Avoid—increased risk of lactic acidosis
Methadone	*see* Opioid Analgesics
Methionine	May precipitate coma
Methocarbamol	Manufacturer advises caution
Methotrexate	Dose-related toxicity—avoid in non-malignant conditions (e.g. psoriasis)
Methotrimeprazine	*see* Antipsychotics
Methoxsalen	Avoid or reduce dose
Methyldopa	Manufacturer advises caution in history of liver disease; avoid in active liver disease
Methysergide	Avoid
Metoclopramide	Reduce dose
Metolazone	*see* Thiazides
Metoprolol	Reduce oral dose
Metronidazole	In severe liver disease reduce total daily dose to one-third, and give once daily
Mexiletine	Avoid (or reduce dose) in severe liver disease
Mianserin	*see* Antidepressants, Tricyclic (and related)
Miconazole	Avoid
Minocycline	*see* Tetracyclines
Mirtazapine	Manufacturer advises caution
Mitoxantrone	Manufacturer advises caution in severe hepatic impairment
Mivacurium	Reduce dose
Mizolastine	Manufacturer recommends avoid in significant hepatic impairment
Moclobemide	Reduce dose in severe liver disease
Modafinil	Halve dose in severe liver disease
Moexipril	*see* ACE Inhibitors
Monoamine Oxidase Inhibitors	*see* MAOIs
Morphine	*see* Opioid Analgesics
Moxonidine	Avoid in severe liver disease
Nabumetone	*see* NSAIDs
Nalbuphine	*see* Opioid Analgesics
Nalidixic Acid	*see* Quinolones
Nandrolone	*see* Anabolic Steroids
Naproxen	*see* NSAIDs
Naratriptan	Max. 2.5 mg in 24 hours in moderate hepatic impairment; avoid if severe
Nateglinide	Manufacturer advises caution in moderate hepatic impairment; avoid in severe impairment—no information available
Nebivolol	No information available—manufacturer advises avoid
Nefazodone	Reduce dose
Nelfinavir	No information available—manufacturer advises caution
Neomycin	Absorbed from gastro-intestinal tract in liver disease—increased risk of ototoxicity
Nevirapine	No information available—manufacturer advises avoid

Drug	Comment
Nicardipine	Reduce dose
Nicoumalone	*see* Anticoagulants, Oral
Nifedipine	Reduce dose
Nimodipine	Elimination reduced in cirrhosis—monitor blood pressure
Nisoldipine	Formulation not suitable in hepatic impairment
Nitrazepam	*see* Anxiolytics and Hypnotics
Nitrofurantoin	Cholestatic jaundice and chronic active hepatitis reported
Nitroprusside	Avoid in severe liver disease
Nizatidine	Manufacturer advises caution
Norethisterone	*see* Progestogens
Norfloxacin	*see* Quinolones
Norgestimate	*see* Progestogens
Norgestrel	*see* Progestogens
Nortriptyline	*see* Antidepressants, Tricyclic
NSAIDs	Increased risk of gastro-intestinal bleeding and can cause fluid retention; avoid in severe liver disease; aceclofenac, initially 100 mg daily; celecoxib, halve initial dose in moderate liver disease; rofecoxib max. 12.5 mg daily in mild hepatic impairment
Oestrogens	Avoid; *see also* Contraceptives, Oral
Ofloxacin	*see* Quinolones
Olanzapine	Consider initial dose of 5 mg daily
Omeprazole	In liver disease not more than 20 mg daily should be needed
Ondansetron	Reduce dose; not more than 8 mg daily in severe liver disease
Opioid Analgesics	Avoid or reduce dose—may precipitate coma
Oral Contraceptives	*see* Contraceptives, Oral
Oxazepam	*see* Anxiolytics and Hypnotics
Oxcarbazepine	No dosage adjustment required in mild to moderate hepatic impairment; no information in severe impairment
Oxprenolol	Reduce dose
Oxybutynin	Manufacturer advises caution
Oxycodone	*see* Opioid Analgesics
Oxypertine	*see* Antipsychotics
Oxytetracycline	*see* Tetracyclines
Paclitaxel	Avoid in severe liver disease
Pancuronium	Possibly slower onset, higher dose requirement and prolonged recovery time
Pantoprazole	Max. 20 mg daily in severe hepatic impairment and cirrhosis—monitor liver function (discontinue if deterioration)
Papaveretum	*see* Opioid Analgesics
Paracetamol	Dose-related toxicity—avoid large doses
Paroxetine	*see* Antidepressants, SSRI
Peginterferon alfa	Avoid in severe hepatic impairment
Pentazocine	*see* Opioid Analgesics

Drug	Comment
Pericyazine	*see* Antipsychotics
Perindopril	*see* ACE Inhibitors
Perphenazine	*see* Antipsychotics
Pethidine	*see* Opioid Analgesics
Phenazocine	*see* Opioid Analgesics
Phenelzine	*see* MAOIs
Phenindione	*see* Anticoagulants, Oral
Phenobarbital	May precipitate coma
Phenoperidine	*see* Opioid Analgesics
Phenothiazines	*see* Antipsychotics
Phenylbutazone	*see* NSAIDs
Phenytoin	Reduce dose to avoid toxicity
Pholcodine	*see* Opioid Analgesics
Pilocarpine	Reduce initial oral dose in moderate or severe cirrhosis
Pimozide	*see* Antipsychotics
Pioglitazone	Avoid
Piperazine	Manufacturer advises avoid
Pipotiazine	*see* Antipsychotics
Piracetam	Avoid
Piroxicam	*see* NSAIDs
Polythiazide	*see* Thiazides
Pravastatin	*see* Statins
Prazosin	Initially 500 micrograms daily; increased with caution
Prednisolone	Side-effects more common
Primidone	Reduce dose; may precipitate coma
Procainamide	Avoid or reduce dose
Procarbazine	Avoid in severe hepatic impairment
Prochlorperazine	*see* Antipsychotics
Progesterone	*see* Progestogens
Progestogens	Avoid; *see also* Contraceptives, Oral
Promazine	*see* Antipsychotics
Promethazine	Avoid—may precipitate coma in severe liver disease; hepatotoxic
Propafenone	Reduce dose
Propantheline	Manufacturer advises caution
Propiverine	Avoid
Propranolol	Reduce oral dose
Propylthiouracil	Reduce dose
Pyrazinamide	Avoid—idiosyncratic hepatotoxicity more common; *see also* p. 286
Quetiapine	Manufacturer advises initial dose of 25 mg daily, increased daily in steps of 25–50 mg
Quinapril	*see* ACE Inhibitors
Quinolones	Hepatic dysfunction reported; *nalidixic acid* partially conjugated in liver; reduce dose of *ofloxacin* in severe liver disease
Quinupristin [ingredient]	*see* Synercid ®
Rabeprazole	Manufacturer advises caution in severe hepatic dysfunction
Raloxifene	Manufacturer advises avoid

Drug	Comment
Raltitrexed	Caution in mild or moderate disease; avoid if severe
Ramipril	*see* ACE Inhibitors
Ranitidine	Increased risk of confusion; reduce dose
Reboxetine	Initial dose 2 mg twice daily, increased according to tolerance
Remifentanil	*see* Opioid Analgesics
Repaglinide	Manufacturer advises avoid in severe liver disease
Reviparin	Manufacturer advises avoid in severe hepatic impairment
Ribavirin	No dosage adjustment required; avoid oral administration in severe hepatic dysfunction or decompensated cirrhosis
Rifabutin	Reduce dose in severe hepatic impairment
Rifampicin	Impaired elimination; monitor liver function; avoid or do not exceed 8 mg/kg daily; *see also* p. 286
Riluzole	Avoid
Risperidone	Manufacturer advises initial dose of 500 micrograms twice daily increased in steps of 500 micrograms twice daily to 1–2 mg twice daily
Ritonavir	Avoid in severe hepatic impairment
Rivastigmine	No information available—manufacturer advises avoid in severe liver disease
Rizatriptan	Reduce dose to 5 mg in mild to moderate liver disease; avoid in severe liver disease
Rocuronium	Reduce dose
Rofecoxib	*see* NSAIDs
Ropinirole	Avoid in severe hepatic impairment
Ropivacaine	Manufacturer advises caution in severe liver disease
Rosiglitazone	Avoid
Saquinavir	Plasma concentration possibly increased; manufacturer advises caution with *Fortovase®* in moderate hepatic impairment and with *Invirase®* in severe impairment; avoid *Fortovase®* in severe impairment
Sertraline	*see* Antidepressants, SSRI
Sibutramine	Increased plasma-sibutramine concentration; manufacturer advises caution in mild to moderate hepatic impairment; avoid if severe impairment
Sildenafil	Initial dose 25 mg; manufacturer advises avoid in severe hepatic impairment
Simvastatin	*see* Statins
Sirolimus	Monitor blood-sirolimus trough concentration
Sodium Aurothiomalate	*see* Gold
Sodium Bicarbonate	*see* Antacids

Drug	Comment
Sodium Fusidate	*see* Fusidic Acid
Sodium Nitroprusside	*see* Nitroprusside
Sodium Phenylbutyrate	Manufacturer advises caution
Sodium Valproate	*see* Valproate
Stanozolol	*see* Anabolic Steroids
Statins	Avoid in active liver disease or unexplained persistent elevations in serum transaminases
Stilboestrol (diethylstilboestrol)	*see* Oestrogens
Sulindac	*see* NSAIDs
Sulphonylureas	Increased risk of hypoglycaemia in severe liver disease; avoid or use small dose; can produce jaundice
Sulpiride	*see* Antipsychotics
Sumatriptan	Manufacturer advises 50 mg oral dose
Suxamethonium	Prolonged apnoea may occur in severe liver disease due to reduced hepatic synthesis of pseudocholinesterase
Synercid®	Plasma concentration possibly increased; manufacturer advises caution in mild to moderate liver disease; avoid in severe liver disease
Tacrolimus	Reduce dose
Tamsulosin	Avoid in severe hepatic impairment
Tegafur with uracil	*see* Uftoral®
Telmisartan	20–40 mg once daily in mild or moderate impairment; avoid in severe hepatic impairment or biliary obstruction
Temazepam	*see* Anxiolytics and Hypnotics
Tenoxicam	*see* NSAIDs
Terbinafine	Reduce dose
Terfenadine	Avoid—risk of arrhythmias
Testosterone	*see* Androgens
Tetracyclines	Avoid (or use with caution)
Theophylline	Reduce dose
Thiazides	Avoid in severe liver disease; hypokalaemia may precipitate coma (potassium-sparing diuretic can prevent); increased risk of hypomagnesaemia in alcoholic cirrhosis
Thiopental	Reduce dose for induction in severe liver disease
Thioridazine	*see* Antipsychotics
Tiagabine	Maintenance dose 5–10 mg 1–2 times daily initially in mild to moderate hepatic impairment; avoid in severe impairment
Tiaprofenic acid	*see* NSAIDs
Tibolone	Avoid in severe liver disease
Ticlopidine	Manufacturer advises caution; discontinue if hepatitis or jaundice develop
Timentin®	Cholestatic jaundice, see p. 265
Tinzaparin	*see* Heparin

Drug	Comment
Tirofiban	Caution in mild to moderate liver disease; avoid in severe liver disease—increased risk of bleeding
Tizanidine	Avoid in severe liver disease
Tolbutamide	*see* Sulphonylureas
Tolfenamic Acid	*see* NSAIDs
Tolterodine	Reduce dose to 1 mg twice daily
Topotecan	Avoid in severe hepatic impairment
Torasemide	*see* Loop Diuretics
Toremifene	Elimination decreased in hepatic impairment—avoid if severe
Tramadol	*see* Opioid Analgesics
Trandolapril	*see* ACE Inhibitors
Tranylcypromine	*see* MAOIs
Trazodone	*see* Antidepressants, Tricyclic (and related)
Tretinoin (oral)	Reduce dose
Tribavirin	*see* Ribavirin
Triclofos	*see* Anxiolytics and Hypnotics
Trifluoperazine	*see* Antipsychotics
Trimeprazine	*see* Alimemazine
Trimetrexate	Manufacturer advises caution; interrupt treatment if severe abnormalities in liver function tests (consult product literature)
Trimipramine	*see* Antidepressants, Tricyclic
Triprolidine	Sedation inappropriate in severe liver disease—avoid
Trospium	Manufacturer advises avoid—no information available
Uftoral®	Manufacturer advises avoid in severe hepatic impairment
Ursodeoxycholic acid	Avoid in chronic liver disease (but used in primary biliary cirrhosis)
Valproate	Avoid if possible—hepatotoxicity and hepatic failure may occasionally occur (usually in first 6 months); *see also* p. 234
Valsartan	Halve dose in mild to moderate hepatic impairment; avoid if severe
Venlafaxine	Halve dose in moderate hepatic impairment; avoid if severe
Verapamil	Reduce oral dose
Verteporfin	Avoid in severe hepatic impairment
Vinblastine	Dose reduction may be necessary
Vincristine	Dose reduction may be necessary
Vindesine	Dose reduction may be necessary
Vinorelbine	Dose reduction may be required in significant hepatic impairment
Warfarin	*see* Anticoagulants, Oral
Xipamide	*see* Thiazides
Zafirlukast	Manufacturer advises avoid
Zalcitabine	Further impairment of liver function may occur
Zaleplon	*see* Anxiolytics and Hypnotics

Drug	Comment
Zidovudine	Accumulation may occur
Zoledronic acid	Manufacturer advises caution in severe hepatic impairment—limited information available
Zolmitriptan	Max. 5mg in 24 hours in moderate or severe hepatic impairment
Zolpidem	*see* Anxiolytics and Hypnotics
Zopiclone	*see* Anxiolytics and Hypnotics
Zotepine	Initial dose 25 mg twice daily, increased gradually according to response (max. 75 mg twice daily); monitor liver function at weekly intervals for first 3 months
Zuclopenthixol	*see* Antipsychotics

Appendix 3: Renal impairment

The use of drugs in patients with reduced renal function can give rise to problems for several reasons:

- failure to excrete a drug or its metabolites may produce toxicity;
- sensitivity to some drugs is increased even if elimination is unimpaired;
- many side-effects are tolerated poorly by patients in renal failure;
- some drugs cease to be effective when renal function is reduced.

Many of these problems can be avoided by reducing the dose or by using alternative drugs.

Principles of dose adjustment in renal impairment

The level of renal function below which the dose of a drug must be reduced depends on whether the drug is eliminated entirely by renal excretion or is partly metabolised, and on how toxic it is.

For many drugs with only minor or no dose-related side-effects very precise modification of the dose regimen is unnecessary and a simple scheme for dose reduction is sufficient.

For more toxic drugs with a small safety margin dose regimens based on glomerular filtration rate should be used. For those where both efficacy and toxicity are closely related to plasma concentrations recommended regimens should be seen only as a guide to initial treatment; subsequent treatment must be adjusted according to clinical response and plasma concentration.

The total daily maintenance dose of a drug can be reduced either by reducing the size of the individual doses or by increasing the interval between doses. For some drugs, if the size of the maintenance dose is reduced it will be important to give a loading dose if an immediate effect is required. This is because when a patient is given a regular dose of any drug it takes more than five times the half-life to achieve steady-state plasma concentrations. As the plasma half-life of drugs excreted by the kidney is prolonged in renal failure it may take many days for the reduced dosage to achieve a therapeutic plasma concentration. The loading dose should usually be the same size as the initial dose for a patient with normal renal function.

Nephrotoxic drugs should, if possible, be avoided in patients with renal disease because the consequences of nephrotoxicity are likely to be more serious when the renal reserve is already reduced.

Use of dosage table

Dose recommendations are based on the severity of renal impairment. This is expressed in terms of glomerular filtration rate (GFR), usually measured by the **creatinine clearance**. The serum-creatinine concentration can usually be used instead as a measure of renal function but is only a rough guide unless corrected for age, weight, and sex. Nomograms are available for making the correction and should be used where accuracy is important.

For prescribing purposes renal impairment is arbitrarily divided into 3 grades (definitions vary for grades of renal impairment; therefore, where the product literature does not correspond with this grading, values for creatinine clearance or another measure of renal function are included):

Grade	GFR	Serum creatinine (approx.)
Mild	20–50 mL/minute	150–300 µmol/litre
Moderate	10–20 mL/minute	300–700 µmol/litre
Severe	<10 mL/minute	> 700 µmol/litre

Note. Conversion factors are:
Litres/24 hours = mL/minute × 1.44
mL/minute = Litres/24 hours × 0.69

DIALYSIS. For prescribing in patients on continuous ambulatory peritoneal dialysis (CAPD) or haemodialysis, consult specialist literature.

Renal function declines with age; many elderly patients have a glomerular filtration rate below 50 mL/minute which, because of reduced muscle mass, may not be indicated by a raised serum creatinine. It is wise to assume at least mild impairment of renal function when prescribing for the elderly.

The following table may be used as a guide to drugs which are known to require a reduction in dose in renal impairment, and to those which are potentially harmful or are ineffective. Drug prescribing should be kept to the minimum in all patients with severe renal disease.

If even mild renal impairment is considered likely on clinical grounds, renal function should be checked before prescribing **any** drug which requires dose modification.

Table of drugs to be avoided or used with caution in renal impairment

Products introduced or amended since publication of BNF No. 42 (September 2001) are underlined.

Drug and degree of impairment	Comment
Abacavir	
Severe	Avoid
Abciximab	
Severe	Avoid—increased risk of bleeding
Acamprosate	
Mild	Avoid; excreted in urine
Acarbose	
Moderate to severe	Manufacturer advises avoid—no information available

Drug and degree of impairment	Comment
ACE Inhibitors	
Mild to moderate	Use with caution and monitor response (see also p. 91). Hyperkalaemia and other side-effects more common. Initial doses: captopril 12.5 mg twice daily, cilazapril 500 micrograms once daily, enalapril 2.5 mg once daily, imidapril 2.5 mg once daily (avoid if creatinine clearance less than 30 mL/minute), moexipril 3.75 mg once daily, perindopril 2 mg once daily (2 mg once daily on alternate days in moderate impairment), quinapril 2.5 mg once daily, ramipril 1.25 mg once daily, trandolapril 500 micrograms once daily
Acebutolol	*see* Beta-blockers
Aceclofenac	*see* NSAIDs
Acemetacin	*see* NSAIDs
Acenocoumarol (nicoumalone)	*see* Anticoagulants, Oral
Acetazolamide	
Mild	Avoid; metabolic acidosis
Aciclovir	
Mild	Reduce intravenous dose
Moderate to severe	Reduce dose
Acipimox	
Mild	Reduce dose; avoid if creatinine clearance less than 30 mL/minute
Acitretin	
Mild	Avoid; increased risk of toxicity
Aclarubicin	Manufacturer advises caution
Acrivastine	
Moderate	Avoid; excreted by kidney
Adrenergic Neurone Blockers	
Moderate to severe	Avoid; increased postural hypotension; decrease in renal blood flow
Alendronic Acid	
Mild	Manufacturer advises avoid if creatinine clearance less than 35 mL/minute
Alfentanil	*see* Opioid Analgesics
Alfuzosin	Start at 2.5 mg twice daily and adjust according to response
Alimemazine (trimeprazine)	
Severe	Avoid
Allopurinol	
Moderate	100–200 mg daily; increased toxicity; rashes
Severe	100 mg on alternate days (max. 100 mg daily)
Almotriptan	
Severe	Max. 12.5 mg in 24 hours

Drug and degree of impairment	Comment
Alprazolam	*see* Anxiolytics and Hypnotics
Alteplase	
Moderate	Risk of hyperkalaemia
Altretamine	
Mild	Nephrotoxic; if renal function deteriorates reduce dose or discontinue
Aluminium Salts	
Severe	Aluminium is absorbed and may accumulate
	Note. Absorption of aluminium from aluminium salts is increased by citrates, which are contained in many effervescent preparations (such as effervescent analgesics)
Amantadine	
Mild to moderate	Reduce dose; avoid in elderly if creatinine clearance less than 60 mL/minute
Severe	Avoid
Amfebutamone	*see* Bupropion
Amifostine	Manufacturer advises avoid
Amikacin	*see* Aminoglycosides
Amiloride	*see* Diuretics, Potassium-sparing
Aminoglycosides	
Mild	Reduce dose; monitor serum concentrations; *see also* section 5.1.4
Amisulpride	
Mild	Manufacturer advises use half normal dose
Moderate	Manufacturer advises use one-third of normal dose
Severe	Manufacturer advises dose reduction and intermittent treatment
Amobarbital	
Severe	Reduce dose; active metabolite accumulates
Amoxicillin	
Severe	Reduce dose; rashes more common
Amphotericin	
Mild	Use only if no alternative; nephrotoxicity may be reduced with use of complexes
Ampicillin	
Severe	Reduce dose; rashes more common
Amprenavir	
Mild to moderate	Use oral solution with caution due to high propylene glycol content
Severe	Avoid oral solution
Amsacrine	Reduce dose
Analgesics	*see* Opioid Analgesics and NSAIDs
Anastrozole	
Moderate to severe	Avoid—no information available

Drug and degree of impairment	Comment
Anticoagulants, Oral	
Severe	Avoid
Antipsychotics	
Severe	Start with small doses; increased cerebral sensitivity; *see also* Amisulpride, Clozapine, Olanzapine, Quetiapine, Risperidone and Sulpiride
Anxiolytics and Hypnotics	
Severe	Start with small doses; increased cerebral sensitivity
Apomorphine	
Severe	Use with caution; max. sublingual dose 2 mg
Aspirin	
Severe	Avoid; sodium and water retention; deterioration in renal function; increased risk of gastro-intestinal bleeding
Atenolol	*see* Beta-blockers
Atosiban	No information available
Atovaquone	Manufacturer advises caution—monitor more closely
Auranofin	*see* Gold
Aurothiomalate	*see* Gold
Azapropazone	*see* NSAIDs (excreted by kidney)
Azathioprine	
Severe	Reduce dose
Azithromycin	
Moderate to severe	No information available
Aztreonam	
Moderate	Reduce dose
Baclofen	
Mild	Use smaller doses (e.g. 5 mg daily); excreted by kidney
Balsalazide	
Moderate to severe	Manufacturer advises avoid
Bambuterol	
Mild	Reduce dose
Bendrofluazide	*see* Thiazides
Bendroflumethiazide (bendrofluazide)	*see* Thiazides
Benorilate [aspirin-paracetamol ester]	*see* Aspirin
Benperidol	*see* Antipsychotics
Benzodiazepines	*see* Anxiolytics and Hypnotics
Benzylpenicillin	
Severe	Max. 6 g daily; neurotoxicity—high doses may cause convulsions

Drug and degree of impairment	Comment
Beta-blockers	
Mild	Start with 2.5 mg of nebivolol; reuce dose of celiprolol if creatinine clearance less than 40 mL/minute
Moderate	Start with small dose of acebutolol (active metabolite accumulates); reduce dose of atenolol, nadolol, pindolol, sotalol (all excreted unchanged); avoid celiprolol if creatinine clearance less than 15 mL/minute
Severe	Start with small dose; higher plasma concentrations after oral administration; may reduce renal blood flow and adversely affect renal function in severe impairment; manufacturer advises avoid celiprolol and sotalol
Betaxolol	*see* Beta-blockers
Bezafibrate	
Mild	Reduce dose
Bicarbonate	*see* Sodium Bicarbonate
Bismuth Chelate	*see* Tripotassium Dicitratobismuthate
Bisoprolol	*see* Beta-blockers
Bleomycin	
Moderate	Reduce dose
Bumetanide	
Moderate	May need high doses
Buprenorphine	*see* Opioid Analgesics
Bupropion	Manufacturer recommends 150 mg daily
Candesartan	
Moderate	Halve initial dose
Severe	Avoid
Capecitabine	
Mild	Use three-quarters of starting dose if creatinine clearance 30–50 mL/minute; avoid if creatinine clearance less than 30 mL/minute
Capreomycin	
Mild	Reduce dose; nephrotoxic; ototoxic
Captopril	*see* ACE Inhibitors
Carbamazepine	Manufacturer advises caution
Carbenoxolone	
Moderate	Avoid; fluid retention
Carboplatin	
Mild	Reduce dose and monitor haematological parameters and renal function
Moderate to severe	Avoid
Cefaclor	No dose adjustment required—manufacturer advises caution
Cefadroxil	
Moderate	Reduce dose
Cefalexin	
Severe	Max. 500 mg daily
Cefamandole	
Mild	Reduce dose

Drug and degree of impairment	Comment
Cefazolin	
Mild	Reduce dose
Cefixime	
Moderate	Reduce dose
Cefotaxime	
Severe	Loading dose of 1 g then use half normal dose
Cefoxitin	
Mild	Reduce dose
Cefpirome	
Mild	Usual initial dose, then use half normal dose
Moderate to severe	Usual initial dose, then use one-quarter normal dose
Cefpodoxime	
Mild	Reduce dose
Cefprozil	Usual initial dose, then use half normal dose
Cefradine	
Ceftazidime	
Mild	Reduce dose
Ceftriaxone	
Severe	Reduce dose; also monitor plasma concentration if both severe renal and hepatic impairment
Cefuroxime	
Moderate to severe	Reduce parenteral dose
Celecoxib	*see* NSAIDS
Celiprolol	*see* Beta-blockers
Certoparin	*see* Heparin
Cetirizine	
Moderate	Use half normal dose
Cetrorelix	
Moderate	Manufacturer advises avoid
Chloral Hydrate	*see* Anxiolytics and Hypnotics
Chloramphenicol	
Severe	Avoid unless no alternative; dose-related depression of haematopoiesis
Chlordiazepoxide	*see* Anxiolytics and Hypnotics
Chloroquine	
Mild to moderate	Reduce dose (but for malaria prophylaxis see section 5.4.1)
Severe	Avoid (but for malaria prophylaxis see section 5.4.1)
Chlorpromazine	*see* Antipsychotics
Chlorpropamide	Avoid
Chlortetracycline	*see* Tetracyclines
Chlortalidone	*see* Thiazides
Chlorthalidone	*see* Thiazides
Ciclosporin	*see* pp. 423–4 (*see also* p. 552 if used in atopic dermatitis or psoriasis and p. 491 if used in rheumatoid arthritis)
Cidofovir	
Mild	Avoid; nephrotoxic
Cilastatin [ingredient]	*see* Primaxin®
Cilazapril	*see* ACE Inhibitors

Drug and degree of impairment	Comment
Cimetidine	
Mild to moderate	600–800 mg daily; occasional risk of confusion
Severe	400 mg daily
Ciprofibrate	
Moderate	100 mg on alternate days
Severe	Avoid
Ciprofloxacin	
Moderate	Use half normal dose
Cisplatin	
Mild	Avoid if possible; nephrotoxic and neurotoxic
Citalopram	
Moderate to severe	No information available
Citrates	Absorption of aluminium from aluminium salts is increased by citrates, which are contained in many effervescent preparations (such as effervescent analgesics)
Cladribine	Regular monitoring recommended
Clarithromycin	
Moderate to severe	Use half normal dose
Clavulanic acid [ingredient]	*see* Co-amoxiclav, *Timentin*®
Clobazam	*see* Anxiolytics and Hypnotics
Clodronate sodium	
Mild to moderate	Use half normal dose and monitor serum creatinine
Severe	Avoid
Clomethiazole	*see* Anxiolytics and Hypnotics
Clopamide	*see* Thiazides
Clopidogrel	Manufacturer advises caution
Clorazepate	*see* Anxiolytics and Hypnotics
Clozapine	
Mild to moderate	Initial dose 12.5 mg daily increased slowly
Severe	Avoid
Co-amoxiclav	
Moderate to severe	Reduce dose
Codeine	*see* Opioid Analgesics
Colchicine	
Moderate	Reduce dose
Severe	Avoid or reduce dose if no alternative
Colistin	
Mild	Reduce dose; nephrotoxic; neurotoxic
Co-trimoxazole	
Mild	Use half normal dose if creatinine clearance 15–30 mL/minute; avoid if creatinine clearance less than 15 mL/minute and if plasma-sulphamethoxazole concentration cannot be monitored
Cyclopenthiazide	*see* Thiazides
Cyclophosphamide	Reduce dose

Drug and degree of impairment	Comment
Cycloserine	
Mild to moderate	Reduce dose
Severe	Avoid
Cyclosporin	*see* Ciclosporin
Dacarbazine	
Mild to moderate	Dose reduction may be required
Severe	Avoid
Dalfopristin [ingredient]	*see* Synercid ®
Dalteparin	*see* Heparin
Danaparoid	*see* Heparin
Daunorubicin	
Mild to moderate	Reduce dose
Debrisoquine	*see* Adrenergic Neurone Blockers
Demeclocycline	*see* Tetracyclines
De-Nol®, De-Noltab®	
Severe	Avoid
Desflurane	
Moderate	Reduce dose
Desloratadine	
Severe	Manufacturer advises caution
Desmopressin	Antidiuretic effect may be reduced
Dexketoprofen	*see* NSAIDs
Dextromethorphan	*see* Opioid Analgesics
Dextromoramide	*see* Opioid Analgesics
Dextropropoxyphene	*see* Opioid Analgesics
Diamorphine	*see* Opioid Analgesics
Diazepam	*see* Anxiolytics and Hypnotics
Diazoxide	
Severe	75–150 mg i/v; increased sensitivity to hypotensive effect
Diclofenac	*see* NSAIDs
Didanosine	
Mild	Reduce dose; consult product literature
Diflunisal	*see* NSAIDs (excreted by kidney)
Digitoxin	
Severe	Max. 100 micrograms daily
Digoxin	
Mild	Reduce dose; toxicity increased by electrolyte disturbances
Dihydrocodeine	*see* Opioid Analgesics
Diltiazem	Start with smaller dose
Diphenoxylate	*see* Opioid Analgesics
Dipipanone	*see* Opioid Analgesics
Disodium Etidronate	*see* Etidronate Disodium
Disodium Pamidronate	*see* Pamidronate Disodium
Disopyramide	
Mild	100 mg every 8 hours *or* 150 mg every 12 hours
Moderate	100 mg every 12 hours
Severe	150 mg every 24 hours

Note. Sustained release preparations may be unsuitable; monitor plasma-disopyramide concentrations

Drug and degree of impairment	Comment
Diuretics, Potassium-sparing	
Mild	Monitor plasma K⁺; high risk of hyperkalaemia in renal impairment; amiloride excreted by kidney unchanged
Moderate	Avoid
Doxycycline	*see* Tetracyclines
Enalapril	*see* ACE Inhibitors
Enflurane	
Severe	Avoid
Enoxaparin	*see* Heparin
Enoximone	Consider dose reduction
Ephedrine	
Severe	Avoid; increased CNS toxicity
Eprosartan	
Mild	Halve initial dose
Eptifibatide	
Mild	Avoid if creatinine clearance less than 30 mL/minute
Ergometrine	
Severe	Manufacturer advises avoid
Ergotamine	
Moderate	Avoid; nausea and vomiting; risk of renal vasoconstriction
Erythromycin	
Severe	Max. 1.5 g daily (ototoxicity)
Esmolol	*see* Beta-blockers
Esomeprazole	
Severe	Manufacturer advises caution
Estramustine	Manufacturer advises caution
Ethambutol	
Mild	Reduce dose; if creatinine clearance less than 30 mL/minute monitor plasma-ethambutol concentration; optic nerve damage
Etidronate Disodium	
Mild	Max. 5 mg/kg daily; excreted by kidney
Moderate	Avoid
Etodolac	*see* NSAIDs
Exemestane	Manufacturer advises caution
Famciclovir	
Mild to moderate	Reduce dose
Famotidine	
Severe	Reduce dose
Fenbufen	*see* NSAIDs
Fenofibrate	
Mild	134 mg daily
Moderate	67 mg daily
Severe	Avoid
Fenoprofen	*see* NSAIDs
Fentanyl	*see* Opioid Analgesics
Flecainide	
Mild	Max. initial dose 100 mg daily
Flucloxacillin	
Severe	Reduce dose

Drug and degree of impairment	Comment
Fluconazole	
Mild to moderate	Usual initial dose then halve subsequent doses
Flucytosine	Reduce dose and monitor plasma-flucytosine concentration—consult product literature
Fludarabine	
Mild	Reduce dose; avoid if creatinine clearance less than 30 mL/minute
Flunitrazepam	*see* Anxiolytics and Hypnotics
Fluoxetine	
Mild to moderate	Reduce dose (give on alternate days)
Severe	Avoid
Flupenthixol	*see* Antipsychotics
Fluphenazine	*see* Antipsychotics
Flurazepam	*see* Anxiolytics and Hypnotics
Flurbiprofen	*see* NSAIDs
Fluvastatin	
Severe	Avoid
Fluvoxamine	
Moderate	Start with smaller dose
Foscarnet	
Mild	Reduce dose; consult product literature
Fosinopril	*see* ACE Inhibitors
Fosphenytoin	Consider 10–25% reduction in dose or infusion rate (except initial dose for status epilepticus)
Frusemide	*see* Furosemide
Furosemide (frusemide)	
Moderate	May need high doses; deafness may follow rapid i/v injection
Fybogel Mebeverine®	
Severe	Avoid; contains 7 mmol potassium per sachet
Gabapentin	
Mild	Reduce dose; consult product literature
Galantamine	
Severe	Avoid
Gallamine	
Moderate	Avoid; prolonged paralysis
Ganciclovir	
Mild	Reduce dose; consult product literature
Ganirelix	
Moderate or severe	Manufacturer advises avoid
Gaviscon®	
Severe	Avoid; high sodium content
Gemcitabine	Manufacturer advises caution
Gemeprost	Manufacturer advises avoid
Gemfibrozil	
Severe	Start with 900 mg daily
Gentamicin	*see* Aminoglycosides
Gestrinone	
Severe	Avoid

Drug and degree of impairment	Comment
Glatiramer	No information available—manufacturer advises caution
Glibenclamide	
Severe	Avoid
Gliclazide	
Mild to moderate	Reduce dose
Severe	Avoid if possible; if no alternative reduce dose and monitor closely
Glimepiride	
Severe	Avoid
Glipizide	
Mild to moderate	Increased risk of hypoglycaemia; avoid if hepatic impairment also present
Severe	Avoid
Gliquidone	Avoid in renal failure
Gold (auranofin, aurothiomalate)	
Mild	Avoid; nephrotoxic
Guanethidine	*see* Adrenergic Neurone Blockers
Haloperidol	*see* Antipsychotics
Heparin	
Severe	Risk of bleeding increased
Hetastarch	
Severe	Avoid; excreted by kidney
Hydralazine	
Mild	Reduce dose if creatinine clearance less than 30 mL/minute
Hydrochlorothiazide	*see* Thiazides
Hydroflumethiazide	*see* Thiazides
Hydromorphone	*see* Opioid Analgesics
Hydroxychloroquine	
Mild to moderate	Reduce dose; only on prolonged use
Severe	Avoid
Hydroxyzine	Use half normal dose
Hypnotics	*see* Anxiolytics and Hypnotics
Ibuprofen	*see* NSAIDs
Idarubicin	
Mild	Reduce dose
Ifosfamide	
Mild	Avoid if serum creatinine concentration greater than 120 micromol/litre
Imidapril	*see* ACE Inhibitors
Imipenem	*see* *Primaxin®*
Indapamide	*see* Thiazides
Indometacin	*see* NSAIDs
Indoramin	Manufacturer advises caution
Inosine Pranobex	
Mild	Avoid; metabolised to uric acid
Insulin	
Severe	May need dose reduction; insulin requirements fall; compensatory response to hypoglycaemia is impaired
Interferon alfa	
Mild to moderate	Close monitoring required
Severe	Avoid

Drug and degree of impairment	Comment
Interferon beta	No information available—monitoring advised
Irinotecan	No information available
Isoniazid	
Severe	Max. 200mg daily; peripheral neuropathy
Isotretinoin	
Mild	Avoid; increased risk of toxicity
Itraconazole	Bioavailability of oral formulations possibly reduced; avoid intravenous infusion if creatinine clearance less than 30 mL/minute
Kaletra®	Avoid oral solution due to propylene glycol content; use capsules with caution in severe impairment
Ketoprofen	*see* NSAIDs
Ketorolac	*see* NSAIDs
Lamotrigine	
Moderate to severe	Metabolite may accumulate
Lamivudine	
Mild	Reduce dose; consult product literature
Leflunomide	
Moderate to severe	Manufacturer advises avoid—no information available
Lepirudin	
Mild to moderate	Manufacturer advises reducing initial dose by 50% and subsequent doses by 50–85%
Severe	Avoid or stop infusion (unless APTT is below therapeutic levels when alternate day administration may be considered)
Lercanidipine	
Severe	Avoid
Levetiracetam	
Mild to moderate	Max. 2 g daily if creatinine clearance 50–79 mL/minute; max. 1.5 g daily if creatinine clearance 30–49 mL/minute; max. 1 g daily if creatinine clearance less than 30 mL/minute
Severe	0.5–1 g daily (as a single dose) in end-stage disease
Levocabastine	
Severe	Manufacturer advises avoid
Levocetirizine	
Mild to moderate	5mg on alternate days if creatinine clearance 30–50mL/minute; 5mg every 3 days if creatinine clearance less than 30mL/minute
Severe	Avoid
Levofloxacin	
Mild	Usual initial dose, then use half normal dose
Moderate to severe	Reduce dose; consult product literature

Drug and degree of impairment	Comment
Levomepromazine (methotrimeprazine)	*see* Antipsychotics
Linezolid	Manufacturer advises metabolites may acumulate if creatinine clearance less than 30 mL/minute
Lisinopril	*see* ACE Inhibitors
Lithium	
Mild	Avoid if possible or reduce dose and monitor plasma concentration carefully
Moderate	Avoid
Lopinavir [ingredient]	*see* Kaletra®
Loprazolam	*see* Anxiolytics and Hypnotics
Lorazepam	*see* Anxiolytics and Hypnotics
Lormetazepam	*see* Anxiolytics and Hypnotics
Lornoxicam	see NSAIDs
Losartan	
Moderate to severe	Start with 25 mg once daily
Loxapine	*see* Antipsychotics
Lymecycline	*see* Tetracyclines
Magnesium Salts	
Moderate	Avoid or reduce dose; increased risk of toxicity; magnesium carbonate mixture and magnesium trisilicate mixture also have high sodium content
Malarone®	
Mild	Avoid if creatinine clearance less than 30 mL/minute
Mefenamic Acid	*see* NSAIDs
Meloxicam	*see* NSAIDs
Melphalan	Reduce dose initially; avoid high doses in moderate to severe impairment
Meprobamate	*see* Anxiolytics and Hypnotics
Meptazinol	*see* Opioid Analgesics
Mercaptopurine	
Moderate	Reduce dose
Meropenem	
Mild	Increase dose interval to every 12 hours
Moderate	Use half normal dose every 12 hours
Severe	Use half normal dose every 24 hours
Mesalazine	
Moderate	Use with caution
Severe	Manufacturer advises avoid
Metformin	
Mild	Avoid; increased risk of lactic acidosis
Methadone	*see* Opioid Analgesics
Methenamine	
Mild	Avoid; ineffective
Methocarbamol	Manufacturer advises caution
Methotrexate	
Mild	Reduce dose; accumulates; nephrotoxic
Moderate	Avoid

Drug and degree of impairment	Comment
Methotrimeprazine	*see* Antipsychotics
Methyldopa	
Moderate	Start with small dose; increased sensitivity to hypotensive and sedative effect
Methysergide	Avoid
Metoclopramide	
Severe	Avoid or use small dose; increased risk of extrapyramidal reactions
Metolazone	*see* Thiazides
Metoprolol	*see* Beta-blockers
Midazolam	*see* Anxiolytics and Hypnotics
Milrinone	
Mild	Reduce dose and monitor response
Minocycline	*see* Tetracyclines
Mirtazapine	Manufacturer advises caution
Mivacurium	
Severe	Reduce dose; prolonged paralysis
Modafinil	
Severe	Use half normal dose
Moexipril	*see* ACE Inhibitors
Morphine	*see* Opioid Analgesics
Moxonidine	
Mild	Max. single dose 200 micrograms and max. daily dose 400 micrograms
Moderate to severe	Avoid
Nabumetone	*see* NSAIDs
Nadolol	*see* Beta-blockers
Nalbuphine	*see* Opioid Analgesics
Nalidixic Acid	
Moderate to severe	Use half normal dose; ineffective in renal failure because concentration in urine is inadequate
Naproxen	*see* NSAIDs
Naratriptan	
Moderate	Max. 2.5 mg in 24 hours
Severe	Avoid
Narcotic Analgesics	*see* Opioid Analgesics
Nebivolol	*see* Beta-blockers
Nefazodone	
Severe	Reduce dose
Nelfinavir	No information available—manufacturer advises caution
Neomycin	
Mild	Avoid; ototoxic; nephrotoxic
Neostigmine	
Moderate	May need dose reduction
Netilmicin	*see* Aminoglycosides
Nevirapine	No information available—manufacturer advises avoid
Nicardipine	
Moderate	Start with small dose
Nicotine	
Severe	May affect clearance of nicotine or its metabolites
Nicoumalone	*see* Anticoagulants, Oral

Drug and degree of impairment	Comment
Nimodipine	Manufacturer advises caution with intravenous administration
Nitrazepam	*see* Anxiolytics and Hypnotics
Nitrofurantoin	
Mild	Avoid; peripheral neuropathy; ineffective because of inadequate urine concentrations
Nitroprusside	
Moderate	Avoid prolonged use
Nizatidine	
Mild	Use half normal dose
Moderate	Use one-quarter normal dose
Norfloxacin	
Mild to moderate	Use half normal dose if creatinine clearance less than 30 mL/minute
NSAIDs	
Mild	Use lowest effective dose and monitor renal function; sodium and water retention; deterioration in renal function possibly leading to renal failure; deterioration also reported after topical use
Moderate to severe	Avoid if possible
Ofloxacin	
Mild	Usual initial dose, then use half normal dose
Moderate	Usual initial dose, then 100 mg every 24 hours
Olanzapine	Consider initial dose of 5 mg daily
Olsalazine	
Moderate	Use with caution
Severe	Manufacturer advises avoid
Opioid Analgesics	
Moderate to severe	Reduce doses or avoid; increased and prolonged effect; increased cerebral sensitivity
Oxaliplatin	
Mild	Manufacturer advises avoid if creatinine clearance less than 30 mL/minute
Oxazepam	*see* Anxiolytics and Hypnotics
Oxcarbazepine	
Mild	Initial dose 300 mg daily if creatinine clearance less than 30 mL/minute; increase according to response at intervals of at least 1 week
Oxpentifylline	*see* Pentoxifylline
Oxprenolol	*see* Beta-blockers
Oxybutynin	Manufacturer advises caution
Oxycodone	*see* Opioid Analgesics
Oxypertine	*see* Antipsychotics
Oxytetracycline	*see* Tetracyclines
Pamidronate Disodium	
Moderate to severe	Max. infusion rate 20 mg/hour
Pancuronium	
Severe	Prolonged duration of block
Pantoprazole	Max. 40 mg daily
Papaveretum	*see* Opioid Analgesics

Drug and degree of impairment	Comment
Paroxetine	
Moderate	Usual initial dose; small increments if necessary
Peginterferon alfa	Close monitoring required—reduce dose if necessary
Penicillamine	
Mild	Avoid if possible or reduce dose; nephrotoxic
Pentamidine	
Mild	Reduce dose; consult product literature
Pentazocine	*see* Opioid Analgesics
Pentoxifylline (oxpentifylline)	
Mild	Reduce dose by 30–50% if creatinine clearance less than 30 mL/minute
Pericyazine	*see* Antipsychotics
Perindopril	*see* ACE Inhibitors
Perphenazine	*see* Antipsychotics
Pethidine	*see* Opioid Analgesics
Phenazocine	*see* Opioid Analgesics
Phenindione	*see* Anticoagulants, Oral
Phenobarbital	
Severe	Avoid large doses
Phenoperidine	*see* Opioid Analgesics
Phenothiazines	*see* Antipsychotics
Phenylbutazone	*see* NSAIDs
Pholcodine	*see* Opioid Analgesics
Pilocarpine	Manufacturer advises caution with tablets
Pimozide	*see* Antipsychotics
Pindolol	*see* Beta-blockers
Piperacillin	
Adult:	
Mild	Max. daily dose 16 g if creatinine clearance is 40–80 mL/minute
Moderate	Max. daily dose 12 g if creatinine clearance is 20–40 mL/minute
Severe	Max. daily dose 8 g if creatinine clearance is less than 20 mL/minute
Child 1 month–12 years:	
Moderate to severe	Reduce dose; consult product literature
Piperazine	
Severe	Reduce dose; neurotoxic
Pipotiazine	*see* Antipsychotics
Piracetam	
Mild	Use half normal dose
Moderate	Use one-quarter normal dose
Severe	Avoid
Piroxicam	*see* NSAIDs
Polythiazide	*see* Thiazides
Potassium Salts	
Moderate	Avoid routine use; high risk of hyperkalaemia
Povidone–iodine	
Severe	Avoid regular application to inflamed or broken mucosa

Drug and degree of impairment	Comment
Pramipexole	
Mild	Initially 88 micrograms twice daily; if renal function declines, reduce dose further
Moderate to severe	Initially 88 micrograms daily; if renal function declines, reduce dose further
Pravastatin	
Moderate to severe	Start at lower end of dosage range
Prazosin	
Moderate to severe	Initially 500 micrograms daily; increase with caution
Primaxin®	
Mild	Reduce dose
Primidone	
Severe	Avoid large doses
Probenecid	
Moderate	Avoid; ineffective and toxicity increased
Procainamide	
Mild	Avoid or reduce dose
Procarbazine	
Severe	Avoid
Prochlorperazine	*see* Antipsychotics
Proguanil	
Mild	100 mg once daily
Moderate	50 mg on alternate days
Severe	50 mg once weekly; increased risk of haematological toxicity
Promazine	*see* Antipsychotics
Propantheline	Manufacturer advises caution
Propiverine	
Severe	Avoid
Propranolol	*see* Beta-blockers
Propylthiouracil	
Mild to moderate	Use three-quarters normal dose
Severe	Use half normal dose
Pseudoephedrine	
Severe	Avoid; increased CNS toxicity
Pyridostigmine	
Moderate	Reduce dose; excreted by kidney
Quetiapine	Manufacturer advises initial dose of 25 mg daily; increased daily in steps of 25–50 mg
Quinapril	*see* ACE Inhibitors
Quinine	Reduce parenteral maintenance dose for malaria treatment *see* section 5.4.1
Quinupristin [ingredient]	*see* Synercid®
Raloxifene	
Severe	Avoid
Raltitrexed	
Mild	Reduce dose and increase dosing interval
Moderate to severe	Avoid
Ramipril	*see* ACE Inhibitors
Ranitidine	
Severe	Use half normal dose; occasional risk of confusion

Drug and degree of impairment	Comment
Ranitidine Bismuth Citrate	
Severe	Avoid
Reboxetine	Initial dose 2 mg twice daily, increased according to tolerance
Regulan®	
Severe	Avoid; contains 6.4 mmol potassium per sachet
Reviparin	
Severe	Manufacturer advises avoid
Ribavirin	
Mild	Avoid oral treatment
Rifabutin	
Mild	Use half normal dose if creatinine clearance less than 30 mL/minute
Riluzole	No information available—manufacturer advises avoid
Risedronate Sodium	
Mild	Manufacturer advises avoid if creatinine clearance less than 30 mL/minute
Risperidone	Manufacturer advises initial dose of 500 micrograms twice daily increased in steps of 500 micrograms twice daily to 1–2 mg twice daily
Ritonavir [ingredient]	*see Kaletra®*
Rivastigmine	Manufacturer advises caution
Rizatriptan	
Mild to moderate	Reduce dose to 5 mg
Severe	Avoid
Rocuronium	
Moderate	Reduce dose; prolonged paralysis
Rofecoxib	*see NSAIDs*
Ropinirole	
Severe	Avoid
Rosiglitazone	
Severe	Manufacturer advises avoid—no information available
Salicylates	*see Aspirin*
Salt Substitutes	
Moderate	Avoid routine use; high risk of hyperkalaemia
Saquinavir	
Severe	Dose adjustment possibly required
Sertraline	Manufacturer advises caution
Sibutramine	
Mild to moderate	Manufacturer advises caution
Severe	Avoid
Sildenafil	
Mild	Initial dose 25 mg if creatinine clearance less than 30 mL/minute
Simvastatin	
Moderate to severe	Doses above 10 mg daily should be used with caution

Drug and degree of impairment	Comment
Sirolimus	Adjust immunosuppressant regimen in patients with raised serum-creatinine
Sodium Aurothiomalate	*see Gold*
Sodium Bicarbonate	
Severe	Avoid; specialised role in some forms of renal disease
Sodium Clodronate	*see Clodronate Sodium*
Sodium Nitroprusside	*see Nitroprusside*
Sodium Phenylbutyrate	Manufacturer advises caution
Sodium Salts	
Severe	Avoid
Sodium valproate	*see Valproate*
Solpadeine®	
Severe	Avoid; contains 18.5 mmol sodium per tablet
Solpadol®	
Severe	Avoid; contains 18.6 mmol sodium per tablet
Sotalol	*see Beta-blockers*
Spironolactone	*see Diuretics, Potassium-sparing*
Stavudine	
Mild	20 mg twice daily (15 mg if <60 kg)
Moderate to severe	20 mg once daily (15 mg if <60 kg)
Streptomycin	*see Aminoglycosides*
Sucralfate	
Severe	Avoid; aluminium is absorbed and may accumulate
Sulfadiazine	
Severe	Avoid; high risk of crystalluria
Sulfametopyrazine	*see Sulphonamides*
Sulfasalazine	
Moderate	Risk of toxicity including crystalluria—ensure high fluid intake
Severe	Avoid
Sulfinpyrazone	
Moderate	Avoid; ineffective as uricosuric
Sulindac	*see NSAIDs*
Sulphonamides	
Moderate	Ensure high fluid intake; rashes and blood disorders; crystalluria a risk
Sulphonylureas	*see under* individual drugs
Sulpiride	
Moderate	Avoid if possible, or reduce dose
Synercid®	Manufacturer advises caution
Tacalcitol	Monitor serum calcium concentration
Tamsulosin	
Severe	Manufacturer advises caution
Tazobactam [ingredient]	*see Tazocin®*

Drug and degree of impairment	Comment
Tazocin®	
Adult:	
Mild	Max 4.5g every 8 hours if creatinine clearance 20–80 mL/minute
Moderate to severe	Max. 4.5 g every 12 hours
Child under 12 years:	Consult product literature
Teicoplanin	
Mild	On day 4 use half normal dose if creatinine clearance is 40–60 mL/minute and use one-third normal dose if creatinine clearance is less than 40 mL/minute
Telmisartan	
Severe	Avoid
Temazepam	*see* Anxiolytics and Hypnotics
Tenoxicam	*see* NSAIDs
Terbinafine	
Mild	Use half normal dose
Terfenadine	
Mild	Use half normal dose if creatinine clearance less than 40 mL/minute
Tetracyclines	
Mild	Avoid tetracyclines except doxycycline or minocycline which may be used cautiously (avoid excessive doses)
Thiazides and Related Diuretics	
Moderate	Avoid; ineffective (metolazone remains effective but risk of excessive diuresis)
Thioridazine	*see* Antipsychotics
Tiaprofenic Acid	*see* NSAIDs
Ticarcillin [ingredient]	*see* Timentin®
Ticlopidine	
Mild	Consider dose reduction; discontinue if haemorrhagic or blood complication occur
Tiludronic Acid	
Moderate to severe	Avoid
Timentin®	
Moderate to severe	Reduce dose
Timolol	*see* Beta-blockers
Tinzaparin	
Severe	May need dose reduction
Tioguanine	
Moderate	Reduce dose
Tirofiban	
Mild	Use half normal dose if creatinine clearance less than 30 mL/minute

Drug and degree of impairment	Comment
Tizanidine	
Mild	Initially 2 mg once daily if creatinine clearance less than 25 mL/minute; increase once-daily dose gradually according to response before increasing frequency
Tobramycin	*see* Aminoglycosides
Tolbutamide	
Mild to moderate	Reduce dose
Severe	Avoid if possible; if no alternative reduce dose and monitor closely
Tolfenamic Acid	*see* NSAIDs
Tolterodine	Manufacturer advises caution
Topiramate	
Moderate to severe	Longer time to steady-state plasma concentrations
Topotecan	
Moderate	Reduce dose
Severe	Avoid
Torasemide	
Moderate	May need high doses
Tramadol	*see* Opioid Analgesics
Trandolapril	*see* ACE Inhibitors
Tranexamic acid	
Mild	Reduce dose
Tretinoin (oral)	
Mild	Reduce dose
Triamterene	*see* Diuretics, Potassium-sparing
Tribavirin	*see* Ribavirin
Triclofos	*see* Anxiolytics and Hypnotics
Trifluoperazine	*see* Antipsychotics
Trimeprazine	*see* Alimemazine
Trimethoprim	
Mild	Use half normal dose after 3 days if creatinine clearance 15–30 mL/minute
Moderate to severe	Use half normal dose if creatinine clearance less than 15 mL/minute—avoid if creatinine clearance less than 10 mL/minute (unless plasma-trimethoprim concentration monitored)
Trimetrexate	
Mild	Manufacturer advises caution; interrupt treatment if serum creatinine concentration greater than 221 micromol/litre
Tripotassium Dicitrato-bismuthate	
Severe	Avoid
Trisodium Edetate	
Mild	Avoid
Trospium	
Mild to moderate	Reduce dose to 20 mg once daily or 20 mg on alternate days if creatinine clearance 10–30 mL/minute
Severe	Avoid

Drug and degree of impairment	Comment
Tylex®	
Moderate to severe	Avoid effervescent tablets; contain 13.6 mmol sodium per tablet
Valaciclovir	*see* Aciclovir
Valproate	
Mild to moderate	Reduce dose
Severe	Alter dosage according to free serum valproic acid concentration
Valsartan	
Moderate to severe	Start with 40 mg once daily
Vancomycin	
Mild	Reduce dose—monitor plasma-vancomycin concentration and renal function regularly
Vecuronium	
Severe	Reduce dose; duration of block possibly prolonged
Venlafaxine	
Moderate	Use half normal dose
Severe	Avoid
Vigabatrin	
Mild	Excreted by kidney—lower maintenance dose may be required
Warfarin	see Anticoagulants, Oral
Xipamide	*see* Thiazides
Zafirlukast	
Moderate to severe	Manufacturer advises caution
Zalcitabine	
Mild to moderate	750 micrograms every 12 hours
Severe	750 micrograms daily
Zidovudine	
Severe	Reduce dose; manufacturer advises oral dose of 300–400 mg daily in divided doses or intravenous dose of 1 mg/kg 3–4 times daily
Zoledronic Acid	Manufacturer advises avoid if serum creatinine above 400 micromol/litre, unless benefit outweighs risk
Zopiclone	*see* Anxiolytics and Hypnotics
Zotepine	Initial dose 25 mg twice daily, increased gradually according to response (max. 75 mg twice daily)
Zuclopenthixol	*see* Antipsychotics

Appendix 4: Pregnancy

Drugs can have harmful effects on the fetus at any time during pregnancy. It is important to bear this in mind when prescribing for a woman of *childbearing age*.

During the *first trimester* drugs may produce congenital malformations (teratogenesis), and the period of greatest risk is from the third to the eleventh week of pregnancy.

During the *second* and *third trimesters* drugs may affect the growth and functional development of the fetus or have toxic effects on fetal tissues; and drugs given shortly before term or during labour may have adverse effects on labour or on the neonate after delivery.

The following list includes drugs which may have harmful effects in pregnancy and indicates the trimester of risk. It is based on human data but information on *animal* studies has been included for some newer drugs when its omission might be misleading.

> Drugs should be prescribed in pregnancy only if the expected benefit to the mother is thought to be greater than the risk to the fetus, and all drugs should be avoided if possible during the first trimester. Drugs which have been extensively used in pregnancy and appear to be usually safe should be prescribed in preference to new or untried drugs; and the smallest effective dose should be used.
>
> Few drugs have been shown conclusively to be teratogenic in man but no drug is safe beyond all doubt in early pregnancy. Screening procedures are available where there is a known risk of certain defects.
>
> Absence of a drug from the list does not imply safety.
>
> It should be noted that the BNF provides independent advice and may not always agree with the product literature.
>
> Information on drugs and pregnancy is also available from the National Teratology Information Service (telephone: (0191) 232 1525).

Table of drugs to be avoided or used with caution in pregnancy

Products introduced or amended since publication of BNF No. 42 (September 2001) are <u>underlined</u>.

Drug (trimester of risk)	Comment
Abacavir	Manufacturer advises avoid (toxicity in *animal* studies)
Abciximab	Manufacturer advises use only if potential benefit outweighs risk—no information available
Acamprosate	Manufacturer advises avoid
Acarbose	Manufacturer advises avoid; insulin is normally substituted in all diabetics

Drug (trimester of risk)	Comment
ACE Inhibitors (1, 2, 3)	Avoid; may adversely affect fetal and neonatal blood pressure control and renal function; also possible skull defects and oligohydramnios; toxicity in *animal* studies
Acebutolol	*see* Beta-blockers
Aceclofenac	*see* NSAIDs
Acemetacin	*see* NSAIDs
Acenocoumarol (nicoumalone)	*see* Anticoagulants, Oral
Acetazolamide	*see* Diuretics
Aciclovir	Experience limited—manufacturers advise use only when potential benefit outweighs risk; limited absorption from topical aciclovir preparations
Acipimox	Manufacturer advises avoid
Acitretin (1, 2, 3)	Teratogenic; effective contraception must be used for at least 1 month before treatment, during treatment, and for at least 2 years after stopping
Aclarubicin	Avoid (toxicity in *animal* studies); *see also* section 8.1
Acrivastine	*see* Antihistamines
Adapalene	Manufacturer advises teratogenicity in *animal* studies and recommends effective contraception during treatment
Alclometasone	*see* Corticosteroids
Alcohol (1, 2)	*see* 5HT₁ Agonists
Alcohol (1, 2)	Regular daily drinking is teratogenic (fetal alcohol syndrome) and may cause growth retardation; occasional single drinks are probably safe
(3)	Withdrawal syndrome may occur in babies of alcoholic mothers
Alendronic Acid	*see* Bisphosphonates
Alfentanil	*see* Opioid Analgesics
Alimemazine (trimeprazine)	*see* Antihistamines
Allopurinol	Toxicity not reported; manufacturer advises avoid; use only if no safer alternative and disease carries risk for mother or child
Almotriptan	*see* 5HT₁ Agonists
Alpha-blockers (post-synaptic)	No evidence of teratogenicity; manufacturers advise use only when potential benefit outweighs risk
Alprazolam	*see* Benzodiaepines
Alprostadil (urethral application only)	Manufacturer advises barrier contraception if partner pregnant
Alteplase	*see* Streptokinase
Altretamine	Avoid (teratogenic and embryotoxic in *animal* studies); *see also* section 8.1
Amantadine	Avoid; toxicity in *animal* studies

Drug (trimester of risk)	Comment
Amfebutamone	*see* Bupropion
Amifostine	Manufacturer advises avoid—no information available
Amikacin	*see* Aminoglycosides
Amiloride	*see* Diuretics
Aminoglutethimide	Avoid; toxicity in *animal* studies and may affect fetal sexual development
Aminoglycosides (2, 3)	Auditory or vestibular nerve damage; risk greatest with streptomycin; probably very small with gentamicin and tobramycin, but avoid unless essential (if given, serum-aminoglycoside concentration monitoring essential)
Aminophylline	*see* Theophylline
Amiodarone (2, 3)	Possible risk of neonatal goitre; use only if no alternative
Amisulpride	Manufacturer advises avoid
Amitriptyline	*see* Antidepressants, Tricyclic
Amlodipine	*see* Calcium-channel Blockers
Amobarbital	*see* Barbiturates
Amorolfine	Systemic absorption very low, but manufacturer advises avoid—no information available
Amoxapine	*see* Antidepressants, Tricyclic
Amphotericin	Not known to be harmful but manufacturers advise avoid unless potential benefit outweighs risk
Amprenavir	Avoid oral solution due to high propylene glycol content; manufacturer advises use capsules only if potential benefit outweighs risk
Amsacrine	Avoid (teratogenic and toxic in *animal* studies); may reduce fertility; *see also* section 8.1
Anabolic Steroids (1, 2, 3)	Masculinisation of female fetus
Anaesthetics, General (3)	Depress neonatal respiration
Anaesthetics, Local (3)	With large doses, neonatal respiratory depression, hypotonia, and bradycardia after paracervical or epidural block; neonatal methaemoglobinaemia with prilocaine and procaine
Analgesics	*see* Opioid Analgesics, Nefopam, NSAIDs and Paracetamol
Androgens (1, 2, 3)	Masculinisation of female fetus
Anticoagulants Heparin (1, 2, 3)	Osteoporosis has been reported after prolonged use; multidose vials may contain benzyl alcohol—some manufacturers advise avoid
Anticoagulants Oral (1, 2, 3)	Congenital malformations; fetal and neonatal haemorrhage *See also* section 2.8.2

Drug (trimester of risk)	Comment
Antidepressants, SSRI	Manufacturers advise use only if potential benefit outweighs risk (no evidence of teratogenicity)
Antidepressants, Tricyclic (and related) (3)	Tachycardia, irritability, and muscle spasms in neonate reported with imipramine
Antiepileptics	Benefit of treatment outweighs risk to fetus; risk of teratogenicity greater if more than one drug used; **important**: *see also* carbamazepine, ethosuximide, phenobarbital, phenytoin, valproate, vigabatrin, and pp. 227–8
Antihistamines	No evidence of teratogenicity; embryotoxicity in *animal* studies with high doses of hydroxyzine and loratadine; manufacturers of azatidine, cetirizine, desloratadine, hydroxyzine, loratadine, mizolastine and terfenadine advise avoid
Antimalarials (1, 3)	Benefit of prophylaxis and treatment in malaria outweighs risk; **important**: *see also* individual drugs and p. 312 and p. 313
Antipsychotics	*See also* amisulpride, clozapine, olanzapine, quetiapine, risperidone, zotepine
(3)	Extrapyramidal effects in neonate occasionally reported
Apomorphine	Avoid
Aspirin (3)	Impaired platelet function and risk of haemorrhage; delayed onset and increased duration of labour with increased blood loss; avoid analgesic doses if possible in last few weeks (low doses probably not harmful); with high doses, closure of fetal ductus arteriosus *in utero* and possibly persistent pulmonary hypertension of newborn; kernicterus in jaundiced neonates
Atenolol	*see* Beta-blockers
Atorvastatin	*see* Statins
Atosiban	For use in premature labour *see* section 7.1.3
Atovaquone	Manufacturer advises avoid unless potential benefit outweighs risk—no information available
Atracurium	Does not cross placenta in significant amounts but manufacturer advises use only if potential benefit outweighs risk
Atropine	Not known to be harmful; manufacturer advises caution
Auranofin	*see* Gold
Aurothiomalate	*see* Gold

Drug (trimester of risk)	Comment
Azapropazone	*see* NSAIDs
Azatadine	*see* Antihistamines
Azathioprine	*see* pp. 421–2
Azelastine	*see* Antihistamines
Azithromycin	Not known to be harmful but manufacturer advises use only if adequate alternatives not available
Aztreonam	Manufacturer advises avoid—no information available
Baclofen	Manufacturer advises use only if potential benefit outweighs risk (toxicity in *animal* studies)
Balsalazide	Manufacturer advises avoid
Bambuterol	*see* section 3.1 [text]
Barbiturates (3)	Withdrawal effects in neonate; *see also* Phenobarbital
Basiliximab	Avoid; adequate contraception must be used during treatment and for 8 weeks after last dose
Beclometasone	*see* Corticosteroids
Bendrofluazide	*see* Diuretics
Bendroflumethi-azide (bendrofluazide)	*see* Diuretics
Benorilate [aspirin-paracet-amol ester]	*see* Aspirin
Benperidol	*see* Antipsychotics
Benserazide [ingredient]	*see* Madopar®
Benzodiazepines	Avoid regular use (risk of neonatal withdrawal symptoms); use only if clear indication such as seizure control (high doses during late pregnancy or labour may cause neonatal hypothermia, hypotonia and respiratory depression)
Beta-blockers	May cause intra-uterine growth restriction, neonatal hypoglycaemia, and bradycardia; risk greater in severe hypertension *See also* section 2.5
Betamethasone	*see* Corticosteroids
Betaxolol	*see* Beta-blockers
Bethanechol	Manufacturer advises avoid—no information available
Bezafibrate	*see* Fibrates
Bismuth Chelate	Manufacturer advises avoid on theoretical grounds
Bisoprolol	*see* Beta-blockers
Bisphosphonates	Manufacturers advise avoid
Bleomycin	Avoid (teratogenic and carcinogenic in *animal* studies); *see also* section 8.1
Botulinum Toxin	Manufacturers advise avoid
Brinzolamide	Manufacturer advises avoid unless essential
Brompheniramine	*see* Antihistamines
Buclizine	*see* Antihistamines
Budesonide	*see* Corticosteroids

Drug (trimester of risk)	Comment
Bumetanide	*see* Diuretics
Bupivacaine	*see* Anaesthetics, Local
Buprenorphine	*see* Opioid Analgesics
Bupropion (amfebutamone)	Manufacturer advises avoid—no information available
Buserelin	Avoid
Buspirone	Manufacturer advises avoid (toxicity in *animal* studies)
Busulfan	Avoid (teratogenic in *animals*); manufacturer advises effective contraception during administration to men or women; *see also* section 8.1
Cabergoline	Once regular ovulatory cycles have been achieved manufacturer advises discontinuation for one month before intended conception (although no evidence of teratogenicity)
Calcitonin (salmon) (salcatonin)	Manufacturer advises avoid unless potential benefit outweighs risk (toxicity in *animal* studies)
Calcipotriol	Manufacturer advises avoid if possible
Calcium Folinate	Manufacturer advises use only if potential benefit outweighs risk
Calcium Levofolinate	*see* Calcium Folinate
Calcium-channel Blockers	May inhibit labour and manufacturers advise that diltiazem and some dihydropyridines are teratogenic in *animals,* but risk to fetus should be balanced against risk of uncontrolled maternal hypertension
Candesartan	As for ACE Inhibitors
Capecitabine	Avoid (teratogenic in *animal* studies); *see also* section 8.1
Capreomycin	Manufacturer advises use only if potential benefit outweighs risk—teratogenic in *animal* studies
Captopril	*see* ACE Inhibitors
Carbamazepine (1)	Risk of teratogenesis including increased risk of neural tube defects (counselling and screening and adequate folate supplements advised, e.g. 5 mg daily); *see also* Antiepileptics and pp. 227–8
(3)	May possibly cause vitamin K deficiency and risk of neonatal bleeding; if vitamin K not given at birth, neonate should be monitored closely for signs of bleeding
Carbenoxolone (3)	Avoid; causes sodium retention with oedema
Carbimazole (2, 3)	Neonatal goitre and hypo-thyroidism; has been associated with aplasia cutis of the neonate
Carbocisteine (1)	Manufacturers advises avoid

Drug (trimester of risk)	Comment
Carboplatin	Avoid (teratogenic and embryotoxic in *animal* studies); *see also* section 8.1
Carmustine	Avoid (teratogenic and embryotoxic in *animals*); manufacturer advises effective contraception during administration to men or women; *see also* section 8.1
Carnitine	No evidence of teratogenicity in *animal* studies; consider serious consequence of discontinuing treatment
Carvedilol	*see* Beta-blockers
Celecoxib	Manufacturer advises avoid (teratogenic in *animal* studies); *see also* NSAIDS
Celiprolol	*see* Beta-blockers
Cephalosporins	Not known to be harmful
Certoparin	*see* Anticoagulants (Heparin)
Cetirizine	*see* Antihistamines
Chloral hydrate	Avoid
Chlorambucil	Avoid; manufacturer advises effective contraception during administration to men or women; *see also* section 8.1
Chloramphenicol (3)	Neonatal 'grey syndrome'
Chlordiazepoxide	*see* Benzodiazepines
Chlormethine (mustine)	Avoid; *see also* section 8.1
Chloroquine	*see* Antimalarials
Chlorphenamine (chlorphenir-amine)	*see* Antihistamines
Chlorpheniramine	*see* Antihistamines
Chlorpromazine	*see* Antipsychotics
Chlorpropamide	*see* Sulphonylureas
Chlortalidone	*see* Diuretics
Chlortetracycline	*see* Tetracyclines
Ciclosporin	*see* p. 421
Cidofovir	Avoid (toxicity in *animal* studies); effective contraception required during and for 1 month after treatment; also men should avoid fathering a child during and for 3 months after treatment
Cilastatin [ingredient]	*see* Primaxin®
Cilazapril	*see* ACE Inhibitors
Cimetidine	Manufacturer advises avoid unless essential
Cinnarizine	*see* Antihistamines
Ciprofibrate	*see* Fibrates
Ciprofloxacin	*see* Quinolones
Cisatracurium	Manufacturer advises avoid—no information available
Cisplatin	Avoid (teratogenic and toxic in *animal* studies); *see also* section 8.1
Citalopram	*see* Antidepressants, SSRI
Cladribine	Avoid (teratogenic in *animal* studies); *see also* section 8.1

Drug (trimester of risk)	Comment
Clarithromycin	Not known to be harmful but manufacturer advises avoid unless potential benefit outweighs risk
Clemastine	*see* Antihistamines
Clindamycin	Not known to be harmful
Clobazam	*see* Benzodiazepines
Clobetasol	*see* Corticosteroids
Clobetasone	*see* Corticosteroids
Clodronate Sodium	*see* Bisphosphonates
Clomethiazole	Avoid if possible—especially during first and third trimesters
Clomifene	Possible effects on fetal development
Clomipramine	*see* Antidepressants, Tricyclic
Clonazepam	*see* Antiepileptics
Clopidogrel	Manufacturer advises avoid—no information available
Clorazepate	*see* Benzodiazepines
Clozapine	Manufacturer advises avoid
Co-amoxiclav	No evidence of teratogenicity but manufacturer advises avoid unless essential
Co-cyprindiol (1, 2, 3)	Feminisation of male fetus (due to cyproterone)
Codeine	*see* Opioid Analgesics
Colistin (2, 3)	Avoid—possible risk of fetal toxicity
Contraceptives, Oral	Epidemiological evidence suggests no harmful effects on fetus
Corticosteroids	Benefit of treatment, e.g. in asthma, outweighs risk (see also CSM advice, section 6.3.2); risk of intra-uterine growth retardation on prolonged or repeated systemic treatment; corticosteroid cover required by mother during labour; monitor closely if fluid retention
Co-trimoxazole	
(1)	Teratogenic risk (trimethoprim a folate antagonist)
(3)	Neonatal haemolysis and methaemoglobinaemia; fear of increased risk of kernicterus in neonates appears to be unfounded
Crisantaspase	Avoid; *see also* section 8.1
Cromoglicate	Not known to be harmful; *see also* section 3.1 [text]
Cyclizine	*see* Antihistamines
Cyclopenthiazide	*see* Diuretics
Cyclophosphamide	Avoid (manufacturer advises effective contraception during and for at least 3 months after administration to men or women); *see also* section 8.1
Cycloserine	Manufacturer advises use only if potential benefit outweighs risk—crosses the placenta
Cyclosporin	*see* Ciclosporin, p. 421
Cyproheptadine	*see* Antihistamines

Drug (trimester of risk)	Comment
Cyproterone [ingredient]	see Co-cyprindiol
Cytarabine	Avoid (teratogenic in *animal* studies); *see also* section 8.1
Dacarbazine	Avoid (carcinogenic and teratogenic in *animal* studies); ensure effective contraception during and for at least 6 months after administration to men or women; *see also* section 8.1
Daclizumab	Avoid
Dactinomycin	Avoid (teratogenic in *animal* studies); *see also* section 8.1
Dalfopristin [ingredient]	see Synercid®
Dalteparin	see Anticoagulants (Heparin)
Danaparoid	Insufficient information available
Danazol (1, 2, 3)	Avoid; has weak androgenic effects and virilisation of female fetus reported
Dantron (danthron)	Manufacturer advises avoid— no information available
Dapsone (3)	Neonatal haemolysis and methaemoglobinaemia; folic acid 5 mg daily should be given to mother
Darbepoetin	No evidence of harm in *animal* studies—manufacturer advises caution
Daunorubicin	Avoid (teratogenic and carcinogenic in *animal* studies); *see also* section 8.1
Debrisoquine	see Guanethidine
Deferiprone	Manufacturer advises avoid— teratogenic and embryotoxic in *animal* studies
Deflazacort	see Corticosteroids
Demeclocycline	see Tetracyclines
Desferrioxamine	Teratogenic in *animal* studies; manufacturer advises use only if potential benefit outweighs risk
Desflurane	see Anaesthetics, General
Desmopressin	Small oxytocic effect in third trimester
Desogestrel	see Contraceptives, Oral
Desonide	see Corticosteroids
Desoximetasone	see Corticosteroids
Dexamethasone	see Corticosteroids
Dexamfetamine	Manufacturer advises avoid (retrospective evidence of uncertain significance suggest- ing possible embryotoxicity)
Dexketoprofen	see NSAIDs
Dextran	Avoid—reports of anaphylaxis in mother causing fetal anoxia, neurological damage and death
Dextromethorphan	see Opioid Analgesics
Dextromoramide	see Opioid Analgesics
Dextropropoxy- phene	see Opioid Analgesics
Diamorphine	see Opioid Analgesics
Dianette®	see Co-cyprindiol

Drug (trimester of risk)	Comment
Diazepam	see Benzodiazepines
Diazoxide (2, 3)	Prolonged use may produce alopecia and impaired glucose tolerance in neonate; inhibits uterine activity during labour
Diclofenac	see NSAIDs
Didanosine	Manufacturer advises use only if potential benefit outweighs risk—no information available
Diethylstilbestrol (1)	High doses associated with vaginal carcinoma, urogenital abnormalities, and reduced fertility in female offspring
Diflucortolone	see Corticosteroids
Diflunisal	see NSAIDs
Digoxin	May need dosage adjustment
Dihydrocodeine	see Opioid Analgesics
Diloxanide	Manufacturer advises avoid— no information available
Diltiazem	see Calcium-channel Blockers
Diphenhydramine	see Antihistamines
Diphenoxylate	see Opioid Analgesics
Diphenylpyraline	see Antihistamines
Dipipanone	see Opioid Analgesics
Dipyridamole	Not known to be harmful
Disodium Etidronate	see Bisphosphonates
Disodium Pamidronate	see Bisphosphonates
Disopyramide (3)	May induce labour
Distigmine	Manufacturer advises avoid (may stimulate uterine contractions)
Disulfiram (1)	High concentrations of acetaldehyde which occur in presence of alcohol may be teratogenic
Diuretics	Not used to treat hypertension in pregnancy
(1)	Manufacturers advise avoid acetazolamide and torasemide (toxicity in *animal* studies)
(3)	Thiazides may cause neonatal thrombocytopenia
Docetaxel	Avoid (toxicity and reduced fertility in *animal* studies); manufacturer advises effective contraception during and for at least 3 months after administration; *see also* section 8.1
Docusate sodium	Not known to be harmful— manufacturer advises caution
Domperidone	Manufacturer advises avoid
Dornase alfa	No evidence of teratogenicity; manufacturer advises use only if potential benefit outweighs risk
Dosulepin (dothiepin)	see Antidepressants, Tricyclic
Dothiepin	see Antidepressants, Tricyclic
Doxazosin	see Alpha-blockers (post- synaptic)

Drug (trimester of risk)	Comment
Doxepin	*see* Antidepressants, Tricyclic
Doxorubicin	Avoid (teratogenic and toxic in *animal* studies); manufacturer of liposomal product advises effective contraception during and for at least 6 months after administration to men or women; *see also* section 8.1
Doxycycline	*see* Tetracyclines
Doxylamine	*see* Antihistamines
Dydrogesterone	Not known to be harmful
Econazole	Not known to be harmful
Edrophonium	Manufacturer advises use only if potential benefit outweighs risk
Efavirenz	Manufacturer advises use only if potential benefit outweighs risk—no information available
Eformoterol	*see* Formoterol
Enalapril	*see* ACE Inhibitors
Enflurane	*see* Anaesthetics, General
Enoxaparin	Manufacturer advises avoid unless no safer alternative
Enoximone	Manufacturer advises use only if potential benefit outweighs risk
Entacapone	Manufacturer advises avoid— no information available
Ephedrine	Increased fetal heart rate reported with parenteral ephedrine
Epirubicin	Avoid (carcinogenic in *animal* studies); *see also* section 8.1
Epoetin	No evidence of harm; benefits probably outweigh risks of anaemia and of transfusion in pregnancy
Eprosartan	*as for* ACE Inhibitors
Eptifibatide	Manufacturer advises use only if potential benefit outweighs risk—no information available
Ergotamine (1, 2, 3)	Oxytocic effects on the pregnant uterus
Erythromycin	Not known to be harmful
Esmolol	*see* Beta-blockers
Esomeprazole	Manufacturer advises caution— no information available
Etanercept	Manufacturer advises avoid— no information available
Ethambutol	Not known to be harmful *see also* p. 283
Ether	*see* Anaesthetics, General
Ethinylestradiol	*see* Contraceptives, Oral
Ethionamide (1)	May be teratogenic
Ethosuximide (1)	May possibly be teratogenic; *see* Antiepileptics
Etidronate Disodium	*see* Bisphosphonates
Etodolac	*see* NSAIDs
Etomidate	*see* Anaesthetics, General
Etoposide	Avoid (teratogenic in *animal* studies); *see also* section 8.1
Etynodiol	*see* Contraceptives, Oral

Drug (trimester of risk)	Comment
Famciclovir	*see* Aciclovir
Famotidine	Manufacturer advises avoid unless potential benefit outweighs risk
Fansidar®	
(1)	Possible teratogenic risk (pyrimethamine a folate antagonist)
(3)	Neonatal haemolysis and methaemoglobinaemia; fear of increased risk of kernicterus in neonates appears to be unfounded *see also* Antimalarials
Felodipine	*see* Calcium-channel Blockers
Fenbufen	*see* NSAIDs
Fenofibrate	*see* Fibrates
Fenoprofen	*see* NSAIDs
Fenoterol	*see* section 3.1 [text]
Fentanyl	*see* Opioid Analgesics
Fenticonazole	Manufacturer advises avoid unless essential
Fexofenadine	*see* Antihistamines
Fibrates	Embryotoxicity in *animal* studies—manufacturers advise avoid
Filgrastim	Toxicity in *animal* studies; manufacturer advises use only if potential benefit outweighs risk
Finasteride (1, 2, 3)	Avoid unprotected intercourse (see section 6.4.2). May cause feminisation of male fetus
Flavoxate	Manufacturer advises avoid unless no safer alternative
Flecainide	Manufacturer advises toxicity in *animal* studies
Fluclorolone	*see* Corticosteroids
Fluconazole	Manufacturer advises avoid— multiple congenital abnormalities reported with long-term high doses
Flucytosine	Teratogenic in *animal* studies; manufacturer advises use only if potential benefit outweighs risk
Fludarabine	Avoid (embryotoxic and teratogenic in *animal* studies); manufacturer advises effective contraception during and for at least 6 months after administration to men or women; *see also* section 8.1
Fludroxycortide (flurandrenolone)	*see* Corticosteroids
Flumazenil	Manufacturer advises avoid unless potential benefit outweighs risk
Flunisolide	*see* Corticosteroids
Flunitrazepam	*see* Benzodiazepines
Fluocinolone	*see* Corticosteroids
Fluocinonide	*see* Corticosteroids
Fluocortolone	*see* Corticosteroids
Fluorouracil	Avoid (teratogenic); *see also* section 8.1

Drug (trimester of risk)	Comment
Fluoxetine	*see* Antidepressants, SSRI
Flupentixol	*see* Antipsychotics
Fluphenazine	*see* Antipsychotics
Flurandrenolone	*see* Corticosteroids
Flurazepam	*see* Benzodiazepines
Flurbiprofen	*see* NSAIDs
Fluticasone	*see* Corticosteroids
Fluvastatin	*see* Statins
Fluvoxamine	*see* Antidepressants, SSRI
Follitropin alfa and beta	Avoid
Fomivirsen	Manufacturer advises use only if potential benefit outweighs risk—no information available
Formoterol (eformoterol)	Manufacturers advise use only if potential benefit outweighs risk; *see also* section 3.1 [text]
Foscarnet	Manufacturer advises avoid
Fosinopril	*see* ACE Inhibitors
Fosphenytoin	*see* Phenytoin
Framycetin	*see* Aminoglycosides
Frusemide	*see* Diuretics
Furosemide (frusemide)	*see* Diuretics
Fusidic acid	*see* Sodium Fusidate
Gabapentin	*see* Antiepileptics
Galantamine	No information available
Gamolenic Acid	Manufacturer advises caution (but no teratogenic effects in *animals*)
Ganciclovir	Avoid—teratogenic risk; *see also* p. 307
Gemcitabine	Avoid (teratogenic in *animal* studies); *see also* section 8.1
Gemfibrozil	*see* Fibrates
Gentamicin	*see* Aminoglycosides
Gestodene	*see* Contraceptives, Oral
Gestrinone (1, 2, 3)	Avoid
Glatiramer	Manufacturer advises avoid unless potential benefit outweighs risk
Glibenclamide	*see* Sulphonylureas
Gliclazide	*see* Sulphonylureas
Glimepiride	*see* Sulphonylureas
Glipizide	*see* Sulphonylureas
Gliquidone	*see* Sulphonylureas
Gold	
Auranofin	Manufacturer advises teratogenicity in *animal* studies; effective contraception should be used during and for at least 6 months after treatment
Aurothiomalate (1, 2, 3)	Manufacturer advises avoid
Goserelin	Manufacturer advises avoid in pregnancy—exclude pregnancy before treatment and use non-hormonal contraceptives during treatment
Granisetron	Manufacturer advises use only when compelling reasons—no information available

Drug (trimester of risk)	Comment
Griseofulvin	Avoid (fetotoxicity and teratogenicity in *animals*); effective contraception required during and for at least 1 month after administration (**important**: effectiveness of oral contraceptives reduced, see p. 387); also men should avoid fathering a child during and for at least 6 months after administration
Growth Hormone	*see* Somatropin
Guanethidine (3)	Postural hypotension and reduced uteroplacental perfusion; should not be used to treat hypertension in pregnancy
Haem arginate (human hemin)	Manufacturer advises avoid unless essential
Halcinonide	*see* Corticosteroids
Haloperidol	*see* Antipsychotics
Halothane	*see* Anaesthetics, General
Heparin	*see* Anticoagulants
Hexachlorophene	Manufacturer advises avoid
5HT$_1$ Agonists	Limited experience—manufacturers advise avoid unless potential benefit outweighs risk
Human menopausal gonadotrophins	Avoid
Hydralazine (1, 2)	Manufacturer advises avoid before third trimester; no reports of serious harm following use in third trimester
Hydrochloro-thiazide	*see* Diuretics
Hydrocortisone	*see* Corticosteroids
Hydroflumethiazide	*see* Diuretics
Hydromorphone	*see* Opioid Analgesics
Hydroxycarbamide (hydroxyurea)	Avoid (teratogenic in *animal* studies); manufacturer advises effective contraception before and during administration; *see also* section 8.1
Hydroxychloro-quine	Avoid for rheumatic disease
Hydroxyprogest-erone	Manufacturer advises use only if strictly indicated—genital malformations and other defects reported in male and female fetuses
Hydroxyurea	*see* Hydroxycarbamide
Hydroxyzine	*see* Antihistamines
Hyoscine butylbromide	Manufacturer advises use only if potential benefit outweighs risk
Ibuprofen	*see* NSAIDs
Idarubicin	Avoid (teratogenic and toxic in *animal* studies); *see also* section 8.1
Idoxuridine	Teratogenic in *animal* studies
Ifosfamide	Avoid (teratogenic and carcinogenic in *animals*); manufacturer advises adequate contraception during and for at least 6 months after administration to men or women; *see also* section 8.1

Drug (trimester of risk)	Comment
Imatinib	Manufacturer advises avoid unless potential benefit outweighs risk *see also* section 8.1
Imidapamil	*see* ACE inhibitors
Imiglucerase	Manufacturer advises use only if potential benefit outweighs risk—no information available
Imipenem [ingredient]	*see Primaxin®*
Imipramine	*see* Antidepressants, Tricyclic
Imiquimod	No evidence of teratogenicity or toxicity in *animal* studies; manufacturer advises caution
Immunosuppressants	*see* section 8.1
Indapamide	*see* Diuretics
Indinavir	Manufacturer advises use only if potential benefit outweighs risk—no information available; theoretical risk of hyperbilirubinaemia in neonate if used at term
Indometacin	*see* NSAIDs
Infliximab	Avoid; manufacturer advises adequate contraception during and for at least 6 months after last dose
Insulin (1, 2, 3)	Insulin requirements should be assessed frequently by an experienced diabetic physician
Interferons	Manufacturers recommend avoid unless compelling reasons
Iodine and Iodides (2, 3)	Neonatal goitre and hypothyroidism
Radioactive iodine (1, 2, 3)	Permanent hypothyroidism—avoid
Iodoform	*see* Povidone–iodine
Ipratropium	Not known to be harmful; see section 3.1
Irbesartan	As for ACE Inhibitors
Irinotecan	Avoid (teratogenic and toxic in *animal* studies); manufacturer advises effective contraception during and for at least 3 months after administration; *see also* section 8.1
Iron (parenteral)	Avoid in early pregnancy
Isocarboxazid	*see* MAOIs
Isoflurane	*see* Anaesthetics, General
Isoniazid	Not known to be harmful; *see also* p. 283
Isotretinoin (1, 2, 3)	Teratogenic; effective contraception must be used for at least 1 month before oral treatment, during treatment and for at least 1 month after stopping; also avoid topical treatment
Isradipine	*see* Calcium-channel Blockers

Drug (trimester of risk)	Comment
Itraconazole	Manufacturer advises use only in life-threatening situations (toxicity at high doses in *animal* studies); ensure effective contraception during treatment and until the next menstrual period following end of treatment
Kaletra®	Avoid oral solution due to high propylene glycol content; manufacturer advises use capsules only if potential benefit outweighs risk (toxicity in *animal* studies)
Ketamine	*see* Anaesthetics, General
Ketoconazole	Manufacturer advises teratogenicity in *animal* studies; packs carry a warning to avoid in pregnancy
Ketoprofen	*see* NSAIDs
Ketorolac	*see* NSAIDs
Ketotifen	*see* Antihistamines
Labetalol	*see* Beta-blockers
Lacidipine	*see* Calcium-channel Blockers
Lactitol (1)	Manufacturer advises avoid—insufficient evidence of safety
Lactulose	Not known to be harmful
Lamivudine	Manufacturer advises avoid during first trimester—no information available
Lamotrigine	*see* Antiepileptics
Lanreotide	Manufacturer advises avoid—growth retardation in *animal* studies
Lansoprazole	Manufacturer advises avoid
Latanoprost	Manufacturer advises avoid
Leflunomide	Avoid—active metabolite teratogenic in *animal* studies; effective contraception essential during treatment and for at least 2 years after treatment in women and at least 3 months after treatment in men (*see also* Leflunomide section 10.1.3)
Lenograstim	Toxicity in *animal* studies; manufacturer advises use only if potential benefit outweighs risk
Lepirudin	Avoid
Lercanidipine	*see* Calcium-channel blockers
Levetiracetam	Toxicity in *animal* studies—manufacturer advises use only if potential benefit outweighs risk; *see also* Antiepileptics
Levobupivacaine (1)	Manufacturer advises avoid if possible—toxicity in *animal* studies; *see also* Anaesthetics, local
Levocabastine	*see* Antihistamines
Levocetirizine	*see* Antihistamines
Levodopa	Manufacturers advise toxicity in *animal* studies
Levofloxacin	*see* Quinolones
Levomepromazine (methotrimeprazine)	*see* Antipsychotics

Drug (trimester of risk)	Comment
Levonorgestrel	*see* Contraceptives, Oral
Levothyroxine (thyroxine)	Monitor maternal serum-thyrotrophin concentration—dosage adjustment may be necessary
Lidocaine (lignocaine)	*see* Anaesthetics, Local
Lignocaine	*see* Anaesthetics, Local
Linezolid	Manufacturer advises use only if potential benefit outweighs risk—no information available
Liothyronine	Does not cross the placenta in significant amounts; monitor maternal thyroid function tests—dosage adjustment may be necessary
Lisinopril	*see* ACE Inhibitors
Lithium	
(1)	Avoid if possible (risk of teratogenicity, including cardiac abnormalities)
(2,3)	Dose requirements increased (but on delivery return to normal abruptly); close monitoring of serum-lithium concentration advised (risk of toxicity in neonate)
Lofepramine	*see* Antidepressants, Tricyclic
Loperamide	Manufacturers advise avoid—no information available
Lopinavir [ingredient]	*see* Kaletra®
Loprazolam	*see* Benzodiazepines
Loratadine	Embryotoxic in *animal* studies; *see also* Antihistamines
Lorazepam	*see* Benzodiazepines
Lormetazepam	*see* Benzodiazepines
Lornoxicam	*see* NSAIDs
Losartan	As for ACE Inhibitors
Lymecycline	*see* Tetracyclines
Madopar®	*see* Levodopa
Magnesium sulphate (3)	Not known to be harmful for short-term intravenous administration in eclampsia but excessive doses cause neonatal respiratory depression
Malarone®	Manufacturer advises avoid unless essential
Maloprim®	
(1)	Possible teratogenic risk (pyrimethamine a folate antagonist)
(3)	Neonatal haemolysis and methaemoglobinaemia (due to dapsone); adequate folate supplements should be given to mother; *see also* Antimalarials
MAOIs (including moclobemide) (1, 2, 3)	No evidence of harm but manufacturers advise avoid unless compelling reasons
Maprotiline	*see* Antidepressants, Tricyclic (and related)
Mebendazole	Manufacturer advises toxicity in *animal* studies

Drug (trimester of risk)	Comment
Mebeverine	Not known to be harmful; manufacturers advise caution
Medroxyprogesterone acetate	Avoid—genital malformations and cardiac defects reported in male and female fetuses
Mefenamic Acid	*see* NSAIDs
Mefloquine (1)	Manufacturer advises teratogenicity in *animal* studies, but *see* p. 312 and p. 313
Meloxicam	*see* NSAIDs
Melphalan	Avoid (manufacturer advises adequate contraception during administration to men or women); *see also* section 8.1
Menadiol (3)	Neonatal haemolytic anaemia, hyperbilirubinaemia and increased risk of kernicterus in jaundiced infants
Menotrophin	Avoid
Meprobamate	Manufacturer advises avoid if possible
Meptazinol	*see* Opioid Analgesics
Mercaptamine	Manufacturer advises avoid
Mercaptopurine	Avoid (teratogenic); *see also* section 8.1
Meropenem	Manufacturer advises use only if potential benefit outweighs risk—no information available
Mesalazine	Negligible quantities cross placenta
Mesna	Not known to be harmful; *see also* section 8.1
Mesterolone	*see* Androgens
Mestranol	*see* Contraceptives, Oral
Metaraminol	May reduce placental perfusion—manufacturer advises use only if potential benefit outweighs risk
Metformin (1, 2, 3)	Avoid; insulin is normally substitued in all diabetics
Methadone	*see* Opioid Analgesics
Methocarbamol	Manufacturer advises avoid unless potential benefit outweighs risk
Methotrexate	Avoid (teratogenic; fertility may be reduced during therapy but this may be reversible); manufacturer advises effective contraception during and for at least 6 months after administration to men or women; *see also* section 8.1
Methotrimeprazine	*see* Antipsychotics
Methyldopa	Not known to be harmful
Methylphenidate	Limited experience; manufacturer advises avoid unless potential benefit outweighs risk
Methylprednisolone	*see* Corticosteroids
Methysergide	Manufacturer advises avoid
Metoclopramide	Not known to be harmful but manufacturer advises use only when compelling reasons
Metolazone	*see* Diuretics
Metoprolol	*see* Beta-blockers

Drug (trimester of risk)	Comment
Metronidazole	Manufacturer advises avoidance of high-dose regimens
Metyrapone	Avoid (may impair biosynthesis of fetal-placental steroids)
Mianserin	*see* Antidepressants, Tricyclic (and related)
Miconazole	Manufacturer advises avoid unless essential
Midazolam	*see* Benzodiazepines
Mifepristone	Manufacturer advises that if treatment fails, essential that pregnancy be terminated by another method
Milrinone	Manufacturer advises use only if potential benefit outweighs risk
Minocycline	*see* Tetracyclines
Minoxidil (3)	Neonatal hirsutism reported
Misoprostol (1, 2, 3)	Avoid—potent uterine stimulant (has been used to induce abortion) and may be teratogenic
Mitomycin	Avoid (teratogenic in *animal* studies); *see also* section 8.1
Mitoxantrone (mitozantrone)	Avoid; manufacturer advises effective contraception during and for at least 6 months after administration to men or women; *see also* section 8.1
Mitozantrone	*see* Mitoxantrone
Mivacurium	Manufacturer advises avoid— no information available
Mizolastine	Manufacturer advises avoid; *see also* Antihistamines
Moclobemide	*see* MAOIs
Modafinil	Manufacturer advises avoid
Moexipril	*see* ACE Inhibitors
Molgramostim	Toxicity in *animal* studies— manufacturer advises avoid unless potential benefit outweighs risk
Montelukast	Manufacturer advises avoid unless essential
Morphine	*see* Opioid Analgesics
Movicol®	Manufacturer advises use only if essential—no information available
Moxonidine	Manufacturer advises avoid— no information available
Moxisylyte (thymoxamine)	Manufacturer advises avoid
Mupirocin	Manufacturer advises avoid unless potential benefit outweighs risk—no information available
Mustine	*see* Chlormethine
Mycophenolate Mofetil	Manufacturer advises avoid— toxicity in *animal* studies; effective contraception required during and for 6 weeks after discontinuation of treatment
Nabumetone	*see* NSAIDs

Drug (trimester of risk)	Comment
Nadolol	*see* Beta-blockers
Nafarelin	Avoid
Nalbuphine	*see* Opioid Analgesics
Nalidixic acid	*see* Quinolones
Naloxone	Manufacturer advises use only if potential benefit outweighs risk
Nandrolone	*see* Anabolic Steroids
Naproxen	*see* NSAIDs
Naratriptan	*see* $5HT_1$ Agonists
Narcotic Analgesics	*see* Opioid Analgesics
Nateglinide	Manufacturer advises avoid— toxicity in *animal* studies; insulin is normally substituted in all diabetics
Nebivolol	*see* Beta-blockers
Nedocromil	*see* section 3.1 [text]
Nefazodone	No information available— manufacturer advises use only if clearly needed
Nefopam	No information available— manufacturer advises avoid unless no safer treatment
Nelfinavir	No information available— manufacturer advises use only if potential benefit outweighs risk
Neomycin	*see* Aminoglycosides
Neostigmine	Manufacturer advises use only if potential benefit outweighs risk
Netilmicin	*see* Aminoglycosides
Nevirapine	Although manufacturers advise avoid, may be appropriate to use if clearly indicated; *see also* p. 300
Nicardipine	*see* Calcium-channel Blockers
Nicorandil	Manufacturer advises use only if potential benefit outweighs risk—no information available
Nicotine (1,2,3)	Avoid
Nicoumalone	*see* Anticoagulants, Oral
Nifedipine	*see* Calcium-channel Blockers
Nimodipine	*see* Calcium-channel Blockers
Nisoldipine	*see* Calcium-channel Blockers
Nitrazepam	*see* Benzodiazepines
Nitrofurantoin (3)	May produce neonatal haemolysis if used at term
Nitrous oxide	*see* Anaesthetics, General
Nizatidine	Manufacturer advises avoid unless essential
Noradrenaline (norepinephrine) (1, 2, 3)	Avoid—may reduce placental perfusion
Norethisterone	Masculinisation of female fetuses and other defects reported; *see also* Contraceptives, Oral
Norfloxacin	*see* Quinolones
Norgestimate	*see* Contraceptives, Oral
Nortriptyline	*see* Antidepressants, Tricyclic

Drug (trimester of risk)	Comment
NSAIDs	Most manufacturers advise avoid (or avoid unless potential benefit outweighs risk); ketorolac contra-indicated during pregnancy, labour and delivery
(3)	With regular use closure of fetal ductus arteriosus *in utero* and possibly persistent pulmonary hypertension of the newborn.Delayed onset and increased duration of labour
Nystatin	No information available, but absorption from gastro-intestinal tract negligible
Octreotide (1, 2, 3)	Possible effect on fetal growth; manufacturer advises use only if potential benefit outweighs risk
Oestrogens	*see* Contraceptives, Oral
Ofloxacin	*see* Quinolones
Olanzapine	Manufacturer advises use only if potential benefit outweighs risk
Olsalazine	Manufacturer advises avoid unless potential benefit outweighs risk
Omeprazole	Manufacturer advises toxicity in *animal* studies
Ondansetron	No information available; manufacturer advises avoid unless potential benefit outweighs risk
Opioid Analgesics (3)	Depress neonatal respiration; withdrawal effects in neonates of dependent mothers; gastric stasis and risk of inhalation pneumonia in mother during labour
Orlistat	Manufacturer advises avoid—no information available
Orphenadrine	Manufacturer advises caution
Oxaliplatin	Manufacturer advises avoid—no information available; *see also* section 8.1
Oxazepam	*see* Benzodiazepines
Oxcarbazepine (1)	Risk of teratogenesis including increased risk of neural tube defects (counselling and screening and adequate folate supplements advised, e.g. 5 mg daily); *see also* Antiepileptics and pp. 227–8
(3)	Because of neonatal bleeding tendency associated with some antiepileptics, manufacturer advises prophylactic vitamin K$_1$ for mother before delivery (as well as for neonate)
Oxitropium	Toxicity in *animal* studies—manufacturer advises use only if potential benefit outweighs risk
Oxprenolol	*see* Beta-blockers

Drug (trimester of risk)	Comment
Oxybutynin	Manufacturer advises avoid unless potential benefit outweighs risk—toxicity in *animal* studies
Oxycodone	*see* Opioid Analgesics
Oxypertine	*see* Antipsychotics
Oxytetracycline	*see* Tetracyclines
Paclitaxel	Avoid (toxicity in *animal* studies); *see also* section 8.1
Pamidronate Disodium	*see* Bisphosphonates
Pancreatin	Not known to be harmful
Pancuronium	Manufacturer advises avoid unless potential benefit outweighs risk—no information available
Pantoprazole	Manufacturer advises avoid unless potential benefit outweighs risk—fetotoxic in *animals*
Papaveretum	*see* Opioid Analgesics
Paracetamol	Not known to be harmful
Paraldehyde	Manufacturer advises avoid unless essential—crosses the placenta
Paroxetine	*see* Antidepressants, SSRI
Penicillamine (1, 2, 3)	Fetal abnormalities reported rarely; avoid if possible
Penicillins	Not known to be harmful
Pentamidine isetionate	Manufacturer advises avoid unless essential
Pentazocine	*see* Opioid Analgesics
Pentostatin	Avoid (teratogenic in *animal* studies); manufacturer advises that men should not father children during and for 6 months after administration; *see also* section 8.1
Pergolide	Manufacturer advises use only if potential benefit outweighs risk
Pericyazine	*see* Antipsychotics
Perindopril	*see* ACE Inhibitors
Perphenazine	*see* Antipsychotics
Pethidine	*see* Opioid Analgesics
Phenelzine	*see* MAOIs
Phenindione	*see* Anticoagulants, Oral
Phenobarbital (1, 3)	Congenital malformations. May possibly cause vitamin K deficiency and risk of neonatal bleeding; if vitamin K not given at birth, neonate should be monitored closely for signs of bleeding; *see also* Antiepileptics
Phenothiazines	*see* Antipsychotics
Phentolamine	No information available

Drug (trimester of risk)	Comment
Phenytoin (1, 3)	Congenital malformations (screening advised); adequate folate supplements should be given to mother (e.g. folic acid 5 mg daily). May possibly cause vitamin K deficiency and risk of neonatal bleeding; if vitamin K not given at birth, neonate should be monitored closely for signs of bleeding. Caution in interpreting plasma concentrations—bound may be reduced but free (i.e. effective) unchanged; *see also* Antiepileptics
Pholcodine	*see* Opioid Analgesics
Phytomenadione	Manufacturer advises use only if potential benefit outweighs risk—no specific information available
Pilocarpine	Avoid—smooth muscle stimulant; toxicity in *animal* studies
Pimozide	*see* Antipsychotics
Pindolol	*see* Beta-blockers
Pioglitazone	Manufacturer advises avoid—toxicity in *animal* studies; insulin is normally substituted in all diabetics
Piperazine	No clinical evidence of harm but packs sold to the general public carry a warning to avoid in pregnancy except on medical advice
Piperacillin	*see* Penicillins
Pipotiazine	*see* Antipsychotics
Piracetam	Manufacturer advises avoid
Piroxicam	*see* NSAIDs
Podophyllotoxin	Avoid
Podophyllum resin (1, 2, 3)	Avoid—neonatal death and teratogenesis have been reported
Polystyrene Sulphonate Resins	Manufacturers advise use only if potential benefit outweighs risk—no information available
Polythiazide	*see* Diuretics
Povidone–iodine (2, 3)	Sufficient iodine may be absorbed to affect the fetal thyroid
Pramipexole	Manufacturer advises use only if potential benefit outweighs risk—no information available
Pravastatin	*see* Statins
Prazosin	*see* Alpha-blockers (post-synaptic)
Prednisolone	*see* Corticosteroids
Prilocaine (3)	Neonatal methaemoglobinaemia; *see also* Anaesthetics, Local
Primaquine (3)	Neonatal haemolysis and methaemoglobinaemia; *see also* Antimalarials
Primaxin®	Manufacturer advises avoid unless potential benefit outweighs risk (toxicity in *animal* studies)

Drug (trimester of risk)	Comment
Primidone	*see* Phenobarbital
Procaine (3)	Neonatal methaemoglobinaemia; *see also* Anaesthetics, Local
Procarbazine	Avoid (teratogenic in *animal* studies and isolated reports in humans); *see also* section 8.1
Prochlorperazine	*see* Antipsychotics
Progesterone	Not known to be harmful
Proguanil	Adequate folate supplements should be given to mother; *see also* Antimalarials
Promazine	*see* Antipsychotics
Promethazine	*see* Antihistamines
Propafenone	Manufacturer advises avoid—no information available
Propantheline	Manufacturer advises avoid—no information available
Propiverine	Manufacturer advises avoid (retardation of skeletal development in *animals*)
Propofol	*see* Anaesthetics, General
Propranolol	*see* Beta-blockers
Propylthiouracil (2, 3)	Neonatal goitre and hypothyroidism
Protionamide (1)	May be teratogenic
Pseudoephedrine	Not known to be harmful
Pyrazinamide	Manufacturer advises use only if potential benefit outweighs risk; *see also* p. 283
Pyridostigmine	Manufacturer advises use only if potential benefit outweighs risk
Pyrimethamine (1)	Theoretical teratogenic risk (folate antagonist); adequate folate supplements should be given to mother; *see also* Antimalarials
Quetiapine	Manufacturer advises use only if potential benefit outweighs risk
Quinagolide	Manufacturer advises discontinue when pregnancy confirmed unless medical reason for continuing
Quinapril	*see* ACE Inhibitors
Quinine (1)	High doses are teratogenic; but in malaria benefit of treatment outweighs risk
Quinolones (1, 2, 3)	Avoid—arthropathy in *animal* studies; safer alternatives available
Quinupristin [ingredient]	*see* Synercid®
Rabeprazole	Manufacturer advises avoid—no information available
Raltitrexed	Pregnancy must be excluded before treatment; ensure effective contraception during and for at least 6 months after administration to men or women; *see also* section 8.1
Ramipril	*see* ACE Inhibitors

Drug (trimester of risk)	Comment
Ranitidine	Manufacturer advises avoid unless essential, but not known to be harmful
Ranitidine bismuth citrate	Safety not established
Rasburicase	Manufacturer advises avoid—no information available
Razoxane	Avoid (teratogenic in *animal* studies); *see also* section 8.1
Reboxetine	Manufacturer advises avoid (and discontinue if pregnancy occurs)—no information available
Remifentanil	No information available; *see also* Opioid Analgesics
Repaglinide	Manufacturer advises avoid; insulin is normally substituted in all diabetics
Reteplase	*see* Streptokinase
Reviparin	Manufacturer advises avoid—no information available
Ribavirin	Avoid; teratogenicity in *animal* studies; ensure effective contraception during oral administration and for 4 months after treatment in women and 7 months after treatment in men; *see also* Ribavirin section 5.3
Rifabutin	Manufacturer advises avoid—no information available
Rifampicin	
(1)	Manufacturers advise very high doses teratogenic in *animal* studies; *see also* p. 283
(3)	Risk of neonatal bleeding may be increased
Riluzole	No information available; manufacturer advises avoid
Risedronate sodium	*see* Bisphosphonates
Risperidone	Manufacturer advises use only if potential benefit outweighs risk
Ritodrine	For use in premature labour see section 7.1.3
Ritonavir	Manufacturer advises use only if potential benefit outweighs risk—no information available;
Rituximab	Avoid unless potential benefit to mother outweighs risk of B-lymphocyte depletion in fetus—effective contraception required during and for 12 months after treatment
Rivastigmine	Manufacturer advises use only if potential benefit outweighs risk
Rizatriptan	*see* 5HT$_1$ Agonists
Rocuronium	Manufacturer advises avoid unless potential benefit outweighs risk
Ropivacaine	Safety not established but not known to be harmful
Rofecoxib	*see* NSAIDs

Drug (trimester of risk)	Comment
Rosiglitazone	Manufacturer advises avoid—toxicity in *animal* studies; insulin is normally substituted in all diabetics
Salbutamol	For use in asthma see section 3.1 [text]
(3)	For use in premature labour see section 7.1.3
Salcatonin	*see* Calcitonin (salmon)
Salicylates	*see* Aspirin
Salmeterol	*see* section 3.1 [text]
Saquinavir	Manufacturer advises use only if potential benefit outweighs risk
Sertraline	*see* Antidepressants, SSRI
Sevelamer	Manufacturer advises use only if potential benefit outweighs risk
Sevoflurane	*see* Anaesthetics, General
Sibutramine	Manufacturer advises avoid—toxicity in *animal* studies
Silver Sulfadiazine	*see* Sulphonamides
Simvastatin	*see* Statins
Sirolimus	Manufacturer advises avoid (toxicity in *animal* studies); effective contraception must be used during treatment and for 12 weeks after stopping
Sodium Aurothiomalate	*see* Gold
Sodium Clodronate	*see* Bisphosphonates
Sodium Cromoglicate	*see* Cromoglicate
Sodium Fusidate	Not known to be harmful; manufacturer advises use only if potential benefit outweighs risk
Sodium phenylbutyrate	Avoid (toxicity in *animal* studies); manufacturer advises adequate contraception during administration
Sodium Valproate	*see* Valproate
Somatropin	Discontinue if pregnancy occurs—no information available but theoretical risk
Sotalol	*see* Beta-blockers
Spironolactone	Manufacturers advise toxicity in *animal* studies
Stanozolol	*see* Anabolic Steroids
Statins	Avoid—congenital anomalies reported; decreased synthesis of cholesterol possibly affects fetal development
Stavudine	No information available
Streptokinase (1, 2, 3)	Possibility of premature separation of placenta in first 18 weeks; theoretical possibility of fetal haemorrhage throughout pregnancy; avoid postpartum use—maternal haemorrhage
Streptomycin	*see* Aminoglycosides
Sulfadiazine	*see* Sulphonamides
Sulfadoxine	*see* Sulphonamides
Sulfametopyrazine	*see* Sulphonamides

Drug (trimester of risk)	Comment
Sulfasalazine (3)	Theoretical risk of neonatal haemolysis; adequate folate supplements should be given to mother
Sulindac	*see* NSAIDs
Sulphonamides (3)	Neonatal haemolysis and methaemoglobinaemia; fear of increased risk of kernicterus in neonates appears to be unfounded
Sulphonylureas (3)	Neonatal hypoglycaemia; insulin is normally substituted in all diabetics; if oral drugs are used therapy should be stopped at least 2 days before delivery
Sulpiride	*see* Antipsychotics
Sumatriptan	*see* 5HT₁ Agonists
Suxamethonium	Mildly prolonged maternal paralysis may occur
Synercid®	Manufacturer advises avoid unless potential benefit outweighs risk—no information available
Tacalcitol	Manufacturer advises avoid unless no safer alternative—no information available
Tacrolimus	Avoid; manufacturer advises toxicity in *animal* studies
Tamoxifen	Avoid—possible effects on fetal development; effective contraception must be used during treatment and for 2 months after stopping
Tazarotene	Avoid; effective contraception required
Tazobactam [ingredient]	*see* Tazocin®
Tazocin®	Manufacturer advises use only if potential benefit outweighs risk
Tegafur with uracil	*see* Uftoral®
Teicoplanin	Manufacturer advises use only if potential benefit outweighs risk
Telmisartan	As for ACE Inhibitors
Temazepam	*see* Benzodiazepines
Temozolomide	Avoid (teratogenic and embryotoxic in *animal* studies); manufacturer advises adequate contraception during administration; *see also* section 8.1; also men should avoid fathering a child during and for at least 6 months after treatment
Tenecteplase	*see* Streptokinase
Tenoxicam	*see* NSAIDS
Terazosin	*see* Alpha-blockers (post-synaptic)
Terbinafine	Manufacturer advises use only if potential benefit outweighs risk—no information available
Terbutaline	For use in asthma *see* section 3.1 [text]
(3)	For use in premature labour *see* section 7.1.3

Drug (trimester of risk)	Comment
Terfenadine	*see* Antihistamines
Testosterone	*see* Androgens
Tetrabenazine	Inadequate information but no evidence of harm
Tetracyclines	
(1)	Effects on skeletal development in *animal* studies
(2, 3)	Dental discoloration; maternal hepatotoxicity with large parenteral doses
Theophylline (3)	Neonatal irritability and apnoea have been reported
Thiazides (3)	May cause neonatal thrombocytopenia; *see also* Diuretics
Thiopental	*see* Anaesthetics, General
Thioridazine	*see* Antipsychotics
Thiotepa	Avoid (teratogenic and embryotoxic in *animals*); *see also* section 8.1
Thymoxamine	*see* Moxisylyte
Thyroxine	*see* Levothyroxine
Tiagabine	Manufacturer advises avoid unless potential benefit outweighs risk
Tiaprofenic Acid	*see* NSAIDs
Ticlodipine	Manufacturer advises avoid unless essential—toxicity in *animal* studies
Tiludronic Acid	*see* Bisphosphonates
Timolol	*see* Beta-blockers
Tinidazole	Manufacturer advises avoid in first trimester
Tinzaparin	Manufacturer advises avoid unless no safer alternative
Tioconazole	Manufacturer advises avoid
Tioguanine	Avoid (teratogenicity reported when men receiving tioguanine have fathered children); ensure effective contraception during administration to men or women; *see also* section 8.1
Tirofiban	Manufacturer advises use only if potential benefit outweighs risk—no information available
Tizanidine	Manufacturer advises use only if potential benefit outweighs risk—no information available
Tobramycin	*see* Aminoglycosides
Tocopheryl Acetate (1, 2, 3)	No evidence of safety of high doses
Tolbutamide	*see* Sulphonylureas
Tolfenamic Acid	*see* NSAIDs
Tolterodine	Manufacturer advises avoid—toxicity in *animal* studies
Topiramate	Manufacturer advises avoid unless potential benefit outweighs potential risk; *see also* Antiepileptics
Topotecan	Avoid (teratogenicity and fetal loss in *animal* studies); *see also* section 8.1
Torasemide	*see* Diuretics

Drug (trimester of risk)	Comment
Tramadol	No information available; *see also* Opioid Analgesics
Trandolapril	*see* ACE Inhibitors
Tranexamic acid	No evidence of teratogenicity in *animal* studies; manufacturer advises use only if potential benefit outweighs risk
Tranylcypromine	*see* MAOIs
Trastuzumab	Avoid unless potential benefit outweighs risk
Trazodone	*see* Antidepressants, Tricyclic (and related)
Treosulfan	Avoid; *see also* section 8.1
Tretinoin (1, 2, 3)	Teratogenic; effective contraception must be used for at least 1 month before oral treatment, during treatment and for at least 1 month after stopping; also avoid topical treatment
Triamcinolone	*see* Corticosteroids
Triamterene	*see* Diuretics
Tribavirin	*see* Ribavirin
Triclofos	Avoid
Trifluoperazine	*see* Antipsychotics
Trilostane (1, 2, 3)	Interferes with placental sex hormone production
Trimeprazine	*see* Alimemazine
Trimetaphan (3)	Avoid; risk of paralytic ileus in newborn
Trimethoprim (1)	Teratogenic risk (folate antagonist); manufacturers advise avoid
Trimetrexate	Avoid (fetotoxicity and teratogenicity in *animals*); avoid conception for at least 6 months after administration to woman or man
Trimipramine	*see* Antidepressants, Tricyclic
Tripotassium Dicitratobismuthate	*see* Bismuth Chelate
Triprolidine	*see* Antihistamines
Tropisetron	Manufacturer advises toxicity in *animal* studies
Trospium	Manufacturer advises caution—no information available
Uftoral®	Avoid; manufacturer advises effective contraception during and for 3 months after administration to men or women
Urofollitropin	Avoid
Ursodeoxycholic acid	No evidence of harm but manufacturer advises avoid
Vaccines (live) (1)	Theoretical risk of congenital malformations, but need for vaccination may outweigh possible risk to fetus (*see also* p. 578); avoid MMR and Rubella vaccines but see p. 592
Valaciclovir	*see* Aciclovir

Drug (trimester of risk)	Comment
Valproate (1, 3)	Increased risk of neural tube defects (counselling and screening advised—**important**: see also pp. 227–8); neonatal bleeding (related to hypofibrinaemia) and neonatal hepatotoxicity also reported; *see also* Antiepileptics
Valsartan	As for ACE Inhibitors
Vancomycin	Manufacturer advises use only if potential benefit outweighs risk—plasma-vancomycin concentration monitoring essential to reduce risk of fetal toxicity
Vasopressin	Oxytocic effect in third trimester
Vecuronium	Manufacturer advises avoid unless potential benefit outweighs risk—no information available
Venlafaxine	Manufacturer advises avoid—no information available
Verapamil	*see* Calcium-channel Blockers
Verteporfin	Manufacturer advises use only if potential benefit outweighs risk (teratogenic in *animal* studies)
Vigabatrin	Congenital anomalies reported—manufacturer advises avoid unless potential benefit outweighs risk; *see also* Antiepileptics
Vinblastine	Avoid (limited experience suggests fetal harm; teratogenic in *animal* studies); *see also* section 8.1
Vincristine	Avoid (teratogenicity and fetal loss in *animal* studies); *see also* section 8.1
Vindesine	Avoid (teratogenic in *animal* studies); *see also* section 8.1
Vinorelbine	Avoid (teratogenicity and fetal loss in *animal* studies); *see also* section 8.1
Vitamin A (1)	Excessive doses may be teratogenic; *see also* p. 464
Vitamin D	High doses teratogenic in *animals* but therapeutic doses unlikely to be harmful
Warfarin	*see* Anticoagulants, Oral
Xipamide	*see* Diuretics
Zafirlukast	Manufacturer advises use only if potential benefit outweighs risk
Zalcitabine	Limited information available; use only if potential benefit outweighs risk
Zaleplon	Manufacturer advises avoid in early pregnancy—no information available; risk of neonatal withdrawal symptoms if used in late pregnancy
Zanamivir	Manufacturer advises use only if potential benefit outweighs risk—no information available

Drug (trimester of risk)	Comment
Zidovudine	Limited information available; manufacturer advises use only if clearly indicated; *see also* p. 300
Zinc sulphate	Safety not established—crosses the placenta
Zoledronic acid	Manufacturer advises avoid—toxicity in *animal* studies
Zolmitriptan	*see* 5HT$_1$ Agonists
Zolpidem	*see* Benzodiazepines
Zopiclone	*see* Benzodiazepines
Zotepine	Manufacturer advises avoid unless potential benefit outweighs risk
Zuclopenthixol	*see* Antipsychotics

Appendix 5: Breast-feeding

Administration of some drugs (e.g. ergotamine) to nursing mothers may cause toxicity in the infant, whereas administration of others (e.g. digoxin) has little effect. Some drugs inhibit lactation (e.g. bromocriptine).

Toxicity to the infant can occur if the drug enters the milk in pharmacologically significant quantities. The concentration in milk of some drugs (e.g. iodides) may exceed those in the maternal plasma so that therapeutic doses in the mother may cause toxicity to the infant. Some drugs inhibit the infant's sucking reflex (e.g. phenobarbital). Drugs in breast milk may, at least theoretically, cause hypersensitivity in the infant even when concentrations are too low for a pharmacological effect.

The following table lists drugs:
- which should be used with caution or which are contra-indicated in breast-feeding for the reasons given above;
- which, on present evidence, may be given to the mother during breast-feeding, because they appear in milk in amounts which are too small to be harmful to the infant;
- which are not known to be harmful to the infant although they are present in milk in significant amounts.

For many drugs insufficient evidence is available to provide guidance and it is advisable to administer only essential drugs to a mother during breast-feeding. Because of the inadequacy of information on drugs in breast milk the following table should be used only as a guide; absence from the table does not imply safety.

Table of drugs present in breast milk

Products introduced or amended since publication of BNF No. 42 (September 2001) are underlined.

Drug	Comment
Abacavir	Breast-feeding not advised in HIV infection
Abciximab	Manufacturer advises avoid—no information available
Acamprosate	Manufacturer advises avoid
Acarbose	Manufacturer advises avoid
Acebutolol	see Beta-blockers
Aceclofenac	Manufacturer advises avoid—no information available
Acemetacin	Manufacturer advises avoid
Acetazolamide	Amount too small to be harmful
Acetohexamide	see Sulphonylureas
Aciclovir	Significant amount in milk after systemic administration—not known to be harmful but manufacturer advises caution
Acipimox	Manufacturer advises avoid
Acitretin	Avoid
Aclarubicin	see Cytotoxic Drugs
Acrivastine	see Antihistamines

Drug	Comment
Adapalene	Manufacturer advises avoid (if used, avoid application to chest)—no information available
Alcohol	Large amounts may affect infant and reduce milk consumption
Alendronic Acid	No information available
Alfacalcidol	see Vitamin D
Alimemazine (trimeprazine)	see Antihistamines
Allopurinol	Present in milk
Almotriptan	Present in milk in animal studies—withhold breast-feeding for 24 hours
Alprazolam	see Benzodiazepines
Altretamine	see Cytotoxic Drugs
Alverine	Manufacturer advises avoid—little information available
Amantadine	Avoid; present in milk; toxicity in infant reported
Amethocaine	see Tetracaine
Amfebutamone	see Bupropion
Amifostine	No information available
Amiloride	Manufacturer advises avoid—no information available
Aminoglutethimide	Avoid
Aminophylline	see Theophylline
Amiodarone	Avoid; present in milk in significant amounts; theoretical risk from release of iodine; see also Iodine
Amisulpride	Manufacturer advises avoid—no information available
Amitriptyline	see Antidepressants, Tricyclic
Amlodipine	Manufacturer advises avoid—no information available
Amobarbital	see Barbiturates
Amorolfine	Manufacturer advises avoid—no information available
Amoxapine	see Antidepressants, Tricyclic
Amphetamines	Significant amount in milk. Avoid
Amphotericin	No information available
Amprenavir	Breast-feeding not advised in HIV infection
Amsacrine	see Cytotoxic Drugs
Androgens	Avoid; may cause masculinisation in the female infant or precocious development in the male infant; high doses suppress lactation
Anthraquinones	Avoid; large doses may cause increased gastric motility and diarrhoea (particularly cascara and dantron)
Anticoagulants, Oral	Risk of haemorrhage; increased by vitamin-K deficiency; warfarin appears safe but phenindione should be avoided; manufacturer of acenocoumarol (nicoumalone) recommends prophylactic vitamin-K for the infant (consult product literature)

Drug	Comment
Antidepressants, SSRI	*see* individual entries
Antidepressants, Tricyclic (and related)	Amount of tricyclic antidepressants (including related drugs such as mianserin and trazodone) too small to be harmful but most manufacturers advise avoid; accumulation of doxepin metabolite may cause sedation and respiratory depression
Antihistamines	Significant amount of some antihistamines present in milk; although not known to be harmful manufacturers of alimemazine, azatadine, cetirizine, cyproheptadine, desloratadine, fexofenadine, hydroxyzine, loratadine, mizolastine, and terfenadine advise avoid; adverse effects in infant reported with clemastine
Antipsychotics	Although amount excreted in milk probably too small to be harmful, *animal* studies indicate possible adverse effects of these drugs on developing nervous system therefore avoid unless absolutely necessary; *see also* amisulpride, chlorpromazine, clozapine, olanzapine, quetiapine, risperidone, sulpiride, zotepine
Apomorphine	Manufacturer advises avoid—no information available
Aspirin	Avoid—possible risk of Reye's syndrome; regular use of high doses could impair platelet function and produce hypoprothrombinaemia in infant if neonatal vitamin K stores low
Atenolol	*see* Beta-blockers
Atorvastatin	Manufacturer advises avoid—no information available
Atosiban	Small amounts present in milk
Atracurium	No information available
Atropine	Small amount present in milk—manufacturer advises caution
Atovaquone	Manufacturer advises avoid—no information available
Auranofin	*see* Gold
Aurothiomalate	*see* Gold
Azapropazone	Avoid—small amounts in milk
Azatadine	*see* Antihistamines
Azathioprine	*see* Cytotoxic Drugs
Azithromycin	Manufacturer advises use only if no suitable alternative—no information available
Aztreonam	Amount probably too small to be harmful—manufacturer advises avoid
Baclofen	Amount too small to be harmful
Balsalazide	Manufacturer advises avoid
Barbiturates	Avoid if possible (*see also* phenobarbital); large doses may produce drowsiness
Basiliximab	Avoid
Beclometasone	*see* Corticosteroids
Bendrofluazide	*see* Thiazides

Drug	Comment
Bendroflumethiazide (bendrofluazide)	*see* Thiazides
Benperidol	*see* Antipsychotics
Benzodiazepines	Present in milk—avoid if possible
Beta-blockers and Labetalol	Monitor infant; possible toxicity due to beta-blockade but amount of most beta-blockers excreted in milk too small to affect infant; acebutolol, atenolol, nadolol, and sotalol are present in greater amounts than other beta-blockers; manufacturers advise avoid celiprolol and nebivolol
Betamethasone	*see* Corticosteroids
Betaxolol	*see* Beta-blockers
Bethanechol	Manufacturer advises avoid
Bezafibrate	Manufacturer advises avoid—no information available
Bisoprolol	*see* Beta-blockers
Bleomycin	*see* Cytotoxic Drugs
Botulinum Toxin	Manufacturers advise avoid
Bromocriptine	Suppresses lactation
Brompheniramine	*see* Antihistamines
Buclizine	*see* Antihistamines
Budesonide	*see* Corticosteroids
Bumetanide	Manufacturer advises avoid if possible—no information available
Bupivacaine	Amount too small to be harmful
Buprenorphine	Amount too small to be harmful; manufacturer advises contra-indicated in the treatment of opioid dependence
Bupropion (amfebutamone)	Present in milk—manufacturer advises avoid
Buserelin	Small amount present in milk—manufacturer advises avoid
Busulfan	*see* Cytotoxic Drugs
Butobarbital	*see* Barbiturates
Cabergoline	Suppresses lactation
Caffeine	Regular intake of large amounts can affect infant
Calciferol	*see* Vitamin D
Calcipotriol	No information available
Calcitonin (salmon) (salcatonin)	Avoid; inhibits lactation in *animals*
Calcitriol	*see* Vitamin D
Calcium Folinate	Manufacturer advises caution—no information available
Calcium Levofolinate	*see* Calcium Folinate
Candesartan	Manufacturer advises avoid—no information available
Capecitabine	Discontinue breast-feeding
Capreomycin	Manufacturer advises caution—no information available
Captopril	Excreted in milk—manufacturers advise avoid
Carbamazepine	Amount probably too small to be harmful but severe skin reaction reported in 1 infant
Carbenoxolone	Manufacturer advises avoid—no information available

Drug	Comment
Carbimazole	Amounts in milk may be sufficient to affect neonatal thyroid function therefore lowest effective dose should be used (*see also* section 6.2.2)
Carbocisteine	No information available
Carboplatin	*see* Cytotoxic Drugs
Carisoprodol	Concentrated in milk; no adverse effects reported but best avoided
Carmustine	*see* Cytotoxic Drugs
Carvedilol	*see* Beta-blockers
Cascara	*see* Anthraquinones
Celecoxib	Manufacturer advises avoid—no information available
Celiprolol	*see* Beta-blockers
Cephalosporins	Excreted in low concentrations
Cetirizine	*see* Antihistamines
Cetrorelix	Manufacturer advises avoid
Chloral Hydrate	Sedation in infant—manufacturer advises avoid
Chlorambucil	*see* Cytotoxic Drugs
Chloramphenicol	Use another antibiotic; may cause bone-marrow toxicity in infant; concentration in milk usually insufficient to cause 'grey syndrome'
Chlordiazepoxide	*see* Benzodiazepines
Chlormethine (mustine)	*see* Cytotoxic Drugs
Chloroquine	Amount probably too small to be harmful when used for malaria prophylaxis; inadequate for reliable protection against malaria, see section 5.4.1; avoid breast-feeding when used for rheumatic diseases
Chlorphenamine (Chlorpheniramine)	*see* Antihistamines
Chlorpheniramine	*see* Antihistamines
Chlorpromazine	Drowsiness in infant reported; *see* Antipsychotics
Chlorpropamide	*see* Sulphonylureas
Chlortalidone	*see* Thiazides
Chlortetracycline	*see* Tetracyclines
Ciclosporin (cyclosporin)	Present in milk—manufacturer advises avoid
Cidofovir	Manufacturer advises avoid
Cilastatin [ingredient]	*see* Primaxin®
Cilazapril	No information available—manufacturer advises avoid
Cimetidine	Significant amount—not known to be harmful but manufacturer advises avoid
Ciprofibrate	Manufacturer advises avoid—present in milk in *animal* studies
Ciprofloxacin	Avoid—high concentrations in breast milk
Cisatracurium	No information available
Cisplatin	*see* Cytotoxic Drugs
Citalopram	Present in milk—manufacturer advises avoid
Cladribine	*see* Cytotoxic Drugs
Clarithromycin	Excreted in milk

Drug	Comment
Clavulanic acid (in co-amoxiclav, Timentir®)	Trace amounts in milk
Clemastine	*see* Antihistamines
Clindamycin	Amount probably too small to be harmful but bloody diarrhoea reported in 1 infant
Clobazam	*see* Benzodiazepines
Clodronate Sodium	No information available
Clomethiazole	Amount too small to be harmful
Clomifene	May inhibit lactation
Clomipramine	*see* Antidepressants, Tricyclic
Clomocycline	*see* Tetracyclines
Clopidogrel	Manufacturer advises avoid
Clorazepate	*see* Benzodiazepines
Clozapine	Manufacturer advises avoid
Co-amoxiclav	Trace amounts in milk
Codeine	Amount too small to be harmful
Colchicine	Present in milk but no adverse effects reported; manufacturers advise avoid because of risk of cytotoxicity
Colecalciferol	*see* Vitamin D
Contraceptives, Oral	Avoid combined oral contraceptives until weaning or for 6 months after birth (adverse effects on lactation); progestogen-only contraceptives do not affect lactation (start 3 weeks after birth or later)
Corticosteroids	Systemic effects in infant unlikely with maternal dose of prednisolone up to 40 mg daily; monitor infant's adrenal function with higher doses
Cortisone Acetate	*see* Corticosteroids
Co-trimoxazole	Small risk of kernicterus in jaundiced infants and of haemolysis in G6PD-deficient infants (due to sulfamethoxazole)
Cough mixtures containing iodides	Use alternative cough mixtures; *see* Iodine
Crisantaspase	*see* Cytotoxic Drugs
Cromoglicate	Unlikely to be present in milk
Cyclopenthiazide	*see* Thiazides
Cyclophosphamide	Discontinue breast-feeding during and for 36 hours after stopping treatment
Cycloserine	Amount too small to be harmful
Cyclosporin	*see* Ciclosporin
Cyproheptadine	*see* Antihistamines
Cyproterone Acetate	Caution; possibility of anti-androgen effects in neonate
Cytarabine	*see* Cytotoxic Drugs
Cytotoxic Drugs	Discontinue breast-feeding
Daclizumab	Avoid
Dactinomycin	*see* Cytotoxic Drugs
Dalfopristin [ingredient]	*see* Synercid®
Dalteparin	No information available
Danaparoid	No information available
Danazol	No data available but avoid because of possible androgenic effects in infant
Dantron	*see* Anthraquinones

Drug	Comment
Dapsone	Haemolytic anaemia; although significant amount in milk, risk to infant very small unless infant is G6PD deficient
Darbepoetin	Manufacturer advises avoid—no information available
Daunorubicin	*see* Cytotoxic Drugs
Deferiprone	Manufacturer advises avoid—no information available
Deflazacort	*see* Corticosteroids
Demeclocycline	*see* Tetracyclines
Desferrioxamine	Manufacturer advises use only if potential benefit outweighs risk—no information available
Desmopressin	Not known to be harmful
Desogestrel	*see* Contraceptives, Oral
Dexamethasone	*see* Corticosteroids
Dexamfetamine	*see* Amphetamines
Dexketoprofen	Manufacturer advises avoid—no information available
Dextromoramide	No information available—manufacturer advises avoid
Dextropropoxyphene	Amount too small to be harmful
Diamorphine	Therapeutic doses unlikely to affect infant; withdrawal symptoms in infants of dependent mothers; breast-feeding no longer considered best method of treating dependence in offspring of dependent mothers and should be stopped
Diazepam	*see* Benzodiazepines
Diclofenac	Amount too small to be harmful
Didanosine	Breast-feeding not advised in HIV infection
Diflunisal	Manufacturer advises avoid
Digoxin	Amount too small to be harmful
Dihydrocodeine	Manufacturer advises use only if potential benefit outweighs risk
Dihydrotachysterol	*see* Vitamin D
Diloxanide	Manufacturer advises avoid
Diltiazem	Significant amount—no evidence of harm but avoid unless no safer alternative
Diphenhydramine	*see* Antihistamines
Diphenylpyraline	*see* Antihistamines
Dipyridamole	Small amount present in milk—manufacturer advises caution
Disodium Etidronate	No information available
Disodium Pamidronate	Manufacturer advises avoid
Disopyramide	Present in milk—use only if essential and monitor infant for antimuscarinic effects
Distigmine bromide	No information available
Docetaxel	*see* Cytotoxic Drugs
Docusate sodium	Present in milk following oral administration—manufacturer advises caution; rectal administration not known to be harmful
Domperidone	Amount probably too small to be harmful
Dornase alfa	Amount probably too small to be harmful—manufacturer advises caution

Drug	Comment
Dosulepin (dothiepin)	*see* Antidepressants, Tricyclic
Dothiepin	*see* Antidepressants, Tricyclic
Doxazosin	Accumulates in milk—manufacturer advises avoid
Doxepin	*see* Antidepressants, Tricyclic
Doxorubicin	*see* Cytotoxic Drugs
Doxycycline	*see* Tetracyclines
Doxylamine	*see* Antihistamines
Dydrogesterone	Present in milk—no adverse effects reported
Edrophonium	Amount probably too small to be harmful
Efavirenz	Breast-feeding not advised in HIV infection
Eformoterol	*see* Formoterol
Enalapril	Amount probably too small to be harmful
Enoxaparin	Manufacturer advises avoid—no information available
Enoximone	Manufacturer advises caution—no information available
Entacapone	Manufacturer advises avoid—no information available
Ephedrine	Irritability and disturbed sleep reported
Epirubicin	*see* Cytotoxic Drugs
Epoetin	Manufacturers advise avoid—no information available
Eprosartan	Manufacturer advises avoid unless potential benefit outweighs risk
Ergocalciferol	*see* Vitamin D
Ergotamine	Avoid; ergotism may occur in infant; repeated doses may inhibit lactation
Erythromycin	Only small amounts in milk
Esmolol	*see* Beta-blockers
Esomeprazole	Manufacturer advises avoid—no information available
Etamsylate	Significant amount but not known to be harmful
Etanercept	Manufacturer advises avoid—no information available
Ethambutol	Amount too small to be harmful
Ethinylestradiol	*see* Contraceptives, Oral
Ethosuximide	Avoid—significant amount in milk; hyperexcitability and poor suckling reported
Etodolac	Manufacturer advises avoid
Etoposide	*see* Cytotoxic Drugs
Etynodiol	*see* Contraceptives, Oral
Famciclovir	Manufacturer advises avoid unless potential benefit outweighs risk—present in milk in *animal* studies
Famotidine	Present in milk—not known to be harmful but manufacturer advises avoid
Fansidar®	Small risk of kernicterus in jaundiced infants and of haemolysis in G6PD-deficient infants (due to sulfadoxine)
Felodipine	Appears in milk
Fenbufen	Small amount present in milk—manufacturer advises avoid
Fenofibrate	Manufacturer advises avoid—no information available

Drug	Comment
Fenoprofen	Amount too small to be harmful
Fentanyl	Manufacturer advises avoid
Fenticonazole	Manufacturer advises avoid unless essential—present in milk in *animal* studies
Fexofenadine	*see* Antihistamines
Filgrastim	No information available—manufacturer advises avoid
Flavoxate	Manufacturer advises caution—no information available
Flecainide	Significant amount but not known to be harmful
Fluconazole	Manufacturer advises avoid—present in milk
Flucytosine	Manufacturer advises avoid
Fludarabine	*see* Cytotoxic Drugs
Flunitrazepam	*see* Benzodiazepines
Fluorouracil	*see* Cytotoxic Drugs
Fluoxetine	Present in milk—manufacturer advises avoid
Flupentixol	*see* Antipsychotics
Fluphenazine	*see* Antipsychotics
Flurazepam	*see* Benzodiazepines
Flurbiprofen	Amount too small to be harmful
Fluticasone	*see* Corticosteroids
Fluvastatin	Manufacturer advises avoid
Fluvoxamine	Present in milk—manufacturer advises avoid
Follitropin alfa and beta	Avoid
Fomepizole	Manufacturer advises caution—no information available
Fomivirsen	Breast-feeding not advised in HIV infection
Formoterol (eformoterol)	Manufacturers advise avoid
Fosinopril	Present in milk—manufacturer advises avoid
Fosphenytoin	*see* Phenytoin
Frusemide	*see* Furosemide
Furosemide (frusemide)	Amount too small to be harmful
Fusidic acid	*see* Sodium fusidate
Gabapentin	Present in milk—manufacturer advises avoid
Galantamine	No information available
Ganciclovir	Avoid; *see also* p. 307
Gemcitabine	*see* Cytotoxic Drugs
Gemfibrozil	Manufacturer advises avoid—no information available
Gestodene	*see* Contraceptives, Oral
Gestrinone	Manufacturer advises avoid
Glatiramer	Manufacturer advises caution—no information available
Glibenclamide	*see* Sulphonylureas
Gliclazide	*see* Sulphonylureas
Glimepiride	*see* Sulphonylureas
Glipizide	*see* Sulphonylureas
Gliquidone	*see* Sulphonylureas
Glymidine	*see* Sulphonylureas
Gold (auranofin, aurothiomalate)	Caution—excreted in milk; theoretical possibility of rashes and idiosyncratic reactions
Goserelin	Manufacturer advises avoid
Granisetron	Manufacturer advises avoid—no information available
Growth Hormone	*see* Somatropin

Drug	Comment
Haem arginate	Manufacturer advises avoid unless essential—no information available
Haloperidol	*see* Antipsychotics
Halothane	Excreted in milk
Hepatitis A Vaccine	No information available
Human menopausal gonadotrphins	Avoid
Hydralazine	Present in milk but not known to be harmful; monitor infant
Hydrochloro-thiazide	*see* Thiazides
Hydrocortisone	*see* Corticosteroids
Hydroflumethiazide	*see* Thiazides
Hydromorphone	Manufacturer advises avoid—no information available
Hydroxycarbamide (hydroxyurea)	*see* Cytotoxic Drugs
Hydroxychloro-quine	Avoid—risk of toxicity in infant
Hydroxyproges-terone	No information available
Hydroxyurea	*see* Cytotoxic Drugs
Hydroxyzine	*see* Antihistamines
Hyoscine	Amount too small to be harmful
Ibuprofen	Amount too small to be harmful but some manufacturers advise avoid (including topical use)
Idarubicin	*see* Cytotoxic Drugs
Idoxuridine	May possibly make milk taste unpleasant
Ifosfamide	*see* Cytotoxic Drugs
Imatinib	*see* Cytotoxic Drugs
Imidapril	Manufacturer advises avoid—no information available
Imiglucerase	No information available
Imipenem [ingredient]	*see* Primaxin®
Imipramine	*see* Antidepressants, Tricyclic
Imiquimod	Manufacturer advises no information available
Indapamide	No information available—manufacturer advises avoid
Indinavir	Breast-feeding not advised in HIV infection
Indometacin	Amount probably too small to be harmful but convulsions reported in one infant—manufacturers advise avoid
Infliximab	Avoid; manufacturer advises avoid for at least 6 months after last dose
Insulin	Amount too small to be harmful
Interferons	Manufacturers advise avoid unless potential benefit outweighs risk—no information available
Iodine	Stop breast-feeding; danger of neonatal hypothyroidism or goitre; appears to be concentrated in milk
Radioactive iodine	Breast-feeding contra-indicated after therapeutic doses. With diagnostic doses withhold breast-feeding for at least 24 hours
Ipratropium	Amount probably too small to be harmful

Drug	Comment
Irbesartan	Manufacturer advises avoid—no information available
Irinotecan	*see* Cytotoxic Drugs
Isoniazid	Monitor infant for possible toxicity; theoretical risk of convulsions and neuropathy; prophylactic pyridoxine advisable in mother and infant
Isotretinoin	Avoid
Itraconazole	Small amounts present in milk—may accumulate; manufacturer advises avoid unless potential benefit outweighs risk
Kaletra®	Breast-feeding not advised in HIV infection
Ketoconazole	Manufacturer advises avoid
Ketoprofen	Amount probably too small to be harmful but manufacturer advises avoid unless essential
Ketorolac	Avoid
Ketotifen	*see* Antihistamines
Labetalol	*see* Beta-blockers
Lacidipine	Manufacturer advises avoid—no information available
Lamivudine	Present in milk—Manufacturer advises avoid; breast-feeding not advised in HIV infection
Lamotrigine	Present in milk but limited data suggest no harmful effects on infants
Lanreotide	Manufacturer advises avoid—growth retardation in *animal* studies
Lansoprazole	Manufacturer advises avoid unless essential—present in milk in *animal* studies
Latanoprost	May be present in milk—manufacturer advises avoid
Leflunomide	Present in milk—manufacturer advises avoid
Lenograstim	Manufacturer advises avoid—no information available
Lepirudin	Avoid
Lercanidipine	Manufacturer advises avoid
Levetiracetam	Manufacturer advises avoid—present in milk in *animal* studies
Levobupivacaine	Likely to be present in milk but risk to infant minimal
Levocabastine	Amount too small to be harmful
Levocetirizine	*see* Antihistamines
Levodopa	No information available
Levofloxacin	Manufacturer advises avoid
Levomepromazine (methotrimeprazine)	*see* Antipsychotics
Levonorgestrel	*see* Contraceptives, Oral
Levothyroxine (thyroxine)	Amount too small to affect tests for neonatal hypothyroidism
Lidocaine (lignocaine)	Amount too small to be harmful
Lignocaine	*see* Lidocaine
Linezolid	Manufacturer advises avoid—present in milk in *animal* studies
Liothyronine	Amount too small to affect tests for neonatal hypothyroidism
Lisinopril	No information available—manufacturer advises caution
Lisuride	May suppress lactation

Drug	Comment
Lithium salts	Present in milk and risk of toxicity in infant—manufacturers advise avoid
Lofepramine	*see* Antidepressants, Tricyclic
Loperamide	Amount probably too small to be harmful
Lopinavir [ingredient]	*see* *Kaletra*®
Loprazolam	*see* Benzodiazepines
Loratadine	*see* Antihistamines
Lorazepam	*see* Benzodiazepines
Lormetazepam	*see* Benzodiazepines
Lornoxicam	Manufacturer advises avoid—present in milk in *animal* studies
Losartan	Manufacturer advises avoid—no information available
Lymecycline	*see* Tetracyclines
Macrogols	Manufacturers advise use only if essential—no information available
Malarone®	Manufacturer advises avoid; *see also* atovaquone and proguanil
Maloprim®	Haemolytic anaemia (due to dapsone); risk to infant very small
Maprotiline	*see* Antidepressants, Tricyclic (and related)
Mebendazole	No information available
Mebeverine	Amount too small to be harmful
Medroxyprogesterone Acetate	Present in milk—no adverse effects reported
Mefenamic Acid	Amount too small to be harmful, but manufacturer advises avoid
Mefloquine	Present in milk but risk to infant minimal
Meloxicam	No information available—manufacturer advises avoid
Melphalan	*see* Cytotoxic Drugs
Menotrophin	Avoid
Meprobamate	Avoid; concentration in milk may exceed maternal plasma concentrations fourfold and may cause drowsiness in infant
Meptazinol	Manufacturer advises use only if potential benefit outweighs risk
Mercaptamine	Manufacturer advises avoid
Mercaptopurine	*see* Cytotoxic Drugs
Meropenem	Manufacturer advises avoid unless potential benefit justifies potential risk
Mesalazine	Diarrhoea reported but manufacturers advise negligible amounts detected in breast milk
Mestranol	*see* Contraceptives, Oral
Metaraminol	Manufacturer advises caution—no information available
Metformin	Avoid (risk of lactic acidosis); also present in milk in *animal* studies
Methadone	Withdrawal symptoms in infant; breast-feeding permissible during maintenance but dose should be as low as possible and infant monitored to avoid sedation
Methotrexate	*see* Cytotoxic Drugs
Methotrimeprazine	*see* Antipsychotics

Drug	Comment
Methyldopa	Amount too small to be harmful
Methylphenidate	No information available—manufacturer advises avoid
Methylprednisolone	see Corticosteroids
Methysergide	Manufacturer advises avoid
Metoclopramide	Small amount present in milk; manufacturer advises avoid
Metolazone	see Thiazides
Metoprolol	see Beta-blockers
Metronidazole	Significant amount in milk; manufacturer advises avoid large single doses
Metyrapone	Manufacturer advises avoid—no information available
Mexiletine	Amount too small to be harmful
Mianserin	see Antidepressants, Tricyclic (and related)
Miconazole	Manufacturer advises caution—no information available
Midazolam	see Benzodiazepines
Mifepristone	No information available—manufacturer advises stop breast-feeding for 14 days after administration
Milrinone	Manufacturer advises caution—no information available
Minocycline	see Tetracyclines
Minoxidil	Present in milk but not known to be harmful
Mirtazapine	Manufacturer advises avoid—present in milk in *animal* studies
Misoprostol	No information available—manufacturer advises avoid
Mitomycin	see Cytotoxic Drugs
Mitoxantrone (mitozantrone)	see Cytotoxic Drugs
Mitozantrone	see Cytotoxic Drugs
Mizolastine	see Antihistamines
Moclobemide	Amount too small to be harmful, but patient leaflet advises avoid
Modafinil	Manufacturer advises avoid—no information available
Moexipril	Manufacturer advises avoid—no information available
Molgramostim	Manufacturer advises avoid (potential for adverse effects in infant)—no information available
Montelukast	Manufacturer advises avoid unless essential
Morphine	Therapeutic doses unlikely to affect infant; withdrawal symptoms in infants of dependent mothers; breast-feeding not best method of treating dependence in offspring and should be stopped
Moxonidine	Present in milk—manufacturer advises avoid
Mupirocin	Manufacturer advises avoid unless potential benefit outweighs risk—no information available
Mustine	see Cytotoxic Drugs
Mycophenolate Mofetil	No information available—manufacturer advises avoid
Nabumetone	No information available—manufacturer advises avoid

Drug	Comment
Nadolol	see Beta-blockers
Nafarelin	Manufacturer advises avoid—no information available
Nalbuphine	Manufacturer advises caution—no information available
Nalidixic Acid	Risk to infant very small but one case of haemolytic anaemia reported
Naloxone	No information available
Naproxen	Amount too small to be harmful but manufacturers advise avoid
Naratriptan	Manufacturer advises caution—no information available
Nateglinide	Manufacturer advises avoid—present in milk in *animal* studies
Nebivolol	see Beta-blockers
Nefazodone	Manufacturer advises avoid—no information available
Nelfinavir	Breast-feeding not advised in HIV infection
Neostigmine	Amount probably too small to be harmful; monitor infant
Nevirapine	Breast-feeding not advised in HIV infection
Nicardipine	Manufacturer advises avoid
Nicorandil	No information available—manufacturer advises avoid
Nicotine	Avoid—present in milk
Nicoumalone	see Anticoagulants, Oral
Nifedipine	Amount too small to be harmful but manufacturers advise avoid
Nimodipine	No information available
Nisoldipine	Manufacturer advises avoid—no information available
Nitrazepam	see Benzodiazepines
Nitrofurantoin	Only small amounts in milk but could be enough to produce haemolysis in G6PD-deficient infants
Nizatidine	Amount too small to be harmful
Nonoxynol-9	Present in milk in *animal* studies
Norethisterone	Higher doses may suppress lactation and alter milk composition—use lowest effective dose; see also Contraceptives, Oral
Norfloxacin	No information available—manufacturer advises avoid
Norgestimate	see Contraceptives, Oral
Nortriptyline	see Antidepressants, Tricyclic
NSAIDs	see individual entries
Nystatin	No information available, but absorption from gastro-intestinal tract negligible
Octreotide	Manufacturer advises avoid unless essential—no information available
Oestrogens	Avoid; adverse effects on lactation; see also Contraceptives, Oral
Ofloxacin	Manufacturer advises avoid
Olanzapine	Manufacturer advises avoid—no information available
Olsalazine	Manufacturer advises avoid
Omeprazole	Manufacturer advises avoid—no information available

Drug	Comment
Ondansetron	Manufacturer advises avoid—no information available
Opioid Analgesics	*see* individual entries
Orlistat	Manufacturer advises avoid—no information available
Orphenadrine	Present in milk—manufacturer advises avoid
Oxaliplatin	*see* Cytotoxic Drugs
Oxazepam	*see* Benzodiazepines
Oxcarbazepine	Present in milk—manufacturer advises avoid
Oxitropium	Amount probably too small to be harmful—manufacturer advises caution
Oxprenolol	*see* Beta-blockers
Oxybutynin	Present in milk—manufacturer advises avoid
Oxycodone	Present in milk—manufacturer advises avoid
Oxypertine	*see* Antipsychotics
Oxytetracycline	*see* Tetracyclines
Paclitaxel	*see* Cytotoxic Drugs
Pancuronium	Manufacturer advises avoid unless potential benefit outweighs possible risk—no information available
Pantoprazole	Manufacturer advises avoid unless potential benefit outweighs risk—small amount present in milk in *animal* studies
Papaveretum	*see* Morphine
Paracetamol	Amount too small to be harmful
Paraldehyde	Manufacturer advises avoid unless essential—present in milk
Paroxetine	Manufacturer advises avoid unless potential benefit outweighs possible risk
Peginterferon alfa	*see* Interferons
Penicillins	Trace amounts in milk
Pentamidine isetionate	Manufacturer advises avoid unless essential
Pentazocine	Small amount present in milk—manufacturer advises caution
Pentostatin	*see* Cytotoxic Drugs
Pergolide	May suppress lactation
Pericyazine	*see* Antipsychotics
Perindopril	Manufacturer advises avoid—no information available
Perphenazine	*see* Antipsychotics
Phenindione	*see* Anticoagulants, Oral
Phenobarbital	Avoid when possible; drowsiness may occur but risk probably small; one report of methaemoglobinaemia with phenobarbital and phenytoin
Phentolamine	No information available
Phenylbutazone	Avoid—small amounts in milk
Phenytoin	Small amount present in milk; manufacturer advises avoid—*but see* section 4.8.1
Phytomenadione	Present in milk
Pilocarpine	Manufacturer advises avoid—no information available
Pimozide	*see* Antipsychotics
Pindolol	*see* Beta-blockers
Pioglitazone	Manufacturer advises avoid—present in milk in *animal* studies

Drug	Comment
Piperacillin	*see* Penicillins
Piperazine	Present in milk—manufacturer advises avoid breast-feeding for 8 hours after dose (express and discard milk during this time)
Piracetam	Manufacturer advises avoid
Piroxicam	Amount too small to be harmful
Pizotifen	Amount probably too small to be harmful, but patient information leaflet advises avoid
Polythiazide	*see* Thiazides
Povidone-iodine	Avoid; iodine absorbed from vaginal preparations is concentrated in milk
Pramipexole	May suppress lactation; manufacturer advises avoid—present in milk in *animal* studies
Pravastatin	Small amount excreted in milk—manufacturer advises avoid
Prazosin	Amount probably too small to be harmful
Prednisolone	*see* Corticosteroids
Primaxin®	Present in milk—manufacturer advises avoid
Primidone	*see* Phenobarbital
Probenecid	No information available
Procarbazine	*see* Cytotoxic Drugs
Prochlorperazine	*see* Antipsychotics
Procainamide	Present in milk—manufacturer advises avoid
Progesterone	Manufacturers advise avoid—present in milk
Proguanil	*see* Chloroquine
Promazine	*see* Antipsychotics
Promethazine	*see* Antihistamines
Propafenone	Manufacturer advises avoid—no information available
Propantheline	May suppress lactation
Propiverine	Manufacturer advises avoid—present in milk in *animal* studies
Propofol	Manufacturer advises avoid—no information available
Propranolol	*see* Beta-blockers
Propylthiouracil	Monitor infant's thyroid status but amounts in milk probably too small to affect infant; high doses might affect neonatal thyroid function
Protirelin	Breast enlargement and leaking of milk reported
Pseudoephedrine	Amount too small to be harmful
Pyrazinamide	Amount too small to be harmful
Pyridostigmine	Amount probably too small to be harmful
Pyrimethamine	Significant amount—avoid administration of other folate antagonists to infant
Quetiapine	Manufacturer advises avoid—no information available
Quinagolide	Suppresses lactation
Quinapril	No information available—manufacturer advises caution
Quinidine	Significant amount but not known to be harmful
Quinupristin [ingredient]	*see* Synercid®

Drug	Comment
Rabeprazole	Manufacturer advises avoid—no information available
Raltitrexed	*see* Cytotoxic Drugs
Ramipril	Manufacturer advises avoid—no information available
Ranitidine	Significant amount but not known to be harmful
Ranitidine Bismuth Citrate	Manufacturer advises avoid—no information available
Rasburicase	Manufacturer advises avoid—no information available
Razoxane	*see* Cytotoxic Drugs
Reboxetine	Manufacturer advises avoid—no information available
Remifentanil	Manufacturer advises caution—present in milk in *animal* studies
Repaglinide	Manufacturer advises avoid
Reteplase	Manufacturer advises avoid breast-feeding for 24 hours after dose (express and discard milk during this time)
Reviparin	No information available
Ribavirin	Avoid—no information available
Rifabutin	Manufacturer advises avoid—no information available
Rifampicin	Amount too small to be harmful
Riluzole	Manufacturer advises avoid—no information available
Risedronate sodium	Manufacturer advises avoid
Risperidone	Manufacturer advises avoid—no information available
Ritonavir	Breast-feeding not advised in HIV infection
Rituximab	Avoid
<u>Rivastigmine</u>	Present in milk in *animal* studies—manufacturer advises avoid
Rizatriptan	Present in milk in *animal* studies—withhold breast-feeding for 24 hours
Rocuronium	Manufacturer advises avoid unless potential benefit outweighs risk—present in milk in *animal* studies
Rofecoxib	Manufacturer advises avoid—present in milk in *animal* studies
Rosiglitazone	Manufacturer advises avoid (present in milk in *animal* studies)
Salbutamol	Probably present in milk—manufacturer advises avoid unless potential benefit outweighs risk
Salcatonin	*see* Calcitonin (salmon)
Saquinavir	Breast-feeding not advised in HIV infection
Secobarbital	*see* Barbiturates
Senna	*see* Anthraquinones
Sertraline	Present in milk but not known to be harmful in short-term use
Sevelamer	Manufacturer advises use only if potential benefit outweighs risk
Sibutramine	Manufacturer advises avoid—no information available
Silver sulfadiazine	*see* Sulphonamides
Simvastatin	Manufacturer advises avoid—no information available

Drug	Comment
Sirolimus	Discontinue breast-feeding
Sodium Clodronate	No information available
Sodium Cromoglicate	*see* Cromoglicate
Sodium fusidate	Present in milk—manufacturer advises caution
Sodium phenylbutyrate	Manufacturer advises avoid—no information available
Sodium Valproate	*see* Valproate
Somatropin	No information available
Sotalol	*see* Beta-blockers
Stavudine	Breast-feeding not advised in HIV infection
Sulfadiazine	*see* Sulphonamides
Sulfametopyrazine	*see* Sulphonamides
Sulfasalazine	Small amounts in milk (1 report of bloody diarrhoea and rashes); theoretical risk of neonatal haemolysis especially in G6PD-deficient infants
Sulfinpyrazone	No information available
Sulindac	No information available
Sulphonamides	Small risk of kernicterus in jaundiced infants particularly with long-acting sulphonamides, and of haemolysis in G6PD-deficient infants
Sulphonylureas	Theoretical possibility of hypoglycaemia in infant
<u>Sulpiride</u>	Best avoided; present in milk; *see also* Antipsychotics
Sumatriptan	Present in milk—withhold breast-feeding for 24 hours
Synercid®	Manufacturer advises avoid—no information available
Tacalcitol	Manufacturer advises avoid application to breast area—no information available
Tacrolimus	Avoid—present in milk
Tamoxifen	Manufacturer advises avoid—no information available
Tazarotene	Manufacturer advises avoid—present in milk in *animal* studies
Tazobactam [ingredient]	*see Tazocin*®
Tazocin®	Present in milk—manufacturer advises use only if potential benefit outweighs risk
Tegafur with uracil	*see* Cytotoxic drugs
Teicoplanin	No information available
Telmisartan	Manufacturer advises avoid—no information available
Temazepam	*see* Benzodiazepines
Temozolamide	*see* Cytotoxic Drugs
Tenecteplase	Manufacturer advises avoid breast-feeding for 24 hours after dose (express and discard milk during this time)
Tenoxicam	No information available
Terazosin	No information available
Terbinafine	Present in milk—manufacturer advises avoid
Terbutaline	Amount too small to be harmful
Terfenadine	*see* Antihistamines
Terlipressin	Not known to be harmful
Tetrabenazine	Manufacturer advises avoid
Tetracaine (amethocaine)	No information available

Drug	Comment
Tetracyclines	Avoid (although absorption and therefore discoloration of teeth in infant probably usually prevented by chelation with calcium in milk)
Theophylline	Present in milk—irritability in infant reported; modified-release preparations preferable
Thiamine	Severely thiamine-deficient mothers should avoid breast-feeding as toxic methylglyoxal excreted in milk
Thiazides	Amount too small to be harmful; large doses may suppress lactation
Thioridazine	*see* Antipsychotics
Thiotepa	*see* Cytotoxic Drugs
Thyroxine	*see* Levothyroxine
Tiagabine	Manufacturer advises avoid unless potential benefit outweighs risk
Tiaprofenic Acid	Amount too small to be harmful
Ticlopidine	Manufacturer advises avoid unless essential—present in milk in *animal* studies
Tiludronic Acid	Manufacturer advises avoid—no information available
Timolol	*see* Beta-blockers
Tinidazole	Present in milk—manufacturer advises avoid breast-feeding during and for 3 days after stopping treatment
Tinzaparin	Manufacturer advises avoid—no information available
Tioguanine	*see* Cytotoxic Drugs
Tirofiban	Manufacturer advises avoid—no information available
Tizanidine	Manufacturer advises use only if potential benefit outweighs risk—no information available
Tolbutamide	*see* Sulphonylureas
Tolfenamic Acid	Amount too small to be harmful
Tolterodine	Manufacturer advises avoid—no information available
Topiramate	Manufacturer advises avoid
Topotecan	*see* Cytotoxic Drugs
Torasemide	No information available
Tramadol	Amount probably too small to be harmful, but manufacturer advises avoid
Trandolapril	Manufacturers advise avoid
Tranexamic acid	Small amount present in milk—antifibrinolytic effect in infant unlikely
Trastuzumab	Avoid breast-feeding during treatment and for six months after
Trazodone	*as for* Antidepressants, Tricyclic
Treosulfan	*see* Cytotoxic Drugs
Tretinoin	Avoid
Triamcinolone	*see* Corticosteroids
Tribavirin	*see* Ribavirin
Trifluoperazine	*see* Antipsychotics
Trimeprazine	*see* Antihistamines
Trimethoprim	Present in milk—short-term use not known to be harmful

Drug	Comment
Trimetrexate	Manufacturer advises termination of breast-feeding; also breast-feeding not advised in HIV infection
Trimipramine	*see* Antidepressants, Tricyclic
Triprolidine	*see* Antihistamines
Tropisetron	No information available
Trospium	Manufacturer advises caution—no information available
Urofollitrophin	Avoid
Ursodeoxycholic acid	Not known to be harmful but manufacturer advises avoid
Valaciclovir	No information available; *see also* Aciclovir
Valproate	Amount too small to be harmful
Valsartan	Manufacturer advises avoid—no information available
Vancomycin	Present in milk—significant absorption following oral administration unlikely
Vasopressin	Not known to be harmful
Vecuronium	No information available
Venlafaxine	Manufacturer advises avoid—no information available
Verapamil	Amount too small to be harmful
Verteporfin	No information available—manufacturer advises avoid breast-feeding for 48 hours after administration
Vigabatrin	Present in milk—manufacturer advises avoid
Vinblastine	*see* Cytotoxic Drugs
Vincristine	*see* Cytotoxic Drugs
Vindesine	*see* Cytotoxic Drugs
Vinorelbine	*see* Cytotoxic Drugs
Vitamin A	Theoretical risk of toxicity in infants of mothers taking large doses
Vitamin D (and related compounds)	Caution with high doses; may cause hypercalcaemia in infant
Warfarin	*see* Anticoagulants, Oral
Xipamide	No information available
Zafirlukast	Present in milk—manufacturer advises avoid
Zalcitabine	Breast-feeding not advised in HIV infection
Zaleplon	Present in milk—manufacturer advises avoid
Zanamivir	Manufacturer advises avoid—no information available
Zidovudine	Breast-feeding not advised in HIV infection
Zoledronic acid	Manufacturer advises avoid—no information available
Zolmitriptan	Manufacturer advises caution—present in milk in *animal* studies
Zolpidem	Small amounts present in milk—manufacturer advises avoid
Zopiclone	Present in milk—manufacturer advises avoid
Zotepine	Manufacturer advises avoid
Zuclopenthixol	*see* Antipsychotics

Appendix 6: Intravenous Additives

INTRAVENOUS ADDITIVES POLICIES. A local policy on the addition of drugs to intravenous fluids should be drawn up by a multi-disciplinary team in each Health Authority and issued as a document to the members of staff concerned.

Centralised additive services are provided in a number of hospital pharmacy departments and should be used in preference to making additions on wards.

The information that follows should be read in conjunction with local policy documents.

Guidelines

1. Drugs should only be added to infusion containers when constant plasma concentrations are needed or when the administration of a more concentrated solution would be harmful.
2. In general, only one drug should be added to any infusion container and the components should be compatible. Ready-prepared solutions should be used whenever possible. Drugs should not normally be added to blood products, mannitol, or sodium bicarbonate. Only specially formulated additives should be used with fat emulsions or amino-acid solutions (section 9.3).
3. Solutions should be thoroughly mixed by shaking and checked for absence of particulate matter before use.
4. Strict asepsis should be maintained throughout and in general the giving set should not be used for more than 24 hours (for drug admixtures).
5. The infusion container should be labelled with the patient's name, the name and quantity of additives, and the date and time of addition (and the new expiry date or time). Such additional labelling should not interfere with information on the manufacturer's label that is still valid. When possible, containers should be retained for a period after use in case they are needed for investigation.
6. It is good practice to examine intravenous infusions from time to time while they are running. If cloudiness, crystallisation, change of colour, or any other sign of interaction or contamination is observed the infusion should be discontinued.

Problems

MICROBIAL CONTAMINATION. The accidental entry and subsequent growth of micro-organisms converts the infusion fluid pathway into a potential vehicle for infection with micro-organisms, particularly species of Candida, Enterobacter, and Klebsiella. Ready-prepared infusions containing the additional drugs, or infusions prepared by an additive service (when available) should therefore be used in preference to making extemporaneous additions to infusion containers on wards etc. However, when this is necessary strict aseptic procedure should be followed.

INCOMPATIBILITY. Physical and chemical incompatibilities may occur with loss of potency, increase in toxicity, or other adverse effect. The solutions may become opalescent or precipitation may occur, but in many instances there is no visual indication of incompatibility. Interaction may take place at any point in the infusion fluid pathway, and the potential for incompatibility is increased when more than one substance is added to the infusion fluid.

Common incompatibilities. Precipitation reactions are numerous and varied and may occur as a result of pH, concentration changes, 'salting-out' effects, complexation or other chemical changes. Precipitation or other particle formation must be avoided since, apart from lack of control of dosage on administration, it may initiate or exacerbate adverse effects. This is particularly important in the case of drugs which have been implicated in either thrombophlebitis (e.g. diazepam) or in skin sloughing or necrosis caused by extravasation (e.g. sodium bicarbonate and certain cytotoxic drugs). It is also especially important to effect solution of colloidal drugs and to prevent their subsequent precipitation in order to avoid a pyrogenic reaction (e.g. amphotericin).

It is considered undesirable to mix beta-lactam antibiotics, such as semi-synthetic penicillins and cephalosporins, with proteinaceous materials on the grounds that immunogenic and allergenic conjugates could be formed.

A number of preparations undergo significant loss of potency when added singly or in combination to large volume infusions. Examples include ampicillin in infusions that contain glucose or lactates, chlormethine hydrochloride (mustine hydrochloride) in isotonic saline and gentamicin/carbenicillin combinations. The breakdown products of dacarbazine have been implicated in adverse effects.

Blood. Because of the large number of incompatibilities, drugs should not normally be added to blood and blood products for infusion purposes. Examples of incompatibility with blood include hypertonic mannitol solutions (irreversible crenation of red cells), dextrans (rouleaux formation and interference with cross-matching), glucose (clumping of red cells), and oxytocin (inactivated).

If the giving set is not changed after the administration of blood, but used for other infusion fluids, a fibrin clot may form which, apart from blocking the set, increases the likelihood of microbial growth.

Intravenous fat emulsions may break down with coalescence of fat globules and separation of phases when additions such as antibacterials or electrolytes are made, thus increasing the possibility of embolism. Only specially formulated products such as

Vitlipid N® (section 9.3) may be added to appropriate intravenous fat emulsions.

Other infusions that frequently give rise to incompatibility include amino acids, mannitol, and sodium bicarbonate.

Bactericides such as chlorocresol 0.1% or phenylmercuric nitrate 0.001% are present in some injection solutions. The total volume of such solutions added to a container for infusion on one occasion should not exceed 15 mL.

Method

Ready-prepared infusions should be used whenever available. **Potassium chloride** is usually available in concentrations of 20, 27, and 40 mmol/litre in sodium chloride intravenous infusion (0.9%), glucose intravenous infusion (5%) or sodium chloride and glucose intravenous infusion. **Lidocaine hydrochloride (lignocaine hydrochloride)** is usually available in concentrations of 0.1 or 0.2% in glucose intravenous infusion (5%).

When addition is required to be made extemporaneously, any product reconstitution instructions such as those relating to concentration, vehicle, mixing, and handling precautions should be strictly followed using an aseptic technique throughout. Once the product has been reconstituted, addition to the infusion fluid should be made immediately in order to minimise microbial contamination and, with certain products, to prevent degradation or other formulation change which may occur; e.g. reconstituted ampicillin injection degrades rapidly on standing, and also may form polymers which could cause sensitivity reactions.

It is also important in certain instances that an infusion fluid of specific pH be used (e.g. **furosemide (frusemide)** injection requires dilution in infusions of pH greater than 5.5).

When drug additions are made it is important to mix thoroughly; additions should not be made to an infusion container that has been connected to a giving set, as mixing is hampered. If the solutions are not thoroughly mixed a concentrated layer of the additive may form owing to differences in density. **Potassium chloride** is particularly prone to this 'layering' effect when added without adequate mixing to infusions packed in non-rigid infusion containers; if such a mixture is administered it may have a serious effect on the heart.

A time limit between addition and completion of administration must be imposed for certain admixtures to guarantee satisfactory drug potency and compatibility. For admixtures in which degradation occurs without the formation of toxic substances, an acceptable limit is the time taken for 10% decomposition of the drug. When toxic substances are produced stricter limits may be imposed. Because of the risk of microbial contamination a maximum time limit of 12 hours should be imposed for additions made elsewhere than in hospital pharmacies offering central additive service.

Certain injections must be protected from light during continuous infusion to minimise oxidation, e.g. amphotericin, dacarbazine, and sodium nitroprusside.

Dilution with a small volume of an appropriate vehicle and administration using a motorised infusion pump is advocated for preparations such as heparin where strict control over administration is required. In this case the appropriate dose may be dissolved in a convenient volume (e.g. 24 to 48 mL) of sodium chloride intravenous infusion (0.9%).

Use of table

The table lists preparations given by three methods:
continuous infusion,
intermittent infusion, and
addition via the drip tubing.

Drugs for **continuous infusion** must be diluted in a large volume infusion. Penicillins and cephalosporins are not usually given by continuous infusion because of stability problems and because adequate plasma and tissue concentrations are best obtained by intermittent infusion. Where it is necessary to administer them by continuous infusion, detailed literature should be consulted.

Drugs that are both compatible and clinically suitable may be given by **intermittent infusion** in a relatively small volume of infusion over a short period of time, e.g. 100 mL in 30 minutes. The method is used if the product is incompatible or unstable over the period necessary for continuous infusion; the limited stability of ampicillin or amoxicillin in large volume glucose or lactate infusions may be overcome in this way.

Intermittent infusion is also used if adequate plasma and tissue concentrations are not produced by continuous infusion as in the case of drugs such as carbenicillin, dacarbazine, gentamicin, and ticarcillin.

An in-line burette may be used for intermittent infusion techniques in order to achieve strict control over the time and rate of administration, especially for infants and children and in intensive care units. Intermittent infusion may also make use of the 'piggy-back' technique provided that no additions are made to the primary infusion. In this method the drug is added to a small secondary container connected to a Y-type injection site on the primary infusion giving set; the secondary solution is usually infused within 30 minutes.

Addition via the drip tubing is indicated for a number of cytotoxic drugs in order to minimise extravasation. The preparation is added aseptically *via* the rubber septum of the injection site of a fast-running infusion. In general, drug preparations intended for a bolus effect should be given directly into a separate vein where possible. Failing this, administration may be made *via* the drip tubing provided that the preparation is compatible with the infusion fluid when given in this manner.

Table of drugs given by intravenous infusion

> Covers addition to *Glucose intravenous infusion* 5 and 10%, *Sodium chloride intravenous infusion* 0.9%, *Compound sodium chloride intravenous infusion* (Ringer's solution), and *Compound sodium lactate intravenous infusion* (Hartmann's solution). Compatibility with glucose 5% and with sodium chloride 0.9% indicates compatibility with *Sodium chloride and glucose intravenous infusion*. Infusion of a large volume of hypotonic solution should be avoided therefore care should be taken if water for injections is used. The information in the Table relates to the proprietary preparations indicated; for other preparations suitability should be checked with the manufacturer

Abciximab (*ReoPro®*)
Continuous *in* Glucose 5% *or* Sodium chloride 0.9%
> Withdraw from vial, dilute in infusion fluid and give *via* infusion pump through a non-pyrogenic low protein-binding 0.2 or 0.22 micron filter

Acetylcysteine (*Parvolex®*)
Continuous *in* Glucose 5%
> See Emergency Treatment of Poisoning

Aciclovir (as sodium salt) (*Zovirax IV®*; *Aciclovir IV*, Faulding DBL; *Aciclovir IV*, Genus; *Aciclovir Sodium*, Zurich)
Intermittent *in* Sodium chloride 0.9% *or* Sodium chloride and glucose *or* Compound sodium lactate
> For *Zovirax IV®*, *Aciclovir IV* (Genus) and *Aciclovir Sodium* (Zurich) initially reconstitute to 25 mg/mL in water for injections or sodium chloride 0.9% then dilute to not more than 5 mg/mL with the infusion fluid; to be given over 1 hour; alternatively, may be administered in a concentration of 25 mg/mL using a suitable infusion pump and given over 1 hour; for *Aciclovir IV* (Faulding DBL) dilute to not more than 5 mg/mL with infusion fluid; give over 1 hour

Aclarubicin (as hydrochloride) (*Aclacin®*)
Intermittent *in* Glucose 5% *or* Sodium chloride 0.9%
> Dissolve initially in 10 mL water for injections or sodium chloride 0.9% then dilute with 200–500 mL infusion fluid to a concentration of 200–500 micrograms/mL; give over 30–60 minutes and protect from light during administration; pH of glucose infusion should be between 5 and 6

Alemtuzumab (*MabCampath®*)
Intermittent *in* Glucose 5% *or* Sodium chloride 0.9%
> Add requisite dose through a low protein binding 5-micron filter to 100 mL infusion fluid; infuse over 2 hours

Alfentanil (as hydrochloride) (*Rapifen® preparations*)
Continuous *or* intermittent *in* Glucose 5% *or* Sodium chloride 0.9% *or* Compound sodium lactate

Alprostadil (*Prostin VR®*)
Continuous *in* Glucose 5% *or* Sodium chloride 0.9%
> Add directly to the infusion solution avoiding contact with the walls of plastic containers

Alteplase (*Actilyse®*)
Continuous *or* intermittent *in* Sodium chloride 0.9%
> Dissolve in water for injections to a concentration of 1 mg/mL and infuse intravenously; alternatively dilute the solution further in the infusion fluid to a concentration of not less than 200 micrograms/mL; not to be infused in glucose solution

Amifostine (*Ethyol®*)
Intermittent *in* Sodium chloride 0.9%

Amikacin sulphate (*Amikin®*)
Intermittent *in* Glucose 5% *or* Sodium chloride 0.9% *or* Compound sodium lactate
> To be given over 30 minutes

Aminophylline
Continuous *in* Glucose 5% *or* Sodium chloride 0.9% *or* Compound sodium lactate

Amiodarone hydrochloride (*Cordarone X®*)
Continuous *or* intermittent *in* Glucose 5%
> Suggested initial infusion volume 250 mL given over 20–120 minutes; for repeat infusions up to 1.2 g in max. 500 mL; infusion in extreme emergency see section 2.3.2; should not be diluted to less than 600 micrograms/mL; incompatible with sodium chloride infusion

Amoxicillin (as sodium salt) (*Amoxil®*)
Intermittent *in* Glucose 5% *or* Sodium chloride 0.9%
> Reconstituted solutions diluted and given without delay; suggested volume 100 mL given over 30–60 minutes
via drip tubing *in* Glucose 5% *or* Sodium chloride 0.9% *or* Ringer's solution *or* Compound sodium lactate
Continuous infusion not usually recommended

Amphotericin (colloidal) (*Amphocil®*)
Intermittent *in* Glucose 5%
> Initially reconstitute with water for injections (50 mg in 10 mL, 100 mg in 20 mL), shaking gently to dissolve (fluid may be opalescent) then dilute to a concentration of 625 micrograms/mL (1 volume of reconstituted solution with 7 volumes of infusion fluid); give at a rate of 1–2 mg/kg/hour or slower if not tolerated (initial test dose 2 mg of a 100 microgram/mL solution over 10 minutes); incompatible with sodium chloride or other electrolyte solutions, flush existing intravenous line with glucose 5% or use separate line

Amphotericin (lipid complex) (*Abelcet®*)
Intermittent *in* Glucose 5%
> Allow suspension to reach room temperature, shake gently to ensure no yellow settlement, withdraw requisite dose (using 17–19 gauge needle) into one or more 20-mL syringes; replace needle on syringe with a 5-micron filter needle provided (fresh needle for each syringe) and dilute to a concentration of 1 mg/mL (2 mg/mL in fluid restriction); preferably give *via* an infusion pump at a rate of 2.5 mg/kg/hour (initial test dose of 1 mg given over 15 minutes); an in-line filter (pore size no less than 15 micron) may be used; do not use sodium chloride or other electrolyte solutions, flush existing intravenous line with glucose 5% or use separate line

Amphotericin (liposomal) (*AmBisome®*)
Intermittent *in* Glucose 5%
> Reconstitute each vial with 12 mL water for injections and shake vigorously to produce a preparation containing 4 mg/mL; withdraw requisite dose from vial and introduce into infusion fluid through the 5 micron filter provided to produce a final concentration of 0.2–2 mg/mL; infuse over 30–60 minutes (initial test dose 1 mg over 10 minutes); incompatible with sodium chloride solutions, flush existing intravenous line with glucose 5% or use separate line

Amphotericin (as sodium deoxycholate complex) (*Fungizone®*)

Intermittent *in* Glucose 5%

Reconstitute each vial with 10 mL water for injections and shake immediately to produce a 5 mg/mL colloidal solution; dilute further in infusion fluid to a concentration of 100 micrograms/mL; pH of the glucose must not be below 4.2 (check each container—see product literature for details of buffer); infuse over 2–4 hours, or longer if not tolerated (initial test dose 1 mg over 20–30 minutes); begin infusion immediately after dilution and protect from light; incompatible with sodium chloride solutions, flush existing intravenous line with glucose 5% or use separate line

Ampicillin sodium (*Penbritin®*)

Intermittent *in* Glucose 5% *or* Sodium chloride 0.9%

Reconstituted solutions diluted and given without delay; suggested volume 100 mL given over 30–60 minutes *via* drip tubing *in* Glucose 5% *or* Sodium chloride 0.9% *or* Ringer's solution *or* Compound sodium lactate

Continuous infusion not usually recommended

Amsacrine (*Amsidine®*)

Intermittent in Glucose 5%

Reconstitute with diluent provided and dilute to suggested volume 500 mL; give over 60–90 minutes; use glass syringes; incompatible with sodium chloride infusion

Atenolol (*Tenormin®*)

Intermittent *in* Glucose 5% *or* Sodium chloride 0.9%

Suggested infusion time 20 minutes

Atosiban (*Tractocile®*)

Continuous *in* Glucose 5% *or* Sodium chloride 0.9% *or* Compound sodium lactate

Withdraw 10 mL infusion fluid from 100-mL bag and replace with 10 mL atosiban concentrate (7.5 mg/mL) to produce a final concentration of 750 micrograms/mL

Atracurium besilate (*Tracrium®*)

Continuous *in* Glucose 5% *or* Sodium chloride 0.9% *or* Compound sodium lactate

Stability varies with diluent

Azathioprine (as sodium salt) (*Imuran®*)

Intermittent *in* Sodium chloride 0.9% *or* Sodium chloride and glucose

Reconstitute 50 mg with 5–15 mL water for injections; dilute with 20–200 mL infusion fluid

Aztreonam (*Azactam®*)

Intermittent *in* Glucose 5% *or* Sodium chloride 0.9% *or* Ringer's solution *or* Compound sodium lactate

Dissolve initially in water for injections (1 g per 3 mL) then dilute to a concentration of less than 20 mg/mL; to be given over 20–60 minutes

Basiliximab (*Simulect®*)

Intermittent *in* Glucose 5% *or* Sodium chloride 0.9%

Reconstitute with 5 mL water for injections then dilute to at least 50 mL with infusion fluid and give over 20–30 minutes

Benzylpenicillin sodium (*Crystapen®*)

Intermittent *in* Glucose 5% *or* Sodium chloride 0.9%

Suggested volume 100 mL given over 30–60 minutes

Continuous infusion not usually recommended

Betamethasone (as sodium phosphate) (*Betnesol®*)

Continuous *or* intermittent *or* via drip tubing *in* Glucose 5% *or* Sodium chloride 0.9%

Bleomycin sulphate

Intermittent *in* Sodium chloride 0.9%

To be given slowly; suggested volume 200 mL

Bumetanide (*Burinex®*)

Intermittent *in* Glucose 5% *or* Sodium chloride 0.9%

Suggested volume 500 mL given over 30–60 minutes

Calcitonin (salmon)/Salcatonin (*Forcaltonin®, Miacalcic®*)

Intermittent *in* Sodium chloride 0.9%

Diluted solution given without delay; dilute in 500 mL and give over at least 6 hours; glass or hard plastic containers should not be used; approx. 20% loss of potency on dilution (take into account when calculating dose)

Calcium folinate (*Calcium Leucovorin®, Refolinon®*)

Intermittent *in* Sodium chloride 0.9%

Calcium Leucovorin® can also be infused in Glucose 5 and 10% or Compound sodium lactate

Protect from light

Calcium gluconate

Continuous *in* Glucose 5% *or* Sodium chloride 0.9%

Avoid bicarbonates, phosphates, or sulphates

Calcium levofolinate (*Isovorin®*)

Intermittent *in* Glucose 5 and 10% *or* Sodium chloride 0.9% *or* Compound sodium lactate

Protect from light

Carboplatin (*Paraplatin®*)

Intermittent *in* Glucose 5% *or* Sodium chloride 0.9%

Final concentration as low as 500 micrograms/mL; give over 15–60 minutes

Carmustine (*BiCNU®*)

Intermittent *in* Glucose 5% *or* Sodium chloride 0.9%

Reconstitute with solvent provided; give over 1–2 hours

Cefamandole (as nafate) (*Kefadol®*)

Intermittent *or* via drip tubing *in* Glucose 5 and 10% *or* Sodium chloride 0.9%

Continuous infusion not usually recommended

Cefazolin (as sodium salt) (*Kefzol®*)

Intermittent *or* via drip tubing *in* Glucose 5 and 10% *or* Sodium chloride 0.9% *or* Compound sodium lactate

Reconstitute initially with water for injections; dilute to 50–100 mL with infusion fluid

Cefotaxime (as sodium salt) (*Claforan®*; *Cefotaxime Injection*, Genus)

Intermittent *in* Glucose 5% *or* Sodium chloride 0.9% *or* Compound sodium lactate *or* Water for injections

Suggested volume 40–100 mL given over 20–60 minutes

Cefoxitin (as sodium salt) (*Mefoxin®*)

Intermittent *or via* drip tubing in Glucose 5 and 10% *or* Sodium chloride 0.9%

Reconstitute initially with water for injections

Cefradine (*Velosef®*)

Continuous *or* intermittent *in* Glucose 5 and 10% *or* Sodium chloride 0.9% *or* Ringer's solution *or* Compound sodium lactate

Reconstitute 500 mg with 5 mL water for injections or glucose 5% or sodium chloride 0.9% then dilute with infusion fluid

Ceftazidime (as pentahydrate) (*Fortum®*, *Kefadim®*)

Intermittent *or via* drip tubing *in* Glucose 5 and 10% *or* Sodium chloride 0.9% *or* Compound sodium lactate

Dissolve 2 g initially in 10 mL (3 g in 15 mL) infusion fluid; for *Fortum®* dilute further to a concentration of 40 mg/mL; for *Kefadim®* dilute further to a concentration of 20 mg/mL; give over up to 30 minutes

Ceftriaxone (as sodium salt) (*Rocephin®*; *Ceftriaxone Injection*, Genus)

Intermittent *or via* drip tubing *in* Glucose 5 and 10% *or* Sodium chloride 0.9%

Reconstitute 2-g vial with 40 mL infusion fluid; give intermittent infusion over at least 30 minutes (60 minutes in neonates); not to be given with infusion fluids containing calcium

Cefuroxime (as sodium salt) (*Zinacef®*)

Intermittent *or via* drip tubing *in* Glucose 5% *or* Sodium chloride 0.9% *or* Compound sodium lactate

Dissolve initially in water for injections (at least 2 mL for each 250 mg, 15 mL for 1.5 g); suggested volume 50–100 mL given over 30 minutes

Chloramphenicol (as sodium succinate) (*Kemicetine®*)

Intermittent *or via* drip tubing *in* Glucose 5% *or* Sodium chloride 0.9%

Chlormethine hydrochloride/Mustine hydrochloride (Abbott)

via drip tubing *in* Glucose 5% *or* Sodium chloride 0.9%

Chloroquine sulphate (*Nivaquine®*)

Continuous *in* Sodium chloride 0.9%

See also section 5.4.1

Ciclosporin (*Sandimmun®*)

Continuous *in* Glucose 5% *or* Sodium chloride 0.9%

Dilute to a concentration of 50 mg in 20–100 mL; give over 2–6 hours; not to be used with PVC equipment

Cidofovir (*Vistide®*)

Intermittent *in* Sodium chloride 0.9%

Dilute requisite dose with 100 mL infusion fluid; infuse over 1 hour

Cimetidine (*Tagamet®*)

Continuous *or* intermittent *in* Glucose 5% *or* Sodium chloride 0.9%

For intermittent infusion suggested volume 100 mL given over 30–60 minutes

Cisatracurium (*Nimbex®*, *Nimbex Forte®*)

Continuous *in* Glucose 5% *or* Sodium chloride 0.9%

Solutions of 2 mg/mL and 5 mg/mL may be infused undiluted; alternatively dilute with infusion fluid to a concentration of 0.1–2 mg/mL

Cisplatin (*Cisplatin*, Pharmacia & Upjohn; *Cisplatin injection solution*, Faulding DBL)

Intermittent *in* Sodium chloride 0.9% *or* Sodium chloride and glucose

Reconstitute initially with water for injections to produce 1 mg/mL solution then dilute in 2 litres infusion fluid; give over 6–8 hours

Cladribine (*Leustat®*)

Continuous *in* Sodium chloride 0.9%

Dilute with 100–500 mL; glucose solutions are unsuitable

Clarithromycin (*Klaricid® I.V.*)

Intermittent *in* Glucose 5% *or* Sodium chloride 0.9% *or* Ringer's solution *or* Compound sodium lactate

Dissolve initially in water for injections (500 mg in 10 mL) then dilute to a concentration of 2 mg/mL; give over 60 minutes

Clindamycin (as phosphate) (*Dalacin® C Phosphate*)

Continuous *or* intermittent *in* Glucose 5% *or* Sodium chloride 0.9%

Give over at least 10–60 minutes (1.2 g over at least 60 minutes; higher doses by continuous infusion)

Clomipramine hydrochloride (*Anafranil®*)

Intermittent *in* Glucose 5% *or* Sodium chloride 0.9%

See product literature for details of initial dose to test tolerance; suggested volume 125–500mL given over 45–180 minutes

Clonazepam (*Rivotril®*)

Intermittent *in* Glucose 5 and 10% *or* Sodium chloride 0.9%

Suggested volume 250 mL

Co-amoxiclav (*Augmentin®*)

Intermittent *in* Sodium chloride 0.9% *or* Water for injections; see also package leaflet

Suggested volume 50–100 mL given over 30–40 minutes and completed within 4 hours of reconstitution

via drip tubing *in* Glucose 5% *or* Sodium chloride 0.9%

Co-fluampicil (as sodium salts) (*Magnapen®*)

Intermittent *in* Glucose 5% *or* Sodium chloride 0.9%

Reconstituted solutions diluted and given without delay; suggested volume 100 mL given over 30–60 minutes

via drip tubing *in* Glucose 5% *or* Sodium chloride 0.9% *or* Ringer's solution *or* Compound sodium lactate

Colistimethate sodium (*Colomycin®*)

Continuous *or* intermittent *in* Glucose 5% *or* Sodium chloride 0.9% *or* Ringer's solution

Max. 6 hours between addition and completion of administration

Co-trimoxazole (*Septrin® for infusion*)

Intermittent *in* Glucose 5 and 10% *or* Sodium chloride 0.9% *or* Ringer's solution

Dilute contents of 1 ampoule (5 mL) to 125 mL, 2 ampoules (10 mL) to 250 mL or 3 ampoules (15 mL) to 500 mL; suggested duration of infusion 60–90 minutes (but may be adjusted according to fluid requirements); if fluid restriction necessary, 1 ampoule (5 mL) may be diluted with 75 mL glucose 5% and infused over max. 60 minutes

Cyclophosphamide (*Endoxana®*)

Intermittent *or via* drip tubing *in* Glucose 5% *or* Sodium chloride 0.9% *or* Water for injections

For intermittent infusion suggested volume 50–100 mL given over 5–15 minutes

via drip tubing in Glucose 5%

Cyclosporin *see* Ciclosporin

Cytarabine (*Cytosar®*)

Continuous *or* intermittent *or via* drip tubing *in* Glucose 5% *or* Sodium chloride 0.9%

Reconstitute *Cytosar®* with water for injections or with infusion fluid; check container for haze or precipitate during administration

Dacarbazine (*DTIC-Dome®; Dacarbazine,* Medac)

Intermittent *in* Glucose 5% *or* Sodium chloride 0.9%

Reconstitute initially with water for injections then for *DTIC-Dome®* dilute in 125–250 mL infusion fluid; for *Dacarbazine* (Medac) dilute in 200–300 mL infusion fluid; give over 15–30 minutes; protect infusion from light

Daclizumab (*Zenapax®*)

Intermittent *in* Sodium chloride 0.9%

Dilute requisite dose in 50 mL infusion fluid; infuse over 15 minutes

Dactinomycin (*Cosmegen Lyovac®*)

Intermittent *or via* drip tubing *in* Glucose 5% *or* Sodium chloride 0.9%

Reconstitute with water for injections

Danaparoid sodium (*Orgaran®*)

Continuous *in* Glucose 5% *or* Sodium chloride 0.9%

Daunorubicin (as hydrochloride) (*Cerubidin®*)

via drip tubing *in* Sodium chloride 0.9%

Reconstitute vial with 4 mL water for injections to give 5 mg/mL solution; dilute requisite dose with infusion fluid to a concentration of 1 mg/mL; give over 20 minutes

Daunorubicin (liposomal) (*DaunoXome®*)

Intermittent *in* Glucose 5%

Dilute to a concentration of 0.2–1 mg/mL; give over 30–60 minutes; incompatible with sodium chloride solutions; in-line filter not recommended (if used, pore size should be no less than 5 micron)

Desferrioxamine mesilate (*Desferal®*)

Continuous *or* intermittent *in* Glucose 5% *or* Sodium chloride 0.9%

Dissolve initially in water for injections (500 mg in 5 mL) then dilute with infusion fluid

Desmopressin (*DDAVP®*)

Intermittent *in* Sodium chloride 0.9%

Dilute with 50 mL and give over 20 minutes

Dexamethasone sodium phosphate (*Decadron®; Dexamethasone,* Faulding DBL; *Dexamethasone,* Organon)

Continuous *or* intermittent *or via* drip tubing *in* Glucose 5% *or* Sodium chloride 0.9%

Dexamethasone (Organon) can also be infused in Ringer's solution *or* Compound sodium lactate

Diamorphine hydrochloride (*Diamorphine Injection,* CP)

Continuous *in* Glucose 5% *or* Sodium chloride 0.9%

Glucose is preferred as infusion fluid

Diazepam (solution) (*Valium®*)

Continuous *in* Glucose 5% *or* Sodium chloride 0.9%

Dilute to a concentration of not more than 40 mg in 500 mL; max. 6 hours between addition and completion of administration; adsorbed to some extent by the plastics of the infusion set

Diazepam (emulsion) (*Diazemuls®*)

Continuous *in* Glucose 5 and 10%

May be diluted to a max. concentration of 200 mg in 500 mL; max. 6 hours between addition and completion of administration; adsorbed to some extent by the plastics of the infusion set

via drip tubing *in* Glucose 5 and 10% *or* Sodium chloride 0.9%

Adsorbed to some extent by the plastics of the infusion set

Diclofenac sodium (*Voltarol®*)

Continuous *or* intermittent *in* Glucose 5% *or* Sodium chloride 0.9%

Dilute 75 mg with 100–500 mL infusion fluid (previously buffered with 0.5 mL sodium bicarbonate 8.4% solution *or* with 1 mL sodium bicarbonate 4.2% solution); for intermittent infusion give 25–50 mg over 15–60 minutes or 75 mg over 30–120 minutes; for continuous infusion give at a rate of 5 mg/hour

Digoxin (*Lanoxin®*)

Intermittent *in* Glucose 5% *or* Sodium chloride 0.9%

To be given over at least 2 hours

Digoxin-specific antibody fragments (*Digibind®*)

Intermittent *in* Sodium chloride 0.9%

Dissolve initially in water for injections (4 mL/vial) then dilute with the sodium chloride 0.9% and give through a 0.22 micron sterile, disposable filter over 30 minutes

Dinoprostone (*Prostin E2®*)

Continuous *or* intermittent *in* Glucose 5% *or* Sodium chloride 0.9%

Disodium folinate (*Sodiofolin®*)

Intermittent *in* Sodium chloride 0.9%

Protect from light

Avoid bicarbonate containing infusions

Disodium pamidronate (*Aredia®*)

Continuous *in* Sodium chloride 0.9%

Reconstitute initially with water for injections (15 mg in 5 mL, 30 mg or 90 mg in 10 mL); dilute with infusion fluid to a concentration of not more than 60 mg in 250 mL; give at a rate not exceeding 1 mg/minute; not to be given with infusion fluids containing calcium

Disopyramide (as phosphate) (*Rythmodan®*)

Continuous *or* intermittent *in* Glucose 5% *or* Sodium chloride 0.9% *or* Ringer's solution *or* Compound sodium lactate

Max. rate by continuous infusion 20–30 mg/hour (or 400 micrograms/kg/hour)

Dobutamine (as hydrochloride) (*Dobutrex®, Posiject®*)

Continuous *in* Glucose 5% *or* Sodium chloride 0.9%

Dilute to a concentration of 0.5–1 mg/mL and give *via* a controlled infusion device; give higher concentration (max. 5 mg/mL) with infusion pump; incompatible with bicarbonate

Docetaxel (*Taxotere®*)

Intermittent *in* Glucose 5% *or* Sodium chloride 0.9%

Stand docetaxel vials and diluent at room temperature for 5 minutes; add diluent to produce a concentrate containing 10 mg/mL and allow to stand for a further 5 minutes; dilute the requisite dose with at least 250 mL infusion fluid to a final concentration not exceeding 740 micrograms/mL; infuse over 1 hour

Dopamine hydrochloride (*Intropin®*)

Continuous *in* Glucose 5% *or* Sodium chloride 0.9% *or* Compound sodium lactate

Dilute to a concentration of 1.6 mg/mL; incompatible with bicarbonate

Dopexamine hydrochloride (*Dopacard®*)

Continuous *in* Glucose 5% *or* Sodium chloride 0.9%

Dilute to a concentration of 400 or 800 micrograms/mL; max. concentration *via* large peripheral vein 1 mg/mL, concentrations up to 4 mg/mL may be infused *via* central vein; give *via* infusion pump or other device which provides accurate control of rate; contact with metal should be minimised; incompatible with bicarbonate

Doxorubicin hydrochloride (*Doxorubicin Rapid Dissolution, Doxorubicin Solution*) (both Pharmacia & Upjohn)

via drip tubing *in* Glucose 5% *or* Sodium chloride 0.9%

Reconstitute *Doxorubicin Rapid Dissolution* with water for injections or sodium chloride 0.9% (10 mg in 5 mL, 50 mg in 25 mL); give over 2–3 minutes

Doxorubicin hydrochloride (liposomal) (*Caelyx®*)

via drip tubing *in* Glucose 5%

Dilute up to 90 mg in 250 mL infusion fluid and over 90 mg in 500 mL infusion fluid

Enoximone (*Perfan®*)

Continuous *or* intermittent *in* Sodium chloride 0.9% *or* Water for injections

Dilute to a concentration of 2.5 mg/mL; incompatible with glucose solutions; use only plastic containers or syringes

Epirubicin hydrochloride (*Pharmorubicin® Rapid Dissolution, Pharmorubicin® Solution*)

via drip tubing *in* Sodium chloride 0.9%

Reconstitute *Pharmorubicin® Rapid Dissolution* with sodium chloride 0.9% or with water for injections (10 mg in 5 mL, 20 mg in 10 mL, 50 mg in 25 mL); give over 3–5 minutes

Epoprostenol (*Flolan®*)

Continuous *in* Sodium chloride 0.9%

Reconstitute with the solvent provided (pH 10.5) to make a concentrate; use this concentrate within 12 hours and store at 2–8°C; dilute with not more than 6 times the volume of sodium chloride 0.9% before use

Erythromycin (as lactobionate)

Continuous *or* intermittent *in* Glucose 5% (neutralised with sodium bicarbonate) *or* Sodium chloride 0.9%

Dissolve initially in water for injections (1 g in 20 mL) then dilute to a concentration of 1 mg/mL for continuous infusion and 1–5 mg/mL for intermittent infusion; give intermittent infusion over 20–60 minutes

Esmolol hydrochloride (*Brevibloc®*)

Continuous *or* intermittent *in* Glucose 5% *or* Sodium chloride 0.9%

Dilute to a concentration of 10 mg/mL; for continuous infusion use a suitable infusion control device; incompatible with bicarbonate

Ethanol

Continuous *in* Glucose 5% *or* Sodium chloride 0.9% *or* Ringer's solution *or* Compound sodium lactate

Dilute to a concentration of 5–10%

Etoposide (*Eposin®; Vepesid®; Etoposide*, APS)

Intermittent *in* Sodium chloride 0.9%

For *Vepesid®* dilute to a concentration of not more than 250 micrograms/mL and give over not less than 30 minutes; for *Etoposide* (APS) dilute with either sodium chloride 0.9% or glucose 5% to a concentration of 200 micrograms/mL and give over 30–60 minutes; for *Eposin®* dilute with either sodium chloride 0.9% or glucose 5% to a concentration of 200–400 micrograms/mL and give over at least 30 minutes; check container for haze or precipitate during infusion

Etoposide (as phosphate) (*Etopophos®*)

Intermittent *in* Glucose 5% *or* Sodium chloride 0.9%

Reconstitute with 5–10 mL of either water for injections or with infusion fluid then dilute further with infusion fluid to a concentration as low as 100 micrograms/mL and give over 5 minutes to 3.5 hours

Filgrastim (*Neupogen®*)

Continuous *or* intermittent *in* Glucose 5%

For a filgrastim concentration of less than 1 500 000 units/mL (15 micrograms/mL) albumin solution (human serum albumin) is added to produce a final albumin concentration of 2 mg/mL; should not be diluted to a filgrastim concentration of less than 200 000 units/mL (2 micrograms/mL) and should not be diluted with sodium chloride solution

Flecainide acetate (*Tambocor®*)

Continuous *or* intermittent *in* Glucose 5% *or* Sodium chloride 0.9% *or* Compound sodium lactate

Minimum volume in infusion fluids containing chlorides 500 mL

Flucloxacillin (as sodium salt) (*Floxapen®*)

Intermittent *in* Glucose 5% *or* Sodium chloride 0.9%

Suggested volume 100 mL given over 30–60 minutes

via drip tubing *in* Glucose 5% *or* Sodium chloride 0.9% *or* Ringer's solution *or* Compound sodium lactate

Continuous infusion not usually recommended

Fludarabine phosphate (*Fludara®*)

Intermittent *in* Sodium chloride 0.9%

Reconstitute each 50 mg with 2 mL water for injections and dilute requisite dose in 100 mL; give over 30 minutes

Flumazenil (*Anexate®*)

Continuous *in* Glucose 5% *or* Sodium chloride 0.9%

Fluorouracil (as sodium salt)

Continuous *or* intermittent *or via* drip tubing *in* Glucose 5% *or* Sodium chloride 0.9%

Give intermittent infusion over 30–60 minutes *or* over 4 hours

Foscarnet sodium (*Foscavir®*)

Intermittent *in* Glucose 5% *or* Sodium chloride 0.9%

Dilute to a concentration of 12 mg/mL for infusion into peripheral vein (undiluted solution *via* central venous line only); infuse over at least 1 hour

Fosphenytoin Sodium (*Pro-Epanutin®*)

Intermittent *in* Glucose 5% *or* Sodium chloride 0.9%

Dilute to a concentration of 1.5–25 mg (phenytoin sodium equivalent)/mL

Furosemide/Frusemide (as sodium salt) (*Lasix®*)

Continuous *in* Sodium chloride 0.9% *or* Ringer's solution

Infusion pH must be above 5.5 and rate should not exceed 4 mg/minute; glucose solutions are unsuitable

Fusidic acid (as sodium salt) (*Fucidin®*)

Continuous *in* Glucose 5% (but see below) *or* Sodium chloride 0.9%

Reconstitute with the buffer solution provided and dilute to 500 mL; give through central venous line over 2 hours (or over 6 hours if superficial vein used); incompatible in solution of pH less than 7.4

Ganciclovir (as sodium salt) (*Cymevene®*)

Intermittent *in* Glucose 5% *or* Sodium chloride 0.9% *or* Ringer's solution *or* Compound sodium lactate

Reconstitute initially in water for injections (500 mg/ 10 mL) then dilute to not more than 10 mg/mL with infusion fluid (usually 100 mL); give over 1 hour

Gemcitabine (*Gemzar®*)

Intermittent *in* Sodium chloride 0.9%

Reconstitute initially with sodium chloride 0.9% (200 mg in at least 5 mL, 1 g in at least 25 mL); may be diluted further with infusion fluid; give over 30 minutes

Gentamicin (as sulphate) (*Cidomycin®*)

Intermittent *or via* drip tubing *in* Glucose 5% *or* Sodium chloride 0.9%

Suggested volume for intermittent infusion 50–100 mL given over 20 minutes

Glyceryl trinitrate (*Nitrocine®, Nitronal®, Tridil®*)

Continuous *in* Glucose 5% *or* Sodium chloride 0.9%

For *Tridil®* dilute to a concentration of not more than 400 micrograms/mL; for *Nitrocine®* suggested infusion concentration 100 micrograms/mL; incompatible with polyvinyl chloride infusion containers such as *Viaflex®* or *Steriflex®*; use glass or polyethylene containers or give *via* a syringe pump

Granisetron (as hydrochloride) (*Kytril®*)

Intermittent *in* Glucose 5% *or* Sodium chloride 0.9% *or* Compound sodium lactate

Dilute 3 mL in 20–50 mL infusion fluid (up to 3 mL in 10–30 mL for children); give over 5 minutes

Haem arginate (*Normosang®*)

Intermittent *in* Sodium chloride 0.9%

Dilute requisite dose in 100 mL infusion fluid in glass bottle and give over at least 30 minutes *via* large antebrachial vein; administer within 1 hour after dilution

Heparin sodium

Continuous *in* Glucose 5% *or* Sodium chloride 0.9%

Administration with a motorised pump advisable

Hydralazine hydrochloride (*Apresoline®*)

Continuous *in* Sodium chloride 0.9% *or* Ringer's solution

Suggested infusion volume 500 mL

Hydrocortisone (as sodium phosphate) (*Efcortesol®*)

Continuous *or* intermittent *or via* drip tubing *in* Glucose 5% *or* Sodium chloride 0.9%

Hydrocortisone (as sodium succinate) (*Efcortelan Soluble®, SoluCortef®*)

Continuous *or* intermittent *or via* drip tubing *in* Glucose 5% *or* Sodium chloride 0.9%

Idarubicin hydrochloride (*Zavedos®*)

via drip tubing *in* Sodium chloride 0.9%

Reconstitute with water for injections; give over 5–10 minutes

Ifosfamide (*Mitoxana®*)

Continuous *or* intermittent *or via* drip tubing *in* Glucose 5% *or* Sodium chloride 0.9%

For continuous infusion, suggested volume 3 litres given over 24 hours; for intermittent infusion, give over 30–120 minutes

Imiglucerase (*Cerezyme®*)

Intermittent *in* Sodium chloride 0.9%

Initially reconstitute with 5.1 mL water for injections to give 40 units/mL solution; dilute requisite dose in 100–200 mL infusion fluid and give over 1–2 hours *or* at a rate not exceeding 1 unit/kg/minute; administer within 3 hours after reconstitution

Imipenem with cilastatin (as sodium salt) (*Primaxin®*)

Intermittent *in* Sodium chloride 0.9% *or* Sodium chloride and glucose

Dilute to a concentration of 5 mg (as imipenem)/mL; infuse 250–500 mg (as imipenem) over 20–30 minutes, 1 g over 40–60 minutes

Continuous infusion not usually recommended

Infliximab (*Remicade®*)

Intermittent *in* Sodium chloride 0.9%

Reconstitute 100 mg with 10 mL water for injections (swirling gently to dissolve—avoid vigorous agitation) and dilute to 250 mL with infusion fluid; give through an in-line filter (1.2 micron or less) over at least 2 hours at a rate not exceeding 2 mL/minute

Insulin (soluble)

Continuous *in* Sodium chloride 0.9% *or* Compound sodium lactate

Adsorbed to some extent by plastics of infusion set; see also section 6.1.3; ensure insulin is not injected into 'dead space' of injection port of the infusion bag

Interferon alfa-2b (*IntronA®*)

Intermittent *in* Sodium chloride 0.9%

For *IntronA®* solution, dilute requisite dose in 50 mL infusion fluid and administer over 20 minutes; not to be diluted to less than 300 000 units/mL

For *IntronA®* powder, reconstitute with 1 mL water for injections; dilute requisite dose in 100 mL infusion fluid and administer over 20 minutes; not to be diluted to less than 100 000 units/mL

Irinotecan hydrochloride (*Campto®*)

Intermittent *in* Glucose 5% *or* Sodium chloride 0.9%

Dilute requisite dose in 250 mL infusion fluid; give over 30–90 minutes

Isoprenaline hydrochloride (*Saventrine IV®*)

Continuous *in* Glucose 5% *or* Sodium chloride and glucose

Dilute in a large-volume infusion; suggested minimum volume 500 mL; pH of the infusion must be below 5

Isosorbide dinitrate (*Isoket 0.05%®, Isoket 0.1%®*)

Continuous *in* Glucose 5% *or* Sodium chloride 0.9%

Adsorbed to some extent by polyvinyl chloride infusion containers; preferably use glass or polyethylene containers or give *via* a syringe pump; *Isoket 0.05%®* can alternatively be administered undiluted using a syringe pump with a glass or rigid plastic syringe

Itraconazole (*Sporanox®*)

Intermittent *in* Sodium chloride 0.9%

Dilute 250 mg in 50 mL infusion fluid and infuse only **60 mL** through an in-line filter (0.2 micron) over 60 minutes

Ketamine (as hydrochloride) (*Ketalar®*)

Continuous *in* Glucose 5% *or* Sodium chloride 0.9%

Dilute to 1 mg/mL; microdrip infusion for maintenance of anaesthesia

Labetalol hydrochloride (*Trandate®*)

Intermittent *in* Glucose 5% *or* Sodium chloride and glucose

Dilute to a concentration of 1 mg/mL; suggested volume 200 mL; adjust rate with in-line burette

Lenograstim (*Granocyte®*)

Intermittent *in* Sodium chloride 0.9%

Initially reconstitute with 1 mL water for injection provided (do not shake vigorously) then dilute with up to 50 mL infusion fluid for each vial of *Granocyte-13* or up to 100 mL infusion fluid for *Granocyte-34*; give over 30 minutes

Lepirudin (*Refludan®*)

Continuous *in* Glucose 5% *or* Sodium chloride 0.9%

Reconstitute initially with water for injections *or* sodium chloride 0.9% then dilute to a concentration of 2 mg/mL with infusion fluid

Magnesium sulphate

Continuous *in* Glucose 5% *or* Sodium chloride 0.9%

Suggested concentration up to 200 mg/mL

Melphalan (*Alkeran®*)

Intermittent *or via* drip tubing *in* Sodium chloride 0.9%

Reconstitute with the solvent provided then dilute with infusion fluid; max. 90 minutes between addition and completion of administration; incompatible with glucose infusion

Meropenem (*Meronem®*)

Intermittent *in* Glucose 5 and 10% *or* Sodium chloride 0.9%

Dilute in 50–200 mL infusion fluid and give over 15–30 minutes

Mesna (*Uromitexan®*)

Continuous *or via* drip tubing *in* Glucose 5% *or* Sodium chloride 0.9%

Metaraminol (as tartrate) (*Aramine®*)

Continuous *or via* drip tubing *in* Glucose 5% *or* Sodium chloride 0.9%

Suggested volume 500 mL

Methotrexate (as sodium salt) (*Methotrexate, Lederle*)

Continuous *or via* drip tubing *in* Glucose 5% *or* Sodium chloride 0.9% *or* Compound sodium lactate *or* Ringer's solution

Dilute in a large-volume infusion; max. 24 hours between addition and completion of administration

Methylprednisolone (as sodium succinate) (*Solu-Medrone®*)

Continuous *or* intermittent *or via* drip tubing *in* Glucose 5% *or* Sodium chloride 0.9%

Reconstitute initially with water for injections; doses up to 250 mg should be given over at least 5 minutes, high doses over at least 30 minutes

Metoclopramide hydrochloride (*Maxolon High Dose®*)

Continuous *or* intermittent *in* Glucose 5% *or* Sodium chloride 0.9% *or* Compound sodium lactate

Continuous infusion recommended; loading dose, dilute with 50–100 mL and give over 15–20 minutes; maintenance dose, dilute with 500 mL and give over 8–12 hours; for intermittent infusion dilute with at least 50 mL and give over at least 15 minutes

Mexiletine hydrochloride (*Mexitil®*)

Continuous *in* Glucose 5% *or* Sodium chloride 0.9%

Milrinone (*Primacor®*)

Continuous *in* Glucose 5% *or* Sodium chloride 0.9%

Dilute to a suggested concentration of 200 micrograms/mL

Mitoxantrone/Mitozantrone (as hydrochloride) (*Novantrone®, Onkotrone®*)

Intermittent *or via* drip tubing *in* Glucose 5% *or* Sodium chloride 0.9%

For administration *via* drip tubing suggested volume at least 50 mL given over at least 3–5 minutes; for intermittent infusion (*Onkotrone®* only), dilute with 50–100 mL and give over 15–30 minutes

Mivacurium (as chloride) (*Mivacron®*)

Continuous *in* Glucose 5% *or* Sodium chloride 0.9%

Dilute to a concentration of 500 micrograms/mL; may also be given undiluted

Molgramostim (*Leucomax®*)

Intermittent *in* Glucose 5% *or* Sodium chloride 0.9%

Reconstitute each vial with 1 mL water for injections; dilute with 25–100 mL infusion fluid to a concentration of not less than 80 000 units/mL; give over 4–6 hours; infusion through low protein binding 0.2 or 0.22 micron filter recommended; some infusion sets (e.g. *Port-A-Cath®*) adsorb molgramostim and should not be used

Mycophenolate mofetil (as hydrochloride) (*CellCept®*)

Intermittent *in* Glucose 5%

Reconstitute each 500-mg vial with 14 mL glucose 5% and dilute the contents of 2 vials in 140 mL infusion fluid; give over 2 hours

Naloxone (*Min-I-Jet® Naloxone Hydrochloride, Narcan®*)

Continuous *in* Glucose 5% *or* Sodium chloride 0.9%

Dilute to a concentration of 4 micrograms/mL

Netilmicin (as sulphate) (*Netillin®*)

Intermittent *or via* drip tubing *in* Glucose 5 and 10% *or* Sodium chloride 0.9%

For intermittent infusion suggested volume 50–200 mL given over 90–120 minutes

Nimodipine (*Nimotop®*)

via drip tubing *in* Glucose 5% *or* Sodium chloride 0.9% *or* Ringer's solution

Not to be added to infusion container; administer *via* an infusion pump through a Y-piece into a central catheter; incompatible with polyvinyl chloride giving sets or containers; protect infusion from light

Nizatidine (*Axid®*)

Continuous *or* intermittent *in* Glucose 5% *or* Sodium chloride 0.9% *or* Compound sodium lactate

For continuous infusion, dilute 300 mg in 150 mL and give at a rate of 10 mg/hour; for intermittent infusion, dilute 100 mg in 50 mL and give over 15 minutes

Noradrenaline acid tartrate/Norepinephrine bitartrate (*Levophed®*)

Continuous *in* Glucose 5% *or* Sodium chloride and glucose

Give *via* controlled infusion device; for administration *via* syringe pump, dilute 4 mg noradrenaline acid tartrate (2 mL solution) with 48 mL; for administration *via* drip counter dilute 40 mg (20 mL solution) with 480 mL; give through a central venous catheter; incompatible with alkalis

Omeprazole (as sodium salt) (*Losec®*)

Intermittent *in* Glucose 5% *or* Sodium chloride 0.9%

Reconstitute with infusion fluid and dilute to 100 mL; give over 20–30 minutes

Ondansetron (as hydrochloride) (*Zofran®*)

Continuous *or* intermittent *in* Glucose 5% *or* Sodium chloride 0.9% *or* Ringer's solution

For intermittent infusion, dilute 32 mg in 50–100 mL and give over at least 15 minutes

Oxaliplatin (*Eloxatin®*)

Continuous *in* Glucose 5%

Reconstitute with water for injections or glucose 5% to a concentration of 5 mg/mL; dilute with 250–500 mL infusion fluid and give over 2–6 hours

Oxytocin (*Syntocinon®*)

Continuous *in* Glucose 5% *or* Sodium chloride 0.9% *or* Compound sodium lactate *or* Ringer's solution

Preferably given *via* a variable-speed infusion pump in a concentration appropriate to the pump; if given by drip infusion for *induction or enhancement of labour*, dilute 5 units in 500 mL infusion fluid; for *postpartum uterine haemorrhage* dilute 5–30 units in 500 mL; if high doses given for prolonged period (e.g. for inevitable or missed abortion or for postpartum haemorrhage), use low volume of an electrolyte-containing infusion fluid (not Glucose 5%) given at higher concentration than for induction or enhancement of labour; close attention to patient's fluid and electrolyte status essential

Paclitaxel (*Taxol®*)

Continuous *in* Glucose 5% *or* Sodium chloride 0.9%

Dilute to a concentration of 0.3–1.2 mg/mL and give through an in-line filter (0.22 micron or less) over 3 hours; not to be used with PVC equipment (short PVC inlet or outlet on filter may be acceptable)

Pantoprazole (as sodium sequihydrate) (*Protium®*)

Intermittent *in* Glucose 5 and 10% *or* Sodium chloride 0.9%

Reconstitute 40 mg with 10 mL sodium chloride 0.9% and dilute to 100 mL with infusion fluid

Pentamidine isetionate (*Pentacarinat®*)

Intermittent *in* Glucose 5% *or* Sodium chloride 0.9%

Dissolve initially in water for injections (300 mg in 3–5 mL) then dilute in 50–250 mL; give over at least 60 minutes

Pentostatin (*Nipent®*)

Intermittent *in* Glucose 5% *or* Sodium chloride 0.9%

Reconstitute initially with 5 mL water for injections to produce a 2 mg/mL solution; dilute requisite dose in 25–50 mL infusion fluid (final concentration 180–330 micrograms/mL) and give over 20–30 minutes

Phenoxybenzamine hydrochloride

Intermittent *in* Sodium chloride 0.9%

Dilute in 200–500 mL infusion; give over at least 2 hours; max. 4 hours between dilution and completion of administration

Phentolamine mesilate (*Rogitine®*)

Intermittent *in* Glucose 5% *or* Sodium chloride 0.9%

Phenylephrine hydrochloride

Intermittent *in* Glucose 5% *or* Sodium chloride 0.9%

Dilute 10 mg in 500 mL infusion fluid

Phenytoin sodium (*Epanutin®*)

Intermittent *in* Sodium chloride 0.9%

Flush intravenous line with Sodium chloride 0.9% before and after infusion; dilute in 50–100 mL infusion fluid (final concentration not to exceed 10 mg/mL) and give through an in-line filter (0.22–0.50 micron) at a rate not exceeding 50 mg/minute (neonates, give at a rate of 1–3 mg/kg/minute); complete administration within 1 hour of preparation

Phytomenadione (in mixed micelles vehicle) (*Konakion® MM*)

Intermittent *in* Glucose 5%

Dilute with 55 mL; may be injected into lower part of infusion apparatus

Piperacillin (as sodium salt) (*Pipril®*)

Intermittent *in* Glucose 5% *or* Sodium chloride 0.9% *or* Water for injections

Reconstitute each 1 g with 5 mL water for injections; dilute requisite dose to at least 50 mL with infusion fluid and give over 20–40 minutes

Piperacillin with tazobactam (as sodium salts) (*Tazocin®*)

Intermittent *in* Glucose 5% *or* Sodium chloride 0.9% *or* Water for injections

Reconstitute initially with water for injections or sodium chloride infusion 0.9% (2.25 g in 10 mL, 4.5 g in 20 mL) then dilute to at least 50 mL with infusion fluid; give over 20–30 minutes

Potassium chloride

Continuous *in* Glucose 5% *or* Sodium chloride 0.9%

Dilute in a large-volume infusion; mix thoroughly to avoid 'layering', especially in non-rigid infusion containers; use ready-prepared solutions when possible

Procainamide hydrochloride (*Pronestyl®*)

Continuous *or* intermittent *in* Glucose 5%

For maintenance, dilute to a concentration of *either* 2 mg/mL and give at a rate of 1–3 mL/minute *or* 4 mg/mL and give at a rate of 0.5–1.5 mL/minute

Propofol (emulsion) (*Diprivan®*)

via drip tubing *in* Glucose 5% *or* Sodium chloride 0.9%

To be administered *via* a Y-piece close to injection site

Continuous *in* Glucose 5%

Dilute to a concentration not less than 2 mg/mL; administer using suitable device to control infusion rate; use glass or PVC containers (if PVC bag used it should be full—withdraw volume of infusion fluid equal to that of propofol to be added); give within 6 hours of preparation; propofol may alternatively be infused undiluted using a suitable infusion pump

Quinine dihydrochloride

Continuous *in* Sodium chloride 0.9%

To be given over 4 hours; see also section 5.4.1

Quinupristin with dalfopristin (*Synercid®*)

Intermittent *in* Glucose 5%

Reconstitute 500 mg with 5 mL water for injections or glucose 5%; gently swirl vial without shaking to dissolve; allow to stand for at least 2 minutes until foam disappears; dilute requisite dose in 100 mL infusion fluid and give over 60 minutes *via* central venous catheter (in an emergency, first dose may be diluted in 250 mL infusion fluid and given over 60 minutes *via* peripheral line); flush line with glucose 5% before and after infusion; incompatible with sodium chloride solutions

Raltitrexed (*Tomudex®*)

Intermittent *in* Glucose 5% *or* Sodium chloride 0.9%

Reconstitute with water for injections; dilute requisite dose in 50–250 mL infusion fluid and give over 15 minutes

Ranitidine (as hydrochloride) (*Zantac®*)

Intermittent *in* Glucose 5% *or* Sodium chloride 0.9% *or* Compound sodium lactate

Rasburicase (*Fasturtec®*)

Intermittent *in* Sodium chloride 0.9%

Reconstitute with solvent provided; gently swirl vial without shaking to dissolve; dilute requisite dose to 50 mL with infusion fluid and give over 30 minutes

Remifentanil (*Ultiva®*)

Intermittent *or via* drip tubing *in* Glucose 5% *or* Sodium chloride 0.9% *or* Water for injections

Reconstitute with infusion fluid to a concentration of 1 mg/mL then dilute further to a concentration of 20–250 micrograms/mL (50 micrograms/mL recommended for general anaesthesia)

Rifampicin (*Rifadin®, Rimactane®*)

Intermittent *in* Glucose 5 and 10% *or* Sodium chloride 0.9% *or* Ringer's solution

Reconstitute with solvent provided then dilute with 250 mL (*Rimactane®*) or 500 mL (*Rifadin®*) infusion fluid; give over 2–3 hours

Ritodrine hydrochloride (*Yutopar®*)

Continuous *in* Glucose 5%

Give *via* controlled infusion device, preferably a syringe pump; if syringe pump available dilute to a concentration of 3 mg/mL; if syringe pump not available dilute to a concentration of 300 micrograms/mL; close attention to patient's fluid and electrolyte status essential

Rituximab (*MabThera®*)

Intermittent *in* Glucose 5% *or* Sodium chloride 0.9%

Dilute to 1–4 mg/mL and gently invert bag to avoid foaming

Rocuronium bromide (*Esmeron®*)

Continuous *or via* drip tubing *in* Glucose 5% *or* Sodium chloride 0.9%

Salbutamol (as sulphate) (*Ventolin® For Intravenous Infusion*)

Continuous *in* Glucose 5%

For *bronchodilatation* dilute 5 mg with 500 mL glucose 5% or sodium chloride 0.9%; for *premature labour* dilute with glucose 5% to a concentration of 200 micrograms/mL for use in a syringe pump *or* for other infusion methods (preferably *via* controlled infusion device), dilute to a concentration of 20 micrograms/mL; close attention to patient's fluid and electrolyte status essential

Sodium calcium edetate (*Ledclair®*)

Continuous *in* Glucose 5% *or* Sodium chloride 0.9%

Dilute to a concentration of not more than 3%; suggested volume 250–500 mL given over at least 1 hour

Sodium clodronate (*Bonefos® Concentrate, Loron®*)

Continuous *in* Sodium chloride 0.9%

Dilute 300 mg in 500 mL and give over at least 2 hours or 1.5 g in 500 mL and give over at least 4 hours; *Bonefos® Concentrate* can also be diluted in Glucose 5%

Sodium nitroprusside (*Faulding DBL*)

Continuous *in* Glucose 5%

Reconstitute 50 mg with 2–3 mL glucose 5% then dilute immediately with 250–1000 mL infusion fluid; preferably infuse *via* infusion device to allow precise control; protect infusion from light

Sodium valproate (*Epilim®*)

Continuous *or* intermittent *in* Glucose 5% *or* Sodium chloride 0.9%

Reconstitute with solvent provided then dilute with infusion fluid

Sotalol hydrochloride (*Sotacor®*)

Continuous *or* intermittent *in* Glucose 5% *or* Sodium chloride 0.9%

Dilute to a concentration of between 0.01–2 mg/mL

Streptokinase (*Kabikinase®*; *Streptase®*; *Streptokinase*, Braun)

Continuous *or* intermittent *in* Glucose 5% *or* Sodium chloride 0.9%

Reconstitute *Kabikinase®* with water for injections, *Streptase®* with sodium chloride 0.9%, and *Streptokinase* (Braun) with either water for injections or sodium chloride 0.9% then dilute further with infusion fluid

Sulfadiazine sodium

Continuous *in* Sodium chloride 0.9%

Suggested volume 500 mL; ampoule solution has a pH of over 10

Suxamethonium chloride (*Anectine®*)

Continuous *in* Glucose 5% *or* Sodium chloride 0.9%

Tacrolimus (*Prograf®*)

Continuous *in* Glucose 5% *or* Sodium chloride 0.9%

Dilute concentrate in infusion fluid to a final concentration of 4–100 micrograms/mL; give over 24 hours; incompatible with PVC

Teicoplanin (*Targocid®*)

Intermittent *in* Glucose 5% *or* Sodium chloride 0.9% *or* Compound sodium lactate

Reconstitute initially with water for injections provided; infuse over 30 minutes

Continuous infusion not usually recommended

Terbutaline sulphate (*Bricanyl®*)

Continuous *in* Glucose 5%

For *bronchodilatation* dilute 1.5–2.5 mg with 500 mL glucose 5% or sodium chloride 0.9% and give over 8–10 hours; for *premature labour* dilute in glucose 5% and give *via* controlled infusion device preferably a syringe pump; if syringe pump available dilute to a concentration of 100 micrograms/mL; if syringe pump not available dilute to a concentration of 10 micrograms/mL; close attention to patient's fluid and electrolyte status essential

Ticarcillin sodium with clavulanic acid (*Timentin®*)

Intermittent *in* Glucose 5% *or* Water for injections

Suggested volume glucose 5%, 50–150 mL (depending on dose) or water for injections, 25–100 mL; given over 30–40 minutes

Tirofiban (*Aggrastat®*)

Continuous *in* Glucose 5% *or* Sodium chloride 0.9%

Withdraw 50 mL infusion fluid from 250-mL bag and replace with 50 mL tirofiban concentrate (250 micrograms/mL) to give a final concentration of 50 micrograms/mL

Tobramycin (as sulphate) (*Nebcin®*)

Intermittent *or via* drip tubing *in* Glucose 5% *or* Sodium chloride 0.9%

For adult intermittent infusion suggested volume 50–100 mL (children proportionately smaller volume) given over 20–60 minutes

Topotecan (as hydrochloride) (*Hycamtin®*)

Intermittent *in* Glucose 5% *or* Sodium chloride 0.9%

Reconstitute 4 mg with 4 mL water for injections then dilute to a final concentration of 25–50 micrograms/mL; give over 30 minutes

Tramadol hydrochloride (*Zydol®*)

Continuous *or* intermittent *in* Glucose 5% *or* Sodium chloride 0.9% *or* Ringer's solution *or* Compound sodium lactate

Tranexamic acid (*Cyklokapron®*)

Continuous *in* Glucose 5% *or* Sodium chloride 0.9% *or* Ringer's solution

Trastuzumab (*Herceptin®*)

Intermittent *in* Sodium chloride 0.9%

Reconstitute each 150-mg vial with 7.2 mL water for injections to produce a 21 mg/mL solution, swirl vial gently to avoid excessive foaming and allow to stand for approximately 5 minutes; dilute requisite dose in 250 mL infusion fluid

Treosulfan (*Treosulfan*) (Medac)

Intermittent *in* Water for injections

Infusion suggested for doses above 5 g; dilute to a concentration of 5 g in 100 mL

Trimetaphan camsilate (Cambridge)

Intermittent *in* Sodium chloride 0.9% *or* Sodium chloride and glucose

Dilute to a concentration of 0.05–0.1% (0.25% if fluid restriction necessary)

Trimethoprim (as lactate) (*Monotrim®*)

via drip tubing *in* Glucose 5% *or* Sodium chloride 0.9% *or* Compound sodium lactate *or* Ringer's solution

Trimetrexate (*Neutrexin®*)

Intermittent *in* Glucose 5%

Reconstitute each 25 mg with 2 mL glucose 5% or water for injections; dilute further with infusion fluid to a concentration of 0.25–2 mg/mL; infuse over 60–90 minutes; incompatible with solutions containing sodium chloride or other electrolytes, flush intravenous line with glucose 5%

Trisodium edetate (*Limclair®*)

Continuous *in* Glucose 5% *or* Sodium chloride 0.9%

Dilute to a concentration of 10 mg/mL; give over 2–3 hours

Tropisetron (as hydrochloride) (*Navoban®*)

Intermittent *or via* drip tubing *in* Glucose 5% *or* Sodium chloride 0.9% *or* Ringer's solution

Suggested concentration for infusion 50 micrograms/mL

Vancomycin (as hydrochloride) (*Vancocin®*)

Intermittent *in* Glucose 5% *or* Sodium chloride 0.9%

Reconstitute each 500 mg with 10 mL water for injections and dilute with infusion fluid to a concentration of up to 5 mg/mL (10 mg/mL in fluid restriction but increased risk of infusion-related effects); give over at least 60 minutes (rate not to exceed 10 mg/minute for doses over 500 mg); use continuous infusion only if intermittent not feasible

Vasopressin, synthetic (*Pitressin®*)

Intermittent *in* Glucose 5%

Suggested concentration 20 units/100 mL given over 15 minutes

Vecuronium bromide (*Norcuron®*)

Continuous *in* Glucose 5% *or* Sodium chloride 0.9% *or* Ringer's solution

Reconstitute with the solvent provided

Verteporfin (*Visudyne®*)

Intermittent *in* Glucose 5%

Reconstitute each 15 mg with 7 mL water for injections to produce a 2 mg/mL solution then dilute requisite dose with infusion fluid to a final volume of 30 mL and give over 10 minutes; protect from light and administer within 4 hours of reconstitution. Incompatible with sodium chloride infusion

Vinblastine sulphate (*Velbe®*)

via drip tubing *in* Sodium chloride 0.9%

Reconstitute with sodium chloride 0.9%; give over approx. 1 minute

Vincristine sulphate (*Oncovin®*)

via drip tubing *in* Glucose 5% *or* Sodium chloride 0.9%

Vindesine sulphate (*Eldisine®*)

via drip tubing *in* Glucose 5% *or* Sodium chloride 0.9%

Reconstitute with sodium chloride 0.9%; give over 1–3 minutes

Vinorelbine (*Navelbine®*)

Intermittent *in* Glucose 5% *or* Sodium chloride 0.9%

Dilute in 125 mL infusion fluid; give over 20–30 minutes

Vitamins B & C (*Pabrinex® I/V High potency*)

Intermittent *or via* drip tubing *in* Glucose 5% *or* Sodium chloride 0.9%

Ampoule contents should be mixed, diluted, and administered without delay; give over 10 minutes (see CSM advice, section 9.6.2)

Vitamins, multiple

(*Cernevit®*)

Intermittent *in* Glucose 5% *or* Sodium chloride 0.9%

Dissolve initially in 5 mL water for injections (or infusion fluid)

(*Multibionta®*)

Intermittent *in* Glucose 5% *or* Sodium chloride 0.9%

Dilute 10 mL in not less than 250 mL of infusion fluid (adults); see also section 9.3

(*Solivito N®*)

Intermittent *in* Glucose 5 and 10%

Suggested volume 500–1000 mL given over 2–3 hours; see also section 9.3

Zidovudine (*Retrovir®*)

Intermittent *in* Glucose 5%

Dilute to a concentration of 2 mg/mL or 4 mg/mL and give over 1 hour

Zoledronic acid (*Zometa®*)

Intermittent *in* Glucose 5% *or* Sodium chloride 0.9%

Reconstitute 4-mg vial with 5 mL water for injections, then dilute with 50 mL infusion fluid; infuse over 15 minutes

Appendix 7: Borderline substances

In certain conditions some foods (and toilet preparations) have characteristics of drugs and the Advisory Committee on Borderline Substances advises as to the circumstances in which such substances may be regarded as drugs. Prescriptions issued in accordance with the Committee's advice and endorsed 'ACBS' will normally not be investigated.

> General Practitioners are reminded that the ACBS recommends products on the basis that they may be regarded as drugs for the management of specified conditions. Doctors should satisfy themselves that the products can safely be prescribed, that patients are adequately monitored and that, where necessary, expert hospital supervision is available.

Foods which may be prescribed on FP10 (GP10 in Scotland)

Note. This is a list of food products which the ACBS has approved. The clinical condition for which the product has approval follows each entry.

Foods included in this Appendix may contain cariogenic sugars and patients should be advised to take appropriate oral hygiene measures.

Aglutella® (Ultrapharm)
Rice, low protein. Net price 500 g = £3.95. For inherited metabolic disorders, renal or liver failure requiring a low-protein diet
Alcoholic Beverages *see under* Rectified Spirit
Alembicol D® (Alembic Products)
Fractionated coconut oil. Net price 5 kg = £125.55. For steatorrhoea associated with cystic fibrosis of the pancreas, intestinal lymphangiectasia, surgery of the intestine, chronic liver disease, liver cirrhosis, other proven malabsorption syndromes; in a ketogenic diet in the management of epilepsy; type 1 hyperlipoproteinaemia
Aminex® (Gluten Free Foods Ltd)
Low-protein. Biscuits, net price 200 g = £3.75. Cookies, 150 g = £3.75. Rusks, 200 g = £3.75. For inherited metabolic disorders, renal or liver failure requiring a low-protein diet
Amino Acid Modules (SHS)
XLEU Faladon, powder, essential and non-essential amino acids 93%, except leucine. Net price 200 g = £49.59. For isovaleric acidaemia
XMET Homidon, powder, essential and non-essential amino acids 93%, except methionine. Net price 200 g = £49.59. For homocystinuria or hypermethioninaemia
XMTVI Asadon, powder, essential and non-essential amino acids 93%, except methionine, threonine, and valine, with trace amounts of isoleucine. Net price 200 g = £49.59. For methylmalonic acidaemia or propionic acidaemia
XPTM Tyrosidon, powder, essential and non-essential amino acids 93%, except methionine, phenylalanine, and tyrosine. Net price 200 g = £49.59. For tyrosinaemia type I where plasma concentrations are above normal
XPHEN TYR Tyrosidon, powder, essential and non-essential amino acids 93%, except phenylalanine and tyrosine. Net price 200 g = £52.07. For tyrosinaemia where plasma methionine concentrations are normal

Aminogran® (UCB Pharma)
Food Supplement, powder, containing all essential amino acids except phenylalanine, for use with mineral mixture (see below), net price 500 g = £42.77. Tablet (≡ 1 g powder), net price 60-tab pack = £9.00. For the dietary management of phenylketonuria. Tablets not to be prescribed for any child under 8 years
Mineral Mixture, powder, containing all appropriate minerals for use with the above food supplement and other synthetic diets. Net price 250 g = £7.24. For phenylketonuria and as a mineral supplement in synthetic diets
Analog® (SHS)
Note. Analog products are generally intended for use in children up to 1 year, see also Flavour Sachets, for use with unflavoured amino acid and peptide products from SHS
MSUD Analog, powder, essential and non-essential amino acids 15.5% except isoleucine, leucine and valine, with carbohydrate, fat, vitamins, minerals, and trace elements. Net price 400 g = £24.00. For maple syrup urine disease
XLeu Analog, powder, essential and non-essential amino acids 15.5% except leucine, with carbohydrate, fat, vitamins, minerals, and trace elements. Net price 400 g = £24.00. For isovaleric acidaemia
Ingredients: include arachis oil (peanut oil)
XLys Analog, powder, essential and non-essential amino acids 15.5% except lysine, with carbohydrate, fat, vitamins, minerals, and trace elements. Net price 400 g = £24.00. For hyperlysinaemia
XLys, Try Low Analog, powder, essential and non-essential amino acids 15.5% except lysine, and low tryptophan, with carbohydrate, fat, vitamins, minerals, and trace elements. Net price 400 g = £24.00. For type 1 glutaric aciduria
XMet Analog, powder, essential and non-essential amino acids 15.5% except methionine, with carbohydrate, fat, vitamins, minerals, and trace elements. Net price 400 g = £24.00. For hypermethioninaemia; homocystinuria
XMTVI Analog, powder, essential and non-essential amino acids 15.5% except methionine, threonine, valine and low isoleucine, with carbohydrate, fat, vitamins, minerals, and trace elements. Net price 400 g = £24.00. For methylmalonic acidaemia or propionic acidaemia
XP Analog, powder, essential and non-essential amino acids 15.5% except phenylalanine, with carbohydrate, fat, vitamins, minerals, and trace elements. Net price 400 g = £18.45. For phenylketonuria
XP LCP Analog, powder, essential and non-essential amino acids except phenylalanine 15.5%, with carbohydrate, fat, vitamins, minerals and trace elements. Gluten- and lactose-free. Net price 400 g = £20.99. For phenylketonuria in infants and children under 2 years of age
XPhen, Tyr Analog, powder, essential and non-essential amino acids 15.5% except phenylalanine and tyrosine, with carbohydrate, fat, vitamins, minerals and trace elements. Net price 400 g = £24.00. For tyrosinaemia
XPTM Analog, powder, essential and non-essential amino acids 15.5% except phenylalanine, tyrosine and methionine, with carbohydrate, fat, vitamins, minerals and trace elements. Net price 400 g = £24.00. For tyrosinaemia
Aproten® (Ultrapharm)
Gluten-free. Flour. Net price 300 g = £1.84. For gluten-sensitive enteropathies including steatorrhoea due to gluten sensitivity, coeliac disease, and dermatitis herpetiformis
Low protein. Low Na⁺ and K⁺. Net prices: biscuits 180 g (36) = £2.80; bread mix 250 g = £2.00; cake mix 300 g = £2.10; crispbread 260 g = £3.95; pasta (anellini, ditalini, rigatini, spaghetti) 500 g = £3.95; tagliatelle 250 g =

£2.10. For inherited metabolic disorders, renal or liver failure requiring a low-protein diet

L-Arginine (SHS)

Powder, net price 100 g = £7.44. For use as a supplement in urea cycle disorders other than arginase deficiency, such as hyperammonaemia types I and II, citrullaemia, arginosuccinic aciduria, and deficiency of N-acetyl glutamate synthetase

Arnott® (Ultrapharm)

Rice Cookies, gluten-free. Net price 200 g = £1.68. For gluten-sensitive enteropathies including steatorrhoea due to gluten sensitivity, coeliac disease, and dermatitis herpetiformis

Barkat® (Gluten Free Foods Ltd)

Gluten-free. Bread mix, net price 500 g = £4.12. Rice bread (sliced), brown or white, 450 g = £2.79. Rice pizza crust, brown or white, 150 g = £2.21. For gluten-sensitive enteropathies including steatorrhoea due to gluten sensitivity, coeliac disease, and dermatitis herpetiformis

Bi-Aglut® (Novartis Consumer Health)

Gluten-free. Biscuits, net price 180 g = £2.60. Crackers, 150 g = £2.15. Cracker toast, 240 g = £3.60. Pastas (fusilli, macaroni, penne, spaghetti), 500 g = £4.86; Lasagne, 250 g = £2.56. For gluten-sensitive enteropathies including steatorrhoea due to gluten sensitivity, coeliac diseases, and dermatitis herpetiformis

Calogen® (SHS)

Emulsion, arachis oil (peanut oil) 50% in water, net price, 250 mL = £3.85 (natural flavour), £4.05 (strawberry flavour); 1 litre = £15.51 (natural flavour), £15.85 (butterscotch flavour). For disease-related malnutrition, malabsorption states or other conditions requiring fortification with a high-fat supplement with or without fluid and electrolyte restrictions

Caloreen® (Nestlé Clinical)

Powder, water-soluble dextrins, 390 kcal/100 g, with less than 1.8 mmol of Na⁺ and 0.3 mmol of K⁺/100 g. Gluten-, lactose-, and fructose-free. Net price 500 g = £3.02. For disease-related malnutrition, malabsorption states or other conditions requiring fortification with a high or readily available carbohydrate supplement

Calshake® (Fresenius Kabi)

Powder, protein 4 g, carbohydrate 58 g, fat 20.4 g, energy 1809 kJ (432 kcal)/87 g. Gluten-free. Strawberry, vanilla and banana flavours, net price 87-g sachet = £1.77; also available chocolate flavour (protein 4 g, carbohydrate 58 g, fat 20.4 g, fibre 1.6 g, energy 1809 kJ (432 kcal)/90 g = £1.77. For disease-related malnutrition, malabsorption states or other conditions requiring fortification with a fat/carbohydrate supplement

Calsip® (Fresenius Kabi)

Liquid, maltodextrin 50%. Flavours: apple, pineapple, neutral. Net price 200-mL carton = 93 p. For disease-related malnutrition, malabsorption states or other conditions requiring fortification with a high or readily available carbohydrate supplement

Caprilon® (SHS)

Powder, protein 11.8%, carbohydrate 55.1%, fat 28.3% (medium chain triglycerides 21.9%). Low in lactose, gluten- and sucrose-free. Used as a 12.7% solution. Net price 420 g = £11.46. For disorders in which a high intake of MCT is beneficial

Carobel, Instant® (Cow & Gate)

Powder, carob seed flour. Net price 45 g = £2.63. For thickening feeds in the treatment of vomiting

Casilan 90® (Heinz)

Powder, whole protein, containing all essential amino acids, 90% with less than 0.1% Na⁺. Net price 250 g = £5.13. For biochemically proven hypoproteinaemia

Clara's Kitchen® (Gluten Free Foods Ltd)

Gluten-free. Bread mix, net price 500 g = £3.53; hi-fibre bread mix, 500 g = £3.53. For gluten-sensitive enteropathies including steatorrhoea due to gluten-sensitivity, coeliac disease and dermatitis herpetiformis.

Clinutren® (Nestlé Clinical)

Clinutren Dessert, protein 12 g, carbohydrate 19 g, fat 3.3 g, energy 650 kJ (160 kcal)/125 g with vitamins and minerals. Gluten-free. Flavours: caramel, chocolate, peach or vanilla, net price 4 × 125-g pot = £4.20. For use

as a nutritional supplement prescribed on medical grounds for: short bowel syndrome, intractable malabsorption, pre-operative preparation of undernourished patients, proven inflammatory bowel disease, following total gastrectomy, dysphagia, bowel fistulas, disease-related malnutrition, continuous ambulatory peritoneal dialysis (CAPD), haemodialysis. Not to be prescribed for any child under 1 year; use with caution for children under 5 years

Clinutren Fruit, protein 8 g, carbohydrate 54 g, fat less than 0.4 g, energy 1040 kJ (250 kcal)/200 mL with vitamins and minerals. Gluten-free. Low-lactose. Flavours: grapefruit, orange, pear-cherry, or raspberry-blackcurrant, net price 4 × 200-mL cup = £6.00. For use as a nutritional supplement prescribed on medical grounds for: short-bowel syndrome, intractable malabsorption, pre-operative preparation of undernourished patients, proven inflammatory bowel disease, following total gastrectomy, dysphagia, bowel fistulas, disease-related malnutrition. Not to be prescribed for any child under 1 year; use with caution for children up to 5 years

Clinutren ISO, protein 7.6 g, carbohydrate 28 g, fat 6.6 g, energy 840 kJ (200 kcal)/200 mL with vitamins and minerals. Gluten-free. Flavours: chocolate, coffee, strawberry-raspberry or vanilla, net price 4 × 200-mL pot = £4.72. For indications see *Clinutren Fruit*

Clinutren 1.5, protein 11 g, carbohydrate 42 g, fat 10 g, energy 1260 kJ (300 kcal)/200 mL with vitamins and minerals. Gluten-free; clinically lactose-free. Flavours: apricot, banana, chocolate, coffee, strawberry-raspberry or vanilla, net price 4 × 200-mL pot = £5.60. For indications see *Clinutren Fruit*

Clinutren Thickener, powder, modified maize starch, gluten-free, net price 300 g = £4.53. Thickening of foods and fluids in dysphagia. Not to be used for children under 3 years

Clinutren Thickened Drinks, liquid, modified maize starch, gluten-free. Flavours: orange, peppermint, and tea, net price 4 × 125 g = £1.96. Thickening of foods and fluids in dysphagia. Not to be used for children under 3 years

Comminuted Chicken Meat (SHS)

Suspension (aqueous). Net price 150 g = £2.32. For carbohydrate intolerance in association with possible or proven intolerance of milk; glucose and galactose intolerance

Complan® Ready to Drink (Heinz)

Liquid, protein 8.7 g, carbohydrate 35 g, fat 8.3 g, energy 1050 kJ (250 kcal)/230 mL, with vitamins and minerals. Gluten-free. Flavours: chocolate, strawberry, vanilla, net price 230-mL carton = £1.00. For use as a sole source of nutrition or as a nutritional supplement prescribed on medical grounds for: short-bowel syndrome, intractable malabsorption, pre-operative preparation of undernourished patients, proven inflammatory bowel disease, following total gastrectomy, dysphagia, bowel fistulas, disease-related malnutrition. Not to be prescribed for any child under 1 year; use with caution for children under 5 years

Corn flour and corn starch For hypoglycaemia associated with glycogen-storage disease

Dextrose *see* Glucose

Dialamine® (SHS)

Powder, essential amino acids 30%, with carbohydrate 62%, energy 1500 kJ (360 kcal)/100 g, with ascorbic acid, minerals, and trace elements. Flavour: orange. Net price 200 g = £23.31. For oral feeding where essential amino acid supplements are required; e.g. chronic renal failure, hypoproteinaemia, wound fistula leakage with excessive protein loss, conditions requiring a controlled nitrogen intake, and haemodialysis

Dietary Specialities (Nutrition Point)

Gluten-free. Bread mix (brown or white), net price 500 g = £4.75; corn bread mix, 500 g = £4.50; cake mix (white), 750 g = £4.75; white or fibre mix, 500 g = £4.75. For gluten-sensitive enteropathies, coeliac disease, and dermatitis herpetiformis

Duobar® (SHS)

Bar, protein-free (phenylalanine nil added), carbohydrate 49.9 g, fat 49.9 g, energy 2692 kJ (648 kcal)/100 g. Low sodium and potassium. Strawberry, toffee, or natural flavours. Net price 45-g bar = £1.16. For disease-related malnutrition, malabsorption states or other conditions requiring fortification with fat/carbohydrate supplement

Duocal® (SHS)

Liquid, emulsion providing carbohydrate 23.4 g, fat 7.1 g, energy 661 kJ (158 kcal)/100 mL. Low-electrolyte, gluten-, lactose-, and protein-free. Net price 250 mL = £2.55; 1 litre = £9.08

MCT Powder, carbohydrate 74 g, fat 23.2 g (of which MCT 83%), energy 2042 kJ (486 kcal)/100 g. Low electrolyte, gluten-, protein- and lactose-free. Net price 400 g = £14.32

Super Soluble Powder, carbohydrate 72.7 g, fat 22.3 g, energy 2061 kJ (492 kcal)/100 g. Low electrolyte, gluten-, protein-, and lactose-free. Net price 400 g = £11.48

All for disease-related malnutrition, malabsorption states or other conditions requiring fortification with fat/carbohydrate supplement

Elemental 028® (SHS)

Note. see also Flavour Sachets, for use with unflavoured amino acid and peptide products from SHS

028 Powder, amino acids 12%, carbohydrate 70.5–72%, fat 6.64%, energy 1544–1568 kJ (364–370 kcal)/100 g with vitamins and minerals. For preparation with water before use. Net price 100-g box (orange flavoured or plain) = £3.82

028 Extra powder, amino acids 15%, carbohydrate 59%, fat 17.45%, energy 1860 kJ(443 kcal)/100 g, with vitamins, minerals, and trace elements. For preparation with water before use. Net price 100 g (plain) = £4.44; also available orange-flavoured (carbohydrate 55%, energy 1793 kJ (427 kcal)/100 g), 100 g = £4.55

028 Extra liquid, amino acids 7.5 g, carbohydrate 27.5 g, fat 8.7 g, energy 896 kJ (215 kcal)/250 mL, with vitamins, minerals, and trace elements. Flavours: grapefruit, orange and pineapple, summer fruits. Net price 250-mL carton = £2.37

All for use as the sole source of nutrition or as a nutritional supplement prescribed on medical grounds for: short-bowel syndrome, intractable malabsorption, proven inflammatory bowel disease, bowel fistulas. Not to be prescribed for any child under 1 year; use with caution for children up to 5 years

Emsogen® (SHS)

Powder, amino acids 15%, carbohydrate 60%, fat 16.4%, energy 1839 kJ (438 kcal)/100 g, with vitamins, minerals, and trace elements. For preparation with water before use. Net price 100 g = £4.68; also available orange-flavoured (carbohydrate 55%, energy 1754 kJ (418 kcal)/100 g), 100 g = £4.68. For use as the sole source of nutrition or as a nutritional supplement prescribed on medical grounds for short-bowel syndrome, intractable malabsorption, proven inflammatory bowel disease, bowel fistulas. Not to be prescribed for any child under 1 year; use with caution for children up to 5 years

Ener-G® (General Dietary)

Gluten-free. Cookies (vanilla flavour), net price 435 g = £3.98. Rice bread (sliced), brown, 474 g = £4.28; white, 456 g = £4.28. Rice loaf, 612 g = £4.28. Tapioca bread (sliced), 480 g = £4.28. Rice pasta (macaroni, shells, small shells, and lasagne), 454 g = £3.98; spaghetti, 447 g = £3.98; tagliatelle, 400 g = £3.98; vermicelli, 300 g = £3.98; cannelloni, 284 g = £3.98. Brown rice pasta: lasagne, 454 g = £3.98; macaroni, 454 g = £3.98; spaghetti, 447 g = £3.98. For gluten-sensitive enteropathies including steatorrhoea due to gluten sensitivity, coeliac disease, and dermatitis herpetiformis

Low protein egg replacer, carbohydrate 94 g, energy 1574 kJ (376 kcal)/100 g. Egg-, gluten- and lactose-free, net price 454 g = £3.38. For phenylketonuria, similar amino acid abnormalities, renal failure, liver failure and liver cirrhosis

Low protein rice bread, net price 600 g = £4.39. For inherited metabolic disorders, renal or liver failure requiring a low-protein diet

Energivit® (SHS)

Powder, protein-free, carbohydrate 66.7 g, fat 25 g, energy 2059 kJ (492 kcal)/100 g with vitamins, minerals and trace elements, net price 400 g = £14.66. For infants requiring additional energy, vitamins, minerals and trace elements following a protein restricted diet

Enfamil® (Mead Johnson)

AR (Anti-Reflux), powder, protein 13 g, fat 26 g, carbohydrate 56 g, energy 2124 kJ (508 kcal)/100 g with vitamins, minerals and trace elements, net price 400 g = £2.55. For significant reflux disease. For use not in excess of a 6-month period. Not to be used in conjunction with any other thickener or antacid product.

Lactofree, powder, protein 11.9 g, fat 28 g, carbohydrate 56 g, energy 2176 kJ (520 kcal)/100g with vitamins, minerals and trace elements. Lactose- and sucrose-free, net price 400 g = £3.22. For proven lactose intolerance

Enlive® (Abbott)

Liquid, protein 9.6 g, carbohydrate 65.4 g, energy 1274 kJ (300 kcal)/240 mL, with vitamins, minerals and trace elements. Fat- and gluten-free; clinically lactose-free. Flavours: apple, fruit punch, grapefruit, lemon and lime, orange, peach, pineapple, strawberry. Net price 240-mL Tetrapak® = £1.63. For use as a nutritional supplement prescribed on medical grounds for: short-bowel syndrome, intractable malabsorption, pre-operative preparation of patients who are undernourished, proven inflammatory bowel disease, dysphagia, bowel fistulas, disease-related malnutrition. Not to be prescribed for any child under 1 year; use with caution for children up to 5 years

Enrich® (Abbott)

Liquid with dietary fibre, providing protein 9.4 g, carbohydrate 34.9 g, fat 8.8 g, fibre 3.4 g, energy 1079 kJ (256 kcal)/250 mL with vitamins and minerals. Lactose- and gluten-free. Vanilla and chocolate flavours. Net price 250-mL can = £2.20. For use as the sole source of nutrition or as a nutritional supplement prescribed on medical grounds for: short-bowel syndrome, intractable malabsorption, pre-operative preparation of patients who are undernourished, proven inflammatory bowel disease, following total gastrectomy, dysphagia, disease-related malnutrition. Not to be prescribed for any child under 1 year; use with caution for children up to 5 years

Enrich Plus® (Abbott)

Liquid with dietary fibre, providing protein 12.5 g, carbohydrate 43 g, fat 9.84 g, fibre 2.5 g, energy 1285 kJ (305 kcal)/200 mL with vitamins and minerals. Lactose- and gluten-free. Vanilla, chocolate, raspberry and banana flavours. Net price 200-mL tetrapak = £1.71. For use as a nutritional supplement for patients with disease-related malnutrition, continuous ambulatory peritoneal dialysis (CAPD), short-bowel syndrome, intractable malabsorption, dysphagia, proven inflammatory bowel disease, bowel fistulas, gastrectomy , and pre-operative preparation of undernourished patients. Not to be prescribed for any child under 1 year; use with caution for children up to 5 years

Ensure® (Abbott)

Liquid, protein 10.0 g, fat 8.4 g, carbohydrate 33.9 g, energy 1057 kJ (251 kcal)/250 mL with minerals and vitamins, lactose- and gluten-free. Vanilla, chocolate, coffee, eggnog, nut, chicken, mushroom, and asparagus flavours. Net price 250-mL can = £1.87

Powder, same composition as Ensure liquid when reconstituted. Vanilla flavour. Net price 400 g = £11.39

Both for use as the sole source of nutrition or as a nutritional supplement prescribed on medical grounds for: short-bowel syndrome, intractable malabsorption, pre-operative preparation of patients who are undernourished, proven inflammatory bowel disease, following total gastrectomy, dysphagia, bowel fistulas, disease-related malnutrition. Neither to be prescribed for any child under 1 year; use with caution for children up to 5 years

Ensure Plus® (Abbott)

Liquid, protein 12.5 g, fat 10.0 g, carbohydrate 40.0 g, with vitamins and minerals, lactose- and gluten-free, energy 1260 kJ (300 kcal)/200 mL. Vanilla flavour. Net price 250-mL can = £2.03; 500-mL ready-to-hang = £3.81; 1-litre ready-to-hang = £7.63; 1.5-litre ready-to-hang = £11.44. Caramel, chocolate, strawberry, banana, fruit of the forest, raspberry, orange, coffee, black currant, peach, vanilla or neutral flavours. Net price 200-mL Tetrapak® = £1.56. As a nutritional supplement prescribed on medical grounds for: short-bowel syndrome, intractable malabsorption, pre-operative preparation of patients who are undernourished, proven inflammatory bowel disease, following total gastrectomy, dysphagia, bowel fistulas, disease-related malnutrition, continuous ambulatory peritoneal dialysis (CAPD), and haemodialysis. Not to be prescribed for any child under 1 year; use with caution for children up to 5 years

Entera® *see* **Fresubin® Energy**

Farley's Soya Formula (Farley)

Powder, providing protein 2%, carbohydrate 7%, fat 3.8% with vitamins and minerals when reconstituted. Gluten-, sucrose-, and lactose-free. Net price 450 g = £3.79. For proven lactose and associated sucrose intolerance in pre-school children, galactokinase deficiency, galactosaemia, and cow's milk protein intolerance

Fate® (Fate)

Low protein. All-purpose mix, net price 500g = £4.85; Cake mix, 2 x 250g = £4.85; Chocolate flavour cake mix, 2 x 250g = £4.85. For inherited metabolic disorders, renal or liver failure requiring a low-protein diet

Flavour Sachets (SHS)

Powder, flavours: cherry-vanilla, grapefruit, harvest fruits, lemon-lime, net price 20 x 5-g sachets = £7.69. For use with SHS unflavoured amino acid and peptide products

Foodlink Complete (Foodlink)

Powder, protein 21.9 g, carbohydrate 57.3 g, fat 13.3 g, energy 1838 kJ (436.5 kcal)/100 g with vitamins and minerals. Flavours: banana, chocolate, natural or strawberry, net price 450-g carton = £3.75; also available, vanilla flavour with fibre (protein 19.5 g, carbohydrate 60.2 g, fat 12.3 g, fibre 8 g, energy 1804 kJ (428 kcal)/100 g = £3.75. As a nutritional supplement prescribed on medical grounds for: short-bowel syndrome, intractable malabsorption, pre-operative preparation of undernourished patients, proven inflammatory bowel disease, following total gastrectomy, dysphagia, bowel fistulas, disease-related malnutrition. Not to be prescribed for any child under 1 year; use with caution for children up to 5 years

Formance® (Abbott)

Semi-solid, protein 4 g, carbohydrate 27 g, fat 5 g, energy 711 kJ (170 kcal)/113 g with vitamins and minerals. Gluten-free. Vanilla, chocolate, and butterscotch flavours. Net price 113-g pot = £1.37. As a nutritional supplement prescribed on medical grounds for: short-bowel syndrome, intractable malabsorption, pre-operative preparation of patients who are undernourished, proven inflammatory bowel disease, following total gastrectomy, dysphagia, bowel fistulas, disease-related malnutrition, continuous ambulatory peritoneal dialysis (CAPD), and haemodialysis. Not to be prescribed for any child under 1 year; use with caution for children up to 5 years

Forticreme® (Nutricia Clinical)

Semi-solid, protein 10 g, carbohydrate 19 g, fat 5 g, energy 680 kJ (161 kcal)/100 g with vitamins and minerals. Gluten-freee. Vanilla, chocolate, coffee and forest fruit flavours, net price 4 × 125-g pot = £5.60. As a nutritional supplement prescribed on medical grounds for: short-bowel syndrome, intractable malabsorption, pre-operative preparation of patients who are undernourished, proven inflammatory bowel disease, following total gastrectomy, dysphagia, bowel fistulas, disease-related malnutrition, continuous ambulatory peritoneal dialysis (CAPD) and haemodialysis. Not to be prescribed for any child under 3 years; use with caution for children aged 3 to 5 years

Fortifresh® (Nutricia Clinical)

Liquid, protein 12 g, carbohydrate 37.4 g, fat 11.6 g, energy 1260 kJ (300 kcal)/200 mL with vitamins, minerals and trace elements. Gluten-free. Flavours: black currant, peach and orange, and raspberry, net price 200 mL carton = £1.50. For use as a nutritional supplement prescribed on medical grounds for: intractable malabsorption, pre-operative preparation of patients who are undernourished, inflammatory bowel disease, dysphagia, disease-related malnutrition. Not to be prescribed for any child under 3 years; use with caution for children aged 3 to 5 years

Fortijuce® (Nutricia Clinical)

Liquid, protein 8 g, carbohydrate 67 g, energy 1270 kJ (300 kcal)/200 mL, with vitamins, minerals and trace elements. Fat-free. Flavours: apricot, blackcurrant, lemon and lime, peach and orange, pineapple, apple and pear, forest fruits. Net price 200-mL carton = £1.50. As a nutritional supplement prescribed on medical grounds for: short-bowel syndrome, intractable malabsorption, pre-operative preparation of patients who are undernourished, proven inflammatory bowel disease, following total gastrectomy, dysphagia, bowel fistulas, disease-related malnutrition. Not to be prescribed for any child under 3 years; use with caution for children up to 5 years

Fortimel® (Nutricia Clinical)

Liquid, protein 20 g, carbohydrate 20.8 g, fat 4.2 g, energy 840 kJ (200 kcal)/200 mL with vitamins and minerals. Gluten-free. Vanilla, strawberry, and forest fruits flavours. Net price 200-mL carton = £1.26. As a nutritional supplement prescribed on medical grounds for: short-bowel syndrome, intractable malabsorption, pre-operative preparation of patients who are undernourished, proven inflammatory bowel disease, following total gastrectomy, dysphagia, bowel fistulas, disease-related malnutrition. Not to be prescribed for any child under 3 years; use with caution for children up to 5 years

Fortini® (Nutricia Clinical)

Liquid, protein 3.4 g, carbohydrate 18.8 g, fat 6.8 g, energy 630 kJ (150 kcal)/100 mL with vitamins, minerals and trace elements. Gluten- and lactose-free. Flavours: strawberry or vanilla, net price 200-mL tetrapak® = £2.24. For use as a nutritional supplement prescribed on medical grounds for: disease-related malnutrition and growth failure. Not to be prescribed for any child under 1 year

Fortini® Multifibre (Nutricia Clinical)

Liquid, protein 3.4 g, carbohydrate 18.8 g, fat 6.8 g, fibre 1.5 g, energy 630 kJ (150 kcal)/100 mL with vitamins, minerals and trace elements. Gluten- and lactose-free. Flavours: banana, chocolate, strawberry, and vanilla, net price 200-mL tetrapak® = £2.35. For indications see Fortini liquid

Fortisip® (Nutricia Clinical)

Liquid, protein 12 g, carbohydrate 36.8 g, fat 11.6 g, energy 1260 kJ (300 kcal)/200 mL, with vitamins, minerals and trace elements. Gluten-free; clinically lactose-free. Vanilla, banana, chocolate, orange, strawberry, tropical fruits, toffee, and neutral flavours; also available chicken and mushroom flavours (protein 10 g, carbohydrate 36 g, fat 13 g, energy 1260 kJ (300 kcal)/200 mL, with vitamins, minerals and trace elements), net price 200 mL = £1.50. As a nutritional supplement prescribed on medical grounds for: short-bowel syndrome, intractable malabsorption, pre-operative preparation of patients who are undernourished, proven inflammatory bowel disease, following total gastrectomy, dysphagia, bowel fistulas, disease-related malnutrition. Not to be prescribed for any child under 3 years; use with caution for children aged 3 to 5 years

Fortisip® Multi Fibre (Nutricia Clinical)

Liquid, protein 12 g, carbohydrate 36.8 g, fat 11.6 g, fibre 4.5 g, energy 1260 kJ (300 kcal)/200 mL, with vitamins, minerals and trace elements. Gluten-free, clinically lactose-free. Banana, orange, strawberry, vanilla flavours; also available chocolate flavour (protein 10 g, carbohydrate 36 g, fat 13 g, fibre 4.5 g, energy 1260 kJ (300 kcal)/200 mL, net price 200 mL = £1.55. As a nutritional supplement prescribed on medical grounds for:

short-bowel syndrome, intractable malabsorption, pre-operative preparation of undernourished patients, proven inflammatory bowel disease, following total gastrectomy, dysphagia, disease-related malnutrition. Not to be prescribed for any child under 3 years; use with caution for children aged 3 to 5 years

Frebini® (Fresenius Kabi)

Liquid, protein 12.5 g, carbohydrate 67.5 g, fat 20 g, energy 2100 kJ (500 kcal)/500 mL, with vitamins, minerals and trace elements. Flavour: neutral, net price 200-mL bottle = £1.89. For use as the sole source of nutrition or as a nutritional supplement prescribed on medical grounds for short-bowel syndrome, intractable malabsorption, pre-operative preparation of patients who are undernourished, proven inflammatory bowel disease, following total gastrectomy, dysphagia, bowel fistulas, disease-related malnutrition and/or growth failure. Not to be prescribed for any child under 1 year

Fresubin® (Fresenius Kabi)

Energy, liquid, protein 11.3 g, carbohydrate 37.6 g, fat 11.66 g, energy 1260 kJ (300 kcal)/200 mL, with vitamins and minerals. Net price 200-mL carton = £1.50 (flavours: vanilla, strawberry, butterscotch, blackcurrant, banana, orange, pineapple, chocolate-mint, vegetable cream, and neutral); 500-mL bottle = £3.69 (flavour: neutral); 500-mL EasyBag® = £3.77; 1-litre EasyBag® = £7.48. For use as sole source of nutrition or as a nutritional supplement prescribed on medical grounds for: short-bowel syndrome, intractable malabsorption, pre-operative preparation of undernourished patients, proven inflammatory bowel disease, following total gastrectomy, dysphagia, bowel fistulas, disease-related malnutrition. Not to be prescribed for any child under 1 year; use with caution for children under 5 years

Energy Fibre, sip feed, protein 11.3 g, carbohydrate 37.6 g, fat 11.6 g, fibre 5 g, energy 1260 kJ (300 kcal)/ 200 mL, with vitamins, minerals and trace elements. Gluten-free; clinically lactose-free. Flavours: banana, cappucino, chocolate, lemon, strawberry, vanilla. Net price 200-mL carton = £1.65. For indications see *Fresubin®* Energy

Energy Fibre, tube feed, protein 28 g, carbohydrate 94 g, fat 29 g, fibre 10 g, energy 3150 kJ (750 kcal)/500 mL, with vitamins, minerals and trace elements. Gluten-free; clinically lactose-free. Unflavoured, net price 500-mL EasyBag® = £3.88; 1-litre EasyBag® = £7.76. For indications see *Fresubin®* Energy

Liquid, protein 7.6 g, carbohydrate 27.6 g, fat 6.8 g, energy 840 kJ (200 kcal)/200 mL with vitamins and minerals. Gluten-free, low lactose and cholesterol. Net price 200-mL carton (nut, peach, black currant, chocolate, mocha, and vanilla flavours) = £1.43; 500-mL bottle (neutral flavour) = £2.85; 500-mL EasyBag® = £2.90; 1-litre EasyBag® = £5.80. For use as the sole source of nutrition or as a nutritional supplement prescribed on medical grounds for: short-bowel syndrome, intractable malabsorption, pre-operative preparation of patients who are undernourished, proven inflammatory bowel disease, following total gastrectomy, dysphagia, bowel fistulas, disease-related malnutrition, and Refsum's disease. Not to be prescribed for any child under 1 year; use with caution for children up to 5 years

Fresubin HP Energy® (Fresenius Kabi)

Liquid, protein 37.5 g, carbohydrate 85 g, fat 30 g, energy 3150 kJ (750 kcal)/500 mL with vitamins, minerals, and trace elements. Gluten-free and low lactose. Vanilla flavour. Net price 500-mL bottle = £3.67; 500-mL EasyBag® = £3.72; 1-litre EasyBag® = £7.44. As a nutritional supplement prescribed on medical grounds for: short-bowel syndrome, intractable malabsorption, pre-operative preparation of patients who are undernourished, proven inflammatory bowel disease, following total gastrectomy, dysphagia, bowel fistulas, disease-related malnutrition, continuous ambulatory peritoneal dialysis (CAPD), and haemodialysis. Not to be prescribed for any child under 1 year; use with caution for children up to 5 years

Fresubin® 1000 (Fresenius Kabi)

Liquid, tube feed, protein 5.5 g, carbohydrate 12.5 g, fat 3.1 g, fibre 2 g, energy 420 kJ (100 kcal)/100mL with vitamins, minerals and trace elements. Gluten-free, clinically lactose-free, net price 1-litre EasyBag® = £8.20. For use as the sole source of nutrition or as a nutritional supplement prescribed on medical grounds for: short-bowel syndrome, intractable malabsorption, pre-operative preparation of undernourished patients, proven inflammatory bowel disease, following total gastrectomy, dysphagia, bowel fistulas, disease-related malnutrition. Not to be prescribed for any child under 1 year; use with caution for children up to 5 years of age

Fresubin® 1200 Complete (Fresenius Kabi)

Liquid, tube feed, protein 4 g, carbohydrate 10 g, fat 2.7 g, fibre 2 g, energy 336 kJ (80 kcal)/100 mL with vitamins, minerals and trace elements. Gluten-free, clinically lactose-free, net price 1.5-litre EasyBag® = £10.20. For use as the sole source of nutrition or as a nutritional supplement prescribed on medical grounds for: short-bowel syndrome, intractable malabsorption, pre-operative preparation of undernourished patients, proven inflammatory bowel disease, following total gastrectomy, bowel fistulas, disease-related malnutrition. Not to be prescribed for any child under 5 years of age

Fresubin® Original Fibre (Fresenius Kabi)

Liquid with dietary fibre, protein 19 g, carbohydrate 69 g, fat 17 g, energy 2100 kJ (500 kcal)/500 mL, with vitamins and minerals. Flavour: neutral. Net price 500-mL bottle = £3.38; 500-mL EasyBag® = £3.51; 1-litre EasyBag® = £7.03. For use as sole source of nutrition or as a nutritional supplement prescribed on medical grounds for: short-bowel syndrome, intractable malabsorption, pre-operative preparation of patients who are undernourished, proven inflammatory bowel disease, following total gastrectomy, dysphagia, disease-related malnutrition. Not to be prescribed for any child under 2 years; use with caution for children up to 5 years

Fructose (laevulose). For proven glucose/galactose intolerance

Galactomin® (SHS)

Formula 17, powder, protein 14.5 g, fat 25.9 g, carbohydrate 56.9 g, mineral salts 3.4 g/100 g. Used as a 13.1% solution with additional vitamins in place of milk. Net price 400 g = £10.55. For proven lactose intolerance in preschool children, galactosaemia and galactokinase deficiency

Formula 19, powder, protein 14.6 g, fat 30.8 g, carbohydrate 49.7 g (fructose as carbohydrate source), mineral salts 2.1 g/100 g, with vitamins. Used as a 12.9% solution in place of milk. Net price 400 g = £27.80. For glucose plus galactose intolerance

Generaid® (SHS)

Powder, whey protein and additional branched-chain amino acids (protein equivalent 81%). Net price 200 g (unflavoured) = £20.39. See also Flavour Sachets. For patients with chronic liver disease and/or porto-hepatic encephalopathy

Plus Powder, whey protein and additional branched-chain amino acids (protein equivalent 11%) carbohydrate 62%, fat 19% with vitamins, minerals and trace elements. Net price 400 g = £14.16. For children over 1 year with hepatic disorders

Glucose (dextrose monohydrate). Net price 100 g = 16p. For glycogen storage disease and sucrose/isomaltose intolerance

Glutafin® (Nutricia Dietary)

Gluten-free. White loaf (sliced or unsliced), net price 400 g = £2.46; part-baked, 400 g = £2.76. Multigrain white loaf (sliced or unsliced), 400 g = £2.76. Fibre loaf (sliced or unsliced), 400 g = £2.46; part-baked, 400 g = £2.76. Fibre rolls (part-baked), 4 = £2.76; long, 2 = £2.76. Multigrain fibre loaf (sliced or unsliced), 400 g = £2.76. White rolls, 4 = £2.76; part-baked, 4 = £2.76; part-baked, long, 2 = £2.76. Multigrain fibre rolls, 4 = £2.76. Mixes (bread, white, multigrain white, fibre, multigrain fibre and pastry), 500 g = £4.83. Biscuits, savoury, 125 g = £1.53; 150 g = £2.10. Biscuits, digestive, sweet or tea, 150 g = £1.53. Biscuits, 200 g = £3.21.

Cake mix, 500 g = £4.83. Crackers, 200 g = £2.49. High fibre crackers, 200 g = £2.09. Pasta (penne, shells, spirals, spaghetti), 500 g = £4.88; (lasagne, tagliatelle), 250 g = £2.56. Pizza bases, 2 × 110 g = £3.46. For gluten-sensitive enteropathies including steatorrhoea due to gluten sensitivity, coeliac disease, and dermatitis herpetiformis

Glutano® (Gluten Free Foods Ltd)

Gluten-free. Biscuits, net price 125 g = £1.58. Crackers, 150 g = £1.58. Flour mix, 750 g = £4.12. Pasta (animal shapes, macaroni, spaghetti, spirals, tagliatelle), 250 g = £1.58. White sliced bread (par-baked), 300 g = £1.86. Wholemeal bread (sliced or par-baked), 500 g = £2.24. Baguette or rolls (par-baked), 200 g = £1.49. For gluten-sensitive enteropathies including steatorrhoea due to gluten sensitivity, coeliac disease, and dermatitis herpetiformis

InfaSoy® (Cow & Gate)

Powder, carbohydrate 7.1%, fat 3.6%, and protein 1.8% with vitamins and minerals when used as a 12.7% solution. Net price 450 g = £3.77; 900 g = £7.23. For proven lactose and associated sucrose intolerance in preschool children, galactokinase deficiency, galactosaemia, and proven whole cow's milk sensitivity

Infatrini® (Nutricia Clinical)

Liquid, protein 2.6 g, carbohydrate 10.3 g, fat 5.4 g, energy 420 kJ (100 kcal)/100 mL with vitamins, minerals and trace elements. Gluten-free. Net price 100 mL = 85p. For use as a sole source of nutrition or as a nutritional supplement prescribed on medical grounds for: failure to thrive, disease-related malnutrition and malabsorption. Manufacturer advises suitable for infants up to 1 year or 8 kg body weight

Instant Carobel® see *Carobel, Instant®*

Isomil® (Abbott)

Powder, protein 1.8%, carbohydrate 6.9%, fat 3.7% with vitamins and minerals when reconstituted. Lactose-free. Net price 400 g = £3.38. For proven lactose intolerance in preschool children, galactokinase deficiency, galactosaemia, and proven whole cow's milk sensitivity

Isosource® (Novartis Consumer Health)

Energy, liquid, protein 28.5 g, carbohydrate 100 g, fat 31 g, energy 3300 kJ (800 kcal)/500 mL with vitamins, minerals and trace elements. Gluten-free; clinically lactose-free. Net price 500-mL bottle = £3.05, 500-mL flexible pouch = £3.05. For indications see *Isosource Standard*

Fibre, liquid, protein 19 g, carbohydrate 68 g, fat 17 g, fibre 7 g, energy 2110 kJ (500 kcal)/500 mL with vitamins, minerals and trace elements. Gluten-free; clinically lactose-free. Net price 500-mL bottle = £2.90, 500-mL flexible pouch = £2.90, 1-litre flexible pouch = £6.15, 1.5-litre flexible pouch = £8.70. For indications see *Isosource Standard*

Standard, liquid, protein 20.5 g, carbohydrate 71 g, fat 17.5 g, energy 2205 kJ (525 kcal)/500 mL with vitamins minerals and trace elements. Gluten-free; clinically lactose-free. Net price 500-mL bottle = £2.60, 500-mL flexible pouch = £2.60, 1-litre flexible pouch = £5.51, 1.5-litre flexible pouch = £7.80. For use as a sole source of nutrition or as a nutritional supplement prescribed on medical grounds for: short-bowel syndrome, intractable malabsorption, pre-operative preparation of undernourished patients, proven inflammatory bowel disease, following total gastrectomy, dysphagia, bowel fistulas, disease-related malnutrition. Not to be prescribed for any child under 1 year; use with caution for children up to 5 years

Jevity® (Abbott)

Liquid, protein 4 g, fat 3.5 g, carbohydrate 14.8 g, dietary fibre 1.1 g, energy 441 kJ (106 kcal)/100 mL, with vitamins and minerals. Gluten-, lactose-, and sucrose-free. Net price 500-mL ready-to-hang = £3.31, 1-litre ready-to-hang = £6.62, 1.5-litre ready-to-hang = £9.93. For use as the sole source of nutrition or as a nutritional supplement prescribed on medical grounds for: short-bowel syndrome, intractable malabsorption, pre-operative preparation of patients who are undernourished, proven inflammatory bowel disease, bowel fistulas, following total gastrectomy, dysphagia, disease-related malnutrition. Not to be prescribed for any child under 1 year; use with caution for children up to 5 years

Plus liquid, protein 5.6 g, carbohydrate 16.1 g, fat 3.9 g, dietary fibre 1.2 g, energy 504 kJ (120 kcal)/100 mL, with vitamins and minerals. Gluten- and lactose-free. Net price 500-mL ready-to-hang = £3.88, 1-litre ready-to-hang = £7.94, 1.5-litre ready-to-hang = £11.92. For indications see under *Jevity®*. Not to be prescribed for any child under 10 years

Juvela® (SHS)

Gluten-free. Harvest mix, fibre mix, and flour mix, net price 500 g = £5.09. Bread (whole or sliced), 400-g loaf = £2.47; part-baked loaf (with or without fibre) 400 g = 2.76. Fibre bread (sliced and unsliced), 400-g loaf = £2.41. Bread rolls, 5 × 85 g = £3.31, fibre bread rolls, 5 × 85 g = £3.31, part-baked rolls (with or without fibre), 5 × 75 g = £3.42. Crispbread, 210 g = £3.28. Digestive biscuits, 160 g = £2.01. Pasta (fusilli, macaroni, spaghetti), 500 g = £4.84; (lasagne), 250 g = £2.54. Pizza bases, 2 × 180 g = £6.09. Savoury biscuits, 110 g = £1.92. Digestive biscuits, 160 g = £2.16. Tea biscuits, 160 g = £2.16. For gluten-sensitive enteropathies including steatorrhoea due to gluten sensitivity, coeliac disease, and dermatitis herpetiformis

Low Protein. Mix, net price 500 g = £5.40. Bread (whole or sliced), 400-g loaf = £2.53. Bread rolls, 5 × 70 g = £3.15. Biscuits, orange and cinnamon flavour, 125 g = £5.28; chocolate chip, 130 g = £5.28. For inherited metabolic disorders, renal or liver failure requiring a low-protein diet

Kindergen® (SHS)

Powder, protein 7.5 g, carbohydrate 60.5 g, fat 26.1 g, energy 2060 kJ (492 kcal)/100 g with vitamins and minerals. Net price 400 g = £18.44. For complete nutritional support or supplementary feeding for infants and children with chronic renal failure who are receiving peritoneal rapid overnight dialysis

Leucine-Free Amino Acid Mix see *Amino Acid Modules*

Lifestyle® (Ultrapharm)

Gluten-free. Brown bread (sliced and unsliced), net price 400 g = £2.38. White bread (sliced and unsliced), 400 g = £2.38. High fibre bread (unsliced), 400 g = £2.38. Bread rolls, 400 g = £2.38. For gluten-sensitive enteropathies including steatorrhoea due to gluten sensitivity, coeliac disease, and dermatitis herpetiformis

Liquigen® (SHS)

Emulsion, medium chain triglycerides 52%. Net price 250 mL = £5.89; 1 litre = £24.69. For steatorrhoea associated with cystic fibrosis of the pancreas; intestinal lymphangiectasia, surgery of the intestine; chronic liver disease and liver cirrhosis; other proven malabsorption syndromes; ketogenic diet in the management of epilepsy; type I hyperlipoproteinaemia

Locasol® (SHS)

Powder, protein 14.6 g, carbohydrate 56.5 g, fat 26.1 g, mineral salts 1.9 g, not more than 55 mg of Ca^{2+}/100 g and vitamins. Used as a 13.1% solution in place of milk. Net price 400 g = £14.67. For calcium intolerance

Loprofin® (SHS)

Low protein. Sweet biscuits, net price 150 g = £1.70; chocolate cream-filled biscuits, 125 g = £1.70; cookies (chocolate chip or cinnamon), 100 g = £4.70; wafers (orange, vanilla, or chocolate), 100 g = £1.64. Breakfast cereal, 375 g = £5.25. Egg replacer, 250 g = £9.84. Egg-white replacer, 100 g = £6.34. Bread (sliced or whole), 400-g loaf = £2.53. Rolls (part-baked) 4 × 65 g = £2.66. Mix, 500 g = £5.38. Crackers, 150 g = £2.31. Herb crackers, 150 g = £2.31. Pasta (macaroni, pasta spirals, spaghetti), 500 g = £5.60. Pasta (vermicelli), 250 g = £2.80. For inherited metabolic disorders, renal or liver failure requiring a low-protein diet

PKU Drink, protein 0.4 g (phenylalanine 10 mg), lactose 9.4 g, fat 2 g, energy 165 kJ (40 kcal)/100 mL. Net price 200-mL Tetrapak® = 50p. For phenylketonuria

Low protein drink (Milupa)
Powder, protein 0.4%, carbohydrate 5.1%, fat 2% when reconstituted. Net price 400 g = £6.91. For inherited disorders of amino acid metabolism in childhood
Note. Termed *Milupa® lpd* by manufacturer

Maxamaid® (SHS)
Note. Maxamaid products are generally intended for use in children aged 1 to 8 years, see also Flavour Sachets, for use with unflavoured amino acid and peptide products from SHS
MSUD Maxamaid, powder, essential and non-essential amino acids 30% except isoleucine, leucine, and valine, with carbohydrate, fat less than 0.5%, vitamins, minerals, and trace elements. Net price 500 g = £61.70. For maple syrup urine disease
XLeu Maxamaid, powder, essential and non-essential amino acids 28.6% except leucine, with carbohydrate, fat less than 0.5%, vitamins, minerals, and trace elements. Net price 500 g = £61.70. For isovaleric acidaemia
XLys Maxamaid, powder, essential and non-essential amino acids 30% except lysine, with carbohydrate, fat less than 0.5%, vitamins, minerals, and trace elements. Net price 500 g = £61.70. For hyperlysinaemia
XLys, Low Try, Maxamaid, powder, essential and non-essential amino acids 30% except lysine, with carbohydrate, fat less than 0.5%, vitamins, minerals, and trace elements. Net price 500 g = £61.70. For type 1 glutaric aciduria
XMet Maxamaid, powder, essential and non-essential amino acids 30% except methionine, with carbohydrate, fat less than 0.5%, vitamins, minerals, and trace elements. Net price 500 g = £61.70. For hypermethioninaemia, homocystinuria
XMTVI Maxamaid, powder, essential and non-essential amino acids 30% except methionine, threonine, valine and low isoleucine, with carbohydrate, fat less than 0.5%, vitamins, minerals, and trace elements. Net price 500 g = £61.70. For methylmalonic acidaemia or propionic acidaemia
XP Maxamaid, essential and non-essential amino acids 30% except phenylalanine, with carbohydrate, vitamins, minerals, and trace elements. Net price powder (unflavoured), 500 g = £37.24; (orange-flavoured), 500 g = £37.24. For phenylketonuria. Not to be prescribed for children under 2 years
XP Maxamaid Concentrate, powder, essential and non-essential amino acids 65% except phenylalanine, with carbohydrate, fat less than 0.5%, vitamins, minerals, and trace elements. Unflavoured. Net price 500 g = £99.15. For phenylketonuria. Not to be prescribed for children under 2 years
XPhen, Tyr Maxamaid, powder, essential and non-essential amino acids 30% except phenylalanine and tyrosine, with carbohydrate, fat less than 0.5%, vitamins, minerals, and trace elements. Unflavoured. Net price 500 g = £61.70. For tyrosinaemia

Maxamum® (SHS)
Note. Maxamum products are generally intended for use in children aged over 8 years
MSUD Maxamum, powder, essential and non-essential amino acids 47% except isoleucine, leucine, and valine, with carbohydrate, fat less than 0.5%, vitamins, minerals, see also Flavour Sachets. Net price 500 g = £98.92. For maple syrup urine disease
XMet Maxamum, powder, essential and non-essential amino acids 47% except methionine, with carbohydrate, fat less than 0.5%, vitamins, minerals, and trace elements. Unflavoured, see also Flavour Sachets. Net price 500 g = £98.92. For hypermethioninaemia, homocystinuria
XMTVI Maxamum, powder, essential and non-essential amino acids 47% except methionine, threonine, valine, and low isoleucine, with carbohydrate, fat less than 0.5%, vitamins, minerals, and trace elements. Unflavoured, see also Flavour Sachets. Net price 500 g = £98.92. For methylmalonic acidaemia or propionic acidaemia

XP Maxamum, powder, essential and non-essential amino acids 47% except phenylalanine, with carbohydrates, vitamins, minerals, and trace elements. Flavours: orange, unflavoured, see also Flavour Sachets. Net price 500 g = £57.55. For phenylketonuria. Not to be prescribed for children under 8 years

Maxijul® (SHS)
Liquid, carbohydrate 50%, with potassium 0.004%, sodium 0.023%. Gluten-, lactose-, and fructose-free. Flavours: black currant, lemon and lime, orange, and natural. Net price 200 mL =£1.01
LE Powder, modification of *Maxijul®* with lower concentrations of sodium and potassium. Net price 200 g = £3.55, 2 kg = £24.73
Super Soluble Powder, glucose polymer, potassium 0.004%, sodium 0.046%. Gluten-, lactose-, and fructose-free. Net price 4 × 132-g sachet pack = £3.98, 200 g = £1.68, 2.5 kg = £14.54, 25 kg = £99.64
All for disease-related malnutrition; malabsorption states or other conditions requiring fortification with high or readily available carbohydrate supplement

Maxipro Super Soluble® (SHS)
Powder, whey protein and additional amino acids (protein equivalent 80%). Net price 200 g = £7.96; 1 kg = £31.86. For biochemically proven hypoproteinaemia. Not to be prescribed for any child under 1 year; unsuitable as a sole source of nutrition

Maxisorb® (SHS)
Powder, protein 12 g, carbohydrate 9 g, fat 6 g, energy 579 kJ (138 kcal)/30 g with minerals. Vanilla, strawberry and chocolate flavours. Net price 5 × 30-g sachets = £3.34. For biochemically proven hypoproteinaemia. Not to be prescribed for any child under 1 year; use with caution for children up to 5 years

MCT Oil
Triglycerides from medium chain fatty acids. For steatorrhoea associated with cystic fibrosis of the pancreas; intestinal lymphangiectasia; surgery of the intestine; chronic liver disease and liver cirrhosis; other proven malabsorption syndromes; in a ketogenic diet in the management of epilepsy; in type I hyperlipoproteinaemia
Available from Mead Johnson (net price 950 mL = £12.18); SHS (net price 500 mL = £9.33)

MCT Pepdite® (SHS)
Powder, essential and non-essential amino acids, peptides, medium chain triglycerides, monoglyceride of sunflower oil, with carbohydrate, fat, vitamins, minerals, and trace elements. Flavour Sachets available.
MCT Pepdite 0–2. Net price 400 g = £12.97
MCT Pepdite 1+. Net price 400 g = £12.97
Both for disorders in which a high intake of medium chain triglyceride is beneficial

Metabolic Mineral Mixture® (SHS)
Powder, essential mineral salts. Net price 100 g = £8.02. For mineral supplementation in synthetic diets

Methionine-Free Amino Acid Mix *see* Amino Acid Modules

Methionine, Threonine, Valine-Free and Isoleucine-Low Amino Acid Mix *see* Amino Acid Modules

Milupa® lpd *see under* Low Protein Drink

Milupa® PKU2 and PKU3 *see under* PKU2 and PKU3

Modulen IBD® (Nestlé)
Powder, protein 18 g, carbohydrate 54 g, fat 23 g, energy 2040 kJ (500 kcal)/100 g with vitamins, minerals and trace elements. Net price 400 g = £9.72. For use as the sole source of nutrition during the active phase of Crohn's disease and for nutritional support during the remission phase in patients who are malnourished. Not to be prescribed for any child under one year; use with caution for young children up to 5 years

Monogen® (SHS)
Powder, protein 11.4 g, carbohydrate 68 g, fat 11.4 g (of which MCT 93%), energy 1772 kJ (420 kcal)/100 g, with vitamins, minerals and trace elements. Net price 400 g = £12.77. For long-chain acyl-CoA dehydrogenase deficiency (LCAD), carnitine palmitoyl transferase deficiency (CPTD), primary and secondary lipoprotein lipase deficiency

MSUD Aid III® (SHS)

Powder, containing full range of amino acids except iso-leucine, leucine, and valine, with vitamins, minerals, and trace elements. Net price 500 g = £123.98. For maple syrup urine disease and related conditions where it is necessary to limit the intake of branched chain amino acids

Neocate® (SHS)

Advance, powder, essential and non-essential amino acids, carbohydrate, fat, vitamins, minerals and trace elements. Milk protein-, soy- and lactose-free. Net price 100 g = £3.87. For proven whole protein intolerance, short-bowel syndrome, intractable malabsorption, and other gastrointestinal disorders where an elemental diet is specifically indicated

Powder, essential and non-essential amino acids, malto-dextrin, fat, vitamins, minerals, and trace elements. Net price 400 g = £18.73. For proven whole protein intoler-ance, short-bowel syndrome, intractable malabsorption, and other gastrointestinal disorders where an elemental diet is specifically indicated

Nepro® (Abbott)

Liquid, protein 16.6 g, carbohydrate 60.2 g, fat 26 g, energy 1988 kJ (474 kcal)/237 mL with vitamins and minerals. Net price 237-mL can = £2.28. For patients with chronic renal failure who are on haemodialysis or continuous ambulatory peritoneal dialysis (CAPD), or patients with cirrhosis or other conditions requiring a high energy, low fluid, low electrolyte diet

Nestargel® (Nestlé)

Powder, carob seed flour 96.5%, calcium lactate 3.5%. Net price 125 g = £2.99. For thickening feeds in the treatment of vomiting

Novasource® Forte (Novartis Consumer Health)

Liquid, protein 30 g, carbohydrate 91.5 g, fat 29.5 g, fibre 11 g, energy 3155 kJ (750 kcal) 500 mL with vitamins, minerals and trace elements. Gluten-free; low-lactose, net price 500-mL flexible pouch = £3.85. For use as a sole source of nutrition or as a nutritional supplement prescribed on medical grounds for: short-bowel syndrome, intractable malabsorption, pre-operative preparation of undernourished patients, proven inflamm-atory bowel disease, following total gastrectomy, dys-phagia, bowel fistulas, disease-related malnutrition, neoplasia-related cachexia. Not to be prescribed for any child under 1 year; use with caution for children up to 5 years

Novasource® GI Control® (Novartis Consumer Health)

Liquid, protein 4.1 g, carbohydrate 14.2 g, fat 3.5 g, fibre 2.2 g, energy 440 kJ (100 kcal)/100 mL with vitamins minerals and trace elements. Gluten-free; clinically lact-ose-free, net price 500-mL bottle = £3.87, 500-mL flexi-ble pouch = £3.87, 1.5-litre flexible pouch = £11.61. For use as a sole source of nutrition or as a nutritional sup-plement prescribed on medical grounds for: short-bowel syndrome, intractable malabsorption, pre-operative preparation of undernourished patients, proven inflamm-atory bowel disease, following total gastrectomy, dys-phagia, bowel fistulas, disease-related malnutrition. Not to be prescribed for any child under 1 year; use with cau-tion for children up to 5 years

Nutilis® (Nutricia Clinical)

Powder, modified maize starch, gluten- and lactose-free. Net price 225 g = £3.49. For thickening of foods in dys-phagia. Not to be prescribed for children under 3 years

Nutramigen® (Mead Johnson)

Powder, protein 13%, carbohydrate 62%, fat 18% with vitamins and minerals. Gluten-, sucrose-, and lactose-free. Net price 425 g = £7.44. For disaccharide and/or whole protein intolerance where additional medium chain triglyceride is not indicated

Nutrini® (Nutricia Clinical)

Liquid, protein 5.5 g, carbohydrate 24.6 g, fat 8.8 g, energy 840 kJ (200 kcal)/200 mL. Gluten- and sucrose-free; clinically lactose-free. Net price 200-mL bottle = £1.82, 500-mL collapsible pack = £4.55. For use as the sole source of nutrition or as a nutritional supplement prescribed on medical grounds for: short-bowel

syndrome, intractable malabsorption, pre-operative preparation of undernourished patients, dysphagia, bowel fistulas, disease-related malnutrition and/or growth failure. Not to be prescribed for any child under 1 year

Extra, liquid, protein 8.2 g, carbohydrate 37 g, fat 13.4 g, energy 1260 kJ (300 kcal)/200 mL. Gluten- and sucrose-free; clinically lactose-free. Net price 200-mL bottle = £2.24, 500-mL collapsible pack = £5.70. For use as the sole source of nutrition or as a nutritional supplement prescribed on medical grounds for: disease-related mal-nutrition and growth failure

Multi Fibre, liquid, protein 5.5 g, carbohydrate 24.6 g, fat 8.8 g, fibre 1.5 g, energy 840 kJ (200 kcal)/200 mL. Glu-ten- and sucrose-free; clinically lactose-free. Net price 200-mL bottle = £2.02, 500-mL collapsible pack = £5.05. For indications see *Nutrini Liquid*

Nutrison® (Nutricia Clinical)

Energy, liquid, protein 30 g, carbohydrate 92 g, fat 29 g, energy 3200 kJ (750 kcal)/500 mL with vitamins, miner-als and trace elements. Gluten- and sucrose-free; clini-cally lactose-free. Net price 500-mL bottle = £3.45; 500-mL pack = £3.81; 1-litre pack = £6.90; 1-litre pack = £10.35. As a nutritional supplement prescribed on medi-cal grounds for: short-bowel syndrome, intractable mal-absorption, pre-operative preparation of undernourished patients, proven inflammatory bowel disease, following total gastrectomy, dysphagia, bowel fistulas, disease-related malnutrition. Not to be prescribed for any child under 1 year; use with caution for children up to 5 years

Multi Fibre, liquid, protein 20 g, carbohydrate 61.5 g, fat 19.5 g, fibre 7.5 g, energy 2100 kJ (500 kcal)/500 mL with vitamins, minerals and trace elements. Gluten- and sucrose-free; clinically lactose-free. Net price 500-mL bottle = £3.20; 500-mL pack = £3.52; 1-litre pack = £6.40; 1.5-litre pack = £9.60. For indications see *Nutri-son Standard* excluding bowel fistulas. Not to be pre-scribed for any child under 1 year; use with caution for children up to 5 years

Soya, liquid, protein 20 g, carbohydrate 61.5 g, fat 19.5 g, energy 2100 kJ (500 kcal)/500 mL, with vitamins, miner-als and trace elements. Gluten- and sucrose-free; clini-cally lactose-free. Net price 500-mL bottle = £3.43; 1-litre pack = £6.85. For indications see *Nutrison Standard*

Standard, liquid, protein 20 g, carbohydrate 61.5 g, fat 19.5 g, energy 2125 kJ (500 kcal)/500 mL, with vitamins, minerals and trace elements. Gluten- and sucrose-free; clinically lactose-free. Net price 500-mL bottle = £2.94; 500-mL pack = £3.26; 1-litre pack = £5.74; 1.5-litre pack = £8.61. For use as the sole source of nutrition or as a nutritional supplement prescribed on medical grounds for: short-bowel syndrome, intractable malabsorption, pre-operative preparation of undernourished patients, proven inflammatory bowel disease, following total gastrectomy, dysphagia, bowel fistulas, disease-related malnutrition. Not to be prescribed for any child under 1 year; use with caution for children up to 5 years

Nutrison MCT® (Nutricia Clinical)

Liquid, protein 25 g, carbohydrate 61.5 g, fat 16.5 g, energy 2095 kJ (500 kcal)/500 mL with vitamins, miner-als and trace elements. Gluten- and fructose-free, clini-cally lactose-free. Vanilla flavour. Net price 500-mL bottle = £3.13; 1-litre pack = £6.25. For indications see *Nutrison Energy*. Not to be prescribed for any child under 1 year; use with caution for children up to 5 years

Organ® (Community)

Gluten-free. Pasta: lasagne (corn, rice and maize), 150 g = £1.99; shells (split pea and soya), 200 g = £1.39; spa-ghetti (corn, rice, rice and maize), 250 g = £1.31; spirals (buckwheat, corn, rice, rice and millet, rice and maize), 250 g = £1.31, spirals (organic brown rice), 250 g = £1.68. Crispbread (corn or rice), 200 g = £1.46. Pizza and pastry mix, 375 g = £1.84. For gluten-sensitive enteropathies including steatorrhoea due to gluten sensi-tivity, coeliac disease, and dermatitis herpetiformis

Osmolite® (Abbott)

Liquid, protein 10.0 g, carbohydrate 33.9 g, fat 8.5 g, energy 1060 kJ (252 kcal)/250 mL with vitamins and min-erals. Gluten- and lactose-free. Net price 250-mL can =

£1.51; 500-mL bottle = £2.91, 1-litre bottle = £5.82, 1.5-litre bottle = £8.73. For use as the sole source of nutrition or as a nutritional supplement prescribed on medical grounds for: short-bowel syndrome, intractable malabsorption, pre-operative preparation of undernourished patients, proven inflammatory bowel disease, following total gastrectomy, bowel fistulas, disease-related malnutrition, dysphagia. Not to be prescribed for any child under 1 year; use with caution for children up to 5 years

Plus, liquid, protein 5.6 g, carbohydrate 15.8 g, fat 3.9 g, energy 508 kJ (121 kcal)/100 mL with vitamins, minerals and trace elements. Gluten-free and clinically lactose-free. Net price 500-mL ready-to-hang = £3.50, 1-litre ready-to-hang = £6.99, 1.5-litre ready-to-hang = £10.48. For indications see *Osmolite Liquid.*

Paediasure® (Abbott)

Liquid, protein 7 g, carbohydrate 27.9 g, fat 12.5 g, energy 1054 kJ (252 kcal)/250 mL with vitamins and minerals. Gluten-free, clinically lactose-free. Flavours: vanilla (can, ready-to-hang and tetrapaks), strawberry, chocolate and banana (tetrapaks). Net price 250-mL can = £2.26, 500-mL ready-to-hang = £4.52, 200-mL tetrapaks = £1.81. For use as the sole source of nutrition or as a nutritional supplement prescribed on medical grounds for: short-bowel syndrome, intractable malabsorption, pre-operative preparation of undernourished patients, dysphagia, bowel fistulas, and disease-related malnutrition and/or growth failure. Not to be prescribed for any child under 1 year

Liquid with fibre, protein 7 g, carbohydrate 27.9 g, fat 12.5 g, fibre 1.3 g, energy 1054 kJ (252 kcal)/250 mL with vitamins and minerals. Gluten-free, clinically lactose-free. Flavours: vanilla (can, ready-to-hang and tetrapak), strawberry (tetrapak). Net price 250-mL can = £2.57, 500-mL ready-to-hang = £5.14, 200-mL tetrapak = £2.06. For indications see *Paediasure Liquid.*

Paediasure® Plus (Abbott)

Liquid, protein 4.2 g, carbohydrate 16.7 g, fat 7.5 g, energy 632 kJ (151 kcal)/100 mL with vitamins and minerals. Gluten-free, clinically lactose-free. Vanilla flavoured, net price 500-mL ready-to-hang = £5.75. For indications see *Paediasure liquid*

Paediatric Seravit® (SHS)

Powder, vitamins, minerals, low sodium and potassium, and trace elements. Net price 200 g (unflavoured) = £11.31; pineapple flavour, 200 g = £12.04. For vitamin and mineral supplementation in restrictive therapeutic diets in infants and children

Pepdite® (SHS)

Powder, peptides, essential and non-essential amino acids, with carbohydrate, fat, vitamins, minerals, and trace elements. Flavour Sachets available.

Pepdite. Providing 1925 kJ (472 kcal)/100 g. Net price 400 g = £12.15

Pepdite 1+. Providing 1787 kJ (439 kcal)/100 g. Net price 400 g = £12.51

Both for disaccharide and/or whole protein intolerance, or where amino acids or peptides are indicated in conjunction with medium chain triglycerides

Peptamen® (Nestlé Clinical)

Liquid, protein 4 g, carbohydrate 12.7 g, fat 3.7 g, energy 420 kJ (100 kcal)/100 mL, with vitamins, minerals and trace elements. Lactose- and gluten-free. Flavours: unflavoured (can), vanilla (cup, see also *Flavour Sachets*). Net price 375-mL can = £3.69, 200-mL cup = £2.25; 500-mL (Dripac-Flex) = £4.57, 1-litre = £8.23. For use as the sole source of nutrition or as a nutritional supplement prescribed on medical grounds for: short-bowel syndrome, intractable malabsorption, proven inflammatory bowel disease, bowel fistulas. Not to be prescribed for any child under 1 year; use with caution for children up to 5 years

Flavour Sachets for use with *Peptamen Liquid* 200-mL cup. Flavours: banana, chocolate, coffee, lemon and lime, strawberry. Net price 18-sachet pack = £5.62

Pepti-Junior® (Cow & Gate)

Powder, protein 15.3 g, fat 28.3 g, carbohydrate 55.1 g, energy 2140 kJ (507 kcal)/100 g with vitamins and minerals. Used as a 13.1% solution in place of milk. Net

price 450 g = £8.22. For disaccharide and/or whole protein intolerance or where amino acids and peptides are indicated in conjunction with medium chain triglycerides

Peptisorb® (Nutricia Clinical)

Liquid, protein 20 g, carbohydrate 88 g, fat 8.5 g, energy 2100 kJ (500 kcal)/500 mL with vitamins, minerals and trace elements. Gluten-free. Net price 500-mL bottle = £4.88; 500-mL pack = £4.88; 1-litre pack = £8.83. For use as the sole source of nutrition or as a nutritional supplement prescribed on medical grounds for: short-bowel syndrome, intractable malabsorption, proven inflammatory bowel disease, bowel fistulas. Not to be prescribed for any child under 1 year; use with caution for children up to 5 years

Perative® (Abbott)

Liquid, providing protein 15.8 g, carbohydrate 42 g, fat 8.8 g, energy 1308 kJ (310 kcal)/237 mL, with vitamins and minerals. Gluten-free, unflavoured. Net price 237-mL can = £2.68, 500-mL ready-to-hang = £5.36, 1-litre ready-to-hang = £10.72. For use as a nutritional supplement prescribed on medical grounds for: short-bowel syndrome, intractable malabsorption, pre-operative preparation of patients who are undernourished, proven inflammatory bowel disease, following total gastrectomy, bowel fistulas, disease-related malnutrition. Not to be prescribed for any child under 5 years

Phenylalanine, Tyrosine and Methionine-Free Amino Acid Mix see Amino Acid Modules

Phlexy-10® Exchange System (SHS)

Bar, essential and non-essential amino acids except phenylalanine 8.33 g, carbohydrate 20.5 g, fat 4.5 g/42-g bar. Citrus fruit flavour. Net price per bar = £3.92

Capsules, essential and non-essential amino acids except phenylalanine 500 mg/capsule. Net price 200-cap pack = £27.32

Drink Mix, powder, containing essential and non-essential amino acids except phenylalanine 10 g, carbohydrate 6.8 g/20-g sachet. Blackcurrant and apple flavour. Net price 20-g sachet = £2.74

All for phenylketonuria

Phlexyvits® (SHS)

Powder, vitamins, minerals and trace elements, net price 30 x 7-g sachets = £47.70 For use as a vitamin and mineral component of restricted therapeutic diets in older children from the age of around 11 years and over and adults with phenylketonuria and similar amino acid abnormalities

PK Aid 4® (SHS)

Powder, containing essential and non-essential amino acids except phenylalanine. Net price 500 g = £91.61. For phenylketonuria

PKU 2® (Milupa)

Granules, containing essential and non-essential amino acids except phenylalanine; with vitamins, minerals, trace elements, 7.1% sucrose. Flavour: vanilla. Net price 500 g = £44.75. For phenylketonuria

PKU 3® (Milupa)

Granules, containing essential and non-essential amino acids except phenylalanine, vitamins, minerals, and trace elements, with 3.4% sucrose. Flavour: vanilla. Net price 500 g = £44.75. For phenylketonuria, not recommended for child under 8 years

PKU-gel® (Vitaflo)

Powder, protein (containing essential and non-essential amino acids, phenylalanine-free) 10.1 g, carbohydrate 8.6 g, fat 0.03 g, energy 285.5 kJ (68 kcal)/20 g with vitamins, minerals and trace elements. Orange or unflavoured, net price 25 x 20 g sachets = £58.00. For use as part of the low-protein dietary management of phenylketonuria in children aged 1 to 10 years. Not recommended for children under 1 year of age.

Pleniday® (Brewhurst)

Gluten-free. Bread: loaf (sliced) net price 350 g = £1.79; country loaf (sliced), 500g = £2.85; rustic loaf (par-baked baguette), 400g = £2.09; petit pan, 2 x 150g = £2.02. Pasta (penne, rigate), 250g = £1.50. For gluten-sensitive enteropathies including steatorrhoea due to gluten sensitivity, coeliac disease, and dermatitis herpetiformis

Polial® (Ultrapharm)

Biscuits. Gluten- and lactose-free. Net price 200-g pack = £2.85. For gluten-sensitive enteropathies including steatorrhea due to gluten sensitivity, coeliac disease, and dermatitis herpetiformis

Polycal® (Nutricia Clinical)

Powder, glucose, maltose, and polysaccharides, providing 1615 kJ (380 kcal)/100 g. Net price 400 g = £2.94

Liquid , glucose polymers providing carbohydrate 61.9 g/100 mL. Low-electrolyte, protein-free. Flavours: apple, black currant, lemon, orange, and neutral. Net price 200 mL = £1.16

Both for disease-related malnutrition; malabsorption states or other conditions requiring fortification with a high or readily available carbohydrate supplement

Polycose® (Abbott)

Powder, glucose polymers, providing carbohydrate 94 g, energy 1598 kJ (376 kcal)/100 g. Net price 350-g can = £3.30. For disease-related malnutrition; malabsorption states or other conditions requiring fortification with a high or readily available carbohydrate supplement

Pregestimil® (Mead Johnson)

Powder, protein 12.8%, carbohydrate 61.6%, fat 18.3% with vitamins and minerals. Gluten-, sucrose-, and lactose-free. Net price 450 g = £8.49. For disaccharide and/or whole protein intolerance or where amino acids or peptides are indicated in conjunction with medium chain triglycerides

Prejomin® (Milupa)

Granules, protein 13.5 g, carbohydrate 57 g, fat 24 g, energy 2085 kJ (497 kcal)/100 g, with vitamins and minerals. Gluten-free. For preparation with water before use. Net price 400 g = £9.35. For disaccharide and/or whole protein intolerance where additional medium chain triglyceride is not indicated

Pro-Cal® (Vitaflo)

Powder, protein 13.5 g, carbohydrate 26.8 g, fat 56.2 g, energy 2788 kJ (667 kcal)/100 g, net price 25 x 15 g sachets = £10.10, 510 g = £9.21, 1.5 kg = £19.07, 12.5 kg = £140, 25 kg = £250. For disease-related malnutrition, malabsorption states or other conditions requiring fortification with a fat/carbohydrate supplement. Not to be prescribed for any child under 1 year; use with caution for young children up to 5 years

Promin® (Firstplay Dietary)

Low protein. Pasta (alphabets, macaroni, shells, shortcut spaghetti, spirals); Pasta tricolour (alphabets, shells, spirals), net price 250 g = £2.65. Pasta meal, 500 g = £5.30. Pasta imitation rice, 500 g = £5.30. For inherited metabolic disorders, renal or liver failure requiring a low-protein diet

ProMod® (Abbott)

Powder, protein 75 g, carbohydrate 7.5 g, fat 6.9 g/100 g. Gluten-free. Net price 275-g can = £8.82. For biochemically proven hypoproteinaemia

Prosobee® (Mead Johnson)

Powder, protein 15.6%, carbohydrate 51.4%, fat 27.9% with vitamins and minerals. Gluten-, sucrose-, and lactose-free. Net price 400 g = £3.51

For proven lactose and associated sucrose intolerance in pre-school children, galactokinase deficiency, galactosaemia, and proven whole cow's milk sensitivity

Protenplus® (Fresenius Kabi)

Liquid, protein 20 g, carbohydrate 19 g, fat 5.2 g, energy 840 kJ (200 kcal)/200 mL, with vitamins, minerals, and trace elements. Gluten-free. Vanilla, strawberry, and chocolate flavours. Net price 200-mL carton = £1.25. As a nutritional supplement prescribed on medical grounds for: short-bowel syndrome, intractable malabsorption, pre-operative preparation of patients who are undernourished, proven inflammatory bowel disease, following total gastrectomy, dysphagia, bowel fistulas, disease-related malnutrition, continuous ambulatory peritoneal dialysis (CAPD) and haemodialysis. Not to be prescribed for any child under 1 year; use with caution for young children up to 5 years

Protifar® (Nutricia Clinical)

Powder, protein 88.5%. Low lactose, gluten- and sucrose-free. Net price 225 g = £5.90. For biochemically proven hypoproteinaemia

Provide® (Fresenius Kabi)

Xtra Liquid, protein 3.75 g, carbohydrate 27.5 g, energy 525 kJ (125 kcal)/100 mL with vitamins, minerals and trace elements. Gluten-free. Blackcurrant, cherry, citrus cola, lemon & lime, melon, orange & pineapple flavour. Net price 200-mL carton = £1.52.

As a nutritional supplement prescribed on medical grounds for: short-bowel syndrome, intractable malabsorption, pre-operative preparation of patients who are undernourished, proven inflammatory bowel disease, following total gastrectomy, dysphagia, bowel fistulas, disease-related malnutrition. Not to be prescribed for any child under 1 year; use with caution for children up to 5 years

QuickCal® (Vitaflo)

Powder, protein 4.6 g, carbohydrate 17 g, fat 77 g, energy 3260 kJ (780 kcal)/100 g, net price 25 x 13 g sachets = £9.05, 520 g = £7.38, 1.5 kg = £15.24, 25 kg = £208.50. For disease-related malnutrition, malabsorption states or other conditions requiring fortification with a fat/carbohydrate supplement. Not to be prescribed for any child under 1 year; use with caution for young children up to 5 years

Rectified Spirit. Where the therapeutic qualities of alcohol are required rectified spirit (suitably flavoured and diluted) should be prescribed

Renamil® (Syner-Med)

Powder, protein 4.7 g, carbohydrate 70.2 g, fat 18.7 g, 1984 kJ (468 kcal)/100 g, with vitamins and minerals. Net price 1 kg = £25.40. For chronic renal failure. Not suitable for infants and children under 1 year

Renapro® (Syner-Med)

Powder, whey protein providing protein 92 g, carbohydrate less than 300 mg, fat 500 mg, 1562 kJ (367 kcal)/100 g. Net price 20 g sachet = £2.22. For dialysis and hypoproteinaemia. Not suitable for infants and children under 1 year

Resource® Benefiber® (Novartis Consumer Health)

Powder, soluble dietary fibre, carbohydrate 47.5 g, fibre 195 g, energy 808 kJ (190 kcal)/250 g with minerals. Gluten-free; low lactose, net price 250 g pack = £7.75. As a nutritional supplement prescribed on medical grounds for: short-bowel syndrome, intractable malabsorption, pre-operative preparation of undernourished patients, proven inflammatory bowel disease, following total gastrectomy, bowel fistulas, disease-related malnutrition. Not to be prescribed for children under 5 years

Resource® Energy Dessert (Novartis Consumer Health)

Semi-solid, protein 6 g, carbohydrate 26.5 g, fat 7.8 g, energy 839 kJ (200 kcal)/125 g with vitamins, minerals, and trace elements. Gluten-free; low lactose. Flavours: caramel, chocolate, or vanilla, net price 125-g cup = £1.29. For use as a nutritional supplement prescribed on medical grounds for: disease-related malnutrition, short-bowel syndrome, intractable malabsorption, proven inflammatory bowel disease, bowel fistulas, dysphagia, pre-operative preparation of undernourished patients, after total gastrectomy, continuous ambulatory peritoneal dialysis (CAPD), haemodialysis. Not to be prescribed for any child under 1 year; use with caution for children up to 5 years

Resource ® Protein Extra (Novartis Consumer Health)

Liquid, protein 18.8 g, carbohydrate 31.2 g, fat 5.6 g, energy 1057 kJ (250 kcal)/200 mL with vitamins, minerals and trace elements. Gluten-free; low lactose. Flavours: apricot, chocolate, summer fruits, or vanilla. Net price 200-mL carton = £1.22. For use as a nutritional supplement prescribed on medical grounds for: disease-related malnutrition, short-bowel syndrome, intractable malabsorption, proven inflammatory bowel disease, bowel fistulas, dysphagia, pre-operative preparation of undernourished patients, after total gastrectomy. Not to be prescribed for any child under 1 year; use with caution for children up to 5 years

Resource® Shake (Novartis Consumer Health)

Liquid, protein 8.9 g, carbohydrate 39.6 g, fat 12.3 g, energy 1280 kJ (305 kcal)/175 mL with vitamins, minerals and trace elements. Gluten-free; low lactose. Flavours: banana, chocolate, lemon, strawberry, summer fruits, toffee, or vanilla. Net price 175-mL carton = £1.46. For use as a nutritional supplement prescribed on medical grounds for: disease-related malnutrition, short-bowel syndrome, intractable malabsorption, proven inflammatory bowel disease, bowel fistulas, dysphagia, pre-operative preparation of undernourished patients, after total gastrectomy. Not to be prescribed for any child under 1 year; use with caution for children up to 5 years

Resource® Thickened Drink (Novartis Consumer Health)

Liquid, carbohydrate 25 g, energy: orange 437 kJ (102 kcal); apple 428 kJ (101 kcal)/114 mL. Syrup and custard consistencies. Gluten-free; clinically lactose free, net price 12 x 114 mL cups = £6.00. For dysphagia. Not suitable for children under 1 year

Resource® Thickened Squash (Novartis Consumer Health)

Liquid, syrup consistency: carbohydrate 16.9 g, energy 287 kJ (68 kcal) /100 mL; custard consistency: carbohydrate 17.8 g, energy 303 kJ (71 kcal) /100 mL. Gluten-free; clinically lactose-free. Orange and lemon flavour, net price 1.89-litre bottle = £3.50. For dysphagia. Not suitable for children under 1 year of age

Resource® ThickenUp® (Novartis Consumer Health)

Powder, modified maize starch. Gluten- and lactose-free, net price 225 g = £3.75. For thickening of foods in dysphagia. Not to be prescribed for children under 1 year

Rite-Diet® Gluten-free (Nutricia Dietary)

Gluten-free. White bread (sliced or unsliced), 400 g = £2.46. White loaf (part-baked), 400 g = £2.76. Fibre bread (sliced or unsliced), 400 g = £2.46. Fibre loaf (part-baked), 400 g = £2.76. White rolls, 4 = £2.50; (part-baked) long, 2 = £2.76. Fibre rolls, 4 = £2.50; (part-baked) long, 2 = £2.76. Flour mix (white or fibre), 500 g = £4.83. For gluten-sensitive enteropathies including steatorrhoea due to gluten sensitivity, coeliac disease, and dermatitis herpetiformis

Rite-Diet® Low-protein (SHS)

Low protein. Baking mix. Net price 500 g = £5.23. Flour mix. 400 g = £4.83. For inherited metabolic disorders, renal or liver failure requiring a low-protein diet

Scandishake® Mix (SHS)

Powder, protein 11.7 g, carbohydrate 66.8 g, fat 30.4 g, energy 2457 kJ (588 kcal)/serving (serving = 1 sachet reconstituted with 240 mL whole milk). Flavours: chocolate, strawberry, vanilla, and unflavoured. Net price 85 g sachet = £1.82. For disease-related malnutrition; malabsorption states or other conditions requiring fortification with a fat/carbohydrate supplement

Schar® (Schär)

Gluten-free. Bread. Net price 250 g = £1.41. Baguette (french bread), 400 g = £2.39. Bread rolls, 150 g = £1.41. Lunch rolls, 150 g = £1.21. White bread buns, 200 g = £1.41. Bread mix, 1 kg = £4.00. Cake mix, 500 g = £3.95. Flour mix, 1 kg = £3.50. Cracker toast, 150 g = £1.72. Crackers, 200 g = £1.86. Crispbread, 250 g = £2.82. Pasta (fusilli, penne, rigati), 500 g = £2.20; (rings, shells, strands) 250 g = £1.40; lasagne, 250 g = £2.80; macaroni pipette, 500 g = £2.20; spaghetti, 500 g = £2.20. Pizza bases, 300 g (2 × 150 g) = £3.78. Biscuits, 175 g = £1.72. Savoy biscuits, 180 g = £1.72. For gluten-sensitive enteropathies including steatorrhoea due to gluten sensitivity, coeliac disease, and dermatitis herpetiformis

SHS Modjul® Flavour System (SHS)

Powder, black currant, orange, pineapple, and savoury tomato flavours. Net price 100 g = £7.69. For use with any unflavoured products based on peptides or amino acids

SMA High Energy® (SMA Nutrition)

Liquid, protein 2 g, carbohydrate 9.8 g, fat 4.9 g, energy 382 kJ (91 kcal)/100mL, with vitamins and minerals. Net price 250 mL = £1.75. For disease-related malnutrition, malabsorption, and growth failure

SMA LF® (SMA Nutrition)

Powder, protein 1.5 g, carbohydrate 7.2 g, fat 3.6 g, energy 282 kJ (67 kcal)/100 mL, with vitamins and minerals. Net price 430 g = £3.99. For proven lactose intolerance

Sno-Pro® (SHS)

Drink, protein 220 mg (phenylalanine 12.5 mg), carbohydrate 8 g, fat 3.8 g, energy 280 kJ (67 kcal)/100 mL. Net price 200 mL = 77p. For phenylketonuria, chronic renal failure, and other inborn errors of metabolism

Sondalis® (Nestlé Clinical)

Sondalis Fibre, protein 3.8 g, carbohydrate 12.5 g, fat 3.9 g, fibre 1.5 g, energy 420 kJ (100 kcal)/100 mL with vitamins, minerals and trace elements. Gluten-free; clinically lactose-free. Flavour: neutral. Net price 500 mL (Dripac-Flex) = £3.20, 1 litre = £6.20. For use as a sole source of nutrition or as a nutritional supplement prescribed on medical grounds for: short bowel syndrome, intractable malabsorption, pre-operative preparation of undernourished patients, proven inflammatory bowel disease, following total gastrectomy, dysphagia, bowel fistulas, disease-related malnutrition. Not to be prescribed for any child under 1 year; use with caution for children under 5 years.

Sondalis ISO, protein 3.8 g, carbohydrate 12.5 g, fat 3.9 g, energy 420 kJ (100 kcal)/100 mL with vitamins, minerals and trace elements. Gluten-free; clinically lactose-free. Flavour: neutral. Net price 500 mL (Dripac-Flex) = £2.80, 1 litre = £5.60. For indications see *Sondalis Fibre*

Sondalis 1.5, protein 5.6 g, carbohydrate 18.8 g, fat 6 g, energy 640 kJ (150 kcal)/100 mL with vitamins, minerals and trace elements. Gluten-free; clinically lactose-free. Flavour: neutral. Net price 500 mL (Dripac-Flex) = £3.20, 1 litre = £5.70. For indications see *Sondalis Fibre*

Sondalis Junior, powder, protein 13.9 g, carbohydrate 62.2 g, fat 18.3 g, energy 1950 kJ (467 kcal)/100 g with vitamins, minerals and trace elements. Gluten-free; clinically lactose-free. Flavour: vanilla, net price 400 g = £9.72. For use as a sole source of nutrition or as a nutritional supplement prescribed on medical grounds for: short bowel syndrome, intractable malabsorption, pre-operative preparation of undernourished patients, proven inflammatory bowel disease, following total gastrectomy, dysphagia, bowel fistulas, disease-related malnutrition, and growth failure in children aged 1-6 years. Not to be prescribed for any child under 1 year

Sunnyvale® (Everfresh)

Mixed grain bread, gluten-free. Net price 400 g = £1.73. For gluten-sensitive enteropathies including steatorrhoea due to gluten sensitivity, coeliac disease and dermatitis herpetiformis

Suplena® (Abbott)

Liquid, protein 7.1 g, carbohydrate 60.7 g, fat 22.7 g, energy 1994 kJ (476 kcal)/237 mL. Flavour: vanilla. Net price 237-mL can = £2.28. For patients with chronic or acute renal failure who are not undergoing dialysis; chronic or acute liver disease with fluid restriction; other conditions requiring a high-energy, low-protein, low-electrolyte, low-volume enteral feed

Survimed OPD® (Fresenius Kabi)

Liquid, protein 22.5 g, carbohydrate 75 g, fat 13 g, energy 2100 kJ (500 kcal)/500 mL, with vitamins, minerals, and trace elements. Gluten-free; low lactose. Net price 500-mL bottle = £4.80; 500-mL EasyBag® = £4.85. As a nutritional supplement prescribed on medical grounds for: short-bowel syndrome, intractable malabsorption, pre-operative preparation of patients who are undernourished, proven inflammatory bowel disease, following total gastrectomy, dysphagia, bowel fistulas, disease-related malnutrition. Not to be prescribed for any child under 1 year; use with caution for children up to 5 years

Thick and Easy® (Fresenius Kabi)

Powder. Modified maize starch. Net price 225-g can = £3.90; 100 × 8-g sachets = £25.00; 4.54 kg = £66.94. For thickening of foods in dysphagia. Not to be prescribed for children under 1 year except in cases of failure to thrive

Thickened Juices, liquid, modified food starch. Flavours: apple, cranberry and orange. Net price 1.35-litre bottle = £3.50. For dysphagia. Not suitable for infants and children under 1 year

Thixo-D® (Sutherland)
Powder, modified maize starch, gluten-free. Net price
375-g tub = £5.79. For thickening of foods in dysphagia.
Not to be prescribed for children under 1 year except in
cases of failure to thrive

Tinkyada® (General Dietary)
Gluten-free. Brown rice pasta (elbows, fettucini, fusilli,
penne, shells, spaghetti, spirals). Net price 454 g =
£3.00. For gluten-sensitive enteropathies including steatorrhoea due to gluten-sensitivity, coeliac disease and
dermatitis herpetiformis

Tritamyl® (Gluten Free Foods Ltd)
Gluten-free. Flour, net price 1 kg = £5.60. Brown bread
mix, 1 kg = £5.60. White bread mix, 1 kg = £5.60. For
gluten-sensitive enteropathies including steatorrhoea
due to gluten sensitivity, coeliac disease and dermatitis
herpetiformis

Trufree® (Nutricia Dietary)
Gluten-free, wheat-free flours. For gluten-sensitive enteropathies including steatorrhoea due to gluten sensitivity,
coeliac disease, and dermatitis herpetiformis
No. 1, net price 1 kg = £5.87. *No. 4 white,* 1 kg = £5.79.
No. 5 brown, 1 kg = £5.79. *No. 6 plain,* 1 kg = £5.24. *No.
7 self-raising,* 1 kg = £5.63

L-Tyrosine (SHS)
Powder, net price 100 g = £11.16. For use as a supplement in maternal phenylketonurics who have low
plasma tyrosine concentrations

Ultra® (Ultrapharm)
Gluten-free. Baguette, net price 400 g = £2.39. Bread, net
price 400 g = £2.39. High-fibre bread, 500 g = £3.26.
Crackerbread, 100 g = £1.72. Pizza base, net price 400 g
= £2.57. For gluten-sensitive enteropathies including
steatorrhoea due to gluten sensitivity, coeliac disease
and dermatitis herpetiformis
Low protein. PKU bread, 400 g = £2.10. PKU flour, 500 g
= £2.98. PKU biscuits, 200 g = £2.15. PKU cookies, 250 g
= £2.25. PKU pizza base, 400 g = £2.15. PKU savoy biscuits, 150 g = £2.00. For inherited metabolic disorders,
renal or liver failure requiring a low-protein diet

Valpiform® (General Dietary)
Gluten-free. Bread mix, net price 1 kg = £6.73. Country
loaf, 400 g = £3.75. Pastry mix, 1 kg = £6.73. Petites
baguettes, 320 g = £2.73. For gluten-sensitive enteropathies including steatorrhoea due to gluten sensitivity,
coeliac disease, and dermatitis herpetiformis
Low protein. Shortbread biscuits, net price 120 g = £4.06.
Cookies with chocolate nuggets, 150 g = £5.25. For
inherited metabolic disorders, renal or liver failure
requiring a low-protein diet

Vita-Bite® (Vitaflo)
Bar, protein 30 mg (less than 2.5 mg phenylalanine),
carbohydrate 15.35 g, fat 8.4 g, energy 572 kJ (137 kcal)/
25-g. Chocolate flavoured, net price 25 g = 71p. For
inherited metabolic disorders, renal or liver failure
requiring a low-protein diet. Not recommended for any
child under 1 year

Vitajoule® (Vitaflo)
Powder, glucose polymers, providing carbohydrate 96 g,
energy 1610 kJ (380 kcal)/100 g. Net price 125 g = 95p,
200 g = £1.50, 500 g = £2.78, 2.5 kg = £13.75, 25 kg =
£91.00. For disease-related malnutrition; malabsorption
states or other conditions requiring fortification with a
high or readily available carbohydrate supplement

Vitamins and Minerals. Only for use in the management
of actual or potential vitamin or mineral deficiency; not
to be prescribed as dietary supplements or 'pick-me-ups'

Vitapro® (Vitaflo)
Powder, whole milk proteins, containing all essential
amino acids, 75%. Net price 250 g = £5.43, 2 kg =
£42.84. For biochemically proven hypoproteinaemia

Vitaquick® (Vitaflo)
Powder. Modified maize starch. Net price 100 g = £2.46,
300 g = £5.19; 2 kg = £26.50; 6 kg = £70.92. For thickening of foods in dysphagia. Not to be prescribed for
children under 1 year except in cases of failure to thrive

Vitasavoury® (Vitaflo)
Powder, protein 12 g, carbohydrate 24 g, fat 54 g, energy
2610 kJ (630 kcal)/100 g, net price 10 x 50 g sachets =

£12.60, 12 x 33 g ready cups = £10.56. Flavours:
chicken, leek and potato, mushroom. As a nutritional
supplement for disease-related malnutrition, malabsorption states or other conditions requiring fortification
with a fat/carbohydrate supplement. Not to be prescribed
for any child under 1 year; use with caution for young
children up to 5 years

Wysoy® (Wyeth)
Powder, carbohydrate 6.9%, fat 3.6%, and protein 2.1%
with vitamins and minerals when reconstituted. Net
price 430 g = £3.98; 860 g = £7.58. For proven lactose
and associated sucrose intolerance in preschool children,
galactokinase deficiency, galactosaemia and proven
whole cow's milk sensitivity

Conditions for which foods may be prescribed on FP10 (GP10 in Scotland)

Note. This is a list of clinical conditions for which the
ACBS has approved food products. It is essential to check
the list of products (above) for availability.

**Amino acid metabolic disorders and similar protein
disorders:** see histidinaemia; homocystinuria; maple
syrup urine disease; phenylketonuria; low-protein products; synthetic diets; tyrosinaemia.

Bowel fistulas:
Complete foods: Complan Ready-to-Drink; Elemental
028 and 028 Extra; Emsogen; Enrich and Enrich Plus;
Ensure; Ensure Powder; Foodlink Complete; Frebini;
Fresubin Energy, Fresubin Energy Fibre (sip and tube
feed), Fresubin Liquid and Sip Feeds, Fresubin 1000,
and Fresubin 1200 Complete; Isosource Energy, Stand-
ard, Fibre; Jevity and Plus; Novasource Forte and GI
Control; Nutrini standard, Extra, and Multifibre; Nutri-
son Multi Fibre, Pepti Liquid, Soya and Standard;
Osmolite Liquid and Plus; Paediasure Liquid and Liquid
with fibre; Peptamen; Sondalis Fibres, ISO and 1.5.
Nutritional supplements: Clinutren Dessert, Fruit, ISO
and 1.5; Enlive; Ensure Plus; Formance; Forticreme;
Fortifresh; Fortijuce; Fortimel; Fortisip; Fortisip Multi
Fibre; Fresubin HP Energy; Modulen IBD; Nutrison
Energy, MCT and Pepti Powder; Perative; Provide Xtra;
Resource Shake; Survimed OPD.

Calcium intolerance: Locasol.

Carbohydrate malabsorption: See also synthetic
diets; malabsorption states.
(a) Disaccharide intolerance: Caloreen; Calsip; Duocal
Super Soluble and Duocal Liquid; Maxijul LE, Liquid,
Super Soluble; Nutramigen; Nutrison Soya; Pepdite;
Pepti-Junior; Polycal liquid and powder; Polycose powder; Pregestimil; Prejomin; Pro-Cal; QuickCal; Vitajoule; Vitasavoury. See also lactose intolerance; lactose
with associated sucrose intolerance.
(b) Glucose and galactose intolerance: Comminuted
Chicken Meat (Cow & Gate); Fructose; Galactomin Formula 19 (fructose formula).
(c) Isomaltose intolerance: Glucose (dextrose).
(d) Lactose intolerance: Comminuted chicken meat
(SHS); Enfamil Lactofree; Farley's Soya Formula; Galactomin Formula 17; InfaSoy; Isomil powder; Nutramigen; Nutrison Soya; Pepdite; Pregestimil; Prejomin;
Prosobee; SMA LF; Wysoy.
(e) Lactose with associated sucrose intolerance: Comminuted Chicken Meat (SHS); Farley's Soya Formula;
Galactomin Formula 17; InfaSoy; Nutramigen; Nutrison
Soya; Pepti-Junior; Pregestimil; Prejomin; Prosobee;
Wysoy.
(f) Sucrose intolerance: Glucose (dextrose) and see also
synthetic diets; malabsorption states; lactose with associated sucrose intolerance.
Note. Lactose or sucrose intolerance is defined as a condition of
intolerance to an intake of the relevant disaccharide confirmed by
demonstrated clinical benefit of the effectiveness of the disac-
charide-free diet, and presence of reducing substances and/or
excessive acid in the stools, a low concentration of the corresponding disaccharidase enzyme on intestinal biopsy, or by breath
tests or lactose tolerance tests

Carnitine palmitoyl transferase deficiency (CPTD): Monogen

Coeliac disease: see gluten-sensitive enteropathies.

Continuous Ambulatory Peritoneal Dialysis (CAPD): see dialysis.

Cystic fibrosis: see malabsorption states.

Dermatitis Herpetiformis: see gluten-sensitive enteropathies.

Dialysis (nutritional supplements for haemodialysis or continuous ambulatory peritoneal dialysis (CAPD) patients): Clinutren Dessert; Enrich Plus; Ensure Plus; Formance; Forticreme; Fresubin HP Energy; Kindergen; Nepro; Protenplus; Renapro; Resource Energy Dessert, Suplena.

Disaccharide intolerance: see carbohydrate malabsorption.

Dysphagia:

Complete foods: Complan ready-to-drink; Enfamil AR; Enrich and Enrich Plus; Ensure; Ensure Powder; Foodlink Complete; Frebini; Fresubin Energy, Fresubin Energy Fibre (sip and tube feed), Fresubin Isofibre; Fresubin Liquid and Sip Feeds, Fresubin 1000, and Fresubin 1200 Complete; Isosource Energy, Fibre and Standard; Jevity and Plus; Novasource GI Control, and Forte; Nutrini Fibre and Standard; Nutrison Multi Fibre, Soya and Standard; Osmolite Liquid and Plus; Paediasure Liquid, Liquid with fibre and Plus; Sondalis Fibres, ISO, Junior and 1.5.

Nutritional supplements: Clinutren Dessert, Fruit, ISO and 1.5; Clinutren Thickened Drinks, Enlive; Ensure Plus; Formance; Forticreme; Fortifresh; Fortijuice; Fortimel; Fortisip; Fortisip Multi Fibre; Fresubin HP Energy; Isosource Energy, Fibre and Standard; Nutrison Energy and MCT; Protenplus; Provide Xtra; Resource Energy Dessert; Resource Benefiber, Protein Extra, ThickenUp, Thickened Squash, and Shake; Survimed OPD.

Thickeners: Clinutren Thickener, Nutilis; Thick & Easy powder and thickened juices; Thixo-D; Vitaquick.

Note. Dysphagia is defined as that associated with intrinsic disease of the oesophagus, e.g. oesophagitis; neuromuscular disorders, e.g. multiple sclerosis and motor neurone disease; major surgery and/or radiotherapy for cancer of the upper digestive tract; protracted severe inflammatory disease of the upper digestive tract, e.g. Stevens-Johnson syndrome and epidermolysis bullosa

Epilepsy (ketogenic diet in): Alembicol D; Liquigen; Medium-Chain Triglyceride Oil (MCT).

Flavouring (for use with any unflavoured SHS product based on peptides or amino acids): SHS Flavour Modjul; Flavour Sachets

Galactokinase deficiency and galactosaemia: Farley's Soya Formula; Galactomin Formula 17; InfaSoy; Isomil powder; Prosobee; Wysoy.

Gastrectomy (total):

Complete foods: Complan ready-to-drink; Enrich; Enrich Plus; Ensure; Ensure Powder; Foodlink Complete; Frebini; Fresubin Energy, Fresubin Energy Fibre (sip and tube feed), Fresubin Isofibre, Fresubin Liquid and Sip Feeds, Fresubin 1000, and Fresubin 1200 Complete; Isosource Energy, Fibre and Standard; Jevity and Plus; Novasource GI Control, and Forte; Nutrini Multi Fibre, Soya and Standard; Osmolite Liquid and Plus; Sondalis Fibres, ISO, Junior and 1.5.

Nutritional supplements: Clinutren Dessert, Fruit, ISO and 1.5; Enlive; Ensure Plus; Formance; Fortijuice; Fortimel; Fortipudding; Fortisip; Fortisip Multi Fibre; Fresubin HP Energy; Nutrison Energy and MCT; Perative; Protein Forte; Provide Xtra; Resource Benefiber; Resource Energy Dessert, Protein Extra, and Shake; Survimed OPD.

Glucose/galactose intolerance: see carbohydrate malabsorption.

Glutaric aciduria: XLys, Low Try Maxamaid

Gluten-sensitive enteropathies: Aproten flour; Arnott gluten-free rice cookies; Barkat gluten-free bread mix, brown or white rice bread (unsliced), Brown or white rice pizza crust; Bi-Aglut biscuits, crackers, cracker toast, lasagne, pasta (fusilli, macaroni, penne, spaghetti); Dietary Specialities Mixes: brown or white bread, corn bread, white cake, white or fibre; Ener-G brown and white rice bread, gluten-free tapioca bread, rice loaf, gluten-free rice pasta (cannelloni, lasagna, macaroni, shells, small shells, spaghetti, tagliatelli, vermicelli); brown rice pasta (lasagna, macaroni, spaghetti); Glutafin bread, multigrain white loaf (sliced or unsliced), white or part-baked), rolls (white or part-baked), fibre bread, mixes (white, multigrain white, fibre, multigrain fibre), biscuits (digestive, savoury, sweet (without chocolate or sultanas), tea), crackers, high fibre crackers and pasta (lasagne, penne, spirals, spaghetti), pizza bases; Glutano gluten-free biscuits, crackers, crispbread, flour mix, pastas (animal shapes, macaroni, spaghetti, spirals, tagliatelle), shortcake rings, wholemeal bread (sliced or par-baked), baguette or rolls (par-baked), white sliced bread (par-baked); Juvela gluten-free harvest mix, loaf and high-fibre loaf (sliced and unsliced), bread rolls, fibre bread rolls, part-baked rolls with or without fibre, crispbread, mix and fibre mix; digestive biscuits, savoury biscuits and tea biscuits, pastas, pizza bases; Lifestyle gluten-free bread rolls, brown and white bread, high-fibre bread and rolls; Liga gluten-free rusks (Jacobs); Pleniday bread and pastas; Polial gluten-free biscuits; Rite-Diet gluten-free fibre rolls, high-fibre bread (sliced and unsliced), white bread (sliced and unsliced), white rolls, part-baked fibre loaf and long rolls; Schar gluten-free bread, bread mix, brown bread ertha, bread rolls and buns, crackers, cake mix, cracker toast, crispbread, flour mix, french bread (baguette), pasta (fusilli, lasagne, macaroni pipette penne, rigati, rings, shells, spaghetti), pizza base, biscuits, savoy biscuits, white bread buns, wholemeal flour mix; Sunnyvale gluten-free bread; Tinkyada gluten-free brown rice pasta (elbows, fettucini, fusilli, penne, shells, spaghetti, spirals); Tritamyl flour, brown bread mix and white bread mix; Trufree gluten-free flours No. 1, No. 4 white, No. 5 brown, No. 6 plain, No. 7 self-raising, No. 8 special dietary; Ultra gluten-free baguette, bread, bread rolls, high-fibre bread, crackerbread, pizza base; Valpiform bread mix, country loaf, pastry mix, petites baguettes

Glycogen storage disease: Caloreen; Corn Flour or Corn Starch; Glucose (dextrose); Maxijul LE, Liquid (orange flavour), and Super Soluble; Polycal Liquid and powder; Polycose; Pro-Cal; QuickCal; Vitajoule; Vitasavoury.

Growth Failure (disease related): Fortini, Fortini Multifibre; Frebini; Infatrini; Nutrini Extra, Multifibre and Standard; Paediasure Liquid and Liquid with fibre and Plus; SMA High Energy; Sondalis Junior; Survimed OPD.

Haemodialysis: see dialysis.

Histidinaemia: see low-protein products; synthetic diets.

Homocystinuria: Analog XMet; Methionine-Free Amino Acid Mix; XMet Maxamaid; XMet Maxamum, and see also low-protein products; synthetic diets.

Hyperlipoproteinaemia type I: Alembicol D; Liquigen; Medium Chain Triglyceride Oil.

Hyperlysinaemia: Analog XLys; XLys Maxamaid

Hypermethioninaemia: Analog XMet; Methionine-Free Amino Acid Mix; XMet Maxamaid; XMet Maxamum.

Hypoglycaemia: Corn Flour or Corn Starch; and see also glycogen storage disease.

Hypoproteinaemia: Casilan 90; Dialamine; Maxipro Super Soluble; Maxisorb; ProMod; Protifar; Renapro; Vitapro.

Inflammatory Bowel Disease:

Complete foods: Elemental 028; Elemental 028 Extra; Emsogen; Enrich; Ensure; Ensure Powder; Foodlink Complete; Frebini; Fresubin Energy, Fresubin Energy Fibre (sip and tube feed), Fresubin Liquid and Sip Feeds, Fresubin 1000, and Fresubin 1200 Complete; Isosource Energy, Fibre and Standard; Jevity and Plus; Novasource GI Control, and Forte; Nutrini Extra, and Fibre; Nutrison Multi Fibre, Soya and Standard; Osmolite Liquid and Plus; Peptamen, Sondalis Fibres, ISO, Junior and 1.5.

Nutritional supplements: Clinutren Dessert, ISO, Fruit and 1.5; Enlive; Ensure Plus; Formance; Forticreme;

Fortifresh; Fortijuce; Fortimel; Fortipudding; Fortisip; Fortisip Multi Fibre; Fresubin HP Energy; Nutrison Energy, MCT and Pepti Powder; Perative; Protein Forte; Provide Xtra; Resource Benefiber, Dessert Energy, Protein Extra, and Shake; Survimed OPD.

Intestinal lymphangiectasia: see malabsorption states.

Intestinal surgery: see malabsorption states

Isomaltose intolerance: see carbohydrate malabsorption.

Isovaleric acidaemia: Leucine-Free Amino Acid Mix; XLeu Analog; XLeu Maxamaid.

Lactose intolerance: see carbohydrate malabsorption.

Lipoprotein lipase deficiency (primary and secondary): Monogen

Liver failure: Aglutella low-protein rice; Alembicol D; Aminex low-protein biscuits, cookies and rusks; Aproten products (anellini, biscuits, bread mix, cake mix, crispbread, ditalini, rigatini, spaghetti, tagliatelle); Ener-G low protein egg replacer, rice bread; Generaid; Generaid Plus; Juvela low-protein (chocolate chip, orange, and cinnamon flavour) cookies, loaf (sliced and unsliced), bread rolls, mix; Liquigen; Loprofin egg replacer, egg white replacer; Loprofin low-protein bread (sliced and unsliced), bread rolls (part-baked), white rolls, fibre bread (sliced and unsliced), mix, breakfast cereal, pasta (macaroni, penne, spaghetti long, pasta spirals, vermicelli), sweet biscuits, chocolate cream-filled biscuits, crackers, cookies (chocolate chip, cinnamon), wafers (orange, chocolate, vanilla); Medium Chain Triglyceride Oil; Nepro; Promin low-protein pasta (alphabets, macaroni, shells, shortcut spaghetti, spirals), pasta tricolour (alphabets, shells, spirals), pasta meal, Rite-Diet low-protein baking mix, flour mix; Suplena; Ultra low-protein, canned bread (brown and white); Ultra PKU biscuits, bread, cookies, flour, pizza base and savoy biscuits; Valpiform cookies with chocolate nuggets, shortbread biscuits; Vita-Bite

Long chain acyl-CoA dehydrogenase deficiency (LCAD): Monogen

Low-protein products: Aglutella low-protein rice; Aminex low-protein biscuits, cookies and rusks; Aproten products (anellini, biscuits, bread mix, cake mix, crispbread, ditalini, rigatini, spaghetti, tagliatelle); Ener-G low protein egg replacer, rice bread; Juvela low-protein (chocolate chip, orange, and cinnamon flavour) cookies, loaf (sliced and unsliced), mix, bread rolls; Loprofin egg replacer, egg white replacer; Loprofin low-protein bread (sliced and unsliced), mix, rolls (part-baked), fibre bread (sliced or unsliced), herb crackers, pasta (macaroni, penne, spaghetti long, pasta spirals, vermicelli); sweet biscuits, chocolate cream-filled biscuits, crackers, cookies (chocolate chip, cinnamon), wafers (orange, chocolate, vanilla); breakfast cereal; PKU-Gel; Promin low-protein pasta (alphabets, macaroni, shells, shortcut spaghetti, spirals), pasta tricolour (alphabets, shells, spirals), pasta meal, pasta imitation rice; Rite-Diet low-protein flour mix, baking mix; Ultra low-protein, canned bread (brown and white); Ultra PKU biscuits, bread, cookies, flour, pizza base and savoy biscuits; Valpiform cookies with chocolate nuggets, shortbread biscuits; Vita-Bite

Malabsorption states: (see also gluten-sensitive enteropathies; liver failure; carbohydrate malabsorption; intestinal lymphangiectasia; milk intolerance and synthetic diets; includes short-bowel syndrome. It should be noted that hyperosmolar feeds should be **avoided** if the short bowel ends in a stoma or the short bowel is anastomosed to the colon.

(a) Protein sources: Caprilon Formula; Comminuted Chicken Meat (Cow & Gate); Duocal Super Soluble and Liquid; Maxipro Super Soluble; Maxisorb; MCT Pepdite; Neocate; Neocate Advance; Pepdite.

(b) Fat sources: Alembicol D; Calogen; Caprilon Formula; Liquigen; MCT Pepdite; Medium Chain Triglyceride Oil; Pro-Cal; QuickCal; Vitasavoury.

(c) Carbohydrate: Caloreen; Calsip; Maxijul LE, Liquid, and Super Soluble; Novasource GI Control, and Forte; Nutrini Extra and Multifibre, Polycal Liquid and Pow-

der; Polycose; Pro-Cal; QuickCal; Resource Benefiber; Vitajoule; Vitasavoury.

(d) Fat/carbohydrate sources: Calshake; Duobar; Duocal Liquid, MCT, and Super Soluble; Scandishake; SPS Energy Bar.

(e) Complete Feeds. For use as the sole source of nutrition or as a nutritional supplement prescribed on medical grounds: Caprilon Formula; Complan Ready-to-Drink; Elemental 028; Elemental 028 Extra; Emsogen; Enrich; Ensure; Ensure Powder; Frebini; Fresubin Energy, Fresubin Energy Fibre (sip and tube feed), Fresubin Liquid and Sip Feeds, Fresubin 1000, and Fresubin 1200 Complete; Isosource Energy, Fibre and Standard; Jevity and Plus; MCT Pepdite; Novasource GI Control, and Forte; Nutrini, Extra and Fibre; Nutrison Multi Fibre, Pepti Liquid, Soya and Standard; Osmolite Liquid and Plus; Paediasure Liquid, Liquid with fibre and Plus; Pepdite; Peptamen; Pepti-Junior; Pregestimil; SMA High Energy; Sondalis Fibres, ISO, Junior and 1.5.

(f) Nutritional supplements. Nutritional supplements prescribed on medical grounds: Clinutren Dessert, Fruit, ISO and 1.5; Enlive; Enrich Plus; Ensure Bar and Plus; Formance; Forticreme; Fortifresh; Fortijuce; Fortimel; Fortisip; Fortisip Multi Fibre; Fresubin HP Energy; Nutrison Energy, MCT, and Pepti Powder; Perative; Protenplus; Provide Xtra; Resource Shake and Benefiber; Survimed OPD.

(g) Minerals: Aminogran Mineral Mixture; Metabolic Mineral Mixture.

(h) Vitamins: As appropriate, and see synthetic diets.

(i) Vitamins and Minerals: Energivity, Paediatric Seravit

Malnutrition (disease-related):

Complete foods: Calogen; Caloreen; Calshake; Calsip; Complan Ready-to-Drink; Duobar; Duocal Liquid, MCT, and Super Soluble; Enrich and Plus; Ensure; Ensure Powder; Foodlink Complete; Frebini; Fresubin Energy, Fresubin Energy Fibre (sip and tube feed), Fresubin Liquid and Sip Feeds, Fresubin 1000, and Fresubin 1200 Complete; Infatrini; Isosource Energy, Fibre and Standard; Jevity and Plus; Maxijul LE, Liquid and Super Soluble; Novasource GI Control and Forte; Nutrini Extra, Fibre and Standard; Nutrison Multi Fibre, Soya and Standard; Osmolite Liquid and Plus; Paediasure Liquid, Liquid with fibre and Plus; Polycal Liquid and Powder; Polycose; Scandishake; SMA High Energy; Sondalis Fibres, ISO and 1.5; Vitajoule.

Nutritional supplements: Clinutren Dessert, Fruit, ISO and 1.5; Enlive; Ensure Plus; Formance; Forticreme; Fortifresh; Fortijuce; Fortimel; Fortini, Fortini Multifibre, Fortipudding; Fortisip; Fortisip Multi Fibre; Fresubin HP Energy; Nutrison Energy and MCT; Perative; Provide Xtra; Pro-cal; QuickCal; Resource Benefiber, Dessert Energy, Protein Xtra, and Shake; Survimed OPD; Vitasavoury

Maple syrup urine disease: Analog MSUD; MSUD Maxamaid; MSUD Maxamum; MSUD Aid III, and see also low-protein products; synthetic diets.

Methylmalonic acidaemia: Analog XMet, Thre, Val, Isoleu; XMet, Thre, Val, Isoleu Maxamaid; XMet, Thre, Val, Isoleu Maxamum; Methionine, Threonine, Valine-Free and Isoleucine-Low Amino Acid Mix.

Milk protein sensitivity: Comminuted Chicken Meat (SHS); Farley's Soya Formula; InfaSoy; Isomil powder; Nutramigen; Prosobee; Wysoy, and see also synthetic diets.

Nutritional support for adults

A. **Nutritionally complete feeds.** For use as the sole source of nutrition or as a necessary nutritional supplement prescribed on medical grounds:

(i) Gluten-Free: Foodlink Complete; Fortifresh; Fresubin Liquid and Sip Feeds; Nutrison Energy, Multi Fibre and Standard; Sondalis 1S0 and Junior.

(ii) Lactose- and Gluten-Free: Enrich; Ensure, Ensure Powder; Fresubin Isofibre; Nutrison Soya; Osmolite Liquid and Plus, Sondalis 1.5.

(iii) Containing fibre: Enrich; Fresubin Energy fibre (tube and sip feed), Fresubin Isofibre; Isosource Fibre; Jevity; Novasource GI Control, and Forte; Nutrini Extra and

Fibre; Nutrison Multi Fibre; Paediasure with Fibre; Sondalis Fibre.

(iv) Elemental Feeds: Elemental 028; Elemental 028 Extra; Emsogen; Peptamen, Peptisorb.

B. **Nutritional source supplements**: see synthetic diets; malabsorption states.

(a) General supplements. Necessary nutritional supplements prescribed on medical grounds: Clinutren range; Enlive; Enrich Plus; Ensure Plus; Foodlink Complete; Formance; Forticreme; Fortijuce; Fortimel; Fortini, Fortini MultiFibre; Fortisip; Fortisip Multi Fibre; Fresubin HP Energy; Fresubin 1000, and 1200 Complete; Maxisorb; Nutrison Energy and MCT; Perative; Protein Forte; Provide Xtra; Resource Shake; Survimed OPD.

(b) Carbohydrates: lactose-free and gluten-free; Caloreen*; Calsip, Maxijul LE*, Liquid, and Super Soluble; Polycal*; Polycal Liquid*; Polycose; Pro-Cal; Quick-Cal; Resource Benefiber; Vitajoule; Vitasavoury.
*Have low electrolyte content.

(c) Fat: Alembicol D; Calogen; Liquigen; MCT Oil.

(d) Fat/carbohydrate sources: Calshake; Duobar; Duocal Liquid, MCT Powder and Super Soluble (low-electrolyte content); Scandishake, SPS Energy Bar.

(e) Nitrogen sources: Casilan 90 (whole protein based, low-sodium); Maxipro Super Soluble (whey protein based, low-sodium); Maxisorb; Pro-Mod (whey protein based, low-sodium).

(f) Minerals: Aminogran Mineral Mixture; Metabolic Mineral Mixture.

Phenylketonuria: Aglutella low-protein rice; Aminex low-protein biscuits, cookies and rusks; Aminogran Food Supplement (powder and tablets) and Mineral Mixture; Analog LCP; Analog XP; Aproten products (annellini, biscuits, bread mix, cake mix, crispbread, ditalini, rigatini, spaghetti, tagliatelle); Ener-G low protein egg replacer; Juvela low-protein loaf (sliced and unsliced), bread rolls, cookies (chocolate chip, orange, and cinnamon flavour), mix; Lofenalac; Loprofin egg replacer; Loprofin low-protein bread (sliced and unsliced), breakfast cereal, rolls (part-baked), rolls (white), fibre bread (sliced and unsliced), mix and pasta (macaroni, penne, spaghetti long, pasta spirals, vermicelli), sweet biscuits, chocolate cream-filled biscuits, crackers, cookies (chocolate chip, cinnamon), wafers (orange, chocolate, vanilla); Loprofin PKU drink; Metabolic Mineral Mixture; Milupa PKU2 and PKU3; Phlexy-10 exchange system; Phlexyvits; PK Aid 4; PKU-Gel; Promin low-protein pasta (alphabets, macaroni, shells, shortcut spaghetti, spirals), pasta tricolour (alphabets, shells, spirals), pasta meal; Rite-Diet low-protein baking mix, flour mix; Sno-Pro; L-Tyrosine supplement; Ultra low-protein, canned white bread; Ultra PKU biscuits, bread, cookies, flour, pizza base, savoy biscuits; Valpiform cookies, shortbread biscuits; XP Maxamaid XP Concentrate Maxamaid; XP Maxamum; and see low-protein products and synthetic diets

Propionic acidaemia: Analog XMet, Thre, Val, Isoleu; XMet, Thre, Val, Isoleu Maxamaid; XMet Thre, Val, Isoleu Maxamum; Methionine, Threonine, Valine-Free and Isoleucine-Low Amino Acid Mix.

Protein intolerance: see amino acid metabolic disorders, low-protein products, milk protein sensitivity, synthetic diets, and whole protein sensitivity.

Refsum's Disease: Fresubin Liquid and Sip Feeds.

Renal dialysis: see Dialysis.

Renal failure: Aglutella low-protein rice; Aminex low-protein biscuits, cookies and rusks; Aproten products (annellini, biscuits, bread mix, cake mix, crispbread, ditalini, rigatini, spaghetti, tagliatelle); Dialamine; Ener-G low protein egg replacer, rice bread; Juvela low-protein (chocolate chip, orange, and cinnamon flavour) cookies, loaf (sliced and unsliced), bread rolls and flour mix; Kindergen; Loprofin egg replacer, egg white replacer, Loprofin bread (sliced and unsliced), breakfast cereal, rolls (part-baked), rolls (white), fibre bread (sliced and unsliced), mix and pasta (macaroni, penne, spaghetti long, pasta spirals, vermicelli), sweet biscuits, chocolate cream-filled biscuits, crackers, cookies (chocolate chip, cinnamon), wafers (orange, chocolate,

vanilla); Nepro; Promin low-protein pasta (alphabets, macaroni, shells, shortcut spaghetti, spirals), pasta tricolour (alphabets, shells, spirals), pasta meal; Renamil; Rite-Diet low-protein flour mix, baking mix, Sno-Pro Drink; Suplena; Ultra low-protein, canned bread (brown and white); Ultra PKU bread, biscuits, cookies, flour, pizza base and savoy biscuits; Valpiform cookies with chocolate nuggets, shortbread biscuits, Vita-Bite

Short-bowel syndrome: see Malabsorption states.

Sicca Syndrome: Glandosane; Luborant; Oralbalance; Saliva Orthana; Salivace; Saliveze; Salivix.

Sucrose intolerance: see Carbohydrate malabsorption.

Synthetic diets:

(a) Fat: Alembicol D; Calogen; Liquigen; Medium Chain Triglyceride Oil; Pro-Cal; QuickCal; Vitasavoury.

(b) Carbohydrate: Caloreen; Calsip; Maxijul LE, Liquid, Super Soluble; Polycal; Polycal Liquid; Polycose powder; Pro-Cal; QuickCal; Vitajoule; Vitasavoury.

(c) Fat/carbohydrate sources: Calshake; Duobar; Duocal Liquid, MCT Powder and Super Soluble (low-electrolyte content); Scandishake.

(d) Minerals: Aminogran Mineral Mixture; Metabolic Mineral Mixture.

(e) Protein sources: see malabsorption states, complete feeds.

(f) Vitamins: as appropriate and see malabsorption states, nutritional support for adults.

(g) Vitamins and Minerals: Paediatric Seravit; Phlexyvits.

Tyrosinaemia: Analog XPhen, Tyr; Analog XPhen, Tyr, Met; XPhen, Tyr Maxamaid; XPTM Tyrosidon; XPT Tyrosidon.

Urea cycle disorders: L-Arginine supplement

Vomiting in infancy: Instant Carobel, Nestargel.

Whole protein sensitivity: Caprilon Formula; MCT Pepdite; Neocate; Neocate Advance; Nutramigen; Pepdite; Pepti-Junior; Pregestimil; Prejomin.
Note. Defined as intolerance to whole protein, proven by at least two withdrawal and challenge tests, as suggested by an accurate dietary history

Xerostomia: Glandosane; Luborant; Oralbalance Dry Mouth Saliva Replacement Gel; Saliva Orthana; Salivace; Saliveze; Salivix.

Conditions for which toilet preparations may be prescribed on FP10 (GP10 in Scotland)

Note. This is a list of clinical conditions for which the ACBS has approved toilet preparations. For details of the preparations see Chapter 13.

Birthmarks: see disfiguring skin lesions.

Dermatitis: Aveeno Bath Oil; Aveeno Cream; Aveeno Colloidal; Aveeno Colloidal Baby; E45 Emollient Bath Oil; E45 Emollient Wash Cream; E45 Lotion; Vaseline Dermacare Cream and Lotion.

Dermatitis herpetiformis: see gluten-sensitive enteropathies.

Disfiguring skin lesions (birthmarks, mutilating lesions, scars, vitiligo): Covermark classic foundation and finishing powder; Dermablend Cover Creme, Leg and Body Cover, and Setting Powder; Dermacolor Camouflage cream and fixing powder; Keromask masking cream and finishing powder; Veil Cover cream and Finishing Powder. (Cleansing Creams, Cleansing Milks, and Cleansing Lotions are excluded.)

Eczema: see dermatitis.

Photodermatoses (skin protection in): Ambre Solaire Total Screen for Sun Intolerant skin SPF 60; Coppertone Ultrashade 23; Delph Sun Lotion SPF 15, SPF 20, SPF 25, and SPF 30; E45 Sun Block SPF 25, and 50; RoC Total Sunblock Cream SPF 25; Spectraban 25, and Ultra; Sunsense Ultra; Uvistat Sun Block Cream Factor 20, and Ultrablock Suncream Factor 30.

Pruritus: see dermatitis.

Appendix 8: Wound management products and elastic hosiery

A8.1 Wound dressings

An overview of the management of *chronic wounds* (including venous ulcers and pressure sores) and the role of different dressings is given below as is the NICE guidance on difficult-to-heal surgical wounds; the notes do not deal with the management of clean surgical wounds which usually heal very rapidly. The correct dressing for wound management depends not only on the type of wound but also on the stage of the healing process. The principal stages of healing are:
- cleansing, removal of debris;
- granulation, vascularisation;
- epithelialisation.

Greater understanding of the requirements of a surgical dressing, including recognition of the benefits of maintaining a moist environment for wound healing, has improved the management of chronic wounds.

The ideal dressing needs to ensure that the wound remains:
- moist with exudate, but not macerated;
- free of clinical infection and excessive slough;
- free of toxic chemicals, particles or fibres;
- at the optimum temperature for healing;
- undisturbed by the need for frequent changes;
- at the optimum pH value.

As wound healing passes through its different stages, variations in dressing type may be required to satisfy better one or other of these requirements. Depending on the type of wound or the stage of the healing process, the functions of dressings may be summarised as follows:

Type of wound	Role of dressing
Dry, necrotic, black	Moisture retention or rehydration
Yellow, sloughy	If dry, moisture retention or rehydration
	If moist, fluid absorption
	Possibly odour absorption
	Possibly antimicrobial activity
Clean, exuding (granulating)	Fluid absorption
	Thermal insulation
	Possibly odour absorption
	Possibly antimicrobial activity
Dry, low exudate (epithelialising)	Moisture retention or rehydration
	Low adherence
	Thermal insulation

A decrease in pain and reduction in healing time is achieved to a marked extent with **alginate**, **foam**, **hydrogel** and **hydrocolloid** dressings and also to an important extent with **vapour-permeable films** and **membranes**; dressings such as dry gauze have little place. Practices such as the use of irritant cleansers may be harmful and are largely obsolete; removal of debris and dressing remnants should need minimal irrigation with physiological saline.

Alginate, **foam**, **hydrogel** and **hydrocolloid** dressings are designed to absorb wound exudate and thus to control the state of hydration of a wound. All are claimed to be effective, but as yet there have been few trials able to establish a clear advantage for any particular product. The choice between different dressings may therefore often depend not only on the type and stage of the wound, but also on personal experience, availability of the dressing, patient preference or tolerance and site of the wound.

> **NICE guidance (debriding agents for difficult-to-heal surgical wounds).** The National Institute for Clinical Excellence has stated that alginate, foam, hydrocolloid, hydrogel, and polysaccharide (as beads or paste) dressings as well as maggots may reduce pain from difficult-to-heal surgical wounds. There is insufficient evidence to support one debriding agent over another and choice should be based on patient acceptability (including factors such as comfort and odour control), type and location of the wound, and total cost (including time for changing the dressings).

A8.1.1 Alginate dressings

The gelling characteristics of alginate dressings vary according to the product used. Some products only gel to a limited extent to form a partially gelled sheet that can be lifted off; others form an amorphous gel that can be rinsed off with water or physiological saline. A secondary covering is needed. They are highly absorbent and are therefore suitable for moderately or heavily exuding wounds, but not for eschars or for dry wounds.

Algisite® M Calcium alginate fibre, sterile, flat non-woven dressing, net price 5 cm × 5 cm = 76p, 10 cm × 10 cm = £1.57, 15 cm × 20 cm = £4.21 (S&N Hlth)

Uses: moderately to heavily exuding wounds

Algisite® M Rope, net price 2 cm × 30 cm = £2.80 (S&N Hlth)

Uses: moderately to heavily exuding cavity wounds

Algosteril® Calcium alginate dressing. Net price 5 cm × 5 cm, 1 = 75p; 10 cm × 10 cm, 1 = £1.72; 10 cm × 20 cm, 1 = £2.91 (Beiersdorf)

Uses: moderately to heavily exuding wounds

Algosteril® Rope, net price 2 g, 30 cm = £3.05 (Beiersdorf)

Uses: moderately to heavily exuding cavity wounds

Kaltostat® (Alginate Dressing, BP 1993, type C). Calcium alginate fibre, flat non-woven pads, 5 cm × 5 cm, net price = 78p; 7.5 cm × 12 cm = £1.70; 10 cm × 20 cm = £3.31; 15 cm × 25 cm = £5.69; (NHS) 30 cm × 60 cm = £24.68 (ConvaTec)

Uses: moderately to heavily exuding wounds

Kaltostat® Wound Packing, net price 2 g = £3.11 (ConvaTec)

Uses: moderately to heavily exuding cavity wounds

Melgisorb® Calcium sodium alginate fibre, sterile, highly absorbent, gelling dressing, flat non-woven pads, net price 5 cm × 5 cm = 75p, 10 cm × 10 cm = £1.56, 10 cm × 20 cm = £2.93 (Mölnlycke)

Uses: moderately to heavily exuding wounds including leg ulcers, dermal lesions and traumatic wounds

Melgisorb® Cavity, calcium sodium alginate fibre, sterile, highly absorbent, gelling filler ribbon, net price 32 cm × 2.2 cm, 3 pieces (2 g) = £2.90 (Mölnlycke)

Uses: moderately to heavily exuding cavity wounds, fistulas, sinuses, pressure sores and deep leg ulcers

SeaSorb® (Alginate Dressing, BP 1993), calcium sodium alginate fibre, sterile, highly absorbent, gelling dressing, 4 cm × 6 cm = 76p; 10 cm × 10 cm = £1.58; 15 cm × 15 cm = £3.27 (Coloplast)

Uses: heavily exuding wounds including leg ulcers and pressure sores

SeaSorb® Filler, calcium sodium alginate fibre, highly absorbent, gelling filler, 2 g = £3.11 (Coloplast)

Uses: moderately to heavily exuding cavity wounds, fistulas, sinus drainage, decubitus and deep leg ulcers

Sorbalgon® Calcium alginate dressing, net price 5 cm × 5 cm = 70p, 10 cm × 10 cm = £1.47 (Hartman)

Uses: for medium to heavily exuding wounds

Sorbalgon T®, calcium alginate cavity dressing, net price 2 g, 32 cm = £3.00 (Hartman)

Uses: for medium to heavily exuding wounds

Sorbsan® (Alginate Dressing, BP 1993, type A). Calcium alginate fibre, highly absorbent, flat non-woven pads, 5 cm × 5 cm, net price = 70p; 10 cm × 10 cm = £1.50; 10 cm × 20 cm = £2.85 (Maersk)

Uses: moderately to heavily exuding wounds

Sorbsan® Plus, alginate dressing bonded to a secondary absorbent viscose pad, net price 7.5 cm × 10 cm = £1.51; 10 cm × 15 cm = £2.67; 10 cm × 20 cm = £3.41; 15 cm × 20 cm = £4.73 (Maersk)

Uses: moderately to heavily exuding shallow wounds and ulcers

Sorbsan® Surgical Packing, 30 cm (2 g) = £3.11 (Maersk)

Sorbsan® Ribbon, 40 cm (with 12.5-cm probe) = £1.81 (Maersk)

Uses: moderately to heavily exuding cavity wounds

Sorbsan® SA NHS calcium alginate fibre, highly absorbent flat non-woven pads for wound contact bonded to adhesive semi-permeable polyurethane foam. Net price 9 cm × 11 cm = £2.24 (Maersk)

Uses: moderately to lightly exuding shallow wounds

Tegagen® (Alginate Dressing, BP 1993, type B). Net price 5 cm × 5 cm = 71p; 10 cm × 10 cm = £1.50 (3M)

Uses: for leg ulcers, pressure sores, second degree burns, post-operative wounds, fungating carcinomas

Tegagen® Rope, net price 2 cm × 30 cm = £2.50 (3M)

Uses: moderately to heavily exudating cavity wounds

A8.1.2 Foam dressings

Foam dressings vary from products that are suitable for lightly exuding wounds to highly absorbent structures for heavily exuding wounds. They may also be used as secondary dressings. In hypergranulating (or overgranulating) tissue (which may arise from the use of occlusive dressings such as hydrocolloids), changing to a more permeable product such as a foam dressing may be beneficial.

Polyurethane Foam Dressing, BP 1993 Absorbent foam dressing of low adherence, sterile, 7.5 cm × 7.5 cm, net price = 93p; 10 cm × 10 cm = £1.11; 10 cm × 17.5 cm = £1.72; 15 cm × 20 cm = £2.32; other sizes (NHS) 10 cm × 25 cm = £4.71; 25 cm × 30 cm = £11.15 (SSL—Lyofoam®)

Uses: treatment of burns, decubitus ulcers, donor sites, granulating wounds

Allevyn® (Drug Tariff title: Polyurethane Foam Film Dressing, Drug Tariff specification 47) Hydrophilic polyurethane dressing, foam sheets with trilaminate structure, non-adherent wound contact layer, foam based central layer, bacteria- and water-proof outer layer (S&N Hlth)

Allevyn® (without adhesive border), 5 cm × 5 cm = £1.04; 9 cm × 9 cm = £2.88 NHS ; 10 cm × 10 cm = £2.06; 10 cm × 20 cm = £3.32; 20 cm × 20 cm = £5.54

Uses: light to moderately exuding wounds

Allevyn® Adhesive (with adhesive border), 7.5 cm × 7.5 cm = £1.23; 12.5 cm × 12.5 cm = £2.21; 17.5 cm × 17.5 cm = £4.36; 12.5 cm × 22.5 cm = £3.44; 22.5 cm × 22.5 cm = £6.35

Uses: light to moderately exuding wounds

Allevyn® LM (without adhesive border), 5 cm × 5 cm = 93p; 10 cm × 10 cm = £1.68; 10 cm × 20 cm = £2.88; 15 cm × 20 cm = £3.59

Uses: light to moderately exuding wounds

Allevyn® Cavity, circular, 5 cm diameter = £3.40; 10 cm = £8.10; tubular 9 cm × 2.5 cm = £3.29; 12 cm × 4 cm = £5.80

Uses: moderately to heavily exuding cavity wounds including deep pressure sores and leg ulcers, surgical inisions and excisions such as pilonidal sinus excisions

Allevyn® Heel (without adhesive border), shaped, 10.5 cm × 13.5 cm = £4.14

Uses: light to moderately exuding heel wounds

Allevyn® Sacrum (with adhesive border), shaped, 17 cm × 17 cm = £3.25; 22 cm × 22 cm = £4.76

Uses: light to moderately exuding sacral wounds

Askina® Transorbent Sterile, adhesive, polyurethane foam film dressing (with a hydrocolloid layer), net price, 5 cm × 7 cm = 91p, 10 cm × 10 cm = £1.72, 15 cm × 15 cm = £3.16, 20 cm × 20 cm = £5.05 (Braun)

Avance®

Silver impregnated polyurethane foam film dressing (SSL)

Avance® (without adhesive border), 10 cm × 10 cm = £2.55; 10 cm × 17 cm = £4.06; 15 cm × 20 cm = £5.61

Avance®A (with adhesive border), 9 cm × 9 cm = £2.14; 12 cm × 12 cm = £3.55; 15 cm × 15 cm = £4.35; 13 cm (sacral) = £3.20

Uses: for exudating wounds

Biatain® Sterile, polyurethane foam film dressing, non-adhesive, net price 10 cm × 10 cm = £1.97; 15 cm × 15 cm = £3.62; 20 cm × 20 cm = £5.40; circular, 5 cm diameter = £1.02; 8 cm diameter = £1.42; with hydrocolloid adhesive border 12 cm × 12 cm = £2.13; 18 cm × 18 cm = £4.27; 23 cm × 23 cm (sacral) = £3.65; 19 cm × 20 cm (heel) = £4.26; 6 cm diameter = £1.45 (Coloplast)

Uses: moderate to heavily exuding, leg ulcers, pressure sores, diabetic ulcers

Cavi-Care® Soft, conforming cavity wound dressing prepared by mixing thoroughly for 15 seconds immediately before use and allowing to expand its volume within the cavity. Net price 20 g = £16.03 (S&N Hlth)

Uses: in the management of open post-operative granulating cavity wounds (with no underlying tracts or sinuses) such as pilonidal sinus excision, dehisced surgical wounds, hydradenitis suppurativa wounds, perianal wounds, perineal wounds, pressure sores

FlexiPore® Sterile, semi-permeable, polyurethane foam film adhesive dressing. Net price, 10 cm × 10 cm = £1.73; 20 cm × 20 cm = £5.06; 6 cm × 7 cm = 93p; 10 cm × 30 cm = £3.60; 15 cm × 20 cm = £3.70 (TSL)

Uses: treatment of light to moderately exuding wounds, leg ulcers, pressure sores

Lyofoam® Polyurethane foam dressing, sterile—see also Polyurethane Foam Dressing, BP (1993) and section A8.1.7 (*Lyofoam C®*) (SSL)

Lyofoam Extra® extra absorbent polyurethane foam dressing, non-adhesive, net price 10 cm × 10 cm = £1.85; 17.5 cm × 10 cm = £3.12; 20 cm × 15 cm = £4.04; 25 cm × 10 cm = £3.78; (𝐍𝐇𝐒) 30 cm × 25 cm = £14.35; with adhesive border, 9 cm × 9 cm = £1.16; 15 cm × 15 cm = £2.17; 22 cm × 22 cm = £4.29; 30 cm × 30 cm = £6.23; sacral, 15 cm × 13 cm = £1.78; 22 cm × 26 cm = £3.38 (SSL)

Lyofoam K® (with adhesive border), 9 cm × 9 cm = £1.24 (SSL)

Uses: treatment of light to moderately exuding wounds

Spyrosorb® (Drug Tariff title: Polyurethane Foam Film Dressing, Drug Tariff specification 47, type 1). Sterile, semipermeable, absorbent polyurethane membrane with polyurethane film and hydrophilic adhesive. Net price 10 cm × 10 cm = £2.09; 20 cm × 20 cm = £5.96 (S&N Hlth).

Uses: light to moderately exuding wounds

Tielle® (Drug Tariff title: Polyurethane Foam Film Dressing with Adhesive Margin, Drug Tariff specification 47). Semi-permeable, foamed gel with non-woven wicking layer and polyurethane backing layer. Net price 11 cm × 11 cm = £2.10; 15 cm × 15 cm = £3.43; 18 cm × 18 cm = £4.37; 7 cm × 9 cm = £1.13; 15 cm × 20 cm = £4.29; *Tielle® Sacrum* 18 cm × 18 cm = £3.17 (J&J)

Uses: light to moderately exuding wounds, leg ulcers

Tielle® Lite (Drug Tariff title: Polyurethane Foam Film Dressing), net price 11 cm × 11 cm = £2.01; 7 cm × 9 cm = £1.07; 8 cm × 15 cm = £2.48; 8 cm × 20 cm = £2.62 (J&J)

Uses: light to non-exuding wounds

Tielle® Plus (Drug Tariff title: Polyurethane Foam Film Dressing with Adhesive Border), net price 11 cm × 11 cm = £2.32; 15 cm × 15 cm = £3.79; 15 cm × 20 cm = £4.75; 15 cm × 15 cm (sacrum) = £2.81 (J&J)

Tielle® Plus Borderless (Drug Tariff title: Polyurethane Foam Film Dressing without Adhesive Border), net price 11 cm × 11 cm = £2.79 (J&J)

Uses: moderate to heavily exuding wounds

A8.1.3 Hydrogel dressings

Hydrogel dressings are most commonly supplied as an amorphous, cohesive material that can take up the shape of a wound. A secondary covering is needed. These dressings are generally used to donate liquid to dry sloughy wounds and facilitate autolytic debridement but they may also have the ability to absorb limited amounts of exudate. Hydrogel sheets are also available which have a fixed structure; such products have limited fluid handling capacity. Hydrogel sheets are best avoided in the presence of infection.

Aquaform® (Drug Tariff specification 50) Hydrogel containing modified starch copolymer. Net price 15 g = £1.74 (Maersk)

Uses: for dry, sloughy or necrotic wounds, lightly exuding wounds, granulating wounds

Debrisan®

Beads, dextranomer. Net price 60-g castor = £29.01 (Pharmacia)

Uses: for exudative and infected wounds, decubital ulcers, leg ulcers, hand burns, surgical wounds, post-traumatic wounds, sprinkle onto wound to a thickness of at least 3 mm and cover with appropriate dressing, renew before saturation occurs (usually once or twice daily)

Paste, dextranomer in a soft paste basis. Net price 10-g pouch = £4.99 (Pharmacia)

Uses: for exudative and infected wounds, decubital ulcers, leg ulcers, surgical wounds, post-traumatic wounds, apply to a thickness of at least 3 mm and cover with appropriate dressing, renew before saturation occurs (usually once or twice daily)

Geliperm® Gel sheets in wet form, 10 cm × 10 cm = £2.15, 12 cm × 13cm = £4.88 (𝐍𝐇𝐒); 12 cm × 26 cm = £8.73 (𝐍𝐇𝐒) (Geistlich)

Uses: wound and ulcer dressing, burns, donor sites

GranuGel® (Drug Tariff Specification 50). Net price 15 g = £1.91 (ConvaTec)

Uses: dry, sloughy or necrotic wounds, lightly exuding wounds, granulating wounds

Hydrosorb®

Absorbent, transparent, hydrogel sheets containing polyurethane polymers covered with a semi-permeable film (Hartmann)

Hydrosorb®, 5 cm × 7.5 cm = £1.74, 10 cm × 10 cm = £2.74; 20 cm × 20 cm = £6.60

Hydrosorb® comfort (with adhesive border, waterproof), 4.5 cm × 6.5 cm = £1.60; 7.5 cm × 10 cm = £2.50; 12.5 cm × 12.5 cm = £3.60

Uses: second degree burns, donor sites; chronic wounds where granulation is unsatisfactory, including leg ulcers, pressure sores

Intrasite Conformable® (Drug Tariff specification 50). Soft and easily moulded non-woven dressing impregnated with Intrasite gel, net price 10 cm × 10 cm = £1.46; 10 cm × 20 cm = £1.96; 10 cm × 40 cm = £3.51 (S&N Hlth)

Uses: for dry, sloughy or necrotic wounds, lightly exudating wounds; granulating wounds

Intrasite® Gel (Drug Tariff specification 50). A ready-mixed hydrogel containing modified carmellose polymer applied directly into the wound. Net price 8-g sachet = £1.46; 15-g sachet = £1.95; ([NHS]) 25-g sachet = £4.11 (S&N Hlth)

Uses: for dry, sloughy or necrotic wounds; lightly exuding wounds; granulating wounds

Iodoflex®

Paste, iodine 0.9% as cadexomer–iodine in a paste basis with gauze backing, net price 5-g unit = £3.90; 10-g = £7.80; 17-g = £12.34 (S&N Hlth)

Uses: for treatment of chronic exuding wounds, such as leg ulcers, apply to wound surface, remove gauze backing and cover; renew when saturated (usually 2–3 times weekly, daily for heavily exuding wounds); max. single application 50 g, max. weekly application 150 g; max. duration up to 3 months in any single course of treatment

Cautions; Contra-indications: avoid in thyroid disorders, in those receiving lithium, in pregnancy and breast-feeding and use in children; caution in patients with severe renal impairment or history of thyroid disorders; iodine may be absorbed particularly if large wounds treated

Iodosorb®

Ointment, iodine 0.9% as cadexomer–iodine in an ointment basis, net price 10 g = £4.31; 20 g = £8.62 (S&N Hlth)

Powder, iodine 0.9% as cadexomer–iodine microbeads, net price 3-g sachet = £1.84 (S&N Hlth)

Uses: for treatment of chronic exuding wounds, such as leg ulcers, apply to wound surface to depth of approx. 3 mm and cover; renew when saturated (usually 2-3 times weekly, daily for heavily exuding wounds); max. single application 50 g, max. weekly application 150 g; max. duration up to 3 months in any single course of treatment

Cautions; Contra-indications: avoid in thyroid disorders, in those receiving lithium, in pregnancy and breast-feeding, and use in children; caution in patients with severe renal impairment or history of thyroid disorders; iodine may be absorbed particularly if large wounds treated

Novogel® Sterile, glycerol-based hydrogel sheets, net price 10 cm × 10 cm = £2.80; 30 cm × 30 cm, standard = £11.85, thin = £11.19; 5 cm × 7.5 cm = £1.78; 15 cm × 20 cm = £5.34; 20 cm × 40 cm = £10.18; 7.5 cm diameter = £2.54 (Ford)

Uses: diabetic wounds, burns, leg ulcers, decubitus ulcers, donor sites

Nu-Gel® (Drug Tariff specification 50). A ready-mixed hydrogel containing alginate, applied directly into wound and covered with secondary dressing. Net price 15 g = £1.85 (J&J)

Uses: dry, sloughy or necrotic, lightly exuding or granulating wounds

Purilon® Gel (Drug Tariff specification 50). Net price 8 g = £1.42, 15 g = £1.88 (Coloplast)

Uses: for dry, sloughy or necrotic wounds; lightly exuding wounds; granulating wounds

Sterigel® (Drug Tariff Specification 50). A ready-mixed hydrogel, applied directly into wound and covered with secondary dressing. Net price 8 g = £1.43; 15 g = £1.88 (SSL)

Uses: dry, sloughy or necrotic, lightly exuding or granulating wounds

Hydrocolloid dressings

Hydrocolloid dressings are usually presented as an absorbent layer on a vapour-permeable film or foam. Because of their impermeable nature, hydrocolloid dressings facilitate rehydration and autolytic debridement of dry, sloughy, or necrotic wounds; they are also suitable for promoting granulation. Fibrous dressings made from modified carmellose fibres resemble alginate dressings (e.g. *Aquacel*®); these are not occlusive.

Aquacel® , Soft sterile non-woven pad containing hydrocolloid fibres, net price 5 cm × 5 cm = 95p; 10 cm × 10 cm = £2.27; 15 cm × 15 cm = £4.28 (ConvaTec)

Uses: moderately to heavily exuding wounds

Aquacel® Ribbon, 2 cm × 45 cm = £2.28 (ConvaTec)

Uses: moderately to heavily exuding cavity wounds

Askina® **Biofilm Transparent** Sterile, semi-permeable, polyurethane film dressing with hydrocolloid adhesive, net price, 10 cm × 10 cm = 95p; 15 cm × 15 cm = £2.15, 20 cm × 20 cm = £2.81 (Braun)

Biofilm S® [NHS] Hydrocolloid dressing with polyurethane-polyester backing; also in powder form for direct application into wound, 10 cm × 10 cm, net price = £1.65; 20 cm × 20 cm = £5.70; *Biofilm*® powder, 1 sachet = £1.82 (Braun)

CombiDERM® Dressing with hydrocolloid adhesive border and absorbent wound contact pad, net price 10 cm × 10 cm = £1.34; 14 cm × 14 cm = £1.87; 15 cm × 18 cm (triangular) = £3.22; 20 cm × 20 cm = £3.58; 20 cm × 23 cm (triangular) = £4.32 (ConvaTec)

Uses: chronic exuding wounds such as leg ulcers, pressure sores; postoperative wounds

CombiDERM N® Hydrocolloid absorbent dressing, net price 7.5 cm × 7.5 cm = £1.05; 14 cm × 14 cm = £1.87; 15 cm × 25 cm = £3.82

Uses: chronic wounds (e.g. leg ulcers and diabetic ulcers) and exuding wounds (e.g. biopsies), and surgical wounds

Comfeel® Soft elastic pad consisting of carmellose sodium particles embedded in adhesive mass; smooth outer layer and polyurethane film backing; available as sheets, powder in plastic blister units and paste for direct application into the wound: Ulcer dressing, net price 10 cm × 10 cm = £2.25; 15 cm × 15 cm = £4.50; 20 cm × 20 cm = £6.89; other sizes ([NHS]): 4 cm × 6 cm = £1.15; powder 6 g = £3.90; paste 12-g sachet = £1.50; 50 g = £5.78 (Coloplast)

Comfeel® **Plus** Hydrocolloid dressings containing carmellose sodium and calcium alginate. Contour dressing 6 cm × 8 cm = £1.82; 9 cm × 11 cm = £3.17; Ulcer Dressing, 4 cm × 6 cm = £1.00; 10 cm × 10 cm = £2.35; 15 cm × 15 cm = £4.68; 18 cm × 20 cm (triangular) = £4.64; 20 cm × 20 cm = £7.02; Transparent Dressing, 5 cm × 7 cm = 55p; 9 cm × 14 cm = £2.00; 15 cm × 20 cm = £2.78; [NHS] Pressure Relieving Dressing, 7 cm × 7 cm = £4.05; 10 cm × 10 cm = £4.05; 15 cm × 15 cm = £8.36 (Coloplast)

Cutinova® *Foam,* net price 5 cm × 6 cm = £1.03; 10 cm × 10 cm = £2.21; 15 cm × 20 cm = £4.02 (Beiersdorf)

Uses: moderately exuding wounds, burns, decubitus ulcers, and leg ulcers

Cutinova® Cavity Sterile, highly absorbent polyurethane dressing consisting of a vapour-permeable foam matrix, net price 5 cm × 6 cm = £1.53; 10 cm × 10 cm = £2.54; 15 cm × 20 cm = £5.09 (Beiersdorf)

Uses: heavily exuding deep wounds, including deep leg ulcers, decubitus ulcers, abscesses; management of post-operative wounds including pilonidal sinus excision

Cutinova® Hydro Sterile, highly absorbent semi-transparent two-layered polyurethane dressing with vapour-permeable foam matrix on a semi-permeable film backing, net price 5 cm × 6 cm = £1.02; 10 cm × 10 cm = £2.05; 15 cm × 20 cm = £4.34 (Beiersdorf)

Uses: moderately to heavily exuding wounds including burns and decubitus ulcers

Cutinova® Thin [NHS] Sterile, highly absorbent, semi-transparent two-layered polyurethane dressing with two-layered vapour-permeable foam matrix on a semi-permeable film backing, net price 5 cm × 6 cm = £1.16; 10 cm × 10 cm = £1.87; 15 cm × 20 cm = £5.13 (Beiersdorf)

Uses: lightly exuding wounds including abrasions, burns, decubitus ulcers, donor sites, skin protection and post-operative wounds

DuoDERM® Extra Thin (formerly Granuflex® ExtraThin), 5 cm × 10 cm = 62p; 7.5 cm × 7.5 cm = 65p; 10 cm × 10 cm = £1.08; 15 cm × 15 cm = £2.30; [NHS] 5 cm × 20 cm = £1.38 (ConvaTec)

Uses: for minimally exuding wounds, such as abrasions, minor burns or minor surgery

Granuflex® Hydrocolloid wound contact layer bonded to plastic foam layer, with outer semipermeable polyurethane film, net price 10 cm × 10 cm = £2.29; 15 cm × 15 cm = £4.35; 15 cm × 20 cm = £4.72; 20 cm × 20 cm = £6.55; [NHS] 20 cm × 30 cm = £11.15 (ConvaTec)

Granuflex® Paste ([NHS]), net price 30 g = £2.68 (ConvaTec)

Granuflex® Bordered Dressing, 6 cm × 6 cm = £1.43; 10 cm × 10 cm = £2.73; 15 cm × 15 cm = £5.17; triangular dressing, 10 cm × 13 cm = £3.23; 15 cm × 18 cm = £5.03 (ConvaTec)

Uses: chronic ulcers, pressure sores, open wounds, debridement of wounds; powders, gel, and pastes used with sheet dressings to fill deep or heavily exuding wounds

Hydrocoll® Hydrocolloid dressing with adhesive border and absorbent wound contact pad, net price 5 cm × 5 cm = 87p; 7.5 cm × 7.5 cm = £1.43; 10 cm × 10 cm = £2.08; 15 cm × 15 cm = £3.91; Contour dressing, 6 cm × 14 cm = £1.83; Sacral dressing, 15 cm × 18 cm = £3.11; Basic dressing without adhesive border, 10 cm × 10 cm = £2.11; 15 cm × 20 cm = £4.49; 20 cm × 20 cm = £6.19; Thin film dressing, 7.5 cm × 7.5 cm = 60p; 10 cm × 10 cm = 99p, 15 cm × 15 cm = £2.24 (Hartmann)

Uses: light to medium exuding wounds

Replicare Ultra® Sterile, adhesive hydrocolloid dressing with outer semipermeable polyurethane film backing, net price 10 cm × 10 cm = £2.13, 15 cm × 15 cm = £4.24, 20 cm × 20 cm = £6.26; Sacral dressing, 15 cm × 18 cm = £4.02 (S&N Hlth)

Uses: lightly to moderately exuding wounds such as leg ulcers, pressure sores; postoperative wounds; superficial burns

Tegasorb® Hydrocolloid dressing with adhesive border, net price 10 cm × 12 cm (oval) = £2.09; 13 cm × 15 cm (oval) = £3.90; without adhesive border 10 cm × 10 cm = £2.13; 15 cm × 15 cm = £4.12 (3M)

Uses: chronic wounds such as leg ulcers and pressure sores

Tegasorb® Thin. Sterile, semi-adhesive, clear film dressing with hydrocolloid and adhesive border, net price 10 cm × 12 cm (oval) = £1.39; 13 cm × 15 cm (oval) = £2.60; without adhesive border 10 cm × 10 cm = £1.42; 15 cm × 15 cm = £2.75 (3M)

Uses: low to moderately exuding wounds including leg ulcers, abrasions, burns, and donor sites

■ Keloid dressings

Silicone gel sheets are used to reduce and prevent hypertrophic and keloid scarring. They should not be used on open wounds. Application times should be increased gradually. Silicone sheets can be washed and reused.

Cica-Care® Soft, self-adhesive, semi-occlusive silicone gel sheet with backing. Net price, 6 cm × 12 cm = £12.01; 15 cm × 12 cm = £23.40 (S&N Hlth)

Mepiform® Self-adhesive silicone gel sheet with polyurethane film backing, net price 5 cm × 7.5 cm = £3.03; 10 cm × 18 cm = £12.30; 4 cm × 30 cm = £8.66 (Mölnlycke)

Silgel® Silicone gel sheet, net price 10 cm × 10 cm =£13.50; 20 cm × 20 cm = £40.00; 40 cm × 40 cm = £144.00; 10 cm × 5 cm = £7.50; 15 cm × 10 cm = £19.50; 30 cm × 5 cm = £19.50; 10 cm × 30 cm = £31.50; 25 cm × 15 cm (submammary) = £21.12; 46 cm × 8.5 cm (abdominal) = £39.46; 5 cm diameter (circular) = £4.00 (Nagor)

Silgel® STC-SE silicone gel, net price, 20-mL tube = £19.00 (Nagor)

■ Hyaluronic acid

Hyalofill®

Hyalofill-F, [NHS] flat, non-woven, absorbent fibrous fleece of *Hyaff* (an ester of hyaluronic acid), net price 5 cm × 5 cm = £9.47, 10 cm × 10 cm = £26.25 (ConvaTec)

Uses: for treatment of chronic or acute wounds, place on surface of lesion and cover with sterile dressing, renew daily or when saturated (at least every 2–3 days)

Hyalofill-R, [NHS] absorbent fibrous rope of *Hyaff* (an ester of hyaluronic acid), net price, 500 mg = £26.25 (ConvaTec)

Uses: for treatment of chronic or acute wounds, position gently inside cavity and cover with sterile dressing, renew daily or when saturated (at least every 2–3 days)

A8.1.5 Vapour-permeable films and membranes

Vapour-permeable films and membranes allow the passage of water vapour and oxygen but not of water or micro-organisms, and are suitable for mildly exuding wounds. They are highly conformable, convenient to use, provide a moist healing environment, and some may permit constant observation of the wound. However, water vapour loss may occur at a slower rate than exudate is generated, so that fluid accumulates under the dressing, which can lead to tissue maceration and to wrinkling at the adhesive contact site (with risk of bacterial entry). Newer versions have increased gaseous permeability; some also contain water-soluble antimicrobials. Despite these advances vapour-permeable films and membranes remain suitable for large heavily exuding wounds and are probably not suitable for chronic leg ulcers. They are most commonly used as secondary dressings over alginates or gels; they are also sometimes used to protect fragile skin of patients at risk of developing minor skin damage.

Vapour-permeable Adhesive Film Dressing, BP 1993 (Semi-permeable Adhesive Dressing) Sterile, extensible, waterproof, water vapour-permeable polyurethane film coated with synthetic adhesive mass; transparent. Supplied in single-use pieces.

Alldress®, net price 10 cm × 10 cm = 78p, 15 cm × 15 cm = £1.70, 15 cm × 20 cm = £2.10 (Mölnlycke); *Askina Derm®*, 6 cm × 7 cm = 36p, 10 cm × 12 cm = £1.00, 15 cm × 20 cm = £2.29 (Braun); *Bioclusive®*, 10.2 cm ×

12.7 cm = £1.36 (J&J); *Cutifilm*®, 5 cm × 7.5 cm = 40p, 7.5 cm × 10 cm = 66p, 10 cm × 14 cm = £1.13 (Beiersdorf); *Hydrofilm*®, 6 cm × 9 cm = 48p, 10 cm × 15 cm = £1.27, 12 cm × 25 cm = £2.29 (Hartman); *Mefilm*®, 6 cm × 7 cm = 39p, 10 cm × 12.7 cm = £1.04, 10 cm × 25 cm = £2.03, 15 cm × 21.5 cm = £2.58 (Mölnlycke); *Mepore*® *Ultra*, 6 cm × 7 cm = 25p, 9 cm × 10 cm = 55p, 9 cm × 15 cm = 82p, 9 cm × 25 cm = £1.37 (Mölnlycke); *OpSite*® *Flexigrid*, 6 cm × 7 cm = 32p, 12 cm × 12 cm = 91p, 15 cm × 20 cm = £2.30, 12 cm × 25 cm = £2.98 (NHS), 10 cm × 12 cm = £1.92 (NHS), *OpSite*® *Plus*, 5 cm × 5 cm = 25p, 9.5 cm × 8.5 cm = 71p, 10 cm × 12 cm = 97p, 10 cm × 30 cm = £1.63, 35 cm × 10 cm = £2.70 (S&N Hlth); *Tegaderm*®, 6 cm × 7 cm = 38p, 12 cm × 12 cm = £1.23, 15 cm × 20 cm = £2.34 (3M)

Uses: postoperative dressing, donor sites, i/v sites, superficial decubitus ulcers, amputation stumps, stoma care; protective cover to prevent skin breakdown

Arglaes® NHS Sterile, semi-permeable, self-adhesive, clear, controlled release polyurethane film dressing containing silver. Net price 6 cm × 8 cm = 99p; 10 cm × 12 cm = £1.99; 15 cm × 25 cm = £3.99 (Maersk)

Uses: flat moist wounds including cuts and abrasions; burns and scalds; superficial pressure areas; surgical wounds

Omiderm® NHS Sterile, water-vapour permeable polyurethane film (plain and meshed versions). Net price 5 cm × 7 cm = £1.30; 8 cm × 10 cm = £2.31; meshed = £3.09; 18 cm × 10 cm = £4.20; meshed = £6.18; 60 cm × 10 cm = £15.50; 21 cm × 31 cm = £15.86; meshed = £21.26; meshed, 23 cm × 39 cm = £31.55 (Chemical Search)

Uses: ulcers; donor sites; superficial and partial thickness burns; meshed: donor sites, skin grafts

A8.1.6 Low adherence dressing and wound contact materials

Low adherence dressings and wound contact materials are used as interface layers under secondary absorbent dressings.

Tulle dressings are manufactured from cotton or viscose fibres which are impregnated with white or yellow soft paraffin to prevent the fibres from sticking, but this is only partly successful and it may be necessary to change the dressings frequently. The paraffin reduces absorbency of the dressing. Dressings with a reduced content of soft paraffin (i.e. *Paratulle*® and *Unitulle*®) are less liable to interfere with absorption; those containing the traditional amount (such as *Jelonet*®) have been considered more suitable for skin graft transfer.

Medicated tulle dressings are not generally recommended for wound care. **Framycetin gauze dressing** is associated with a high incidence of hypersensitivity and absorption (with systemic toxicity) may follow exposure to large amounts. Although hypersensitivity is less likely with **chlorhexidine gauze dressing**, its antibacterial efficacy has not been established.

Povidone–iodine fabric dressing is a knitted viscose dressing with povidone–iodine incorporated in a hydrophilic polyethylene glycol basis; this facilitates diffusion of the iodine into the wound and permits removal of the dressing by irrigation. The iodine has a wide spectrum of antimicrobial activity but it is rapidly deactivated by wound exudate; systemic absorption of iodine may occur.

Perforated film absorbent dressings overcome the problems of adherence but they are suitable only for wounds with mild to moderate amounts of exudate; they are **not** appropriate for leg ulcers or for other lesions that produce large quantities of viscous exudate.

Knitted viscose primary dressing is an alternative to tulle dressings for exuding wounds; it is sometimes used as the initial layer of multi-layer compression bandaging.

Absorbent Perforated Dressing with Adhesive Border Low adherence dressing consisting of viscose and rayon absorbent pad with adhesive border.
Cosmopor E®, net price 5 cm × 7.2 cm = 7p, 6 cm × 10 cm = 13p, 8 cm × 10 cm = 15p, 6 cm × 15 cm = 17p, 8 cm × 15 cm = 24p, 8 cm × 20 cm = 32p, 10 cm × 20 cm = 39p, 10 cm × 25 cm = 48p, 10 cm × 35 cm = 67p (Hartmann)
Medipore®+*Pad*, net price 5 cm × 7.2 cm = 7p, 10 cm × 10 cm = 14p, 10 cm × 15 cm = 23p, 10 cm × 20 cm = 35p, 10 cm × 25 cm = 43p, 10 cm × 35 cm = 60p (3M)
Mepore®, net price 6 cm × 7 cm = 9p, 9 cm × 10 cm = 18p, 9 cm × 15 cm = 30p, 9 cm × 20 cm = 36p, 9 cm × 25 cm = 51p, 9 cm × 30 cm = 58p, 9 cm × 35 cm = 63p (Mölnlycke)
Primapore®, net price 6 cm × 8.3 cm = 15p, 8 cm × 10 cm = 16p, 8 cm × 15 cm = 27p, 10 cm × 20 cm = 35p, 10 cm × 25 cm = 40p, 10 cm × 30 cm = 51p, 12 cm × 35 cm = 84p (S&N Hlth)
Sterifix®, net price 5 cm × 7 cm = 17p, 7 cm × 10 cm = 28p, 10 cm × 14 cm = 50p (Hartman)
Uses: lightly exuding and post-operative wounds

Absorbent Perforated Plastic Film Faced Dressing (Drug Tariff specification 9). Low-adherence dressing consisting of 3 layers.
Cutilin®, net price 5 cm × 5 cm = 12p, 10 cm × 10 cm = 20p, 10 cm × 20 cm = 38p (Beiersdorf)
Interpose®, net price 5 cm × 5 cm = 9p, 10 cm × 10 cm = 15p, 10 cm × 20 cm = 32p (Frontier)
Melolin®, net price 5 cm × 5 cm = 14p, 10 cm × 10 cm = 22p, 20 cm × 10 cm = 43p (S&N Hlth)
Release ®, net price 5 cm × 5 cm = 13p, 10 cm × 10 cm = 21p, 20 cm × 10 cm = 39p (J&J)
Skintact®, net price 5 cm × 5 cm = 10p, 10 cm × 10 cm = 17p, 20 cm × 10 cm = 34p (Robinson)
Solvaline N®, net price 5 cm × 5 cm = 9p, 10 cm × 10 cm = 16p, 10 cm × 20 cm = 32p (Vernon-Carus)
Where no size specified by the prescriber, the 5 cm × 5 cm size to be supplied
Uses: dressing for post-operative and low exudate wounds; low adherence property and low absorption capacity

Knitted Viscose Primary Dressing, BP 1993 Warp knitted fabric manufactured from a bright viscose monofilament. Net price 9.5 cm × 9.5 cm = 31p; 9.5 cm × 19 cm = 59p (J&J—*N-A Dressing*®); 9.5 cm × 9.5 cm = 25p (Parema—*Paratex*®); 9.5 cm × 9.5 cm = 26p; 12.5 cm × 14.5 cm = 39p (Robinsons—*Robinson Primary*®); 9.5 cm × 9.5 cm = 27p (SSL—*Setoprime*®; S&N—*Tricotex*®); silicone-coated, 9.5 cm × 9.5 cm = 30p; 9.5 cm × 19 cm = 56p (J&J—*N-A Ultra*®)
Uses: low adherence wound contact layer for use on ulcerative and other granulating wounds with superimposed absorbent pad

Paraffin Gauze Dressing, BP 1993 (Tulle Gras). Fabric of leno weave, weft and warp threads of cotton and/or viscose yarn, impregnated with white or yellow soft paraffin, sterile, 10 cm × 10 cm, net price (light loading) = 25p; (normal loading) = 33p (most suppliers including Vernon-Carus—*Paranet*® (light loading); SSL—*Paratulle*® (light loading); Hoechst Marion Roussel—*Unitulle*® (light loading); S&N Hlth—*Jelonet*® (normal loading))
Uses: treatment of abrasions, burns, and other injuries of skin, and ulcerative conditions; postoperatively as penile and vaginal dressing and for sinus packing; heavier loading for skin graft transfer

Chlorhexidine Gauze Dressing, BP 1993 Fabric of leno weave, weft and warp threads of cotton and/or viscose yarn, impregnated with ointment containing chlorhexidine acetate, sterile, 5 cm × 5 cm, net price = 24p, 10 cm × 10 cm = 49p (S&N Hlth—*Bactigras®*)

Framycetin Gauze Dressing, BP 1993 PoM

Fabric of leno weave, weft and warp threads of cotton, impregnated with ointment containing framycetin sulphate 1% in white soft paraffin containing 10% wool fat, sterile, net price 10 cm × 10 cm = 25p (Hoechst Marion Roussel—*Sofra-Tulle ®*)

Cautions: large areas (risk of ototoxicity); see also cautions in section 13.10.1

Uses: wide range of infected lesions

Povidone–iodine Fabric Dressing (Drug Tariff specification 43). Knitted viscose primary dressing impregnated with povidone–iodine ointment 10%, net price 5 cm × 5 cm = 28p; 9.5 cm × 9.5 cm = 42p (J&J—*Inadine®*); 5 cm × 5 cm = 25p, 9.5 cm × 9.5 cm = 37p (SSL—*Poviderm®*)

Uses: wound contact layer for abrasions and superficial burns

Atrauman®

Non-adherent knitted polyester primary dressing impregnated with neutral triglycerides, 5 cm × 5 cm = 23p, 7.5 cm × 10 cm = 24p, 10 cm × 10 cm = 54p (Hartmann)

Uses: abrasions, burns, and other injuries of skin, and ulcerative conditions; postoperatively for granulating wounds

Melolite® NHS Absorbent fabric pad covered on both sides by polyethylene net, net price 5 cm × 7.5 cm =7p, 10 cm × 7.5 cm = 10p, 15 cm × 7.5 cm = 14p, 20 cm × 7.5 cm = 18p (S&N Hlth)

Uses: primary dressing over clean sutured wounds, lacerations, and abrasions

Mepilex® Low adherence silicone dressing with polyurethane foam film backing, net price 10 cm × 10 cm = £2.18, 10 cm × 20 cm = £3.59, 15 cm × 15 cm = £4.05, 20 cm × 20 cm = £5.99; with silicone adhesive border (*Mepilex® Border*) 7.5 cm × 7.5 cm = £1.28, 10 cm × 10 cm = £2.32, 15 cm × 15 cm = £3.79, 15 cm × 20 cm = £4.75 (Mölnlycke)

Uses: pressure sores, venous ulcers, diabetic ulcers, donor sites, dermal lesions, traumatic wounds; should be covered with simple absorbent secondary dressing

Mepitel® Non-adherent silicone dressing. Net price 5 cm × 7.5 cm = £1.49, 7.5 cm × 10 cm = £2.61, 10 cm × 18 cm = £5.62, 20 cm × 30 cm = £14.21 (Mölnlycke)

Uses: leg ulcers, decubitus ulcers, burns, fixation of skin grafts; should be covered with simple absorbent secondary dressing

Mesorb® Cellulose wadding pad with gauze wound contact layer and non-woven repellent backing, net price 10 cm × 10 cm = 52p, 10 cm × 15 cm = 67p, 10 cm × 20 cm = 83p, 15 cm × 20 cm = £1.18, 20 cm × 25 cm = £1.86, 20 cm × 30 cm = £2.11 (Mölnlycke)

Uses: post-operative use for heavily exuding wounds

* **Surgipad®** NHS Absorbent pad of absorbent cotton and viscose in sleeve of non-woven viscose fabric, sterile, net price pouch 12 cm × 10 cm = 18p, 20 cm × 10 cm = 25p, 20 cm × 20 cm = 30p, 40 cm × 20 cm = 41p; non-sterile, net price pack 12 cm × 10 cm = 5p, 20 cm × 10 cm = 10p, 20 cm × 20 cm = 17p, 40 cm × 20 cm = 28p (J&J)

Uses: for heavily exuding wounds requiring frequent dressing changes

* NHS Except in Sterile Dressing Pack with Non-woven Pads

---

denotes preparations that are considered to be less suitable for prescribing (see p. vi)

Odour absorbent dressings

These dressings have an important role in absorbing the odour of infected wounds. Some dressings may also benefit wound healing by binding bacteria, but this effect awaits confirmation.

Actisorb® Silver 200 (formerly Actisorb® Plus) Knitted fabric of activated charcoal, with one-way stretch, with silver residues, within spun-bonded nylon sleeve. Net price 6.5 cm × 9.5 cm = £1.45, 10.5 cm × 10.5 cm = £2.28, 10.5 cm × 19 cm = £4.14 (J&J)

CarboFLEX® Dressing in 5 layers: wound-facing absorbent layer containing alginate and hydrocolloid; water-resistant second layer; third layer containing activated charcoal; non-woven absorbent fourth layer; water-resistant backing layer. Net price 10 cm × 10 cm = £2.59, 8 cm × 15 cm = £3.11; 15 cm × 20 cm = £5.90 (ConvaTec)

Carbonet® NHS Activated charcoal dressing, net price 10 cm × 10 cm = £2.92, 10 cm × 20 cm = £5.70 (S&N Hlth)

Carbopad® VC Activated charcoal non-absorbent dressing, net price 10 cm × 10 cm = £1.59, 10 cm × 20 cm = £2.15 (Vernon-Carus)

CliniSorb® Odour Control Dressings Layer of activated charcoal cloth between viscose rayon with outer polyamide coating. Net price 10 cm × 10 cm = £1.57, 10 cm × 20 cm = £2.09, 15 cm × 25 cm = £3.36 (CliniMed)

Lyofoam C® Lyofoam sheet with layer of activated charcoal cloth and additional outer envelope of polyurethane foam. Net price 10 cm × 10 cm = £2.59, 15 cm × 20 cm = £5.90, 25 cm × 10 cm = £5.30 (SSL)

Dressing packs

The role of dressing packs is very limited. They are used to provide a clean or sterile working surface; packs shown below include cotton wool balls, but they are not recommended for use on wounds.

Sterile Dressing Pack (Drug Tariff specification 10). Contains gauze and cotton tissue pad, gauze swabs, absorbent cotton wool balls, absorbent paper towel, water repellent inner wrapper. Net price per pack = 73p (*Vernaid®*)

Sterile Dressing Pack with Non-woven Pads (Drug Tariff specification 35). Contains non-woven fabric covered dressing pad, non-woven fabric swabs, absorbent cotton wool balls, absorbent paper towel, water repellent inner wrapper. Net price per pack = 73p (*Vernaid®*)

Surgical absorbents

Surgical absorbent dressings, applied directly to the wound, have many disadvantages, since they adhere to the wound, shed fibres into it, and dehydrate it; they also permit leakage of exudate ('strike through') with an associated risk of infection. Surgical absorbents may be used as secondary absorbent layers in the management of heavily exuding wounds.

Absorbent Cotton, BP Carded cotton fibres of not less than 10 mm average staple length, available in rolls and balls, 25 g, net price = 61p; 100 g = £1.39; 500 g = £4.69 (most suppliers). 25-g pack to be supplied when weight not stated

Uses: general purpose cleansing and swabbing, preoperative skin preparation, application of medicaments; supplementary absorbent pad to absorb excess wound exudate

Absorbent Cotton, Hospital Quality As for absorbent cotton but lower quality materials, shorter staple length etc. 100 g, net price = 97p; 500 g = £3.05 (most suppliers)

Drug Tariff specifies to be supplied only where specifically ordered

Uses: suitable only as general purpose absorbent, for swabbing, and routine cleansing of incontinent patients; not for wound cleansing

Gauze and Cotton Tissue, BP 1988 Consists of absorbent cotton enclosed in absorbent cotton gauze type 12 or absorbent cotton and viscose gauze type 2. 500 g, net price = £5.94 (most suppliers, including Robinsons—*Gamgee Tissue*® (blue label))

Uses: absorbent and protective pad, as burns dressing on non-adherent layer

Gauze and Cotton Tissue (Drug Tariff specification 14). Similar to above. 500 g, net price = £4.34 (most suppliers, including Robinsons—*Gamgee Tissue*® (pink label))

Drug Tariff specifies to be supplied only where specifically ordered

Uses: absorbent and protective pad, as burns dressing on non-adherent layer

Absorbent Lint, BPC Cotton cloth of plain weave with nap raised on one side from warp yarns. 25 g, net price = 76p; 100 g = £2.32; 500 g = £9.77 (most suppliers). 25-g pack supplied where no quantity stated

Note. Not recommended for wound management

Absorbent Cotton Gauze, BP 1988 Cotton fabric of plain weave, in rolls and as swabs (see below), usually Type 13 light, sterile. 90 cm (all) × 1 m, net price = 92p; 3 m = £1.91; 5 m = £2.98; 10 m = £5.71 (most suppliers). 1-m packet supplied when no size stated

Uses: pre-operative preparation, for cleansing and swabbing

Note. Drug Tariff also includes unsterilised absorbent cotton gauze, 25 m roll, net price = £13.08

Cellulose Wadding, BP 1988 Delignified wood pulp bleached white, in multiple laminate form. 500 g, net price = £2.39 (most suppliers)

Uses: absorbing large volumes of fluid

Absorbent Muslin, BP 1988 [DHS] Fabric of plain weave, warp threads of cotton, weft threads of cotton and/or viscose

Uses: wet dressing, soaked in 0.9% sterile sodium chloride solution

Absorbent Cotton Ribbon Gauze, BP 1993 [DHS] Cotton fabric of plain weave in ribbon form with fast selvedge edges

Uses: post-surgery cavity packing for sinus, dental, throat cavities etc.

Absorbent Cotton and Viscose Ribbon Gauze, BP 1993 Woven fabric in ribbon form with fast selvedge edges, warp threads of cotton, weft threads of viscose or combined cotton and viscose yarn, sterile. 5 m (both) × 1.25 cm, net price = 69p; 2.5 cm = 76p

Uses: post-surgery cavity packing for sinus, dental, throat cavities etc.

Gauze Swab, BP 1988 Consists of absorbent cotton gauze type 13 light or absorbent cotton and viscose gauze type 1 folded into squares or rectangles of 8-ply with no cut edges exposed, sterile, 7.5 cm × 7.5 cm, net price 5-pad packet = 33p; non-sterile, 10 cm × 10 cm 100-pad packet = £5.36 (most suppliers)

Filmated Gauze Swab, BP 1988 As for Gauze Swab, but with thin layer of Absorbent Cotton enclosed within, non-sterile, 10 cm × 10 cm, net price 100-pad packet = £7.36 (Vernon-Carus—*Cotfil*®)

Uses: general swabbing and cleansing

Non-woven Fabric Swab (Drug Tariff specification 28). Consists of non-woven fabric folded 4-ply; alternative to gauze swabs, type 13 light, sterile, 7.5 cm × 7.5 cm, net price 5-pad packet = 21p; non-sterile, 10 cm × 10 cm, 100-pad packet = £2.51 (J & J—*Topper 8*®); 100-pad pack = £2.43 (CliniMed)

Uses: general purpose swabbing and cleansing; absorbs more quickly than gauze

Filmated Non-woven Fabric Swab (Drug Tariff specification 29). Film of viscose fibres enclosed within non-woven viscose fabric folded 8-ply, non-sterile, 10 cm × 10 cm, net price 100-pad packet = £5.45 (J & J—*Regal*®)

Uses: general purpose swabbing and cleansing

A8.2 Bandages and adhesives

According to their structure and performance bandages are used for dressing retention, for support, and for compression.

A8.2.1 Non-extensible bandages

Bandages made from non-extensible woven fabrics have generally been replaced by more conformable products therefore their role is now extremely limited. Triangular calico bandage has a role as a sling.

Open-wove Bandage, BP 1988 Cotton cloth, plain weave, warp of cotton, weft of cotton, viscose, or combination, one continuous length. Type 1, 5 m (all): 2.5 cm, net price = 30p; 5 cm = 49p; 7.5 cm = 70p; 10 cm = 91p (most suppliers) 5 m × 5 cm supplied when size not stated

Uses: protection and retention of absorbent dressings; support for minor strains, sprains; securing splints

Triangular Calico Bandage, BP 1980 Unbleached calico rt. angle triangle. 90 cm × 90 cm × 1.27 m, net price = £1.10 (most suppliers)

Uses: sling

Domette Bandage, BP 1988 [DHS] Fabric, plain weave, cotton warp and wool weft (hospital quality also available, all cotton). 5 m (all): 5 cm, net price = 54p; 7.5 cm = 81p; 10 cm = £1.08; 15 cm = £1.61 (Robert Bailey)

Uses: protection and support where warmth required

Multiple Pack Dressing No. 1 (Drug Tariff). Contains absorbent cotton, absorbent cotton gauze type 13 light (sterile), open-wove bandages (banded). Net price per pack = £3.41

A8.2.2 Light-weight conforming bandages

Lightweight conforming bandages are used for dressing retention, with the aim of keeping the dressing close to the wound without inhibiting movement or restricting blood flow. The elasticity of **conforming-stretch bandages** (also termed contour bandages) is greater than that of **cotton conforming bandages**.

Cotton Conforming Bandage, BP 1988 Cotton fabric, plain weave, treated to impart some elasticity to warp and weft. 3.5 m (all):

type A, 5 cm, net price = 62p, 7.5 cm = 77p, 10 cm = 95p, 15 cm = £1.30 (S&N Hlth—*Crinx*®)
type B, 5 cm = 62p, 7.5 cm = 80p, 10 cm = 97p, 15 cm = £1.28 (J&J—*Kling*®)

Knitted Polyamide and Cellulose Contour Bandage, BP 1988 Fabric, knitted warp of polyamide filament, weft of cotton or viscose, fast edges, one continuous length. 4 m stretched (all): 5 cm = 18p, 7 cm = 23p, 10 cm = 25p, 15 cm = 44p (Parema—*K-Band*®); 5 cm = 13p, 7 cm = 18p, 10 cm = 19p, 15 cm = 35p (Bailey—*Knit Fix*®)

Polyamide and Cellulose Contour Bandage, BP 1988 (formerly Nylon and Viscose Stretch Bandage). Fabric, plain weave, warp of polyamide filament, weft of cotton or viscose, fast edges, one continuous length. 4 m stretched (all): Robinsons—*Stayform*®(5 cm = 31p, 7.5 cm = 39p, 10 cm = 44p, 15 cm = 74p); SSL—*Slinky*® (net price 5 cm = 39p, 7.5 cm = 57p, 10 cm = 68p, 15 cm = 97p); S&N Hlth—*Easifix*® (5 cm = 34p, 7.5 cm = 41p, 10 cm = 47p, 15 cm = 81p)

Conformimg Bandage (Synthetic) Fabric, plain weave, warp of polyamide, weft of viscose. 4 m stretched (all); Hartmann—*Peha-crepp*®*E* (6 cm = 13p, 8 cm = 15p, 10 cm = 18p, 12 cm = 22p)

A8.2.3   Tubular bandages

Tubular bandages are available in different forms, according to the function required of them. Some are used under orthopaedic casts and some are suitable for protecting areas to which creams or ointments (other than those containing potent corticosteroids) have been applied. The conformability of the elasticated versions makes them particularly suitable for retaining dressings on difficult parts of the body or for soft tissue injury, but their use as the only means of applying pressure to an oedematous limb or to a varicose ulcer is not appropriate, since the pressure they exert is inadequate. Compression hosiery (section A8.3.1) reduces the recurrence of venous leg ulcers and should be considered after wound healing.

Cotton Stockinette, Bleached, BP 1988 Knitted fabric, cotton yarn, tubular, 1 m × 2.5 cm, net price = 29p; 5 cm = 45p; 7.5 cm = 55p; 6 m × 10 cm = £3.73 (J&J, SSL)
Uses: 1 m lengths, basis (with wadding) for Plaster of Paris bandages etc. ; 6 m length, compression bandage

Elasticated Tubular Bandage, BP 1993 (formerly Elasticated Surgical Tubular Stockinette). Knitted fabric, elasticated threads of rubber-cored polyamide or polyester with cotton or cotton and viscose yarn, tubular. Lengths 50 cm and 1 m, widths 6.25 cm, 6.75 cm, 7.5 cm, 8.75 cm, 10 cm, 12 cm (other sizes 🅝🅗🅢); Easigrip—*EasiGRIP*®; Sigma—*Sigma ETB*®; S&N Hlth—*Tensogrip*®; JLB—*Textube*®; SSL—*Tubigrip*®. Where no size stated by prescriber the 50 cm length should be supplied and width endorsed
Uses: retention of dressings on limbs, abdomen, trunk

Elasticated Surgical Tubular Stockinette, Foam padded (Drug Tariff specification 25). Fabric as for Elasticated Tubular Bandage with polyurethane foam lining. Heel, elbow, knee, small, net price = £2.54, medium = £2.74, large = £2.93; sacral, small, medium, and large (all) = £13.09 (SSL—*Tubipad*®)
Uses: relief of pressure and elimination of friction in relevant area; porosity of foam lining allows normal water loss from skin surface

Elasticated Viscose Stockinette (Drug Tariff specification 46). Lightweight plain-knitted elasticated tubular bandage, net price 3.5 cm (small limb), length 1 m = 76p; 5 cm (medium limb), length 1 m = 84p, 3 m = £2.39; 5 m = £4.09; 7.5 cm (large limb), length 1 m = £1.12, 3 m = £3.15, 5 m = £5.49; 10.75 cm (child trunk), length 1 m = £1.76, 3 m = £5.49, 5 m = £8.80; 17.5 cm (adult trunk), length 1 m = £2.22 (SSL—*Tubifast*®)
Uses: retention of dressings

Elastic Net Surgical Tubular Stockinette (Drug Tariff Specification 26). Lightweight elastic open-work net tubular fabric.
type A : arm/leg, 40 cm × 1.8 cm (size C), net price = 37p; thigh/head, 60 cm × 2.5 cm (size E) = 66p; trunk (adult), 60 cm × 4.5 cm (size F) = 97p; trunk (OS adult) 60 cm × 5.4 cm (size G) = £1.31 (SSL—*Netelast*®)

Ribbed Cotton and Viscose Surgical Tubular Stockinette, BP 1988 Knitted fabric of 1:1 ribbed structure, singles yarn spun from blend of two-thirds cotton and one-third viscose fibres, tubular. Length 5 m (all):
type A (lightweight): arm/leg (child), arm (adult) 5 cm, net price = £2.12; arm (OS adult), leg (adult) 7.5 cm = £2.78; leg (OS adult) 10 cm = £3.69; trunk (child) 15 cm = £5.31; trunk (adult) 20 cm = £6.13; trunk (OS adult) 25 cm = £7.33 (SSL)
type B (heavyweight): sizes as for type A, net price £2.12–£7.33 (Sallis—*Eesiban*®)
Drug Tariff specifies various combinations of sizes to provide sufficient material for part or full body coverage
Uses: protective dressings with tar-based and other non-steroid ointments

Tubular Gauze Bandage, Seamless 🅝🅗🅢 Unbleached cotton yarn, positioned with applicators. 20 m roll (all): 00, net price = £2.40; 01 = £2.75; 12 = £3.70; 34 = £5.40; 56 = £7.40; 78 = £8.70; T1 = £11.15; T2 = £14.40 (SSL—*Tubegauz*®)
Uses: retention of dressings on limbs, abdomen, trunk

A8.2.4   Support bandages

Light support bandages, which include the various forms of crepe bandage, are used in the prevention of oedema; they are also used to provide support for mild sprains and joints but their effectiveness has not been proven for this purpose. Since they have limited extensibility, they are able to provide light support without exerting undue pressure. For a warning against injudicious compression see section A8.2.5.

Crepe Bandage, BP 1988 Fabric, plain weave, warp of wool threads and crepe-twisted cotton threads, weft of cotton threads; stretch bandage. 4.5 m stretched (all): 5 cm, net price = 87p; 7.5 cm = £1.22; 10 cm = £1.61; 15 cm = £2.33 (most suppliers)
Uses: light support system for strains, sprains, compression over paste bandages for varicose veins

Cotton Crepe Bandage light support bandage, 4.5 m stretched (all): 5 cm, net price = 48p; 7.5 cm = 67p; 10 cm =87p; 15 cm = £1.27 (Millpledge–*Hospicrepe 239*)

Cotton Crepe Bandage, BP 1988 Fabric, plain weave, warp of crepe-twisted cotton threads, weft of cotton and/ or viscose threads; stretch bandage. 4.5 m stretched (both): 7.5 cm, net price = £2.74; 10 cm = £3.52; other sizes 🅝🅗🅢 (most suppliers)
Uses: light support system for strains, sprains, compression over paste bandages for varicose ulcers

Cotton, Polyamide and Elastane Bandage Fabric, cotton, polyamide, and elastane; light support bandage (Type 2). 4.5 m stretched (all): 5 cm, net price = 64p, 7.5 cm = 92p, 10 cm = £1.18, 15 cm = £1.72 (S&N Hlth —*Soffcrepe*®); 4.5 m stretched, 10 cm = net price = £1.14 (SSL—*Setocrepe*®)
Uses: light support for sprains and strains; retention of dressings

Cotton Stretch Bandage, BP 1988 Fabric, plain weave, warp of crepe-twisted cotton threads, weft of cotton threads; stretch bandage, lighter than cotton crepe. 4.5 m stretched (all): 5 cm, net price = 56p; 7.5 cm = 78p; 10 cm = £1.04; 15 cm = £1.48 (Millpledge—*Hospicrepe 233*)
Uses: light support system for strains, sprains, compression over paste bandages for varicose veins

Cotton Suspensory Bandage (Drug Tariff). Type 1: cotton net bag with draw tapes and webbing waistband; net price small, medium, and large (all) = £1.52, extra large = £1.61. Type 2: cotton net bag with elastic edge and webbing waistband; small = £1.67, medium = £1.73, large = £1.79, extra large = £1.86. Type 3: cotton net bag with elastic edge and webbing waistband with elastic

insertion; small, medium, and large (all) = £1.81; extra large = £1.88. Type supplied to be endorsed
Uses: support of scrotum

Knitted Elastomer and Viscose Bandage Knitted fabric, viscose and elastomer yarn. Type 2: light support bandage, 4.5 m stretched (all): 5 cm, net price = 49p, 7 cm = 69p, 10 cm = 91p, 15 cm = £1.30 (Parema—*K-Lite*®)
Uses: light support for sprains and strains

Type 3a: light compression bandage, 6 m stretched, 10 cm, net price = £2.46; 15 cm = £2.67; 8 m stretched, 10 cm = £3.15 (SSL—*Elset*®); 12 m stretched, 15 cm = £5.29 (SSL—*Elset*®S); 6 m stretched, 10 cm, net price = £1.42; 8.7 m stretched, 10 cm = £2.01 (Parema—*K-Plus*®); 8.7 m stretched, 10 cm = £3.44 (S&N Hlth—*Litepress*®)
Uses: light compression for varicose ulcers

A8.2.5 High compression bandages

High compression products are used to provide the high compression needed for the management of gross varices, post-thrombotic venous insufficiency, venous leg ulcers, and gross oedema in average-sized limbs. Their use calls for an expert knowledge of the elastic properties of the products and experience in the technique of providing careful graduated compression. Inappropriate application can lead to uneven and inadequate pressures or to hazardous levels of pressure. In particular, injudicious use of compression in limbs with arterial disease has been reported to cause severe skin and tissue necrosis (in some instances calling for amputation). Doppler testing is required before treatment with compression.

■ High compression bandages (Drug Tariff specification 52)

PEC High Compression Bandage (Drug Tariff). Polyamide, elastane, and cotton compression (high) extensible bandage, 3.5 m unstretched (both): 7.5 cm, net price = £2.59; 10 cm = £3.34 (SSL—*Setopress*®)
Uses: high compression for varicose ulcers

VEC High Compression Bandage (Drug Tariff). Viscose, elastane, and cotton compression (high) extensible bandage, 3 m unstretched (both); 7.5 cm, net price = £2.52; 10 cm = £3.24 (S&N—*Tensopress*®)
Uses: high compression for varicose ulcers

High Compression Bandage (Drug Tariff). Cotton, viscose, nylon, and Lycra® extensible bandage, 3 m (unstretched), 10 cm = £3.24 (ConvaTec—*SurePress*®)
Uses: high compression for venous leg ulcers

■ Short Stretch Compression Bandage
Short stretch bandages help to reduce oedema and promote healing of venous leg ulcers. They are also used to reduce swelling associated with lymphoedema. They are applied at full stretch over padding (*see* Sub-compression Wadding Bandage below) which protects areas of high pressure and sites at high risk of pressure damage.

Actiban® , net price (all 5 m), 8 cm = £3.00; 10 cm = £3.22; 12 cm = £3.92 (Activa)
Uses: venous leg ulcers and lympoedema

Actico® , cohesive, net price 6 m × 10 cm = £3.04 (Activa)
Uses: venous leg ulcers, lymphoedema

Comprilan® , net price (all 5 m) 6 cm = £2.54; 8 cm = £3.08; 10 cm = £3.50; 12 cm = £4.08 (Beiersdorf)
Uses: venous leg ulcers and lymphoedema

Rosidal K® , net price (all 5 m) 8 cm = £3.08; 10 cm = £3.36; 12 cm = £4.08; ◖NHS◗ 6 cm = £2.95 (Vernon-Carus)
Uses: venous leg ulcers and lymphoedema

Silkolan® , net price (all 5 m) 8 cm = £3.10; 10 cm = £3.50 (Parema)
Uses: venous leg ulcers and lymphoedema

Tensolan K® , net price (all 5 m) 8 cm = £3.16; 10 cm = £3.62; 12 cm = £3.99 (S&N Hlth)
Uses: venous leg ulcers and lymphoedema

Varex® short stretch , net price 5 m x 10 cm = £3.27 (SSL)
Uses: venous leg ulcers and lymphoedema

■ Sub-compression Wadding Bandage

Cellona® Undercast Padding , net price 2.75 m unstretched (all): 7.5 cm = 37p; 10 cm = 46p; 15 cm = 59p; ◖NHS◗ 20 cm = 97p (Vernon-Carus)

Flexi-Ban® , padding, net price 3.5 m unstretched, 10 cm = 46p (Activa)

K-Soft® , net price 3.5 m unstretched, 10 cm = 41p (Parema)

Ortho-Band Plus® , net price 10 cm × 3.5 cm unstretched = 40p (Millpledge)

Soffban® Natural , net price 3.5 m unstretched, 10 cm = 61p (S&N Hlth)

Softexe® , net price 3.5 m unstretched, 10 cm = 60p (SSL)

Sohfast® , soft absorbent bandage, net price 3.5 m unstretched, 10 cm = 42p (Robinsons)

SurePress® , absorbent padding, net price 3 m unstretched, 10 cm = 49p (ConvaTec)

Velband® , absorbent padding, net price 4.5 m unstretched, 10 cm = 72p (J&J)

A8.2.6 Extra-high performance compression bandages

These bandages are capable of applying pressures even higher than those of high compression bandages, therefore the same stringent warnings apply. Their use is reserved for the largest and most oedematous limbs. Extra-high performance compression bandages are poorly tolerated by patients.

Elastic Web Bandage, BP 1993 (also termed Blue Line Webbing). Characteristic fabric woven ribbon fashion, warp threads of cotton and rubber with mid-line threads coloured blue; weft threads of cotton or combined cotton and viscose; may be dyed skin colour; with or without foot loop. Per m (both) 7.5 cm, net price = 75p; 10 cm = £1.07; with foot loop (Drug Tariff specification 2a) 7.5 cm = £4.32 (Marlow, SSL)
Uses: provision of support and high compression over large surface

Elastic Web Bandage without Foot Loop (also termed Red Line Webbing) (Drug Tariff specification 2b) (Scott-Curwen). Characteristic fabric woven ribbon fashion, warp threads of cotton and rubber with mid-line threads coloured red, weft threads of cotton or combined cotton and viscose. 7.5 cm × 2.75 m (2.5 m unstretched), net price = £3.42; 7.5 cm × 3.75 m (3.5 m unstretched) = £4.13
Uses: provision of support and high compression over large surfaces

Heavy Cotton and Rubber Elastic Bandage, BP 1993 Heavy version of above with one end folded as foot loop; fastener also supplied. 1.8 m unstretched × 7.5 cm, net price = £11.59 (Marlow, SSL, S&N Hlth—*Elastoweb*®).
Uses: provision of high even compression over large surface

Adhesive bandages

Elastic adhesive bandages are used to provide compression in the treatment of varicose veins and for the support of injured joints; they should no longer be used for the support of fractured ribs and clavicles. They have also been used with **zinc paste bandage** in the treatment of venous ulcers, but they can cause skin reactions in susceptible patients and may not produce sufficient pressures for healing (significantly lower than those provided by other compression bandages).

Elastic Adhesive Bandage, BP 1993 Woven fabric, elastic in warp (crepe-twisted cotton threads), weft of cotton and/or viscose threads spread with adhesive mass containing zinc oxide. 4.5 m stretched (all): 5 cm, net price = £3.23; 7.5 cm = £4.67; 10 cm = £6.22 (Robinsons—*Flexoplast®*; S&N Hlth—*Elastoplast®* Bandage). 7.5 cm width supplied when size not stated
Uses: compression for chronic leg ulcers; compression and support for swollen or sprained joints

Cohesive bandages

Cohesive bandages adhere to themselves, but not to the skin, and are useful for providing support for sports use where ordinary stretch bandages might become displaced and adhesive bandages are inappropriate. Care is needed in their application, however, since the loss of ability for movement between turns of the bandage to equalise local areas of high tension carries the potential for creating a tourniquet effect. They should not be used if arterial disease is suspected.

■ Cohesive extensible bandages

These elastic bandages adhere to themselves and not to skin; this prevents slipping during use.
Uses: support of sprained joints; outer layer of multi-layer compression bandaging

Coban® Net price 6 m stretched, 10 cm = £2.80; other sizes NHS 4.5 m stretched (all): 2.5 cm = £1.23; 5 cm = £1.72; 7.5 cm = £2.58; 10 cm = £3.44; 15 cm = £5.15 (3M)

Cohfast® Latex-free, net price 6.3 m stretched, 10 cm = £2.82; other sizes NHS 4.5 m stretched (both): 5 cm = £1.28; 7.5 cm = £1.98 (Robinson)

Co-Plus® Net price 6.3 m stretched, 10 cm (flesh-coloured, white or mixed) = £2.85; other sizes NHS , 6.3 m stretched (all): 2.5 cm (flesh-coloured or white) = £1.14; 5 cm (flesh-coloured or white)= £1.76; 7.5 cm (flesh-coloured, white or mixed) = £2.60; 15 cm (flesh-coloured or white) = £5.20 (S&N Hlth)

Secure® Forte NHS Net price 4.5 m stretched, 6 cm = £2.43; 8 cm = £3.24; 10 cm = £4.33 (J&J)

Medicated bandages

Zinc Paste Bandage remains one of the standard treatments for leg ulcers and can be left on undisturbed for up to a week; it is often used in association with compression for treatment of venous ulcers.

Zinc paste bandages are also used with **coal tar** and **ichthammol** in chronic lichenified skin conditions such as chronic eczema (ichthammol often being preferred since its action is considered to be milder).They are also used with **calamine** in milder eczematous skin conditions (but the inclusion of **clioquinol** may lead to irritation in susceptible subjects).

Zinc Paste Bandage, BP 1993 Cotton fabric, plain weave, impregnated with suitable paste containing zinc oxide; requires additional bandaging. Net price 6 m × 7.5 cm = £3.22 (SSL—*Steripaste®* (15%), *excipients: include* polysorbate 80); £3.17 (SSL—*Zincaband®* (15%), *excipients: include* hydroxybenzoates); £3.20 (S&N Hlth—*Viscopaste PB7®* (10%), *excipients: include* hydroxybenzoates)

Zinc Paste and Calamine Bandage (Drug Tariff specification 5). Cotton fabric, plain weave, impregnated with suitable paste containing calamine and zinc oxide; requires additional bandaging. Net price 6 m × 7.5 cm = £3.28 (SSL—*Calaband®*)

Zinc Paste, Calamine, and Clioquinol Bandage, BP 1993 Cotton fabric, plain weave, impregnated with suitable paste containing calamine, clioquinol, and zinc oxide; requires additional bandaging. Net price 6 m × 7.5 cm = £3.28 (SSL—*Quinaband®*, *excipients: include* hydroxybenzoates)

Zinc Paste and Ichthammol Bandage, BP 1993 Cotton fabric, plain weave, impregnated with suitable paste containing zinc oxide and ichthammol; requires additional bandaging. Net price 6 m × 7.5 cm = £3.18 (SSL—*Ichthaband®*(15/2%), *excipients: include* hydroxybenzoates; S&N Hlth—*Ichthopaste®*(6/2%), *excipients:* none as listed in section 13.1.3)
Uses: see section 13.5

■ Medicated stocking

Zipzoc® Sterile rayon stocking impregnated with ointment containing zinc oxide 20%. Net price 4-pouch carton = £13.33; 10-pouch carton = £33.33 (S&N Hlth)
Uses: chronic leg ulcers; can be used under appropriate compression bandages or hosiery in chronic venous insufficiency

Multi-layer compression bandaging

Although multi-layer compression bandaging 'kits' are not prescribable as such on the NHS, individual components of the 'kit' are prescribable; see also Sub-compression Wadding Bandage, section A8.2.5.

Hospifour® (Millpledge)

Hospifour # 1 (Ortho-Band Plus®—see Sub-compression Wadding Bandage); Hospifour # 2 (*Hospicrepe 239®*— see Cotton Crepe Bandage); Hospifour # 4 (*AAA-Flex®*), net price 10 cm × 6.3 m (stretched) = £1.93

K-Four® (Parema)

K-Four # 1 (*K-Soft®*—see Sub-compression Wadding Bandage); *K-Four* # 2 (*K-Lite®*—see Knitted Elastomer and Viscose Bandage); *K-Four* # 3 (*K-Plus®*—see Knitted Elastomer and Viscose Bandage); *K-Four* # 4 (*Ko-Flex®*), net price 10 cm × 6 m (unstretched) = £2.75

Profore® (S&N Hlth.)

Profore® wound contact layer (*Tricotex®*—see Knitted Viscose Primary Dressing); *Profore®* #1 (*Softban® Natural*—see Sub-compression Wadding bandage); *Profore®* #2 (*Soffcrepe®*—see Cotton, Polyamide and Elastane Bandage); *Profore®* #3 (*Litepress®*—see Knitted Elastomer and Viscose Bandage); *Profore®* #4 (*Co-Plus®*—see Cohesive bandages); *Profore® Plus* (*Tensopress®*—see VEC High Compression Bandage); *Profore® Lite* (low compression) NHS = £5.23

System 4 (33L)

System 4 wound contact layer (*Setoprime®*—see Knitted Viscose Primary Dressing); *System 4 #1* (*Softexe®*—see Sub-compression Wadding Bandage); *System 4 #2* (*Setocrepe®*—see Cotton, Polyamide and Elastane Bandage); *System 4 #3* (*Elset®*—see Knitted Elastomer and Viscose Bandage); *System 4 #4* (*Coban®*—see Cohesive bandages)

Ultra Four (Robinsons)

Ultra Four #1 (Robinsons—*Sohfast®*—see Sub-compression Wadding Bandage); *Ultra Four #2* (Parema—*K-Lite®*—see Knitted Elastomer and Viscose Bandage); *Ultra Four #3* (Parema—*K-Plus®*—see Knitted Elastomer and Viscose Bandage); *Ultra Four #4* (Robinsons—*Cohfast®*—see Cohesive bandages)

A8.2.11 Surgical adhesive tapes

Adhesive tapes are useful for retaining dressings on joints or awkward body parts. These tapes, particularly those containing rubber, can cause irritant and allergic reactions in susceptible patients; synthetic adhesives have been developed to overcome this problem, but they, too, may sometimes be associated with reactions. Adhesive tapes that are occlusive may cause skin maceration. Care is needed not to apply these tapes under tension, to avoid creating a tourniquet effect. If applied over joints they need to be orientated so that the area of maximum extensibility of the fabric is in the direction of movement of the limb.

Permeable adhesive tapes

Zinc Oxide Adhesive Tape, BP 1988 (Zinc Oxide Plaster). Fabric, plain weave, warp and weft of cotton and/or viscose, spread with an adhesive containing zinc oxide. 5 m (all): 1.25 cm, net price = 82p; 2.5 cm = £1.19; 5 cm = £2.01; 7.5 cm = £3.02 (most suppliers)
Uses: securing dressings and immobilising small areas

Permeable Woven Synthetic Adhesive Tape, BP 1988 Non-extensible closely woven fabric, spread with a polymeric adhesive. 5 m (all): 1.25 cm, net price = 68p; 2.5 cm = 99p; 5 cm = £1.72 (Beiersdorf—*Leukosilk®*)
Uses: securing dressings for patients with skin reactions to other plasters and strapping, which require use for long periods

Elastic Adhesive Tape, BP 1988 (Elastic Adhesive Plaster). Woven fabric, elastic in warp (crepe-twisted cotton threads), weft of cotton and/or viscose threads, spread with adhesive mass containing zinc oxide. 1.5 m stretched × 2.5 cm, net price = 77p; 4.5 m stretched × 2.5 cm = £1.45 (Robinsons—*Flexoplast®*; S&N—*Elastoplast®*).
Uses: securing dressings
For 5 cm width, see Elastic Adhesive Bandage

Permeable Non-woven Synthetic Adhesive Tape, BP 1988 Backing of paper-based or non-woven textile material spread with a polymeric adhesive mass. 5 m (all): BioDiagnostics—*Scanpor®* (net price 1.25 cm = 39p, 2.5 cm = 63p, 5 cm = £1.09); Beiersdorf—*Leukopor®* (1.25 cm = 45p, 2.5 cm = 70p, 5 cm = £1.23); 3M—*Micropore®* (1.25 cm = 58p, 2.5 cm = 86p, 5 cm = £1.52); Hartmann—*Albufilm®* (1.25 cm = 61p, 2.5 cm = 94p, 5 cm = £1.73; *Albupore®* (1.25 cm = 45p, 2.5 cm = 72p, 5 cm = £1.24). Where no brand stated by prescriber, net price of tape supplied not to exceed 39p (1.25 cm), 63p (2.5 cm), £1.09 (5 cm)
Uses: securing dressings; skin closures for small incisions for patients with skin reactions to other plasters and strapping, which require use for long periods

Permeable, Apertured Non-Woven Synthetic Adhesive Tape, BP 1988 Non-woven fabric with a polyacrylate adhesive. 5 m (all): 2.5 cm, net price = 83p; 5 cm = £1.48; 10 cm = £2.36; 15 cm = £3.22; 20 cm = £4.12; 30 cm = £5.91 (Mölnlycke—*Mefix®*)
Uses: securing dressings

Occlusive adhesive tapes

Impermeable Plastic Adhesive Tape, BP 1988 Extensible water-impermeable plastic film spread with an adhesive mass. 2.5 cm × 3 m, net price = £1.15; 2.5 cm × 5 m = £1.72; 5 cm × 5 m = £2.18; 7.5 cm × 5 m = £3.17 (Robinsons; SSL; S&N Hlth)
Uses: securing dressings; covering site of infection where exclusion of air, water, and water vapour is required

Impermeable Plastic Synthetic Adhesive Tape, BP 1988 Extensible water-impermeable plastic film spread with a polymeric adhesive mass. 5 m (both): net price, 2.5 cm = £1.63; 5 cm = £3.12 (3M—*Blenderm®*)
Uses: isolating wounds from external environment; covering sites where total exclusion of water and water vapour required; securing dressings and appliances

A8.2.12 Adhesive dressings

Adhesive dressings (also termed 'island dressings') have a limited role for minor wounds only. The inclusion of an antiseptic is not particularly useful and may cause skin irritation in susceptible subjects.

Permeable adhesive dressings

Elastic Adhesive Dressing, BP 1993 [DHS] Wound dressing or dressing strip, pad attached to piece of extension plaster, leaving suitable adhesive margin; both pad and margin covered with suitable protector; pad may be dyed yellow and may be impregnated with suitable antiseptic (see below); extension plaster may be perforated or ventilated
Uses: general purpose wound dressing
Note. Permitted antiseptics are aminoacridine hydrochloride (aminacrine hydrochloride), chlorhexidine hydrochloride (both 0.07–0.13%), chlorhexidine gluconate (0.11–0.20%); domiphen bromide (0.05–0.25%)

Permeable Plastic Wound Dressing, BP 1993 [DHS] Consisting of an absorbent pad, which may be dyed and impregnated with a suitable antiseptic (see under Elastic Adhesive Dressing), attached to a piece of permeable plastic surgical adhesive tape, to leave a suitable adhesive margin; both pad and margin covered with suitable protector (most suppliers)
Uses: general purpose wound dressing, permeable to air and water

Vapour permeable adhesive dressings

Vapour-permeable Waterproof Plastic Wound Dressing, BP 1993 (former Drug Tariff title: Semi-permeable Waterproof Plastic Wound Dressing). Consists of absorbent pad, may be dyed and impregnated with suitable antiseptic (see under Elastic Adhesive Dressing), attached to piece of semipermeable waterproof surgical adhesive tape, to leave suitable adhesive margin; both pad and margin covered with suitable protector. 8.5 cm × 6 cm, net price = 32p (S&N Hlth—*Elastoplast Airstrip®*)
Uses: general purpose waterproof wound dressing, permeable to air and water vapour

Occlusive adhesive dressings

Impermeable Plastic Wound Dressing, BP
1993 NHS Consists of absorbent pad, may be dyed and impregnated with suitable antiseptic (see under Elastic Adhesive Dressing), attached to piece of impermeable plastic surgical adhesive tape, to leave suitable adhesive margin; both pad and margin covered with suitable protector (most suppliers)

Uses: protective covering for wounds requiring an occlusive dressing

A8.2.13   Skin closure dressings

Skin closure strips are used as an alternative to sutures for minor cuts and lacerations.

Skin closure strips, sterile
Leukostrip®, 6.4 mm × 76 mm, 3 strips per envelope. Net price 10 envelopes = £5.18 (Beiersdorf)
Steri-strip®, 6 mm × 75 mm, 3 strips per envelope. Net price 12 envelopes = £8.37; NHS 3 mm × 75 mm, 12 envelopes = £8.37; 12 mm × 100 mm, 12 envelopes = £10.89 (3M)

Drug Tariff specifies that these are specifically for personal administration by the prescriber

A8.3   Elastic hosiery

Before elastic hosiery can be dispensed, the quantity (single or pair), article (including accessories), and compression class (I, II or III) must be specified by the prescriber; all dispensed articles must state on the packaging that they conform with Drug Tariff technical specification No. 40, for further details see Drug Tariff.

Note. Graduated compression tights are NHS.

A8.3.1   Graduated compression hosiery

Class 1 Light Support
Hosiery, compression at ankle 14–17 mm Hg, thigh length or below knee with knitted in heel. Net price per pair, circular knit (standard), thigh length = £6.57, below knee = £6.00; light weight elastic net (made-to-measure), thigh length = £17.58, below knee = £13.72

Uses: superficial or early varices, varicosis during pregnancy

Class 2 Medium Support
Hosiery, compression at ankle 18–24 mm Hg, thigh length or below knee with knitted in heel. Net price per pair, circular knit (standard), thigh length = £9.76, below knee = £8.77, (made-to-measure), thigh length = £32.60, below knee = £20.39; net (made-to-measure), thigh length = £17.58, below knee = £13.72; flat bed (made-to-measure, only with closed heel and open toe), thigh length = £32.60, below knee = £20.39

Uses: varices of medium severity, ulcer treatment and prophylaxis, mild oedema, varicosis during pregnancy

Class 3 Strong Support
Hosiery, compression at ankle 25–35 mm Hg, thigh length or below knee with open or knitted in heel. Net price per pair, circular knit (standard), thigh length = £11.56, below knee = £9.94, (made-to-measure) thigh length = £32.60, below knee = £20.39; flat bed (made-to-measure, only with open heel and open toe), thigh length = £32.60, below knee = £20.39

Uses: gross varices, post thrombotic venous insufficiency, gross oedema, ulcer treatment and prophylaxis

A8.3.2   Accessories

Suspender
Suspender, for thigh stockings, net price = 57p, belt (specification 13), = £4.37, fitted (additional price) = 57p

A8.3.3   Anklets

Class 2 Medium Support
Anklets, compression 18–24 mm Hg, circular knit (standard and made-to-measure), net price per pair = £5.75; flat bed (standard and made-to-measure) = £11.94; made-to-measure = £11.29

Uses: soft tissue support

Class 3 Strong Support
Anklets, compression 25–35 mm Hg, circular knit (standard and made-to-measure), net price per pair = £8.02; flat bed (standard) = £8.02; made-to-measure = £11.94

Uses: soft tissue support

A8.3.4   Knee caps

Class 2 Medium Support
Kneecaps, compression 18-24 mm Hg, circular knit (standard and made-to-measure), net price per pair = £5.75; flat bed (standard and made-to-measure) = £11.94; made-to-measure = £9.38

Uses: soft tissue support

Class 3 Strong Support
Kneecaps, compression 25-35 mm Hg, circular knit (standard and made-to-measure), net price per pair = £7.66; flat bed (standard) = £7.66; made-to-measure = £11.94

Uses: soft tissue support

Appendix 9: Cautionary and advisory labels for dispensed medicines

Numbers following the preparation entries in the BNF correspond to the code numbers of the cautionary labels that pharmacists are recommended to add when dispensing. It is also expected that pharmacists will counsel patients when necessary.

Counselling needs to be related to the age, experience, background, and understanding of the individual patient. The pharmacist should ensure that the patient understands how to take or use the medicine and how to follow the correct dosage schedule. Any effects of the medicine on driving or work, any foods or medicines to be avoided, and what to do if a dose is missed should also be explained. Other matters, such as the possibility of staining of the clothes or skin by a medicine should also be mentioned.

For some preparations there is a special need for counselling, such as an unusual method or time of administration or a potential interaction with a common food or domestic remedy, and this is indicated where necessary.

ORIGINAL PACKS. Most preparations are now dispensed in unbroken original packs (see Patient Packs, p. vii) that include further advice for the patient in the form of patient information leaflets. Label 10 may be used where appropriate. More general leaflets advising on the administration of preparations such as eye drops, eye ointments, inhalers, and suppositories are also available.

SCOPE OF LABELS. In general no label recommendations have been made for injections on the assumption that they will be administered by a healthcare professional or a well-instructed patient. The labelling is not exhaustive and pharmacists are recommended to use their professional discretion in labelling new preparations and those for which no labels are shown.

Individual labelling advice is not given on the administration of the large variety of antacids. In the absence of instructions from the prescriber, and if on enquiry the patient has had no verbal instructions, the directions given under 'Dose' should be used on the label.

It is recognised that there may be occasions when pharmacists will use their knowledge and professional discretion and decide to omit one or more of the recommended labels for a particular patient. In this case counselling is of the utmost importance. There may also be an occasion when a prescriber does not wish additional cautionary labels to be used, in which case the prescription should be endorsed 'NCL' (no cautionary labels). The exact wording that is required instead should then be specified on the prescription.

Pharmacists label medicines with various wordings in addition to those directions specified on the prescription. Such labels include 'Shake the bottle', 'For external use only', and 'Store in a cool place', as well as 'Discard . . . . days after opening' and 'Do not use after . . . .', which apply particularly to antibiotic mixtures, diluted liquid and topical preparations, and to eye-drops. Although not listed in the BNF these labels should continue to be used when appropriate; indeed, 'For external use only' is a legal requirement on external liquid preparations, while 'Keep out of the reach of children' is a legal requirement on all dispensed medicines. Care should be taken not to obscure other relevant information with adhesive labelling.

It is the usual practice for patients to take standard tablets with water or other liquid and for this reason no separate label has been recommended.

The label or labels for each preparation are recommended after careful consideration of the information available. However, it is recognised that in some cases this information may be either incomplete or open to a different interpretation. The Executive Editor will therefore be grateful to receive any constructive comments on the labelling suggested for any preparation.

Recommended label wordings

Wordings which can be given as separate warnings are labels 1–19 and labels 29–33. Wordings which can be incorporated in an appropriate position in the directions for dosage or administration are labels 21–28. A label has been omitted for number 20.

If separate labels are used it is recommended that the wordings be used without modification. If changes are made to suit computer requirements, care should be taken to retain the sense of the original.

I   Warning. May cause drowsiness

To be used on *preparations for children* containing antihistamines, or other preparations given to children where the warnings of label 2 on driving or alcohol would not be appropriate.

2   Warning. May cause drowsiness. If affected do not drive or operate machinery. Avoid alcoholic drink

To be used on *preparations for adults that can cause drowsiness*, thereby affecting the ability to drive and operate hazardous machinery; label 1 is more appropriate for children. *It is an offence to drive while under the influence of drink or drugs.*

Some of these preparations only cause drowsiness in the first few days of treatment and some only cause drowsiness in higher doses.

In such cases the patient should be told that the advice applies until the effects have worn off. However many of these preparations can produce a slowing of reaction time and a loss of mental concentration that can have the same effects as drowsiness.

Avoidance of alcoholic drink is recommended because the effects of CNS depressants are enhanced by alcohol. Strict prohibition however could lead to some patients not taking the medicine. Pharmacists should therefore explain the risk and encourage compliance, particularly in patients who may think they already tolerate the effects of alcohol (see also label 3). Queries from patients with epilepsy regarding fitness to drive should be referred back to the patient's doctor.

Side-effects unrelated to drowsiness that may affect a patient's ability to drive or operate machinery safely include *blurred vision, dizziness, or nausea*. In general, no label has been recommended to cover these cases, but the patient should be suitably counselled.

3 Warning. May cause drowsiness. If affected do not drive or operate machinery

To be used on *preparations containing monoamine-oxidase inhibitors*; the warning to avoid alcohol and dealcoholised (low alcohol) drink is covered by the patient information leaflet.

Also to be used as for label 2 but where alcohol is not an issue.

4 Warning. Avoid alcoholic drink

To be used on *preparations where a reaction such as flushing may occur if alcohol is taken* (e.g. metronidazole and chlorpropamide). Alcohol may also enhance the hypoglycaemia produced by some oral antidiabetic drugs but routine application of a warning label is not considered necessary.

5 Do not take indigestion remedies at the same time of day as this medicine

To be used with label 25 on *preparations coated to resist gastric acid* (e.g. enteric-coated tablets). This is to avoid the possibility of premature dissolution of the coating in the presence of an alkaline pH.

Label 5 also applies to drugs such as ketoconazole *where the absorption is significantly affected by antacids*; the usual period of avoidance recommended is 2 to 4 hours.

6 Do not take indigestion remedies or medicines containing iron or zinc at the same time of day as this medicine

To be used on *preparations containing ciprofloxacin and some other quinolones, doxycycline, lymecycline, minocycline, and penicillamine*. These drugs chelate calcium, iron and zinc and are less well absorbed when taken with calcium-containing antacids or preparations containing iron or zinc. These incompatible preparations should be taken 2–3 hours apart.

7 Do not take milk, indigestion remedies, or medicines containing iron or zinc at the same time of day as this medicine

To be used on *preparations containing norfloxacin or tetracyclines that chelate, calcium, iron, magnesium, and zinc* and are thus less available for absorption; these incompatible preparations should be taken 2–3 hours apart. Doxycycline, lymecycline and minocycline are less liable to form chelates and therefore only require label 6 (see above).

8 Do not stop taking this medicine except on your doctor's advice

To be used on *preparations that contain a drug which is required to be taken over long periods without the patient necessarily perceiving any benefit* (e.g. antituberculous drugs).

Also to be used on *preparations that contain a drug whose withdrawal is likely to be a particular hazard* (e.g. clonidine for hypertension). Label 10 (see below) is more appropriate for corticosteroids.

9 Take at regular intervals. Complete the prescribed course unless otherwise directed

To be used on *preparations where a course of treatment should be completed* to reduce the incidence of relapse or failure of treatment.

The preparations are antimicrobial drugs given by mouth. Very occasionally, some may have severe side-effects (e.g. diarrhoea in patients receiving clindamycin) and in such cases the patient may need to be advised of reasons for stopping treatment quickly and returning to the doctor.

10 Warning. Follow the printed instructions you have been given with this medicine

To be used particularly on *preparations containing anticoagulants, lithium and oral corticosteroids*. The appropriate treatment card should be given to the patient and any necessary explanations given.

This label may also be used on other preparations to remind the patient of the instructions that have been given.

11 Avoid exposure of skin to direct sunlight or sun lamps

To be used on *preparations that may cause phototoxic or photoallergic reactions* if the patient is exposed to ultraviolet radiation. Many drugs other than those listed (e.g. phenothiazines and sulphonamides) may on rare occasions cause reactions in susceptible patients. Exposure to high intensity ultraviolet radiation from sunray lamps and sunbeds is particularly likely to cause reactions.

12 Do not take anything containing aspirin while taking this medicine

To be used *on preparations containing probenecid and sulfinpyrazone* whose activity is reduced by aspirin.

Label 12 should not be used for anticoagulants since label 10 is more appropriate.

13 Dissolve or mix with water before taking

To be used on *preparations that are intended to be dissolved in water* (e.g. soluble tablets) or *mixed with water* (e.g. powders, granules) before use. In a few cases other liquids such as fruit juice or milk may be used.

14 This medicine may colour the urine

To be used on *preparations that may cause the patient's urine to turn an unusual colour.* These include phenolphthalein (alkaline urine pink), triamterene (blue under some lights), levodopa (dark reddish), and rifampicin (red).

15 Caution flammable: keep away from fire or flames

To be used on *preparations containing sufficient flammable solvent to render them flammable if exposed to a naked flame.*

16 Allow to dissolve under the tongue. Do not transfer from this container. Keep tightly closed. Discard eight weeks after opening

To be used on *glyceryl trinitrate tablets* to remind the patient not to transfer the tablets to plastic or less suitable containers.

17 Do not take more than . . . in 24 hours

To be used on *preparations for the treatment of acute migraine* except those containing ergotamine, for which label 18 is used. The dose form should be specified, e.g. tablets or capsules.

It may also be used on preparations for which no dose has been specified by the prescriber.

18 Do not take more than . . . in 24 hours or

. . . in any one week

To be used on preparations containing ergotamine. The dose form should be specified, e.g. tablets or suppositories.

19 Warning. Causes drowsiness which may continue the next day. If affected do not drive or operate machinery. Avoid alcoholic drink

To be used on *preparations containing hypnotics (or some other drugs with sedative effects) prescribed to be taken at night.* On the rare occasions (e.g. nitrazepam in epilepsy) when hypnotics are prescribed for daytime administration this label would clearly not be appropriate. Also to be used as *an alternative to the label 2 wording* (the choice being at the discretion of the pharmacist) *for anxiolytics prescribed to be taken at night.*

It is hoped that this wording will convey adequately the problem of residual morning sedation after taking 'sleeping tablets'.

21 . . . with or after food

To be used on *preparations that are liable to cause gastric irritation,* or *those that are better absorbed with food.*

Patients should be advised that a *small amount of food is sufficient.*

22 . . . half to one hour before food

To be used on some preparations *whose absorption is thereby improved.* Most oral antibacterials require label 23 instead (see below).

23 . . . an hour before food or on an empty stomach

To be used on *oral antibacterials whose absorption may be reduced by the presence of food and acid in the stomach.*

24 . . . sucked or chewed

To be used on *preparations that should be sucked or chewed.*

The pharmacist should use discretion as to which of these words is appropriate.

25 . . . swallowed whole, not chewed

To be used on *preparations that are enteric-coated or designed for modified-release.*

Also to be used on *preparations that taste very unpleasant or may damage the mouth* if not swallowed whole.

26 . . . dissolved under the tongue

To be used on *preparations designed for sublingual use.* Patients should be advised to hold under the tongue and avoid swallowing until dissolved. The buccal mucosa between the gum and cheek is occasionally specified by the prescriber.

27 . . . with plenty of water

To be used on *preparations that should be well diluted* (e.g. chloral hydrate), *where a high fluid intake is required* (e.g. sulphonamides), or *where water is required to aid the action* (e.g. methylcellulose). The patient should be advised that 'plenty' means at least 150 mL (about a tumblerful). In most cases fruit juice, tea, or coffee may be used.

28 To be spread thinly . . .

To be used on *external preparations* that should be applied sparingly (e.g. corticosteroids, dithranol).

29 Do not take more than 2 at any one time. Do not take more than 8 in 24 hours

To be used on containers of dispensed *solid dose preparations containing paracetamol for adults when the instruction on the label indicates that the dose can be taken on an 'as required' basis.* The dose form should be specified, e.g. tablets or capsules.

This label has been introduced because of the serious consequences of overdosage with paracetamol.

30 Do not take with any other paracetamol products

To be used on all containers of dispensed *preparations containing paracetamol.*

31 Contains aspirin and paracetamol. Do not take with any other paracetamol products

To be used on all containers of dispensed *preparations containing aspirin and paracetamol (e.g. benorilate).*

32 Contains aspirin
To be used on containers of dispensed *preparations containing aspirin when the name on the label does not include the word 'aspirin'*.

33 Contains an aspirin-like medicine
To be used on containers of dispensed *preparations containing aspirin derivatives*.

Products and their labels

Products introduced or amended since publication of BNF No. 42 (September 2001) are underlined.
Proprietary names are in *italic*.
C = counselling advised; see BNF = consult product entry in BNF

Abacavir, C, hypersensitivity reactions, see BNF
Acamprosate, 21, 25
Acarbose, C, administration, see BNF
Accolate, 23
Acebutolol, 8
Aceclofenac, 21
Acemetacin, 21, C, driving
Acenocoumarol, 10 anticoagulant card
Acetazolamide, 3
Acetazolamide m/r, 3, 25
Achromycin, 7, 9, 23, C, posture
Aciclovir susp and tabs, 9
Acipimox, 21
Acitretin, 10 patient information leaflet, 21
Acrivastine, C, driving, alcohol, see BNF
Actinac, 28
Actonel, C, administration, food and calcium, see BNF
Acupan, 2, 14 (urine pink)
Adalat LA, 25
Adalat Retard, 25
Adcal, 24
Adcal-D₃, 24
Adcortyl with Graneodin, 28
Adcortyl with Graneodin, 28
Adipine MR, 21, 25
Adizem preps, 25
AeroBec, 8, C, dose
AeroBec Forte, 8, 10 steroid card, C, dose
Aerocrom, 8
Aerolin Autohaler, C, dose, see BNF
Agenerase caps, 5
Agenerase oral solution, 4, 5
Airomir, C, dose, change to CFC-free inhaler, see BNF
Akineton, 2
Albendazole, 9
Alclometasone external preps, 28
Aldara, 10 patient information leaflet
Aldomet, 3, 8
Alendronic acid, C, administration, see BNF
Alfuzosin, 3, C, dose, see BNF
Alfuzosin m/r, 3, 25, C, dose, see BNF
Alimemazine, 2
Allegron, 2
Allopurinol, 8, 21, 27
Almogran, 3
Almotriptan, 3
Alphosyl HC, 28
Alphaderm, 28
Alprazolam, 2
Altretamine, 21
Alvedon, 30

Alvercol, 25, 27, C, administration, see BNF
Amantadine, C, driving
Aminophylline m/r, see preps
Amiodarone, 11
Amisulpride, 2
Amitriptyline, 2
Amitriptyline m/r, 2, 25
Amobarbital, 19
Amorolfine, 10 patient information leaflet
Amoxapine, 2
Amoxicillin, 9
Amoxicillin chewable tabs, 9, 10 patient information leaflet
Amoxicillin dispersible sachets, 9, 13
Amoxil, 9
Amoxil dispersible sachets, 9, 13
Amoxil paed susp, 9, C, use of pipette
Amphotericin loz, 9, 24, C, after food
Amphotericin mixt (g.i.), 9, C, use of pipette
Amphotericin mixt (mouth), 9, C, use of pipette, hold in mouth, after food
Amphotericin tabs, 9
Ampicillin, 9, 23
Amprenavir caps, 5
Amprenavir oral solution, 4, 5
Amytal, 19
Anafranil, 2
Anafranil m/r, 2, 25
Androcur, 21
Andropatch, C, administration, see BNF
Angettes-75, 32
Angiopine MR, 25
Angiopine 40 LA, 21, 25
Angitil SR, 25
Angitil XL, 25
Anhydrol Forte, 15
Anquil, 2
Antabuse, 2, C, alcohol reaction, see BNF
Antacids, see BNF dose statements
Antepsin, 5
Anthranol preps, 28
Anticoagulants, oral, 10 anticoagulant card
Antihistamines (see individual preparations)
Antipressan, 8
Anturan, 12, 21
Apomorphine sublingual tabs, C, driving
Arava, 4
Aromasin, 21
Arpicolin, C, driving
Artane, C, before or after food, driving, see BNF
Arythmol, 21, 25

Arthrotec, 21, 25
Asacol tabs, 5, 25, C, blood disorder symptoms, see BNF
Asacol enema and supps, C, blood disorder symptoms, see BNF
Asasantin Retard, 21, 25
Ascorbic acid, effervescent, 13
Ascorbic acid tabs (500mg), 24
Asendis, 2
Asmabec preps, 8, 10 steroid card (high-dose preparations only), C, dose
Asmasal, C, dose, see BNF
Aspav, 2, 13, 21, 32
Aspirin and papaveretum dispersible tabs, 2, 13, 21, also 32 (if 'aspirin' not on label)
Aspirin dispersible tabs, 13, 21, also 32 (if 'aspirin' not on label)
Aspirin effervescent, 13, also 32 (if 'aspirin' not on label)
Aspirin e/c, 5, 25, also 32 (if 'aspirin' not on label)
Aspirin m/r, 25, also 32 (if 'aspirin' not on label)
Aspirin supps, 32 (if 'aspirin' not on label)
Aspirin tabs, 21, also 32 (if 'aspirin' not on label)
Aspirin, paracetamol and codeine tabs, 21, 29, also 31 (if 'aspirin' and 'paracetamol' not on label)
Astemizole, C, driving, alcohol, see BNF
Atarax, 2
Atenolol, 8
Ativan, 2 or 19
Atorvastatin, C, muscle effects, see BNF
Atovaquone, 21
Atrovent inhalations, C, dose, see BNF
Augmentin susp and tabs, 9
Augmentin Duo, 9
Augmentin dispersible tabs, 9, 13
Auranofin, 21, C, blood disorder symptoms, see BNF
Aureocort, 28
Avloclor, 5, C, malaria prophylaxis, see BNF
Avomine, 2
Azapropazone, 11, 21, C, photosensitivity, see BNF
Azatadine, 2
Azathioprine, 21
Azithromycin caps, 5, 9, 23
Azithromycin susp and tabs, 5, 9

New British Approved Names (see p. x) used throughout this Appendix

Clozapine, 2, 10 patient information leaflet

Clozaril, 2, 10 patient information leaflet

Coal tar paint, 15

Co-amoxiclav, 9

Co-amoxiclav dispersible tabs, 9, 13

Cobadex, 28

Co-beneldopa, 14 (urine reddish), 21

Co-beneldopa dispersible tabs, 14 (urine reddish), 21, C, administration, see BNF

Co-beneldopa m/r, 5, 14 (urine reddish), 25

Co-Betaloc, 8

Co-Betaloc SA, 8, 25

Co-careldopa, 14 (urine reddish), 21

Co-careldopa m/r, 14 (urine reddish), 25

Co-codamol caps and tabs, 29, 30

Co-codamol dispersible tabs, 13, 29, 30

Co-codamol sachets, 2,13, 30

Co-codaprin dispersible tabs, 13, 21, 32

Co-codaprin tabs, 21, 32

Codafen Continus, 2, 21, 25

Codalax, 14 (urine red)

Co-danthramer, 14 (urine red)

Co-danthrusate, 14 (urine red)

Codeine phosphate syr and tabs, 2

Co-dergocrine, 22

Co-dydramol, 21, 29, 30

Co-fl; uampicil, 9, 22

Cogentin, 2

Colazide, 21, 25

Colestid, 13, C, avoid other drugs at same time, see BNF

Colestipol preps, 13, C, avoid other drugs at same time, see BNF

Colestyramine, 13, C, avoid other drugs at same time, see BNF

Collodion, flexible, 15

Colofac, C, administration, see BNF

Colofac MR, 25, C, administration, see BNF

Colpermin, 5, 25

Combivent, C, dose

Co-methiamol, 29, 30

Comtess, 14 (urine reddish-brown)

Condyline, 15

Convulex, 8, 25, C, blood or hepatic disorder symptoms (see BNF), driving (see BNF)

Co-prenozide, 8, 25

Co-proxamol, 2, 10 patient information leaflet, 29, 30

Coracten preps, 25

Cordarone X, 11

Corgard, 8

Corgaretic, 8

Coroday MR, 25

Corticosteroid external preps, 28

Corticosteroid tabs, 10 steroid card, 21

Corticosteroid injections (systemic), 10 steroid card

Cortisone tab, 10 steroid card, 21

Cortisyl, 10 steroid card, 21

Cosalgesic, 2, 10 patient information leaflet, 29, 30

Co-tenidone, 8

Co-triamterzide, 14 (urine blue in some lights), 21

Co-trimoxazole mixts and tabs, 9

Co-trimoxazole dispersible tabs, 9, 13

Creon preps, C, administration, see BNF

Crixivan, C, administration, see BNF

Cromogen Easi-Breathe, 8

Cuplex, 15

Cyclizine, 2

Cyclophosphamide, 27

Cycloserine caps, 2, 8

Cymevene, 21

Cyproheptadine, 2

Cyprostat, 21

Cyproterone, 21

Cystrin, 3

┌─────────────────────────────┐
│ **New British Approved Names** │
│ (see p. x) used throughout this │
│ Appendix │
└─────────────────────────────┘

Daktacort, 28

Daktarin oral gel, 9, C, hold in mouth, after food

Dalacin C, 9, 27, C, diarrhoea, see BNF

Dalmane, 19

Dantrium, 2

Dantrolene, 2

Dapsone, 8

DDAVP tabs and intranasal, C, fluid intake, see BNF

Decadron tabs, 10 steroid card, 21

Deflazacort, 5, 10 steroid card

Deltacortril e/c, 5, 10 steroid card, 25

Deltastab inj, 10 steroid card

Demeclocycline, 7, 9, 11, 23

De-Noltab, C, administration, see BNF

Depixol, 2

Depo-Medrone (systemic), 10 steroid card

Dermestril, C, administration, see BNF

Dermovate cream and oint, 28

Dermovate scalp application, 15, 28

Dermovate-NN, 28

Deseril, 2, 21

Desmopressin tabs and intranasal, C, fluid intake, see BNF

Desmospray, C, fluid intake, see BNF

Desmotabs, C, fluid intake, see BNF

Desoximetasone external preps, 28

Destolit, 21

Deteclo, 7, 9, 11, 23, C, posture

Detrunorm, 3

Detrusitol, m/r, 25

Dexamethasone inj, 10 steroid card

Dexamethasone tabs, 10 steroid card, 21

Dexamfetamine, C, driving

Dexedrine, C, driving

Dexketoprofen, 22

Dextromoramide, 2

Dextropropoxyphene, 2

DF118 Forte, 2, 21

DHC Continus, 2, 25

Diamorphine preps, 2

Diamox tabs, 3

Diamox SR, 3, 25

Diazepam, 2 *or* 19

Diclofenac dispersible tabs, 13, 21

Diclofenac e/c, 5, 25

Diclofenac m/r, 21, 25

Dicloflex Retard, 21, 25

Diclomax 75 mg SR and Retard, 21, 25

Diconal, 2

Didanosine e/c caps, 25, C, administration

Didanosine tabs, 23, C, administration

Didronel, C, food and calcium, see BNF

Didronel PMO, 10 patient leaflet, C, food and calcium, see BNF

Diflucan 50 and 200mg, 9

Diflucan susp, 9

Diflucortolone external preps, 28

Diflunisal, 21, 25, C, avoid aluminium hydroxide

Digoxin elixir, C, use of pipette

Dihydrocodeine, 2, 21

Dihydrocodeine m/r, 2, 25

Dihydroergotamine, nasal spray, 18, C, dosage

Dilcardia SR, 25

Diloxanide, 9

Diltiazem, 25

Dilzem preps, 25

Dimeticone, see paediatric prep

Dimotane, 2

Dimotane LA, 2, 25

Dimotane Plus, 2

Dimotane Plus, Paediatric, 1

Dindevan, 10 anticoagulant card, 14 (urine pink or orange)

Dioderm, 28

Dipentum, 21, C, blood disorder symptoms, see BNF

Diphenhydramine, 2

Diphenylpyraline m/r, 2, 25

Diprosalic, 28

Diprosone, 28

Dipyridamole MR, 21, 25

Dipyridamole, 22

Dirythmin SA, 25

Disipal, C, driving

Disodium etidronate, C, food and calcium, see BNF

Disopyramide m/r, 25

Disprin CV, 25, 32

Disprol, 30

Distaclor, 9

Distaclor MR, 9, 21, 25

Distalgesic, 2, 10 patient information leaflet, 29, 30

Distamine, 6, 22, C, blood disorder symptoms, see BNF

Distigmine, 22

Disulfiram, 2, C, alcohol reaction, see BNF

Dithranol preps, 28

Dithrocream preps, 28

Dithrolan, 28

Ditropan, 3

Diumide-K Continus, 25, 27, C, posture, see BNF

Dolmatil, 2

Dolobid, 21, 25, C, avoid aluminium hydroxide
Doloxene, 2
Doloxene Compound, 2, 21, 32
Domperamol, 17, 30
Doralese, 2
Dostinex, 21, C, hypotensive reactions, see BNF
Dosulepin, 2
Doxazosin m/r, 25
Doxepin, 2
Doxepin topical, 2, 10 patient information leaflet
Doxycycline caps, 6, 9, 11, 27, C, posture, see BNF
Doxycycline dispersible tabs, 6, 9, 11, 13
Doxycycline tabs, 6, 11, 27, C, posture, see BNF
Dozic, 2
Driclor, 15
Droleptan, 2
Dromadol XL, 2, 25
Droperidol, 2
Dulcolax tabs, 5, 25
Dumicoat, 10 patient information leaflet
Duofilm, 15
Duovent inhalations, C, dose
Durogesic, 2
Duromine, 25, C, driving
Dutonin, 3
Dyazide, 14 (urine blue in some lights), 21
Dyspamet tabs, C, administration, see BNF
Dytac, 14 (urine blue in some lights), 21
Dytide, 14 (urine blue in some lights), 21

Econacort, 28
Edronax, C, driving
Efcortelan external preps, 28
Efcortesol, 10 steroid card
Efexor, 21, C, driving, skin reactions, see BNF
Efexor XL, 21, 25, C, driving, skin reactions, see BNF
Elantan preps, 25
Elleste Solo MX patches, C, administration, see BNF
Elocon, 28
Emcor preps, 8
Emeside, 8, C, blood disorder symptoms (see BNF), driving (see BNF)
Emflex, 21, C, driving
En-De-Kay mouthwash, C, food and drink, see BNF
Endoxana, 27
Entacapone, 14 (urine reddish-brown)
Entocort CR, 5, 10 steroid card, 22, 25
Epanutin caps, 8, 27, C, administration, blood or skin disorder symptoms (see BNF), driving (see BNF)
Epanutin Infatabs, 8, 24, C, blood or skin disorder symptoms (see BNF), driving (see BNF)
Epanutin susp, 8, C, administration, blood or skin disorder symptoms (see BNF), driving (see BNF)

Epilim Chrono, 8, 25, C, blood or hepatic disorder symptoms (see BNF), driving (see BNF)
Epilim e/c tabs, 5, 8, 25, C, blood or hepatic disorder symptoms (see BNF), driving (see BNF
Epilim crushable tabs, liquid and syrup, 8, C, blood or hepatic disorder symptoms (see BNF), driving (see BNF)
Eprosartan, 21
Epogam, C, administration, see BNF
Equagesic, 2, 21, 32
Equanil, 2
Ergotamine, 18, C, dosage
Erymax, 5, 9, 25
Erythrocin, 9
Erythromycin caps, 5, 9, 25
Erythromycin ethyl succinate, 9
Erythromycin ethyl succinate gran, 9, 13
Erythromycin stearate tabs, 9
Erythromycin tabs, 5, 9, 25
Erythroped, 9
Erythroped A tabs, 9
Esomeprazole, 25
Estracombi, C, administration, see BNF
Estracyt, 23, C, dairy products, see BNF
Estraderm MX, C, administration, see BNF
Estraderm TTS, C, administration, see BNF
Estradiol vaginal ring, 10 patient information leaflet
Estrapak-50, C, administration, see BNF
Estramustine, 23, C, dairy products, see BNF
Estring, 10 patient information leaflet
Estriol, 25
Ethambutol, 8
Ethosuximide, 8, C, blood disorder symptoms (see BNF), driving (see BNF)
Etidronate, C, food and calcium, see BNF
Etodolac m/r, 25
Etonogestrel implant, C, see patient information leaflet
Etoposide caps, 23
Eumovate external preps, 28
Eurax-Hydrocortisone, 28
Evorel preps, C, administration, see BNF
Exelon caps, 21, 25
Exelon solution, 21
Exemestane, 21

Famciclovir, 9
Famvir, 9
Farlutal 500-mg tabs, 27
Fasigyn, 4, 9, 21, 25
Faverin, C, driving, see BNF
Fefol, 25
Fefol-Vit, 25
Felbinac foam, 15
Feldene caps, 21
Feldene dispersible tabs, 13, 21
Feldene Melt, 10 patient information leaflet, 21
Felodipine m/r, 25
Fematrix, C, administration, see BNF
Femapak, C, administration, see BNF

FemSeven, C, administration, see BNF
Fenbid, 25
Fenbufen, 21
Fenofibrate, 21
Fenofibrate m/r, 21, 25
Fenoprofen, 21
Fenopron, 21
Fentanyl patch, 2
Fentazin, 2
Feospan, 25
Ferrograd, 25
Ferrograd C, 25
Ferrograd Folic, 25
Ferrous salts m/r see preps
Ferrous sulphate paed mixt, 27
Fexofenadine, C, driving, see BNF
Filair, 8, C, dose
Filair Forte, 8, 10 steroid card, C, dose
Flagyl S, 4, 9, 23
Flagyl supps, 4, 9
Flagyl tabs, 4, 9, 21, 25, 27
Fleet Phospho-soda, 10 patient information leaflet, C, administration
Flixotide, 8, 10 steroid card (high-dose preparations only), C, dose
Flixotide Evohaler, 8, C, dose, change to CFC-free inhaler (see BNF), 10 steroid card (250-*Evohaler* only)
Flomax MR, 25
Florinef, 10 steroid card
Floxapen, 9, 23
Fluanxol, 2, C, administration, driving, see BNF
Flucloxacillin, 9, 23
Fluconazole 50 and 200mg, 9
Fluconazole susp, 9
Fludrocortisone, 10 steroid card
Fludroxycortide external preps, 28
Flunitrazepam, 19
Fluocinolone external preps, 28
Fluocinonide external preps, 28
Fluocinolone scalp lotion, 15, 28
Fluocortolone external preps, 28
Fluorigard mouthwash, C, food and drink, see BNF
Fluoxetine, C, driving, see BNF
Flupentixol, see preps
Fluphenazine, 2
Flurazepam, 19
Flurbiprofen, 21
Flurbiprofen m/r, 21, 25
Fluticasone inhalations, 8, 10 steroid card (high-dose preparations only), C, dose
Fluticasone inhalations (CFC-free), 8, C, dose, change to CFC-free inhaler (see BNF), 10 steroid card (high-dose preparations only)
Fluvastatin, C, muscle effects, see BNF
Fluvastatin m/r, 25, C, muscle effects, see BNF
Fluvoxamine, C, driving, see BNF
Foradil, C, dose, see BNF
Formoterol fumarate, C, dose, see BNF
Fortagesic, 2, 21, 29, 30
Fortipine LA 40, 21, 25
Fortovase, 21
Fortral caps and tabs, 2, 21
Fortral supps, 2
Fosamax, C, administration, see BNF

Franol, 21
Franol Plus, 21
Frisium, 2 *or* 19, 8, C, driving (see BNF)
Froben, 21
Froben SR, 21, 25
Frusene, 14 (urine blue in some lights), 21
Fucibet, 28
Fucidin susp, 9, 21
Fucidin tabs, 9
Fucidin H, 28
Full Marks lotion, mousse, 15
Fungilin loz, 9, 24, C, after food
Fungilin susp (g.i.), 9, C, use of pipette
Fungilin susp (mouth), 9, C, use of pipette, hold in mouth, after food
Fungilin tabs, 9
Furadantin, 9, 14 (urine yellow or brown), 21
Furamide, 9
Fybogel, 13, C, administration, see BNF
Fybogel Mebeverine, 13, 22, C, administration, see BNF
Fybozest Orange, 13, C, administration, see BNF
Gabapentin, 3, 5, 8, C, driving (see BNF)
Gabitril, 21
Galake, 21, 29, 30
Galantamine, 21
Gamanil, 2
Gamolenic acid in evening primrose oil, C, administration, (see BNF)
Ganciclovir, 21
Gastrobid Continus, 25
Glucobay, C, administration, see BNF
Glucophage, 21
Glyceryl trinitrate patch, see preps
Glyceryl trinitrate m/r, 25
Glyceryl trinitrate tabs, 16
Gregoderm, 28
Griseofulvin, 9, 21, C, driving
Grisovin, 9, 21, C, driving
GTN 300 mcg, 16
Guar gum, 13, C, adminstration, see BNF
Guarem, 13, C, administration, see BNF

New British Approved Names (see p. x) used throughout this Appendix

Haelan, 28
Halciderm Topical, 28
Halcinonide external preps, 28
Haldol, 2
Half-Inderal LA, 8, 25
Half-Securon SR, 25
Half-Sinemet CR, 14 (urine reddish), 25
Haloperidol, 2
HeliClear, 5, 9, 25
HeliMet, 4, 5, 9, 25, 27
Heminevrin, 19
Hexalen, 21
Hiprex, 9
Hydergine, 22
Hydrocortisone inj, 10 steroid card
Hydrocortisone external preps, 28
Hydrocortisone tabs, 10 steroid card, 21
Hydrocortisone butyrate external preps, 28

Hydrocortisone butyrate scalp lotion, 15, 28
Hydrocortistab inj, 10 steroid card
Hydrocortone, 10 steroid card, 21
Hydromorphone caps, 2, C, administration, see BNF
Hydromorphone m/r, 2, C, administration, see BNF
Hydroxychloroquine, 5, 21
Hydroxyzine, 2
Hyoscine, 2 (patches, 19)
Hypolar Retard, 25
Hypovase, 3, C, dose, see BNF
Hytrin, 3, C, dose, see BNF
Ibumousse, 15
Ibuprofen, 21
Ibuprofen gran, 13, 21
Ibuprofen m/r, 25, 27
Ibuspray, 15
Idarubicin caps, 25
Imazin XL, 25, 32
Imdur, 25
Imigran, 3, 10 patient information leaflet
Imipramine, 2
Imiquimod, 10 patient information leaflet
Imodium Plus, 24
Implanon, C, see patient information leaflet
Imunovir, 9
Imuran, 21
Indapamide m/r, 25
Inderal, 8
Inderal-LA, 8, 25
Inderetic, 8
Inderex, 8, 25
Indinavir, C, administration, see BNF
Indocid caps and susp, 21, C, driving
Indocid-R, 21, 25, C, driving
Indolar SR, 21, 25, C, driving
Indometacin caps and mixt, 21, C, driving
Indometacin m/r, see preps
Indometacin supps, C, driving
Indomod, 25, C, driving
Indoramin, 2
Industrial methylated spirit, 15
Infacol, C, use of dropper
Inosine pranobex, 9
Insulin, C, see BNF
Intal Spincaps and inhalers, 8
Invirase, 21
Iodine Solution, Aqueous, 27
Ionamin, 25, C, driving
Ipratropium inhalations, C, dose, see BNF
Isib 60XL, 25
Ismo Retard, 25
Ismo tabs, 25
Isocarboxazid, 3, 10 patient information leaflet
Isocard, 10 patient information leaflet, C, administration, see BNF
Isodur XL, 25
Isogel, 13, C, administration, see BNF
Isoket Retard, 25
Isomide CR, 25
Isoniazid elixir and tabs, 8, 22
Isordil (sublingual), 26
Isosorbide dinitrate m/r, 25
Isosorbide mononitrate, 25
Isosorbide mononitrate m/r, 25
Isotard XL, 25
Isotrate, 25

Isotretinoin, 10 patient information card, 21
Isotretinoin gel, 10 patient information leaflet
Isotrex, 10 patient information leaflet
Isotrexin, 10 patient information leaflet
Ispagel, 13, C, administration, see BNF
Ispaghula, 13, C, administration, see BNF
Itraconazole caps, 5, 9, 21, 25
Itraconazole liq, 9, 23
Junifen, 21
Kaletra, 21
Kalspare, 14 (urine blue in some lights), 21
Kalten, 8
Kapake tabs, 2, 29, 30
Kapake sachets, 2, 13, 30
Kay-Cee-L, 21
Keflex, 9
Kelfizine W tabs, 9, 13
Kemadrin, C, driving
Kenalog (systemic), 10 steroid card
Keppra, 8
Keral, 22
Kerlone, 8
Ketoconazole tabs and susp, 5, 9, 21
Ketoprofen caps, 21
Ketoprofen CR, 21, 25
Ketoprofen m/r caps, 21, 25
Ketotifen, 2, 8, 21
Ketorolac tabs, 17, 21
Ketovail, 21, 25
Kinidin Durules, 25
Klaricid, 9
Klaricid sachets, 9, 13
Klaricid XL, 9, 21, 25
Klean-Prep, C, administration, see BNF
Kloref, 13, 21
Konakion tabs, 24
Konsyl, 13, C, administration, see BNF

Labetalol, 8, 21
Lacidipine, 21 no longer required
Lactitol, C, administration, see BNF
Lamictal dispersible tabs, 8, 13, C, driving (see BNF)
Lamictal tabs, 8, 13, C, driving (see BNF)
Lamisil, 9
Lamotrigine dispersible tabs, 8, 13, C, driving (see BNF)
Lamotrigine tabs, 8, 13, C, driving (see BNF)
Lamprene, 8, 14 (urine red), 21
Lanoxin-PG elixir, C, use of pipette
Lansoprazole caps, 5, 25
Lansoprazole susp, 5, 13
Largactil, 2, 11
Lariam, 21, 25, 27, C, driving, malaria prophylaxis, see BNF
Lasikal, 25, 27, C, posture, see BNF
Lasix + K, 25, 27, C, posture, see BNF
Lederfen, 21
Ledermycin, 7, 9, 11, 23
Leflunomide, 4
Lentizol, 2, 25
Lercanidipine, 22
Lescol, C, muscle effects, see BNF
Lescol XL, 25, C, muscle effects, see BNF
Levetiracetam, 8

Mycobutin, 8, 14 (urine orange-red), C, soft lenses
Mynah, 8, 23
Myocrisin inj, C, blood disorder symptoms, see BNF
Myotonine Chloride, 22
Mysoline, 2, 8, C, driving (see BNF)
Nabilone, 2, C, behavioural effects, see BNF
Nabumetone, 21, 25
Nabumetone susp, 21
Nadolol, 8
Nafarelin spray, 10 patient information leaflet, C, nasal decongestants, see BNF
Naftidrofuryl, 25, 27
Nalcrom, 22, C, administration, see BNF
Nalidixic acid, 9, 11
Napratec, 21
Naprosyn EC, 5, 25
Naprosyn S/R, 25
Naprosyn tabs and susp, 21
Naproxen e/c, 5, 25
Naproxen m/r, 25
Naproxen tabs and susp, 21
Naramig, 3
Naratriptan, 3
Nardil, 3, 10 patient information leaflet
Narphen, 2
Natrilix SR, 25
Navoban, 23
Nedocromil sodium inhalation, 8
Nefazodone, 3
Nefopam, 2, 14 (urine pink)
Negram, 9, 11, 23
Nelfinavir tabs, 21
Nelfinavir powder, 21, C, administration, see BNF
Neo-Medrone, 28
Neo-Mercazole, C, blood disorder symptoms, see BNF
Neo-NaClex-K, 25, 27, C, posture, see BNF
Neoral, C, administration, see BNF
Neotigason, 10 patient information leaflet, 21
Nerisone, 28
Nerisone Forte, 28
Neulactil, 2
Neurontin, 3, 5, 8, C, driving (see BNF)
Nevirapine, C, hypersensitivity reactions, see BNF
Nexium, 25
Nicardipine m/r, 25
Nicorette Microtab, 26
Nicotine (lozenges), 24
Nicotine (sublingual), 26
Nicotinell lozenges, 24
Nicotinic acid tabs, 21
Nidazol, 4, 9, 21, 25, 27
Nifedipine m/r, see preps
Nifedipress MR, 25
Nifedotard, 25
Nifelease, 25
Niferex elixir, C, infants, use of dropper
Nisoldipine, 22, 25
Nitrazepam, 19
Nitrofurantoin, 9, 14 (urine yellow or brown), 21
Nitrofurantoin m/r, 9, 14 (urine yellow or brown), 21, 25
Nivaquine, 5, C, malaria prophylaxis, see BNF

Nizoral, 5, 9, 21
Nootropil, 3
Norfloxacin, 7, 9, 23, C, driving
Noritate, 10 patient information leaflet
Normacol preps, 25, 27, C, administration, see BNF
Normax, 14 (urine red)
Normison, 19
Norprolac, 21, C, hypotensive reactions, see BNF
Nortriptyline, 2
Norvir, 21, C, administration see BNF
Nozinan, 2
Nuelin, 21
Nuelin SA preps, 25
Nurofen for children, 21
Nu-Seals Aspirin, 5, 25, 32
Nutrizym preps, C, administration, see BNF
Nuvelle TS, C, administration, see BNF
Nycopren, 5, 25
Nystadermal 28
Nystaform-HC, 28
Nystan pastilles, 9, 24, C, after food
Nystan susp (g.i.), 9, C, use of pipette
Nystan susp (mouth), 9, C, use of pipette, hold in mouth, after food
Nystan tabs, 9
Nystatin mixt (g.i.), 9, C, use of pipette
Nystatin mixt (mouth), 9, C, use of pipette, hold in mouth, after food
Nystatin pastilles, 9, 24, C, after food
Nystatin tabs, 9

New British Approved Names (see p. x) used throughout this Appendix

Occlusal, 15
Ocusert Pilo, C, method of use
Oestrogel, C, administration, see BNF
Ofloxacin, 6, 9, 11, C, driving
Olanzapine tabs, 2
Olanzapine orodispersible tabs, 2, C, administration, see BNF
Olbetam, 21
Olsalazine, 21, C, blood disorder symptoms, see BNF
Omeprazole, C, administration, see BNF
Ondansetron (freeze-dried tablets), C, administration, see BNF
Opilon, 3
Opium tincture, 2
Optimax, 3
Optimine, 2
Oramorph preps, 2
Oramorph SR, 2, 25
Orap, 2
Orbenin, 9, 23
Orelox, 5, 9, 21
Orovite Complement B6, 25
Orphenadrine, C, driving
Orudis caps, 21
Oruvail, 21, 25
Ostram, 13
Ovestin, 25
Oxazepam, 2
Oxerutins, 21
Oxis, C, dose, see BNF
Oxitropium, C, dose

Oxivent, C, dose
Oxprenolol, 8
Oxprenolol m/r, 8, 25
Oxybutynin, 3
Oxycodone caps and liq, 2
Oxycodone m/r, 2, 25
OxyContin, 2, 25
OxyNorm, 2
Oxypertine, 2
Oxytetracycline, 7, 9, 23
Palladone, 2, C, administration, see BNF
Palladone SR, 2, C, administration, see BNF
Paludrine, 21, C, malaria prophylaxis, see BNF
Panadol tabs, 29, 30
Panadol Soluble, 13, 29, 30
Panadol susp, 30
Pancrease preps, C, administration, see BNF
Pancreatin, C, administration, see BNF
Pancrex gran, 25, C, dose, see BNF
Pancrex V Forte tabs, 5, 25, C, dose, see BNF
Pancrex V caps, 125 caps and pdr, C, administration, see BNF
Pancrex V tabs, 5, 25, C, dose, see BNF
Pantoprazole, 25
Paracetamol liq and supps, 30
Paracetamol tabs, 29, 30
Paracetamol tabs, soluble, 13, 29, 30
Paradote, 29, 30
Paramax sachets, 13, 17, 30
Paramax tabs, 17, 30
Pariet, 25
Parlodel, 21, C, hypotensive reactions, see BNF
Parnate, 3, 10 patient information leaflet
Paroven, 21
Paroxetine, 21, C, driving, see BNF
Penbritin caps, 9, 23
Penicillamine, 6, 22, C, blood disorder symptoms, see BNF
Pentasa tabs and gran, C, administration, blood disorder symptoms, see BNF
Pentasa enema and supps, C, blood disorder symptoms, see BNF
Pentazocine caps and tabs, 2, 21
Pentazocine supps, 2
Pentoxifylline m/r, 21, 25
Peppermint oil caps, 5, 22, 25
Percutol, C, administration, see BNF
Pergolide, C, hypotensive reactions, see BNF
Periactin, 2
Pericyazine, 2
Periostat, 6, 11, 27, C, posture, see BNF
Permethrin dermal cream, 10 patient information leaflet
Perphenazine, 2
Persantin, 22
Persantin Retard, 21, 25
Pethidine, 2
Phenazocine, 2
Phenelzine, 3, 10 patient information leaflet
Phenergan, 2

Phenindione, 10 anticoagulant card, 14 (urine pink or orange)

Phenobarbital elixir and tabs, 2, 8, C, driving (see BNF)

Phenothrin lotion, mousse, 15

Phenoxymethylpenicillin, 9, 23

Phentermine m/r, 25, C, driving

Phenylbutazone, e/c, 5, 21, 25, C, blood disorder symptoms, see BNF

Phenytoin caps and tabs, 8, 27, C, administration, blood or skin disorder symptoms (see BNF), driving (see BNF)

Phenytoin chewable tabs, 8, 24, C, blood or skin disorder symptoms (see BNF), driving (see BNF)

Phenytoin susp, 8, C, administration, blood or skin disorder symptoms (see BNF), driving (see BNF)

Phosex, 25

Phosphate-Sandoz, 13

Phyllocontin Continus, 25

Physeptone, 2

Physiotens, 3

Phytomenadione, 24

Picolax, 10 patient information leaflet, 13, C, solution, see BNF

Pilocarpine tabs, 21, 27, C, driving

Pimozide, 2

Pindolol, 8

Piperazine powder, 13

Piracetam, 3

Piriton, 2

Piroxicam caps and tabs, 21

Piroxicam dispersible tabs, 13, 21

Pivmecillinam, 9, 21, 27, C, posture, see BNF

Pizotifen, 2

Plaquenil, 5, 21

Plendil, 25

Podophyllin paint cpd, 15, C, application, see BNF

Ponstan, 21

Potaba caps and tabs, 21

Potaba Envules, 13, 21

Potassium chloride m/r, see preps

Potassium citrate mixt, 27

Potassium effervescent tabs, 13, 21

Pramipexole, C, hypotensive reactions, driving, see BNF

Pranoxen Continus, 25

Pravastatin, C, muscle effects, see BNF

Praxilene, 25, 27

Prazosin, 3, C, dose, see BNF

Precortisyl, 10 steroid card, 27

Precortisyl Forte, 10 steroid card, 21

Prednesol, 10 steroid card, 13, 21

Prednisolone inj, 10 steroid card

Prednisolone tabs, 10 steroid card, 21

Prednisolone e/c, 5, 10 steroid card, 25

Preservex, 21

Prestim, 8

Priadel liq, 10 lithium card, C, fluid and salt intake, see BNF

Priadel tabs, 10 lithium card, 25, C, fluid and salt intake, see BNF

Primidone, 2, 8, C, driving (see BNF)

Prioderm lotion, 15

Pripsen, 13

Pro-Banthine, 23

Probenecid, 12, 21, 27

Procarbazine, 4

Prochlorperazine, 2

Prochlorperazine buccal tabs, 2, C, administration, see BNF

Prochlorperazine sachets, 2, 13

Procyclidine, C, driving

Prograf, 23, C, driving, see BNF

Proguanil, 21, C, malaria prophylaxis, see BNF

Progynova TS preps, C, administration, see BNF

Promazine, 2

Promethazine, 2

Propaderm, 28

Propafenone, 21, 25

Propantheline, 23

Propiverine hydrochloride, 3

Propranolol, 8

Propranolol m/r, 8, 25

Prothiaden, 2

Protionamide, 8, 21

Protium, 25

Prozac, C, driving, see BNF

Psorin, 28

Pulmicort, 8, 10 steroid card, C, dose

Pulmicort LS, 8, C, dose

Pulmicort Respules, 8, 10 steroid card, C, dose

Pylorid, C, discoloration (tongue and faeces), see BNF

Pyrazinamide, 8

Pyrogastrone liquid, 21

Pyrogastrone tabs, 21, 24

Questran preps, 13, C, avoid other drugs at same time, see BNF

Quetiapine, 2

Quinagolide, 21, C, hypotensive reactions, see BNF

Quinidine m/r, 25

Quinocort, 28

Quinoderm with Hydrocortisone, 28

Qvar preps, 8, 10 steroid card (high-dose preparations only), C, dose

Rabeprazole, 25

Ranitidine bismuth citrate, C, discoloration (tongue and faeces), see BNF

Ranitidine effervescent tabs, 13

Rapamune, C, administration

Rebetol, 21

Reboxetine, C, driving

Regulan, 13, C, administration, BNF

Regurin, 23

Relifex, 21, 25

Relifex susp, 21

Remedeine , 2, 21, 29, 30

Remedeine effervescent tabs, 2, 13, 21, 29, 30

Reminyl, 2

Renagel, 21

Requip, 21, C, driving, see BNF

Resonium A, 13

Restandol, 21, 25

Retrovir syrup, C, use of oral syringe

Revanil, 21, C, hypotensive reactions, see BNF

Rheumacin SR, 21, 25, C, driving

Rheumox, 11, 21, C, photosensitivity, see BNF

Rhumalgan, 5, 25

Ridaura, 21, C, blood disorder symptoms, see BNF

Rifabutin, 8, 14 (urine orange-red), C, soft lenses

Rifadin, 8, 14 (urine orange-red), 22, C, soft lenses

Rifampicin caps and mixt, 8, 14 (urine orange-red), 22, C, soft lenses

Rifater, 8, 14 (urine orange-red), 22, C, soft lenses

Rifinah, 8, 14 (urine orange-red), 22, C, soft lenses

Rilutek, C, blood disorders, driving

Rimactane, 8, 14 (urine orange-red), 22, C, soft lenses

Rimactazid, 8, 14 (urine or-ange-red), 22, C, soft lenses

Risedronate sodium, C, administration, food and calcium, see BNF

Risperdal, 2

Risperidone, 2

Ritonavir, 21, C, administration, see BNF

Rivastigmine, 21, 25

Rivotril, 2, 8, C, driving (see BNF)

Rizatriptan tabs, 3

Rizatriptan wafers, 3, C, administration

Roaccutane, 10 patient information card, 21

Robaxin, 2

Rohypnol, 19

Ronicol Timespan, 25

Ropinirole, 21, C, driving, see BNF

Rowachol, 22

Rowatinex caps, 25

Rozex, 10 patient information leaflet

Rythmodan Retard, 25

Sabril sachets, 3, 8, 13, C, driving (see BNF)

Sabril tabs, 3, 8, C, driving (see BNF)

Safapryn, 5, 25

Safapryn-Co, 5, 25

Salactol, 15

Salagen, 21, 27, C, driving

Salazopyrin, 14 (urine orange-yellow), C, blood disorder symptoms and soft lenses, see BNF

Salazopyrin EN-tabs, 5, 14 (urine orange-yellow), 25, C, blood disorder symptoms and soft lenses, see BNF

Salbulin, C, dose, change to CFC-free inhaler, see BNF

Salbutamol inhalations, C, dose, see BNF

Salbutamol inhalations (CFC-free), C, dose, change to CFC-free inhaler, see BNF

Salbutamol m/r, 25

Salicylic acid collodion, 15

Salicylic acid lotion, 15

Salmeterol, C, dose, see BNF

Salofalk, 5, 25, C, blood disorder symptoms, see BNF

Salts 'SPR' plaster remover, 15

Sandimmun, C, administration, see BNF

Sandrena, C, administration, see BNF

Sando-K, 13, 21

Sandocal, 13

SangCya, C, administration, see BNF

Sanomigran, 2

Saquinavir, 21

Scopoderm TTS, 19, C, administration, see BNF

Secadrex, 8

Secobarbital, 19

Seconal, 19

Sectral, 8

Securon SR, 25

Selegiline (freeze-dried tablets), C, administration, see BNF

Selexid, 9, 21, 27, C, posture, see BNF

Semprex, C, driving, alcohol, see BNF

Septrin susp and tabs, 9

Septrin dispersible tabs, 9, 13

Serc, 21

Serenace, 2

Seretide, 8, 10, steroid card (250- and 500-*Accuhaler* only), C, dose

Seretide Evohaler, 8, C, dose, change to CFC-free inhaler (see BNF), 10 steroid card (250-*Evohaler* only)

Serevent, C, dose, see BNF

Seroquel, 2

Seroxat liq and tabs, 21, C, driving, see BNF

Sertraline, C, driving, see BNF

Sevredol, 2

Sevelamer, 21

Simvastatin, C, muscle effects, see BNF

Sinemet CR, 14 (urine reddish), 25

Sinemet preps, 14 (urine reddish), 21

Sinequan, 2

Singulair chewable tabs, 23, 24

Sinthrome, 10 anticoagulant card

Sirolimus, C, administration

Skelid, C, food and calcium

Slofedipine XL, 25

Slo-Indo, 21, 25, C, driving

Slo-Phyllin, 25 or C, administration, see BNF

Sloprolol, 8, 25

Slow Sodium, 25

Slow-Fe, 25

Slow-Fe Folic, 25

Slow-K, 25, 27, C, posture, see BNF

Slow-Trasicor, 8, 25

Slozem, 25

Sodium Amytal, 19

Sodium aurothiomalate, C, blood disorder symptoms, see BNF

Sodium cellulose phosphate, 13, 21, C, may be sprinkled on food

Sodium chloride m/r, 25

Sodium chloride tabs, 13

Sodium chloride and glucose oral pdr, cpd, 13

Sodium clodronate, C, food and calcium, see BNF

Sodium cromoglicate (oral), 22, C, administration, see BNF

Sodium cromoglicate inhalations, 8

Sodium fusidate susp, 9, 21

Sodium fusidate tabs, 9

Sodium picosulfate pdr, 10 patient information leaflet, 13, C, see BNF

Sodium valproate e/c, 5, 8, 25, C, blood or hepatic disorder symptoms (see BNF), driving (see BNF)

Sodium valproate m/r, 8, 25, C, blood or hepatic disorder symptoms (see BNF), driving (see BNF)

Sodium valproate crushable tabs, liquid and syrup, 8, C, blood or hepatic disorder symptoms (see BNF), driving (see BNF)

Solian, 2

Solpadol caplets, 2, 29, 30

Solpadol Effervescent, 2, 13, 29, 30

Solu-Cortef, 10 steroid card

Solu-Medrone, 10 steroid card

Solvazinc, 13, 21

Somnite, 19

Sonata, 2

Soneryl, 19

Sotacor, 8

Sotalol, 8

Sparine, 2

Sporanox caps, 5, 9, 21, 25

Sporanox liq, 9, 23

Stelazine syrup and tabs, 2

Stelazine Spansule, 2, 25

Stemetil, 2

Stemetil Eff, 2, 13

Sterculia, C, administration, see BNF

Stiedex, 28

Stilnoct, 19

Stugeron, 2

Stugeron Forte, 2

Subutex, 2, 26

Sucralfate, 5

Sudafed Plus, 2

Suleo-M, 15

Sulfadiazine, 9, 27

Sulfametopyrazine, 9, 13

Sulfasalazine, 14 (urine orange-yellow), C, blood disorder symptoms and soft lenses, see BNF

Sulfasalazine e/c, 5, 14 (urine orange-yellow), 25, C, blood disorder symptoms and soft lenses, see BNF

Sulfinpyrazone, 12, 21

Sulindac, 21

Sulpiride, 2

Sulpitil, 2

Sulpor, 2

Sumatriptan, 3, 10 patient information leaflet

Suprax, 9

Supralip, 21, 25

Suprecur, C, nasal decongestants, see BNF

Suprefact nasal spray, C, nasal decongestants, see BNF

Surgam tabs, 21

Surgam SA, 25

Surgical spirit, 15

Surmontil, 2

Suscard Buccal, C, administration, see BNF

Sustac, 25

Symmetrel, C, driving

Synalar external preps, 28

Synarel, 10 patient information leaflet, C, nasal decongestants, see BNF

Synflex, 21

Syscor MR, 22, 25

New British Approved Names (see p. x) used throughout this Appendix

---

Tacrolimus, 23, C, driving, see BNF

Tagamet effervescent tabs, 13

Tamsulosin m/r, 25

Tarka, 25

Tarivid, 6, 9, 11, C, driving

Tavanic, 6, 9, 25, C, driving

Tavegil, 2

Tegretol Chewtabs, 3, 8, 21, 24, C, blood, hepatic or skin disorder symptoms (see BNF), driving (see BNF)

Tegretol liq, supps and tabs, 3, 8, C, blood, hepatic or skin disorder symptoms (see BNF), driving (see BNF)

Tegretol Retard, 3, 8, 25, C, blood, hepatic or skin disorder symptoms (see BNF), driving (see BNF)

Telfast, C, driving, see BNF

Temazepam, 19

Temgesic, 2, 26

Temodal, 23, 25

Temozolamide, 23, 25

Tenben, 8

Tenif, 8, 25

Tenoret 50, 8

Tenoretic, 8

Tenormin, 8

Tenoxicam tabs, 21

Tensipine MR, 21, 25

Terazosin, 3, C, dose, see BNF

Terbinafine, 9

Terbutaline inhalations, C, dose, see BNF

Terbutaline m/r, 25

Terfenadine, C, driving, alcohol

Teril CR, 3, 8, 25, C, blood, hepatic or skin disorder symptoms (see BNF), driving (see BNF)

Terra-Cortril oint, 28

Terra-Cortril Nystatin, 28

Terramycin, 7, 9, 23

Testosterone patch, C, administration, see BNF

Testosterone undecanoate caps, 21, 25

Tetrabenazine, 2

Tetracycline, 7, 9, 23, C, posture

Tetracycline mouthwash, see BNF

Tetralysal preps, 6, 9

Teveten, 21

Theo-Dur, 25

Theophylline, 21

Theophylline m/r, see preps

Thioridazine, 2

Tiabendazole, 3, 21, 24

Tiagabine, 21

Tiaprofenic acid tabs, 21

Tiaprofenic acid m/r, 25

Ticlid, 21

Ticlopidine, 21

Tilade, 8

Tildiem preps, 25

Tiloryth, 5, 9, 25

Tiludronic acid, C, food and calcium

Timodine, 28

Timolol, 8

Timonil Retard, 3, 8, 25, C, blood, hepatic or skin disorder symptoms (see BNF), driving (see BNF)

Tinidazole tabs, 4, 9, 21, 25

Tizanidine, 2

Tofranil, 2

Tolterodine m/r, 25

Topamax Sprinkle, 3, 8, C, administration, driving (see BNF)
Topamax tabs, 3, 8, C, driving (see BNF)
Topiramate Sprinkle caps, 3, 8, C, administration, driving (see BNF)
Topiramate tabs, 3, 8, C, driving (see BNF)
Toradol tabs, 17, 21
Tramadol, 2
Tramadol m/r, 2, 25
Tramadol sachets, 2, 13
Tramadol soluble, 2, 13
Tramake, 2
Tramake Insts, 2, 13
Trandate, 8, 21
Tranxene, 2 or 19
Tranylcypromine, 3, 10 patient information leaflet
Trasicor, 8
Trasidrex, 8, 25
Traxam foam, 15
Trazodone, 2, 21
Trazodone m/r, 2, 21, 25
Trental m/r, 21, 25
Treosulfan, 25
Tretinoin caps, 21
Tri-Adcortyl external preps, 28
Triamcinolone inj, 10 steroid card
Triamcinolone tabs, 10 steroid card, 21
Triamterene, 14 (urine blue in some lights), 21
Triapin preps, 25
Tribavirin caps, 21
Triclofos sodium, 19
Trientine, 6, 22
Trifluoperazine, 2
Trifyba, C, administration, see BNF
Trihexyphenidyl, C, before or after food, driving, see BNF
Trilostane, 21
Trimethoprim mixt and tabs, 9
Trimipramine, 2
Trimopan, 9
Trimovate, 28
Tripotassium dicitratobismuthate, C, administration, see BNF
Triprolidine m/r, 2, 25
Triptafen preps, 2
Trizivir, C, hypersensitivity reactions, see BNF
Tropisetron, 23
Tropium, 2
Trospium chloride, 23
Tryptophan, 3
Tuinal, 19
Tylex caps, 2, 29, 30
Tylex effervescent tabs, 2, 13, 29, 30
Typhoid vaccine, oral, 23, 25, C, administration, see BNF

Ubretid, 22
Ucerax, 2
Ultralanum Plain, 28
Uniphyllin Continus, 25
Univer, 25
Uprima, C, driving
Urdox, 21
Uriben, 9, 11
Ursodeoxycholic acid, 21
Ursogal, 21
Ursofalk, 21
Utinor, 7, 9, 23, C, driving

New British Approved Names (see p. x) used throughout this Appendix

---

Valaciclovir, 9
Valium, 2 or 19
Vallergan, 2
Valoid, 2
Valproic acid, 8, 25, C, blood or hepatic disorder symptoms (see BNF), driving (see BNF)
Valtrex, 9
Vancocin caps, 9
Vancomycin caps, 9
Velosef, 9
Venlafaxine, 21, C, driving, skin reactions
Venlafaxine m/r, 21, 25, C, driving, skin reactions
Ventide, 8, C, dose, see BNF
Ventmax SR, 25
Ventodisks, C, dose, see BNF
Ventolin Evohaler, C, dose, change to CFC-free inhaler, see BNF
Ventolin inhalations, C, dose, see BNF
Vepesid caps, 23
Verapamil m/r, 25
Verapress, 25
Vertab SR, 25
Vesanoid, 21
Viazem XL, 25
Vibramycin caps, 6, 9, 11, 27, C, posture, see BNF
Vibramycin-D, 6, 9, 11, 13
Videx, 23, C, administration, see BNF
Videx e/c caps, 25, C, administration
Videx tabs, 23, C, administration
Vigabatrin sachets, 3, 8, 13, C, driving (see BNF)
Vigabatrin tabs, 3, 8, C, driving (see BNF)
Vioform-Hydrocortisone, 28
Viracept tabs, 21
Viracept powder, 21, C, administration, see BNF
Viramune, C, hypersensitivity reactions, see BNF
Visclair, 5, 22, 25
Viskaldix, 8
Visken, 8
Vivotif, 23, 25, C, administration, see BNF
Volmax, 25
Voltarol dispersible tabs, 13, 21
Voltarol tabs, 5, 25
Voltarol 75mg SR and Retard, 21, 25

Warfarin, 10 anticoagulant card
Warfarin WBP, 10 anticoagulant card
Warticon, 15
Welldorm, 19, 27
Wellvone, 21

Xanax, 2
Xatral, 3, C, dose, see BNF
Xatral XL, 3, 25, C, dose, see BNF
Xepin, 2, 10 patient information leaflet
Xismox XL, 25
Xyzal, C, driving

Zaditen, 2, 8, 21
Zadstat supps, 4, 9
Zafirlukast, 23
Zaleplon, 2
Zamadol, 2
Zamadol SR, 2, 25
Zanaflex, 2
Zanidip, 22
Zantac effervescent tabs, 13
Zarontin, 8, C, blood disorder symptoms (see BNF), driving (see BNF)
Zavedos caps, 25
Zelapar, C, administration, see BNF
Zemtard XL, 25
Ziagen, C, hypersensitivity reactions, see BNF
Zidovudine syrup, C, use of oral syringe
Zimovane, 19
Zinamide, 8
Zinc sulphate, see preps
Zinnat sachets, 9, 13, 21
Zinnat susp, 9, 21
Zinnat tabs, 9, 21, 25
Zirtek, C, driving, alcohol, see BNF
Zispin, 2, 25
Zithromax caps, 5, 9, 23
Zithromax susp and tabs, 5, 9
Zocor, C, muscle effects, see BNF
Zofran Melt, C, administration, see BNF
Zoleptil, 2
Zolmitriptan orodispersible tabs, C, administration, see BNF
Zolpidem, 19
Zomig Rapimelt, C, administration, see BNF
Zomorph, 2, 25
Zopiclone, 19
Zotepine, 2
Zoton caps, 5, 25
Zoton susp, 5, 13
Zovirax susp and tabs, 9
Zuclopenthixol, 2
Zydol, 2
Zydol soluble, 2, 13
Zydol SR, 2, 25
Zydol XL, 2, 25
Zyloric, 8, 21, 27
Zyomet, 10 patient information leaflet
Zyprexa tabs, 2
Zyprexa Velotab, 2, C, administration, see BNF
Zyvox tabs, 9, 10 patient information leaflet

Dental Practitioners' Formulary

List of Dental Preparations

The following list has been approved by the appropriate Secretaries of State, and the preparations therein may be prescribed by dental practitioners on form FP10D (GP14 in Scotland).

Sugar-free versions, where available, are preferred.

Aciclovir Cream, BP
Aciclovir Oral Suspension, BP, 200 mg/5 mL
Aciclovir Tablets, BP, 200 mg
Amoxicillin Capsules, BP
Amoxicillin Oral Powder, DPF[1]
Amoxicillin Oral Suspension, BP
Amphotericin Lozenges, BP
Amphotericin Oral Suspension, BP
Ampicillin Capsules, BP
Ampicillin Oral Suspension, BP
Artificial Saliva, DPF[2]
Ascorbic Acid Tablets, BP
Aspirin Tablets, Dispersible, BP[3]
Azithromycin Oral Suspension, 200 mg/5 mL, DPF
Benzydamine Mouthwash, BP 0.15%
Benzydamine Oromucosal Spray, BP 0.15%
Carbamazepine Tablets, BP
Carmellose Gelatin Paste, DPF
Cefalexin Capsules, BP
Cefalexin Oral Suspension, BP
Cefalexin Tablets, BP
Cefradine Capsules, BP
Cefradine Oral Solution, DPF
Chlorhexidine Gluconate 1% Gel, DPF
Chlorhexidine Mouthwash, BP
Chlorhexidine Oral Spray, DPF
Chlorphenamine Tablets/Chlorpheniramine Tablets, BP
Choline Salicylate Dental Gel, BP
Clindamycin Capsules, BP
Diazepam Oral Solution, BP, 2 mg/5 mL
Diazepam Tablets, BP
Diflunisal Tablets, BP
Dihydrocodeine Tablets, BP, 30 mg
Doxycycline Capsules, BP, 100 mg
Doxycycline Tablets, 20 mg, DPF
Ephedrine Nasal Drops, BP
Erythromycin Ethyl Succinate Oral Suspension, BP
Erythromycin Ethyl Succinate Tablets, BP
Erythromycin Stearate Tablets, BP
Erythromycin Tablets, BP
Fluconazole Capsules, 50 mg, DPF
Fluconazole Oral Suspension, 50 mg/5 mL, DPF
Hydrocortisone Cream, BP, 1%
Hydrocortisone Lozenges, BPC[2]
Hydrocortisone and Miconazole Cream, DPF
Hydrocortisone and Miconazole Ointment, DPF
Hydrogen Peroxide Mouthwash, BP

Ibuprofen Oral Suspension, BP, sugar-free
Ibuprofen Tablets, BP
Lidocaine 5% Ointment/Lignocaine 5% Ointment, DPF
Menthol and Eucalyptus Inhalation, BP 1980[4]
Metronidazole Oral Suspension, DPF
Metronidazole Tablets, BP
Miconazole Oromucosal Gel, BP
Mouthwash Solution-tablets, DPF
Nitrazepam Tablets, BP
Nystatin Ointment, BP
Nystatin Oral Suspension, BP
Nystatin Pastilles, BP
Oxytetracycline Tablets, BP
Paracetamol Oral Suspension, BP[5]
Paracetamol Tablets, BP
Paracetamol Tablets, Soluble, BP
Penciclovir Cream, DPF
Pethidine Tablets, BP
Phenoxymethylpenicillin Oral Solution, BP
Phenoxymethylpenicillin Tablets, BP
Povidone–Iodine Mouthwash, BP, 1%
Promethazine Hydrochloride Tablets, BP
Promethazine Oral Solution, BP
Sodium Chloride Mouthwash, Compound, BP
Sodium Fluoride Oral Drops, BP
Sodium Fluoride Tablets, BP
Sodium Fusidate Ointment, BP
Sodium Perborate Mouthwash, DPF
Temazepam Oral Solution, BP
Temazepam Tablets, BP
Tetracycline Capsules, BP
Tetracycline Tablets, BP
Thymol Glycerin, Compound, BP 1988[4]
Triamcinolone Dental Paste, BP
Vitamin B Tablets, Compound, Strong, BPC
Zinc Sulphate Mouthwash, DPF

> Preparations in this list which are not included in the BP or BPC are described on next page

1. Amoxicillin Dispersible Tablets are no longer available
2. Supplies may be difficult to obtain
3. The BP directs that when soluble aspirin tablets are prescribed, dispersible aspirin tablets should be dispensed
4. This preparation does not appear in subsequent editions of the BP
5. The BP directs that when Paediatric Paracetamol Oral Suspension or Paediatric Paracetamol Mixture is prescribed and no strength stated Paracetamol Oral Suspension 120 mg/5 mL should be dispensed

Details of DPF preparations

Preparations on the List of Dental Preparations which are specified as DPF are described as follows in the DPF.

Although brand names have sometimes been included for identification purposes preparations on the list should be prescribed by non-proprietary name.

Amoxicillin Oral Powder PoM (proprietary product: *Amoxil Sachets SF*), amoxicillin (as trihydrate) 750 mg[1] and 3 g sachet
  1. 750-mg sachets are no longer available

Artificial Saliva, (proprietary product: *Luborant*) consists of sorbitol 1.8 g, carmellose sodium (sodium carboxymethylcellulose) 390 mg, dibasic potassium phosphate 48.23 mg, potassium chloride 37.5 mg, monobasic potassium phosphate 21.97 mg, calcium chloride 9.972 mg, magnesium chloride 3.528 mg, sodium fluoride 258 micrograms/60 mL, with preservatives and colouring agents

Azithromycin Oral Suspension 200 mg/5 mL PoM (proprietary product: *Zithromax*); azithromycin (as dihydrate) 200 mg/5 mL when reconstituted with water

Carmellose Gelatin Paste (proprietary product: *Orabase Oral Paste*), gelatin, pectin, carmellose sodium, 16.58% of each in a suitable basis

Cefradine Oral Solution PoM (proprietary product: *Velosef Syrup*), cefradine 250 mg/5 mL when reconstituted with water

Chlorhexidine Gluconate 1% Gel (proprietary product: *Corsodyl Dental Gel*), chlorhexidine gluconate 1%

Chlorhexidine Oral Spray (proprietary product: *Corsodyl Oral Spray*), chlorhexidine gluconate 0.2%

Doxycycline Tablets 20 mg PoM (proprietary product: *Periostat*), doxycycline (as hyclate) 20 mg

Fluconazole Capsules 50 mg PoM (proprietary product: *Diflucan*), fluconazole 50 mg

Fluconazole Oral Suspension 50 mg/5 mL PoM (proprietary product: *Diflucan*), fluconazole 50 mg/5 mL when reconstituted with water

Hydrocortisone and Miconazole Cream PoM (proprietary product: *Daktacort Cream*), hydrocortisone 1%, miconazole nitrate 2%

Hydrocortisone and Miconazole Ointment PoM (proprietary product: *Daktacort Ointment*), hydrocortisone 1%, miconazole nitrate 2%

Lidocaine 5% Ointment/Lignocaine 5% Ointment (proprietary product: *Xylocaine Ointment*), lidocaine 5% in a suitable basis

Metronidazole Oral Suspension PoM (proprietary product: *Flagyl S*), metronidazole (as benzoate) 200 mg/5 mL

Mouthwash Solution-tablets consist of tablets which may contain antimicrobial, colouring and flavouring agents in a suitable soluble effervescent basis to make a mouthwash suitable for dental purposes

Penciclovir Cream PoM (proprietary product: *Vectavir Cream*), penciclovir 1%

Sodium Perborate Mouthwash (proprietary product: *Bocasan Mouthwash*), sodium perborate 68.6%

Zinc Sulphate Mouthwash consists of zinc sulphate lotion, BP. Directions for use: dilute 1 part with 4 parts of warm water
Note. May be difficult to obtain

Nurse Prescribers' Formulary

Nurse Prescribers' Formulary Appendix (Appendix NPF). List of preparations approved by the Secretary of State which may be prescribed on form FP10P (form GP10(N) in Scotland, form HS21(N) in Northern Ireland) by Nurses for National Health Service patients

Medicinal Preparations

Almond Oil Ear Drops, BP
Arachis Oil Enema, NPF
[1]Aspirin Tablets, Dispersible, 300 mg, BP
Bisacodyl Suppositories, BP (includes 5-mg and 10-mg strengths)
Bisacodyl Tablets, BP
Cadexomer–Iodine Ointment, NPF
Cadexomer–Iodine Paste, NPF
Cadexomer–Iodine Powder, NPF
Catheter Maintenance Solution, Chlorhexidine, NPF
Catheter Maintenance Solution, Mandelic Acid, NPF
Catheter Maintenance Solution, Sodium Chloride, NPF
Catheter Maintenance Solution, 'Solution G', NPF
Catheter Maintenance Solution, 'Solution R', NPF
Choline Salicylate Dental Gel, BP
Clotrimazole Cream 1%, BP
Co-danthramer Capsules, NPF
Co-danthramer Capsules, Strong, NPF
Co-danthramer Oral Suspension, NPF
Co-danthramer Oral Suspension, Strong, NPF
Co-danthrusate Capsules, BP
Co-danthrusate Oral Suspension, NPF
Crotamiton Cream, BP
Crotamiton Lotion, BP
Dextranomer Beads, NPF
Dextranomer Paste, NPF
Dimeticone barrier creams containing at least 10%
Docusate Capsules, BP
Docusate Enema, NPF
Docusate Enema, Compound, BP
Docusate Oral Solution, BP
Docusate Oral Solution, Paediatric, BP
Econazole Cream 1%, BP
Emollients as listed below:
  Alcoderm® Cream
  Alcoderm® Lotion
  Aqueous Cream, BP
  Arachis Oil, BP
  Cetraben® Emollient Cream
  Dermamist®
  Diprobase® Cream
  Diprobase® Ointment
  Doublebase®
  E45® Cream
  Emulsifying Ointment, BP
  Epaderm®
  Hydromol® Cream
  Hydrous Ointment, BP
  Keri® Therapeutic Lotion
  LactiCare® Lotion
  Lipobase®
  Liquid and White Soft Paraffin Ointment, NPF
  Neutrogena® Dermatological Cream
  Oilatum® Cream
  Paraffin, White Soft, BP
  Paraffin, Yellow Soft, BP
  Ultrabase®
  Unguentum M®

Preparations on this list which are not included in the BP or BPC are described on p. 764

Emollient Bath Additives as listed below:
  Alpha Keri® Bath Oil
  [2]Balneum®
  [3]Dermalo® Bath Emollient
  Diprobath®
  Hydromol® Emollient
  Oilatum® Emollient
  Oilatum® Fragrance Free
  Oilatum® Gel
Folic Acid 400 micrograms/5 mL Oral Solution, NPF
Folic Acid Tablets 400 micrograms, BP
Glycerol Suppositories, BP
Ispaghula Husk Granules, BP
Ispaghula Husk Granules, Effervescent, BP
Ispaghula Husk Oral Powder, BP
Lactitol Powder, NPF
Lactulose Solution, BP
Lidocaine Gel/Lignocaine Gel, BP
Lidocaine Ointment/Lignocaine Ointment, NPF
Lidocaine and Chlorhexidine Gel/Lignocaine and Chlorhexidine Gel, BP
Macrogol Oral Powder, Compound, NPF
Magnesium Hydroxide Mixture, BP
Magnesium Sulphate Paste, BP
Malathion alcoholic lotions containing at least 0.5%
Malathion aqueous lotions containing at least 0.5%
Mebendazole Oral Suspension, NPF
Mebendazole Tablets, NPF
Methylcellulose Tablets, BP
Miconazole Cream 2%, BP
Miconazole Oromucosal Gel, BP
Mouthwash Solution-tablets, NPF
Nicotine Inhalation Cartridge for Oromucosal Use, NPF
Nicotine Lozenge, NPF
Nicotine Medicated Chewing Gum, NPF
Nicotine Nasal Spray, NPF
Nicotine Sublingual Tablets, NPF
Nicotine Transdermal Patches, NPF
Nystatin Oral Suspension, BP
Nystatin Pastilles, BP
Olive Oil Ear Drops, BP
Paracetamol Oral Suspension, BP (includes 120 mg/5 mL and 250 mg/5 mL strengths—both of which are available as sugar-free formulations)
[1]Paracetamol Tablets, BP
[1]Paracetamol Tablets, Soluble, BP (includes 120-mg and 500-mg tablets)
Permethrin Cream, NPF
Permethrin Cream Rinse, NPF
Phenothrin Alcoholic Lotion, NPF
Phenothrin Aqueous Lotion, NPF
Phenothrin Foam Application, NPF
Phosphates Enema, BP
Piperazine and Senna Powder, NPF
Povidone–Iodine Solution, BP
Senna Granules, Standardised, BP
Senna Oral Solution, NPF
Senna Tablets, BP
Senna and Ispaghula Granules, NPF
Sodium Bicarbonate Ear Drops, BP
Sodium Chloride Solution, Sterile, BP
Sodium Citrate Compound Enema, NPF
Sodium Picosulfate Elixir, NPF
Sterculia Granules, NPF
Sterculia and Frangula Granules, NPF
Streptokinase and Streptodornase Topical Powder, NPF
Thymol Glycerin, Compound, BP 1988
[4]Titanium Ointment, NPF
Zinc and Castor Oil Ointment, BP
Zinc Oxide and Dimeticone Spray, NPF
Zinc Oxide Impregnated Medicated Stocking, NPF

---

1. Max. 96 tablets; max. pack size 32 tablets
2. Except pack sizes that are not to be prescribed under the NHS (see Part XVIIIA of the Drug Tariff, Part XI of the Northern Ireland Drug Tariff)
3. Formerly Emmolate® Bath Oil
4. Incorporated into BP 2001 (effective 1 December 2001)

Appliances and Reagents (including Wound Management Products)

Applicators, Vaginal as listed in Part IXA of the Drug Tariff (Part 3 of the Scottish Drug Tariff, not prescribable by nurses in Northern Ireland)

Atomizers, Hand Operated as listed in Part IXA of the Drug Tariff (Part 3 of the Scottish Drug Tariff, not prescribable by nurses in Northern Ireland)

Auto Inflation Device (for treatment of glue ear) as listed in Part IXA of the Drug Tariff (Part 3 of the Scottish Drug Tariff, Part III of the Northern Ireland Drug Tariff)

Breast Reliever as listed in Part IXA of the Drug Tariff (Part 3 of the Scottish Drug Tariff, not prescribable by nurses in Northern Ireland)

Breast Shields as listed in Part IXA of the Drug Tariff (not prescribable by nurses in Scotland or Northern Ireland)

Chemical Reagents

The following as listed in Part IXR of the Drug Tariff (Part 9 of the Scottish Drug Tariff, Part II of the Northern Ireland Drug Tariff):

Detection Tablets for Glycosuria

Detection Tablets for Ketonuria

Detection Strips for Glycosuria

Detection Strips for Ketonuria

Detection Strips for Proteinuria

Detection Strips for Blood Glucose

Reagent solutions (Gerhardt's Reagent and Ammonia Solution, Strong, BP) (not prescribable by nurses in Northern Ireland)

Catheter Accessories as listed in Part IXA of the Drug Tariff (Part 3 of the Scottish Drug Tariff, Part III of the Northern Ireland Drug Tariff)

Catheter Maintenance Solutions as listed in Part IXA of the Drug Tariff (Part 3 of the Scottish Drug Tariff, Part III of the Northern Ireland Drug Tariff)

Catheters, Urethral Sterile as listed under Catheters in Part IXA of the Drug Tariff (Part 3 of the Scottish Drug Tariff, Part III of the Northern Ireland Drug Tariff)

Chiropody Appliances as listed in Part IXA of the Drug Tariff (Part 2 of the Scottish Drug Tariff (except for Corn Plasters), not prescribable by nurses in Northern Ireland)

Contraceptive Devices as listed in Part IXA of the Drug Tariff (Part 3 of the Scottish Drug Tariff, Part III of the Northern Ireland Drug Tariff (fertility (ovulation) thermometers only))

Douches (with vaginal and rectal fittings) as listed in Part IXA of the Drug Tariff (Part 3 of the Scottish Drug Tariff, not prescribable by nurses in Northern Ireland)

Droppers as listed in Part IXA of the Drug Tariff (Part 3 of the Scottish Drug Tariff, not prescribable by nurses in Northern Ireland)

Elastic Hosiery including accessories as listed in Part IXA of the Drug Tariff (Part 4 of the Scottish Drug Tariff, Part III of the Northern Ireland Drug Tariff)

Eye Baths as listed in Part IXA of the Drug Tariff (Part 3 of the Scottish Drug Tariff, not prescribable by nurses in Northern Ireland)

Eye drops Dispensers as listed in Part IXA of the Drug Tariff (Part 3 of the Scottish Drug Tariff, Part III of the Northern Ireland Drug Tariff)

Eye Shades as listed in Part IXA of the Drug Tariff (Part 3 of the Scottish Drug Tariff, not prescribable by nurses in Northern Ireland)

Finger Cots as listed in Part IXA of the Drug Tariff (Part 3 of the Scottish Drug Tariff, not prescribable by nurses in Northern Ireland)

Finger Stalls as listed in Part IXA of the Drug Tariff (Part 3 of the Scottish Drug Tariff, not prescribable by nurses in Northern Ireland)

Hypodermic Equipment as listed in Part IXA of the Drug Tariff (Part 3 of the Scottish Drug Tariff, Part III of the Northern Ireland Drug Tariff (with some exceptions))

Incontinence Appliances as listed in Part IXB of the Drug Tariff (Part 5 of the Scottish Drug Tariff, Part III of the Northern Ireland Drug Tariff)

Inhaler, Spare Tops as listed in Part IXA of the Drug Tariff (Part 3 of the Scottish Drug Tariff, not prescribable by nurses in Northern Ireland)

Insufflators as listed in Part IXA of the Drug Tariff (Part 3 of the Scottish Drug Tariff, not prescribable by nurses in Northern Ireland)

Iodine Brush as listed under Brushes in Part IXA of the Drug Tariff (Part 3 of the Scottish Drug Tariff, not prescribable by nurses in Northern Ireland)

Irrigation Fluids as listed in Part IXA of the Drug Tariff (Part 2 of the Scottish Drug Tariff, Part III of the Northern Ireland Drug Tariff)

Latex Foam, Adhesive as listed in Part IXA of the Drug Tariff (not prescribable by nurses in Scotland or Northern Ireland)

Lubricating Jelly as listed in Part IXA of the Drug Tariff (Part 2 of the Scottish Drug Tariff, not prescribable by nurses in Northern Ireland)

Nasal Device (nasal dilator) as listed in Part IXA of the Drug Tariff (Part 3 of the Scottish Drug Tariff, Part III of the Northern Ireland Drug Tariff)

Nipple Shields, Plastic as listed in Part IXA of the Drug Tariff (Part 3 of the Scottish Drug Tariff, not prescribable by nurses in Northern Ireland)

Peak Flow Meters as listed in Part IXA of the Drug Tariff (Part 3 of the Scottish Drug Tariff, not prescribable by nurses in Northern Ireland)

Pessaries as listed in Part IXA of the Drug Tariff (Part 3 of the Scottish Drug Tariff, Part III of the Northern Ireland Drug Tariff (with some exceptions))

Protectives as listed in Part IXA of the Drug Tariff (Part 2 of the Scottish Drug Tariff, Part III of the Northern Ireland Drug Tariff (EMA Disposable Film Gloves only))

Rectal Dilators as listed in Part IXA of the Drug Tariff (Part 3 of the Scottish Drug Tariff, not prescribable by nurses in Northern Ireland)

Saliva Stimulating Tablets as listed in Part IXA of the Drug Tariff (Part 3 of the Scottish Drug Tariff, not prescribable by nurses in Northern Ireland)

In the Drug Tariff Appliances and Reagents which may **not** be prescribed by Nurses are annotated ⊗

(Nx in the Scottish Drug Tariff and N̸ in the Northern Ireland Drug Tariff)

Stoma Appliances and Associated Products as listed in Part IXC of the Drug Tariff (Part 6 of the Scottish Drug Tariff, Part III of the Northern Ireland Drug Tariff)

Suprapubic Belts (replacements only) as listed in Part IXA of the Drug Tariff (Part 3 of the Scottish Drug Tariff, not prescribable by nurses in Northern Ireland)

Suprapubic Catheters as listed in Part IXA of the Drug Tariff (Part 3 of the Scottish Drug Tariff, not prescribable by nurses in Northern Ireland)

Synovial Fluid as listed in Part IXA of the Drug Tariff (Part 3 of the Scottish Drug Tariff, not prescribable by nurses in Northern Ireland)

Syringes (Bladder/Irrigating, Ear, Enema, Spare Vaginal Pipes) as listed in Part IXA of the Drug Tariff (Part 3 of the Scottish Drug Tariff, not prescribable by nurses in Northern Ireland)

Tapeless IV Holders as listed in Part IXA of the Drug Tariff (Part 2 of the Scottish Drug Tariff, not prescribable by nurses in Northern Ireland)

Test Tubes as listed in Part IXA of the Drug Tariff (Part 3 of the Scottish Drug Tariff, not prescribable by nurses in Northern Ireland)

Tracheostomy and Laryngectomy Appliances as listed in Part IXA of the Drug Tariff (Part 2 of the Scottish Drug Tariff, not prescribable by nurses in Northern Ireland)

Trusses as listed in Part IXA of the Drug Tariff (Part 3 of the Scottish Drug Tariff, not prescribable by nurses in Northern Ireland)

Urine Sugar Analysis Equipment as listed in Part IXA of the Drug Tariff (Parts 3 and 9 of the Scottish Drug Tariff, Part III of the Northern Ireland Drug Tariff)

Wound Management and Related Products (including bandages, dressings, gauzes, lint, stockinette, etc)

The following as listed in Part IXA of the Drug Tariff (Part 2 of the Scottish Drug Tariff, Part III of the Northern Ireland Drug Tariff):

In the Drug Tariff Appliances and Reagents which may **not** be prescribed by Nurses are annotated Ⓝ

(Nx in the Scottish Drug Tariff and ✗ in the Northern Ireland Drug Tariff)

Absorbent Cellulose Dressing with Fluid Repellent Backing
Absorbent Cottons
Absorbent Cotton Gauzes
Absorbent Cotton and Viscose Ribbon Gauze, BP 1988
Absorbent Dressing Pads, Sterile
Absorbent Lint, BPC
Absorbent Perforated Dressing with Adhesive Border
Absorbent Perforated Plastic Film Faced Dressing
Arm Slings
Belladonna Adhesive Plaster BP 1980
Boil Dressing Pack
Boric Acid Lint BPC 1963
Cellulose Wadding, BP 1988
Chlorhexidine Gauze Dressing, BP
Conforming Bandage (Synthetic)
Cotton Conforming Bandage, BP 1988
Cotton Crêpe Bandage, BP 1988

Cotton Crêpe Bandage, Hospicrepe 239
Cotton, Polyamide and Elastane Bandage
Cotton Stretch Bandage, BP 1988
Crêpe Bandage, BP 1988
Elastic Adhesive Bandage, BP
Elastic Diachylon Bandage, Ventilated BPC
Elastic Web Bandages
Elastomer and Viscose Bandage, Knitted
Gauze and Cotton Tissues
Heavy Cotton and Rubber Elastic Bandage, BP
High Compression Bandages (Extensible)
Knitted Polyamide and Cellulose Contour Bandage, BP 1988
Knitted Viscose Primary Dressing, BP, Type 1
Multi-layer Compression Bandaging
Multiple Pack Dressing No. 1
Open-wove Bandage, BP 1988, Type 1
Paraffin Gauze Dressing, BP
Plaster of Paris Bandage BP 1988
Polyamide and Cellulose Contour Bandage, BP 1988
Polyester Primary Dressing with Neutral Triglycerides, Knitted
Povidone–Iodine Fabric Dressing, Sterile
Short Stretch Compression Bandage
Skin Adhesive, Sterile
Skin Closure Strips, Sterile
Standard Dressings
Sterile Dressing Packs
Stockinettes
Sub-compression Wadding Bandage
Surgical Adhesive Tapes
Surgical Sutures (absorbable and non-absorbable)
Suspensory Bandages, Cotton
Swabs
Tapeless Dressing Holders
Triangular Calico Bandage, BP 1980
Vapour-permeable Adhesive Film Dressing, BP (including with absorbent pad)
Vapour-permeable Waterproof Plastic Wound Dressing, BP, Sterile
Wound Drainage Pouch
Wound Management Dressings (including activated charcoal, alginate, capillary-action, cavity, hydrocolloid, hydrogel, foam and silicone)
Zinc Paste Bandages (including both plain and with additional ingredients)

Nurse Prescribers' Extended Formulary. Subject to parliamentary procedure, from April 2002 nurses who have received specific preparation and training will be able to prescribe from the Nurse Prescribers' Extended Formulary which includes certain prescription-only medicines. Details, including the list of prescription-only medicines, may be found on the Department of Health website at: www.doh.gov.uk/nurseprescribing

Details of NPF preparations

Preparations on the Nurse Prescribers' Formulary which are not included in the BP or BPC are described as follows in the Nurse Prescribers' Formulary.

Although brand names have sometimes been included for identification purposes the non-proprietary names shown on the list should be used for prescribing purposes.

Arachis Oil Enema (proprietary product: *Fletchers' Arachis Oil Retention Enema*), arachis oil

Cadexomer–Iodine Ointment (proprietary product: *Iodosorb Ointment*), cadexomer–iodine containing iodine 0.9% in an ointment basis

Cadexomer–Iodine Paste PoM (proprietary product: *Iodoflex*), cadexomer–iodine containing iodine 0.9% in a paste basis

Cadexomer–Iodine Powder PoM (proprietary product: *Iodosorb Powder*), cadexomer–iodine containing iodine 0.9%

Catheter Maintenance Solution, Chlorhexidine (proprietary products: *Uro-Tainer Chlorhexidine; Uriflex C*), chlorhexidine 0.02%

Catheter Maintenance Solution, Mandelic Acid (proprietary product: *Uro-Tainer Mandelic Acid*), mandelic acid 1%

Catheter Maintenance Solution, Sodium Chloride (proprietary products: *Uro-Tainer Sodium Chloride; Uriflex-S*), sodium chloride 0.9%

Catheter Maintenance Solution, 'Solution G' (proprietary products: *Uro-Tainer Suby G, Uriflex G*), citric acid 3.23%, magnesium oxide 0.38%, sodium bicarbonate 0.7%, disodium edetate 0.01%

Catheter Maintenance Solution, 'Solution R' (proprietary products: *Uro-Tainer Solution R, Uriflex R*), citric acid 6%, gluconolactone 0.6%, magnesium carbonate 2.8%, disodium edetate 0.01%

Co-danthramer Capsules PoM co-danthramer 25/200 (dantron 25 mg, poloxamer '188' 200 mg)

Co-danthramer Capsules, Strong PoM co-danthramer 37.5/500 (dantron 37.5 mg, poloxamer '188' 500 mg)

Co-danthramer Oral Suspension PoM (proprietary product: *Codalax*), co-danthramer 25/200 in 5 mL (dantron 25 mg, poloxamer '188' 200 mg/5 mL)

Co-danthramer Oral Suspension, Strong PoM (proprietary product: *Codalax Forte*), co-danthramer 75/1000 in 5 mL (dantron 75 mg, poloxamer '188' 1 g/5 mL)

Co-danthrusate Oral Suspension PoM (proprietary product: *Normax*), co-danthrusate 50/60 (dantron 50 mg, docusate sodium 60 mg/5 mL)

Dextranomer Beads (proprietary product: *Debrisan Beads*), dextranomer

Dextranomer Paste (proprietary product: *Debrisan Paste*), dextranomer in a soft paste basis

Dimeticone barrier creams (proprietary products: *Conotrane Cream*, dimeticone '350' 22%; *Siopel Barrier Cream*, dimeticone '1000' 10%; *Vasogen Barrier Cream*, dimeticone 20%), dimeticone 10–22%

Docusate Enema (proprietary product: *Norgalax Micro-enema*) docusate sodium 120 mg in 10 g

Folic Acid Oral Solution 400 micrograms/5 mL (proprietary product: *Folicare*), folic acid 400 micrograms/5 mL

Lactitol Powder, lactitol 10 g/sachet

Lidocaine Ointment/Lignocaine Ointment, lidocaine 5%

Liquid and White Soft Paraffin Ointment, liquid paraffin 50%, white soft paraffin 50%

Macrogol Oral Powder, Compound (proprietary product: *Movicol*), macrogol '3350' (polyethylene glycol '3350') 13.125 g, sodium bicarbonate 178.5 mg, sodium chloride 350.7 mg, potassium chloride 46.6 mg/sachet

Malathion alcoholic lotions (proprietary products: *Prioderm Lotion; Suleo-M Lotion*), malathion 0.5% in an alcoholic basis

Malathion aqueous lotions (proprietary products: *Derbac-M Liquid; Quellada M Liquid*), malathion 0.5% in an aqueous basis

Mebendazole Oral Suspension PoM (proprietary product: *Vermox*), mebendazole 100 mg/5 mL

[1] **Mebendazole Tablets** PoM (proprietary products: *Ovex, Vermox*), mebendazole 100 mg

1. PoM exemption, see p. 323

Mouthwash Solution-tablets consist of tablets which may contain antimicrobial, colouring and flavouring agents in a suitable soluble effervescent basis to make a mouthwash

[2] **Nicotine Inhalation Cartridge for Oromucosal Use** (proprietary products: *Nicorette® Inhalator, Boots® Nicotine Inhalator*), nicotine 10 mg

2. For use with inhalation mouthpiece; to be prescribed as either a starter pack (6 cartridges with inhalator device and holder) or refill pack (42 cartridges with inhalator device)

Nicotine Lozenge nicotine (as bitartrate) 1 mg (proprietary product: *Nicotinell® Mint Lozenge*) or nicotine (as polacrilex) 2 mg or 4 mg (proprietary product: *NiQuitin CQ® Lozenges*)

Nicotine Medicated Chewing Gum (proprietary products: *Nicorette® Gum, Nicorette® Plus Gum, Nicotinell® Gum, Nicotinell® Plus Gum, Boots® Nicotine Gum*), nicotine 2 mg or 4 mg

Nicotine Nasal Spray (proprietary product: *Nicorette® Nasal Spray*), nicotine 500 micrograms/metered spray

[3] **Nicotine Sublingual Tablets** (proprietary product: *Nicorette® Microtab*), nicotine (as a cyclodextrin complex) 2 mg

3. To be prescribed as either a starter pack (2 x 15-tablet discs with dispenser) or refill pack (7 x 15-tablet discs)

[4] **Nicotine Transdermal Patches**
Releasing in each 16 hours, nicotine approx. 5 mg, 10 mg, or 15 mg (proprietary product: *Nicorette® Patch*) or releasing in each 24 hours nicotine approx. 7 mg, 14 mg, or 21 mg (proprietary products: *Nicotinell TTS®, NiQuitin CQ®, Boots® NRT Patch*)

4. Prescriber should specify the brand to be dispensed

Permethrin Cream (proprietary product: *Lyclear Dermal Cream*), permethrin 5%

Permethrin Cream Rinse (proprietary product: *Lyclear Cream Rinse*), permethrin 1%

Phenothrin Alcoholic Lotion (proprietary product: *Full Marks Lotion*), phenothrin 0.2% in a basis containing isopropyl alcohol

Phenothrin Aqueous Lotion (proprietary product: *Full Marks Liquid*), phenothrin 0.5% in an aqueous basis

Phenothrin Foam Application (proprietary product: *Full Marks Mousse*), phenothrin 0.5% in an alcoholic basis

Piperazine and Senna Powder (proprietary product: *Pripsen Oral Powder*), piperazine phosphate 4 g, sennosides 15.3 mg/sachet

Senna Oral Solution (proprietary product: *Senokot Syrup*), sennosides 7.5 mg/5 mL

Senna and Ispaghula Granules (proprietary product: *Manevac Granules*), senna fruit 12.4%, ispaghula 54.2%

Sodium Citrate Compound Enema (proprietary products: *Micolette Micro-enema; Micralax Micro-enema; Relaxit Micro-enema*), sodium citrate 450 mg with glycerol, sorbitol and an anionic surfactant

Sodium Picosulfate Elixir (proprietary products: *Dulcolax Liquid, Laxoberal* NHS), sodium picosulfate 5 mg/5 mL

Sterculia Granules (proprietary product: *Normacol Granules*), sterculia 62%

Sterculia and Frangula Granules (proprietary product: *Normacol Plus Granules*), sterculia 62%, frangula (standardised) 8%

Streptokinase and Streptodornase Topical Powder PoM (proprietary product: *Varidase Topical*), streptokinase 100 000 units, streptodornase 25 000 units

Titanium Ointment (proprietary product: *Metanium Ointment*), titanium dioxide 20%, titanium peroxide 5%, titanium salicylate 3%

Zinc Oxide and Dimeticone Spray (proprietary product: *Sprilon*), dimeticone 1.04%, zinc oxide 12.5% in a pressurised aerosol unit

Zinc Oxide Impregnated Medicated Stocking (proprietary product: *Zipzoc*), sterile rayon stocking impregnated with ointment containing zinc oxide 20%

Index of manufacturers

'Special-order' manufac-
turers—see p. 776

Abbott
Abbott Laboratories Ltd,
Abbott House, Norden Rd,
Maidenhead, Berks SL6 4XE.
Tel: (01628) 773 355
Fax: (01628) 644 185

Activa
Activa Health Care,
Units 26/27, Imex Business Park,
Shobnall Rd, Burton-on-Trent
Staffs DE14 2AU.
Tel: (01283) 540 957
Fax: (01283) 845 361
healthcare@activa.uk.com

A&H
Allen & Hanburys Ltd,
see GSK

Adams Hlth.
Adams Healthcare Ltd,
Lotherton Way,
Garforth, Leeds LS25 2JY.
Tel: (0113) 232 0066
Fax: (0113) 287 1317

Akita
Akita Pharmaceuticals Ltd,
Manx House,
Spectrum Business Estate,
Maidstone, Kent ME15 9YP.
Tel: (01622) 766 389
Fax: (01622) 679 977

Alcon
Alcon Laboratories (UK) Ltd,
Pentagon Park, Boundary Way,
Hemel Hempstead, Herts
HP2 7UD.
Tel: (01442) 341 234
Fax: (01442) 341 200

Alembic Products
Alembic Products Ltd,
River Lane, Saltney,
Chester, Cheshire CH4 8RQ.
Tel: (01244) 680 147
Fax: (01244) 680 155

ALK-Abelló
ALK-Abelló (UK) Ltd,
2 Tealgate, Hungerford,
Berks RG17 0YT.
Tel: (01488) 686 016
Fax: (01488) 685 423

Allergan
Allergan Ltd,
Coronation Rd, High Wycombe,
Bucks HP12 3SH.
Tel: (01494) 444 722
Fax: (01494) 473 593

Allergy
Allergy Therapeutics Ltd,
Dominion Way, Worthing,
West Sussex BN14 8SA.
Tel: (01903) 844 702
Fax: (01903) 844 744
infoservices@allergytherapeutics.com

Alliance
Alliance Pharmaceuticals Ltd,
Avonbridge House, Bath Rd,
Chippenham, Wilts SN15 2BB.
Tel: (01249) 466 966
Fax: (01249) 466 977
info@alliancepharma.co.uk

Alpha
Alpha Therapeutic UK Ltd,
Thetford House, Roman Way,
Thetford, Norfolk IP24 1XB.
Tel: (01842) 821 104
Fax: (01842) 821 105

Alpharma
Alpharma Ltd,
Whiddon Valley, Barnstaple,
Devon EX32 8NS.
Tel: (01271) 311 257
Fax: (01271) 311 329
med.info@alpharma.co.uk

Amgen
Amgen Ltd,
240 Cambridge Science Park,
Milton Rd, Cambridge
CB4 0WD.
Tel: (01223) 420 305
Fax: (01223) 426 314

Anglian
Anglian Pharma plc,
Titmore Court, Titmore Green,
Little Wymondley, Hitchin,
Herts SG4 7XJ.
Tel: (01438) 743 070
Fax: (01438) 743 080
mail@anglianpharma.plc.uk

Anpharm
see Antigen

Anstead
Anstead International,
Radford House, Radford Way,
Billericay, Essex CM12 0DE.
Tel: (01277) 630 063
Fax: (01277) 631 356

Antigen
Antigen Pharmaceuticals (UK),
Antigen House,
82 Waterloo Rd, Hillside,
Southport PR8 4QW.
Tel: (01704) 562 777
Fax: (01704) 562 888

APS
Approved Prescription Services
Ltd,
Brampton Rd, Hampden Park,
Eastbourne, East Sussex
BN22 9AG.
Tel: (01323) 501 111
Fax: (01323) 520 306

Ardern
Ardern Healthcare Ltd,
Pipers Brook Farm, Eastham,
Tenbury Wells, Worcs
WR15 8NP.
Tel: (01584) 781 777
Fax: (01584) 781 788
info@ardernhealthcare.com

Arun
Arun Pharmaceuticals UK Ltd,
Delta House,
Southwood Crescent,
Southwood Business Park,
Farnborough, Hants GU14 0NL.
Tel: (01252) 543 862
Fax: (01252) 547 845

AS Pharma
AS Pharma Ltd,
PO Box 5227, Milton Keynes,
Bucks MK1 1XW.
Tel: (01908) 371 025
Fax: (01908) 378 315

Ashbourne
Ashbourne Pharmaceuticals Ltd,
Victors Barns, Hill Farm,
Brixworth, Northampton
NN6 9DQ.
Tel: (01604) 883 100
Fax: (01604) 881 640

ASTA Medica
ASTA Medica Ltd,
168 Cowley Rd, Cambridge
CB4 0DL.
Tel: (01223) 423 434
Fax: (01223) 420 943

AstraZeneca
AstraZeneca UK Ltd,
Horizon Place,
600 Capability Green, Luton,
Beds LU1 3LU.
Tel: 0800 7830 033
Fax: (01582) 838 003
medical.informationgb@astrazeneca.com

Athena
Athena Neurosciences
see Elan

Aurum
Aurum Pharmaceuticals Ltd,
Bampton Rd, Harold Hill,
Romford,
Essex RM3 8UG.
Tel: (01708) 386 660
Fax: (01708) 384 032

Aventis Behring
Aventis Behring Ltd,
Aventis House, Market Place,
Haywards Heath RH16 1DB.
Tel: (01444) 447 400
Fax: (01444) 447 401
medinfo@aventis.com

Aventis Pasteur
Aventis Pasteur MSD Ltd,
Mallards Reach, Bridge Ave,
Maidenhead, Berks SL6 1QP.
Tel: (01628) 773 737
Fax: (01628) 671 722

Aventis Pharma
Aventis Pharma Ltd,
Aventis House,
50 Kings Hill Ave, Kings Hill,
West Malling, Kent ME19 4AH.
Tel: (01732) 584 000
Fax: (01732) 584 080

Axcan
Axcan Pharma Ltd,
Borough Rd, Godalming,
Surrey GU7 2AB.
Tel: (01438) 860 782
Fax: (01438) 860 927

Ayrton Saunders
Ayrton Saunders Ltd,
Reeds Lane, Moreton,
Wirral CH46 1QW.
Tel: (0151) 677 8000
Fax: (0151) 606 8614

Bailey, Robert

Robert Bailey UK Ltd,
Whinleys Estate, Church Lane,
Clarborough, Retford,
Notts DN2 9NA.
Tel: (01777) 869 888
Fax: (01777) 869 444

Bard

Bard Ltd,
Forest House, Brighton Rd,
Crawley, West Sussex
RH11 9BP.
Tel: (01293) 527 888
Fax: (01293) 552 428

Bartholomew Rhodes

Bartholomew Rhodes,
Manor House, Victors Barns,
Northampton Rd, Brixworth,
Northampton NN6 9DQ.
Tel: (01604) 882 626
Fax: (01604) 883 199

Bausch & Lomb

Bausch & Lomb UK Ltd,
106 London Rd,
Kingston-upon-Thames,
Surrey KT2 6TN.
Tel: (020) 8781 2900
Fax: (020) 8781 2901

Baxter

Baxter Healthcare Ltd,
Caxton Way, Thetford, Norfolk
IP24 3SE.
Tel: (01842) 767 189
Fax: (01842) 767 099

Baxter Anaesthesia

Baxter Anaesthesia,
Unit 31 Wellington Business
Park, Dukes Ride,
Crowthorne, Berks RG45 6LS.
Tel: (01344) 759 300
Fax: (01344) 759 330

Baxter BioScience

Wallingford Rd,
Compton, Newbury,
Berks RG20 7QW.
Tel: (01635) 206 345
Fax: (01635) 206 373

Bayer

Bayer plc,
Pharmaceutical Division,
Bayer House, Strawberry Hill,
Newbury, Berks RG14 1JA.
Tel: (01635) 563 000
Fax: (01635) 563 393
medical.operations@bayer.co.uk

Bayer Consumer Care

see Bayer

Bayer Diagnostics

Bayer plc,
Diagnostics Division,
Bayer House,
Strawberry Hill,
Newbury, Berks RG14 1JA.
Tel: (01635) 563 000
Fax: (01635) 563 393

BCM Specials

BCM Specials Manufacturing,
D10 First 114,
Nottingham NG90 2PR.
Tel: 0800 952 1010
Fax: 0800 085 0673
bcm-specials@bcm-ltd.co.uk

Beacon

Beacon Pharmaceuticals Ltd,
85 High St, Tunbridge Wells
TN1 1YG.
Tel: (01892) 506 958
Fax: (01892) 610 397

Becton Dickinson

Becton Dickinson UK Ltd,
Between Towns Rd,
Cowley, Oxford,
Oxon OX4 3LY.
Tel: (01865) 748 844
Fax: (01865) 717 313

Beiersdorf

Beiersdorf UK Ltd,
Yeomans Drive, Blakelands,
Milton Keynes,
Bucks MK14 5LS.
Tel: (01908) 211 444
Fax: (01908) 211 555

Bell

Bell, Sons & Co Ltd,
PO Box 62, Tanhouse Lane,
Widnes, Cheshire WA8 0SA.
Tel: (0151) 424 8352
Fax: (0151) 420 7574

Bell and Croyden

John Bell and Croyden,
54 Wigmore St, London
W1H 0AU.
Tel: (020) 7935 5555
Fax: (020) 7935 9605

Bencard

see GSK

Berk

Berk Pharmaceuticals,
see APS

BHR

BHR Pharmaceuticals Ltd,
41 Centenary Business Centre,
Hammond Close,
Attleborough Fields, Nuneaton,
Warwickshire CV11 6RY.
Tel: (024) 7635 3742
Fax: (024) 7632 7812
info@bhr.co.uk

Bio Diagnostics

Bio Diagnostics Ltd,
Upton Industrial Estate,
Rectory Rd, Upton-upon-Severn,
Worcs WR8 0XL.
Tel: (01684) 592 262
Fax: (01684) 592 501

Biocare

Biocare International Inc.
Belvoir House, Chapel St,
Haconby, Lincs
PE10 0UP.
Tel: (01778) 570441
Fax: (01778) 570441

Biogen

Biogen Ltd,
5d Roxborough Way,
Foundation Park, Maidenhead,
Berks SL6 3UD.
Tel: (01628) 501 000
Fax: (01628) 501 010

Bioglan

Bioglan Laboratories Ltd,
5 Hunting Gate, Hitchin,
Herts SG4 0TJ.
Tel: (01462) 438 444
Fax: (01462) 421 242

Biomatrix

Biomatrix UK Ltd,
Lamb House, Church St,
Chiswick,
London W4 2PD.
Tel: (020) 8987 8830
Fax: (020) 8994 7083

Bio-Medical

Bio-Medical Services,
BMS Laboratories Ltd,
River View Rd, Beverley,
North Humberside HU17 0LD.
Tel: (01482) 860 228
Fax: (01482) 872 042

Biomet Merck

Biomet Merck Ltd,
Waterton Industrial Estate,
Bridgend, South Wales
CF31 3XA.
Tel: (01656) 655 221
Fax: (01656) 645 454

Biorex

Biorex Laboratories Ltd,
2 Crossfield Chambers,
Gladbeck Way, Enfield,
Middx EN2 7HT.
Tel: (020) 8366 9301
Fax: (020) 8367 4627

Biosurgical Research

Biosurgical Research Unit,
Surgical Materials Testing
Laboratory,
Princess of Wales Hospital,
Coity Rd, Bridgend,
Mid Glamorgan,
South Wales CF31 1RQ.
Tel: (01656) 752 820
Fax: (01656) 752 830
maggots@smtl.co.uk

Blackwell

Blackwell Supplies Ltd,
Medcare House,
Centurion Close,
Gillingham Business Park,
Gillingham, Kent ME8 0SB.
Tel: (01634) 877 620
Fax: (01634) 877 621

Blake

Thomas Blake & Co,
The Byre House, Fearby,
Nr. Masham, North Yorkshire
HG4 4NF.
Tel: (01765) 689 042
Fax: (01765) 689 042
sales@veilcover.com

BOC

BOC Gases,
Priestly Rd, Worsley, Manchester
M28 2UT.
Tel: 0800 111 333
Fax: 0800 111 555

Boehringer Ingelheim

Boehringer Ingelheim Ltd,
Ellesfield Ave, Bracknell, Berks
RG12 8YS.
Tel: (01344) 424 600
Fax: (01344) 741 444

Boots

Boots The Chemists,
Medical Services, D90 East FO8,
Nottingham NG90 1BS.
Tel: (0115) 959 5168
Fax: (0115) 959 2565

Borg

Borg Medicare, PO Box 99,
Hitchin, Herts SG5 2GF.
Tel: (01462) 442 993
Fax: (01462) 441 293

Boston

Boston Hospital Products,
Unit 1-3 Waymills, Whitchurch,
Shropshire SY13 1QN.
Tel: (01948) 664 487
Fax: (01948) 663 099
boston@enterprise.net

BPL

Bio Products Laboratory,
Dagger Lane, Elstree, Herts
WD6 3BX.
Tel: (020) 8258 2200
Fax: (020) 8258 2604

BR

BR Pharmaceuticals Ltd,
51a Broom Mill Estate,
Coal Hill Lane, Farsley, Leeds,
West Yorkshire LS28 5NA.
Tel: (0113) 256 5836
Fax: (0113) 255 7093

Braun

B. Braun (Medical) Ltd,
Brookdale Rd,
Thorncliffe Park Estate,
Chapeltown,
Sheffield S35 2PW.
Tel: (0114) 225 9000
Fax: (0114) 225 9111
enquiry@bbmuk.demon.co.uk

Braun Biotrol

see Braun

Bray

Bray Health & Leisure,
1 Regal Way, Faringdon,
Oxon SN7 7BX.
Tel: (01367) 240 736
Fax: (01367) 242 625
solportltd@btinternet.com

Brewhurst

Brewhurst Health Food Supplies
Ltd, Abbot Close,
Oyster Lane, Byfleet,
Surrey KT14 7JP.
Tel: (01932) 334 501
Fax: (01932) 351 7131

Bristol-Myers Squibb

Bristol-Myers Squibb
Pharmaceuticals Ltd,
141–149 Staines Rd, Hounslow,
Middx TW3 3JA.
Tel: (020) 8572 7422
Fax: (020) 8754 3789
medical.information@bms.com

Britannia

Britannia Pharmaceuticals Ltd,
41–51 Brighton Rd, Redhill,
Surrey RH1 6YS.
Tel: (01737) 773 741
Fax: (01737) 762 672
medicalservices@forumgroup.co.uk

Brodie & Stone

Brodie and Stone plc,
51 Calthorpe St,
London WC1X 0HH.
Tel: (020) 7278 9597
Fax: (020) 7278 2458
mailbox@brodieandstone.com

BSIA

see Torbet

Cambridge

Cambridge Laboratories,
Deltic House, Kingfisher Way,
Silverlink Business Park,
Wallsend,
Tyne & Wear NE28 9NX.
Tel: (0191) 296 9369
Fax: (0191) 296 9368
enquiries@camb-labs.com

Cangene

Cangene Europe Ltd
Action International House
Crabtree Office Village,
Eversly Way, Egham,
Surrey TW20 8RY
Tel: (01784) 471 990
Fax: (01784) 473 071

Castlemead

Castlemead Healthcare Ltd,
PO Box 57, Ware SG10 6LL.
Tel: (01462) 454 452
Fax: (01462) 435 684

Celltech

Celltech Pharmaceuticals Ltd,
208 Bath Rd, Slough,
Berks SL1 3WE.
Tel: (01753) 534 655
Fax: (01753) 447 605

CeNeS

CeNeS Pharmaceuticals,
Compass House, Vision Park,
Chivers Way, Histon,
Cambridge CB4 9ZR.
Tel: (0870) 241 3674
Fax: (01223) 266 467
medinfo@cenes.co.uk

Cephalon

Cephalon UK Ltd,
11-13 Frederick Sanger Rd,
Surrey Research Park,
Guildford, Surrey GU2 7YD.
Tel: 0800 783 4869
Fax: (01483) 453 324
medinfo@cephalon.com

Ceuta

Ceuta Healthcare Ltd,
Hill House, 41 Richmond Hill,
Bournemouth, Dorset, BH2 6HS.
Tel: (01202) 780 558
Fax: (01202) 780 559

Chauvin

Chauvin Pharmaceuticals Ltd,
Ashton Rd, Harold Hill,
Romford,
Essex RM3 8SL.
Tel: (01708) 383 838
Fax: (01708) 371 316

Chemical Search

Chemical Search International
Ltd,
29th floor, 1 Canada Square,
Canary Wharf,
London E14 5DY.
Tel: (020) 7712 1758
Fax: (020) 7712 1759
info@chemicalsearch.co.uk

Chemidex

Chemidex Pharma Ltd,
Chemidex House,
Egham Business Village,
Crabtree Rd, Egham,
Surrey TW20 8RB.
Tel: (01784) 477 167
Fax: (01784) 471 776
info@chemidex.co.uk

Chiron

Chiron UK Ltd,
PathoGenesis House, Park Lane,
Cranford, Hounslow TW5 9RR.
Tel: (020) 8580 4000
Fax: (020) 8580 4001

CHS

Cambridge Healthcare Supplies
Ltd,
Unit 14D, Rackheath Industrial
Estate, Rackheath,
Norwich NR13 6LH.
Tel: (01603) 735 200)
Fax: (01603) 735 217

Chugai

Chugai Pharma UK Ltd,
Mulliner House, Flanders Rd,
Turnham Green,
London W4 1NN.
Tel: (020) 8987 5680
Fax: (020) 8987 5661

Clement Clarke

Clement Clarke International Ltd,
Airmed House, Edinburgh Way,
Harlow, Essex CM20 2TT.
Tel: (01279) 414 969
Fax: (01279) 456 304
resp@clement-clarke.com

CliniMed

CliniMed Ltd,
Cavell House, Knaves Beech
Way, Loudwater, High
Wycombe, Bucks HP10 9QY.
Tel: (01628) 850 100
Fax: (01628) 850 331
enquiries@clinimed.demon.co.uk

Codan

Codan Ltd,
Eastheath Ave,
Wokingham, Berks RH41 2PR.
Tel: (0118) 978 3663
Fax: (0118) 877 6274

Colgate-Palmolive

Colgate-Palmolive Ltd,
Guildford Business Park,
Middleton Rd, Guildford, Surrey
GU2 5LZ.
Tel: (01483) 302 222
Fax: (01483) 303 003

CollaGenex

CollaGenex International Ltd,
The Old Stable Block,
7 Buttermarket, Thame,
Oxon OX9 3EW.
Tel: (01844) 218 989
Fax: (01844) 218 795

Coloplast

Coloplast Ltd,
Peterborough Business Park,
Peterborough PE2 6FX.
Tel: (01733) 392 000
Fax: (01733) 233 348

Community

Community Foods Ltd,
Micross, Brent Terrace,
London NW2 1LT.
Tel: (020) 8450 9411
Fax: (020) 8208 1803
email@communityfoods.co.uk

Concord

Concord Pharmaceuticals Ltd,
PO Box 5970,
Dunmow, Essex CM6 1FY.
Tel: 0845 602 0137
Fax: 0870 241 2335
enquiries@concord-pharma.com

ConvaTec

ConvaTec Ltd,
Harrington House, Milton Rd,
Ickenham, Uxbridge, Middx
UB10 8PU.
Tel: (01895) 628 400
Fax: (01895) 628 456

Co-Pharma

Co-Pharma Ltd,
Unit 4, Metro Centre,
Tolpits Lane, Watford,
Herts WD1 8SS.
Tel: (01923) 255 580
Fax: (01923) 255 581
sales@co-pharma.co.uk

Cow & Gate

see Nutricia Clinical
Tel: (01225) 768 381
Fax: (01225) 768 847

CP

CP Pharmaceuticals Ltd,
Ash Rd North, Wrexham
Industrial Estate, Wrexham,
Clwyd LL13 9UF.
Tel: (01978) 661 261
Fax: (01978) 660 130
mail@cppharma.co.uk

Crawford

Crawford Pharmaceuticals,
Furtho House,
20 Towcester Rd,
Milton Keynes MK19 6AQ.
Tel: (01908) 262 346
Fax: (01908) 567 730

Crookes

Crookes Healthcare Ltd,
D80 Building,
Nottingham NG90 1LP.
Tel: (0115) 953 9922
Fax: (0115) 968 8722
pauline.flanagan@crookes.co.uk

Cupal

Cupal Ltd,
see SSL

Cusi

Cusi Ophthalmic Generics,
Pentagon Park, Boundary Way,
Hemel Hempstead, Herts
HP2 7UD.
Tel: (01442) 341 326
Fax: (01442) 341 281

DDD

DDD Ltd,
94 Rickmansworth Rd, Watford,
Herts WD1 7JJ.
Tel: (01923) 229 251
Fax: (01923) 220 728

DDSA

DDSA Pharmaceuticals Ltd,
310 Old Brompton Rd,
London SW5 9JQ.
Tel: (020) 7373 7884
Fax: (020) 7370 4321

De Vilbiss

De Vilbiss Health Care UK Ltd,
High St, Wollaston,
West Midlands DY8 4PS.
Tel: (01384) 446 688
Fax: (01384) 446 699

De Witt

E. C. De Witt & Co Ltd,
Tudor Rd, Manor Park, Runcorn,
Cheshire WA7 1SZ.
Tel: (01928) 579 029
Fax: (01928) 579 712
ecdewitt@ecdewitt.com

Dental Health

Dental Health Products Ltd,
60 Boughton Lane,
Maidstone,
Kent ME15 9QS.
Tel: (01622) 749 222
Fax: (01622) 744 672

Dermal

Dermal Laboratories Ltd,
Tatmore Place, Gosmore,
Hitchin, Herts SG4 7QR.
Tel: (01462) 458 866
Fax: (01462) 420 565

DermaPharm

DermaPharm Ltd,
Penrhyn House,
10 St Mark's Hill, Surbiton,
Surrey KT6 4PW.
Tel: (020) 8399 3040
Fax: (020) 8399 0808
info@dermapharm.co.uk

Dexcel

Dexcel Pharma Ltd,
Bishop Crewe House,
North St, Daventry,
Northants NN11 5PN.
Tel: (01327) 312 266
Fax: (01327) 312 262
DexcelPharma@compuserve.com

DF

Duncan, Flockhart & Co Ltd,
see GSK

DiagnoSys

DiagnoSys Medical,
Cams Hall, Fareham,
Hants PO16 8AB.
Tel: 0800 085 8808
Fax: (01329) 227 599

Disetronic

Disetronic Medical Systems Ltd,
Stoneleigh Deer Park,
Stareton,
Nr Kenilworth CV8 2LY.
Tel: (012476) 531 338
Fax: (012476) 531 345
info@disetronic.co.uk

Dista

Dista Products Ltd,
see Lilly

Dominion

Dominion Pharma Ltd,
Dominion House,
Lion Lane,
Haslemere,
Surrey GU27 1JL.
Tel: (01428) 661 078
Fax: (01428) 661 075
dominion@dompharm.com

Dowelhurst

Dowelhurst Ltd,
1 Hawkes Drive,
Heathcote Industrial Estate,
Warwick CV34 6LX.
Tel: (01926) 461 600
Fax: (01926) 461 626

DuPont

see Bristol-Myers Squibb

Durbin

Durbin plc,
240 Northolt Rd,
South Harrow,
Middx HA2 8TL.
Tel: (020) 8869 6500
Fax: (020) 8869 6565
info@durbin.co.uk

Easigrip

Easigrip Ltd,
Unit 13, Scar Bank,
Millers Rd, Warwick,
Warwickshire CV34 5DB.
Tel: (01926) 497 108
Fax: (01926) 497 109

Eastern

Eastern Pharmaceuticals Ltd,
Coomb House, 7 St Johns Rd,
Isleworth, Middx TW7 6NA.
Tel: (020) 8569 8174
Fax: (020) 8569 8175

Eisai

Eisai Ltd,
3 Shortlands, Hammersmith,
London W6 8EE.
Tel: (020) 8600 1400
Fax: (020) 8600 1401
Lmedinfo@eisai.net

Elan

Elan Pharma Ltd,
Abel Smith House,
Gunnels Wood Rd, Stevenage,
Herts SG1 2FG.
Tel: (01438) 765 100
Fax: (01438) 765 008
Medinfo@Elanuk.com

Eldon

Eldon Laboratories,
2–4 Pooley Close,
Newcastle-upon-Tyne NE5 2TF.
Tel: 0800 616 132
Fax: 0800 163 961

Elida Fabergé

Elida Fabergé Ltd,
Coal Rd, Seacroft, Leeds
LS14 2AR.
Tel: (0113) 222 5000
Fax: (0113) 222 5362

Entaco

Entaco Ltd,
Royal Victoria Works,
Birmingham Rd, Studley,
Warwickshire B80 7AP.
Tel: (01527) 852 306
Fax: (01527) 857 447

Epiderm

Epiderm Ltd,
Copthorne House, Mill Lane,
Burgh-on-Bain,
Market Rasen LN8 6JZ.
Tel: (01507) 313 777
Fax: (01507) 313 888

Evans Vaccines

Evans Vaccines Ltd,
Gaskill Rd, Speke,
Liverpool L24 9GR.
Tel: (0151) 705 5000
Fax: (0151) 705 5018

Everfresh

Everfresh Natural Foods,
Gatehouse Close, Aylesbury,
Bucks HP19 3DE.
Tel: (01296) 425 333
Fax: (01296) 422 545

Exelgyn

Exelgyn Laboratories,
PO Box 4511,
Henley-on-Thames, Oxon
RG9 1XH.
Tel: (0800) 731 6120
Fax: (01491) 577 443

Fabre

Pierre Fabre Ltd,
Hyde Abbey House,
23 Hyde St, Winchester,
Hampshire SO23 7DR.
Tel: (01962) 856 956
Fax: (01962) 844 014
PFabreUK@aol.com

Farillon

Farillon Ltd,
Ashton Rd, Romford,
Essex RM3 8UE.
Tel: (01708) 379 000
Fax: (01708) 376 554

Farley

Farley Health Products,
Mint Bridge Rd, Kendal,
Cumbria LA9 6NL.
Tel: (01539) 723 815
Fax: (01539) 730 376
Farleys_Heinz@Heinz.co.uk

Fate

Fate Special Foods,
Unit E2,
Brook Street Business Centre,
Brook St, Tipton,
West Midlands DY4 9DD.
Tel: (01215) 224 433
Fax: (01215) 224 433

Faulding DBL

Faulding Pharmaceuticals plc,
Queensway,
Leamington Spa CV31 3RW.
Tel: (01926) 820 820
Fax: (01926) 821 049

Fenton

Fenton Pharmaceuticals Ltd,
4J Portman Mansions,
Chiltern St,
London W1U 6NS.
Tel: (020) 7224 1388
Fax: (020) 7486 7258
fent.pharm@lineone.net

Ferraris

Ferraris Medical Ltd,
Ferraris House, Aden Rd,
Enfield, Middx EN3 7SE.
Tel: (020) 8805 9055
Fax: (020) 8805 9065
ferraris@globalnet.co.uk

Ferring

Ferring Pharmaceuticals UK,
The Courtyard,
Waterside Drive, Langley,
Berks SL3 6EZ.
Tel: (01753) 214 800
Fax: (01753) 214 801

Firstplay Dietary

Firstplay Dietary Foods Ltd,
338 Turncroft Lane, Offerton,
Stockport, Cheshire SK1 4BP.
Tel: (0161) 474 7576
Fax: (0161) 474 7576

Florizel

Florizel Ltd,
PO Box 138,
Stevenage SG2 8YN.
Tel: (01462) 436 156
Fax: (01462) 457 402

Flynn

Flynn Pharma Ltd,
7 Serlby Court, Addison Rd,
London W14 8EE.
Tel: (01462) 458 974
Fax: (01462) 450 755

Foodlink

Foodlink (UK) Ltd,
2B Plymouth Rd, Plympton,
Plymouth PL7 4JR.
Tel: (01752) 344 544
Fax: (01752) 342 412
Foodlink@compuserve.com

Ford

Ford Medical Associates Ltd,
2 Bridport Way, Braintree,
Essex CM7 9FJ.
Tel: (01376) 343 061
Fax: (01376) 339 014
tmf@globalnet.co.uk

Forest

Forest Laboratories Europe,
Bourne Rd, Bexley DA5 1NX.
Tel: (01322) 550 550
Fax: (01322) 555 469
medinfo@forest-labs.co.uk

Fournier

Fournier Pharmaceuticals Ltd,
22-23 Progress Business Centre,
Whittle Parkway, Slough
SL1 6DG.
Tel: (01753) 740 400
Fax: (01753) 740 444

Fox

C. H. Fox Ltd,
22 Tavistock St,
London WC2E 7PY.
Tel: (020) 7240 3111
Fax: (020) 7379 3410

FP

Family Planning Sales Ltd,
28 Kelburne Rd, Cowley,
Oxford OX4 3SZ.
Tel: (01865) 772 486
Fax: (01865) 748 746

Fresenius Kabi

Fresenius Kabi Ltd,
Hampton Court, Tudor Rd,
Manor Park, Runcorn,
Cheshire WA7 1UF
Tel: (01928) 594 200
Fax: (01928) 594 320

Frontier

Frontier Multigate Ltd,
Newbridge Rd Industrial Estate,
Blackwood, South Wales
NP12 2YL.
Tel: (01495) 233 050
Fax: (01495) 233 055
multigate@frontier-group.co.uk

Fujisawa

Fujisawa Ltd,
C P House, 1st Floor,
97–107 Uxbridge Rd,
Ealing, London W5 5TL.
Tel: (020) 8840 9520
Fax: (020) 8840 9521
balwant.heer@fujisawa.co.uk

Futuna

Futuna Ltd,
229 Preston Rd,
Clayton-le-Woods
Preston PR6 7PT.
Tel: (0870) 601 2037
Fax: (0870) 601 2036

Gainor Medical

Gainor Medical Europe,
Unit 7F, Mobbs Miller House,
Christchurch Rd,
Northampton NN3 3XE.
Tel: (01604) 638 340
Fax: (01604) 636 901
irenesharrock@aol.com

Galderma

Galderma (UK) Ltd,
Galderma House,
Church Lane, Kings Langley,
Herts WD4 8JP.
Tel: (01923) 291 033
Fax: (01923) 291 060

Galen

Galen Ltd,
Seagoe Industrial Estate,
Craigavon, Northern Ireland
BT63 5UA.
Tel: (028) 3833 4974
Fax: (028) 3835 0206

Garnier

Laboratoires Garnier,
Golden Ltd,
PO Box 5, Pontyclun, Glam
CF7 8XW.
Tel: (01443) 233 724
Fax: (01443) 233 726

GBM

GBM Healthcare Ltd,
Beechlawn House,
Hurtmore Rd, Godalming,
Surrey GU7 2RA.
Tel: (01483) 860 881
Fax: (01483) 425 715
mba_gbm@compuserve.com

Geistlich

Geistlich Pharma,
Newton Bank, Long Lane,
Chester CH2 2PF.
Tel: (01244) 347 534
Fax: (01244) 319 327

General Dietary

General Dietary Ltd,
PO Box 38,
Kingston upon Thames,
Surrey KT2 7YP.
Tel: (020) 8336 2323
Fax: (020) 8942 8274

Generics

Generics (UK) Ltd,
Albany Gate, Darkes Lane,
Potters Bar,
Herts EN6 1AG.
Tel: (01707) 853 000
Fax: (01707) 643 148

Genus

Genus Pharmaceuticals,
Benham Valence,
Newbury,
Berks RG20 8LU.
Tel: (01635) 568 400
Fax: (01635) 568 401
enquiries@genuspharma.com

Genzyme

Genzyme Biosurgery,
4620 Kingsgate, Cascade Way,
Oxford Business Park South,
Oxford OX4 2SU.
Tel: (01865) 405 200
Fax: (01865) 774 172

Gilead

Gilead Sciences,
The Flowers Building,
Granta Park, Great Abington
Cambridge CB1 6GT.
Tel: (01223) 897 300
Fax: (01223) 897 282

GlaxoSmithKline

see GSK

GlaxoWellcome

see GSK

Glenwood

Glenwood Laboratories Ltd,
Jenkins Dale, Chatham,
Kent ME4 5RD.
Tel: (01634) 830 535
Fax: (01634) 831 345
g.wooduk@virgin.net

Gluten Free Foods

Gluten Free Foods Ltd,
270 Centennial Park,
Centennial Ave,
Elstree, Borehamwood,
Herts WD6 3SS.
Tel: (020) 8953 4444
Fax: (020) 8953 8285
info@glutenfree-foods.co.uk

Goldshield

Goldshield Pharmaceuticals Ltd,
NLA Tower,
12–16 Addiscombe Rd, Croydon
CR0 0XT.
Tel: (020) 8649 8500
Fax: (020) 8686 0807

Grifols

Grifols UK Ltd,
72 St Andrews Rd,
Cambridge CB4 1GS.
Tel: (01223) 446 900
Fax: (01223) 446 911

GSK

GlaxoSmithKline,
Stockley Park West, Uxbridge,
Middx UB11 1BT.
Tel: 0800 221 441
Fax: (020) 8990 4328
customercontactuk@gsk.com

GSK Consumer Healthcare

GlaxoSmithKline Consumer
Healthcare,
Wallis House, Brentford,
Middx TW8 9BD.
Tel: (020) 8560 5151

Hansam

Hansam Healthcare Ltd,
PO Box 23876,
London SE15 4WT.
Tel: 0870 241 3019

Hartmann

Paul Hartmann Ltd,
Unit P2, Parklands,
Heywood Distribution Park,
Pilsworth Rd, Heywood,
Lancs OL10 2TT.
Tel: (01706) 363 200
Fax: (01706) 363 201

Hawgreen

Hawgreen Ltd,
PO Box 157,
Hatfield AL10 8ZP.
Tel: (01462) 441 831
Fax: (01462) 435 868

Heinz

H.J. Heinz Company Ltd,
South Building, Hayes Park,
Hayes UB4 8AL
Tel: (020) 8573 7757
Fax: (020) 8848 2325
Farleys_Heinz@Heinz.co.uk

Helios

Helios Healthcare Ltd,
PO Box 36, Old Warden,
Biggleswade SG18 9UP.
Tel: (01462) 441 834
Fax: (01462) 435 417

Henleys

Henleys Medical Supplies Ltd,
Brownfields, Welwyn Garden
City, Herts AL7 1AN.
Tel: (01707) 333 164
Fax: (01707) 334 795

Hillcross

AAH Pharmaceuticals Ltd,
Sapphire Court,
Walsgrave Triangle,
Coventry CV2 2TX.
Tel: (024) 7643 2000
Fax: (024) 7643 2001

HK Pharma

HK Pharma Ltd,
PO Box 105,
Hitchin, Herts SG5 2GG.
Tel: (01462) 433 993
Fax: (01462) 450 755

Hoechst Marion Roussel

see Aventis Pharma

Horizon

Horizon Lifecare Ltd,
Millbank House,
171–185 Ewell Rd, Surbiton,
Surrey KT6 6AX.
Tel: (020) 8410 0755
Fax: (020) 8410 9000
info@horizonlifecare.com

Hypoguard

Hypoguard Ltd,
Dock Lane, Melton, Woodbridge,
Suffolk IP12 1PE.
Tel: (01394) 387 333
Fax: (01394) 380 152
enquiries@hypoguard.com

ICN

ICN Pharmaceuticals Ltd,
Cedarwood,
Chineham Business Park,
Crockford Lane,
Basingstoke,
Hants RG24 8WD.
Tel: (01256) 374 607
Fax: (01256) 707 334
icnuk@icnpharm.com

IDIS

IDIS World Medicines,
171–185 Ewell Rd, Surbiton,
Surrey KT6 6AX.
Tel: (020) 8410 0700
Fax: (020) 8410 0800
idis@idis.co.uk

Infai

Infai UK Ltd,
University of York Science Park,
University Rd, Heslington,
York YO1 5DG.
Tel: (01904) 435 228
Fax: (01904) 435 112
infai@infaiuk.ymn.co.uk

Intrapharm

Intrapharm Laboratories Ltd,
60 Boughton Lane,
Maidstone, Kent ME15 9QS.
Tel: (01622) 749 222
Fax: (01622) 744 672
sales@intrapharmlabs.com

Invicta

see Pfizer

Ipsen

Ipsen Ltd,
1 Bath Rd, Maidenhead,
Berks SL6 4UH
Tel: (01628) 771 417
Fax: (01628) 770 199

IVAX

IVAX Pharmaceuticals UK Ltd,
IVAX Quays, Albert Basin,
Royal Docks,
London E16 2QJ.
Tel: (08705) 020 304
Fax: (08705) 323 334

J&J

Johnson & Johnson Ltd,
Foundation Park, Roxborough
Way, Maidenhead,
Berks SL6 3UG.
Tel: (01628) 822 222
Fax: (01628) 821 222

J&J Medical

Johnson & Johnson Medical,
Coronation Rd, Ascot, Berks
SL5 9EY.
Tel: (01344) 871 000
Fax: (01344) 872 599

J&J MSD

Johnson & Johnson MSD,
Enterprise House, Station Rd,
Loudwater, High Wycombe,
Bucks HP10 9UF.
Tel: (01494) 450 778
Fax: (01494) 450 487

Janssen-Cilag

Janssen-Cilag Ltd,
PO Box 79, Saunderton,
High Wycombe, Bucks
HP14 4HJ.
Tel: (01494) 567 567
Fax: (01494) 567 568

JHC

JHC Healthcare Ltd,
The Maltings, Bridge St,
Hitchin, Herts SG5 2DE.
Tel: (01462) 432 533
Fax: (01462) 432 535

JLB

B. Braun JLB Ltd,
Unit 2A, St Columb Industrial
Estate, St Columb Major,
Cornwall TR9 6SF.
Tel: (01637) 880 065
Fax: (01637) 881 549

K/L

K/L Pharmaceuticals Ltd,
25 Macadam Place, South
Newmoor Industrial Estate,
Irvine KA11 4HP.
Tel: (01294) 215 951
Fax: (01294) 221 600

Kent

Kent Pharmaceuticals Ltd,
Wotton Rd, Ashford, Kent
TN23 6LL.
Tel: (01233) 638 614
Fax: (01233) 646 899

Kestrel
Kestrel Healthcare Ltd,
Network House, Basing View,
Basingstoke RG21 4HG.
Tel: (01256) 307 580
Fax: (01256) 307 590

King
King Pharmaceuticals Ltd
3 Ash Street,
Leicester LE5 0DA.
Tel: (01462) 434366
Fax: (01462) 450 755

Kyowa Hakko
Kyowa Hakko UK Ltd,
258 Bath Rd, Slough,
Berks SL1 4DX.
Tel: (01753) 566 020
Fax: (01753) 566 030

LAB
Laboratories for Applied
Biology,
91 Amhurst Park, London
N16 5DR.
Tel: (020) 8800 2252
Fax: (020) 8809 6884

Lagap
Lagap Pharmaceuticals Ltd,
Woolmer Way, Bordon, Hants
GU35 9QE.
Tel: (01420) 478 301
Fax: (01420) 474 427

Lamberts
Lamberts (Dalston) Ltd,
PO Box 883, Oxford OX4 3RR.
Tel: (01865) 717 300
Fax: (01865) 748 746

Lederle
see Wyeth

Leo
Leo Pharmaceuticals,
Longwick Rd, Princes
Risborough, Bucks
HP27 9RR.
Tel: (01844) 347 333
Fax: (01844) 342 278
medical-info.uk@leo-pharma.com

LifeScan
LifeScan,
Enterprise House, Station Rd,
Loudwater, High Wycombe,
Bucks HP10 9UF.
Tel: (01494) 450 423
Fax: (01494) 463 299

Lilly
Eli Lilly & Co Ltd,
Dextra Court, Chapel Hill,
Basingstoke, Hants RG21 5SY.
Tel: (01256) 315 000
Fax: (01256) 315 858

Lincoln
Lincoln Medical Ltd,
37/39 Burton St,
Melton Mowbray,
Leics LE13 1AF.
Tel: (01722) 410 443
Fax: (01664) 411 991
johndmm@lincolnmedical.co.uk

Link
Link Pharmaceuticals Ltd,
Bishops Weald House,
Albion Way, Horsham,
West Sussex RH12 1AH.
Tel: (01403) 272 451
Fax: (01403) 272 455

Loveridge
J.M. Loveridge,
Southbrook Rd,
Southampton,
Hampshire SO15 1BH.
Tel: (023) 8022 8411

Lundbeck
Lundbeck Ltd,
Lundbeck House, Caldecotte
Lake Business Park, Caldecotte,
Milton Keynes, Bucks MK7 8LF.
Tel: (01908) 649 966
Fax: (01908) 647 888

3M
3M Health Care Ltd,
3M House, Morley St,
Loughborough,
Leics LE11 1EP.
Tel: (01509) 611 611
Fax: (01509) 237 288

Maersk
Maersk Medical Ltd,
Thornhill Rd,
North Moons Moat, Redditch,
Worcs B98 9NL.
Tel: (01527) 642 22
Fax: (01527) 592 111

Mandeville
Mandeville Medicines,
Stoke Mandeville Hospital,
Ayelsbury, Bucks HP21 8AL.
Tel: (01296) 394 142
Fax: (01296) 397 223

Manx
Manx Pharma,
Unit 2 Spectrum Business Estate,
Parkwood,
Maidstone, Kent ME15 9YP.
Tel: (01622) 766 389
Fax: (01622) 761 435

Marlow
J. G. Marlow & Sons Ltd,
Pelham St Mills,
Pelham St, Derby DE22 3UG.
Tel: (01332) 344 148
Fax: (01332) 360 695

Martindale
Martindale Pharmaceuticals Ltd,
Bampton Rd, Harold Hill,
Romford, Essex RM3 8UG.
Tel: (01708) 386 660
Fax: (01708) 384 032

MASTA
MASTA,
Moorfield Rd, Yeadon,
Leeds LS19 7BN.
Tel: (0113) 238 7500
Fax: (0113) 238 7501
medical@masta.org

Mead Johnson
Mead Johnson Nutritional
see Bristol-Myers Squibb

Medac
Medac (UK),
13 Lynedoch Crescent,
Glasgow G3 6EQ.
Tel: (0141) 332 8464
Fax: (0141) 332 8619

Medic-Aid
Medic-Aid Ltd,
Heath Place, Bognor Regis,
West Sussex PO22 9SL.
Tel: (01243) 840 888
Fax: (01243) 846 100
info@medic-aid.com

Medigas
Medigas Ltd,
Enterprise Drive, Four Ashes,
Wolverhampton WV10 7DF.
Tel: (01902) 791 944
Fax: (01902) 791 125

MediSense
MediSense,
Abbott Laboratories Ltd,
Mallory House,
Vanwall Business Park,
Maidenhead, Berks SL6 4UD.
Tel: (01628) 678 900
Fax: (01628) 678 805

Medix
see Clement Clarke

MedLogic
MedLogic Global Ltd,
Western Wood Way,
Language Science Park,
Plympton, Plymouth,
Devon PL7 5BG.
Tel: (01752) 209 955
Fax: (01752) 209 956

Menarini
A. Menarini Pharmaceuticals UK
Ltd,
Menarini House, Mercury Park,
Wycombe Lane, Wooburn Green,
Bucks HP10 0HH.
Tel: (01628) 856 400
Fax: (01628) 856 402

Menarini Diagnostics
A. Menarini Diagnostics,
Wharfedale Rd,
Winnersh, Wokingham,
Berks RG41 5RA.
Tel: (0118) 944 4100
Fax: (0118) 944 4111

Mepra-pharm
see Co-Pharma

Merck
Merck Pharmaceuticals,
Harrier House, High St,
West Drayton, Middx,
UB7 7QG.
Tel: (01895) 452 200
Fax: (01895) 452 296
medinfo@merckpharma.co.uk

Merck Sharp & Dohme
see MSD

Merck Consumer Health
see Seven Seas

Millpledge
Millpledge Healthcare,
Whinleys Estate, Clarborough,
Retford, Notts DN22 9NA.
Tel: (01777) 708 440
Fax: (01777) 860 020
sales@millpledge.u-net.com

Milupa
Milupa Ltd,
Whitehorse Business Park,
Trowbridge,
Wilts BA14 0XB.
Tel: (01225) 711 511
Fax: (01225) 711 970

Mölnlycke
Mölnlycke Healthcare Ltd,
Southfields Rd, Dunstable,
Beds LU6 3EJ.
Tel: 0870 606 0766
Fax: 0870 608 1888
info.uk@molnlyckehc.com

MSD

Merck Sharp & Dohme Ltd,
Hertford Rd, Hoddesdon, Herts
EN11 9BU.
Tel: (01992) 467 272
Fax: (01992) 451 066

Nagor

Nagor Ltd,
PO Box 21, Global House,
Isle of Man Business Park,
Douglas,
Isle of Man IM99 1AX.
Tel: (01624) 625 556
Fax: (01624) 661 656
enquiries@nagor.com

Napp

Napp Pharmaceuticals Ltd,
Cambridge Science Park,
Milton Rd, Cambridge
CB4 0GW.
Tel: (01223) 424 444
Fax: (01223) 424 441

Nestlé

Nestlé UK Ltd,
St. George's House, Croydon
CR9 1NR.
Tel: (020) 8686 3333
Fax: (020) 8686 6072

Nestlé Clinical

Nestlé Clinical Nutrition,
St. George's House, Park Lane,
Croydon,
Surrey CR9 1NR.
Tel: (020) 8667 5130
Fax: (020) 8667 5616

Network

Network Health & Beauty,
Network House,
41 Invincible Rd, Farnborough,
Hants GU14 7QU.
Tel: (01252) 533 333
Fax: (01252) 533 344
networkm@globalnet.co.uk

Neutrogena

see J&J

Nordic

see Ferring.
Tel: (020) 8898 8665

Norgine

Norgine Ltd,
Chaplin House, Moorhall Rd,
Harefield, Middx UB9 6NS.
Tel: (01895) 826 600
Fax: (01895) 825 865

Novartis

Novartis Pharmaceuticals UK,
Frimley Business Park,
Frimley, Camberley,
Surrey GU16 5SG.
Tel: (01276) 698 370
Fax: (01276) 698 449

Novartis Consumer Health

Novartis Consumer Health,
Wimblehurst Rd, Horsham,
West Sussex RH12 5AB.
Tel: (01403) 210 211
Fax: (01403) 323 939

Novartis Ophthalmics

Novartis Ophthalmics,
Delta House,
Southwood Crescent,
Southwood, Farnborough,
Hants GU14 0NL.
Tel: (01276) 692 255
Fax: (01252) 524 424

Novo Nordisk

Novo Nordisk Ltd,
Broadfield Park, Brighton Rd,
Crawley, West Sussex RH11 9RT.
Tel: (01293) 613 555
Fax: (01293) 613 535
novocare@novonordisk.com

Nutricia Clinical

Nutricia Clinical Care,
Nutricia Ltd, White Horse
Business Park, Trowbridge,
Wiltshire BA14 0XQ.
Tel: (01225) 711 677
Fax: (01225) 711 798

Nutricia Dietary

Nutricia Dietary Care,
see Nutricia Clinical
Tel: (01225) 711 801
Fax: (01225) 711 567

Nutrition Point

Nutrition Point Ltd,
13 Taurus Park,
Westbrook, Warrington,
Cheshire WA5 5ZT.
Tel: (07041) 544 044
Fax: (07041) 544 055
info@nutritionpoint.ltd.uk

Octapharma

Octapharma Ltd,
6 Elm Court, Copse Drive,
Meriden Green,
Coventry CV5 9RG.
Tel: (01676) 521 000
Fax: (01676) 521 200
octapharma@octapharma.co.uk

Omron

Omron Healthcare (UK) Ltd,
18-20 The Business Park,
Henfield, West Sussex BN5 9SL.
Tel: (01273) 495 033
Fax: (01273) 495 123
info@omronhealthcare.co.uk

Opus

see Trinity

Oral B Labs

Oral B Laboratories Ltd,
Gillette Corner,
Great West Rd, Isleworth,
Middx TW7 5NP.
Tel: (020) 8847 7800
Fax: (020) 8847 7828

Orbis

Orbis Consumer Products Ltd,
Unit 31, Northfields Industrial
Estate,
Beresford Ave, Wembley,
Middx HA0 1NW.
Tel: (020) 8902 3736
Fax: (020) 8902 4723

Organon

Organon Laboratories Ltd,
Cambridge Science Park, Milton
Rd, Cambridge, CB4 0FL.
Tel: (01223) 432 700
Fax: (01223) 424 368

Orion

Orion Pharma (UK) Ltd,
1st Floor, Leat House,
Overbridge Square, Hambridge
Lane, Newbury, Berks
RG14 5UX.
Tel: (01635) 520 300
Fax: (01635) 34994

Orphan Europe

Orphan Europe (UK) Ltd,
32 Bell St, Henley-on-Thames,
Oxon RG9 2BH.
Tel: (01491) 414 333
Fax: (01491) 414 443
info.uk@orphan-europe.com

Owen Mumford

Owen Mumford Ltd,
Brook Hill, Woodstock, Oxford
OX20 1TU.
Tel: (01993) 812 021
Fax: (01993) 813 466

Oxford Pharmaceuticals

Oxford Pharmaceuticals Ltd,
Masters House, Sandridge Close,
Harrow, Middx HA1 1XD.
Tel: (020) 8861 0788
Fax: (020) 8427 1994

Oxygen Therapy Co Ltd

The Oxygen Therapy Co Ltd,
Dumballs Rd, Cardiff
CF1 6JE.
Tel: 0800 373 580

Paines & Byrne

Paines & Byrne Ltd,
Yamanouchi House, Pyrford Rd,
West Byfleet,
Surrey KT14 6RA.
Tel: (01932) 355 405
Fax: (01932) 353 458

Pantheon

Pantheon Healthcare Ltd,
Studio 8, 48 Tierney Rd,
London SW2 4QS.
Tel: (0845) 602 0137

Parema

Parema Ltd,
Sullington Rd, Shepshed,
Loughborough,
Leics LE12 9JJ.
Tel: (01509) 502 051
Fax: (01509) 650 898

Pari

Pari Medical Ltd,
Enterprise House, Station
Approach, West Byfleet,
Surrey KT14 6NE.
Tel: (01932) 341 122
Fax: (01932) 341 134

Parke-Davis

see Pfizer

Parkside

Parkside Healthcare,
12 Parkside Ave,
Salford M7 4HB.
Tel: (0161) 795 2792
Fax: (0161) 795 4076

PathoGenesis

PathoGenesis Ltd,
PathoGenesis House,
Park Lane, Cranford,
Hounslow TW5 9RR.
Tel: (020) 8580 4000
Fax: (020) 8580 4001

Peckforton

Peckforton Pharmaceuticals Ltd,
Crewe Hall, Crewe,
Cheshire CW1 6UL.
Tel: (01270) 582 255
Fax: (01270) 582 299

Penn

Penn Pharmaceutical Services
Ltd,
Units 23 & 24 Tafarnaubach
Industrial Estate, Tredegar,
Gwent, NP22 3AA.
Tel: (01495) 711 222
Fax: (01495) 711 225
penn@pennpharm.co.uk

Pfizer

Pfizer Ltd,
Walton Oaks, Dorking Rd,
Tadworth,
Surrey KT20 7NS.
Tel: (01737) 331 111
Fax: (01737) 332 507

Pfizer Consumer

Pfizer Consumer Healthcare,
Lambert Court, Chestnut Ave,
Eastleigh, Hants SO53 3ZQ
Tel: (023) 8064 1400
Fax: (023) 8062 9726

Pharmacia & Upjohn

see Pharmacia

Pharmacia

Pharmacia Ltd,
Davy Ave, Knowlhill,
Milton Keynes,
Bucks MK5 8PH.
Tel: (01908) 661 101
Fax: (01908) 690 091

Pharmagenix

Pharmagenix Ltd,
Manx House,
Spectrum Business Estate,
Maidstone, Kent ME15 9YP.
Tel: (01622) 766 389
Fax: (01622) 761 435

Pharma-Global

Pharma-Global Ltd,
SEQ Ltd, Nerin House,
26 Ridgeway St, Douglas,
Isle of Man IM1 1EL.
Tel: (01624) 613 997
Fax: (01624) 613 998

Pharmark

Pharmark Ltd,
7 Windermere Rd, West
Wickham, Kent BR4 9AN.
Tel: (020) 8688 5895

Phoenix

Phoenix Pharma,
Glevum Works, Upton St,
Gloucester GL1 4LA.
Tel: (01452) 522 255
Fax: (01452) 306 051
enquiries@phoenixpharma.com

Pickles

J. Pickles Healthcare,
Beech House, 62 High St,
Knaresborough, N. Yorks
HG5 0EA.
Tel: (01423) 867 314
Fax: (01423) 869 177

Procter & Gamble

Procter & Gamble UK,
The Heights, Brooklands,
Weybridge, Surrey KT13 0XP.
Tel: (01932) 896 000
Fax: (01932) 896 200

Procter & Gamble Pharm.

Procter & Gamble
Pharmaceuticals UK Ltd,
Lovett House, Lovett Rd, Staines,
Middx TW18 3AZ.
Tel: (01784) 495 000
Fax: (01784) 495 253

Provalis

Provalis Healthcare Ltd,
Newtech Square,
Deeside Industrial Park,
Deeside, Flintshire CH5 2NT.
Tel: (01244) 288 888
Fax: (01244) 280 342

Ranbaxy

Ranbaxy (UK) Ltd,
6th Floor, CP House,
97-107 Uxbridge Rd,
Ealing, London W5 5TL.
Tel: (020) 8280 1600
Fax: (020) 8280 1616

Rand Rocket

Rand Rocket Ltd,
ABCare House, Hownsgill
Industrial Park, Consett,
County Durham DH8 7NU.
Tel: (01207) 591 099
Fax: (01207) 591 098

R & C

see Reckitt Benckiser

Reckitt Benckiser

Reckitt Benckiser Healthcare,
Dansom Lane,
Hull HU8 7DS.
Tel: (01482) 326 151
Fax: (01482) 582 526
miu@reckittbenckiser.com

Regent

Regent-GM Laboratories Ltd,
861 Coronation Rd, Park Royal,
London NW10 7PT.
Tel: (020) 8961 6868
Fax: (020) 8961 9311
info@regent-gm.com

Rhône-Poulenc Rorer

see Aventis Pharma

Richmond

Richmond Pharmaceuticals Ltd
Coomb House, 7 St John's Rd,
Isleworth,
Middx TW7 6NA
Tel: (020) 8569 8174
Fax: (020) 8569 8175

Robinsons

Robinson Healthcare Ltd,
Waterside, Walton, Chesterfield,
Derbyshire S40 1YF.
Tel: (01246) 220 022
Fax: (01246) 505 115
enquiries@robinsoncare.com

Roche

Roche Products Ltd,
40 Broadwater Rd,
Welwyn Garden City,
Herts AL7 3AY.
Tel: (01707) 366 000
Fax: (01707) 338 297
medinfo.uk@roche.com

Roche Consumer Health

see Roche
Tel: (01707) 366 000
Fax: 0800 394 353

Roche Diagnostics

Roche Diagnostics Ltd,
Bell Lane, Lewes,
East Sussex BN7 1LG.
Tel: (01273) 480 444
Fax: (01273) 480 266

Rosemont

Rosemont Pharmaceuticals Ltd,
Rosemont House, Yorkdale
Industrial Park, Braithwaite St,
Leeds LS11 9XE.
Tel: (0113) 244 1999
Fax: (0113) 246 0738

Rowa

Rowa Pharmaceuticals Ltd,
Bantry, Co Cork, Ireland.
Tel: (00 353 27) 50077
Fax: (00 353 27) 50417
rowa@rowa-pharma.ie

Rybar

see Shire

Sallis

E. Sallis Ltd,
Vernon Works, Waterford St,
Basford, Nottingham
NG6 0DH.
Tel: (0115) 978 7841
Fax: (0115) 942 2272

Salts

Salt & Son Ltd,
Lord St,
Birmingham B7 4DS.
Tel: (0121) 359 5123
Fax: (0121) 359 0830
salt@salts.co.uk

Sangstat

Imtix Sangstat (UK) Ltd,
42 Thames St, Windsor,
Berks SL4 1PR.
Tel: (01753) 625 704
Fax: (01753) 625 701

Sankyo

Sankyo Pharma UK Ltd,
Sankyo House, Repton Place,
White Lion Rd, Amersham,
Bucks HP7 9LP.
Tel: (01494) 766 866
Fax: (01494) 766 557

Sanofi-Synthelabo

Sanofi-Synthelabo,
One Onslow St, Guildford,
Surrey GU1 4YS.
Tel: (01483) 505 515
Fax: (01483) 535 432

Schär

Dr Schär,
PO Box 126,
Worcester WR5 2ZN.
Tel: 0808 100 0483
Fax: (01905) 357 899
info@schaer.com

Schering Health

Schering Health Care Ltd,
The Brow, Burgess Hill,
West Sussex RH15 9NE.
Tel: (01444) 232 323
Fax: (01444) 246 613
medicalinformation@schering.co.uk

Schering-Plough

Schering-Plough Ltd,
Shire Park, Welwyn Garden City,
Herts AL7 1TW.
Tel: (01707) 363 636
Fax: (01707) 363 763

Schwarz
Schwarz Pharma Ltd,
Schwarz House, East St,
Chesham, Bucks HP5 1DG.
Tel: (01494) 797 500
Fax: (01494) 773 934

Scotia
Scotia Pharmaceuticals Ltd,
Scotia House,
Castle Business Park,
Stirling FK9 4TZ.
Tel: (01786) 895 100
Fax: (01786) 895 450
medenq@scotia-holdings.com

Searle
see Pharmacia

Serono
Serono Pharmaceuticals Ltd,
Bedfont Cross, Stanwell Rd,
Feltham, Middx TW14 8NX.
Tel: (020) 8818 7200
Fax: (020) 8818 7222
serono_uk@serono.com

Servier
Servier Laboratories Ltd,
Fulmer Hall, Windmill Rd,
Fulmer, Slough SL3 6HH.
Tel: (01753) 662 744
Fax: (01753) 663 456

Seven Seas
Seven Seas Ltd,
Hedon Rd, Marfleet, Hull
HU9 5NJ.
Tel: (01482) 375 234
Fax: (01482) 374 345

Shire
Shire Pharmaceuticals Ltd,
Hampshire International
Business Park,
Chineham, Basingstoke,
Hants RG24 8EP.
Tel: (01256) 894 000
Fax: (01256) 894 708

SHS
SHS International Ltd,
100 Wavertree Boulevard,
Liverpool L7 9PT.
Tel: (0151) 228 8161
Fax: (0151) 230 5365
seve@shsint.co.uk

Sigma
Sigma Pharmaceuticals plc,
PO Box 233, Watford, Herts
WD2 4EW.
Tel: (01923) 250 201
Fax: (01923) 241 726

Sinclair
Sinclair Pharmaceuticals Ltd,
Borough Rd, Godalming, Surrey
GU7 2AB.
Tel: (01483) 426 644
Fax: (01483) 860 927

S&N Hlth.
Smith & Nephew Healthcare Ltd,
Healthcare House, Goulton St,
Hull HU3 4DJ.
Tel: (01482) 222 200
Fax: (01482) 222 211
advice@smith-nephew.com

SMA Nutrition
see Wyeth

SmithKline Beecham
see GSK

SNBTS
Scottish National Blood
Transfusion Service,
Protein Fractionation Centre,
Ellen's Glen Rd,
Edinburgh EH17 7QT.
Tel: (0131) 536 5700
Fax: (0131) 536 5781

Solvay
Solvay Healthcare Ltd,
Mansbridge Rd, West End,
Southampton SO18 3JD.
Tel: (023) 8046 7000
Fax: (023) 8046 5350
medinfo.shl@solvay.com

Sovereign
Sovereign Medical,
Sovereign House, Miles Gray Rd,
Basildon,
Essex SS14 3FR.
Tel: (01268) 535 200
Fax: (01268) 535 299

Specials Laboratory
The Specials Laboratory Ltd,
Royal Victoria Infirmary,
Queen Victoria Rd,
Newcastle-upon-Tyne NE1 4LP.
Tel: (0191) 261 0555
Fax: (0191) 261 0555

Special Products
Special Products Ltd,
Orion House, 49 High St,
Addlestone, Surrey KT15 1TU.
Tel: (01932) 820 666
Fax: (01932) 850 444
graham.march@specprod.co.uk

Squibb
see Bristol-Myers Squibb

SSL
SSL International plc,
Toft Hall, Knutsford,
Cheshire WA16 9PD.
Tel: (01565) 624 000
Fax: (01565) 624 001
medical.information@ssl-international.com

Stafford-Miller
see GSK

STD Pharmaceutical
STD Pharmaceutical Products
Ltd,
Fields Yard, Plough Lane,
Hereford HR4 0EL.
Tel: (01432) 353 684
Fax: (01432) 371 314
enquiries@stdpharm.co.uk

Sterling Health
see GSK Consumer Healthcare

Sterwin
Sterwin Medicines
PO Box 611,
Guildford,
Surrey GU1 4YS.
Tel: (01483) 554 101
Fax: (01483) 554 810

Stiefel
Stiefel Laboratories (UK) Ltd,
Holtspur Lane, Wooburn Green,
High Wycombe, Bucks
HP10 0AU.
Tel: (01628) 524 966
Fax: (01628) 810 021
general@stiefel.co.uk

Strakan
Strakan Ltd,
Buckholm Mill,
Buckholm Mill Brae,
Galashiels TD1 2HB.
Tel: (01896) 668 060
Fax: (01896) 668 061
medinfo@strakan.com

Sussex
Sussex Pharmaceutical Ltd,
Charlwoods Rd,
East Grinstead,
Sussex RH19 2HL.
Tel: (01342) 311 311
Fax: (01342) 313 078

Sutherland
Sutherland Health Ltd,
Unit 1, Rivermead, Pipers Way,
Thatcham, Berks RG19 4EP.
Tel: (01635) 874 488
Fax: (01635) 877 622

Swedish Orphan Int AB
Swedish Orphan International
AB,
PO Box 351,
The Grove, Pipers Lane,
Harpenden AL5 1ZP.
Tel: (01582) 769 616
Fax: (01582) 764 326

Syner-Med
Syner-Med (Pharmaceutical
Products) Ltd,
Airport House, Purley Way,
Croydon, Surrey CR0 0XZ.
Tel: (020) 8410 6400
Fax: (020) 8410 6409
synermedpp@aol.com

Takeda
Takeda UK Ltd,
Takeda House, Mercury Park,
Wycombe Lane,
Wooburn Green, High Wycombe,
Bucks HP10 0HH
Tel: (01628) 537 900
Fax: (01628) 526 615

Taro
Taro Pharmaceuticals (UK) Ltd,
Riverside House, Station Rd,
Bishops Stortford,
Herts CM23 3AJ.
Tel: (01279) 859 100
Fax: (01279) 859 179

Teva
Teva Pharmaceuticals Ltd,
Barclays House,
1 Gatehouse Way,
Aylesbury,
Bucks HP19 8DB.
Tel: (01296) 719 768
Fax: (01296) 719 769
info@tevapharma.co.uk

Thornton & Ross
Thornton & Ross Ltd,
Linthwaite Laboratories,
Huddersfield HD7 5QH.
Tel: (01484) 842 217
Fax: (01484) 847 301
mail@thorntonross.co.uk

Tillomed
Tillomed Laboratories Ltd,
3 Howard Rd,
Eaton Socon, St Neots,
Cambs PE19 3ET.
Tel: (01480) 402 400
Fax: (01480) 402 402

Timesco
Timesco of London,
Timesco House,
1 Knights Rd, London E16 2AT.
Tel: (020) 7511 1234
Fax: (020) 7511 7888

Torbet
Torbet Laboratories Ltd,
Unit 14D,
Rackheath Industrial Estate,
Rackheath, Norwich NR13 6LH.
Tel: (01603) 735 200
Fax: (01603) 735 217

Trinity
Trinity Pharmaceuticals Ltd,
The Old Exchange,
12 Compton Rd, Wimbledon,
London SW19 7QD.
Tel: (020) 8944 9443
Fax: (020) 8947 9325

TSL
Tissue Science Laboratories plc,
Victoria House,
Victoria Rd, Aldershot,
Hants GU11 1EJ.
Tel: (01252) 333 002
Fax: (01252) 333 010
enquiries@tissuescience.com

Tudor
Tudor Health Care Ltd,
Martindale House, The Green,
Ruddington, Nottingham
NG11 6HH.
Tel: (0115) 940 5393
Fax: (0115) 940 5388
tudorhealthcare@compuserve.com

Tyco
Tyco Healthcare,
154 Fareham Rd, Gosport,
Hants PO13 0AS.
Tel: (01329) 224 000

Typharm
Typharm Ltd,
Unit 14D,
Rackheath Industrial Estate,
Rackheath, Norwich NR13 6LH.
Tel: (01603) 735 200
Fax: (01603) 735 217

UCB Pharma
UCB Pharma Ltd,
3 George St, Watford,
Herts WD1 8UH.
Tel: (01923) 211 811
Fax: (01923) 229 002

Ultrapharm
Ultrapharm Ltd,
Centenary Business Park,
Henley-on-Thames,
Oxon RG9 1DS.
Tel: (01491) 578 016
Fax: (01491) 570 001
orders@glutenfree.co.uk

UniChem
UniChem Ltd,
UniChem House, Cox Lane,
Chessington, Surrey KT9 1SN.
Tel: (020) 8391 2323
Fax: (020) 8974 1707

Unigreg
Unigreg Ltd,
Enterprise House,
181–189 Garth Rd, Morden,
Surrey SM4 4LL.
Tel: (020) 8330 1421
Fax: (020) 8330 6812
admin@unigreg.co.uk

Univar
see Anstead

Universal
Universal Hospital Supplies,
313 Chase Rd,
London N14 6JH.
Tel: (020) 8920 6207
Fax: (020) 8882 6571

Vernon-Carus
Vernon-Carus Ltd,
Penwortham Mills, Preston,
Lancs PR1 9SN.
Tel: (01772) 744 493
Fax: (01772) 748 754
mail@vernon-carus.co.uk

Vitaflo
Vitaflo Ltd,
11 Century Building,
Brunswick Business Park,
Liverpool L3 4BL.
Tel: (0151) 709 9020
Fax: (0151) 709 9727
vitaflo@vitaflo.co.uk

Vitaline
Vitaline Pharmaceuticals UK Ltd,
Rx Court, 5 Church St,
Aylesbury, Bucks HP20 2QP.
Tel: (01296) 420 600
Fax: (01296) 420 700

Vitalograph
Vitalograph Ltd,
Maids Moreton, Buckingham
MK18 1SW.
Tel: (01280) 822 811
Fax: (01280) 823 302
sales@vitalograph.co.uk

Wallace Mfg
Wallace Manufacturing Chemists
Ltd,
Wallace House,
New Abbey Court,
51–53 Stert St, Abingdon,
Oxon OX14 3JF.
Tel: (01235) 538 700
Fax: (01235) 538 800
info@alinter.co.uk

Wanskerne
Wanskerne Ltd,
31 High Cross St, St. Austell,
Cornwall PL25 4AN.
Tel: (01726) 69500
Fax: (01726) 69135

Ward
Ward Surgical Appliance Co Ltd,
57A Brightwell Ave, Westcliffe-
on-Sea, Essex SS0 9EB
Tel: (01702) 354 064
Fax: (01702) 354 064

Warner Lambert
see Parke-Davis

W-L
Warner Lambert UK Ltd,
see Parke-Davis

Wyeth
Wyeth Laboratories,
Huntercombe Lane South,
Taplow, Maidenhead,
Berks SL6 0PH.
Tel: (01628) 604 377
Fax: (01628) 666 368

Wynlit
Wynlit Laboratories,
153 Furzehill Rd,
Borehamwood,
Herts WD6 2DR
Tel: 07903 370 130
Fax: (020) 8292 6117

Wyvern
Wyvern Medical Ltd,
PO Box 17, Ledbury,
Herefordshire HR8 2ES.
Tel: (01531) 631 105
Fax: (01531) 634 844

Yamanouchi
Yamanouchi Pharma Ltd,
Yamanouchi House, Pyrford Rd,
West Byfleet, Surrey
KT14 6RA.
Tel: (01932) 342 291
Fax: (01932) 353 458

Zeal
G. H. Zeal Ltd,
Deer Park Rd,
London SW19 3UU.
Tel: (020) 8542 2283
Fax: (020) 8543 7840
scientific@zeal.co.uk

Zurich
see Trinity

'Special-order' Manufacturers

The following **companies** manufacture 'special-order' products: BCM Specials, Eldon Laboratories, Mandeville, Martindale, Oxford Pharmaceuticals, Phoenix, Rosemont, Special Products, The Specials Laboratory (see Index of Manufacturers for contact details).

Hospital manufacturing units also manufacture 'special-order' products, details may be obtained from any of the centres listed below.

It should be noted that when a product has a licence *the Department of Health recommends that the licensed product should be ordered* unless a specific formulation is required.

England

East Anglian and Oxford

Mr G. Hanson,
Production Manager,
Pharmacy Manufacturing Unit,
The Ipswich Hospital NHS Trust,
Heath Rd,
Ipswich IP4 5PD.
Tel: (01473) 703 603
Fax: (01473) 703 609
con.hanson@ipsh-tr.anglox.nhs.uk

London

Mr M. Lillywhite,
Regional Technical Pharmacist,
St. Bartholomew's Hospital,
West Smithfield, London,
EC1A 7BE.
Tel: (020) 7601 7475/7491
Fax: (020) 7601 7486

Mr P. Forsey,
Production Manager,
Guy's and St. Thomas' Hospital
Trust,
St. Thomas' Hospital,
Lambeth Palace Rd
London SE1 7EH.
Tel: (020) 7922 8316
Fax: (020) 7960 5644
paul.forsey@gstt.sthames.nhs.uk

Mr C. Evans,
Production Manager,
Pharmacy Department,
St. George's Hospital,
Blackshaw Rd, Tooting,
London SW17 0QT.
Tel: (020) 8725 1770
Fax: (020) 8725 3690

Mr Alan Krol,
Director of Commercial Services,
Pharmacy Department,
Moorfields Eye Hospital NHS
Trust, City Rd,
London EC1V 2PD.
Tel: (020) 7566 2363
Fax: 0800 328 8191 or
(020) 7566 2367
alan.krol@moorfields.nhs.uk

North West

Mr M.D. Booth,
Production & Aseptic Services
Manager,
Stockport Pharmaceuticals,
Stepping Hill Hospital,
Poplar Grove,
Stockport, Cheshire SK2 7JE.
Tel: (0161) 419 5657
Fax: (0161) 419 5664

Northern

Mr C Adams,
Principal Pharmacist,
Pharmacy Manufacturing Unit,
Newcastle General Hospital,
Westgate Rd,
Newcastle-upon-Tyne NE4 6BE.
Tel: (0191) 273 8811 ext 22689
Fax: (0191) 226 0620
adams.fam@virgin.net

South Western

Mr C. W. Lewis,
Principal Pharmacist,
Manorpark Pharmaceuticals,
Blackberry Hill Hospital,
Manor Rd, Bristol BS16 2EW.
Tel: (0117) 975 4852
Fax: (0117) 958 6676
chriswlewis@compuserve.com

Trent

Mr R. W. Brookes,
Production Pharmacist,
Royal Hallamshire Hospital,
Glossop Rd,
Sheffield S10 2JF.
Tel: (0114) 271 3104
Fax: (0114) 271 2783
roger.brookes@sth.nhs.uk

Wessex

Ms G. Middlehurst,
Production Manager
Regional Manufacturing Unit,
Queen Alexandra Hospital,
Cosham, Portsmouth,
Hants PO6 3LY.
Tel: (02392) 286 335
Fax: (02392) 378 288
gillian.middlehurst@porthosp.nhs.uk

West Midlands

Mr A. Broad,
Principal Pharmacist,
Sterile Fluids Manufacturing
Unit,
Queen Elizabeth Medical Centre,
Edgbaston,
Birmingham B15 2TH.
Tel: (0121) 627 2326
Fax: (0121) 627 2168
Alan.Broad@university-b.wmids.nhs.uk

Mr P. G. Williams,
Principal Pharmacist,
Pharmacy Manufacturing Unit,
Queens Hospital,
Burton Hospitals NHS Trust,
Belvedere Rd,
Burton-on-Trent DE13 0RB
Tel: (01283) 566 333/511 511
Extn 5138
Fax: (01283) 593 036
paul.williams@queens.
    burtonh-tr.wmids.nhs.uk

Yorkshire

Dr J. Harwood,
Production Manager,
Pharmacy Manufacturing Unit,
Huddersfield Royal Infirmary,
Lindley, Huddersfield,
West Yorks HD3 3EA.
Tel: (01484) 342 421
Fax: (01484) 342 074
john.harwood@cht.nhs.uk

Northern Ireland

Mrs S. M. Millership,
Principal Pharmacist,
Central Pharmaceutical
Production Unit,
CSA Distribution Centre,
77 Boucher Cres, Belfast
BT12 6HU.
Tel: (028) 9055 3407

Scotland

Mr J. A. Cook,
Principal Pharmacist—
Production,
Tayside Pharmaceuticals,
Ninewells Hospital,
Dundee DD1 9SY.
Tel: (01382) 632 273
Fax: (01382) 632 060

Wales

Mr C. Powell
Principal Pharmacist,
Pharmacy Department,
University Hospital of Wales,
Heath Park, Cardiff CF14 4XW.
Tel: (029) 2074 4828
Fax: (029) 2074 3114
colin.powell@UHW-
TR.wales.nhs.uk

Index

Where an entry is followed by more than one page reference, the principal reference is printed in **bold** type. Proprietary (trade) names are printed in italic type.

Flurbiprofen, 480
    diabetic neuropathy, 338
    eye, 517
    postoperative pain, 606
    rheumatic disease, 475, **480**
    sore throat, 528, 529
Flutamide, 432, **433**
Fluticasone propionate
    asthma, 144, 145, **148**
    nasal allergy, 525
    nasal polyps, 525
    skin, 546
Flu/Vac/SA, 587
Flu/Vac/Split, 586, 587
Fluvastatin, 127, **128**
Fluvirin, 587
Fluvoxamine, 194, **196**
FML, 507
Foam dressings, 734
Folate deficiency, 440
Folate rescue, 407
Folic acid, 440, **441**
    iron and, 438
    pregnancy, 438, 440
Folicare, 441
Folinic acid rescue, 407
Folinic acid *see* Calcium folinate,
    407, 440
Folinic acid *see* Disodium folinate,
    407, **408**
Follicle-stimulating hormone, 362
Follitropin, 362
Fomepizole, 27
Fomivirsen, **505**, 506
Foodlink Complete, 721
Foods for special diets, 459
    ACBS, 718
    vitamin supplements, 470
Foradil, 137
Forcaltonin, 368
Forceval, 470
Forceval Protein Powder, 459
Formaldehyde, 558
Formance, 721
Formoterol, 131, **137**, 147
Formulary
    Dental, 759
    Nurse, 761
Forticreme, 721
Fortifresh, 721
Fortijuce, 721
Fortimel, 721
Fortini preparations, 721
Fortipine preparations, 106
Fortisip preparations, 721
Fortovase, 305
Fortral, 220
Fortum, 269
Fosamax preparations, 368
Foscarnet, 306, **308**
    infusion table, 712
Foscavir, 308
Fosfestrol, 428, **429**
Fosinopril, 93
    see also ACE inhibitors
Fosphenytoin, 238
    infusion table, 712
Frador, 529
Fragmin, 114
Fragrances, excipient, 535

Framycetin
    ear [ingredient], 520
    eye, 503, **504**
    skin, 564
        dressing, 738, 739
Franol preparations, 164
FreAmine-III—discontinued
Frebini, 722
Freeway Lite, 143
Fresh frozen plasma, 124
Freshly prepared, 2
Fresubin preparations, 722
Frisium, 236
Froben preparations, 480
Froop, 67
Froop-Co, 69
Fru-Co, 69
Fructose, 455
    ACBS, 722
    presence of, 2
Frumil preparations, 68, 69
Frusemide *see* Furosemide, **66**, 67
Frusene, 69
Frusol, 67
FSH *see* Follicle-stimulating horm-
    one, 362
FTU *see* Fingertip unit, 541
Fucibet, 544
Fucidin, 278
    skin, 565
Fucidin H, 542
Fucithalmic, 504
Full Marks, 571
Fuller's earth, 28
Fungal infections, 293
    anogenital, 384
    eye, 505
    oral, 530
    skin, 565
Fungilin, 295
    mouth, 530
Fungizone, 295
Furadantin, 293
Furosemide, **66**, 67
    infusion table, 712
Fusafungine, 527
Fusidic acid, 278
    eye, 503, **504**
    infusion table, 712
    skin, 542, 544, 563, **565**
Fybogel, 51
Fybogel Mebeverine, 36
Fybozest Orange, 126

G6PD deficiency, 444
    drugs to be avoided in, 445
Gabapentin, 228, **230**
    diabetic neuropathy, 338
    neuropathic pain, 221
    postherpetic neuralgia, 222
    trigeminal neuralgia, 222
Gabitril, 234
Galactokinase deficiency, ACBS,
    730
Galactomin, 722
Galactorrhoea, 371
Galactosaemia, ACBS, 730
Galactose intolerance, ACBS, 729
Galake, 211
Galantamine, 252, **253**

Galcodine, 162, 164
Galenamet, 39
Galenamox, 262
Galenphol, 162, 164
Galfer, 437
Galfer FA, 438
Galfloxin, 261
Gallamine, 609
Galloway's, 164
Gallstones, 59
Galpamol, 212
Galprofen, 477
Galpseud, 164, 165
Gamanil, 191
Gamgee Tissue, blue label, 740
Gamgee Tissue, pink label, 740
Gammabulin, 595
Gamolenic acid, 548
    breast pain, 375
    eczema, 548
Ganciclovir, 306, **307**
    eye, 505, 506
    infusion table, 712
Ganda, 511
Ganglion-blocking drugs, 97
Ganirelix, 372, **373**
Garamycin
    ear, 522
    eye, 504
Gardenal Sodium, 232
Gardnerella vaginalis, 288
Gargles, 531
Gas cylinders, 600
Gas-gangrene, 259
    prophylaxis, 258
Gastrectomy
    ACBS, 730
    iron therapy, 436
    vitamin B_{12}, 440
Gastric emptying, poisoning and,
    21
Gastrobid Continus, 206
Gastrocote, 33
Gastro-enteritis, 45, 255
Gastroflux, 205
Gastro-intestinal system
    electrolytes, 447
Gastro-oesophageal reflux disease,
    30, 31, 38
Gaucher's disease, 471
Gauze and cotton tissue, 740
Gauze swabs, 740
    filmated, 740
Gauze, cotton ribbon, absorbent,
    740
    viscose and, 740
Gaviscon preparations, 33, 34
    infant, 33
G-CSF, 445, 446
Gelatin infusion, 453, **454**
Gelcosal—discontinued
Gelcotar—discontinued
Geliperm, 735
Gelofusine, 454
Gels, definition, 534
GelTears, 515
Gelusil, 34
Gemcitabine, 413, **414**
    infusion table, 712

In Confidence

COMMITTEE ON SAFETY OF MEDICINES

MEDICINES CONTROL AGENCY

MCA

SUSPECTED ADVERSE DRUG REACTIONS

If you are suspicious that an adverse reaction may be related to a drug or combination of drugs please complete this Yellow Card. Please report all adverse reactions for black triangle (▼) drugs and only serious adverse reactions for established drugs. For additional reporting advice please see page 10 of the BNF or the MCA website www.open.gov.uk/mca/mcahome.htm. Do not be put off reporting because some details are not known.

PATIENT DETAILS   Patient Initials: _____   Sex: M / F   Weight if known (kg): _____

Age (at time of reaction): _____   Identification (Your Practice / Hospital Ref.)*: _____

SUSPECTED DRUG(S)

Give brand name of drug and batch Number if known	Route	Dosage	Date started	Date stopped	Prescribed for

SUSPECTED REACTION(S)   Outcome

Please describe the reaction(s) and any treatment given: Recovered ☐

Recovering ☐

Continuing ☐

Other ☐

Date reaction(s) started: _____   Date reaction(s) stopped: _____   ☐ ☐

Do you consider the reaction to be serious?   Yes / No

If *yes*, please indicate why the reaction is considered to be serious (please tick all that apply):

Patient died due to reaction ☐   Involved or prolonged inpatient hospitalisation

Life threatening ☐   Involved persistent or significant disability or incapacity

Congenital abnormality ☐   Medically significant; please give details:

* This is to enable you to identify the patient in any future correspondence concerning this report

Please attach additional pages if necessary

OTHER DRUGS (including self-medication & herbal remedies)

Did the patient take any other drugs in the last 3 months prior to the reaction? Yes / No

If *yes*, please give the following information if known:

Drug (Brand, if known)	Route	Dosage	Date started	Date stopped	Prescribed for

Additional relevant information e.g. medical history, test results, known allergies, rechallenge (if performed), suspected drug interactions. For congenital abnormalities please state all other drugs taken during pregnancy and the date of the last menstrual period.

REPORTER DETAILS
Name and Professional Address:

CLINICIAN (if not the reporter)
Name and Professional Address:

Post code: _____ Tel No: _____

Post code: _____ Tel No: _____

Speciality: _____

Speciality: _____

Signature: _____ Date: _____

If you would like information about other adverse reactions associated with the suspected drug, please tick this box ☐

Send to **Medicines Control Agency, CSM FREEPOST, LONDON SW8 5BR** or if you are in one of the following NHS regions:

to **CSM Mersey, FREEPOST, Liverpool L3 3AB**   or **CSM West Midlands, FREEPOST SW2991, Birmingham B18 7BR**

or **CSM Northern, FREEPOST 1085, Newcastle upon Tyne NE1 1BR**   or **CSM Wales, FREEPOST, Cardiff CF4 1ZZ**

COMMITTEE ON SAFETY OF MEDICINES

MEDICINES CONTROL AGENCY

In Confidence

SUSPECTED ADVERSE DRUG REACTIONS

If you are suspicious that an adverse reaction may be related to a drug or combination of drugs please complete this Yellow Card. Please report all adverse reactions for black triangle (▼) drugs and only serious adverse reactions for established drugs. For additional reporting advice please see page 10 of the BNF or the MCA website www.open.gov.uk/mca/mcahome.htm. Do not be put off reporting because some details are not known.

PATIENT DETAILS   Patient Initials: _____   Sex: M / F   Weight if known (kg): _____

Age (at time of reaction): _____   Identification (Your Practice / Hospital Ref.)*: _____

SUSPECTED DRUG(S)

Give brand name of drug and batch Number if known	Route	Dosage	Date started	Date stopped	Prescribed for

SUSPECTED REACTION(S)

Please describe the reaction(s) and any treatment given:

Outcome

☐ Recovered

☐ Recovering

☐ Continuing

☐ Other

Date reaction(s) started: _____   Date reaction(s) stopped: _____

Do you consider the reaction to be serious?   Yes / No

If yes, please indicate why the reaction is considered to be serious (please tick all that apply):

☐ Patient died due to reaction   ☐ Involved or prolonged inpatient hospitalisation

☐ Life threatening   ☐ Involved persistent or significant disability or incapacity

☐ Congenital abnormality   Medically significant; please give details:

* This is to enable you to identify the patient in any future correspondence concerning this report

Please attach additional pages if necessary

OTHER DRUGS (including self-medication & herbal remedies)

Did the patient take any other drugs in the last 3 months prior to the reaction?   Yes / No

If *yes*, please give the following information if known:

Drug (Brand, if known)	Route	Dosage	Date started	Date stopped	Prescribed for

Additional relevant information e.g. medical history, test results, known allergies, rechallenge (if performed), suspected drug interactions. For congenital abnormalities please state all other drugs taken during pregnancy and the date of the last menstrual period.

REPORTER DETAILS

Name and Professional Address: _____

CLINICIAN (if not the reporter)

Name and Professional Address: _____

Post code: _____   Tel No: _____

Post code: _____   Tel No: _____

Speciality: _____

Speciality: _____

Signature: _____   Date: _____

If you would like information about other adverse reactions associated with the suspected drug, please tick this box ☐

Send to **Medicines Control Agency, CSM FREEPOST, LONDON SW8 5BR** or if you are in one of the following NHS regions:

to **CSM Mersey, FREEPOST, Liverpool L3 3AB**

or **CSM West Midlands, FREEPOST SW2991, Birmingham B18 7BR**

or **CSM Northern, FREEPOST 1085, Newcastle upon Tyne NE1 1BR**

or **CSM Wales, FREEPOST, Cardiff CF4 1ZZ**

COMMITTEE ON SAFETY OF MEDICINES

In Confidence

SUSPECTED ADVERSE DRUG REACTIONS

MEDICINES CONTROL AGENCY

MCA

If you are suspicious that an adverse reaction may be related to a drug or combination of drugs please complete this Yellow Card. Please report all adverse reactions for black triangle (▼) drugs and only serious adverse reactions for established drugs. For additional reporting advice please see page 10 of the BNF or the MCA website www.open.gov.uk/mca/mcahome.htm. Do not be put off reporting because some details are not known.

PATIENT DETAILS	Patient Initials:		Sex: M / F	Weight if known (kg):
Age (at time of reaction):	Identification (Your Practice / Hospital Ref.)*:			

SUSPECTED DRUG(S)

Give brand name of drug and batch Number if known	Route	Dosage	Date started	Date stopped	Prescribed for

SUSPECTED REACTION(S)

Outcome

Please describe the reaction(s) and any treatment given:

☐ Recovered
☐ Recovering
☐ Continuing
☐ Other

Date reaction(s) started: _____ Date reaction(s) stopped: _____

Do you consider the reaction to be serious?   Yes / No

If yes, please indicate why the reaction is considered to be serious (please tick all that apply):

☐ Patient died due to reaction ☐ Involved or prolonged inpatient hospitalisation
☐ Life threatening ☐ Involved persistent or significant disability or incapacity
☐ Congenital abnormality ☐ Medically significant; please give details:

* This is to enable you to identify the patient in any future correspondence concerning this report

Please attach additional pages if necessary

OTHER DRUGS (including self-medication & herbal remedies)

Did the patient take any other drugs in the last 3 months prior to the reaction? Yes / No

If yes, please give the following information if known:

Drug (Brand, if known)	Route	Dosage	Date started	Date stopped	Prescribed for

Additional relevant information e.g. medical history, test results, known allergies, rechallenge (if performed), suspected drug interactions. For congenital abnormalities please state all other drugs taken during pregnancy and the date of the last menstrual period.

REPORTER DETAILS
Name and Professional Address:

CLINICIAN (if not the reporter)
Name and Professional Address:

Post code: _____   Tel No: _____

Speciality:

Signature: Date:

Post code: _____   Tel No: _____

Speciality:

If you would like information about other adverse reactions associated with the suspected drug, please tick this box ☐

Send to **Medicines Control Agency, CSM FREEPOST, LONDON SW8 5BR** or if you are in one of the following NHS regions:

to **CSM Mersey, FREEPOST, Liverpool L3 3AB**   or **CSM West Midlands, FREEPOST SW2991, Birmingham B18 7BR**

or **CSM Northern, FREEPOST 1085, Newcastle upon Tyne NE1 1BR**   or **CSM Wales, FREEPOST, Cardiff CF4 1ZZ**

COMMITTEE ON SAFETY OF MEDICINES

SUSPECTED ADVERSE DRUG REACTIONS

MEDICINES CONTROL AGENCY

In Confidence

MCA

If you are suspicious that an adverse reaction may be related to a drug or combination of drugs please complete this Yellow Card. Please report all adverse reactions for black triangle (▼) drugs and only serious adverse reactions for established drugs. For additional reporting advice please see page 10 of the BNF or the MCA website www.open.gov.uk/mca/mcahome.htm. Do not be put off reporting because some details are not known.

PATIENT DETAILS	Patient Initials: _____	Sex: M / F	Weight if known (kg): _____
Age (at time of reaction): _____	Identification (Your Practice / Hospital Ref.)*: _____		

SUSPECTED DRUG(S)

Give brand name of drug and batch Number if known	Route	Dosage	Date started	Date stopped	Prescribed for

SUSPECTED REACTION(S)

Please describe the reaction(s) and any treatment given:

	Outcome
	Recovered ☐
	Recovering ☐
	Continuing ☐
	Other ☐

Date reaction(s) started: _____   Date reaction(s) stopped: _____

Do you consider the reaction to be serious?   Yes / No

If yes, please indicate why the reaction is considered to be serious (please tick all that apply):

Patient died due to reaction	☐	Involved or prolonged inpatient hospitalisation	☐
Life threatening	☐	Involved persistent or significant disability or incapacity	☐
Congenital abnormality	☐	Medically significant; please give details:	

* This is to enable you to identify the patient in any future correspondence concerning this report

Please attach additional pages if necessary

OTHER DRUGS (including self-medication & herbal remedies)

Did the patient take any other drugs in the last 3 months prior to the reaction?   Yes / No

If yes, please give the following information if known:

Drug (Brand, if known)	Route	Dosage	Date started	Date stopped	Prescribed for

Additional relevant information e.g. medical history, test results, known allergies, rechallenge (if performed), suspected drug interactions. For congenital abnormalities please state all other drugs taken during pregnancy and the date of the last menstrual period.

REPORTER DETAILS Name and Professional Address:	**CLINICIAN (if not the reporter)** Name and Professional Address:
Post code: Tel No:	Post code: Tel No: Speciality:
Speciality:	If you would like information about other adverse reactions associated with the suspected drug, please tick this box ☐
Signature: Date:	

Send to **Medicines Control Agency, CSM FREEPOST, LONDON SW8 5BR** or if you are in one of the following NHS regions:

to **CSM Mersey, FREEPOST, Liverpool L3 3AB**   or **CSM West Midlands, FREEPOST SW2991, Birmingham B18 7BR**

or **CSM Northern, FREEPOST 1085, Newcastle upon Tyne NE1 1BR**   or **CSM Wales, FREEPOST, Cardiff CF4 1ZZ.**

Joint British Societies Coronary Risk Prediction Chart

British Cardiac Society - British Hypertension Society - British Hyperlipidaemia Association - British Diabetic Association

NO DIABETES

MEN

CHD risk <15% over next 10 years
CHD risk 15-30% over next 10 years
CHD risk >30% over next 10 years

CHD risk over next 10 years

SBP = systolic blood pressure mmHg
TC : HDL = serum total cholesterol to
HDL cholesterol ratio.

How to use the Coronary Risk Prediction Charts for Primary Prevention

These charts are for estimating coronary heart disease (CHD) risk (non-fatal MI, coronary death and new angina pectoris) for individuals who have **not** already developed CHD or other major atherosclerotic disease. They are an aid to making clinical decisions about how intensively to intervene on lifestyle and whether to use antihypertensive and lipid lowering medication, but should **not replace clinical judgment**.

- The use of these charts is not appropriate for patients who have existing diseases which already put them at high risk. Such diseases are:

  - CHD or other major atherosclerotic disease
  - Familial hypercholesterolaemia or other inherited dyslipidaemias
  - Renal dysfunction including diabetic nephropathy

(Continued over)

NO DIABETES

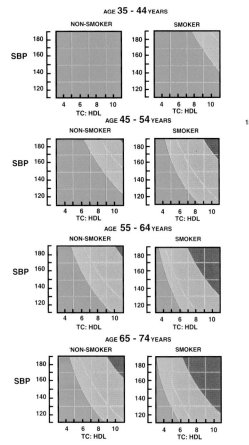

WOMEN

AGE 35 - 44 YEARS

NON-SMOKER / SMOKER

SBP — 180, 160, 140, 120
TC: HDL — 4, 6, 8, 10

■ CHD risk <15% over next 10 years
■ CHD risk 15-30% over next 10 years
■ CHD risk >30% over next 10 years

AGE 45 - 54 YEARS

NON-SMOKER / SMOKER

CHD risk over next 10 years
15%   20%   30%

AGE 55 - 64 YEARS

NON-SMOKER / SMOKER

SBP = systolic blood pressure mmHg
TC : HDL = serum total cholesterol to
HDL cholesterol ratio.

AGE 65 - 74 YEARS

NON-SMOKER / SMOKER

- The charts should not be used to decide whether to introduce antihypertensive medication when blood pressure is persistently at or above 160/100 or when target organ damage due to hypertension is present. In both cases antihypertensive medication is recommended regardless of CHD risk.

- To estimate an individual's absolute 10 year risk of developing CHD choose the table for his or her gender, diabetes (yes/no), smoking status (smoker/non-smoker) and age. Within this square define the level of risk according to the point where the coordinates for systolic blood pressure and the ratio of total cholesterol to high density lipoprotein (HDL) cholesterol meet. If no HDL cholesterol result is available, then assume this is 1.00mmol/l and the lipid scale can be used for total serum cholesterol alone. Diabetes refers to type 2 diabetes. See later notes, if patient has type 1 diabetes or impaired fasting glucose.

- Higher risk individuals are defined as those whose 10 year CHD risk exceeds 15%, which is equivalent to a combined risk of CHD and stroke (cardiovascular risk) of >20% over the same period. As a minimum those at highest CHD risk (>30% red) should be targeted and treated now. When resources allow others with a CHD risk of >15% (orange) should be progressively targeted.

- Smoking status should reflect lifetime exposure to tobacco and not simply tobacco use at the time of assessment. For example, those who have given up smoking within 5 years should be

(Continued over

MEN

AGE **35 - 44** YEARS

CHD risk <15% over next 10 years
CHD risk 15-30% over next 10 years
CHD risk >30% over next 10 years

CHD risk over next 10 years
15%   20%   30%

SBP = systolic blood pressure mmHg
TC : HDL = serum total cholesterol to
          HDL cholesterol ratio.

regarded as current smokers for the purposes of the charts. Ex-smokers with prolonged or heavy exposure more than 5 years ago may continue to be at higher risk than life-long non-smokers.

- The initial blood pressure and the first random (non-fasting) total cholesterol and HDL cholesterol can be used to estimate an individual's risk. However, the decision on using drug therapy should generally be based on repeat risk factor measurements over a period of time.

- These charts (and all other currently available methods of CHD risk prediction) are based on groups of people with untreated levels of blood pressure, total cholesterol and HDL cholesterol. In patients already receiving antihypertensive therapy in whom the decision is to be made about whether to introduce lipid-lowering medication or vice versa the charts can act as a guide, but unless recent pre-treatment risk factor values are available it is generally safest to assume that CHD risk is higher than that predicted by current levels of blood pressure or lipids on treatment.

- CHD risk is also higher than indicated in the charts for:-
    - Those with a family history of premature CHD (male first degree relatives aged <55 years and female first degree relatives aged <65 years) which increases the risk by a factor of approximately 1.5
    - Those with raised triglyceride levels
    - Women with premature menopause

(Continued over)

DIABETES

WOMEN

AGE 35 - 44 YEARS

AGE 45 - 54 YEARS

AGE 55 - 64 YEARS

AGE 65 - 74 YEARS

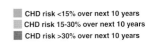

CHD risk <15% over next 10 years
CHD risk 15-30% over next 10 years
CHD risk >30% over next 10 years

CHD risk over next 10 years
15%   20%   30%

SBP = systolic blood pressure mmHg
TC : HDL = serum total cholesterol to
            HDL cholesterol ratio.

- Those who are not yet diabetic, but have impaired fasting glucose (6.1-6.9mmol/l)
- Patients with Type 1 diabetes in whom the risk is often greater than predicted by the total cholesterol to HDL cholesterol ratio. It may be more accurate to ignore HDL cholesterol in them and use the lipid scale for total serum cholesterol alone, but direct evidence for this is currently lacking.
- As the person approaches the next age category. Risk increases exponentially with age so the risk will be closer to the higher decennium for the last four years of each decade.

• In ethnic minorities the risk charts should be used with caution because they have not been validated in these populations. For example, in people originating from the Indian subcontinent it is safest to assume that the CHD risk is higher than predicted from the charts.

• An individual can be shown on the chart the direction in which his or her risk of CHD can be reduced by changing smoking status, blood pressure or cholesterol, but it should be borne in mind that the estimate of risk is for a group of people with similar risk factors and that within that group there will be considerable variation in risk. The charts are primarily to assist in directing intervention to those who typically stand to benefit most.

ADULT ADVANCED LIFE SUPPORT

Precordial thump
if appropriate

Basic Life Support
if appropriate

Check responsiveness → Open airway Check breathing → Give 2 effective breaths → Check for signs of a circulation → Compress chest Continue CPR

Attach defibrillator-monitor

Assess rhythm

± Check pulse

VF / VT

Non VF / VT

Defibrillate x 3 as necessary

During CPR
Correct reversible causes*

If not already
Check electrode/paddle positions & contact

Attempt/verify airway & O₂ i.v. access

Give epinephrine (adrenaline) every 3 min

Consider amiodarone atropine/pacing buffers

CPR 1 min

CPR 3 min
1 min if immediately after defibrillation

Potentially reversible causes

Hypoxia
Hypovolaemia
Hyper/hypokalaemia & metabolic disorders
Hypothermia

Tension pneumothorax
Tamponade
Toxic/therapeutic disorders
Thrombo-embolic & mechanical obstruction

Precordial thump
if appropriate

Call for help
Fill in local emergency No.

☎ ....

Fetch
1. Defibrillator
2. Oxygen
3. Resuscitation equipment

Place electrodes/paddles correctly

If flat trace, check switches, connections and gain

Give oxygen

Secure airway

Secure IV access

© 2001
ations courtesy of Laerdal
45 ERC rev D

European Resuscitation Council In co-operation with

Available from:
LAERDAL MEDICAL LTD.
Laerdal House, Orpington, Kent BR6 OHX,
Tel. 01689 876634, Fax. 01689 873800

Approximate conversions and units

lb	kg	stones	kg	mL	fl oz
1	0.45	1	6.35	50	1.8
2	0.91	2	12.70	100	3.5
3	1.36	3	19.05	150	5.3
4	1.81	4	25.40	200	7.0
5	2.27	5	31.75	500	17.6
6	2.72	6	38.10	1000	35.2
7	3.18	7	44.45		
8	3.63	8	50.80		
9	4.08	9	57.15		
10	4.54	10	63.50		
11	4.99	11	69.85		
12	5.44	12	76.20		
13	5.90	13	82.55		
14	6.35	14	88.90		
		15	95.25		

Prescribing in children

Age	Ideal body-weight		Height		Body-surface
	kg	lb	cm	inch	m²
Newborn*	3.5	7.7	50	20	0.23
1 month*	4.2	9	55	22	0.26
3 months*	5.6	12	59	23	0.32
6 months	7.7	17	67	26	0.40
1 year	10	22	76	30	0.47
3 years	15	33	94	37	0.62
5 years	18	40	108	42	0.73
7 years	23	51	120	47	0.88
12 years	39	86	148	58	1.25
Adult					
Male	68	150	173	68	1.80
Female	56	123	163	64	1.60

* The figures relate to full term and not preterm infants who may need reduced dosage according to their clinical condition.

Length

1 metre (m)	= 1000 millimetres (mm)
1 centimetre (cm)	= 10 mm
1 inch (in)	= 25.4 mm
1 foot (ft) =12 inches	= 304.8 mm

Mass

1 kilogram (kg)	= 1000 grams (g)
1 gram (g)	= 1000 milligrams (mg)
1 milligram (mg)	= 1000 micrograms
1 microgram	= 1000 nanograms
1 nanogram	= 1000 picograms

Volume

1 litre	= 1000 millilitres (mL)
1 millilitre (1 mL)	= 1000 microlitres
1 pint	≈ 568 mL

Other units

1 kilocalorie (kcal)	= 4186.8 joules (J)
1000 kilocalories (kcal)	= 4.1868 megajoules (MJ)
1 megajoule (MJ)	= 238.8 kilocalories (kcal)
1 millimetre of mercury (mmHg)	= 133.3 pascals (Pa)
1 kilopascal (kPa)	= 7.5 mmHg (pressure)

Plasma-drug concentrations in the BNF are expressed in mass units per litre (e.g. mg/litre). The approximate equivalent in terms of amount of substance units (e.g. micromol/litre) is given in brackets.

Recommended wording of cautionary and advisory labels

For details see Appendix 9

1 Warning. May cause drowsiness

2 Warning. May cause drowsiness. If affected do not drive or operate machinery. Avoid alcoholic drink

3 Warning. May cause drowsiness. If affected do not drive or operate machinery

4 Warning. Avoid alcoholic drink

5 Do not take indigestion remedies at the same time of day as this medicine

6 Do not take indigestion remedies or medicines containing iron or zinc at the same time of day as this medicine

7 Do not take milk, indigestion remedies, or medicines containing iron or zinc at the same time of day as this medicine

8 Do not stop taking this medicine except on your doctor's advice

9 Take at regular intervals. Complete the prescribed course unless otherwise directed

10 Warning. Follow the printed instructions you have been given with this medicine

11 Avoid exposure of skin to direct sunlight or sun lamps

12 Do not take anything containing aspirin while taking this medicine

13 Dissolve or mix with water before taking

14 This medicine may colour the urine

15 Caution flammable: keep away from fire or flames

16 Allow to dissolve under the tongue. Do not transfer from this container. Keep tightly closed. Discard 8 weeks after opening

17 Do not take more than ... in 24 hours

18 Do not take more than ... in 24 hours or ... in any one week

19 Warning. Causes drowsiness which may continue the next day. If affected do not drive or operate machinery. Avoid alcoholic drink

21 ... with or after food

22 ... half to one hour before food

23 ... an hour before food or on an empty stomach

24 ... sucked or chewed

25 ... swallowed whole, not chewed

26 ... dissolved under the tongue

27 ... with plenty of water

28 To be spread thinly ...

29 Do not take more than 2 at any one time. Do not take more than 8 in 24 hours

30 Do not take with any other paracetamol products

31 Contains aspirin and paracetamol. Do not take with any other paracetamol products

32 Contains aspirin

33 Contains an aspirin-like medicine